Pulmonary Diseases and Disorders

Second Edition

Volume 2

ALFRED P. FISHMAN, M.D.

William Maul Measey Professor of Medicine
Director, Cardiovascular-Pulmonary Division, Department of Medicine
Hospital of the University of Pennsylvania

McGraw-Hill Book Company

New York St Louis San Francisco Colorado Springs Oklahoma City Auckland
Bogotá Caracas Hamburg Lisbon London Madrid Mexico Milan Montreal
New Delhi Panama Paris San Juan São Paulo Singapore Sydney Tokyo Toronto

PULMONARY DISEASES AND DISORDERS

Copyright © 1988, 1980 by McGraw-Hill, Inc. All rights reserved. Printed in the United States of America. Except as permitted under the United States Copyright Act of 1976, no part of this publication may be reproduced or distributed in any form or by any means, or stored in a data base or retrieval system, without the prior written permission of the publisher.

1234567890 KGPKGP 8921098

ISBN 0-07-079982-2 (set)
ISBN 0-07-021132-9 (v. 1)
ISBN 0-07-021133-7 (v. 2)
ISBN 0-07-021122-1 (v. 3)

This book was set in Melior by York Graphic Services, Inc.
The editors were J. Dereck Jeffers and Muza Navrozov;
the production supervisor was Robert R. Laffler;
the cover was designed by Edward R. Schultheis;
the page layout was done by Till & Till, Inc.;
the index was prepared by Irving Tullar.
Arcata Graphics/Kingsport was printer and binder.

Library of Congress Cataloging-in-Publication Data

Pulmonary diseases and disorders.

    Bibliography: p.
    Includes index.
    1. Lungs—Diseases. I. Fishman, Alfred P.
[DNLM: 1. Lung Diseases. WF 600 P981]
RC756.P826 1988   616.2′4   87-26166
ISBN 0-07-079982-2 (set)

Front cover: Lateral view of resin cast of left human lung, with airways (yellow), pulmonary arteries (red), and pulmonary veins (blue) filled out to fine lobular branches. *(Courtesy of Dr. H. C. Walter Weber, Department of Anatomy, University of Bern, Switzerland.)*

TO THE MEMORY OF FLORIE

NOTICE

Medicine is an ever-changing science. As new research and clinical experience broaden our knowledge, changes in treatment and drug therapy are required. The editors and the publisher of this work have checked with sources believed to be reliable in their efforts to provide information that is complete and generally in accord with the standards accepted at the time of publication. However, in view of the possibility of human error or changes in medical sciences, neither the editors, nor the publisher, nor any other party who has been involved in the preparation or publication of this work warrants that the information contained herein is in every respect accurate or complete. Readers are encouraged to confirm the information contained herein with other sources. For example and in particular, readers are advised to check the product information sheet included in the package of each drug they plan to administer to be certain that the information contained in this book is accurate and that changes have not been made in the recommended dose or in the contraindications for administration. This recommendation is of particular importance in connection with new or infrequently used drugs.

Contents

APPENDIXES

PART 8 **NONINFECTIOUS DISORDERS OF THE
         PULMONARY PARENCHYMA**

PART 9 **PULMONARY CIRCULATORY DISORDERS**

PART 14 **MYCOBACTERIAL DISEASES OF THE LUNGS**

VOLUME 3
PAGES 1793–2564

PART 15 **CANCER OF THE LUNGS**

Contributors

Masazumi Adachi, M.D., Sc.D.
Professor of Pathology, State University of New York, Health Science Center of Brooklyn; Director of Laboratories, Kingsbrook Jewish Medical Center, Brooklyn, New York

Zalman S. Agus, M.D.
Professor of Medicine, Chief, Renal-Electrolyte Section, Department of Medicine, University of Pennsylvania School of Medicine, Philadelphia, Pennsylvania

Abass Alavi, M.D.
Professor of Radiology, Division of Nuclear Medicine, Department of Radiology Hospital of the University of Pennsylvania, Philadelphia, Pennsylvania

Steven M. Albelda, M.D.
Assistant Professor of Medicine, Cardiovascular-Pulmonary Division, Hospital of the University of Pennsylvania, Philadelphia, Pennsylvania

Murray D. Altose, M.D.
Chief, Pulmonary Medicine, Cleveland Metropolitan General Hospital, Cleveland, Ohio

Nicholas R. Anthonisen, M.D., Ph.D.
Professor and Head, Section of Respiratory Diseases, The University of Manitoba, Winnipeg, Manitoba, Canada

Donald Armstrong, M.D.
Chief, Infectious Disease Service, Memorial Sloan-Kettering Cancer Center, New York, New York

Jeffrey Askanazi, M.D.
Associate Professor of Anesthesiology, Albert Einstein College of Medicine, The Bronx, New York

Marianne Bachofen, M.D.
Department of Anesthesiology, Inselpital, Bern, Switzerland

Joseph H. Bates, M.D.
Chief, Medical Services, John L. McClellan Veterans Administration Memorial Hospital, Little Rock, Arkansas

John Bienenstock, M.D.
Professor of Medicine and Pathology; Chairman, Department of Pathology, Molecular Virology and Immunology Program, McMaster University, Health Sciences Centre, Hamilton, Ontario, Canada

Alan L. Bisno, M.D.
Professor of Medicine, Department of Medicine, University of Miami School of Medicine; Chief, Medical Service, Veterans Administration Medical Center, Miami, Florida

Edward R. Block, M.D.
Professor of Medicine, Division of Pulmonary Medicine, University of Florida College of Medicine; Associate Chief of Staff for Research, Gainesville Veterans Administration Medical Center, Gainesville, Florida

Alvin L. Bowles, Sr., M.D.
Director, Pulmonary Ward, Harper Hospital, Detroit, Michigan

Joseph D. Brain, S.D. in Hyg.
Cecil K. and Philip Drinker Professor of Environmental Physiology and Director, Respiratory Biology Program, Department of Environmental Science and Physiology, Harvard University School of Public Health, Boston, Massachusetts

Kenneth L. Brigham, M.D.
Joe & Morris Werthan Professor of Investigative Medicine; Director, Center for Lung Research, Department of Medicine, Vanderbilt University School of Medicine, Nashville, Tennessee

Peter H. Burri, M.D.
Professor of Anatomy, Institute of Anatomy, University of Bern, Bern, Switzerland

Jerome O. Cantor, M.D.
Assistant Professor of Pathology, Department of Pathology, College of Physicians and Surgeons of Columbia University, New York, New York

Desmond N. Carney, M.D., Ph.D.
Consultant Medical Oncologist, Mater Hospital, Dublin, Ireland

Edwin H. Cassem, S.J., M.D.
Chief, Psychiatric Consultation Service, Massachusetts General Hospital; Associate Professor of Psychiatry Harvard Medical School, Boston, Massachusetts

Randall D. Cebul, M.D.
Associate Professor of Medicine, Henry J. Kaiser Family Foundation Faculty Scholar and Chief, Division of General Medicine, Cleveland Metropolitan General Hospital, Case Western Reserve University, Cleveland, Ohio

Neil S. Cherniack, M.D.
Professor of Medicine and Physiology, Case Western Reserve University; Director, Pulmonary Division, University Hospitals, Cleveland, Ohio

Sanford Chodosh, M.D.
Chief of Medicine and Pulmonary, Veterans Administration Outpatient Clinic; Associate Professor of Medicine, Boston University School of Medicine, Boston, Massachusetts

Jacob Churg, M.D.
Professor Emeritus and Consultant, Department of Pathology, Mount Sinai School of Medicine, New York, New York; Pathologist, Department of Pathology, Barnert Memorial Hospital Center, Patterson, New Jersey; Clinical Professor of Pathology, Department of Pathology, University of Medicine and Dentistry of New Jersey, Newark, New Jersey

James M. Clark, M.D., Ph.D.
Clinical Associate Professor of Pharmacology, Institute for Environmental Medicine, University of Pennsylvania, Philadelphia, Pennsylvania

William D. Claypool, M.D.
Assistant Professor of Medicine, Section of Respiratory and Critical Care Medicine, Department of Medicine, The University of Illinois College of Medicine at Chicago, Chicago, Illinois

Jordan J. Cohen, M.D.
Associate Chairman and Professor of Medicine, University of Chicago Pritzker School of Medicine; Chairman, Department of Medicine, Michael Reese Hospital and Medical Center, Chicago, Illinois

Martin H. Cohen, M.D.
Chief, Oncology Section, Veterans Administration Medical Center; Professor of Medicine, George Washington University Medical Center, Washington, D.C.

Robert W. Colman, M.D.
Professor of Medicine and Director, Thrombosis Research Center; Chief, Hematology-Oncology Section, Temple University School of Medicine, Philadelphia, Pennsylvania

George W. Counts, M.D.
Professor of Medicine, Department of Medicine, University of Washington School of Medicine, Fred Hutchinson Cancer Research Center, Harborview Medical Center, Seattle, Washington

James D. Cox, M.D.
Professor and Chairman, Department of Radiation Oncology, The Presbyterian Hospital in the City of New York, Columbia-Presbyterian Medical Center, New York, New York

Ronald G. Crystal, M.D.
Chief, Pulmonary Branch, National Heart, Lung and Blood Institute, National Institutes of Health, Bethesda, Maryland

Ronald P. Daniele, M.D.
Professor of Medicine and Pathology, Cardiovascular-Pulmonary Division, Department of Medicine, Hospital of the University of Pennsylvania, Philadelphia, Pennsylvania

Arthur M. Dannenberg, Jr., M.D., Ph.D.
Professor (Experimental Pathology), Department of Environmental Health Sciences, Immunology, and Infectious Diseases and Department of Epidemiology, School of Hygiene and Public Health, joint appointment in Department of Pathology, School of Medicine, The Johns Hopkins University, Baltimore, Maryland

Paul T. Davidson, M.D.
Director, Tuberculosis Control, Los Angeles County Department of Health Services, Public Health Programs, Rancho Los Amigos Medical Center, Downey, California

Scott F. Davies, M.D.
Director, Division of Pulmonary Medicine, Hennepin County Medicine Center; Associate Professor of Medicine, University of Minnesota School of Medicine, Minneapolis, Minnesota

Roger M. Des Prez, M.D.
Professor of Medicine, Vanderbilt University Medical School; Chief, Medical Service, Veterans Administration Medical Center, Nashville, Tennessee

Burton F. Dickey, M.D.
Assistant Professor of Medicine, Pulmonary Division, Boston University School of Medicine, Boston, Massachusetts

R. Gordon Douglas, Jr., M.D.
Chairman, Department of Medicine, Cornell University Medical College; Physician-in-Chief, The New York Hospital, New York, New York

Norman H. Edelman, M.D.
Professor of Medicine and Physiology; Chief, Division of Pulmonary and Critical Care Medicine, Department of Medicine, UMDNJ-Robert Wood Johnson Medical School, Academic Health Science Center, New Brunswick, New Jersey

Paul J. Edelson, M.D.
Associate Professor of Pediatrics and Microbiology, Cornell University Medical College; Director, Division of Pediatric Infectious Diseases and Immunology, The New York Hospital, New York, New York

Paul H. Edelstein, M.D.
Associate Professor of Pathology and Laboratory Medicine and Director of Clinical Microbiology, Hospital of the University of Pennsylvania, Philadelphia, Pennsylvania

Gary R. Epler, M.D.
Chairman, Department of Medicine, New England Baptist Hospital; Associate Clinical Professor of Medicine, Boston University School of Medicine, Boston, Massachusetts

David M. Epstein, M.D.
Associate Professor of Radiology, Department of Radiology, University of Pennsylvania, Philadelphia, Pennsylvania

Paul E. Epstein, M.D.
Chief, Pulmonary Division, The Graduate Hospital; Clinical Associate Professor of Medicine, University of Pennsylvania, Philadelphia, Pennsylvania

Robert J. Fallat, M.D.
Director, Division of Pulmonary Medicine, Pacific Presbyterian Medical Center; Associate Clinical Professor of Medicine, University of California, San Francisco, San Francisco, California

George M. Feldman, M.D.
Assistant Professor of Medicine, Renal-Electrolyte Section, Department of Medicine, Hospital of the University of Pennsylvania, Philadelphia, Pennsylvania

Victor J. Ferrans, M.D., Ph.D.
Chief, Section on Ultrastructure, Pathology Branch, National Heart, Lung, and Blood Institute, National Institutes of Health, Bethesda, Maryland

Isaiah J. Fidler, D.V.M., Ph.D
Professor and Chairman, Department of Cell Biology, The University of Texas System Cancer Center; M. D. Anderson Hospital and Tumor Institute, Texas Medical Center, Houston, Texas

Gregory A. Filice, M.D.
Staff Physician, Infectious Disease Section, Veterans Administration Medical Center; Assistant Professor of Medicine, University of Minnesota, Minneapolis, Minnesota

Robert B. Filuk, M.D.
Assistant Professor of Medicine, Stanford University, Palo Alto, California

Sydney M. Finegold, M.D.
Associate Chief of Staff for Research and Development, Veterans Administration Wadsworth Medical Center; Professor of Medicine, UCLA School of Medicine, Los Angeles, California

Aron B. Fisher, M.D.
Professor of Physiology and Medicine and Director, Institute for Environmental Medicine, University of Pennsylvania School of Medicine, Philadelphia, Pennsylvania

Alfred P. Fishman, M.D.
William Maul Measey Professor of Medicine and Director, Cardiovascular-Pulmonary Division, Department of Medicine, Hospital of the University of Pennsylvania, Philadelphia, Pennsylvania

Jay A. Fishman, M.D.
Assistant in Medicine, Massachusetts General Hospital; Instructor in Medicine, Harvard Medical School, Boston, Massachusetts; Visiting Scientist, Yale University School of Medicine, New Haven, Connecticut

William J. Fulkerson, Jr., M.D.
Assistant Professor of Medicine, Duke University Medical Center, Durham, North Carolina

Jack D. Fulmer, M.D.
Director of Pulmonary Research and Professor of Medicine, Division of Pulmonary and Critical Care Medicine, Department of Medicine, The University of Alabama at Birmingham; Staff Physician, Veterans Administration Medical Center, Birmingham, Alabama

John N. Galgiani, M.D.
Associate Professor of Medicine, University of Arizona College of Medicine; Chief, Section of Infectious Diseases, Veterans Administration Medical Center, Tucson, Arizona

Stuart M. Garay, M.D.
Assistant Clinical Professor of Medicine, Department of Medicine, New York University School of Medicine, New York, New York

Jack Gauldie, Ph.D.
Professor of Pathology, Department of Pathology, McMaster University Health Sciences Centre, Hamilton, Ontario, Canada

Ralph T. Geer, M.D.
Associate Professor of Anesthesia and Internal Medicine, Department of Anesthesia, Hospital of the University of Pennsylvania, Philadelphia, Pennsylvania

Warren B. Gefter, M.D.
Associate Professor of Radiology, Department of Radiology, University of Pennsylvania, Philadelphia, Pennsylvania

Jon P. Gockerman, M.D.
Associate Professor of Medicine, Hematology-Oncology Division, Duke University Medical Center, Durham, North Carolina

Roberta M. Goldring, M.D.
Professor of Medicine, Department of Medicine, New York University School of Medicine, New York, New York

Michael A. Grippi, M.D.
Assistant Professor of Medicine and Director, Respiratory Services, Cardiovascular Pulmonary Division, Department of Medicine, Hospital of the University of Pennsylvania, Philadelphia, Pennsylvania

Frederick L. Grover, M.D.
Professor of Surgery, Division of Cardiothoracic Surgery, The University of Texas Health Science Center, San Antonio, Texas

Kenneth R. Hande, M.D.
Associate Professor of Medicine and Pharmacology, Vanderbilt University Medical School; Chief, Medical Oncology, Veterans Administration Medical Center, Nashville, Tennessee

John Hansen-Flaschen, M.D.
Assistant Professor of Medicine, Department of Medicine; Cardiovascular-Pulmonary Division, Hospital of the University of Pennsylvania, Philadelphia, Pennsylvania

Edward F. Haponik, M.D.
Associate Professor of Medicine, Division of Pulmonary and Critical Care Medicine School of Medicine in New Orleans, Louisiana State University Medical Center, New Orleans, Louisiana

P. Kent Harman, M.D.
Chief, Cardiac Surgery, St. Charles Medical Center, Bend, Oregon

Jean E. Hawkins, Ph.D.
Director, Reference Laboratory for Tuberculosis and Other Mycobacterial Diseases, Veterans Administration Medical Center, West Haven, Connecticut

Donald Heath, D.Sc., M.D., Ph.D.
George Holt Professor of Pathology, University of Liverpool, Liverpool, United Kingdom

Joan C. Hendricks, V.M.D., Ph.D.
Assistant Professor of Medicine, Department of Clinical Studies, University of Pennsylvania, School of Veterinary Medicine, Philadelphia, Pennsylvania

Ian T. T. Higgins, M.D.
Professor Emeritus of Epidemiology and of Environmental and Industrial Health, School of Public Health, University of Michigan, Ann Arbor, Michigan

Michael P. Hlastala, M.D.
Professor of Medicine and Physiology and Biophysics, Division of Respiratory Diseases, University of Washington School of Medicine, Seattle, Washington

Peter W. Hochachka, Ph.D.
Professor of The Faculties of Science and Medicine, Department of Zoology and Sports Medicine Division, The University of British Columbia, Vancouver, British Columbia, Canada

Fred D. Holford, M.D.
Associate Professor of Medicine, Cardiology Division, University of Colorado Health Sciences Center, Denver, Colorado

Cyrus C. Hopkins, M.D.
Assistant Professor of Medicine, Harvard Medical School; Hospital Epidemiologist and Physician, Infection Control Unit, Massachusetts General Hospital, Boston, Massachusetts

Leonard D. Hudson, M.D.
Professor of Medicine and Head, Division of Pulmonary and Critical Care Medicine, Department of Medicine, University of Washington, Seattle, Washington

Renato V. Iozzo, M.D.
Assistant Professor of Pathology, Department of Pathology, University of Pennsylvania School of Medicine, Philadelphia, Pennsylvania

Larry K. Jackson, M.D.
Associate Professor of Medicine, Division of Pulmonary and Critical Care Medicine, The University of Alabama at Birmingham School of Medicine; Chief, Pulmonary Section, Veterans Administration Medical Center, Birmingham, Alabama

Brian V. Jegasothy, M.D.
Professor and Chairman, Department of Dermatology, University of Pittsburgh, Pittsburgh, Pennsylvania

Alan H. Jobe, M.D., Ph.D.
Professor of Pediatrics, Harbor-UCLA Medical Center, UCLA School of Medicine, Torrance, California

Waldemar G. Johanson, Jr., M.D.
Professor and Chairman, Department of Internal Medicine, The University of Texas Medical Branch at Galveston, Galveston, Texas

Carol Johnson Johns, M.D.
Associate Professor of Medicine and Assistant Dean and Director of Continuing Education, The Johns Hopkins University School of Medicine; Active Staff Physician, The Johns Hopkins Hospital, Baltimore, Maryland

Bruce E. Johnson, M.D.
Investigator, NCI-Navy Medical Oncology Branch, National Cancer Institute and Naval Hospital, Bethesda, Maryland

Norman L. Jones, M.D.
Professor of Medicine, Ambrose Cardiorespiratory Unit, McMaster University, Hamilton, Ontario, Canada

Robert N. Jones, M.D.
Professor of Medicine, Tulane University School of Medicine, New Orleans, Louisiana

Anna-Luise A. Katzenstein, M.D.
Professor of Pathology, Division of Surgical Pathology, Department of Pathology, The University of Alabama at Birmingham, Birmingham, Alabama

A. B. Kay, M.D., Ph.D.
Professor and Director, Department of Allergy and Clinical Immunology, The Cardiothoracic Institute, Brompton Hospital, London, England

Homayoun Kazemi, M.D.
Chief, Pulmonary Unit, Massachusetts General Hospital; Professor of Medicine, Harvard Medical School, Boston, Massachusetts

Mark A. Kelley, M.D.
Associate Professor of Medicine, Cardiovascular-Pulmonary Division; Vice Chairman, Department of Medicine, Hospital of the University of Pennsylvania, Philadelphia, Pennsylvania

Jeffrey A. Kern, M.D.
Assistant Professor of Medicine, Cardiovascular-Pulmonary Division, Department of Medicine, Hospital of the University of Pennsylvania, Philadelphia, Pennsylvania

Gary T. Kinasewitz, M.D.
Associate Professor of Medicine, Physiology, and Biophysics and Director, Cardiopulmonary Research Center, Department of Medicine, Louisiana State University Medical Center, Shreveport, Louisiana

Jerome I. Kleinerman, M.D.
Professor and Vice Chairman, Department of Pathology, Case Western Reserve University School of Medicine, and Director, Department of Pathology, Cleveland Metropolitan General Hospital, Cleveland, Ohio

Lewis R. Kline, M.D.
Assistant Professor of Medicine, Cardiovascular-Pulmonary Division, Department of Medicine, Hospital of the University of Pennsylvania, Philadelphia, Pennsylvania

Robert A. Klocke, M.D.
Professor of Medicine and Physiology; Chief, Pulmonary Division, Department of Medicine, State University of New York at Buffalo, Buffalo, New York

Michael I. Kotlikoff, V.M.D., Ph.D.
Assistant Professor, Department of Animal Biology, University of Pennsylvania School of Veterinary Medicine, Philadelphia, Pennsylvania

Ann V. Krupinski, B.S., R.CPT
Chief Technician, Pulmonary Diagnostic Services, Cardiovascular-Pulmonary Division, Department of Medicine, Hospital of the University of Pennsylvania, Philadelphia, Pennsylvania

Charles Kuhn III, M.D.
Professor of Pathology, Brown University, Division of Biology and Medicine; Pathologist-in-Chief, Memorial Hospital of Rhode Island, Pawtucket, Rhode Island

Paul Kvale, M.D.
Head, Division of Pulmonary and Critical Care Medicine, and Director, Laser Center, Henry Ford Hospital, Detroit, Michigan

Paul N. Lanken, M.D.
Associate Professor of Medicine, Cardiovascular-Pulmonary Division, Department of Medicine, University of Pennsylvania School of Medicine, and Director, Medical Intensive Care Unit, Hospital of the University of Pennsylvania, Philadelphia, Pennsylvania

Kenneth V. Lieberman, M.D.
Assistant Professor of Pediatrics and Chief, Division of Pediatric Nephrology, Mount Sinai School of Medicine, New York, New York

Glen A. Lillington, M.D.
Division of Pulmonary and Critical Care Medicine, Department of Internal Medicine, University of California, Davis, School of Medicine, Davis, California

H. Kim Lyerly, M.D.
Assistant in Surgery, Department of Surgery, Duke University Medical Center, Durham, North Carolina

Rob Roy MacGregor, M.D.
Chief, Infectious Diseases Section, and Professor of Medicine, University of Pennsylvania School of Medicine, Philadelphia, Pennsylvania

Peter T. Macklem, M.D.
Professor and Chairman, Department of Medicine, McGill University; Physician-in-Chief, Royal Victoria Hospital, Montreal, Canada

Nicolaos E. Madias, M.D.
Associate Professor of Medicine, Tufts University School of Medicine; Chief, Division of Nephrology, New England Medical Center Hospitals, Boston, Massachusetts

Adel A. F. Mahmoud, M.D., Ph.D.
The John H. Hord Professor of Medicine and Chairman, Department of Medicine, Case Western Reserve University; Physician-in-Chief, University Hospitals of Cleveland, Cleveland, Ohio

Lars Malm, M.D.
Assistant Professor, Department of Oto-Rhino-Laryngology, University of Lund, Malmö General Hospital, Malmö, Sweden

Robert L. Mayock, M.D.
Professor of Medicine, Cardiovascular-Pulmonary Division, Department of Medicine, University of Pennsylvania School of Medicine, Philadelphia, Pennsylvania

E. R. McFadden, Jr., M.D.
Argyl J. Beams Professor of Medicine, Case Western Reserve University; Director, Asthma and Allergic Disease Center, University Hospitals of Cleveland, Cleveland, Ohio

David S. McKinsey, M.D.
Clinical Assistant Professor of Medicine, Department of Medicine, University of Missouri-Kansas City; Assistant Director, Department of Infectious Diseases, Research Medical Center, Kansas City, Missouri

Myron R. Melamed, M.D.
Chairman, Department of Pathology, Memorial Hospital for Cancer and Allied Diseases, New York, New York

Robert B. Mellins, M.D.
Professor of Pediatrics, Department of Pediatrics, and Director, Pediatric Pulmonary Division, College of Physicians & Surgeons of Columbia University, New York, New York

Louis F. Metzger, A.B., R.CPT
Associate Director/Technical Affairs, Pulmonary Diagnostic Services, Cardiovascular-Pulmonary Division, Department of Medicine, Hospital of the University of Pennsylvania, Philadelphia, Pennsylvania

Richard D. Meyer, M.D.
Professor of Medicine and Director, Division of Infectious Diseases, Department of Medicine, Cedars-Sinai Medical Center, UCLA School of Medicine, Los Angeles, California

R. Drew Miller, M.D.
Professor of Medicine, Mayo Medical School; Consultant, Division of Thoracic Diseases and Internal Medicine, Mayo Clinic and Foundation, Rochester, Minnesota

Wallace T. Miller, M.D.
Professor and Vice Chairman, Department of Radiology, Hospital of the University of Pennsylvania, Philadelphia, Pennsylvania

Richard P. Millman, M.D.
Assistant Professor of Medicine, Brown University School of Medicine; Director, Pulmonary Function and Sleep Apnea Laboratories, Providence, Rhode Island

John D. Minna, M.D.
Professor of Medicine, Uniformed Services University of the Health Sciences; Branch Chief, NCI-Navy Medical Oncology Branch, National Cancer Institute and Naval Hospital, Bethesda, Maryland

Wm. Keith C. Morgan, M.D.
Professor of Medicine, Chest Disease Unit, University Hospital, University of Western Ontario, London, Ontario, Canada

Adrian R. Morrison, D.V.M., Ph.D.
Professor of Anatomy, Laboratories of Anatomy, Department of Animal Biology, University of Pennsylvania School of Veterinary Medicine, Philadelphia, Pennsylvania

Clifton F. Mountain, M.D.
Professor of Surgery, Department of Thoracic Surgery, The University of Texas System Cancer Center; M. D. Anderson Hospital and Tumor Institute, Texas Medical Center, Houston, Texas

James L. Mullen, M.D.
Director, Nutrition Support Service, and Associate Professor of Surgery, Department of Surgery, Hospital of the University of Pennsylvania, Philadelphia, Pennsylvania

Albert G. Mulley, Jr., M.D., M.P.P.
Chief, General Internal Medicine Unit, Massachusetts General Hospital; Assistant Professor of Medicine, Harvard Medical School, Boston, Massachusetts

David M. F. Murphy, M.D.
Chairman, Department of Pulmonary Medicine, Deborah Heart and Lung Center, Browns Mills, New Jersey

Henry W. Murray, M.D.
Chief, Division of Infectious Diseases, The New York Hospital—Cornell Medical Center; Associate Professor of Medicine, Department of Medicine, Cornell University Medical College, New York, New York

Allen R. Myers, M.D.
Professor of Medicine, Department of Medicine, Temple University School of Medicine, Philadelphia, Pennsylvania

Chuzo Nagaishi, M.D.
Emeritus Professor of Kyoto University, Honorary President, Japanese Association for Thoracic Surgery, Takatsuki City, Osaka Prefecture, Japan

Thomas W. Nash, M.D.
Assistant Professor of Medicine, Divisions of Pulmonary and General Medicine, Department of Medicine, Cornell University Medical College, The New York Hospital—Cornell Medical Center, New York, New York

Harold C. Neu, M.D.
Professor of Medicine and Pharmacology, Department of Medicine, and Chief, Division of Infectious Diseases, Department of Medicine, College of Physicians and Surgeons of Columbia University, New York, New York

Richard H. Ochs, M.D.
Associate Director of Laboratories, Department of Pathology, Bryn Mawr Hospital, Bryn Mawr, Pennsylvania

Yoshio Okada, M.D.
Professor and Head, Second Department of Surgery, Shiga University of Medical Science, Otsu, Shiga Ken, Japan

Gerald N. Olsen, M.D.
Professor of Medicine and Director, Pulmonary and Critical Care Medicine, University of South Carolina School of Medicine, Columbia, South Carolina

Allan I. Pack, M.D., Ph.D.
Associate Professor of Medicine, Cardiovascular-Pulmonary Division, Department of Medicine, Hospital of the University of Pennsylvania, Philadelphia, Pennsylvania

Harold I. Palevsky, M.D.
Assistant Professor of Medicine, Cardiovascular-Pulmonary Division, Department of Medicine, Hospital of the University of Pennsylvania, Philadelphia, Pennsylvania

Michael G. Pearson, M.R.C.P.
Consultant Physician, Mersey Regional Thoracic Unit, Fazakerley Hospital, Liverpool, England

Theodore L. Phillips, M.D.
Professor and Chairman, Department of Radiation Oncology, and Research Associate, Laboratory of Radiobiology, University of California, San Francisco, San Francisco, California

Alan K. Pierce, M.D.
Professor of Medicine, Pulmonary Disease Division, Department of Internal Medicine, The University of Texas Health Science Center at Dallas, Dallas, Texas

Janet E. Price, Ph.D.
Assistant Biologist, Department of Cell Biology, The University of Texas System Cancer Center; M. D. Anderson Hospital and Tumor Institute, Texas Medical Center, Houston, Texas

Donald F. Proctor, M.D.
Professor Emeritus, Environmental Health Sciences, Otolaryngology, and Anesthesiology, The Johns Hopkins Medical Institutions, Baltimore, Maryland

Lynne M. Reid, M.D.
S. Burt Wolbach Professor of Pathology, Harvard Medical School; Pathologist-in-Chief, The Children's Hospital, Boston, Massachusetts

Bruce A. Reitz, M.D.
Professor of Surgery and Cardiac Surgeon-in-Charge, Department of Surgery, The Johns Hopkins Hospital, Baltimore, Maryland

Daniel G. Remick, M.D.
Instructor in Pathology, Department of Pathology, The University of Michigan Medical School, Ann Arbor, Michigan

Herbert Y. Reynolds, M.D.
Professor of Internal Medicine and Head, Pulmonary Section, Yale University School of Medicine, New Haven, Connecticut

Hal B. Richerson, M.D.
Professor of Medicine, Department of Internal Medicine, and Director, Division of Allergy/Immunology, The University of Iowa Hospitals and Clinics, Iowa City, Iowa

Andrew L. Ries, M.D.
Associate Professor of Medicine, Pulmonary and Critical Care Division, University of California, San Diego, San Diego, California

Henrique Rigatto, M.D.
Professor of Pediatrics, Department of Pediatrics, and Director, Neonatal Research, University of Manitoba Health Sciences Centre, Winnipeg, Manitoba, Canada

J. C. Rosenberg, M.D., Ph.D.
Chief, Department of Surgery, Hutzel Hospital, Detroit Medical Center; Professor of Surgery, Wayne State University School of Medicine, Detroit, Michigan

Edward C. Rosenow III, M.D.
Professor of Medicine, Thoracic Diseases and Internal Medicine, Mayo Clinic, Rochester, Minnesota

E. J. Ross, M.D., Ph.D.
Emeritus Professor of Endocrinology, Department of Clinical Pharmacology, University College London and The Middlesex Hospital Medical School, The Rayne Institute, London, England

Milton D. Rossman, M.D.
Assistant Professor of Medicine, Cardiovascular-Pulmonary Division, Department of Medicine, Hospital of the University of Pennsylvania, Philadelphia, Pennsylvania

Charis Roussos, M.D., M.Sc., Ph.D.
Professor of Medicine, Director, Critical Care Division, Royal Victoria Hospital, McGill University, Montreal, Canada

Robert H. Rubin, M.D.
Chief of Infectious Disease for Transplantation, Massachusetts General Hospital; Associate Professor of Medicine, Harvard Medical School, Boston, Massachusetts

Ronald N. Rubin, M.D.
Associate Professor of Medicine and Thrombosis Research, Thrombosis Research Center; Deputy Chairman, Department of Internal Medicine, Temple University School of Medicine, Philadelphia, Pennsylvania

David C. Sabiston, Jr., M.D.
James B. Duke Professor of Surgery and Chairman, Department of Surgery, Duke University Medical Center, Durham, North Carolina

Steven A. Sahn, M.D.
Professor of Medicine and Director, Division of Pulmonary and Critical Care Medicine, Medical University of South Carolina, Charleston, South Carolina

George A. Sarosi, M.D.
Professor and Vice Chairman, Department of Internal Medicine, and Director, Division of General Medicine, University of Texas Health Science Center at Houston, Houston, Texas

Thomas F. Scanlin, M.D.
Director, Cystic Fibrosis Center, The Children's Hospital of Philadelphia; Professor of Pediatrics, University of Pennsylvania School of Medicine, Philadelphia, Pennsylvania

Ralph Scicchitano, M.D., Ph.D.
Instructor in Medicine, Department of Medicine, McMaster University Health Sciences Centre, Hamilton, Ontario, Canada

Robert M. Senior, M.D.
Professor of Medicine, Washington University School of Medicine; Director, Respiratory and Critical Care Division, The Jewish Hospital of St. Louis, St. Louis, Missouri

Elizabeth F. Sherertz, M.D.
Associate Professor of Medicine, Division of Dermatology, University of Florida; Chief, Dermatology Section, Veterans Administration Medical Center, Gainesville, Florida

Dennis A. Silage, Ph.D.
Associate Professor, Department of Electrical Engineering, Temple University; Lecturer, Cardiovascular-Pulmonary Division, Department of Medicine, Hospital of the University of Pennsylvania, Philadelphia, Pennsylvania

James R. Snapper, M.D.
Associate Professor of Medicine, Center for Lung Research, Department of Medicine, and Senior Investigator, the Center for Lung Research, Vanderbilt University School of Medicine, Nashville, Tennessee

Walter E. Stamm, M.D.
Professor of Medicine, University of Washington School of Medicine; Head, Infectious Diseases Division, Harborview Medical Center, Seattle, Washington

William W. Stead, M.D.
Professor of Medicine, University of Arkansas for Medical Sciences; Director, Tuberculosis Program, Division of Health Maintenance, Arkansas Department of Health, Little Rock, Arkansas

James A. Strauchen, M.D.
Associate Professor of Pathology and Associate Professor of Neoplastic Diseases, Mount Sinai School of Medicine, City University of New York, New York, New York

Lotte Strauss, M.D.†
Professor of Pathology, Department of Pathology, Mount Sinai School of Medicine, New York, New York

Morton N. Swartz, M.D.
Chief, Infectious Disease Unit, Department of Medicine, Massachusetts General Hospital, Boston, Massachusetts

J. Peter Szidon, M.D.
Professor of Medicine, Pulmonary Medicine Section, Rush Presbyterian-St. Lukes Medical Center, Chicago, Illinois

Ira B. Tager, M.D., M.P.H.
Associate Professor of Medicine, University of California, San Francisco, Veterans Administration Medical Center, San Francisco, California

†Deceased.

George H. Talbot, M.D.
Assistant Professor of Medicine, Infectious Diseases Section, Department of Medicine, Hospital of the University of Pennsylvania, Philadelphia, Pennsylvania

C. Richard Taylor, Ph.D.
Alexander Agassiz Professor of Zoology, Museum of Comparative Zoology, Harvard University, Cambridge, Massachusetts

Joseph F. Tomashefski, Jr., M.D.
Assistant Professor of Pathology, Department of Pathology, Cleveland Metropolitan General Hospital School of Medicine, Case Western Reserve University, Cleveland, Ohio

Nils Gunnar Toremalm, M.D.
Professor, Department of Oto-Rhino-Laryngology, University of Lund, Malmö General Hospital, Malmö, Sweden

J. Kent Trinkle, M.D.
Professor of Surgery and Head, Division of Cardiothoracic Surgery, The University of Texas Health Science Center, San Antonio, Texas

Gerard M. Turino, M.D.
John H. Keating, Sr., Professor of Medicine, College of Physicians and Surgeons of Columbia University; Director, Department of Medicine, St. Luke's-Roosevelt Hospital Center, New York, New York

Margaret Turner-Warwick, D.M., Ph.D.
Dean, The Cardiothoracic Institute; Professor of Medicine, Department of Thoracic Medicine, Brompton Hospital, London, England

Michael G. Velchik, M.D.
Assistant Professor of Radiology, Division of Nuclear Medicine, Hospital of the University of Pennsylvania, Philadelphia, Pennsylvania

Bruno W. Volk, M.D.
Professor in Residence, Department of Pathology, University of California at Irvine, Irvine, California

Elizabeth E. Wack, M.D.
Clinical Instructor in Medicine, Department of Internal Medicine, University of Arizona College of Medicine, Tucson, Arizona

Peter D. Wagner, M.D.
Professor of Medicine, Section of Physiology, Department of Medicine, University of California, San Diego, School of Medicine, La Jolla, California

Ko-Pen Wang, M.D.
Associate Professor of Medicine and Otolaryngology and Director, Bronchoscopy Research and Training Program, The Johns Hopkins University School of Medicine, Baltimore, Maryland

Peter A. Ward, M.D.
Professor and Chairman, Department of Pathology, The University of Michigan Medical School, Ann Arbor, Michigan

Lawrence G. Wayne, Ph.D.
Chief, Tuberculosis Research Laboratory, Veterans Administration Medical Center, Long Beach, California

John G. Weg, M.D.
Professor of Internal Medicine, Division of Pulmonary and Critical Care Medicine, University of Michigan Medical Center, Ann Arbor, Michigan

Ewald R. Weibel, M.D.
Professor of Anatomy, Department of Anatomy, University of Bern, Bern, Switzerland

Hans Weill, M.D.
Schlieder Foundation Professor of Pulmonary Medicine, Pulmonary Diseases Section, Department of Medicine, Tulane University School of Medicine, New Orleans, Louisiana

Arnold N. Weinberg, M.D.
Professor of Medicine, Harvard Medical School; Physician, Infectious Disease Unit, Massachusetts General Hospital; Director, Medical Department, Massachusetts Institute of Technology, Boston and Cambridge, Massachusetts

Emmanuel Weitzenblum, M.D.
Professor of Pulmonology, Pulmonary Function Laboratory, Department of Pulmonary, Pavillon Laennec, University Hospital, Strasbourg, France

Michael J. Welsh, M.D.
Professor of Medicine, Pulmonary Division and Laboratory of Epithelial Transport, Department of Internal Medicine, The University of Iowa College of Medicine, Iowa City, Iowa

M. Henry Williams, Jr., M.D.
Professor of Medicine, Pulmonary Division, Albert Einstein College of Medicine of Yeshiva University, The Bronx, New York

Curtis B. Wilson, M.D.
Member, Department of Immunology, Research Institute of Scripps Clinic, La Jolla, California

Richard H. Winterbauer, M.D.
Head, Chest and Infectious Diseases Section, Department of Medicine, Virginia Mason Clinic, Seattle, Washington

Theodore E. Woodward, M.D.
Professor of Medicine Emeritus, Department of Medicine, University of Maryland School of Medicine and Hospital, Veterans Administration Medical Center, Baltimore, Maryland

Raymond Yesner, M.D.
Professor of Pathology Emeritus and Director, Autopsy Division, Department of Pathology, Yale University School of Medicine, New Haven, Connecticut

Peter M. Yurchak, M.D.
Associate Clinical Professor of Medicine, Harvard Medical School, Massachusetts General Hospital, Cardiac Unit, Boston, Massachusetts

Muhammad B. Zaman, M.D.
Associate Attending Pathologist, Department of Pathology, Memorial Sloan-Kettering Cancer Center, New York, New York

Warren M. Zapol, M.D.
Anesthetist, Department of Anesthesia, Massachusetts General Hospital; Professor of Anesthesia, Harvard Medical School, Boston, Massachusetts

Preface

The original edition seems to have done what it set out to do. Clinicians were afforded a panoramic view of diseases and disorders of the lungs with an eye toward how the lungs interrelate with other parts of the body, all within the framework of medicine in general. Each entity was considered in terms of the mechanisms responsible for the disturbances, always grasping for therapeutic handles by which the pathologic process might be reversed but often forced to acknowledge that empiricism remained the order of the day. Finally, to ensure balanced perspective, each disease or disorder was depicted critically through the eyes of a seasoned expert.

Why a second edition? In a word, to update and to improve.

THE NEED TO UPDATE

In the eight years since the original edition, new clinical entities have surfaced, concepts and practice of chest medicine have undergone considerable revision, and the scientific underpinnings have shifted ground. In the parlance of Kuhn, many of these changes represent "normal" science and medicine in evolution, entirely in keeping with existing paradigms. Among these are improved preventive measures, such as vaccination against the pneumococcal and influenza virus; fuller exploitation of invasive diagnostic methods, notably bronchoscopy and cardiac catheterization; increasing substitution of noninvasive techniques, such as oximetry, for more traumatic

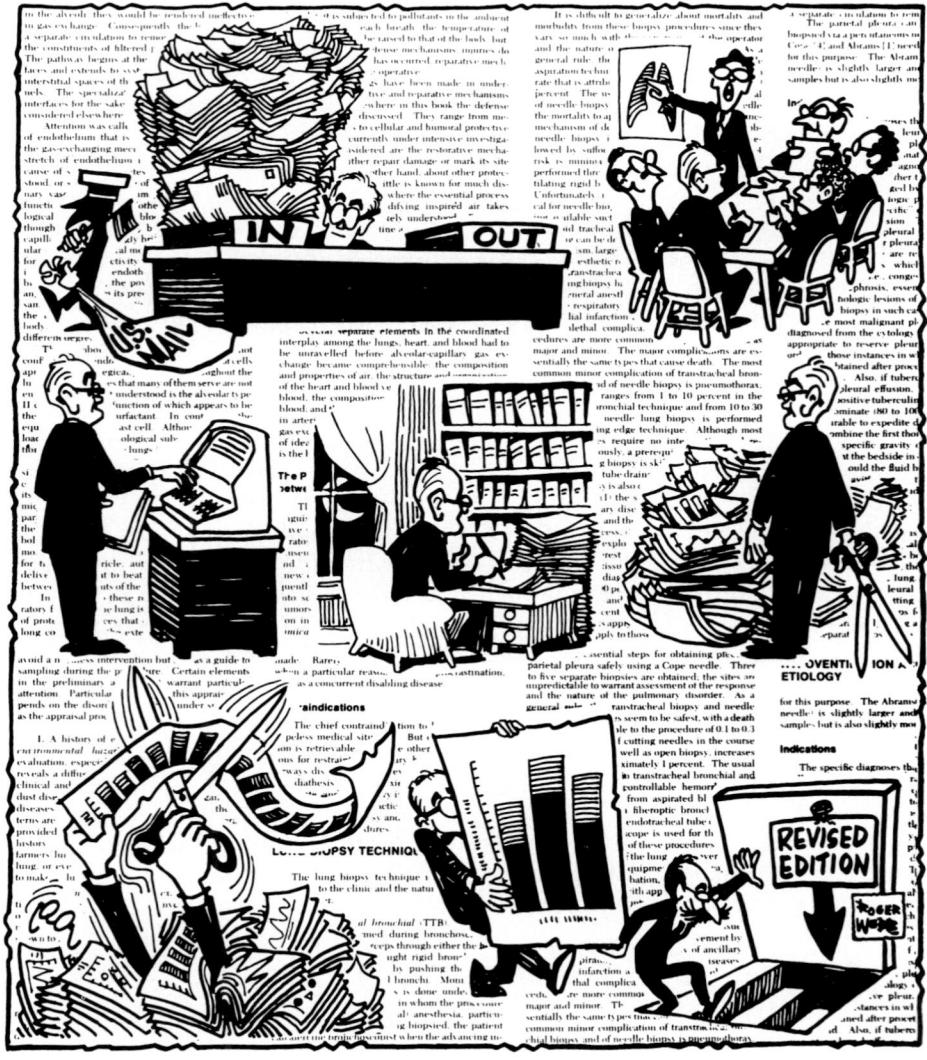

procedures; and new therapeutic modalities, ranging as widely as from antibiotics and replacement of surfactant to chemo- and radiation therapy. A strong case could also be made for "critical care medicine" as a natural outgrowth of normal progress in pulmonary medicine.

In addition to normal progress, the last seven years have been punctuated by the advent of new clinical entities, concepts, and techniques that can no longer be accommodated within traditional patterns of thinking. For example, the immunosuppressive disorders, exemplified in the extreme by AIDS, constitute a revolution in science and medicine that calls for new paradigms about mechanisms of injury and defense and for fresh approaches in management. On a much lesser scale, computed tomography and nuclear magnetic resonance have sent quivers of diagnostic anticipation among pulmonary specialists. And in the wings are impending breakthroughs in the basic sciences that hold promise of bright, new therapeutic modalities: no longer is it fantasy to imagine the identification of the genetic defect responsible for cystic fibrosis or reversing the biochemical defect in α_1-antitrypsin deficiency.

Part of the updating is to signal a broadening of the scientific underpinnings of chest medicine. A decade ago, the weight of chest medicine rested squarely on pathology, physiology, anatomy and, to a lesser extent, biochemistry. As a result, structure-function relationships have become the bedrock of pulmonary medicine. But since then the weight has shifted to include cell biology, molecular biology and molecular genetics, on the one hand, and integrative and developmental biology, on the other. These extensions are evident throughout the book, from chapters devoted to immune mechanisms and mediators to those concerned with sleep disorders.

IMPROVING THE BOOK

In addition to ensuring that its contents are current and comprehensive, and in mobilizing a stellar cast of authors, a considerable effort has been made to enhance the retrieval of the information that it contains. In addition to a precise index, an outline now precedes each chapter and an enlarged, selected, and annotated bibliography points the way to additional references. Regrouping of the chapters helps to identify categories of pulmonary disease, to define essentials and to avoid needless duplication. Fresh illustrations depict lesions and relationships that would be tedious and difficult to define in words. Since many readers had found them useful in teaching, a large effort was made to mobilize proper pictures and to reproduce them well.

THE BOOK AS PART OF A CONTINUING TRADITION

The editor was introduced to chest medicine in the 1950s at the Bellevue Hospital in New York City. At that time, J. Burns Amberson headed the Chest Service; Dickinson W. Richards was Chief of Medicine; André Cournand directed the Cardiopulmonary Laboratory. The setting was replete with seasoned chest physicians and imaginative but disciplined clinical investigators. The patients were seriously ill and needed help. The place was like a beehive: all doors were open; every crowded laboratory was busy. Looking back, Amberson, Cournand, and Richards had created a medical and scientific oasis that centered around pulmonary diseases. It is the animating spirit of these three individuals that sparks the present book.

INDEBTEDNESS TO MANY

As in the original edition, the editor owes much to many. The first acknowledgment has to be to the physicians, scientists, and educators who wrote the individual chapters that make up this book. They also deserve credit for putting up with the editor. Suzanne Markloff was my right hand, gently but firmly steering authors, manuscripts, and all around her in the proper direction. Betsy Ann Bozzarello helped create an environment in which the book could be produced, acting as a buffer, on the one hand, and as an implementor, on the other. Whenever we got into trouble, which was often, Daniel Barrett pitched in to help us meet deadlines. Throughout, Roger Webb sustained all of us with a gentle sense of humor (see the figure, page xxvii) and provided drawings that helped in the formidable task of linking the disparate sections of the book into a cohesive text.

The publisher enjoyed the first edition and did all imaginable to help in preparing the second. Robert McGraw was unstinting in the effort to surpass the original work in form and format. Dereck Jeffers and Muza Navrozov helped in the never-ending pursuit of the "final inch," sometimes surging out front, occasionally falling back to push, but always at hand.

Encouragement and indulgence from my family sustained the effort: to Linda, who understood and helped all the way; to Hannah, who took it all in her wobbly stride; to Mark and Jay, who were always there when needed; to Gayle and Martha for a new dimension.

Alfred P. Fishman

Noninfectious Disorders of the Pulmonary Parenchyma

Chapter 56

Aspiration Diseases of the Lungs

Paul E. Epstein

Aspiration pneumonia comprises a diverse group of disorders that are linked by the common factor of soiling of the lower respiratory tract by foreign, nongaseous substances. While this term effectively conveys the concept of accidental inhalation of potentially damaging material, it fails to distinguish between solid and liquid, caustic and bland, or infected and sterile. Unfortunately, the term *aspiration pneumonia* has been used in the clinical literature to denote at least three separate syndromes: aspiration of gastric acid, aspiration of particulate matter, and pulmonary infection resulting from aspiration. Some clinicians find it useful to distinguish between *aspiration pneumonitis*, an inflammatory response to aspirated material that is *not* associated with infection, and *aspiration pneumonia*, to imply the addition of infection to the aspiration pneumonitis.

Most often, nongaseous challenges of the lungs come from the gastrointestinal tract as a result of reflux or regurgitation.

NORMAL PROTECTIVE MECHANISMS

An important function of the upper respiratory tract is to separate the flow of gas from the flow of liquids and solids. Although free bidirectional flow of gases must occur for the lungs to function properly, unidirectional flow of liquids and solids is the norm. The anatomic and neurophysiological mechanisms that support this normal function are important to understand. During quiet breathing the oropharynx is relaxed and the epiglottis is in a low resting position. The vocal cords are open and air enters the unobstructed trachea. A highly coordinated sequence of neuromuscular events occurs during swallowing: the pharyngeal palate moves upward and backward, closing off access to the nasopharynx. The epiglottis is tilted downward into the hypopharynx, protecting the glottic opening, and the vocal chords close. Pharyngeal constrictor muscles push the bolus to be swallowed through the hypopharynx, pharyngoesophageal segment, and cervical esophagus. In the adult, and probably in the infant as well, swallowing and breathing are mutually exclusive events. Once a bolus of liquid or solid has entered the esophagus, waves of secondary peristalsis are observed.

Although initiation of swallowing is a voluntary event, its coordination is a centrally mediated reflex involving striated muscle fibers. Distention of the esophagus also produces secondary waves of peristalsis that are mediated by local reflex arcs. Peristaltic waves generated by these mechanisms tend to empty the esophagus into the stomach and to discourage reflux into the pharynx. The upper esophageal sphincter, made up of the cricopharyngeus and inferior pharyngeal constrictor muscles, also resists reflux by maintaining its tone as a result of constant firing of the vagal constrictor fibers. At the distal end of the esophagus the lower esophageal sphincter also maintains a high resting tone exceeding that found in the stomach or the esophagus. In humans, the vagus may exert a modest effect on the lower esophageal sphincter, but the high resting tone of the sphincter is probably predominantly myogenic in origin.

Reversal of flow in the upper gastrointestinal tract, whether in the form of vomiting or gastroesophageal reflux, challenges the protective mechanisms described above. A variety of pathologic and iatrogenic circumstances can interfere with the coordination of neuromuscular events and predispose to the occurrence of aspiration.

CLINICAL SETTINGS IN WHICH ASPIRATION OCCURS

Although vomiting and gastroesophageal reflux are common events, clinically significant aspiration usually occurs only if the normal protective mechanisms should fail. Three broad categories of failure have been recognized: (1) depression of reflex protection, (2) alteration in anatomic structures, and (3) iatrogenic causes.

Depression of Reflex Protection

Depression of consciousness automatically blunts the reflex response to aspiration. The most common setting for depression of reflex protection occurs during surgical anesthesia (Fig. 56-1). The risk of aspiration during surgery is particularly high when the operative procedure is an emergency and the patient has not had adequate time for the stomach to empty. In these circumstances, an upper abdominal operation entails the greatest danger, since manipulation of the stomach often leads to regurgitation of partially digested food and gastric juice. The sensorium is also depressed by alcohol and by narcotic drugs. Intoxication with these substances frequently leads to vomiting that is complicated by a loss of the protective gag reflex. Drug addicts suffering from overdosage often arrive at the hospital with central nervous depression and secondary aspiration pneumonitis (see Chapter 90). Various types of abnormalities in the central nervous system also predispose to aspiration of gastric contents (Fig. 56-2). Patients with myasthenia gravis or the Guillain-Barré syndrome are particularly vulnerable to aspiration since bulbar neuropathy, and the laryngeal incompetence that it produces, are common, severe, and prolonged. A cuffed endotracheal tube or a tracheostomy is often required in these patients to prevent soiling of the lungs. Seizure disorders and cerebrovascular accidents frequently combine the triple threats of loss of consciousness, vomiting, and discoordination of swallowing reflexes, thereby impairing the protective role of the larynx and glottis. Also, impairment of protective body movements, such as automatic turning and bending during vomiting, predisposes to aspiration.

Anatomic Changes

Alterations in laryngeal and esophageal anatomy also predispose to aspiration of foreign materials. Tracheobronchial fistulas—congenital, traumatic, or neoplastic—can lead to spillage of swallowed material into the lungs. Bilateral vocal cord paralysis (Fig. 56-3) enables soiling of the lower respiratory tract by saliva as well as by other liquids and solids swallowed during meals. Esophageal dilatation and failure of the esophagus to empty as a result of achalasia frequently leads to regurgitation and aspiration (Fig. 56-4). Similarly, a carcinoma of the esophagus may produce soiling of the lower respiratory tract either by regurgitation due to overfilling or by the production of a tracheoesophageal fistula (Fig. 56-5). Other types of esophageal disease, such as a Zenker's diverticulum or scleroderma of the esophagus, also predispose to aspiration pneumonia.

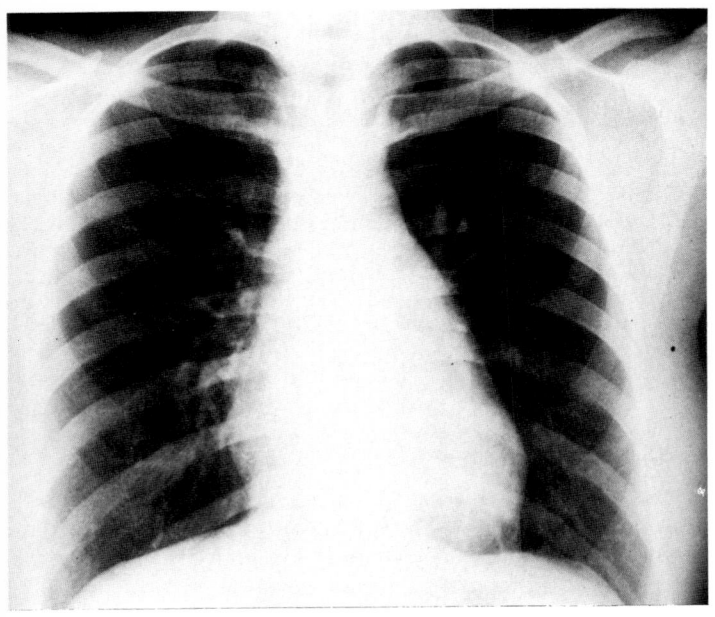

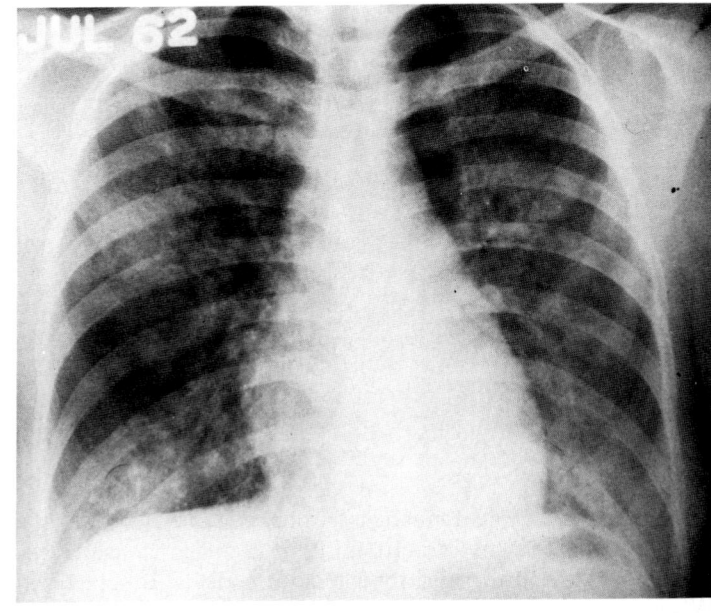

A   B

FIGURE 56-1   Aspiration during surgical anesthesia.   *A.* Preoperative chest radiograph of a 26-year-old woman about to undergo emergency appendectomy.   *B.* Postoperative chest radiograph. During surgery, the anesthesiologist suspected that the patient had aspirated gastric contents. Follow-up radiograph shows diffuse aspiration pneumonia.

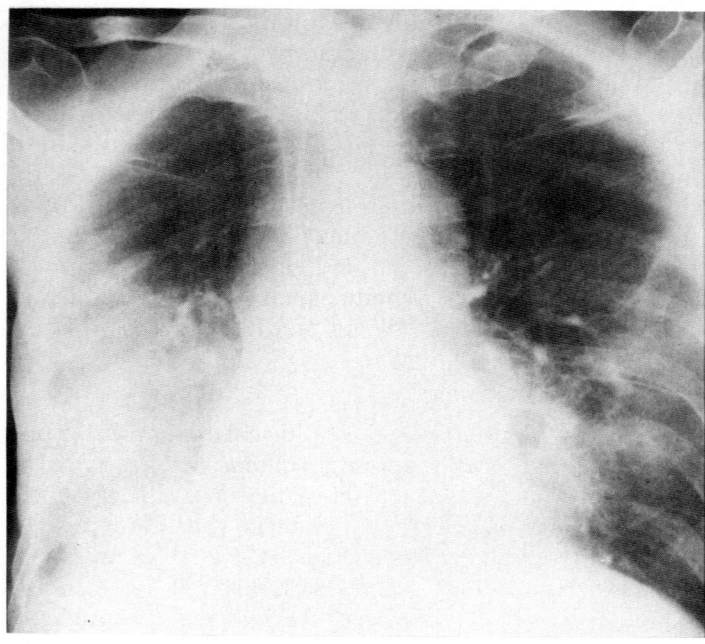

A

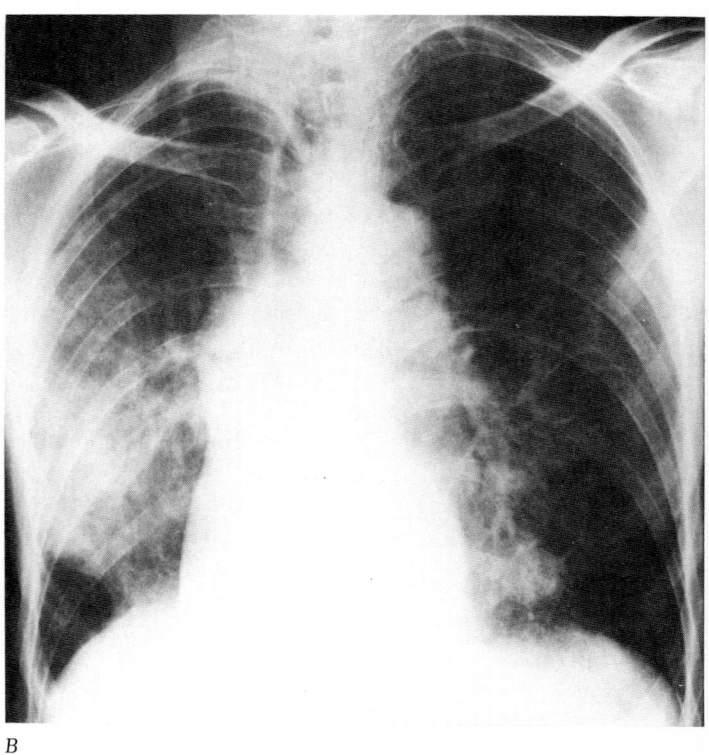

B

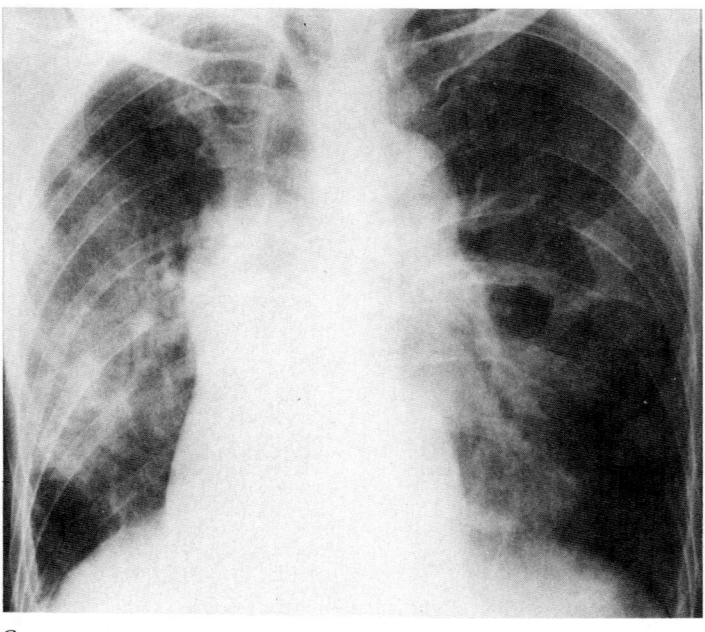

C

FIGURE 56-2 Recurrent aspiration pneumonitis in a 65-year-old man with neurologic deficit due to multiple sclerosis. Gag reflex could not be elicited on repeated testing. *A.* Bilateral lower lobe infiltrates are present, resulting from observed aspiration of food. *B.* Three weeks later, the left lung had cleared significantly. A new patch of aspiration pneumonitis is seen at the left base in the cardiophrenic angle. The right lung process has partially cleared. *C.* Two months later, the right mid-lung process has stabilized, indicating scar formation. A new infiltrate is seen at the right apex.

Iatrogenic Factors

The introduction of a nasogastric tube disturbs laryngeal function; glottic movement is impaired by the physical presence of the tube and by irritation evoked by the tube. When the tube is used for feeding, the combination of gastric distention, pharyngeal reflexes, and depressed laryngeal guarding predisposes to aspiration of gastric contents.

TYPES OF ASPIRATION

The consequences of aspiration depend importantly on the nature, as well as the quantity, of material inhaled into the airways and parenchyma.

Solid Material

A chunk of food lodged above the vocal cords, blocking the glottic opening, is a dire emergency. While eating, the

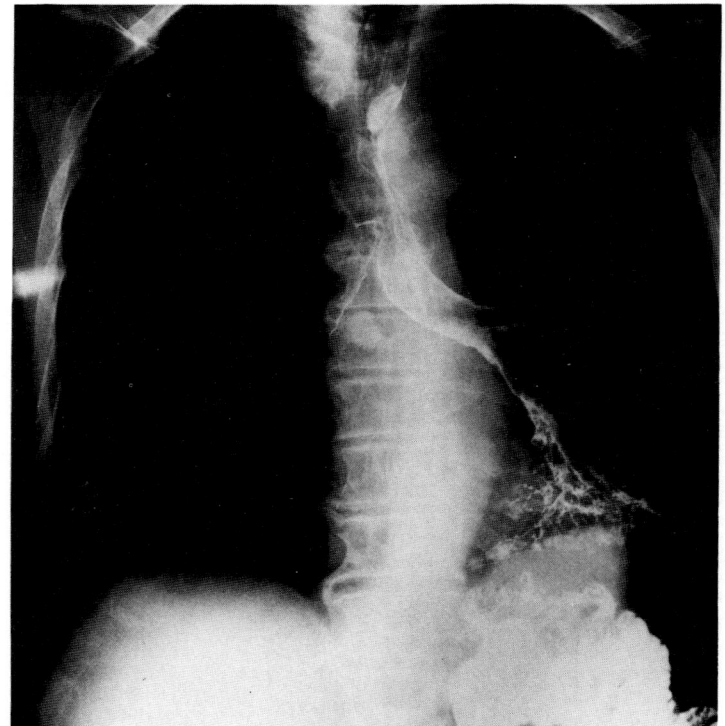

FIGURE 56-3   Bilateral vocal cord paralysis. Barium swallow demonstrates massive aspiration of barium into the lungs.

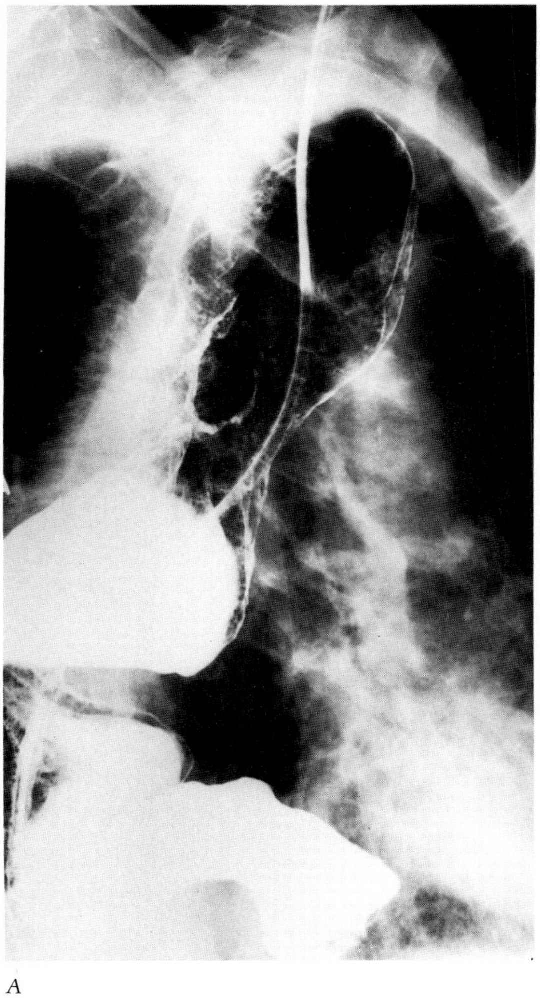

A

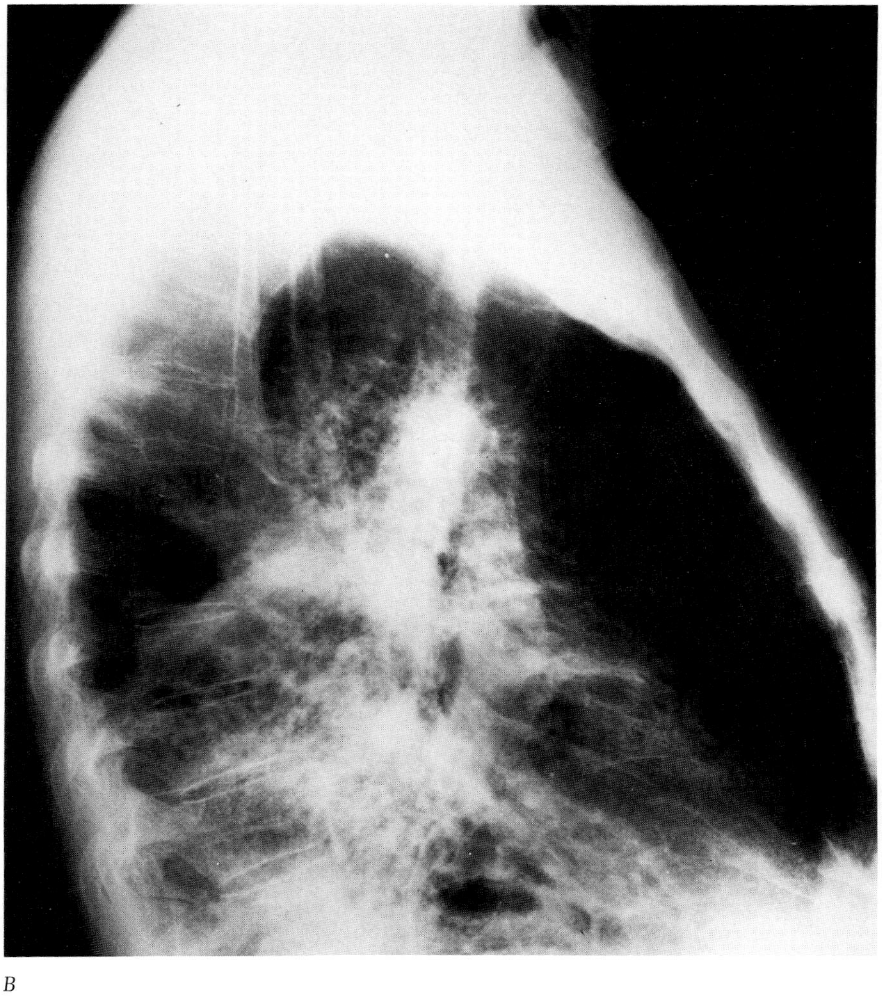

B

FIGURE 56-4   Achalasia of the esophagus.   A. Barium swallow on a patient with long-standing achalasia who noted rapid weight loss. Endoscopic biopsy demonstrated carcinoma of the esophagus. Barium swallow with nasogastric tube in place shows severe dilatation of the esophagus.   B. Lateral chest radiograph of the same patient shows posterior and basal pulmonary infiltrates caused by chronic aspiration of esophageal contents.

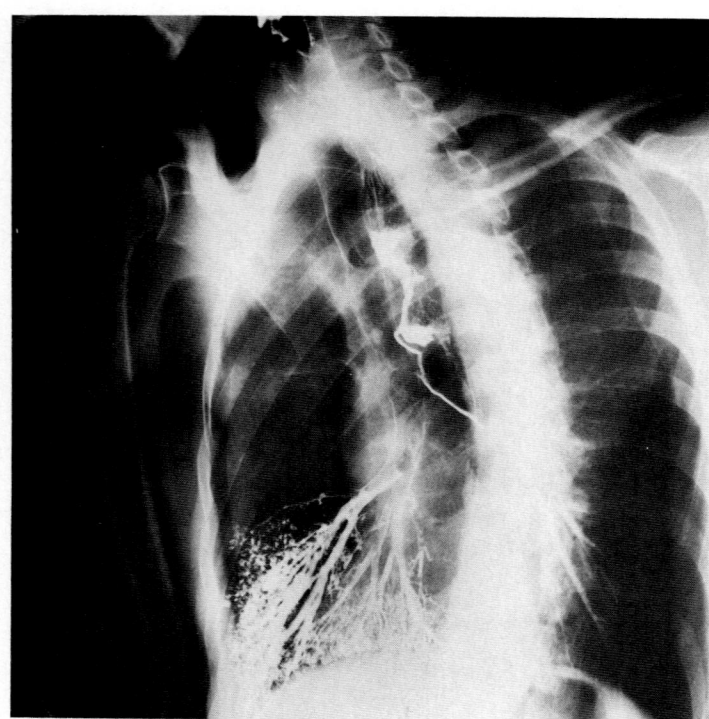

FIGURE 56-5 Aspiration pneumonitis in association with carcinoma of the esophagus in a 49-year-old man. After several episodes of aspiration had occurred while eating, a barium swallow (shown here) was performed. The radiograph shows ingested barium flowing from the esophagus into the tracheobronchial tree through a carcinomatous fistula.

victim suddenly interrupts the conversation by beginning to choke and to gasp desperately for breath. Sometimes the individual is suspected of being in the throes of a heart attack or stroke. The picture is actually that of acute asphyxia; cyanosis and air hunger predominate. Arterial hypercapnia and hypoxemia drive the ventilation, but breathing efforts are ineffective. Very quickly, unless the obstruction is relieved, the central nervous stimulation of respiration gives way to respiratory depression which, coupled with exhaustion, ends in asphyxia and death.

The only effective therapy is to remove the obstruction which often acts like a check valve, allowing air to exit but not to enter. One popular approach is a "bear hug" from behind—the Heimlich maneuver—to dislodge the solid particle. Although it can be executed too forcefully, fracturing ribs and diaphragm in the process, as a rule it is uncomplicated and often lifesaving. If it is suspected that pieces of the material have broken off to enter the bronchi, rigid bronchoscopy is in order once the catastrophic episode is over.

Another familiar type of aspirated solid particle is a peanut or seed that lodges in a major bronchus (Fig. 56-6). Dry vegetable fibers, such as the peanut, tend to be retained in the bronchial lumen, becoming hydrated and swollen, gradually impacting and not only obstructing the lumen but also interfering with local cleansing mechanisms. The manifestations range from acute coughing and chest pain immediately after the foreign body is aspirated,

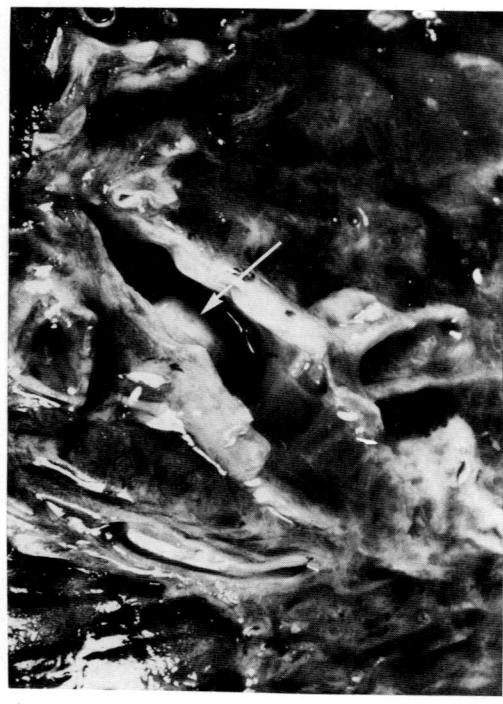

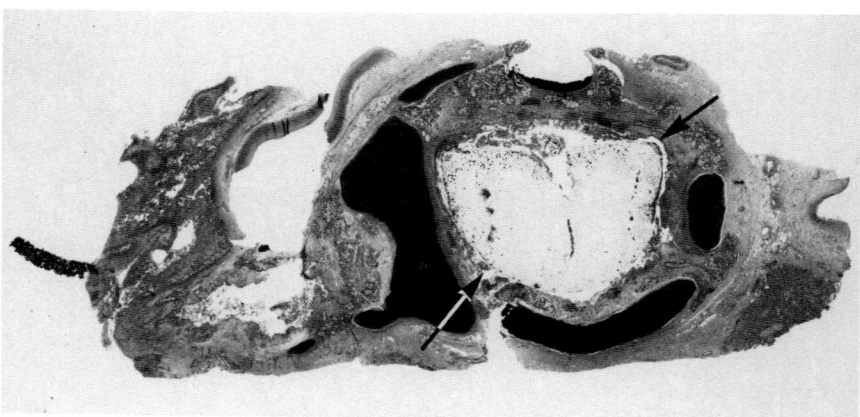

B

A

FIGURE 56-6 Bronchial obstruction caused by aspiration of a peanut in a 45-year-old man. A. Gross specimen of the resected right lower lobe with the bronchus opened. Lying within the bronchial lumen is an aspirated peanut (arrow). B. Low-power cross-sectional view of a bronchus that was totally obstructed by vegetable fibers (arrows). ×3 (Courtesy of Dr. Ray Mark.)

to gradual atelectasis that evolves over days, to a chronic localized cholesterol pneumonia as the cells of the foreign body desquamate, and in time to bronchiectasis that extends distally from the site of obstruction. Treatment depends on the time between inhalation and recognition: early on, the material can be removed through a rigid bronchoscope. Once the stage of pulmonary infiltrate is reached, bronchiectasis becomes the predominant problem. If the diagnosis of aspirated foreign body is made and the obstruction removed by bronchoscopy, medical management occasionally succeeds. However, often the nature of the underlying process remains obscure until the segment is removed surgically.

Gastric Contents

Vomiting by an individual with inadequate function of the glottic opening is the most common cause of aspira-

tion. The material that enters the tracheobronchial tree can be categorized as either semisolid, liquid, or feculent; its nature depends on the clinical state of the patient just prior to the episode. The effects of aspirating solid material were described in the previous section. In this section, the consequences of aspirating liquid gastric contents are considered.

Aspiration occurs either overtly or silently. During the first 1 to 3 h after aspiration, the patient usually appears to be clinically well. Subsequently, dyspnea and tachypnea appear and rapidly intensify; cyanosis, tachycardia, and systemic hypotension then develop.

On the chest radiograph, the pulmonary parenchyma usually appears to be normal immediately after the episode. However, soon after the aspiration (Fig. 56-7), often coincident with the onset of symptoms, a diffuse, confluent, alveolar infiltrate appears in the areas affected by the aspiration. The area of the lung that is involved on the

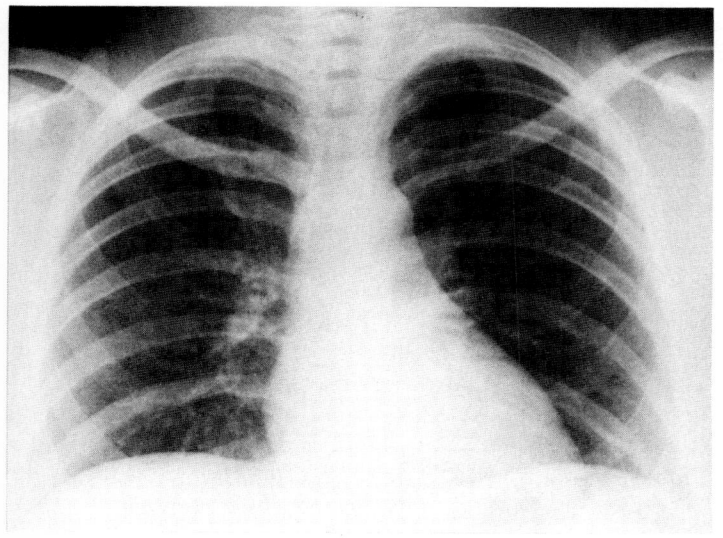

A

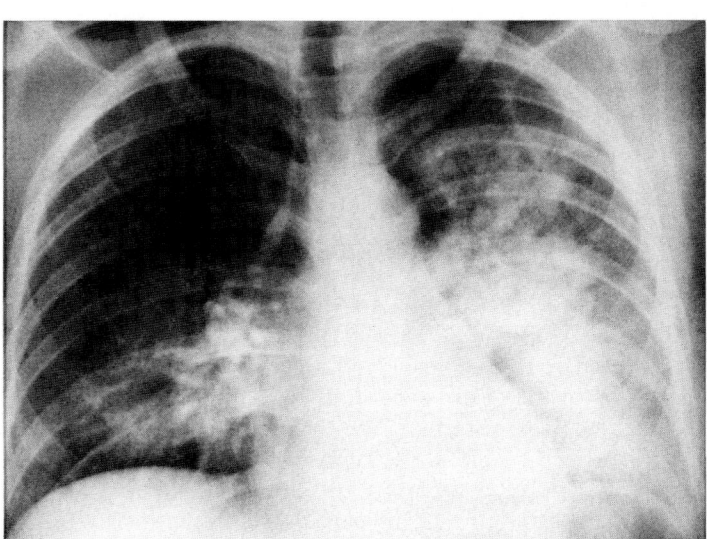

B

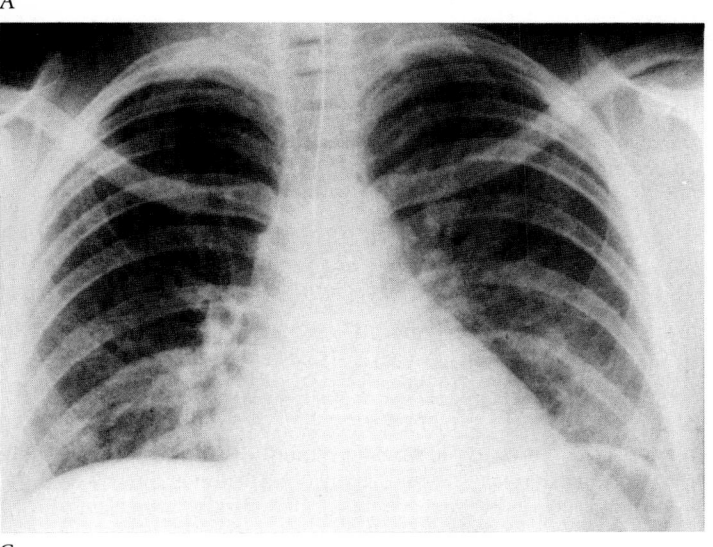

C

FIGURE 56-7 Aspiration pneumonitis in a 38-year-old woman following abdominal surgery for management of a ruptured tubal pregnancy. *A.* Preoperatively. Normal chest radiograph. *B.* Two hours postoperatively. Despite the intraoperative use of a cuffed endotracheal tube, her clinical course and chest radiograph suggested aspiration of gastric acid. *C.* Three days postoperatively. Remarkable clearing of the infiltrate has occurred in this short time span.

chest radiograph depends on the position of the patient at the time that vomiting occurred. Most often the infiltrate involves the posterior and inferior portions of the lungs. However, since the deposition of fluid depends on gravity, the patient's position during the vomiting determines the site of pneumonitis. The right lung is often more severely affected than the left lung because of the straighter disposition of the right main-stem bronchus. The apexes of the lungs are rarely involved, except after large volumes of acid are aspirated.

The acute radiographic changes are not distinctive. They usually resemble the patterns of pulmonary edema, but a variety of other disease processes are often mimicked. Indeed, unless the vomiting episode has been witnessed, the radiographic changes are usually attributed to left ventricular failure, i.e., hemodynamic pulmonary edema. The lack of cardiomegaly, the inability to demonstrate reorientation of the vascular pattern toward the apexes, and the asymmetric appearance of the infiltrate are sometimes helpful in differentiating aspiration pneumonitis from hemodynamic pulmonary edema. If aspiration has been massive, progressive changes ("white out") evolve on the chest radiograph. These changes are indistinguishable from those of the adult respiratory distress syndrome.

PATHOPHYSIOLOGY OF ASPIRATING GASTRIC CONTENTS

In 1946, Mendelson described a distinctive clinical entity in 40 obstetric patients that he attributed to the aspiration of acid gastric contents (Fig. 56-8). He surmised that the syndrome of dyspnea, tachypnea, cyanosis, tachycardia, and systemic hypotension that had occurred in his patients soon after surgery (cesarean section) was due to aspirated hydrochloric acid.

Since then, it has become increasingly evident that the type and severity of the damage depends heavily on the character of the aspirate: not only the pH of the aspiration liquid but also the presence or absence of particulate matter and the size of the particles are important determinants of the subsequent pathophysiological sequence.

Small Volumes of Fluids

In an attempt to evaluate the effects of aspiration on large airways, Wynne et al. performed scanning electron microscopy on tracheal samples from mice that had undergone experimental instillation of small volumes of various test fluids, including normal saline (pH 5.9), hydrochloric acid (pH 1.5), filtered acidic canine gastric juice (pH 1.5), or filtered neutralized canine gastric juice (pH 5.9). Although the tracheal mucosa of the saline-treated animals

showed no changes, both the HCl-treated and the acidic gastric juice-treated (pH 1.5) groups showed prompt and complete loss of ciliated and nonciliated respiratory epithelial cells. Regeneration of nearly normal epithelium occurred within 7 days after instilling the HCl but was only about 50 percent completed 7 days after instilling the acidic gastric juice (pH 1.5). Animals that received a bolus of gastric juice at high pH (5.9) also showed mucosal damage, but the damage was more moderate and healing was similarly delayed.

These studies, using small quantities of test fluids, made several important points. Damage to the mucosa of the large airways occurs promptly at the time of acid aspiration; the damage ranges in severity from mild to hemorrhagic and affects primarily subsegmental bronchi. Although the pH of the aspirated fluid was a critical determinant of the severity of damage, it was not the only important factor; other constituents of gastric juice appear to have the ability to injure respiratory epithelium and to retard healing. Aspiration of small volumes of gastric contents is generally considered to be a common event, one that occurs in most people during normal sleep. Even when the volume is small enough to be unnoticed because it does not reach the alveoli, the loss of ciliated respiratory epithelial cells of the large airways may injure the defense mechanisms of the lung, particularly in patients with preexisting pulmonary disease. However, convincing demonstration of an increased incidence of respiratory tract infections as a result of repeated small volume aspiration has not yet been presented.

An important feature of the response to acid aspiration is reflex bronchospasm. This has been observed clinically since the earliest observations of aspiration pneumonia, but the underlying mechanism has been elucidated only recently by Boyle et al. who found that the introduction of minute amounts of hydrochloric acid into the trachea of cats elicits more than a fourfold increase in mean inspiratory and expiratory pressures and in total lung resistance. The amount of acid instilled (0.05 ml) was intentionally kept small to ensure that lower respiratory tract structures were not affected. Introduction of a similar volume of saline into the trachea failed to elicit bronchospasm. Although each animal subjected to acid in the trachea experienced a large increase in total pulmonary resistance, the change was transient and returned to baseline values within 1 min. That the vagus nerve played a role in producing these changes was confirmed by performing bilateral cervical vagotomy—which abolished the airway response. This vagally mediated reflex has also been implicated in the causation of asthma in patients with reflux esophagitis. Although it was once believed that esophageal irritation could, per se, cause vagally mediated bronchospasm, experimental evidence suggests that tracheal irritation is a far more likely initiating mechanism.

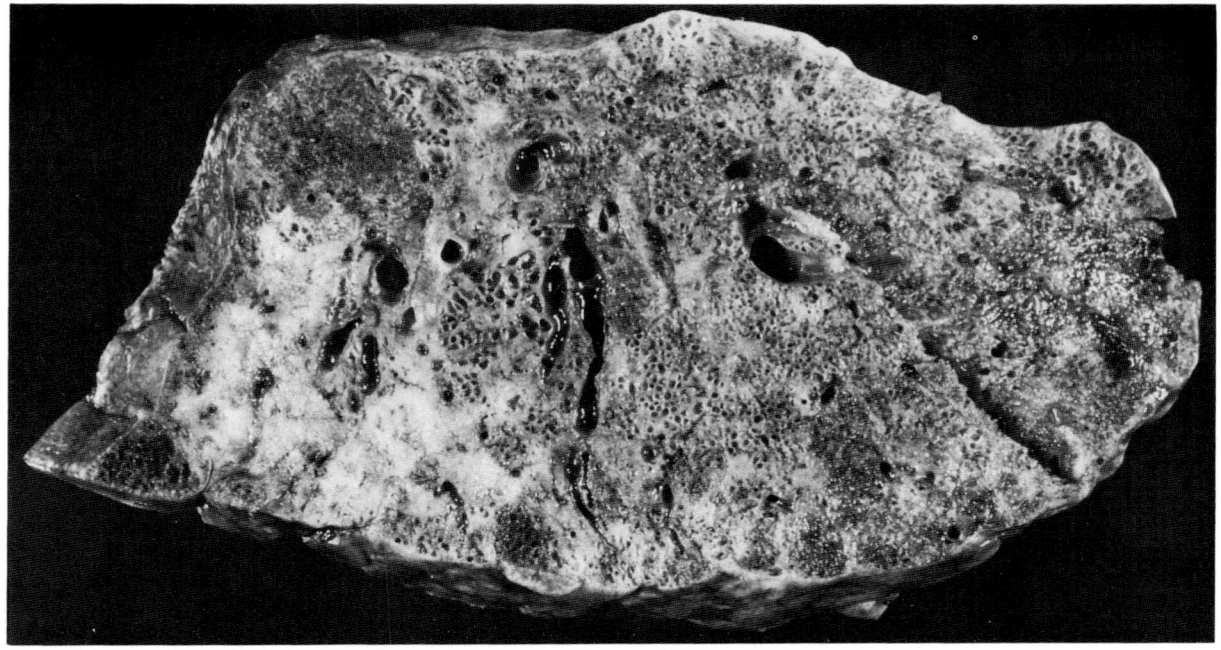

A

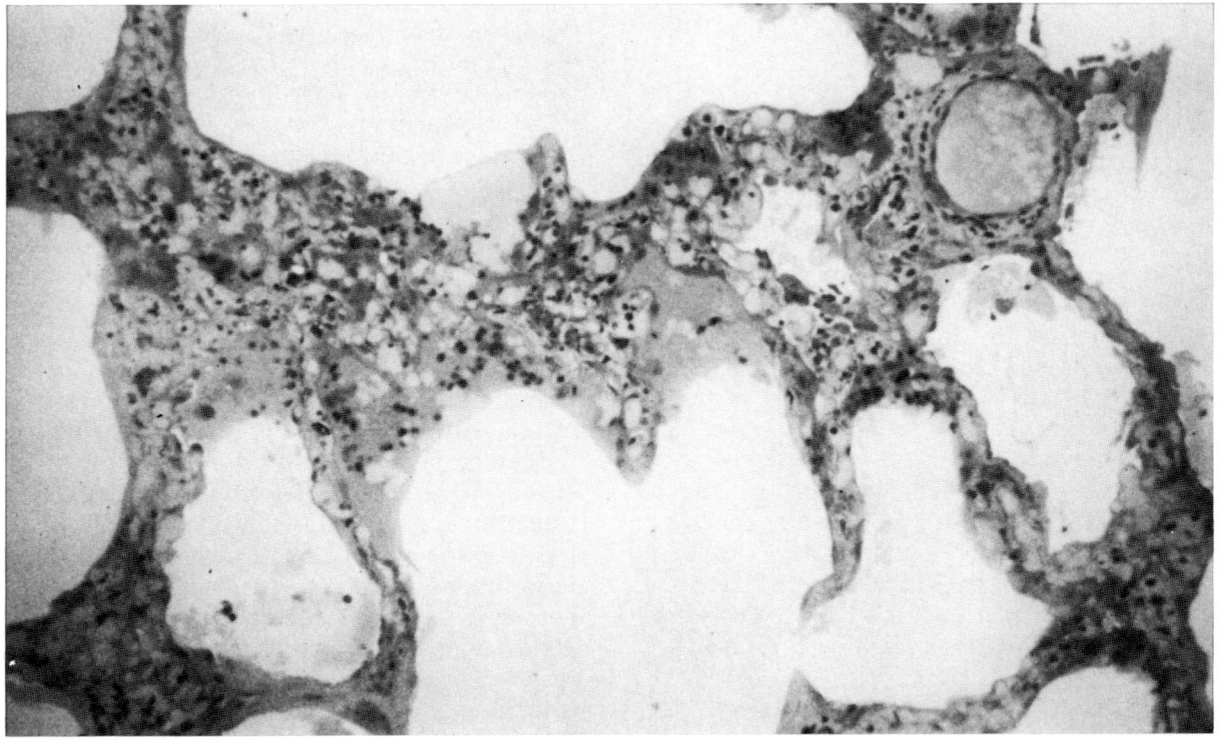

B

FIGURE 56-8 Late effects of gastric acid aspiration. *A*. Gross specimen of lung at autopsy shows severe tissue destruction with cystic degeneration and focal bronchopneumonia at the base. *B*. Microscopic section of the same lung shows interstitial fibrosis and loss of normal alveolar architecture. H&E, ×160.

Larger Volumes of Fluids

Larger volumes of aspirated material evoke greater disturbances than those described above. Most experimental models of aspiration pneumonia have used between 1.5 and 3.0 ml/kg of body weight of liquids. When volumes of this magnitude are used, the nature of the response depends largely on the pH of the liquids instilled or aspirated. Both clinical and experimental observations suggest that the liquid is rapidly spread distally to the alveoli. In fact, using methylene blue as a tracer, staining of the pleura can be observed within 12 to 18 s of aspiration. When hydrochloric acid of pH less than 2.5 is instilled, the alveolar epithelial cells are rapidly destroyed; both type I and type II pneumocytes are lost and pre-formed surfactant is instantaneously inactivated.

In humans, the damage has been found to involve the entire alveolar capillary barrier, including the basement membranes and the capillary endothelial cells. Damage to these structures causes major changes in the permeability of pulmonary blood vessels and results in a massive shift of plasma constituents and of the formed elements of the blood into the alveoli. Contact between the aspirated material and the tracheobronchial mucous proteins, as well as the proteins in the exudate, rapidly buffers the acid entering the lungs. Within 10 min of aspirating fluid of pH 1.5, the measured pH rises to 3.5, a level generally recognized as causing no further caustic damage. Nonetheless, initial contact with highly acidic liquid has been shown to increase vascular permeability in a predictable fashion. Experimental models, using intravascular loads of colloid materials of varying molecular weight and size, have shown that the speed and magnitude of extracapillary leakage varies inversely with the pH up to the limiting value of 2.5; above this value, pulmonary alveolar-capillary permeability does not seem to increase. Although it is reasonable to attribute the increase in alveolar-capillary permeability entirely to the mechanical consequences of cell damage and death, the possibility exists that histamine, released by mast cells in the lungs as a response to the presence of acid, may also contribute to the leakiness of the alveolar-capillary barrier. Determination of histamine concentrations in the alveoli in experimental models of aspiration have shown appreciable increments in animals exposed to liquid of below pH 2.5.

THE LEAKY ALVEOLAR-CAPILLARY BARRIER

Pulmonary arterial pressures increase dramatically in both patients and experimental animals early in the course of acid aspiration, presumably for diverse reasons, such as hypoxia, mechanical alterations in the parenchyma evoked by edema and the inflammatory process, local atelectasis, congestion and thromboses in the pulmonary microvessels, and the local release of vasoactive substances by damaged tissue. The end result is a leaky

alveolar-capillary barrier. Any increase in hydrostatic pressure tends to worsen the leak and to promote alveolar flooding. The accumulation of excess water in the lungs is reflected in the increase in lung weight. Pulmonary angiography performed following acid aspiration has demonstrated severe vascular narrowing in the region of pulmonary damage. As intravascular volume is depleted by the exudation of fluid into the lungs, both systemic and pulmonary artery pressures fall.

The permeability changes described above, complicated by increments in pulmonary microcirculatory pressures, decrease pulmonary compliance presumably due to interstitial and alveolar edema and flooding. Abnormal relationships between alveolar ventilation and blood flow derange alveolar-capillary gas exchange, resulting in arterial hypoxemia, without hypercapnia, due to venous admixture. Shunting of blood through unventilated areas of lung after aspiration of gastric contents is often quite large. The clinical picture of diffuse alveolar-capillary damage, "permeability" pulmonary edema, and arterial hypoxemia that is refractory to treatment, accompanied by the characteristic whiting out of the lungs on the chest radiograph, often leads to the clinical diagnosis of adult respiratory distress syndrome.

Ingredients Other Than Fluids

Early studies of aspiration pneumonia stressed the importance of low pH as the primary determinant of injury to the respiratory tract. It was thought that aspiration of liquid with a pH greater than 2.5 would cause only transient physiological derangement, approximating that caused by a similar volume of saline. This concept has since been challenged by a variety of experimental observations: (1) aspiration of partially digested foodstuffs elicits inflammatory reactions in the lungs even when pH is as high as 3.5; (2) fecal contamination of the aspirated material is lethal, no matter what the pH; (3) the presence of food in the aspirate virtually abolishes the acute inflammatory reaction caused by the aspiration of acid but complicates the situation by adding the element of mechanical obstruction of the airways that, in turn, interferes with gas exchange (as manifested by acute arterial hypoxemia and hypercapnia); (4) the delayed response (48 h) to aspiration of small food particles of beef and vegetables caught in bronchioles is an inflammatory process, often confluent and occasionally hemorrhagic, in which polymorphonuclear leukocytes and macrophages center around the retained material; many, but not all of the abnormalities in gas exchange in this "late" stage are attributable to the mechanical trapping and inflammatory response in the bronchioles; and (5) the physiological effect of aspirating nonparticulate material of high pH is gone within 48 h.

These experimental observations correlate quite well with clinical experience in that aspiration of gastric con-

tents usually produces a dramatic acute onset but may then either resolve quickly or evolve into the adult respiratory distress syndrome. In clinical settings, it is difficult to be certain about the pH of vomitus reaching the lungs, since proteinaceous tracheobronchial secretions rapidly buffer the aspirated material. Estimates of acidity of the aspirate in humans, based on samples of gastric contents procured by nasogastric tube as quickly as possible after aspiration, indicate that the syndrome that follows aspiration of gastric fluid of high pH resolves rapidly. Recurrent aspiration of particulate matter produces a finely granular infiltrate on the chest radiograph that can only be inferred to represent a bronchiolar inflammatory process.

CLINICAL ASSESSMENT

Clinical assessment of patients suspected of having aspirated gastric contents must take into account the medical background of the individual, the setting in which the event has taken place, and the pathophysiology of the illness. The diagnosis is not difficult if the event has been witnessed by medical personnel. However, since aspiration frequently occurs in patients with altered states of consciousness, the diagnosis must also be suspected in neurologically impaired or anesthetized patients who suddenly develop respiratory distress. Frequently, regurgitation and aspiration occur silently, and the only clues to the correct diagnosis are the onset of a typical clinical pattern of respiratory distress associated with a characteristically abnormal chest radiograph.

Assessment begins with examination of the oropharynx for vomitus. Nasotracheal suctioning may also provide evidence for the diagnosis if food particles are recovered as the suction catheter traverses the nasopharynx or as it enters the trachea itself. Microscopic examination of the aspirated material is sometimes helpful in demonstrating vegetable or meat fibers. The patient is usually tachypneic and restless, and cyanosis is common. Fever is often mild or moderate, even in the presence of infection. Auscultatory changes frequently include a cacophony of coarse rhonchi or wheezes and rales. These adventitious sounds reflect the presence of foreign matter in the tracheobronchial tree, and vagally mediated bronchospastic response to airway invasion, and the presence of edema fluid in the distal airways. Examination of the chest radiograph reveals an alveolar infiltrate in the dependent segments of the lungs. When aspiration has occurred in the supine position, the affected areas are the posterior segment of the upper lobe and the superior and posterior basal segments of the lower lobe. The right lung is involved more often than the left lung because of the straighter course between the trachea and right main bronchus. It should be emphasized that other lung segments may be predominantly involved because of the body posi-

tion at the time of regurgitation or because the volume of aspirated material is large. Segmental or lobar collapse indicates the presence of large food particles that have occluded major bronchi.

Arterial blood-gas analysis is critically important in both the initial assessment and in following the course of the illness. Arterial hypoxemia is a constant feature of clinically significant aspiration pneumonia, and its intensity often determines the outcome of the illness. Clinically, hypercapnia is uncommon; when it does occur, it suggests aspiration of moderate-sized particulate matter from the stomach. The state of fluid balance is initially assessed by observing the stability of the systemic arterial blood pressure, the tendency to orthostasis, and the output of urine. However, in view of the necessity to expand the intravascular volume aggressively in patients with underlying medical disorders who are suspected of having aspirated, many clinicians also introduce a Swan-Ganz catheter into the pulmonary artery for hemodynamic monitoring. This allows measurement of pulmonary capillary wedge pressure to prevent overloading the left ventricle as well as pulmonary artery pressure, and oxygen saturation of mixed venous blood as an estimate of oxygen extraction by the tissues. Once the disease is established, and the need for more sophisticated monitoring equipment arises, the patient is moved to the intensive-care unit setting.

TREATMENT

Four concerns dictate the response of the clinician to the diagnosis of aspiration pneumonia: (1) maintenance of adequate oxygenation, (2) maintenance of adequate intravascular volume, (3) promotion of reparative processes, and (4) avoidance or treatment of infection. Therapeutic measures to deal with these concerns often overlap. The sine qua non for effective treatment is to avoid severe arterial hypoxemia.

Bronchoscopy

As in other causes of acute respiratory failure, the physician must ensure a clear airway before other methods in support of oxygenation are considered. If mechanical removal of particulate matter from the respiratory tract is required, rigid bronchoscopy is performed. Although fiberoptic bronchoscopy is simple and allows diagnostic assessment of the tracheobronchial tree, it is inefficient and incomplete in removing particulate matter.

Although large- and moderate-sized particles should be removed at bronchoscopy, it is probably counterproductive to lavage the tracheobronchial tree with large amounts of fluid in an attempt to remove small particles because of the likelihood of dispersing the aspirate into

peripheral portions of the lung. Moreover, the use of alkaline lavage fluids is inappropriate since buffering of aspirated gastric contents by tracheobronchial secretions and exudate is virtually complete within 10 to 15 min of the acute event. Nor are exogenous alkalinizing agents used, since they may, per se, cause damage.

Respiratory Therapy

The primary goal of management after aspiration is to avoid intolerable levels of arterial hypoxemia. As a rule, the mainstay for accomplishing this goal is supplemental oxygen. In experimental studies involving aspiration of hydrochloric acid, intermittent positive pressure breathing, with or without positive end-expiratory pressure (PEEP), has improved mortality statistics. However, the clinical situation is often less severe than the experimental, so that maintenance of arterial oxygenation can often be accomplished by supplemental oxygen alone, as long as exposure for days to concentrations greater than 50 percent is avoided (see Chapter 151). In essence, if adequate arterial oxygenation (arterial O_2 saturations greater than 80 percent) can be maintained without endotracheal intubation and mechanical ventilation, the trauma and risks entailed in these procedures should be avoided. Conversely, if the situation deteriorates to the level of the adult respiratory distress syndrome, more vigorous intervention in the intensive-care setting is generally required (see Chapter 143).

Fluid Management

Damage to the alveolar-capillary membrane caused by aspiration of gastric acid can produce a massive shift of fluid from the intravascular space into the interstitium and alveoli. A rapid onset of systemic hypotension and of hemoconcentration after aspiration attests to the magnitude of the shift. Although the onset of hypotension calls for the immediate restoration of intravascular volume, the literature is not as certain about whether crystalloids or colloids should be used in replacement therapy.

Presumably, the rationale for infusing colloids has been to raise the intravascular colloid osmotic pressure, thereby promoting the reversal of pulmonary edema. However, this rationale is faulty in that it presupposes that the capillary barrier remains semipermeable, i.e., impermeable to albumin. In severe instances of aspiration injury, the concentration of albumin in fluid from the airways has proved to be the same as in plasma, i.e., large parts of the alveolar barrier have become completely leaky to albumin. In these severe instances, it is difficult to imagine how infusion of albumin can decrease pulmonary edema. Conversely, if alveolar-capillary barriers do retain their integrity in certain parts of the lungs, albumin reaching these areas could promote the reabsorption of pulmonary edema fluid.

With few exceptions, experimental studies have failed to establish a therapeutic advantage of albumin—either in the intact animal or in the isolated lobe. Moreover, the early studies that did favor albumin are flawed in that they did not maintain rigid hemodynamic control of the pulmonary circulation; relatively small elevations of pulmonary artery pressure in acid-damaged lungs can cause a major increase in fluid exudation.

Clinical experience tends to confirm that crystalloid fluid replacement is at least as effective as colloid. The volume status of the patient must be monitored carefully to ensure that vascular pressures in the pulmonary microcirculation do not increase appreciably to enhance transduction into the leaky lungs. Because of the dire consequences of subjecting damaged vessels to increased microvascular pressures, a Swan-Ganz catheter to monitor pulmonary wedge pressures is virtually mandatory in managing seriously ill patients.

Corticosteroids

Corticosteroids have been used clinically in the management of aspiration pneumonia since 1955. The theoretical basis for the use of steroids rests on their anti-inflammatory and lysosomal membrane stabilizing properties. Despite initial optimism, the consensus reached during the past decade is that steroids are ineffective in the management of aspiration pneumonia—either acutely or chronically.

Infection and Antibiotics

Invasion of the respiratory tract by foreign materials is often followed by infection. The fact that the lower respiratory tract is ordinarily sterile is testimony to the efficiency of the mechanical and immunologic defenses of the lung. Aspiration of gastric contents imposes an unusual, and frequently overwhelming, burden on the defense mechanisms by presenting a large bacterial inoculum at the same time that mucociliary function is damaged and leukocyte access is impeded. Nonetheless, it is often difficult to diagnose the onset of infection following aspiration since radiographic infiltrates, fever, cough, and leukocytosis result from the damage caused by the presence of acid in the lung whether or not infection has taken place.

In fact, infection does not appear to be a primary, or early, event in aspiration of gastric contents. Instead, infection usually occurs several days later when reparative processes have begun. Its presence is heralded by a recrudescence of fever, increase in the production of sputum that turns purulent, and extension of infiltrate on the chest radiograph. The organisms responsible for the pulmonary infection depend heavily on the setting in which aspiration takes place. Since the presence of hydrochloric acid usually renders the stomach contents sterile, most

organisms causing pulmonary infection originate from the oral cavity through which the gastric contents travel en route to the lungs: in patients who have not been chronically ill, anaerobic organisms predominate in the mouth, although aerobic species are also present in lesser numbers; in patients who have been hospitalized for a long while, either because of chronic illness or acute, severe illness, the oral cavity is often colonized by gram-negative organisms, changing the available flora from which infectious organisms may be recruited.

Four clinical presentations are characteristic of anaerobic, or mixed, pleuropulmonary infections due to aspiration of gastric contents: (1) pneumonia, (2) lung abscess, (3) necrotizing pneumonia, and (4) empyema—the last

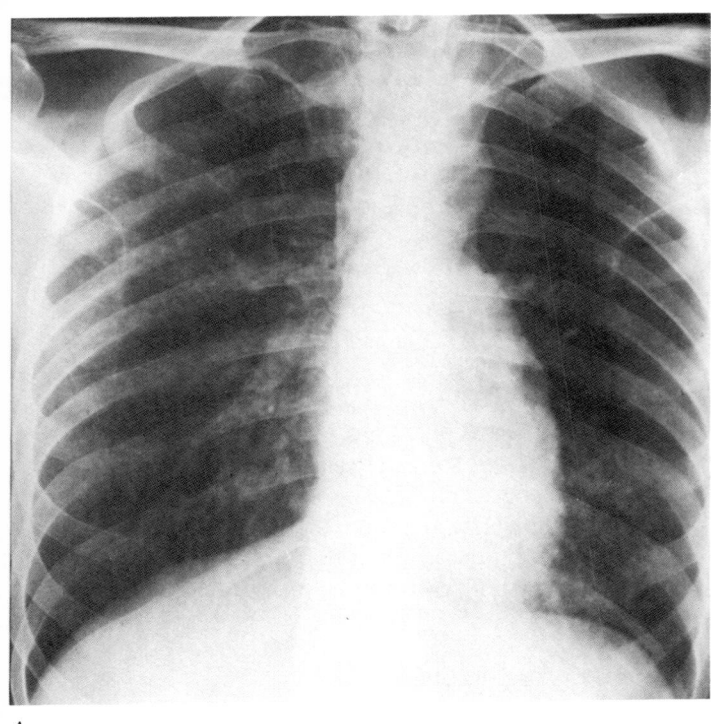

A

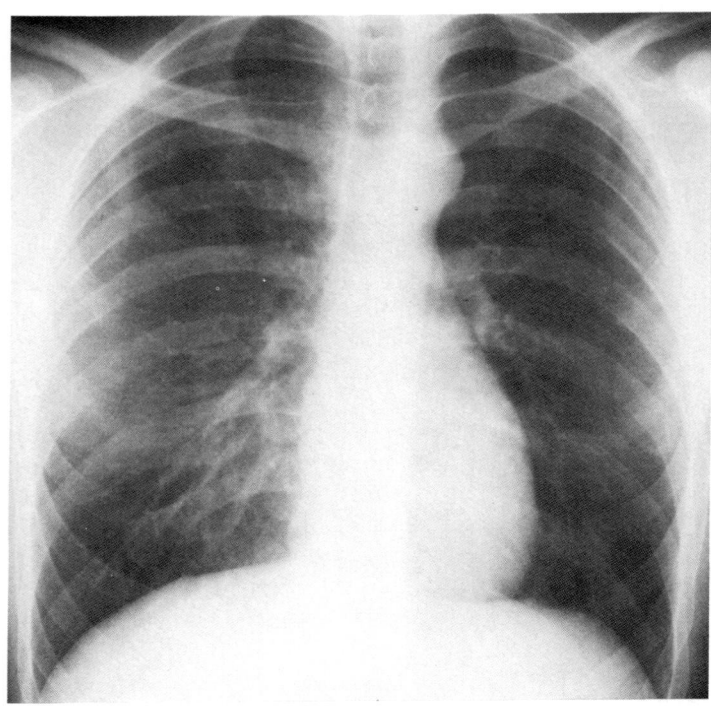

B

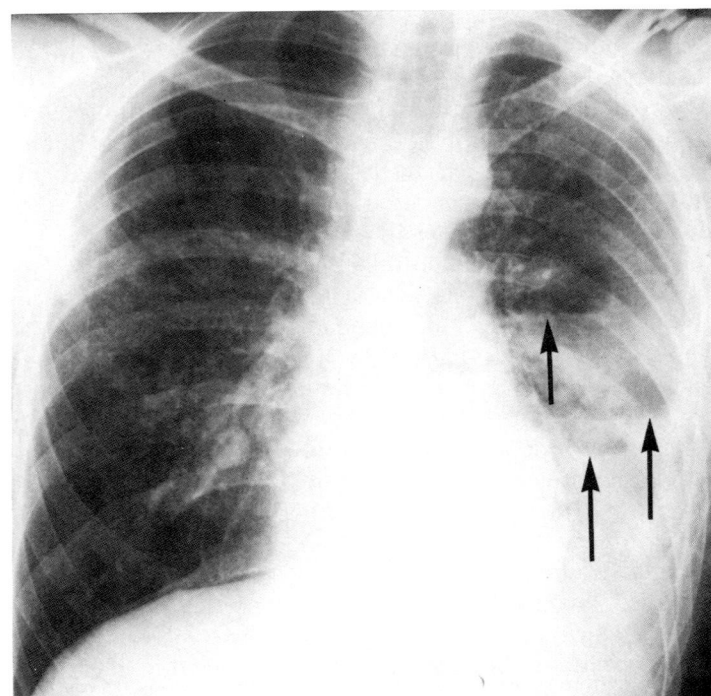

C

FIGURE 56-9 Necrotizing pneumonia following aspiration of gastric contents. *A.* Normal chest radiograph of a 27-year-old man admitted to the hospital for evaluation of a seizure disorder. *B.* Two days later, after a seizure, a patchy bronchopneumonic infiltrate can be seen in both lungs. *C.* One week later, multiple air-fluid levels (arrows) and empyema can be seen in the left hemithorax, indicating the presence of a necrotizing pneumonia.

usually occurring in association with one of the others (Figs. 56-9 and 56-10). In 54 patients with postaspiration pulmonary infections, Bartlett et al. found anaerobes alone in 25, both anaerobes and aerobes in 25, and aerobes alone in only 4 patients; community-acquired infections were more apt to be with anaerobes alone, whereas hospital-acquired infections were more likely to be with both anaerobes and aerobes. Anaerobic isolates included *Bacteroides melaninogenicus, Fusobacterium nucleatum, Peptostreptococcus, Bacteroides fragilis,* and microaerophilic streptococci. Aerobic (or facultative) bacteria included *Staphylococcus aureus, Diplococcus pneumoniae,* enteric gram-negative bacilli, and *Pseudomonas.*

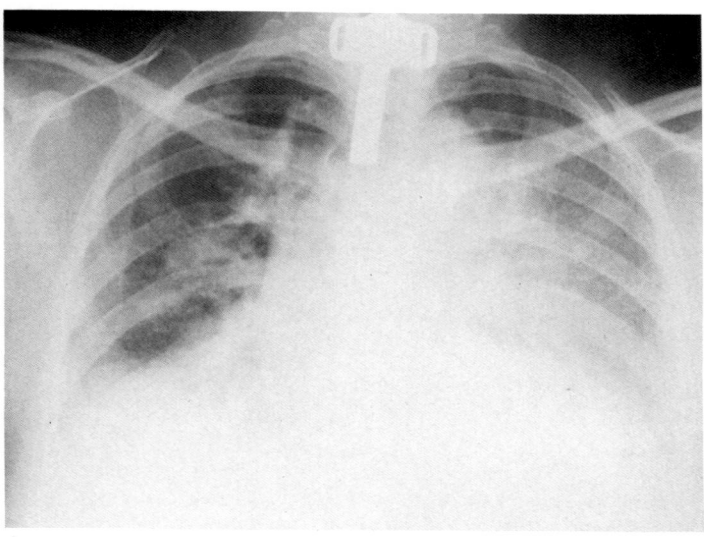

A

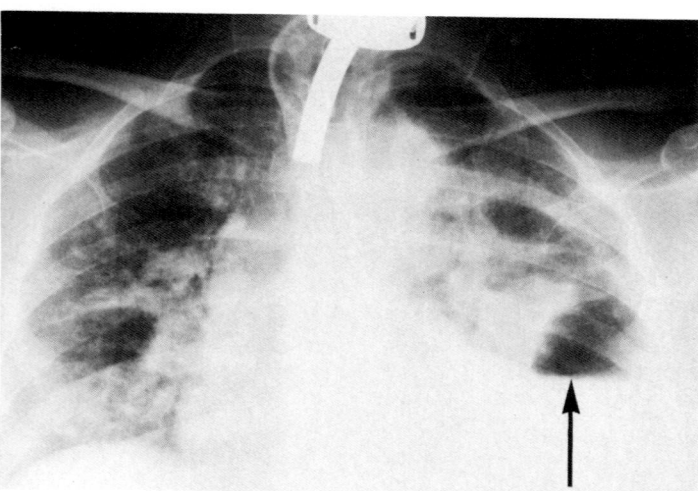

B

FIGURE 56-10 Lung abscess resulting from aspiration of gastric contents. *A.* Chest radiograph of a 48-year-old woman who was admitted to the hospital in a comatose state after having ingested 10 g of glutethimide (Doriden). Two hours before this radiograph was taken, she had vomited and aspirated her gastric contents. *B.* Five days later, a large cavity (arrow) with an air-fluid level is present in the lung.

Antibiotics continue to be used widely in patients who have aspirated. However, the administration of antibiotics before the onset of overt infection has little or no demonstrably beneficial effect on the subsequent course of the illness. In fact, studies have suggested that despite prophylactic antibiotics, infection can occur and is sometimes complicated by the emergence of resistant organisms. These findings suggest that the appropriate course of action would be to observe the postaspiration patient carefully for evidence of infection, to identify the process, i.e., pneumonia, lung abscess, necrotizing pneumonia, and/or empyema, to isolate the responsible organism, to select proper antibiotics based on bacteriologic results, and to incorporate antibiotics, as needed, in the overall management program.

PREVENTION

Although the pathophysiology of aspiration pneumonia has been greatly clarified in recent years, this understanding has not improved the clinical outlook for patients with this disorder. The mortality rate is still of the order of 55 to 70 percent. Desperate interventions, such as the use of the membrane oxygenator in severe aspiration pneumonia, have proved fruitless, in large measure because of the extensive and irreversible damage to the pulmonary parenchyma (Fig. 56-8).

Prevention is, therefore, more apt to be rewarding than treatment of consequences of severe aspiration pneumonia. Some predisposing causes such as substance abuse and cerebrovascular disease are beyond the control of the physician; others can be modified. For example, careful preoperative preparation has decreased the incidence of this syndrome markedly. The use of smaller nasogastric feeding tubes that produce less disruption of esophageal sphincter action is another reasonable measure. Even with small-bore nasogastric tubes in place, care must be taken not to overfill the stomach in the course of daily feeding, and gastric residuum should be assessed frequently.

The possibility of aspiration at the time of parturition deserves special mention. Since gastric emptying is frequently delayed at the onset of labor, a variety of therapeutic maneuvers have been recommended to decrease the likelihood of aspirating acidic material. Administration of antacids prior to delivery has been shown to be reliable in raising gastric pH above 2.5, but no studies have been done to show that this strategy actually decreases the incidence of aspiration pneumonia. Furthermore, a potential danger to the prepartum, or preoperative, administration of antacids is that aspiration of these materials may also produce an inflammatory response in the lung. Consequently, another pharmacologic

approach has been advocated to decrease gastric acid production, i.e., the administration of cimetadine, either orally or parenterally, before parturition or surgery. This technique has proved successful in increasing gastric pH. In principle, by combining the administration of cimetadine with metoclopramide, an agent that promotes gastric emptying, the prospect of avoiding aspiration in surgical or obstetrical patients would be expected to improve. However, this approach has not yet been sufficiently tested to establish its efficacy.

BIBLIOGRAPHY

Awe WC, Fletcher WS, Jacob SW: The pathophysiology of aspiration pneumonitis. Surgery 16:232–239, 1966.
  The response to intratracheal instillation of hydrochloric acid at various pH levels was tested in 50 dogs. Hemodynamic parameters, plasma volume, and arterial blood gases were monitored. Severe and prolonged abnormalities were noted with instillation of fluid of below pH 3. Treatment with steroids and saline lavage did not favorably influence the course. Positive pressure respiration improved the blood-gas abnormalities.

Bannister WK, Sattilaro AJ, Otis RD: Therapeutic aspects of aspiration pneumonitis in experimental animals. Anesthesiology 22:440–443, 1961.
  This study demonstrates that lavage of the bronchi following aspiration is not helpful in management of the subsequent lung damage.

Bartlett JG, Finegold SM: Anaerobic infections of the lung and pleural space. Am Rev Respir Dis 110:56–77, 1974.
  State-of-the-art discussion of the infectious complications of aspiration of gastric contents with specific emphasis on anaerobic infections.

Bartlett JG, Gorbach SL, Finegold SM: The bacteriology of aspiration pneumonia. Am J Med 56:202–207, 1974.
  Prospective study of 54 cases of pulmonary infection following aspiration of gastric contents demonstrates the predominance of anaerobic organisms in nonhospitalized patients. The common occurrence of aerobic and facultative bacteria, particularly enteric gram-negative bacilli and pseudomonads, was demonstrated in patients whose disease developed in the hospital.

Booth DJ, Zuidema GD, Cameron JL: Aspiration pneumonia: Pulmonary arteriography after experimental aspiration. J Surg Res 12:48–52, 1972.
  Pulmonary angiography was performed before and after the instillation of hydrochloric acid into the right main-stem bronchus. Marked vasospasm and thrombosis of the pulmonary artery branches occurred in untreated animals. In animals treated with positive pressure ventilation the vascular changes did not occur.

Boyle JT, Tuchman DN, Altschuler SM, Nixon TE, Pack AI, Cohen S: Mechanisms for the association of gastroesophageal reflux and bronchospasm. Am Rev Respir Dis 131(suppl):S16–S20, 1985.
  Tracheal and esophageal instillation of hydrochloric acid showed that tracheal irritation was much more powerful than esophageal irritation in the production of reflex bronchospasm.

Buchman SR, Sugarman HJ, Tatum JL, Wright TP, Blocher CR, Hirsch JI: Failure of methylprednisolone, ibuprofen or prostacyclin to reduce HCl induced pulmonary albumin leak in dogs. Surgery 92:163–170, 1984.
  The effect of various anti-inflammatory agents on HCl-induced pulmonary albumin leak was tested in dogs using a gamma scintigraphic technique. None of the anti-inflammatory agents was effective in preventing protein leak across the damaged capillary membrane. Prostacyclin appeared to worsen the abnormality.

Donner MW: Radiologic evaluation of swallowing. Am Rev Respir Dis 131(suppl):S20–S23, 1979.
  Diagnostic imaging procedures were used to analyze the muscular sequence during swallowing.

Gates S, Huang T, Cheney FW: Effects of methylprednisolone on resolution of acid aspiration pneumonitis. Arch Surg 118:1262–1265, 1983.
  Using a canine model of acid aspiration the authors found no therapeutic value of methylprednisolone administration over the 4-day course of the experiment.

Glauser FL, Millen JE, Falls R: Effective acid aspiration on pulmonary alveolar epithelial membrane permeability. Chest 76:201–205, 1979.
  An in vivo model of aspiration pneumonitis using a liquid-filled canine lung measured movement of substances of specific molecular size across the pulmonary alveolar epithelial membrane as a response to injury by acidic solutions. Permeability increased markedly at pH 1.5 and 2.5 but not with pH 3.5 or above. Increased levels of histamine were found in the acid-damaged lungs.

Glauser FL, Millen JE, Falls R: Increased alveolar epithelial permeability with acid aspiration. The effects of high dose steroids. Am Rev Respir Dis 120:1119–1123, 1979.
> *Using the liquid-filled dog lung model, changes in alveolar epithelial permeability were measured in response to acid solutions. Pretreatment or posttreatment with methylprednisolone produced no improvement in the increased permeability associated with acid aspiration.*

Greenfield LJ, Singleton RP, McCaffree DR, Coalson JJ: Pulmonary effects of experimental graded aspiration of hydrochloric acid. Annals Surg 170:74–86, 1969.
> *A canine model of aspiration pneumonitis was used to evaluate the respiratory and hemodynamic changes produced by instillation of acid into the trachea. Hemoconcentration, increased lung weight, severe hypoxia, decreased cardiac output, and increased pulmonary vascular resistance were noted. In addition, rapid loss of surfactant activity occurred after acid instillation.*

Hamelberg W, Bosomworth PP: Aspiration pneumonitis: Experimental studies and clinical observations. Anesthes Analges (Cleve) 43:669–677, 1964.
> *Experimental instillation of hydrochloric acid stained with methylene blue showed rapid distribution of the instilled liquid to the pleura within a period of 12 to 18 s.*

Hausman W, Lunt RL: Problems of treatment of peptic aspiration pneumonia following obstetric anesthesia (Mendelson's syndrome). J Obstet Gynecol Brit Comm 62:509–512, 1955.
> *Description of the first clinical use of corticosteroids in the management of aspiration pneumonia.*

Hodgkinson R, Glassenberg R, Joyce TH, Coombs DW, Ostheimer GW, Gibbs CP: Comparison of cimetadine (Tagamet) with antacid for safety and effectiveness in reducing gastric acidity before elective Caesarean section. Anesthes 59:86–90, 1983.
> *One hundred twenty-six women undergoing cesarean section received either cimetadine or antacid in a randomized, double-blind, multicenter trial. Both cimetadine and antacid were successful in raising the gastric pH to over 2.5.*

Johanson WG, Harris GD: Aspiration pneumonia, anaerobic infections and lung abscess. Med Clin North Am 64:385–394, 1980.
> *The authors present a review of aspiration syndromes with specific regard to infectious complications.*

Lewis RT, Burgess JH, Hampson LG: Cardiorespiratory studies in critical illness: Changes in aspiration pneumonitis. Arch Surg 103:335–340, 1971.
> *Cardiorespiratory studies in 18 patients with acid aspiration pneumonitis were correlated with the clinical course. Hypoxemia was improved by intermittent positive pressure breathing with oxygen. The pneumonitis was noninfective at the onset, and prophylactic antibiotic administration did not prevent subsequent pulmonary infection.*

Lode H: Initial therapy in pneumonia. Clinical, radiographic, and laboratory data important for the choice. Am J Med 80:70–74, 1986.
> *Clinical signs and symptoms, as well as radiographic infiltrations, are of considerable value in community-acquired pneumococcal and aspiration pneumonia. In hospital-acquired pneumonia, the situation is more complex.*

Manchikanti L, Marrero TC, Roush JR: Preanesthetic cimetadine and metoclopromide for acid aspiration prophylaxis in elective surgery. Anesthesiology: 61:48–54, 1984.
> *One hundred fifty patients were randomly allocated to groups receiving metoclopromide, cimetadine, or both in variant dosage schedules. Both cimetadine and metoclopromide favorably modified the risk factors in all the experimental groups.*

Marrie TJ, Durant H, Kwan C: Nursing home-acquired pneumonia. A case-control study. J Am Geriatr Soc 34:697:702, 1986.
> *Aspiration pneumonia was more common among patients with nursing home-acquired pneumonia (p < .001), and Hemophilus influenza pneumonia more common among the patients with community-acquired infection (p < .01).*

Mendelson CL: The aspiration of stomach contents into the lungs during obstetrical anesthesia. Am J Obstet Gynecol 52:191–205, 1946.
> *Classic description of the effects of aspiration of gastric contents in patients and experimental demonstration in animals that the syndrome was due to hydrochloric acid.*

Nanjo S, Bhattacharya J, Staub NC: Concentrated albumin does not affect lung edema formation after acid instillation in the dog. Am Rev Respir Dis 128:884–889, 1983.
> *Acute pulmonary edema caused by hydrochloric acid aspiration was observed in a canine model. Administration of human serum albumin produced no benefit in the prevention or treatment of the pulmonary edema.*

Nelson S, Laughon BE, Summer WR, Eckhaus MA, Bartlett JG, Jakab GJ: Characterization of the pulmonary inflammatory response to an anaerobic bacterial challenge. Am Rev Respir Dis 133:212–217, 1986.
> *After experimental tracheal inoculation in mice, B. gingivalis causes marked inflammation in the lung that progresses to severe bronchopneumonia and lung abscess.*

Peitzman AB, Shires GT, Illner H, Shires GT: Pulmonary acid injury: Effects of positive end-expiratory pressure and crystalloid versus colloid fluid resuscitation. Arch Surg 117:662–668, 1982.
> *A canine model of aspiration pneumonitis was used to study the effect of positive end-expiratory pressure breathing and crystalloid-versus-colloid fluid repletion. PEEP improved oxygenation but did not alter progression of the injury. Cardiac output and oxygen transfer were improved by plasma volume repletion while receiving PEEP, but colloid administration was no better than crystalloid in achieving this result. Colloid did not modify the progression of the injury.*

Peitzman AB, Shires GT, Illner H, Shires GT: The effect of intravenous steroids on alveolar capillary membrane permeability in pulmonary acid injury. J Trauma 22:347–352. 1982.
> *A canine model of acid-induced aspiration pneumonitis demonstrated that pulmonary acid injury resulted in a marked increase in alveolar capillary permeability to albumin, smaller solutes, and water which was not ameliorated by the administration of methylprednisolone.*

Ristagno RL, Kornstein MJ, Hansen-Flaschen JH: Diagnosis of occult meat aspiration by fiberoptic bronchoscopy. Am J Med 80:154–156, 1986.
> *Cytologic examination of bronchial washings from a patient with a persistent localized pulmonary infiltrate revealed large numbers of striated muscle fibers reflecting recent food aspiration.*

Teabeaut JR: Aspiration of gastric contents. Am J Pathol 28:51–62, 1952.
> *A critical influence of pH on the development of aspiration pneumonitis was demonstrated in an animal model.*

Toung TJ, Cameron JL: Cimetadine as a preoperative medication to reduce the complications of aspiration of gastric contents. Surgery 87:205–208, 1980.
> *Comparative study of three groups of 28 patients receiving cimetadine or atropine or glycopyrrolate showed that cimetadine was more effective than the other two medications in raising the gastric pH above 2.5. Ninety-nine percent of the patients receiving cimetadine has gastric pH above that level, while the other two drugs were 29 and 54 percent effective, respectively.*

Toung TJ, Cameron JL, Kimura T, Permutt S: Aspiration pneumonia: Treatment with osmotically active agents. Surgery 89:588–593, 1981.
> *Using an ex vivo perfused ventilation canine pulmonary lobe, the effects of mannitol, dextran, and albumin were tested in aspiration pneumonitis caused by the instillation of hydrochloric acid. Only albumin administration was successful in preventing weight gain in the experimental lobe and in stabilizing the pulmonary artery and end-inspiratory pressures.*

Wynne JW, Demarco FJ, Hood CI: Physiological effects of corticosteroids in food stuff aspiration. Arch Surg 116:46–49, 1981.
> *A canine model of aspiration of gastric contents containing small food particles was used to evaluate the effect of intravenous methylprednisolone on physiological and histologic abnormalities. The authors conclude that steroids are of no benefit in the treatment of foodstuff-induced aspiration pneumonia.*

Wynne JW, Modell JH: Respiratory aspiration of stomach contents. Ann Intern Med 87:466–474, 1977.
> *Thorough clinical review of the pathophysiology of the various syndromes associated with aspiration of stomach contents is presented. Both diagnostic and therapeutic aspects of the problem are also reviewed.*

Wynne JW, Ramphal R, Hood CI: Tracheal mucosal damage after aspiration: A scanning electron microscope study. Am Rev Respir Dis 124:728–732, 1981.
> *A mouse model of aspiration of gastric contents was used to evaluate tracheal damage caused by hydrochloric acid and gastric juice of various pH levels. Scanning electron micrographs showed that gastric contents caused marked damage to the tracheal mucosa that is more severe when the pH of the gastric content is low. In addition, gastric juice may contain substances that delay healing.*

Chapter *57*

Pulmonary Alveolar Proteinosis

William D. Claypool

Pulmonary alveolar proteinosis (PAP) is a syndrome which results from the abnormal accumulation of surfactant phospholipids and proteins in the alveolar spaces. It is an uncommon disorder that affects primarily males and was first described by Rosen et al. in 1958. Although it has been difficult to prove cause and effect, the disorder has occurred in individuals who have experienced different kinds of insult to the lungs. The material that fills the alveolar spaces is protein-lipid in nature, granular and eosinophilic, and it stains positive with the PAS stain (Fig. 57-1). Within the material are found lamellated concentric structures that are counterparts of the cytoplasmic inclusions that characterize alveolar type II cells (see Chapter 2). In most respects, the material in the alveoli is qualitatively similar to normal surfactant. Because of the excess of this material in the alveolar spaces, profound alterations occur in gas exchange, exercise tolerance and probably in alveolar antimicrobial defenses. Appropriate therapy, directed at mechanically removing this material from the alveoli, greatly alleviates symptoms and signs of the disease.

NORMAL SURFACTANT TURNOVER

Alveolar type II cells (granular pneumocytes) secrete the complex material that lines the epithelial surfaces of the lungs and is necessary for maintaining the expanded state that is prerequisite for the lungs to operate. The phospholipid components are now known to be critical for the effectiveness of surfactant as an "antiatelectasis" factor.

Less clear are the functions of other protein components of surfactant. However, both serum proteins and surfactant-specific apoproteins have been identified, some of the latter possibly serving as an important modulator of the recycling of the phospholipids between alveoli and the type II cells as part of the normal turnover of surfactant.

PATHOGENESIS

Pulmonary alveolar proteinosis is a disorder of surfactant homeostasis. Most evidence suggests that it is due to decreased removal of alveolar surfactant rather than to an increase in its production. The turnover of the components of surfactant may be quite rapid. In juvenile experimental animals, the bulk of the surfactant phospholipids recycle—from alveolar spaces through the type II epithelial cells which synthesize them—at turnover times that are measured in hours. In addition, local mechanisms in-

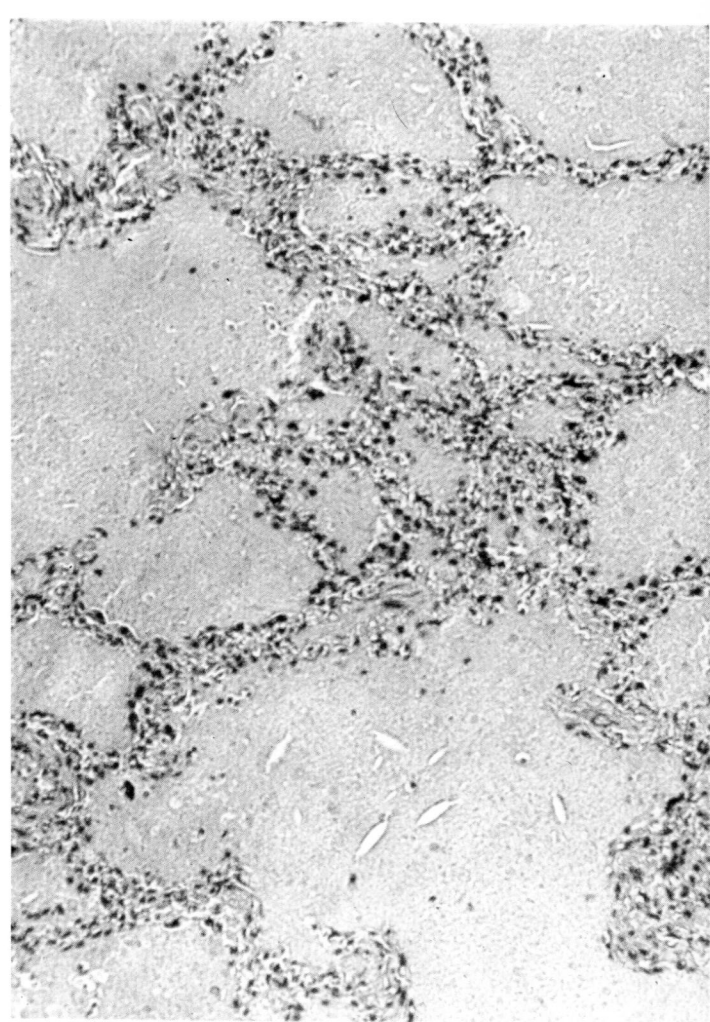

FIGURE 57-1 Light microscopy showing airspaces filled with slightly granular PAS-positive material.

volving surfactant apoproteins may increase the turnover of surfactant phospholipids by the type II epithelial cells. Most of the breakdown and removal of surfactant appears to be accomplished by the type II cells; the alveolar macrophages are less involved. Other mechanisms, such as the ciliary escalator of the airways or the lymphatics, contribute little to the breakdown and removal of the constituents of surfactant.

There are several steps in the intra-alveolar and intracellular regulation of the quantity of surfactant in the alveolar spaces. Interference with the cycle, particularly in the return phase, by diverse stimuli ranging from inorganic particulates, fibrogenic dusts, and wood products to viral infections and antimetabolic chemotherapy, could lead to a decrease in the uptake of the surfactant phospholipid from the alveolar spaces at the level of the surfactant apoproteins or the apoprotein-phospholipid product. However, it should be noted that, although insults to the lungs such as these are common, the clinical syndrome of pulmonary alveolar proteinosis is a distinctly uncommon disorder.

PATHOLOGY

The usual appearance of PAP that is unassociated with other diseases of the lung, i.e., classic or primary PAP, is that of a dense collection of periodic acid-Schiff (PAS)-positive material within the alveolar spaces, whereas the interstitium is normal (Fig. 57-2). The PAP material is biochemically similar to normal surfactant except for more

serum proteins and more specific immunoglobulins than are generally present in normal surfactant. In addition, the material within the alveoli contains normal surfactant apoproteins and possibly surfactant-specific proteins. Compared with normal surfactant, these proteins are either altered or their precursors are overabundant.

In "secondary" PAP, or alveolar phospholipidosis, interstitial thickening of the lung is associated with less homogeneous distribution of surfactant-specific apoproteins. Among the physical insults associated with PAP are inhaled silica and aluminum dust. Amphiphilic cationic drugs, such as chlorphentermine, can induce alveolar phospholipidosis in animals; amiodarone lung toxicity in humans also has some features of a lung phospholipidosis. The phospholipidosis due to amphiphilic drugs involves more than the alveolar spaces since abnormal lipid accumulation is seen in the liver, kidneys, and occasionally in the brain of experimental animals. The extent to which these animal models of phospholipidosis resemble biochemically the human forms of PAP is unclear.

CLINICAL FEATURES

The symptoms of patients with PAP are similar to those of other patients with a progressive restrictive lung disease. As a rule, they complain of a nonproductive cough, progressive dyspnea on exertion, and fatigue. Depending on the severity of the disorder, some experience weight loss, hemoptysis, chest pain, and fevers.

Most patients with PAP are usually between 20 and

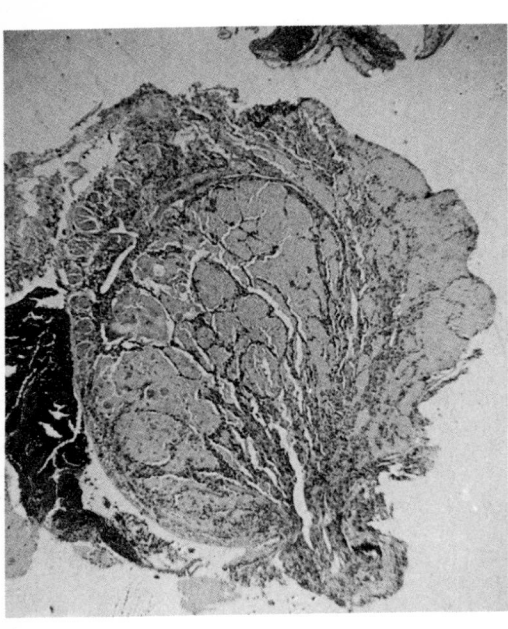
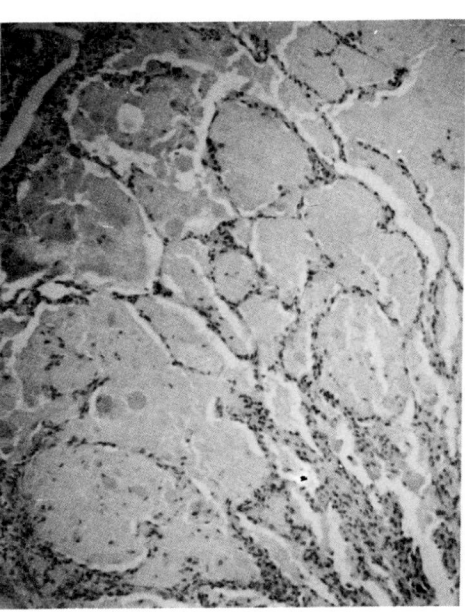
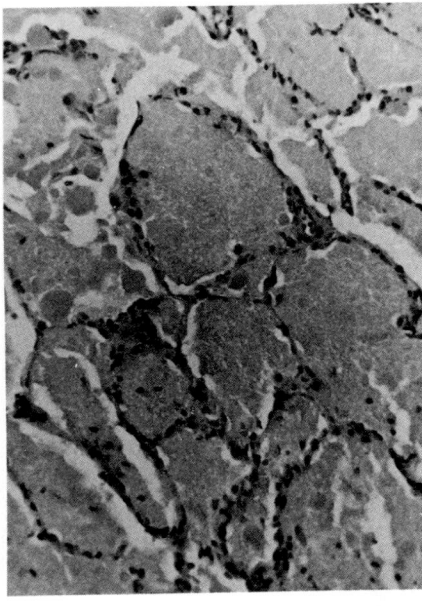

A B C

FIGURE 57-2 Light microscopy at increasing magnifications of a transbronchial biopsy specimen showing dense alveolar filling with the PAS-positive alveolar proteinosis material. (Original magnifications: $A = \times 21$; $B = \times 53$; $C = \times 132$.) The alveolar septa are normal. (*Courtesy of Dr. Dean Schraufnagel.*)

50 years old, but the disorder also affects infants and the elderly. The incidence in males is about four times that of females. PAP has also been reported in siblings.

Opportunistic pulmonary infections, particularly with *Nocardia*, which were described in untreated or incompletely treated PAP, now seem to occur less often, possibly because of interventions that ameliorate the disease. Moreover, the purported association of alveolar proteinosis with neoplasms has not withstood the test of close scrutiny and a larger experience.

The clinical signs are usually confined to the lungs, primarily in the form of diffuse crackles on lung auscultation. However, patients with severe and long-standing hypoxemia often develop cyanosis, clubbing of the digits, evidence of pulmonary hypertension and, occasionally, overt cor pulmonale.

The chest radiograph in pulmonary alveolar proteinosis is often distinctive (Fig. 57-3): a "bat wing" pattern of parenchymal involvement, within which radiographic evidence of alveolar or nodular infiltrates is unassociated with mediastinal adenopathy, is clearly discernible. However, the radiographic patterns vary considerably. Therefore, the diagnosis of PAP should be considered in the patient with a history of chronic insidious dyspnea in whom the chest radiograph shows bilateral alveolar or nodular infiltrates without mediastinal adenopathy and without the Kerley B lines of interstitial pulmonary edema.

Other laboratory features helpful in the diagnosis of PAP are concentric reductions in lung volumes and in the diffusing capacity. In addition, arterial hypoxemia, an increase in the shunt fraction ($\dot{Q}s/\dot{Q}T$), and an increase in the concentration of lactic dehydrogenase (LDH) in the serum are characteristic findings. Although most patients with pulmonary alveolar proteinosis produce no sputum, the common myelin figures of phospholipid whorls have been found in electron micrographs of sputum produced by some patients with PAP.

Histologic examination of lung tissue is generally required to clinch the diagnosis of PAP. Often tissue obtained by transbronchial biopsy using a flexible bronchoscope suffices for the diagnosis, especially if all the other signs and symptoms of the disorder are present. But, if doubt remains about the diagnosis, open lung biopsy is necessary. This is especially true if there is a question of secondary-versus-primary alveolar proteinosis. This distinction should be made because the so-called secondary proteinosis with pulmonary fibrosis may not respond as readily to a therapeutic bronchoalveolar lavage.

DIAGNOSTIC PROCEDURES

In patients with a productive cough, it is occasionally possible to identify the alveolar phospholipid of PAP in the expectorated sputum or to visualize by electron micros-

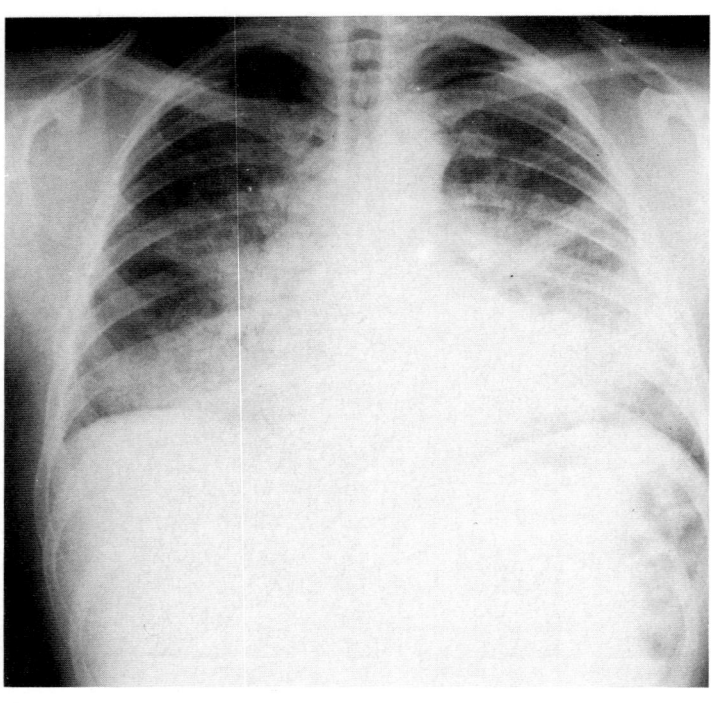 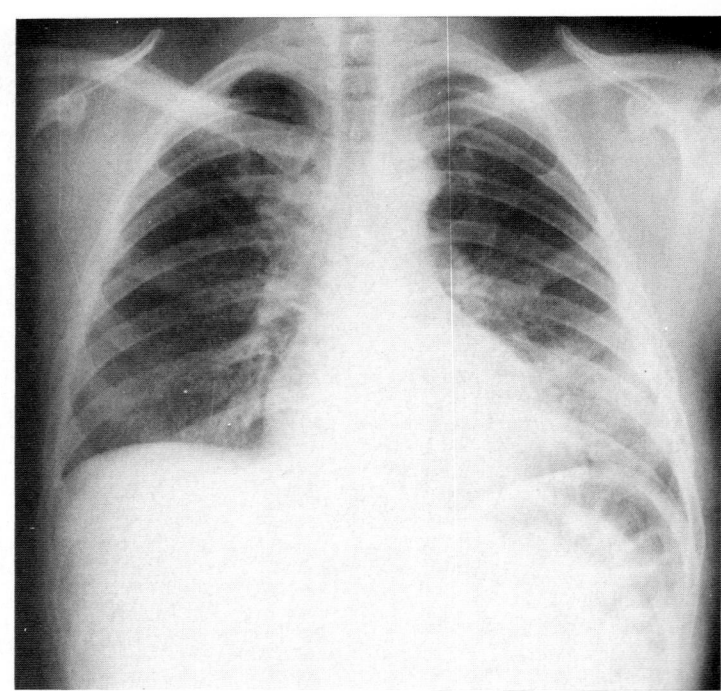

A   *B*

FIGURE 57-3   The initial radiograph *(A)* shows evidence of diffuse airspace consolidation. Two weeks later, after bronchopulmonary lavage therapy of both lungs *(B)*, the airspace consolidation has cleared considerably. *(Courtesy of Dr. M. Altose.)*

copy the distinctive lamellar appearance of a phospho-lipid-aqueous mixture (after proper fixing and staining with osmium tetroxide) (Fig. 57-4). But, as a rule, patients with PAP do not produce sputum. In these individuals, segmental bronchial lavage, using a flexible fiberoptic bronchoscope, can retrieve lipid-laden macrophages and disclose lipid in the alveolar spaces; by appropriate staining and histologic examination of material from the turbid washings, this material can be shown to be phospholipid in nature. However, this approach generally does not distinguish PAP from other disorders, such as *Pneumocystis carinii* pneumonia, uremic pneumonitis, immunosuppressive therapy for hematologic malignancy or pulmonary edema, the pathology of which can mimic that of PAP.

The possibility has been raised that PAP may be distinguishable from secondary alveolar proteinosis by staining for surfactant-specific apoprotein. However, when all is said and done, segmental lavage is generally an uncertain basis for distinguishing between PAP and secondary alveolar proteinosis so that lung biopsy is still the surest way to establish the diagnosis.

THERAPY

Once the diagnosis of PAP has been established, the physician is faced with the choice of whether to observe the patient in the hope of a spontaneous remission or to intervene therapeutically. Pivotal for this decision is the exercise tolerance of the patient and the disability produced by the disease. The following considerations enter into the decision: spontaneous remission with full resolution of all signs and symptoms does occur in up to a quarter of patients and, depending on symptoms, there may be no danger in waiting to see if this remission will occur. However, if the patient is symptomatic, or if there are signs of end-organ damage due to longstanding hypoxemia, then therapeutic intervention is in order.

The therapeutic alternatives that have been tried in patients with PAP include the inhalation of enzymatic or mucolytic agents, limited bronchoalveolar lavage through a flexible fiberoptic bronchoscope, and bronchoalveolar lavage of one whole lung after the patient has been anesthetized and intubated. The earlier therapeutic interventions, such as inhalation treatments using aerosolized

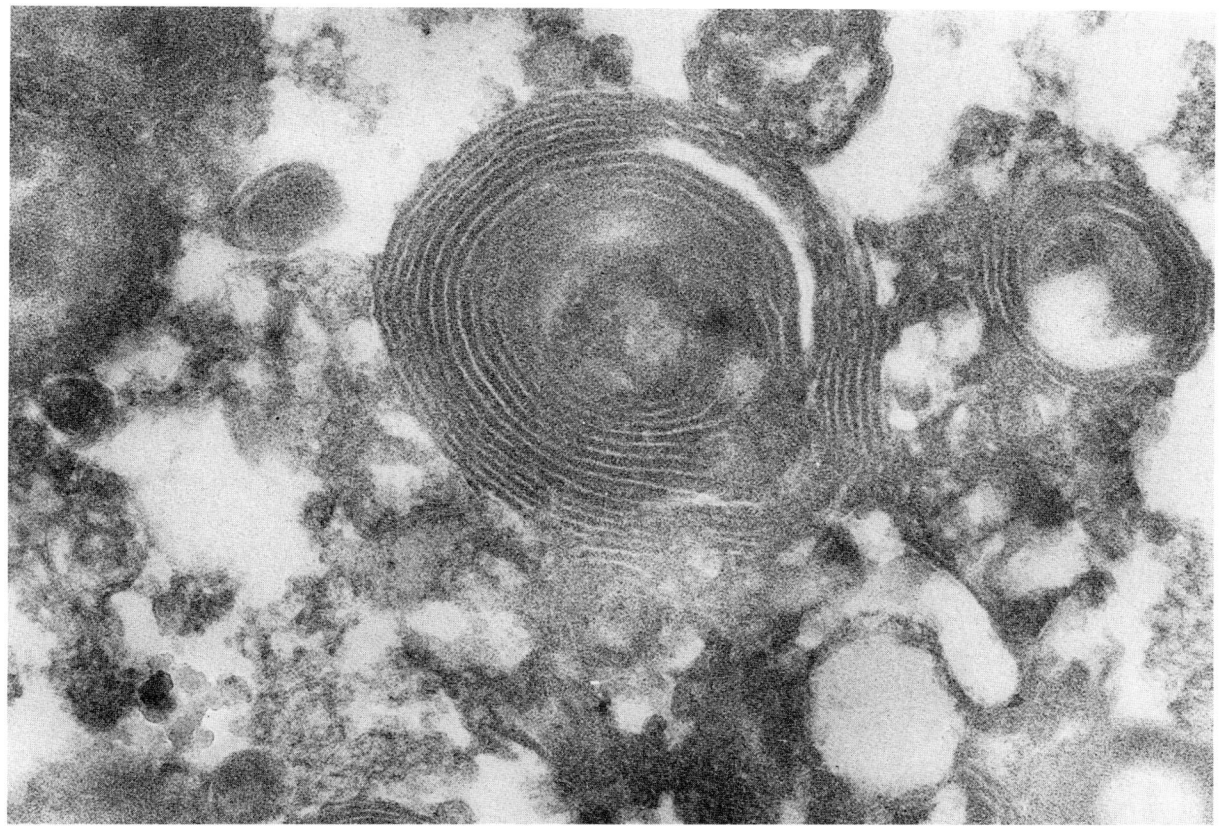

FIGURE 57-4 Electron micrograph of material removed by bronchoalveolar lavage. Tightly packed membranes are arranged concentrically as in the lamellar bodies of type II cells (×65,000). *(Courtesy of Dr. M. Altose.)*

acetylcystine or trypsin, have been largely abandoned because they often caused fever, bronchospasm, and bronchitis; moreover, even if these complications did not occur, this approach was ineffective because these agents probably did not penetrate to the distal airways where the bulk of the PAP material is lodged. Similarly, the use of flexible fiberoptic bronchoscopy to perform bronchoalveolar lavage also proved to have serious drawbacks: if topical anesthesia was used, time constrained the duration and volume of the lavage; if general anesthesia was used, then the small suction channel of the bronchoscope limited the amount of lavage fluid that could be used. As a logical evolution, the preferred treatment has become the use of a split-lumen endotracheal-endobronchial tube for intubating the patient after general anesthesia has been induced. This "lung separator" makes it possible to lavage one lung at a time, using large volumes of fluid. The technique of bronchoalveolar lavage of a whole lung affords a safe and effective method for mechanically removing the phospholipid material from alveolar spaces. For optimal results, the procedure should be performed by a team including a physician experienced in bronchospirometry and with intubation.

Bronchoalveolar Lavage of a Whole Lung

Baseline studies, performed before whole-lung lavage is undertaken, serve to quantify the extent of the patient's disorder, to measure the degree of impairment, and to track the postlavage course of the patient (Fig. 57-5). The tests include determination of the static lung volumes, the diffusing capacity for carbon monoxide ($D_{L_{CO}}$), the fraction of the cardiac output that is shunted ($\dot{Q}s/\dot{Q}T$) while the patient breathes 100% O_2, and the arterial blood gases (P_{O_2}, P_{CO_2}). In addition, the level of lactic dehydrogenase in the serum is determined since it is usually abnormally high in these patients before treatment and provides a useful test for monitoring after therapy. The pretreatment combination of a high serum LDH and a shunt of 15 percent or more supports the diagnosis of pulmonary alveolar proteinosis, although these may also be seen in patients with *P. carinii* pneumonia.

Bronchoalveolar lavage is generally done twice, separated by an interval of 3 to 7 days. Large volumes of fluid are involved; e.g., at least 50 L of warm, sterile saline is at hand before the procedure starts. By using an axially rotating Stryker frame table, the patient can be lavaged in both the supine and prone positions. Blood pressure, body temperature, and arterial oxygenation are monitored continuously.

A rapid-acting barbiturate administered intravenously is used for anesthesia and is followed by a neuromuscular blocking agent to induce paralysis and to enable controlled ventilation. The patient is intubated with a split-lumen endotracheal tube for separate ventilation and lavage of the two lungs. Great care is taken to ensure *complete* separation.

Once the tube is in the proper place, bronchospirometry is performed to identify the lung to be lavaged. As a rule, the more severely affected lung is lavaged during the first procedure, while the other lung is ventilated; only under special circumstances are both lungs lavaged simultaneously. During the phasic emptying of the lavaged lung, arterial oxygenation drops as fluid-filled alveoli are perfused, thereby creating the effect of a large shunt.

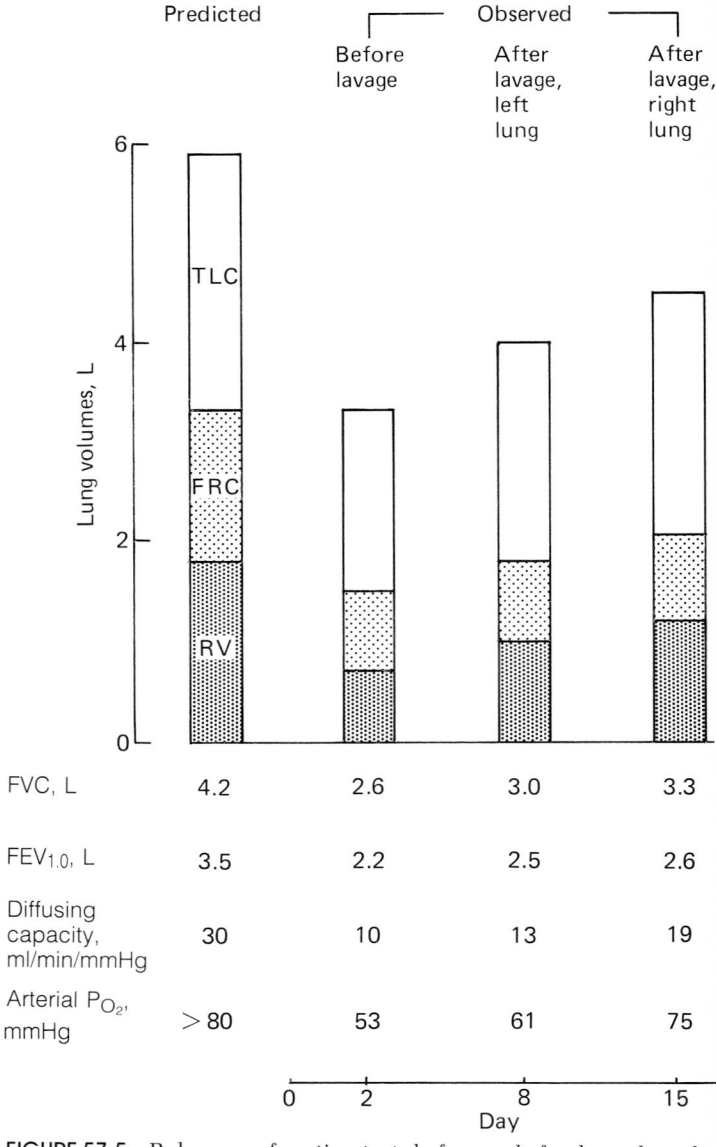

	Predicted	Before lavage	After lavage, left lung	After lavage, right lung
FVC, L	4.2	2.6	3.0	3.3
FEV$_{1.0}$, L	3.5	2.2	2.5	2.6
Diffusing capacity, ml/min/mmHg	30	10	13	19
Arterial P$_{O_2}$, mmHg	>80	53	61	75

FIGURE 57-5 Pulmonary function tests before and after bronchopulmonary lavage. After lavage, improvement occurs in all lung volumes, diffusing capacity, and arterial P_{O_2}. (*Courtesy of Dr. M. Altose.*)

The total volume of saline that is infused and recovered is determined frequently, with the operator always on guard for leakage into the opposite lung or ipsilateral pleural space. An esophageal stethoscope is useful for prompt detection of a spill into the opposite lung. Of the 45 to 50 L used for lavage, as a rule 500 to 1500 ml of fluid is retained in the lung. Characteristically, there is a striking decrease in turbidity as the lavage proceeds, ranging from cloudy fluid at the outset to virtually clear fluid at the end.

After the lavage has been completed, the tracheobronchial lumen has been cleared of residual lavage fluid and the patient has been extubated, a chest radiograph is done, checking for a large hydropneumothorax. The radiographic pattern in the lavaged lung at this juncture is that of diffuse alveolar opacification (even though arterial oxygenation is improving). If the initial lavage is uncomplicated, lavage of the contralateral lung is performed 3 to 7 days later. The patient is generally ready for discharge within 2 days after the second lavage. Some patients remit completely after this combined lavage; others experience repeated relapses that require the procedure to be repeated. At present, there is no way to identify the patient who will require chronic lavage.

As noted previously, the material lavaged from the alveolar spaces is quite similar in lipid and protein composition to that of normal surfactant. However, the concentration of total protein is higher, the increase in the fraction of immunoglobulin protein exceeds that of the other proteins, and surfactant-specific nonserum glycoproteins are present. The implications of these abnormalities with respect to pathogenesis are unclear.

PROGNOSIS

Although it is difficult to predict the long-term outlook for a particular patient, most of the patients who undergo whole-lung lavage for PAP that is unassociated with pulmonary fibrosis experience an improvement in pulmonary function and in exercise performance. However, it is still not possible to predict who will require a repeat lavage. Nor is it possible to identify patients who will require multiple lavages, each providing less benefit, and who will develop increasing pulmonary fibrosis. It is widely held that patients who smoke or who are around inhalational irritants tend to have fewer spontaneous remissions, have more relapses, and develop pulmonary fibrosis or permanent respiratory disability.

CONCLUSION

Pulmonary alveolar proteinosis is a disease of uncertain etiology that represents a disorder of lung surfactant homeostasis. It may not be due to a single specific etiologic insult. Treatment is supportive; it does not address the underlying etiologies or cellular pathophysiology of this disorder. Nonetheless, for patients with the disease, whole-lung lavage affords the prospect of palliation and permanent reversal of the disorder. Current research is directed toward achieving a better understanding of surfactant homeostasis and identifying a common abnormality in the processing of surfactant in the lungs of these patients.

BIBLIOGRAPHY

Bell DY, Hook GER: Pulmonary alveolar proteinosis: Analysis of airway and alveolar proteins. Am Rev Respir Dis 119:979–990, 1979.
> *Extensive description of the protein species of PAP lavage material showing increases in immunoglobulins over other serum proteins and the presence of two proteins not found in the serum.*

Claypool WD, Rogers RM, Matuschak GM: Update on the clinical diagnosis, management, and pathogenesis of pulmonary alveolar proteinosis (phospholipidosis). Chest 85:550–558, 1984.
> *Comprehensive, well-referenced review of the physiology and treatment of PAP relating it to the basic science advances in surfactant reprocessing.*

Claypool WD, Wang DL, Chander A, Fisher AB: An ethanol/ether soluble apoprotein from rat lung surfactant augments liposome uptake by isolated granular pneumocytes. J Clin Invest 74:677–684, 1984.
> *Demonstration that surfactant apoproteins can augment the reuptake of phospholipid liposomes by isolated pulmonary type II cells.*

Crawford SW, Mecham RP, Sage H: Structural characteristics and intermolecular organization of human pulmonary-surfactant-associated proteins. Biochem J 240:107–114, 1986.
> *A study of the intermolecular organization and structural relationships of the pulmonary-surfactant-associated proteins in the bronchoalveolar lavage fluid obtained from a patient with alveolar proteinosis.*

Hallman M, Epstein BL, Gluck L: Analysis of labeling and clearance of lung surfactant phospholipids in rabbits: Bidirectional surfactant flux between lamellar bodies and alveolar lavage. J Clin Invest 68:742–751, 1981.
   Demonstrates the reuptake of surfactant materials from the alveolar space into the pulmonary parenchyma and demonstrates that alveolar macrophages contribute relatively little to the rapid clearance of alveolar surfactant phospholipid.

Hook GE, Gilmore LB, Talley FA: Dissolution and reassembly of tubular myelin-like multilamellated structures from the lungs of patients with pulmonary alveolar proteinosis. Lab Invest 55:194–208, 1986.
   Specific proteins present in the insoluble accumulations from the lungs of patients with pulmonary alveolar proteinosis can spontaneously form tubular myelin-like multilamellated structures under in vitro conditions.

Hruban A: Pulmonary changes induced by amphiphilic drugs. Environ Health Perspect 16:111–118, 1976.
   General overview of the systemic and pulmonary abnormalities caused by several types of cationic amphiphilic drugs used both in experimental animal models and in clinical settings.

Jacobs H, Jobe A, Ikegami M, Conaway D: The significance of reutilization of surfactant phosphatidylcholine. J Biol Chem 258:4159–4165, 1983.
   Demonstrates the magnitude and rapidity of type II cell reaccumulation of surfactant in juvenile animals. The turnover time of greater than 90 percent of surfactant phosphatidylcholine through the type II cell lamellar body is approximately 10 h.

Kao D, Wasserman KG, Costley D, Benfield JR: Advances in the treatment of pulmonary alveolar proteinosis. Am Rev Respir Dis 111:361–363, 1975.
   Demonstrates the importance of chest percussion during whole-lung lavage.

King RJ, Clements JA: Lipid synthesis of surfactant turnover in the lungs, in Fishman AP, Fisher AB (eds), *Handbook of Physiology, sect 3: The Respiratory System, vol I: Circulation and Nonrespiratory Functions.* Bethesda, MD, American Physiological Society, 1985, pp 309–336.
   A review of the lipid composition of lung tissue, the metabolic pathways of lipids in lung tissue, and the regulation of surfactant metabolism.

Marchlinski FE, Gansler TS, Waxman HL, Josephson ME: Amiodarone pulmonary toxicity. Ann Intern Med 97:839–845, 1982.
   Demonstration that amiodarone pulmonary toxicity may be associated with an abnormality in phospholipid processing similar to that seen with other cationic amphiphilic drugs.

Martin RJ, Rogers RM, Myers NM: Pulmonary alveolar proteinosis: Shunt fraction and lactic acid dehydrogenase concentration as aids to diagnosis. Am Rev Respir Dis 117:1059–1062, 1978.
   Shows that the LDH is elevated and the measured $\dot{Q}s/\dot{Q}T$ is greater than 12 percent in all their patients with PAP. The diagnosis should be suspected by these two findings in any patient with diffuse lung disease.

Prakash UBS, Barham SS, Carpenter HA, Dines DE, Marsh HM: Pulmonary alveolar phospholipoproteinosis: Experience with 34 cases and a review. Mayo Clin Proc 62:499–518, 1987.
   A review of the clinical features of alveolar proteinosis based on the Mayo Clinic experience.

Rogers RM, Levin DC, Gray BA, Mosely LW: Physiologic effects of bronchopulmonary lavage in alveolar proteinosis. Am Rev Respir Dis 118:225–264, 1978.
   Important overview of the expected physiological alterations evoked by whole-lung lavage therapy in PAP.

Rosen SH, Castleman B, Liebow AA, Enzinger FM, Hunt RTN: Pulmonary alveolar proteinosis. N Engl J Med 258:1123–1142, 1958.
   Original pathologic and historical description of 24 cases of PAP collected from several centers. This article remains one of the most important contributions to the understanding of this disorder.

Ross GF, Ohning BL, Tannenbaum D, Whitsett JA: Structural relationships of the major glycoproteins from human alveolar proteinosis surfactant. Biochim Biophys Acta 911:294–305, 1987.
   Two major collagenase-sensitive polypeptides, alveolar proteinosis peptides of 34 kilodaltons (APP-34) and those of 62 kilodaltons (APP-62), were isolated and purified from bronchoalveolar lavage of patients with alveolar proteinosis.

Sahu S, Lynn WS: Characterization of a high-molecular-weight glycoprotein isolated from the pulmonary secretions of patients with alveolar proteinosis. Biochem J 177:153–158, 1979.
   Description of a 250,000 MW protein which may be a precursor to other surfactant-specific apoproteins. The elevation of this precursor protein may be a clue to a unifying mechanistic abnormality in PAP.

Selecky PA, Wasserman K, Benfield JR, Lippmann M: The clinical and physiological effect of whole-lung lavage in pulmonary alveolar proteinosis. Ann Thorac Surg 24:451–461, 1977.

A well organized review of an extensive longitudinal experience with a treated population of patients with PAP.

Singh G, Katyal SL, Bedrossian CWM, Rogers RM: Pulmonary alveolar proteinosis—staining for surfactant specific apoprotein in alveolar proteinosis and in conditions simulating it. Chest 83:82–86, 1983.

Using immunoperoxidase staining of surfactant-specific apoproteins, the authors show differences in the alveolar staining of primary versus secondary PAP.

Chapter 58

The Pulmonary Lymphatic System

Chuzo Nagaishi / Yoshio Okada

The structure of the lymphatic system of the lung is, in principle, not much different from that of other organs. It consists of the lymphatics belonging to the vascular system and the lymph nodes located sporadically along the lymph vessels. In a broad sense, the extravascular fluid pathway system designated by Kihara as the *tissue fluid pathway* also belongs to the lymphatic system.

OVERVIEW OF THE PULMONARY LYMPHATIC SYSTEM

By injecting dye solution into the subpleural lymphatics, fine networks of lymphatics are disclosed. Most of these fine lymphatics are devoid of valves; they consist of capillaries surrounded by single layers of endothelium (Fig. 58-1). From the lymph capillary networks, dye passes to lymphatics that bear valves; the valves prevent the spread of dye into surrounding lymph capillary networks. Several lymphatics join together to form collecting lymphatics. In the collecting lymphatics the valves are in dense arrangement. As long as the valves are competent, they act to divert the flow of lymph retrogradely to the collecting lymphatics; in this way, flow is directed to the first lymph node and carried from it to the venous junction. Most of the lymph from the lungs flows through the bronchomediastinal lymphatic trunk into the right subclavian vein and some through the thoracic duct into the left subclavian vein.

According to our observations during thoracotomy, dye solution injected into the pulmonary lymph capillaries appears in the right bronchomediastinal trunk 20 to 30 min after injection. The amount of lymph flow varies from individual to individual and is greatly influenced by manipulations of the thorax, e.g., operative procedures. However, protein content and lymphocyte count are relatively stable: the protein content is on the order of 6.0 g/dl; the lymphocyte count is on the order of 3000/mm³.

Fundamentally, the structure of the regional lymph nodes in the lung is also the same as that of other organs. In the lymph fluid from the lung is dusts absorbed from the respiratory tract. The histiocytes in the sinuses of the lymph nodes engulf these foreign particles and deposit them in the sinuses. Accordingly, with increasing age, anthracosis in the regional lymph nodes of the lungs becomes more evident. The resulting fibrosis of the lymph nodes may decrease lymph node function.

In rabbits and rats, lymphocytes infiltrate into certain regions of the bronchial epithelium. According to Kihara, this system of "bronchial associated lymphoid tissue" is a part of the extravascular fluid pathway system by which substances are transported from the trachea into the lymphatics. The role played by this system in the immune mechanisms of the body is considered in detail elsewhere in this book.

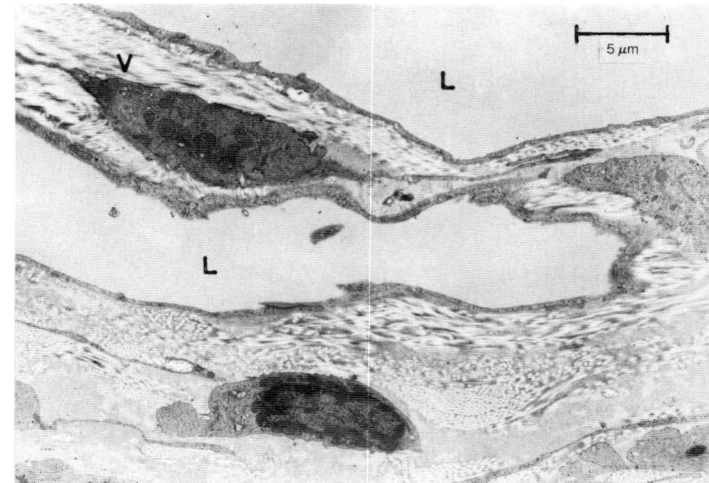

FIGURE 58-1 Electron-microscope appearance of lymph vessels in the bronchial wall of a rat. A valve is present in the center. Fibroblasts and collagen fibers can be observed in the valve. L = lumen of the lymphatics; V = valve.

INTRAPULMONARY LYMPHATICS

In the age of Mascagni (1781) and Cruikshank (1790), the pulmonary lymphatics were divided into two groups, superficial and deep. Subsequently, Miller and others reclassified the pulmonary lymphatics according to their location as follows (Fig. 58-2):

1. Superficial
2. Deep
   a. In the interlobular connective tissue
   b. Related to the pulmonary veins
   c. Related to the bronchi
      i. In the submucosal layer
      ii. In the adventitia
   d. Related to the pulmonary arteries

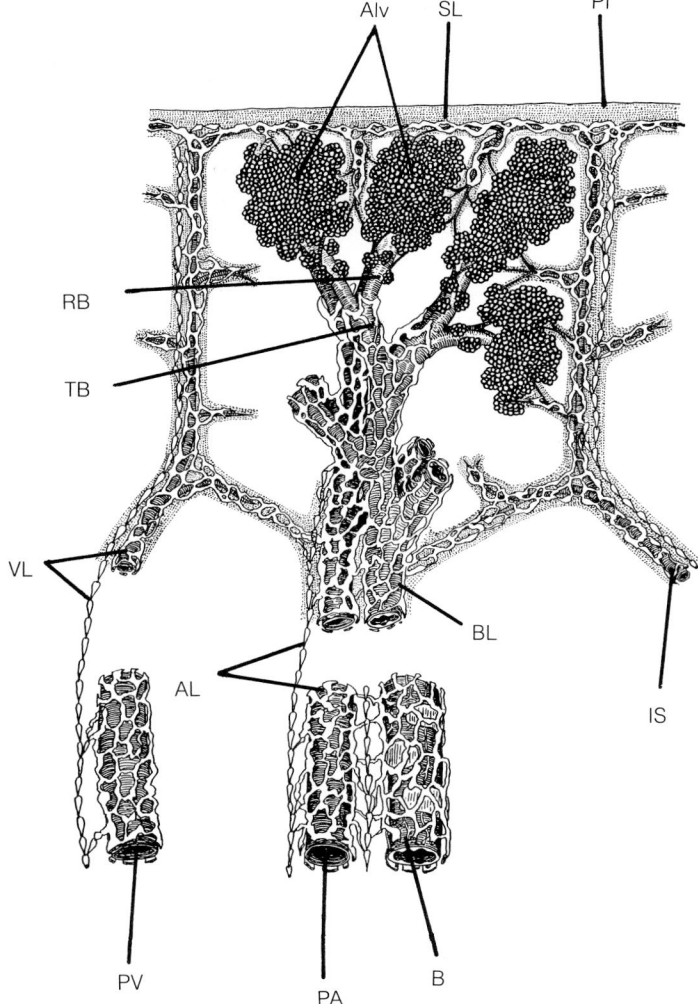

FIGURE 58-2 Distribution of lymphatics in the lung. AL = lymphatics and collecting lymphatics related to the pulmonary artery; Alv = alveolar region; B = bronchus; BL = lymphatics related to the bronchus; IS = interlobular septa; PA = pulmonary artery; Pl = pulmonary pleura; PV = pulmonary vein; RB = respiratory bronchiole; SL = septal lymphatics; TB = terminal bronchiole; VL = venous lymphatics.

Embryologically, Kempmeier (1828) and others observed that the pulmonary lymphatics in humans originate from the thoracic duct, the right bronchomediastinal lymphatic trunk, and the retroperitoneal lymphatic bursa. These lymphatics extend to the hilus early in gestation to form a lymphatic plexus. At about 3 months of gestation, the perihilar lymphatic plexus starts to penetrate into the lung along the bronchus, pulmonary artery, and vein. By the end of the first half of fetal life, the pulmonary lymphatics extend to all regions noted above, and their distribution is almost complete. In the second half of fetal life, the lymph capillary networks become denser, and the lymphatics and collecting lymphatics develop valves.

Subpleural Lymphatics

Fine lymphatic networks can be observed in the pulmonary pleura. These lymphatics are in the deepest layer of the pulmonary pleura, i.e., the interstitial layer (Fig. 58-3). Although the diameters of the vessels are variable, most subpleural lymphatics in humans are capillaries. From these minute vessels, lymph flows via the lymphatics into the collecting lymphatics en route toward the hilus. As a rule, the collecting lymphatics of the subpleural lymphatics run along the pulmonary lobules and the boundaries of the pulmonary segments. Most penetrate directly into the lung without detouring onto the surface of the lung; with the lung they follow branches of the pulmonary veins into the hilus.

Interlobular Lymphatics

The interlobular lymphatics are located near the center of the interlobular connective tissue, and most of them are capillaries (Fig. 58-4). These lymph capillaries form fine networks in the interlobular connective tissue and anastomose densely with the lymphatics that accompany

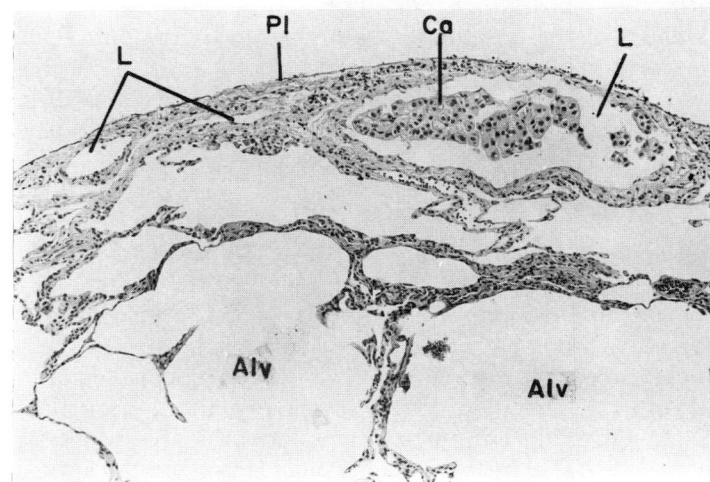

FIGURE 58-3 Subpleural lymphatics in lymphangitic carcinomatosis of adults. Dilated lymphatics with malignant cells inside and two fine lymph vessels can be observed. Alv = alveolus; Ca = malignant cells; L = lymphatics; Pl = pleura.

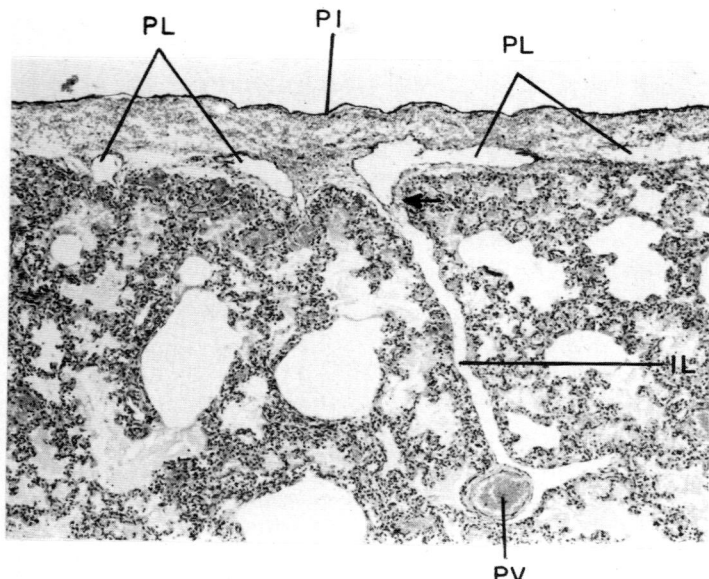

FIGURE 58-4 Lymphatics in interlobular connective tissue related to pulmonary venous branch. The lung is that of a fetus near term. Lymph in the region flows from the subpleural region to the interlobular septum. Arrow points to a valve. IL = lymphatics in interlobular connective tissue; PL = subpleural lymphatics; Pl = pleura; PV = pulmonary venous branch.

the pulmonary veins. The interlobular lymphatics are devoid of independent collecting lymphatics; they join with those of the pulmonary veins to extend toward the hilus via the collecting lymphatics.

Lymphatics Related to the Pulmonary Veins

Well-developed lymphatics are found in tissue along branches of the pulmonary veins; lymphatic networks are seen in the vicinity of the large branches of pulmonary veins. Lymphatics related to the pulmonary veins also anastomose with subpleural lymphatics and interlobular lymphatics.

For many years, disputes continued about the existence of lymphatics in the alveolar regions of the lungs. However, using histologic and electron-microscopic studies, we have been unable to find lymphatics in the alveolar wall. The confusion seems to have arisen because lymphatics related to the interlobular venules are adjacent to the alveolar wall; frequently these lymphatics are mistakenly thought to be within the alveolar wall rather than adjacent to it.

In the subpleural zone, venules run from the interlobular portion toward the pulmonary pleura. The lymphatics related to the pulmonary veins run from the interlobular portion to the pulmonary pleura, i.e., from inside the lung toward the surface.

Lymphatics Related to the Bronchi

In small bronchi that are devoid of cartilage, only a single layered lymphatic network is observed. In the large bron-

chi with cartilage in their walls, single-layered networks of lymphatics are seen in the submucosa and adventitia. The submucosal lymphatics (Fig. 58-5) are small, whereas those in the adventitia are large; anastomoses between the submucosal and adventitial plexi run between the cartilages of the bronchi.

Peripherally, lymphatics related to bronchi extend to the vicinity of terminal bronchioles; they are not observed in the alveolar region.

Lymphatics Related to the Pulmonary Arteries

Well-developed lymphatics surround the pulmonary artery. As a rule, these lymphatics are more developed than those related to the bronchi; they also extend further toward the periphery, i.e., to the most peripheral portion of the terminal bronchiole (Fig. 58-6).

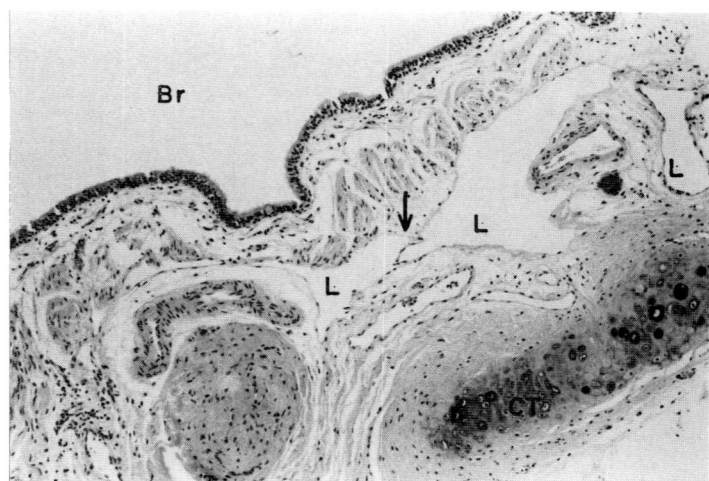

FIGURE 58-5 Lymphatics in bronchial submucosal layer (human). Arrow indicates a valve. Br = bronchial lumen; L = lymphatics.

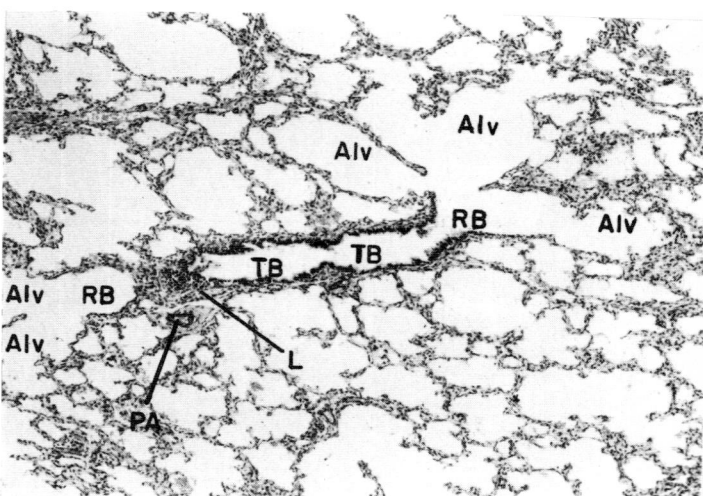

FIGURE 58-6 Lymphatics related to a peripheral branch of the pulmonary artery in a child. Alv = alveolar region; L = lymphatics; PA = pulmonary arterial branch; RB = respiratory bronchiole; TB = terminal bronchiole.

Lymphatics in the vicinity of the pulmonary artery form fine networks that surround the pulmonary artery and anastomose densely with lymphatics in the bronchial adventitia. They drain into the collecting lymphatics which run along the pulmonary artery toward the hilus. Lymphatics related to the bronchi drain toward the hilus via the collecting lymph vessels surrounding the pulmonary artery.

Lymph Flow of the Intrapulmonary Lymphatics

The subpleural lymphatics, interlobular lymphatics, and lymphatics related to the pulmonary veins anastomose freely. The lymph in these lymphatics flows primarily into collecting lymphatics surrounding the pulmonary veins toward the hilus.

The lymphatics related to the bronchi and those related to the pulmonary artery intermingle; flow from both

is chiefly via the collecting lymphatics surrounding the pulmonary artery toward the hilus.

In view of the above, lymph from the lungs can be roughly classified into two systems (Fig. 58-7): *interstitial,* or *interstitial-venous,* lymph flow and *parenchymal,* or *bronchoarterial,* lymph flow. Each system is independent except for communications at certain junctures.

Lymphatics of Animals

The distribution of lymphatics in the lung differs according to species. In the human and bovine lung, interlobular septa are prominent as are the interstitial and parenchymal lymphatics. However, in the dog, rabbit, and rat, in which interlobular septa are absent, the interstitial lymphatics are poorly developed except for the subpleural lymphatics. However, even in these animals parenchymal lymphatics are well developed, particularly those relating to the pulmonary artery in the rabbit and the rat.

REGIONAL LYMPH NODES AND EFFERENT LYMPH FLOWS OF THE LUNG

Development of Regional Lymph Nodes of the Lung

About the third month of gestation, lymph nodes start to develop in the human hilus. As shown in Fig. 58-8, the process begins with infiltration of lymphocytes into the lymphatic plexus of the hilus. As infiltration continues, areas surrounding the infiltrated portion form a marginal sinus.

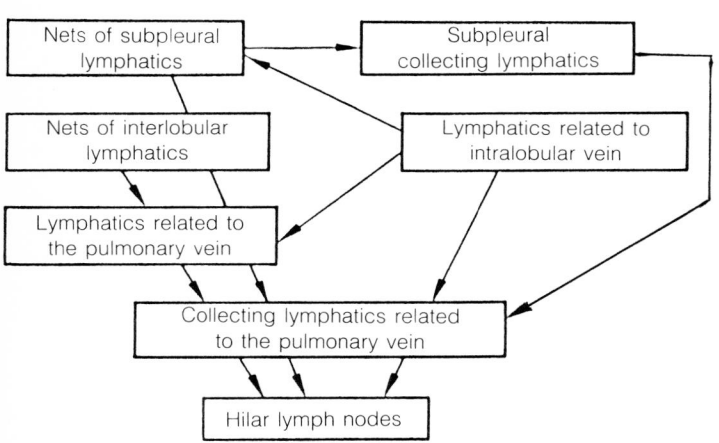

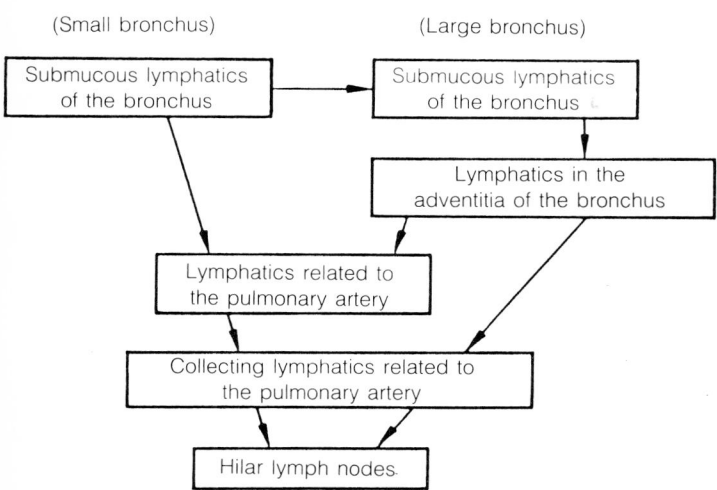

FIGURE 58-7 Lymph flow system in the lung.

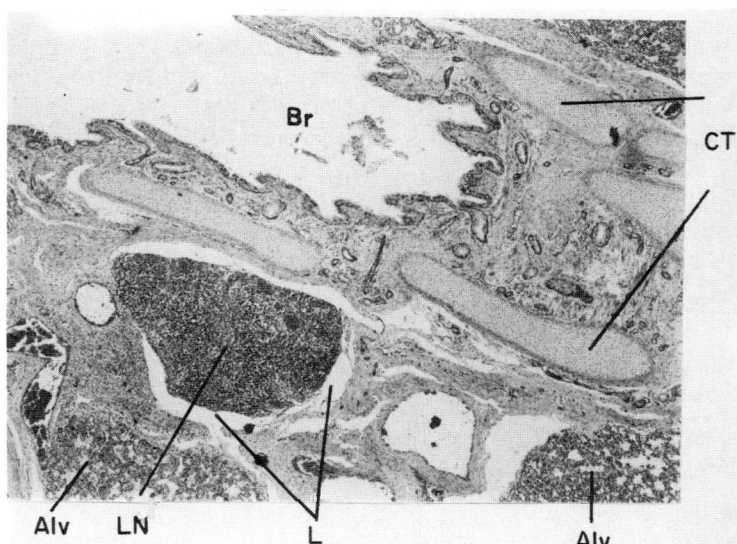

FIGURE 58-8 Origin of the hilar lymph node in the fetus. Lymph nodes surrounded by lymphatics around the bronchus. Alv = alveolar region; Br = bronchial lumen; CT = cartilage; L = lymphatics; LN = lymph node (origin).

By the end of fetal life, a lymph node-like substance appears and differentiation into cortical and medullary regions takes place. The development of a germinal center within lymph nodes is a sign of maturity; it is not seen in the fetus. These observations indicate that the hilar lymph nodes continue to differentiate, develop, and mature after birth.

Distribution of Regional Lymph Nodes of the Lung

Figure 58-9 is a topographic schema of the regional lymph nodes of the lung derived from observations made during thoracotomy and from experiments conducted by injecting dye solution into the pulmonary lymphatics. The numbers on this chart are in accord with the recommendations of the Japanese Lung Cancer Society for the nomenclature of the regional lymph nodes. This approach facilitates the description of metastases of lung cancers.

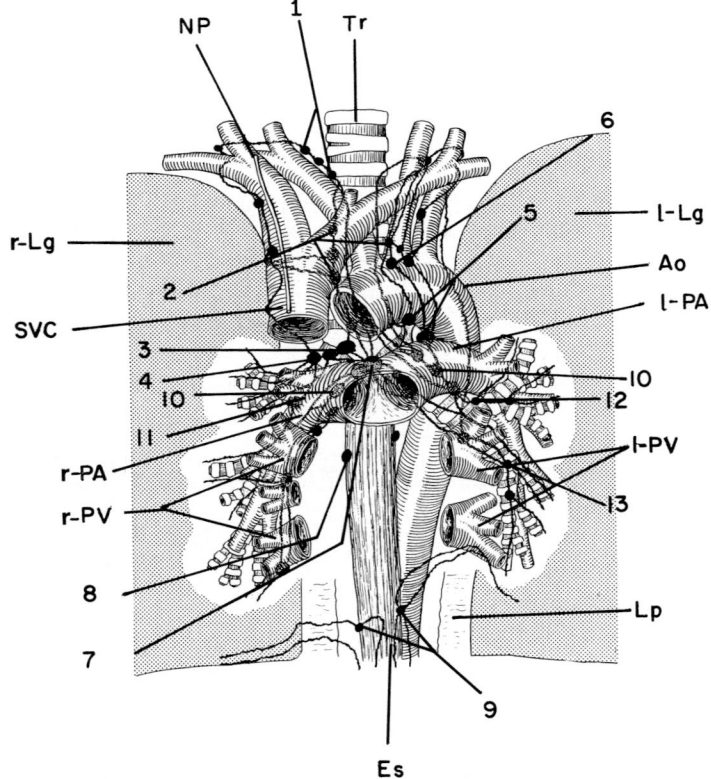

FIGURE 58-9 Regional lymph nodes of the lung. Ao = aorta; Es = esophagus; l-Lg = left lung; Lp = pulmonary ligament; l-PA = left pulmonary artery; l-PV = left pulmonary vein; NP = phrenic nerve; r-Lg = right lung; r-PA = right pulmonary artery; r-PV = right pulmonary vein; SVC = superior vena cava; Tr = trachea; 1 = superior regional lymph node; 2 = paratracheal lymph node; 3 = pretracheal lymph node; 4 = tracheobronchial lymph node; 5 = Botallo's duct (ductus arteriosus); 6 = paraaortic lymph node; 7 = subcarinal lymph node; 8 = paraesophageal lymph node; 9 = pulmonary ligament lymph node; 10 = main bronchus lymph node; 11 = interlobar lymph node; 12 = lobar lymph node; 13 = segmental lymph node.

MEDIASTINAL LYMPH NODES

Superior Mediastinal Lymph Nodes (No. 1)
These lymph nodes are the highest mediastinal lymph nodes. They are located in the upper one-third of the trachea within the thorax, i.e., where the left and right innominate veins join.

Paratracheal Lymph Nodes (No. 2)
These are groups of lymph nodes located on both sides of the trachea. In general, those on the right side are larger than those on the left. The right side consists of around 5 to 10 nodes.

Pretracheal Lymph Nodes (No. 3)
These lymph nodes are located in the lower two-thirds of the trachea. Those located at the anterior tracheal bifurcation are particularly well developed.

Retrotracheal Lymph Nodes (No. 3p)
These lymph nodes are located in the posterior wall of the trachea.

Tracheobronchial Lymph Nodes (No. 4)
These lymph nodes are located where the trachea and principal bronchus form an obtuse angle. Those on the right side are medial to the azygos vein; those on the left are within the aortic arch. Generally, those on the right are well developed.

Subaortic Lymph Nodes (No. 5)
Well-developed lymph nodes are found between the aortic arch and the trunk of the pulmonary artery in relation to the ductus arteriosus. These are Botallo's duct lymph nodes. The group consists of three to five lymph nodes and are among the best developed regional lymph nodes in the left lung.

Paraaortic Lymph Nodes (No. 6)
These lymph nodes are adjacent to the exterior portion of the ascending aorta. They are called the aortic arch lymph nodes.

Subcarinal Lymph Nodes (No. 7)
This group of lymph nodes located directly below the bifurcation of the trachea is also referred to as sub-bifurcation lymph nodes. The efferent lymph flow from both lungs crosses between these nodes.

Paraesophageal Lymph Nodes (No. 8)
These are lymph nodes located adjacent to the esophagus at a level below that of the tracheal bifurcation.

Pulmonary Ligament Lymph Nodes (No. 9)
These lymph nodes are located in the pulmonary ligament. The nodes at the lower border of the inferior pulmonary vein also belong to this group.

HILAR LYMPH NODES

Lymph nodes identified in Fig. 58-9 by numbers 10 to 13 are often called bronchopulmonary nodes.

Main Bronchus Lymph Nodes (No. 10)

These lymph nodes occur at both the superior and inferior margins of the main bronchus: the superior nodes drain to the tracheobronchial lymph nodes on the proximal side, the inferior nodes to the tracheal bifurcation nodes on the proximal side. The boundary between the two nodes is not distinct.

Interlobar Lymph Nodes (No. 11)

These are located between the divisions of the lobes. On the right side, they are classified into superior and middle lobar nodes (11s) and middle and inferior lobar node (11f).

Lobar Lymph Nodes (No. 12)

These lymph nodes are in the vicinity of the lobar bronchi.

INTRAPULMONARY LYMPH NODES

Segmental Lymph Nodes (No. 13)

These lymph nodes are located around segmental bronchi.

Efferent Lymph Flow of the Lung

Efferent lymph that originates in the roots of the respective pulmonary lobes runs to lymph nodes Nos. 4, 5, and 7. On the right side, the route is paratracheal, ascending along the right side of the trachea; on the left, the route is along the right innominate (brachiocephalic) vein. The lymph from these routes may flow independently into the right venous junction or drain into the bronchomediastinal lymphatic trunks and from them into the right venous junction; about one-half of the flow runs directly into a trunk vessel and the other half has to traverse two or three vessels before reaching the venous junction. Therefore, in order to obtain relatively pure lymph, the right bronchomediastinal lymphatic trunk is recommended. The left route consists of (1) the paratracheal route that ascends along the left side of the trachea and (2) the aortic arch route that crosses the aortic arch and then ascends on its left side. The lymph from these routes empties into the thoracic duct, which terminates in the left venous junction. As a rule, the routes of lymph flow are variable, but there are two main routes of efferent lymph flow originating in the pulmonary lobes.

THE RIGHT LUNG

Most of the lymph originating in the right upper lobe flows into lymph nodes Nos. 10 and 4. Some passes through the brachiocephalic venous route and some flows via Nos. 3a and 2, i.e., the right tracheal route, to the right venous junction.

Most of the lymph from the right middle and lower lobes flows into nodes Nos. 7 and 3. In addition to lymph originating from the right upper lobe, lymph from the middle and lower lobes runs via the right tracheal or brachiocephalic venous route into the vein at the right venous junction. Occasionally, lymph originating from the basal portion of the right lower lobe passes through the pulmonary ligament and runs into node No. 8; some may pass via branches along the esophagus toward the peritoneal cavity.

THE LEFT LUNG

Most of the lymph orginating in the left upper lobe runs into nodes Nos. 10 and 5 and, from there, via the left tracheal or aortic arch route, into the vein at the left venous junction. Most of the lymph originating in the left lower lobe drains into node No. 7. But, in the proximal region, as well as from the right lung, lymph flows into the vein at the right venous junction via either the right tracheal or brachiocephalic venous route.

In the left lower lobe, some of the lymphatics originating in the basal portion run through the pulmonary ligament and penetrate on node No. 8, reaching the peritoneal cavity along the esophagus. However, on the right side, such lymphatics are not always present. The presence of these lymphatics on one side provides no assurance that they also exist on the other side.

Therefore, it is understandable that when superclavicular lymph node biopsy is done in a patient with a lung cancer, the right side is preferable for biopsy. In contrast, in patients with abdominal or digestive tract cancers, the preferred side of biopsy is the left supraclavicular lymph node, i.e., Virchow's node.

LYMPHATICS OF SEVERAL INTRATHORACIC ORGANS

Figure 58-10 shows the pathway of efferent lymphatics in several organs in the thorax.

Lymphatics of the Diaphragm

In the diaphragm, lymphatic networks are observed in the subpleural and subperitoneal regions.

The lymphatics originating in a very small, anterior part of the diaphragm run anteriorly and enter, at the anterior border of the diaphragm, the anterior diaphragmatic lymph nodes that are located on either side of the sternum. The lymphatics originating in these nodes ascend along the internal mammary vessels of the same side and pass the parasternal lymph node to join the vein at the venous junction.

The lymphatics draining other parts of the diaphragm run toward the central portion of the diaphragm and then along the esophagus, aorta, or inferior vena cava into the peritoneal cavity. The lymphatic that runs along the

In view of the above, cases of lung cancer with invasion of the diaphragm, particularly in the posterior region, bear a high risk of metastasis to the abdominal lymph nodes. In 254 autopsied cases of lung cancer, 210 had metastasis on the abdominal lymph nodes.

Lymphatics of the Parietal Pleura

The lymphatics of the parietal pleura form fine networks that drain into collecting lymph nodes; the latter are arranged in parallel in the intercostal spaces.

The direction of lymph flow in the intercostal spaces varies with the location: lymph originating in front of the anterior axillary line passes anteriorly through the anterior intercostal lymph node and into the internal mammary lymphatics on the same side. As in the case of lymph from the anterior portion of the diaphragm, the anteriorly derived lymph flows through the parasternal lymph node and into the vein at the venous junction.

In contrast, lymph originating behind the posterior axillary line flows posteriorly into the thoracic duct, traversing either the posterior intercostal lymph nodes that are sparse and located in the posterior region of the intercostal space or the prevertebral lymph nodes.

When operating on a patient with lung cancer in whom invasion of the chest wall has occurred, the direction of lymph flow must be taken into account in deciding the extent of resection. Because of the abundant anastomoses between lymph vessels in the intercostal spaces, extensive resection of the upper and lower neighboring intercostal spaces is recommended.

Lymphatics of the Heart

The lymphatic drainage of the heart is via two collecting lymphatics: one lymphatic runs along the left coronary artery, passes the root of the trunk of the pulmonary artery running from the left posteriorly, and then joins the lymph nodes of the heart. In many instances, these lymphatics join others coming from the lungs in the region of the tracheal bifurcation. Lymph originating in the cardiac lymph node also flows into the left tracheobronchial lymph node No. 4. Other collecting lymphatics, primarily those along the right coronary artery, pass on the right of the origin of the aorta and run into the lymph node in the region of the tracheal bifurcation where they join the lymphatics from the lung. Therefore, lymphatics from the heart join lymphatics from the lungs at the tracheal bifurcation. From there, cardiac and pulmonary drainage are via the same lymphatics and enter the systemic venous system at the venous junction.

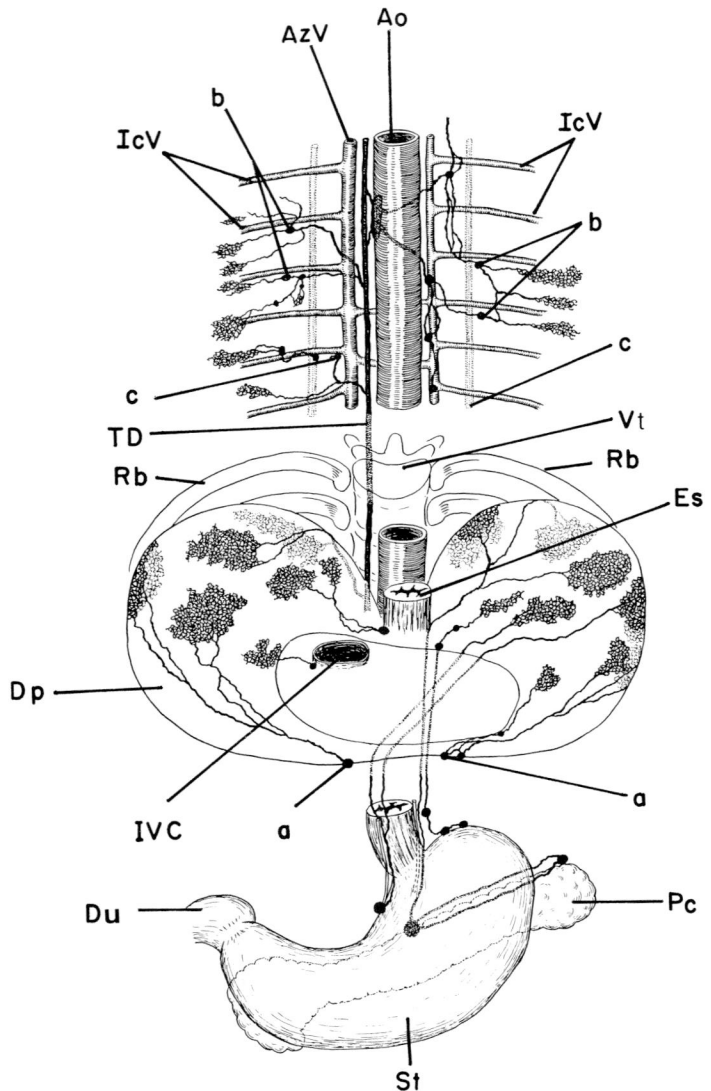

FIGURE 58-10 Lymphatics of several organs in the thorax. Ao = aorta; AzV = azygos vein; Dp = diaphragm; Du = duodenum; Es = esophagus; IcV = intercostal vein; IVC = inferior vena cava; Pc = pancreas; Rb = rib; St = stomach; TD = thoracic duct; Vt = vertebra; a = anterior diaphragmatic lymph node; b = posterior intercostal lymph node; c = prevertebral lymph node.

esophagus to enter the lymph node in the region of the cardia is most often observed. Some diaphragmatic lymphatics descend along the posterior surface of the stomach to reach the lymph nodes located along the superior border of the pancreas or enter the nodes in the tail of the pancreas. Those that descend from the aortic hiatus join the thoracic duct in the peritoneal cavity.

BIBLIOGRAPHY

Albelda SM, Hansen-Flaschen JH, Lanken PN, Fishman AP: Effects of increased ventilation on lung lymph flow in unanesthetized sheep. J Appl Physiol 60:2063–2070, 1986.
An increase in spontaneous minute ventilation increased lymph flow from the lungs in tracheostomized, unanesthetized, spontaneously breathing sheep.

Gnepp DR. Lymphatics, in Staub NC, Taylor AE (eds), *Edema.* New York, Raven Press, 1984, pp 263–298.
A comprehensive review of the organization and functional anatomy of the lymphatic system in the lungs. Extensive bibliography.

Harmsen AG, Mason MJ, Muggenburg BA, Gillett NA, Jarpe MA, Bice DE: Migration of neutrophils from lung to tracheobronchial lymph node. J Leukocyte Biol 41:95–103, 1987.
Neutrophils are similar to pulmonary alveolar macrophages (PAM) in their ability to phagocytize particles in the lung and then migrate to the TBLN.

Kihara T: Das extravaskuläre Saftbahnensystem. Okajimas Folia Anat 28:601, 1951.
Originally described by Kihara, the extravascular fluid pathway refers to the fluid pathway between the blood vessels and the lymph vessels. In a broad sense, it can be considered a part of the lymphatic system.

Lauweryns JM, Baert JH: Alveolar clearance and the role of the pulmonary lymphatics. Am Rev Respir Dis 115:625–683, 1977.
Report on the anatomy of pulmonary lymphatics, macrophages of the lungs, and other fine structures. The focus is on the clearance system by which foreign substances are removed from the lungs.

Miller WS: The Lung, 2d ed. Springfield, Ill, Charles C Thomas, 1947.
A classic report on the structure of the lung. The chapter on the lymphatic system deals with research on the pulmonary lymphatics up to the first half of this century.

Nagaishi C, Nagasawa N, Yamashita Y, Okada Y, Inaba N: *Functional Anatomy and Histology of the Lung.* Baltimore, MD, University Park Press, 1972.
In Nagaishi's Department of Thoracic Surgery, Kyoto University, morphologic, functional, and other fundamental studies on the chest have been performed since 1948. This magnificently illustrated book represents a dynamic approach to the structure of the lungs.

Ottaviani G: Richerche anatomiche sui vasi linfatici del polmone umane. Morph Kahrb 82:453, 1938.
Detailed observation on the development of the lymphatic system in the human lung during fetal life. Valuable for the understanding of the course of development of the lymphatic system in the human lung.

Rouviere H: *Anatomy of the Human Lymphatic System.* Ann Arbor, Mich, Edwards, 1938.
Detailed investigation of the lymphatics of the lung and of the routes of efferent lymph flow.

Staub NC: Pulmonary edema. Physiol Rev 54:687–811, 1974.
The morphology of the pulmonary lymphatic system, the dynamics of pulmonary lymph flow, and the movements of tissue fluids are described in detail.

Stein MG, Mayo J, Muller N, Aberle DR, Webb WR, Gamsu G: Pulmonary lymphangitic spread of carcinoma: appearance on CT scans. Radiology 162:371–375, 1987.
Chest computed tomography (CT), including high-resolution CT with thin (1.5-mm) sections was used to evaluate proved (pathologically or clinically) lymphangitic spread (LS) of tumor in 12 patients.

Taylor AE, Parker JC: Pulmonary interstitial spaces and lymphatics, in Fishman AP, Fisher AB (eds), *Handbook of Physiology,* sect 3: Respiration, vol I: Circulation and Nonrespiratory Functions. Bethesda, MD, American Physiological Society, 1985, pp 167–230.
An excellent review of the structure and composition of the pulmonary interstititium and of the forces responsible for the movement of fluid through it.

Chapter 59

Lung Lymph Composition and Flow in Normal and Abnormal States

Kenneth L. Brigham / James R. Snapper

Lymph Flow from the Lungs
  Safety Factors against Pulmonary Edema
  Permeability of the Pulmonary Microcirculation

Protein Concentration of Pulmonary Lymph
  Molecular Sieving

Pulmonary Lymph and Fluid Balance

Humoral and Cellular Mediators in Pulmonary Lymph

Metabolites of Arachidonic Acid

Cellular Constituents of Pulmonary Lymph

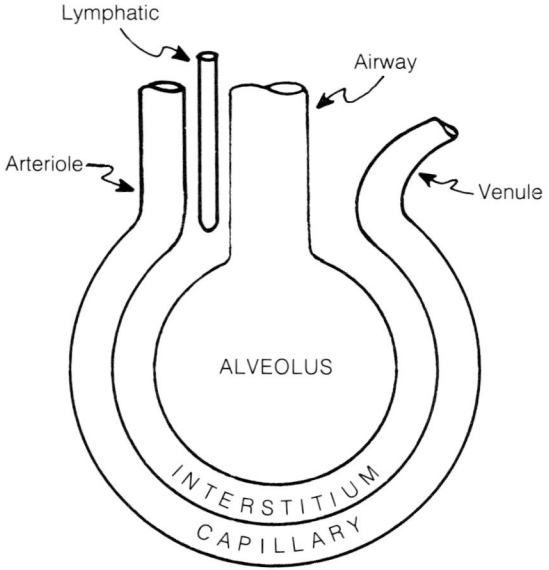

FIGURE 59-1 Conceptual diagram of a lung fluid exchange unit. *(From Brigham, Parker, Roselli, Hobson, Harris, 1982.)*

The lungs are plentifully endowed with lymphatics. Terminal lymphatics begin somewhere around small airways (apparently not reaching the level of alveoli), progressively coalescing as they traverse through the lung to emerge at the hili and enter hilar and mediastinal lymph nodes. Efferent lymphatics from the lymph nodes enter the venous system.

Figure 59-1 is a diagram of relationships among terminal lung lymphatics, microvessels, and airspaces. The terminal lymphatics in the vicinity of the small airways are located within the connective tissue sheath that surrounds airways and arterial vessels. Small pulmonary veins traverse the lung separately from airways and arteries, but are also surrounded by a potential space that is bounded by connective tissue. Not shown are the lymphatics that accompany the pulmonary veins. Interstitial pulmonary edema, the early stage of fluid accumulation in the lung, is the collection of fluid in the potential spaces around blood vessels and airways to produce cuffs. Alveolar pulmonary edema occurs when fluid crosses both the capillary endothelium and the alveolar epithelium.

As in other organs, the pulmonary lymphatics presumably collect fluid filtered from exchange vessels in the lungs and return it to the circulation. If this is true, then in a steady state (that is, when fluid is not accumulating in the lung) the flow of lymph from the lung will equal the net amount of fluid being filtered across exchange vessels. In addition, many investigators have presupposed that the protein concentration in lung lymph equals that in the microvascular filtrate. Based on these two assumptions, it is possible to evaluate microvascular function in the lung by measuring lymph flow from the lungs and the protein concentrations of the lymph.

The assumption that protein concentration in the lymph reflects protein concentration in the microvascular filtrate has been questioned. On the one hand, measurements of exchange of macromolecules across the lymphatics and lymph nodes, as well as comparisons of protein concentrations in lymph and in pulmonary interstitial fluid, suggest that proteins do not change concentration during transit through lymphatics. On the other hand are two types of evidence: (1) morphologic, suggesting that terminal lymphatics may sieve proteins as the interstitial fluid enters them; and (2) physiological, suggesting that fluid may exchange across the walls of lymphatics, thereby having the potential for altering solute concentrations in lymph. Although the question remains unresolved, it is now common practice to infer microvascular function from measurements of lymph flow and protein concentration in the lung (as well as in other organs).

The sampling of lymph from the lungs has also proved useful in determining how fluid and solutes that have accumulated within the lungs are cleared.

Collecting pulmonary lymph that is uncontaminated by systemic lymph is difficult. In the 1940s, Cecil Drinker cannulated the right lymphatic duct in dogs and assumed that the lymph originated primarily from the lungs. The preparation that he devised has been used extensively, with modifications, over the years. But, several investiga-

tors have shown that substantial fractions of right lymphatic duct lymph in dogs may derive from sources other than the lung. Staub and coworkers, taking advantage of the unique lymphatic anatomy of the sheep, developed a preparation in which the efferent duct from a large mediastinal node (the caudal mediastinal lymph node) was cannulated and nonpulmonary contributions to the node were surgically resected. Physiological studies suggest that lymph collected in this preparation is primarily from the lung, and the preparation is now in wide use for evaluating lung fluid balance. More recently, others have developed a similar preparation in goats whose pulmonary lymphatic anatomy appears to be similar to that of sheep. Although published physiological data seem to support the assumption that the pulmonary lymph preparation in the sheep provides primarily lymph from the lungs, questions about systemic contributions to lymph collected from such preparations continue to be raised.

Some investigators have also succeeded in cannulating small lymphatics at the hilus of the lung in dogs. Such a preparation has the advantage of assuring that the lymph collected is solely from the lung; it also has the advantage of collecting lymph prior to its passage through lymph nodes. However, data from such preparations are generally similar to those collected from the other preparations described above.

Lymph from the lungs has been used to measure more than lung lymph flow and protein concentrations. Several reports have suggested that the concentration of potential humoral mediators of lung injury are higher in pulmonary lymph than in blood plasma. Lung lymph also contains leukocytes and occasionally erythrocytes. The concentrations and types of cells can change during lung injury and edema formation. Such findings suggest that lung lymph is useful in evaluating the importance of endogenous humoral and cellular mediators of lung injury.

LYMPH FLOW FROM THE LUNGS

Lymph flows from the normal lung. This means that under normal conditions the net Starling forces in the microcirculation of the lungs are positive in the direction of filtrations. This conclusion differs from the interpretation of their data advanced by Guyton and Lindsey in the late 1950s.

Guyton and Lindsey elevated left atrial pressure in dogs and found no accumulation of water in the lungs until left atrial pressure exceeded plasma oncotic pressure. From these data they concluded that hydrostatic pressure in the exchange vessels of the lungs and the plasma oncotic pressure were the only forces affecting filtration. Since plasma oncotic pressure is normally higher than microvascular pressure in the lung, this would mean that under normal circumstances the net forces favor ab-

sorption and that there could be no filtration and, hence, no lymph flow. The answer to this dilemma is provided by more recent data that show clearly that interstitial oncotic pressure is normally high, making a substantial contribution to the Starling forces; as a result, the sum of those forces is slightly positive, favoring filtration.

Safety Factors against Pulmonary Edema

Since, as Guyton and Lindsey showed, hydrostatic pressures can be elevated substantially in the lung circulation without increasing lung water, there must be some safety factors that protect the lungs against edema in the face of modest increments in hydrostatic pressure. One of these safety factors is an increase in the flow of lymph from the lungs. Although few direct data exist concerning interstitial hydrostatic pressure, interstitial hydrostatic pressure probably increases as interstitial edema forms. Increased interstitial hydrostatic pressure may also serve as a safety factor since, if it increases, the gradient of hydrostatic transcapillary pressures that favor the formation of edema would automatically be decreased.

As an important route for removal of pulmonary edema fluid, the pulmonary lymphatics presumably constitute an important protective safety factor. But pulmonary lymphatics are not the only route by which fluid is removed from the lungs; edema fluid can be reabsorbed via the pulmonary vasculature. Transplantation of the lungs would be impossible if alternative routes of fluid removal did not exist: pulmonary lymphatics are interrupted on the donor lungs and are not surgically reanastomosed. Insurmountable pulmonary edema is not a regular complication of lung transplantation, even though minor interstitial edema does occur; the pulmonary lymphatics presumably reanastomose within a few weeks. An increase in central venous pressure theoretically interferes with lymphatic drainage by increasing hydrostatic pressure downstream from the lymphatics. But even though an increase in central venous pressure may contribute importantly to the formation of a pleural effusion in right ventricular failure, its importance in pulmonary edema is less clear. Lymphatic spread of tumor can cause a regional radiographic picture of interstitial pulmonary edema. The role of pulmonary lymphatics in the removal of recently filtered fluid is compared with their role in chronic interstitial edema later in this chapter.

The flow of lymph from the lungs increases with each increase in hydrostatic pressures in the pulmonary circulation. The normal relationship between the steady-state flow of lymph from the lungs and pulmonary microvascular pressure is shown in Fig. 59-2; the water content of the lungs is also shown as a function of pulmonary microvascular pressure. Modest increases in pressures in the pulmonary circulation cause lymph flow from the lungs to increase, but water does not accumulate in the lungs. The

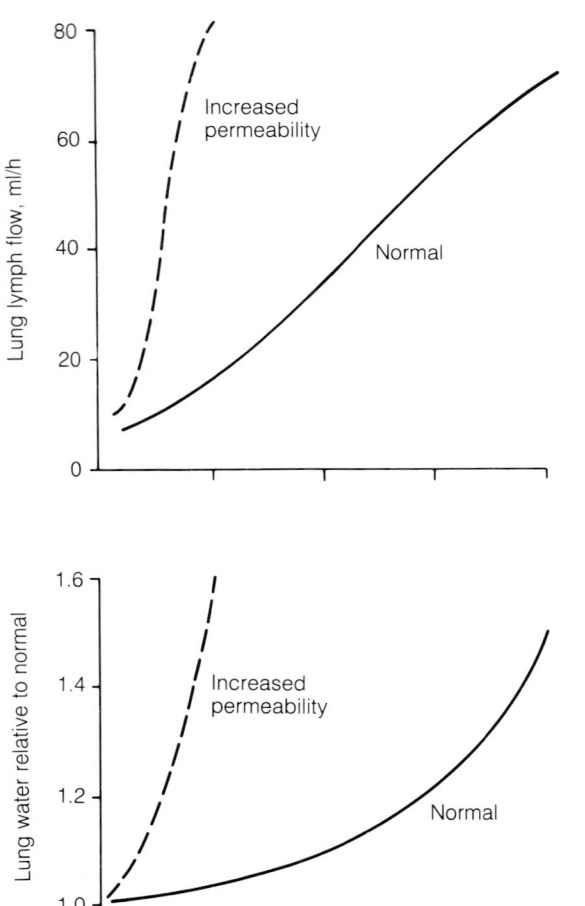

FIGURE 59-2 Idealized relationships between pulmonary lymph flow *(upper)* and lung water *(lower)* to hydrostatic pressure in the left atrium. Normal conditions are shown by solid lines and increased microvascular permeability by dashed lines.

pressure at which water begins to accumulate in the lungs must be a point at which the net filtration of fluid outstrips the capacity of lymphatics to drain away the excess filtered fluid. In practice it is difficult to demonstrate a maximum lymph flow from the lungs.

Permeability of the Pulmonary Microcirculation

Although the term permeability has a very precise meaning in the dynamics of fluid and solute transport across membranes, the term is commonly used in a general sense to mean how easily fluid and solutes cross the walls of microvessels. In that sense, increased permeability simply means that the walls of lung microvessels leak excessive fluid and protein.

As would be suspected, when permeability is high, lymph flow from the lungs is higher than normal for a given pressure. The relationship between pulmonary lymph flow and microvascular pressure during increased permeability is also shown schematically in Fig. 59-2; so is the relationship between the water content of the lungs and pulmonary microvascular pressure during increased permeability. Compared to the normal responses to increased pressure, both curves are shifted to the left and the slopes are steeper: lymph flow from the lungs increases as a much steeper function of pressure, and water accumulates in the lungs at low pressures, even in the normal range. Thus, the protective mechanism (safety factor) of increasing lymph flow is severely stressed when permeability is high and presumably is saturated at a low pressure, permitting the accumulation of fluid in the lungs.

It is generally believed that the group of diseases known collectively in humans as the adult respiratory distress syndrome (ARDS) results, at least in part, from increased permeability in the pulmonary microcirculation. This belief is based on the clinical finding that extensive pulmonary edema occurs without increase in pulmonary vascular pressures and upon the fact that several experimental models designed to simulate clinical circumstances in which ARDS occurs cause an increase in pulmonary vascular permeability. If this is true, relationships between lymph flow from the lungs, an index of transvascular filtration, and pulmonary vascular pressures have clinical implications. The steep slope of that relationship (Fig. 59-2) implies that reducing vascular pressures would exert a profound effect on transvascular filtration rate when permeability is increased. The steep slope of the relationship between lymph flow from the lungs and microvascular pressure forms the rationale for therapies aimed at maintaining low pulmonary vascular pressures in patients with ARDS.

If increased interstitial hydrostatic pressure is an important safety factor, this protective effect may be diminished in patients with acute injury to the lungs. Experimental evidence suggests that the normally "tight" alveolar epithelial barrier, as well as the capillary endothelium, becomes more permeable in these patients. If this occurs, edema fluid can pass freely from the interstitium to the alveolar space without significant increases in interstitial hydrostatic pressure. Thus, this protective safety factor may be lost in patients with ARDS.

Lymph flow from the lungs is generally viewed as passive, the direction of flow being maintained away from the lungs by a series of valves in the larger lymphatics. This probably is an oversimplification since the lymphatics have an intrinsic capability of pumping; they may also be subjected to external forces that tend to pump lymph through the valves away from the lungs. The importance of such mechanisms, and factors which may affect them, are poorly understood. It is probable that these factors are of only minor importance as a protective safety factor in the exchange of fluid and solutes in the lungs.

PROTEIN CONCENTRATION OF PULMONARY LYMPH

Under normal hemodynamic conditions, the protein concentration of lung lymph is high, approximately two-thirds of the concentration in plasma. As indicated above, this high concentration partially accounts for the net Starling forces that favor filtration in the pulmonary microcirculation under baseline circumstances when hydrostatic pressures are low. Also, under normal conditions, relationships between protein concentrations in lung lymph and plasma are a function of protein molecular size. This relationship, shown in Fig. 59-3, demonstrates sieving of proteins between plasma and pulmonary lymph as a function of the molecular size of the proteins. Such data have encouraged characterization of the barrier between plasma and lymph as a porous membrane, thereby enabling quantitative inferences about the barrier, since the mathematics that describes transport through porous media is well understood.

As lymph flow from the lungs increases in response to increasing hydrostatic pressure in the exchange vessels of the lungs, the concentration of proteins in this lymph falls (Fig. 59-4). In experimental animals this relationship is highly reproducible. If the concentration of protein in lymph from the lungs does reflect the concentration around exchange vessels, then the decreasing concentration of protein in the lymph as pressure increases modestly would represent a negative feedback mechanism that

acts to reduce the net sum of filtration forces, thereby protecting against excessive filtration in response to increased hydrostatic pressure. This mechanism is believed to be an additional safety factor protecting against hydrostatic edema.

As shown in Fig. 59-4, lymph protein concentration approaches a minimum value at about four to five times the baseline lymph flow from the lungs. Four- to fivefold increases in lung lymph flow are produced by left atrial pressures of about 30 cmH$_2$O in experimental animals. This is approximately the same pressure that Guyton and Lindsey, and others, have found to be a threshold for fluid accumulation in the lungs. This coincidence implies that decreasing interstitial protein concentration (and thus, oncotic pressure) is an important protective mechanism. When interstitial protein concentration can decrease no further, the lungs become susceptible to edema.

Molecular Sieving

From what is known about the movement of fluid and solutes through semipermeable membranes, it would be predicted that sieving of macromolecules according to their molecular size would be exaggerated in response to mechanical increases in pressure. That is what happens in the lungs as illustrated in Fig. 59-5. This figure shows that although concentrations of all lymph proteins (with respect to concentrations in plasma) decrease as hydrostatic

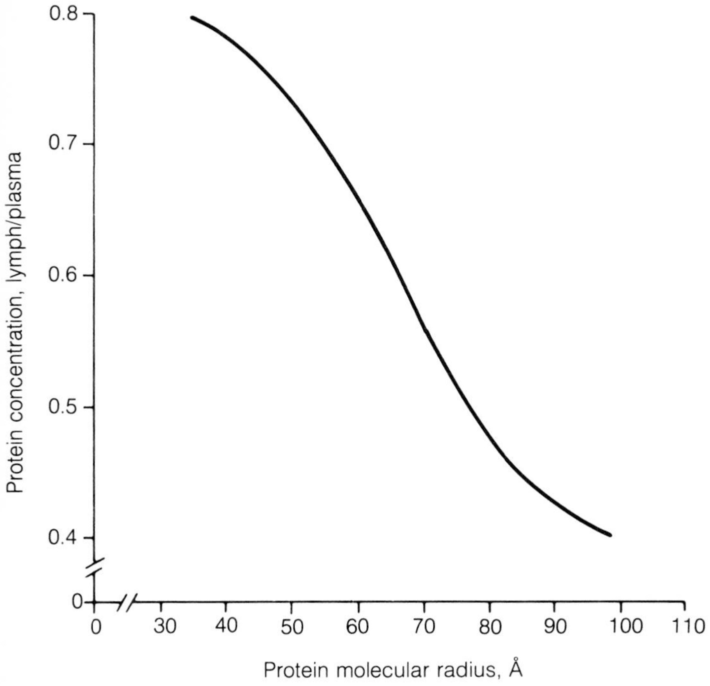

FIGURE 59-3 Total protein concentration in lung lymph relative to plasma concentration as a function of protein size. Sieving of proteins by size is operative under normal baseline conditions. (*From Brigham, Parker, Roselli, Hobson, Harris, 1982.*)

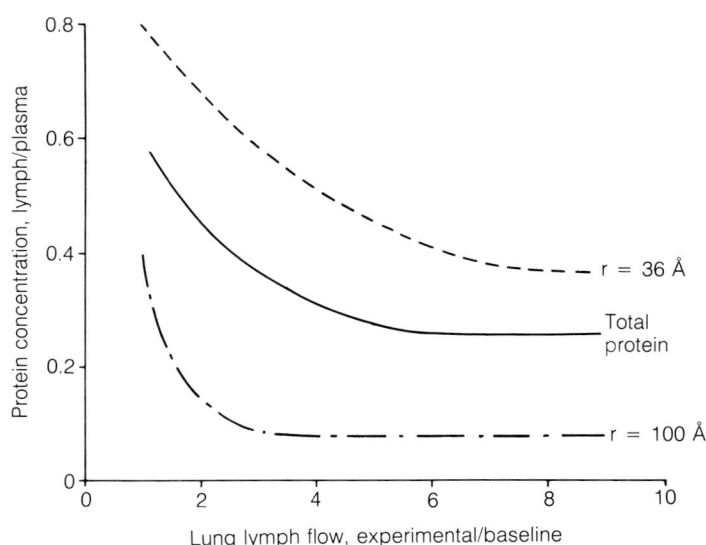

FIGURE 59-4 The ratio of protein concentration in pulmonary lymph to protein concentration in plasma as a function of steady-state lung lymph flow. Lung lymph flow was increased by increasing left atrial pressure. Data for total protein, albumin (r = 36 Å), and a larger protein (r = 100 Å) are shown. Minimal lymph/plasma concentrations are approached at four- to sixfold increases in lymph flow and lymph/plasma concentrations are lower for larger proteins than for smaller ones. (*From Brigham, Parker, Roselli, Hobson, Harris, 1982.*)

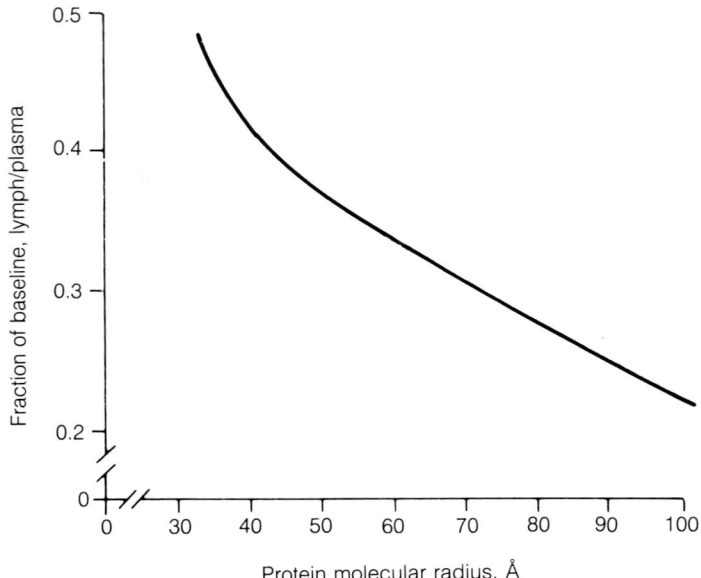

FIGURE 59-5 Relative washdown of different size proteins caused by increasing left atrial pressure. The smallest protein (r = 36 Å) washed down to 48 percent of its baseline value whereas the larger protein (r = 100 Å) washed down to 20 percent of its baseline value. This demonstrates exaggerated sieving of proteins between plasma and lung lymph in response to increased pressure. *(From Brigham, Parker, Roselli, Hobson, Harris, 1982.)*

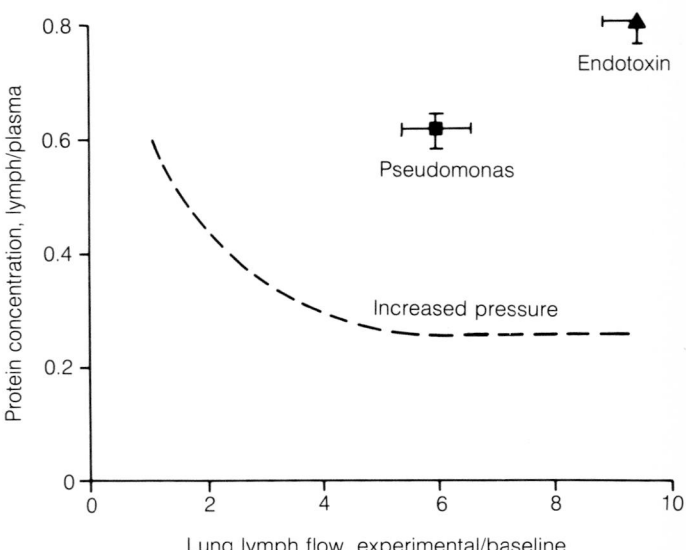

FIGURE 59-6 Relationships between the ratio of protein concentration in pulmonary lymph to protein concentration in plasma and pulmonary lymph flow. Responses to increased left atrial pressure are contrasted with responses to increased lung vascular permeability produced by infusion of either *Pseudomonas* bacteria or *E. coli* endotoxin. *(From Brigham et al: Lymphology 12:177–190, 1979.)*

pressure increases, the concentration of larger proteins decreases more than that of the smaller ones. This exaggerated sieving in response to elevated hydrostatic pressures lends credence to the concept that the barrier between plasma and lung lymph behaves as a porous membrane.

When vascular permeability in the lungs increases, the effects on the protein concentration in lymph from the lungs depend on how severe a permeability change has occurred; if permeability became infinite, the concentrations of protein in lymph and plasma would be equal for molecules of all sizes. Most experimental evidence suggests that such severe alterations in vascular permeability do not occur in the lungs. Indeed, they would probably not be compatible with life.

In contrast to the relationship that exists between the protein concentration in lymph and the rate of lymph flow when lymph flow is increased by increasing pressure, very large increases in lymph flow can occur with no decrease in lymph protein concentration during a steady state of increased permeability (Fig. 59-6). This may be one explanation for the particularly devastating effects of pulmonary edema due to increased permeability: the loss of the normal protective mechanism of decreasing interstitial protein concentration as filtration increases undoubtedly renders the lungs more susceptible to edema.

Even when the permeability of the plasma to lymph barrier in the lungs increases, sieving of proteins persists: concentrations of proteins in lymph still decrease with increasing molecular size (Fig. 59-7). If the assumptions

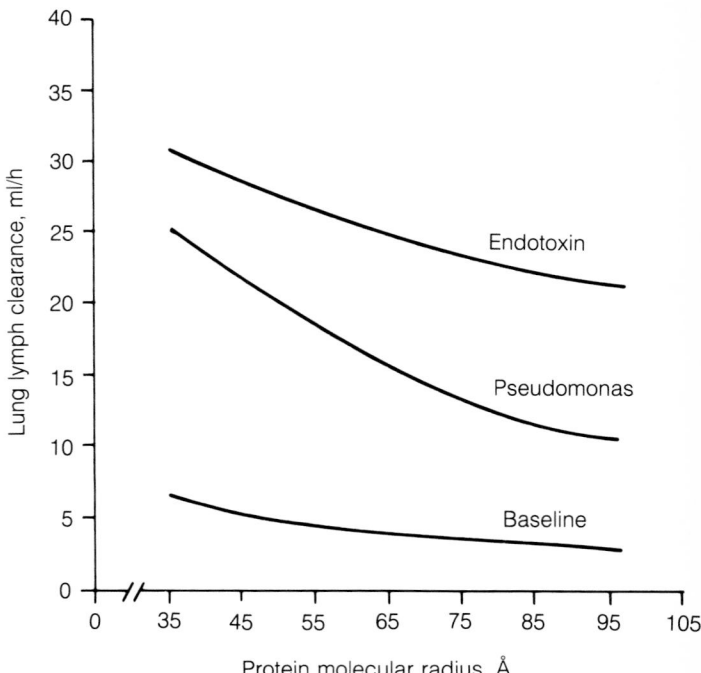

FIGURE 59-7 Lung lymph clearance (lymph flow × lymph/plasma concentration) of proteins as a function of protein size at baseline and during increased vascular permeability produced by infusion of either *Pseudomonas* bacteria or *E. coli* endotoxin. Protein molecular sieving persists during increased permeability. *(From Brigham et al: Lymphology 12:177–190, 1979.)*

upon which inferences from lymph data are made about microvascular function are true, this means that changes in permeability sufficient to produce large increases in filtration (Fig. 59-2) can occur even though the sieving properties of the plasma to lymph barrier are not eliminated; thus, the structural changes that occur in the walls of exchange vessels in the lungs when permeability is increased may be subtle. This conclusion is substantiated by morphologic studies in several experimental conditions: not always do such studies demonstrate structural alterations in the microvessels of the lungs consistent with the physiological changes of increased vascular permeability. Wholesale destruction of microvessel walls in the lung need not necessarily be implied even when edema due to increased permeability is severe.

PULMONARY LYMPH AND FLUID BALANCE

If the anatomic relationships schematized in Fig. 59-1 are correct and if they are static, it would be expected that lymph flow from the lungs would equal the net filtration rate of fluid across the pulmonary microvessels. Also, when transvascular filtration rate would outstrip the capacity of lymphatics, fluid would accumulate in the lung; lymph flow would then remain high even if transvascular filtration were to decrease to normal, the lymphatics acting as an exit route for edema fluid. However, the functional relationships between lymphatics and fluid accumulated in the lungs are not that simple.

In edematous lungs, a general relationship exists between the flow of lymph and the amount of edema (Fig. 59-8). However, under certain circumstances, lymph flow from the lungs returns to near normal even though excess interstitial fluid (edema) is still present. This unexpected finding may reflect the existence of extravascular fluid compartments in the lungs that do not have ready access to the pulmonary lymphatics. In animals given large quantities of saline to cause pulmonary edema, Gee and associates found that the rate of lymph flow related more closely to the rate of transvascular filtration than to the total amount of edema. These results imply that lymphatics may not be a major route for clearing excess fluid from the lungs once it has accumulated.

In pulmonary edema produced in dogs by infusing alloxan, Gee and coworkers have also shown that the solute concentrations in pulmonary lymph derive primarily from the microvascular filtrate and that the concentrations of solutes in pulmonary lymph may differ greatly from the solute concentrations in interstitial cuffs around vessels and airways (Fig 59-9). After edema had developed, they infused Evans blue dye. They took lung biopsies after allowing time for the Evans blue to exit the vascular space and enter the pulmonary interstitial space. As Fig. 59-9 shows, dye was not present in the cuffs of edema fluid even though the lymphatics were darkly stained with the dye. This disparity suggests that preexistent edema fluid was not a major component of lymph and that

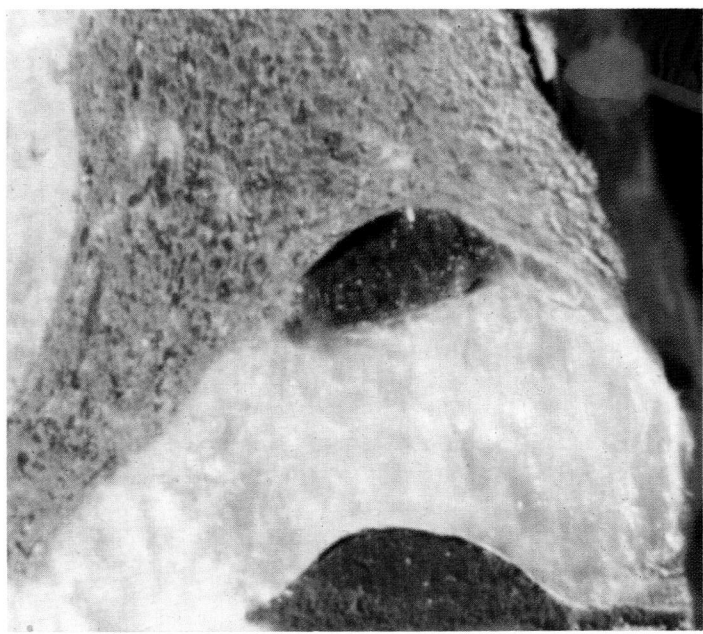

FIGURE 59-9 Photomicrograph of a fresh frozen lung biopsy from a dog with edema caused by alloxan infusion. After edema had developed, a dye (Evans blue) was given intravenously, and sufficient time for the dye to exit the intravascular space was allowed before the biopsy. The picture shows a large cuff of white edema fluid around a pulmonary vein, 1.5 mm in diameter. In the periphery of the cuff is a lymphatic with dark blue contents. That the dye is in lymphatics but not in the edema cuff suggests that lymph is more representative of fluid being filtered from microvessels than of edema fluid accumulated in the lung. ×25. *(Gee, Havill, 1980.)*

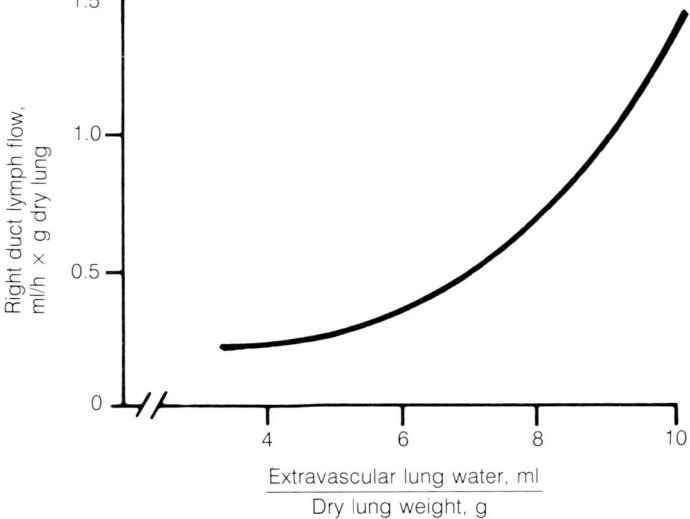

FIGURE 59-8 Relationship between lung lymph flow and lung water in dogs during pulmonary edema caused by infusing alpha naphthylthiourea. *(From Pine, Beach, Cottrell, Scola, Turino, 1976.)*

solutes filtered from microvessels may enter lymphatics without equilibrating in the interstitial edema fluid. How established interstitial edema fluid is removed is not clear, but these studies suggest that pulmonary lymphatics may not be the major route for this removal. The relationship between lung lymph and edema fluid in alveoli appears to be similar: the pulmonary lymphatics may not be the major route for clearing pulmonary edema fluid from alveoli.

HUMORAL AND CELLULAR MEDIATORS IN PULMONARY LYMPH

If pulmonary lymph samples the interstitial space at the level of the microcirculation, then mediators released at that level should appear in lymph. One criterion for whether a given mediator originated in the lung would be that its concentration in pulmonary lymph exceed the concentration in simultaneously collected plasma from peripheral blood. The absence of mediators in pulmonary lymph does not exclude the possibility that such mediators are produced and released by the lungs and that they exert important effects. But the presence of mediators in pulmonary lymph in higher concentrations than in plasma would strongly suggest their production in, or release from, the lungs, or both. Although concentrations of several potential humoral mediators have been measured in pulmonary lymph, this section deals only with the cyclooxygenase and lipoxygenase metabolites of arachidonic acid.

Interpretation of alterations in the cellular constituents of lung lymph are even more difficult than those related to humoral mediators. Lymph from the lungs normally contains larger numbers of lymphocytes, probably T lymphocytes, and very few granulocytes or erythrocytes. The total concentration of cells may decrease while edema is forming, whereas cells such as granulocytes and erythrocytes may appear for the first time. These new cell types may enter lung lymph from the pulmonary or bronchial circulations or directly from lymph nodes located between the pulmonary lymphatics and the sites of collection. The decrease in total cell concentration can result from simple dilution, sequestration within the interstitial space or lymphatics, or migration from the vascular or alveolar spaces.

METABOLITES OF ARACHIDONIC ACID

There are several reasons to suspect that metabolites of arachidonic acid may be important endogenous mediators of lung injury. For example, thromboxane A_2 is a potent smooth-muscle constrictor, prostacyclin is the most potent known pulmonary vasodilator, and several prosta-

glandins are bronchoconstrictors; lipoxygenase products of arachidonate are granulocyte chemotaxins and airway constrictors, and may increase microvascular permeability. In addition, several eicosanoids are released in response to a variety of stimuli that damage the lungs.

Figure 59-10 shows the concentrations in pulmonary lymph of both cyclooxygenase [thromboxane B_2 (the stable metabolite of the active thromboxane A_2), 6-keto-prostaglandin $F_{1\alpha}$ (the stable metabolites of prostacyclin), and prostaglandin E_2] and lipoxygenase [5- and 12-hydroxyeicosatetraenoic acid (5- and 12-HETE) and leukotriene B_4] products of arachidonate before, and after, the infusion of *Escherichia coli* endotoxin into unanesthetized sheep. The differences in the timing of the increases in the concentrations of cyclooxygenase and lipoxygenase products in the lymph from the lungs may prove relevant to the pathogenesis of the lung injury in this animal model. Though not shown, the actual concentrations of the arachidonate metabolites were higher than those obtained simultaneously from plasma, strongly suggesting production in the lungs.

CELLULAR CONSTITUENTS OF PULMONARY LYMPH

There is growing evidence that a number of insults to the lungs that damage microvessels require the presence of circulating granulocytes and that the injury probably results from activation of granulocytes in vivo, pulmonary leukostasis, and local damage to the microvascular endothelium by products of activated granulocytes. Experi-

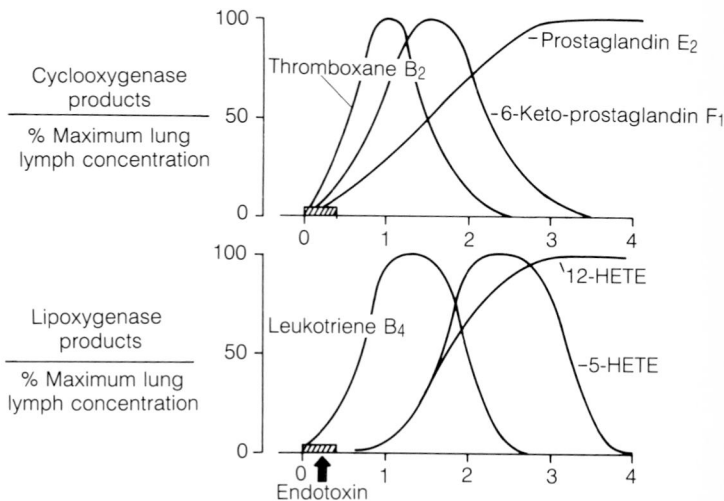

FIGURE 59-10 Lung lymph concentrations of cyclooxygenase (*upper panel*) and lipoxygenase (*lower panel*) products of arachidonate following *E. coli* endotoxemia in unanesthetized sheep. The vertical axes are percent maximal lung lymph concentrations of the various arachidonate metabolites, and the horizontal axes are time in hours after endotoxemia.

mental situations in which this sequence of events has been implicated include responses to infusion of complement-activated plasma, pulmonary vascular injury following extensive pulmonary microembolism, pulmonary vascular injury following endotoxemia, and pulmonary oxygen toxicity. At least during the development of pulmonary oxygen toxicity, it appears that alveolar macrophages produce granulocyte chemotaxins that may be responsible for attracting granulocytes to the lung. In addition, when granulocytes are activated, they produce granulocyte chemotaxins (notably leukotriene B_4) that may perpetuate activation of granulocytes and pulmonary leukostasis. If these processes are occurring at the level of the pulmonary microcirculation, then one might expect granulocyte chemotaxins to appear in lymph from the lungs.

Figure 59-11 shows that this is so: in unanesthetized sheep, chemotactic activity increases in lymph from the lungs coincident with the onset of physiological evidence of pulmonary oxygen toxicity and reaches very high levels as toxicity progresses. The changes in chemotactic activity in lung lymph are much greater than in the arterial blood plasma. As with arachidonate products discussed above, these data strongly implicate the lung itself as the origin of granulocyte chemotaxins in the course of the

development of pulmonary oxygen toxicity. Such findings are consistent with an important role for activators of granulocytes in damage to the lungs that occurs as a result of prolonged breathing of high concentrations of oxygen. Such measurements in other conditions in which pulmonary lung injury occurs may help to elucidate the pathogenesis of those abnormalities.

Figure 59-12 shows the changes in the concentrations of total lymph leukocytes in lymph from the lungs and the percentage of granulocytes in this lymph in response to the infusion of phorbol myristate acetate in unanesthetized sheep. The relationship between changes such as these in lymph from the lungs and lung injury has yet to be proven. It may be possible, in the future, to relate changes in the cellular constituents of lung lymph to inflammatory changes in the lungs themselves and, ultimately, to the pathogenesis of lung injury.

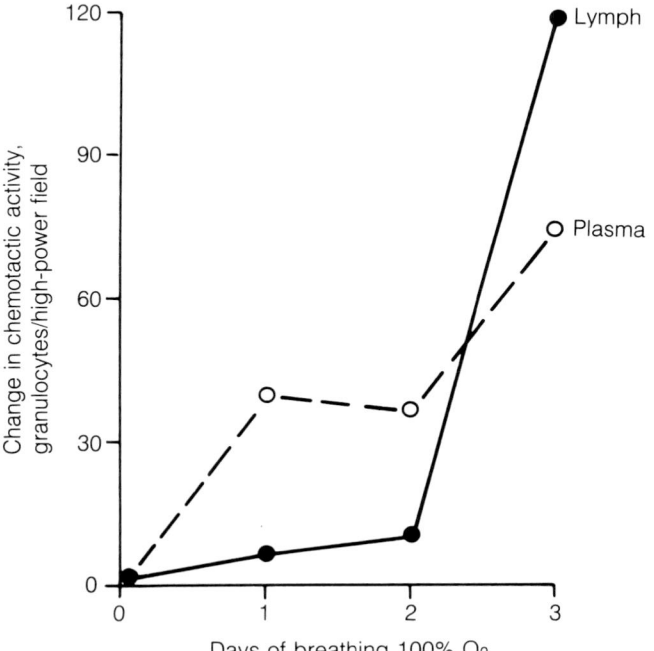

FIGURE 59-11 Effects of breathing 100% oxygen on granulocyte chemotactic activity in lung lymph and blood plasma in a sheep. Chemotactic activity reached much higher levels in lymph than in plasma, although levels in both increased. (*Newman, unpublished observations.*)

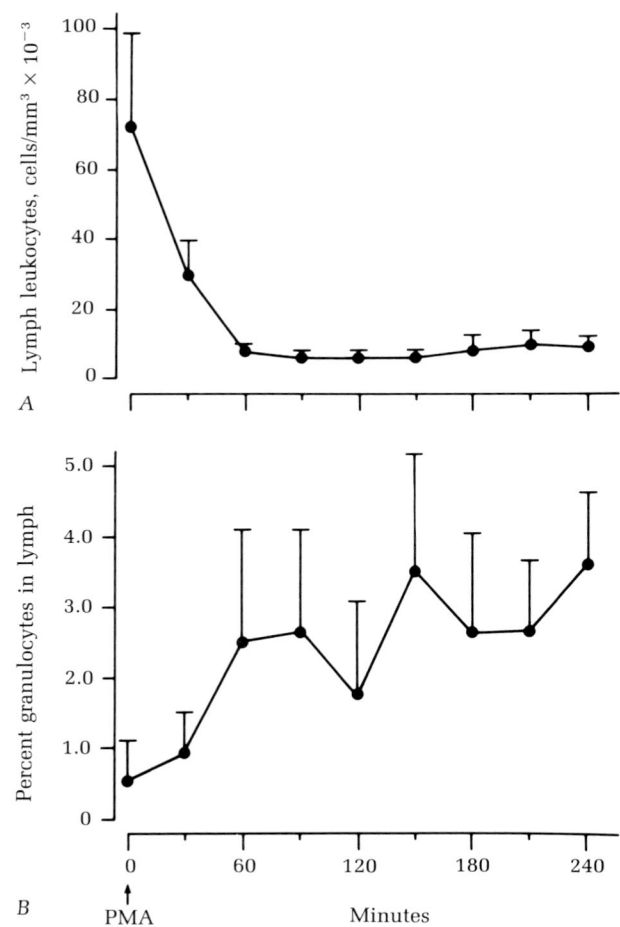

FIGURE 59-12 Lung lymph total leukocyte (*A*) and percent granulocyte (*B*) counts following phorbol myristate acetate in awake sheep. The horizontal axes are time in minutes after phorbol myristate acetate (PMA). (*Modified after Dyer, Snapper: J Appl Physiol 60:576–589, 1986.*)

BIBLIOGRAPHY

Brigham KL: Lung lymph composition and flow in experimental pulmonary edema, in Fishman AP, Renkin EM (eds), *Pulmonary Edema*. Bethesda, MD, American Physiological Society, 1979, pp 161–173.
> *An overview by measurements of lung lymph flow and protein composition in experiments that entailed manipulation of forces affecting transmicrovascular fluid and solute exchange.*

Brigham KL, Parker RE, Roselli RJ, Hobson J, Harris TR: Blood to lymph transport of macromolecules in the pulmonary circulation. Ann Acad Sci 384:246–264, 1982.
> *Discusses the basic principles of macromolecular transports as assessed through lung lymph.*

Carter RD, Joyner WL, Renkin EM: Effects of histamine and some other substances on molecular selectivity of the capillary wall to plasma protein and dextran. Microvasc Res 7:31–48, 1974.
> *Discusses the effects of alterations in capillary permeability on transport in a systemic vascular bed using the dog paw model.*

Conhaim RL, Lai-Fook SJ, Staub NC: Sequence of perivascular liquid accumulation in liquid-inflated dog lung lobes. J Appl Physiol 60:513–520, 1986.
> *In 9 isolated dog lung lobes filled with liquid to total lung capacity and rapidly frozen in liquid N_2, the filling pattern and model analyses suggest that liquid entered the interstitium from an airspace site associated with arteries of ~0.1–1.0 mm in diameter, spread to adjacent sites, and eventually reached the lobe hilum.*

Cottrell TS, Levine OR, Senior RM, Wiener J, Spiro D, Fishman AP: Electron-microscopic alteration at the alveolar level in pulmonary edema. Circ Res 21:783–797, 1967.
> *Describes the ultrastructure of the lung with pulmonary edema formation.*

Drake RE, Allen SJ, Williams JP, Laine GA, Gabel JC: Lymph flow from edematous dog lungs. J Appl Physiol 62:2416–2420, 1987.
> *The resistance of the extrapulmonary art of the lung lymph system limits the maximum flow of lymph from edematous lungs.*

Dyer EL, Snapper JR: The role of circulating granulocytes in sheep lung injury produced by phorbol myristate acetate. J Appl Physiol 60:576–589, 1986.
> *Describes alterations in the cellular constituents of lung lymph during lung injury and altered lung fluid and solute exchange.*

Erdmann AJ III, Vaughn TR Jr, Brigham KL, Woolverton WC, Staub NC: Effect of increased vascular pressure on lung fluid balance in unanesthetized sheep. Circ Res 37:271–284, 1975.
> *Original description of the effects of increased left atrial pressure on lung fluid and solute exchange using the sheep lung lymph preparation.*

Garlick DG, Renkin EM: Transport of large molecules from plasma to interstitial fluid and lymph in dogs. Am J Physiol 219:1595–1605, 1970.
> *Describes the basic transport of fluid and solutes in a systemic capillary bed using the dog paw preparation.*

Gee MH, Havill AM: The relationship between pulmonary perivascular cuff fluid and lung lymph in the dog with edema. Microvasc Res 19:209–216, 1980.
> *Demonstrates that edema fluid which has accumulated in perivascular cuffs is not rapidly removed via pulmonary lymphatics.*

Gee MH, Spath JA Jr: The dynamics of the lung fluid filtration system in dogs with edema. Circ Res 46:796–801, 1980.
> *Further studies of the dynamics of the various interstitial compartments in the clearance of edema fluid from the lungs.*

Gorin AB, Hasagawa G, Hollinger M, Sperry J, Zuckerman J: Release of angiotensin converting enzyme by the lung of *Pseudomonas* bacteremia in sheep. J Clin Invest 68:163–170, 1981.
> *Demonstrates that angiotensin converting enzyme is released into lung lymph during septicemia.*

Guyton A, Lindsey A: Effects of elevated left atrial pressure and decreased plasma protein concentration on the development of pulmonary edema. Circ Res 7:649–657, 1959.
> *A study of the effects of prolonged increase of left atrial pressure on the development of pulmonary edema in dogs showed that Starling's law of capillary fluid exchange applies to the pulmonary circulation.*

Harris TR, Roselli RJ: A multiple pore model of lung transvascular exchange: Description of transport with increased vascular pressure. J Appl Physiol 50:1–14, 1981.
  Describes a model that helps to explain the transport of macromolecules of different sizes in the pulmonary circulation.

Lauweryns JM: The blood and lymphatic microcirculation of the lung. Pathol Annu 6:365–415, 1971.
  Describes the ultrastructure of the pulmonary lymphatics.

Meyer E: Acute and chronic clearance of lung fluid, protein and cells, in Kirkpatrick CH (ed), *Lung Water and Solute Exchange*, vol 7, Lung Biology in Health and Disease. New York, Dekker, 1978, pp 277–321.
  Describes the basic physiology including the time course and routes for clearance of alveolar pulmonary edema fluid.

Newman JH, Fulkerson WJ, Kobayashi T, English D, Meyrick B, Brigham KL: Effects of methylprednisolone on lung oxygen toxicity in awake sheep. J Appl Physiol 60:1386–1392, 1986.
  In lung-lymph fistula sheep, methylprednisolone did not affect either the time course or magnitude of gas exchange abnormality, lymph flow and composition, loss of hypoxic vasoconstriction, lung granulocyte accumulation, or postmortem lung water caused by 100% O_2 breathing.

Newman JH, Loyd JE, English DK, Ogletree ML, Fulkerson WJ, Brigham KL: Effects of 100% oxygen on lung vascular function in awake sheep. J Appl Physiol 54:1379–1386, 1983.
  Describes the changes in chemotactic activity observed in lung lymph with oxygen toxicity.

Pine MB, Beach PM, Cottrell TS, Scola M, Turino GM: The relationship between right duct lymph flow and extravascular lung water in dogs given alpha-naphthylthiourea. J Clin Invest 58:482–492, 1976.
  Describes the relationship between filtration and lung water in increased permeability pulmonary edema.

Renkin EM: Lymph as a measure of the composition of interstitial fluid, in Fishman AP, Renkin EM (eds), *Pulmonary Edema*. Bethesda, MD, American Physiological Society, 1979, pp 145–160.
  A consideration of the distribution of large-molecular solutes, especially the plasma proteins, in lymph and interstitial fluid.

Sloop CH, Dory L, Roheim PS: Interstitial fluid lipoproteins. J Lipid Res 28:225–237, 1987.
  All density classes of plasma lipoproteins are present in lymph. In peripheral lymph, the lymph/plasma concentration ratios of lipoproteins vary from 0.03 for VLDL-sized particles to 0.2 for HDL. Lymph from lung and myocardium contains proportionately more lipoproteins than does peripheral lymph: their lymph/plasma concentration ratios vary from 0.1 to 0.6.

Staub NC: Pulmonary edema. Physiol Rev 54:687–811, 1974.
  A basic review of the physiological factors involved in pulmonary edema formation.

Chapter 60
Pulmonary Edema

Alfred P. Fishman

Pulmonary edema is a consequence of high pressures in the pulmonary microcirculation (predominantly capillaries) or an increase in the permeability of the alveolar-capillary barrier (generally of its endothelial aspect) or a combination of both high pressures and increased alveolar-capillary permeability. To understand the pathophysiology of these three categories of pulmonary edema, it is helpful to keep in mind the normal turnover of water and macromolecules in the lungs.

NORMAL WATER AND MACROMOLECULAR TURNOVER IN THE LUNGS

Gas exchange in the lungs occurs across thin, moist membranes. For these surfaces to operate effectively, they must be continuously cleared of excess water, proteins, and debris. The requirement is satisfied largely by the existence of a separate circulation for water and proteins that begins at the alveolar-capillary level; at this site, an extract of plasma enters the interstitial space from where it will be returned to the systemic circulation via pulmonary lymphatics. Only when the capacity of this drainage system for removing water from the lungs is exceeded does excess water accumulate, i.e., does pulmonary edema form.

Brief surges of excess water in the lungs are regular features of daily life. For example, sudden, vigorous exertion, as during running for a bus, increases the water content of the lungs briefly by transiently increasing pulmonary capillary pressures. The excess water is accommodated in the interstitium until it is drained from the lungs. The level at which excess water in the lungs becomes evident depends on the type of edema and the method of assessment, e.g., physical findings, radiographs, direct determinations of lung water, and the experience of the observer.

The Water Content of the Lungs

The water content of the lungs, exclusive of that within blood vessels, is estimated to be of the order of 300 to 400 ml. Thus, the extravascular water volume is about the same as, or a little less than, the intravascular blood volume of the lungs. About 100 ml of this volume is in the immediate surroundings of the alveolar capillaries, i.e., the volume of fluid around the alveolar capillaries is about the same as that within them. And, like the capillary blood volume, it is spread as a thin film over a large surface area, i.e., more than 70 m². Should edema exceed the bounds of the interstitial space, the gas compartment of the lungs affords an enormous compartment for accumulation of excess water, e.g., about 2500 ml at functional residual capacity (FRC) in the adult, 70-kg male.

Starling's Equation

Clinical as well as physiological thinking about water exchange in the lungs is conditioned by Starling's equation (Fig. 60-1). The barrier between blood and the pericapillary interstitial space, i.e., the pulmonary capillary endothelium, is assumed to be semipermeable. Interstitial forces, both hydrostatic (P_{if}) and osmotic (π_{if}), feature prominently in the balance of forces across the semipermeable barrier. Unfortunately, the interstitial forces are not directly quantifiable; in contrast, the hydrostatic pressure in the pulmonary capillaries (Pc) and the oncotic pressure of the plasma (π_{pl}) can be accurately determined. Despite the inaccessibility of the pericapillary interstitial space, considerable information relating to the formation of pulmonary edema can be obtained clinically by determining the intravascular pressures, per se, i.e., the mean capillary pressure (Pc) and the osmotic pressure of the plasma proteins (oncotic pressures) (π_{if}) (Fig. 60-2).

Normally, the mean pulmonary capillary pressure is of the order of 7 to 10 mmHg; pulmonary capillary pressure is pulsatile, reaching peaks of 20 to 30 mmHg during exercise. In contrast, the plasma oncotic pressure is steady at about 25 mmHg. Therefore, the oncotic pressure due to plasma proteins acts as a safety factor so that the lungs tend to remain moist but unflooded since, except during peak pulsatility, net balance of intraluminal forces during each cardiac cycle protects against transudation from lumen into interstitium. Other safety factors are the compliance of the interstitial spaces, surfactant lining the alveoli, and the topographic distribution of hydrostatic

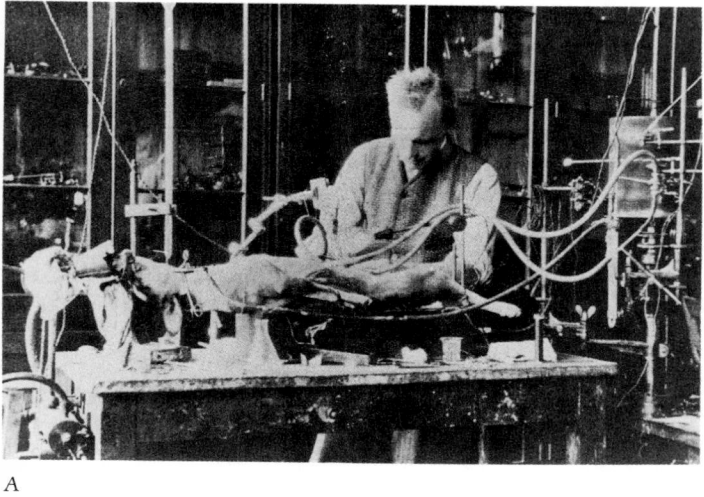

A

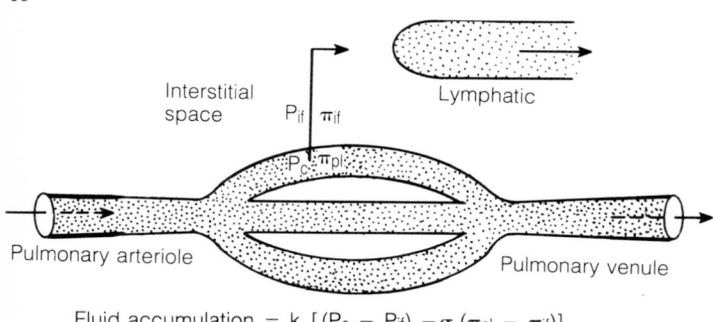

Interstitial
space P_{if} π_{if} Lymphatic

P_c, π_{pl}

Pulmonary arteriole   Pulmonary venule

Fluid accumulation = k [$(P_c - P_{if}) - \sigma (\pi_{pl} - \pi_{if})$]

     k = filtration coefficient

     P_c = capillary hydrostatic pressure

     P_{if} = pericapillary hydrostatic pressure

     σ = reflection coefficient

     π_{pl} = colloid osmotic pressure of plasma

     π_{if} = colloid osmotic pressure of

B   pericapillary fluid

FIGURE 60-1 Starling's law of transcapillary exchange. *A.* E. H. Starling at work on a dog experiment. *(From Fishman and Richards, 1964.)* *B.* Schematic representation of forces influencing transcapillary exchange. The balance of forces shown in the equation generally favors fluid filtration into the interstitial space. Excess fluid and protein in the interstitial space is returned via pulmonary lymphatics to the systemic circulation.

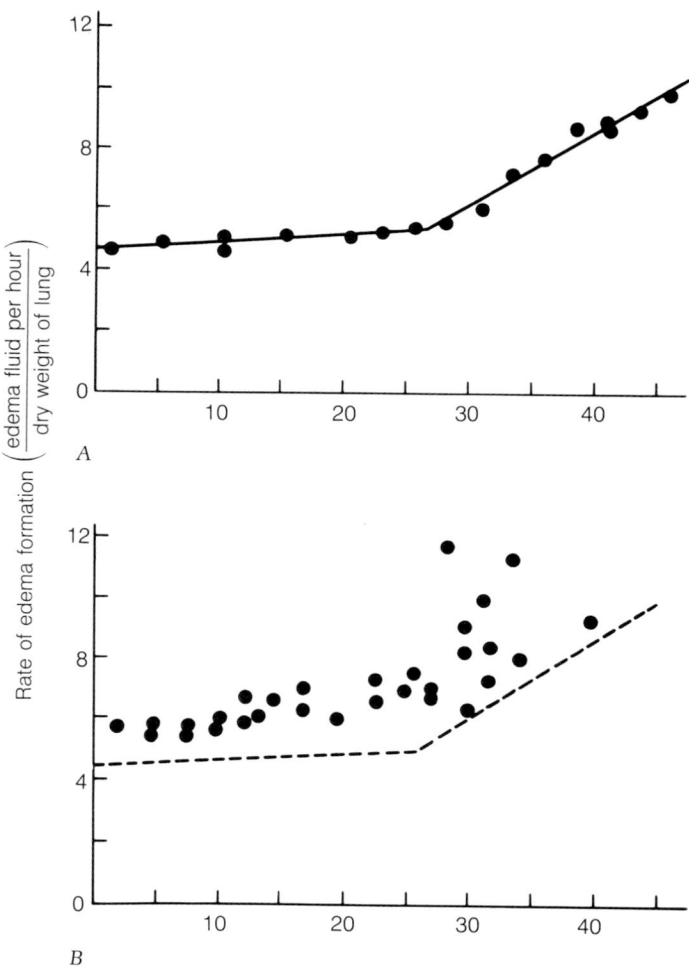

FIGURE 60-2 Fluid loss into lungs as a function of capillary pressure and plasma protein concentration. *A.* While oncotic pressure of plasma proteins was normal, progressive increments in left atrial pressure caused an abrupt increase in fluid loss at a threshold value of about 25 mmHg. *B.* Acute hypoproteinemia (solid dots) induced by plasmapheresis decreased the threshold. *(After Guyton and Lindsey, 1959.)*

pressures under the influence of gravity; the latter tends to keep the apices more edema-free than the bases.

An acute increase in hydrostatic pressure in the pulmonary microcirculation causes water to accumulate in the lungs in a curvilinear fashion (Fig. 60-2); the process is enhanced by a concomitant decrease in plasma oncotic pressure. Hypoproteinemia, per se, does not cause pulmonary edema but does facilitate its formation. Rarely is it possible to implicate a solitary abnormality in either of the interstitial pressures, hydrostatic or oncotic, in the pathogenesis of pulmonary edema except in the case of a large and precipitous decrease in pericapillary interstitial pressure, as is occasionally produced inadvertently by a

rapid and forceful aspiration of a chronic pneumothorax or by a strenuous inspiration during intense bronchospasm.

Nomenclature of the Water-Exchanging Vessels

Starling's hypothesis presupposes a uniformly semipermeable capillary membrane. However, ultrastructural studies suggest that permeability of the capillary barrier may vary along the length of the capillary. Moreover, the exchange of water and proteins in the pulmonary circulation takes place not only across anatomic capillaries but also across venular and probably arteriolar vessels that also lack organized media in their walls. To take these vessels into account, some investigators choose to refer to

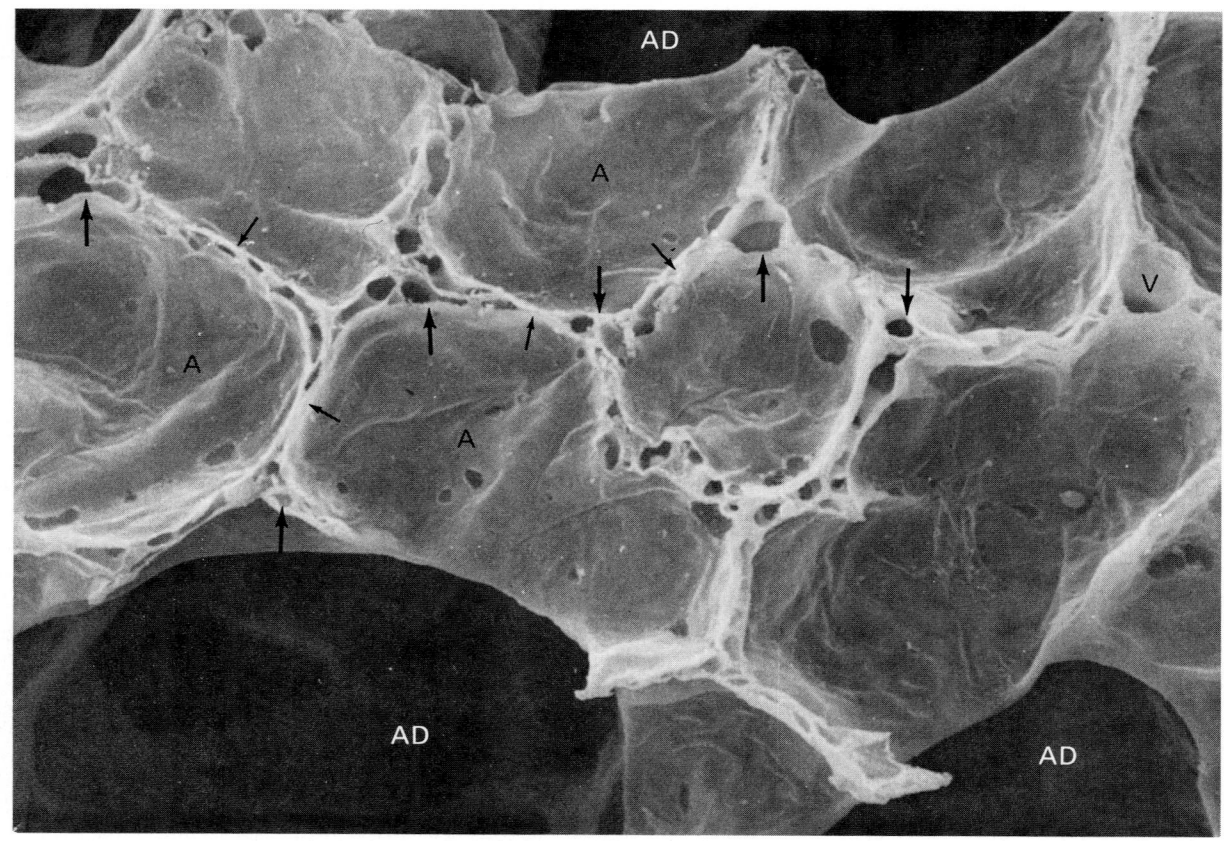

A

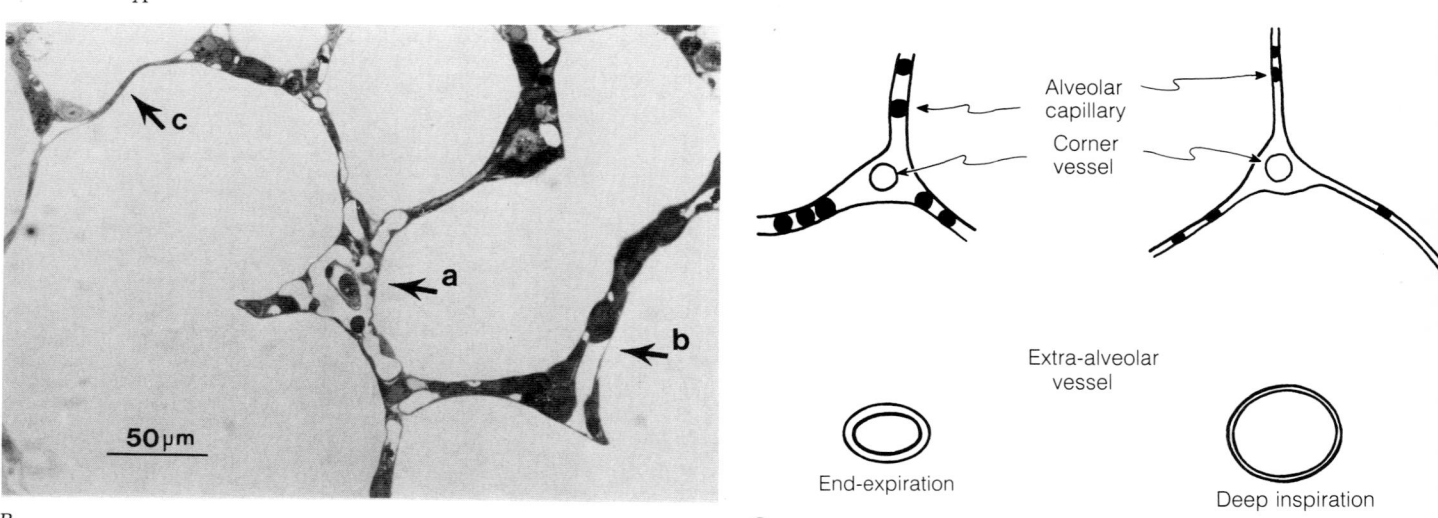

B   C

FIGURE 60-3 Effects of breathing on different types of pulmonary microvessels. A. Scanning electron micrograph of rabbit lung inflated by air to 80 percent of total lung capacity. Fixed by vascular perfusion. Bold arrows point to widened capillaries in "corners" where three alveolar septa join; fine arrows point to narrowed capillaries in the plane of the septum. A = alveolus; AD = alveolar duct; V = small pre- or postcapillary vessel. ×522. *(Unpublished observation of J. Gil, H. Bachofen, P. Gehr, and E. R. Weibel. Micrograph courtesy of E. R. Weibel.)* B. Capillaries inside a bundle of capillaries (a) in corner presumably connect small arteries with small veins and are protected against excess alveolar pressure. Arrangement is due to reversible pleating of alveolar walls. Some septal capillaries (b) are open but flattened, whereas others (c) are derecruited. Normal rabbit lung fixed under zone 2 conditions by vascular perfusion of OsO_4 into the pulmonary artery. Thin epoxy section. *(Courtesy of J. Gil.)*   C. A deep inspiration narrows alveolar vessels, widens extra-alveolar vessels, but leaves corner vessels unaffected. Accordingly, blood flow continues through corner vessels unaffected by respiration.

the water- and protein-exchanging vessels as *microvascular* instead of *capillary*.

However, in this chapter, traditional usage of *pulmonary capillary* is retained for two reasons: (1) the bulk of water exchange in the lungs does take place across the walls of pulmonary capillaries; and (2) the designation *microvascular* obscures important functional differences among the minute vessels of the lungs which include not only the traditional pulmonary microcirculation made up of pulmonary arterioles, capillaries, and venules but also *extra-alveolar vessels* (Fig. 60-3) which are thick-walled *microvessels* that contribute little, if at all, to fluid exchange, and *bronchial venules* that seem to engage in water and macromolecular exchange only under special circumstances (Fig. 60-4). Of special interest are the extra-alveolar vessels lodged in alveolar corners (Fig. 60-3) which remain open after blood flow through alveolar capillaries has been arrested by high alveolar pressures, e.g., when alveolar pressure exceeds pulmonary arterial pressure by more than 10 cmH₂O.

Functional Anatomy of the Water-Circulatory Apparatus

Most fluid exchange in the lungs takes place in the vicinity of gas exchange. The capillaries across the walls of which these exchanges occur are anatomically indistinguishable from muscle capillaries. However, they are distinctive in the eccentric way in which they are incorporated into the alveolar septum. Because of this unusual arrangement, the alveolar-capillary barrier seems to consist of two distinct and separate functional areas: a *thin side*, which seems designed for gas exchange, and a *thick side*, which seems to be built for water exchange while also providing a connective-tissue support for the capillary (Fig. 60-5). On the thin side, where the basement membranes of the alveolar epithelium and of the pulmonary capillary are fused, there is no interstitial space; conversely, on the thick side, the two basement membranes are separated by a matrix of collagen and elastic fibers, a ground substance of polymerized hyaluronic acid and other mucopolysaccharides, and the peripheral extensions of fibroblasts. The first evidence of interstitial edema is widening of the thick side by the excess water (Fig. 60-5).

The alveolar capillaries drain toward extra-alveolar vessels located in alveolar corners formed by the junction of several alveoli (Fig. 60-3). Because of the geometric configuration of the alveolar junctions and the Laplace relationship, interstitial hydrostatic pressures are more negative at alveolar corners (where the smaller radii of curvature generate the higher local recoil pressures) than elsewhere in the alveolar-capillary interstitium. The gradients of hydrostatic pressure created by the varying radii of curvature favor the movement of interstitial fluid formed across alveolar-capillary walls toward the lymphatic endings in the vicinity of terminal bronchioles; once within lymphatics, the interstitial fluid is moved on toward hilar lymphatics for return to systemic veins. It

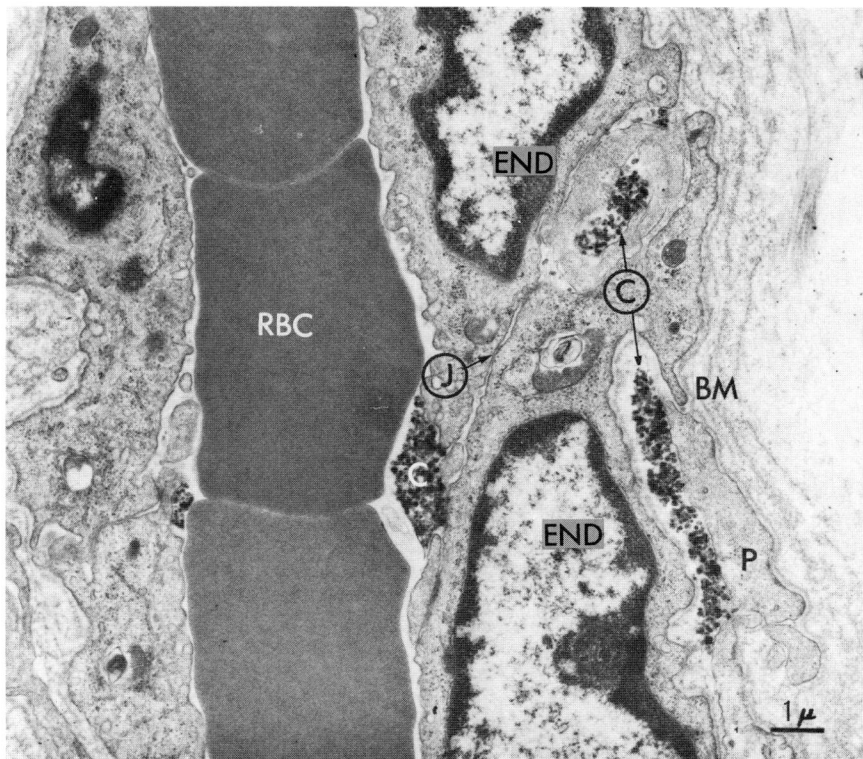

FIGURE 60-4 Pulmonary edema caused by bronchial venular leakage. Ten minutes after the subpleural injection of histamine, carbon (C) that had been injected intravenously is shown on both sides of the endothelial cells. Some carbon remains in the capillary lumen, which contains red blood cells (RBC). This carbon is in the vicinity of an endothelial cleft and junction (J). Carbon has also entered the interstitial space, where it is between the endothelium (END) and a pericyte (P). Uranyl acetate and lead citrate. BM = basement membrane. ×7400. *(From Pietra, Szidon, Leventhal, Fishman, 1971.)*

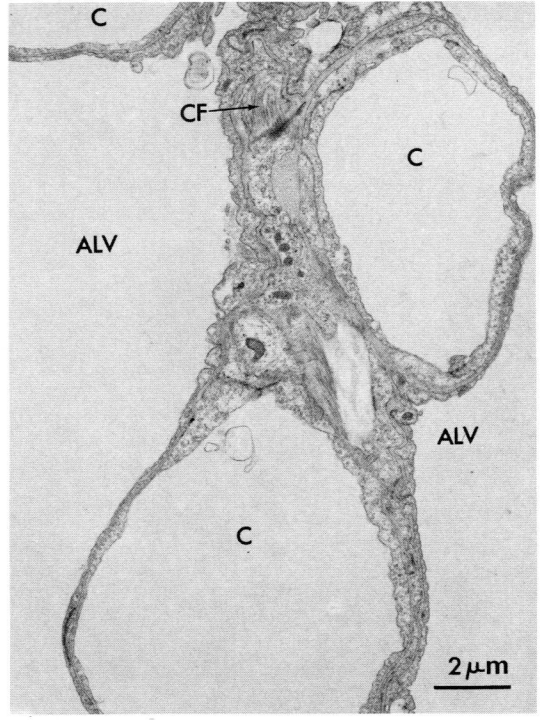
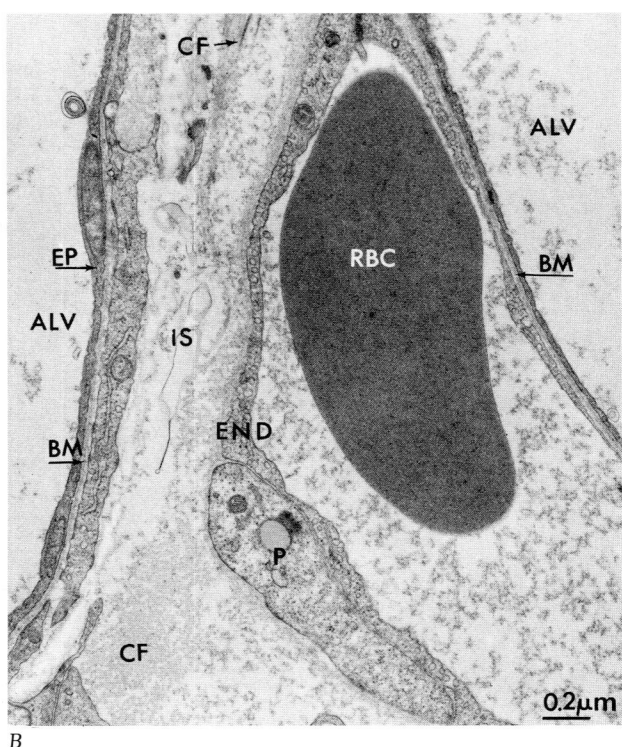

A

B

FIGURE 60-5 Alveolar-capillary interfaces. *A.* Edge-on view of the alveolar-capillary membrane. Electron micrograph showing three capillaries (C) suspended in the septum between alveoli (ALV). On the right side of the middle capillary, the alveolar septum is thin; the opposite side is thick, containing supporting elements, including collagen fibers (CF), in the interstitial space between the capillary and alveolar basement membranes. Uranyl acetate and lead citrate. ×5700. *B.* Interstitial pulmonary edema. The interstitial space (IS) of the thick portion of the alveolar septum has been considerably widened by edema fluid during hemodynamic pulmonary edema, whereas the opposite thin part, containing the fused basement membranes (BM), remains unchanged in thickness. In the alveoli, surrounding the red blood cell (RBC) in the capillary and staining the collagen fibers (CF) of the interstitial space, is the stroma-free hemoglobin (not reacted with benzidine) that was injected as a tracer. Uranyl acetate and lead citrate. END = endothelium; EP = epithelial cells; P = pericyte. ×6840. *(From Fishman, 1972.)*

should be kept in mind that upsets in the interstitial hydrostatic gradients can derange this sequence. For example, during positive pressure breathing, inordinately high airway pressures can cause extra-alveolar vessels to leak fluid into the interstitium instead of acting as drainage vessels for excess alveolar interstitial fluid.

Fluid propelled toward the hilus by successive gradients in interstitial pressure accumulates in peribronchiolar "sumps." Since excess pericapillary fluid is difficult to discern histologically, it was once believed that cuffs of peribronchiolar fluid seen histologically originated from vessels in the immediate vicinity of the bronchioles. However, ultrastructural studies using electron-dense tracers subsequently showed that pulmonary edema originates more distally, i.e., from pulmonary capillaries and possibly from the thin-walled arterioles and venules with which the capillaries connect. It should be kept in mind that, in the pulmonary circulation, the terminal arterioles and venules are thin-walled and muscle-poor. Because of their structural resemblance to capillaries, it seems likely

that these minute vessels can also engage in fluid exchange according to Starling's forces that operate across their walls.

ULTRASTRUCTURAL ANATOMY

It is widely held that water- and fat-soluble molecules can traverse the entire endothelial surface, whereas macromolecules, such as plasma proteins, can cross the endothelial barrier only via pinocytotic vesicles or via interendothelial clefts which are narrowed in spots to form pores. Until the advent of electron microscopy, it was not possible to relate the physiological concept of "pores" to the anatomic makeup of the alveolar-capillary barrier (Fig. 60-6). Since then, interendothelial pores have been identified and shown to correspond to physiological predictions that they are about 40 to 50 Å wide; pores of this size would be expected to be exceedingly effective in preventing the escape of lipid-insoluble macromolecules from the capillary lumina (Fig. 60-6). A large increase in pulmonary capillary pressure enlarges the pores, thereby

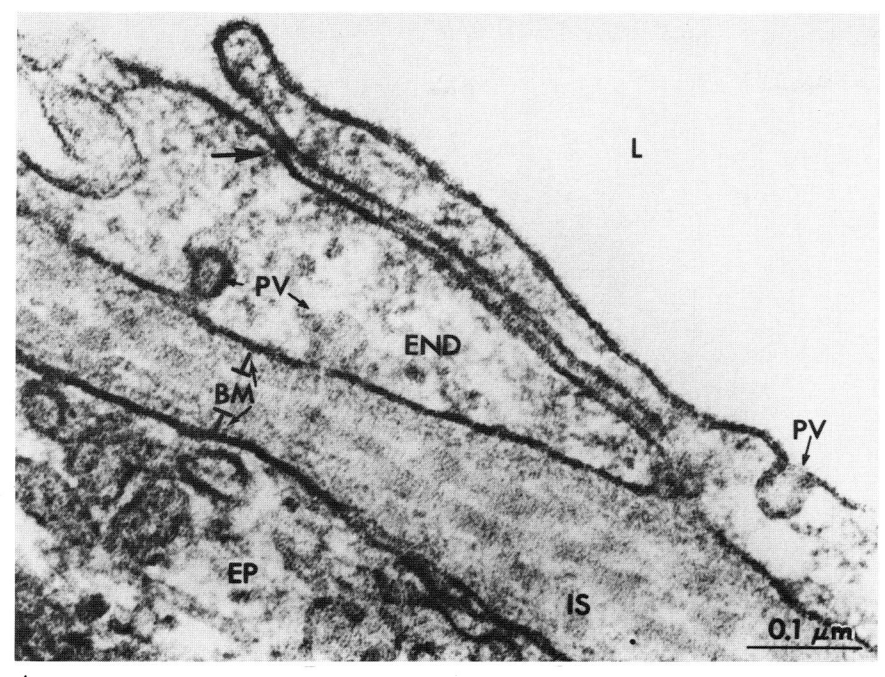

A

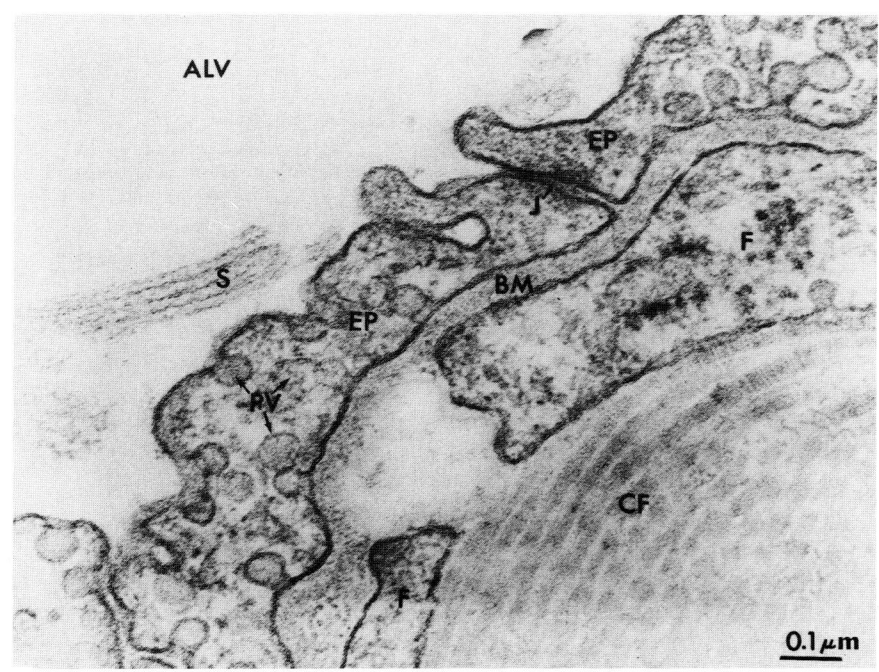

B

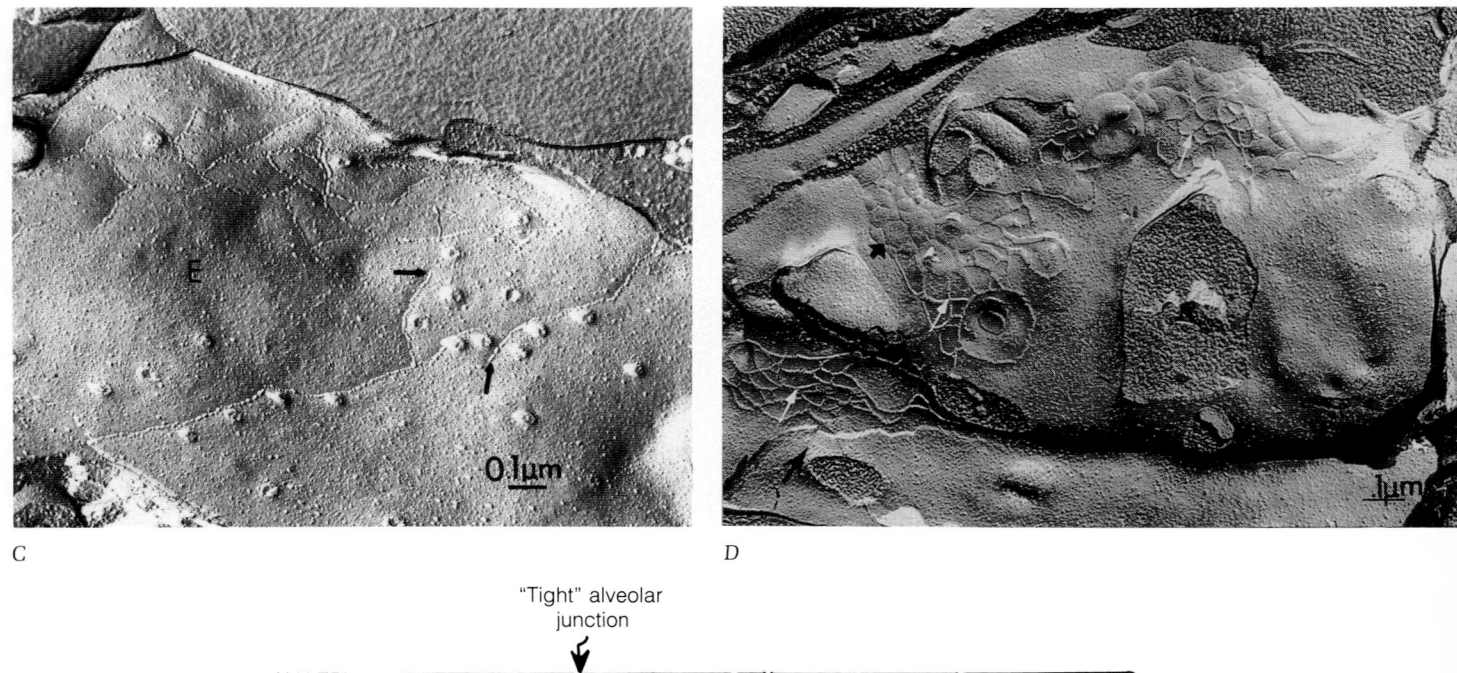

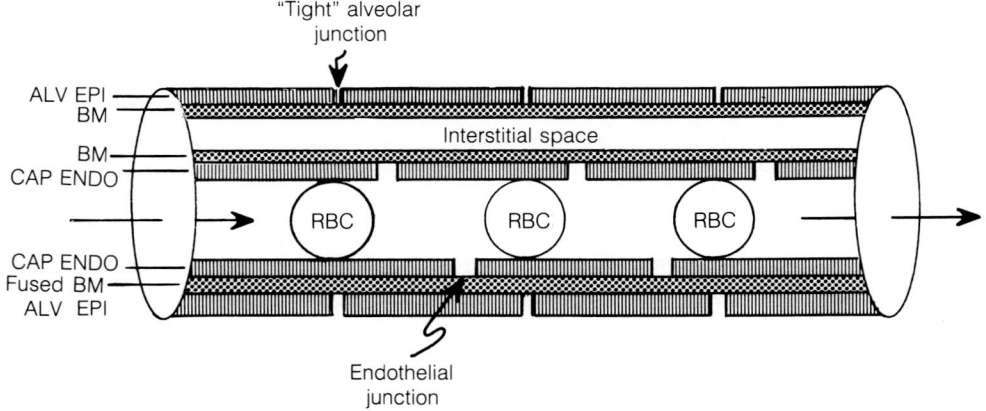

C   D

E

FIGURE 60-6 The alveolar-capillary barrier. *Facing page: A.* Ultrastructure. The capillary lumen (L) is lined by endothelial cells that are separated by an intercellular cleft leading to the interstitial space (IS) on the thick side of the alveolar septum. The interstitial space is bordered by epithelial and endothelial basement membranes (BM). The arrow points to a junction in the cleft. Pinocytotic vesicles (PV) are shown in the endothelial cells (END). *B.* The alveolar surface (ALV) lined by epithelial cells (EP). The junction (J) is indicated in the intercellular cleft. A fibroblast (F) and collagen fibers (CF) are shown in the interstitial space. The epithelial junctions have been shown experimentally to be tighter than the endothelial junctions. *C.* Freeze-fracture replica of an endothelial junction revealing two to three rows of particles (arrows) over shallow grooves in the exoplasmic face. Discontinuous nature of particles suggests the presence of potential pathways between junctional strands. Large arrow indicates direction of shadowing. ×59,640. *D.* Freeze-fracture replica of an epithelial junction revealing an intricate network of solid ridges on the protoplasmic face (white arrows) and grooves on exoplasmic face (black arrow). This arrangement suggests strong interactions between components of the cell membrane at the level of the junction and the presence of a tight seal between adjacent cells. ×40,900. *E.* Schematic representation of both faces of the alveolar-capillary barrier. Thick side of the barrier, with interstitial space separating the two basement membranes, is above; thin side, with fused basement membranes, is below. ALV EPI = alveolar epithelium; BM = basement membrane; CAP ENDO = capillary endothelium; RBC = red blood cell in capillary lumen. *(From Fishman and Pietra, in Fishman and Renkin, 1979.)*

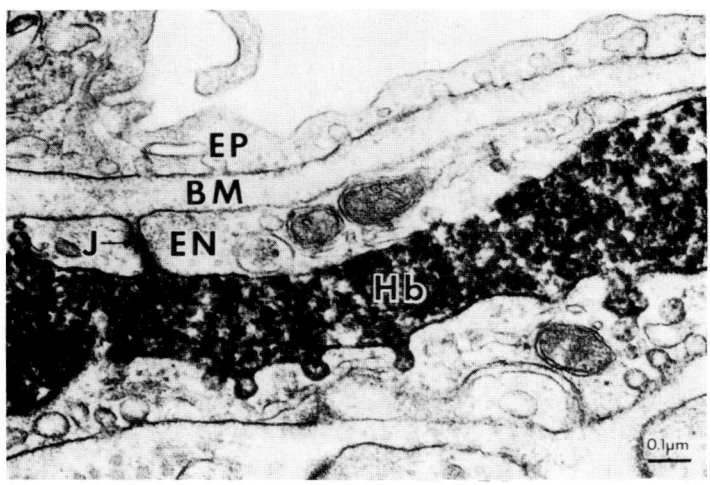

A

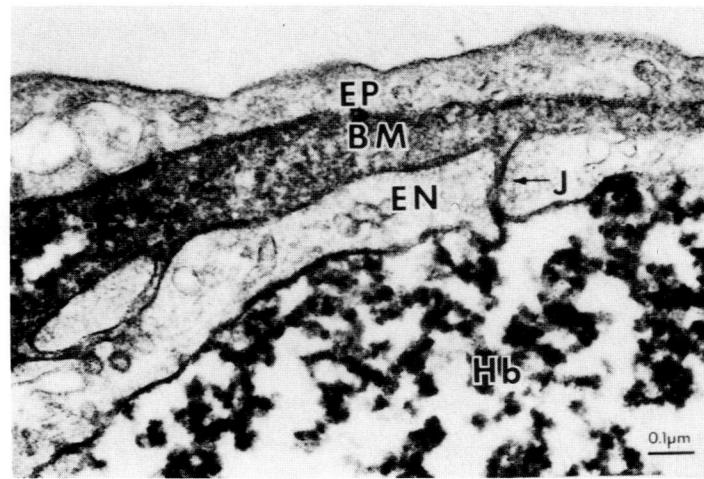

B

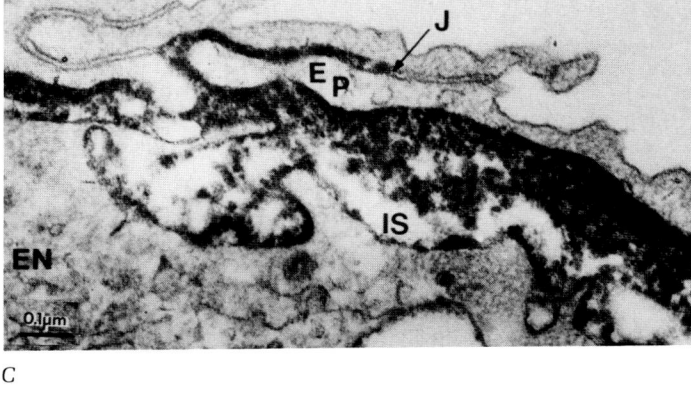

C

FIGURE 60-7 Stretched pores. Ultrastructural demonstration. *A.* Normal pulmonary arterial pressure. After perfusing the dog lung with stroma-free hemoglobin (Hb) for 20 min, electron-dense hemoglobin fills the lumen of the capillary. None of the electron-dense tracer has escaped from the capillary lumen. Instead, the hemoglobin (about the same size as serum albumin) is arrested at the junctions (J) between endothelial cells (EN). The basement membrane (BM) and alveolar epithelium (EP) are free of black tracer (hemoglobin reacted with peroxidase). *B.* Pulmonary capillary hypertension. Same as *A* but perfusion at 50 mmHg. Hemoglobin (Hb) extends from the capillary lumen, through the junction (J) between endothelial cells (EN) into the basement membrane (BM). The epithelium (E_P) is devoid of the tracer. *C.* Pulmonary capillary hypertension. Continued perfusion at 50 mmHg. Illustrated is a segment of the alveolar-capillary barrier containing a distinct interstitial space (IS). The hemoglobin tracer extends from the interstitial space between alveolar epithelial cells (EP) to be arrested at the junction (J). It does not penetrate the alveolar space (A). EN = endothelial cells. *(Modified after Pietra, Szidon, Leventhal, Fishman, 1969.)*

enabling macromolecules to pass from capillary lumens to pericapillary interstitial spaces via interendothelial junctions (Fig. 60-7).

Small pores cannot account fully for the passage of macromolecules from capillary lumen to interstitium, particularly of those larger than albumin. To deal with this discrepancy, "large pores" have traditionally been invoked, and pinocytotic vesicles have been judged to operate as their anatomic equivalents (Fig. 60-8). However, the situation is obviously more complicated than can be explained by large and small pores. For example, it has now been shown that the endothelial surface is topped by domains of electrostatic charges that undoubtedly influence the passage of charged macromolecules from plasma to interstitium (Fig. 60-8).

For experimental purposes, the reflection coefficient in the Starling equation is generally assumed to be one, i.e., that plasma proteins do not traverse the endothelium. However, in reality, proteins do cross via pores and pinocytotic vesicles. Indeed, the mean lymph-plasma ratio for plasma proteins is normally about 0.75. Also, the proteins appear to be sieved, largely on the basis of molecular charge and somewhat on the basis of electrostatic charge. As a result, the lymph-plasma ratio is heavily weighted by the smaller proteins.

THE LYMPHATICS

The final stage in this removal of excess water from the lungs is accomplished by an extensive network of lymphatics, i.e., the third (water) circulation of the lungs. This network begins as fine lymphatic capillaries in the vicinity of the terminal bronchioles and arborizes its way through the lungs to empty into systemic extrathoracic veins (see Chapter 58). This network proliferates in states of chronic pulmonary congestion and edema; the emptying of lymphatics into systemic veins is impeded by high systemic venous pressures. Although unidirectional valves in normal muscular lymphatics, lymphatic contractions, and ventilatory movements sustain forward flow when systemic venous pressures become high, it is

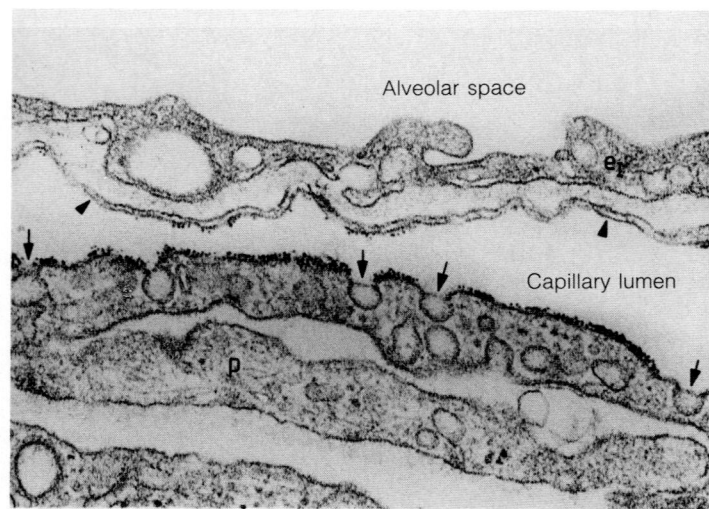

FIGURE 60-8 Pinocytotic vesicles and electrostatic domains in the mouse lung. Three minutes after intravascular perfusion of cationized ferritin, the charged particles are seen to be bound almost continuously on the luminal surface of the "thick" side of the alveolar capillary. However, the cationized ferritin does not bind to the pinocytotic vesicles and their diaphragms (arrows). On the opposite ("thin") side of the capillary which contains no pinocytotic vesicles, binding of cationic ferritin to endothelium is scarce or absent (arrowheads). Microdomains of different electrostatic charge or charge density on the endothelial surface are evident as local variations in the accumulation of cationic ferritin. e_I = type I epithelial cell; P = pericyte. ×51,240. (Courtesy of Dr. M. Simionescu.)

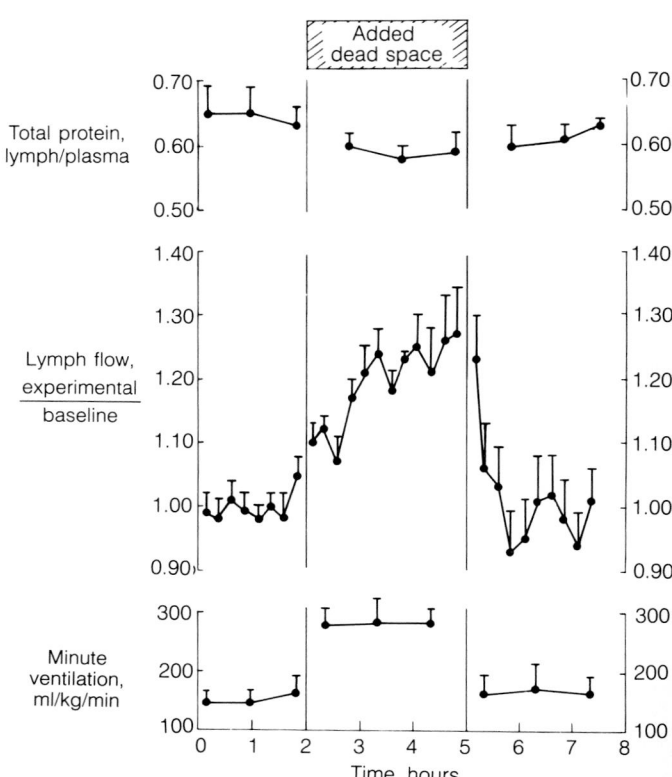

FIGURE 60-9 An increase in ventilation produced in the unanesthetized sheep by increasing dead space (middle panel). Along with the increase in ventilation, lymph flow increased and the lymph-plasma ratio of total proteins decreased. Removal of the dead space reversed the changes. (From Albelda, Hansen-Flaschen, Lanken, Fishman, 1986.)

not known if lymphatic valves remain competent when the lymphatic circulation proliferates. An increase in rate and depth of ventilation increases lymph flow, presumably because of a combination of a decrease in pericapillary pressure and massage of the large lymphatics as a result of the increased respiratory movements (Fig. 60-9). Although the pulmonary lymphatics proliferate remarkably in states of chronic pulmonary congestion and edema, it is not known if their valves become incompetent as the lymphatics dilate.

In a normal adult resting quietly, lymphatic flow is estimated to be about 20 ml/h. The major role of the pulmonary lymphatics is to return protein, rather than water, to the systemic circulation. Local obstruction of lymphatics promotes the accumulation of excess water and proteins in the vicinity (Fig. 60-10). As noted above, the protein concentration of lung lymph formed through normal vascular walls is ordinarily quite high, i.e., about two-thirds of the concentration in plasma. Without lymphatic drainage to return this protein to plasma, the oncotic pressures responsible for transcapillary flux of water would be seriously compromised.

SURFACTANT

The layer of surfactant that lines the alveoli is an important antiedema (as well as antiatelectasis) factor (Fig.

60-11). The nature of this lining is considered elsewhere in this book (see Chapters 2, 15, and 57).

J RECEPTORS

Paintal originally posited that juxtacapillary receptors (J receptors), juxtaposed to bundles of collagen fibers in alveolar-capillary septa, act as stretch receptors when stimulated by swelling of the adjacent collagen fibers as excess water accumulated in the pericapillary interstitial spaces. Although receptors for interstitial swelling do seem to exist, it is now questionable whether they are juxtacapillary in location. Instead, recent evidence favors relocation of the receptors to the interstitium surrounding bronchioles rather than capillaries.

THE INTEGRATED SYSTEM

Based on the individual components of the water- and protein-exchanging system considered above, it is possible to envisage the circulation that mobilizes excess water and proteins from the interstitial spaces of the lungs (Fig. 60-12). According to this schema, stimulation of the J receptors stimulates breathing, thereby promoting drainage

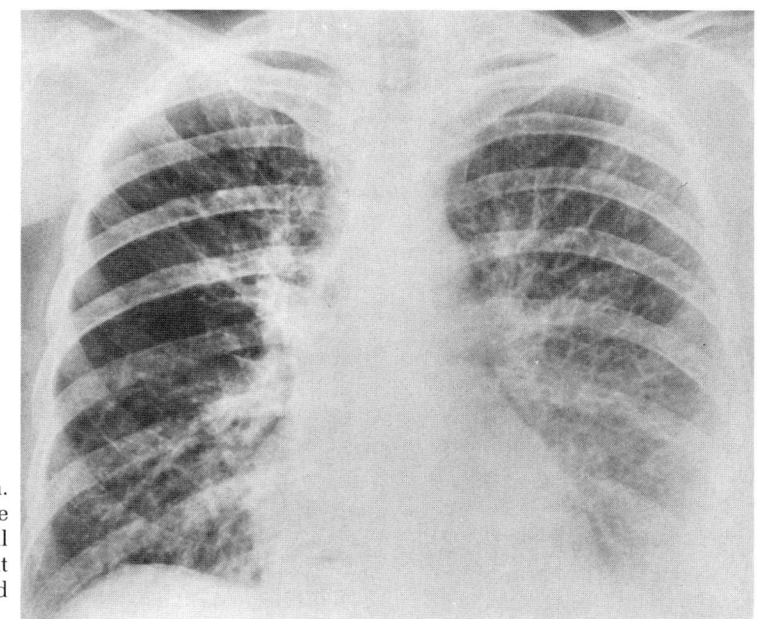

A

FIGURE 60-10 Lymphangitic spread of metastatic carcinoma. *A.* Lymphangitic spread of metastatic carcinoma of the breast. The extensive racemose pattern is more marked on the right. *B.* Renal cell carcinoma (left kidney) metastatic to the lungs. *C.* Same patient as *B.* Lymphatic containing metastatic cells. Surrounding the filled lymphatic are alveoli containing edema fluid.

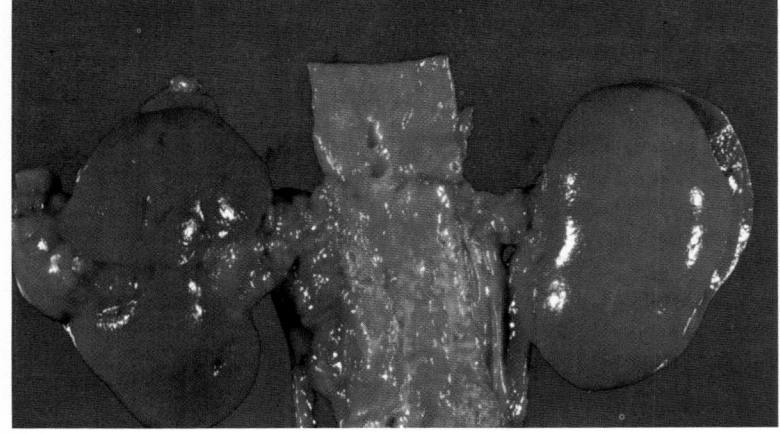

B

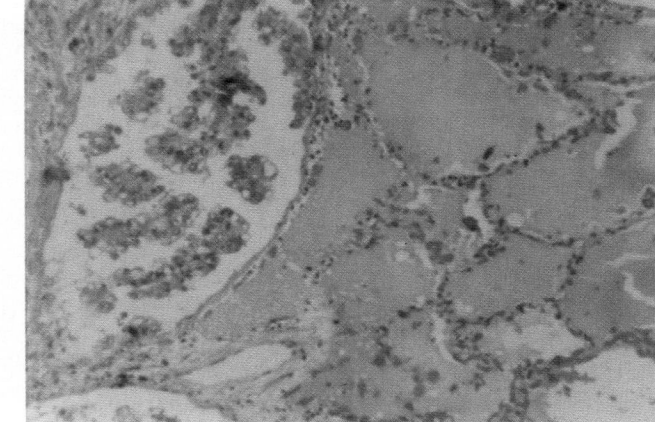

C

of fluid from the gas-exchanging surfaces toward the pulmonary lymphatics. Apparently, the J-reflex system is also part of a large control system which relaxes the muscles of the extremities while the ventilation is being stimulated. Teleologically, the larger reflex system can be interpreted as designed to slow physical activity, thereby decreasing water accumulation in the lungs (Fig. 60-12).

EXCESS WATER IN THE LUNGS

Definition of Pulmonary Edema

Pulmonary edema is defined as excess water in the lungs. A wide variety of etiologies can cause excess water to accumulate in the lungs (Table 60-1). As a rule, except when the alveolar-capillary barrier is damaged via the airways, a stage of interstitial edema precedes alveolar edema. Alve-

olar edema tends to aggravate and perpetuate pulmonary edema in two ways: (1) by eliminating the surfactant layer, it promotes alveolar collapse, i.e., atelectasis; and (2) by lifting off the surfactant layer (Fig. 60-11), it also upsets the Starling forces in favor of further accumulation of fluid in the alveoli.

General Aspects

Before considering particular types of pulmonary edema, certain general aspects merit consideration.

CLINICAL RECOGNITION

Physiologists are fond of saying that lung water has to increase by about 30 percent before the presence of excess water can be reliably detected. Unfortunately, this is a modest estimate that is probably truer in the laboratory

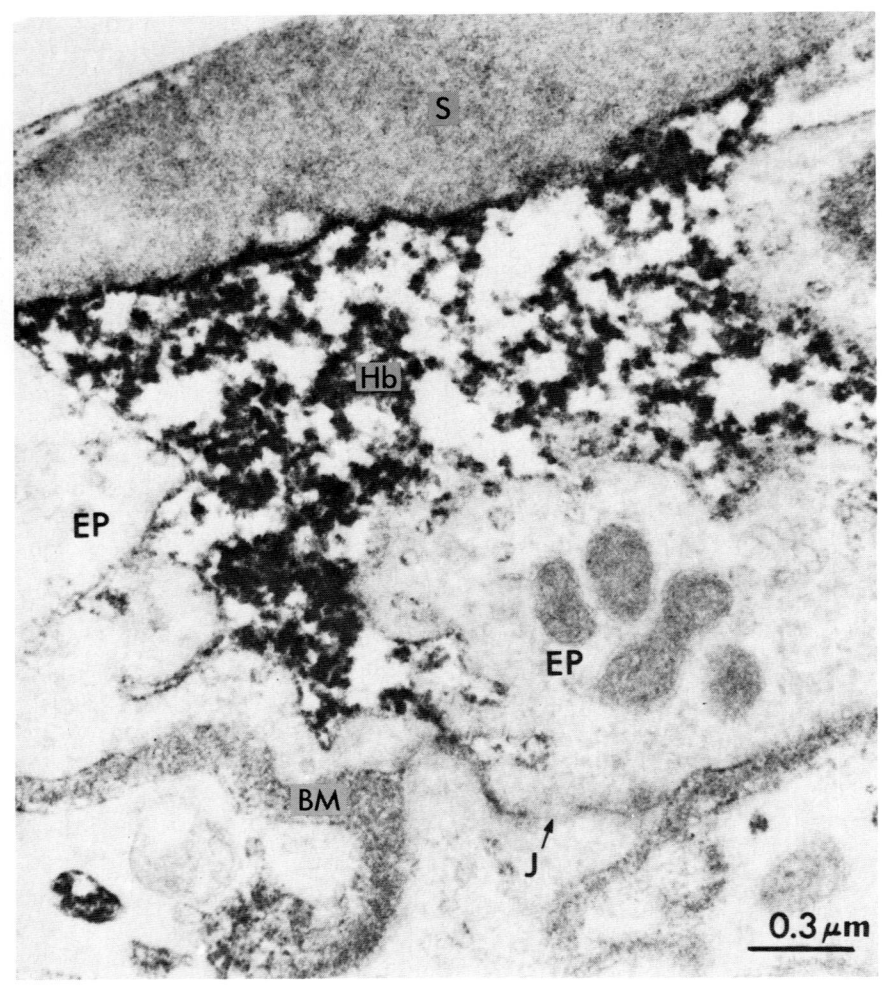

FIGURE 60-11 Surfactant displaced in pulmonary edema. The layer of surfactant (S) has been lifted from the alveolar epithelium (EP) by edema fluid containing stroma-free hemoglobin as an electron-dense marker (Hb). BM = basement membrane. J = junction. *(From Pietra, Szidon, Leventhal, Fishman, 1969.)*

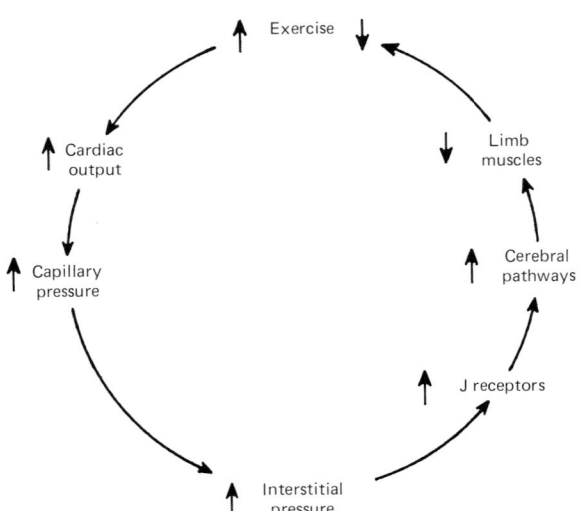

FIGURE 60-12 J receptors during exercise. At the start of exercise (↑ exercise), hemodynamic changes lead to stimulation of J receptors by way of an increase in interstitial pressure. The central component of the reflex causes a decrease in the tone of the limb muscles, prompting a decrease in exercise (top, ↓). *(Courtesy of M. Kalia.)*

setting than at the bedside. In clinical circumstances, underlying cardiac or pulmonary factors often complicate the picture. Also, in certain types of edema, the excess water accumulates most visibly around central structures, e.g., "butterfly" pulmonary edema, whereas in the others the first abnormalities are manifest at the lung bases, e.g., left ventricular failure. Therefore, clinicians are more inclined to say that pulmonary edema first becomes manifest when lung water has increased by 300 percent rather than by 30 percent.

Basal rales are the traditional hallmarks of early pulmonary edema. But, in reality, by the time that rales become audible, excess water has overflowed from alveoli into terminal bronchioles; it is in the bronchioles that the rales of pulmonary edema are generated. An earlier sign that is often disregarded is rapid shallow breathing, a consequence of waterlogged, stiff lungs and of stimulation of the breathing by J receptors.

Chest Radiography

The radiograph is a powerful instrument for detecting and monitoring pulmonary edema (Table 60-2). The principal

types encountered clinically, i.e., cardiogenic, permeability, and overhydration, have certain distinctive features.

In *chronic cardiogenic pulmonary edema*, the radiographic constellation includes abnormalities in the cardiac silhouette, enlargement, blurring and increased density of the hilar regions, the presence of septal (Kerley) lines, redistribution of pulmonary blood flow toward the

TABLE 60-1
Examples of Diverse Etiologies of Pulmonary Edema

Intact alveolar-capillary barrier
  Hemodynamic
    Cardiogenic, e.g., left ventricular failure
    Overhydration, e.g., uremia
    High altitude
    Neurogenic
  Precipitous drop in interstitial pressure
    Reexpansion of chronic pneumothorax
    Strenuous inspiration during bronchospasm

Leaky alveolar-capillary barrier
  Adult respiratory distress syndrome
  Toxic inhalants
  Gastric aspiration
  Postradiation pneumonitis
  Hypersensitivity pneumonitis

Abnormal lymphatic drainage
  Lymphangitic carcinomatosis
  Pulmonary fibrosis, e.g., silicosis
  Systemic venous hypertension

Uncertain
  Narcotic overdosage
  Pulmonary emboli
  Postcardiopulmonary bypass
  Postchronic embolectomy

apices, widening of interlobar fissures, peribronchial and perivascular cuffs, and pleural effusions (Fig. 60-13).

In *permeability edema*, typified by the adult respiratory distress syndrome on the one hand and the inhalation of noxious fumes on the other (Fig. 60-14), the cardiac silhouette is generally normal in size and contour, the pattern of pulmonary blood flow and the hilar regions are generally normal, widespread and patchy infiltrates are present with frequent air bronchograms, and the pulmonary edema is often peripheral in distribution; peribronchial and perivascular cuffing are uncommon as is pleural effusion.

Finally, in *overhydration pulmonary edema*, a common occurrence in uremia, the hilar regions are enlarged, the pattern of blood flow is normal, the edema is preferentially central in distribution, and the lung fields show a generalized, mild haziness (Fig. 60-15). Overlap among all these radiographic categories of pulmonary edema is common.

Worthy of emphasis are two aspects of the clinical detection of pulmonary edema: (1) radiographic evaluation remains the most reliable and expedient tool for early detection of pulmonary edema, i.e., while the edema is still interstitial, and for monitoring the course of pulmonary edema; and (2) clinical recognition that relies on physical examination and detection of rales is counting on the production of adventitious sounds of air passage in terminal bronchioles, i.e., on overflowing alveolar edema.

DISTRIBUTION OF PULMONARY EDEMA

The patterns of pulmonary edema are shaped not only by their etiologies and pathogenetic mechanisms, i.e., hemodynamic, permeability, or overhydration, but also by mechanical factors, notably regional variations in compliance, by lung disease and by the differential effects of gravity on blood, lung tissue that contains air, and air.

TABLE 60-2
Radiographic Features of Different Types of Pulmonary Edema*

	Extrapulmonary Signs		Pulmonary Signs			
	Heart	Pleura	Pulmonary Vasculature	Hili	Interstitium	Topography of Edema
Chronic hemodynamic†	Abnormal	Effusions common	Redistribution favoring apices; prominent pulmonary veins	Enlarged, blurred, air bronchograms	Kerley B and septal lines	Widespread edema to periphery
Permeability	ND	ND	ND	ND	ND	"White-out"
Overload	Enlarged	Effusions common	Generous vasculature throughout	Enlarged, blurred, air bronchograms	Kerley B and septal lines	Variable: from butterfly to widespread

*Radiographs taken in conventional upright position.

†In acute left ventricular failure, the pulmonary vasculature is full from top to bottom—as in the case of volume overload—but different from the redistribution pattern of chronic congestive heart failure.

NOTE: ND = not distinctive.

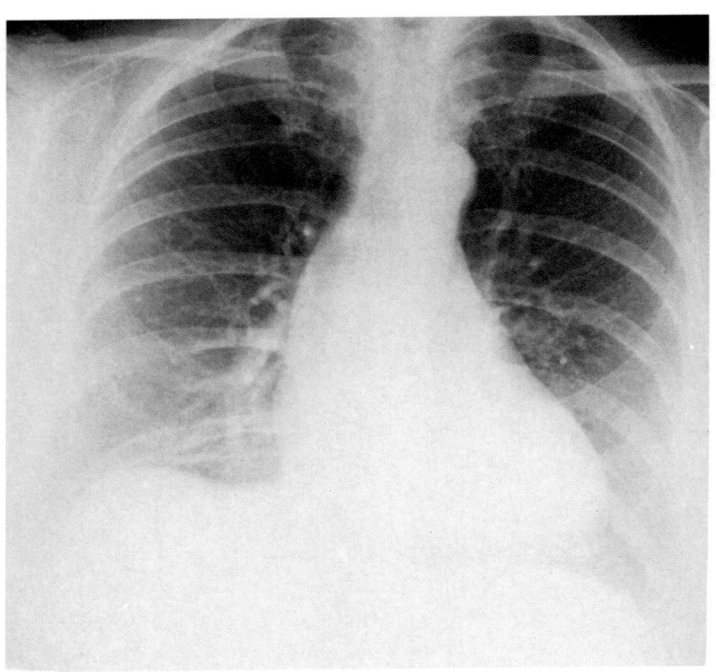
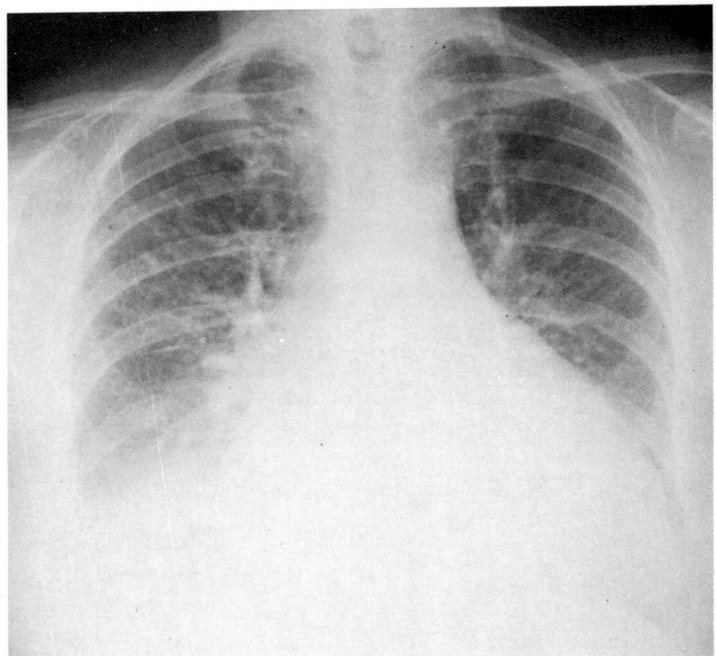

A

B

FIGURE 60-13 Chronic hemodynamic (cardiogenic) pulmonary edema in a 62-year-old woman. A. The cardiac silhouette is abnormally large. Pulmonary vascular markings toward the apices are unduly prominent. Interstitial edema is prominent. Pleural effusions are present bilaterally. B. Three years later. Progressive cardiomegaly, pulmonary congestion and edema, and bilateral pleural effusions.

Distortions in normal architecture produced by local disease modify normal patterns.

In the normal lung, the balance among vascular hydrostatic, alveolar, and blood pressure is such that blood flow and pressure are greater at the bases than at the apices. Left to its own devices, edema follows a gravity-dependent pattern. Differences in interstitial compliance also direct excess fluid to intralobar septa (Fig. 60-16). Familiar manifestations of excess interstitial fluid are the Kerley B lines that are seen radiographically at the periphery of the lung as linear streaks that run parallel to the domes of the diaphragm.

Excess pleural fluid is a common concomitant of hemodynamic pulmonary edema. As a rule, this extrapulmonary fluid is easy to recognize. However, excess fluid in an interlobar fissure can occasionally be mistaken for a carcinoma of the lung unless its contour and location are appreciated (Fig. 60-17).

Lung disease, past or present, influences where excess fluid accumulates. When an inflammatory process, such as that caused by *Pneumocystis*, is widespread and indolent, excess fluid accumulates through the lungs in the vicinity of capillaries. In contrast, a local scar, as in silicosis, or local lymphatic invasion by tumor favors accumulation of excess fluid around affected sites.

As indicated above, gravity strongly affects the distribution of excess fluid (Fig. 60-15). Therefore, the body position of the patient before the chest radiograph is taken often shapes the pattern that the edema will assume. In general, once edema has formed, it tends to gravitate toward the dependent parts of the lungs, usually the lung bases where hydrostatic pressures are highest. In turn, accumulation of excess fluid at the bases tends to redirect fluid toward the apices as perivascular pressures increase. In time, persistent edema at the lung bases tends to redistribute the blood flow not so much by excess fluid as by perivascular fibrosis that is presumably due to the accumulation of large and irritating plasma proteins in the pericapillary interstitial space.

PULMONARY FUNCTION TESTS

Stiff, edematous lungs do a great deal of work and expend considerable energy in breathing because of excess water in the extravascular compartment and engorgement of the vascular compartments. Both the excess water and blood are accommodated at the expense of the alveolar air volume. Alveoli tend to become inoperative because of flooding and to close because of displacement of surfactant (Fig. 60-11). One important consequence of the stiffened, congested, and edematous lungs is rapid, shallow breathing and inability to fill the lungs normally with air during a maximum inspiration.

Preoccupation with interstitial and alveolar edema should not obscure the fact that various other derange-

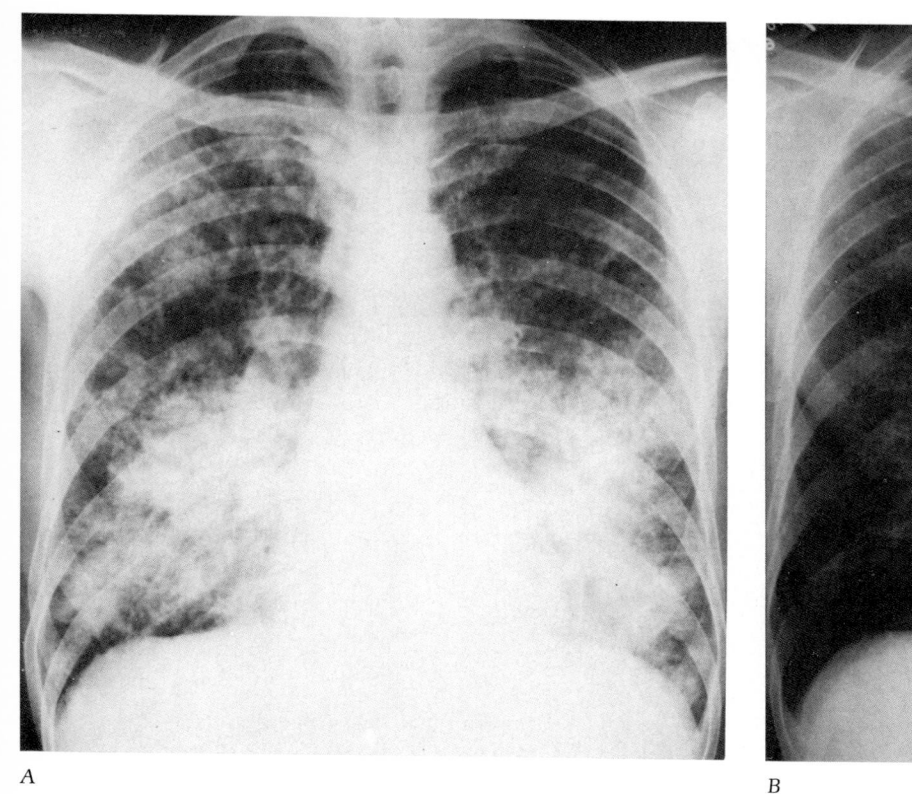

A

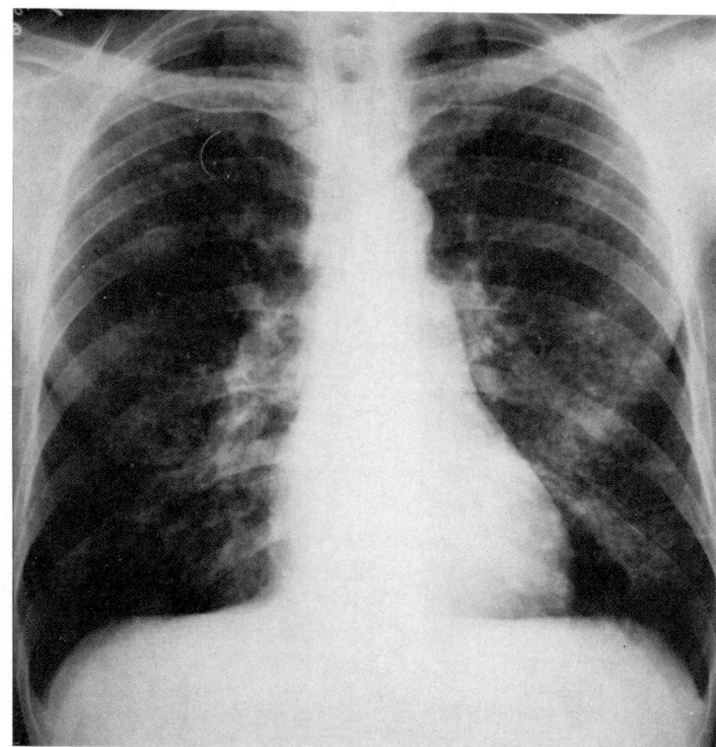

B

C

FIGURE 60-14 Pulmonary edema after inhaling nitrogen dioxide.
A. A few hours after inhalation. Butterfly pulmonary edema.
B. One month later. C. Three months after the inhalation. *(Courtesy
of Dr. H. Weill.)*

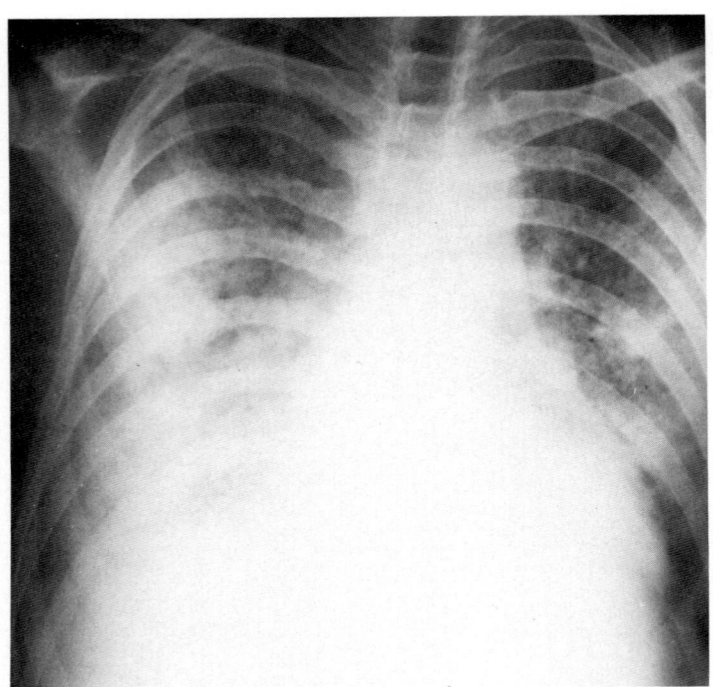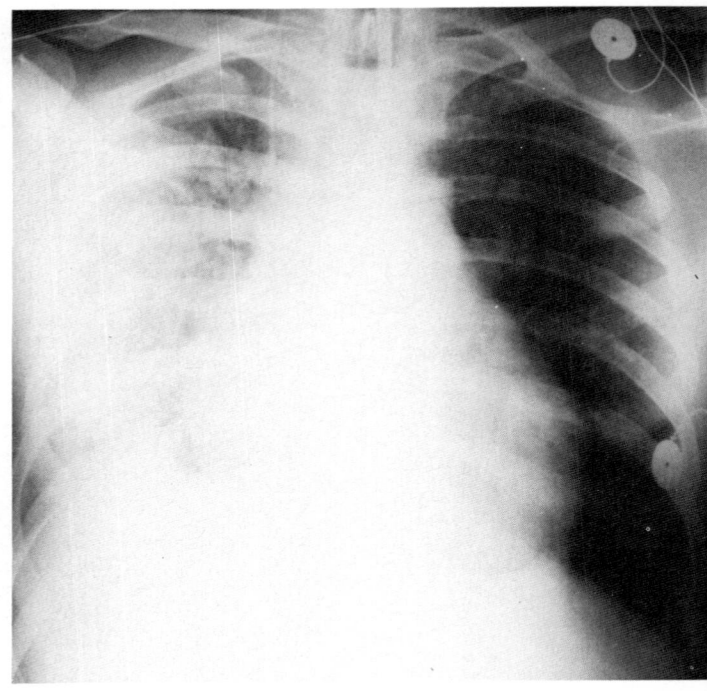

A   B

FIGURE 60-15 Overhydration pulmonary edema. A. Conventional upright chest radiograph showing widespread pulmonary edema. B. After 3 h of lying on the right side. The excess fluid has shifted toward the dependent side.

ments operating simultaneously may be contributing importantly to the clinical syndrome associated with hemodynamic (cardiogenic) pulmonary edema: (1) if left ventricular failure is part of biventricular failure (congestive heart failure), high systemic venous pressures impede the emptying of pulmonary lymphatics; (2) widespread increase of venous pressure also affects bronchial veins, leading to congestion and submucosal edema of the airways, thereby contributing to cough, asthma, and possibly to hemoptysis; and (3) a low cardiac output may compromise oxygen delivery to the diaphragm and other respiratory muscles, thereby contributing to their fatigue.

Serial determinations of the vital capacity have proved useful in following the course of resolving or worsening pulmonary edema. Other lung volumes, or determinations of pulmonary compliance, airway resistance, and the work of breathing, generally add little to the practical information provided by the vital capacity (Fig. 60-18). For a while, the closing volume was advocated for the early detection of excess water in the lungs. The original idea was that this measurement could detect premature closure of small airways because excess water would accumulate around terminal bronchioles and compress them; as a result, closing volume should enlarge (Fig. 60-19). However, it now turns out that because the very small airways are tightly embedded in the pulmonary pa-

renchyma (Fig. 60-19), excess fluid accumulates only around larger bronchioles and bronchi. Nor are small arterioles and arteries compressed by excess interstitial fluid even though edema fluid does accumulate around them in cuffs. The explanation for the increase in airway resistance that occurs in pulmonary edema has now swung away from compression of small vessels and airways by peribronchovascular fluid to edema within alveoli and airways.

Blood-Gas Tensions

Pulmonary edema that is sufficient to be discernible on the chest radiograph is regularly associated with mild arterial hypoxemia (60 to 80 mmHg), often with hypocapnia. However, an acute episode of severe pulmonary edema sometimes causes hypercapnia (arterial $P_{CO_2} > 45$ mmHg). For example, hypercapnia is not uncommon in the pulmonary edema that accompanies an acute episode of severe left ventricular failure that occurs after a massive myocardial infarction.

One way to picture relationships between pulmonary edema and abnormalities in blood-gas levels is shown in Fig. 60-15: (1) during interstitial and early alveolar edema, which is spotty in distribution, reflex hyperventilation from the stiff lungs—presumably because of the J receptors—promotes hypocapnia; (2) should the edema fluid

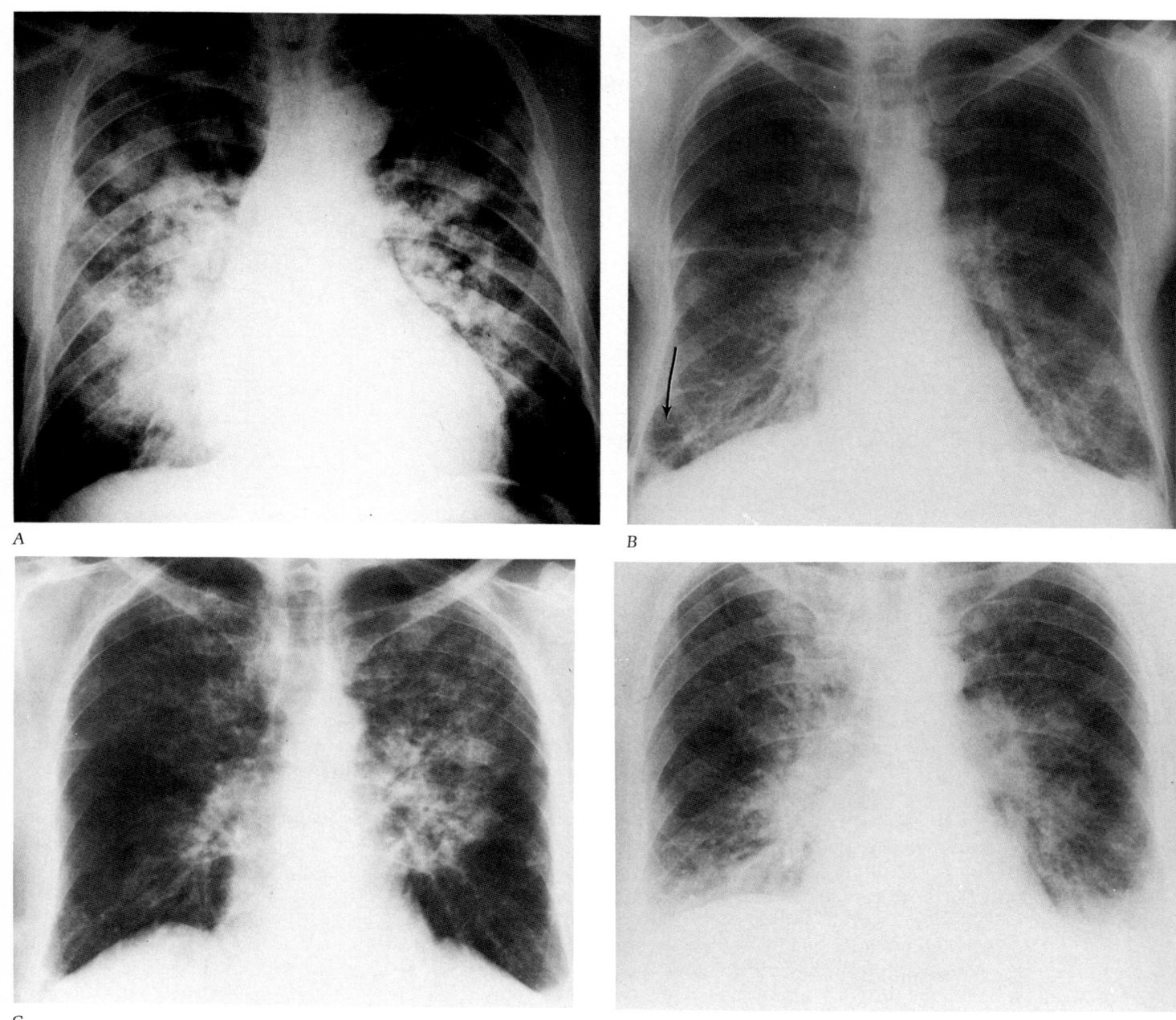

A   *B*

C   *D*

FIGURE 60-16   Patterns of hemodynamic pulmonary edema. *A.* Hemodynamic pulmonary edema. Butterfly pattern following acute myocardial infarction and left ventricular failure. Compare with permeability pulmonary edema in Fig. 60-14.   *B.* Pulmonary edema following acute mitral valvular insufficiency after ruptured chordae tendinae. Edema is most marked at the lung bases, the hilar regions show blurred bronchovascular markings, and fluid has accumulated in septa. The arrow points to a Kerley B line. Kerley A and C lines are also present. *C* and *D.* Chest radiographs in same patient as in *B*, taken at weekly intervals before surgical replacement of mitral valve.

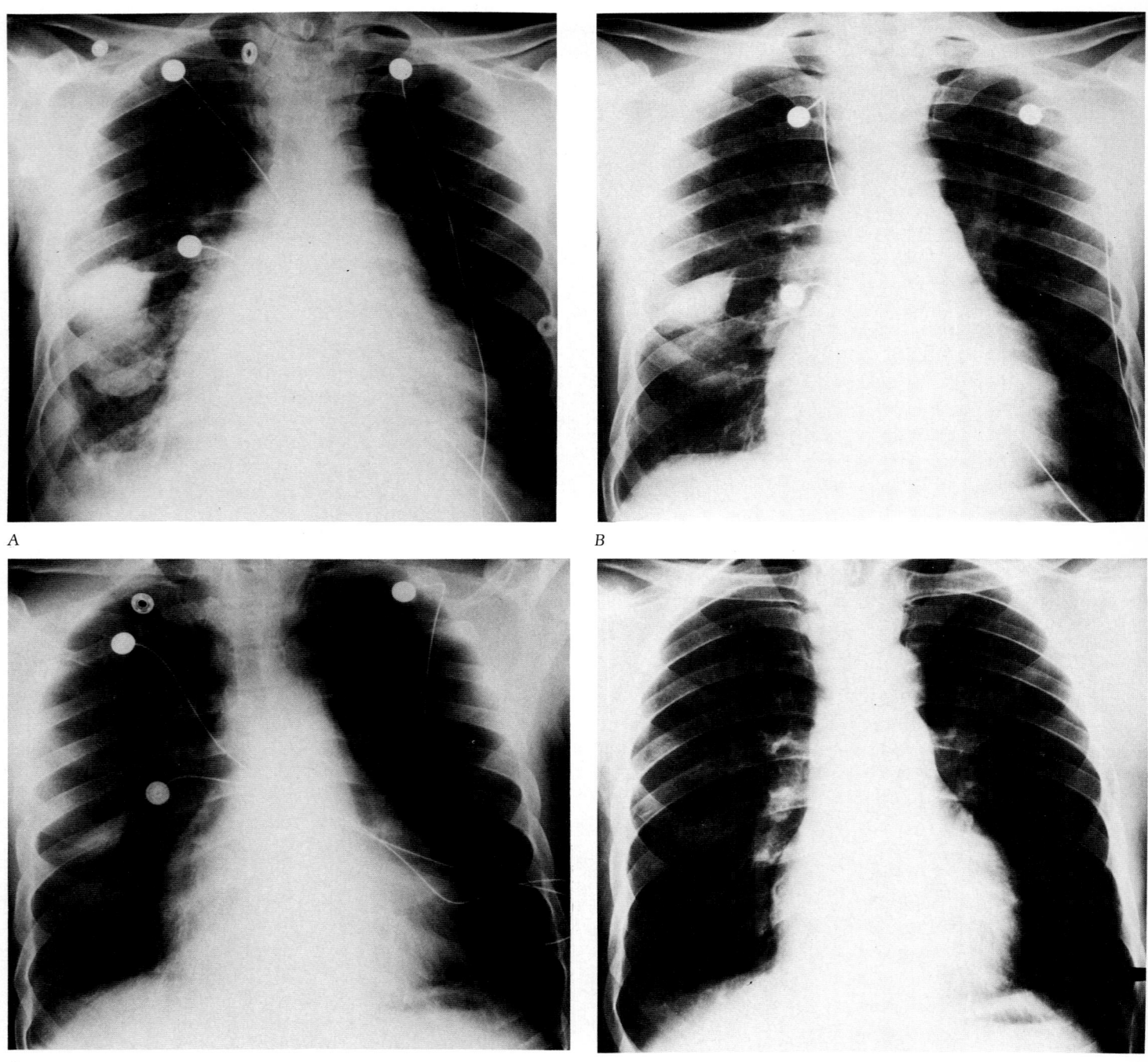

FIGURE 60-17 Vanishing tumor in congestive heart failure. A cardiotonic program led to disappearance of the tumor. *A.* On admission for shortness of breath. Cardiomegaly in association with a tumor in the vicinity of the interlobar fissure. An infiltrate is also present in the right lower lobe. *B.* Three days later. The cardiac silhouette is smaller, the infiltrate in the right lower lobe is virtually gone, and the tumor is smaller and sharply demarcated. *C.* Four days after admission. The contour and location are distinctive. *D.* Eleven days after admission. Cardiac silhouette is normal and the tumor is gone.

flood the alveoli and mount the airways to reach terminal bronchioles, the level of arterial P_{CO_2} will be determined by the balance between hyperventilation of unaffected alveoli and ventilation-perfusion abnormalities in the others; and (3) if alveolar ventilation cannot be sustained at a high level, either because of fatigue of the respiratory muscles or because of respiratory depression, hypercap-

nia ensues. Respiratory depression is induced primarily by narcotics or sedatives, but it also follows overzealous administration of diuretics, such as ethacrynic acid, which induces metabolic alkalosis by depleting the body of hydrogen ions. According to the schema of Fig. 60-20, hypercapnia indicates a late stage of pulmonary edema. Indeed, it is unlikely to occur until pulmonary edema is extensive and severe and has reached the stage of bronchiolar flooding. Metabolic acidosis becomes superimposed on respiratory acidosis when the stage of severe ventilatory depression and arterial hypoxemia is reached.

QUANTITATIVE ASSESSMENT

The traditional clinical hallmarks of pulmonary edema—dyspnea, orthopnea, rales, frothy fluid in airways and radiographic changes—represent an advanced, rather than an incipient, state of excess water in the lungs. These practical limitations have excited interest in methods that would enable reliable determination, in vivo, of the water content of the lungs. However, none of the techniques currently available are either sufficiently accurate or reliable for clinical use on the one hand or sufficiently informative to warrant their expense or trouble on the other.

Double Indicator-Dilution Technique

Despite reservations about clinical utility, there is a large literature that the clinician has to face about lung water and its determination. The traditional approach is an application of the double indicator-dilution technique. Using a simultaneous injection of tritiated water and Evans blue (T-1824) as markers, the extravascular content of water in the lungs has been measured in animals and in human beings (Fig. 60-21). The method measures the

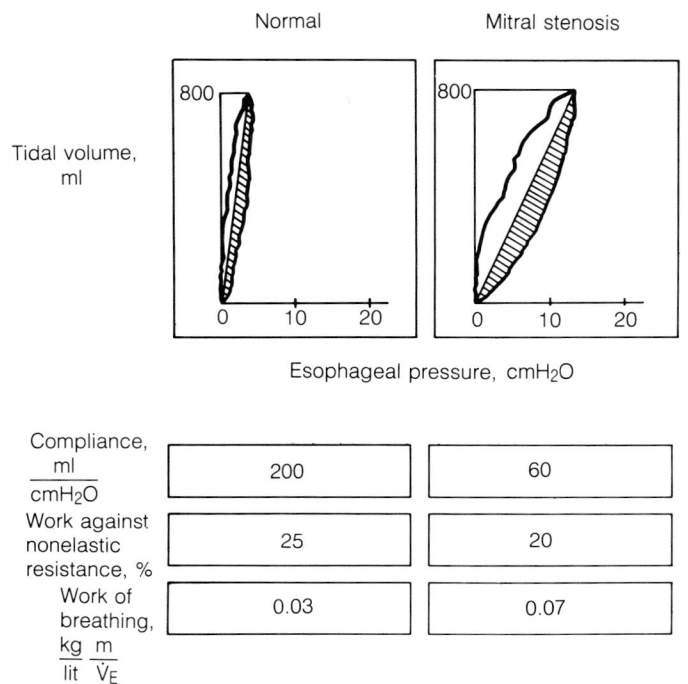

FIGURE 60-18 Mechanics of breathing in mitral stenosis. The stiff lungs are responsible for the characteristic breathing pattern of rapid frequency and small tidal volumes.

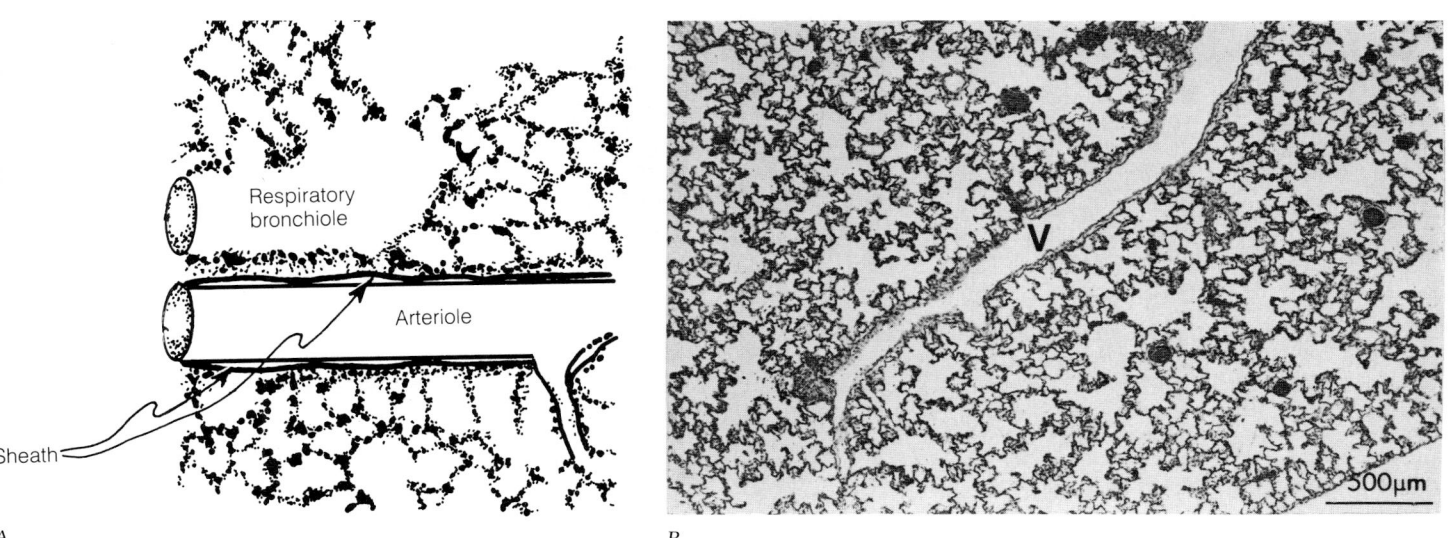

A   B

FIGURE 60-19 Perivascular sheaths. A. Pulmonary arteriole. The fascial sheath extends along the wall of a pulmonary arteriole. (*Adapted from Hayek. From Fishman, 1986.*) B. Large extra-alveolar vein. The loose connective tissue sheath surrounds the vein (V). (*Courtesy J. Gil. From Fishman, 1985.*)

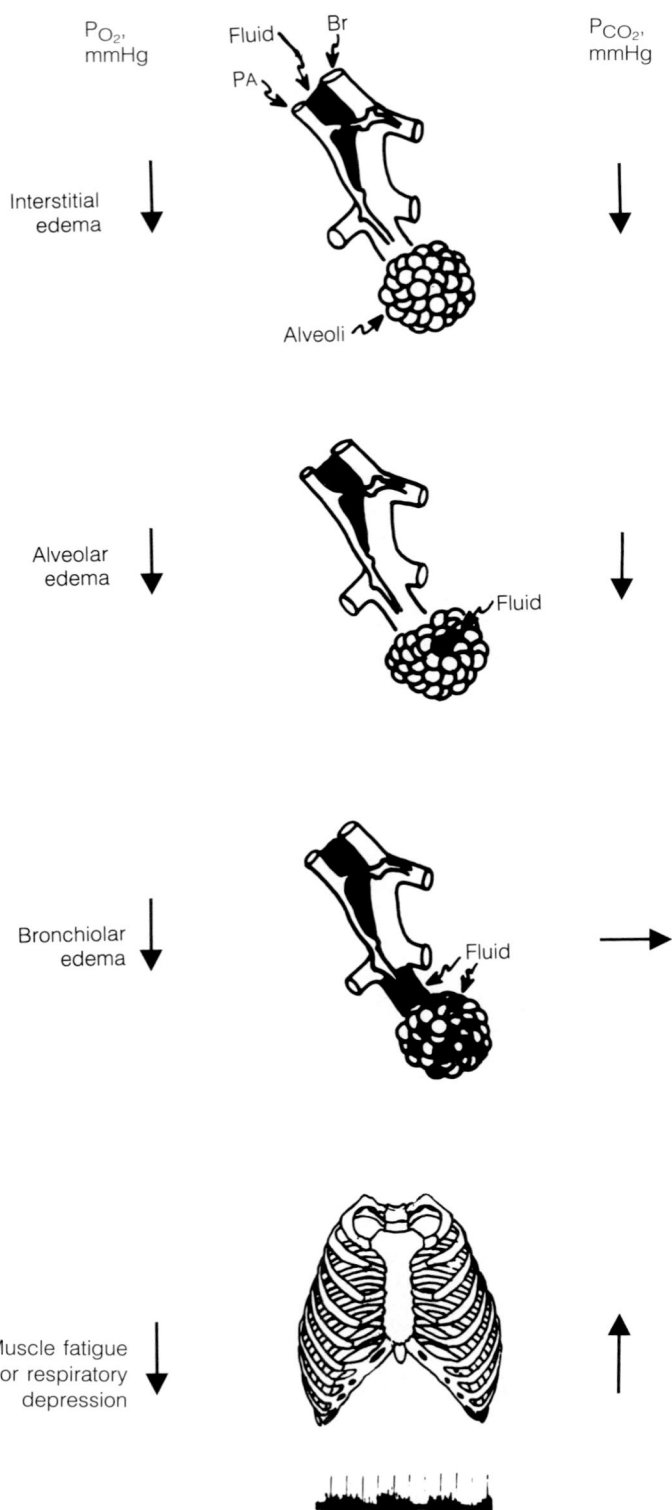

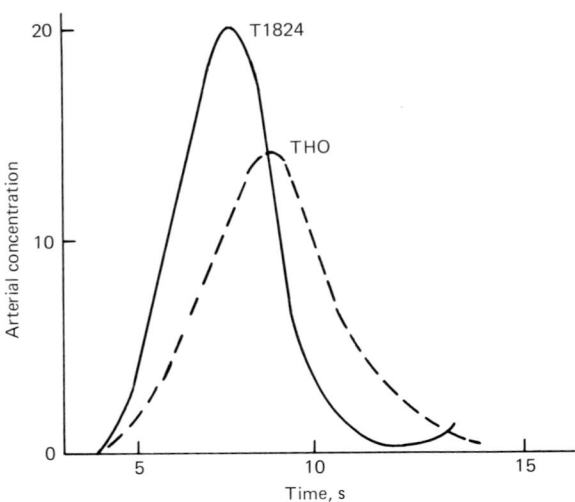

FIGURE 60-21 The double indicator-dilution technique of Chinard and Enns for determining the extravascular water volume of the lungs. T1824 is the tracer for the intravascular volume; tritiated water (THO) measures the total water volume. The difference between the THO volume and the T1824 is the extravascular water volume of the lungs.

FIGURE 60-20 Arterial blood-gas levels in pulmonary edema. The thickness of each arrow indicates qualitatively the degree to which the respective blood-gas tension changes. Alveolar P_{CO_2}, starting low in interstitial and alveolar edema, reverses as bronchiolar edema increases and becomes abnormally high as respiratory muscles fatigue.

water content of those parts of the lungs that are perfused. Therefore, in upright human beings, it does not take into full account the water content of the apexes of the lungs, particularly in states of systemic and pulmonary hypotension (e.g., shock) in which the normal hypoperfusion of the apexes is exaggerated. The indicator-dilution method is also cumbersome and least reproducible in states associated with low cardiac output, pulmonary congestion, and pulmonary edema. In essence, it is more of a research, than a clinical, tool.

Other methods currently under exploration are even more cumbersome and on weaker footing with regard to practicality, accuracy, and reproducibility. They are products of the recent surge in high technology. Among these are Compton Scatter Microwave, computed tomography, nuclear magnetic resonance, and positron emission tomography.

Types of Pulmonary Edema

As indicated at the outset of this chapter, pulmonary edema develops from either high pressure in the pulmonary microcirculation (hemodynamic pulmonary edema) or increased permeability of the microvessels (permeability pulmonary edema) or a combination of the two. Permeability pulmonary edema is strongly influenced by fluctuations in pulmonary capillary pressures: an increase in pulmonary capillary pressure can add a large component of hemodynamic pulmonary edema to that originating in leaky vessels. The combination of permeability and hemodynamic pulmonary edema is a common problem in the intensive-care setting where infusions are a regular fea-

ture and systemic hypotension is often combatted by attempts at expanding the circulating blood volume by administering fluids intravenously.

HEMODYNAMIC (CARDIOGENIC) PULMONARY EDEMA

Clinically, hemodynamic pulmonary edema is generally cardiogenic in origin and occurs in two forms: acute and chronic. The acute form is exemplified by the rapid accumulation of excess water in the lungs after an acute myocardial infarction or after rupture of chordae tendinae. The chronic form is typified by the persistent pulmonary edema that accompanies chronic left ventricular failure or chronic mitral valvular disease.

Acute

An abrupt onset of incompetence of the left side of the heart, as caused by acute mitral regurgitation or left ventricular failure, causes left atrial and pulmonary venous pressure to increase and pulmonary capillary pressures to increase concomitantly; as a result, a plasma filtrate passes into the pulmonary interstitial space. The radiographic pattern corresponds to the sites of formation of the edema fluid since readjustments due to gravity have not yet had time to occur. Not infrequently, a butterfly pattern is seen; this pattern has prompted the unproven idea that the pulmonary circulation can be viewed as consisting of "cortical" and "medullary" components. As interstitial fluid accumulates quickly, the respiratory rate increases reflexly. Expansion of the pulmonary interstitial volume at the expense of the plasma volume is reflected in progressive hemoconcentration; if the filtrate is poor in protein, the plasma protein concentration and the colloid osmotic pressure increase along with the red cell mass. As a rule, the lymph-plasma ratio of proteins < 1.0. Some degree of arterial hypoxemia is a regular occurrence; acute hypercapnia represents severe pulmonary edema that is often life-threatening if progressive. Lactic acidosis is a common concomitant of arterial hypoxemia and hypercapnia in low-output states, such as after acute myocardial infarction.

Chronic

In states of protracted hemodynamic pulmonary edema, the lungs are the seat of chronic passive congestion and edema. Under the influence of gravity, fluid deposits in the interstitium of the dependent parts of the lungs, almost invariably the lung bases. In time, chronic stasis, the trapping of large proteins into the interstitial space, and the ensuing fibrosis redirect pulmonary blood flow from the bases toward the apices. Lymphatics undergo remarkable proliferation. Exercise causes an inordinate increase in blood volume since the left ventricle cannot keep pace with the augmented systemic venous return; as a result, pressures increase everywhere in the pulmonary circulation (Fig. 60-22). If pressures increase abruptly and inordinately so that interendothelial pores are stretched beyond their usual sieving function, the composition of the resulting hemodynamic edema may resemble that of permeability edema. In the extreme, if the burst in pulmonary capillary pressure should cause flooding of the airways, fluid collected from the trachea would be expected to approximate plasma in composition.

PERMEABILITY PULMONARY EDEMA

In permeability pulmonary edema, the fluid-exchanging vessels become leaky for water and proteins. Unfortunately, this defect has little diagnostic value since there is no easy way to measure it clinically. Instead, permeability pulmonary edema is generally said to exist when radiographic evidence of pulmonary edema coexists with insufficient hemodynamic basis to account for it. As a rule, a pulmonary wedge pressure < 15 mmHg suffices to exclude a hemodynamic basis.

Large quantities of both water and proteins escape

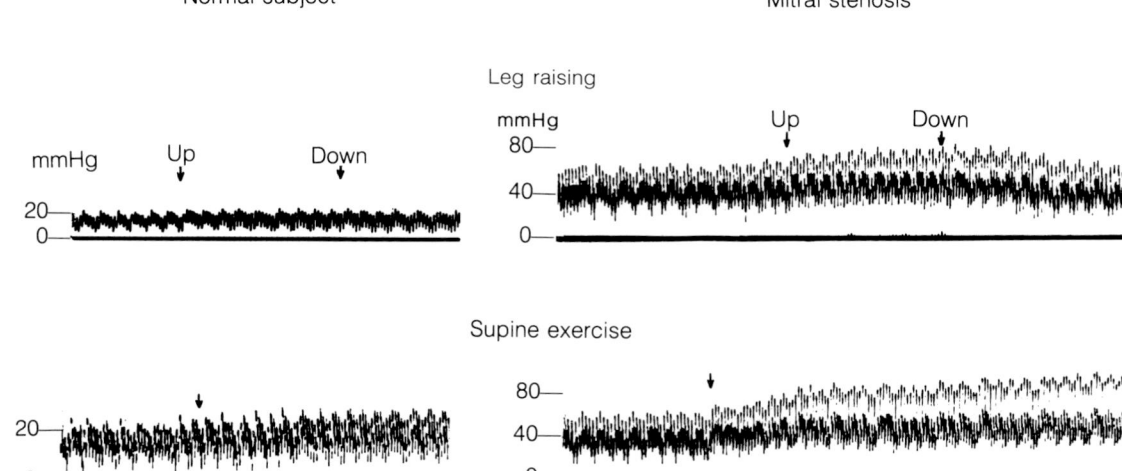

FIGURE 60-22 The effects of increasing blood volume on pulmonary arterial pressures. *Left.* In the normal subject, neither leg raising (upper ↓) nor supine exercise (lower ↓) raises pulmonary arterial pressure appreciably. *Right.* In contrast, in the patient with mitral stenosis, simply raising the legs passively (upper ↓) or supine exercise (lower ↓) raises the pulmonary arterial pressure. The increase persists until the intervention stops.

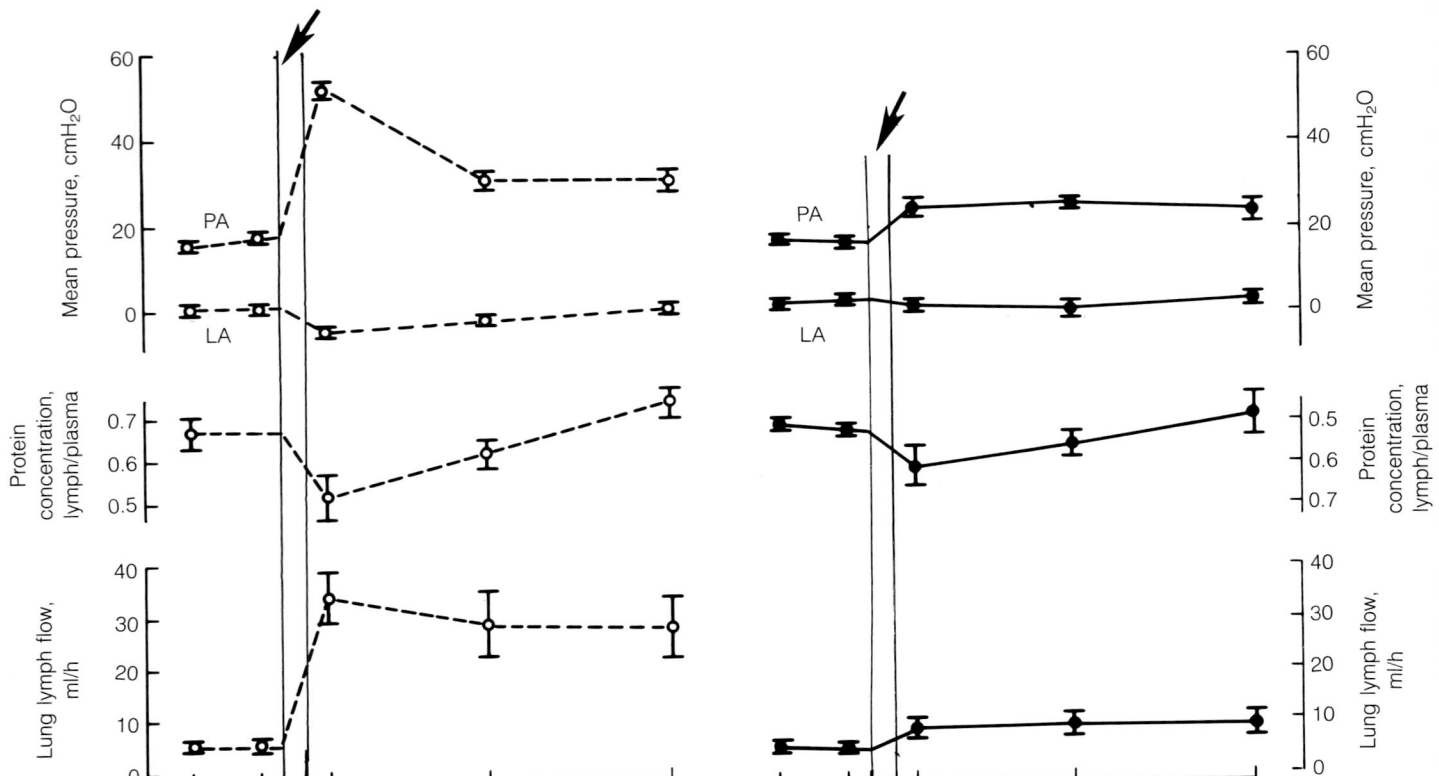

FIGURE 60-23 Infusion of *E. coli* endotoxin in sheep. *Left.* The administration of endotoxin (arrows) causes an abrupt rise in pulmonary arterial pressure along with a sharp decrease in the lymph-plasma protein ratio as lymph flow increases. The secondary effect is reflected in the rising lymph-plasma protein ratio characteristic of an increase in permeability. *Right.* Combined therapy with methylprednisolone and meclofenamate abolishes the initial pulmonary pressor response due to cyclooxygenase inhibition, whereas the steroid attenuates the later permeability response. PA = pulmonary artery; LA = left atrium. The statistical symbols indicate mean ±SEM (standard error of the mean), N = 6. *(Modified after Newman, 1985.)*

through the damaged capillary vessels. With reference to Starling's equation, the filtration coefficient for water (κ) increases and the reflection coefficient (σ) decreases; i.e., hindrance to the exit of plasma proteins from the vessel decreases. Accordingly, in contrast to the composition of the interstitial fluid of early hemodynamic pulmonary edema, the interstitial fluid of permeability pulmonary edema is rich in proteins, i.e., concentrations that are 50 to 80 percent of plasma proteins are not unusual.

Permeability pulmonary edema is a prominent feature of the adult respiratory distress syndrome. Also, gram-negative bacterial sepsis is the most common clinical antecedent of the adult respiratory distress syndrome. This clinical experience has prompted the development and intensive use of gram-negative bacterial endotoxin to create permeability pulmonary edema in sheep (Fig. 60-23). Other experimental models include oxygen toxicity in the rat and sheep, alloxan or oleic acid administered intravenously in dogs, chelating agents in the rabbit, α-naphthylthiourea in rats, and *Pseudomonas* bacteria in sheep. Relatively few attempts have been made to reproduce clinical permeability edema using exposures to irritant gases, e.g., chlorine and nitrogen dioxide.

Arachidonic acid metabolites have been intensively investigated as potential mediators of the hemodynamic and permeability consequences of the diffuse pulmonary injury caused by the intravenous infusion of endotoxin. Elsewhere (Chapter 28) is considered the complicated array of effects elicited by endotoxin, particularly its role in stimulating the role of cachectin (tumor necrosis factor). The sequence of changes following the infusion of endotoxin is distinctive (Fig. 60-23): soon after the infusion starts, pulmonary arterial pressure climbs rapidly to a peak; at this time, levels of thromboxane B_2 in pulmonary lymph also peak. As pulmonary arterial pressure begins to fall, a prostacyclin metabolite appears. Then a stage of increased pulmonary vascular permeability sets in, and lipoxygenase products appear. Using blockers of metabolites in the cyclooxygenase pathway, the pulmonary hypertensive response can be abolished without affecting the subsequent increase in permeability.

Although there is little doubt that arachidonic acid metabolites are produced in the course of lung injury, it has proved difficult to quantify, or to picture in sequence, the roles played by the various products of arachidonic acid metabolism, since the cascade entails alternative

pathways and ephemeral intermediaries. For example, lipoxygenase products, once believed to be involved pathogenetically in increasing permeability after infusing endotoxin, have since been exonerated; the leukotrienes C_4 and D_4 do not increase the filtration coefficient of excised perfused guinea pig lungs. Indeed, recently the alternative has been advanced that intracellular oxygen radicals may be involved in the pathogenesis of the widespread pulmonary endothelial damage that underlies permeability pulmonary edema of different etiologies, e.g., endotoxin or oxygen toxicity.

MISCELLANEOUS

Certain types of pulmonary edema are not readily explained in terms of altered alveolar capillary (microcirculatory) hemodynamics or permeability. Indeed, in certain instances extra-alveolar vessels are known to be at fault (e.g., when high airway pressures are used during mechanical ventilation), whereas in others (e.g., after administering histamine, bradykinin, or endotoxin) the bronchial venules, i.e., the systemic venules of the lungs, become leaky.

Miscellaneous forms of clinical pulmonary edema warrant special consideration since ideas about their pathogenesis strongly influence approaches to their management.

Narcotic Overdosage

Pulmonary edema sometimes complicates an overdosage of heroin or methadone; pulmonary edema due to sedative overdosage, e.g., barbiturates, is much more uncommon. In one distinctive syndrome of narcotic overdosage,

the patient is comatose, severely hypoxemic, and in respiratory acidosis because of severe ventilatory depression. The chest radiograph reveals a nonuniform pattern of pulmonary edema that generally seems to reflect the body position in which the individual was found (Fig. 60-24). Three explanations have been offered for the pulmonary edema: (1) leakage of pulmonary capillaries due to a direct noxious effect of the narcotic or sedative or of a contaminant injected simultaneously, (2) left ventricular failure due to hypoxemia and acidosis that is sufficiently severe to compromise myocardial performance, and (3) decrease in lymph flow from the lungs due to depression of ventilation. None of these is entirely convincing per se. Most impressive is the reversibility of the pulmonary edema: assisted ventilation and restoration of arterial blood gases toward normal are followed in short order by resolution of the infiltrate.

Neurogenic

Pulmonary edema is a common and often serious complication of a variety of injuries to the brain. Among these are generalized seizures, subarachnoid hemorrhage, head trauma, brain tumors, and bacterial meningitis. Because of the heterogeneity of the central nervous insults, the gravity of the intracranial disturbance, and the brittleness of the clinical state, the pathogenesis of this type of pulmonary edema (neurogenic pulmonary edema) is difficult to explore systematically in patients.

Consequently, the pathogenesis of neurogenic pulmonary edema (NPE) has been investigated experimentally (Fig. 60-25) and extrapolations have been made to the human counterparts. Although much has been learned

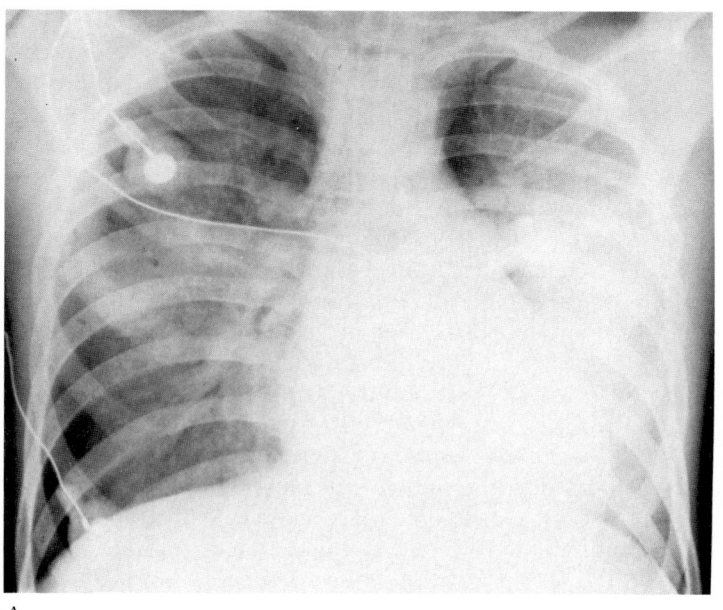 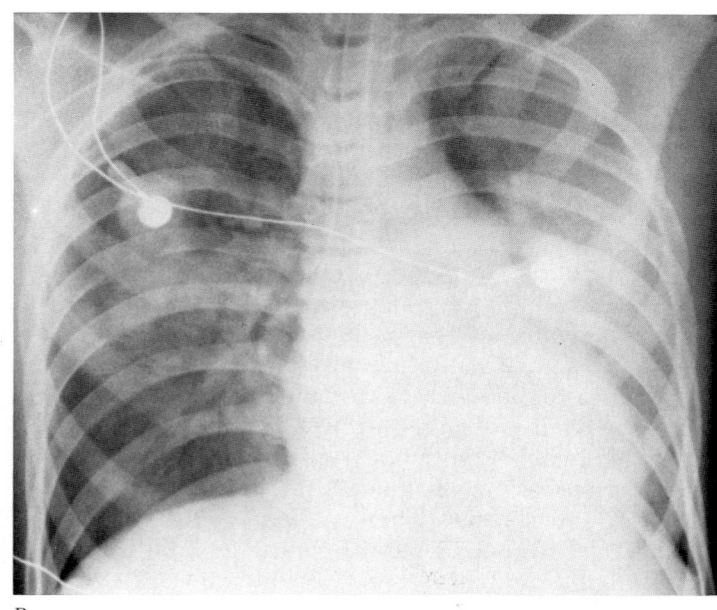

A   B

FIGURE 60-24 Methadone overdosage in a 13-year-old boy. *A.* On admission. Severe pulmonary edema, most marked on left. *B.* Five hours later after assisted ventilation and diuresis. Considerable clearing.

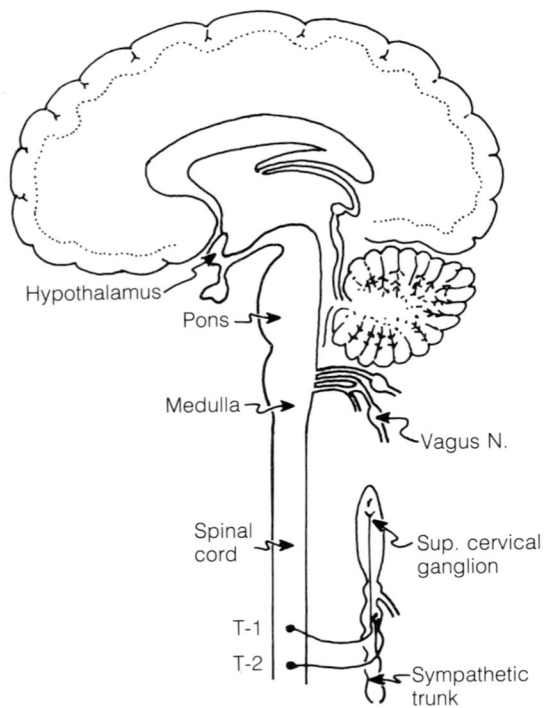

FIGURE 60-25 The hypothalamus and medulla in the pathogenesis of neurogenic pulmonary edema. Stimulation of the hypothalamus or medulla (ventrolateral and upper aspects; nucleus of the tractus solitarius and area postrema) has engaged the autonomic nervous system in massive autonomic discharges that culminate in neurogenic pulmonary edema.

from this approach, large gaps in understanding still remain on several accounts: (1) the difficulty in reproducing the clinical syndromes experimentally; methods used have ranged from large and global increases in intracranial pressure of different durations to specific lesions (e.g., preoptic hypothalamic lesions or bilateral ablation of areas in the nucleus solitarius), intracranial injection of chemical irritants, interruption of reflex inhibitory pathways to the sympathetic nervous system, electrical stimulation of areas in the brain that excite sympathetic neurons, cerebral ischemia, and hypoxia; (2) the wide variety of hemodynamic derangements provoked by the experimental manipulations and their transient nature as compared to the lingering pulmonary edema; and (3) differences in the composition of the edema fluid and pulmonary lymph, both of which are generally judged to contain too much plasma protein for hemodynamic pulmonary edema; i.e., increased permeability contributes to the pulmonary edema. The clinical situation is generally complicated further by the patient's inability to cough or raise secretions and, particularly after trauma, by disturbed pulmonary mechanisms.

One virtually consistent thread throughout these experiments is that neurogenic pulmonary edema is associated with intense and widespread activation of the sympathetic nervous system that, in turn, induces remarkable hemodynamic alterations: systemic and pulmonary vaso-

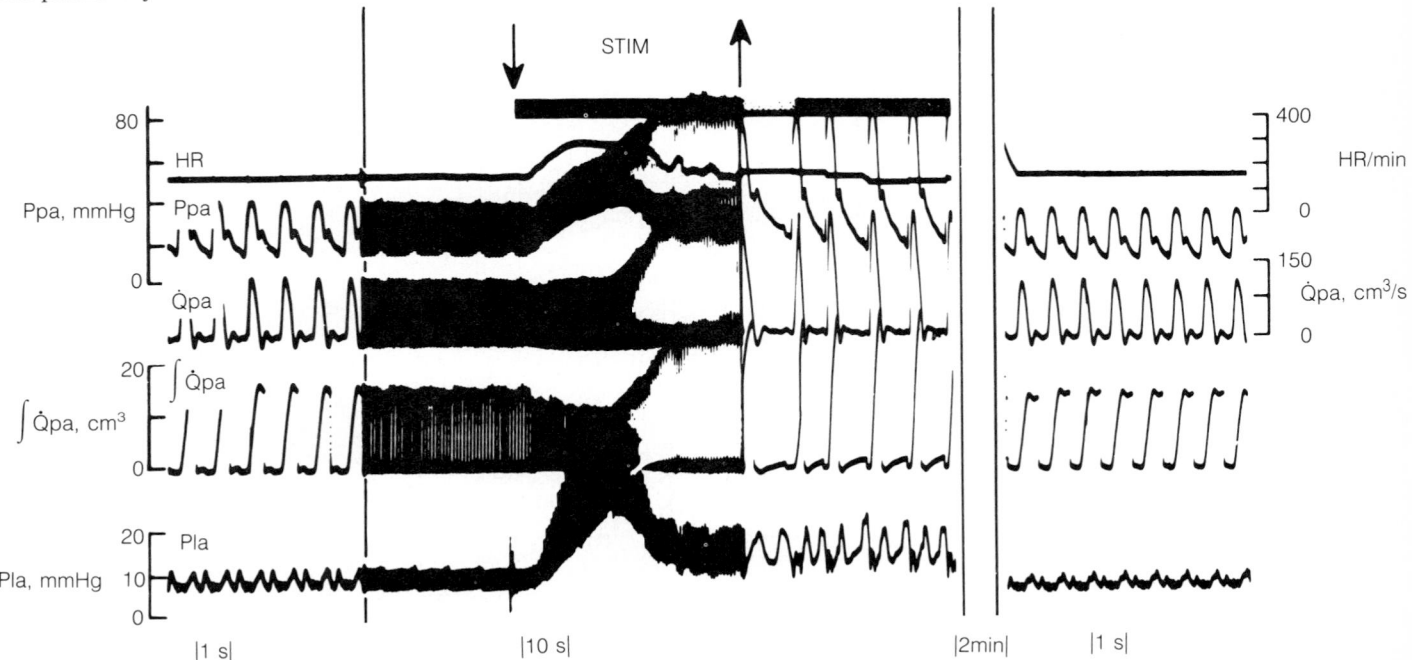

FIGURE 60-26 Hypothalamic stimulation in the dog. During the period of stimulation (STIM ↑), pressures increased dramatically in the pulmonary artery (Ppa) and left atrium (Pla). Concomitantly, right ventricular stroke output (∫Q̇pa) and pulmonary arterial flow (Q̇pa) also increase. In this type of central nervous disturbance, acute left ventricular failure is the dominant hemodynamic upset that leads, in turn, to a striking increase in left atrial pressure (Pla), pulmonary engorgement, pulmonary venous hypertension, and pulmonary edema. The imbalance between the right (normal) and left (failing) ventricles seems more important in increasing pulmonary vascular pressures and volume than does constriction of the capacitance vessels in the two circuits. (Modified from Szidon and Fishman, 1969.)

constriction is intense and involves both the resistance and capacitance vessels of the two circuits (Fig. 60-26). The left ventricle fails because of the inordinate pressure work imposed by the systemic hypertension, and the pulmonary blood volume increases remarkably, largely due to the imbalance between the failing left ventricle and the normal-pumping right ventricle.

This sequence would relegate neurogenic pulmonary edema to the realm of hemodynamic (cardiogenic) pulmonary edema (Fig. 60-27). However, a permeability component (i.e., leaky vessels) is also generally invoked to explain the high concentrations of plasma proteins in edema fluid (collected from the airways) and the high lymph-plasma ratios of plasma proteins. Although it is not possible on the basis of available information to discount completely a "permeability" component mediated by mysterious neurohumoral mechanisms, two alternative explanations have been offered for the proteinaceous edema fluid and lymph: (1) the "stretched pore" phenomenon that could follow a burst of severe pulmonary hyper-

tension, thereby allowing proteins as well as water to escape into the interstitium via interendothelial pores, and (2) damage to endothelium by the abrupt increase in pulmonary vascular pressures.

Clearly, management of neurogenic pulmonary edema depends on the bedside assessment of the respective roles of hemodynamic or permeability factors. Fortunately, as a rule, neurogenic pulmonary edema is generally self-limited and not life-threatening so that treatment is supportive, e.g., enriching the inspired O_2 mixture to avoid serious arterial hypoxemia. However, should the pulmonary situation progress to the equivalent of the adult respiratory distress syndrome—in which permeability factors generally play a large part—the same therapeutic principles apply. However, one word of caution: assisted ventilation, including high-frequency ventilation and positive end-pressure ventilation, runs the risk of raising intracranial pressure. Consequently, great circumspection is required in the use of mechanical ventilation in neurogenic pulmonary edema.

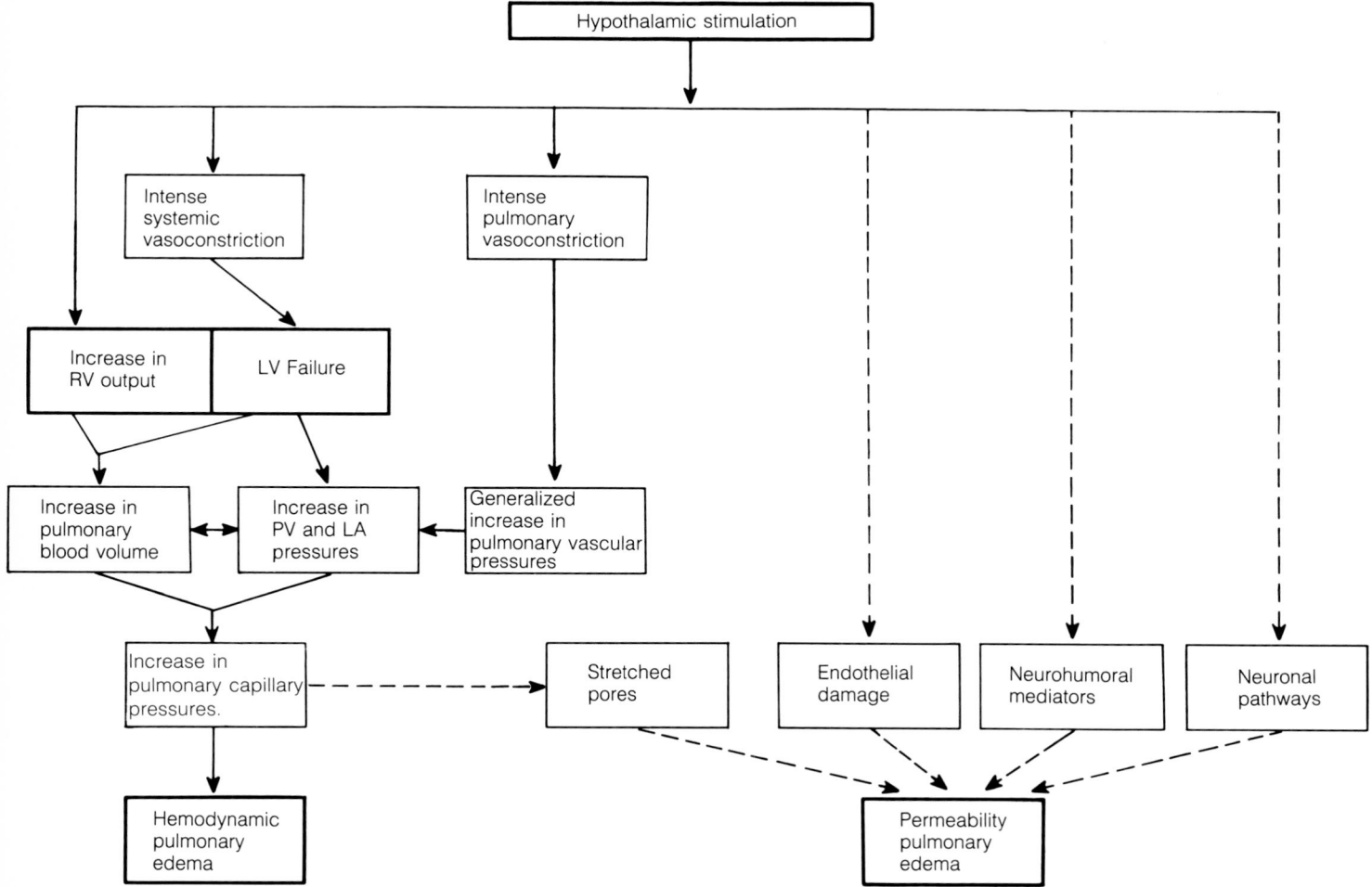

FIGURE 60-27   Postulated pathogenesis of neurogenic pulmonary edema. The edema appears to be predominantly hemodynamic (cardiogenic) in origin but often with a component attributable to increased capillary permeability. It is a matter of speculation whether the increase in permeability is due to stretched pores or endothelial injury. LV = left ventricular; RV = right ventricular; PV = pulmonary venous; LA = left atrial.

Pulmonary Emboli

The quantity of water in the lungs usually increases after pulmonary emboli but rarely to the point of clinical edema. In contrast, removal of a large organized clot is almost invariably followed by pulmonary edema of the affected segment or lobe. The mechanisms responsible for the accumulation of excess water in the lungs after pulmonary emboli are speculative; presumably different mechanisms are operative after a single embolus and after multiple emboli. Proposed mechanisms have ranged from purely mechanical (a burst of pulmonary hypertension and compromise of left ventricular performance by bulging of the interventricular septum) to increased permeability due to an interplay involving the generation of thrombin, platelet aggregation, leukocyte adherence, and activation. Another postulated sequence invokes the release of mediators, e.g., bradykinin and histamine, from mast cells in the vicinity. The nature of the embolic material (fat, clot, air), the size of the embolus and where it lodges, the state of the collateral circulation of the lungs, the repetitiveness of the embolic process, and the complication of pulmonary infarction differ from one experimental circumstance to another and among clinical disorders. Therefore, it seems likely that the pulmonary edema that follows pulmonary embolism probably has different pathogenetic mechanisms.

Uremia

As a rule, pulmonary edema in uremia (Fig. 60-28) is due primarily to overhydration and an expanded circulating blood volume leading to high pulmonary capillary pressures. It is accompanied by other manifestations of a "congested state" in which the heart is overtaxed by the excessive blood volume and anemia but is coping by maintaining a high cardiac output. In addition to warm hands and evidence of a hyperdynamic circulation, the cardiac output is high, pressures throughout the pulmonary circulation are mildly increased, and the pulmonary blood volume is abnormally large. Although the edema appears to be predominantly hemodynamic in origin since pulmonary capillary pressures are increased, the possibility also exists that there is often a "leaky" component due to metabolic abnormalities associated with uremia. However, reduction in the circulating blood volume—as by renal dialysis—promotes clearing of the pulmonary edema.

High Altitude Pulmonary Edema

Although the clinical features of high altitude pulmonary edema are well known, much about its pathogenesis is enigmatic. The clinical aspects can be listed as follows: (1) the disorder is uncommon and occurs in individuals who, for some unexplained reason, are susceptible to pulmonary edema at high altitude; (2) the victim is physically fit, often young, and without evidence of cardiovascular or pulmonary disease; (3) the precipitating factor is a rather rapid transition from low to high altitude (generally higher than 2700 m); (4) exercise and exposure to cold air are enhancing influences; (5) progressive shortness of breath, undue fatigue, and a nonproductive cough that herald the onset are soon followed by the appearance of widespread fluffy infiltrate on the chest radiograph (Fig. 60-29); (6) without treatment the pulmonary edema intensifies, often becoming life-threatening because of the arterial hypoxemia that it induces; and (7) descent to a lower altitude promptly relieves the syndrome.

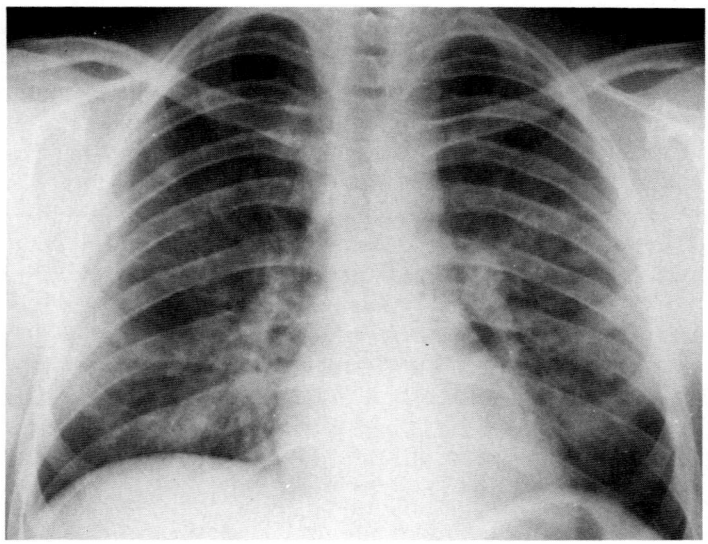

A

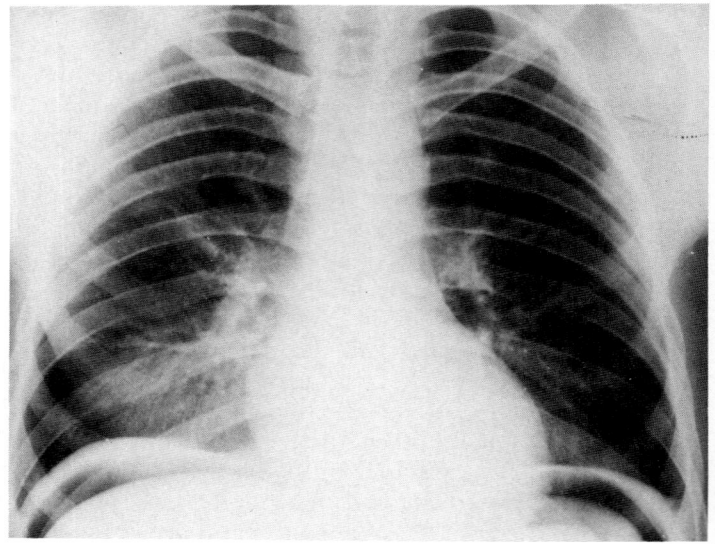

B

FIGURE 60-28 Acute glomerulitis complicated by oliguria, azotemia, acidosis, anemia, and hypertension in a 26-year-old man. *A.* Before dialysis. *B.* After dialysis.

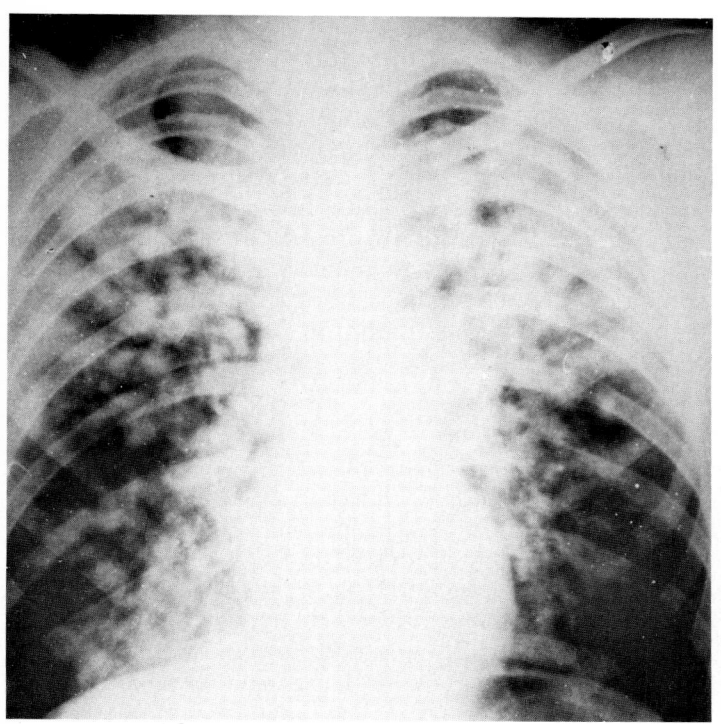
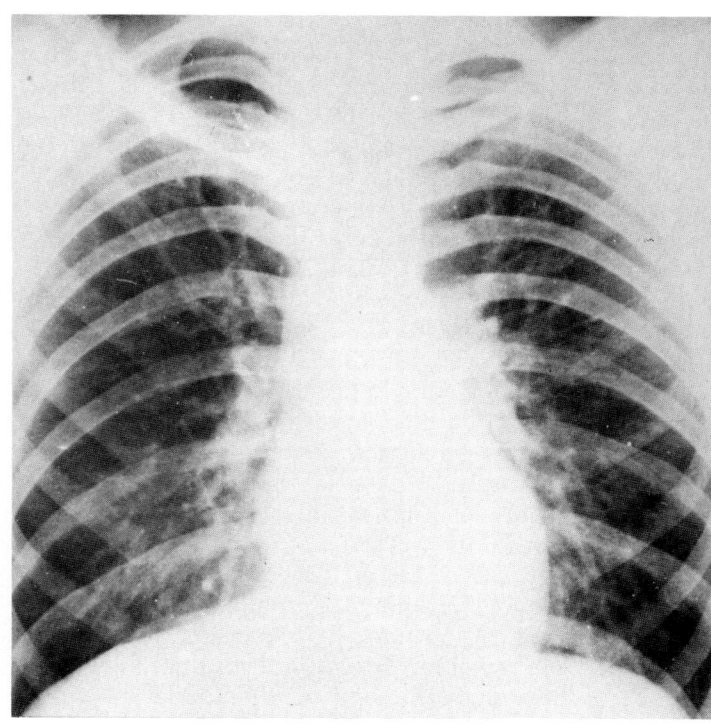

A

B

FIGURE 60-29 High altitude pulmonary edema in a 17-year-old boy born at 14,200 ft (Cerro de Pasco) who returned to altitude after a 2-week stay at sea level (Lima). *A.* Day after return to altitude and vigorous walking. Hospitalized for dyspnea and cough productive of foamy, pink sputum. *B.* Next day. Within 24 h, the pulmonary edema had cleared. *(Courtesy of D. Penaloza.)*

Among the diverse explanations that have been proffered to account for this sequence are increased pulmonary vascular reactivity, a decrease in the ventilatory response to hypoxia, increased pulmonary vascular permeability engendered in some way by hypoxia, mechanical stresses, and fibrin products. However, the more durable explanations for these sequences seem to derive their strength from two assumptions: (1) the victim is constitutionally predisposed to respond to hypoxia with an inordinate degree of pulmonary arterial hypertension, and (2) the vascular resistances throughout the pulmonary arterial tree that are responsible for the hypertension are nonhomogeneously distributed. As a result of this combination of widespread and uneven vasoconstriction, the large increase in pulmonary arterial pressure (caused by intensive generalized precapillary vasoconstriction) is transmitted with little damping to the capillary beds supplied by less-constricted vessels; the result is regional "pulmonary overperfusion" (Fig. 60-30). As a rule, the victim is exercising at altitude: the combination of exercise and hypoxia makes the situation worse by further increasing pulmonary vascular pressures.

It should be underscored that hypoxia, per se, does not cause an increase in pulmonary capillary permeability, perhaps lending strength to the idea that inordinate, nonuniform pulmonary vasoconstriction is the root cause of high altitude pulmonary edema. Whether stretched

pores in the unprotected capillary beds or endothelial damage by sudden exposure to high capillary pressures contribute to the edema is unclear. However, the mechanism is clearly reversible since withdrawal to lower altitude relieves the pulmonary edema.

Drowning
Unless interrupted, drowning culminates in asphyxia and death. Characteristically, the lungs fill with large quantities of water, often mixed with aspirated vomitus. In many respects, the resultant alveolar hypoventilation, arterial hypoxemia, acidosis, and cardiorespiratory arrest may be regarded as a paradigm of extreme pulmonary edema. In principle, near-drowning in freshwater leads to the flow of hypotonic fluid into the systemic circulation followed by hemolysis and hemodilution, whereas near-drowning in saltwater does the opposite, i.e., results in hemoconcentration and decrease in blood volume. Although the biochemical abnormalities associated with fresh- and saltwater near-drowning differ, the central therapeutic goals in both are reversal of the hypoxemia and metabolic acidosis and prevention of brain damage.

Reexpansion
Unilateral pulmonary edema occasionally develops after evacuation of an ipsilateral pneumothorax or pleural effusion. As a rule, it follows application of high negative intrathoracic pressure, but it has also occurred after water

944

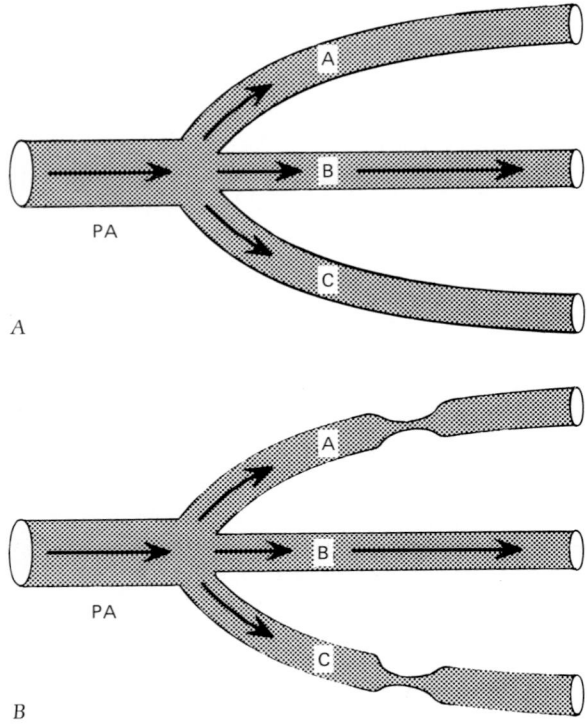

FIGURE 60-30 Schematic representation of the pathogenesis of regional overperfusion. *A.* The precapillary vessels (A, B, and C) are uniform in caliber. *B.* Nonuniform vasoconstriction causes precapillary vessels like A and C to decrease markedly in caliber; the result is an increase in pulmonary arterial pressure. Meanwhile, precapillary B remains widely patent, transmitting the increase in pulmonary arterial pressure to the capillary bed beyond it.

seal drainage. Rapid withdrawal of the air or fluid seems to enhance the prospect of unilateral pulmonary edema, especially in the case of a pneumothorax that has been present for 3 days or more and if the underlying lung has been fully collapsed. Rapid evacuation of a large pleural effusion also seems to predispose to ipsilateral pulmonary edema.

In keeping with the above, prevention is directed at gradually expanding the collapsed lung, particularly if the collapse is 3 days old or more and complete.

Resorption of Excess Fluid

The rate of resolution of pulmonary edema depends on a variety of factors including the nature of the insult, the integrity of alveolar-capillary barriers, and the concentration of proteins in the edema fluid. An increase in minute ventilation, presumably driven reflexly via J receptors in the interstitium, promotes the movement of excess fluid toward central lymphatics. Fluid formed at the level of the alveolar capillaries accumulates in peribronchial sumps; the perivascular pressures direct excess fluid from the pericapillary interstitial spaces toward the interstitium around extra-alveolar minute vessels along favorable pres-

sure gradients. Hemodynamic pulmonary edema often responds to appropriate therapy in hours, whereas the combination of interstitial and alveolar edema usually takes days to clear.

Depending on the nature and the location of the excess fluid, the route for removal may be via lymphatics, pulmonary circulation, or bronchial circulation. For example, protein in interstitial fluid is removed predominantly by lymphatics and possibly by pinocytic transfer from abluminal to luminal aspects of microvessels. Although active transport of electrolytes has also been demonstrated to occur experimentally, the clinical significance of this type of observation is unclear. Nor have the relative contributions of different loci of resorption (alveolar vessels, extra-alveolar vessels, or other microvessels, including bronchial venules) been quantified.

Treatment

Acute pulmonary edema is often a medical emergency, whereas *chronic* pulmonary edema is a cause of disability and restricted activity. One fundamental decision at the start of treatment is whether the edema is predominantly hemodynamic or permeability in nature. A second is whether the situation is life-threatening.

HEMODYNAMIC (CARDIOGENIC) PULMONARY EDEMA

The usual cause of this type of pulmonary edema is either left ventricular failure or mitral valvular disease, i.e., cardiogenic pulmonary edema. Identification and proper management of initiating factors, e.g., acute myocardial infarction, shape the overall direction of treatment (Table 60-3). Some degree of arterial hypoxemia is a regular oc-

TABLE 60-3
Measures Useful in Managing Chronic Hemodynamic Pulmonary Edema

Improve arterial oxygenation
Improve pump performance of the failing ventricle
    Cardiac glycosides (digoxin)
    Other positive inotropic drugs (amrinone)
    Pacemaker for bradycardia or loss of atrioventricular synchrony
Reduce the cardiac workload
    Rest (physical and emotional)
    Vasodilator agents
Control salt and water retention
    Limit dietary sodium intake
    Diuretics
    Mechanical removal of excess fluid
        Phlebotomy
        Dialysis
        Ultrafiltration
    Seek and manage initiating mechanism

currence, but it is generally mild. Normocapnia progressive to hypercapnia generally accompanies levels of arterial P_{O_2} < 50 mmHg and is a sign that the pulmonary edema is severe; at this stage, alveolar fluid has mounted into larger airways. Progressive hypercapnia should be regarded as life-threatening.

Acute

The acute onset of cardiogenic pulmonary edema constitutes a medical emergency in which the immediate therapeutic goals are to (1) allay anxiety, (2) decrease preload, (3) improve oxygenation, and (4) treat causal and precipitating factors. The first three categories are emergency measures; the search for, and treatment of, the underlying condition is deferred until a stable hemodynamic and gas-exchanging state is achieved.

The patient is placed in a sitting position and given humidified 100% O_2 to breathe, by positive pressure mask if possible. Vital signs are monitored frequently, and a cannula is placed in a peripheral vein for ready access. Arterial blood is sampled immediately for P_{O_2}, P_{CO_2}, and pH, and venous blood is drawn for the determinations of urea nitrogen, creatinine, electrolytes, and complete blood count.

Placement of flow-directed pulmonary artery (Swan-Ganz) and arterial lines for monitoring of pressures and arterial blood gases is often advisable. An electrocardiogram and a portable chest radiograph are taken; if a tachycardia has triggered the pulmonary edema, the possibility is weighed of electrical conversion of supraventricular or ventricular tachyarrhythmias that are not due to digitalis excess.

1. *Allay anxiety.* Morphine is the traditional mainstay of therapy in cardiogenic pulmonary edema. It acts by relieving anxiety and pain, in the process slowing the heart rate and decreasing cardiac output toward normal. The usual dosage is 2 to 5 mg administered intravenously over a 3-min period; this dosage can be repeated at 15-min intervals while keeping an eye peeled for respiratory depression. Naloxone is at hand if respiratory depression should ensue. Morphine is not used if intracranial pressure is high, and only circumspectly in patients with chronic pulmonary disease.

2. *Decrease preload.* To decrease systemic venous return (preload), strategies range from rotating tourniquets applied to three of the four extremities, to phlebotomy and intermittent positive pressure breathing. Systemic vasodilators are often used to decrease systemic and pulmonary vascular pressures. Nitroglycerin, 0.3 to 0.6 mg sublingually, is sometimes effective in reducing systemic venous return, but proper dosage is often difficult to judge so that arterial hypotension may be excessive. Nitroprusside given intravenously is generally preferred. It acts by causing systemic vasodilatation, both arterial and venous.

As a rule, a priming dose of 20 μg/min is followed by increments at 5-min intervals of 5 μg/min as long as systemic arterial blood pressure is maintained and until pulmonary edema is symptomatically relieved.

3. *Inotropic agents and diuretics.* Digoxin, 0.5 mg given intravenously, is generally administered for its inotropic effect if the patient has not been receiving digitalis. A diuretic, usually furosemide, is given intravenously, starting with doses of 20 to 40 mg and repeated in increasing doses to achieve a diuresis. The actions of furosemide extend beyond their renal effects, often seeming to dilate systemic veins before the diuresis begins. Digitalis plays only a secondary role in the management of acute cardiogenic pulmonary edema, less for its antiarrhythmic than for its inotropic effects.

Aminophylline is given intravenously when bronchospasm is a prominent feature. It acts not only as a bronchodilator but as an inotropic and diuretic agent. The desirable end point is a blood level of 10 to 20 mg/L. A reasonable starting dose is 5 mg/kg, administered intravenously and *slowly*, e.g., over a 10- to 20-min interval. Older individuals, or those with renal or hepatic disease, should receive a smaller dosage.

4. *Assisted ventilation.* Life-threatening pulmonary edema, manifested by progressive hypoxemia and hypercapnia and the development of a metabolic acidosis, raises the urgent prospect of tracheal intubation and positive pressure breathing. Fortunately, in more than 90 percent of patients, assisted ventilation is not required since arterial hypoxemia, respiratory acidosis, the occasional superimposed metabolic acidosis, and cardiac performance respond quickly to conventional therapeutic measures, that include the breathing of O_2-enriched mixtures. Rarely does the metabolic acidosis, per se, require specific treatment, such as the intravenous administration of sodium bicarbonate. Indeed, administration of bicarbonate runs the risk of upsetting the acid-base balance in the opposite direction, of disturbing potassium balance, of predisposing to arrhythmias, and of aggravating the pulmonary edema by promoting circulatory overload.

The criteria for intubation and assisted ventilation vary from clinic to clinic. Most clinics reserve intubation and assisted ventilation for patients with acute pulmonary edema who are incapable of breathing adequately on their own because of exhaustion or ventilatory depression. This type of deterioration is indicated by progressive arterial hypoxemia and hypercapnia despite the administration of oxygen, morphine, digitalis, and diuretics and the use of ancillary measures, such as rotating tourniquets or phlebotomy. In the few clinics where a team is geared for intubation and assisted ventilation in acute pulmonary edema, criteria for intubation are less stringent than in most.

The effectiveness of positive pressure breathing in pulmonary edema, particularly of positive end-expiratory pressure (PEEP), depends on the balance between its beneficial and harmful consequences: the beneficial effect generally predominates as long as imposed airway pressures are not too high, i.e., >20 to 30 cmH$_2$O (and the patient is normovolemic); under these circumstances, the increase in end-expiratory volume opens airspaces and improves oxygenation. But harmful effects supervene at higher pressures; as perivascular (interstitial) pressures decrease around the minute *extra-alveolar* vessels, transmural vascular pressures increase, thereby promoting fluid leakage.

Older texts attributed the beneficial effects of positive pressure breathing (at levels of 20 to 30 cmH$_2$O) to a reduction in systemic venous return, i.e., similar in many ways to those of a phlebotomy. Although this idea may apply to normal lungs, it encounters difficulty when lungs are edematous, i.e., when imposed airway pressures of 20 to 30 cmH$_2$O are blunted in transmission to pleural spaces and, therefore, do little to impede systemic return or to influence cardiac output unless the patient is hypovolemic. However, in hypovolemic patients with edematous lungs, the fraction of imposed airway pressure reaching the lungs may suffice to impede venous return seriously; the resultant systemic hypotension may then become life-threatening unless positive pressure breathing is discontinued. Mild lower-body positive pressure using military antishock trousers has been suggested as a strategy by which cardiac output and systemic arterial blood pressure can be sustained.

Chronic

As a rule, standard cardiotonic programs are used to relieve hemodynamic pulmonary edema while seeking to reverse or manage initiating mechanisms. These generally consist of measures that improve arterial oxygenation, improve the contractile performance of the heart, reduce cardiac work, and control the retention of excess salt and water (Table 60-2).

PERMEABILITY PULMONARY EDEMA

As a rule, the therapeutic measures described in Chapter 143 for the adult respiratory distress syndrome apply to the management of permeability pulmonary edema. A few aspects warrant special mention.

Adequate arterialization of blood leaving the lungs is the ultimate test of the lungs as a gas exchanger. For this reason, determinations of arterial P$_{O_2}$, P$_{CO_2}$, and pH are central to the management of permeability pulmonary edema. With respect to arterial P$_{O_2}$, a value of 60 to 65 mmHg affords a tolerable level of oxygenation as long as cardiac output remains at near-normal levels. Early in the evolution of pulmonary edema, this level can be achieved by the administration of O$_2$-enriched inspired mixtures, delivered by one of many devices: nasal prongs, Venturi mask, or a mask and reservoir bag. If enrichment (up to 100% O$_2$) fails to maintain arterial P$_{O_2}$ around 60 mmHg, particularly if CO$_2$ retention also ensues, intubation and mechanical ventilation become mandatory. The breathing of O$_2$ mixtures containing more than 50% O$_2$ entails a hazard of aggravating leakage by inflicting additional endothelial damage. But, this risk is not appreciable unless the O$_2$-enriched mixture is continued beyond 4 to 5 days, particularly if the O$_2$ content is lower than 70 percent.

In general, mechanical ventilation improves oxygenation by increasing the mean lung volume and relieves hypercapnia by improving alveolar ventilation. The addition of positive end-expiratory pressure is commonplace in treating permeability pulmonary edema since it often enables lower concentrations of O$_2$ to be used. It acts by preventing alveolar collapse secondary to loss or displacement of surfactant by the alveolar fluid; as a rule, calculated shunts decrease during PEEP. Two problems attend the use of PEEP: (1) barotrauma, particularly if airway pressures exceed 20 to 25 mmHg, and (2) compromise of systemic venous return by transmission of the imposed pressure to the pleura, thereby decreasing cardiac output and O$_2$ delivery to the tissues. Two useful signals that venous return has been compromised are a drop in systemic arterial blood pressure and the development of metabolic acidosis. Volume expansion is sometimes successful in overriding the high airway pressures and in restoring cardiac output, systemic blood pressure and O$_2$ delivery.

Pharmacologic attempts to restore capillary permeability to normal have been of little avail. Corticosteroids and nonsteroid anti-inflammatory drugs (ibuprofen, indomethacin, and meclofenamate) have not proved helpful in preventing or ameliorating the clinical syndrome, although they have shown promise in animal models. Products of arachidonic acid metabolism are being tested, but the results are equivocal. Antioxidant drugs, dimethylsulfoxide and allopurinol, are also being tried on the grounds that intracellular metabolites of oxygen are involved not only in the original injury but in the subsequent phase when stimulated neutrophils attach to the endothelial surface. Pulmonary vasodilators have been used sporadically, but they run the risk of increasing blood flow through airless parts of the lungs.

Although "leaky vessels" are the hallmark of permeability pulmonary edema, not infrequently a hemodynamic component is superimposed particularly by the overzealous administration of fluids intravenously. This situation should be avoided since a goal in management is to sustain the cardiac output for O$_2$ delivery to the tissues at the lowest possible pulmonary capillary pressures.

The use of osmotic agents to withdraw excess fluid

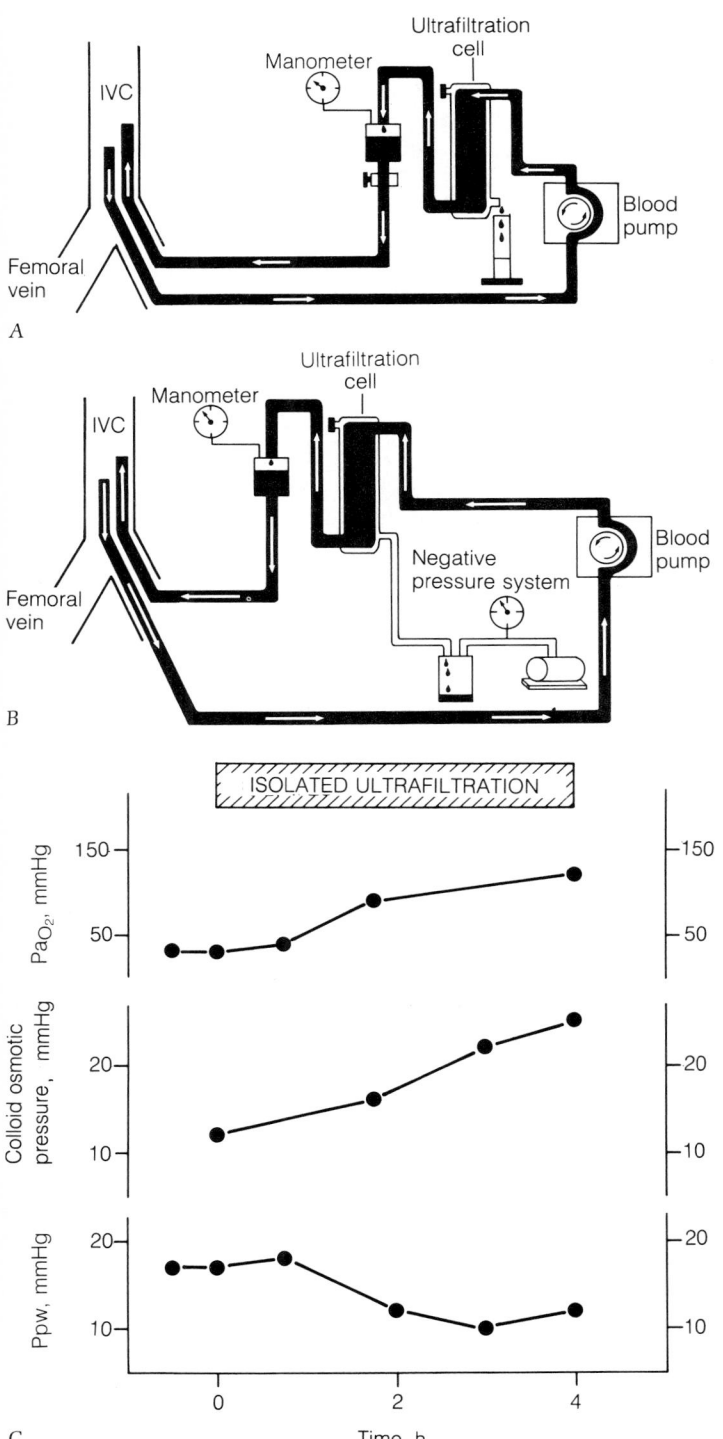

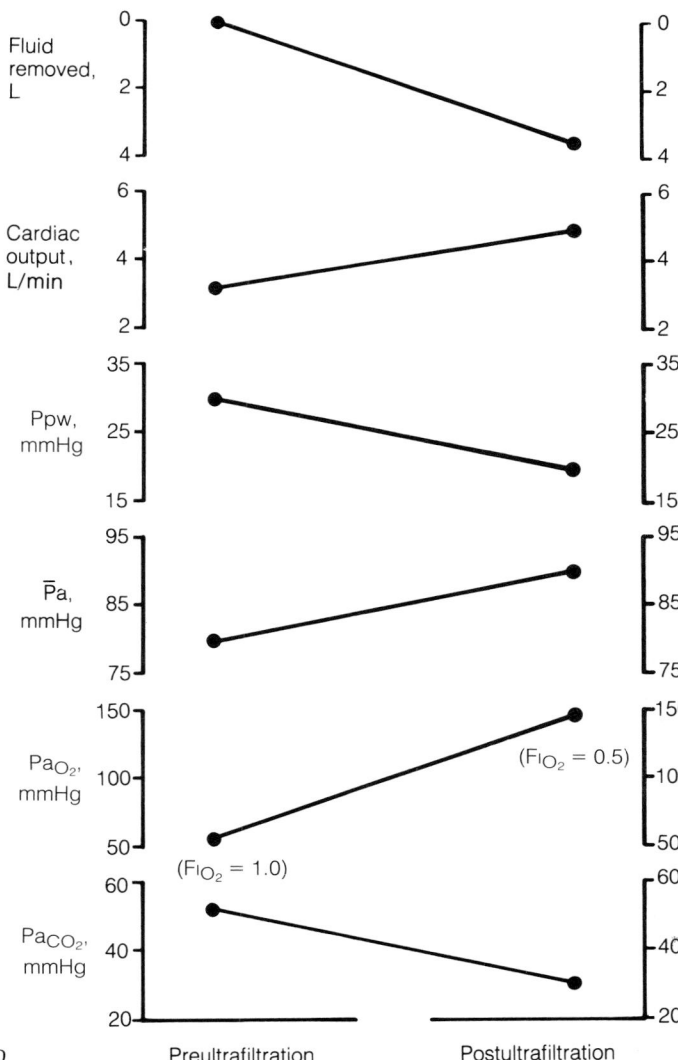

FIGURE 60-31 Ultrafiltration in pulmonary edema. *A.* Positive pressure ultrafiltration. A screw clamp in the line returning blood to the inferior vena cava (IVC) is tightened, increasing filtration pressure within the lumen. *B.* Negative pressure ultrafiltration. The transmembrane pressure is increased by applying negative pressure on the dialysate side of the membrane. *C.* Ultrafiltration in the adult respiratory distress syndrome. Arterial oxygenation increased along with an increase in colloid osmotic pressure and a decrease in pulmonary wedge pressure. *D.* Ultrafiltration in cardiogenic shock and fluid overload. Removal of fluid was accompanied by an increase in cardiac output, a decrease in pulmonary wedge pressure, and improved blood gases. The arterial P_{O_2} increased considerably even though the O_2 content of inspired air was decreased from 100 to 50 percent. *(After Gerhardt, 1980.)*

from the lungs into the pulmonary microcirculation has not been of much help. Both crystalloidal solutions, such as urea and mannitol, and colloidal solutions, particularly of serum albumin, have been tried. Retrospectively, the ineffectiveness of the osmotic agents was preordained since osmotic agents cannot exert their effects across a leaky barrier. Besides being ineffective, once the semipermeable properties of the alveolar-capillary barrier are lost, the use of osmotic agents engenders the danger of circulatory overload. To neutralize this hazard, ingenious attempts were made to combine the intravenous administration of 25% albumin with the simultaneous

administration of a potent diuretic, e.g., furosemide. These were not effective. Finally, resort to high-molecular-weight dextrans (of the order of MW 500,000) was notably futile since these macromolecules poured into the tracheal fluid, reaching virtually the same concentration there as in plasma.

ULTRAFILTRATION

By modifying equipment currently used for renal dialysis (hollow fiber hemofilter) so that the apparatus filters water and solutes out of the circulation instead of relying on diffusion (Fig. 60-31), a fresh approach was developed for the treatment of refractory pulmonary edema. As might be expected from first principles, this approach has proved more effective in hemodynamic pulmonary edema. Although some success has followed its use in the adult respiratory distress syndrome, at present the technique must still be regarded as experimental.

OUTCOME

About one-third of patients with permeability pulmonary edema (largely the adult respiratory distress syndrome) survive. In these, resolution is not always complete. But, it is intriguing that some who do recover almost completely seem to pass through a stage of pulmonary fibrosis that resolves with time.

BIBLIOGRAPHY

Albelda SM, Hansen-Flaschen JH, Lanken PN, Fishman AP: Effects of increased ventilation on lung lymph flow in unanesthetized sheep. J Appl Physiol 60:2063–2070, 1986.
Hyperpnea induces an increase in pulmonary lymph flow by decreasing perimicrovascular interstitial pressure along with an increase in pulmonary pumping. In turn, the increase in pumping is due to the presence of one-way valves in the lymphatics and the influence of respiratory movements on the lymphatics tethered in pulmonary parenchyma.

Albert RK, Greenberg G, Guest RJ, Luchtel D, Henderson WR: Leukotrienes C_4 and D_4 do not increase filtration coefficient of excised perfused guinea pig lungs. J Appl Physiol 62:1–9, 1987.
No increase in pulmonary vascular permeability could be demonstrated after infusing these products of the 5-lipoxygenase pathway of arachidonic acid metabolism. The results suggest that other mediators must be involved in the increase in pulmonary vascular permeability that follows intravenous infusion of endotoxin.

Allen SJ, Drake RE, Jeffrey Katz, Gabel JC, Laine GA: Lowered pulmonary arterial pressure prevents edema after endotoxin in sheep. J Appl Physiol 63:1008–1011, 1987.
Escherichia coli endotoxin causes increased capillary membrane permeability and increased pulmonary arterial pressure (Ppa) in sheep. Reduction of Ppa may limit the amount of pulmonary edema associated with endotoxin.

Basset G, Crone C, Saumon G: Significance of active ion transport in transalveolar water absorption: a study on isolated rat lung. J Physiol Lond 384:311–324, 1987.
The alveolar epithelium performs solute-coupled fluid transport from alveoli to plasma and shows many features that are common to other fluid-transporting epithelia; with an approximate surface area of 100 m² in human beings, it constitutes one of the largest epithelial surfaces in the body.

Beutler B, Cerami A: Cachectin: More than a tumor-necrosis factor. N Engl J Med 316:379, 1987.
Tumor necrosis factor (cachectin) is a mediator of endotoxic shock. This review provides a full perspective of tumor necrosis factor, the pathologic disturbances that it evokes, and the implications for therapy. It obviously relates to "permeability edema" that occurs clinically and also to that produced experimentally by the administration of endotoxin.

Bishop MJ, Chi EY, Cheney FW Jr: Lung reperfusion in dogs causes bilateral lung injury. J Appl Physiol 63:942–950, 1987.
Not only did reperfusion after 48 h of pulmonary arterial occlusion result in marked edema and inflammatory infiltrates in the reperfused lung but it also caused mild edema and inflammation in the contralateral continuously perfused lung. The local and distant injury does not appear to be mediated by xanthine oxidase-produced O_2 radicals.

Brigham KL, Meyrick B, Berry LC Jr, Repine JE: Antioxidants protect cultured bovine lung endothelial cells from injury by endotoxin. J Appl Physiol 63:840–850, 1987.
Using cultured bovine pulmonary endothelial cells, two chemically dissimilar drugs that act intracellularly to decrease concentrations of toxic metabolites of oxygen prevented direct injury of endothelium by Escherichia coli endotoxin.

Cottrell TS, Levine OR, Senior RM, Wieber J, Spiro D, Fishman AP: Electron microscopic alterations at the alveolar level in pulmonary edema. Circ Res 21:783–798, 1967.

The original description of the thin and thick aspects of the alveolar capillary barrier, a pivotal observation for understanding the circulation of water and macromolecules in the lungs.

Cross CE: Oxygen radicals and human disease. Ann Intern Med 107:526–545, 1987.

Oxygen radicals are being implicated in the pathogenesis of many clinical disorders, including certain types of lung injury and edema.

Davies KJA: Protein damage and degradation by oxygen radicals: I. General aspects. J Biol Chem 262:9895–9901, 1987.

The first of a series of four consecutive papers in the same issue that deal with the toxic effects of oxygen radicals on proteins.

Fishman AP: Pulmonary edema: The water-exchanging function of the lung. Circulation 46:390–408, 1972.

A consideration of the pathogenesis of the various types of clinical pulmonary edema in the light of recent physiological, histologic, and ultrastructural insights.

Fishman AP: Pulmonary circulation, in Fishman AP, Fisher AB (eds), *Handbook of Physiology,* sect 3: *The Respiratory System, vol 1: Circulation and Nonrespiratory Functions.* Bethesda, American Physiological Society, 1985, pp 93–165.

A comprehensive overview of the regulation of the pulmonary circulation and of the interplay between structure and function.

Fishman AP, Renkin EM (eds): *Pulmonary Edema.* Washington DC, American Physiological Society, 1979.

A collection of papers devoted to the state of the art in research on mechanisms of pulmonary edema and to their clinical relevance.

Fishman AP, Richards DW (eds): *Circulation of the Blood. Men and Ideas.* New York, Oxford University Press, 1964.

The contributors, all distinguished physiologists, trace the growth of ideas in cardiovascular physiology. Each deals with a particular topic to which he has had deep personal involvement as a scientist.

Gerhardt RE: Ultrafiltration in the management of the adult respiratory distress syndrome, in Fishman AP (ed), *Update: Pulmonary Diseases and Disorders.* New York, McGraw-Hill, 1980, pp 387–395.

A review of the principles and practice of ultrafiltration in the handling of refractory pulmonary edema, uremia, and the adult respiratory distress syndrome.

Glasser SW, Korfhagen TR, Weaver T, Pilot-Matias T, Fox JL, Whitsett JA: cDNA and deduced amino acid sequence of human pulmonary surfactant-associated proteolipid SPL (Phe). Proc Natl Acad Sci USA 84:4007–4011, 1987.

Description of a hydrophobic peptide that is a major protein component of surfactant lipid extracts that may be useful for synthesis of replacement surfactants.

Guyton AC, Lindsey AE: Effect of elevated left atrial pressure and decreased plasma protein concentration on the development of pulmonary edema. Circ Res 7:649–657, 1959.

No edema formed in the lungs of dogs until pulmonary capillary pressure exceeded the colloid osmotic pressure (about 20 mmHg) by 3 mmHg. Induced hypoproteinemia reduced the critical hydrostatic pressure for edema formation. Since normal pulmonary capillary pressure in the dog is about 7 mmHg whereas the oncotic pressure is about 28 mmHg, the safety factor afforded by the plasma proteins is about 21 mmHg.

Holm BA, Notter RH: Effects of hemoglobin and cell membrane lipids on pulmonary surfactant activity. J Appl Physiol 63:1434–1442, 1987.

These experiments show that molecular components in hemorrhagic pulmonary edema can biophysically inactivate endogenous whole lung surfactant and adversely affect lung mechanics. Exogenous surfactant replacement can reverse this process even in the continued presence of inhibitor molecules and thus has potential utility in therapy for adult, as well as neonatal, respiratory distress syndrome.

Lakshminarayan S, Jindal SK, Kirk W, Butler J: Acute increases in anastomotic bronchial systemic to pulmonary blood flow due to generalized lung injury. J Appl Physiol 62:2358–2361, 1987.

There is an acute increase in bronchial-pulmonary blood flow following a generalized lung injury due to the inflammatory response.

Landis EM: The capillary circulation, in Fishman AP, Richards DW (eds), *Circulation of the Blood. Men and Ideas.* Bethesda, American Physiological Society, 1982, pp 355–406.
  A fascinating historical account of the growth of ideas about the structure and function of the capillaries, including the forces involved in the transcapillary exchange of fluids and macromolecules.

Malik AB, Staub NC: *Mechanisms of Lung Microvascular Injury.* New York, The New York Academy of Sciences, 1982.
  A state-of-the-art conference on the pulmonary microcirculation prompted by fresh insights into the pathogenesis of the adult respiratory distress syndrome.

Maron MB: Analysis of airway fluid protein concentration in neurogenic pulmonary edema. J Appl Physiol 62:470–476, 1987.
  Both hemodynamic and increased permeability mechanisms may play a role to varying degrees in the development of this form of NPE.

Matthay MA (ed): Symposium on pulmonary edema. Clin Chest Med 6:299–551, 1985.
  A collection of papers dealing with the mechanisms involved in the formation and resolution of pulmonary edema. Among the topics that are particularly well treated are neurogenic pulmonary edema, the pulmonary edema of high altitude, and the resolution of pulmonary edema.

Michel RP, Zocchi L, Rossi A, Cardinal GA, Ploy-Song-Sang Y, Poulsen RS, Milic-Emili J, Staub NC: Does interstitial lung edema compress airways and arteries? A morphometric study. J Appl Physiol 62:108–115, 1987.
  Based on morphometric studies, the authors conclude that interstitial edema does not compress small airways or arteries. However, other mechanisms, notably alveolar edema and fluid in the airways, may account for the increase in airway resistance.

Minnear FL, Kite C, Hill LA, van der Zee H: Endothelial injury and pulmonary congestion characterize neurogenic pulmonary edema in rabbits. J Appl Physiol 63:335–341, 1987.
  Pulmonary congestion, pulmonary vascular hypertension, and focal endothelial injury contribute to the development of neurogenic pulmonary edema secondary to intracisternal injection of fibrinogen-sodium citrate.

Newman JH: Sepsis and pulmonary edema. Clin Chest Med 6:371–391, 1985.
  This article draws heavily on an extensive experimental experience with endotoxemia to provide a full view of current understanding of permeability pulmonary edema. The experimental insights are reinforced by observations on the adult respiratory distress syndrome.

Ornato JP: The resuscitation of near-drowning victims. JAMA 256:75–77, 1986.
  A guide to sustaining life, providing support for the respiration and circulation, and protecting the central nervous system.

Paintal AS: The mechanism of excitation of type J receptors and the J reflex, in Porter R (ed), *Breathing. Ciba Foundation Symposium.* London, Churchill, 1970, pp 59–76.
  A classic presentation that sparked current interest in the J reflex.

Payen DM, Brun-Buisson CJL, Carli PA, Huet Y, Leviel F, Cinotti L, Chiron B: Hemodynamic, gas exchange and hormonal consequences of LBPP during PEEP ventilation. J Appl Physiol 62:61–70, 1987.
  Application of mild lower-body positive pressure (LBPP) increases cardiac output and O_2 delivery in individuals undergoing mechanical ventilation with PEEP.

Pietra GG, Szidon JP, Leventhal MM, Fishman AP: Hemoglobin as a tracer in hemodynamic pulmonary edema. Science 166:1643–1646, 1969.
  Using stroma-free hemoglobin as an electron-opaque marker, ultrastructural studies showed that endothelial junctions in the pulmonary capillaries act as distensible pores under the influence of hydrostatic pressures.

Pietra GG, Szidon JP, Leventhal MM, Fishman AP: Histamine and interstitial pulmonary edema in the dog. Circ Res 24:323–337, 1971.
  Ultrastructural studies showed that histamine causes bronchial venules to leak while leaving alveolar capillary vessels unaffected.

Pistolesi M, Miniati M, Milne ENC, Guintini C: The chest roentgenogram in pulmonary edema. Clin Chest Med 6:315–344, 1985.
Personal experience and an exhaustive review of the literature provide a critical appraisal of the value of the chest radiograph in cardiogenic, renal, and permeability edema. In clinical disorders, the overall radiographic appearance, rather than any single criterion, is the basis for differential diagnosis and for follow-up.

Staub NC, Taylor AE (eds): Edema. New York, Raven, 1984.
A massive scholarly tome devoted to edema in its broadest sense but with Starling's concept of transvascular liquid balance as the keystone. Chapters on a variety of clinical types of pulmonary edema illustrate the physiological principles and pathophysiological mechanisms.

Stevens JH, O'Hanley P, Shapiro JM, Mihm FG, Satoh PS, Collins JA, Raffin TA: Effects of anti-C5a antibodies on the adult respiratory distress syndrome in septic primates. J Clin Invest 77:1812–1816, 1986.
Treatment with rabbit anti-human C5a des arg antibodies attenuates ARDS and some of the systemic manifestations of sepsis in nonhuman primates.

Szidon JP, Fishman AP: Autonomic control of the pulmonary circulation, in Fishman AP, Hecht HH (eds), The Pulmonary Circulation and Interstitial Space. Chicago, University of Chicago Press, 1969, pp 239–265.
An overview of hemodynamic pulmonary edema based on physiological-anatomic correlations. Neurogenic pulmonary edema is considered to be predominantly hemodynamic with an added component of leaky vessels due to stretched pores.

Taniguchi H, Taki F, Takagi K, Satake T, Sugiyama S, Ozawa T: The role of leukotriene B$_4$ in the genesis of oxygen toxicity in the lung. Am Rev Respir Dis 133:805–808, 1986.
During pure O$_2$ breathing, an increase in LTB$_4$ is responsible for the accumulation of PMN in the lung and that PMN recruitment contributes to lung injury.

Taylor AE, Parker JC: Pulmonary interstitial spaces and lymphatics, in Fishman AP, Fisher AB (eds), Handbook of Physiology, sect 3: The Respiratory System, vol 1: Circulation and Non-Respiratory Functions. Bethesda, American Physiological Society, 1985, pp 167–230.
A comprehensive review of the organization of the pulmonary interstitium, the forces involved in the exchange of substances across the pulmonary vascular endothelium, and the clinical consequences of disorders in pulmonary capillary permeability.

Tracey KJ, Beutler B, Lowry SF, Merryweather J, Wolpe S, Milsark IW, Hariri RJ, Fahey TJ III, Zentella A, Albert JD, Shires GT, Cerami A: Shock and tissue injury induced by recombinant human cachectin. Science 234:470–474, 1986.
Cachectin (tumor necrosis factor), a protein produced in large quantities by endotoxin-activated macrophages, has been implicated as an important mediator of the lethal effect of endotoxin. Recombinant human cachectin infused into rats is capable of inducing many of the deleterious effects of endotoxin.

Wead WB, Cassidy SS, Reynolds RC: Pulmonary edema in dogs fails to cause reflex responses. Am J Physiol 252:H89–H99, 1987.
Contrary to the popular view that pulmonary C-fibers reflexly stimulate the ventilation in pulmonary edema, these experiments in the isolated lung failed to affect respiratory frequency.

Wheeldon EB, Hansen-Flaschen JH: Intravascular macrophages in the sheep lung. J Leukocyte Biol 40:657–661, 1986.
The presence of intravascular macrophages in the sheep lung and their absence in the human lung may account for the more injurious effects of endotoxin in the sheep lung than in the human lung.

Whitsett JA, Pilot T, Clark JC, Weaver TE: Induction of surfactant protein in fetal lung. Effects of cAMP and dexamethasone on SAP-35 RNA and synthesis. J Biol Chem 262:5256–5261, 1987.
Induction of pulmonary surfactant protein (SAP-35) synthesis during organ culture of human fetal lung was associated with increased SAP-35 RNA. SAP-35 synthesis and SAP-35 RNA were inhibited by dexamethasone and enhanced cAMP.

Chapter *61*

Depositional Diseases of the Lung

Richard H. Ochs

Interstitial Depositional Disease
  Whipple's Disease
  Amyloidosis
  Diffuse Pulmonary Calcification

Alveolar Depositional Disease
  Alveolar Hemorrhage Syndromes
  Alveolar Microlithiasis

Depositional disease refers to those conditions in which something is deposited in the lungs in sufficient amount so as to distort normal lung structure and function, sometimes resulting in symptoms or clinical signs of disease. The material deposited in excess can be cells, either inflammatory or neoplastic; extracellular connective tissue elements, either fibrillar, such as collagen, or matrix substance, such as proteoglycans; endogenously derived crystalline material, such as hemosiderin or amyloid; or exogenously derived material, such as inorganic dust. These elements can be deposited singly or in combination.

An additional consideration is where in the lung the material lodges. It can be predominantly in the interstitial space, e.g., the inflammation and scarring of the interstitial pneumonitides; predominantly within alveolar spaces, as is the case with phospholipid accumulation in alveolar proteinosis; or a combination of the two, as in the case of hemosiderin deposition in the pulmonary hemorrhagic syndromes.

INTERSTITIAL DEPOSITIONAL DISEASE

Depositional diseases affecting predominantly the pulmonary interstitium include inflammatory diseases, the interstitial spread of malignant neoplasms, the accumulation of macrophages containing excessive amounts of the products of inborn errors of metabolism or bacterial metabolism, amyloidosis, and diffuse interstitial calcification. In this chapter, emphasis is placed on Whipple's disease, amyloidosis, and diffuse calcification. Excluded from consideration are the interstitial pneumonitides, neoplastic diseases, inborn errors of metabolism, pulmo-

nary edema, acute infectious diseases, and diffuse pulmonary infiltrates in the compromised host, all of which are discussed elsewhere in this text.

By definition, depositional diseases of the pulmonary interstitium involve the expansion of the alveolar interstitial spaces. Although these diseases are designated as interstitial, they often involve injury to the adjacent epithelial and endothelial cells; in some instances, these cells are the initial site of injury. Moreover, involvement of the interstitial compartment frequently extends beyond the alveolar septa to involve connective tissue surrounding, or even within, conducting airways, blood vessels, and the pleura.

Therefore, pulmonary interstitial disease must be regarded as neither confined to the pulmonary interstitium nor limited to alveolar septa. However, since the dominant process does involve the alveolar septa, resulting in derangement of the specialized gas-exchanging surface in the lung, the diffusion barrier for gaseous diffusion is widened and alveolar ventilation and perfusion become mismatched. Chronic alveolar injury leads to gross restructuring of the lung so that gas-exchanging surfaces are lost and the mismatch of ventilation and perfusion is exaggerated.

Some interstitial diseases do not involve an inflammatory infiltrate at any stage of their evolution. Among these are neoplastic infiltrates in the interstitium, such as lymphangitic spread of carcinoma, leukemic and lymphomatous infiltrates, and Kaposi's sarcoma. Nor is there an inflammatory response to interstitial pulmonary amyloidosis, which involves the deposition of an abnormal acellular crystalline material in the pulmonary interstitium. In diffuse pulmonary amyloidosis, the amyloid is derived from a soluble circulating plasma precursor that is presumably produced at an extrapulmonary location. Inflammation is also usually absent in diffuse calcification of the pulmonary interstitium, particularly in patients in whom the deposits are due to derangement of calcium metabolism.

Whipple's Disease

Whipple's disease is a rare disorder that was initially described as a disease of the small intestine that caused diarrhea and malabsorption. Subsequently, the disease was recognized to be systemic in nature and to be caused by infection with an unidentified rod-shaped bacillus demonstrable by electron microscopy. Oddly, the bacillus provokes little inflammatory response. But its presence is associated with the accumulation of foamy macrophages that contain copious amounts of glycoprotein, which can be stained by the periodic acid-Schiff (PAS) reaction. This material may be a product of the bacilli, since they also stain with the PAS reaction.

Although pathologic evidence of pulmonary involvement in patients dying with Whipple's disease is com-

mon, clinical evidence of pulmonary involvement is rare. Whipple's disease of the lung can produce pleuritic chest pain, pleural effusion, nonproductive cough, or a diffuse reticulonodular infiltrate on the chest radiograph that is associated with physiological evidence of restrictive lung disease. On biopsy, there are peribronchial and perivascular collections of the characteristic foamy macrophages, which also accumulate in the pleura. Occasionally, the tunica media of the pulmonary arteries is prominently infiltrated by free, rather than intracellular, bacilli in association with medial degeneration but without vasculitis. In one patient with Whipple's disease, pulmonary hypertension was found. However, it was not clear if the pulmonary hypertension stemmed from infiltration of pulmonary arterial walls or chronic passive congestion secondary to cardiac involvement by Whipple's disease, or if it was unrelated to the Whipple's disease. Antibiotic therapy usually clears the gastrointestinal manifestations, whereas the nongastrointestinal manifestations are usually refractory to therapy.

Amyloidosis

Amyloid refers to one of several insoluble proteins deposited in tissues which have in common: (1) a characteristic amorphous appearance on routine histologic examination, (2) a characteristic fibrillar structure on electron-microscopic examination, and (3) a characteristic physicochemical structure, namely, antiparallel β-pleated sheets. The last feature provides all amyloid substances with a unique affinity for the dye Congo red which renders the amyloid red-orange on microscopic examination. Because of the highly ordered structure of binding sites for the dye, stained amyloid shows birefringence when viewed with cross-polarized lenses, i.e., the amyloid appears yellow or apple green, depending on the orientation of the polarizing lenses to the crystalline axis (Fig. 61-1).

There are several different, chemically unrelated types of amyloid (see below), all of which share the previously mentioned features. Evidence is mounting that, in all forms of amyloidosis, a larger soluble precursor molecule from the blood is cleaved, presumably by macrophages, at the sites of deposition. This results in spontaneous polymerization of the smaller fragments into fibrils, which assume the characteristic structure of amyloid. Once deposited, the amyloid apparently cannot be mobilized from the tissues. As amyloid accumulates in tissues, it can alter the physical structure of organs, producing increased weight and stiffness, as well as impaired nutrition from blood vessels, leading to atrophy of parenchymal cells. The functional consequences can be as diverse as nephrotic syndrome due to involvement of glomeruli and restrictive cardiomyopathy due to involvement of myocardium.

As mentioned previously, there are several different types of amyloid. One appears to be derived from the light chains of immunoglobulins, most often lambda light chains, and is referred to as AL(amyloid light chain)-derived. This is the type of amyloid usually found in association with multiple myeloma and other plasma cell dyscrasias, as well as most instances of systemic amyloidosis which are neither familial nor associated with some chronic inflammatory disorder (previously known as primary amyloidosis). Another amyloid type is known as AA(amyloid associated)-derived. Amino acid sequencing indicates that this AA protein is derived from an acute phase reactant normally found in serum, known as SAA (serum amyloid associated) protein. This is the type of amyloid found in patients with underlying chronic inflammatory disorders such as tuberculosis, osteomyelitis,

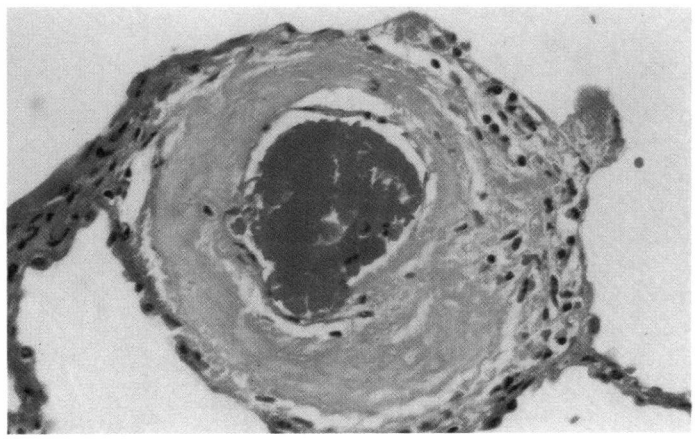

A

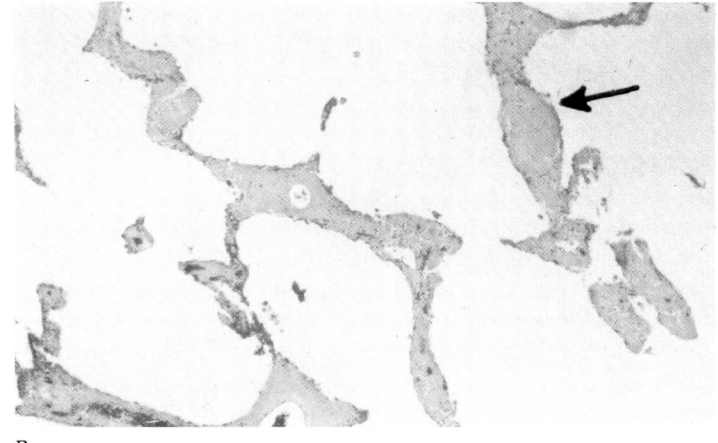

B

FIGURE 61-1 Amyloid deposition. *A.* The typical amorphous appearance of amyloid is seen deposited within the wall of a pulmonary venule. Green birefringence on polarized light examination after staining with Congo red will confirm the amyloid nature of the deposit. H&E, ×700. *B.* Amorphous amyloid in the alveolar interstitial space. Arrow indicates a thickened alveolar septum. H&E, ×420.

and rheumatoid arthritis (previously known as secondary amyloidosis), as well as in patients with familial Mediterranean fever. A third type of amyloid is derived from cleavage of circulating prealbumin and is found in senile cardiac amyloidosis (actually a systemic disorder in which the lung is involved in almost all patients) and other forms of familial amyloidosis, particularly the neurotropic varieties such as Swedish and Portuguese.

Amyloid in the lung can involve the tracheobronchial tree, either as plaques or tumoral masses. Amyloid can also involve the pulmonary parenchyma, either as a solitary nodule or multiple discrete nodules, or as a diffuse interstitial and vascular deposition. Tracheobronchial and nodular parenchymal deposits usually occur in the absence of systemic amyloidosis, while diffuse interstitial and vascular deposits more frequently occur with systemic amyloidosis.

ISOLATED AMYLOID IN THE LOWER RESPIRATORY TRACT

Clinically evident involvement of the tracheobronchial tree by amyloid deposition usually occurs as an isolated phenomenon, i.e., unassociated with systemic amyloidosis. The amyloid most frequently is deposited as multiple submucosal plaques that are readily identifiable at bronchoscopy. This diffuse tracheobronchial deposition is likely to be symptomatic, producing cough, stridor, or hemoptysis. Bronchoscopic biopsy is diagnostic, and endoscopic resection can relieve obstruction. As is the case at other sites of amyloid deposition, vascular involvement can be associated with considerable bleeding following biopsy. It has been postulated that diffuse tracheobronchial amyloid deposition is a precursor of tracheopathia osteoplastica.

Less often, isolated deposition of amyloid in the tracheobronchial tree produces a solitary raised nodular mass that mimics an endobronchial neoplasm. In these instances, the signs and symptoms point to localized bronchial obstruction, with or without hemoptysis. Although diagnosis can be accomplished by bronchoscopic biopsy, removal by conservative surgery is preferable so that an associated neoplasm can be ruled out.

Solitary pulmonary nodules (amyloidomas), as well as multiple amyloid nodules, occur as incidental radiographic findings in asymptomatic individuals. These nodules have no distinctive features: occasionally they contain focal calcifications or cavities.. The diagnosis is usually made after surgical resection. Although the diagnosis has occasionally been made by percutaneous aspiration using a fine needle and by transbronchial biopsy, it is prudent to resect a solitary nodule or one of multiple nodules since, on rare occasions, amyloid deposition occurs within a pulmonary neoplasm. Pathologic examination often reveals an intense associated local inflammatory reaction consisting of plasma cells, macrophages, and multinucleated giant cells. Occasional chemical analyses have revealed that the amyloid in the nodules is immunoglobulin-derived.

The consensus is that both tracheobronchial amyloidosis and nodular parenchymal amyloidosis represent a localized abnormal immune response of bronchial-associated lymphoid tissue (BALT) rather than a systemic immune disorder.

PULMONARY INVOLVEMENT IN SYSTEMIC AMYLOIDOSIS

At autopsy, most patients with systemic amyloidosis, regardless of type (AL-, AA- and prealbumin-derived), have microscopic deposits of amyloid in their lungs. The deposits may be confined to the walls of small blood vessels, to the alveolar septal interstitium, or to both. Rarely is the deposition sufficiently severe to produce clinical disease. Symptomatic patients, usually with either AL-derived amyloid or senile cardiac amyloidosis, exhibit dyspnea, restrictive pulmonary function tests, and either accentuated interstitial markings or reticulonodular infiltrates on the chest radiograph. The diagnosis can be established by transbronchial or open lung biopsy.

Diffuse Pulmonary Calcification

Calcification of the pulmonary parenchyma can occur by a variety of mechanisms. *Dystrophic calcification* refers to the deposition of calcium salts, most often crystalline hydroxyapatite, in dead tissue, such as within the healing granulomas of tuberculosis. This type of calcification is usually localized; its distinctive radiographic features are sometimes helpful diagnostically (see Chapter 35). *Metastatic calcification* refers to the deposition of calcium salts, usually amorphous, in normal tissues (Fig. 61-2). This latter type of calcification occurs in association with some derangement of calcium metabolism, such as hyperparathyroidism, hypervitaminosis D, the milk alkali syndrome, sarcoidosis, increased bone turnover due to multi-

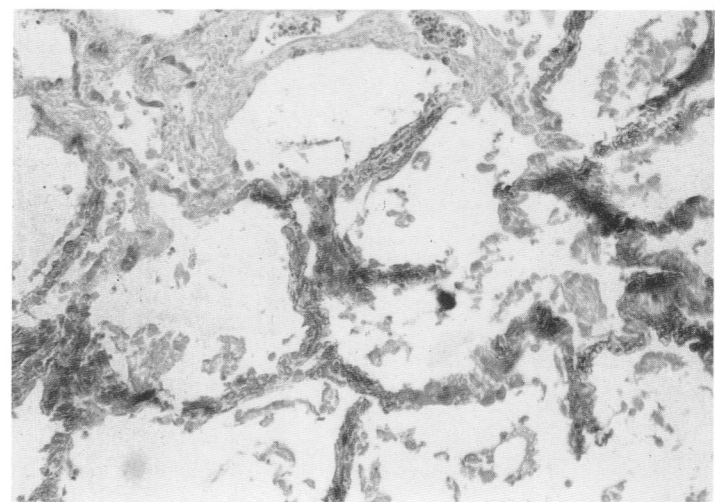

FIGURE 61-2 Metastatic calcification of alveolar septa in a renal dialysis patient. Photomicrograph shows calcium forming a dark red precipitate within the alveolar septa. Alizarin red, ×280.

ple myeloma or metastatic carcinoma, or chronic renal failure.

Although metastatic calcification can occur in almost any tissue of the body, it occurs most often in the lungs, kidneys, stomach, and the walls of blood vessels. Metastatic calcification in the lungs usually affects the interstitium of alveolar septa and the walls of pulmonary vessels, sometimes localizing on elastic fibers. Clinical manifestations of diffuse pulmonary calcification are unusual, occurring most often in patients who are in chronic renal failure, particularly in those on chronic hemodialysis. Radiographically, metastatic calcification usually takes the form of a diffuse interstitial infiltrate. Rarely do the patients manifest dyspnea, arterial hypoxemia, and the pulmonary function tests of restrictive pulmonary disease. The calcific nature of the infiltrate is generally evident on the routine chest radiograph or on the CT scan; recognition is furthered by scanning with either technetium 99m or gallium 67.

The mechanism responsible for diffuse pulmonary calcification is unknown. Although high levels of parathyroid hormone or a marked increase in the calcium-phosphate solubility product do occur in an occasional patient, calcification can occur in the absence of either. Ultrastructural observations of minimal, presumably early, lesions show selective deposition of calcium on elastic fibers, suggesting that they may serve as the initial nidus. In contrast to their apparent role in alveolar microlithiasis, extracellular matrix vesicles do not appear to be involved.

ALVEOLAR DEPOSITIONAL DISEASE

Material can accumulate in alveolar spaces either as part of a localized disease process that produces irregular or nodular infiltrates on the chest radiograph or as a diffuse infiltrate throughout both lungs. Localized alveolar accumulations usually do not produce pulmonary symptoms unless they are quite large, or are superimposed on preexisting lung disease, or cause associated inflammation of the pleura. Bacterial bronchopneumonia often acts in this way; so does a pulmonary neoplasm. Localized alveolar accumulations are considered elsewhere in this book.

Diffuse alveolar filling is likely to produce symptomatic impairment of respiratory function. In alveoli filled with fluid, cells, or debris, gas exchange is impaired. To some extent, local mechanisms, such as pulmonary vasoconstriction, rearrange blood flow in keeping with the alveolar ventilation. But, when alveolar consolidation is extensive, some pulmonary arterial blood inevitably passes through the affected alveolar capillary bed without adequate oxygenation. Massive alveolar filling is usually caused by fluid accumulation, e.g., pulmonary edema, or a mixture of fluid and inflammatory cells, e.g., confluent bacterial pneumonia. Occasionally, the alveolar filling is by neoplastic cells, e.g., bronchioloalveolar cell carcinoma, blood, e.g., diffuse alveolar hemorrhage, or the products of abnormal cell metabolism, e.g., alveolar proteinosis and alveolar microlithiasis. In this chapter, only the alveolar hemorrhage syndromes and alveolar microlithiasis are considered further.

Alveolar Hemorrhage Syndromes

The presence of extravasated blood in pulmonary parenchyma occurs as part of many diseases. The conditions in which extensive intra-alveolar hemorrhage throughout both lungs is due to some form of injury to alveolar septa are shown in Table 61-1. Not listed in this table are the extrapulmonary causes of bleeding into undamaged lung. Some instances of alveolar injury and hemorrhage are immunologic and toxic in etiology; but there are others in which the cause remains enigmatic. The pulmonary hemorrhage may occur as an isolated phenomenon or in association with glomerulonephritis or in association with a systemic disease, such as systemic vasculitis or a connective tissue disease syndrome, most frequently systemic lupus erythematosus.

In order to distinguish one syndrome from another, extrapulmonary manifestations of disease and the laboratory evaluation of possible pathogenic mechanisms must

TABLE 61-1
Causes of Alveolar Hemorrhage

Mechanism	Example
Intact alveolar septa	
Aspiration of blood	Tracheobronchial neoplasm
Passive congestion	Pulmonary veno-occlusive disease
Bleeding diathesis	Disseminated intravascular coagulation
Injured alveolar septa	
Anti-basement membrane antibody	Goodpasture's syndrome
Immune complex deposition	Systemic vasculitis
Toxic	Trimellitic anhydride
Unknown	Idiopathic pulmonary hemosiderosis

be taken into account. Since prognosis and effective therapy differ from syndrome to syndrome, and since some instances of pulmonary hemorrhage are life-threatening, prompt diagnostic evaluation for the institution of proper therapy is often a matter of great urgency.

CLINICAL FEATURES

The cardinal manifestations of diffuse alveolar hemorrhage include hemoptysis, diffuse alveolar infiltrates on the chest radiograph, and anemia. Dyspnea and hypoxemia also occur. The degree of hemoptysis ranges from blood-tinged sputum to massive amounts of pure blood. Although massive hemoptysis is a common manifestation of diffuse alveolar hemorrhage, it is not a regular feature so that life-threatening intrapulmonary hemorrhage can occur in the absence of hemoptysis. The detection of hemosiderin-laden macrophages in the sputum (as by the Prussian blue stain) indicates that blood has been present in the alveolar spaces sufficiently long for it to be broken down by alveolar macrophages. Hemosiderin-laden macrophages are not specific for any particular syndrome, but they do indicate that some intrapulmonary pathologic process includes hemorrhage as a component.

Clinically significant pulmonary hemorrhage is usually associated with extensive pulmonary infiltrates on the chest radiograph. Fresh bleeding produces an alveolar filling pattern which can be difficult to distinguish from pulmonary edema or a pneumonia (e.g., viral) but, as a rule, the shadows are denser. As the intra-alveolar hemorrhage is broken down and resorbed, the infiltrate assumes a finely nodular pattern; in contrast to the rapid resolution of edema, it may take weeks to resolve. Chronic or recurrent hemorrhage may produce fine interstitial fibrosis that is manifested as a reticular pattern on the chest radiograph; a fresh hemorrhage may superimpose an alveolar pattern on the delicate fibrotic pattern. The chest radiograph is a more accurate predictor of the amount, or progression, of alveolar hemorrhage than is the amount of hemoptysis

Clinically significant alveolar hemorrhage is usually sufficient to cause anemia. Therefore, sequential determinations of the concentration of hemoglobin in peripheral blood affords a good monitor for continued or recrudescent bleeding, even when hemoptysis is absent. If the anemia is iron-deficiency in type, and if there is no other obvious reason for the iron deficiency, chronic or repetitive alveolar hemorrhage can be inferred.

As with other alveolar filling processes, alveolar hemorrhage must be extensive to cause dyspnea. Lesser degrees of hemorrhage may, nonetheless, produce sufficient ventilation-perfusion mismatch to cause arterial hypoxemia. Ewan and associates have shown that measurement of carbon monoxide uptake can be a very sensitive and specific indicator of acute pulmonary hemorrhage. Like all alveolar filling processes, alveolar hemorrhage decreases the carbon monoxide diffusing capacity. But, unlike other causes, alveolar hemorrhage is associated with an increase in carbon monoxide uptake by the lung due to the binding of carbon monoxide by intra-alveolar red blood cells in association with a decrease in the delivery of carbon monoxide to arterial blood.

RECOGNIZED SYNDROMES

Goodpasture's Syndrome

This entity was originally described as an association of alveolar hemorrhage with glomerulonephritis (Fig. 61-3). It was later determined that pulmonary and renal damage in many such patients was mediated by antibodies that are specificity directed against a component of glomerular and other capillary basement membranes. While, as noted below, there are other causes of concomitant alveolar hemorrhage and glomerulonephritis, most authorities now reserve the eponym Goodpasture's syndrome for disease mediated by antiglomerular basement membrane antibodies (anti-GBM antibodies) (see Chapter 45).

Goodpasture's syndrome can present with a broad spectrum of clinical findings. The classic case presents with massive hemoptysis and overt glomerulonephritis, often with acute renal failure on presentation. However, some patients present only with hemoptysis, having either subclinical or no renal disease at presentation, only to later develop overt renal disease. Least frequently, patients present with acute glomerulonephritis due to anti-GBM antibody, and only later or perhaps never develop pulmonary hemorrhage. If pulmonary hemorrhage is never manifested, the Goodpasture's eponym should be withheld.

Biopsy of the lung in Goodpasture's syndrome is usually nondiagnostic. Routine light-microscopic examination shows intra-alveolar hemorrhage, usually associated with intra-alveolar hemosiderin-laden macrophages. There is no evidence of vasculitis, interstitial or intra-alveolar inflammation, or necrosis. Nonspecific reparative proliferation of the alveolar lining cells may be present. Only occasionally will immunofluorescence microscopy show diagnostic linear deposits of immunoglobulin and/or complement along alveolar capillary walls. Kidney biopsy in Goodpasture's syndrome is usually diagnostic: whereas conventional light microscopy shows nonspecific focal or diffuse glomerulonephritis—which may be crescentic and which may be necrotizing—immunofluorescence microscopy usually shows linear deposition of immunoglobulin (usually IgG, occasionally IgA) and frequently shows complement deposition as well.

Even without biopsy, the diagnosis of Goodpasture's syndrome can be achieved by detection of anti-GBM antibody in the patient's serum. This is most reliably detected

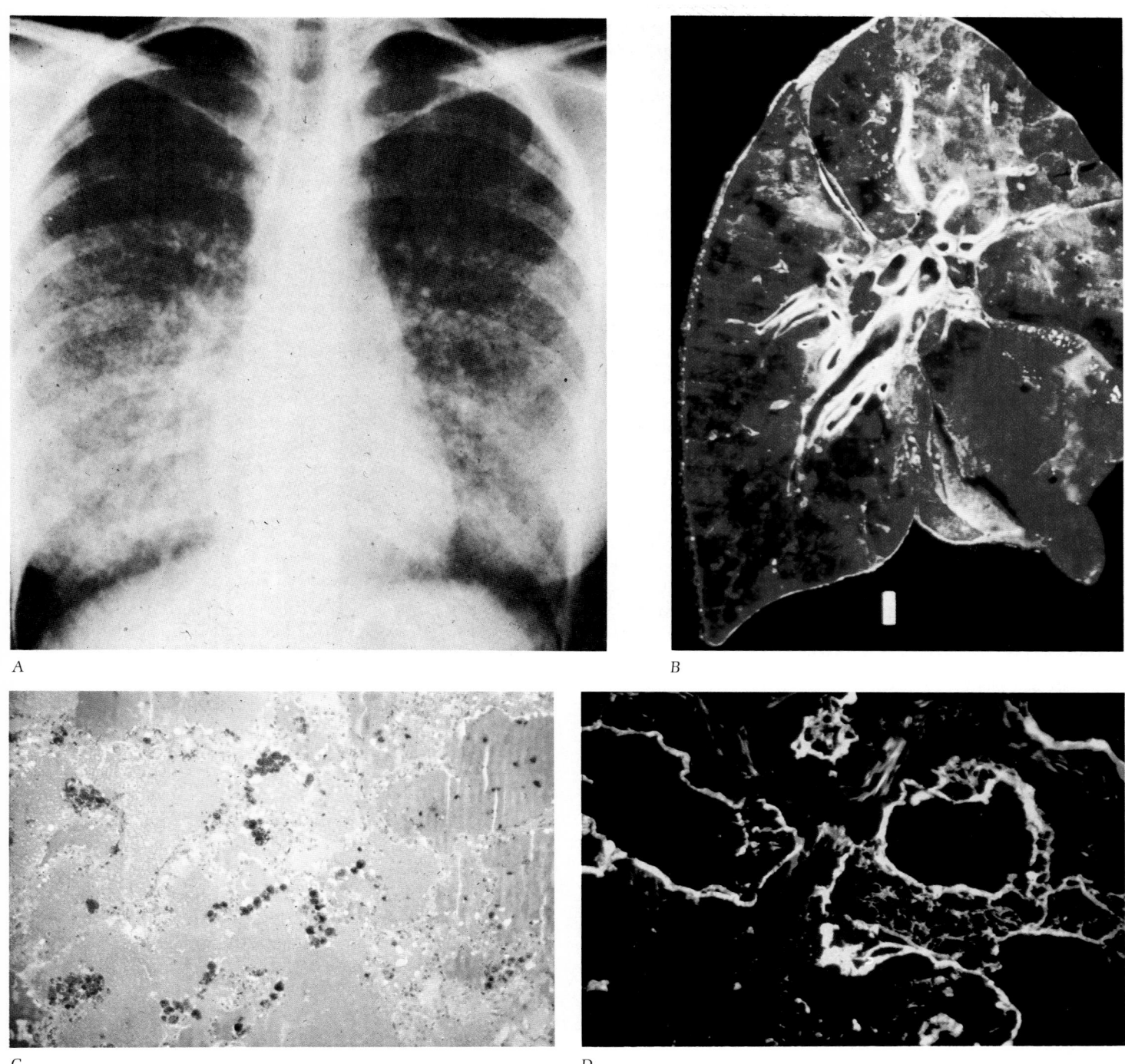

A

B

C

D

FIGURE 61-3   Goodpasture's syndrome.   A. Chest radiograph showing bilateral alveolar infiltrates, predominantly in the mid- and lower lung fields.   B. Autopsy specimen showing cut surface of lung with massive alveolar hemorrhage. *(Courtesy of Dr. Richard Garnett, Reid Memorial Hospital, Richmond, Indiana.)*   C. Photomicrograph of intact alveoli, containing both red blood cells and hemosiderin-laden macrophages. H&E, ×45.   D. Immunofluorescent demonstration of immunoglobulin lining alveolar surfaces in a uniform distribution. Fluoresceinated anti-IgG, ×113.

(97 percent) by radioimmunoassay (RIA) or by enzyme-linked immunosorbent assay (ELISA). If these studies are not immediately available, indirect immunofluorescence (using the patient's serum as the primary antibody and normal human or animal kidney as the substrate) provides a less sensitive (80 percent) but rapid and specific assay.

Even though anti-GBM antibodies are held to be the mediator of tissue damage in Goodpasture's syndrome, the reason for the appearance of the antibody is uncertain. Both pulmonary damage, leading to unmasking or alteration of pulmonary capillary basement membrane antigens, and renal damage, leading to unmasking or alteration of glomerular basement membrane antigens, have been suggested. In the latter instance, backflow of normally shed glomerular basement membrane antigen from urine into the renal interstitium might lead to the production of anti-GBM antibodies. Animal studies have shown that human anti-GBM antibodies show far greater avidity for glomerular basement membrane than for pulmonary capillary basement membrane, and usually localize only in the kidney to produce renal damage. It has been suggested that some additional co-factor or injury responsible for pulmonary localization of the antibody must be operative. Along this line, one study of the smoking history of patients with anti-GBM disease, with and without pulmonary hemorrhage, found that all patients with pulmonary hemorrhage were smokers, while most of the patients without pulmonary hemorrhage were nonsmokers. This intriguing observation remains to be corroborated.

When pulmonary hemorrhage due to Goodpasture's syndrome is life-threatening, the administration of corticosteroids intravenously in high doses and plasmapheresis to lower circulating levels of anti-GBM antibody are lifesaving. This treatment has largely replaced emergency nephrectomy. If the patient does not have advanced renal failure at the time of diagnosis, chronic immunosuppression with some combination of corticosteroids and either azathioprine or cyclophosphamide can prevent progressive renal damage. If irreversible renal failure has already occurred, the patient can eventually be successfully transplanted, once antiglomerular basement membrane antibodies have disappeared from the patient's serum. Elimination of the antibodies can be achieved by immunosuppression alone; or, in some instances, pretransplant nephrectomy may be required.

Alveolar Hemorrhage and Glomerulonephritis Not Due to Anti-GBM Antibody

Fewer than half of the patients with associated alveolar hemorrhage and glomerulonephritis manifest anti-GBM antibodies. Most of those who do *not* manifest anti-GBM antibodies do have evidence of immune complex deposition as the mediator of the tissue injury; although they may exhibit isolated pulmonary and renal disease, usually they have evidence of systemic vasculitis (see below).

The remainder show no evidence of antibody involvement and are regarded as idiopathic. Patients with immune complex-mediated disease appear to benefit from immunosuppressive therapy. This type of therapy is of unproven value in the idiopathic group.

Alveolar Hemorrhage with Systemic Vasculitis and Connective Tissue Disease Syndromes

Clinically significant alveolar hemorrhage is uncommon in multisystem disease. However, it does occur in two contexts: systemic vasculitis and the connective tissue disease syndromes. The systemic vasculitides include a number of well-defined syndromes with varying propensities for involvement of the pulmonary circulation. When the larger pulmonary vessels are involved by inflammation, focal hemorrhage is more likely to be produced. Diffuse alveolar hemorrhage usually implies inflammation of alveolar capillaries ("capillaritis") with disruption of alveolar septa. This has been interpreted by some as a form of interstitial pneumonitis and by others as a primary vascular process. Diffuse alveolar hemorrhage has been reported with both classic (medium-sized artery) polyarteritis nodosa and microscopic (hypersensitivity) polyarteritis nodosa, Churg-Strauss allergic granulomatosis, Wegener's granulomatosis, Henoch-Schönlein purpura, essential mixed cryoglobulinemia, Behçet's disease and, most frequently, necrotizing systemic vasculitis, which does not fit into any of the other recognizable categories. Particularly in the latter cases, clinical and pathologic evidence of extrapulmonary vasculitis, most often involving skin, joints, or peripheral nervous system, is essential to substantiate the diagnosis.

Diffuse alveolar hemorrhage also occurs as a rare complication of certain connective tissue disease syndromes, most often systemic lupus erythematosus, but also rheumatoid arthritis, progressive systemic sclerosis, and mixed connective tissue disease. Particularly in systemic lupus erythematosus, other causes of alveolar hemorrhage must be considered, including infection and coagulopathy. When such causes have been eliminated, alveolar hemorrhage is sometimes found to be associated with capillaritis, with interstitial pneumonitis, or with immunofluorescent or ultrastructural evidence of immune complex deposition in alveolar septa. However, none of these injuries is uniformly associated with pulmonary hemorrhage in systemic lupus erythematosus.

Toxic Alveolar Hemorrhage

At least one toxic agent has been associated with the development of alveolar hemorrhage unassociated with the development of either antiglomerular basement membrane antibody or immune complex-mediated cell injury. Workers exposed to dust or fumes containing trimellitic anhydride (a component of certain plastics, paints, and

epoxy resins) may develop acute onset of dyspnea, hemorrhage, fever, pulmonary infiltrates, and anemia due to alveolar hemorrhage. Pathologic study confirms alveolar hemorrhage without damage to basement membranes or deposits of immune complexes; there is no evidence of renal disease. Patients recover with only supportive therapy when exposure to the causative agent is arrested. Although trimellitic anhydride is known to act as a hapten, provoking antibodies which bind to human serum albumin or red blood cells conjugated with this agent, these antibodies have only been associated with acute rhinitis and asthmatic symptoms in other workers. The antibodies have not been found in the serum of patients with the pulmonary hemorrhage syndrome.

Idiopathic Pulmonary Hemosiderosis

When all the above diseases and syndromes have been excluded as likely possibilities, there still remains a small group of patients who develop recurrent diffuse alveolar hemorrhage in the absence of extrapulmonary disease and with no evidence of an immune etiology. These patients are considered to have *idiopathic pulmonary hemosiderosis*, a diagnosis of exclusion (Fig. 61-4). Clinically, the patients form a heterogeneous group with respect to the onset and course of disease which range from fulminant and fatal, to chronic relapse with eventual chronic pulmonary insufficiency due to interstitial fibrosis, to spontaneous remission with little or no residual deficit. The disease usually affects children and young adults. Pathologic examination reveals nonspecific alveolar hemorrhage without evidence of inflammation, vasculitis, or immune complex deposition. The few available ultrastructural

observations include focal disruption, smudging, or lamination of alveolar capillary basement membranes. Pathogenesis of this condition remains unknown. However, its clinical and morphologic similarity to some cases of alveolar hemorrhage of known immune pathogenesis, its occasional responsiveness to immunosuppressive therapy, its occasional association with coeliac sprue—a presumably immunologic disease of the small intestine—and its frequent association with a nonspecific elevation of serum IgA, all point to an as yet unrecognized immune pathogenesis.

DIAGNOSIS AND MANAGEMENT

When a patient presents with dyspnea that is associated with diffuse alveolar infiltrates on the chest radiograph and either hemoptysis or otherwise unexplained anemia, diffuse alveolar hemorrhage must be suspected. The exclusion of a bleeding diathesis, an extrapulmonary source of aspirated blood, a localized tracheobronchial source of bleeding such as a neoplasm, and the exclusion of necrotizing pulmonary infection, coupled with the demonstration of hemosiderin-laden macrophages in either sputum or bronchoalveolar lavage fluid, confirms the diagnosis. If respiratory impairment is life-threatening, supportive care and empiric high dose intravenous corticosteroid therapy should be initiated even before a specific diagnosis is achieved. Occupational and drug ingestion history, evaluation of renal function, including a search for proteinuria, hematuria, and azotemia, as well as a search for evidence of systemic vasculitis, an assay for serum anti-GBM antibody and other autoantibodies, clarify the etiol-

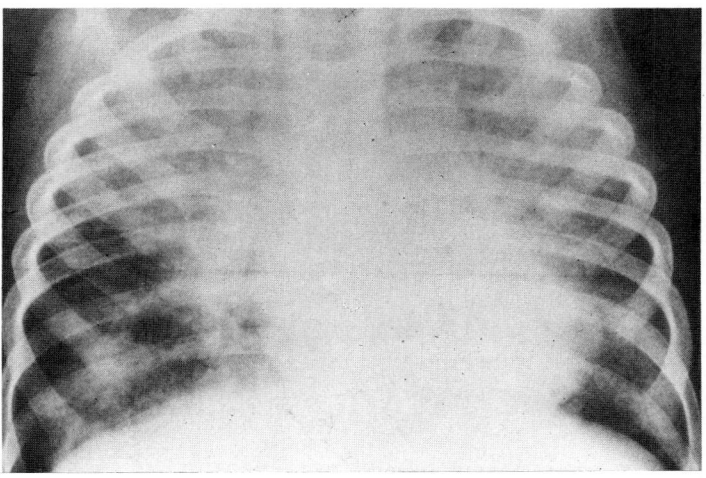

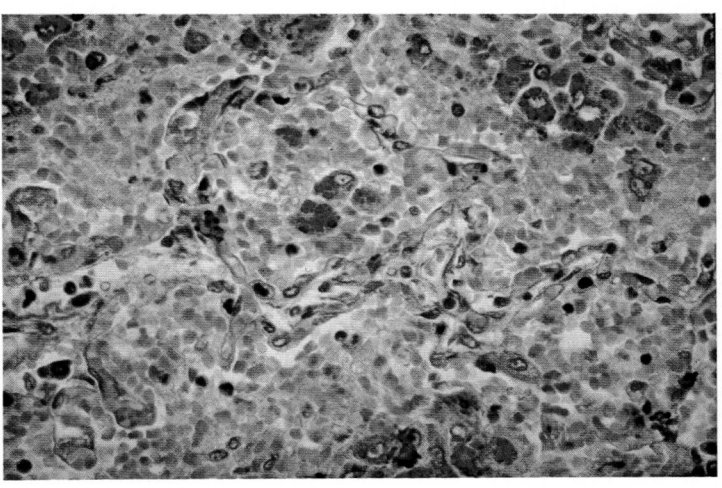

A

B

FIGURE 61-4   Idiopathic pulmonary hemosiderosis in a 21-month-old child with anemia soon after birth. Iron stain of the sputum showed hemosiderin-laden macrophages.   *A.* Chest radiograph showing extensive, bilateral, almost punctate densities throughout both lung fields, most prominent in the perihilar regions where an alveolar filling pattern appears.   *B.* Photomicrograph of lung at autopsy, showing intact alveoli containing degenerating red blood cells and hemosiderin-laden macrophages. Immunofluorescence studies for immunoglobulin and complement deposition were negative. H&E, ×131. *(Courtesy of Department of Pathology, St. Christopher's Hospital for Children, Philadelphia, Pennsylvania.)*

ogy in most patients. Transbronchial and even open lung biopsy is rarely diagnostic, except in cases of Wegener's granulomatosis. If there is evidence of renal involvement, kidney biopsy may clarify either anti-GBM or immune complex pathogenesis.

If the diagnosis proves to be Goodpasture's syndrome, the addition of plasmapheresis and cytotoxic immunosuppression may preserve renal function. If irreversible renal failure occurs, renal transplantation is still possible (see "Goodpasture's Syndrome," above). If the diagnosis proves to be some form of systemic vasculitis or connective tissue disease, immunosuppressive therapy and plasmapheresis may be needed to control pulmonary or extrapulmonary manifestations. If the diagnosis proves to be idiopathic pulmonary hemosiderosis, high dose cortico-

steroid therapy with or without plasmapheresis is useful in controlling acute bleeding, but the long-term effectiveness of these measures in preventing reoccurrence or progression of this disease is unknown.

Alveolar Microlithiasis

This rare disorder usually presents as an abnormal chest radiograph from an asymptomatic patient (Fig. 61-5). The chest radiograph is diagnostic, showing a sandlike micronodulation throughout the lung fields. This is caused by the presence of innumerable minute calcified spherules filling the alveolar spaces. The calcification is usually sufficiently dense that it can be recognized on the routine radiograph. The spherules also bind technetium

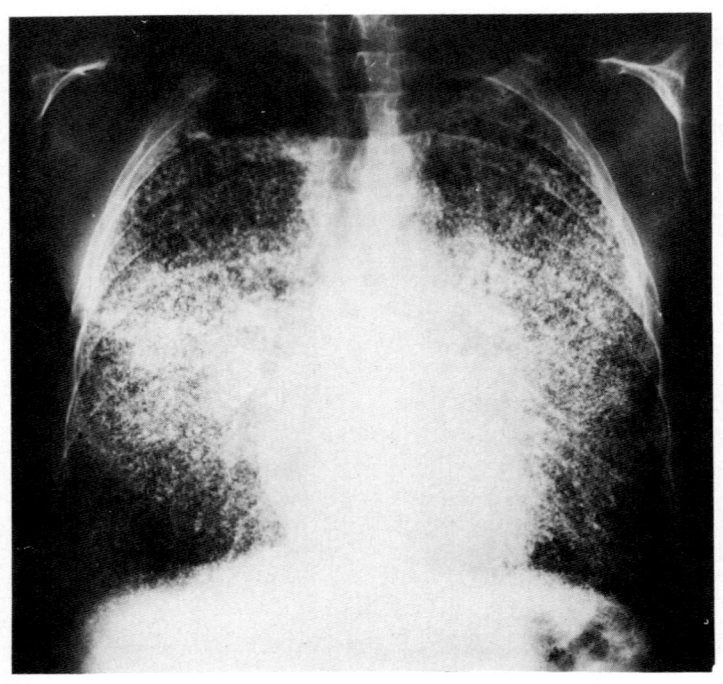

A

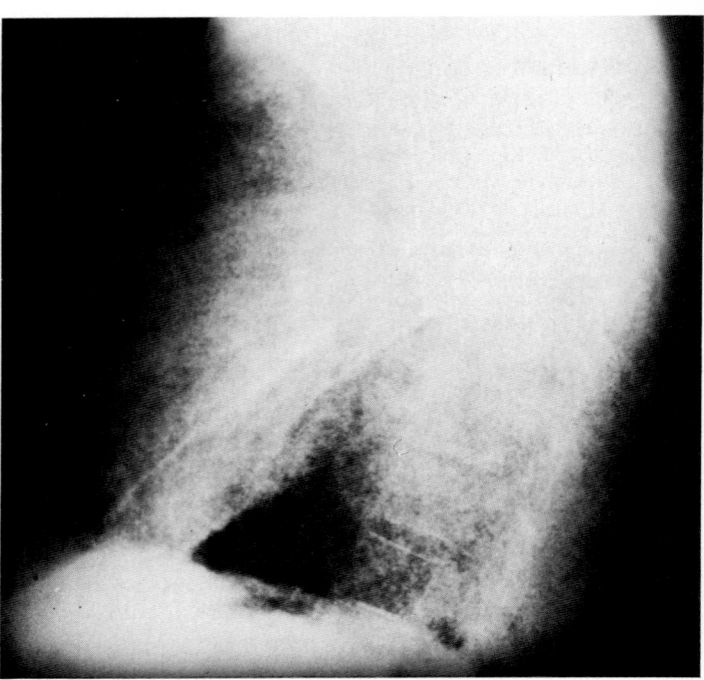

B

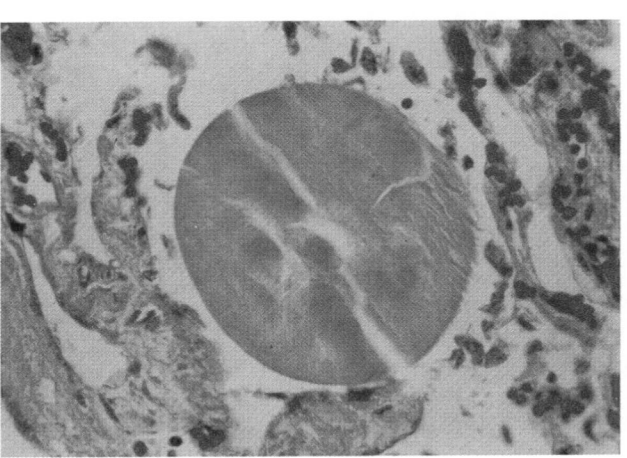

C

FIGURE 61-5 Alveolar microlithiasis in a 46-year-old man admitted for nonpulmonary problems. History included slight dyspnea on exertion and previous episodes of "pneumonia" during 1947, 1950, and 1952. Clinical examination revealed severe restrictive lung disease, pulmonary hypertension, and cor pulmonale. Diagnosis confirmed by lung biopsy. *A* and *B.* Posterior-anterior and lateral chest radiographs demonstrate innumerable, tiny calcified nodules throughout both lung fields. Thin, lucent lines on each side represent normal pleura visualized between the calcified pulmonary parenchyma and the chest wall. Emphysematous blebs in the apices displace the calcifications. *C.* Photomicrograph demonstrating a typical calcospherite in an alveolar space. H&E, ×1120.

99m, which can be a diagnostic adjunct. Although not usually required, bronchoalveolar lavage or biopsy can confirm the diagnosis. Biopsy shows the calcified spherules filling alveolar spaces. They have a concentric lamellated appearance, suggesting that they grow by the addition of successive layers. They contain both calcium and phosphorus. While the microliths are intra-alveolar, one ultrastructural study has suggested that their formation is initiated in the pulmonary interstitium by the deposition in a collagenous matrix of hydroxyapatite crystals produced by extracellular matrix vesicles. These membrane-bound vesicles are derived from mesenchymal cells and have the capacity to concentrate calcium ions and liberate phosphate from membrane phospholipids.

Although usually asymptomatic at the time of presentation, alveolar microlithiasis rarely produces functional abnormalities. When it does, the findings are restrictive pulmonary function tests or exercise-induced pulmonary hypertension. No therapy, including one attempt at therapeutic bronchoalveolar lavage, has proven effective. The etiology of this condition is unknown, but some cases appear familial.

BIBLIOGRAPHY

Albelda SM, Gefter WB, Epstein DM, Miller WT: Diffuse pulmonary hemorrhage: A review and classification. Radiology 154:289–297, 1985.
The radiographic differential diagnosis and clinicopathologic classification of the pulmonary hemorrhagic syndromes are illustrated and summarized.

Bab I, Rosenmann E, Ne'eman Z, Sela J: The occurrence of extracellular matrix vesicles in pulmonary alveolar microlithiasis. Virch Arch (Pathol Anat) 391:357–361, 1981.
Ultrastructural study of a biopsy from one patient suggests that microlith formation is initiated in the pulmonary interstitium.

Barnard NJ, Crocker PR, Blainey AD, Davies RJ, Ell SR, Levison DA: Pulmonary alveolar microlithiasis. A new analytical approach. Histopathology 11:639–645, 1987.
A case of pulmonary alveolar microlithiasis is presented in which x-ray energy spectroscopy and microscopic infrared spectroscopy were used to determine the chemical composition of the microliths.

Bestetti-Bosisio M, Cotelli F, Schiaffino E, Sorgato G, Schmid C: Lung calcification in long-term dialysed patients: A light and electron microscopic study. Histopathology 8:69–79, 1984.
Postmortem examination of 29 hemodialysed patients revealed extensive pulmonary interstitial calcification in four, but this was clinically detectable in only one patient. Ultrastructural study suggested elastic fibers serve as the initial nidus for calcium deposition.

Boyce NW, Holdsworth SR: Pulmonary manifestations of the clinical syndrome of acute glomerulonephritis and lung hemorrhage. Am J Kidney Dis 8:31–36, 1986.
The pulmonary manifestations at the time of initial diagnosis were reviewed in 45 patients with the clinical syndrome of acute glomerulonephritis and lung hemorrhage.

Brown J, Walfredo L, Felton C: Hemodynamic and pulmonary studies in pulmonary alveolar microlithiasis. Am J Med 77:176–178, 1984.
Study of one patient illustrates that compromise of the pulmonary vascular bed by this entity is associated with exercise-induced pulmonary hypertension.

Donaghy M, Rees AJ: Cigarette smoking and lung haemorrhage in glomerulonephritis caused by autoantibodies to glomerular basement membrane. Lancet 2:1390–1392, 1983.
Smoking history was obtained in 47 patients with antibasement membrane-induced glomerulonephritis: 37 of 39 patients with alveolar hemorrhage smoked, whereas 8 of 10 nonsmokers experienced no alveolar hemorrhage. These findings suggest that smoking-induced pulmonary injury is an important cofactor in producing alveolar hemorrhage due to Goodpasture's syndrome.

Ewan PW, Jones HA, Rhodes CG, Hughes JMB: Detection of intrapulmonary hemorrhage with carbon monoxide uptake. N Engl J Med 295:1391–1396, 1976.
Increased ratio of pulmonary uptake to clearance of carbon monoxide following single-breath exposure is shown to be a sensitive marker for detection of alveolar hemorrhage.

Faubert PF, Shapiro WB, Porush JG, Chou S-Y, Gross JM, Bondi E, Gomez-Leon G: Pulmonary calcification in hemodialysed patients detected by Technetium-99m diphosphonate scanning. Kidney Int 18:95–102, 1980.
Twenty-three patients on chronic hemodialysis were prospectively studied by scanning for evidence of pulmonary calcification. Fourteen patients, despite negative chest radiographs, had positive scans; half of these patients showed impaired diffusion capacity, compared to no patients with diffusion defects among those with negative scans.

Haupt HM, Moore GW, Hutchins GM: The lung in systemic lupus erythematosus. Am J Med 71:791–797, 1981.
Review of autopsies of 120 patients with systemic lupus erythematosus at Johns Hopkins Hospital revealed lupus-related pulmonary lesions in 22 patients. However, alveolar hemorrhage could be attributed directly to lupus in only two patients.

Herbert FA, Orford R: Pulmonary hemorrhage and edema due to inhalation of resins containing trimellitic anhydride. Chest 76:546–551, 1979.
Seven patients occupationally exposed to this agent developed symptomatic alveolar hemorrhage. Survey of 29 coworkers suggested five more with pulmonary problems related to trimellitic anhydride.

Hui AN, Koss MN, Hochholzer L, Wehunt WD: Amyloidosis presenting in the lower respiratory tract. Clinicopathologic, radiologic, immunohistochemical, and histochemical studies on 48 cases. Arch Pathol Lab Med 110:212–218, 1986.
A comprehensive study of 48 cases of amyloidosis localized to the lower respiratory tract.

Kisilevsky R: Amyloidosis: A familiar problem in the light of current pathogenetic developments. Lab Invest 49:381–390, 1983.
This literature review highlights common pathogenic mechanisms among the different forms of amyloidosis.

Leatherman JW, Davies SF, Hoidal JR: Alveolar hemorrhage syndromes: Diffuse microvascular lung hemorrhage in immune and idiopathic disorders. Medicine 63:343–361, 1984.
This comprehensive review of diffuse alveolar hemorrhage provides a practical diagnostic and therapeutic approach, as well as outlining the recognized clinical syndromes.

Mark EJ, Ramirez JF: Pulmonary capillaritis and hemorrhage in patients with systemic vasculitis. Arch Pathol Lab Med 109:413–418, 1985.
Pathologic study of 13 patients with extrapulmonary vasculitis of various types and extensive pulmonary hemorrhage showed inflammation and necrosis of alveolar capillaries. These findings may explain the previously reported association between interstitial pneumonitis and alveolar hemorrhage, as in some cases of systemic lupus erythematosus.

Morrison DA, Gay RG, Feldshon D, Sampliner RE: Severe pulmonary hypertension in a patient with Whipple's disease. Am J Med 79:263–267, 1985.
A patient is reported with Whipple's disease and progressive pulmonary hypertension in the absence of cardiac involvement by Whipple's.

Pitkanen P, Westermark P, Cornwell GG: Senile systemic amyloidosis. Am J Pathol 117:391–399, 1984.
Systematic autopsy study of 13 patients with senile cardiac amyloidosis, employing immunohistochemistry with antibodies against the appropriate amyloid protein, showed widespread systemic involvement. Vascular and interstitial deposition was demonstrated in the lungs of all cases studied.

Prakash UBS, Barham SS, Rosenow EC, Brown ML, Payne WS: Pulmonary alveolar microlithiasis. Mayo Clin Proc 58:290–300, 1983.
The Mayo Clinic experience with eight patients is discussed, as well as a review of the literature.

Thompson PJ, Citron KM: Amyloid and the lower respiratory tract. Thorax 38:84–87, 1983.
This literature review provides a systematic overview of both isolated pulmonary amyloidosis and pulmonary involvement in systemic amyloidosis.

Winberg CD, Rose ME, Rappaport H: Whipple's disease of the lung. Am J Med 65:873–880, 1978.
Biopsy of a symptomatic pulmonary infiltrate first led to the diagnosis of Whipple's disease in this widely cited case report.

Chapter 62

Tuberous Sclerosis and Lymphangiomyomatosis

Alfred P. Fishman

These two disorders are considered together because of the possibility that lymphangiomyomatosis is a forme fruste of tuberous sclerosis and because their pulmonary abnormalities are so strikingly similar with respect to morbid anatomy, physiological derangements, and clinical expressions.

TUBEROUS SCLEROSIS

Tuberous sclerosis (Bourneville's disease) is a rare hereditary disease which, when full-blown, is characterized by a distinctive triad of convulsive seizures, mental retardation, and adenoma sebaceum. The clinical features were recognized by von Recklinghausen in 1862, and the histologic appearance was described by Bourneville in 1880. Interest remains high in this disorder because of its uncertain etiology and pathogenesis and the many organs that it affects.

The paucity of information about the molecular and embryologic basis of tuberous sclerosis has resulted in ambiguity about how to classify it with respect to other diseases that it resembles in one aspect or another. About 50 years ago, the designation *phacomatoses* was introduced, originally to include tuberous sclerosis and neurofibromatosis and later Hippel-Lindau disease. However, in recent years, enthusiasm for this designation has waned because there is little reason to implicate a common etiology or pathogenesis for these diverse entities. Instead, the current inclination is to include tuberous sclerosis (and neurofibromatosis) in the larger category of *hamartoses*, which implicates a developmental defect in organization as the basis for the abnormal mixture of tissues. The hamartoses include the Sturge-Weber syndrome, the Peutz-Jeghers syndrome, and a variety of other genetic and sporadic disorders. Although lumped together with others that share an organizational defect, it should be stressed that tuberous sclerosis and neurofibromatosis are clinically and anatomically distinct from each other as well as from the other hamartoses.

Clinical Features

The skin lesions are a prominent diagnostic feature of tuberous sclerosis. The first lesions generally appear in childhood as hypopigmented spots over the trunk. But most distinctive are the lesions of adenoma sebaceum which generally appear in adolescence. These lesions are wartlike and distributed in a butterfly pattern over the cheeks and face. Often they are accompanied by discoloration and thickening of the lower back that resembles pigskin or sharkskin (shagreen patch). Many, but not all, patients manifest mental retardation. The range of mental retardation is broad; in some, mental slowing is barely perceptible; in others, it is severe enough to require institutionalization.

Men and women are about equally affected, and multisystem involvement is quite common. In addition to the skin and the brain abnormalities, visceral tumors of the heart, kidney, gastrointestinal tract, liver, or spleen are also common. Pulmonary involvement is uncommon in tuberous sclerosis, i.e., the lungs are affected in no more than 0.1 percent of all patients with either the full, or the incomplete, form of the disease.

Etiology

About one-half of the cases are sporadic; the others are heredofamilial. Inheritance is via a Mendelian autosomal dominant pattern.

Pathology

The lungs vary greatly in appearance from one part to another; some regions appear normal, whereas others are emphysematous and resemble a honeycomb because of innumerable cystic spaces. Small nodules (hamartomas) are scattered throughout. Where these nodules impinge on small pulmonary veins, areas of capillary congestion and telltale residua of bleeding are seen. Subpleural blebs are common and are probably the source both of pain and of pneumothorax.

A common feature is diffuse pulmonary leiomyomatosis, characterized by proliferation and hypertrophy of

smooth-muscle fibers in the walls of bronchioles and alveoli and around arterioles, capillaries, and lymphatics.

Clinical Manifestations

PULMONARY MANIFESTATIONS

Patients with pulmonary involvement are generally seen by the physician because of either spontaneous pneumothorax, hemoptysis, chest pain, or dyspnea. Patients with tuberous sclerosis in whom the lungs are involved differ in some respects from others in whom the lungs are spared (Table 62-1). More than 80 percent of patients with pulmonary lesions are women. Adenoma sebaceum is frequent (about 80 percent) in patients with pulmonary manifestations of tuberous sclerosis, but epilepsy and mental retardation are relatively uncommon (20 and 46 percent, respectively). Respiratory signs and symptoms rarely occur before 20 years of age, and the patient generally seeks medical advice at about 30 to 35 years of age.

In patients with pulmonary involvement the most common initial complaint referable to the lungs is dyspnea. In many patients, the onset of dyspnea is associated with a spontaneous pneumothorax. Pneumothorax is a complication in almost one-third of patients with pulmonary involvement. Other important presenting complaints are hemoptysis and chest pain. Cyanosis occurs only late in the disease. Pulmonary osteoarthropathy is rare.

Once pulmonary manifestations begin, they tend to progress. Most patients with pulmonary manifestations die of respiratory insufficiency within 5 years after symptoms begin. However, in some, the course is longer, i.e., up to 20 years. The most frequent cardiopulmonary causes of death are cor pulmonale and recurrent pneumothorax. Generally, pulmonary infection is a problem only late in the disease.

The radiographic appearance of the lungs is that of diffuse interstitial infiltration that is most prominent in the bases. In the early stage, the pattern is reticulonodular. As the disease progresses, the infiltrations become honeycombed. In this respect, the radiographic appearance may resemble that of histiocytosis X or of systemic sclerosis.

PULMONARY PERFORMANCE

Pulmonary function has been evaluated in only a few patients. The outstanding abnormalities are those of restrictive lung disease with progressive impairment of diffusion. In time, ventilation-perfusion abnormalities are superimposed. Obstructive disease of the airways is rarely prominent until the disease is far advanced. Hypercapnia is uncommon until the preterminal stages are reached. Pulmonary hypertension and cor pulmonale ensue as arterial hypoxemia becomes persistent, and respiratory insufficiency becomes marked.

THORACIC AND PLEURAL MANIFESTATIONS

Not only the lungs but also the chest cage and pleura may be affected.

Bony Thorax
The ribs and spine are involved in only a few patients. Dense sclerotic patches occur in bone and resemble osteoblastic metastases on the radiograph. Subperiosteal new bone formation and cystic lesions occasionally occur in the ribs.

Pleura
Chylothorax is an exceedingly uncommon complication of tuberous sclerosis with pulmonary fibrosis. In this respect, tuberous sclerosis of the lungs differs sharply from lymphangiomyomatosis (see "Lymphangiomyomatosis") in which chylothorax is common. Nonchylous pleural effusion (exudate) is rare.

Treatment

Corticosteroids have been tried in the attempt to relieve respiratory insufficiency, but to no avail.

LYMPHANGIOMYOMATOSIS (LYMPHANGIOLEIOMYOMATOSIS, LAM)

This is a rare disorder characterized by the proliferation of smooth muscle everywhere in the lungs, resulting in air-

TABLE 62-1
Some Features of Tuberous Sclerosis with and without Involvement of the Lungs

	Without Pulmonary Involvement	With Pulmonary Involvement
Age when first seen, years	<20	30–35
Presenting symptom	Central nervous disorder	Dyspnea
Male-female ratio	1:1	1:5
Mental retardation, % affected	60	40
Epilepsy, % affected	70–90	20

ways and interstitial disease, chylous effusion due to lymphatic obstruction, and recurrent pneumothoraxes. Abdominal proliferation of smooth muscle also occurs in some instances, resulting in chylous effusions when the abdominal lymphatics are affected. Because lymphangiomyomatosis has been seen only in women, generally in their childbearing years, the probability is high that the muscular proliferation is stimulated, in some way, by the sex hormones.

Clinical Features

The usual complaint is dyspnea, generally the result of a pleural effusion. About one-quarter to one-half of these patients develop spontaneous pneumothorax. Hemoptysis is somewhat less common. A few have chylous ascites which either antedates or accompanies the pleural effusion. The disease is generally progressive with repeated pleural effusions, progressive pulmonary infiltration, and honeycombing. Although most patients die within 10 years of onset of pulmonary manifestations, in some instances the disease does stabilize, apparently in response to successful surgical intervention.

The most common radiographic abnormality is pleural effusion. Often the effusion is bilateral. Thoracentesis reveals that the effusion is chylous in nature (Fig. 62-1).

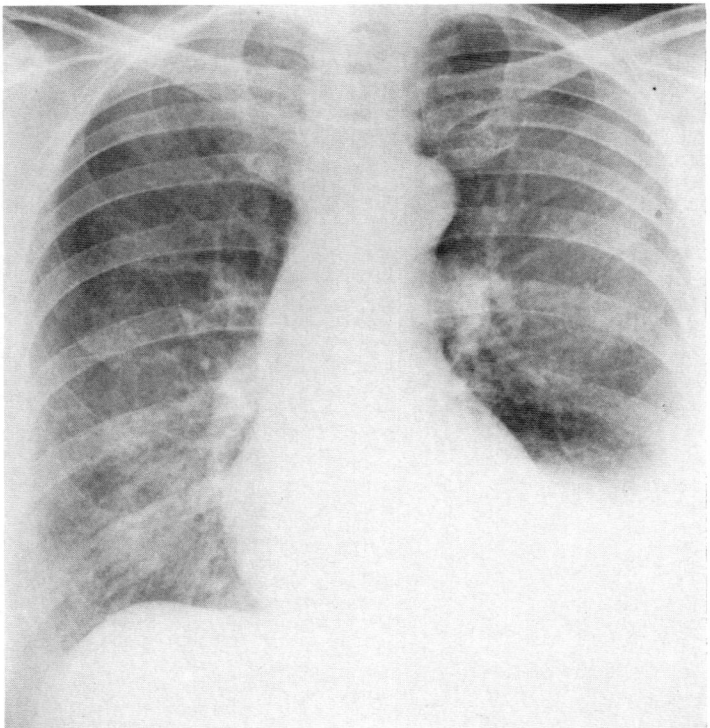

FIGURE 62-1 Chylothorax in a 69-year-old woman with lymphangiomyomatosis. Radiograph taken on admission. A chylothorax is present on the left. Same patient as case 8 in Miller, Cornog, Sullivan, 1971.

The incidence of chylous effusion approaches 80 percent in patients with lymphangiomyomatosis, a value much higher than in patients with other interstitial disorders, e.g., lupus erythematosus, rheumatoid arthritis, or asbestosis. In those who develop pneumothorax, interstitial pulmonary disease is invariably present (Fig. 62-2). The radiographic appearance is that of a fine, reticulonodular infiltrate that affects both lungs diffusely. As the disease progresses, honeycombing ensues. Lymphangiography may be useful in demonstrating the site of lymphatic obstruction and the presence of fistulous communications between paravertebral lymphatics and the pleural space.

Pathology

Nearly all pathologic observations have been made on samples of lung obtained at autopsy or open thoracotomy. Transbronchial biopsy has also been used successfully.

The fundamental abnormality in the lungs is hyperplasia of atypical smooth muscle, particularly along lymphatic channels; the hypertrophied muscle intrudes into the walls of venules and bronchioles and into some airspaces, leading to obstruction of lymphatics, small airways, and veins. Often a tumor mass forms, consisting of the same tissue as in the lungs and involving the thoracic duct. The morphologic feature of the proliferative process is a combination of bundles of atypical smooth muscle interspersed with anastomosing lymphatic channels (Fig. 62-3). Chylothorax is attributed to rupture of lymphatics in the pleura or mediastinum, or to rupture of the obstructed thoracic duct, followed by lymphatic fistulous connections with the pleural space. When ascites is present, a retroperitoneal mass of lymphangiomyomatosis tissue is found in the retroperitoneum.

Distended peribronchial and perivascular lymphatics and interstitial edema contribute to the radiographic evidence of interstitial disease. Thin-walled emphysematous spaces in association with muscular hyperplasia are responsible for a distinctive type of honeycombing (Fig. 62-4). Honeycombing is presumably the source of the pneumothoraxes. Hemoptysis stems from venoocclusive muscular hyperplasia and results in local accumulations of macrophages containing hemosiderin.

Etiology

Lymphangiomyoma is generally held to be of developmental or hamartomatous origin. Whether it is genetically linked is unknown.

Pulmonary Performance

Tests of pulmonary function are abnormal in that they reflect a combination of obstructive disease of the airways and interstitial disease of the lungs, in varying combinations. Thus, when the lungs are extensively involved, air-

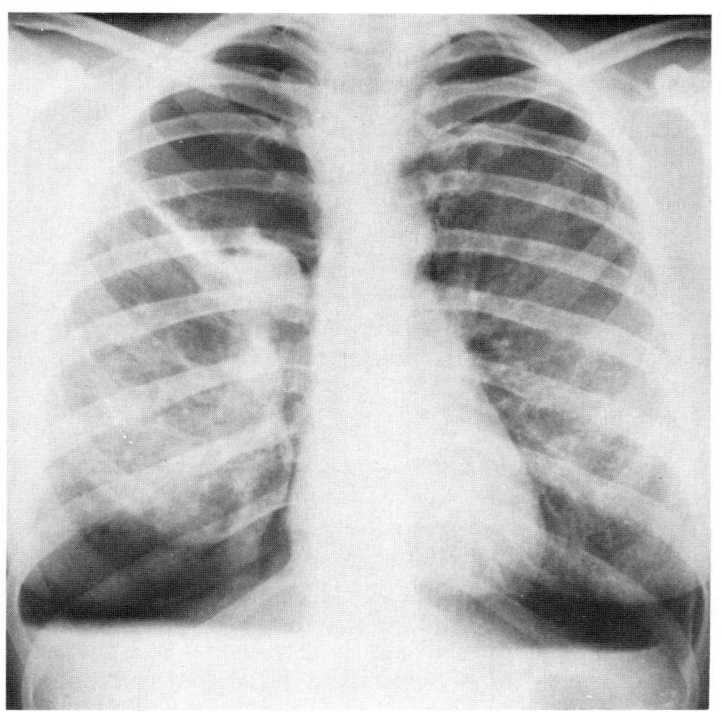

A

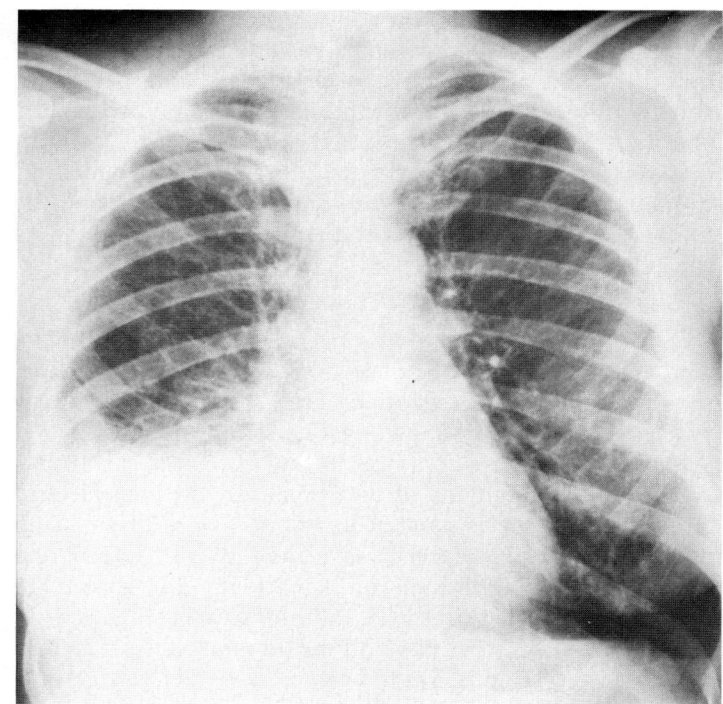

B

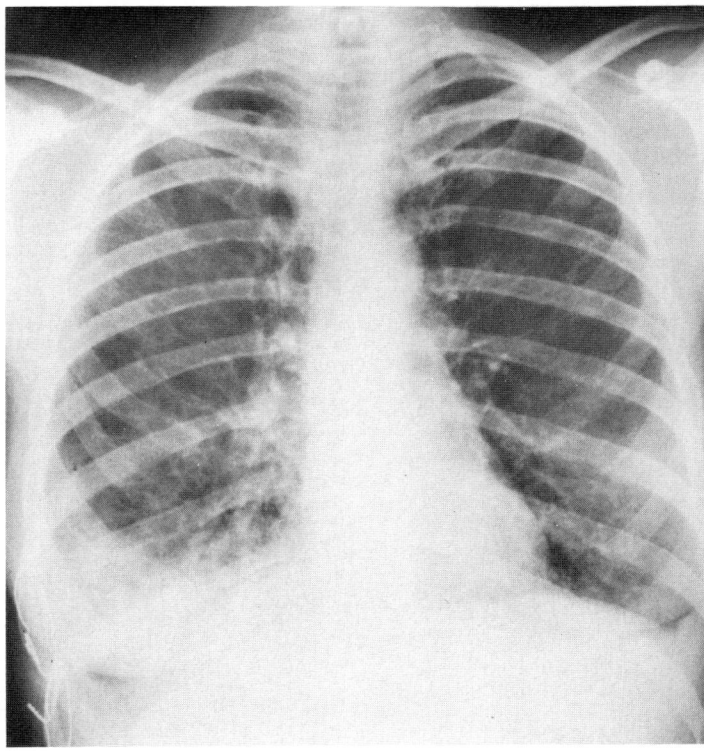

C

FIGURE 62-2 Lymphangiomyomatosis in a 56-year-old woman with retroperitoneal lymphangiomyomatosis found on exploratory laparotomy 5 years before present admission. *A.* On admission. Spontaneous bilateral pneumothoraxes. A diffuse linear interstitial infiltrate is present bilaterally. Bilateral talc poudrage performed. *B.* Three years later. Right chylous effusion. Treated by ligating thoracic duct. Biopsy from region of ligation revealed lymphangiomyoma. *C.* Three months later. Right chylous effusion considerably reduced. Reticulonodular infiltrate bilaterally. Patient subsequently developed left pleural effusion. Same patient as case 20 of Miller, Cornog, Sullivan, 1971.

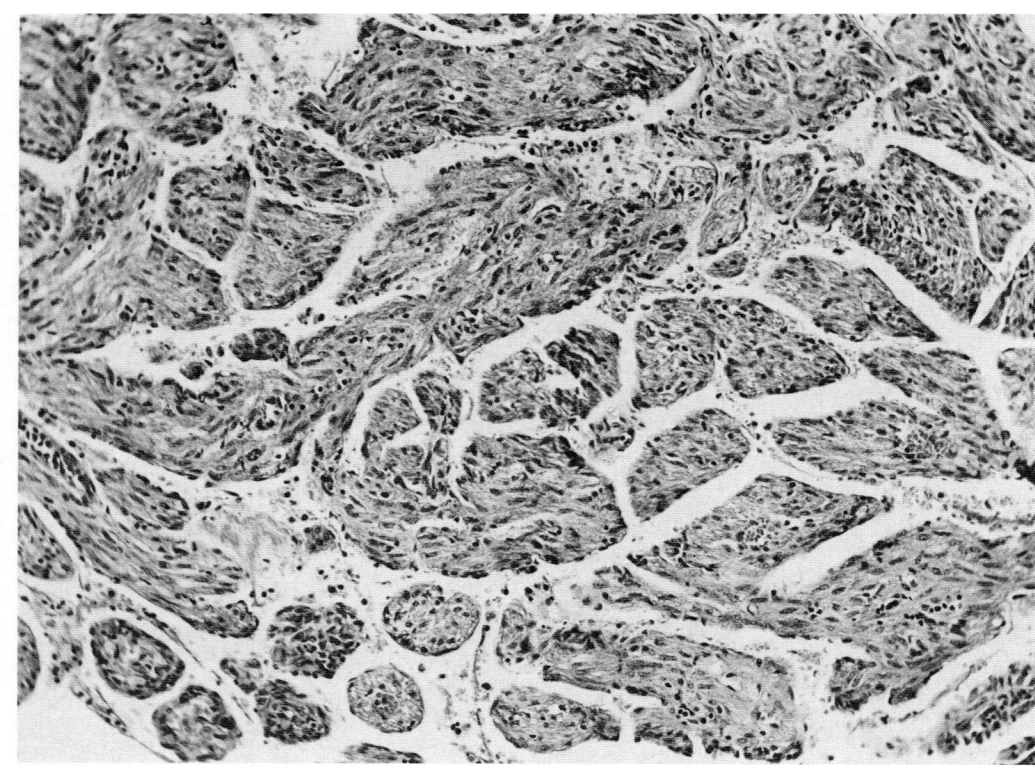

FIGURE 62-3 Histologic appearance of lymphangiomyoma. The typical picture consists of anastomosing cords of cells that enclose freely communicating, endothelial-lined channels. H&E, ×140. *(From Cornog and Enterline, 1966.)*

way resistance and forced expiratory flow are decreased, loss of elastic recoil results in high values for residual volume (RV) and functional residual capacity (FRC), the diffusing capacity is severely curtailed, and arterial hypoxemia due to ventilation blood flow inhomogeneities is marked. In time, recurrent chylothoraxes compromise pulmonary function further by adding a component of restrictive disease imposed by scarring of the visceral pleural surface. In contrast to more conventional forms of interstitial disease (sarcoidosis, scleroderma, idiopathic interstitial fibrosis), the chest radiograph and the total lung capacity (measured by body plethysmograph) are generally normal despite generalized reticulonodular interstitial disease.

Treatment

No medical management has proved to be consistently effective. The troublesome recurrence of chylothorax was once treated by ligation of the thoracic duct. This procedure has been succeeded by the use of sclerosing agents, generally tetracycline, instilled into the pleural space. In a few instances, decortication has been necessary to release a lung encased in cortical scar.

Because the disease affects predominantly women of childbearing age, attempts have been made to treat the disease by oophorectomy. Although progression of the disease appears to slow after this procedure, the functional abnormalities have persisted. A second therapeutic approach is based on the stimulatory effects of estrogens on skeletal and smooth muscle. Large doses of progesterone seemed to arrest the disease, prompting a search for estrogen and progesterone receptors in the lungs of patients with lymphangiomyomatosis and prompting the administration of progesterone when progesterone receptors have been found. In the one or two patients treated to date with progesterone after lung biopsy had shown progesterone receptors to be present, pulmonary function increased modestly, presumably owing to the antiestrogen effects of the progesterone. Based on this limited experience, the optimal therapy now seems to be the use of progesterone or tamoxifen to arrest or possibly ameliorate the pulmonary process and to control recurrent chylothorax by pleurodesis. Whether lung biopsy for progesterone and estrogen receptors will prove to be the proper guide for hormonal manipulation in lymphangiomyomatosis remains to be seen.

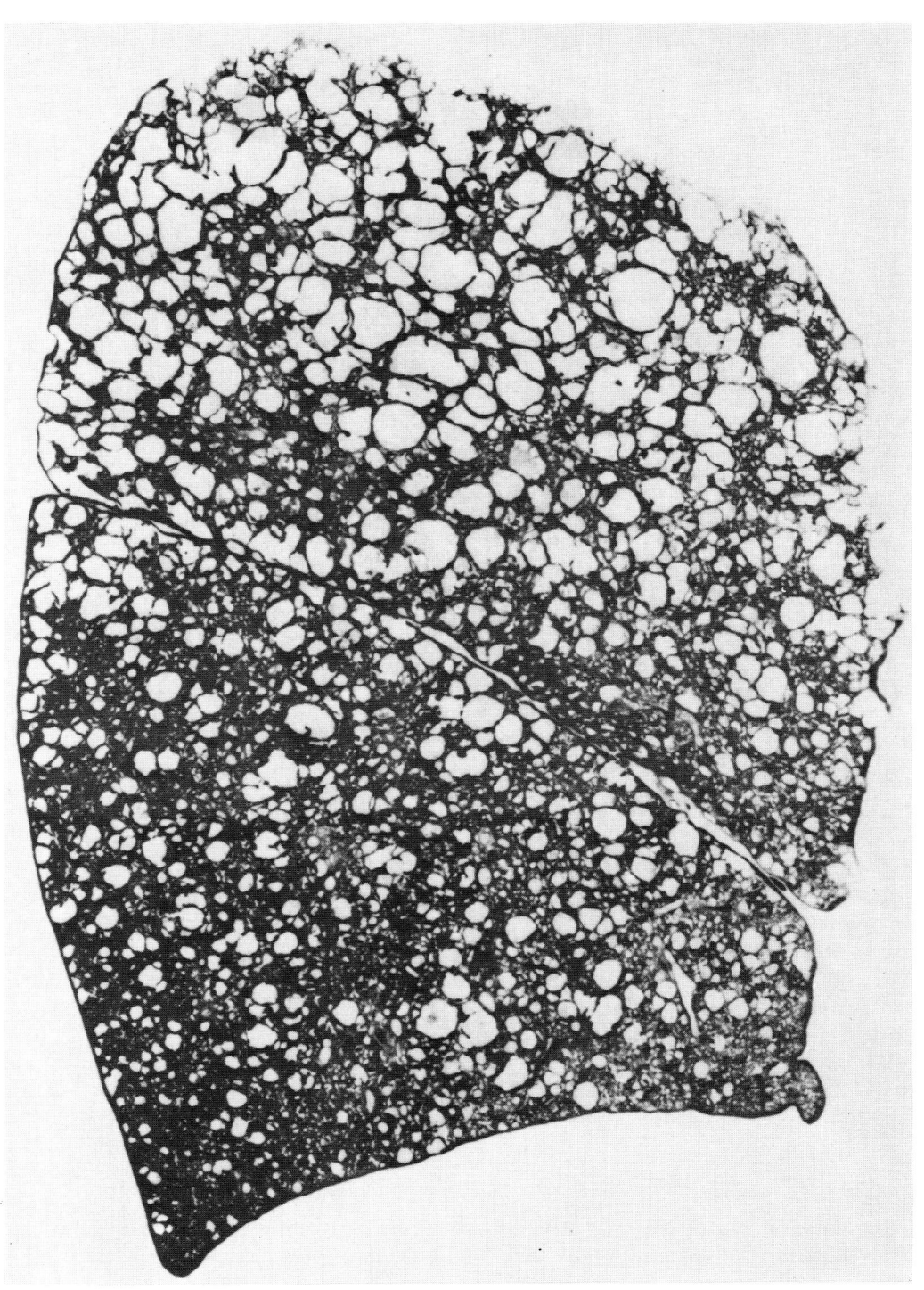

FIGURE 62-4 Lymphangiomyomatosis causing generalized honeycombing. Same patient as case 6 of Cornog and Enterline, 1966.

BIBLIOGRAPHY

Adamson D, Heinrichs WL, Raybin DM, Raffin TA: Successful treatment of pulmonary lymphangiomyomatosis with oophorectomy and progesterone. Am Rev Respir Dis 132:916–921, 1985.

A case report of successful treatment of a patient with severe pulmonary lymphangiomyomatosis by oophorectomy, large doses of progesterone (medroxyprogesterone acetate), and drainage of a chylous pleural effusion and ascites.

Aughenbaugh GL: Thoracic manifestations of neurocutaneous disease. Radiol Clin North Am 22:741–756, 1984.

A review of neurofibromatosis, tuberous sclerosis, and ataxia-telangiectasia with particular reference to their thoracic and radiographic manifestations.

Banner AS: Hormone receptors in lymphangiomyomatosis. Chest 85:3–4, 1984.

An editorial relating to a paper by Brentani et al. (Chest 85:96–99, 1984) in the same issue summarizing the need for proper preparation of biopsy material if hormonal receptors are to be detectable in tissue sections.

Carrington CB, Cugell DW, Gaensler EA, Marks A, Redding RA, Schaaf JT, Tomasian A: Lymphangioleiomyomatosis. Am Rev Respir Dis 116:977–995, 1977.

An analysis of the pathologic, physiological, and radiologic observations in six patients with lymphangiomyomatosis (lymphangioleiomyomatosis). In addition to the telltale signs of chylous effusions and repeated pneumothoraxes in women of childbearing age, the authors stress other diagnostic features of the clinical syndrome, including airflow obstruction, inordinate impairment of gas exchange, and radiographic evidence of enlarged lungs in the face of increasing prominence of interstitial markings.

Cornog JL Jr, Enterline HT: Lymphangiomyoma, a benign lesion of chylliferous lymphatics synonymous with lymphangiopericytoma. Cancer 19:1909–1930, 1966.

A review of the older literature pointing out the ambiguity in nomenclature and settling for lymphangioma. Attention is called to a possible relationship to tuberous sclerosis.

Corrin B, Liebow AA, Friedman PJ: Pulmonary lymphangiomyomatosis. Am J Pathol 79:348–382, 1975.

Pathologic, physiological, clinical, and radiologic correlations are presented on 28 women in the reproductive age group who were found at autopsy to have hyperplasia of atypical smooth muscle along the lymphatics of the lungs, thorax, and abdomen. A possible relationship between tuberous sclerosis and lymphangiomyomatosis is underscored. Chylous effusions and repeated pneumothoraxes in women of childbearing age are impressive signals of the disease.

Dishner W, Cordasco EM, Blackburn J, Demeter S, Levin H, Carey WD: Pulmonary lymphangiomyomatosis. Chest 85:796–799, 1984.

In one patient, clinical improvement occurred after treatment with progesterone even though analysis for steroid receptors was negative.

Fryer AE, Chalmers A, Connor JM, Fraser I, Povey S, Yates AD, Yates JR, Osborne JP: Evidence that the gene for tuberous sclerosis is on chromosome 9. Lancet 1:659–661, 1987.

Linkage analysis was undertaken in 19 families with tuberous sclerosis by use of 26 polymorphic markers. The findings support the assignment of the gene for tuberous sclerosis to the distal long arm of chromosome 9.

Harris JO, Waltuck BL, Swenson EW: Pathophysiology of the lungs in tuberous sclerosis: Case report and literature review. Am Rev Respir Dis 100:379–387, 1969.

A case report focusing on the pathophysiological features including airways obstruction, hyperinflation, air trapping, maldistribution of ventilation and blood flow, and pulmonary hypertension. Diffusion impairment was minimal.

Jao J, Gilbert S, Messer R: Lymphangiomyoma and tuberous sclerosis. Cancer 19:1188–1192, 1972.

A case report in which chylothorax (a prominent feature of lymphangiomyoma) occurred in a patient with the clinical features of tuberous sclerosis (mental deficiency, adenoma sebaceum, and epilepsy). Like tuberous sclerosis, lymphangioma is proposed to be a hamartomatous lesion.

Lack EE, Dolan MR, Finisio J, Grover G, Singh M, Triche TJ: Pulmonary and extrapulmonary lymphangioleiomyomatosis. Report of a case with bilateral renal angiomyolipomas, multifocal lymphangioleiomyomatosis, and a glial polyp of the endocervix. Am J Surg Pathol 10:650–657, 1986.

An extraordinary case of a 33-year-old female who had pulmonary and extrapulmonary lymphangioleiomyomatosis, bilateral renal angiomyolipomas, multifocal lymphangioleiomyomatosis involving the uterus, ovaries, periadrenal vessels, and liver. The classical stigmata of the tuberous sclerosis complex were absent. The multifocal lymphangioleiomyomatosis of the various organs described presents an extremely rare manifestation of this disorder.

Luna CM, Gene R, Jolly EC, Nahmod N, Defranchi HA, Patino G, Elsner B: Pulmonary lymphangiomyomatosis associated with tuberous sclerosis. Treatment with tamoxifen and tetracycline-pleurodesis. Chest 88:473–475, 1985.

    In a patient with both lymphangiomyomatosis and tuberous sclerosis, open lung biopsy provided evidence of steroid receptors for estrogen. Downhill course was arrested by treatment with tamoxifen (and tetracycline pleurodesis for chylothorax).

Malik SK, Pardee N, Martin CJ: Involvement of the lungs in tuberous sclerosis. Chest 58:538–540, 1970.

    A case report of a patient with classic systemic evidence of tuberous sclerosis with radiographic evidence of pulmonary involvement for 19 years. In contrast to report of Harris, Waltuck, Swenson, 1969, progressive diffusion difficulty was a prominent feature.

Milledge RD, Gerald BE, Carter WJ: Pulmonary manifestations of tuberous sclerosis. Am J Roentgenol Radium Ther Nucl Med 98:734–748, 1966.

    A case report, including autopsy findings, of a patient with the typical clinical, radiographic, and pathologic features of tuberous sclerosis.

Miller WT, Cornog JL Jr, Sullivan MA: Lymphangiomyomatosis. A clinical-roentgenologic-pathologic syndrome. Am J Roentgenol Radium Ther Nucl Med 111:565–572, 1971.

    A review of seven patients with lymphangiomyomatosis stressing the radiographic features. The diagnostic value of interstitial lung disease coupled with chylous pleural effusion is underscored.

Moolten SE: Hamartial nature of the tuberous sclerosis complex and its bearing on the tumor problem. Arch Intern Med 69:589–623, 1942.

    Based on a case study, similarities are noted between tuberous sclerosis and a variety of hamartomatous disorders.

Shen A, Iseman MD, Waldron JA, King TE: Exacerbation of pulmonary lymphangioleiomyomatosis by exogenous estrogens. Chest 91:782–785, 1987.

    Estrogen therapy for osteoporosis caused marked deterioration of the pulmonary lymphangioleiomyomatosis.

Part 9

Pulmonary Circulatory Disorders

Chapter 63
The Normal Pulmonary Circulation

The pulmonary circulation is trapped between the two ventricles: at the mercy of the right ventricle at one end and dependent on left ventricular performance at the other. Moreover, the pulmonary circulation is part of the woof and warp of the lungs (Fig. 63-1), strongly influenced by pressures generated at the pleural surfaces; the pleural pressures are transmitted, via the parenchyma, to the consecutive pulmonary vascular segments, affecting some more than others and even, in a few instances, e.g., the extra-alveolar vessels, oppositely. The effectiveness of the transmitted pressures is greatly enhanced by the intrinsic properties and design of the pulmonary circulation: high distensibility, low resistance, and a built-in reserve of recruitable vessels in the uppermost portions of the lungs should the need arise, e.g., as during exercise.

There are passive influences. And, as a rule, they dominate control of the normal pulmonary circulation. This is in strong contrast to the systemic circulation where baroreceptor mechanisms, the autonomic nervous system, and neurohumoral substances hold sway. Instead, control of the pulmonary circulation is vested primarily in the same gases, i.e., O_2 and CO_2, that the lungs were designed to exchange with the external environment. This is not to say that the pulmonary circulation lacks nerves or is not involved with neurohumoral mediators. Indeed, the enormous endothelial expanse of the lungs is almost continuously engaged either in generating or processing biologically active substances. But, when all is said and done, these substances exert little vasomotor influence on the pulmonary circulation, particularly with respect to gas exchange. For example, prostacyclin, a powerful vasodilator, does more to keep initial tone low, i.e., to keep the overall pulmonary circulation vasodilated, than to adjust blood flow to ventilation for the sake of external gas exchange.

PULMONARY HEMODYNAMICS

Common practice in dealing with the pulmonary circulation is to consider its behavior solely in terms of "changes in (calculated) resistance" without taking into account levels of pressure and flow.

This approach overlooks the fact that the relationship between driving pressure ($\bar{P}pa - \bar{P}la$) and pulmonary blood flow ($\dot{Q}t$) is curvilinear, making it difficult to interpret a change in calculated resistance when hemody-

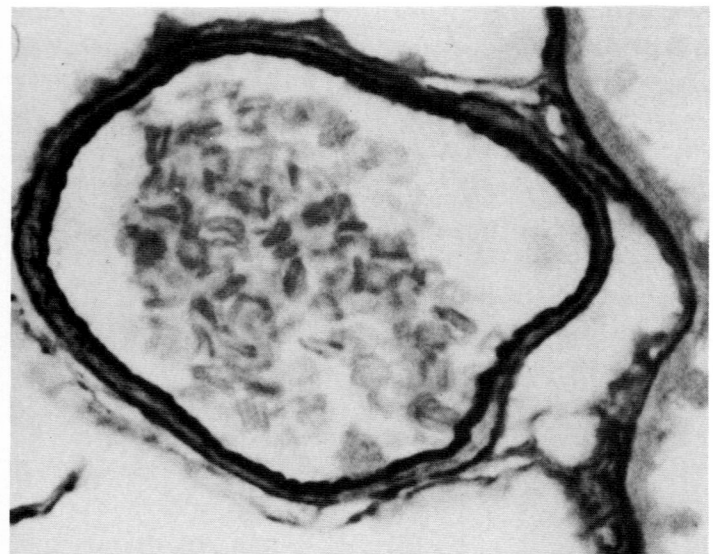

FIGURE 63-1 Muscular pulmonary artery in the rat illustrating the tethering role of the parenchyma surrounding it. Elastic Van Gieson's stain (×1040). (Courtesy of Dr. J. M. Kay.)

namic conditions are changing. Moreover, the common expedient of ignoring left pressure, as during exercise when the catheter tip tends to dislodge, renders the value for calculated resistance meaningless in physical terms. In the sections that follow, each factor in the resistance equation is assessed separately.

Pulmonary Blood Flow (and Oxygen Delivery)

Averaged over several respiratory cycles, the outputs of the two ventricles are approximately the same; although the output of the left ventricle is slightly greater than that of the right ventricle because of the admixture of bronchial venous to pulmonary venous blood, this "anatomic venous admixture" is about 1 to 2 percent of the total left ventricular output.

In humans, the cardiac output is generally determined by some application of the indicator-dilution or Fick principles. For both, reliable determinations require a steady state; the time required to achieve a steady state is generally shorter for the indicator-dilution techniques. Also, in practice, indicator-dilution techniques are easier to apply. As a result, indicator-dilution techniques are quite popular. However, the indicator-dilution technique is not as reliable as the Fick technique unless carefully done, and it is apt to be misleading when cardiac output is low, e.g., as in heart failure. Other techniques for determining the cardiac output, such as those designed to determine pulmonary capillary blood flow, are neither easy to perform nor reliable.

In the steady state, cardiac output is matched to metabolic rate: cardiac output ($\dot{Q}$T) increases by 600 to 800 ml/min per 10-ml increase in oxygen uptake ($\Delta\dot{V}_{O_2}$); during heart failure, $\Delta\dot{Q}$T/$\dot{V}_{O_2}$, falls below normal.

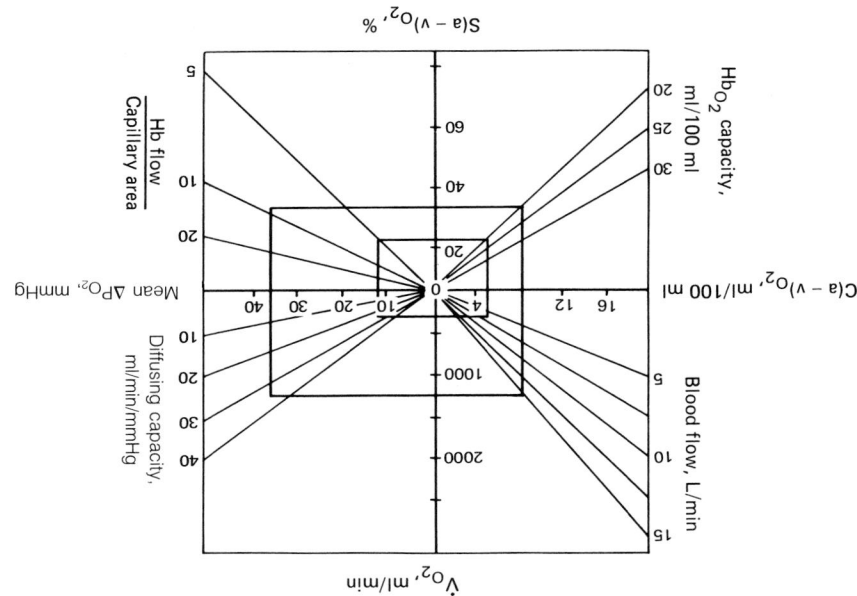

FIGURE 63-2 The Morgan-Murray diagram illustrating the respiratory and circulatory adaptations to changing metabolic needs ($\dot{V}_{O_2}$). Two rectangles are shown, one during exercise (outer rectangle) and the other for conditions at rest (inner rectangle). At rest, $\dot{V}_{O_2}$ = 250 ml/min; during exercise, it increased to 1250 ml/min. Ca_{O_2} = concentration of O_2 in arterial blood; Cv_{O_2} = concentration of O_2 in venous blood; Hb = hemoglobin; Hb_{O_2} = O_2 capacity of hemoglobin; Sa_{O_2} = arterial O_2 saturation; Sv_{O_2} = venous O_2 saturation. (Adapted from Barcroft: Features in the Architecture of Physiologic Function, New York, Hafner, 1972, pp 187–215.)

The primary mission of the coordinated interplay among the respiration, circulation, and blood is to deliver oxygen to tissues and organs in accord with their metabolic needs (Fig. 63-2) and to carry off the carbon dioxide that they generate in the course of metabolism. *Oxygen delivery* is defined as the product of cardiac output and the arterial O_2 content ($\dot{Q}$T × Ca_{O_2}): an increase in O_2 requirement by the tissues, e.g., as during exercise, is ordinarily met either by increasing the cardiac output, widening the arteriovenous O_2 difference, or both. In contrast to the roughly linear relation between oxygen uptake and cardiac output during exercise, the relation between oxygen uptake and the arteriovenous oxygen difference is hyperbolic. The relative contribution of an increase in cardiac output and a widening of the arteriovenous oxygen difference to satisfying the tissue requirements for oxygen depends on how the increase in metabolism is induced, e.g., either by exercise, increase in body temperature, hormones, or drugs.

Polycythemia enhances O_2 delivery by increasing the O_2-carrying capacity of the blood; but, if the increase becomes excessive, complications induced by an increase in red cell mass tend to nullify the advantages of polycythemia for gas exchange. In states of low cardiac output or arterial hypoxemia, O_2 delivery can be enhanced by increasing the oxygen content of arterial blood, e.g., by breathing O_2-enriched inspired air or by mechanical ventilation.

CARDIAC OUTPUT AT REST AND DURING EXERCISE

In order to compare values obtained from individuals of different dimensions, cardiac output is generally expressed in terms of body surface area, i.e., as cardiac

index. In normal adults, lying quietly at rest, supine and in the postprandial state, the cardiac index averages about 3.12 L/min/m² (SD ± 0.40). The corresponding oxygen uptake is 138 ml/min/m² (SD ± 14). Depending on its type and severity, exercise evokes a series of adaptive responses in the respiration, circulation, and metabolism. Part of this integrated response of the respiratory apparatus is an increase in pulmonary blood flow (Fig. 63-2). But, without concomitant changes in the other parameters shown in Fig. 63-1, O_2 delivery would fall short of metabolic need. As a rule, a modest increase in flow elicits a barely perceptible increase in pulmonary arterial pressure, as reserve vessels are recruited to serve as conduits and as open vessels are dilated by the slight increments in transmural pressures.

In unanesthetized human subjects, the treadmill and bicycle ergometer are the conventional devices for achieving calibrated and reproducible levels of exercise. The hemodynamic effects of anxiety, caused by unfamiliarity with the procedure, may dominate the response, not only at rest but during moderate exercise. For this reason, values of $\dot{V}_{O_2}$ at rest are often lower *after* exercise than *before*, i.e., after the threat of the unknown is gone. Quantification of the level of exercise is accomplished either by determining oxygen uptake or by assessing the work load. Tachycardia and the respiratory exchange ratio are often more reliable indices of anxiety than are clinical signs and symptoms.

INTRAPULMONARY DISTRIBUTION OF THE CARDIAC OUTPUT

Matching of blood flow ($\dot{Q}$) to alveolar ventilation ($\dot{V}_A$) is a prime prerequisite for efficiency in gas exchange. Some of the stimuli for local rearrangement of blood flow, e.g., hypoxia, are considered subsequently in this chapter. Other influences relating to $\dot{V}_A/\dot{Q}$ adjustments are considered in a separate chapter (Chapter 13).

Pulmonary Vascular Pressures

As a practical measure, intravascular and intracardiac pressures are generally referred to atmospheric, taking care to eliminate any hydrostatic pressure difference between the intrathoracic site of pressure recording and the external transducer. External landmarks are used to set this "zero hydrostatic level"; most popular is a level 5 cm below the angle of Louis or 10 to 12 cm above the tabletop. Although the use of different reference levels does complicate comparison of data from different laboratories, each serves equally well for comparative measurements in the same individual.

PULMONARY ARTERIAL PRESSURES

Ordinarily, the mean pulmonary arterial pressure is about 10 to 12 mmHg, i.e., of the order of one-eighth of that in the systemic circulation. During systole, pulmonary arterial pressure increases abruptly from diastolic values of 5 to 10 mmHg to 20 to 30 mmHg. Aging is associated with a slight increase in pulmonary arterial pressures.

In contour, the pulmonary arterial pressure resembles that recorded at the root of the aorta (Fig. 63-3). Full-bodied pulmonary arterial curves are more apt to be recorded in pulmonary hypertensive states than when pressures are normotensive; distorting mechanical influences often deform contours markedly when pulmonary arterial pressures are normal or near normal.

PULMONARY CAPILLARY PRESSURES

The pulmonary capillaries are interpolated between pulmonary arterioles and venules in a complicated maze that works remarkably well for gas and water exchange at the expense of accessibility. As a result, direct determinations of pulmonary capillary pressures are not available. Instead, *microcirculatory* pressures (in arterioles, capillaries, and venules) are generally estimated either by determining the left atrial pressure indirectly as the *pulmonary wedge* pressure or by assuming that the microcirculatory, or capillary, pressure is intermediate between the mean pulmonary arterial and the pulmonary wedge pressures.

PULMONARY ARTERIOVENOUS PRESSURE DIFFERENCES

The drop in mean pressure between the pulmonary artery and left atrium is small, of the order of 10 mmHg, i.e., about one-eighth of the pressure drop across the systemic circulation (Fig. 63-4). No consensus yet exists about where most of the pressure drop occurs, i.e., precapillary, capillary, or postcapillary vessels. Micropuncture of subpleural vessels suggests that most of the drop occurs in the pulmonary capillaries. Most of the other studies favor pre- and postcapillary segments about equally. One way to

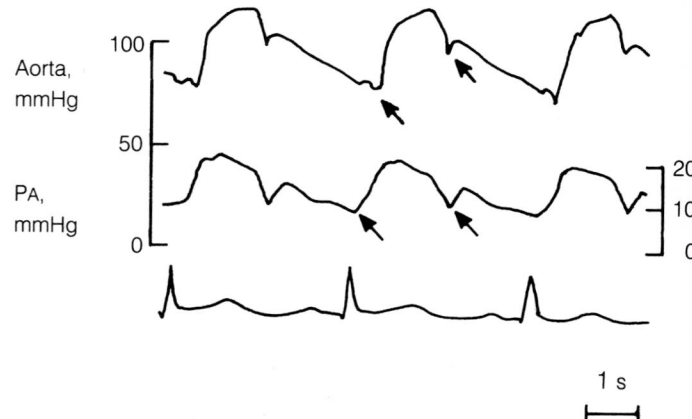

FIGURE 63-3 Simultaneous pressures recorded directly from the root of the aorta and main pulmonary artery (PA) in a human subject. (*Adapted from Fishman: in Hamilton WF, Dow P (eds), Handbook of Physiology, sec 2: Circulation, vol II, Washington DC, American Physiological Society, 1963.*)

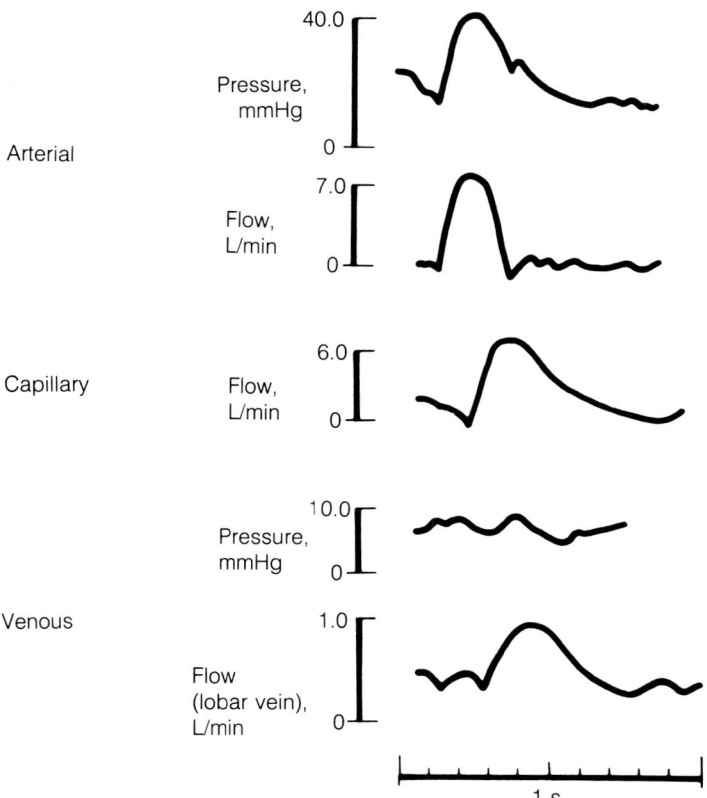

FIGURE 63-4 Schematic representation of pulsatile pressures and flows in consecutive segments of the pulmonary vasculature. Pressure contours between the pulmonary artery and vein undergo considerable transformation so that the pulmonary venous pressure resembles closely the left atrial pressure. In contrast, flow surges ahead under the impulse of the right ventricle retaining its pulsatile contour in the pulmonary veins. *(From Wiener, Morkin, Skalak, Fishman: Circ Res 19:834–850, 1966.)*

account for discrepancies in results is to blame them on the different techniques and preparations. In any event, it is important to recall that, in the normal pulmonary circulation, the pressure drop under scrutiny is small, that artifacts and extraneous influences readily assume inordinate proportions in the low-pressure pulmonary circulation, and that structures comparable to systemic arterioles do not exist. Clearly, these pressure differences assume different proportions and meanings in the hypertensive pulmonary circulation.

LEFT ATRIAL AND PULMONARY WEDGE PRESSURES

In intact unanesthetized humans, the mean left artrial pressure is about 5 to 10 mmHg. During a single respiratory cycle, swings in pressure occur of the order of 3 to 12 mmHg. Because the left atrium is relatively inaccessible in the intact human, pulmonary wedge pressures are generally used as a substitute.

The pulmonary arterial wedge pressure (Pw) is recorded by advancing a cardiac catheter through the right side of the heart and pulmonary arterial tree until it is impacted in a small precapillary vessel. By this procedure, a direct conduit is formed between the catheter lumen, the wedged vessel (usually an artery of the order of 1500 to 3000 Å), the distal pulmonary capillary bed, and the pulmonary veins. The wedged catheter then provides a measure of pressure in the first venous tributary that is open beyond the obstruction; this is also a fairly accurate measure of left atrial pressure as long as the vessels between the wedged catheter and left atrium are open.

Commonly used as an alternative practical approach to estimating left atrial pressure is the inflation of a balloon in one pulmonary artery so that pressures can be recorded distal to the occlusive balloon (Fig. 63-5). The tracing obtained in this way resembles that of the pulmonary arterial wedge pressure.

Various criteria have been advanced to guarantee that a value obtained for Pw is a reliable measure of mean left atrial pressure: Pw less than mean pulmonary arterial and diastolic pressures; fully oxygenated blood withdrawn from the impacted catheter; the characteristic snap of the catheter as it is withdrawn from the wedge position; and

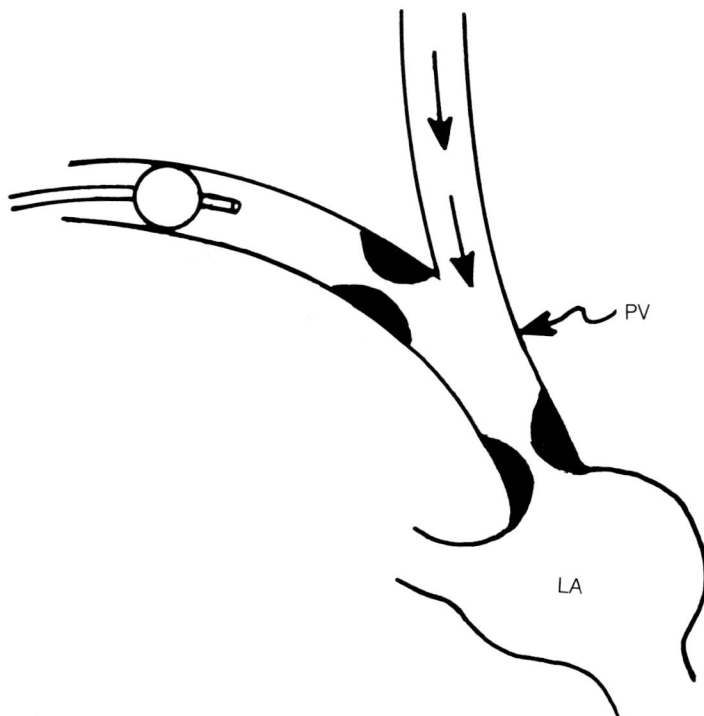

FIGURE 63-5 Meaning of pressure determined distal to an occlusive balloon. After the balloon is inflated, the pressure recorded is that which exists at the conjunction of flowing streams (two arrows) and the static pool beyond the occlusive balloon. Narrowing of pulmonary venule (PV) distal to the occlusive balloon, as by venoconstriction, does not affect the use of the postballoon pressure (or pulmonary wedge pressure) as a measure of left atrial pressure unless obstruction ensues that closes the channel to the left atrium (LA). *(Adapted from Marini: Respiratory Medicine and Intensive Care, Baltimore, Williams & Wilkins, 1981.)*

the distinctive configuration of the wedge tracing. Unfortunately, even when all criteria are met, the Pw may fail to provide a measure of mean left atrial pressure if the catheter fails to be wedged properly or if the tip is wedged in an area where alveolar pressure exceeds pulmonary venous pressure (see subsequent section, "Zones of the Lungs"), or if pulmonary arterial vessels between the catheter tip and the left atrium are occluded, or if the airways and/or the parenchyma of the intervening lung are sufficiently abnormal to generate abnormal perivascular pressures, e.g., by fibrosis or obstructive airways disease.

In brief, when used critically, the pulmonary arterial wedge pressure, or the balloon-occlusion pressure, usually provides a reliable measure of the mean left atrial pressure. However, it cannot be used to determine the *pulmonary capillary pressure*, i.e., the mean luminal pressure in the alveolar capillaries.

TRANSMURAL VERSUS LUMINAL PRESSURES

During each respiratory cycle, all intrathoracic vessels are affected to some extent by the swings in pleural pressure. The pressure that determines the calibers of the vessels is the *transmural pressure*. For the alveolar capillaries, this pressure is calculated as the difference between the luminal pressure in the pulmonary capillaries and the alveolar pressure; for the other pulmonary vessels, the transluminal pressure is determined as the difference between luminal and pleural pressure. The substitution of pleural pressure for perivascular pressure has drawbacks: not only is pleural pressure difficult to measure, but transmission is complex and other forces, such as alveolar surface tension, exert ill-defined effects. In practice, esophageal pressure is generally used as a measure of pleural pressure, and pleural pressure is regarded as equivalent to perivascular pressure.

Whether blood pressure in the pulmonary circulation is referred to atmospheric or to pleural pressure depends on the use to which the results are to be put: the *transmural pressure* described above provides a measure of *distending pressure*; in contrast, for the calculation of pulmonary vascular resistance, blood pressures referred to atmosphere are needed. Also, for the meaningful calculation of pulmonary vascular resistance, left atrial pressure must exceed alveolar pressure, i.e., zone 3 conditions (see below) must be operative.

Pulmonary Blood Volume

In normal humans, the pulmonary blood volume is about 10 percent of the total circulating blood volume. As a rule, it is measured by a variant of the indicator-dilution principle. In the hypothetical human adult male weighing 70 kg, this value is of the order of 400 to 500 ml. This volume is of interest on several pathophysiological accounts: (1) as a determinant of the mechanical behavior of the lungs, (2)

as a reservoir that provides the preload for the left ventricle, (3) as a supply of hemoglobin for alveolar-capillary gas exchange, (4) as a source of water and macromolecules that engage in alveolar-capillary exchange, (5) as a potential mechanism for increasing pulmonary capillary pressures and promoting pulmonary edema, and (6) as a potential mechanism for evoking dyspnea.

CHANGES IN PULMONARY BLOOD VOLUME

Changes in pulmonary blood volume are at the expense of the air volumes. Thus, the vital capacity decreases in acute pulmonary congestion. The pulmonary blood volume varies with body position: it increases when the individual lies down and decreases when the individual stands; it is readily enlarged by intravenous infusions, by immersing the body in water, by inflation of an anti-gravity suit, by negative pressure breathing, and by displacement of blood from the systemic circulation, e.g., as during systemic vasoconstriction. Conversely, the pulmonary blood volume decreases when the individual stands on his (or her) head, after a large venesection, i.e., one that decreases cardiac output, during positive pressure breathing or the Valsalva maneuver, and during systemic vasodilatation.

PARTITION OF THE PULMONARY BLOOD VOLUME

In normal individuals, the pulmonary blood volume appears to be subdivided equally among the pulmonary arteries, capillaries, and veins. In the hypothetical 70-kg man, the pulmonary capillary blood volume can only be estimated: values range from 100 to 200 ml, depending on the method. Upon sitting up, the pulmonary capillary blood volume shares in the overall decrease in pulmonary blood volume; during exercise, as cardiac output goes up, pulmonary capillary blood volume also increases. More of the increase in volume is accomplished by recruiting new capillaries from the reserve than by dilating open vessels. As capillary blood volume enlarges due to recruitment and dilation, the endothelial surface area gas and fluid exchanges enlarge correspondingly.

Pulmonary Vascular Resistance

The term "resistance" is generally used as a measure of the hindrance offered by a vascular bed to the flow of blood through it. In the normal pulmonary circulation, an increase in cardiac output or in pulmonary arterial pressure decreases pulmonary vascular resistance (Fig. 63-6). The decrease is not linear; the pattern of change depends on the vasomotor tone that exists before exercise begins ("initial tone") and on the levels of blood pressures and flow achieved during exercise.

For normal adult lungs, in which the pulmonary circulation is almost maximally dilated, there is no consen-

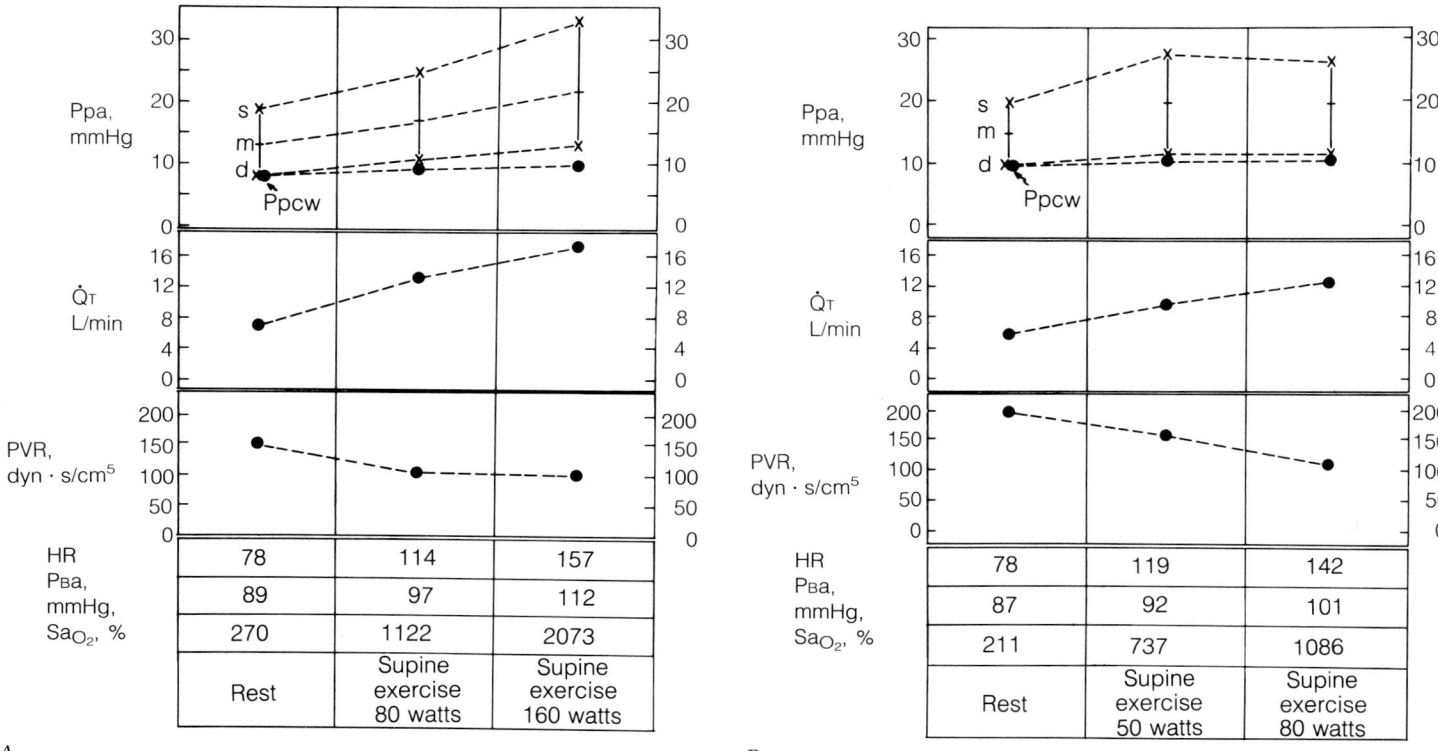

FIGURE 63-6 Pulmonary hemodynamics at rest and during steady-state supine exercise in humans. *A.* Normal males (mean values), average age 23.6 ± 2.1. *B.* Normal females (mean values), average age 23.8 ± 3.9. P$_{Ba}$ = brachial arterial pressure; Q̇$_T$ = cardiac output; d = diastolic pressure; HR = heart rate; m = mean pressure; Ppa = pulmonary arterial pressure; Ppcw = pulmonary capillary wedge pressure; PVR = pulmonary vascular resistance; s = systolic pressure. *(Adapted from Gurtner, Walser, Fässler: Prog Resp Res 9:295–315, 1975.)*

sus about the relative contributions of precapillaries, capillaries, and venules to overall resistance. Indeed, in this relaxed system of consecutive branching tubes, it may well be that the capillaries and venules offer most of the resistance to blood flow. But the small muscular arteries (100 to 1000 μm) and arterioles (<100 μm) are the only vessels that seem capable of appreciable vasoconstriction. Consequently, these precapillary vessels are generally referred to as *resistance vessels* and pictured, by remote analogy, as the principal sites of pulmonary vasomotor activity. That other contractile elements, such as perivascular contractile cells, ever feature prominently in actively changing pulmonary vascular resistance is a remote possibility.

DETERMINATION OF PULMONARY VASCULAR RESISTANCE

Different approaches have been used to detect changes in pulmonary vascular resistance. Physiologists advocate comparisons of the slopes and intercepts of pressure-flow curves as the most meaningful approach. Unfortunately, the many serial measurements needed to construct these curves are not easy to obtain in intact humans.

Instead, clinicians continue to rely heavily on values for pulmonary vascular resistance that are based on the following formula:

$$R = \frac{\overline{Ppa} - \overline{Ppv}}{\dot{Q}}$$

where

R = pulmonary vascular resistance, either R units or dyn · s/cm^5

$\overline{Ppa} - \overline{Ppv}$ = drop in mean pressures across the pulmonary circuit, mmHg. (Pulmonary wedge pressure is generally substituted for $\overline{Ppv}$.)

$\dot{Q}$ = mean pulmonary blood flow, ml/s

The formula and units above express pulmonary vascular resistance in R (resistance) units. For the normal pulmonary circulation, the value for R is about 0.1. Some prefer to express pulmonary vascular resistance in dyne seconds per centimeter^5. To do so, the numerator of the equation is multiplied by 1332. The normal value is then of the order of 100.

All too often in clinical studies, instead of the pressure *difference*, the pulmonary arterial pressure is used in the numerator of the equation. In deference to the omission of outflow pressure (Ppv or Pw), the calculated value is then referred to as "total," i.e., total pulmonary vascular resistance. As noted previously, unfortunately, the value calculated in this way is bereft of either physiological or physical meaning.

Even under ideal circumstances and when all elements of the equation are properly determined, the concept of resistance must be regarded as an operational ratio, rather than taken at face value as a numerical descriptor of a physical state.

INTERPRETATION OF A CHANGE IN CALCULATED PVR

A change in calculated pulmonary vascular resistance (PVR) is generally used to infer that a change has occurred in the calibers of resistance vessels, i.e., in the muscular pulmonary arteries and arterioles. The next step is to judge if the change has been mediated actively or passively. If the hemodynamic state is changing between control and test periods (Fig. 63-7), the most reliable basis for comparing values for resistance is at constant values for either pressure or flow. Even then the possibility has to be weighed that the test period entails a change in the extent of the pulmonary vascular bed. For example, exercise in the upright position may recruit uppermost parts of the pulmonary vascular tree as flow and pressure increase. It then becomes difficult to decide if the decrease in calculated resistance is due to overall increase in the calibers of open vessels, or recruitment of vessels that were previously closed, or both.

One practical approach in humans is to construct *passive* pressure drop-flow curves before an intervention and then see where the test points fall (Fig. 63-7).

In the pulmonary circulation of native residents at high altitude, the muscular media of the small pulmonary arteries and arterioles are thicker and precapillary smooth muscle extends further distally. Because of these anatomic changes, pulmonary vascular resistance is ordinar-

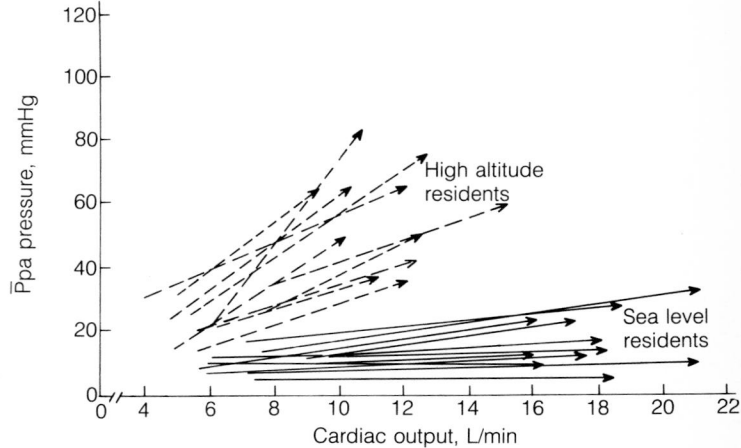

FIGURE 63-8 Relation of mean pulmonary arterial pressure to cardiac output for normal sea level residents and high altitude residents. At any level of cardiac output, the pulmonary arterial pressure is usually higher in the high altitude resident. (*Modified after Voelkel and Reeves, 1979.*)

ily higher at altitude than at sea level (Fig. 63-8) and the precapillary vessels seem to contribute more to overall resistance than at sea level.

PASSIVE MODIFIERS OF PVR

Testing for *active* changes in pulmonary vascular caliber is always haunted by the prospect of overlooked passive changes. Among these, three warrant special mention:

1. An increase in pulmonary arterial or pulmonary venous pressure automatically causes resistance to fall, either by opening segments of the pulmonary microcirculation that were previously closed (recruitment) or by distending resistance vessels that are already open.

2. Lung volumes passively affect pulmonary vascular resistance: calculated pulmonary vascular resistance due to passive influences is lowest at end-expiration (FRC) and increases as lung volumes move in either direction (Table 63-1). This topic is considered in detail in the subsequent section, "The Gas-Exchanging Vessels" (Fig. 63-9).

3. Unless left atrial pressure exceeds alveolar pressure in the portion of the pulmonary vascular bed under consideration, conventional calculation of pulmonary vascular resistance as $(\overline{P}pa - \overline{P}la)/\dot{Q}$ is meaningless since alveolar, rather than left atrial pressure, intervenes to act as the outflow pressure. This topic is considered later in terms of the zones of the lungs. Here it will suffice to indicate that in the upright lung, resistance to blood flow decreases automatically from top to bottom as, under the influence of gravity, dependent vessels open wider the distension of open *vessels*, and vessels previously closed are forced open ("recruited").

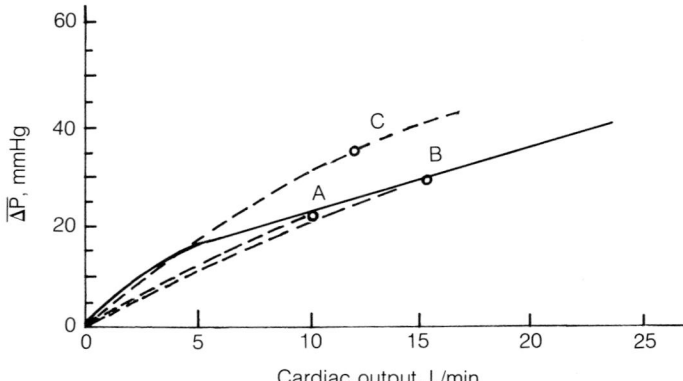

FIGURE 63-7 Use of pulmonary vascular pressure drop-flow curves to detect pulmonary vasomotor activity. The human subject is supine to promote uniform distribution of blood flow during control and test periods. All measurements are made in the steady state. The dashed lines radiating from the origin represent resistance isopleths. The lower solid line is the pressure-flow curve for the individual, based on points obtained at rest and during exercise (points A and B). Point C represents a shift to a higher curve, i.e., an increase in pulmonary vascular resistance. (*Courtesy of D. Silage.*)

CRITICAL CLOSURE

The concept of *critical closure* was originally invoked as a measure of vascular tone. It now seems that this concept is more germane to understanding the recruitment of vessels in the pulmonary circulation than to measuring vasomotricity. Whereas the pressure drop-flow relationship is influenced by the tone of the pulmonary vasculature, the intercept, i.e., the mean critical closing pressure, depends on alveolar pressure, smooth-muscle tone, the innate characteristics of the blood, the alveolar surface tension, and the degree of oxygenation. In both the pulmonary and systemic circulations, this value is determined by observing the transmural pressure at which flow stops as the luminal pressure is decreased. The concept of critical closure raises the prospect that certain strategically

disposed vessels, i.e., the *corner vessels*, may serve as preferential channels that sustain blood flow through the lungs when the driving pressure becomes too low for perfusing alveolar vessels.

PULMONARY VASCULAR IMPEDANCE

The concept of vascular impedance extends the conventional concept of pulmonary vascular resistance by relating pulsatile pressures to pulsatile flows in order to gain information about the geometry and viscoelastic properties of the vessels, their dimensions, the sites of wave reflections, the occurrence of pulmonary vasomotor activity, and the relationship between mechanical performance and energetics of the right ventricle on the one hand and the pulmonary circulation on the other. Little application of this approach has been made to the hypertensive pulmonary circulation.

Induced Changes in Pulmonary Hemodynamics

MECHANICAL VENTILATION

From the hemodynamic point of view, the best analyzed types of mechanical ventilation are *positive pressure* ventilation and *positive end-expiratory* ventilation (PEEP). In the former, airway pressures increase during inflation, returning promptly to atmospheric during expiration; in the

TABLE 63-1

Mechanisms of Increase in Pulmonary Vascular Resistance at Lung Volumes above and below FRC

	High Lung Volumes	Low Lung Volumes
Alveolar capillaries	Compressed	Open
Extra-alveolar vessels	Open	Compressed

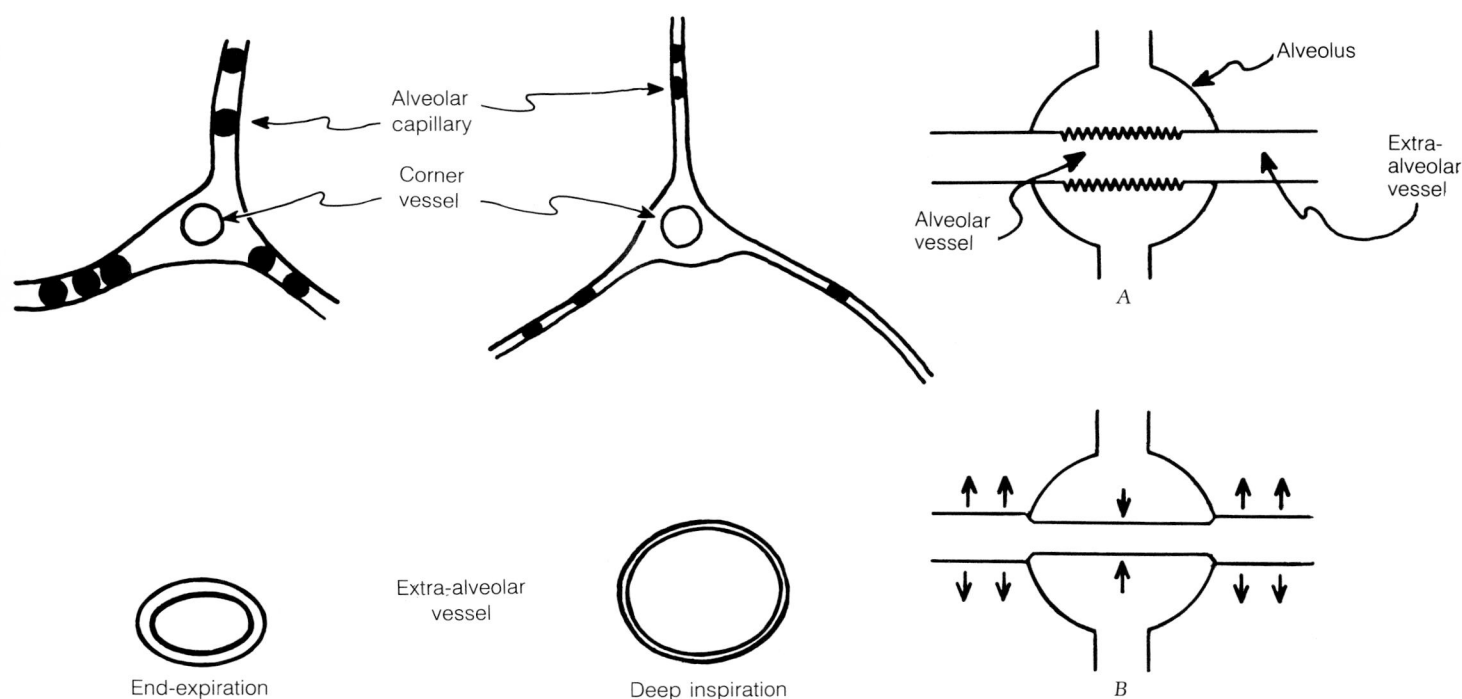

FIGURE 63-9 Schematic representation of the effects of a deep breath on the relative calibers of alveolar capillaries, "corner vessels," and extra-alveolar vessels. *Left.* At end-expiration, the alveolar capillaries (containing red cells) are wide-bored. The relative sizes of corner vessels and of extra-alveolar vessels are also shown. Deep inspiration narrows the alveolar vessels and widens extra-alveolar vessels, leaving corner vessels virtually unchanged in caliber. *Right.* The same phenomenon is shown for alveolar and extra-alveolar vessels: A represents end-expiration and B end-inspiration.

latter, raised airway pressure is sustained throughout the breathing cycle. Terminology used in clinical practice generally focuses on the positive end-expiratory pressure, and the designation PEEP generally refers to continuous positive pressure ventilation rather than solely to positive end-expiratory pressure (Chapter 155).

In normal humans, the imposition of PEEP at a level of 5 cmH$_2$O decreases stroke volume, cardiac output, and central blood volume, leaving heart rate unaffected. Pulmonary arterial pressures (referred to atmospheric pressures) also increase; the increase in alveolar pressure causes more of the lung to be in zone 1 or 2 at the expense of zone 3 (see "Zones of the Lungs") and pulmonary wedge pressures to exceed left atrial pressures. In the hypoperfused upper areas of the lungs, blood flow preferentially traverses alveolar corner vessels, thereby producing high $\dot{V}_A/\dot{Q}$ ratios. At higher levels of PEEP, these hemodynamic effects are exaggerated. Stiffening of the lungs by pulmonary edema requires higher levels of PEEP to produce the same effects, e.g., 15 to 40 cmH$_2$O instead of 5 cmH$_2$O. However, at these levels, the risk of barotrauma to the lungs also increases markedly.

During positive pressure ventilation, intrapleural pressure is positive during inspiration, thereby compressing both alveolar and extra-alveolar vessels as the lung volume increases; resistance to blood flow through both the alveolar and extra-alveolar vessels therefore increases during lung inflation. During PEEP, pleural pressure remains positive during both inspiration and expiration, thereby increasing pulmonary vascular resistance in the alveolar and extra-alveolar vessels throughout the respiratory cycle.

That the cardiac output falls when normal lungs are subjected to PEEP is beyond cavil. But how this decrease is effected remains enigmatic. At least three mechanisms have been proposed: the traditional one implicates a decrease in venous return (preload) to the *right* ventricle. The second entails a decrease in *left* ventricular preload and impairment of both right and left ventricular performance. The third attributes a negative inotropic effect to PEEP mediated by way of cardiovascular inhibitory mechanisms in the brain and the local release of prostaglandins. Clearly, the use of PEEP triggers an intricate resetting of regulatory mechanisms that seems to involve mechanical, reflex and local humoral mechanisms. Which mechanism(s) dominate at any given time may well depend on the experimental and clinical setting.

EXERCISE

Mention has been made above (Fig. 63-6) of the changes in pulmonary vascular pressures, flows, and resistances brought about by exercise. Here it may be useful to underscore that: (1) pulmonary arterial and wedge pressures are difficult to record accurately during exercise because res-

piratory swings are marked and the records are apt to be distorted by artifacts; (2) a "wedged" pulmonary arterial catheter often becomes dislodged during exercise; and (3) especially during strenuous exercise, shifts in the midposition of the lung and changes in compliance often occur and complicate attempts to sort out the mechanisms involved in a change of pressure.

Despite these difficulties in measurement and interpretation, the hemodynamics of the normal pulmonary circulation during light exercise are remarkably predictable: at the start of the exercise, the pulmonary arterial mean pressure (referred to atmosphere) increases abruptly by 3 to 5 mmHg. As exercise continues, a plateau is reached, generally at 1 to 2 mmHg less than peak values; the increase in systolic pressure is greater than the increase in diastolic pressure. Because of the increase in pulsatility and in mean pulmonary arterial pressure, perfusion of the apices improves.

Direct determinations of left atrial pressure during exercise in intact humans or dogs have not been reported. The pulmonary wedge pressure is generally little affected by mild exercise, but intensification of the exercise tends to increase it.

VASOMOTOR REGULATION

Three topics are of special interest with respect to the vasomotor regulation of the pulmonary circulation: (1) the level of initial tone; (2) detection of a vasomotor response, i.e., of an active change in vascular caliber in response to an applied stimulus, e.g., the vasomotor effects of acute hypoxia; and (3) the vasomotor mechanisms underlying an active change in pulmonary vascular tone.

Initial Tone

Whether a pulmonary vessel will constrict or dilate in response to a given stimulus depends, in part, on its initial tone. In the normal adult at sea level, initial tone in the pulmonary circulation is exceedingly low so that the resistance vessels are virtually maximally dilated. As indicated previously, it has been suggested that vasodilator prostaglandins contribute importantly to this low initial tone. Initial tone is higher in the fetus and in the native resident at high altitude than in the adult at sea level.

Hypoxia, as at altitude, and acidosis, as in uremia, increase initial tone. So do experimental manipulations and stress that release biologically active substances into the circulation. Tone of the pulmonary vasculature in the fetus is much greater than in the child or adult: in the fetus, the partially constricted pulmonary circulation responds vigorously to certain vasodilator agents, e.g., bradykinin, whereas the adult pulmonary circulation virtually ignores these substances.

In contrast to the role of high initial tone in increasing responsiveness to pulmonary vasodilators, high initial tone generally blunts the response to pulmonary vasoconstrictors. In essence, the pulmonary circulation operates over a range of calibers that range from fully open to maximally constricted: the more constricted the vessels at the outset, the less their capability of constricting further, e.g., in response to a vasoconstrictor substance. Conversely, the lower the initial tone, i.e., the more dilated the vessel at the outset, the greater the degree of vasoconstriction that a pulmonary vasoconstrictor can evoke. As a corollary, because initial tone is so low in the normal pulmonary circulation at sea level, not much further vasodilatation can be expected from a vasodilating agent, e.g., acetylcholine.

Regulatory Mechanisms

Vasomotor responses can be elicited from the isolated lung devoid of all nervous connections and perfused by artificial fluids. This capability underscores the primary role played by vasomotor mechanisms intrinsic to the lungs in effecting vasomotor control. However, it does not exclude the possibility that extrinsic influences, such as nerves, can contribute important elements of control should the occasion arise, e.g., the "fight or flight reaction" associated with a terrifying experience.

Nervous Control

ADRENERGIC NERVES, RECEPTORS, AND MEDIATORS

The sympathetic nervous system seems to play an appreciable role in adjusting pulmonary vascular tone only in the individual under stress. Cholinergic activity does not appear to be involved at any time in the control of the pulmonary circulation.

The sympathetic innervation to the pulmonary circulation includes α- and β-adrenergic receptors on pulmonary vascular smooth muscle. α-Adrenergic receptors appear to predominate. The α-adrenergic receptors, e.g., norepinephrine, are constrictors whereas the β-adrenergics, e.g., isoproterenol, are dilators. In the normal resting adult at sea level, adrenergic activity is modest and α-adrenergic influences predominate.

VASOMOTOR REFLEXES

Nervous connections from afar mediate certain reflex effects on the pulmonary circulation. A systemic *depressor reflex* is evoked by an abrupt, large increase in pulmonary arterial or venous pressure and elicits modest bradycardia and *systemic* hypotension; sectioning the vagi abolishes this reflex. The *J reflex* begins with the deformation of receptors (formerly pictured as J or juxtacapillary receptors within alveolar walls but now relegated to terminal airways) and evokes tachypnea, bronchoconstriction, and

disinclination to exercise. Reflex realignments of the resistance and compliance characteristics of the pulmonary circulation on the one hand, and of the outputs of the two ventricles on the other, match the behaviors of the two sides of the heart. Stimulation of systemic baro- and chemoreceptors elicits reflex changes in pulmonary vascular tone. The Bainbridge reflex is triggered by distension of the pulmonary venoatrial junction and elicits reflex tachycardia. Finally, it has been proposed that CO_2-sensitive receptors within the lungs can augment ventilation. These reflex patterns demonstrate that the pulmonary circulation is integrated into the regulatory mechanisms of the body in a complex way. They have generally been demonstrated under special experimental conditions. Therefore, it is difficult to predict what roles they play under natural conditions.

Occasionally individuals with pulmonary hypertension (as do deteriorating experimental preparations) show swings in pulmonary arterial pressure reminiscent of Traube-Hering-Mayer waves. Imbalance in central vasomotor control has been held responsible for their genesis. However, the mechanisms responsible for these "vasomotor" waves remain unsettled.

Pharmacologic Agents

Pulmonary vasodilators are currently being tried in the attempt to relieve pulmonary hypertension. Some of these agents, e.g., nifedipine, seem to exert their effects directly on the membrane of smooth-muscle cells of the media; others, notably acetylcholine, seem to work by way of endothelial-smooth-muscle interactions; a third group, i.e., the prostaglandins, seems to depend on the release of biologically active substances as intermediaries.

Among the vasomotor agents that have been tested, three groups stand out: vasoactive amines, polypeptides, and the prostaglandins. These groups can be sorted according to whether they act as pulmonary vasoconstrictors or pulmonary vasodilators.

VASOCONSTRICTORS

Norepinephrine and phenylephrine, potent stimulators of the α-adrenergic system in the pulmonary circulation, consistently elicit pulmonary vasoconstriction. Epinephrine, which possesses α- and β-adrenergic effects, not only evokes less vasoconstriction on a weight-for-weight basis but can also, depending on the preparation, cause vasodilatation.

Angiotensin II, an octapeptide, formed in the lungs by the action of converting enzyme from angiotensin I, a decapeptide, generally, but not invariably, elicits pulmonary vasoconstriction. Small doses (of the order of 0.03 μg/kg/min administered intravenously) suffice to increase pulmonary arterial pressure without discernible effect on the systemic circulation.

Histamine (in doses of the order of 10^{-5} g given intravenously over a 2-min period) elicits more variable responses. Although species difference and the type of experimental preparation seem to influence the outcome, as a rule histamine (like hypoxia) appears to be a powerful pulmonary vasoconstrictor and systemic vasodilator. At one time it was suspected that histamine is an important local mediator in the regulation of the pulmonary circulation. However, this belief appears to be unfounded.

Discrepant effects of histamine on the pulmonary circulation can be rationalized in terms of H_1 and H_2 receptors and their blocking agents: chlorpheniramine to block H_1 receptors selectively; metiamide to block H_2 receptors. The use of these agents suggests that pulmonary vasoconstriction is mediated by H_1 receptors and vasodilatation by H_2 receptors.

Serotonin (in doses of the order of 10^{-5} g given intravenously in a few minutes) is another vasoconstrictive amine that occurs in the mast cells of some species but not others. It is synthesized from dietary tryptophan in the enterochromaffin cells of the gut. The serotonin released by these cells is largely removed by the liver, the excess being almost completely removed by the endothelial cells of the pulmonary circulation. Any serotonin that escapes the metabolic machinery of the liver and lungs is stored as dense granules in circulating platelets. In addition to direct effects on vessels, airways, and platelets, serotonin enhances vasoconstriction and platelet aggregation produced by other vasoactive agents, such as norepinephrine and angiotensin II.

Two separate binding sites have been identified for serotonin: S_1-receptor binding sites that are labeled by serotonin, and S_2-receptor binding sites that are labeled by serotonin antagonists, e.g., spiperone and ketanserin. The physiological and pharmacologic effects of serotonin (vasomotor activity, bronchoconstriction platelet aggregation) appear to be related to the binding of serotonin to the S_2 receptor; no such effects have been attributed to binding to the S_1 receptor.

The distinction between S_1 receptors and S_2 receptors holds great promise for reexamining the role of serotonin in the bronchoconstriction and pulmonary vasoconstriction evoked by pulmonary embolism. In contrast to histamine, which seems to affect both pulmonary arterial and venous components, serotonin seems to constrict predominantly the precapillary vessels.

VASODILATORS

Much of the response to vasodilators appears to depend on the initial tone of the pulmonary resistance vessels.

Isoproterenol

In the normal pulmonary circulation, isoproterenol usually evokes a barely detectable drop in pressure; this modest response has been attributed to low initial tone due either to the paucity of β receptors or to the low level of their activity in the normal state. The vasodilator response is much more impressive in animal preparations in which initial tone is high and in some patients with pulmonary hypertension. It has been suggested that the pulmonary vasodilator effect of isoproterenol when pulmonary vascular tone is high does not depend entirely on pulmonary vascular adrenergic receptors but also on vasodilator prostaglandins. One complicating feature in the use of isoproterenol as a pulmonary vasodilator is its powerful inotropic effect on the heart.

Acetylcholine

The influence of initial tone is even more dramatically illustrated by acetylcholine: this agent elicits virtually no vasodilator response in the normal pulmonary circulation. Conversely, when administered intravenously (in dosages of the order of 0.1 mg/kg/min), it elicits brisk vasodilatation if the pulmonary circulation is in a state of heightened tone, as in the fetus, or in adults during exposure to alveolar hypoxia.

Bradykinin

This pulmonary vasodilator is a member of a family of vasoactive polypeptides. It is inactivated by the same converting enzyme(s) in the lungs that converts angiotensin I to II. Although it is consistently a powerful systemic vasodilator, it is not as predictable as a pulmonary vasodilator, usually evoking pulmonary vasodilatation. The biologic role of bradykinin in regulating the pulmonary circulation is unclear. The possibility has been raised that the origin of bradykinin in the pulmonary vascular endothelium constitutes a source of vasodilator agent for the systemic circulation. Although angiotensin II and bradykinin share a dependency on converting enzyme for their genesis, they act differently on vascular smooth muscle: angiotensin acts without intermediaries, whereas vasoactive prostaglandins are involved in the effects of the kallidins. Indeed, at least in some of the species, the variability in the vasoactive effects of bradykinin and the kallidins has been attributed to variations in the extent to which different prostaglandins are engaged as mediators of the vasodilator response.

VASOACTIVE PROSTAGLANDINS AND THEIR PRECURSORS

In the search for likely candidates as chemical mediators of pulmonary vasomotor activity, arachidonic acid has almost achieved the status of the philosopher's stone because of the multitude of biologically active products that it generates.

Arachidonic acid (eicosatrienoic acid), a 20-carbon polyunsaturated fatty acid, is the precursor of the prostaglandins (Fig. 63-10). It is released from tissues by deacylation of cellular phospholipids. Upon release, it is metabolized by either the cyclooxygenase or lipoxygenase

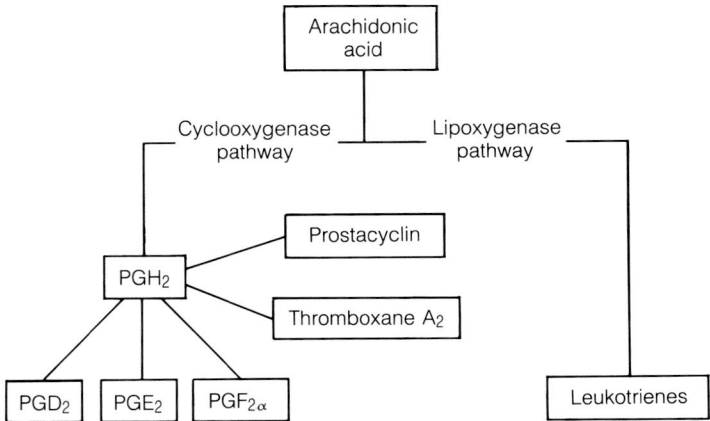

FIGURE 63-10 The arachidonic acid cascade illustrating the two pathways and a few metabolic products capable of pulmonary vasomotor activity. *(From Fishman, 1985.)*

enzyme systems. Because the arachidonic acid metabolites released from membrane lipids are organ- and cell-specific, and because experimental conditions strongly influence the metabolism of arachidonic acid, either the cyclooxygenase or lipoxygenase pathway may predominate. Administered arachidonic acid need not have the same metabolic consequences as that generated endogenously. Nor are physiological and pharmacologic doses and patterns of release apt to be identical. Therefore, it is difficult to predict which pathway will dominate or how experimental circumstances are influencing the biologic effects. As a rule, arachidonic acid injected intravenously elicits pulmonary vasoconstriction largely because of the predominant effect of thromboxane A_2 even though prostacyclin, a potent vasodilator, is also released; leukotrienes do not appear to be operative in this circumstance.

Pharmacologic interruption of one pathway has been used to uncover the effect of metabolites produced by the other. For example, indomethacin, which inhibits prostaglandin synthetase, is a popular agent for blocking the cyclooxygenase pathway in order to disclose the actions exerted by metabolites of the lipoxygenase pathway. Diethylcarbamazine, which interferes with the lipoxygenase pathway, serves the same purpose for the cyclooxygenase pathway. However, specificity of these and other inhibitors for particular sites in the arachidonic acid cascade is rarely complete. Moreover, alternative pathways in the metabolism of arachidonate provide opportunity for subtle experimental quirks to channel the cascade into one pathway or another, thereby covertly shaping the vasomotor response of the pulmonary circulation, not only to prostaglandins, exogenous as well as endogenous, but also to inapparent neurohumoral influences and to biologically active molecules. Finally, considerable species variation exists in the intensity of the vasomotor response to particular products of arachidonic acid metabolism.

Considerable diversity of biologic effects exists among the prostaglandins: (1) certain metabolic products of the cyclooxygenase pathway are pulmonary vasoconstrictors, e.g., $PGF_{2\alpha}$, PGE_2, thromboxane A_2, whereas others are pulmonary vasodilators, e.g., PGE_1, PGI_2; PGE_2, which constricts the adult pulmonary vascular bed, dilates the neonatal pulmonary vascular bed; (2) leukotrienes, generated by the lipoxygenase pathway, include potent pulmonary vasoconstrictors; (3) suspicion is high that the prostaglandins are involved as intermediaries in pulmonary vasomotor responses to other agents such as the kallidins, histamine, and isoproterenol; (4) it is also suspected that a balance between prostaglandin vasodilator activity on the one hand and the constrictor effect of thromboxane A_2 on the other is importantly involved in setting the low initial tone of the normal pulmonary circulation; and (5) hemodynamic (and other mechanical) factors influence both the release of vasoactive prostaglandins (e.g., PGI_2) and the endothelial metabolism of prostaglandins.

Of all the prostaglandins, prostacyclin [prostaglandin I_2, (PGI_2)] is currently attracting most attention as a potent pulmonary (and systemic) vasodilator and antithrombogenic agent. This agent is formed by the action of prostacyclin synthetase on the prostaglandin endoperoxide PGH_2. Shear stress of the endothelium appears to be a potent stimulus to the release of prostacyclin from endothelium. So does bradykinin.

Another major line of experimental interest involving the prostaglandins has been the control of the ductus arteriosus (Fig. 63-11) (see section "The Fetal and Neonatal Pulmonary Circulation"). Despite its embryologic origin (as the distal segment of the left sixth aortic arch) and its location as a bridge between the pulmonary artery and the

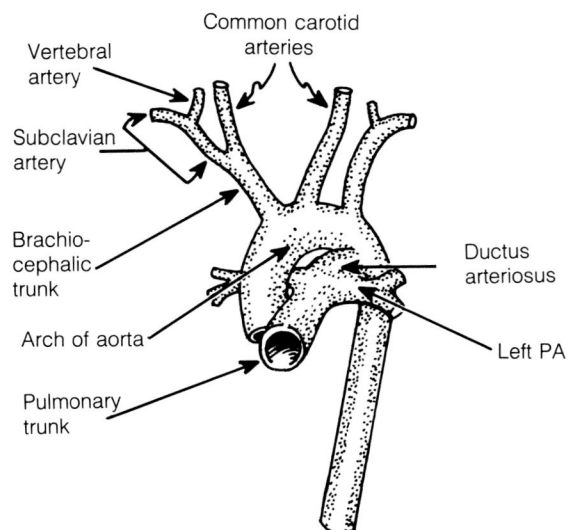

FIGURE 63-11 Relationship between ductus arteriosus and contiguous vessels. PA = pulmonary artery.

descending aorta, the ductus arteriosus leads a vasomotor life of its own, independent of the two circulations that it bridges. For example, immediately postpartum, i.e., upon switching from the hypoxic environment in utero to the air-breathing, oxygen-rich environment of independent neonatal life, the ductus arteriosus contracts vigorously to the point of self-obliteration of its lumen; at the same time, the pulmonary circulation vasodilates.

Closure of the ductus arteriosus immediately after birth depends heavily on prostaglandins in its walls. Conversely, premature closure of the ductus arteriosus, i.e., before birth, as may be caused by transplacental passage of indomethacin taken by the mother, may either cause fetal pulmonary arterial hypertension or interfere with the morphologic development of the pulmonary vascular bed. The vasomotor responses of the ductus arteriosus to prostaglandins and to inhibitors of the cyclooxygenase pathway have been turned to clinical advantage: on the one hand, PGE_2 or PGE_1 has been used to maintain patency of the ductus arteriosus in newborns with congenital heart disease who need continued communication between the pulmonary and systemic circulations; on the other hand, indomethacin, an inhibitor of the prostaglandin synthetase element of the cyclooxygenase pathway, has been used to promote closure of a persistent ductus arteriosus in premature infants.

Interest is high in the role of arachidonic metabolites that damage the lungs and also elicit pulmonary vasoconstriction. Although the mechanisms are complex, one model has indicated that thromboxane, generated by oxygen metabolites from neutrophils, is involved. Another model has shown that infusion of *Escherichia coli* endotoxin or ethchlorvynol is followed by a two-phased response. The first phase, characterized by marked pulmonary hypertension and leukopenia, involves the cyclooxygenase pathway and is associated with the release of thromboxane A_2 (and prostacyclin) into lymph and blood. In the subsequent phase, characterized by a striking increase in pulmonary microvascular permeability, the lipoxygenase pathway is primarily involved. Accordingly, whereas the pulmonary hypertension can be alleviated by administering either indomethacin or imidazole, the subsequent permeability phase is unaffected by cyclooxygenase inhibition, suggesting that the lipoxygenase-derived products are involved in the increase in microvascular permeability. In the adult respiratory distress syndrome, the types of arachidonic acid metabolites have been found to vary greatly and often unpredictably; but, gravely ill patients with sepsis generally do manifest high levels of thromboxane and prostacyclin.

Respiratory Gases and pH

ACUTE HYPOXIA

Acute hypoxia is a powerful pulmonary vasoconstrictor agent (Fig. 63-12). Its intrapulmonary effects on the pulmonary resistance vessels automatically adjust pulmonary capillary blood flow to alveolar ventilation. Alveolar hypoxia, induced by lowering inspired P_{O_2}, is a reliable method for inducing the pulmonary pressor response; whether hypoxemia of the mixed venous or systemic arterial blood has the same effect is unsettled.

In human subjects, acute hypoxia causes an increase in pulmonary arterial pressure without affecting left atrial pressure or usually the cardiac output. The pressor response starts within a few breaths, generally reaching its peak by 3 min, and attenuates gradually as hypoxia continues. Severe acidosis augments the hypoxic pressor response. The site of pulmonary vasoconstriction in response to acute hypoxia is generally considered to be predominantly at the precapillary level, involving the small muscular arteries and arterioles. However, the likelihood remains that smooth muscle anywhere in the pulmonary circulation responds to acute hypoxia by an increase in tone. The vasoconstriction produced by acute hypoxia can be relieved by vasodilators; among these, the vasodilator prostaglandins, such as prostacyclin, appear to be remarkably effective. The role of endothelial-medial interaction in the hypoxic pressor response is currently under investigation.

It was noted above that many of the features of the hypoxic pressor response can be evoked in the isolated lung that lacks innervation and is artificially perfused. However, in the innervated lung, acute hypoxia elicits not only constriction of the resistance vessels but also tensing of the major arteries. The latter effect clearly involves the adrenergic components of the sympathetic nerve supply to the lungs.

How the intrapulmonary effects of acute hypoxia are mediated is still being explored along two major lines: (1) direct and (2) via mediators. The proponents of a direct effect invoke cellular events in pulmonary vascular smooth muscle. However, there is no consensus even in this group: some favor an effect of acute ATP production, whereas others are more impressed with acute hypoxia as a mechanism for increasing the intracellular concentration of calcium ions.

More popular than a direct effect is the idea of a unique, but mysterious, chemical mediator that is released within the lungs during acute hypoxia. Although considerable evidence has been adduced in support of this hypothesis, most is circumstantial and little has survived intense scrutiny. Among the last mediators to be discounted were angiotensin and histamine. Others, such as the vasoactive intestinal polypeptide and substance P, seem to be fading. Currently the focus is on the prostaglandins: not on the cyclooxygenase pathway since its constituents seem to dampen the pulmonary vasoconstriction evoked by acute hypoxia; instead, attention is directed to the leukotrienes, notably leukotriene C_4. At present, it is not possible to implicate any specific prod-

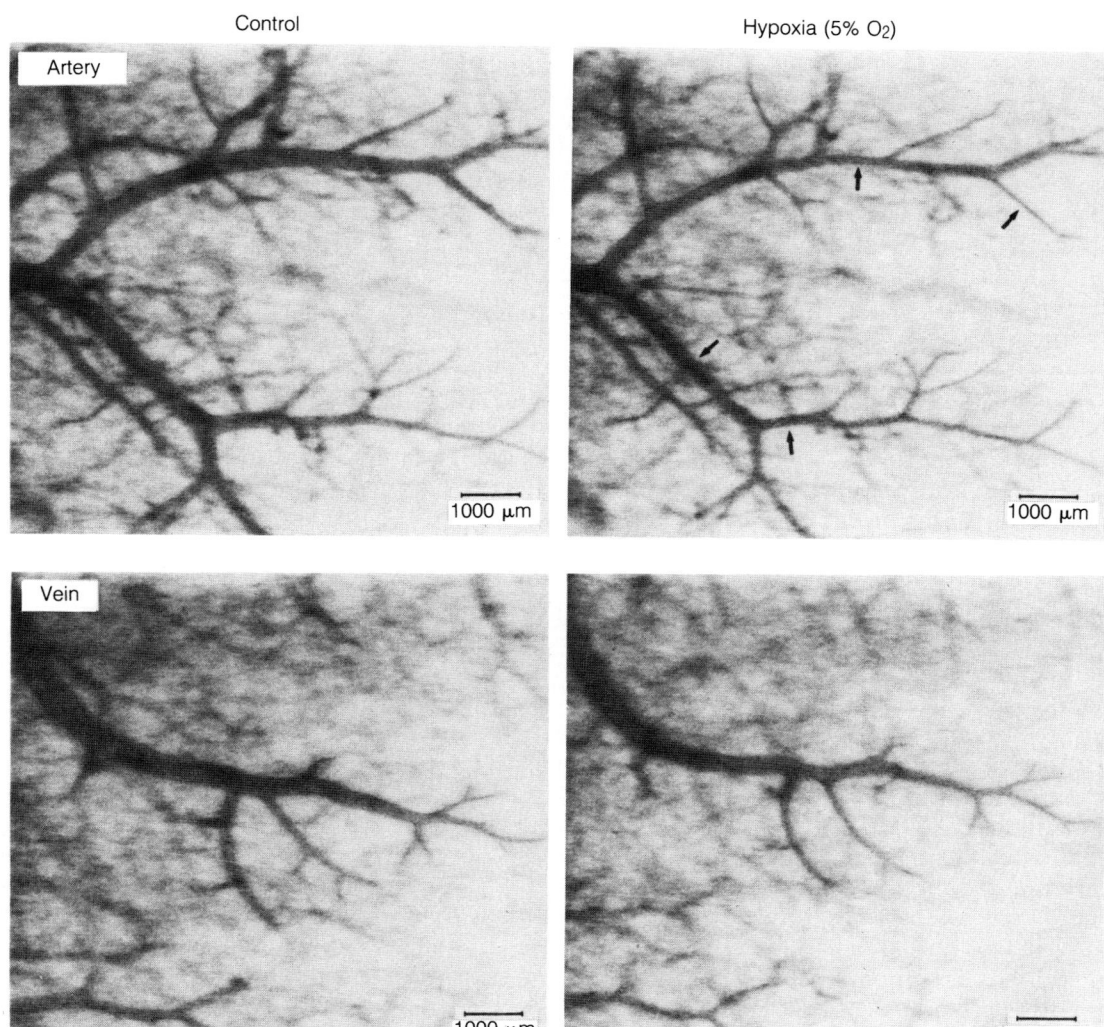

| Control | Hypoxia (5% O₂) |

Artery

1000 μm

1000 μm

Vein

1000 μm

1000 μm

FIGURE 63-12 Direct visualization of the vasoconstrictor effect of acute hypoxia. While breathing 5% O_2 in N_2, the pulmonary precapillary vessels are attenuated by vasoconstriction, whereas the pulmonary veins undergo no appreciable change. *(Courtesy of Dr. I. Ninomiya, National Cardiovascular Research Institute, Osaka, Japan.)*

uct of arachidonic acid metabolism as the unique mediator in the hypoxic pressor response.

The direct action and the mediator hypotheses outlined above are the traditional concepts. As insights into vascular smooth muscle become more penetrating, these two fundamental approaches are being extended in the search for the intimate mechanism: on the one hand, electrophysiological studies are examining the possibility that acute hypoxia decreases the transmembrane potential, thereby bringing the cell closer to its threshold potential for activation; an alternative approach is to seek a link between endothelium and the underlying vascular smooth muscle that could be affected by acute hypoxia. A third intensive effort is directed at the idea that the mechanism of hypoxic pulmonary vasoconstriction involves increased calcium transport into smooth muscle via calcium channels. However, none of these approaches seem to offer the prospect of settling whether direct effects or mediators or both are involved in the hypoxia pressor re-

sponse. All that can be said at present is that how acute hypoxia exerts its pulmonary pressor effect remains an enigma. Whether a complex interplay, or a unique biologic substance, or a combination of the two is responsible remains to be resolved.

Before concluding the hypoxic pressor response, it seems necessary to point out that the above considerations have focused on precapillary vessels even though there are many different contractile elements in the lungs that could contribute to the pressor response to acute hypoxia. These have been mentioned above. But, despite this acknowledgement, constriction of smooth muscle in precapillaries still seems to account for virtually all experimental and clinical observations during acute hypoxia.

In atelectasis, hypoxia appears to be much more responsible for reducing blood flow through the affected area than mechanical influences, such as compression by airless parenchyma and kinking of vessels. However, the interplay among the factors operative during atelectasis is

complicated. For example, should atelectasis cause systemic arterial hypoxemia, systemic reflexes come into play to augment the blood flow through the atelectatic lung.

CHRONIC HYPOXIA

Life at high altitude is associated with chronic hypoxia, arterial hypoxemia, thickening and extension of the muscular layers of the resistance vessels (pulmonary arteries and arterioles), and pulmonary hypertension. What causes the smooth muscle to proliferate and to extend distally is currently under investigation. As in the case of acute hypoxia, chronic hypoxia affects the pulmonary and systemic circulations oppositely, relaxing systemic vascular smooth muscle while eliciting pulmonary vasoconstriction. At Morococha, Peru—an altitude of 4540 m—the ambient P_{O_2} of about 80 mmHg is associated in adults with a mean pulmonary arterial pressure of about 28 mmHg, i.e., about twice the average value of 12 mmHg in sea level residents (Lima) even though cardiac output and pulmonary wedge pressures are the same. During moderate exercise, mean pulmonary arterial pressure increases considerably: at 14,900 ft in the Peruvian Andes, quadrupling the oxygen uptake intensifies arterial hypoxemia, and doubles both the cardiac output (from 3.65 to 7.49 L/min/m²) and the pulmonary arterial pressure (from 41/15, 29 mmHg, to 77/40, 60 mmHg). In individuals suffering from chronic mountain sickness, in which severe arterial hypoxemia and hypercapnia are secondary to alveolar hypoventilation, pulmonary arterial pressures are much higher. Genetic factors seem to influence human susceptibility to pulmonary hypertension at altitude.

Pulmonary arterial pressure and pulmonary vascular resistance decrease somewhat, but not to normal, when native residents of high altitude take up residence at sea level. In large measure, the persistent increase in pulmonary vascular resistance is due to anatomic changes in the pulmonary arterial tree elicited by the chronic hypoxia. The pulmonary arterial and arteriolar walls are thickened by hypertrophy and hyperplasia of the media, which also extend peripherally into precapillary vessels that are ordinarily nonmuscular. Despite this restructuring of precapillary vessels, the pulmonary capillaries and veins remain unchanged. Polycythemia, because it increases blood viscosity, contributes to the pulmonary hypertension associated with chronic hypoxia.

After moving to sea level, the anatomic lesions of hypoxic pulmonary hypertension gradually revert toward normal. However, 2 years after the native resident of high altitude has moved to sea level, a modest increment in cardiac output elicits an inordinate increase in pulmonary arterial pressure, presumably because of residual muscularization of the small pulmonary arteries.

Children born at altitude undergo more gradual involution of pulmonary arterial pressures than do those born

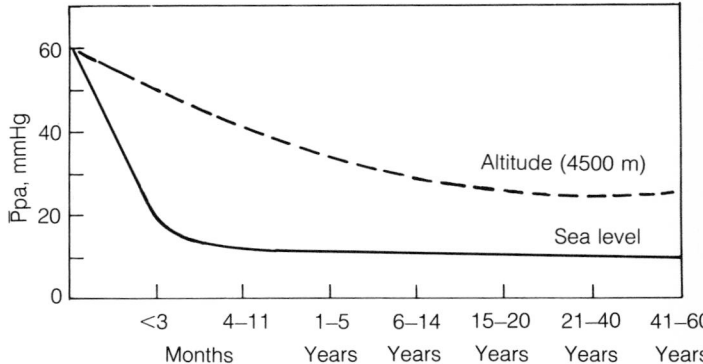

FIGURE 63-13 Patterns of decrease in pulmonary arterial pressure with age, at altitude and at sea level. The observations at altitude were made in the Peruvian Andes, at an elevation of approximately 15,000 ft. *(From Peñaloza, Gamboa: Cardiología Pediátrica. Madrid, Salvat, 1986; see Fishman, 1985.)*

at sea level (Fig. 63-13). Therefore, up to the age of 5 years, children raised at altitude have uniformly higher pulmonary arterial pressures (of the order of 58/32, 44 mmHg) than do older children at altitude (of the order of 41/18, 28 mmHg).

ACUTE HYPERCAPNIA

Enrichment of inspired air with tolerable concentration of CO_2, i.e., 5 to 7 percent, has little effect on the human pulmonary circulation, presumably because of the increase in ventilation that minimizes change in blood pH. However, if the ventilatory response is limited, e.g., during anesthesia, a distinct pressor response is evoked as arterial blood becomes acidotic, i.e., as pH falls to 7.2 or less. The combination of moderate to severe acidosis—no matter how induced—and acute hypoxia elicits a greater response than either alone, i.e., the pressor response to acute hypoxia and acute hypercapnia combined is synergistic.

BLOOD pH

Just as severe acidosis elicits pulmonary vasoconstriction, so does severe alkalosis cause pulmonary vasodilatation. The interplay between hypoxia and acidosis is believed to be of considerable importance in areas of alveolar hypoventilation in which the combination of local acidosis and hypoxia promotes the diversion of blood flow to better ventilated parts of the lungs.

THE PULMONARY CIRCULATION IN GAS EXCHANGE

The pulmonary circulation was designed to operate in concert with alveolar ventilation for the sake of gas exchange. Certain aspects of this interplay warrant special mention: (1) the lungs receive the entire cardiac output,

(2) the pulmonary blood flow is about the same as the alveolar ventilation, and (3) although the respiratory and circulatory processes are phasic, the rates are entirely different, i.e., about 15 breaths and 80 heartbeats per minute at rest. Therefore, matching of air and blood for optimal arterialization of mixed venous blood requires delicate tuning of operations that are not in phase, either at rest or during exercise; no vasomotor nerves or neurohumoral substances are at hand to make the speedy and fine adjustments of alveolar blood flow to alveolar ventilation.

Matching of air and blood for optimal gas exchange involves about 300 million alveoli that bear myriad capillary segments in their walls. The interposition of pulmonary capillaries between contiguous alveoli provides an enormous surface area for gas exchange, about 100 m^2 at rest, that increases further during exercise. The volume of blood in the capillaries at any one instant is of the order of 100 to 200 ml, and red blood cells pass from one end of the gas-exchanging network to the other in about 0.75 s.

Four aspects of the distribution of the pulmonary circulation have attracted special attention with respect to gas exchange: (1) gas-exchanging vessels, (2) effects of gravity, (3) interplay among pressures influencing vascular calibers, and (4) effects of inflation.

The Gas-Exchanging Vessels

As the pulmonary vessels branch their way to the capillaries and then regroup to form venous trunks leading to the left atrium, the consecutive segments are subject to different surrounding pressures. These perivascular pressures strongly influence vascular calibers because intravascular pressures in the pulmonary circulation are low and vessel diameters depend heavily on transmural pressures (intra- minus perivascular pressure). Appreciation of the importance of the different perivascular pressures has encouraged useful distinctions between extra- and intrapulmonary vessels on the one hand and among three types of intrapulmonary vessels on the other.

EXTRAPULMONARY VESSELS

Vessels lying outside the lungs and within the mediastinum are subjected to subcostal pleural pressure modified by local mechanical distortions. Because of the local effects, the pressures surrounding the hilar vessels during inflation are somewhat less negative than subcostal pleural pressures. Extrapulmonary veins are thin-walled and collapsible. Blood flow through them is pulsatile. Their cross section changes shape as left atrial pressure increases, and the waveform of pulmonary venous blood flow is related inversely to left atrial pressure.

INTRAPULMONARY VESSELS

When the lungs are inflated, under conditions designed to simulate the natural state, intrapulmonary arteries and

veins lengthen without appreciable narrowing. However, the effect of lung inflation on the calibers of intrapulmonary vessels is not uniform because of regional differences in pleural pressure, nonuniform transmission of pleural pressures to the walls of consecutive vascular segments, the original vascular dimensions and degree of distension, the physical characteristics of the vascular walls, the anatomic way in which the vessel is incorporated into the surrounding lung, and the level of vascular tone. Depending on the perivascular pressures to which they are exposed, three types of intrapulmonary vessels have been distinguished: alveolar, corner, and extra-alveolar (Fig. 63-9).

ALVEOLAR VESSELS

Alveolar vessels are capillaries that are contained within the walls that separate adjacent alveoli. They are surrounded by interstitium that varies in thickness and in the nature and content of cells, collagen, and elastic fibers. The appearance of the alveolar capillaries depends heavily on the route of fixation. Thus, fixation via the airways—which removes the surfactant lining—causes the capillaries to bulge into the alveoli, whereas fixation by perfusion—so that the lung remains air-filled—eliminates these deformations, widens capillaries unnaturally, and does away with alveolar pleats and folds. As the lung expands, alveolar walls unfold, and the connective tissue elements surrounding them are rearranged. The calibers of the alveolar capillaries depend on the level of lung inflation, and they undergo compression (without change in wall thickness) when alveolar pressures increase. It is clear from the above that impressions of alveolar morphology are meaningful only when full account is taken not only of the route of fixation but also of the way in which the lung was handled during fixation.

As the lungs expand, largely because of the surfactant lining of the alveoli, the alveolar pericapillary pressure is less than the alveolar pressure but higher than the pressure surrounding extra-alveolar vessels. This difference between the interstitial pressures to which alveolar and extra-alveolar vessels are exposed is exaggerated at high levels of lung inflation.

CORNER VESSELS

Corner vessels (Fig. 63-9) are located at sites where three alveoli abut; there they are contained within pleats in the alveolar walls beneath sharp curvatures in the overlying alveolar film of surfactant. They are neither extra-alveolar vessels (see below)—in that they lack a surrounding sleeve of connective tissue—nor conventional components of the pulmonary microcirculation. Their location and anatomic arrangement within pleats seem to offer considerable protection against fluctuations in alveolar pressure. Indeed, blood flow persists in these vessels

when alveolar pressure exceeds pulmonary arterial pressure by 10 cmH$_2$O. Originally pictured as arteriovenous anastomoses, they are now viewed as preferential channels through which blood flow continues in the face of wide swings in alveolar pressure.

EXTRA-ALVEOLAR VESSELS

Extra-alveolar vessels are, by definition, small vessels that are not affected by changes in alveolar pressure but do enlarge during lung inflation (Fig. 63-9). The definition is far more precise for physiologists than for anatomists since the designation *extra-alveolar vessel* appears to include diverse components of the pulmonary microcirculation, notably veins, venules, arteries, and precapillaries.

Despite this morphologic diversity, the key to the physiologic behavior of the extra-alveolar vessels appears to be the connective tissue sheath which they share. Surrounding the extra-alveolar vessels is an interstitial space that is bounded by extensions of the fascial sheaths that envelop the trachea and esophagus. Within the perivascular interstitial space lies loose areolar tissue, collagenous fibers, and lymph vessels that drain lymph from the lung parenchyma; in pulmonary edema, excess fluid (and protein) accumulates within this space. The sheaths extend further peripherally along the pulmonary arteries than the bronchi; for pulmonary arteries, and probably for pulmonary veins, the perivascular sheaths continue peripherally to vessels of the order of 100 μm in diameter. Dilatation of extra-alveolar vessels during inflation is a consequence of a drop in the surrounding interstitial pressure.

The degree to which extra-alveolar vessels widen during inflation depends on their initial calibers which, in turn, vary with lung volume. During deflation to levels below FRC, small arteries and veins tend to close, possibly because of inherent vascular tone abetted by alveolar hypoxia in the poorly expanded regions. At this time, the site of maximum resistance to blood flow shifts proximally in the arterial tree.

Effects of Gravity

A variety of techniques have been used to test the influence of gravity on the topographic distribution of blood delivered to the lungs. Among these have been the intravenous injection of a polysoluble gas, e.g., xenon, the inhalation of a very soluble gas, e.g., carbon dioxide, and the intravenous injection of microaggregated albumin followed by radiographic determination of the distribution of radioactivity. Although interpretation of the results of these different methods is often complicated by individual peculiarities of the techniques coupled with the different types of information that they provide, the results do agree that in the upright lungs, blood flow decreases steadily from the bottom to the top (Fig. 63-14), that gravity is the compelling force, and that an interplay among pulmonary arterial, alveolar, and pulmonary venous pressures is involved. As a consequence of these influences, in a relaxed, seated subject—particularly in one with an elongated thorax—the apices are apt to be poorly perfused, especially in states of pulmonary hypotension or increased alveolar pressure.

Interplay among Pressures Influencing Vascular Calibers

VASCULAR WATERFALL

In 1960, Banister and Torrance demonstrated that the level of alveolar pressure could influence pressure-flow relationships in the pulmonary circulation and drew an analogy between the behavior of the pulmonary arterial,

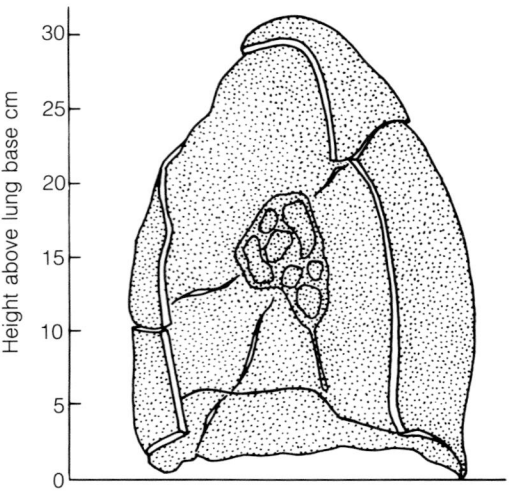

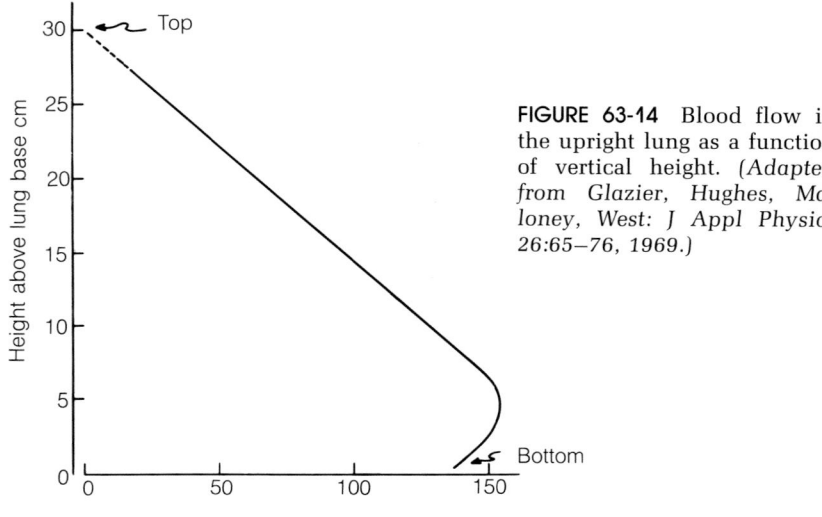

FIGURE 63-14 Blood flow in the upright lung as a function of vertical height. (*Adapted from Glazier, Hughes, Maloney, West: J Appl Physiol 26:65–76, 1969.*)

pulmonary venous, and alveolar pressures and that of a Starling resistor. The crucial point of their demonstration was that when alveolar pressure (chamber pressure) exceeded venous (downstream) pressure, the driving pressure became arterial minus alveolar pressure, and not arterial minus venous pressure. Permutt compared this behavior to that of a waterfall where height does not influence the flow of water over its brink.

ZONES OF THE LUNGS

Recognition of the effects of alveolar pressure on pressure-flow relationships in the pulmonary circulation, coupled with the formulation of the behavior of pulmonary microvessels in terms of the Starling resistor, paved the way for a model of the topographic distribution of blood flow in the lungs under the influence of gravity (Fig. 63-15). As a result, it is now commonplace to use "zones" of blood flow in the lungs as operative shorthand for specifying the interplay between pulmonary arterial, alveolar, and pulmonary venous pressures.

In the normal, upright lung (estimated height of 25 cm at FRC), about 15 cm is above the left atrium and about 10 cm is below. Assuming that the mean pulmonary arterial pressure measured at the level of the left atrium is of the order of 15 cmH$_2$O and that left atrial pressure is about 7 cmH$_2$O, the top few centimeters of the lung will be hypoperfused during most of the cardiac cycle except for flushes of blood during the peak ejection phase of systole. This zone has been designated as zone 1. In the next lower zone (zone 2), blood flow increases regularly with distance down the lung. Below zone 2 is another zone of increasing blood flow (zone 3). Finally, a zone 4 may exist near the base; in the zone, blood flow decreases instead of increases.

Zone 1

In the vertical lung, blood flow in zone 1, where alveolar pressure exceeds arterial pressure (PA > Ppa), is minimal. In this zone, although most alveolar capillaries appear to be attenuated or collapsed, extra-alveolar vessels in the alveolar corners often remain open, once again emphasizing that the extra-alveolar vessels are exposed to different forces than are the alveolar vessels. As noted previously, persistence of blood flow through parts of zone 1 presumably occurs via (corner) vessels.

The apices of upright lungs would be deprived of pulmonary blood flow were it not for the pulsatility of pulmonary arterial blood flow; a flush of blood during systole perfuses the apices even though mean pulmonary arterial pressure is too low to sustain blood flow to the apices.

Zone 2

In zone 2, pulmonary arterial pressure exceeds alveolar pressure which, in turn, exceeds pulmonary venous pressure (Ppa > PA > Ppv) (Fig. 63-15). In this constellation of pressures, blood flow is no longer determined by the usual pressure drop across the pulmonary circulation. Instead, the outflow pressure is alveolar pressure and the driving force is the pulmonary arterial-alveolar pressure difference. This hemodynamic situation in which flow is independent of downstream pressure has been likened to a "vascular waterfall."

Under the influence of gravity, the pulmonary arterial pressure increases by about 1 cmH$_2$O per centimeter distance down the lung, whereas alveolar pressure remains unchanged; the driving pressure and, therefore, the blood flow, increases down this zone. Changing relationships between alveolar and luminal pressures then shift outflow pressures from alveolar to pulmonary venous, and then back. Flow through the capillaries of zone 2 is pictured as

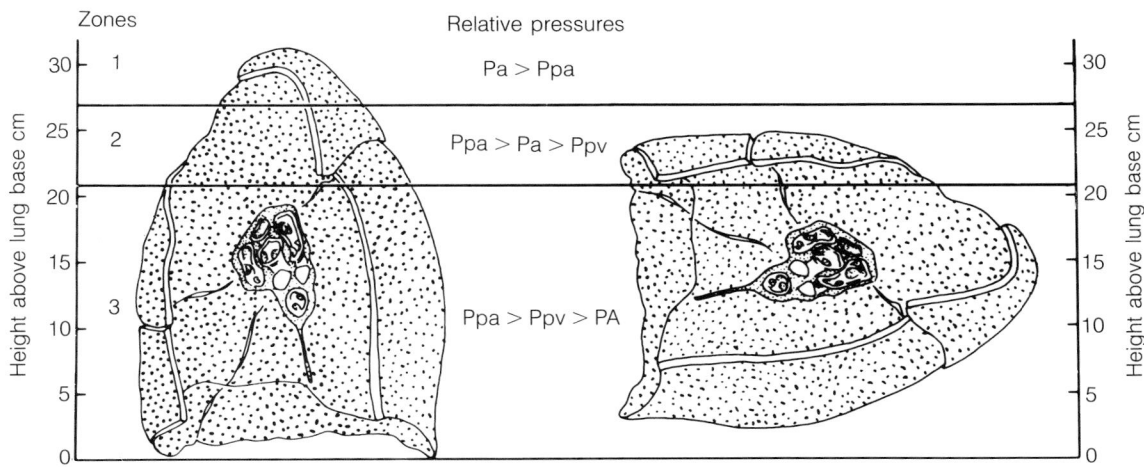

FIGURE 63-15 Zones of the lungs in different body positions as determined by the interplay among pulmonary arterial pressure (Ppa), alveolar pressure (PA) and pulmonary venous pressure (Ppv). In the supine position, the uppermost part of the lung is shown as being in zone 2 and the remainder in zone 3; there is no zone 1 in this position. [Adapted from Hughes: in Widdicombe (ed), Respiratory Physiology II, vol 14. Baltimore, University Park, 1977, pp 135–183.]

intermittent, as through "sluice gates" that open when pulmonary venous pressures exceed alveolar pressures and close when alveolar pressures exceed pulmonary venous pressures.

Zone 3

It is only in this zone that conventional calculations of pulmonary vascular resistance are valid: since pulmonary venous pressure is greater than alveolar pressure (Ppa > Ppv > PA), blood flow is determined by the arteriovenous difference in pressure (since both exceed alveolar pressure) (Fig. 63-15). Resistance to blood flow in zone 3 is less than in zone 2. The driving pressure here remains fixed down to the bottom of the lung because the effect of gravity causes arterial and venous pressures to decrease equally per centimeter of distance as the lung base is approached (Fig. 63-16). Despite the constant driving pressure, flow increases toward the bottom of the lung as resistance decreases. In contrast to zone 2, where the increase in blood flow from top to bottom of the zone is predominantly due to recruitment of vessels that were previously closed, in zone 3 a comparable increase in blood flow is effected largely by distension of patent microvessels, i.e., capillaries.

Zone 4

The upright lung includes in its most dependent part, where vascular pressures are highest, an area of decreased blood flow. The zone of reduced flow (zone 4) disappears on deep inflation. This paradox of high vascular pressures and low blood flow is not explicable in terms of the three-zone model in which pulmonary arterial and pulmonary venous pressures are related to alveolar pressures in predicting distribution of blood flow. The mechanism is believed to reside in the extra-alveolar rather than in the alveolar vessels. Indeed, at residual volume, due to the increase in perivascular pressure and mechanical distortion of extra-alveolar vessels, the distribution of blood flow throughout the lung is attributable to extra-alveolar vessels.

It is worth emphasizing that zones are a functional rather than an anatomic concept; instead of being fixed topographically, they vary in vertical height according to shifts in the relationships between pulmonary arterial, pulmonary venous, and alveolar pressures. For example, positive pressure breathing enlarges zone 2 at the expense of zone 3, and zone 1 at the expense of zone 2. Awareness of the functional nature of these relationships affects the interpretation of changes in calculated pulmonary vascular resistance: for vessels in zone 2, because alveolar pressure rather than pulmonary venous pressure is the outlet pressure, the conventional calculation of pulmonary vascular resistance is meaningless; oppositely, for vessels in zone 3, the calculation is meaningful since pulmonary venous pressure rather than alveolar pressure determines the quantity of blood flow.

Effects of Inflation

It was pointed out above ("Pulmonary Vascular Resistance") that at either very high or low levels of lung inflation—no matter how accomplished—pulmonary vascular resistance increases. Inflation of the collapsed, isolated lung using *negative pressure* first *decreases* resistance and then *increases* resistance as high levels of inflation are reached. These observations can be reconciled by attributing: (1) the *high resistance* at high levels of inflation (alveolar pressure held constant) to narrowing of alveolar capillaries, and (2) the *high resistance* during lung collapse to closure, narrowing, and kinking of alveolar capillaries and extra-alveolar vessels.

Distension and Recruitment. The extent of the alveolar capillary network is quite variable, and the number, size, and shape of the open capillaries depends on the method of fixation for histologic examination as well as on the experimental circumstances. But, some uncertainty still persists about the relative roles played by recruitment (opening of new capillaries) or distension (increase in the caliber of patent capillaries) in enlarging the capillary network.

Not very long ago, pulmonary capillary distension was discounted largely on the basis of extrapolation from the behavior of systemic capillaries. However, attempts to draw analogy between the distensibility of systemic and pulmonary capillaries appear predestined to fail because pulmonary capillaries are suspended in a sea of air and

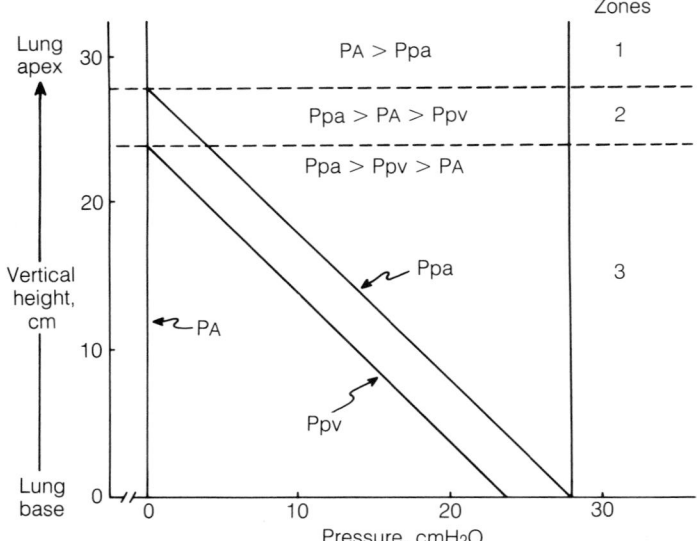

FIGURE 63-16 Parallel courses of pulmonary arterial (Ppa) and pulmonary venous (Ppv) pressures with vertical height. Only in zone 3, in which pulmonary venous pressure (Ppv) exceeds alveolar pressure (PA), does the conventional calculation of pulmonary vascular resistance (using pulmonary venous or left atrial pressure as the outflow pressure) apply.

not imbedded in tissue. Indeed, it has now been amply shown that pulmonary vascular calibers do increase appreciably as transmural pressures are raised. But it has also become evident that the relationship between vascular calibers and transmural pressure is far from simple. Moreover, there is no consensus about the extent to which the alveolar capillary bed is distensible.

How recruitment is effected remains unsettled. When blood flow is minimal (as in zone 1) only few capillaries are open; these are predominantly "corner vessels" lodged within septal pleats. As transmural pressures increase, the extent of the open capillary bed enlarges, primarily by recruitment in zone 2 and by dilatation in zone 3. Some believe that as pulmonary arterial pressure increases, critical opening pressures of different arterioles are successively overcome to open new arteriolar domains to blood flow. Others favor the view that capillaries control their own destinies, i.e., that capillaries per se, rather than arterioles, are responsible for opening new portions of the capillary bed and that both distensibility and recruitment occur at the capillary level.

Despite lingering doubts about the mechanisms involved in the operation of recruitment and distensibility under different conditions, a few generalizations can be made: (1) pulmonary capillaries are more distensible than systemic capillaries, presumably due to the lack of supporting connective tissue in the lung; (2) both recruitment and distensibility are more affected by changes in pulmonary arterial than in pulmonary venous pressure; and (3) recruitment is the predominant mechanism for enlarging the capillary bed in the apices of the lungs in response to pulsatile flow, whereas recruitment and distensibility probably both contribute—although to different degrees, depending on the circumstances—in the more dependent parts of the lungs.

The concepts about recruitment and distensibility outlined above, based on detailed morphologic observations and tube flow, differ from those provided by the sheet flow model which relies heavily on fluid mechanics and in which capillary recruitment is completely discounted. Whether a middle ground exists between these opposite views remains to be seen.

THE FETAL AND NEONATAL PULMONARY CIRCULATION

Before birth, the lungs play no role in gas exchange; this function is served by the placenta. For the sake of their nutrition and role as a metabolic organ, the lungs are provided with a modest blood flow, and most of the blood returning to the right side of the heart is directed toward the systemic circulation by way of the foramen ovale and ductus arteriosus. As a result of this diversion, the lungs before birth receive about 10 to 15 percent of the right ventricular output. After birth, as the lungs assume gas-exchanging functions and fetal connections close, the entire output of the right ventricle perfuses the lungs.

In the fetus approaching term, pulmonary arterial and aortic pressure levels are virtually identical; during gestation, blood pressures in both circuits increase in parallel, while pulmonary blood flow increases dramatically. At the same time, pulmonary vascular resistance decreases progressively as the number of minute vessels increases.

Near term, the small muscular arteries, which constitute the "resistance" vessels, are well endowed with smooth muscle. After birth, the media of the small muscular arteries regress rapidly. However, prolonging hypoxia, as by exposing the newborn to a continued decrease in inspired P_{O_2} for 2 weeks, not only retards the normal involution of pulmonary vascular smooth muscle but also leads to the development of new muscle in peripheral precapillary vessels that would otherwise be expected to be devoid of muscle.

Regulation of the Fetal Pulmonary Circulation

Compared to the adult pulmonary circulation, the fetal circulation affords much more vascular resistance, a higher initial tone and, as has been noted above, a greater vascular reactivity; reactivity increases with gestational age. Also, in contrast to the adult pulmonary circulation, the fetal pulmonary circulation manifests a considerable reactive hyperemia.

Fetal hypoxia, no matter how induced, elicits intense pulmonary vasoconstriction. The magnitude of the response increases as gestation advances, consistent with the idea that pulmonary vascular smooth muscle grows increasingly responsive to hypoxia as gestation advances. In contrast to the adult, the sympathetic nervous system contributes importantly to initial tone and to the pressor response to acute hypoxia. As in the adult, acidosis elicits pulmonary vasoconstriction and greatly enhances the pulmonary pressor response to acute hypoxia; the more severe the acidosis, the greater the pressor and enhancing effects.

Postnatal Pulmonary Vasodilatation

Ventilation of the lungs with air causes a marked drop in pulmonary vascular resistance. Two factors are involved: predominant is the increase in P_{O_2}; a much lesser role is played by physical expansion of the lungs. The mechanism by which relief of hypoxia exerts its vasodilator effect in the fetus is not settled. However, the most likely prospects at present seem to be the prostaglandins. This prospect stems from two types of observations: (1) distension of the lungs of adult animals results in the release of prostaglandins, particularly those of the E series, and (2) indomethacin blunts the continued drop in pulmonary vascular resistance that would be expected to continue for

10 to 20 min after the initial fall. Moreover, in the fetus, prostaglandin synthetase inhibitors enhance the pulmonary pressor response to acute hypoxia.

Attention has been called repeatedly in this section to the marked reactivity of the fetal pulmonary circulation. The purposes served by the marked pulmonary vasoreactivity are not certain. But, since the increase in fetal pulmonary vascular resistance does direct the bulk of the pulmonary arterial inflow to the placenta, brain, and myocardium, the capability for marked pulmonary vasodilatation may be importantly involved in the circulatory rearrangements after birth.

THE BRONCHIAL CIRCULATION

Although popular usage has firmly entrenched the designation *bronchial*, the term is inadequate on two accounts: (1) the systemic blood supply to the lungs originates not only from bronchial arteries but also from the aorta and other intrathoracic arteries, and (2) the systemic arterial blood is delivered not only to the walls of the bronchi but also to the adventitia or large vessels and structures of the lungs.

In the normal lung, the bronchial circulation has the features of a nutrient circulation: it is modest in size, carries arterialized blood, and is distributed primarily to the airways, blood vessels, and supporting structures of the lungs. At the level of the respiratory bronchioles, the bronchial arteries give rise to capillaries which communicate with pulmonary capillaries.

Venous return from the bronchial circulation is via either bronchial or pulmonary veins: from the hilar structures and large bronchi, bronchial venous blood is returned to the *right* atrium via systemic veins; from more peripheral airways and the substance of the lung, bronchial venous blood is returned to the left atrium by two routes: via bronchial-pulmonary capillary anastomoses and by "bronchopulmonary veins" that connect bronchial capillaries to small pulmonary veins. The direction taken by bronchial venous outflow is determined by the relative pressures at the outlet of the two systems. For example, an increase in left atrial pressure detours bronchial venous drainage toward the right, rather than the left, atrium. In some animals, functioning communications exist not only between the bronchial and pulmonary capillary circulations but also between the bronchial arteries and other systemic arteries.

Certain features of the bronchial circulation merit special attention: (1) although difficult to demonstrate and of doubtful functional significance, microscopic anastomoses between bronchial and pulmonary arteries do appear to exist at the precapillary level in the normal lung; (2) the bronchial arteries proliferate remarkably in certain types of lung disease, liver disease, and congenital

heart disease—often in association with clubbing of the digits; (3) the mechanisms responsible for the proliferation of the bronchial circulation are unclear, but certain influences, such as cortisone, retard its expansion, whereas growth hormone stimulates it; (4) the bronchial veins in the submucosa of the airways form a large plexus that runs the entire length of the tracheobronchial tree, sending off communicating branches to a corresponding venous plexus on the other side of the tracheal muscle; (5) the bronchial venules respond to certain vasoactive agents, notably histamine and bradykinin, as do other systemic venules; and (6) the bronchial venous circulation is involved in the pathogenesis of experimental pulmonary edema produced in the dog and sheep by histamine, endotoxin, and bradykinin.

Determination of Bronchial Blood Flow

Because bronchial blood flow in the normal lung is so small, it is difficult to measure accurately by techniques that depend on indicator-dilution or Fick's principles. This task becomes easier when the bronchial circulation increases as after ligation of a major pulmonary artery. In sheep, accurate determinations of bronchial blood flow and responses of the bronchial circulation to diverse stimuli have been quantified by placing an electromagnetic flow probe around a large bronchial artery (*carinal artery*) that supplies bronchial arterial blood to the airways and supporting structures of more than 80 percent of the lungs.

Normal Levels of Bronchial Blood Flow

In the normal human lung, bronchial blood flow is of the order of 1 to 2 percent of the cardiac output. This blood is delivered to the supporting framework of the lungs up to the respiratory bronchioles. Beyond this point, the pulmonary circulation takes over as the nutrient circulation. One likely function of the bronchial circulation is in air conditioning the inspired air. The disposition and architecture of the submucosal bronchial venous plexus seem to constitute an anatomic arrangement that could properly adjust the temperature and water content of air passing to and fro in the airways.

The Bronchial Circulation in Disease

In the normal lung the minute bronchial circulation operates covertly. But, should the pulmonary circulation to an area be compromised or lost—as by ligation or an embolus—the bronchial circulation proliferates far beyond local metabolic need for viability and function. The stimulus for proliferation is unclear. Expansion of the bronchial arterial circulation is clinically marked in two major categories of disease: (1) those involving severe curtailment of pulmonary blood flow, as in congenital pulmonary atresia, and (2) a chronic inflammatory bronchopul-

monary process, such as bronchiectasis, old inflammatory cavities, chronic lung abscess, and lung cancer. Because clubbing of the digits, occasionally accompanied by hypertrophic osteoarthropathy, is also common in these disorders, question is often raised about the relationship between clubbing of the digits and expansion of the collateral circulation to the lungs. In contrast to the disorders of the lungs associated with bronchial arterial blood is chronic mitral stenosis in which hemoptysis usually originates from bronchial veins underlying the tracheobronchial mucosa.

An expanded bronchial arterial circulation can also constitute a hemodynamic burden, i.e., a left-to-right shunt. But, rarely, as in widespread bronchiectasis, do the connections between the bronchial and pulmonary arteries enlarge sufficiently to cause cardiac embarrassment. Should a wedged pulmonary arterial catheter lodge in the vicinity of bronchial-pulmonary arterial anastomoses, the pulmonary wedge pressure is apt to be misleading.

As noted above, bronchial venous blood that drains into the left atrium contributes to anatomic venous admixture. Another source of anatomic venous admixture occurs in some patients with cirrhosis of the liver in whom abnormal anatomic connections allow the passage of portal venous blood into the pulmonary venous system. In an occasional patient with hepatic cirrhosis, the portal-pulmonary blood flow becomes quite large, i.e., about 5 to 15 percent of the cardiac output. Occasionally, these anastomotic channels enlarge sufficiently to be demonstrable during life using indicators or angiography. More often the quantity of blood shunted from the portal to pulmonary venous system is too small to be measured reliably.

Since primary carcinoma of the lungs often receives much of its blood supply from systemic arteries, particularly if the neoplasm obstructs blood flow to the pulmonary artery, attempts have been made to deliver chemotherapeutic agents to the cancerous site via a bronchial artery. This approach has proved ineffective. Also, in some patients in whom life-threatening hemoptysis complicates a carcinoma of the lungs, particulate matter has been injected as bronchial arterial emboli in the hope of occluding the feeder bronchial artery. Unfortunately, selective embolization is, at best, only transiently effective.

BIBLIOGRAPHY

Banister J, Torrance RW: The effects of tracheal pressure upon flow-pressure relations in the vascular bed of isolated lungs. Q J Exp Physiol 45:352–367, 1960.
Analysis of the effects of tracheal pressures on the pulmonary vascular bed and the consequences of the changes in pressure which occur during cardiac and respiratory cycles.

Bhattacharya J, Nanjo S, Staub NC: Micropuncture measurement of lung microvascular pressure during 5-HT infusion. J Appl Physiol 52:634–637, 1982.
Direct determinations of pulmonary vascular pressures using micropuncture techniques applied to pulmonary vessels.

Downing SE, Lee JC: Nervous control of the pulmonary circulation. Annu Rev Physiol 42:199–210, 1980.
A balanced exposition of the contribution of the autonomic nervous system to the regulation of the pulmonary circulation.

Fishman AP: Hypoxia on the pulmonary circulation: How and where it acts. Circ Res 38:221–231, 1976.
A depiction of the possible mechanisms and sites of action of acute hypoxia.

Fishman AP: Pulmonary Circulation, in Fishman AP, Fisher AB (eds), *Handbook of Physiology*, sect 3: *The Respiratory System*, vol 1: *Circulation and Non-Respiratory Functions*. Bethesda, MD, American Physiological Society, 1985, pp 93–166.
A comprehensive overview of the pulmonary circulation. Extensive bibliography.

Furchgott RF: Role of endothelium in responses of vascular smooth muscle. Circ Res 53:557–573, 1983.
A seminal paper that has prompted all sorts of research about endothelial-smooth-muscle communication in vasomotor responses.

Gil J: Organization of microcirculation in the lung. Annu Rev Physiol 42:177–186, 1980.
An important contribution to understanding of the arrangement of the microcirculation of the lungs not only with respect to gas exchange but also to fluid exchange.

Glazier JB, Hughes JMB, Maloney JE, West JB: Measurements of capillary dimensions and blood volume in rapidly frozen lungs. J Appl Physiol 26:65–76, 1969.
An important paper that has worn well as a foundation of current concepts about the zones of the lungs.

Grover RF, Weil JV, Reeves JT: Cardiovascular adaptation to exercise at high altitude. Exer & Sports Sci Rev 14:269–302, 1986.
An extensive review of the normal pulmonary circulations not only at altitude but also at sea level.

Hughes JM: Pulmonary circulation and fluid balance. Int Rev Physiol 14:135–183, 1977.
A review that relates the control of the pulmonary circulation to the water circulation of the lungs.

Magno MG, Fishman AP: Origin, distribution, and blood flow of bronchial circulation in anesthetized sheep. J Appl Physiol 53:272–279, 1982.
The discovery of a large bronchial artery in which blood flow to a defined segment could be accurately measured revitalized interest in the bronchial circulation.

Permutt S, Bromberger-Barnea B, Bane HN: Alveolar pressure, pulmonary venous pressure and the vascular waterfall. Med Thorac 19:239–260, 1962.
This paper should be read by those interested in the concept of vascular waterfall and the zones of the lungs.

Reeves JT, McMurtry IF, Voelkel NF: Possible role for membrane lipids in the function of the normal and abnormal pulmonary circulation. Am Rev Respir Dis 136:196–199, 1987.
One of a series of papers in the same issue dealing with the experimental and hypothetical aspects of the role of membrane lipids (platelet-activating factor and arachidonic acid metabolites) in the regulation of adult and perinatal pulmonary vasomotor tone.

Rudolph AM: Fetal and neonatal pulmonary circulation. Annu Rev Physiol 41:383–395, 1979.
A concise overview of the adjustments in the pulmonary circulation at birth.

Shirai M, Sada K, Ninomiya I: Effects of regional alveolar hypoxia and hypercapnia on microcirculation in small pulmonary vessels in cats. J Appl Physiol 61:440–448, 1986.
Using an x-ray TV system, the authors analyzed the responses to acute hypoxia and hypercapnia in small pulmonary vessels during unilobar hypoxia and hypercapnia in the cat. For a given hypoxic stimulus, the internal diameter of precapillary vessels was constricted to a much greater extent than that of the veins. Not only acute hypoxia, but acute hypercapnia elicited pulmonary vasoconstriction.

Skalak RF, Wiener F, Morkin E, Fishman AP: The energy distribution in the pulmonary circulation. II. Experiments. Phys Med Biol 11:437–449, 1966.
The energetics of the pulmonary circulation based on direct measurements. Provides insight into the synchrony of the two ventricles and applies the law of mass action to the understanding of instant-to-instant changes in pulmonary vascular pressures and flows on the one hand, and the work of the right ventricle on the other.

Szidon JP, Fishman AP: Autonomic control of the pulmonary circulation, in Fishman AP, Hecht H (eds), Pulmonary Circulation and Interstitial Space. Chicago, IL, University of Chicago Press, 1969, pp 239–268.
The role of the autonomic nervous system in promoting the integrated responses of the pulmonary circulation.

Voelkel NF, Chang SW, McDonnell TJ, Westcott JY, Haynes J: Role of membrane lipids in the control of normal vascular tone. Am Rev Respir Dis 136:214–217, 1987.
A consideration of the determinants of pulmonary vascular tone, focusing on membrane lipids (platelet-activating factor) and metabolites of arachidonic acid.

Voelkel N, Reeves JT: Primary pulmonary hypertension, in Moser K (ed), Pulmonary Vascular Diseases. New York, Dekker, 1979, pp 573–628.
A large experience with normal pulmonary hemodynamics at altitude is used as a basis for comparison with the abnormal pulmonary circulation.

West JB: Regional differences in the lung. New York, Academic, 1977, pp 85–165.
A review of some fundamental precepts of the zones of the lungs.

Chapter 64

Pulmonary Hypertension and Cor Pulmonale

Alfred P. Fishman

PULMONARY (ARTERIAL) HYPERTENSION

The pulmonary circulation is a low-resistance, highly distensible circulation. In normal individuals lying supine, systolic pressures are of the order of 15 to 25 mmHg; the corresponding diastolic pressures are 5 to 10 mmHg. The mean driving pressure, i.e., the difference between the mean blood pressure in the pulmonary artery and in the left atrium, is about 10 to 12 mmHg, one-eighth of that in the systemic circulation (Fig. 64-1). Since blood flow (cardiac output) is the same in both circulations, the pulmonary vascular resistance is about eight times less than the systemic vascular resistance. The large aggregate cross-sectional area of the pulmonary circulation is responsible for this low resistance, which is reflected in the sparsity of muscle in the pulmonary resistance vessels, the large run-off of blood from the pulmonary arterial tree during each systole, the large capacity and expansibility of the pulmonary arterial tree, and the large number of minute vessels that are held in reserve.

During exercise, pulmonary blood flow increases. Accompanying this increment in blood flow is a decrease in pulmonary vascular resistance brought about by recruiting new parts of the pulmonary vascular bed and by

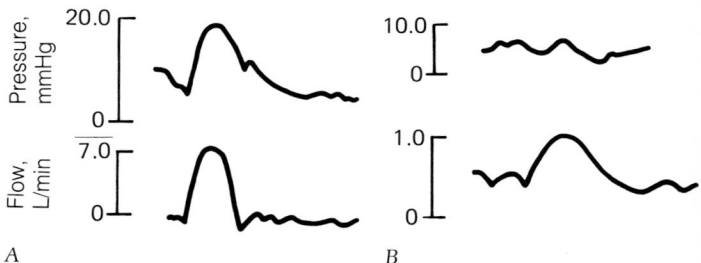

FIGURE 64-1 Schematic representation of pressure and flow pulses in the pulmonary artery (*A*) and vein (*B*).

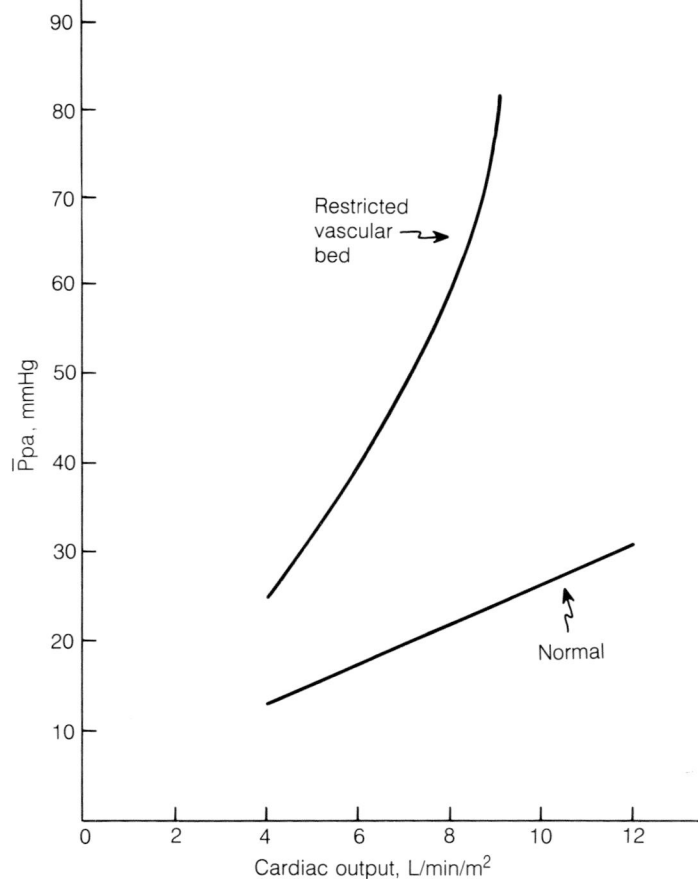

FIGURE 64-2 Pulmonary circulation at sea level, at rest and during exercise. Restriction of the pulmonary arterial tree causes higher pulmonary arterial pressures at any level of blood flow.

widening the calibers of those vessels that were already open. As a result of these accommodations, a considerable increase in pulmonary blood flow elicits only a modest increase in pulmonary arterial pressure (Fig. 64-2).

Normal values for the pulmonary circulation of an adult at sea level are shown in Table 64-1. For the sea-level dweller, pulmonary arterial hypertension (pulmonary hypertension) is said to exist when the level of pulmonary arterial pressure increases by 5 to 10 mmHg, e.g., from 25/10 with a mean of 18 mmHg to 35/15 with a mean of 25 mmHg. However, this level, which for sea-level dwellers would represent a modest increase, is normal for dwellers at high altitude (Fig. 64-3).

TABLE 64-1

Representative Values for the Normal Pulmonary Circulation at Sea Level*

	Rest	Mild Exercise
Pulmonary blood flow, L/min	8	16
Pulmonary vascular pressures, mmHg		
Pulmonary artery	25/10, 18	30/13, 20,
Pulmonary veins	5	8
Pulmonary blood volumes, ml		
Total	250	250
Capillary	60	100

*For an adult male weighing about 70 kg.

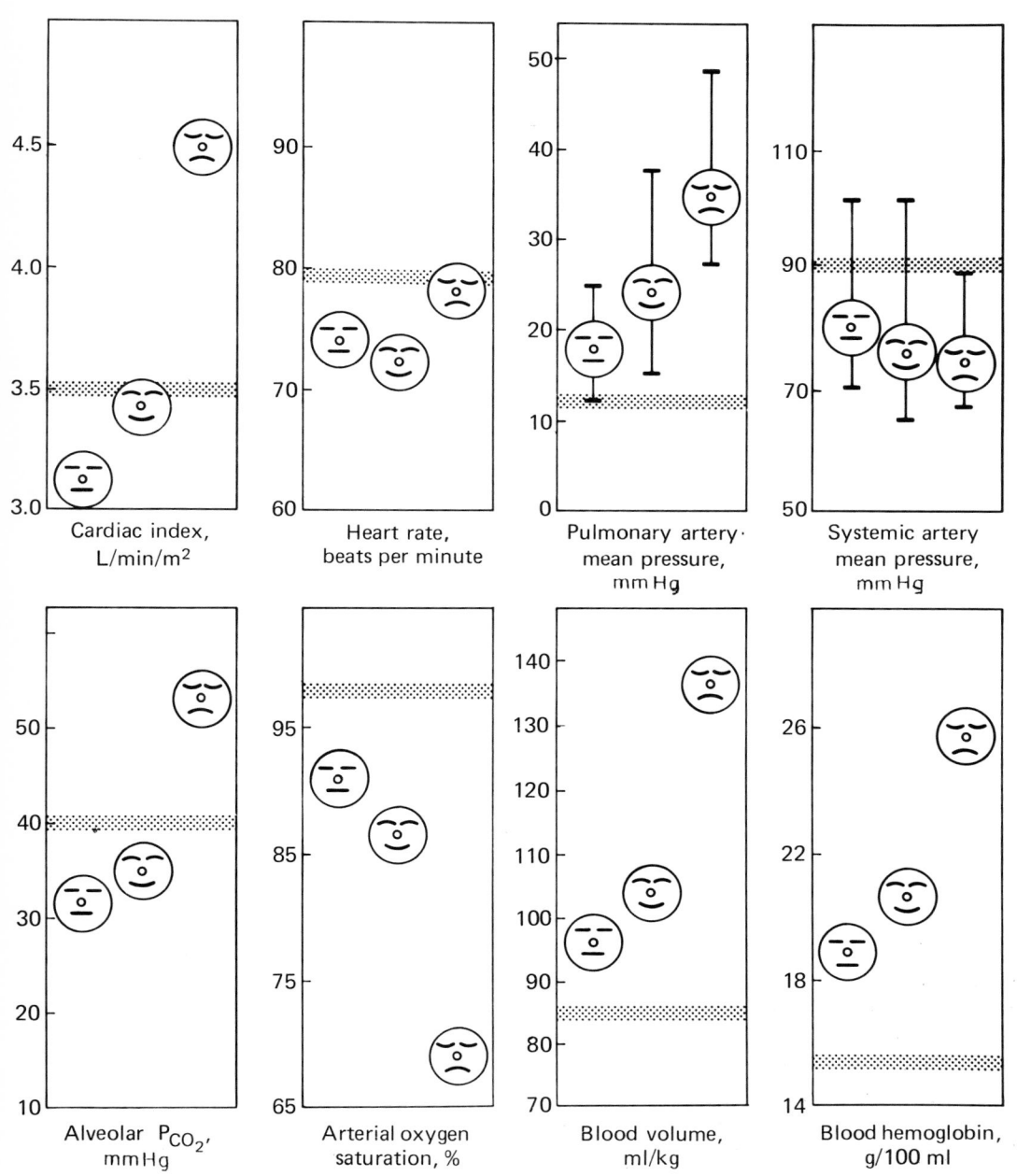

FIGURE 64-3 Schematic representations of respiratory and circulatory measurements of human beings at altitude (14,900 ft). The three circles within each of the eight rectangular boxes represent typical values for the 1-year resident (left circle); the acclimatized native resident (middle circle); the mountain-sick native resident (right circle). (*After Fishman, 1963.*)

TABLE 64-2

Potential Pathogenetic Mechanisms Leading to Pulmonary Arterial Hypertension and Cor Pulmonale

Mechanisms	Example
Primary	
Anatomic decrease in cross-sectional area (vessel destruction; encroachment on lumen by hypertherapy) of the pulmonary resistance vessels	Interstitial fibrosis and granuloma
Vasoconstriction of pulmonary resistance vessels	Hypoxia and acidosis
Contributory	
Large increments in pulmonary blood flow	Exercise
Increased pressures on the left side of the heart and pulmonary veins	Left ventricular failure or pulmonary veno-occlusive disease
Increased viscosity of the blood	Secondary polycythemia of chronic hypoxia
Unproved	
Compression of pulmonary resistance vessels by raised alveolar pressures in their vicinity	Asthmatic bronchitis
Bronchial arterial-pulmonary arterial anastomoses	Expanded bronchial circulation

Pathogenesis of Pulmonary (Arterial) Hypertension

Not only is the normal pulmonary circulation low in resistance and highly distensible, but it is also predominantly passive. There are no baroreceptors comparable to those in the systemic circulation. Also, stimulation of pulmonary vasomotor nerves exerts only modest effects on the pulmonary circulation's capacity, distensibility, and resistance to blood flow. Finally, humoral substances, such as the components of the renin-angiotensin system, do not appear to be involved in sustained pulmonary hypertension.

In principle, six different mechanisms may cause, or contribute to, pulmonary hypertension. They are listed in Table 64-2. Of the six, only the first two (the primary mechanisms) are distinctive for cor pulmonale. Although the others are not unique for cor pulmonale, they do aggravate pulmonary hypertension arising from anatomic curtailment and vasoconstriction of the pulmonary resistance vessels, thereby adding to the burden of the right ventricle. An acute increase in pulmonary arterial pressure is not difficult to produce experimentally. The intravenous injection of all sorts of particulate matter has been shown to elicit pulmonary hypertension. Curiously, this form of pulmonary hypertension rarely lasts for more than minutes; in some mysterious way, the pressure soon falls spontaneously to normal. More extensive embolization usually brings the experiment to an abrupt end because of acute dilatation and failure of the right ventricle or because of ventricular fibrillation. The ability of the right ventricle to compensate for acute increases in afterload is limited. Therefore, the design of experimental models of chronic pulmonary hypertension in animals using emboli must impose serial increments in afterloads if adaptation of the right ventricle is to occur.

Strategies other than embolization have been used to produce more durable types of pulmonary hypertension. Most popular is the use of chronic hypoxia in susceptible animals, e.g., in the cow at high altitude. Another approach has been the use of the drug monocrotaline in rats and, to a lesser extent, in dogs and nonhuman primates. This type of pulmonary hypertension is less consistent than that produced by chronic hypoxia, and generally experimental interstitial disease, such as that produced by injections of Freund's adjuvant, is associated with pulmonary hypertension. Finally, attempts are currently being made to produce pulmonary hypertension experimentally using immune mechanisms to damage the linings of the small vessels. Of all these methods, that of chronic hypoxia is best standardized and understood. One mode of chronic pulmonary hypertension produced by increasing flow into a restricted pulmonary vascular bed is characterized by the appearance of plexiform and angiomatoid vascular lesions. These lesions also occur in certain instances of pulmonary hypertension in humans. Reliable animal models produced by other mechanisms are sorely needed to explore pathogenetic mechanisms and to test for effective vasodilator agents.

The search for mechanisms of pulmonary hypertension is currently being actively pursued. Membrane phenomena at the endothelial surface are one promising line of research. Various mediators, such as histamine, that once had strong advocates, have been succeeded by prostaglandins that are liberated within the lungs. The search is on for receptors and channels, particularly those involving calcium cell-cell communication at the luminal surface of the resistance vessels, along with a succession of "growth" factors that manifest a multiplicity of functions. The occasional coexistence of pulmonary hypertension and cirrhosis of the liver raises the possibility that humoral mediators from afar, which manage to bypass the damaged liver, are responsible. However, relationships along the lung-liver axis are exceedingly complicated. Although it is unlikely that any single mechanism will be able to account for the diverse types of pulmonary hypertension, it does seem reasonable that biochemical events that increase vascular tone and lead to growth and proliferation of pulmonary vascular smooth muscle will prove to be an important common denominator.

ANATOMIC RESTRICTION

In clinical situations, acute reduction in the extent of the normal pulmonary vascular bed rarely suffices, per se, to raise pulmonary arterial pressures to pulmonary hypertensive levels. For example, pneumonectomy in human beings has little effect on pulmonary arterial pressures (Fig. 64-4), and in the dog more than two-thirds of the lungs must be ablated before pulmonary arterial pressures approach hypertensive levels. Even in chronic rarefaction of the lungs, particularly emphysema that is unassociated with chronic bronchitis, the characteristic decrease in the

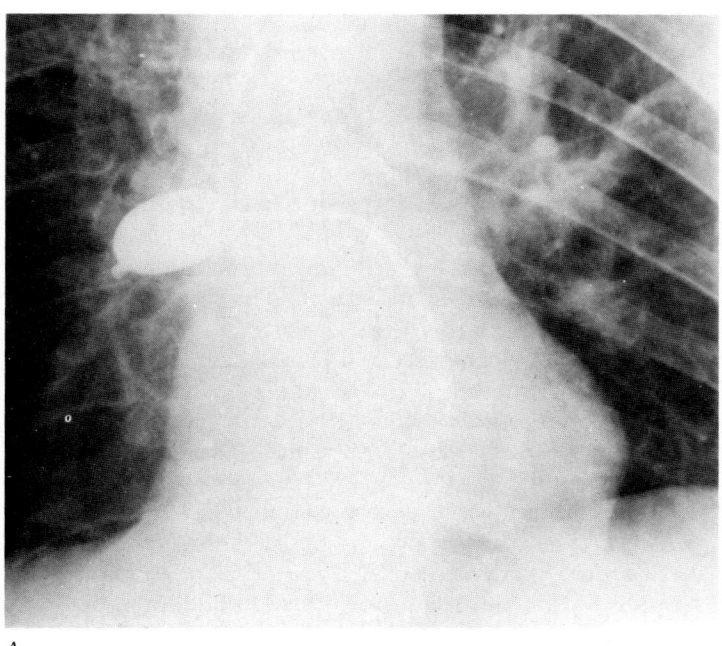

A

FIGURE 64-4 Occlusion of right pulmonary artery by balloon at tip of cardiac catheter. *A.* Balloon inflated in right pulmonary artery. *B.* Oxygen uptake by the two lungs before *(left)*, during *(middle)*, and after *(right)* balloon occlusion of the pulmonary artery. During the occlusion O$_2$ uptake by the right lung ceases, indicating arrest of blood flow through the ipsilateral lung. *C.* The inflation (arrow) causes virtually no change in left pulmonary arterial pressure even though blood flow through the left lung has doubled. RPA = right pulmonary artery: MPA = main pulmonary artery. *(After Fishman, 1963.)*

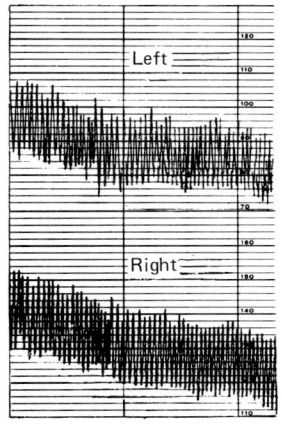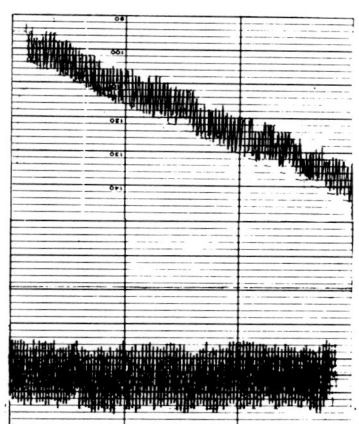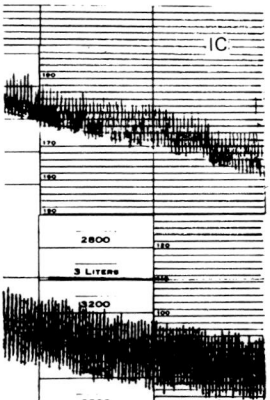

B

RPA

MPA

C

number of minute vessels in the emphysematous areas rarely leads to pulmonary hypertension. Multiple pulmonary emboli cause pulmonary hypertension by obliterating large segments of the pulmonary arterial tree and by increasing resistance to blood flow in many of the vessels that remain open (Fig. 64-5). A decrease in the number of pulmonary blood vessels has been proposed as a contributory mechanism in various forms of human and experimental pulmonary hypertension, such as those caused by congenital heart disease, *Crotalaria*, and chronic hypoxia. By and large, when anatomic restriction leads to pulmonary hypertension, occlusive and amputative vascular disease coexist.

Widespread interstitial lung disease has long been known to be a forerunner of pulmonary hypertension. For example, the original description of *alveolar-capillary block*, a syndrome that focused primarily on diffusion impairment due to thickening of the alveolar-capillary barrier, pictured thickening and obliteration of the alveolar-capillary barrier as the major causes of impaired gas exchange and of pulmonary hypertension. Scleroderma was one of the prototypes. Now it is known that the model of alveolar-capillary block was an oversimplification and that interstitial lung disease is rarely confined to the interstitium. For example, obliterative vascular disease of the resistance vessels often accompanies interstitial disease in scleroderma. Indeed, in some instances, vascular lesions predominate to the point of virtually no interstitial disease.

In the CREST syndrome, a benign variant of progressive systemic sclerosis (characterized by calcinosis, Raynaud's phenomenon, esophageal dysfunction, sclerodactylia, and telangiectasis), pulmonary hypertension is often unaccompanied by pulmonary fibrosis. Raynaud's phenomenon induced by immersing the hand in cold water is not accompanied by vasospasm in the pulmonary circulation. Instead, the cause of the pulmonary hypertension seems to reside in obliterative changes in the small- and medium-sized pulmonary arteries produced by myxomatous changes similar to those that occur in the digital arteries of patients who manifest Raynaud's phenomenon as part of the clinical syndrome of diffuse systemic sclerosis. In other connective tissue disorders, such as lupus erythematosus, combinations of interstitial and intrinsic vascular abnormalities contribute to pulmonary hypertension.

HYPOXIA AND ACIDOSIS

Pulmonary vasoconstriction is an important mechanism for causing hypertension. Hypoxia is the most effective vasoconstrictor; acidosis is next. Both exert their effects within the lungs. In the normal pulmonary circulation, even these "powerful" vasoconstrictors generally elicit only modest increments in pulmonary arterial pressure; i.e., acute hypoxia, induced by breathing a gas mixture consisting of 10% O_2 and the remainder N_2 ("10% O_2 in N_2"), may evoke an increment of 5 to 10 mmHg (Fig. 64-6). However, certain animal species and some inbred human groups seem to be congential hyperreactors.

How hypoxia causes pulmonary arterial smooth muscle to constrict is unclear. Attention is currently focused on two major alternatives (Fig. 64-7): (1) an *indirect*

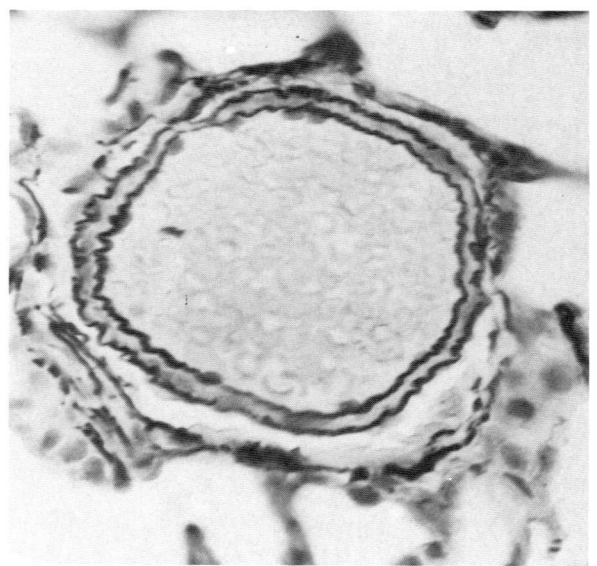

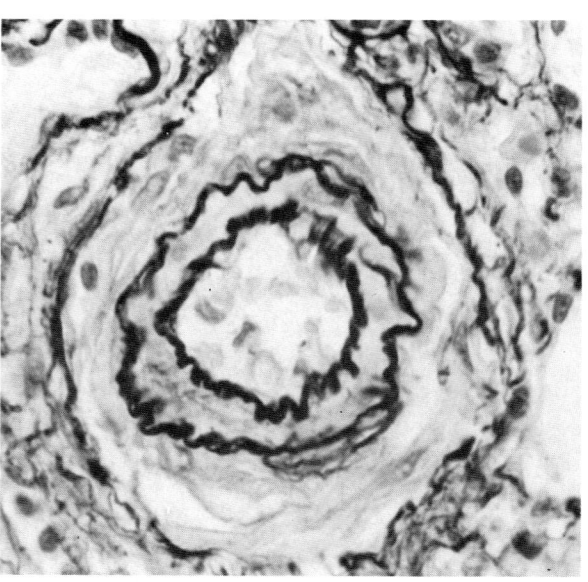

A

B

FIGURE 64-5 Normal and thickened pulmonary resistance vessels. *A.* Pulmonary arteriole showing thin muscular media, double elastic lamina, and widely patent lumen (40 μm). Aldehyde-fuchsin-elastic, ×560. *B.* Pulmonary arteriole from pulmonary hypertensive dog showing marked thickening of the media, decrease in lumen size, and perivascular fibrosis (40 μm). Aldehyde-fuchsin-elastic, ×560. *(Courtesy of Dr. B. Atkinson.)*

method via alveolar hypoxia, which might cause certain cells (e.g., mast cells) in the pulmonary parenchyma to discharge vasoactive substances, e.g., histamine, or (2) a *direct* constrictor effect of hypoxia on pulmonary arterial smooth muscle. Although the mechanism underlying the pressor effect of acute hypoxia is still being explored by physiologists, for practical purposes, the pulmonary hypertensive effect of acute hypoxia can be regarded to be the result of a direct effect of the low P_{O_2} on smooth muscle in the walls of the resistance vessels of the lungs.

Acidosis not only has a direct pressor effect on the pulmonary circulation (Fig. 64-6), but it also reinforces the pressor response to acute hypoxia. In contrast to acute

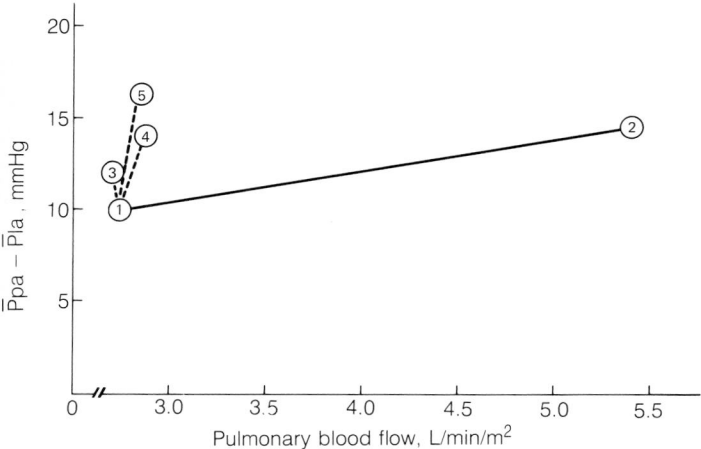

FIGURE 64-6 Schematic representation of pulmonary circulatory response to different stimuli: 1 = ambient air; 2 = exercise; 3 = acidosis (pH = 7.25); 4 = 12% O_2; 5 = combination of 3 and 4.

hypoxia, acute hypercapnia exerts a pressor effect only if it causes acidosis. Therefore, human subjects exposed to acute hypercapnia, e.g., to an inspired gas mixture containing 5% CO_2, generally fail to develop pulmonary hypertension, because the increase in minute ventilation while breathing this concentration of CO_2 maintains arterial pH at near-normal levels.

Chronic hypoxia, no matter how caused, is associated with pulmonary hypertension. Experimental studies of the pulmonary circulation in animals exposed to hypoxia for several weeks show that structural changes begin early and are completely reversible. The most striking change is the de novo muscularization of peripheral small pulmonary arteries which normally have either no smooth muscle or only a partial layer. This peripheral extension of newly formed muscle probably narrows the vascular lumen, thereby contributing to increased vascular resistance. Medium-sized vessels also undergo increase in medial thickness. The reactivity of this new muscle to hypoxia has not yet been established. It seems reasonable, although it is not yet proved, that the human pulmonary circulation chronically exposed to hypoxia undergoes similar changes.

CONTINUED RESIDENCE AT HIGH ALTITUDE

As noted above, at comparable levels of pulmonary blood flow, the pulmonary arterial pressure is consistently higher at altitude (greater than 7000 to 8000 ft) than at sea level. The higher the altitude, the more marked the pulmonary hypertension. At Morococha, Peru (4540-m altitude), mean pulmonary arterial pressure at rest is of the order of 25 mmHg; it more than doubles during moderate

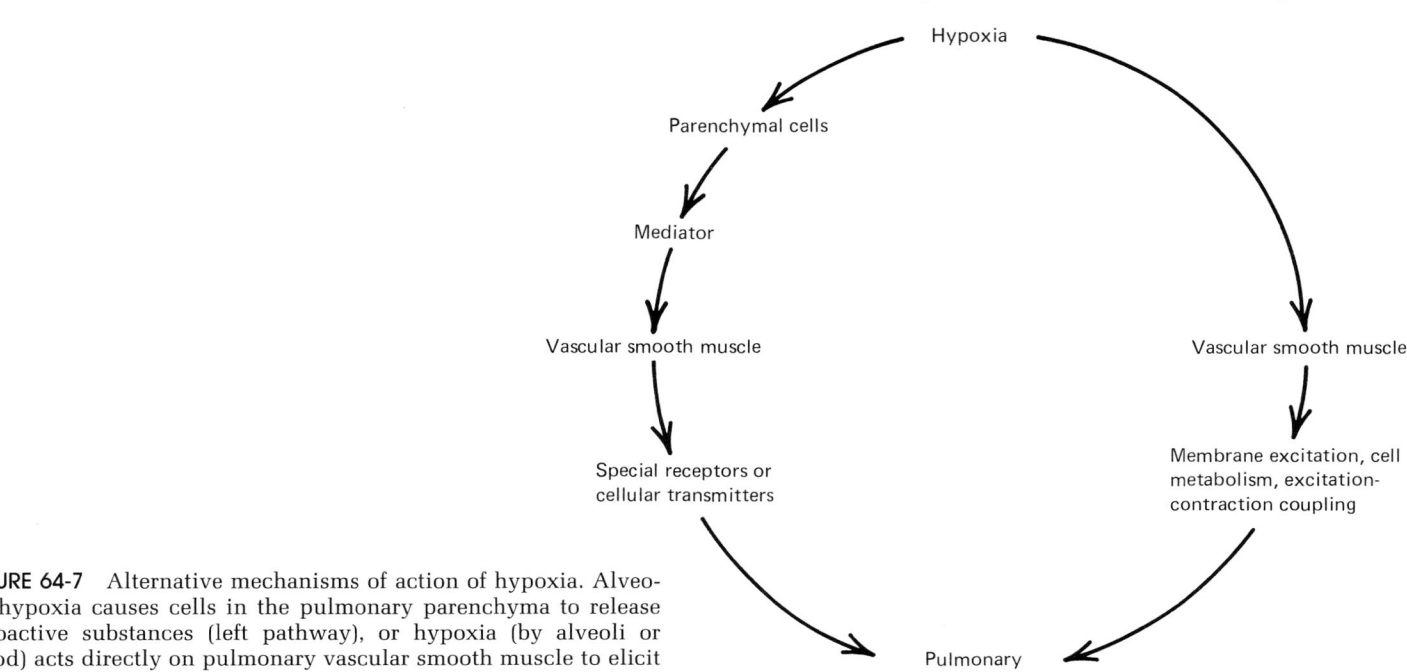

FIGURE 64-7 Alternative mechanisms of action of hypoxia. Alveolar hypoxia causes cells in the pulmonary parenchyma to release vasoactive substances (left pathway), or hypoxia (by alveoli or blood) acts directly on pulmonary vascular smooth muscle to elicit vasoconstriction (right pathway).

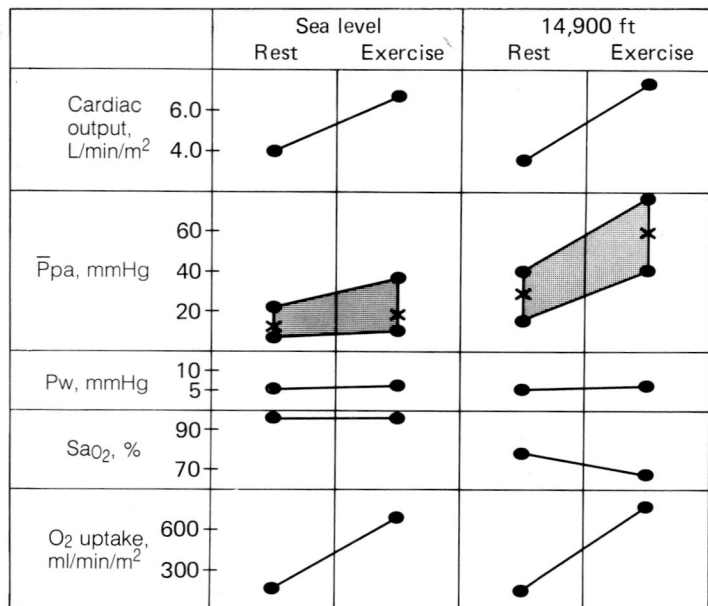

FIGURE 64-8 Comparison of pulmonary circulation at sea level and at altitude (14,900 ft), at rest and during exercise. The same increment in blood flow causes much larger increments in pulmonary arterial pressure at altitude than at sea level.

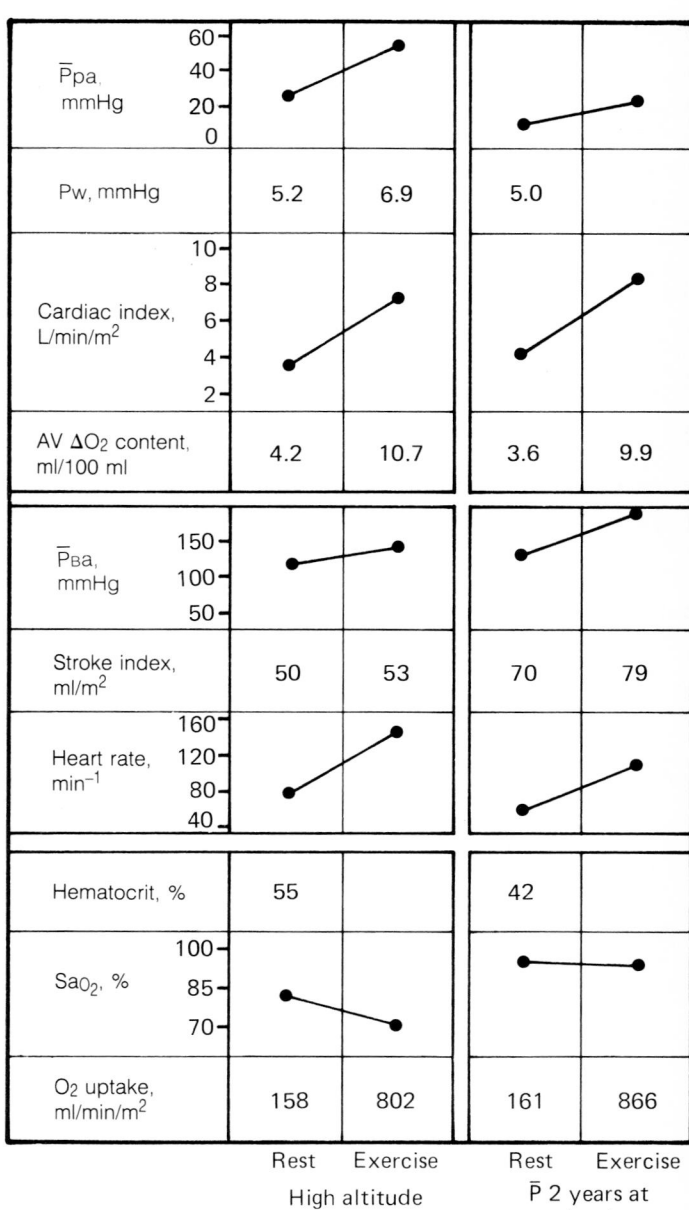

FIGURE 64-9 Return of pulmonary artery pressures to normal after prolonged residence at sea level.

exercise (Fig. 64-8). In comparison to the hearts of sea dwellers, the right ventricle is hypertrophied. Any intensification of the degree of hypoxia, as by pulmonary disease or alveolar hypoventilation, aggravates pulmonary hypertension. Breathing 100% O_2 decreases pulmonary artery pressure in the chronically hypoxic altitude dweller, but not quite to normal.

Although increased muscularization of the pulmonary resistance vessels contributes importantly to the increased resistance to blood flow, increased muscularization per se is not the full explanation. For example, it does not explain why residents at high altitude in South America manifest less hypertension than do people living at a comparable height in the United States. Nor does it indicate why pulmonary vasoconstriction is much more vigorous in some individuals and animals at a given altitude than in others. Finally, evidence has been provided, both in humans and other animals, for genetic predisposition to inordinate pulmonary pressor effects when certain individuals are exposed to hypoxia. Neither the anatomic nor physiological basis for this heightened susceptibility is understood.

Upon changing residence from altitude to sea level, pulmonary artery pressures drop as arterial oxgenation improves. But even after 2 years at sea level, the mean pulmonary artery pressure at rest is somewhat high and increases abnormally, albeit not to the same extent as at altitude (Fig. 64-9).

Whether the higher levels of pulmonary artery pressure at altitude should be regarded as part of an adaptive process or as a penalty is debatable. One possible advantage of the higher pressures is to promote uniformity of pulmonary blood flow by increasing blood flow to the apexes. The improved distribution in pulmonary blood flow, coupled with the increase in ventilation and in diffusing capacity, could enhance the function of the lungs at altitude. However, it is difficult to prove that the increased perfusion of the apexes secondary to an increase in pulmonary arterial pressure materially improves gas exchange in the normal lung at altitude.

MOUNTAIN SICKNESS

Failure to adapt to high altitude may be acute or chronic. Acute mountain sickness (*seroche*) affects the newcomer at altitude; it is unusual below 7000 ft and is almost a regular occurrence over 12,000 ft. Lassitude, headache, nausea, vomiting, and palpitations are disabling, and cyanosis and Cheyne-Stokes breathing are striking. Usually adjustment occurs within 3 to 4 days, and normal activity can be resumed.

Chronic mountain sickness affects native residents at high altitude. The disease is uncommon. The vivid description by Monge is unforgettable:

> At rest, the patient appears reddish or blue and he turns purple at the least effort. In cases of most severe involvement the scleras are intensely colored by the distended capillaries; the eyes being hidden behind edematous and bluish eyelids. The face is blue-violet, almost black, resembling that of an asphyxiated person. The mucous membranes are reddish. The tongue appears larger than normal and full of blood. All the superficial blood vessels appear dilated. Varices are common. Epistaxis is frequent; aphonia is usually noted. The hands show clubbing of fingers. The nails become thick and appear to be inserted like watch glasses. The person resembles an old emphysematous, plethoric patient, walking slowly and heavily. He feels extremely weak and has a marked tendency to sleep. A state of drowsiness is frequently found. Spells of dizziness and fainting occur commonly. Nausea and vomiting at the least effort are noted occasionally; there are spells of diarrhea. Blurring of vision and temporary blindness are frequently observed. Transient deafness occurs. Sometimes the patient suddenly falls into a kind of asphyxial coma for two or three hours, to return later to his pitiful condition. Aphonia, coughing, and repeated bronchitis are present. Also recurring are congestive processes in the lungs with hemoptysis.

Hurtado appreciated that the clinical picture was secondary to severe alveolar hypoventilation. More than one mechanism may produce the same pathetic clinical picture. In some subjects, alveolar hypoventilation appears to be secondary to an unexplained loss of acclimatization that blunts the response of the peripheral arterial chemoreceptors to the hypoxemic stimulus. In others, as in miners, chronic lung disease evokes the same picture by deranging ventilation-perfusion relationships. No matter which of these mechanisms is operative or predominates, the end result is the same: severe arterial hypoxemia, hypercapnia, polycythemia, and severe pulmonary hypertension (Fig. 64-3).

OTHER PULMONARY CIRCULATORY DISORDERS AT ALTITUDE

The incidence of patent ductus arteriosus is higher at altitude than at sea level, and becomes quite high at altitudes greater than 9000 ft. It is still unsettled whether primary pulmonary hypertension is more prevalent at altitude than at sea level. The subject is of interest since hypoxic vasoconstriction is the root cause of pulmonary hypertension at high altitude, and the possibility has been raised that primary hypertension also begins as a vasoconstrictive disorder.

COLLATERAL CIRCULATION

The collateral circulation to the lungs undergoes remarkable proliferation in certain types of congenital heart disease, particularly those involving severe stenosis of the pulmonary outflow tract. It also expands in areas of chronic pulmonary inflammation, such as lung abscess and bronchiectasis (Fig. 64-10). Following ligation of one pulmonary artery, the viability of the lung is maintained by the enlarged collateral circulation. Indeed, the vascularity often appears normal on chest radiographs because of the collateral circulation and retrograde filling of the pulmonary arterial tree by left atrial contractions. However, the collateral circulation has not been shown to be involved in the pathogenesis of pulmonary hypertension.

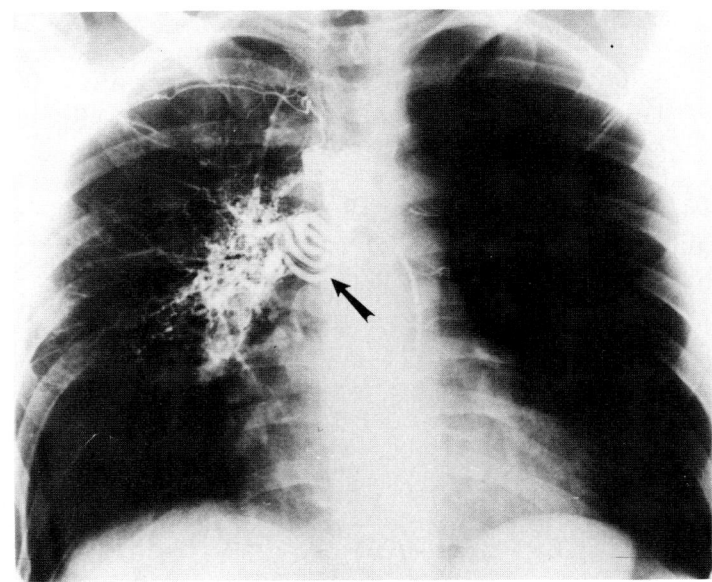

FIGURE 64-10 Anomalous bronchial arteries in a 19-year-old man with recurrent hemoptysis of unknown cause. Conventional chest radiographs revealed chronic inflammatory process, proved not to be due to bronchiectasis, in right middle lobe. Angiography (shown) and thoracotomy displayed two large bronchial arteries originating from the descending thoracic aorta. Also shown (arrow) is the delivery of contrast material to the pulmonary capillary bed via the bronchial arteries. (*Courtesy of Dr. P. Lanken.*)

Diagnosis of Pulmonary (Arterial) Hypertension

Recognizing that pulmonary hypertension exists and then quantifying it is of interest from the point of early detection, intervention, and evaluation of the response to therapy. The problem usually arises in individual patients but occasionally in populations, such as the epidemic of aminorex pulmonary hypertension that occurred in Europe.

The only certain method that is currently available for the diagnosis of pulmonary (arterial) hypertension is by right-sided cardiac catheterization. It is true that when pulmonary arterial pressures begin to approach systemic levels, the diagnosis of pulmonary hypertension can generally be made by a combination of clinical, radiographic, and electrocardiographic observations. Even levels of mean pulmonary arterial pressure of the order of 40 to 50 mmHg are apt to be overlooked unless suspicion is high, e.g., during an epidemic of primary pulmonary hypertension or if a patient seems predisposed to repeated pulmonary embolization.

Because right-sided, cardiac catheterization is impractical as a screening measure and troublesome as a method for follow-up study, reliable, noninvasive techniques—other than chest radiography, electrocardiography, and fluoroscopy—have been sought. The approaches to these new tests have been diverse: perfusion lung scans, hemodynamic correlations between pulmonary capillary blood volume and diffusing capacity, and the ratio of physiological dead space to tidal volume during exercise. However, none of these indirect approaches has proved reliable, particularly at modest levels of pulmonary hypertension when vasodilator therapy is most apt to be successful.

Promising, albeit still in its infancy, is the use of echocardiography for the detection of pulmonary hypertension. Although this technique has not proved useful for determining either the volume of the right ventricle or the thickness of its wall, some are sanguine about its prospects for detecting moderate to severe pulmonary hypertension by recording the speed and patterns of opening and closure of the pulmonary valve. One practical obstacle in implementing this goal is the difficulty in localizing the pulmonary valve when tricuspid insufficiency accompanies right ventricular failure.

Treatment of Pulmonary (Arterial) Hypertension

Relief of pulmonary hypertension is a primary goal in dealing with patients with cor pulmonale, particularly if they develop right ventricular failure. In individuals with impaired gas exchange, in whom hypoxia and acidosis contribute importantly to pulmonary vasoconstriction, relief from these stimuli ameliorates the hypertension. This approach to management of pulmonary hypertension is considered subsequently in the section on cor pulmonale. So is the need to minimize physical activity in order to avoid both the pulmonary hypertensive effects of increasing blood flow into a restricted pulmonary vascular bed and further derangements in gas exchange that increase pressor stimuli, i.e., hypoxia and acidosis.

One form of pulmonary hypertension that can be dramatically reversible is that due to large organized clots lodged in major pulmonary arteries. Although uncommon, surgical removal of the larger occlusive lesions generally results in considerable relief of pulmonary hypertension—often after an intervening bout of pulmonary edema in the area that is once again exposed to pulmonary arterial pressures and blood flow.

Rekindled interest in an old way of treating pulmonary hypertension merits special consideration. For more than 30 years, waves of pharmacologic agents have been advocated for the treatment of pulmonary (arterial) hypertension. Among these have been anticoagulants, agents acting directly on vascular smooth muscle (nitroprusside, hydralazine, and diazoxide), β-adrenergic agonists (isoproterenol), α-adrenergic blockers (phentolamine), inhibitors of the converting enzyme (captopril), calcium channel blockers (verapamil, nifedipine, and diazepam), and prostaglandins (prostaglandin E and prostacyclin). Until the last few years, documentation of success has been sparse, largely in the form of case reports supplemented by clinical trials of short duration. As a rule, little regard was paid to the natural course of the underlying disease or to long-term follow-up. However, despite the continuing search for effective pulmonary vasodilator agents, no pharmacologic agent has proved to be predictably or consistently successful either in relieving symptoms or in affecting the course or the outcome of pulmonary hypertension.

COR PULMONALE

The term *cor pulmonale* denotes right ventricular enlargement (hypertrophy and/or dilatation) secondary to abnormal lungs, chest bellows, or control of breathing (Fig. 64-11). It is generally used as a synonym for pulmonary heart disease. Cor pulmonale may be acute or chronic. In chronic cor pulmonale, hypertrophy generally predominates; in acute cor pulmonale, dilatation is the rule.

The most common cause of acute cor pulmonale is massive embolization of the lungs. Also common are bouts of acute cor pulmonale and respiratory failure that punctuate the natural history of chronic cor pulmonale, particularly as the disorder progresses into its preterminal stages.

Periodically, misgivings are voiced about the value of retaining the term cor pulmonale: pathologists rarely use it; clinicians have difficulty in making the diagnosis. But each challenge reentrenches the term because of several attractive features and prospects: if it were discarded, a

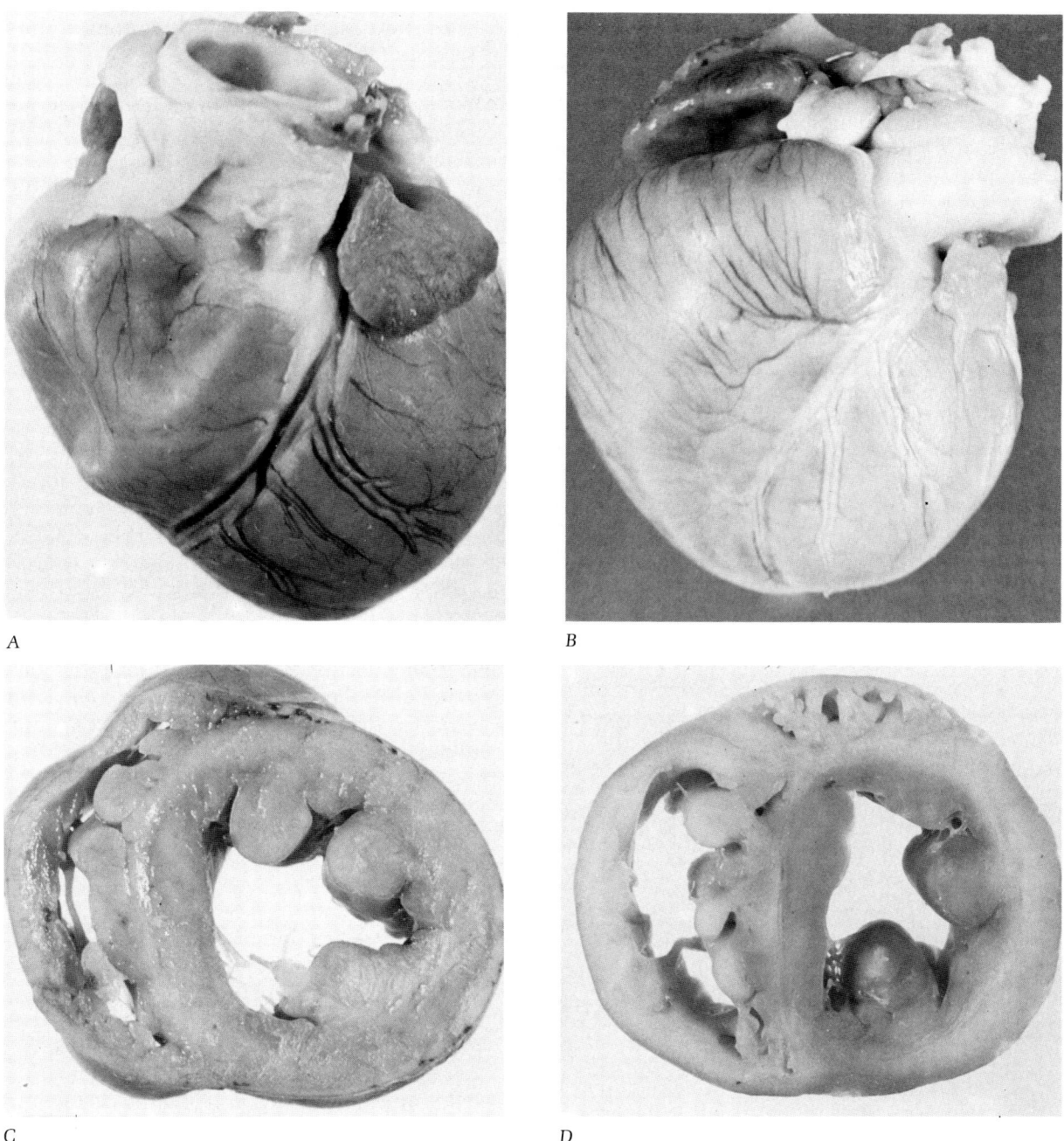

A

B

C

D

FIGURE 64-11 Cor pulmonale in experimental pulmonary arterial hypertension in the dog. A. Normal heart. B. Chronic cor pulmonale secondary to severe pulmonary arterial hypertension. C. Cross section of normal heart to show thin wall of the right ventricular cavity. D. Cross section of heart with chronic cor pulmonale to show hypertrophy of the right ventricular myocardium and enlargement of the right ventricular cavity. (Courtesy of Dr. B. Atkinson.)

large literature, based on a host of clinical, physiological, and anatomic observations made during the last three decades, would be rendered ambiguous, and common denominators in the pathogenesis of pulmonary hypertension would be obscured; conversely, if pathologists could be attracted to the term, the way would open for fresh correlations between morbid anatomy, the natural history of the antecedent disorders, the clinical expressions of cor pulmonale, and the pathogenetic mechanisms that lead to it. Finally, the diagnosis of cor pulmonale is not as elusive as generally imagined once the likelihood of its being present is taken into serious account.

General Features

The categories of pulmonary and ventilatory disorders that often lead to chronic cor pulmonale are indicated in Table 64-3. The common denominator shared by these diverse entities is pulmonary hypertension that stems from a primary disorder of the lungs or respiratory apparatus.

This view of chronic cor pulmonale has several important implications:

1. The disorder of the lungs need not be intrinsic pulmonary disease. Even normal lungs can be responsible if they are not ventilated properly either because the respiratory apparatus does not function properly or the respiratory centers should fail to respond adequately to the stimuli that converge upon them.

2. Although right ventricular hypertrophy generally does account for most of the cardiomegaly in chronic cor pulmonale, some dilatation is almost invariable, particularly by the time that the heart is examined at autopsy. In contrast to the right ventricular enlargement, the left ventricle is generally spared. Occasionally, the left ventricle is enlarged in cor pulmonale or can be shown to operate poorly. In these few instances, it is often difficult to settle whether the involvement of the left ventricle is secondary to the cor pulmonale or if it is a separate disorder. This topic will be considered subsequently.

3. Although pulmonary arterial hypertension invariably precedes cor pulmonale, it is not a synonym for cor pulmonale. Should the pulmonary hypertension be secondary to congenital heart disease or to primary disorders of the left side of the heart, diagnosis of cor pulmonale is automatically excluded.

4. Somewhat paradoxically, recognition by the physician that the patient has cor pulmonale often also provides the first clue to pulmonary hypertension, which otherwise was obscured by manifestations of the underlying disorder.

For the definition of cor pulmonale to be useful, its boundaries have to be sharp. The limits have changed since 20 years ago, when antecedent lung disease was the sine qua non; now the definition also includes those patients in whom the right ventricular enlargement follows alveolar hypoventilation and patients with normal lungs that do not operate adequately, either because of an abnormal chest bellows or a deranged control of breathing. This expansion of the definition was a logical outgrowth of the realization that inadequate performance of any component of the complicated respiratory apparatus can produce the same stimuli, e.g., hypoxia and acidosis, for pulmonary hypertension.

Quite recently the definition was sharpened by restricting the pathogenesis of the antecedent pulmonary hypertension to the precapillary bed. The stimulus for the more restricted definition was a new entity, pulmonary veno-occlusive disease. For two reasons, pulmonary veno-occlusive disease has generally been accepted to lie at the outer fringes, but not within the confines, of cor pulmonale: (1) because pulmonary veno-occlusive disease affects vessels that are distal to the pulmonary capillary bed, pulmonary congestion and edema are characteristic features of this disorder, whereas they are rarely part of the usual pulmonary hypertensive disorders leading to cor pulmonale; and (2) the pathogenesis of pulmonary hypertension in pulmonary veno-occlusive disease, and the right ventricular enlargement that follows, are more closely akin to syndromes elicited by diseases of the left side of the heart, e.g., mitral valvular disease, than to the intrinsic pulmonary disorders, e.g., obstructive airways disease and restrictive lung disease, that usually lead to cor pulmonale. At present, it seems reasonable to regard pulmonary veno-occlusive disease as a landmark that defines the boundary of disorders that are encompassed within the designation cor pulmonale, i.e., its perimeter rather than part of its enclosure.

Some clinicians find it useful to draw analogy between the pulmonary hypertension–cor pulmonale sequence and the systemic hypertension–left ventricular overload sequence. By this analogy, pulmonary arterial hypertension, the load that the right ventricle bears, is distinguished from: (1) cor pulmonale, the adaptive enlargement of the right ventricle in response to the augmented hemodynamic load; and (2) the combination of cor pulmonale and right ventricular failure, a stage representing the failure of the right ventricle to deal adequately with the hemodynamic load.

Depending on exacerbations of the underlying pulmonary disorder, pulmonary arterial hypertension may come and go, or at least improve. This is particularly true in the patient with bronchitis and emphysema who is top-

TABLE 64-3
Categories of Pulmonary Disorders Leading to Chronic Cor Pulmonale

Category	Example
Primary pulmonary hypertension	Idiopathic
Other forms of pulmonary hypertension	
Occlusive disorders of small pulmonary arteries	Multiple pulmonary emboli
Pulmonary interstitial disease	Boeck's sarcoid
Alveolar hypoventilation	
With normal lungs ("general")	Kyphoscoliosis
Ventilation-perfusion abnormalities ("net")	Chronic airways disease

pled into acute respiratory insufficiency by a bout of pneumonia only to return to the brink of pulmonary insufficiency as the acute respiratory infection subsides. If the respiratory infection is brief, and the degree of hypoxia that it evokes is modest, pulmonary arterial hypertension will in turn be moderate and the right ventricle will not enlarge appreciably. However, should respiratory insufficiency persist and pulmonary hypertension be sustained at high levels, the right ventricle will fail and initiate the familiar sequence of salt and water retention, systemic venous congestion, and peripheral edema.

INCIDENCE AND PREVALENCE

It is not possible to provide an accurate picture of the incidence of chronic cor pulmonale and of the morbidity and mortality that it causes because pulmonary insufficiency generally obscures the cardiac disorder during life and because right ventricular hypertrophy is easily overlooked at autopsy.

Less than one-half of patients with chronic bronchitis and emphysema manifest right ventricular enlargement at autopsy. The incidence varies not only from country to country but also according to cities and habits of the population. In the United States, cor pulmonale generally makes up about 6 to 7 percent of all types of adult heart disease. In Delhi, where a large segment of the population lives under conditions of severe air pollution, the incidence has been estimated to be of the order of 16 percent. In Sheffield, England, cor pulmonale constitutes 30 to 40 percent of clinical heart failure. In general, in areas where smoking is rife, air pollution severe, and chronic bronchitis and emphysema prevalent, the incidence of cor pulmonale is high. Men are more often affected than women because of their greater exposure to air pollutants.

Diffuse interstitial lung disease often terminates in cor pulmonale and right ventricular failure. Cor pulmonale is also a common complication of cystic fibrosis of the pancreas in adults. Most disorders, however, affect too little of the lungs, or are too circumscribed in their effects on alveolar-capillary gas exchange, to elicit pulmonary hypertension and cor pulmonale. Tuberculosis, although extensive, is rarely the cause of cor pulmonale, unless both lungs are extensively affected by destruction and conglomerate fibrosis or surgical intervention has deranged the functioning of the chest bellows. Patients who have chronic bronchitis and emphysema or diffuse interstitial fibrosis may be breathless for years without developing cor pulmonale. Allergic asthma is an uncommon antecedent of cor pulmonale. In general, the more extensive the pulmonary derangement, and the more upset the ventilation-perfusion relationships, the more likely is pulmonary hypertension and cor pulmonale to develop.

HEMODYNAMIC FEATURES

The normal right ventricle is a thin-walled, distensible muscular pump that accommodates considerable variations in systemic venous return without large changes in filling pressures. In response to chronic pressure overload imposed by the pulmonary hypertension, the right ventricle hypertrophies. This hypertrophy involves mainly the free ventricular wall rather than the inflow and outflow tracts. Preterminally, a bout of intolerable hypoxia often exaggerates the degree of pulmonary hypertension and imposes an acute afterload on the right ventricle, which accommodates by dilating.

Cor pulmonale without right ventricular failure is associated with a normal cardiac output both at rest and during exercise; the filling pressure (end-diastolic pressure) of the right ventricle is normal (less than 5 mmHg).

Sustained modest pulmonary arterial hypertension, or an episode of pulmonary arterial pressures approximating systemic arterial pressure, causes the right ventricle to fail. This form of heart failure is unusual because the car-·

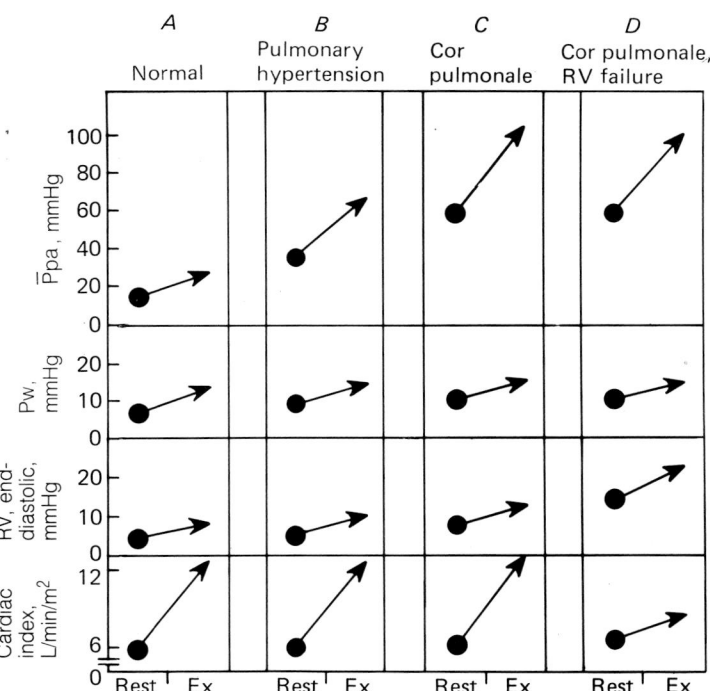

FIGURE 64-12 Schematic representation of evolution of chronic cor pulmonale. Hemodynamic studies at rest and during exercise in a normal subject (A). The stage of pulmonary arterial hypertension (B) is succeeded by cor pulmonale (C) in which the right ventricle performs normally despite pulmonary arterial hypertension but is known to be enlarged because of radiographic and electrocardiographic findings. Once right ventricular failure supervenes (D), cardiac output fails to increase normally during exercise, despite an increase of right ventricular filling pressure (end-diastolic) to abnormally high levels.

diac output often is normal at rest, particularly if hypoxia coexists. However, the hallmark of heart failure is failure of the cardiac output to increase normally during exercise even though right ventricular end-diastolic pressures (filling pressures) reach abnormally high levels (Fig. 64-12). Salt and water retention, expansion of the plasma volume, and systemic venous congestion follow right ventricular failure; the interstitial water content of the lungs also increases. The mechanisms responsible for the salt and water retention in right ventricular failure are still unsettled.

Recovery reverses the water and electrolyte disturbances. Relief of pulmonary hypertension diminishes the load on the right ventricle, its filling pressures return to normal, and the cardiac output once again responds appropriately to the level of exercise. Support of the heart by cardiotonic agents is much less effective than relief of the afterload, i.e., pulmonary hypertension, in restoring adequate cardiac performance.

The left atrial pressure is normal in cor pulmonale except when circulating blood volume is increased or if cor pulmonale is complicated by left ventricular failure.

ROLE OF HYPERCAPNIA

Acute hypercapnia is without direct effect on the pulmonary circulation. However, it does cause and potentiate pulmonary hypertension if it produces acidosis. *Acute* hypercapnia plays an important extracirculatory role in cor pulmonale by stimulating the ventilation, dilating cerebral vessels, and eliciting disturbances in the central nervous system. Other side effects are attributable to increased sympathetic activity. These acute effects are incapacitating.

In contrast, *chronic* hypertension, as occurs in patients with chronic obstructive airways disease, is generally well tolerated. Other pulmonary disorders, such as widespread interstitial fibrosis, are generally free of hypercapnia except preterminally when marked derangements in ventilation-perfusion supervene as the architecture of the lungs is increasingly distorted. The hospitalized patient with cor pulmonale and heart failure is apt to have both acute and chronic hypercapnia. In many instances, particularly those of chronic bronchitis and emphysema, successful treatment restores the patient to the tolerable levels of chronic hypercapnia to which he or she has adapted gradually over the years as the lungs have progressively failed.

THE LEFT VENTRICLE

Left ventricular failure is a serious threat to a patient with cor pulmonale. It exerts its harmful effects by increasing the pulmonary blood volume and promoting the accumu-

lation of extravascular water, thereby decreasing pulmonary compliance and increasing airway resistance; as a result, the work of breathing and gas exchange is further deranged. Experimental observations over the years have encouraged the idea that hypertrophy and failure of the right ventricle can, per se, lead to disorders in left ventricular performance. However, there is no firm clinical support for this notion. Indeed, clinical evidence is against this view. For example, at high altitude, where mild-to-modest pulmonary hypertension is a regular feature of daily life, cardiomegaly is confined to the right ventricle except for the rare patient with chronic mountain sickness who experiences intolerable levels of arterial hypoxemia by virtue of alveolar hypoventilation. Such extreme arterial hypoxemia not only generates severe pulmonary hypertension but also compromises O_2 delivery to the myocardium of both ventricles. In this state of extreme hypoxemia, impaired performance of the left ventricle would not be surprising.

Also, at sea level, it is difficult to demonstrate that left ventricular function is impaired as a result of cor pulmonale. Those who have found abnormalities have not been clear about the mechanism. Few still subscribe to the idea that hypertrophy of the ventricular septum (part of the right ventricle) is responsible for impaired left ventricular performance. Usually the problem is to exclude independent disease of the left ventricle (Fig. 64-13). In elderly people, it is usually reasonable to imagine the concurrence of independent arteriosclerotic disease of the coronary arteries. In the young patient with cor pulmonale and sarcoidosis, the inclination is to attribute the left ventricular dysfunction to granulomatous involvement of the myocardium. On the other hand, there is little doubt that a damaged or overloaded left ventricle from any cause is not apt to prosper in a patient with persistent hypoxemia and acidosis, particularly if they are severe.

CLINICAL FEATURES

It was noted that before the right ventricle fails, the antecedent pulmonary disease may obscure the presence of pulmonary hypertension and right ventricular enlargement. On occasion, chest pain may be the first signal of severe pulmonary hypertension. Not infrequently, the diagnosis of pulmonary hypertension is first entertained because of evidence of right ventricular hypertrophy on the electrocardiogram.

Each pathogenetic sequence culminating in cor pulmonale leaves its own imprint on the clinical manifestations. For example, obstructive disease of the airways is usually associated with hyperinflation of the lungs, which shifts the position of the heart and makes heart sounds less audible. Interstitial disorders of the lungs consistently evoke tachypnea. Nonetheless, all sequences do

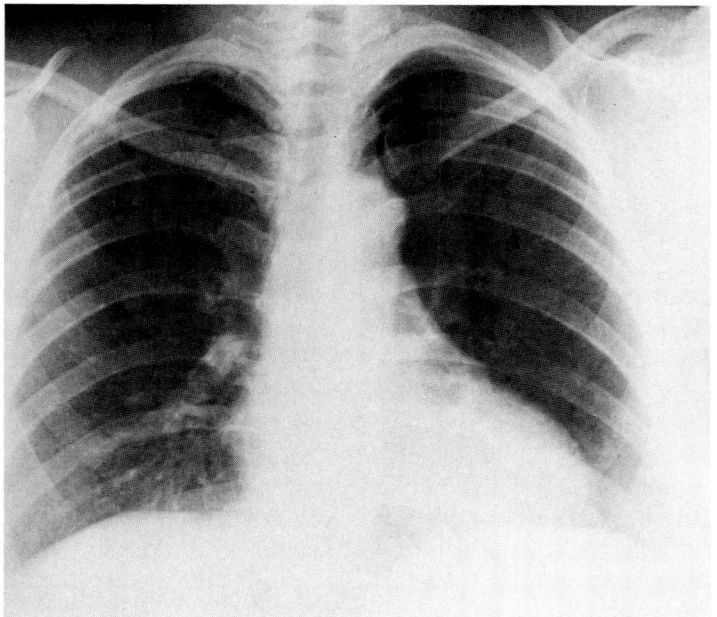

A

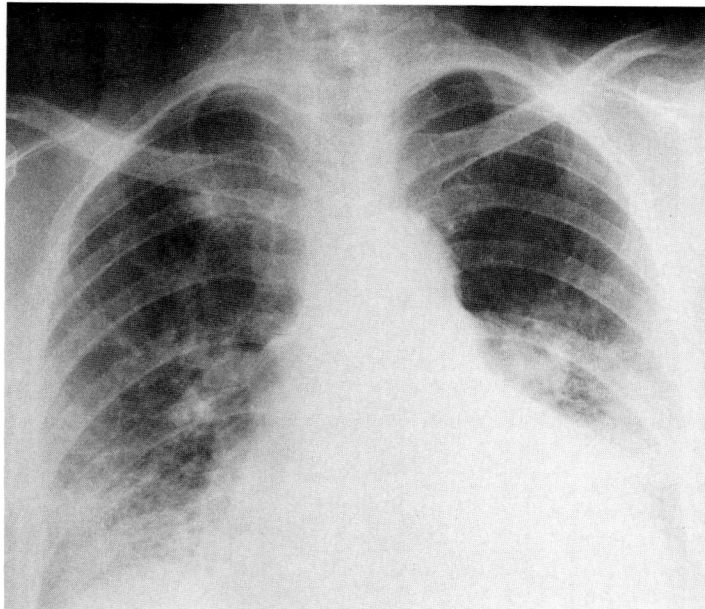

B

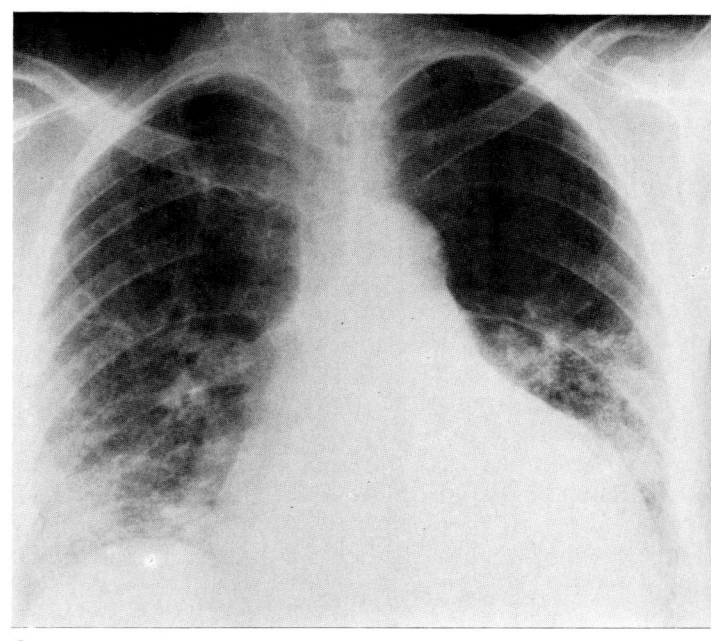

C

FIGURE 64-13 Cor pulmonale, right ventricular failure, and pulmonary edema. *A.* In 1956, enlarged heart, cause unknown. The lungs appear normal. *B.* In 1976, increased cardiomegaly is associated with idiopathic interstitial fibrosis (lung biopsy in 1970) and pulmonary edema. *C.* Four days later. Edema has cleared leaving evidence of interstitial fibrosis.

have certain physical findings in common. Most distinctive is the accentuation of the pulmonary component of the second heart sound; when pulmonary hypertension is severe, this pulmonary component may even be palpable. Rarely is the degree of splitting of the second heart sound helpful, but splitting does tend to be narrower than usual when pulmonary hypertension is severe and to be abnormally wide if right bundle branch block is present.

An important sign of cor pulmonale is a right-sided (ventricular), diastolic (S_3) gallop. In timing, it coincides with the third heart sound; it is accentuated by inspira-

tion. Less helpful is the right atrial gallop (S_4) which occurs immediately before the first heart sound and represents an accentuation of the normal atrial sound; it suggests an increase in the filling pressure of the right side of the heart.

An adjuvant sign that may be helpful once the diagnosis is suspected is a pulmonary ejection click early during systole, best heard along the left sternal border. If pulmonary hypertension is severe—approaching systemic levels—the murmur of functional pulmonic valvular insufficiency may be heard along the left sternal border.

Once the right ventricle has failed to the point of eliciting systemic venous hypertension, tricuspid insufficiency may become manifest.

These evidences of pulmonary hypertension and cor pulmonale are apt to be overlooked unless the predisposing pulmonary abnormality (Table 64-2) is recognized and the patient is subjected to a thorough clinical search for evidence of right ventricular enlargement. Some predisposing conditions are easier to recognize than others. Diffuse pulmonary parenchymal lesions that cast distinctive shadows on the chest radiograph are more easily recognized than is chronic bronchitis, which generally makes no distinctive imprint on the chest radiograph. Not uncommonly, the elderly patient who presents in overt

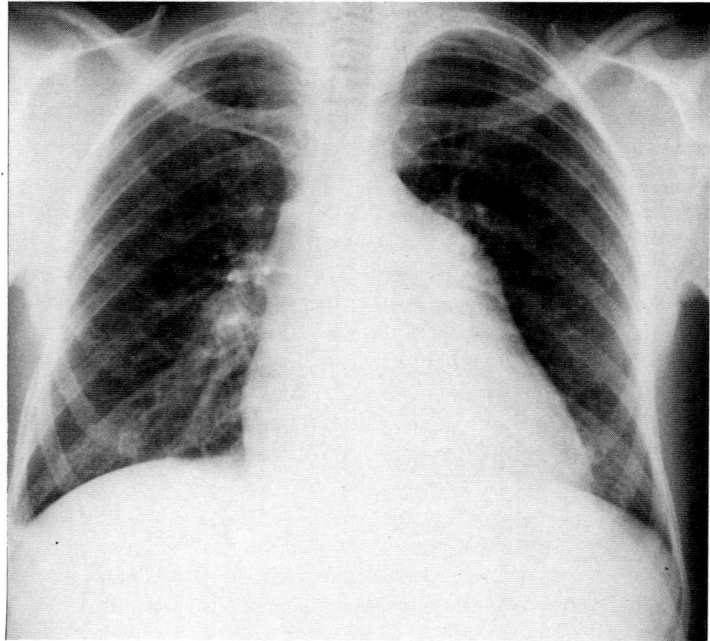

FIGURE 64-14   Multiple pulmonary emboli. The prominent central pulmonary arteries in conjunction with the marked pruning of the peripheral tree reflect the marked pulmonary arterial hypertension.

"congestive heart" failure proves to have cor pulmonale rather than arteriosclerotic heart disease.

In time, tricuspid insufficiency develops. It is manifested by a holosystolic murmur, best heard in the fourth interspace to the left of the sternum; the murmur characteristically increases in intensity during inspiration (as do the third and fourth heart sounds). Distended neck veins pulsate with each heartbeat; the liver often also shows expansile pulsations that are synchronous with the heartbeat. Hydrothorax and ascites are uncommon, even after right ventricular failure has progressed to the stage of hepatomegaly and pedal edema.

When pulmonary hypertension has lasted for years, radiographs show not only the cardiomegaly produced by right ventricular and right atrial enlargement but also evidence of severe pulmonary hypertension: prominence of the central pulmonary arterial trunks in association with attenuation of the peripheral branches of the pulmonary arterial tree (Fig. 64-14). Because physical signs of pulmonary hypertension and right ventricular enlargement are rarely conclusive, heavy reliance is placed on the electrocardiogram to detect right ventricular overload (Fig. 64-15).

ARRHYTHMIAS

Transient arrhythmias often occur in cor pulmonale, particularly during the stage of combined heart failure and respiratory failure. When arterial hypoxemia, hypercapnia, and acidosis coexist and are severe, the arrhythmias may be life-threatening. This combination has been implicated as a cause of sudden death during acute respiratory failure, presumably from ventricular fibrillation. Respiratory alkalosis, a common concomitant of mechanical hyperventilation and hypokalemia, may also trigger a serious arrhythmia.

A transient sinus arrhythmia occasionally signals the onset of a bout of respiratory insufficiency and coexistent arterial hypoxemia and respiratory acidosis. The usual arrhythmia is atrial tachycardia, nodal rhythm, or a wan-

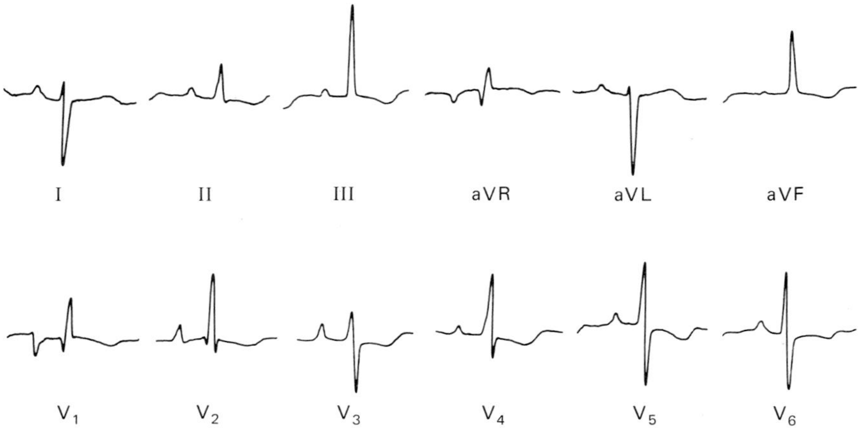

I   II   III   aVR   aVL   aVF

V₁   V₂   V₃   V₄   V₅   V₆

FIGURE 64-15   Twenty-six-year-old woman in whom the first evidence of primary pulmonary hypertension was by electrocardiography. The record shows marked right axis deviation and dominant R waves over the right precordium consistent with right ventricular hypertrophy.

dering pacemaker. Less common is an episode of atrial flutter or fibrillation.

The likelihood of arrhythmia is enhanced by intense adrenergic discharge because of anxiety, central nervous stimulation, or excessive use of bronchodilators. In this setting, digitalis must be administered with extreme caution since it may operate synergistically with the sympathetic stimulation to precipitate a life-threatening arrhythmia.

TREATMENT: GENERAL ASPECTS

Since cor pulmonale is a consequence of pulmonary hypertension, the goal of therapy is to decrease the work load of the right ventricle by decreasing pulmonary arterial pressure. This generally involves restoration of arterial blood-gas tensions toward normal, and, in particular, the relief of arterial hypoxemia. Invariably, success in restoring cardiac competence depends on success in relieving respiratory failure.

In a particular patient, the approach depends on the etiology and state of the underlying pulmonary disorder. Unfortunately, little lasting relief can be expected when anatomic lesions, such as healed multiple pulmonary emboli, are the basis for the pulmonary hypertension. Much more amenable to therapy are pulmonary disorders in which a reversible element can be identified. Most common among these is a state of exaggerated ventilation-perfusion imbalances that has been produced by an upper respiratory infection in a patient with bronchitis and emphysema. Even multiple pulmonary emboli or primary pulmonary hypertension, conditions in which anatomic occlusion of the pulmonary arterial tree is the predominant mechanism, may have a reversible component contributing to pulmonary hypertension. The inclination is strong to administer pulmonary vasodilators to these patients. The reasons for restraint will be considered subsequently.

Of cardinal importance is the prompt achievement of a tolerable level of arterial oxgenation at rest, during exercise, and during sleep, and the institution, when applicable, of adequate treatment for infection. Relief of acute hypercapnia is often critical but should be gradual. Vigorous application of ancillary measures, such as postural drainage and the administration of diuretics and digitalis, should not obscure these two primary goals.

Cor pulmonale, i.e., right ventricular enlargement, usually goes through a long phase of hypertrophy before dilatation and heart failure supervene. Until the hypertrophied right ventricle fails, cor pulmonale requires no cardiotonic program. But, once the right ventricle does fail, cardiotonic measures are in order. Among these measures, bed rest stands out as a necessary strategy to avoid the inevitable increments in pulmonary arterial pressure that occur during daily activity. The usual general measures used to treat left ventricular failure, notably salt restriction, also apply to right ventricular failure. However, overzealous salt restriction is avoided since excessive depletion of serum chlorides will drive up the level of serum bicarbonate, thereby defeating attempts to diminish hypercapnia.

Clinicians who use diuretics, digitalis, and vasodilators almost always have to be more circumspect in treating right ventricular failure than left ventricular failure.

Diuretics

These can be helpful in managing cor pulmonale in heart failure but they must be used cautiously. The lungs share in excess water accumulation of the body; this excess fluid in the lungs further compromises pulmonary gas exchange and may heighten pulmonary vascular resistance. That diuretics can improve alveolar ventilation and arterial oxygenation in cor pulmonale has now been amply demonstrated. But, the use of diuretics engenders hemodynamic side effects that may be troublesome: volume depletion, diminished venous return to the right side of the heart, and a decrease in cardiac output. Another potential complication of powerful diuretics is the production of a hypokalemic metabolic alkalosis, which diminishes the effectiveness of the CO_2 stimulus on the respiratory centers and lessens the ventilatory drive. Also, renal excretion of bicarbonate is compromised when diuretics deplete potassium and chloride. For these reasons, careful monitoring of serum electrolytes, particularly bicarbonate, chloride, and potassium ions, is mandatory once a program of salt depletion, using salt restriction and diuretics, is begun.

Oxygen Therapy

The use of supplemental oxygen in obstructive airways disease is employed to relieve hypoxic pulmonary vasoconstriction, to improve the cardiac output, to lessen sympathetic vasoconstriction, and to alleviate tissue hypoxia. Thus, treatment of pulmonary hypertension is part of an overall program to manage severe obstructive airways disease. Two separate trials, that of the Medical Research Council and of the National Heart, Lung and Blood Institute (Nocturnal Oxygen Therapy Trial), have shown that intellectual function and survival are improved in chronically hypoxemic patients (arterial $P_{O_2} < 55$ mmHg) who have polycythemia (hematocrit > 55 percent), are edematous, and who show P pulmonale on the electrocardiogram, i.e., "blue bloaters" who develop pulmonary hypertension and right ventricular failure. However, to be effective, oxygen must be administered for at least 18 h per day, including at night when arterial hypoxemia and respiratory acidosis intensifies inordinately in these patients. Before the advent of right ventricular failure, supplemental oxygen was administered empirically for patient comfort.

Digitalis

This agent is used by some clinicians to support the failing right ventricle; others shy away from this agent even when right-sided heart failure is blatant. They do so on several accounts: (1) the inotropic effect of digitalis on right ventricular performance is modest; (2) should ventricular output increase into the restricted vascular bed, pulmonary arterial pressure will increase further; and (3) patients with cor pulmonale and right ventricular failure are often hypoxemic and somewhat acidotic, thereby predisposed to arrhythmia. Even small doses of digitalis may serve as the trigger. Digitalis seems to benefit patients with demonstrable left ventricular dysfunction. Heart rate is a poor guide to digitalis dosage because hypoxemia, as well as heart failure, evokes tachycardia. Also predisposing to arrhythmia are hypokalemia induced by diuretics, and medications given to relieve bronchospasm, including isoprenaline and theophylline. In essence, the safest use of digitalis for its cardiotonic effect is when right ventricular failure is unaccompanied by arterial hypoxemia, acid-base upsets, and the administration of bronchodilators, i.e., in disorders other than obstructive airways disease.

Pulmonary Vasodilators

These agents have been tried in both secondary and primary pulmonary hypertension. In both secondary and primary types of pulmonary hypertension, overall success rates have been modest, but occasional instances of dramatic improvement have occurred. At the disappointing end is the experience with severe obstructive airways disease: for example, no demonstrable differences in hemodynamics or survival are evident after 1 year of nifedipine treatment (10 mg three times daily). In contrast is the infrequent but dramatic and enduring decrease in pulmonary arterial pressure along with an increase in cardiac output, improved quality of life, and continued state of good health in primary pulmonary hypertension. These agents are considered in the following pages under the individual categories of disease leading to pulmonary hypertension.

Ancillary Measures

Carbonic anhydrase inhibitors (acetazolamide) were once in vogue for treating patients with chronic hypercapnia. The rationale was to promote diuresis and loss of bicarbonate by the kidney. However, untoward effects, presumably the result of adding metabolic acidosis to the preexisting respiratory acidosis, have led most physicians to abandon the use of acetazolamide as a primary diuretic agent. However, it can be used judiciously to correct the alkalemia induced by excessive diuresis, volume contraction, and hypochloremia.

Phlebotomy also used to be standard treatment for the polycythemia of chronic hypoxia as the hematocrits went above 55 to 60 percent. However, even though repeated, small phlebotomies often result in symptomatic improvement and increased exercise tolerance, it proved difficult to show objective improvement in gas exchange, pulmonary mechanics, or pulmonary arterial pressure after "safe" phlebotomies, i.e., of 250 ml or so; larger phlebotomies were avoided since they occasionally resulted in minor strokes and episodes of hypotension. However, restoring hematocrits gradually, i.e., by repeated 250-ml phlebotomies at intervals of several days or weekly, did decrease pulmonary arterial pressure as hematocrits approached normal levels, i.e., about 50 percent; lower hematocrits offer no further advantage. Therefore, small phlebotomies still have a role when secondary polycythemia becomes severe.

PROGNOSIS

No prospective studies are available concerning the prognosis of chronic cor pulmonale. Observations in the 1950s suggested that once the right ventricle fails and systemic venous congestion ensues, life expectancy is less than 4 years. But the ability to tide these patients over episodes of acute respiratory failure associated with infections and heart failure has improved enormously in the past 5 years. In our own experience, 5- to 10-year survival after the first appearance of peripheral edema is not unusual.

The prognosis for a particular patient with cor pulmonale is inextricably linked to that of the underlying pulmonary disease or disorder. In essence, the circulatory disorders are potentially reversible if the initiating mechanisms can be brought under control. In those patients in whom cor pulmonale is a complication of gradual obliteration of small pulmonary arteries by intrinsic disease (emboli) or of interstitial fibrosis, there is little hope for improvement since the anatomic changes are apt to be fixed, and arterial hypoxemia is rarely striking until it is preterminal. The outlook for longevity is much better in patients with chronic bronchitis and emphysema in whom blood gases can be maintained at near-normal levels.

Underlying Disorders I: Obliterative Pulmonary Vascular Disease (Including Thromboembolism)

This category is considered first because, in principle, it is the more straightforward of the different mechanisms for pulmonary hypertension: anatomic obstruction of the pulmonary microcirculation. There are two distinct subsets to this category: (1) *secondary obliterative pulmonary vascular disease*, when the etiology is identifiable, and (2) *primary pulmonary vascular disease*, when, despite intensive search, the etiology remains unknown. As a rule, in either category, occlusive disease of the small arteries and arterioles of the pulmonary vascular tree is a gradual process, one in which time is marked in years rather than months.

PATHOPHYSIOLOGY: GENERAL ASPECTS

The general features of both secondary and primary pulmonary hypertension arising from intraluminal obstruction are quite similar. Pulmonary arterial pressure often approaches systemic arterial levels, while cardiac output and left atrial pressures remain normal. This increase in pulmonary arterial pressure produced by disease contrasts sharply with the puny effects on the normal pulmonary circulation of experimentally occluding one pulmonary artery (Fig. 64-4) or of inducing acute hypoxia (Fig. 64-5). This contrast underscores the idea that in order to achieve the *sustained* and *severe* pulmonary hypertension that occurs in occlusive pulmonary vascular disease, not only must the pulmonary resistance vessels thicken, often to the point of closure, and the pulmonary arterial tree become curtailed in extent and limited in distensibility, but the right ventricle must undergo hypertrophy.

The common denominator for sustained pulmonary hypertension in these disorders is anatomic occlusion of large portions of the distal pulmonary arterial tree and increased resistance to blood flow through the remaining vessels, which are partially occluded because of either the original injury, e.g., a partially occluding inflammatory process, or recanalization after healing, as in an organized pulmonary embolus (Fig. 64-16). Systemic arterial hypoxemia often adds a reversible component in the form of pulmonary vasoconstriction. Early in the course of obliterative vascular disease, the arterial hypoxemia at rest is mild and contributes little to the pulmonary arterial hypertension. Preterminally, however, as the right ventricle fails, the role of the *anatomic venous admixture*, or *shunt*, increases considerably as the heart fails, and the O_2 content of blood returning to the lung decreases because of the slowed circulation and greater O_2 extraction in peripheral tissues.

CLINICAL FEATURES: GENERAL ASPECTS

Since there is no obstructive disease of the airways and hyperinflation of the lungs to cloud the clinical picture, and no appreciable interstitial lung disease to complicate interpretation, right ventricular enlargement is manifested in pure form. A cardiac thrust can be seen along the left sternal border or lifting the sternum; a fourth heart sound emanates from the hypertrophied ventricle. A prominent *a* wave is discernible in the jugular venous pulse. The pulmonary component of the second heart sound is accentuated, and, as pulmonary arterial pressures reach systemic levels, the murmur of pulmonary valvular insufficiency often appears. Right ventricular failure is accompanied by jugular venous distension and a gallop sound (S_3); the gallop is intensified by a deep inspiration. The liver is enlarged and tender, and a hepatojugular reflex can be elicited. Peripheral edema appears.

SECONDARY OBLITERATIVE PULMONARY VASCULAR DISEASE

The list of etiologies responsible for secondary obliterative pulmonary vascular diseases is long. It ranges from a variety of intrinsic diseases of the lungs, congenital cardiac diseases, and acquired disease of the left side of the heart to thromboembolic disease arising in peripheral veins (Table 64-3). In this section, only widespread disease of the resistance vessels of the lungs, i.e., the pulmonary arterioles and small muscular arteries, will be considered.

Etiology

In the United States, widespread occlusion of small muscular arteries and arterioles by organized clots is the most common cause of secondary obliterative pulmonary vascular disease. As a rule, the clots are definitely organized

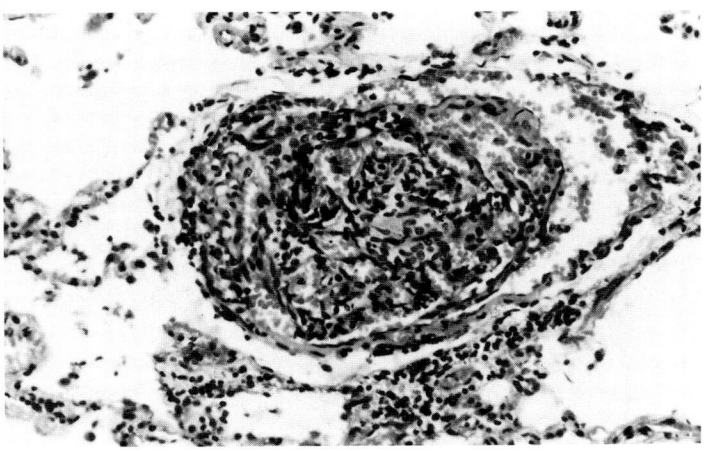
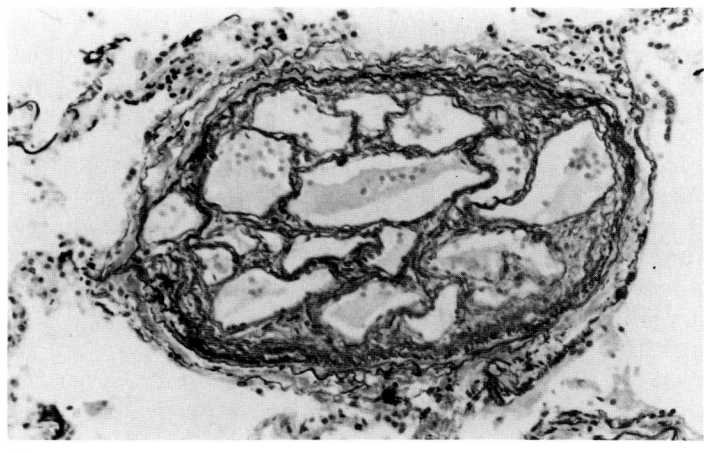

A   *B*

FIGURE 64-16 Contrast between plexiform and thromboembolic occlusions. *A.* Plexiform lesions in a muscular pulmonary artery in a 56-year-old woman with primary pulmonary hypertension. There is an active proliferation of intimal cells with capillarylike channels in between. The branch is dilated. To the left is focal destruction of the arterial wall which contains some lymphocytes and polymorphs. H&E, ×140. *B.* Muscular pulmonary artery in a 63-year-old man with thromboembolic pulmonary hypertension. Many vessels were obstructed by intravascular fibrous septa as remnants of recanalized emboli. Elastic van Gieson stain, ×140. *(Courtesy of Dr. C. A. Wagenvoort.)*

emboli. Occasionally, as in the syndrome of *multiple pulmonary emboli*, local thrombi have been invoked, presumably on the basis of an endothelial clotting disorder in the pulmonary precapillary vessels. More convincing evidence of local thromboses rather than pulmonary emboli exists for sickle cell anemia, which has a propensity for thrombosis in many organs, including the lungs. However, this entity is rarely associated with pulmonary hypertension.

In other parts of the world, such as those in which schistosomiasis is endemic, pulmonary obliterative disease is due to ova which act both mechanically and by local immunoreactions to produce an obliterative vasculitis. Interestingly, a similar phenomenon occurs in the United States in dogs infected with heartworms. An association has been proposed between filariasis and pulmonary hypertension in regions where *Wuchereria bancrofti* is endemic. However, this relationship is still tenuous.

Occasionally, etiologies, such as diet or pharmacologic agents, are highly suspect of causing pulmonary hypertension, but until now the evidence has been more circumstantial than telltale. This was the case with the epidemic of *primary pulmonary hypertension* generally held attributable to the over-the-counter sale of the anorectic agent, aminorex, in Switzerland, Germany, and Austria. Although the agent was suspected, it could not be indicted, and *aminorex pulmonary hypertension* still falls under the purview of primary pulmonary hypertension.

Pathophysiology

Progressive obliteration of the pulmonary arterial tree by multiple pulmonary emboli is the prototype of this group. However, in this disorder the final common pathway of pulmonary hypertension and cor pulmonale can be reached by two different clinical routes: in one, the pulmonary hypertension follows clinically overt thromboembolic disease that usually is either neglected or overlooked until too late (Fig. 64-17); in the other, the clinical picture is indistinguishable from that of primary pulmonary hypertension, and the true nature of the occlusive vascular disease is only discovered at autopsy.

Clinical Features

The natural history of patients with clinically discernible thromboembolic disease is described in Chapter 66. If properly managed with anticoagulant and surgical therapy early in the course of their disease, pulmonary hypertension is usually avoidable.

The category of multiple pulmonary emboli, in which the source and occurrence of pulmonary emboli is inapparent during life, is difficult to detect clinically until severe pulmonary hypertension dominates the scene and the clinical picture is indistinguishable from primary pulmonary hypertension. The typical patient is a young or middle-aged adult—more often a woman than a man—who presents with progressive dyspnea that is first attrib-

uted to "being out of shape" and is later appreciated as a sign of ill-health. Breathlessness on mild exertion is incapacitating; on occasion, the breathlessness is associated with precordial pain. Clinical appraisal indicates the presence of pulmonary hypertension and right ventricular enlargement without evidence of either left ventricular, valvular, or pulmonary disease. Often, despite intensive search, proof that pulmonary embolization has occurred cannot be adduced during life. Indeed, some picture the syndrome of multiple pulmonary vascular emboli as one, in reality, of widespread pulmonary vascular thrombi possibly arising from an endothelial defect of the pulmonary microcirculation.

Tachypnea is a consistent finding. It persists during sleep and is generally associated with tachycardia. This pattern of rapid, shallow breathing is indistinguishable from that arising from stiffened lungs of any cause, e.g., interstitial (and peribronchiolar) pulmonary edema. Vagal afferent impulses are generally believed to be responsible. The result of the rapid, shallow breathing is alveolar and dead-space hyperventilation that, in turn, decreases the P_{CO_2} in arterial blood and in alveolar gas and widens the alveolar-arterial difference in P_{O_2}.

Treatment

The prophylaxis and treatment of thromboembolic episodes that are clinically evident are described elsewhere (Chapter 66).

It has been proposed that in addition to mechanical obstruction, pulmonary vasoconstriction contributes to pulmonary hypertension. Accordingly, in addition to anticoagulants, vasodilators may have a place in managing patients with severe pulmonary hypertension. However, it is important to avoid overlooking candidates for pulmonary endarterectomy in whom dramatic results can be obtained by removing the obstructive organized clots (Fig. 64-17).

The treatment of the syndrome of multiple pulmonary emboli is usually the same as for primary pulmonary hypertension unless evidence can be adduced for recent thromboembolic episodes.

PRIMARY OBLITERATIVE PULMONARY VASCULAR DISEASE (PRIMARY PULMONARY HYPERTENSION)

The description *primary* (arterial) *pulmonary hypertension* has two implications: (1) despite extensive search for etiologic agents, no cause for the hypertension can be found; clearly, the extent of the search will vary from clinic to clinic; and (2) the predominant pulmonary vascular lesions are in the small muscular arteries and arterioles; automatically this caveat eliminates pulmonary veno-occlusive disease in which the small veins and venules are primarily affected. Although primary pulmonary hypertension is a rare disease, interest in it is now uncommonly high on two accounts: (1) a stream of new vasodilator agents has raised the prospect of ameliorating a

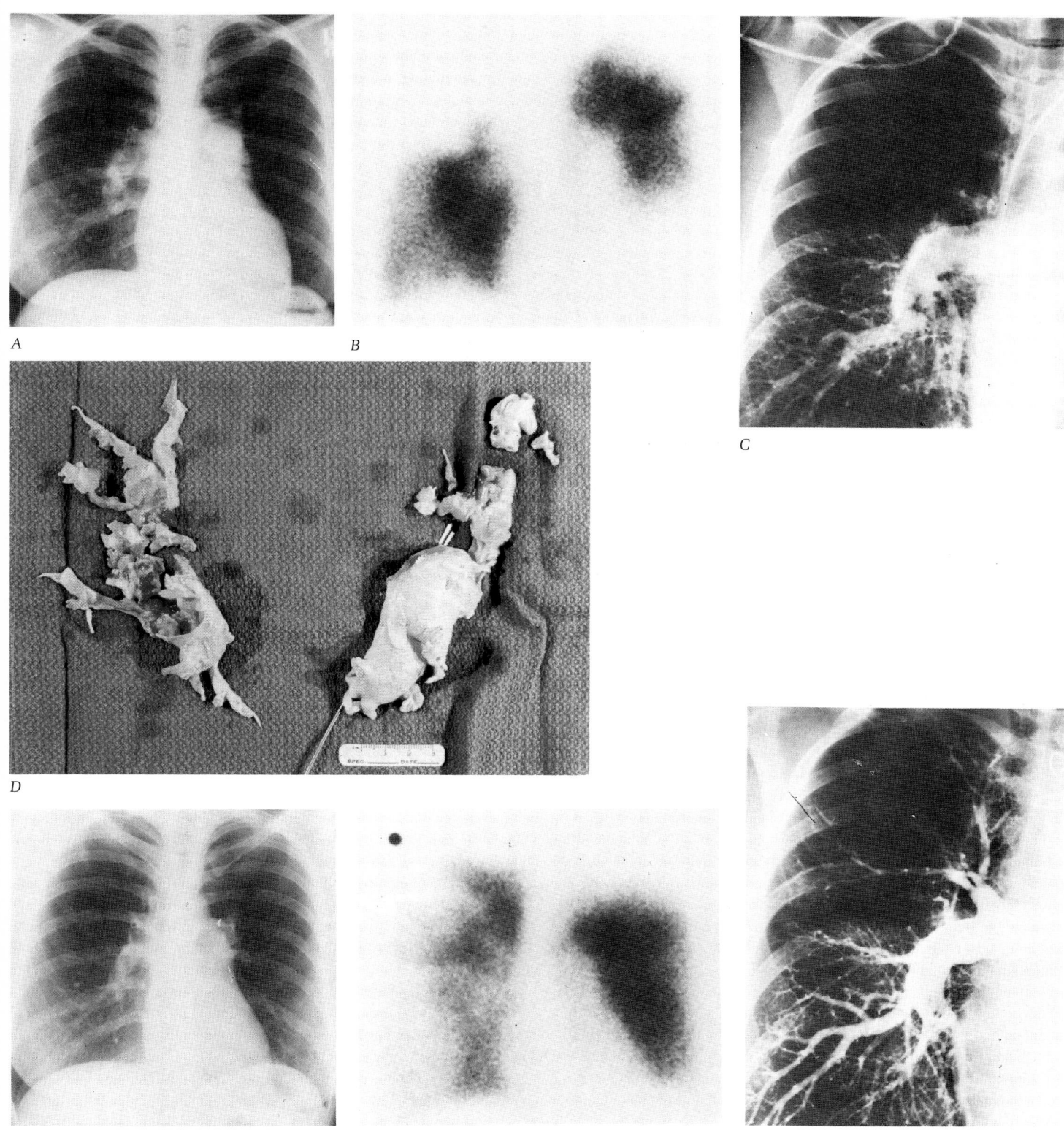

FIGURE 64-17 Chronic pulmonary thromboembolism, before and after surgery, in a 35-year-old woman suspected of having had episodes of pulmonary emboli between 1977 and 1979. Progressive pulmonary hypertension, cor pulmonale, and right ventricular failure. *A.* Preoperative chest radiograph. Pulmonary arterial pressure = 96/78 mmHg; pulmonary wedge pressure = 4 mmHg; cardiac output = 3.1 L/min. The chest radiograph reveals hyperlucency and diminished vasculature in the right upper and left lower lobes. Also cardiomegaly with prominent central pulmonary arteries. *B.* Preoperative perfusion scan. Confirms chest radiograph above. *C.* Preoperative angiogram of right upper lobe showing absence of blood flow. *D.* Organized clot removed by Dr. L. H. Edmunds from the right upper and left lower pulmonary arteries at surgery. *E.* Postoperative (1 year later) chest radiograph. The chest radiograph is virtually normal. Pulmonary arterial pressure = 44/20 mmHg; cardiac output = 5.0 L/min. *F.* Postoperative perfusion scan. Blood is now perfusing the right upper and left lower lobes. *G.* Postoperative angiogram of right upper lobe. Larger vessels that were previously unfilled (see C) now extend to right upper lobe. (*Courtesy of Dr. H. Palevsky.*)

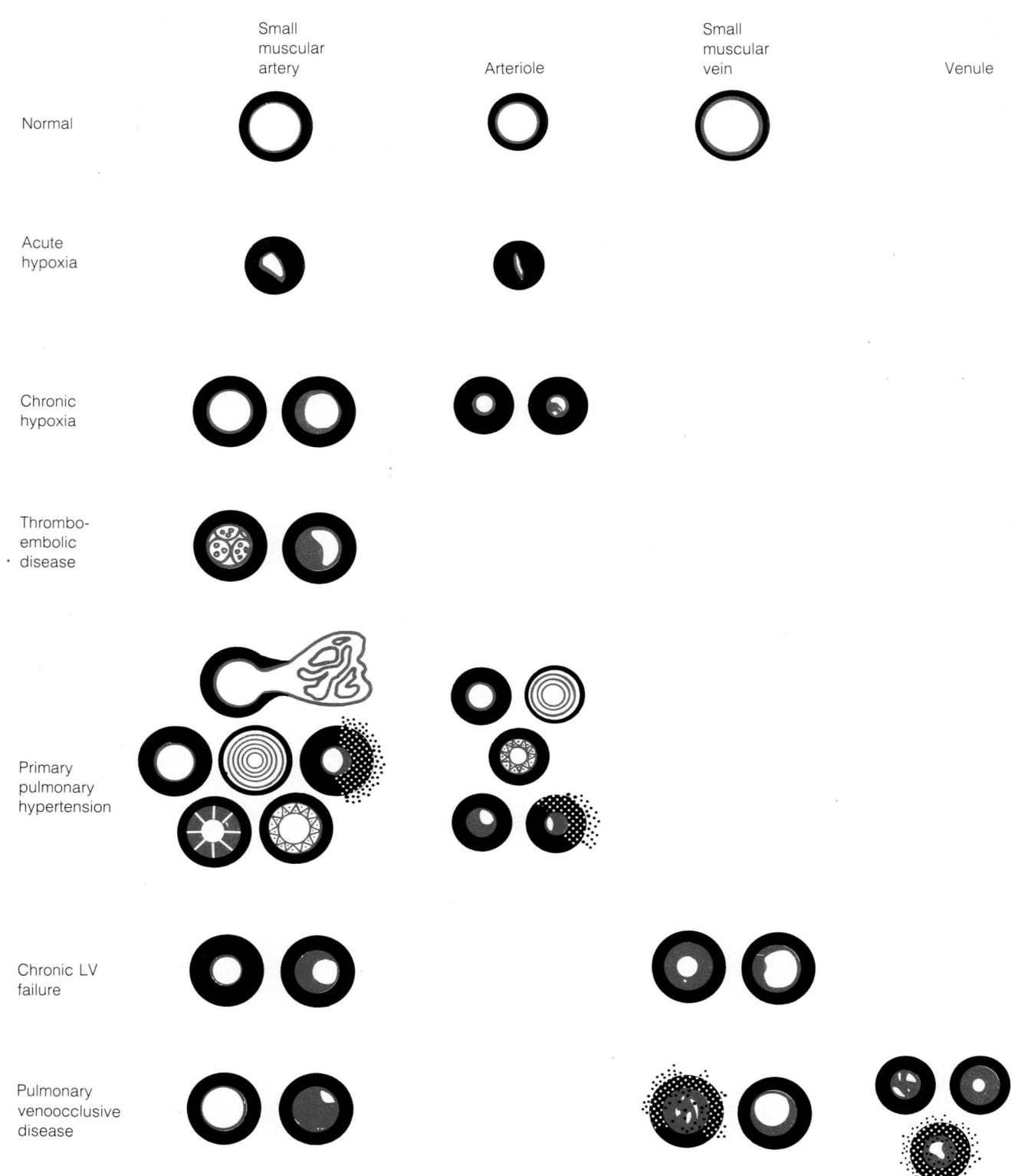

FIGURE 64-18 Spectrum of pulmonary vascular lesions in primary pulmonary hypertension and other pulmonary hypertensive disorders.

disorder that was previously regarded as a prognosis of impending doom, and (2) the creation of a national registry, that now lists about 200 patients on whom data were collected systematically for analysis, has raised the prospect of fresh insights into etiologies, pathogenetic mechanisms, natural history, and management.

As indicated above, the vessels primarily affected are the small muscular arteries and arterioles. In these vessels, the spectrum of lesions is broad, almost invariably affecting both intima and media (Fig. 64-18). For the pathologist, the differential diagnosis usually boils down to eliminating multiple pulmonary emboli as the etiology. There are two basic ground rules for this distinction: (1) the organized clots of multiple pulmonary emboli almost invariably manifest eccentric fibroelastosis, whereas the intimal changes in primary pulmonary hypertension generally feature concentric fibroelastosis; and (2) plexiform and angiomatoid lesions that occur in primary pulmonary hypertension are virtually unknown in multiple pulmonary emboli. However, it should be noted that neither the plexiform nor the angiomatoid lesions are diagnostic of primary pulmonary hypertension. Instead, they probably reflect a healed pulmonary arteritis and can be found in various other disease states, including Eisenmenger's complex, schistosomiasis, and hepatic cirrhosis.

Etiology

By definition, the etiology of primary pulmonary hypertension is unknown. Indeed, it seems likely that multiple etiologies converge on the same pathologic changes in the pulmonary arterial tree (Fig. 64-19). In a few patients, primary pulmonary hypertension seems attributable to sustained pulmonary vasoconstriction from birth, or persistence of the fetal circulation, or amniotic fluid emboli. In others, the coincidence of Raynaud's syndrome and primary pulmonary hypertension has nurtured the ideas of pulmonary vasospasm and collagen vascular disease; this idea has not withstood scrutiny. The familial occurrence of primary pulmonary hypertension has raised the possibility of genetic transmission.

Pathophysiology

In most patients, the vascular disease progresses inexorably, but at different rates. As a rule, the course is briefer, i.e., 1 to 2 years between diagnosis and death, in young women than in older men and women. In some instances, as illustrated by the aminorex epidemic, the disease stops and even reverses.

As expected from the predominant involvement of pulmonary precapillary vessels, despite marked pulmonary arterial hypertension, pulmonary arterial wedge pressure is normal, and the cardiac output is normal or slightly reduced. In severe pulmonary hypertension, right ventricular end-diastolic pressure and mean right atrial pressure become abnormally high: the *a* wave in the right atrium is conspicuous, a reflection of the forceful atrial contraction necessary to fill the hypertrophied right ven-

tricle. As the long-standing overload on the right side of the heart continues, right ventricular failure finally develops.

Systemic arterial hypoxemia, if present, is mild. Late in the disease, many patients develop peripheral cyanosis secondary to reduced cardiac output and peripheral vasoconstriction; central cyanosis also occurs preterminally in some patients because of right-to-left shunting through a patent foramen ovale.

Clinical Features

The first clue is often an abnormal chest radiograph (Fig. 64-20) or an electrocardiograph indicative of right ventricular hypertrophy. Initial complaints, particularly easy fatigability and chest discomfort, are often dismissed as neurotic. Direct determination of pulmonary circulatory pressures by cardiac catheterization is currently the only way to prove the diagnosis.

When the disease is advanced, dyspnea, particularly during exercise, is common. Many patients are tachypneic and complain of nondescript chest pain as well as breathlessness. Other common symptoms are weakness, fatigue, and syncope; the latter is often an ominous manifestation but occasionally disappears spontaneously even though the disease progresses. In time, right-sided heart failure evolves. On occasion, an enlarged pulmonary artery causes hoarseness because of compression of the left recurrent laryngeal nerve.

Patients with severe pulmonary hypertension seem prone to sudden death. Thus, death has occurred unexpectedly during normal activities, cardiac catheterization, and surgical procedures and after the administration of barbiturates or anesthetic agents. In a few instances, bradycardia leading to cardiac arrest has preceded sudden death (Fig. 64-21).

On physical examination, there is no evidence of primary pulmonary or cardiac disease. Otherwise, the cardiac examination is consistent with right ventricular overload, secondary to pulmonary hypertension of any cause.

Early in the evolution of the disease, the chest radiograph appears normal. In time, the central pulmonary arteries become increasingly prominent as the peripheral vessels become attenuated, and the cardiac silhouette enlarges (Fig. 64-20). The electrocardiogram almost invariably shows some evidence of right ventricular overload, usually in conjunction with right atrial involvement.

The minimal criteria for entry of a patient into the National Registry also indicate the mainstays of differential diagnosis: normal pulmonary function tests, except for a moderate reduction in diffusing capacity; right-sided cardiac catheterization to exclude congenital or acquired heart disease; perfusion scans, and angiography if the scan is inconclusive for pulmonary emboli; serologic testing to eliminate collagen vascular disease; liver function tests to detect the coincidence of cirrhosis and pulmonary hypertension.

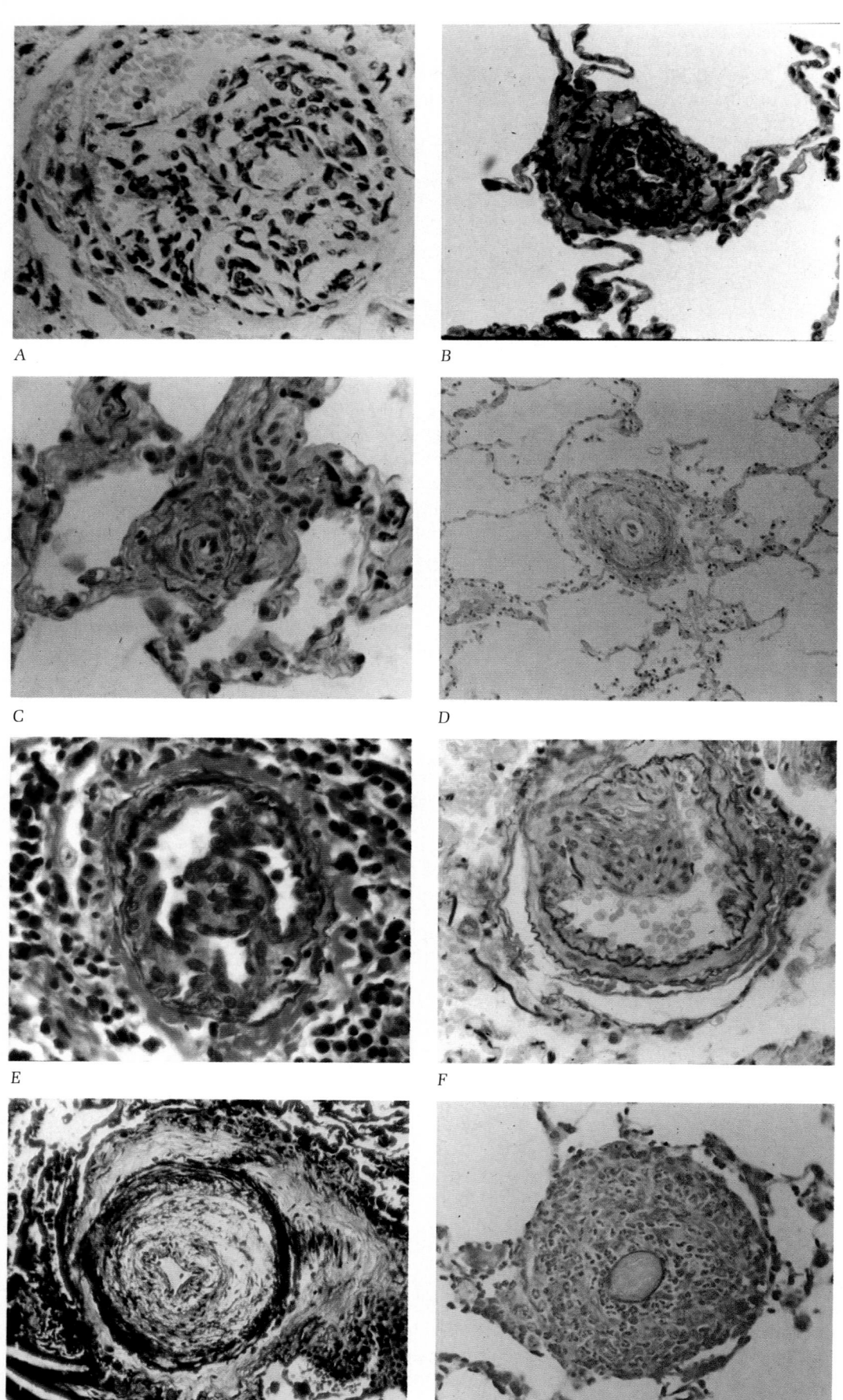

A

B

C

D

E

F

G

H

FIGURE 64-19 Vascular lesions at open lung biopsy in patients referred with clinical diagnosis of primary pulmonary hypertension. In three patients (A, B, G) no etiology was identified histologically; in the other five, etiologies were identified. A. Unexplained pulmonary hypertension. Plexiform lesion. B. Unexplained pulmonary hypertension. Small muscular artery. C. Pericapillary fibrosis. D. Scleroderma. E. Systemic lupus erythematosus. F. Multiple pulmonary emboli. G. Cirrhosis of liver (portal hypertension) and unexplained pulmonary hypertension. H. Schistosomiasis. (A to E courtesy of Dr. G. G. Pietra.)

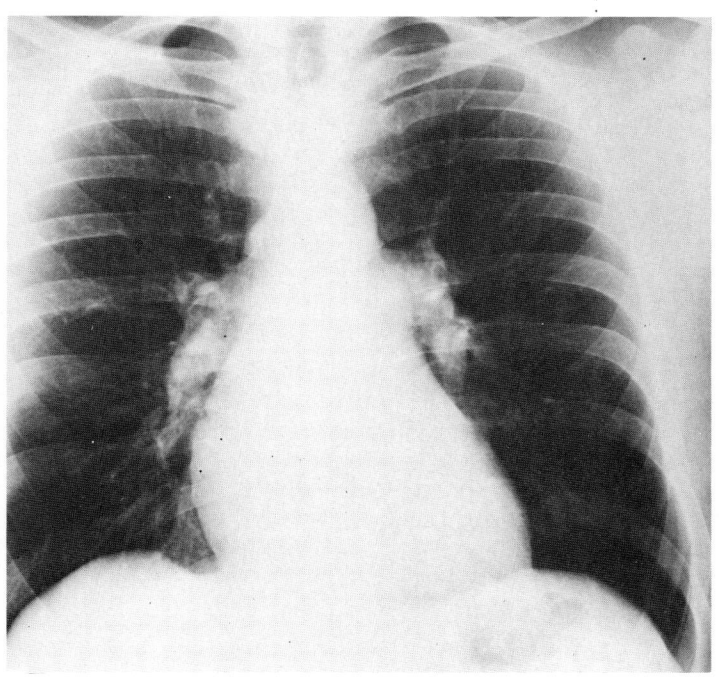
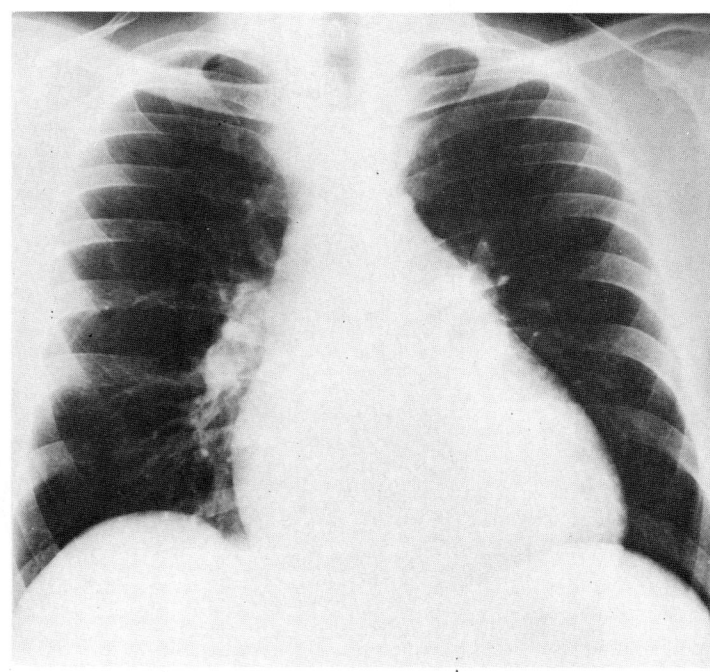

A   B

FIGURE 64-20 Radiographic changes in primary pulmonary hypertension. *A.* Spontaneous enlargement of the cardiac silhouette in a 30-year-old man in the 14 months between chest radiographs associated with increasing dyspnea. *B.* Decrease in the cardiac silhouette in response to chronic pulmonary vasodilator therapy.

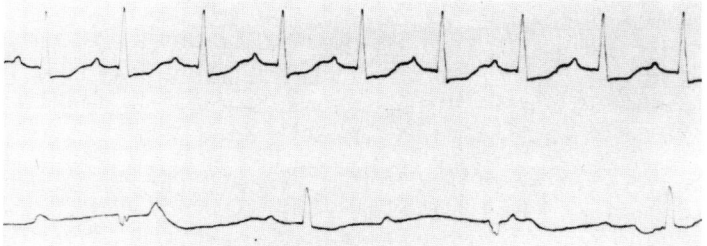

FIGURE 64-21 Primary pulmonary hypertension. Bradycardia and prolongation of atrioventricular conduction, that progressed to atrioventricular dissociation while on bedpan. Associated with syncope.

Treatment
In only one-third of patients who tested acutely for vasodilator response does the desired response occur (Fig. 64-22). The optimal response—a drop in pulmonary arterial pressure and an increase in cardiac output—occurs in far fewer (Fig. 64-23), even though calculated pulmonary vascular resistance may fall; this distinction between a decrease in calculated resistance and in the load borne by the right ventricle (mean pulmonary arterial pressure × cardiac output) has long-term implications with respect to right ventricular failure since the heart will continue to be overburdened if the pulmonary arterial pressure does not fall. Most often, the patient who develops a pulmonary vasodilator response to one agent will do the same with one or more agents even though the mechanisms of induc-

ing vasodilatation are different (Table 64-4). Improved well-being and increased exercise tolerance while taking a pulmonary vasodilator agent almost invariably implies that the cardiac output has improved, generally in response to both pulmonary vasodilatation and an inotropic effect of the agent on the heart.

Underlying Disorders II:
Dietary Pulmonary Hypertension

There is no longer any question that substances taken by mouth can selectively damage the pulmonary circulation. Three instances have been particularly well studied: experimentally induced pulmonary hypertension in animals, using *Crotalaria*, and spontaneous outbreaks in humans caused on the one hand by aminorex and on the other by "toxic oil." Because *plexiform lesions* have been found at autopsy in the human outbreaks, ambiguity has arisen about their relationships to primary pulmonary hypertension. However, it is clear that etiology cannot be inferred from similar anatomic lesions since the same morphology can result from multiple etiologies and pathogenetic mechanisms. For this reason, "dietary pulmonary hypertension" is considered here separately.

CROTALARIA PULMONARY HYPERTENSION

Crotalaria is a genus of annual shrubs that was introduced into southern states from the tropics and subtropics to restore the soil between crops. Unfortunately, *Crotalaria* is

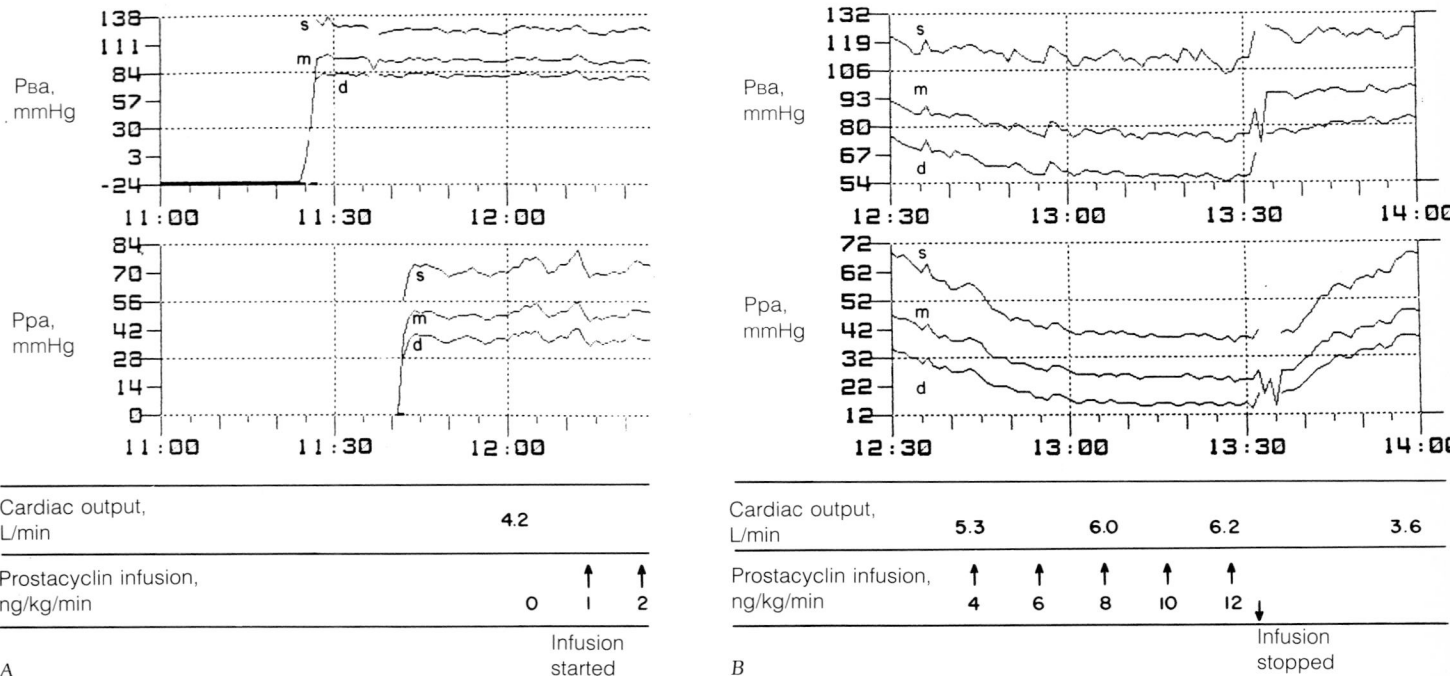

FIGURE 64-22 Prostacyclin infusion in primary pulmonary hypertension. *Left: Control* (11:30–12:15). Infusion started at 12:15. *Right: Test.* Within a few minutes, pulmonary arterial pressures decreased while cardiac output increased. Systemic arterial pressures also fell but much less strikingly. Stopping the infusion (13:30) resulted in a prompt return to control levels. (*Courtesy of Dr. H. Palevsky.*)

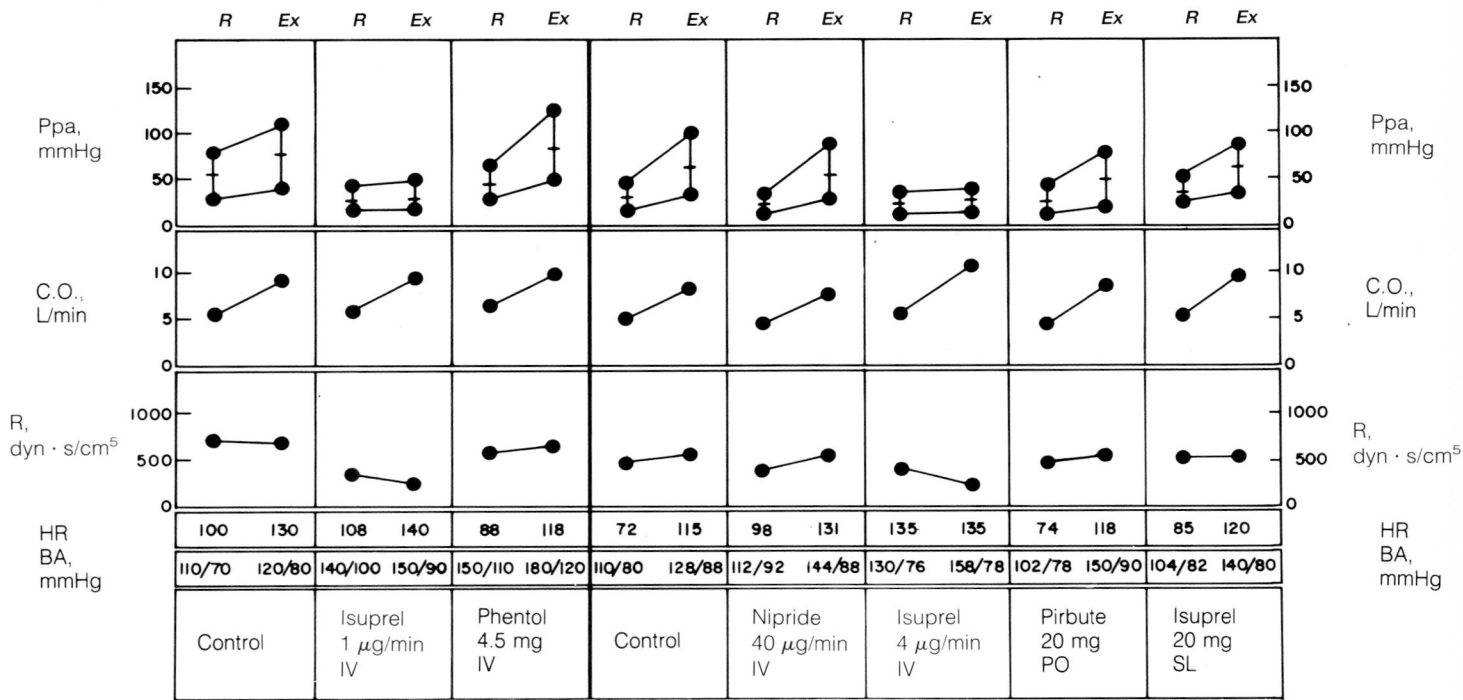

FIGURE 64-23 Repeat vasodilator studies over a 4-month interval. Patient took no medication between trials. Each column contains determinations at rest *(R)* and during exercise *(Ex)*. *Left three columns* (May 5, 1981): During the control period, as cardiac output increased during exercise, the level of pulmonary arterial pressure (systolic, diastolic, and mean) also increased. Isoproterenol (Isuprel) administered intravenously was associated with an unchanged pattern of change in cardiac output, but at lower pulmonary arterial pressures. Pulmonary wedge pressures (not shown) remained normal and unchanged. Calculated resistance fell. Phentolamine did not elicit a vasodilator response. *Right five columns* (September 25, 1981): The vasodilator response to isoproterenol (Isuprel) given intravenously was unchanged. A less impressive response occurred after sodium nitroprusside (Nipride). Oral pirbute and sublingual isoproterenol (Isuprel) (last two columns) did not elicit a pulmonary vasodilator response. C.O. = cardiac output, R = pulmonary vascular resistance, HR = heart rate, BA = brachial artery, IV = intravenous, PO = per os, SL = sublingual.

TABLE 64-4

Two Representative Vasodilator Agents Currently Used in the Management of Pulmonary Hypertension

Agent	Mechanism of Action	Acute Testing for Effectiveness	Usual Maintenance Therapy	Major Side Effects; Comments
Nifedipine	Interferes with calcium fluxes in vascular smooth muscle.	10 mg sublingually repeated once after 15 min. Exercise 15 min later.	Nifedipine 50 mg bid to qid	Systemic vasodilatation and hypotension; flushing, dysesthesias, peripheral edema. Little experience to date.
Hydralazine	Directly on vascular smooth muscle; greater dilator effect on arterioles than on veins; myocardial stimulant.	10 mg IV repeated once after 10 min. Resting hemodynamics followed by exercise 20 min later.	Hydralazine, start with 10 mg qid, increase to 50–75 mg qid.	Flushing, nasal congestion, conjunctivitis, CNS stimulation, drug fever, muscle cramps. Lupuslike syndrome at doses of 200–400 mg/day. Side effects lessened by gradual increase in dosage.

poisonous to humans and animals because of the pyrrolizidine alkaloids that it contains. The major offending pyrrolizidine alkaloid in C. spectabilis is monocrotaline. Other species of the shrub such as C. fulva contain their own distinctive alkaloids, e.g., fulvine. Ingestion of Crotalaria by domestic animals (and humans) leads to incapacitating damage of the liver, lungs, and central nervous system. In the West Indies, where poisoning by C. spectabilis is endemic in the native population, hepatotoxicity predominates. However, the rat and the nonhuman primate (Macaca) manifest primarily the sequelae of pulmonary arterial hypertension, i.e., right heart failure and death.

The pyrrolizidine alkaloid, monocrotaline, does not act directly on the pulmonary circulation of the rat. Instead, monocrotaline apparently has to be converted by the liver to dehydromonocrotaline as a prerequisite for pulmonary vascular toxicity. At autopsy, the pulmonary vascular lesions resemble those produced by severe, long-standing mitral stenosis in humans: medial hypertrophy, necrotizing arteriolitis, and proliferation of mast cells. Moreover, the lesions appear to be morphologically distinct from those of primary pulmonary hypertension, since neither plexiform lesions nor intimal fibrosis are regular features.

These experiments have demonstrated conclusively that substances taken by mouth can cause obliterative vascular lesions in the pulmonary circulation.

Another disorder produced by Crotalaria is occlusion of pulmonary veins and venules, in animals and humans, after the medicinal use of "bush tea" prepared from C. retusa. Bush tea can also produce veno-occlusive disease of the liver. The curious association between vascular involvement in liver and lungs considered in conjunction has invited speculation about how the arrangement of the intestine, liver, and lungs in series ("gut-liver-lung axis") might go awry to allow toxic materials to gain access to, and to inflict damage on, pulmonary vascular endothelium.

AMINOREX PULMONARY HYPERTENSION

Between 1966 and 1968, an epidemic of pulmonary hypertension erupted in Switzerland, Austria, and Germany: in these countries, the incidence of pulmonary hypertension increased 20-fold. In contrast to the pulmonary vascular lesions produced by pyrrolizidine alkaloids in the rat, the pathology in humans was typical of primary pulmonary hypertension, including the plexiform lesions and intimal fibrosis; the liver was spared. By coincidence or as a consequence, the epidemic followed the introduction of an appetite depressant agent, aminorex (2-amino-5-phenyl-2-oxazoline), in November 1965. Aminorex resembles epinephrine and amphetamine in chemical structure; both of these agents release endogenous stores of catecholamines.

After aminorex was banned in 1968, the epidemic subsided. However, the case implicating aminorex as the etiologic agent was only circumstantial.

Although 80 percent of those patients with pulmonary hypertension did give a history of ingesting aminorex, the quantities that were taken were often minimal. Moreover, what about the 20 percent who did not take aminorex? Nonetheless, despite reservations of this kind, most clinicians have interpreted the outbreak of primary pulmonary hypertension to be a consequence of aminorex ingestion. To explain the peculiar pulmonary pressor effect of aminorex in some individuals but not in others, they have invoked some type of predisposition, possibly genetic, as a prerequisite for the obliterative pulmonary vascular lesions. A similar genetic vulnerability has also been invoked to explain sporadic instances of unbridled pulmonary hypertension at altitude and of primary pulmonary hypertension.

Attempts to reproduce dietary pulmonary hypertension by administering aminorex to animals have been uniformly unsuccessful. But, the cumulative experience with aminorex provided several important lessons. Among the more important was the observation that pulmonary hypertension was often reversible, particularly when detected early in its course and before pressures reached systemic levels.

TOXIC OIL SYNDROME

Another episode in the story of dietary pulmonary hypertension unfolded with the occurrence of the "toxic oil syndrome." In May and June 1981, adulterated rapeseed oil, a bootleg pseudo olive oil, sold door-to-door in Spain, caused an extraordinary epidemic of noncardiogenic pulmonary edema. Twenty thousand individuals were affected, and about 375 died. About 2000 went on to sequelae. As a consequence of close surveillance, three stages of the disease have now been identified: early (first 6 months), intermediate (6 months to 2 years), and chronic (persisting to date since 1981). From the outset, it was clear that the damage was widespread, e.g., affecting lungs, liver, skin, nervous system, immune system, muscle, and fat, and that endothelial injury everywhere features prominently in the pathogenesis of the clinical syndromes.

Early

During the first 3 to 4 months after ingesting the toxic oil, the lungs were the seat of noncardiogenic pulmonary edema; pleural effusions were also common. Eosinophilia was striking and consistent. Most patients recovered (without pulmonary fibrosis) in 6 months or less. Pulmonary hypertension did occur but reversed spontaneously.

Intermediate

After the first 6 months, thromboembolic phenomena, affecting gut, spleen, and other viscera, including lungs, supervened. Weight loss and peripheral neuromuscular dystrophies were common. In patients who had pulmonary hypertension, the blood pressures often seemed to be reverting toward normal.

Chronic

In this phase (particularly in years 4 and 5 after the oil was ingested) pulmonary hypertension and cor pulmonale have become increasingly evident. The vascular lesions in the lungs are characterized by intimal fibrosis and proliferation in precapillary vessels in association with organized pulmonary thromboemboli. Plexiform lesions have also been seen. However, neither necrotizing arteritis nor pulmonary fibrosis have been observed.

Unfortunately, the chemical ingredients in the toxic oil responsible for the syndrome remain enigmatic and are unlikely to be uncovered since the bootleggers provided no recipe for the adulterated cooking oil as they went out of business, and reliable samples are now difficult to come by. Nonetheless, the outbreak showed that ingested material—often in small quantities—could cause widespread endothelial injury that involved the lungs. It also underscored the spontaneous reversibility of the pulmonary hypertension (as well as the ineffectiveness of vasodilators tried at different stages in the disease). Most unusual is the sharing of thromboembolism and intimal damage in pathogenesis, a coincidence that is strikingly different from the finding of occasional clots in the pulmonary circulation at autopsy in patients with primary pulmonary hypertension.

Underlying Disorders III: Pulmonary Interstitial (Restrictive) Disease

ETIOLOGY

A wide variety of stimuli evoke pulmonary interstitial fibrosis (Fig. 64-24). The most familiar etiologies in this group are sarcoidosis, asbestosis, and radiation fibrosis. Lymphangitic spread of carcinoma within the lungs produces the same functional effect (Fig. 64-25). The common denominator is a pattern of restrictive lung disease which was originally categorized as *alveolar-capillary block*. Although the original concept of alveolar-capillary block focused excessively on impairment to diffusion through thickened alveolar-capillary membranes, and did not take account of associated derangements in ventilation-perfusion relationships, categorization of these different anatomic disorders according to functional derangements that they produce is still useful in practice.

Progressive fibrosis and infiltration not only thickens and distorts the pulmonary interstitium (Fig. 64-26), replacing the normal mucopolysaccharide matrix with cells and scar tissue, but also entraps the pulmonary blood vessels. As a result, some segments of the pulmonary vascular bed are amputated, others are encased in scar, and the overall distensibility of the pulmonary parenchyma is diminished. In some disorders, honeycombing due to the pulling of scar tissue on normal and less affected lung intensifies the distortions in the pulmonary parenchyma. Some of these interstitial processes affect the small airways indirectly by substituting a surrounding of scar tissue for the normal alveolar ambience; with others, such as sarcoidosis, the disease process not only affects the parenchyma of the lung but also the airways.

PATHOPHYSIOLOGY

The lungs are stiff (poorly compliant) because of the diffuse interstitial disease. Their elastic recoil is correspondingly low. Asbestosis often adds a second mechanism for reducing pulmonary compliance, i.e., encasement of the lung by a thickened pleura. Minute and alveolar ventilation are high, and breathing is rapid and shallow, presumably an adaptation that minimizes the elastic work of breathing.

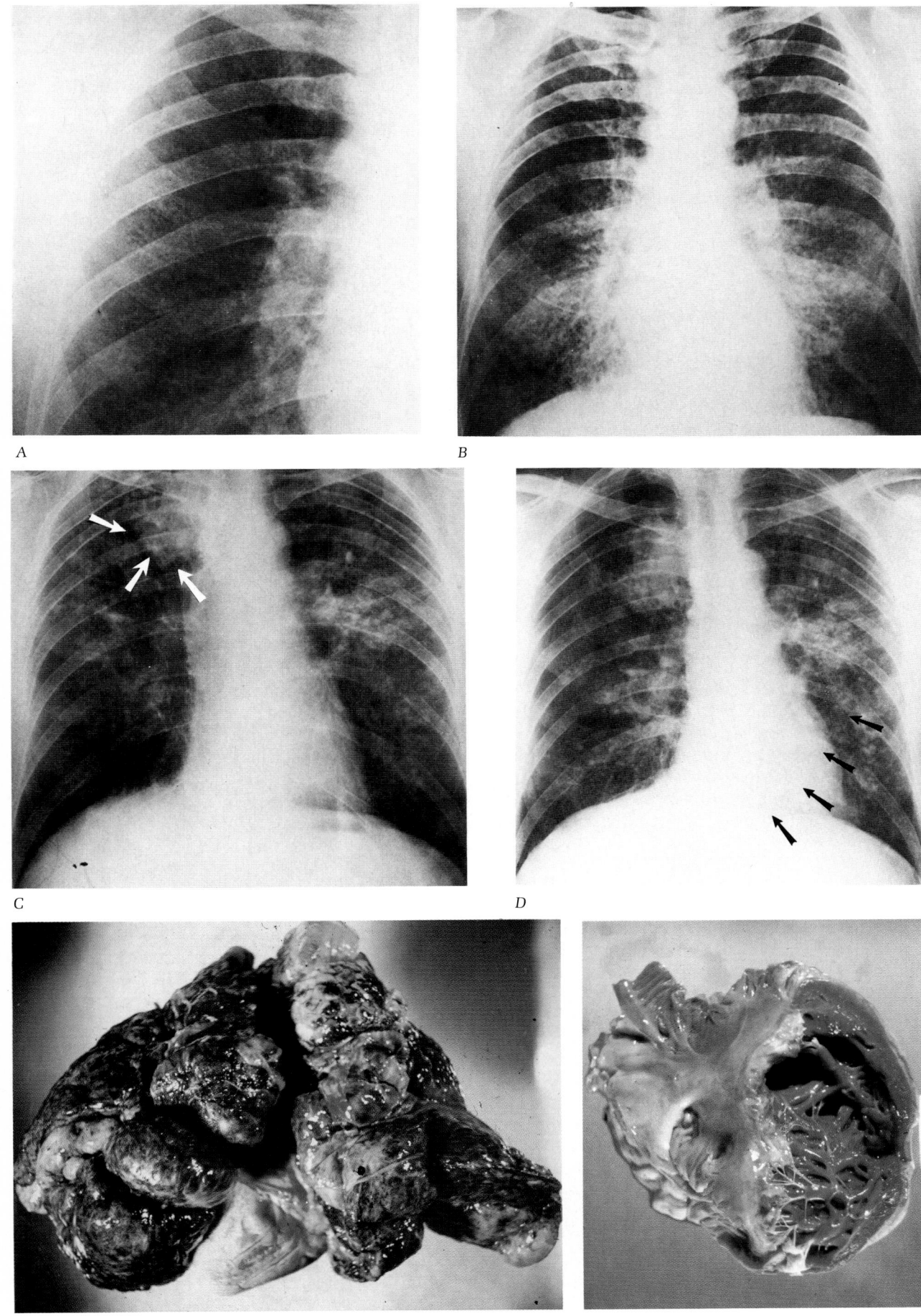

A

B

C

D

E

F

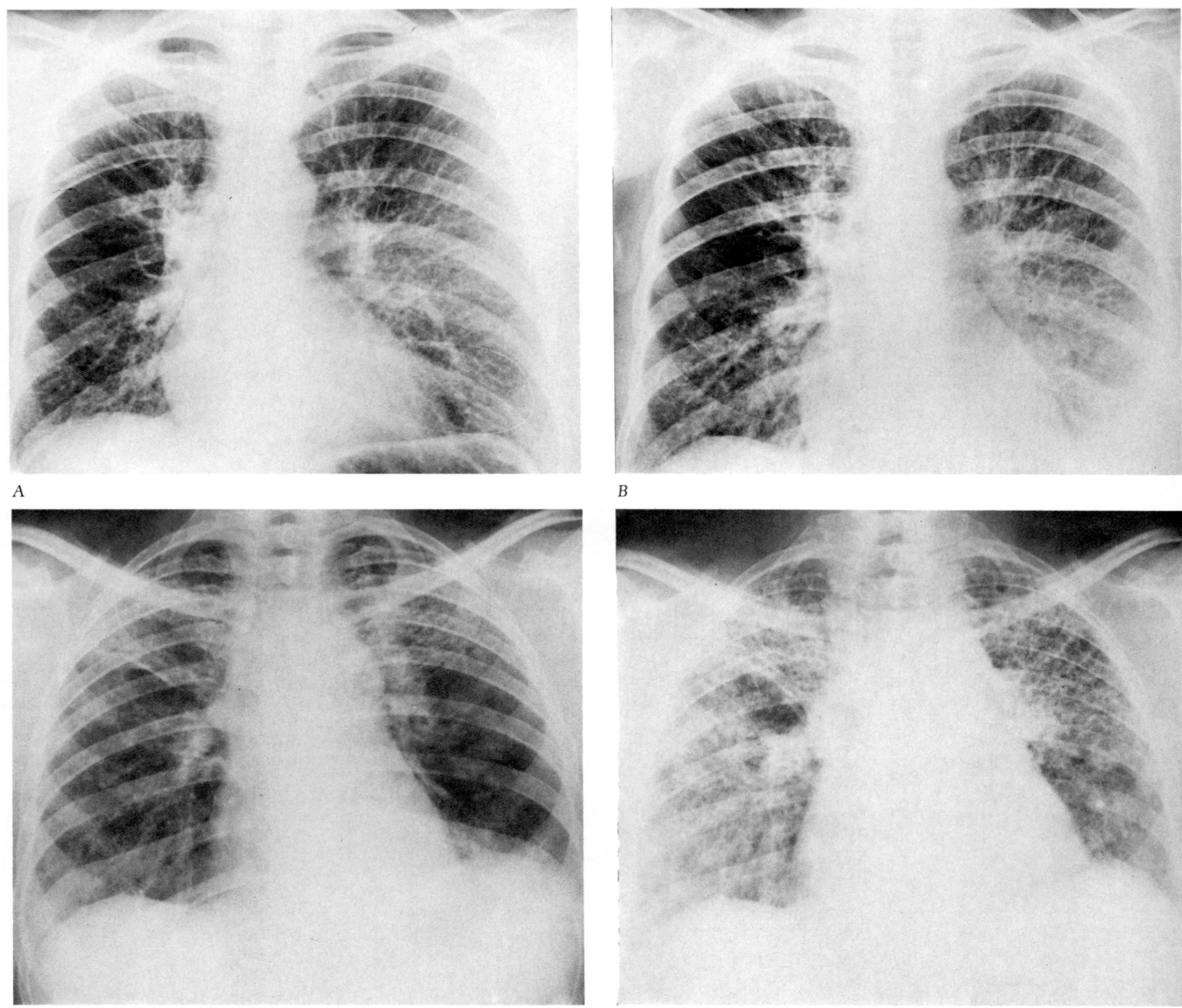

A

B

C

D

FIGURE 64-25   Diffuse interstitial disease.   *A* and *B*. Lymphangitic spread of carcinoma of the breast in a 50-year-old woman. In the 2 years between the chest radiographs, dyspnea and tachypnea had progressed. The pulmonary function tests showed severe impairment of diffusion; the electrocardiogram indicated right ventricular enlargement (cor pulmonale).   *C* and *D*. Sarcoidosis in a 50-year-old man. In the 2 years between the chest radiographs, pulmonary fibrosis had progressed strikingly. At autopsy, pulmonary fibrosis was marked; bronchi were widely dilated and emphysematous areas were juxtaposed to areas of dense fibrosis. Cor pulmonale was confirmed.

◀ **FIGURE 64-24**   Diffuse interstitial disease. Silicosis.   *A*. Simple silicosis. Right upper lobe. Fine nodularity is evidence of early widespread disease. Hilar adenopathy is also present.   *B*. Simple silicosis. The silicotic nodules are larger and more profuse.   *C*. Progressive massive fibrosis and emphysema complicating silicosis. A large shadow is seen in the right upper lobe (arrows). In addition, the upper lobes are slightly contracted, whereas the lower lobes are unusually radiolucent.   *D*. Same patient as in C. Pneumothorax on the right complicates massive fibrosis.   *E*. Progressive massive fibrosis and emphysema complicating silicosis. Large bullae are widespread.   *F*. Cor pulmonale secondary to progressive massive fibrosis. *(A to D after Dauber, 1982; E, F courtesy of Dr. S. Moolten.)*

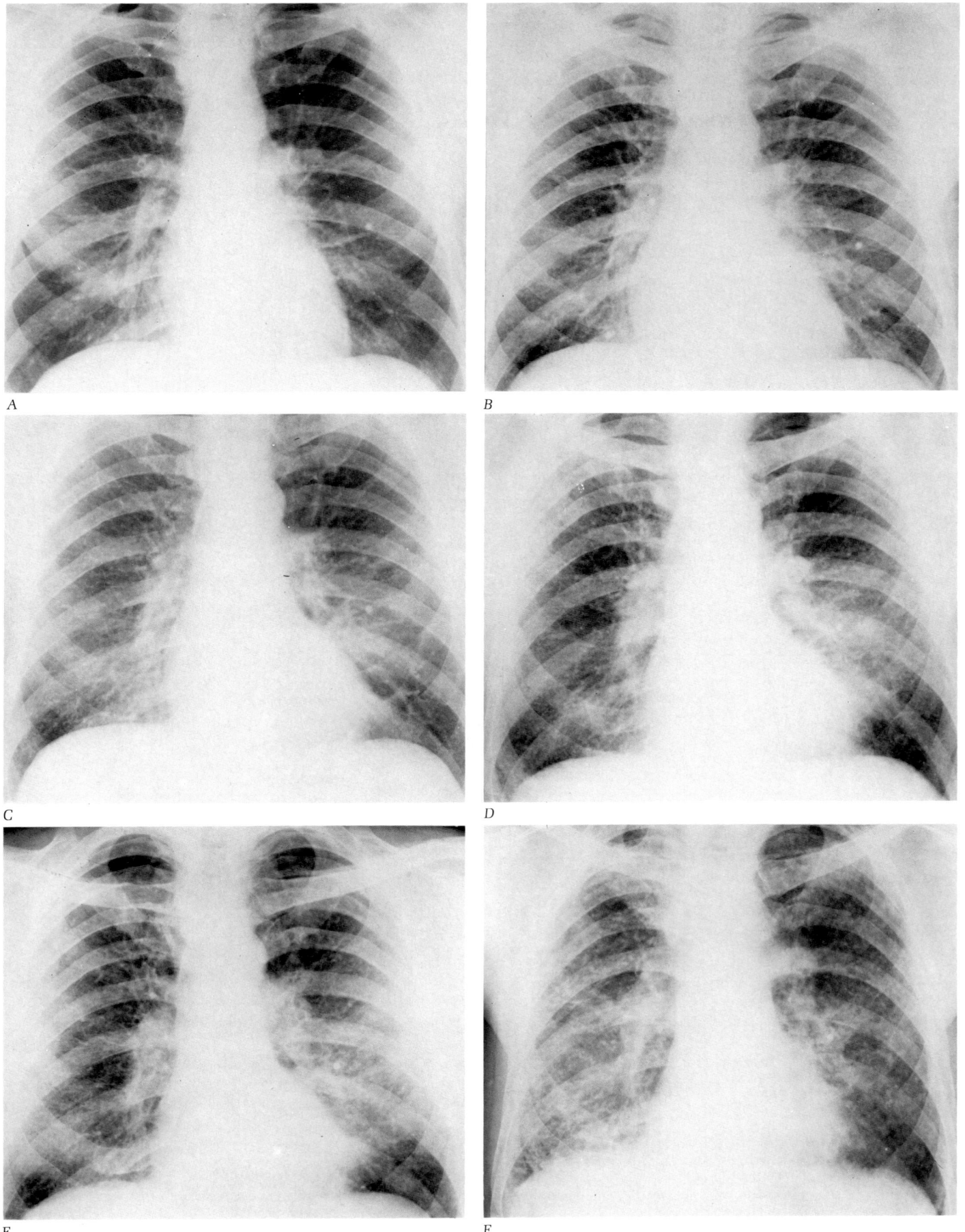

FIGURE 64-26 Pulmonary asbestosis. Consecutive changes over 18 years. The patient had worked in an asbestos plant for 3 years before the first radiograph shown was taken. *A.* 1937. *B.* 1940. *C.* 1944. *D.* 1947. *E.* 1949. *F.* 1955.

Lung volumes undergo gradual, concentric reduction as the interstitial disease progresses. Early in the disease, the blood-gas levels are virtually normal: arterial P_{O_2} is sustained at near-normal levels by chronic alveolar hyperventilation, and arterial P_{CO_2} is only minimally subnormal. But even at this stage, exercise often elicits a precipitous drop in arterial P_{O_2}. When the interstitial process has advanced sufficiently to cast shadows on the chest radiograph (Fig. 64-26), O_2 consumption is abnormally high, in large measure due to the increase in the work of breathing. The arterial P_{CO_2} is still normal or slightly low, reflecting a new balance between the augmented alveolar ventilation and the O_2 consumption. The diffusing capacity decreases progressively with the interstitial fibrosis; even when normal at rest, it often fails to increase normally during graded exercise.

Derangements in alveolar ventilation and blood flow at a microscopic level are present early in interstitial disease, but in time, progressive disease exaggerates the imbalances sufficiently to cause arterial hypoxemia at rest. As long as the arterial hypoxemia remains mild, pulmonary hypertension is generally modest (Fig. 64-27). But as arterial hypoxemia intensifies, the level of pulmonary hypertension also increases, and cor pulmonale begins to evolve. Arterial eucapnia or hypocapnia is gradually succeeded by hypercapnia. Right ventricular failure occurs late in the course of the disease, in association with severe hypoxemia and respiratory acidosis.

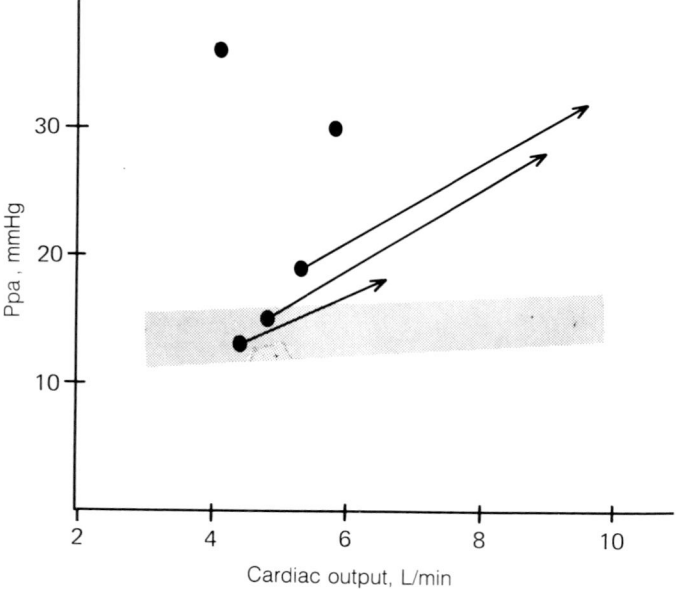

FIGURE 64-27 Pulmonary asbestosis. Hemodynamic observations in five patients. Two of the five had pulmonary hypertension at rest; the other three became pulmonary hypertensive during exercise. ● = at rest; → = exercise. The shaded background indicates the normal pulmonary arterial pressure-flow relationship.

CLINICAL FEATURES

The clinical picture is generally dominated by the underlying disorder until dyspnea and tachypnea become manifest. Cough is rarely a prominent feature. The chest radiograph is particularly diagnostic in disclosing a diffuse reticular or reticulonodular interstitial pattern (Fig. 64-28) that is consistent with either interstitial fibrosis or infiltration, or both.

TREATMENT

The focus of management is on the underlying lung disease, and success in relieving the pulmonary hypertension depends on the extent to which the pulmonary interstitial disease is reversible.

Underlying Disorders IV: Alveolar Hypoventilation Despite Normal Lungs

This topic is considered fully elsewhere in this book. Here it will suffice to consider those aspects germane to pulmonary hypertension.

ETIOLOGY

In patients who develop alveolar hypoventilation even though their lungs are normal, the common pathogenetic denominators are alveolar hypoxia and arterial hypoxemia, often reinforced by respiratory acidosis. In contrast to the "net" alveolar hypoventilation of obstructive airways disease, which is a consequence of ventilation-perfusion imbalances, alveolar hypoventilation in patients with normal lungs is global, affecting the lung everywhere, albeit not necessarily to the same extent. Global alveolar hypoventilation generally stems from an inadequate ventilatory drive or an ineffective chest bellows (Fig. 64-29). In particular, a variety of disorders, ranging from sleep apnea syndrome or a "dead" respiratory center to paralysis of respiratory muscles, kyphoscoliosis, and obesity, can be responsible.

PATHOPHYSIOLOGY

The diverse etiologies share hypoxia and respiratory acidosis as the common pathogenetic mechanism for pulmonary hypertension. However, the routes to hypoxia and acidosis are different. In the sleep apnea syndrome, or in the state of chronic alveolar hypoventilation that follows damage to the respiratory center, e.g., as by encephalitis, the lungs and chest wall are entirely normal. Postpoliomyelitis damage to the respiratory center is often associated with paralyzed respiratory muscles and with damaged nerves to the intercostal muscles. Extreme obesity imposes a mechanical burden upon the respiratory apparatus, chiefly by way of the abdomen, but often the mechanical load is accompanied by another derangement, e.g., an inherently inadequate ventilatory drive, that

(Text continues on page 1033.)

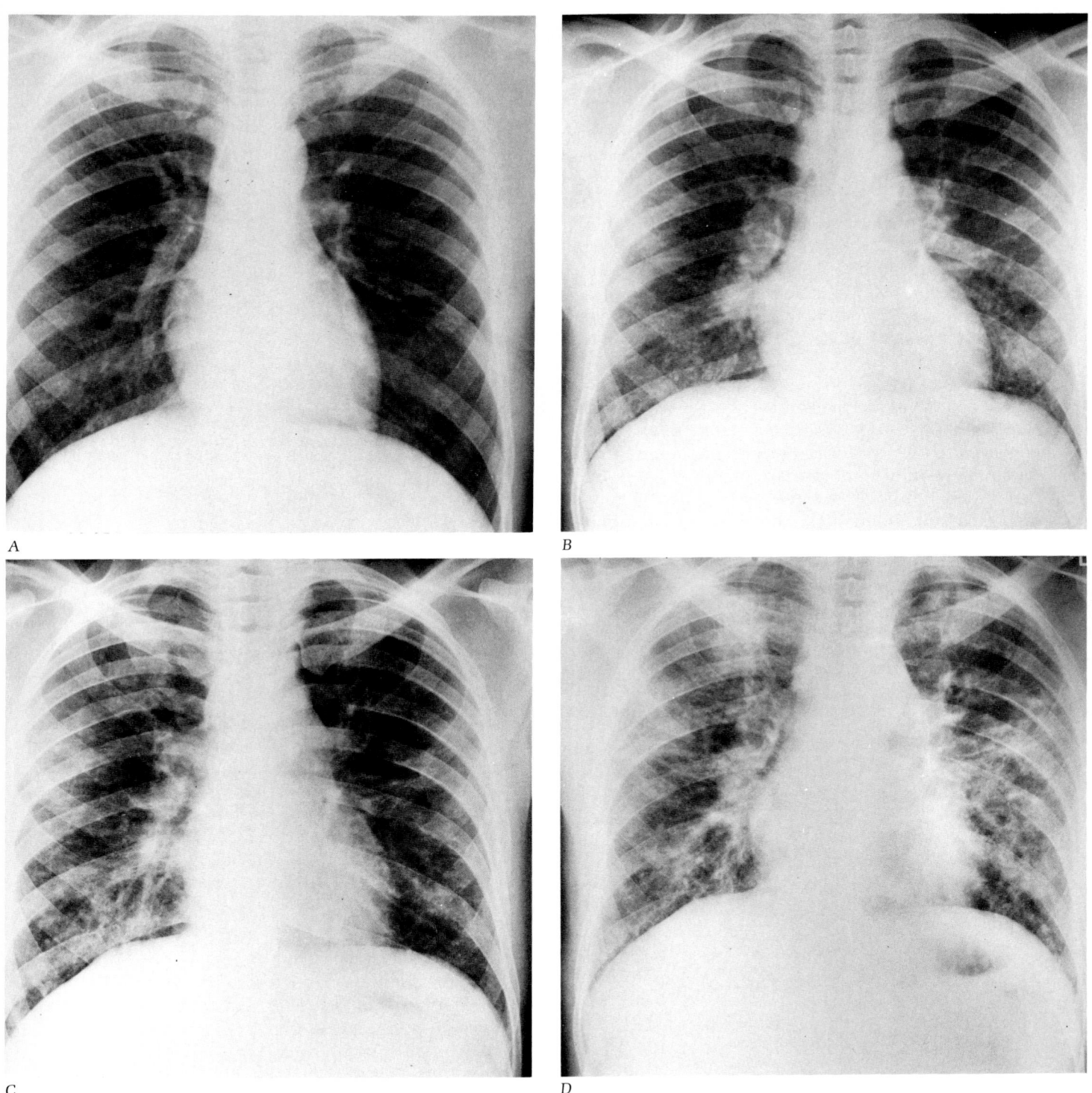

A

B

C

D

FIGURE 64-28 Sarcoidosis. Consecutive stages in evolution of diffuse pulmonary fibrosis which, in time, became associated with ventilation-perfusion abnormalities and cor pulmonale.

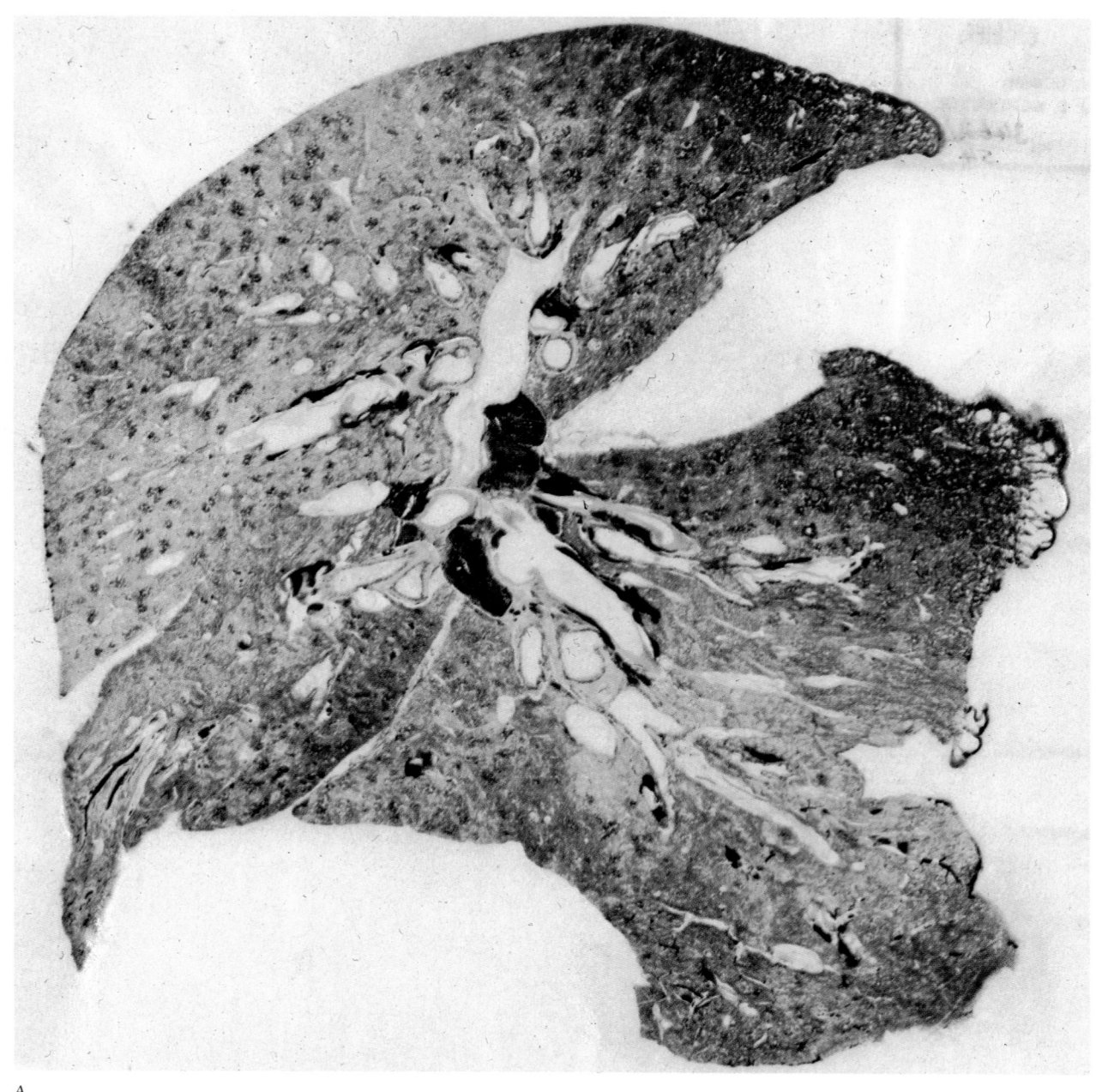

A

FIGURE 64-29 Alveolar hypoventilation secondary to abnormalities in chest wall and pleura. Sagittal sections. A. Kypho-scoliosis.

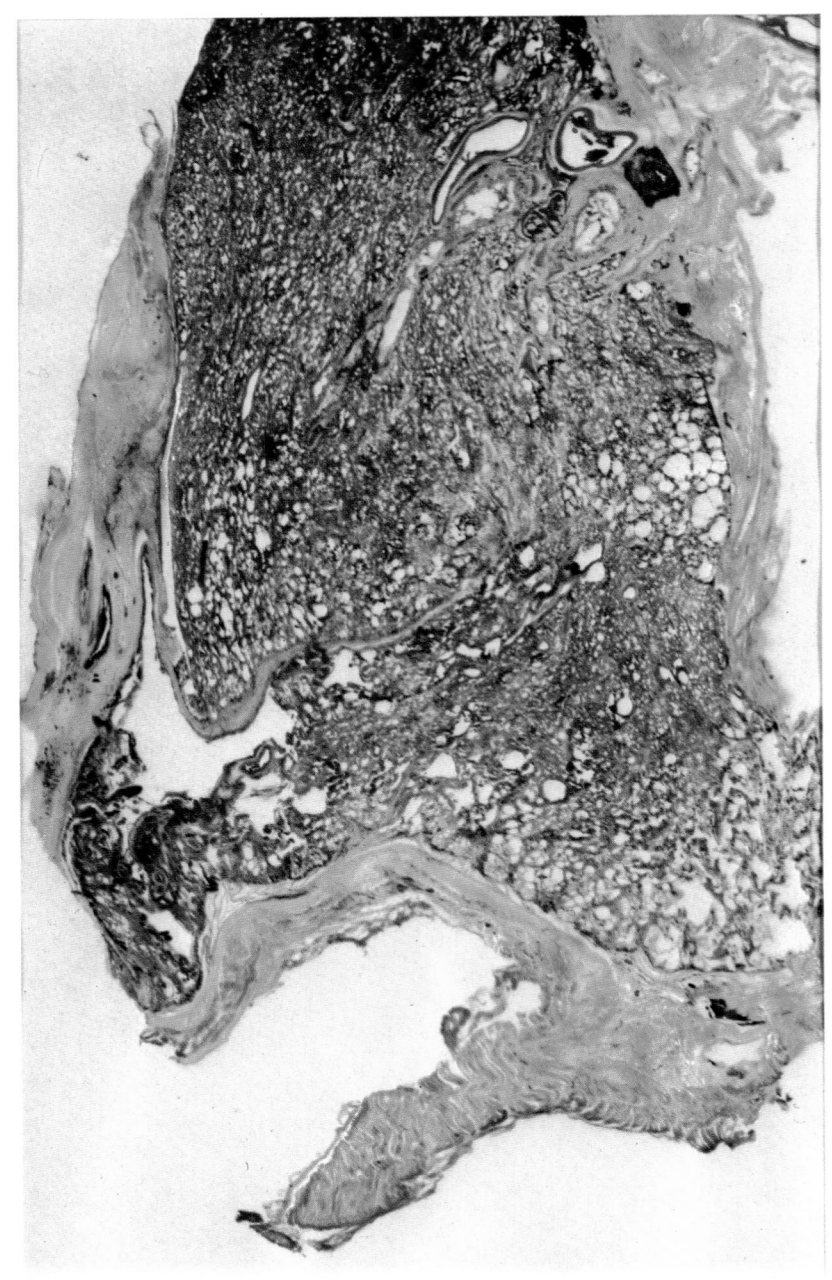

B

FIGURE 64-29 (continued) *B.* Asbestosis. Encasement of lung by thickened pleura. *(A, courtesy of Dr. J. Gough, Cardiff; B, courtesy of Dr. S. Moolten.)*

contributes to the alveolar hypoventilation. In kyphoscoliosis not only is the lung compressed and distorted but the mechanical operation of the chest bellows is compromised and the elastic properties of the lungs and chest wall are abnormal, albeit to different degrees.

Although the routes to hypoxia are different, once the arterial P_{O_2} falls below 40 to 50 mmHg, the pulmonary arterial walls of the patients undergo the same changes as those that occur spontaneously in native dwellers at high altitude: pulmonary arteries and arterioles manifest muscular hypertrophy, and a self-perpetuating mechanism is instituted for pulmonary hypertension. (Fig. 64-30).

CLINICAL FEATURES

These are dominated by the consequences of alveolar hypoxia and hypercapnia and modified by the initiating factors, e.g., kyphoscoliosis. Early in the disorder, when arterial hypoxemia and hypercapnia at rest are minimal, cyanosis may appear during exercise, the result of an inappropriate ventilatory response to increased metabolic demand. During sleep, arterial hypoxemia and hypercapnia intensify, but the blood gases return to near-normal levels during the waking hours. Even at this stage, an upper respiratory infection sometimes topples the subject into acute respiratory failure. On occasion, the first signal of alveolar hypoventilation is right ventricular failure. At that time, cerebral signs of hypercapnia are absent because respiratory acidosis has developed gradually and the kidneys have had time to retain enough bicarbonate.

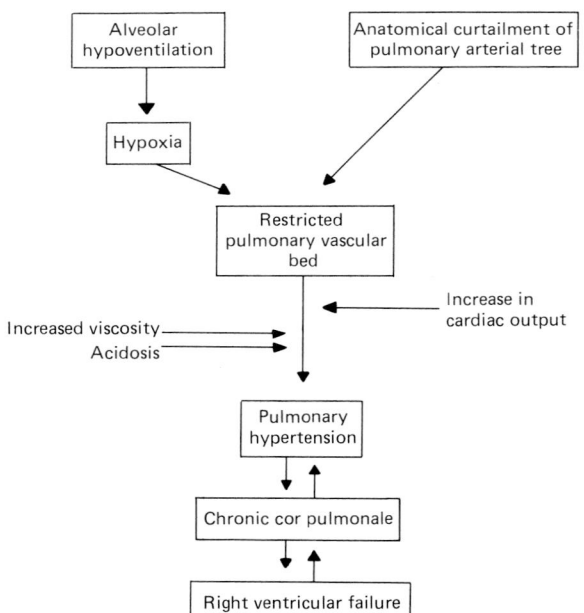

FIGURE 64-30 Evolution of pulmonary hypertension and cor pulmonale in kyphoscoliosis.

TREATMENT

Attention is directed toward relieving arterial hypoxemia and hypercapnia at rest, during sleep and during exercise (Chapter 82). Restoration of blood gases toward normal is effective in relieving pulmonary hypertension.

Underlying Disorders V: Alveolar Hypoventilation Due to Obstructive Airways Disease

ETIOLOGY

Chronic bronchitis and emphysema is the most common cause of pulmonary hypertension and cor pulmonale (Fig. 64-31). As in the alveolar hypoventilation that occurs in patients with normal lungs, the cause of the pulmonary hypertension is hypoxia (alveolar and arterial), usually in conjunction with respiratory acidosis, but the mechanisms leading to the abnormal blood gases are different. Moreover, although chronic bronchitis and emphysema generally coexist, it is the chronic bronchitis that is predominantly responsible for the abnormal blood gases that lead to pulmonary hypertension. Emphysema, per se, probably contributes by amputating segments of the pulmonary vascular bed but does not itself cause pulmonary hypertension even when rarefaction of the lungs is exceedingly extensive.

Cystic fibrosis is another common cause of pulmonary hypertension (Fig. 64-32). Here, too, the root cause is persistent hypoxia resulting from ventilation-perfusion abnormalities.

Cor pulmonale is uncommon in uncomplicated silicosis or tuberculosis. On the other hand, it is not uncommon when silicosis, anthrosilicosis, or long-standing fibrotic tuberculosis is complicated by extensive, conglomerate, massive fibrosis, distorted adjacent parenchyma, shrunken lobes, and bronchitis (Fig. 64-33). The likelihood of cor pulmonale is increased further by chronic pleurisy, fibrothorax, or excisional surgery. In such cases, a combination of anatomic restriction of the vascular bed and disturbances in gas exchange is involved in the pathogenesis of the pulmonary hypertension. Indeed, the disturbances in gas exchange often brought to clinical levels by an acute respiratory infection are the most reversible element of this disorder.

PATHOPHYSIOLOGY

The evolution of cor pulmonale in chronic bronchitis and emphysema depends on whether chronic bronchitis or emphysema predominates. For example, the "pink puffer" only develops pulmonary hypertension incident to a bout of acute respiratory infection; both the respiratory failure and the pulmonary hypertension can be expected to reverse in response to supportive and antibiotic therapy. In contrast, the "blue bloater," who is unremit-

(Text continues on page 1040.)

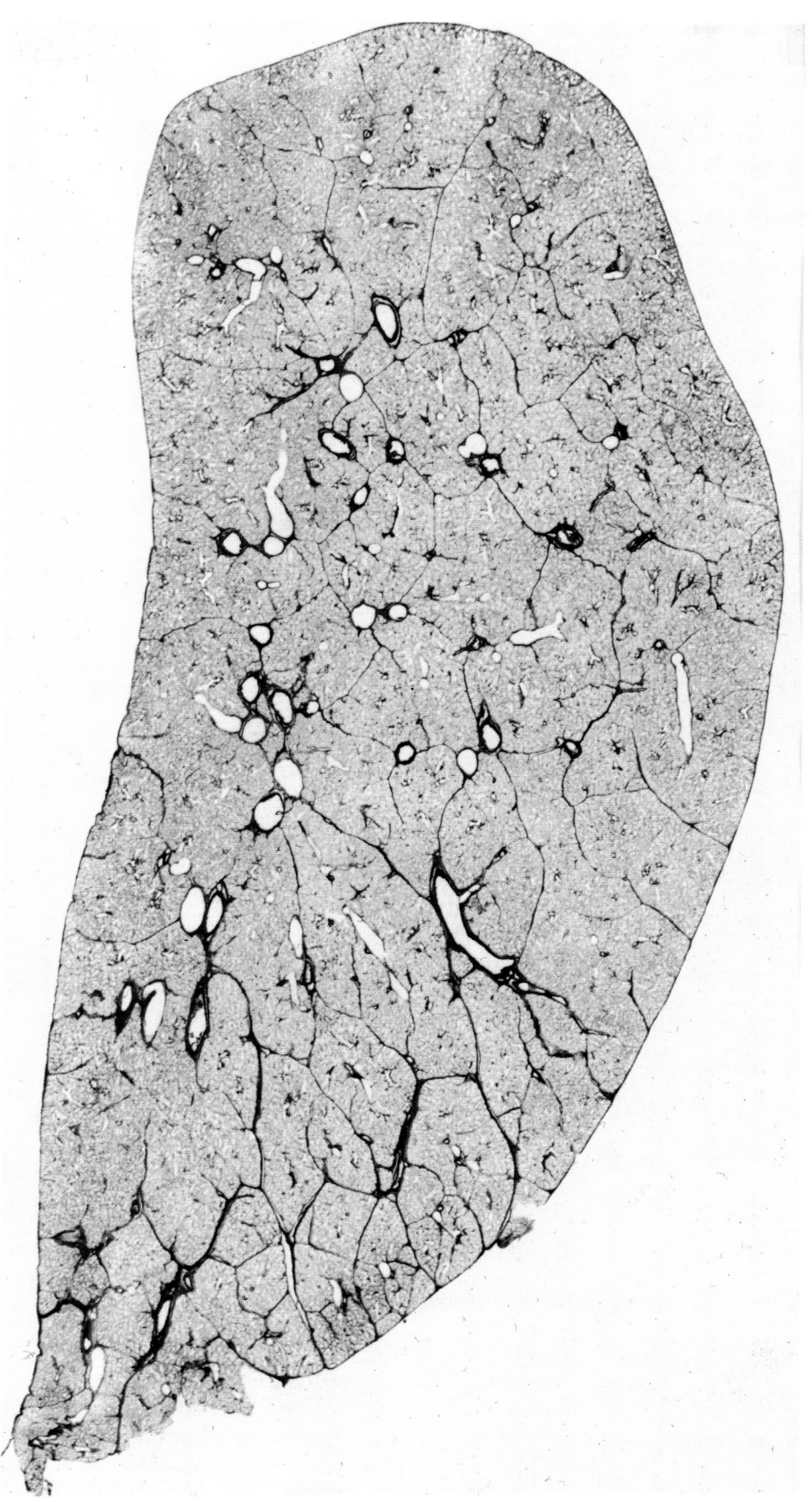

A

FIGURE 64-31 Chronic bronchitis, centri-lobular emphysema, and cor pulmonale. Sagittal sections. *A*. Normal architecture except for pulmonary congestion.

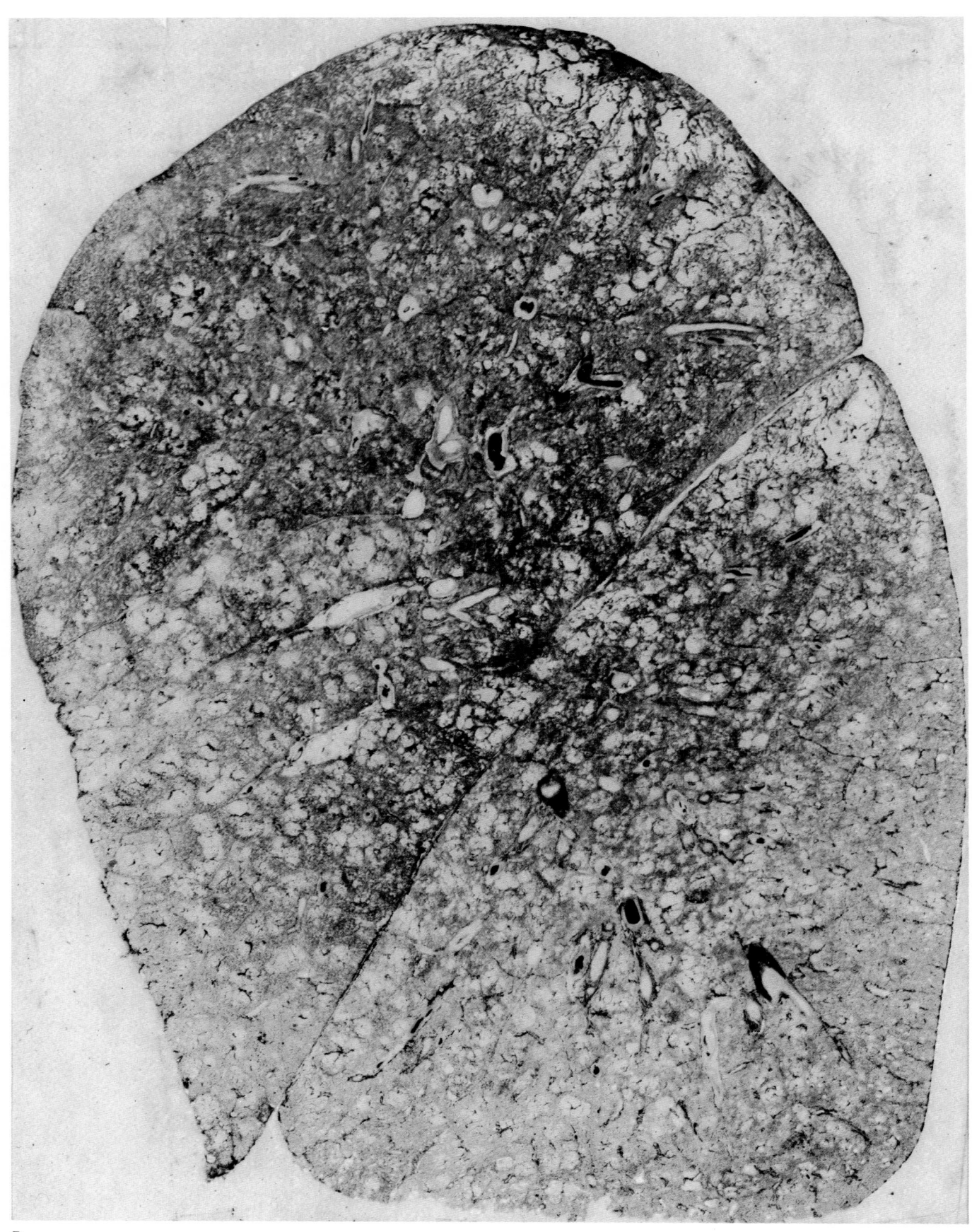

B

FIGURE 64-31 (continued) *B. Centrilobular emphysema. (Courtesy of Dr. S. Moolten.)*

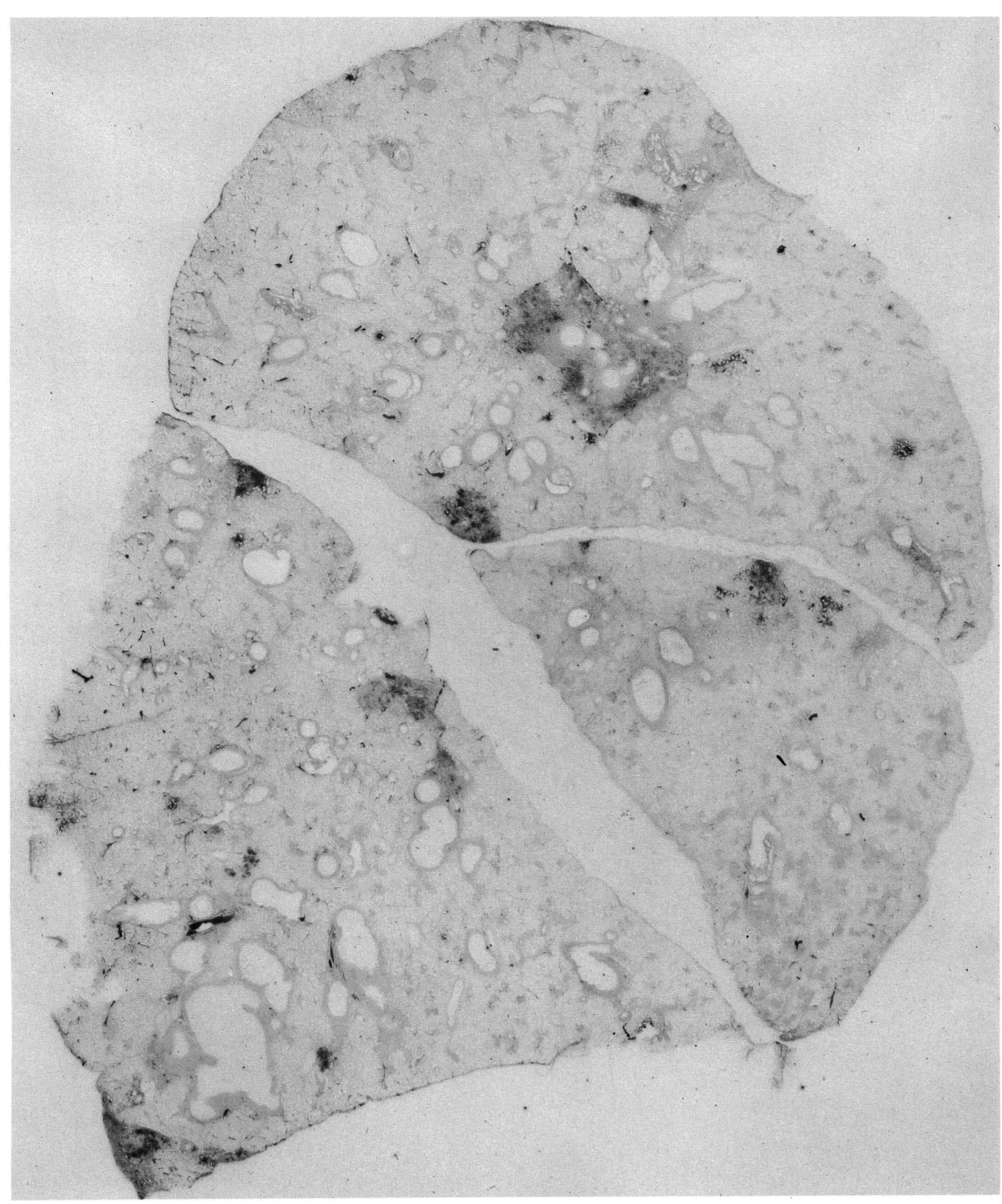

FIGURE 64-32 Cystic fibrosis. Sagittal section. The large airways are dilated and bronchiectatic, whereas the gas-exchanging surface is well preserved. (*Courtesy of Dr. S. Moolten.*)

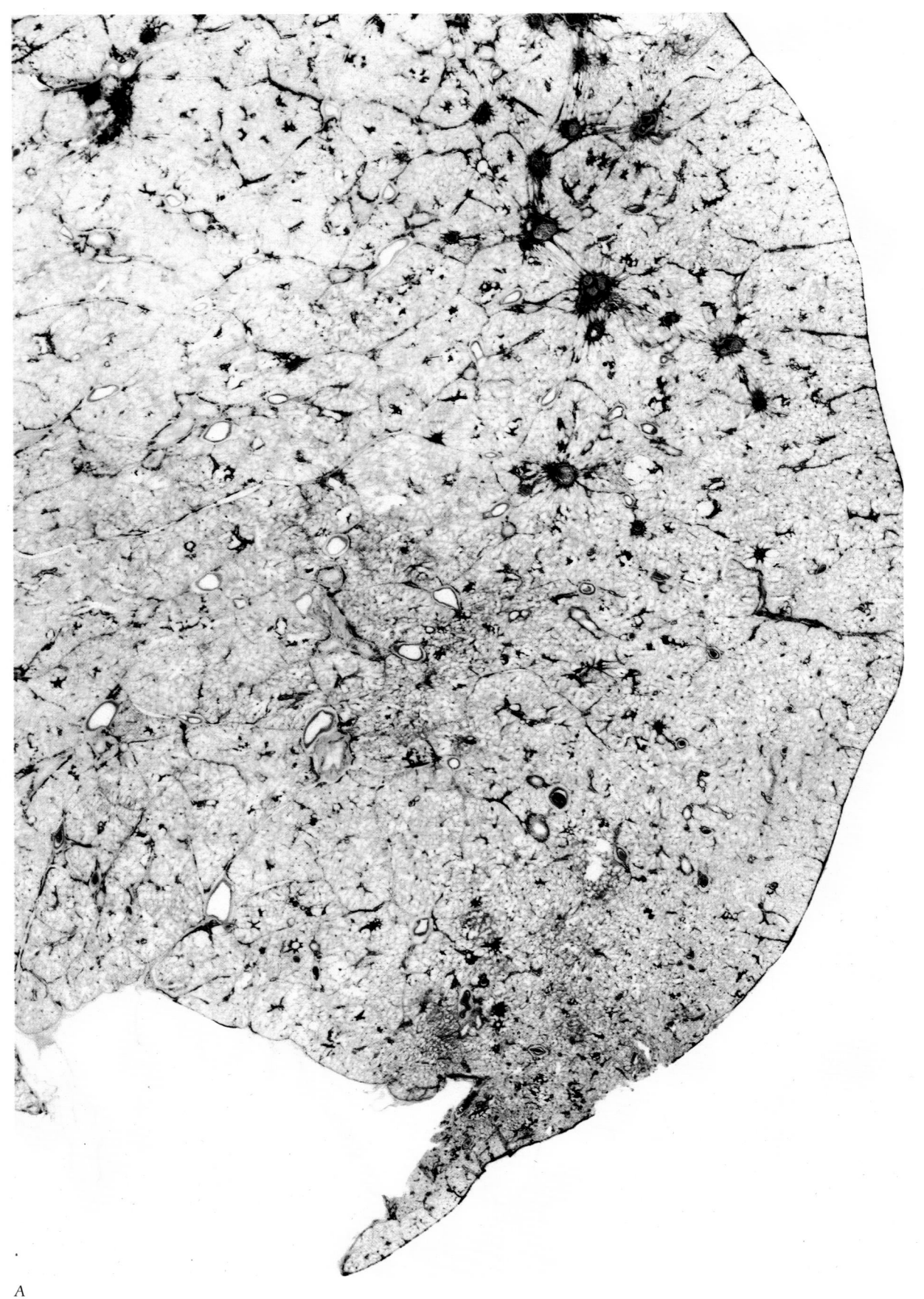

A

FIGURE 64-33 Coal miners' pneumoconiosis. Sagittal sections. *A.* Coal macules (black stars, upper right). The architecture is otherwise virtually normal.

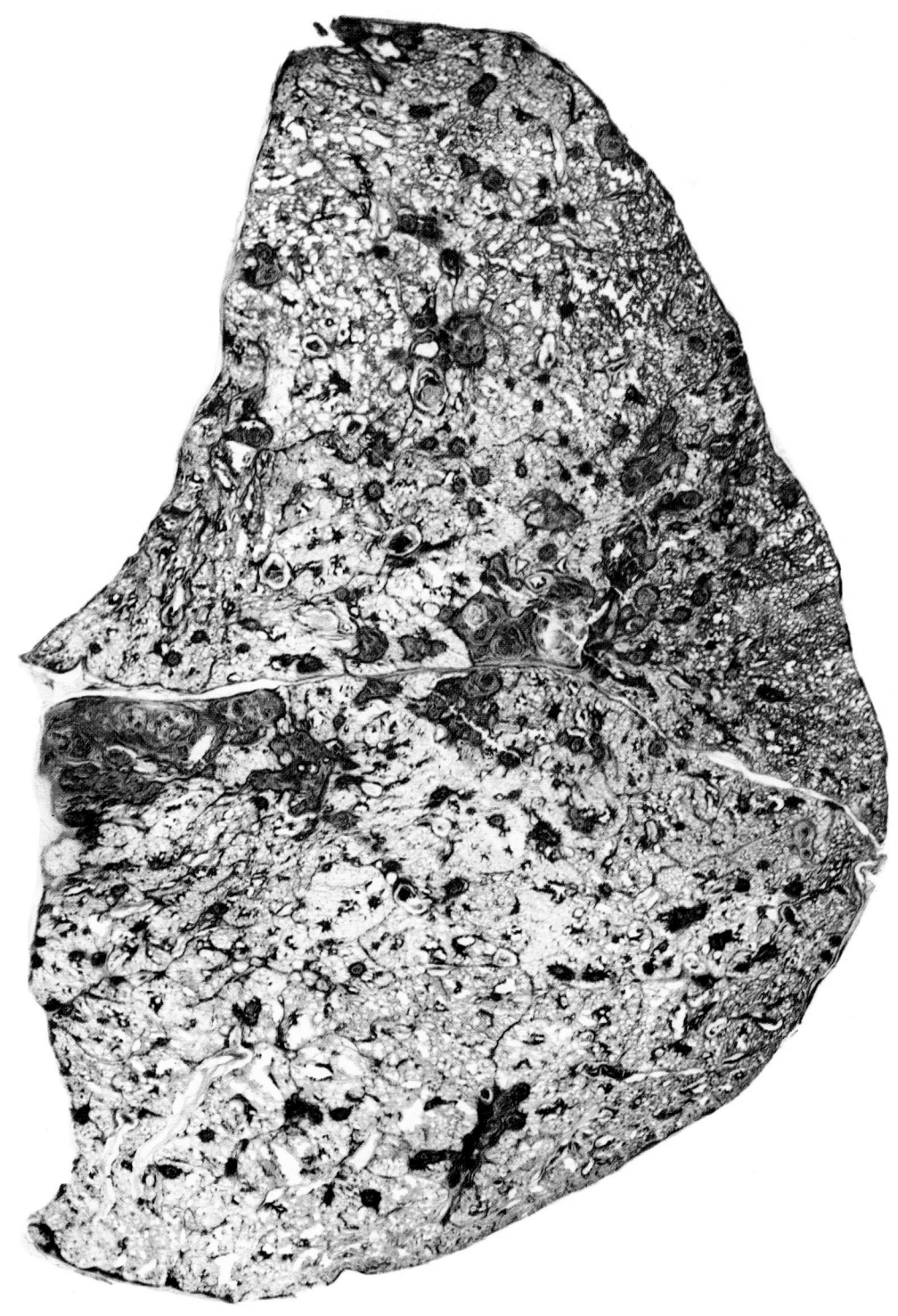

B

FIGURE 64-33 (continued) *B.* Anthracosilicotic nodules, predominantly in vicinity of fissure. Background lung shows centrilobular emphysema.

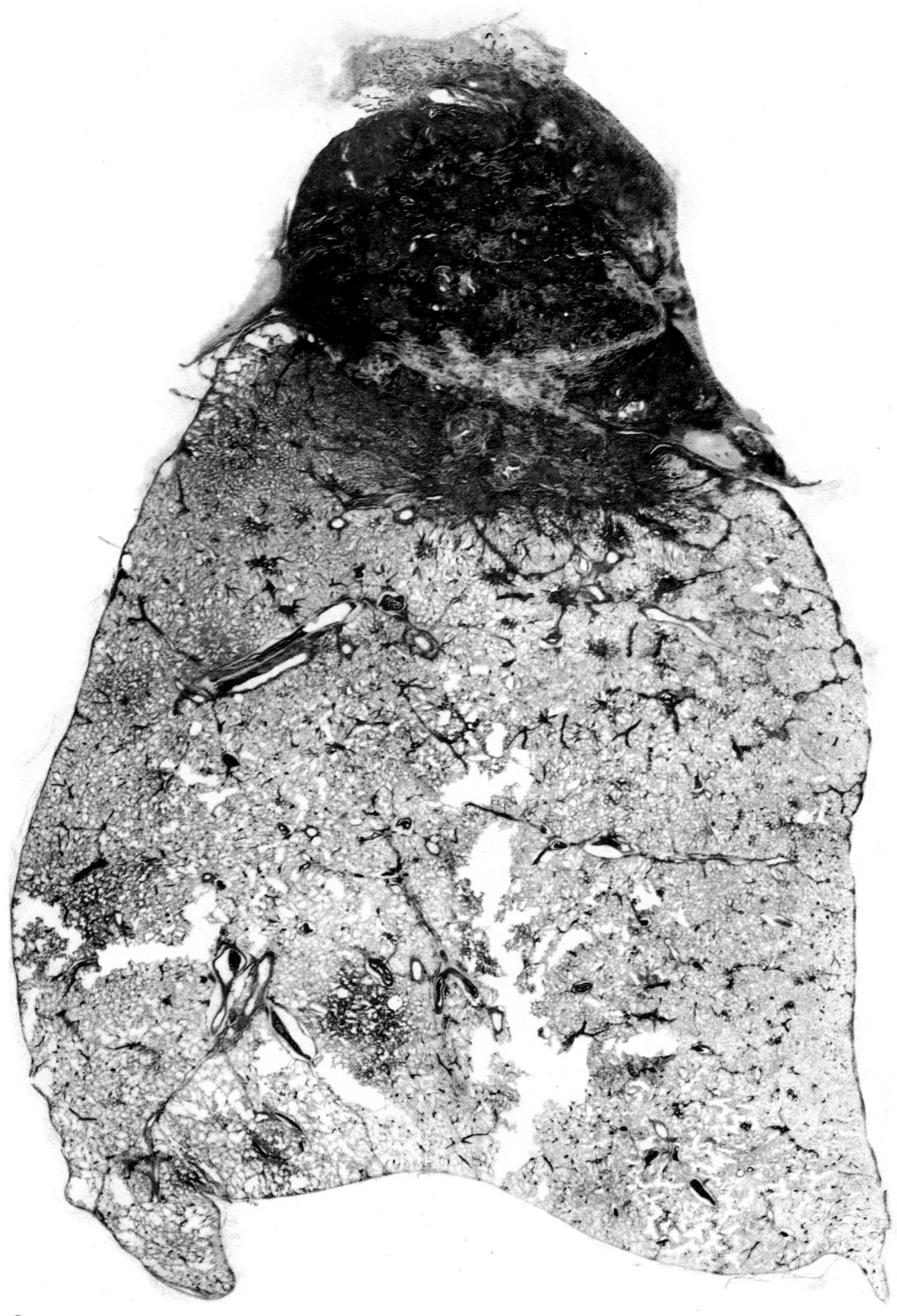

C

FIGURE 64-33 (continued)   *C.* Progressive massive fibrosis. Cor pulmonale is uncommon in *A* unless parenchymal changes are associated with chronic bronchitis (which cannot be seen on these sections). However, cor pulmonale is not uncommon in *B* and *C*, which often derange blood-gas composition severely. *(Courtesy of J. C. Wagner, Cardiff.)*

tingly hypoxic, constantly maintains at least a modest level of pulmonary hypertension that can be markedly exacerbated by an acute respiratory infection (Fig. 64-34).

The origin of the hypoxia in obstructive airways disease is in alveolar ventilation-perfusion abnormalities. These derangements are responsible for the alveolar hypoxia, arterial hypoxemia, and respiratory acidosis that culminate in cor pulmonale.

CLINICAL FEATURES

In chronic bronchitis and emphysema, cor pulmonale and right ventricular failure are encountered in three different settings: in the pink puffer during an acute respiratory infection; in the blue bloater who is chronically refractory to all cardiotonic and pulmonary measures; and in the blue bloater during an acute respiratory infection. Not infrequently, in all three categories a bout of florid right ventricular failure is triggered by an acute respiratory infection. But, during respiratory failure, the level of pulmonary hypertension is rarely as high in the pink puffer as in the blue bloater; the lower level in the pink puffer stems from the long intervals of normal arterial blood-gas levels between respiratory infections which prevent muscular hypertrophy of the resistance vessels of the lung.

During the bout of respiratory failure, the clinical pictures of the pink puffer and the blue bloater are often indistinguishable. However, as the infection subsides, it usually becomes clear whether a patient is predominantly emphysematous or bronchitic (Fig. 64-35).

Hyperinflation of the lungs in patients with chronic cor pulmonale secondary to chronic bronchitis and emphysema often obscures enlargement of the right ventricle. Nonetheless, many characteristic features of right ventricular enlargement can be uncovered if looked for carefully: a rhythmic lift of the sternum with each heartbeat; remote but accentuated pulmonary component of the second heart sound; cardiac pulsations in the epigastrium. Right ventricular failure often occurs in a setting of striking cyanosis, unexplained drowsiness or inappropriate behavior, distended neck veins, warm hands, suffused conjunctivas, hepatomegaly, and edema of the extremities. The gallops (S_3 and S_4) of right ventricular failure are generally present, and the murmur of tricuspid insufficiency can usually be elicited if the patient's sensorium is not too blunted to respond to the command "Take a deep breath." Not only is the liver generally displaced downward by the low diaphragm, it is also enlarged and tender to gentle pressure over the right upper part of the abdomen. Once suspicion is raised that ventilation-perfusion abnormalities are the cause of the clinical picture, an arterial blood sample will confirm that the P_{O_2} is low ($P_{O_2} <$ 40 to 50 mmHg), the P_{CO_2} is high ($P_{CO_2} >$ 50 mmHg), and respiratory acidosis is present. These blood-gas values are

rare in left ventricular disorders unless the patient is in frank pulmonary edema.

Radiography is of greater value in suggesting or in confirming enlargement of the right ventricle in a patient with chronic bronchitis and emphysema than in proving it. The chest radiograph depends on the state of the underlying pulmonary disorder and on the degree of pulmonary hypertension and right ventricular failure. Most characteristic is the combination of "dirty lungs," prominent pulmonary arterial trunks at the hili, and a pruned peripheral arterial tree. Serial radiographs are generally more useful in detecting cardiomegaly than is a single examination (Fig. 64-36).

Electrocardiographic evidence of right ventricular enlargement is often blurred in patients with bronchitis and emphysema because of rotation and displacement of the heart, widened distances between electrodes and the cardiac surface, and the predominance of dilatation over hypertrophy in the cardiac enlargement. P pulmonale is more a reflection of the effects of hypertension on the right ventricle. If a distinctive pattern of right ventricular enlargement does occur, the degree of cardiomegaly must be severe. Because of these limitations, it is not surprising that the standard criteria for right ventricular enlargement have been satisfied in only one-third of patients with chronic bronchitis and emphysema who have been shown to have right ventricular hypertrophy at autopsy.

The electrocardiographic criteria for right ventricular enlargement in patients with obstructive disease of the airways are summarized elsewhere in this book (Chapter 34). One of the more reliable indexes of right ventricular enlargement in these patients had proved to be variability of successive electrocardiograms that accompanies changing degrees of arterial hypoxemia. As the arterial P_{O_2} drops to distinctly subnormal levels (e.g., below 60 to 70 mmHg while awake), T waves tend to become inverted, biphasic, or flat in the right precordial leads (V_1 to V_3), the mean electrical axis of the QRS shifts 30° or more to the right of the patient's usual axis, ST segments become depressed in leads II, III, and aVF, and right bundle branch block (incomplete or complete) often appears. These changes tend to reverse as arterial oxygenation improves.

TREATMENT

In the patient with obstructive airways disease, as in the patient with "general alveolar hypoventilation" (despite normal lungs), the center of attention is the blood gases: relief of arterial hypoxemia and hypercapnia (acidosis) relieves the pulmonary hypertension.

Except for the use of pulmonary vasodilators, the treatment of pulmonary hypertension is an automatic byproduct of managing the obstructive airways disease: antibiotics to clear an acute upper respiratory infection, bronchodilators (notably, but not exclusively, theophyl-

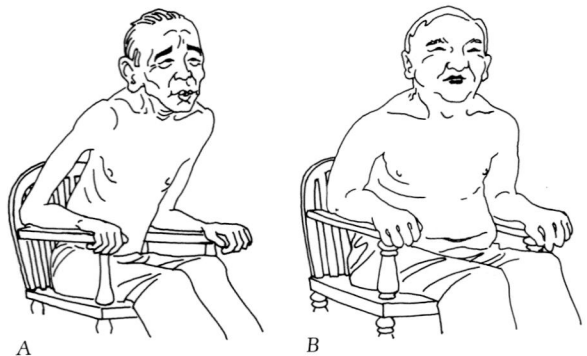

FIGURE 64-34 The pink puffer and the blue bloater. Physical features. The pink puffer (left) is dyspneic and expires through pursed lips using the accessory muscles of respiration. The blue bloater (right) is cyanotic and is not working as hard at breathing as the pink puffer.

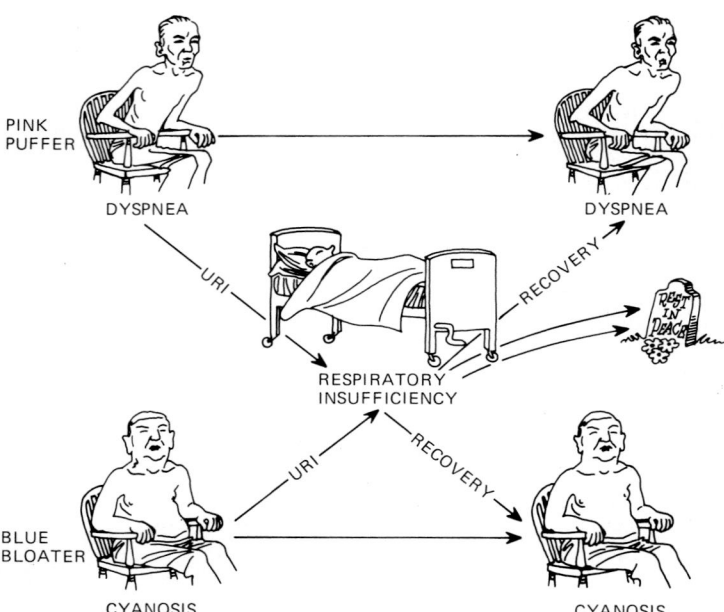

FIGURE 64-35 The pink puffer and the blue bloater. Natural histories. The pink puffer leads a breathless existence which is interrupted by bouts of acute respiratory insufficiency (center) from which he or she may recover completely (upper right) or go on to a stage of persistent cyanosis and respiratory acidosis (lower right). In contrast, the blue bloater generally leads a briefer existence, with more frequent bouts of acute respiratory insufficiency, from which he or she is less apt to recover completely. During the stage of acute respiratory insufficiency, the pink puffer and blue bloater are usually indistinguishable.

line, which not only relaxes muscle tone in the airways but also enhances cardiac and diaphragmatic contractility, increases mucociliary clearance, and exerts a diuretic effect), and supplemental oxygen as necessary. The advent of right ventricular failure calls for a cardiotonic regimen that may include digitalis, diuretics, and supplemen-

tal oxygen (see "Cor Pulmonale: General Features, Treatment," above).

On the grounds that vasoconstriction, presumably other than that evoked by hypoxia and acidosis, is also operative in obstructive airways disease—an unproven assumption—pulmonary vasodilators have been tried as therapeutic agents. As yet, no particular role for them has been identified. Moreover, their use entails certain risks: (1) individual responses to vasodilators are highly variable and unpredictable; (2) in chronic airways obstruction, vasodilators can worsen gas exchange, thereby intensifying arterial hypoxemia; (3) no prolonged beneficial effect has yet been shown on survival; and (4) preoccupation with vasodilators is, in obstructive airways disease, apt to distract from time-honored and proven measures, directed at the underlying pulmonary disease.

PULMONARY VENOUS HYPERTENSION

Pulmonary venous hypertension, especially if severe and protracted, as in chronic mitral valvular disease, left ventricular failure, or mediastinal fibrosis, inevitably elicits pulmonary arterial hypertension. The increment in arterial pressure is not simply passive, i.e., a consequence of back pressure, since it is disproportionately high, suggesting either sustained reflex pulmonary precapillary vasoconstriction or anatomic changes in the precapillary vessels, or both, i.e., possibly reflex at the outset and then anatomic as the pulmonary arterial hypertension continues. That much of the arterial hypertension is anatomic is indicated by the frequent concurrence of medial hypertrophy and fibrosis of the pulmonary muscular arteries on the one hand and of intimal fibrosis on the other. At the same time, the small pulmonary veins become arterialized, including an increase in thickness of the media often in conjunction with intimal fibrosis. The "pulmonocardiac" disorders, i.e., lung disease consequent to cardiac disease, are considered in Chapter 68. Here only one disease affecting predominantly the pulmonary veins is considered.

Pulmonary Veno-occlusive Disease

This is a rare disease, a little more than 100 patients having been reported to date. It affects children and adults, the age range varying from 11 days to 76 years; males are affected somewhat more than females. Most reported cases have been diagnosed at autopsy. The etiology of this disorder is unknown. Indeed, as in the case of primary pulmonary hypertension, the possibility of diverse etiologies is strong.

The pathology is also variable. Although, as a rule, pulmonary veins and venules are predominantly affected, and are partially to fully obstructed by intimal fibrosis,

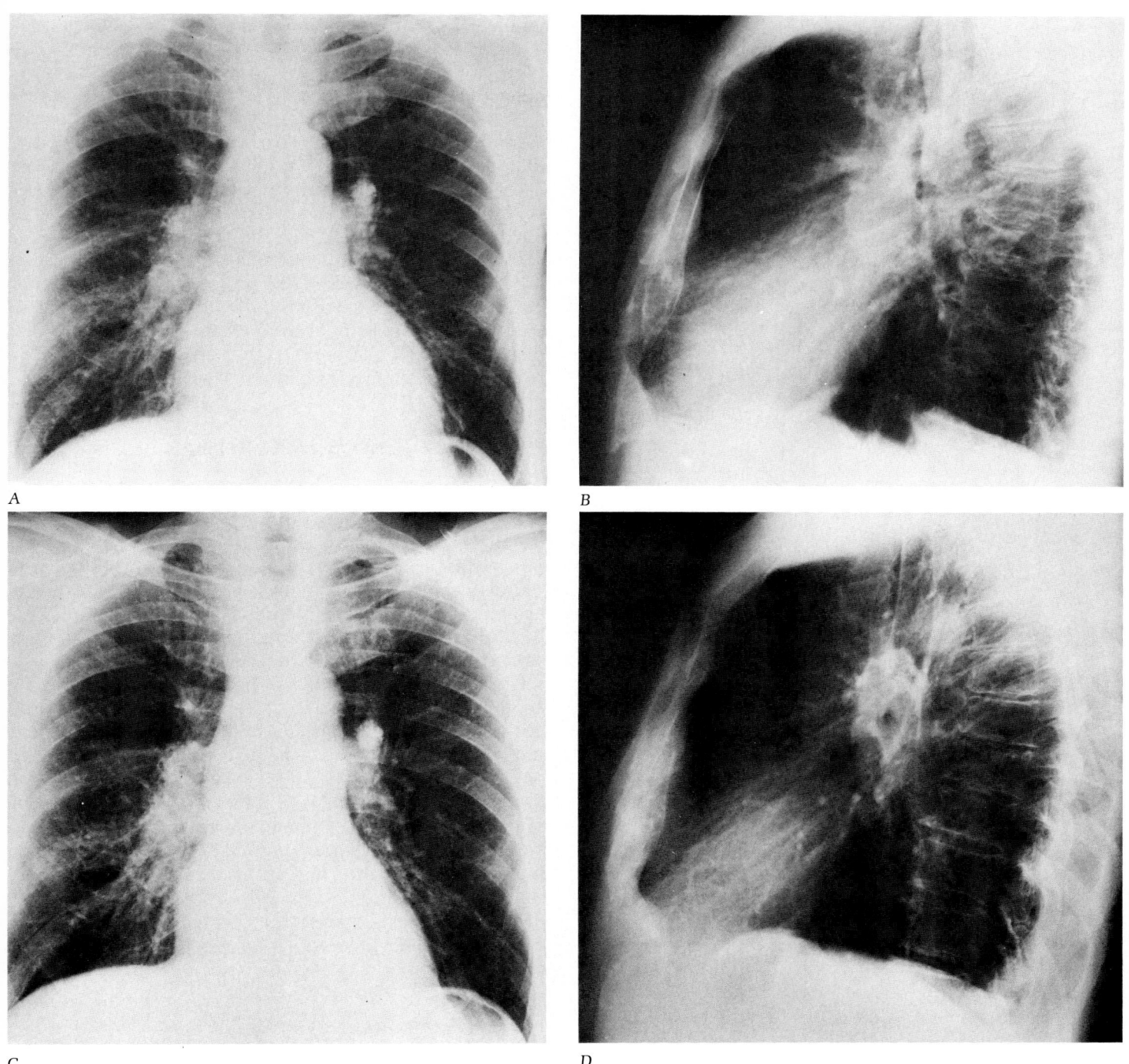

A

B

C

D

FIGURE 64-36 Chronic bronchitis and emphysema. *A* and *B*. Posteroanterior and lateral views during episode of right ventricular failure. *C* and *D*. Posteroanterior and lateral views 3 weeks later, after recovery.

sometimes the precapillary vessels show the same lesions, whereas the intervening capillary bed, with its huge endothelial surface, is spared. Although in situ thrombosis has been suggested as the initiating mechanism of the disorder in the venules, this mechanism is still speculative.

CLINICAL FEATURES

The clinical picture is variable, and the symptoms are usually the same as those of primary (arterial) pulmonary hypertension. But, there is no support for the diagnosis of primary (arterial) pulmonary hypertension from either: (1) the chest radiography (Fig. 64-37), which fails to reveal striking disproportion between the central pulmonary arteries and peripheral pruning of the pulmonary vasculature and is apt to show evidences of chronic pulmonary congestion and edema, or (2) the electrocardiogram, which fails to show convincing evidence of right ventricular overload. Nor is the pulmonary arterial wedge pressure helpful since it is usually normal (in conjunction with pulmonary arterial hypertension), apparently reflecting either pressures in communicating veins in which flow has been arrested or left atrial pressure, or artifacts. The difficulty in interpreting measurements of pulmonary arterial wedge pressure from a single site underscores the need for measurements made in different wedge (or occlusive balloon) positions once the diagnosis of pulmonary veno-occlusive disease is raised. In addition to primary (arterial) pulmonary hypertension, evaluation usually centers around eliminating mitral valvular disease, con-

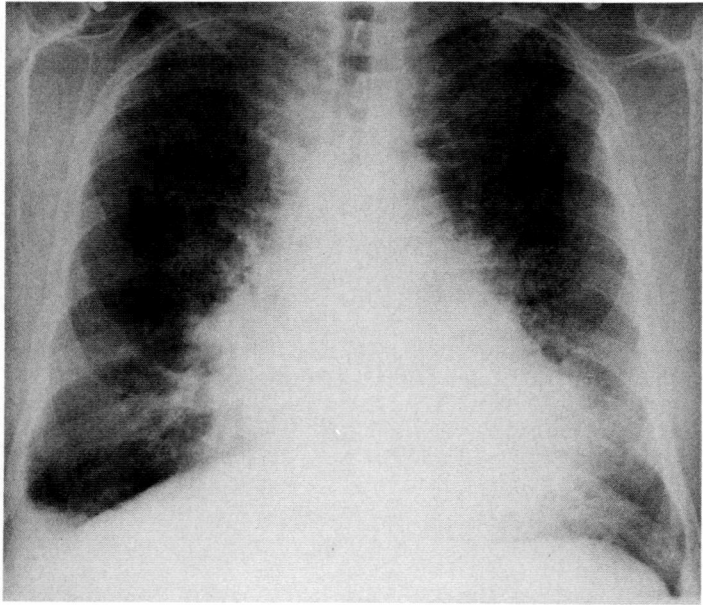

FIGURE 64-37 Pulmonary veno-occlusive disease. Posteroanterior chest radiograph demonstrates pulmonary venous engorgement and edema. Diagnosis established by cardiac catheterization, angiography, and lung biopsy.

genital heart disease, and pulmonary thromboembolic disease.

TREATMENT

Depending on beliefs concerning etiology and pathogenesis, patients have been treated with anticoagulants, platelet-inhibiting agents, or immunosuppressive therapy. An occasional patient has improved while receiving a pulmonary vasodilator, e.g., continued prazosin or hydralazine and isosorbide dinitrate, after showing acute hemodynamic improvement in response to the intravenous infusion of nitroprusside and antiplatelet agents (aspirin and dipyridamole). Unfortunately, experience with treatment is still too limited for meaningful generalizations.

PULMONARY ARTERIOVENOUS FISTULA

Aside from its intrinsic interest as a congenital anomaly, this disorder stands in marked contrast to pulmonary hypertension since the arteriovenous fistulas in the lungs constitute a runoff to prevent appreciable increments in pulmonary arterial pressure.

Pulmonary arteriovenous fistulas are abnormal communications between the pulmonary arteries and the pulmonary veins; the capillary network that normally separates arteries from veins is absent. Two types of pulmonary arteriovenous fistulas occur: (1) congenital, which include those associated with hereditary hemorrhagic telangiectasia (Osler-Rendu-Weber), and (2) those acquired from (a) trauma, (b) schistosomiasis, (c) longstanding hepatic cirrhosis, and (d) carcinoma.

The anomaly is uncommon. Among families with hereditary hemorrhagic telangiectasia, only 15 percent of affected family members have pulmonary arteriovenous fistulas, although about 50 percent of patients with pulmonary arteriovenous fistulas have evidence of other mucocutaneous telangiectases or a family history of hereditary hemorrhagic telangiectasia.

Pulmonary arteriovenous fistulas are local lesions that do not disturb the adjacent pulmonary tissue, i.e., there is no associated atelectasis, bronchiectasis, or pneumonia. Generally, the pulmonary artery supplies all the afferent blood, although, occasionally, when in association with hereditary hemorrhagic telangiectasia, some of the afferent supply may be from a bronchial artery or from other systemic arteries. The lesions are multiple in one-third of the cases and are most frequently found in the lower lobes adjacent to the visceral pleura, although they can also be deep in the parenchyma.

Grossly, the lesions appear as thin-walled aneurysmal sacs connecting the artery and the vein. Thrombotic masses may be present within the aneurysmal sac. Micro-

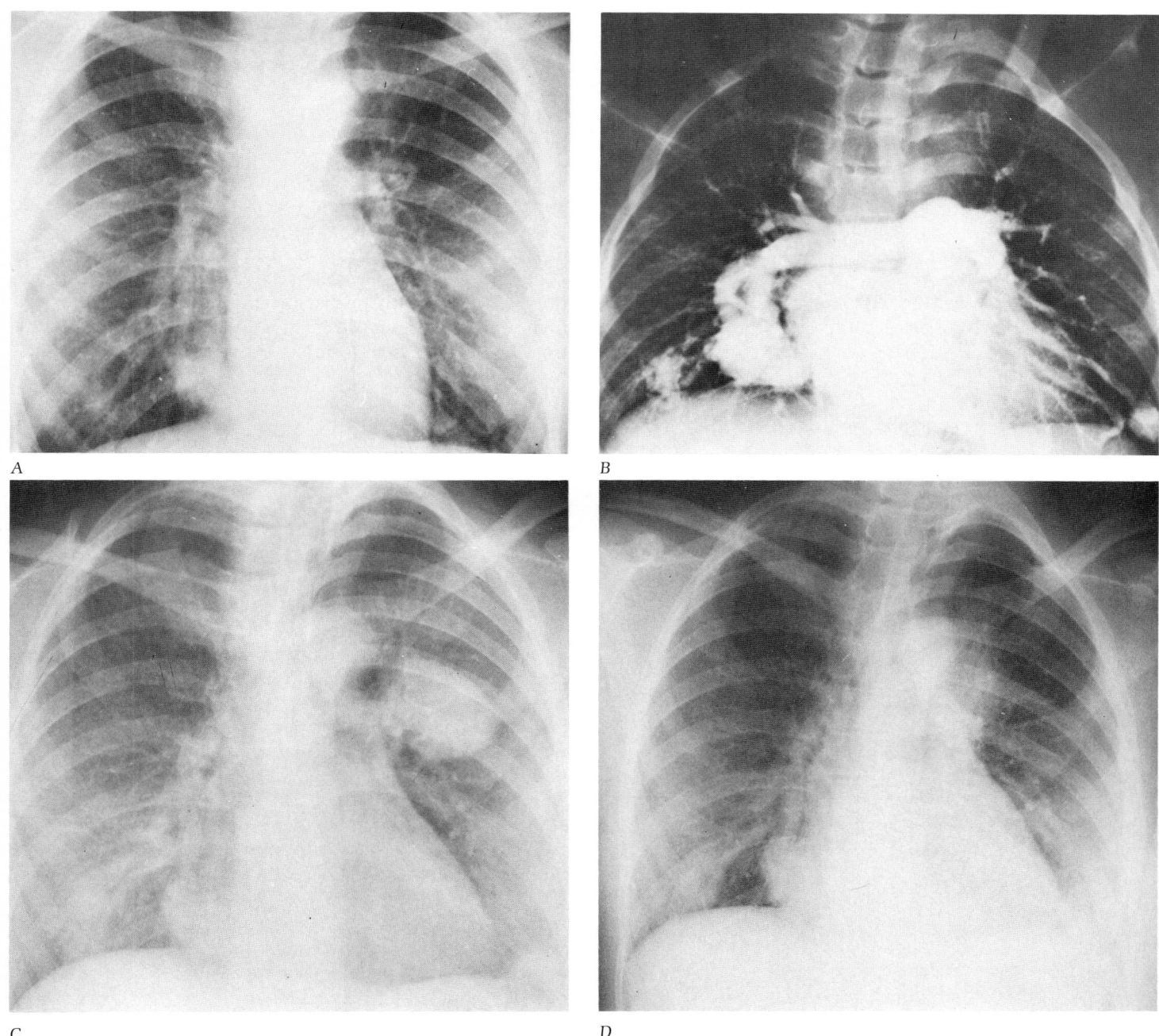

A

B

C

D

FIGURE 64-38 Pulmonary arteriovenous fistulas in a 24-year-old pregnant woman with hereditary hemorrhagic telangiectasia. *A.* Before pregnancy. Small, nodular densities are seen at both bases and in the left hilus. The shunt was estimated to be 49 percent of the cardiac output. *B.* Arteriogram before pregnancy demonstrating arteriovenous fistulas of both lower lobes. *C.* Seven months pregnant, admitted to the hospital with hemoptysis and left hemothorax. The enlargement of the arteriovenous fistulas is striking. The pregnancy was terminated. *D.* Two weeks after termination of pregnancy. The nodular densities have decreased in size. *(From Rossman, 1980.)*

scopically, the sac walls contain various amounts of muscle, fibrous tissues, and occasionally small amounts of calcium.

The pulmonary arteriovenous fistulas act as bypass routes allowing mixed venous blood to escape arterialization in the lungs. Despite the hypoxic stimulus, pulmonary hypertension has not occurred; however, the chronic arterial hypoxemia does evoke erythrocytosis and polycythemia.

Clinical Manifestations

Most patients with pulmonary arteriovenous fistulas are asymptomatic and come to medical attention because of an abnormality found on routine radiography. About half

of the patients complain of dyspnea. Epistaxis is present in 50 percent of patients, usually in association with hereditary hemorrhagic telangiectasia. These patients may also have gastrointestinal bleeding, strokes, brain abscesses, or seizures. Most patients are diagnosed in the third or fourth decade of life.

On physical examination, the patients with dyspnea usually are cyanotic and clubbed. One-third of all patients will have mucocutaneous telangiectases. A characteristic feature of pulmonary arteriovenous fistula is an extracardiac murmur or bruit. Because pulmonary blood flow increases during inspiration, the intensity of the murmur also increases during inspiration and decreases during expiration. Similarly, the Valsalva maneuver, by transiently decreasing pulmonary blood flow, decreases flow through the fistula and decreases, or eliminates, the murmur. As expected, the Müller maneuver (forced inspiration with a closed glottis after full expiration) does the opposite, i.e., increases the murmur. Occasionally, for unexplained reasons, the murmur may be atypical and either increase with expiration or be heard only during diastole.

The most important laboratory examination is chest radiography. A solitary fistula takes the form of a coin lesion, or a bunch of grapes, in the peripheral lung fields (Fig. 64-38). Less than 5 percent of pulmonary arteriovenous fistulas contain calcium demonstrable by radiography. Usually, feeding and draining vessels connect the lesion to the hilus. Tomography is useful in demonstrating the continuity of the hilar vessels and the fistula. Fluoroscopy usually demonstrates the pulsating nature of the mass. Angiography is not usually needed to make the diagnosis but can be used to demonstrate the vascular nature of the lesion and to determine the exact number of fistulas present. Patients with a significant shunt will have a secondary polycythemia, although, if there has been significant bleeding, some patients may actually be anemic. The arterial P_{O_2} is invariably decreased and does not increase appreciably with 100% O_2.

Local complications of the pulmonary arteriovenous fistulas are due to rupture of the aneurysmal sacs with bleeding either into the bronchi causing hemoptysis or into the pleura where it produces a hemothorax. Thrombosis within the pulmonary arteriovenous fistula is common and is occasionally the cause of bland and septic emboli to the central nervous system. Strokes and seizures may result from telangiectases in the central nervous system.

Differential Diagnosis

The radiographic shadows may simulate bronchiectasis, tuberculosis or other granulomatous disease, solitary pulmonary nodules, or metastatic carcinoma. The murmur or bruit must be differentiated from valvular or congenital heart disease. The cause of the cyanosis may erroneously be attributed to congenital heart disease. The normal white blood count, platelets, and spleen help to identify the polycythemia as secondary to hypoxia and not to polycythemia vera.

Treatment

The only available treatment for pulmonary arteriovenous fistulas is excision. Because of the vascular nature of the lesion, wedge resection and lobectomy have been the procedures of choice. Since adjacent lung parenchyma is normal, an attempt is made to preserve as much lung as possible. However, because as many as one-third of the patients have multiple fistulas, recurrence is possible after surgery. Therefore, in all patients with cyanosis and polycythemia, hemoptysis, or rapidly increasing lesions for whom surgery is considered, preoperative pulmonary arteriogram is necessary so that all the fistulas can be identified. Generally, all symptoms due to the pulmonary arteriovenous fistulas are reversed if surgery is successful.

Prognosis

Because the anomaly is uncommon, the natural history is not well understood. Whereas some pulmonary lesions enlarge rapidly, others remain stable or enlarge slightly over a period of years. Serious complications are just as likely to be pulmonary (hemoptysis or hemothorax in about 10 percent) as neurologic (about 10 percent).

BIBLIOGRAPHY

Bergofsky EH, Turino GM, Fishman AP: Cardiorespiratory failure in kyphoscoliosis. Medicine 38:263–317, 1959.
  Classic description. The pathogenesis of hypercapnic respiratory failure in disorders of the chest wall is outlined.

Bjornsson J, Edwards WD: Primary pulmonary hypertension: A histopathologic study of 80 cases. Mayo Clin Proc 60:16–25, 1985.
  Describes the histologic features that seem to form the morphologic substrate for the increase in pulmonary vascular resistance that characterizes primary pulmonary hypertension.

Chitwood WR, Sabiston DC, Wechsler AS: Surgical treatment of unresolved pulmonary embolism. Clin Chest Med 5:507–536, 1984.
> *A review, in historical perspective, of the current use of surgical embolectomy in treating certain patients with long-standing embolic occlusions of major pulmonary arteries.*

Dauber JH: Silicosis, in Fishman AP (ed), *Update: Pulmonary Diseases and Disorders.*, New York, McGraw-Hill, 1982, pp 149–166.
> *A comprehensive review of the manifestations and management of acute and chronic silicosis.*

Edwards WD: Pathology of pulmonary hypertension. Cardiovasc Clin 18:321–359, 1988.
> *A comprehensive review of the various morphologic changes in different types of pulmonary hypertension.*

Enson Y, Thomas HM III, Bosken CH, Wood JA, Leroy EC, Blanc WA, Wigger HJ, Harvey RM, Cournand A: Pulmonary hypertension in interstitial lung disease. Trans Assoc Am Physicians 88:248–255, 1975.
> *Description of hemodynamics in diffuse interstitial lung diseases of miscellaneous etiologies based on extensive personal experience.*

Fishman AP: Dynamics of the pulmonary circulation, in Hamilton WF, Dow P (eds), *Handbook of Physiology, sect 2: Circulation vol II.* Washington, DC, American Physiological Society, 1963, pp 1667–1743.
> *A comprehensive overview of the normal pulmonary circulation as a background for analyzing mechanics that lead to pulmonary hypertension.*

Fishman AP: Dietary pulmonary hypertension. Circ Res 35:657–660, 1974.
> *The implications are discussed of the experimental experiences using Crotalaria to generate pulmonary hypertension and of the epidemic of aminorex pulmonary hypertension in humans.*

Fishman AP: Pulmonary thromboembolism: Pathophysiology and clinical features, in Fishman AP (ed), *Pulmonary Diseases and Disorders.* New York, McGraw-Hill, 1980, pp 809–926.
> *A succinct account of pulmonary thromboembolic disease that calls special attention to the category of multiple pulmonary emboli.*

Fishman AP: Pulmonary circulation, in Fishman AP, Fisher A (eds), *The Handbook of Physiology, sect 3: The Respiratory System, vol I: Circulation and Nonrespiratory Functions.* Bethesda, American Physiological Society, 1985, pp 93–165.
> *A comprehensive survey of the regulation of the pulmonary circulation, particularly useful as a background for considering pathogenesis of clinical pulmonary hypertension. Emphasis is placed on the concept of pulmonary vascular resistance, the interpretation of pulmonary wedge pressures, and the identification of pulmonary vasomotor activity.*

Fishman AP, Pietra GG: Primary pulmonary hypertension. Annu Rev Med 31:421–431, 1980.
> *A review of current understanding of primary pulmonary hypertension with special emphasis on etiology. Comprehensive bibliography.*

Groves BM, Rubin LJ, Frosolono MF, Cato AE, Reeves JT: A comparison of the acute hemodynamic effects of prostacyclin and hydralazine in primary pulmonary hypertension. Am Heart J 110:1200–1204, 1985.
> *Interest in this comparison for those using pulmonary vasodilator agents lies in the hypothesis that hydralazine, which can be taken orally, exerts its effects by way of prostacyclin, for which no oral form is yet available.*

Higenbottam T, Wheeldon D, Wells F, Wallwork J: Long-term treatment of primary pulmonary hypertension with continuous intravenous epoprostenal (prostacyclin). Lancet 1:1046–1047, 1984.
> *This paper describes the first of now seven patients, unmanageable by oral vasodilators, who were treated by continuous infusion of prostacyclin for months up to 2 years. After 1 year of continuous, self-administration of prostacyclin intravenously, the patient remained greatly improved.*

Hughes JD, Rubin LJ: Primary pulmonary hypertension. An analysis of 28 cases and a review of the literature. Medicine (Baltimore) 65:56–72, 1986.
> *A review of primary pulmonary hypertension, including course, prognosis, and response to therapy.*

Hurtado A: Chronic mountain sickness. JAMA 120:1278–1282, 1942.
> *Eight cases of Monge's disease are described with special emphasis on hematologic abnormalities.*

Jones DK, Higenbottam TW, Wallwork J: Treatment of primary pulmonary hypertension intravenous epoprostenol (prostacyclin). Br Heart J 57:270–278, 1987.
> *Ten patients with severe primary pulmonary hypertension and pronounced disability who were unresponsive to oral vasodilators were treated with intravenous epoprostenol (prostacyclin). Continued intravenous infusion of epoprostenol for 1–25 months was associated with subjective and clinical improvement.*

Kilbourne EM, Rigau-Perez JG, Heath CW Jr, Zack MM, Falk H, Martin-Marcos M, de Carlos A: Clinical epidemiology of toxic-oil syndrome. Manifestations of a new illness. N Engl J Med 309:1408–1414, 1983.
> *An epidemiologic investigation linked the occurrence of illness with the ingestion of an unlabeled, illegally marketed cooking oil.*

Long WA, Rubin LJ: Prostacyclin and PGE_1 treatment of pulmonary hypertension. Am Rev Respir Dis 136:773–776, 1987.
> *Prostacyclin and PGE_1 show promise in treatment of many forms of pulmonary hypertension. Although prostacyclin holds greater promise of therapeutic efficacy, it is still an investigational drug for pulmonary hypertension.*

Mathur PN, Powles ACP, Pugsley SO, McEwan MP, Campbell EJM: Effect of digoxin on right ventricular function in severe chronic airflow obstruction. Ann Intern Med 95:283–288, 1981.
> *In 15 patients with cor pulmonale due to severe chronic obstructive airways disease, equilibrium radionuclide angiography showed that after 8 weeks of digoxin, the right ventricular ejection fraction increased only in those in whom both the left and right ejection fractions were initially abnormal.*

Mecham RP, Whitehouse LA, Wrenn DS, Parks WC, Griffin GL, Senior RM, Crouch EC, Stenmark KR, Voelkel NF: Smooth muscle-mediated connective tissue remodeling in pulmonary hypertension. Science 237:423–426, 1987.
> *Smooth-muscle cells in the pulmonary artery play a critical role in evoking the vascular changes of pulmonary hypertension by modifying the phenotype of surrounding cells in the vessel wall.*

Melot C, Hallemans R, Naeije R, Mols P, Lejeune P: Deleterious effects of nifedipine on pulmonary gas exchange in chronic obstructive pulmonary disease. Am Rev Respir Dis 130:612–616, 1984.
> *The immediately preceding paper by Keller et al. in the same issue of the journal, pp 606–611, deals with hydralazine in a similar population.*

Monge MC: Life in the Andes and chronic mountain sickness. Science 95:79–84, 1942.
> *Classic paper discussing chronic mountain sickness in residents of the Andes.*

Moser KM, Spragg KG, Utley J, Daily PO: Chronic thrombotic obstruction of major pulmonary arteries. Ann Intern Med 99:299–305, 1983.
> *Fifteen patients with chronic pulmonary thromboembolism and pulmonary hypertension are reported. Endarterectomy and surgical removal of thrombi produced marked symptom reversal.*

Olson JW, Hacker AD, Altiere RJ, Gillespie MN: Polyamines and the development of monocrotaline-induced pulmonary hypertension. Am J Physiol 247:H682–H685, 1984.
> *Provocative article that explores the role of polyamines as the biochemical link between pulmonary hypertension and thickening of the media in pulmonary hypertension.*

Packer M: Vasodilator therapy for primary pulmonary hypertension. Ann Intern Med 103:258–270, 1985.
> *A comprehensive review of limitations and hazards of this form of therapy.*

Rich S, Brundage BH: High-dose calcium channel-blocking therapy for primary pulmonary hypertension: evidence for long-term reduction in pulmonary arterial pressure and regression of right ventricular hypertrophy. Circulation 76:135–141, 1987.
> *Substantial reductions in pulmonary arterial pressure and pulmonary vascular resistance that are associated with regression of right ventricular hypertrophy are possible in some patients with primary pulmonary hypertension by use of calcium channel-blocking drugs in high doses.*

Rich S, Dantzker DR, Ayres SM, Bergofsky EH, Brundage BH, Detre KM, Fishman AP, Goldring RM, Groves BM, Koerner SK et al: Primary pulmonary hypertension. A national prospective study. Ann Intern Med 107:216–223, 1987.
> *Initial report from the National Registry for Primary Pulmonary Hypertension describing the uniform population of 187 patients entered between 1981–1987.*

Rich S, Kieras K, Hart K, Groves BM, Stobo JD, Brundage BH: Antinuclear antibodies in primary pulmonary hypertension. J Am Coll Cardiol 8:1307–1311, 1986.
> *In patients with primary pulmonary hypertension, 40 percent had positive antinuclear antibodies at titers of 1:80 dilutions or greater.*

Saadjian A, Philip-Joet F, Arnaud A: Hemodynamic and oxygen delivery responses to nifedipine in pulmonary hypertension secondary to chronic obstructive lung disease. Cardiology 74:196–204, 1987.
> *In 24 patients with pulmonary hypertension secondary to severe chronic obstructive lung disease, nifedipine (20 mg sublingually) caused significant improvement in pulmonary hypertension, right ventricular pump function, and increased oxygen delivery to the tissues. In 10 patients, improvement was still apparent after continued oral intake (30 mg/day) for 15 days.*

Salerni R, Rodnan GP, Leon DF, Shaver JA: Pulmonary hypertension in the CREST syndrome variant of progressive systemic sclerosis (scleroderma). Ann Intern Med 86:394–399, 1977.
> *Severe pulmonary hypertension with little or no pulmonary fibrosis is reported in 10 patients with CREST, previously believed to be a benign variant of scleroderma. Intimal fibrosis and myxomatous changes in pulmonary vessels account for pulmonary hypertension.*

Schrijen F, Uffholtz H, Polu JM, Poincelot F: Pulmonary and systemic hemodynamic evolution in chronic bronchitis. Am Rev Respir Dis 117:25–31, 1978.
> *Long-term follow-up of patients with chronic airways obstruction showing the relationship of the blue bloater type to the development of pulmonary hypertension.*

Shuck JW, Oetgen WJ, Tesar JT: Pulmonary vascular response during Raynaud's phenomenon in progressive systemic sclerosis. Am J Med 78:221–227, 1985.
> *In four pulmonary normotensive patients with diffuse interstitial fibrosis and in four with the CREST syndrome, Raynaud's phenomenon could not be elicited by immersing a hand in cold water.*

Terry P: Pulmonary arteriovenous malformation. N Engl J Med 308:1197–1200, 1983.
> *In 10 patients with pulmonary arteriovenous malformations, arterial blood gases, pulmonary function, and pulmonary hemodynamics were determined. Arterial hypoxemia was associated with chronic hyperventilation. Balloon embolization of the malformations was followed by increases in arterial P_{O_2} (from 43 to 64 mmHg).*

Theodore J, Jamieson SW, Burke CM, Reitz BA, Stinson EB, van Kessel A, Dawkins KD, Herran, JJ, Oyer PE, Hunt SA, Shumway NE, Robin ED: Physiologic aspects of human heart-lung transplantation. Chest 86:349–357, 1984.
> *Follow-up studies (up to 27 months) are reported in the first nine survivors who had undergone heart-lung transplantation at Stanford University Medical Center. The transplanted lungs function well in gas exchange soon after transplant and remain normal months after surgery.*

Timms RM, Khaja FU, Williams GW: The nocturnal oxygen therapy trial. Hemodynamic response to oxygen therapy in chronic obstructive pulmonary disease. Ann Intern Med 102:29–36, 1985.
> *A multicenter trial of both 12-h and continuous oxygen therapy on pulmonary hemodynamics in 203 patients with obstructive airways disease and hypoxemia. Continuous prolonged oxygen therapy did improve the hemodynamic abnormalities in some patients, and the hemodynamic response was predictive of survival.*

Trell E: Benign, idiopathic pulmonary hypertension. Acta Med Scand 193:137–143, 1973.
> *Two cases of unusually long duration of idiopathic pulmonary hypertension (about 27 and 40 years, respectively) are presented and discussed with respect to others reported in the literature. No autopsy or biopsy findings.*

Tuxen DV, Powles AC, Mathur PN, Pugsley SO, Campbell EJM: Detrimental effects of hydralazine in patients with chronic airflow obstruction and pulmonary hypertension. Am Rev Respir Dis 129:388–395, 1984.
> *Pulmonary vasodilators can worsen ventilation-perfusion mismatch and aggravate hypoxemia.*

Voelkel N, Reeves JT: Primary pulmonary hypertension, in Moser KM (ed), *Pulmonary Vascular Diseases*. New York, Dekker, 1979, pp 573–628.
> *Excellent clinical and physiological review of current understanding of primary pulmonary hypertension against a background of an extensive personal experience with both this disorder and the pulmonary hypertension of high altitude.*

Wagenvoort CA, Wagenvoort N: *Pathology of Pulmonary Hypertension*. New York, Wiley, 1977.
> *Splendid morphologic treatise on pulmonary hypertension based on years of collecting pathologic material, careful analysis, and intriguing extrapolations from morbid anatomy to etiology and clinical syndromes.*

Weir EK, Reeves JT: *Pulmonary Hypertension*. New York, Futura, 1984.
> *A collection of papers that summarizes the current understanding of pulmonary hypertension and its various subsets. Considerable emphasis is placed on management.*

Chapter 65

Prophylaxis and Treatment of Thromboembolism Based on Pathophysiology of Clotting Mechanisms

Robert W. Colman / Ronald N. Rubin

PROPHYLAXIS OF VENOUS THROMBOEMBOLISM

The coagulation of blood is a physiological mechanism that evolved to keep the vascular space and volume intact. As in most of the body defense systems, inappropriate or excessive activation can result in a *pathologic* and occlusive thrombus which is capable of causing morbid or even lethal organ damage. The factors which predispose to such pathologic thrombosis include intrinsic abnormalities or deficiencies of the blood itself (*hypercoagulability*) as well as vascular changes which affect the blood secondarily. Although more than a century old, the preconditions of *Virchow's triad* (venous stasis, hypercoagulability of blood, and vessel wall injury) still serve as a scaffolding to support a discussion of the etiologies and modes to prevent thromboembolism.

Endothelial injury is an important component in normal hemostasis. Normally the endothelial cell lining of blood vessels forms a continuous protective barrier between the coagulation protein and platelets in the blood and the subendothelial connective tissue. Exposure of blood to components of the vascular basement membrane results in conversion of the contact phase coagulation proteins from inactive zymogen forms into active protease species which then initiate the activation of the entire coagulation pathway. Further, vessel injury with exposure of the subendothelium also results in platelet adhesion and aggregation. Clearly these mechanisms may be

important life-saving responses in the event of trauma with disruption of vascular integrity. However, more subtle injuries to the endothelial cell lining can also occur in instances such as atherosclerosis, exposure to products of cigarette smoke and toxins, and altered hemodynamic stresses and may result in pathologic coagulation with thrombosis forming *within* the lumen of a blood vessel. Many of the chemical and anticoagulant methods of thromboembolism prophylaxis to be discussed below attempt to do so by rendering the coagulation system and platelets less sensitive to activation by preexisting vascular/endothelial injury or by blocking the consequences of the triggered systems.

The second leg of Virchow's triad involves an increased tendency of the blood itself to coagulate (*hypercoagulability*). As time has passed, this general property has been linked to specific protein or formed element excesses and/or deficiencies in blood which result in alterations of the finely balanced clotting mechanism toward excessive coagulation (Fig. 65-1). Many examples have been well documented and explain the increased association of pathologic thromboembolism with certain conditions and disease states. For example, in pregnancy and birth control pill usage, there is an increase of procoagulant factor levels (factors XII, V, VIII, fibrinogen) and simultaneous diminution of plasma protease inhibitors (antithrombin III, CI esterase inhibitor), which probably results in tipping the balance toward enhanced thrombosis and thromboembolic events seen in these populations.

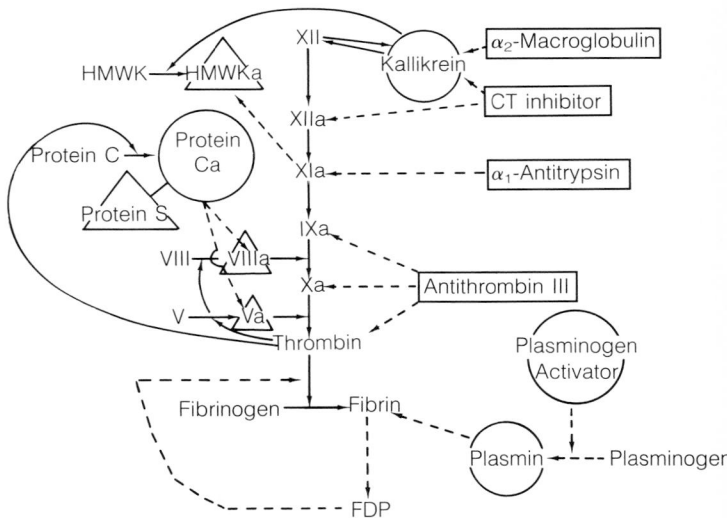

FIGURE 65-1 The control of blood coagulation. Solid arrows indicate activation pathways. An increase in the amount of substrate or in the activity of these pathways promotes blood coagulation and pathologic thrombosis. Dashed arrows indicate inhibitory pathways. A decrease in these substrates or in the activity of these pathways also decreases the inhibition of blood coagulability; hence, the tendency toward blood coagulation and pathologic thrombosis is also increased. □ = plasma protease inhibitors; ○ = fibrinolytic proteins; △ = anticoagulant proteins.

The coagulation system is also excessively activated in certain forms of cancer. Circulating tumor cells and their products have been shown to behave as potent procoagulants which can activate factor X. Thus, there is firm biochemical explanation for the frequent association of thrombosis and hypercoagulability found in such patients. A congenital decrease in fibrinolytic proteins such as plasminogen or anticoagulant proteins C and S may also enhance the tendency toward thrombosis. Excessive platelet sensitivity to agonists such as ADP or epinephrine seem able to tip the hemostatic balance toward excessive thrombosis and cause hypercoagulability. Such "sticky platelets" have been implicated in the excessive thrombotic tendency seen in diabetes, atherosclerosis, and hyperlipoproteinemia. A similar mechanism may also be involved in the thrombotic tendency found in myeloproliferative diseases such as polycythemia vera.

A more firmly established and ever-expanding definition of hypercoagulability has emerged by studying the plasma inhibitors of blood coagulation. This protein system acts as a brake on activated clotting proteins and thus provides localization to the clotting process. In recent years deficiencies in the plasma inhibitor antithrombin III have been elegantly demonstrated and clearly associated with statistically increased numbers of thromboses in affected patients. These entities can occur as familial inherited diseases or as acquired conditions (i.e., nephrotic syndrome with renal loss of antithrombin III).

Again, many of the chemical and anticoagulant means of thrombosis prophylaxis are designed to readjust the balance between hemorrhage versus thrombosis away from excessive clotting. Examples include the use of aspirin as an agent to interfere with normal platelet function, small doses of heparin to inhibit activated factor Xa, and the use of warfarin (Coumadin) to lower the levels of circulating functional factors II, VII, IX and X.

Finally, low blood flow or stasis is the third part of Virchow's triad associated with excessive thrombosis. Stasis allows activated coagulation factors to locally accumulate in high concentrations, decreases hepatic clearance, and therefore favors thrombosis. Two particular areas subject to low blood flow and thrombosis are abnormal dilatations (aneurysms) of large blood vessels and the spaces or sinuses behind the valves found in the deep veins of the leg. In addition to the above anatomy, certain acquired situations also will enhance stasis and pooling of blood. These include congestive heart failure, hip fracture, cerebral vascular accidents, anesthesia, and the postoperative states. Thus, a patient undergoing major surgery may experience stasis in the operating room due to anesthesia. In addition, the surgical patient experiences more stasis in the postoperative state due to diminished ambulation. Hip fracture patients with casted lower extremities are another important example of stasis contributing to pathologic thrombosis. Although many of the chemical and anticoagulant prophylactic methods will "thin" the blood (lower the coagulant capacity) and help prevent clotting in such stasis situations, many of the mechanical means discussed below aim to artificially enhance blood flow and diminish the degree of stasis present and thus diminish thrombosis formation in this way.

Figure 65-1 is a generalized single presentation of the coagulation system with procoagulant and inhibitor interaction points shown. Table 65-1 lists certain common conditions associated with excessive thrombosis with an explanation of the altered pathophysiology which is presumed responsible for the increased association with thrombosis.

Prevention of Stasis

MECHANICAL METHODS USED TO PREVENT THROMBOEMBOLISM

Attempts at mechanical prophylaxis aspire to prevent clots from forming in the deep veins of the legs. Proper nursing has a traditional role in preventing venous stasis. This practice involves diverse measures, such as elevating the patient's legs to enhance venous flow, helping the patient perform leg exercises, and frequently changing the patient's posture.

These measures are generally accepted as useful on clinical grounds but are difficult to validate experimentally, in part because of inevitable differences between patient populations in different studies. Recently, using the technique of ^{125}I-labeled fibrinogen scanning, several separate studies have evaluated the merits of mechanical means of prevention of stasis. These studies have demonstrated that, in controlled trials in patients undergoing abdominal operations, intermittent pneumatic compression of the calf with special boots during and after the surgery was as effective in thrombosis prophylaxis as more commonly used drug treatments and seemed to be less hazardous regarding side effects. Although techniques for intermittent calf compression continue to improve, some patient discomfort is often reported such that not all patient populations at high risk and who are to remain immobile for a long while can utilize these techniques.

CHEMICAL MECHANISMS USED TO PREVENT THROMBOEMBOLISM

Dextran has antithrombotic effects which have been attributed to three separate mechanisms: expansion of the blood volume, which decreases blood viscosity; coating of the vascular endothelium, leading to decreased platelet-vessel wall interaction; and interference with platelet function and polymerization of fibrin. Dextran causes only a modest decrease in venous thrombosis, but its effects can be accomplished without need for laboratory control and with little risk of bleeding. The use of dextran also has a few distinct disadvantages: it has to be given intravenously, it is expensive, and it entails the danger of volume overload, particularly in old people.

TABLE 65-1
Common Conditions Associated with Excessive Thrombosis

Condition	Altered Pathophysiology Resulting in Thrombotic Diathesis
A. Following major thoracic, abdominal, and pelvic surgery	1. Venodilatation and prolonged stasis of blood caused by anesthetic state. 2. Diminished ambulation after surgery further encourages venous stasis and pooling.
B. Spinal cord injury	1. Neuropathic vasodilatation increases venous capacitance of leg veins; impaired ambulation additionally causes stasis.
C. Hip fracture	1. Chemically induced intense venodilatation with endothelium damage and coagulation activation. 2. Mechanical trauma to veins with endothelial damage and coagulation activation. 3. Traction on vessels at surgery with venous stasis. 4. Postoperative state (see A).
D. Post myocardial infarction and cerebrovascular accident	1. Prolonged bed rest with venous stasis.
E. Postpartum state	1. In pregnancy the coagulation pathway is amplified while the fibrinolytic pathway is diminished. This altered balance results in hypercoagulability. 2. Pressure on veins from gravid uterus and trauma of delivery increase venous stasis.
F. Carcinomatosis	1. Tumor cells and/or tumor-related products act as procoagulants which can activate factor X and initiate a hypercoagulable state. 2. Patients often with limited ambulation enhancing venous stasis.
G. Familial deficiency of inhibitor proteins (antithrombin III) fibrinolytic proteins (plasminogen) or anticoagulant proteins (proteins C and S)	1. Absence of inhibitor proteins results in unopposed coagulation activity once clotting pathway activated (see Fig. 65-1). The result is an altered balance markedly favoring thrombosis.

Inhibition of Hypercoagulability

ANTICOAGULANT METHODS USED TO PREVENT THROMBOEMBOLISM

Heparin
Administered parenterally, heparin is the designation for a group of sulfated mucopolysaccharides that exerts an antithrombotic effect only when a naturally occurring α_2-globulin inhibitor, antithrombin III, is present. Antithrombin III inactivates irreversibly the coagulant factors IXa, Xa, and thrombin. Heparin markedly accelerates the rate of inhibition of these activated intermediates (Fig. 65-1).

Because of biologic amplification in the coagulation cascade, the amount of heparin needed to inhibit factor Xa is 1000 times less than that needed to inactivate the thrombin that is formed by factor Xa. Moreover, less heparin is needed to prevent a thrombotic process than to treat it. Prompted by these consideratinos, over 25 large-scale trials of prophylaxis using low-dose (minidose) heparin have been performed since 1971, and nearly all have shown this practice to be effective. In this dosage heparin is almost universally without effect on partial thromboplastin time or clotting time. Low dose heparin acts primarily by inhibiting activation of factor X. The prophylactic therapy is continued until the risk of thromboembolism is judged to be gone.

The recommended dose of heparin for prevention of thromboembolic complications of general surgery is 5000 units administered subcutaneously. The program is begun 2 h before surgery and is administered thereafter every 8 to 12 h until the patient is ambulatory or is discharged (usually 5 to 7 days after operation). Before undertaking this form of treatment, the patient is screened for a hemo-

static disorder that might cause hemorrhage by determining that the partial thromboplastin time and the number of circulating platelets are normal. Drugs that interfere with platelet function (see later in this chapter) are stopped 5 days before surgery. In certain types of patients, low dose heparin has proved to be dangerous or ineffective in protecting against thromboembolism: open prostatectomy, surgical procedures on the hip or knee, spinal epidural block, or surgical procedures on the brain or eye. Most importantly, low dose heparin prophylaxis should not be used as a substitute for adequate anticoagulant therapy for established thromboembolic disease.

Oral Anticoagulants

Coumarin and related compounds are the only effective oral anticoagulants that are currently available. They are vitamin K antagonists that act by competitive inhibition at a hepatic enzymatic site. Vitamin K is necessary for the synthesis of calcium-binding sites in factors II, VII, IX, and X (Fig. 65-2). The anticoagulant effect of coumarin compounds is completely reversed by vitamin K.

The vitamin K antagonists, typified by warfarin, are rapidly absorbed. They are almost completely bound (more than 90 percent) to albumin and are hydroxylated

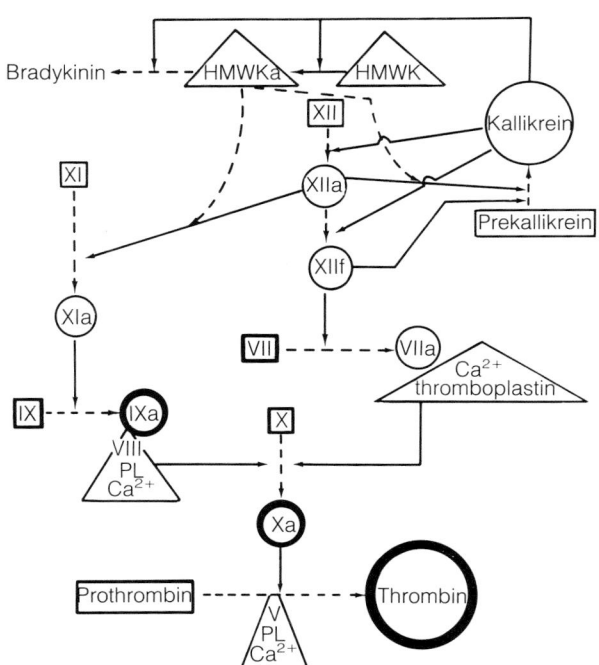

FIGURE 65-2 Site of action of heparin and sodium warfarin on blood coagulation. Solid arrows indicate enzymatic actions; dashed arrows indicate transformation from precursor to active enzyme; brackets indicate enzymatic complexes. Precursors of coagulation factors are designated by Roman numerals or commonly accepted names. Dashed arrows indicate nonenzymatic acceleration of the indicated reactions. □, ▫ = vitamin K-dependent factors, susceptible to functional depression by warfarin; ○ = active enzyme; ● = enzymes inhibited by antithrombin in the presence of heparin; HMWK = high-molecular-weight kininogen.

to inactive compounds by hepatic microsomal enzymes. Once warfarin is begun, the rate of reduction in the levels of factors II, VII, IX, and X in plasma depends on the rate at which they are catabolized, i.e., on their biologic half-lives. Since each is metabolized at a different rate, each protein reaches the therapeutic range (10 to 20 percent of normal plasma concentrations) at a different time: the biologic half-life of factor VII is 6 h, whereas that of prothrombin is 40 h; for factors IX and X, the half-lives lie in between.

Oral anticoagulants have been used for years to prevent venous thrombosis and pulmonary embolism in patients who are known to be at high risk, but there is no unanimity concerning the value of this type of prophylaxis.

A recent, well-done study on patients undergoing knee and hip surgery by Francis and colleagues used small doses of warfarin, beginning 10 to 14 days preoperatively, sufficient to raise the prothrombin time 1.5 to 3.0 s, and then followed after surgery with higher doses to raise the prothrombin time to 1.5 times control values. This "two-step warfarin" program diminished the incidence of venographically proved venous thrombosis from 51 percent in patients treated with dextran to 21 percent in the warfarin group without any increase in bleeding side effects. Thus, this two-step warfarin regimen was highly effective in preventing thrombosis, but did not result in excessive bleeding in these high risk patients. Other studies using warfarin do demonstrate an increased incidence of bleeding, i.e., wound hematomas, compared to heparin regimens. At present, the consensus is that oral anticoagulants are useful in preventing clotting in *high risk* patients. However, the risk of postoperative hemorrhage and the inconvenience of laboratory monitoring have limited the prophylactic use of oral anticoagulants after surgery.

Defibrinating Agents

A totally different group of anticoagulants includes those which prevent the formation of fibrin by removing fibrinogen (the substrate of thrombin) from the circulation. This approach is in marked contrast to that of heparin, which inhibits coagulant enzymes, or of warfarin, which reduces the concentration of enzyme precursors. Two enzymes, ancrod and reptilase, purified from snake venoms, are used. Other coagulation factors, as well as platelets, are not affected by ancrod or reptilase. The effect of ancrod as a prophylactic agent of postoperative venous thrombosis has been only minimally tested. However, when ancrod was given immediately after surgical operation, bleeding occurred in most patients and was severe in 25 percent. Therefore, this form of therapy cannot be used in the first 48 h of the postoperative period.

Antiplatelet Agents

Venous stasis promotes the formation of a fibrin clot. The valve cusp generally serves as a nidus for the formation of

the thrombus which then propagates in the direction of blood flow by the deposition of successive layers of formed elements and fibrin. Even in the earliest venous thrombi, platelet aggregates are mixed with fibrin; it is not possible to tell which comes first. A deposition of platelets in the valve pocket accompanies the increase in blood viscosity during stasis. Since the concentration of thrombin that is required to aggregate platelets is considerably less than for fibrin formation, it is likely that thrombin-induced aggregation of platelets in the valve pocket precedes fibrin formation. Furthermore, activated clotting factors that form in slow and turbulent blood tend to accumulate in the valve pocket.

If platelets do play a significant role in venous thrombosis, a variety of agents are available to inhibit their aggregation and participation in thrombi. For example, the platelet contains cyclic adenosine monophosphate (cAMP) that inhibits platelet aggregation and release of its contents. The amount of cAMP in the cell is determined by its rate of formation by a membrane-bound enzyme, adenyl cyclase, and the rate of destruction by a second group of enzymes, cAMP phosphodiesterases. Two drugs are currently available to inhibit platelet function by increasing intracellular cyclic AMP. The first is dipyridamole (Persantine). In animal trials, this agent has been shown to be a powerful inhibitor of thrombus formation in injured vessels and to decrease platelet adhesiveness. One important mechanism by which this agent acts is by inhibiting cAMP phosphodiesterases, leading to an increase of cAMP in the platelet, and, thereby, to inhibition of platelet aggregation.

Other potent inhibitors of platelet aggregation and release are prostaglandins E_1 and I_2. They also increase cAMP but do so by stimulating adenyl cyclase. Their short half-life in vivo and hemodyamic effects (hypotension) currently limit its practical usefulness.

The most popular group of drugs known to have antiplatelet activity are the nonsteroidal, anti-inflammatory drugs typified by aspirin. Several tablets of aspirin prolong the bleeding time and inhibit prostaglandin synthesis, and thus the platelet release reaction, for as long as 1 week. The acetyl group binds to a platelet enzyme, cyclooxygenase, and thereby inhibits platelet function for its lifetime, an effect unique for this drug. Other drugs, such as phenylbutazone and indomethacin, do not permanently affect the platelet, but their inhibitory effects are similar to aspirin.

What is the evidence for the efficacy of platelet-active drugs in preventing venous thrombosis and pulmonary embolism? Although the above antiplatelet agents, including aspirin and dipyridamole, have been shown to have significant roles in treating thrombotic disorders including transient ischemic attacks and thrombi associated with prosthetic cardiac valves, they have not been shown to have significant efficacy on prophylaxis of deep venous thrombosis in either orthopedic or general surgical patient populations.

Vasoactive Drugs Used to Prevent Thromboembolism

A newer direction for thrombosis prophylaxis utilizes drugs which venoconstrict the capacitance vessels (veins, venules) in the legs. This constriction increases venous flow and return and markedly reduces venous stasis in the leg veins. The prototype group of such drugs contains derivatives of ergotamine which have vasoconstrictive activity on venous smooth muscle but minimal activity on arterial smooth-muscle receptors. In a randomized prospective multicenter study comparing heparin and dihydroergotamine mixtures with placebo, dihydroergotamine plus heparin 5000 units given at 12-h intervals significantly reduced the incidence of postsurgical venous thrombosis, compared to either agent alone or placebo. Ongoing similar studies in orthopedic surgical patients are underway to determine if such agents can add to this situation as well. Thus, these drugs may be able to provide even more complete prophylaxis with less hemorrhagic side effects.

Choice of Agents for Prophylaxis

Of the agents that have been critically evaluated for preventing venous thrombi and pulmonary embolism, five show promise: oral anticoagulants, low-dose heparin, dextran, vasoactive substances (dihydroergotamine), and pneumatic compression. No single approach can be universally applied in all patients. Oral anticoagulants, although associated with a significant risk of bleeding, remain the safest and most effective antithrombotic agent in hip surgery. Low dose heparin is effective in general surgery; in the absence of a preexisting hemostatic problem, it is recommended for all patients over 40 years of age who are about to undergo major surgery. Since patients under 40 rarely have fatal pulmonary embolism, therapeutic measures that entail less risk, such as mechanical calf compression, seem appropriate. Dextrans should probably be reserved for occasional high-risk patients in whom the use of oral anticoagulants or minidose heparin is contraindicated. Vasoactive drugs seem additive to minidose heparin in general surgical patients and are being carefully evaluated for efficacy in orthopedic cases. Thus, the time may be approaching when patients could receive individually tailored regimens for prophylaxis utilizing any or a combination of anticoagulants, venoconstrictors, and mechanical external devices to aid blood flow. As techniques and methods improve, we hope prophylactic benefits will increase while hemorrhage and other side effects, although already infrequent, will shrink to the point of being negligible.

TREATMENT OF THROMBOEMBOLIC DISEASE

Medical Management: Anticoagulants

HEPARIN

At the first convincing sign of deep venous thrombosis, heparin therapy is begun and is usually continued for 7 to 10 days at which time the thrombus is generally either lysed or well organized. Heparin prevents recurrent embolism in all but a tiny fraction of patients.

The dose of heparin that is required depends on the patient's rate of metabolism of the drug, which is quite variable, and on the coagulant activity that must be neutralized. Heparin is metabolized more quickly in pulmonary embolism than in uncomplicated deep venous thrombosis. This explains the frequent finding of large heparin requirements ("heparin resistance") seen early in pulmonary embolism. Thus, in contrast to the prophylactic low dose therapy (5000 units every 8 to 12 h), therapeutic doses for venous thrombosis average 1000 units every hour, whereas in pulmonary embolism doses in the range of 1750 units per hour are often required.

Monitoring the rate of heparin administration is necessary both to ensure adequacy of anticoagulation and to alert against impending bleeding. For monitoring, the activated partial thromboplastin time (aPTT) is the preferred test. Although it correlates well with the clotting time, it is more reproducible. Data suggest that continuous intravenous infusion that is monitored to correspond to an aPTT of 1.5 to 2.5 times control is as effective in preventing further thromboembolism as is a program of intermittent injections every 4 h while effecting an eight- to tenfold reduction in major bleeding. The major problem in continuous infusion is the need for exceedingly close supervision of the infusion rate to prevent over- or underanticoagulation. Usually several tests are required the first day to establish the appropriate dose and then only one a day thereafter. If bleeding occurs, heparin is discontinued; if bleeding is severe, heparin can be rapidly neutralized with protamine. Aspirin and other antiplatelet agents should be avoided during heparin therapy.

ORAL ANTICOAGULANTS

The antithrombotic action of the vitamin K antagonists that function as oral anticoagulants is not fully effective for about 5 days, i.e., the time required for all of the vitamin K-dependent coagulant factors (II, VII, IX, X) to fall to therapeutic levels. Therefore, heparin is continued for 5 days after warfarin is begun to allow time for the oral anticoagulant to become effective. The prothrombin time is used to monitor warfarin therapy. When the blood sample is collected in a tube containing citrate, the desired prothrombin time is 1.5 to 2.0 times the control prothrombin time. Since the risk of recurrent thromboembolism is greatest during the first months after the initial event and gradually subsides over the next 5 months, anticoagulants are usually continued for 3 months after deep venous thrombosis if the patients are ambulatory and symptom-free. However, after pulmonary embolism or if predisposing conditions, such as continued immobilization, continue, 6 months is more appropriate. Should minor bleeding occur, stopping warfarin or administering vitamin K generally suffices; 8 to 24 h is generally required for prothrombin time to return to normal. For more rapid reversal of prothrombin time, as for the case of major bleeding, plasma is transfused; the reversal is then almost immediate. Whenever warfarin is administered, account must be taken of other medications that either enhance or inhibit its effect.

FIBRINOLYTIC AGENTS

Fibrinolytic agents dissolve the fibrin matrix of a clot and therefore are potentially useful for treating, as well as preventing, thromboembolism. Fibrinolysis in vivo is initiated by the release of tissue plasminogen activator of urokinase from endothelial cells. Both activators act on plasminogen to convert it to the active enzyme plasmin. Plasmin is, in turn, neutralized by α_2-antiplasmin, a naturally occurring proteolytic inhibitor. Plasmin that is activated in the gel phase of a clot is protected from the inhibitor and dissolves fibrin.

Two activators, streptokinase, derived from β-hemolytic streptococci, and urokinase, purified from human urine or human kidney cells in culture, have received extensive clinical trials. The two agents differ in their mode of action. Urokinase is a plasminogen activator that directly converts plasminogen to plasmin. It is not antigenic, and the major practical problem in its use has been its very significant expense.

In contrast to urokinase, streptokinase, which is available in large amounts, is antigenic and is neutralized by antibodies remaining from previous streptococcal infections. This problem can be overcome by infusing high concentrations of streptokinase. The usual mode of administration of streptokinase is by intravenous drip for 12 to 24 h; a loading dose is required. The action of the drug in lysing fibrin can be monitored by the demonstration of fibrin degradation products in the blood or, more conveniently, by determining the thrombin time, which should be two to three times normal, or the fibrinogen level, which should at least be halved. Heparin must be administered after a course of fibrinolytic therapy to prevent rethrombosis; it is usually begun after the thrombin time has decreased to below two times normal values. The major side effect of fibrinolytic therapy is bleeding. Since fibrin is necessary for healing of a surgical incision, fibrinolytic therapy is contraindicated for 7 to 10 days after surgery. The fibrinolytic activity can be reversed by administering ϵ-aminocaproic acid.

The place of these two fibrinolytic agents in the therapy of acute major pulmonary embolism has been defined by two carefully controlled cooperative trials under the aegis of the National Heart, Lung, and Blood Institute. Urokinase (for 12 to 24 h) and streptokinase (for 12 h) showed equivalent effects. Both produced greater resolution of pulmonary emboli at 24 h than did the heparin-treated controls, as measured by angiography, radioisotope lung scan, or hemodynamic measurements. However, if treatment was begun after the first week, no differences were found between fibrinolytic therapy and heparin. Mortality was the same after fibrinolytic therapy or heparin. Thus, thrombolytic therapy is probably most useful in patients who are critically ill after massive embolism (usually associated with systemic hypotension). In this group, fibrinolytic therapy with urokinase or streptokinase appears to accomplish a "medical embolectomy." Other potential candidates for thrombolytic therapy are patients who survive large emboli for 24 to 48 h but in whom the emboli are apt to resolve slowly because of associated cardiac or pulmonary disease.

Theoretically, urokinase or streptokinase should, by dissolving clots, be the ideal treatment for venous thrombosis. These agents are particularly effective if given when the clot is forming. In practice, because fibrinolytic therapy is usually administered more than 72 h after the start of thrombosis, it is much less effective. Moreover, fibrinolytic therapy is contraindicated within 7 to 10 days of surgery. These two restrictions automatically exclude a large number of potential candidates.

Another type of fibrinolytic agent has come into focus in recent years. This is the so-called tissue plasminogen activator derived either from tissue culture or in bacteria by genetic engineering recombinant techniques. These activators induce plasminogen to plasmin conversion in the matrix of the fibrin clot. Thus, the plasmin generated is protected from plasma inhibitors and is active only at the site of the thrombus. Theoretically this should result in enhanced efficacy with reduced hemorrhagic side effects because plasma clotting proteins will not be effected by the localized plasmin. These activators have been systematically studied and demonstrate efficacy in lysing acute thrombi associated with acute myocardial infarction. The experience with deep venous thrombosis and pulmonary embolism remains scanty and anecdotal. However, one might expect similiar efficacy for these indications as well, although more definitive experience is required.

DEFIBRINATING AGENTS

The use of defibrinating agents such as ancrod for treating thromboembolism has been limited, and most clinical observations have been uncontrolled. In the three controlled trials of treatment with this defibrinating agent, ancrod prevented further extension of the thrombus to the same extent as heparin but, unlike streptokinase, did not induce thrombolysis. There are two major differences from heparin therapy. First, unlike heparin, which has an immediate effect, ancrod requires about 6 h to decrease fibrinogen levels to approximately 50 mg/100 ml, i.e., to therapeutic levels; heparin is immediately effective. In addition, unlike heparin, ancrod cannot be used for at least 48 h after surgery without causing severe hemorrhage. Thus, ancrod does not appear to have major advantages over heparin in anticoagulant therapy.

OTHER AGENTS

Dextran does not appear to be of any value in the treatment of thromboembolic disease. Aspirin does not yet have an established place in the management of deep vein thrombosis.

Surgical Management

VENOUS THROMBECTOMY

The mechanical removal of thrombi using catheters does not appear to reduce morbidity, prevent damage to valves, or decrease postthrombotic sequelae. Occasionally, in severe cases of phlegmasia cerulea dolens, thrombectomy may prevent venous gangrene. Heparin must be used in these cases after surgical intervention to prevent rethrombosis.

PULMONARY EMBOLECTOMY

Most patients with massive pulmonary embolism die too soon for intervention, i.e., in less than 30 min. Most of those who survive do well on heparin or thrombolytic therapy. In an occasional patient in circulatory collapse, pulmonary embolectomy can be lifesaving if a trained surgical team is on hand for rapid intervention. Sasahara and others have defined specific indications for pulmonary embolectomy which include (1) the presence of massive pulmonary embolism confirmed by pulmonary angiography; (2) failure of accepted and optimal therapy for hypoxemia (oxygen, anticoagulants, or thrombolytic therapy) and for deranged hemodynamics (fluids, pressors) with the patient continuing to be hypotensive (<90 mmHg systolic; urine output < 20 ml/h) and hypoxic (PO_2 < 60 mmHg on maximal oxygen) after 2 h of treatment. The decision for surgery, which will be infrequent, must not be delayed because once severe cardiovascular collapse occurs, surgical mortality excedes 90 percent, whereas in earlier intervention, survivorship of 50 percent can result.

VENOUS INTERRUPTION

Improved medical measures have decreased the necessity of operative treatment. When medical treatment proves ineffective or is contraindicated, surgery is performed on

the inferior vena cava. It must be remembered that once a pulmonary embolism has occurred, the clot already in the lung is *not* addressed by a venous interruption procedure. Venous interruptions, therefore, always are preventive in nature. It is the next embolism that the surgery addresses.

Several major indications are generally cited for partially interrupting the vena cava. Most popular is evidence of recurrent pulmonary embolism despite "adequate" anticoagulation. However, close examination usually reveals that the dosage of heparin or oral anticoagulants was not well controlled.

One accepted indication for ligation of the inferior vena cava is septic thrombophlebitis in the pelvis that is complicated by septic pulmonary emboli. Another is the existence of contraindications to anticoagulant therapy such as an actively bleeding lesion.

A variety of surgical procedures have been applied—ligation, plication leaving fine channels, and the application of clips that partially or totally occlude the vessel. Protection against bland emboli is best achieved by narrowing the inferior vena cava rather than by ligating it; the latter is associated with significant late morbidity. One immediate effect of total interruption of blood flow through the inferior vena cava is edema of the legs, which generally resolves slowly and tends to recur after exercise. Other approaches to elimination of pulmonary emboli

include the "umbrella" or other catheter-borne devices introduced into the inferior vena cava (Fig. 65-2). Currently the most favored vena cava interruption technique involves the transvenous placement of a special coated filter as described by Greenfield and colleagues. Advantages include transvenous method of placement, which avoids laparotomy, and structure and coating, which is supposed to allow for blood flow without need for concurrent anticoagulant therapy to maintain early and late patency. Each of the procedures aimed at the vena cava has its own problems: plication does not prevent small emboli from reaching the lungs, nor does it exclude embolization from the upper border of the deformed vena cava.

Finally, no form of obstruction to the inferior vena cava can guarantee full protection against emboli. Large collateral vessels do develop rapidly and may serve as alternative pathways by which small emboli can reach the lungs; thrombi tend to recur at the site of vena caval distortions; thrombi from areas other than those drained by the inferior vena cava may propagate and be transmitted to the lungs. Accordingly, surgery on the vena cava to prevent clots from moving to the lungs should not be undertaken unless the therapeutic hand is forced, i.e., if medical management and anticoagulant therapy have proved ineffective and if emboli are likely to recur and to be life-threatening.

BIBLIOGRAPHY

Basu D, Gallus A, Hirsh J, Cade J: A prospective study of the value of monitoring heparin treatment with the activated partial thromboplastin time. N Engl J Med 287:324–327, 1973.
   A large study designed to seek a relation between the activated partial thromboplastin time and recurrent thromboembolism during treatment found recurrences to be rare if the aPTT is prolonged to 1.5 or more control values.

Bounameaux H, Vermylen J, Collen D: Thrombolytic treatment with recombinant tissue-type plasminogen activator in a patient with massive pulmonary embolism. Ann Intern Med 103:64–65, 1985.
   The first report of successful clot-selective thrombolysis in a patient with massive pulmonary embolism using recombinant human tissue-type plasminogen activator confirming the efficacy of tPA (tissue plasminogen activator) in this setting.

Colman RW, Oxley L, Gianussa P: Statistical comparison of the automated activated partial thromboplastin time and the clotting time in the regulation of heparin therapy. Am J Clin Pathol 53:904–907, 1970.
   Laboratory study demonstrates the quicker, more efficient aPTT correlates well with the more cumbersome clotting time in the regulation of heparin therapy.

Francis CW, Marder VJ, Evarts CM, Yaukoolbodi S: Two step warfarin therapy. Prevention of postoperative venous thrombosis without excessive bleeding. JAMA 249:374–379, 1983.
   To improve prophylaxis against deep venous thrombosis in orthopedic surgery, two-step anticoagulation with warfarin was used. Initial mild anticoagulation pre- and intraoperatively was followed with more aggressive degrees of anticoagulation with excellent efficacy without enhanced bleeding complications.

Friedman PA: Vitamin K-dependent proteins. N Engl J Med 310:1458–1460, 1984.
   Complete, well referenced editorial review covering warfarin pharmacology and mechanisms of anticoagulation.

Goldhaber SZ, Buring JE, Lipnick RJ, Hubblefield F, Hennekens CH: Interruption of the interior vena cava by clip or filter. Am J Med 76:512–516, 1984.
A discussion of the varying mechanical devices available for interrupting the vena cava. The paper reviews the advantages of each.

Moser G, Krahenbuhl B, Barroussel R: Mechanical versus pharmacological prevention of deep vein thrombosis. Surg Gynecol Obstet 152:448–461, 1981.
A fine review of the varying methods used as prophylaxis for thromboembolism. The paper concludes they are all reasonably similiar in efficacy, and pneumatic compression may be less hazardous.

Moser KM, Lemoine JR: Is embolic risk conditioned by location of deep-vein thrombosis? Ann Intern Med 94:439–447, 1981.
This article stratifies deep venous thrombosis into proximal, involving popliteal and ileofemoral veins, and distal, involving only veins distal to the knee. It is the proximal case which frequently results in pulmonary embolism and postphlebitic syndrome and must be aggressively treated. Distal cases have a more benign prognosis.

Multicenter Trial Committee: Heparin-dihydroergotamine prophylaxis of postoperative deep vein thrombosis. JAMA 251:2966–2971, 1984.
Well-designed prospective study demonstrated that mixtures of heparin and a venoconstricting agent, dihydroergotamine, provided better prophylaxis in postoperative patients than either heparin alone or placebo. This paper introduces such vasoactive drugs into clinical use as deep venous thrombosis prophylaxis.

O'Reilly RA: The pharmacodynamics of the oral anticoagulant drugs. Prog Hemostasis Thrombosis 2:175–213, 1974.
An extensive, complete review article dealing with the entire realm of clinical use of warfarin.

Petitti DB, Strom BL, Melmon KL: Duration of warfarin anticoagulant therapy and the probabilities of recurrent thromboembolism and hemorrhage. Am J Med 81:255–259, 1986.
The longer the warfarin therapy, the higher the risk of medically important complications from therapy. Intensive, long-term warfarin anticoagulation, in patients with a first episode of venous thromboembolism and no predisposing condition, is associated with more toxicity than efficacy and should be abandoned.

Prevention of fatal postoperative pulmonary embolism by low dose of heparin: An international multicentre trial. Lancet 2:45–51, 1975.
Still classic huge study which clearly demonstrated efficacy of minidose heparin in the prevention of postoperative pulmonary embolism. This study demonstrated protection not only against deep venous thrombosis documented by noninvasive methods but also against pathologically demonstrated (autopsy findings) pulmonary embolism.

Rubin RN, Sherry SS: Therapeutic fibrinolysis, in Bayless T, Brain M, Cherniak R (eds), *Current Therapy in Internal Medicine.* Philadelphia, BC Decker Inc., 1984, pp 337–341.
Review article summarizes current indications and uses of thrombolytic therapy in venous (as well as arterial) thromboembolic diseases.

Sasahara A, Barsamian E: Another look at pulmonary embolectomy. Ann Thorac Surg 16:317–323, 1973.
A review of specific indications for pulmonary embolectomy.

Sharma GW: Historical overview of antithrombotic and thrombolytic therapy. Am J Med 83:2–5, 1987.
A review that traces the changing approaches over the years to antithrombotic and thrombolytic therapy. Current attempts to achieve safe and effective thrombolysis focus on recombinant tissue-specific plasminogen activator, antisoylated streptokinase plasminogen activator complex, and pro-urokinase.

Simon TL, Hyers TM, Gaston JP: Heparin pharmacokinetics: Increased pharmacokinetics in pulmonary embolism. Br J Haematol 39:111–118, 1978.
This study measured heparin half-life in deep venous thrombosis and pulmonary embolism in humans. Increased clearance in pulmonary embolism results in enhanced heparin requirements (25 units per kilogram) in pulmonary embolism compared to deep venous thrombosis (15 units per kilogram). This likely explains some of the heparin resistance encountered in acute pulmonary embolism.

Virchow R: Die Verstopfung der Lungenarterie und ihre Folgen. Beitr Exp Pathol Physiol 2:227–380, 1846.
Virchow's original treatise linking thrombosis to the triad of venous stasis, hypercoagulability, and injury to vessel walls.

Chapter *66*

Pulmonary Thromboembolic Disease

Mark A. Kelley / Alfred P. Fishman

The designation *pulmonary (venous) thromboembolism* refers to the migration of a clot (or clots) from systemic veins to the lungs. The term has ominous overtones, more as a harbinger of sudden death from clots still to be released than from the morbidity of the clots already dispatched to the lungs.

Each year, more than 500,000 individuals in the United States are affected by thromboembolism (Fig. 66-1).

Of these, two-thirds have undiagnosed pulmonary emboli that result in a mortality of at least 30 percent. When pulmonary emboli are correctly diagnosed and treated, the mortality falls to less than 10 percent. These data underscore the pressing need for preventing the formation of thrombi in peripheral veins, for early detection of thrombi that do form, for early and zealous management of peripheral thrombi to avoid embolization to the lungs, and for promoting the resolution of pulmonary emboli.

SOURCES OF EMBOLI

Most pulmonary emboli come from deep veins in the legs. A clot that is destined to become an embolus generally begins in the deep veins of the calf and propagates centrally from the sural up the popliteal and femoral and sometimes to the iliac veins—gradually exceeding its restraints until part of the advancing edge dangles precariously in the venous lumen (Fig. 66-2).

An uncommon, but important, source of pulmonary emboli, especially in women, are the pelvic veins. Pelvic thrombi may be bland or septic. Often the pelvic origin of the emboli is suggested by a history of obstetrical difficulty during recent parturition, recent gynecologic surgery, or clinical signs of pelvic pathology. When the emboli are bland, they evoke few systemic disturbances unless they cause pulmonary infarction. In contrast, septic emboli are usually associated with unmistakable evidence of septicemia in conjunction with multiple pulmonary consolidations that often go on to cavitate, as well as with a history of recent pelvic infection, e.g., septic abortion.

Blood clot is not the only material that ends up as pulmonary emboli. Any particulate matter that gains entry to the venous side of the circulation may lodge in the lungs. Fragments of tissue, parasites, liquid droplets, and gases find their way into the veins either by injection or as a consequence of trauma; the particles may be sterile or septic. Drug addicts often embolize the lungs with talc and cotton fibers in the course of a mainline injection. Not only do these particles occlude vessels, but they also excite inflammation in the walls.

Amniotic fluid embolism is a rare but catastrophic complication of pregnancy. Amniotic fluid gains access to the uterine venous circulation either as a result of vigorous uterine contraction after rupture of the membranes or through tears or surgical incisions in the myometrium or endocervix.

A third distinctive clinical picture is elicited by air embolism. The accidental introduction of air into the venous circulation occasionally occurs in the course of intravenous injections, hemodialysis, placement of central venous lines, induction of an artificial pneumothorax or

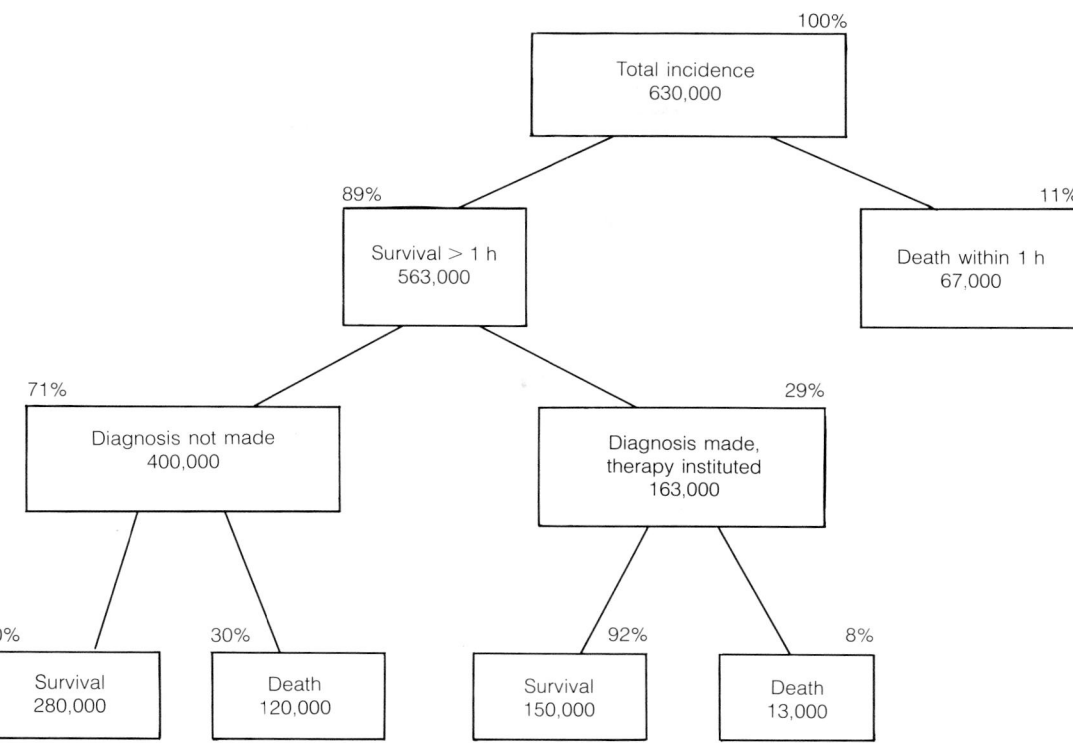

FIGURE 66-1 Estimated incidence and survival statistics for pulmonary embolism in the United States. (*Modified after Dalen and Alpert, 1975.*)

pneumoperitoneum, or after chest injury. The syndromes elicited by fat, amniotic fluid, and air emboli are considered later in this chapter.

FACTORS PREDISPOSING TO VENOUS THROMBOSIS

Virchow identified venous stasis, hypercoagulability, and injury to the venous walls as the factors favoring venous thrombosis.

Stasis

Clinically, venous thrombosis often follows an episode of venous stasis. However, even though stasis is clearly important, it is generally regarded to be a contributory or precipitating factor rather than a primary initiating mechanism. Thus, blood trapped in a vein between two ligatures remains fluid for hours. Moreover, venous thrombosis occurs without preceding stasis in women ingesting oral contraceptives, in individuals with paroxysmal nocturnal hemoglobinuria, and in familial disorders such as dysfibrinogenemias, antithrombin III deficiency, and homocystinuria.

Elderly patients are particularly prone to venous stasis because of limited mobility, cramped postures imposed by disease, prolonged bed rest during illness, slowing of the circulation by congestive heart failure, and deep venous varicosities. Even normal persons, who sit for a long while with knees flexed, as in a long trip by automo-

bile or airplane, occasionally develop a pulmonary embolus when they disembark.

Postoperative patients, especially those who have undergone extensive and prolonged operations on the abdomen and pelvis, are particularly prone to pulmonary embolism. Embolization is so common in this population that much of the available information concerning prophylactic anticoagulation is derived from patients who have undergone surgery.

Hypercoagulability

Although hypercoagulable states might be expected to predispose to venous thrombosis, evidence of hypercoagulability in association with thromboembolism is generally difficult to obtain. Nonetheless, in certain clinical disorders, biochemical disorders do predispose to thrombosis. These disorders fall into two broad categories: (1) those which predispose to venous thrombosis, and (2) those in which restraining mechanisms fail to limit the size of the hemostatic plug.

PREDISPOSING CONDITIONS

Endothelial injury, that can be inflicted in a variety of subtle as well as overt ways, predisposes to clotting. For example, it is now widely held that widespread covert injury of the pulmonary microcirculation can lead to generalized thrombi of the small pulmonary arteries and arterioles; organization of these disseminated thrombi could

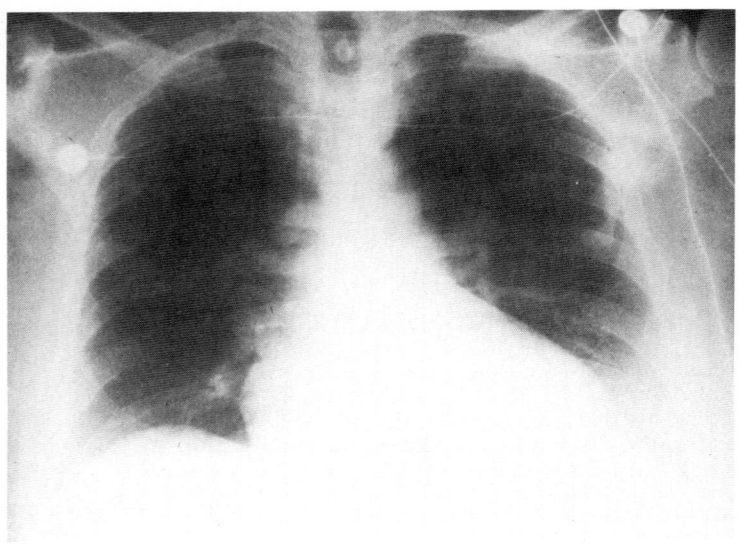

A

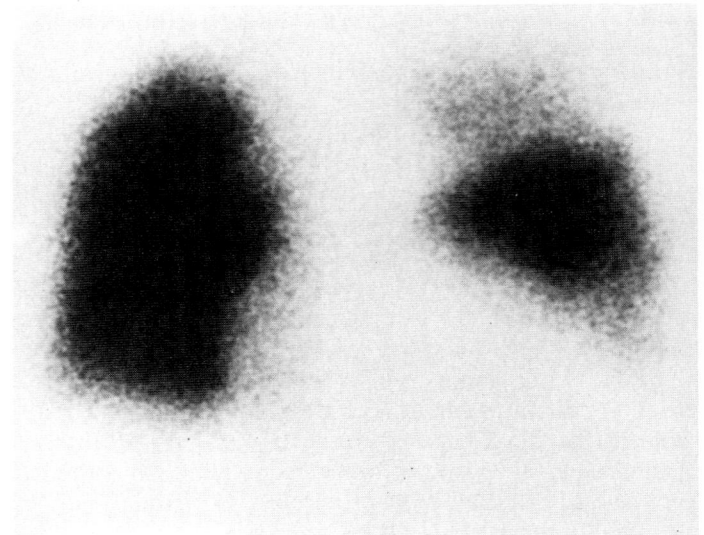

B

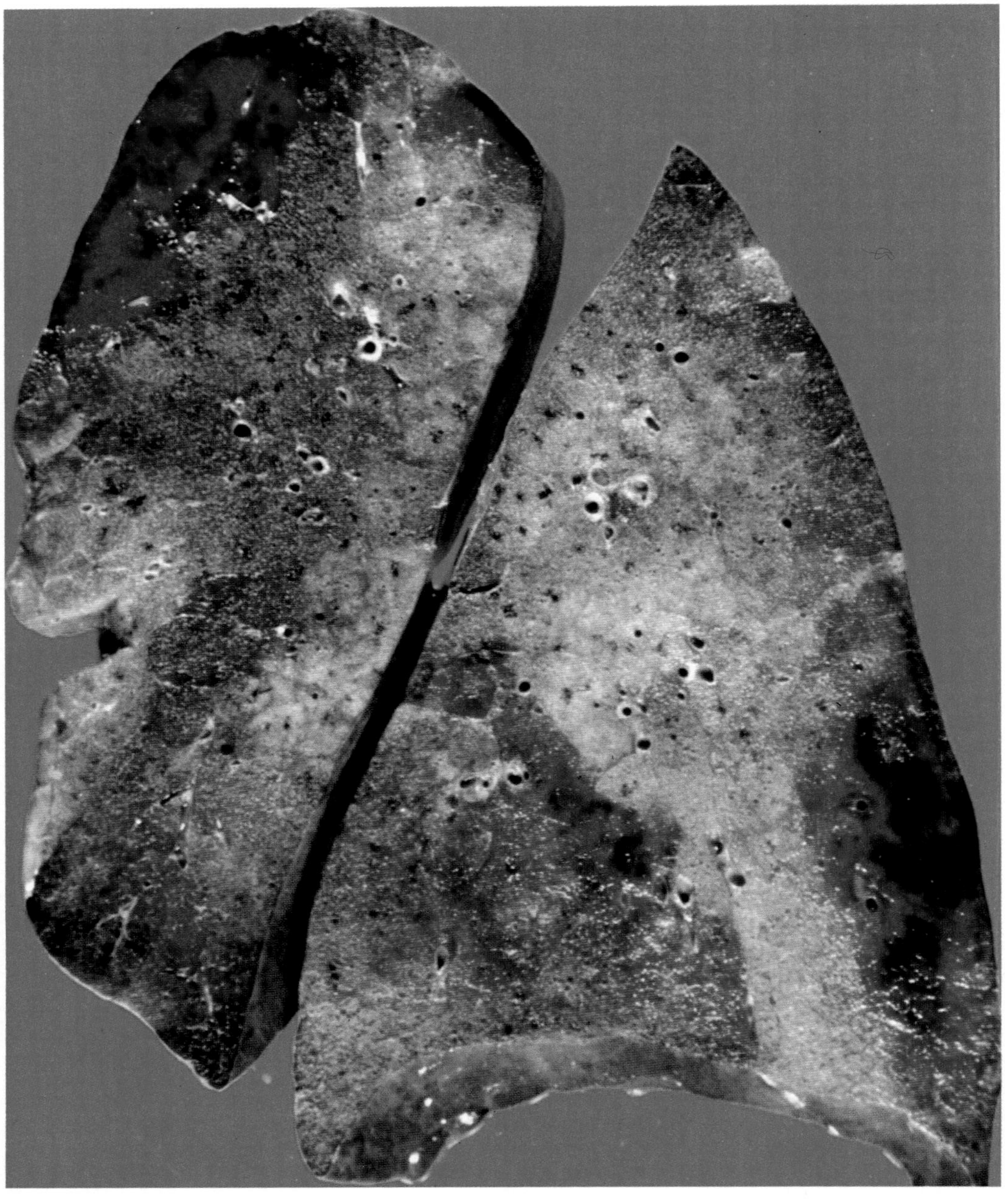

FIGURE 66-2 Fatal pulmonary emboli secondary to deep vein thrombosis. *A.* Portable chest radiograph. Mild cardiomegaly and hazy infiltrate at left base. *B.* Perfusion lung scan. Defect in area of infiltrate and another wedge-shaped defect in left upper lung zone where chest radiograph was clear. *C.* Autopsy. Multiple pleural-based pulmonary infarcts.

then lead to obliterative vascular disease and pulmonary hypertension. This prospect is considered further under the syndrome of "Multiple Pulmonary Emboli," below.

Particular etiologies of widespread endothelial injury have recently been uncovered. Among these are hemocystinemia and autoimmune injury, as in systemic lupus erythematosus. Predominantly, but not exclusively in patients with systemic lupus erythematosus, a lupuslike anticoagulant (LLAC) appears in the blood and, in contrast to what is generally expected of anticoagulants, predisposes to thrombosis. How it does so is unclear, but three mechanisms have been proposed: (1) inhibition of prostacyclin synthesis by endothelium; (2) inhibition of plasminogen activator, thereby decreasing the potential for thrombolysis; and (3) promotion of platelet aggregation due to interaction of the LLAC with the phospholipid in the platelet membranes.

Clot formation is also enhanced by an excessive number of circulating platelets, e.g., essential thrombocytosis, or by damaged platelets, e.g., paroxysmal nocturnal hemoglobinuria or heparin-induced thrombocytopenia. Disseminated intravascular coagulation leads to thrombosis by activating the clotting cascade. The familiar association between malignancy and venous thrombosis has been attributed to low grade disseminated intravascular coagulation.

OVERSHOOT OF THE CLOTTING MECHANISM

Certain circumstances predispose to excessive growth and propagation of a clot. Among these is stasis that retards the elimination of activated coagulant products from the region of a small clot. Hyperviscosity syndromes due to polycythemia or elevated serum proteins can also enhance the propagation of a clot. Other uncommon hematologic abnormalities promoting clot formation include antithrombin III deficiency, congenitally abnormal fibrinogen, and a familial deficiency of tissue plasminogen activator.

The Vessel Wall

Injury to the venous wall, as in a hip fracture, may initiate and perpetuate venous thrombosis. The injury, particularly if accompanied by blood stasis, produces patchy endothelial damage, presumably in response to release of chemotactic substances, such as complement fragments (C′3a and C′5a), plasminogen activator, and kallikrein. The endothelial damage exposes the underlying collagen tissue which, in turn, activates factor XII and prompts the formation of plasmin and the initiation of the fibrinolytic response. Release of kinins increases vascular permeability so that plasma proteins leak into the collagen matrix and activate Hageman factor. Remote substances, from tissue damage elsewhere, also contribute to coagulation in this setting of vascular injury and stasis. This interplay sets the stage for a propagating thrombus.

Since hours usually pass between the time of fracture and orthopedic intervention, a clot is generally present in deep local veins by the time that the patient comes to surgery. The problem then is to prevent its extension and liberation as an embolus to the lungs. This distinction is important with respect to proper anticoagulant therapy.

PHYSIOLOGICAL CONSEQUENCES

The effects of pulmonary emboli range from imperceptible to disastrous. The physiological and clinical impact depends not only on how much of the pulmonary vascular bed is obliterated, the sizes of affected vessels, and the nature of the emboli but also on secondary effects that follow impingement of the emboli in the lungs, i.e., local release of neurohumoral substances, such as serotonin and histamine, arterial hypoxemia that stimulates systemic chemoreceptors, and reflex stimulation of the ventilation and circulation.

Respiratory

The hallmark of embolization of the lungs is rapid, shallow breathing (tachypnea) that results in an increase in minute ventilation; dead-space ventilation invariably increases, and alveolar ventilation generally increases. Intrapulmonary reflexes, involving the vagus nerves, set the ventilatory pattern. Of the three receptor mechanisms in the lungs (stretch, irritant, and juxtacapillary), only the latter two have been shown to play a role in the reflex stimulation of the ventilation by pulmonary emboli.

Occlusion of terminal pulmonary arteries by emboli is associated with constriction of terminal bronchioles. Two mechanisms are held responsible: (1) the release of vasoconstrictive substances from platelet aggregates within the clot and, possibly, from mast cells in the affected lung, and (2) hypocapnia secondary to the increase in alveolar ventilation.

Circulatory

Several factors shape the hemodynamic consequences of acute pulmonary emboli (Fig. 66-3). Emboli that are small in size and few in number usually cause no hemodynamic upset. Conversely, large emboli to major pulmonary arteries, or a large shower of small emboli, often evoke systemic hypotension, bradycardia, pulmonary hypertension, and a decrease in cardiac output. In individuals without cardiopulmonary disease, large increments in pulmonary arterial pressure occur only when more than half of the pulmonary vasculature has been compromised by clot. A much smaller clot burden suffices to evoke pulmonary hypertension in patients with preexistent cardiopulmonary disease in whom pulmonary vascular resistance is often abnormally high before embolization because of their underlying disease.

While the extent of the pulmonary vascular bed occlusion is of major importance, the pathogenesis of the pulmonary hypertension in pulmonary thromboembolism involves more than mechanical amputation of the pulmo-

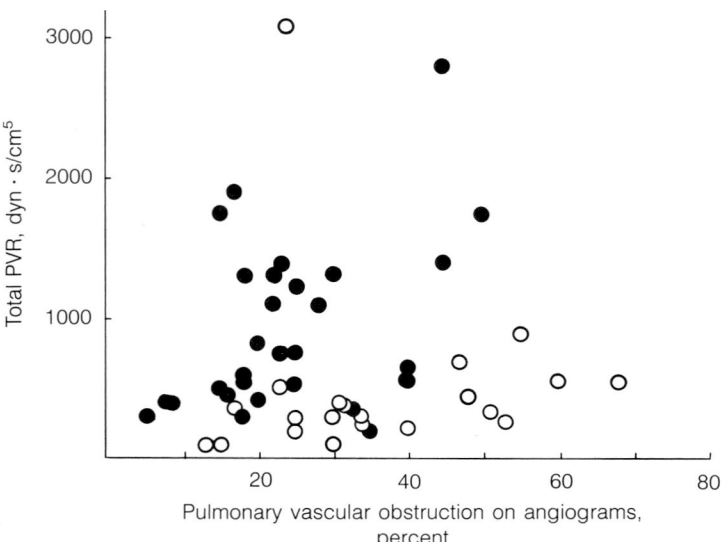

FIGURE 66-3 Hemodynamic consequences of pulmonary embolism and the underlying state of the pulmonary vasculature. Patients in whom the pulmonary vasculature was previously normal (open circles) develop little increase in pulmonary vascular resistance (PVR) until the clot burden exceeds 50 percent. In those with antecedent cardiopulmonary disease (solid circles), the pulmonary vascular resistance increases appreciably with only modest clot burden. (*Modified after Sharma, McIntyre, Sharma, Sasahara, 1984.*)

nary arterial tree and heightened resistance to blood flow. That other influences are operative is suggested by: (1) the difficulty in generating severe and lasting pulmonary hypertension experimentally by occluding major pulmonary arteries; (2) the frequent disparity between the small size of an acute embolus and the transient, inordinate increase in pulmonary arterial pressure suggesting reflex vasoconstriction; and (3) the consistent but unexplained increase in lung water that occasionally results in frank pulmonary edema, particularly in patients with underlying disease of the left ventricle (Fig. 66-4). These discrepancies have prompted a search for additional factors, particularly reflex vasoconstriction and the release of neurohumoral substances. At present, evidence for neurohumoral substances, such as serotonin, is sparse. The consensus is that mechanical limitation of the pulmonary arterial tree, reinforced by reflex pulmonary vasoconstriction, is responsible for pulmonary arterial hypertension after acute embolization. Whether the increase in pulmonary vascular water is due to capillary hyperperfusion or hypertension in the unoccluded parts of the pulmonary circulation or to damage of endothelium by substances released in the clotting process is currently being investigated.

Some emboli cause pulmonary infarction. Why infarction occurs is not clear, but the consensus is that infarction will not occur unless oxygenation is also compromised locally, either by airway disease or by insufficient bronchial collateral circulation. Pulmonary emboli exert different effects in the normal than in the abnormal lung. Chronic congestive heart failure predisposes to infarction, possibly by impeding bronchial venous return to the atria.

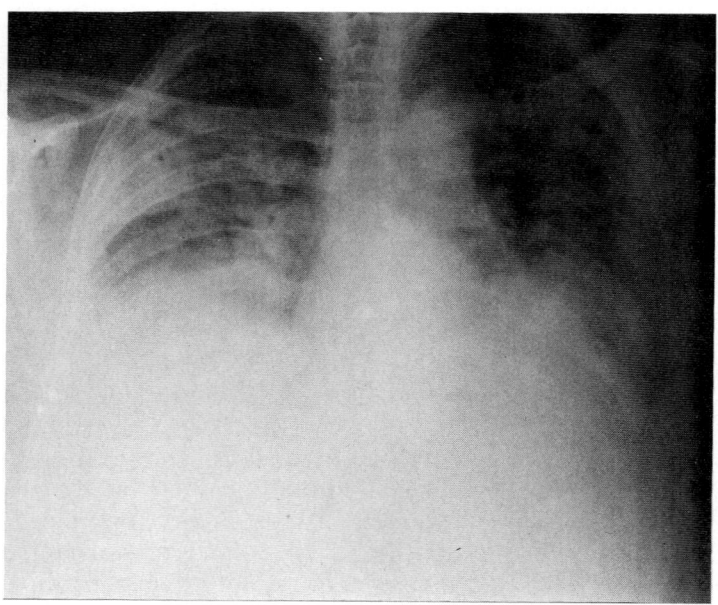

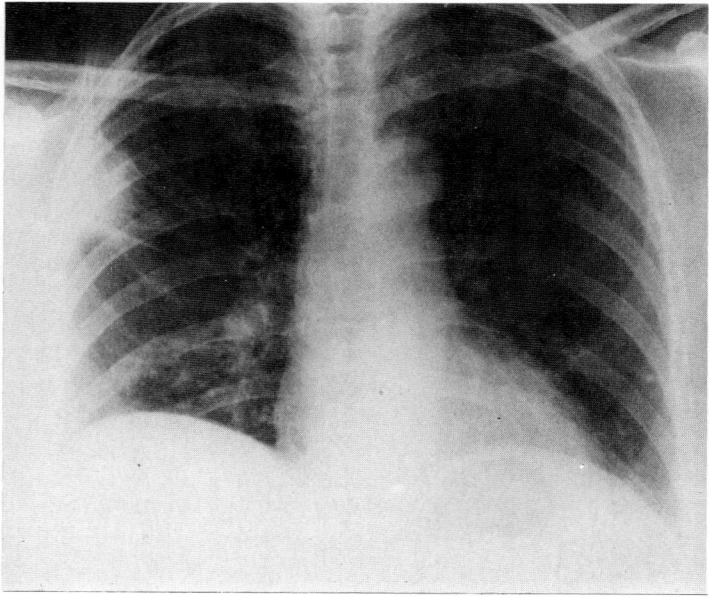

A   *B*

FIGURE 66-4 Bilateral pulmonary edema in a 50-year-old patient with pulmonary embolism. *A.* Upon admission. Overt pulmonary edema. *B.* Ten days later. Chest has cleared except for shadow in right upper lobe that resolved slowly.

Ventilation-Circulation Imbalances

Focal areas of edema and atelectasis often develop in the vicinity of occluded pulmonary arteries. Loss of alveolar surfactant contributes to these changes by promoting alveolar collapse and fluid accumulation. Because of continued blood flow through these hypoventilated, edematous areas of the lung in the vicinity of the occluded artery, arterial hypoxemia ensues. This arterial hypoxemia behaves as though it is predominantly due to "anatomic venous admixture" in that it is only slightly relieved by breathing pure O_2. Venous admixture is sometimes intensified by a low cardiac output, e.g., in massive pulmonary embolism that is associated with low values for mixed venous P_{O_2}. Rarely does pulmonary hypertension cause

sufficient increase in right atrial pressure to reverse flow through a patent foramen ovale.

Because of the upsets between alveolar ventilation and alveolar blood flow, the characteristic features of extensive emboli to the lungs are: (1) increased dead-space ventilation, alveolar ventilation, and venous admixture; (2) arterial hypoxemia and hypocapnia; and (3) widening of the alveolar-arterial difference in P_{O_2} [P(A-a)$_{O_2}$]. Although the physiological dead space often increases in patients with pulmonary emboli because the close of pulmonary vessels interrupts blood flow to many alveoli, attempts at quantification of the amount of clot by using the increment in physiological dead space have proved unreliable. One plausible explanation for the discrepancy is the occurrence of bronchoconstriction in the areas de-

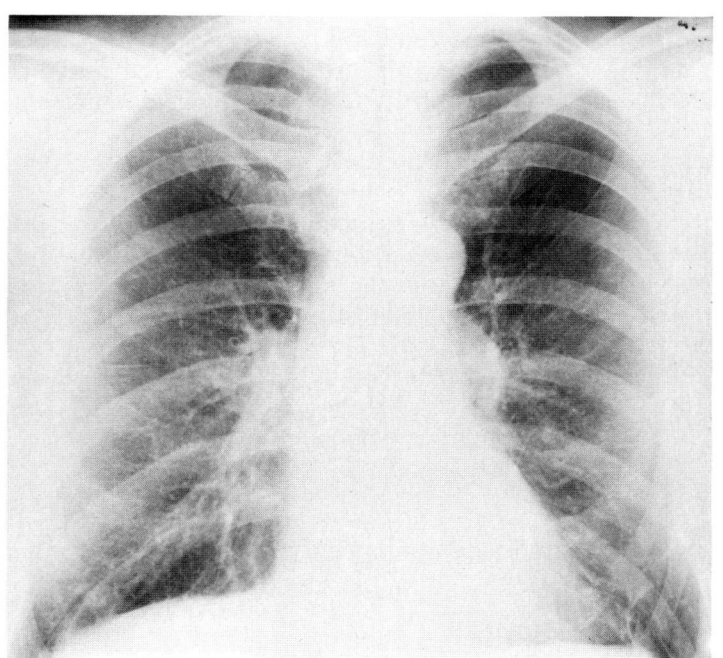

A

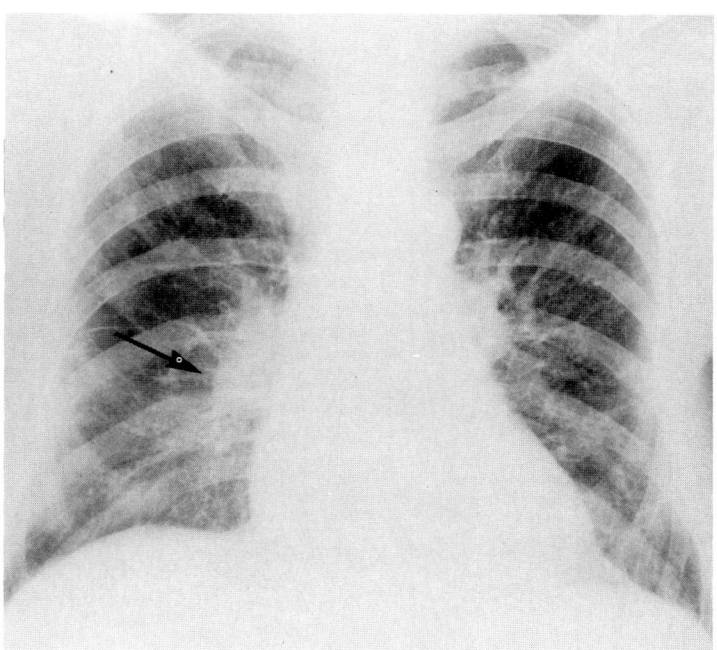

B

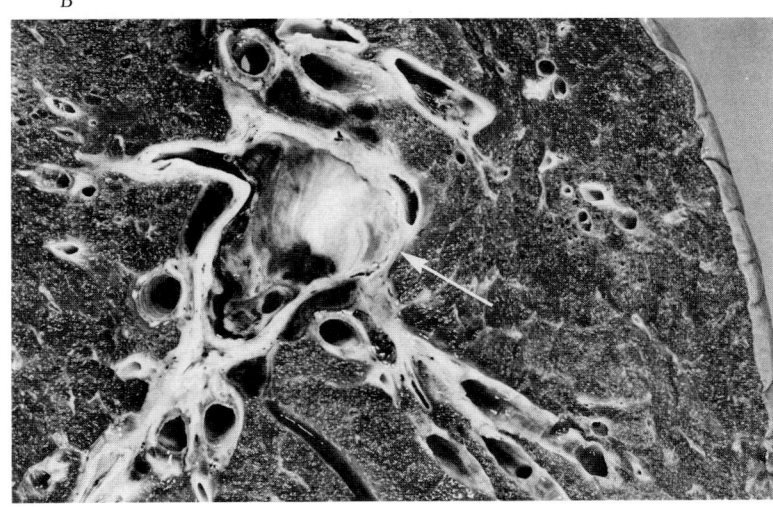

C

FIGURE 66-5   Organization of massive thrombus.   A. 1967, before embolization of right pulmonary artery.   B. 1972, large organized thrombus in right pulmonary artery (arrow). Death followed attempt at surgical removal. Confirmed at autopsy. C. Another patient. Organized thrombus at autopsy (arrow). Patient died of unrelated cause. *(Courtesy of Dr. G. G. Pietra.)*

prived of circulation, thereby partially adjusting the alveolar ventilation to the diminished circulation.

NATURAL HISTORY OF CLOTS IN THE LUNGS

Clots that reach the lungs are dealt with in two general ways: fibrinolysis and organization (Fig. 66-5). In addition, large clots in a major pulmonary artery are often disintegrated by the mechanical pounding that accompanies each cardiac ejection. Overwhelming of the fibrinolytic mechanisms by multiple emboli favors persistence of the clots and their subsequent incorporation into vascular lining. Resolution of infarction (Fig. 66-6) is accomplished either by resumption of blood flow through the occluded vessel, or by expansion of the bronchial collateral circulation, or by increasing alveolar ventilation in the affected area. Usually, all three mechanisms contribute. Resolution of a pulmonary embolus is generally complete if only atelectasis and edema are involved; but if pulmonary infarction occurs, progressive shrinkage and scarring of the affected area generally follow.

CLINICAL MANIFESTATIONS OF DEEP VENOUS THROMBOSIS IN THE LEGS

Because thrombi originate so often in the deep veins of the legs, particularly those of the calf, careful examination of the legs is indispensible in searching for a source of pulmonary emboli. The characteristic signs are swelling of the leg (most often unilateral), duskiness, pain to deep pressure over the gastrocnemius muscle or to dorsiflexion of the foot (Homan's sign), or palpable deep thrombi. Sometimes the superficial veins are dilated as part of the expansion of the collateral venous circulation. Occasionally, the swollen calf is associated with a tender cord in the femoral triangle. Unfortunately, in about one-half of patients in whom the legs are the source of deep venous thrombi, the clinical examination of the legs is normal. Conversely, a clinical examination that suggests the presence of a clot often proves to be erroneous.

CLINICAL MANIFESTATIONS OF PULMONARY EMBOLI

For convenience, four categories of clinical manifestations can be identified. Three of the four categories are acute and run their course in a matter of days: (1) massive occlusion of the pulmonary arterial tree, often by a large embolus that lodges in the central pulmonary arterial tree and arrests blood flow through most of the pulmonary vascular bed; (2) embolism associated with infarction, an uncommon but distinctive clinical disorder; and (3) embolism without pulmonary infarction, the most common type, in which the degree of vascular obstruction is considerably less than massive central occlusion. The remaining category, chronic *multiple pulmonary emboli*, designates a syndrome that is elicited by repeated embolization of the lungs, over months to years, and results in severe progressive pulmonary hypertension.

Acute Massive Occlusion

The extent of the pulmonary vascular tree that is occluded by large emboli varies from patient to patient. Traditionally, the idea of massive occlusion implies that enough of the pulmonary circulation has been compromised for circulatory collapse to ensue (Fig. 66-7). Fortunately, this group is small. The clinical picture is that of shock, i.e., systemic hypotension and impaired perfusion of vital organs. The patient is pale, weak, listless to the point of apathy, sweaty, nauseated, and oliguric; mentation is often impaired. Particularly striking is tachypnea; tachycardia is a regular feature. Autopsy discloses a large embolus in the vicinity of the bifurcation and evidence that blood flow to at least two lobar arteries has been arrested.

Certain clinical signs are associated with this classic but uncommon emergency. Because so much of the pulmonary vascular tree has been occluded by the embolus and because often the patient has an underlying cardiac or pulmonary disorder that predisposed to embolization, pulmonary hypertension is sometimes striking: the acutely dilated pulmonary artery produces a visible or palpable impulse in the second left interspace along the sternal border; the sound of pulmonary valve closure becomes accentuated, sometimes to the point of being palpable; the pulmonary component of the second heart sound often becomes louder than the aortic component, and the second heart sound is narrowly split. Should right ventricular failure supervene, a right ventricular S_3 gallop or a summation gallop and the murmur of tricuspid insufficiency are often heard along the left lower border of the sternum.

Both the clinical manifestations and the electrocardiographic patterns (Fig. 66-8) described above are rarely documented because of the desperate nature of the situation. Much more common are large emboli that compromise the circulation but are not immediately disastrous. Many occlude fewer than two lobar arteries; some seem to be massive at the outset but then fragment and relocate to impact on less and less of the pulmonary vascular tree. In this group, dyspnea, tachypnea, chest pain (usually pleuritic), and anxiety are common features. Fever, sweating and hemoptysis occur less consistently. Systemic hypotension is a consistent feature but is often mild. Depending on the degree of compromise of the pulmonary circulation and the underlying disorder, the signs and symptoms range from those of massive occlusion to those

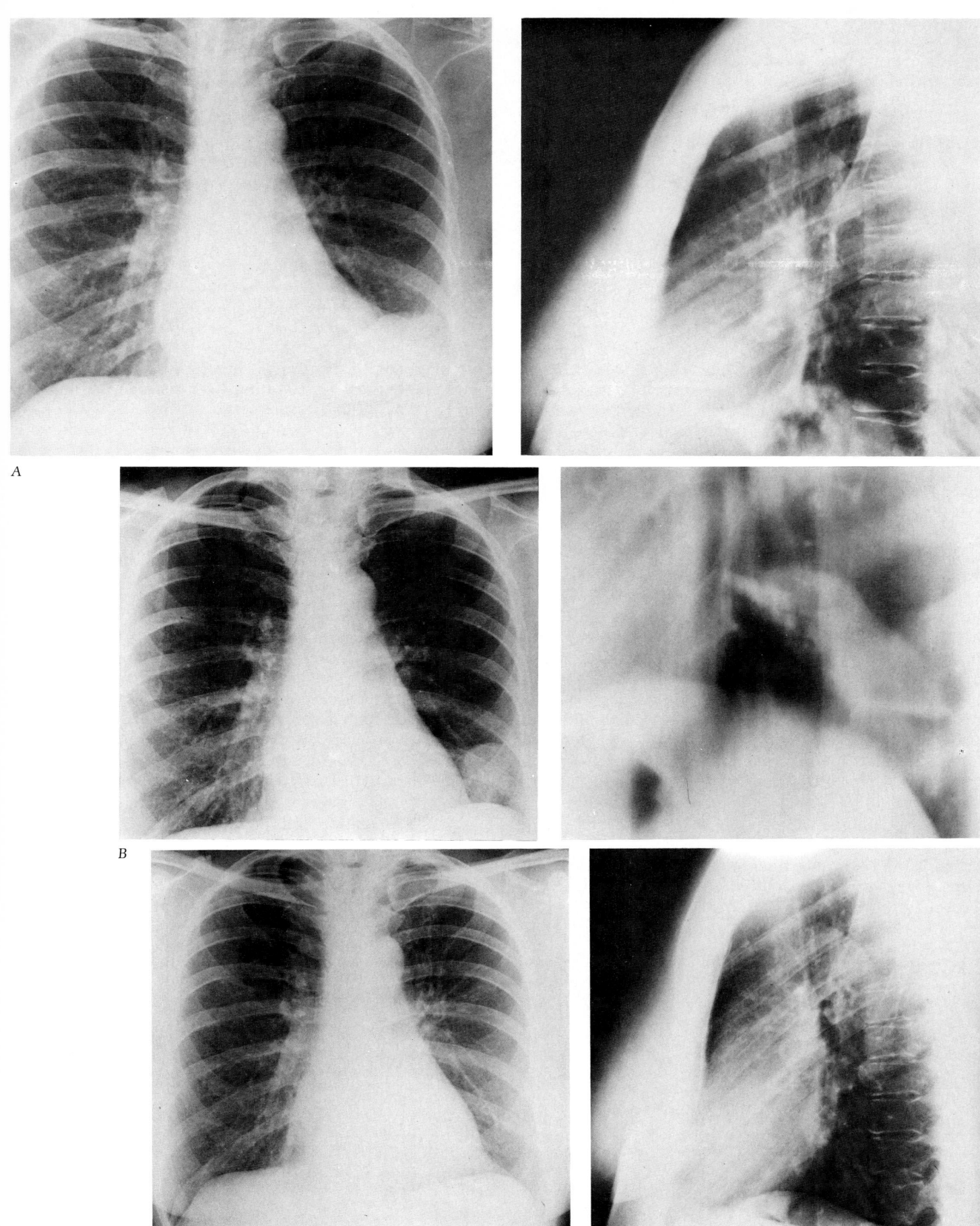

A

B

C

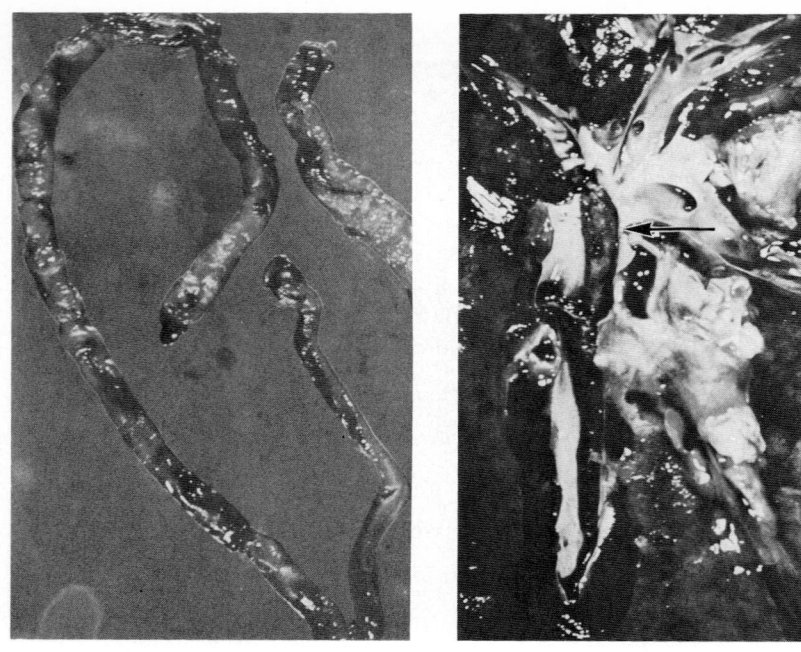

A   B

FIGURE 66-7 Thromboembolism. *A.* Massive venous thrombus. *B.* Venous thrombus lodged in pulmonary artery. *(Courtesy of Dr. G. G. Pietra.)*

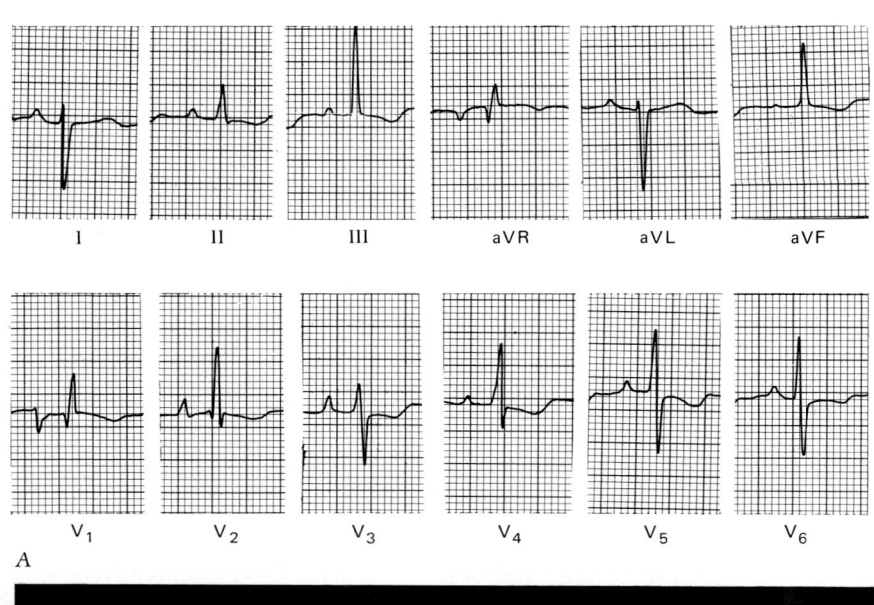

A

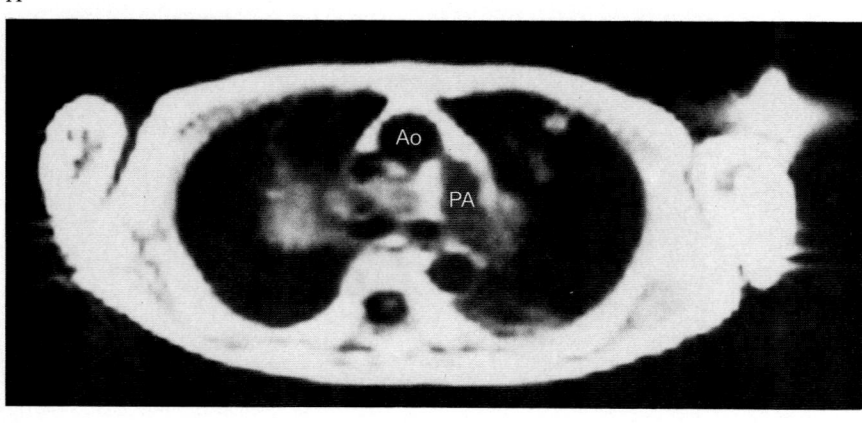

B

FIGURE 66-8 Massive pulmonary embolism. *A.* Electrocardiogram from a 26-year-old woman who experienced a massive pulmonary embolism. Sinus tachycardia. An RS pattern is seen in lead I and a tall R in lead III, accompanied by T-wave inversion in lead III and leads V_1 to V_6. The precordial transition zone is shifted to the left. The QRS pattern suggests incomplete bundle branch block. At autopsy, fresh massive emboli as well as evidence of old emboli were found in the main pulmonary arteries. *B.* Magnetic resonance image (MRI) of a 66-year-old woman with massive pulmonary embolism that totally occluded the left pulmonary artery. This vessel (LPA) projects a gray image associated with little or no blood flow. This contrasts with the black image projected by the lumen of the aorta (Ao) where blood flow is rapid.

◀ **FIGURE 66-6** Resolution of a pulmonary infarct. A 48-year-old woman with known adenocarcinoma of the ovary for 2 years, admitted with a swollen leg. *A.* Posteroanterior and lateral views 19 days after admission. The shadow of the pulmonary infarct blends with that of the left pleural effusion and diaphragm. *B.* Twenty-five days after admission. A discrete nodular shadow, about 4 cm in diameter is seen on the PA view. A lateral body section shows the elliptical appearance of the infarcted area. *C.* Five months after admission. The evidence of pulmonary infarction is gone. *(Courtesy of Dr. S. Eisman.)*

of pulmonary infarction and peripheral emboli. These are considered subsequently.

Rarely in massive occlusion of the central pulmonary arteries does the chest radiograph reveal dilatation and engorgement of the unaffected pulmonary arterial tree, diminished vascularity and increased radiolucency on the affected side, and dilatation of the heart (right ventricle and atrium). However, the affected vessel sometimes shows an abrupt "cutoff" that marks the end of the clot; occasionally, the edge of the embolus is visible. Angiography is much more definitive in defining the nature and extent of the catastrophic event (Fig. 66-9).

Acute Pulmonary Infarction

Only about 10 percent of pulmonary emboli elicit clinical and radiographic evidence of infarction (Fig. 66-6). Pulmonary infarction is generally manifested by acute onset of pleural pain, breathlessness, pleural friction rub, pleural effusion, or hemoptysis. The pleuritic pain is often sharp and localized to the ribs but, depending on the location of the infarct, can be referred to the shoulder or abdomen. As a result of the pain, mobility of one hemithorax may be diminished. Although the severity of the pain and the acuity of onset can simulate that of myocardial ischemia, its pleuritic nature and failure to respond to nitroglycerin are usually helpful in establishing its identity.

Infarcts characteristically are juxtaposed to pleural surfaces (Fig. 66-1). On the chest radiograph, the infarct sometimes appears as a wedge-shaped opacity at the periphery of the lung. However, fresh infarcts are usually much more nonspecific in appearance, often simulating a

bronchopneumonia (Fig. 66-10). Usually several days are required for the nondescript infarcted area to assume a distinctive radiographic appearance (Fig. 66-6). Often the infarct is obscured by a pleural effusion so that only after the effusion has been removed or resorbed does the identity of the infarct become evident. The nature of the pleural fluid that accompanies pulmonary infarction is considered elsewhere (see Chapter 135). A pulmonary infarct in a costophrenic angle bears close resemblance to pleural thickening or free fluid, but often its border is convex toward the hilus (Hampton hump) rather than concave (Fig. 66-11).

Pulmonary Embolism without Infarction

Submassive embolization without infarction is the most common and difficult syndrome to evaluate (Fig. 66-12). Usually emboli are multiple, so that infarcted and noninfarcted areas of occlusion coexist. Emboli that do not cause infarction lack the diagnostic specificity of pulmonary infarction (group II) or of massive embolization (group I) (Fig. 66-13). Instead, the hallmarks of this syndrome are meager: unexplained tachypnea, dyspnea, and tachycardia. The more extensive the embolization, the more apt is breathlessness to be severe and persistent; often this unexplained dyspnea is associated with anxiety and substernal oppression. Tachypnea and tachycardia persist during sleep. Syncope is uncommon, usually occurring in association with a large central clot. Recurrent episodes of breathlessness in individuals predisposed to venous thrombosis should automatically alert the physician not only to the prospect of pulmonary embolization

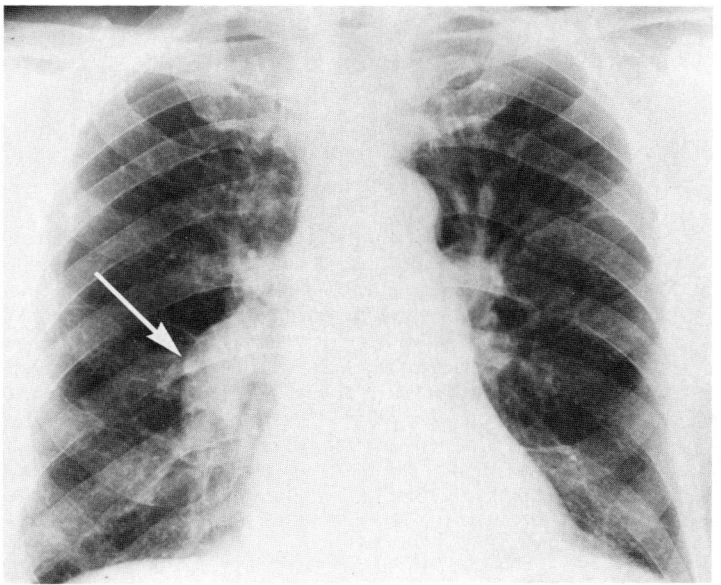

A

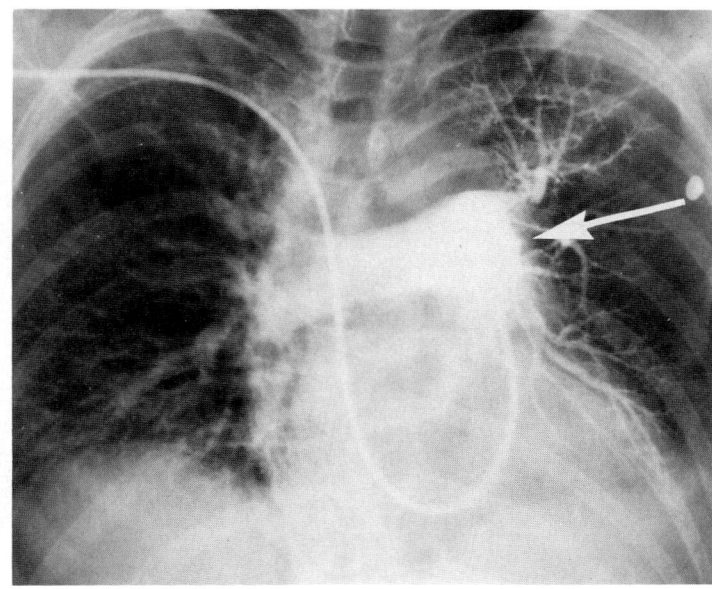

B

FIGURE 66-9   Massive pulmonary embolism.   *A.* Chest radiograph in massive pulmonary embolism. Portable radiograph showing abrupt cutoff of the right pulmonary artery (arrow) and ipsilateral hypovascularity.   *B.* Angiogram (another patient). Arrow indicates abrupt cutoff.

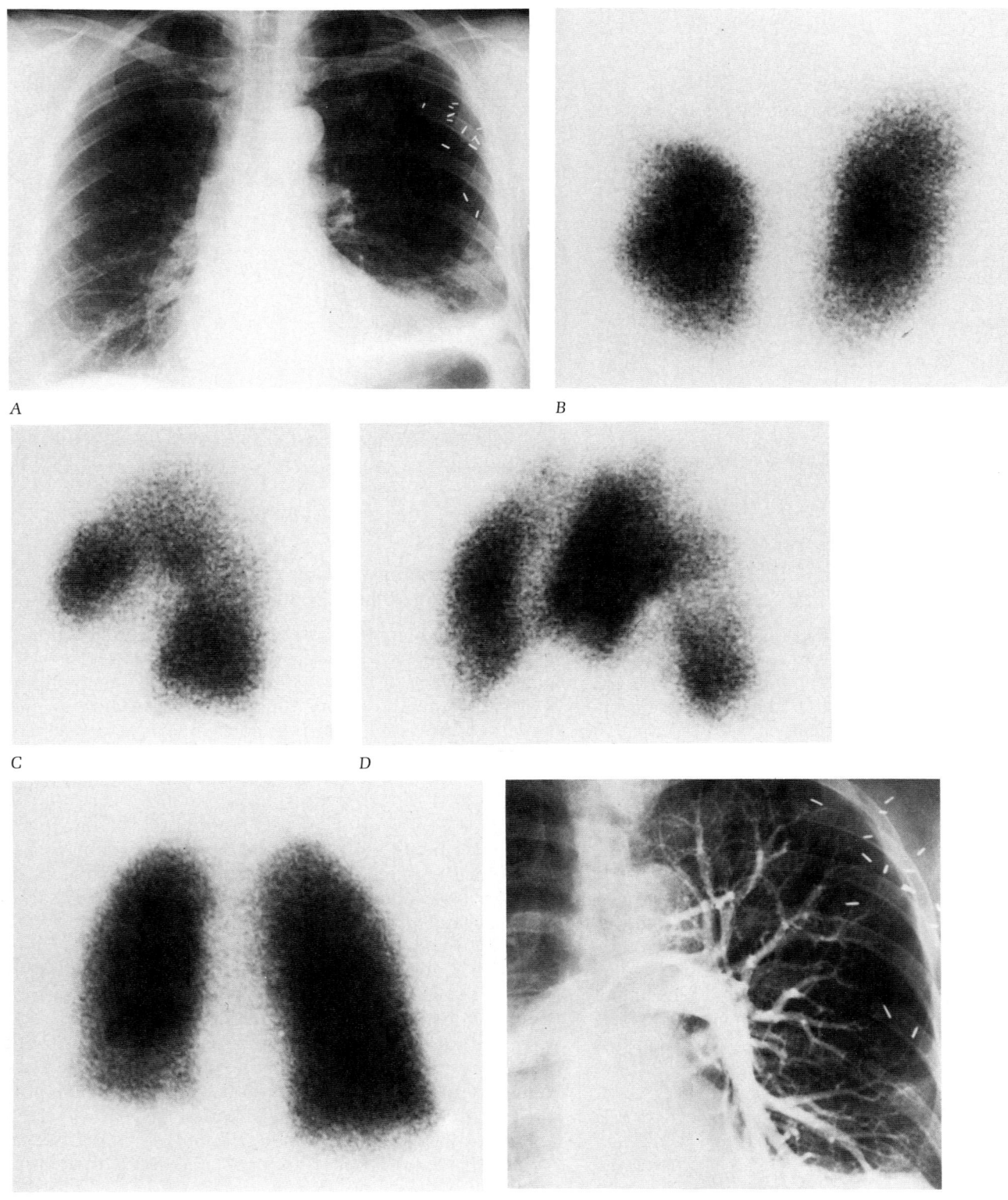

FIGURE 66-10 Pulmonary emboli and infarction. A 66-year-old woman who had a recent left radical mastectomy complained of left pleuritic pain. *A.* Posteroanterior radiograph. Pleural effusion, atelectasis, and pulmonary infiltrate in the left lower lobe. *B, C,* and *D.* Perfusion lung scan. A wedge-shaped defect is present in the left lower lobe on the anterior (*B*), left lateral (*C*), and left anterior oblique (*D*) projections. *E.* Ventilation lung scan (posterior view). Ventilation is decreased at the left base in the area of the abnormality on the chest radiograph. *F.* Selective pulmonary arteriogram. Areas of multiple pulmonary emboli are present in the left lower lobe.

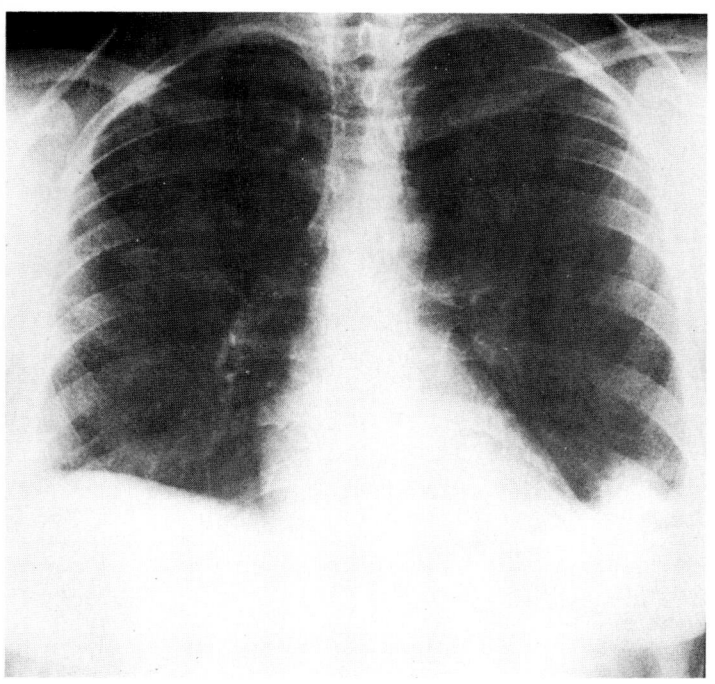

FIGURE 66-11 Hampton hump. A pulmonary infarct presenting as a pleural-based, wedge-shaped parenchymal lesion.

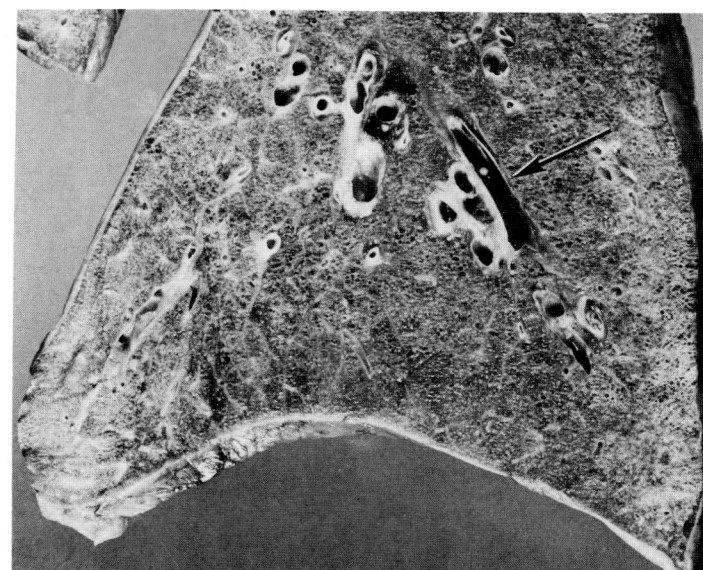

FIGURE 66-12 Pulmonary embolus in a medium-sized vessel without infarction. (Courtesy of Dr. G. G. Pietra.)

but also to the possibility of sudden death. On rare occasions, especially if right atrial pressures are high, e.g., secondary to pulmonary hypertension, a pulmonary embolus traverses a patent foramen ovale to enter the systemic circulation and produce "paradoxical embolization" of a systemic organ, e.g., the brain.

The physical examination is rarely helpful except for tachypnea and tachycardia. Pleuritic pain sometimes occurs even though there is no radiographic evidence of pulmonary infarction; it is intensified by deep breathing or by pressure on the overlying ribs. A few rales are occasionally identified in the area of embolism, often in association with a decrease in breath sounds; a local wheeze sometimes occurs.

The chest radiograph is often normal and is rarely diagnostic. One hemidiaphragm is occasionally elevated, presumably a consequence of ipsilateral pneumoconstriction; platelike areas of atelectasis appear at the lung bases as linear streaks that parallel the diaphragm (Fleischner lines); or large parts of the lung are avascular (Westermark's sign). Taken separately, these radiographic criteria are rarely diagnostic; but, in a candidate for pulmonary embolization, a high diaphragm on one side accompanied by Fleischner lines, an area of distinct hypovascularity, a nondescript area of pulmonary consolidation, or a small pleural effusion lend support to the impression that embolization has occurred. This impression can be reinforced by lung scans, but angiography is often needed to clinch the diagnosis.

Multiple Pulmonary Emboli (Pulmonary Microthromboembolism)

The category of *multiple pulmonary emboli* has traditionally included two different kinds of patients. The first subset consists of those who have had documented episodes of systemic venous thrombosis or pulmonary emboli over the years. The repeated emboli gradually give rise to pulmonary hypertension, and the patients may die suddenly or in cor pulmonale and heart failure (Fig. 66-14).

The second subset consists of individuals who, without a prior history of thrombosis or emboli, gradually become incapacitated, usually over a period of months to years, by insidious breathlessness, nondescript episodes of precordial pain, and mounting anxiety; by biopsy or autopsy, they prove to have widespread occlusive disease due to thrombi or emboli in the minute arteries and arterioles of the lungs. Because of the widespread nature of these lesions in the pulmonary microcirculation, the relative uniformity of their appearance, and the possibility that they represent local thrombi (due to local malfunction of pulmonary vascular endothelium rather than minute emboli), some clinicians and pathologists now refer to their entity as *pulmonary microthromboembolic disease.* The course of individuals in this second group often mimics that of primary pulmonary hypertension, i.e., progressive breathlessness, right ventricular enlargement (cor pulmonale), or even right ventricular failure without discernible cause (Fig. 66-14).

Whereas the first group clearly has peripheral venous thrombosis and pulmonary embolism as its basis, the rea-

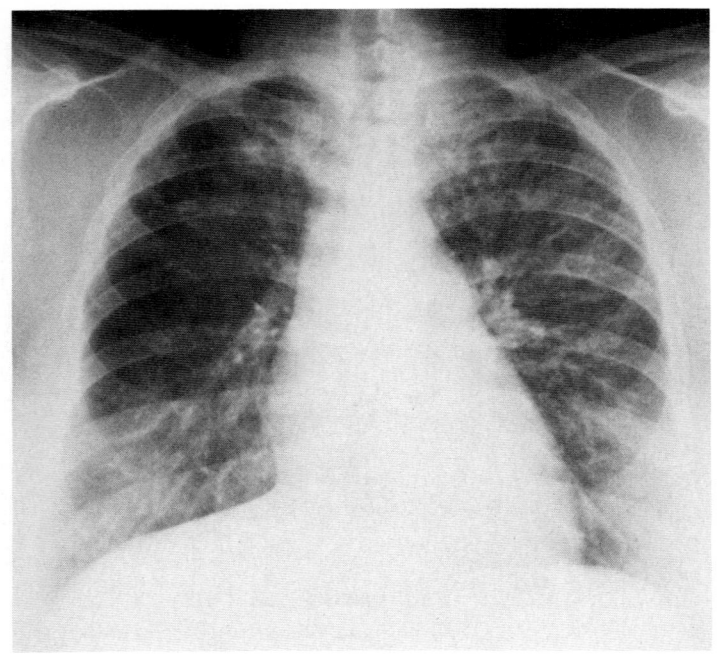

A

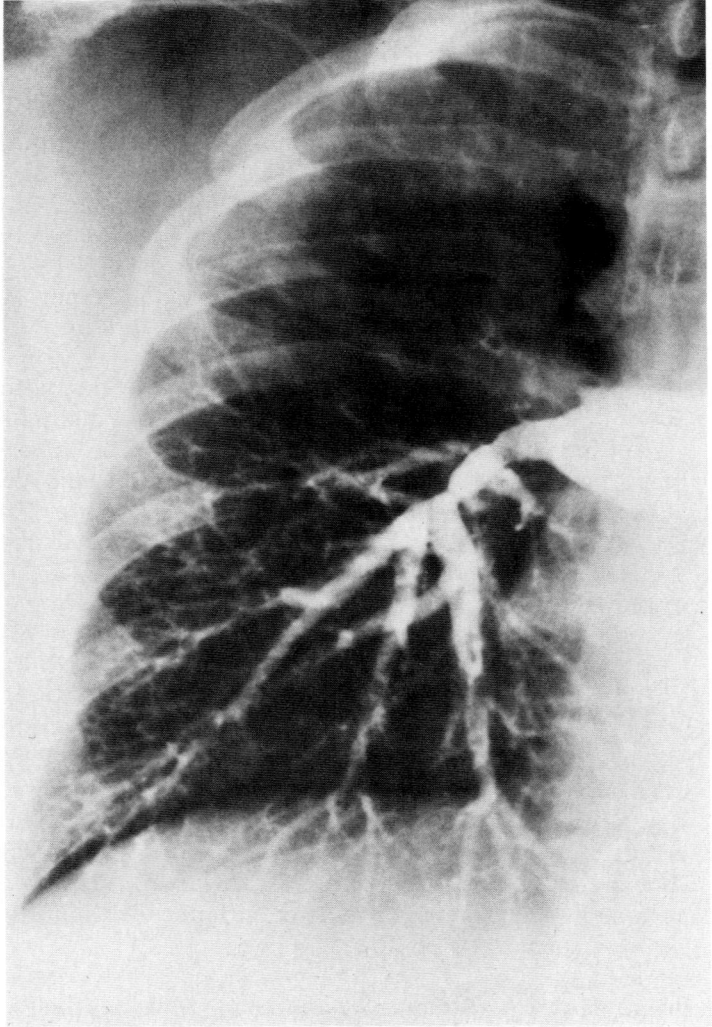

B

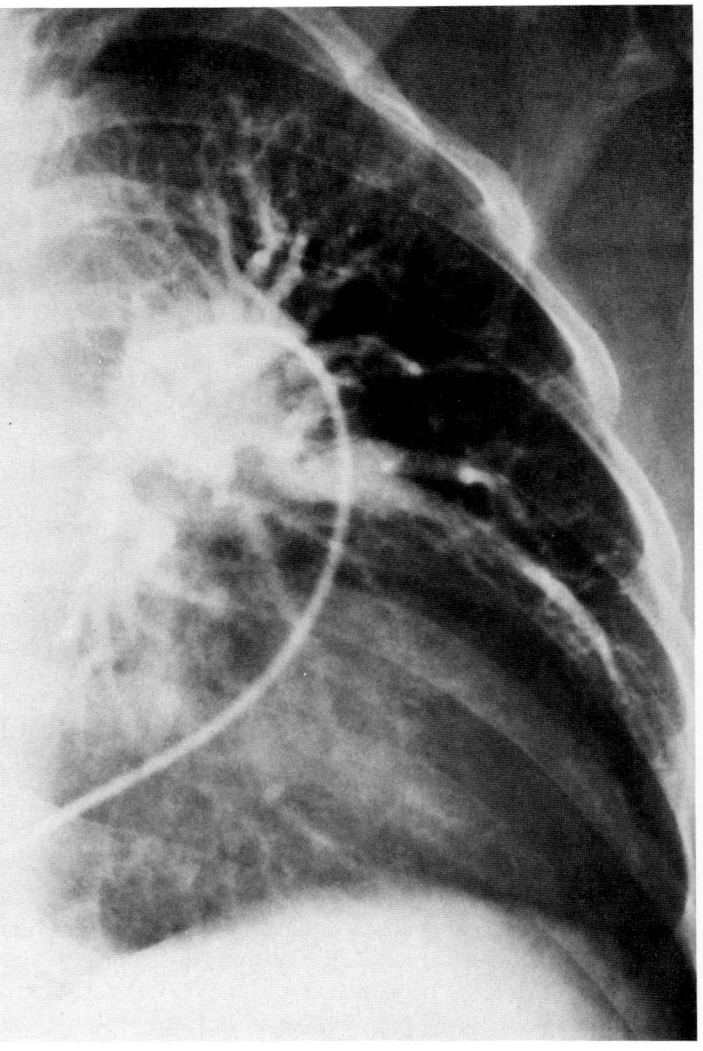

C

FIGURE 66-13 Large pulmonary emboli. A 31-year-old female gymnast admitted for shortness of breath on mild exertion. A. Posteroanterior radiograph. Hyperlucent area with diminished vascular markings over area of right upper lobe. Increased vascularity on left. B. Angiogram. Right lung. Complete lack of blood flow to right upper lobe. C. Angiogram. Left lung. Spotty interruption of blood flow to parts of left upper lobe.

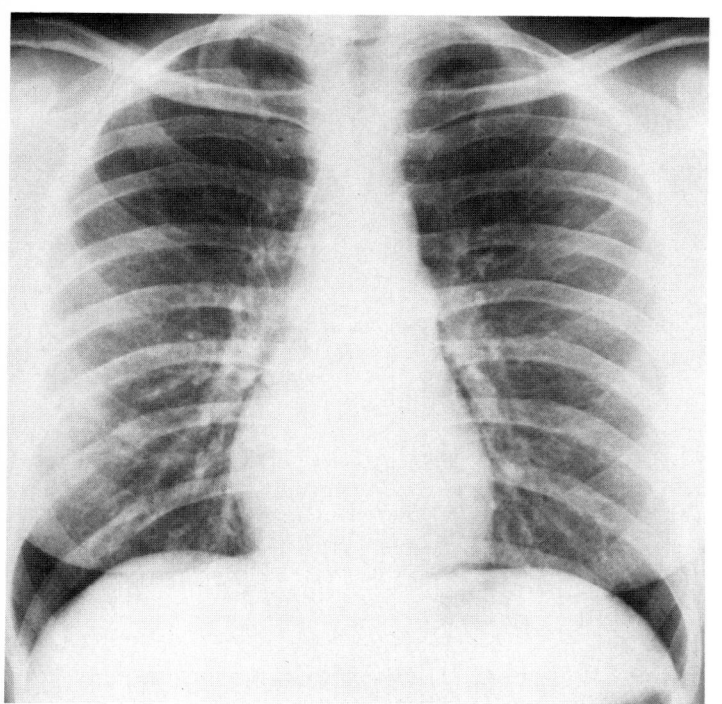

A

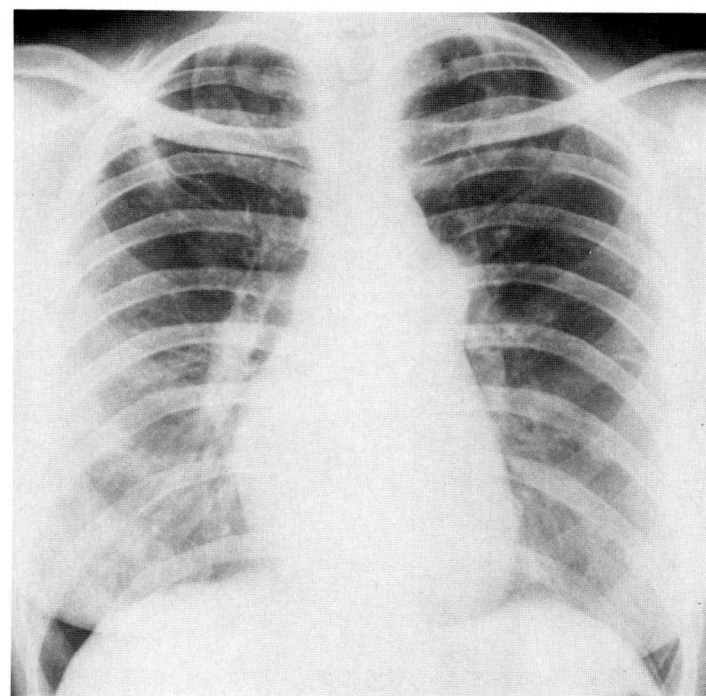

B

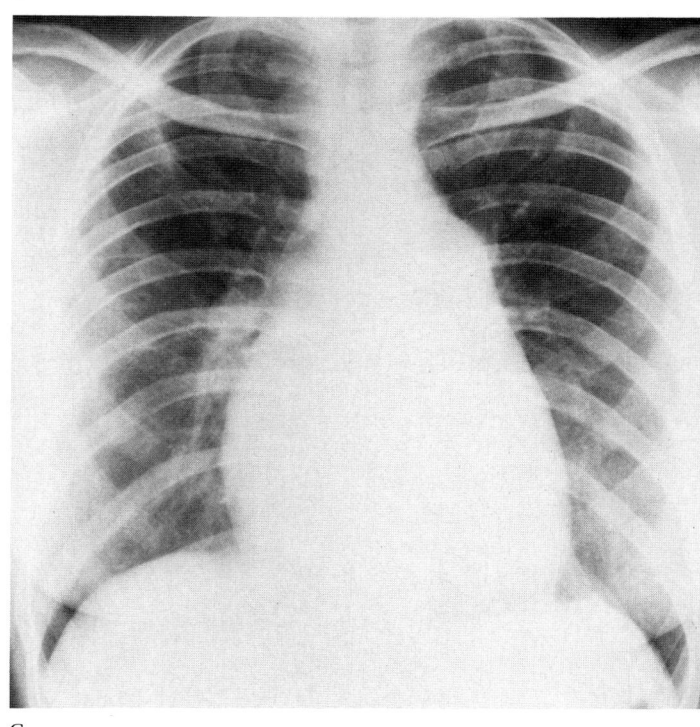

C

FIGURE 66-14 Recurrent pulmonary emboli. A 33-year-old woman who died with clinical diagnosis of "primary pulmonary hypertension." At autopsy widespread occlusion of small pulmonary arteries by organized clot that had undergone variable degrees of recanalization. *A.* On admission for hemoptysis. Cardiac silhouette is within normal limits. *B.* One year later. Cardiac enlargement with prominent central pulmonary artery. *C.* Two years after admission and shortly before death. Cardiomegaly, prominent central pulmonary arteries, and bilateral attenuation of vascular markings.

son for the pulmonary occlusive vascular disease is generally much less evident in those of the second group who lack either clear-cut history or peripheral thromboses or overt emboli and in whom the microcirculation of the lungs is almost exclusively affected. In this group, the likelihood of widespread endothelial damage predisposing to local pulmonary thrombosis is as tenable as the idea of a shower of covert minute emboli. The syndrome of multiple pulmonary emboli generally terminates in a state of chronic pulmonary hypertension. The latter is considered elsewhere in this book (see Chapter 64). Here it is pertinent to note that more than half of patients with the clinical diagnosis of primary pulmonary hypertension show widespread thrombotic occlusion of pulmonary arterioles and small muscular arteries at biopsy or autopsy. In some instances, the organized and fresh clots appear to be complications of a slowed circulation. But, in the majority, pulmonary microthromboemboli appear to have been the cause of the clinically unexplained pulmonary hypertension.

Unresolved Pulmonary Embolism

Although virtually all patients who survive large, proximal pulmonary emboli undergo clinical, hemodynamic, and angiographic resolution of the clot, in rare instances, pulmonary embolism fails to resolve, leaving large segments of the pulmonary arterial tree occluded by organized clot (Fig. 66-5). The diagnosis requires a high degree of suspicion. In a few instances, a large clot organized in a major pulmonary arterial branch has been mistaken for a carcinoma of the lung. Almost invariably, the patients give a history of a previous embolic episode and are incapacitated by dyspnea. Except for the accentuated P_2 of pulmonary hypertension, the physical findings are not helpful. Arterial hypoxemia generally coexists with the pulmonary hypertension. The electrocardiogram is apt to show right ventricular hypertrophy when cor pulmonale supervenes. The chest radiograph often reveals dilated central pulmonary arteries, sometimes with peripheral pruning over affected parts of the lungs. Lung scans suggest, and angiography demonstrates, the nature of the obliterative vascular process. Most are also left with pulmonary hypertension that is a harbinger of cor pulmonale.

In recent years, the condition has proved to be treatable by surgically removing the organized occlusive clot(s), i.e., by thromboendarterectomy rather than embolectomy. Immediately after the occluded vessel is reopened, and for a few days thereafter, the patient is apt to experience "reperfusion" pulmonary edema confined to the vascular bed that has been reopened. The improvement after embolectomy is often dramatic, clearly arresting the previous downhill course. The procedure is technically difficult and, in the most experienced hands, the mortality rate to date is of the order of 10 to 15 percent.

DIAGNOSTIC MEASURES

It has been noted above that, except for massive pulmonary emboli that threaten life because of circulatory collapse, the clot in the lungs is of little therapeutic concern. In time, even an area of infarcted lung will clear spontaneously. Much more important is the threat of a devastating embolus from a clot that may be propagating beyond its restraints in a peripheral deep vein.

Diagnostic measures currently take two directions: the embolus in the lungs and the thrombus in a systemic deep vein.

Pulmonary Emboli

Most important is the identification of the individual who is predisposed to systemic venous thrombosis. The existence of a predisposing mechanism, particularly venous stasis, in a patient with sudden onset of unexplained breathlessness is of utmost diagnostic importance. Other common important predisposing factors are carcinoma (especially of the lung or pancreas), the use of oral contraceptives, prolonged bed rest, recent surgery, trauma, congestive heart failure, and preexisting thromboembolic disease. Unfortunately, proving that embolization has occurred can be difficult: as a rule, neither the clinical appraisal, nor the chest radiograph, nor the conventional laboratory tests prove that pulmonary embolization has, or has not, occurred. Pulmonary angiography is the most reliable of the tests currently available.

CLINICAL SIGNS AND SYMPTOMS

In pulmonary embolism, the diagnostic yield from signs and symptoms is notoriously poor. Tachypnea, pleuritic pain, and hemoptysis are nonspecific. Similarly, a pleural rub, an exaggerated pulmonic component of the second heart sound, and overt phlebitis occur in other clinical disorders.

The mainstay for the diagnosis of pulmonary embolism is a high degree of clinical suspicion. The so-called classic syndrome of acute shortness of breath, pleuritic chest pain, and acute heart failure is rarely seen. More typical is an aggravation of the antecedent dyspnea, the onset of unexplained chest pain or arrhythmia, or the occurrence of a new fever.

LABORATORY DATA

The white blood cell count and serial determinations of enzyme concentrations in serum have proved to be of little value in the diagnosis of pulmonary embolism. The white blood cell count is generally normal or slightly increased; at times it is quite high. Similarly, the triad of an increase in the concentration of lactic dehydrogenase and bilirubin in the serum coupled with a normal concentra-

tion of transaminase, once believed to be suggestive of pulmonary embolism, has proved to be nonspecific.

The determination of the concentrations of fibrin degradation products in serum, although attractive in principle, suffers from a lack of uniformity in standards. Moreover, false-positive results have been encountered in such diverse conditions as surgery, trauma, renal disease, and systemic lupus erythematosus. Until more reliable and specific techniques are developed, studies of this kind have little diagnostic value.

ELECTROCARDIOGRAM

The most common electrocardiographic findings in pulmonary embolism are nonspecific STT wave changes. Except in massive embolization, the pattern of right ventricular strain with an S1/Q3/T3 pattern is unusual. Atrial arrhythmias are common in pulmonary embolism but may be seen in a variety of other disorders. Thus, the electrocardiogram is nonspecific in the diagnosis of pulmonary embolism, and its major value may be in identifying other clinical disorders, e.g., acute myocardial infarction.

ARTERIAL BLOOD GASES

The diagnostic value of arterial blood gases in pulmonary embolism is supportive at best. As a rule, the arterial P_{O_2} is somewhat low, as is the arterial P_{CO_2}. Although arterial blood gases are abnormal in the great majority of patients with pulmonary embolism, similar changes are often seen in conditions that enter into the differential diagnosis of pulmonary embolism. Also, in about 10 to 15 percent of patients with pulmonary embolism, arterial blood gases and alveolar-arterial differences in P_{O_2} are normal. As a rule, these patients are young with a normal pulmonary circulation prior to embolization and with a modest burden of clot after embolization. Thus, in diagnosing pulmonary embolism, arterial blood gases can be weighed only in the balance.

CHEST RADIOGRAPHY

It is uncommon for the chest radiograph in pulmonary embolism to be normal. More typically, the chest radiograph shows either infiltrate, or effusion, or atelectasis, or a combination of the three. Similar findings occur in pneumonia, pleuritis, and congestive heart failure. The classic finding of a peripheral wedge-shaped infarct (Hamptom hump) is uncommon, whereas Westermark's sign, another "classic" sign characterized by hypoperfusion of one lung secondary to massive pulmonary embolism, is rare.

The accuracy of radionuclide lung scans for diagnosing pulmonary embolism is currently being explored as part of a large, multicenter study sponsored by the National Institutes of Health. This study, entitled "Prospec-tive Investigation of Pulmonary Diagnosis" (PIOPED), may shed considerable light on the objectivity of lung scans in diagnosing pulmonary embolism (see Chapter 166).

Studies currently under way indicate that the lung scan is an excellent screening test to *exclude* the diagnosis of pulmonary embolism: no instance has been reported of a normal perfusion scan in an individual who proved to have a pulmonary embolism by angiography or at postmortem.

However, a diagnostic dilemma does arise when perfusion abnormalities are found on the lung scan. Originally, a key criterion for diagnosing ventilation-perfusion scans as being of "high probability" was a normal ventilation scan in the face of perfusion defects. This dictum has since proved to be only partially tenable: in about 25 percent of patients who have pulmonary emboli, ventilation defects correspond in distribution to the perfusion defects. Also, multiple, small nonsegmental perfusion defects (particularly when matched by ventilation defects) were once interpreted confidently as "low probability scans" since the pattern suggested underlying parenchymal lung disease, e.g., chronic obstructive airways disease. However, it has become clear that the same pattern can be produced by emboli that have partially recanalized, thereby reducing the size of scan defects so that they become innocuous in appearance. Pulmonary emboli have been found in up to 20 percent of patients with these "low probability" scan patterns.

The inaccuracy of the abnormal lung scan is unfortunate since lung scans are technically simple, noninvasive, and widely available. However, the only conclusive statement that can now be made is that a normal perfusion scan excludes the diagnosis of pulmonary embolism, whereas an abnormal perfusion scan supports it.

PULMONARY ANGIOGRAPHY

The pulmonary angiogram remains the most accurate diagnostic study in evaluating pulmonary embolism (Fig. 66-15). Two angiographic findings in large vessels are characteristic of pulmonary embolism: a filling defect is the more common and reliable; a *cutoff* of the radiopaque stream is not as convincing. Although angiography in experienced hands has a very low morbidity and mortality, it does entail right heart catheterization with its associated risks. The injection of contrast material intravenously is also inevitably attended by some risk. Nonetheless, angiography generally causes only a minor threat to life compared with the hazards of pulmonary embolization.

When properly done, using magnification and selective injections and views, pulmonary angiography can detect clots as small as 0.5 mm. With rare exceptions, a normal angiogram excludes the diagnosis of embolism in all but the minute vessels of the lungs. Another exception

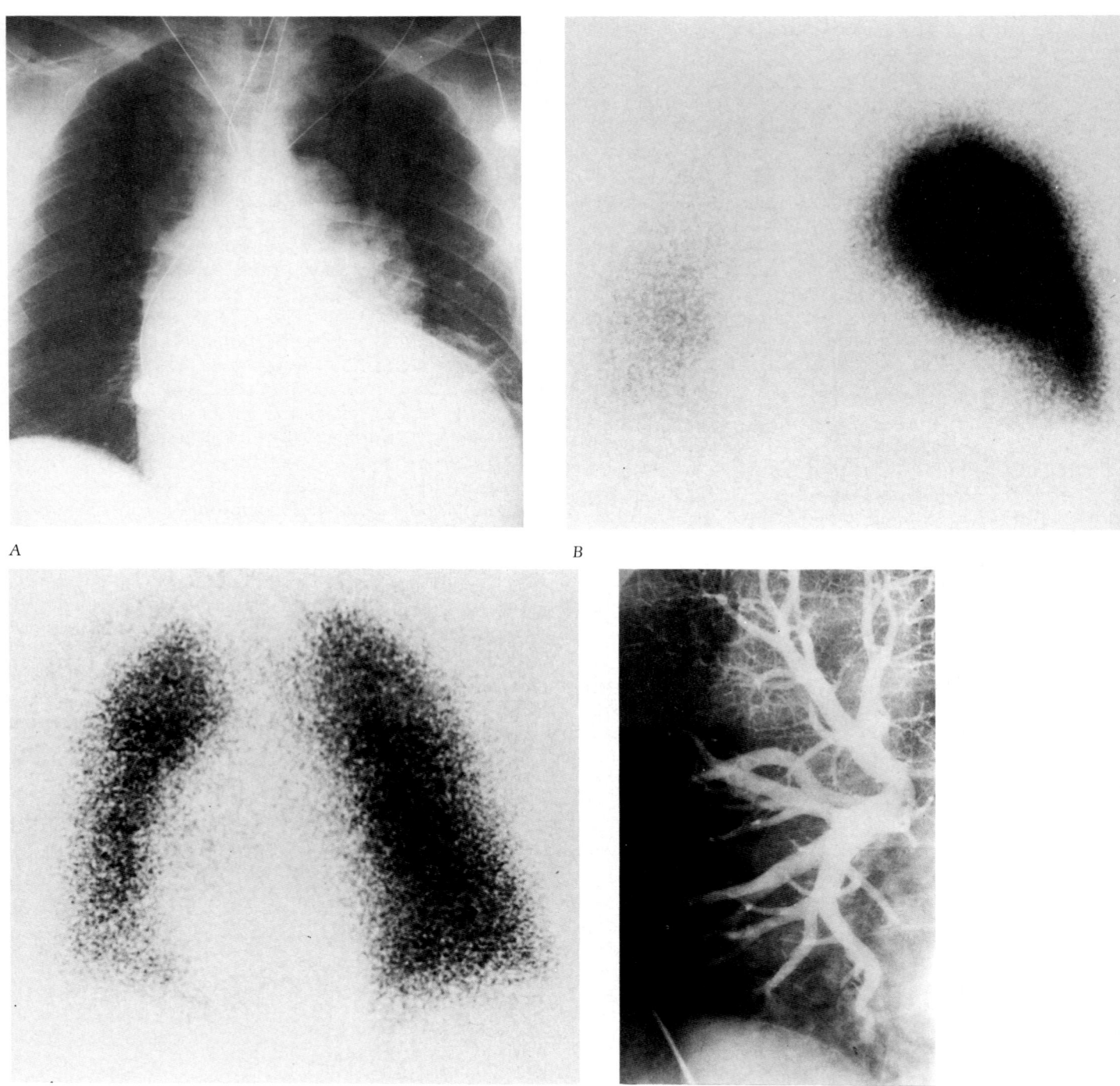

A

B

C

D

FIGURE 66-15 Compression of pulmonary artery simulating massive pulmonary embolism. A 72-year-old man with a history of thoracic aortic aneurysm. Presented with sudden onset of dyspnea. *A.* Chest radiograph cardiomegaly and enlarged thoracic aorta. Lung markings decreased in right lung. *B.* Perfusion lung scan (anterior view). Perfusion to the entire right lung is markedly decreased. *C.* Ventilation scan. No abnormalities attributable to emboli. *D.* Pulmonary arteriogram. No emboli. Extrinsic compression of the right pulmonary artery by the enlarged thoracic aorta.

is incomplete occlusion that allows flow to continue through small pulmonary vessels.

The major flaws of pulmonary angiography are its invasiveness, expense, technical complexity, and limited availability. To reduce these disadvantages, digital subtraction angiography has been developed whereby a bolus of contrast material is injected into a large peripheral vein, and the resultant radiographic image of the pulmonary circulation is enhanced through special computerized techniques. Unfortunately, this method has not proven to be as sensitive as pulmonary angiography and, in most medical centers, its use for the diagnosis of pulmonary embolism has been abandoned.

OTHER DIAGNOSTIC TECHNIQUES

As described in Chapter 36, magnetic resonance imaging (MRI) of the lung is undergoing rapid development (Fig. 66-8B). In theory, this technique would be ideal for studying pulmonary embolism because contrast between flowing blood and clot would be expected to be enhanced. To date, only massive pulmonary emboli have been visualized using MRI (Fig. 66-8B). Definition of the future role of MRI in the diagnosis of pulmonary embolism awaits perfection of techniques for improving resolution and eliminating artifacts.

Another approach to imaging relies on the use of radioactive substances that are incorporated into clots. Certain substances, such as labeled fibrinogen and platelets, require active clot formation for the radionuclide to be incorporated into its substance. Using these techniques, an image can be obtained only after several days, i.e., an impractical delay for the diagnosis of pulmonary embolism.

More recently, a labeled antibody directed against fibrin is being tested. This approach does not require that the clot be forming, since the fibrin protein is found on the surface of most clots, regardless of their age.

TREATMENT

The agents and interventions available for the prevention and treatment of thromboembolism are considered in detail in Chapter 65. Here certain aspects of management will be enlarged upon.

Prophylaxis

A recent Consensus Development Conference on "Prevention of Venous Thrombosis and Pulmonary Embolism," sponsored by the National Heart, Lung and Blood Institute, came to certain conclusions that bear reiteration: (1) screening tests for deep venous thrombosis (^{125}I-fibrinogen uptake and/or venography) are useful markers in suspected pulmonary embolism, (2) many common medical conditions and surgical procedures (Table 66-1) are associated with a high incidence of deep venous thrombosis that predisposes to pulmonary embolism, and (3) prophy-

laxis should be undertaken whenever feasible in these high-risk patient groups.

As a rule, prophylaxis begins with elevation of the foot of the bed, gradient elastic stockings, and external pneumatic compression. Estrogen therapy or the use of contraceptive pills is discontinued before surgery. Low dose heparin (5000 units given subcutaneously every 8 to 12 h, starting 2 h before surgery and continued until the patient is ambulatory) reduces the incidence of deep venous thrombosis in many, but not all, surgical patients.

Low dose heparin has proved effective in preventing deep venous thrombosis in general surgical patients and in moderate- to high-risk gynecologic and obstetrical patients. Protection from the prophylactic use of low dose heparin is more difficult to prove in patients undergoing orthopedic surgery. In patients undergoing elective surgery of the hip or reconstruction of the knee, adjusted-dose heparin or warfarin may be required to treat phlebitis. Low dose heparin (or other anticoagulants) can be hazardous in neurosurgical patients; preventive external leg compression is an effective alternative in this group.

With respect to medical conditions, low dose heparin

TABLE 66-1

Common Surgical Procedures and Medical Conditions Predisposing to Deep Venous Thrombosis and Pulmonary Embolism

Surgical procedures
  General surgery in patients >40 years
  Orthopedic surgery of the lower extremities
  Urologic surgery
  Gynecology and obstetrics
  Neurosurgery
  Trauma*
Medical conditions†
  Low cardiac output states
  Prior thromboembolism
  Obesity
  Polycythemia vera
  Immobilization
  Stroke
  Inflammatory bowel disease
  Paroxysmal nocturnal hemoglobinuria
  Cancer
  Nephrotic syndrome
  Estrogen therapy
  Sepsis
  Lupus anticoagulant

* Especially fractured hip in the elderly and acute injury of the head and spinal cord.

† Other than inherited deficiencies of inhibitors or regulators of coagulation or fibrinolysis.

SOURCE: Based on Consensus Development Conference, National Institutes of Health, March, 1986.

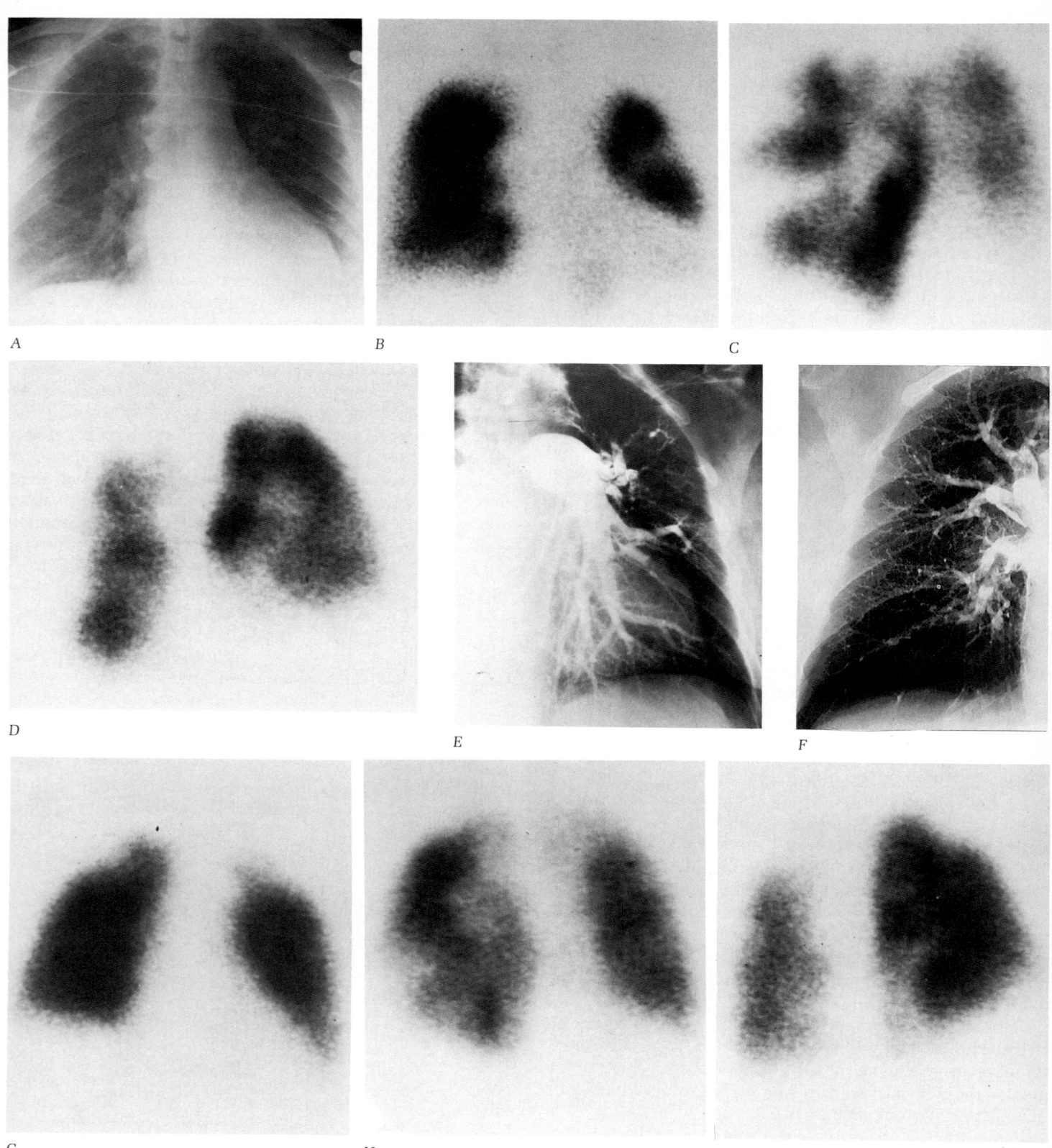

FIGURE 66-16 Streptokinase infusion for large pulmonary emboli. A 72-year-old woman with bilateral ankle fractures. Sudden onset of severe dyspnea. *A.* Portable chest radiograph. Slight cardiomegaly and clear lung fields. *B, C,* and *D.* Perfusion scan. Multiple defects in both lungs, well shown in anterior (*B*), left posterior oblique (*C*), and right posterior oblique (*D*) views. Most defects are in the left lung. Ventilation scan (not shown) was normal. *E* and *F.* Pulmonary arteriogram. Multiple emboli are lodged at branching sites of left (*E*) and right (*F*) pulmonary arteries. *G, H,* and *I.* Four days after a 24-h infusion of streptokinase. The perfusion scan is greatly improved. Only small defects remain in the anterior (*G*), left posterior oblique (*H*), and right posterior oblique (*I*) projections.

is used in low-output states to prevent deep venous thrombosis. In patients who are chronically predisposed to thrombosis because of a slowed circulation, warfarin therapy can be useful.

Fibrinolytic Agents

As noted in Chapter 65, heparin arrests clot formation enabling the endogenous thrombolytic system of the body to slowly dissolve the clot. Fibrinolysis occurs spontaneously when an *endogenous* serum protease, i.e., blood- or tissue-type plasminogen activator (t-PA), binds (with high affinity) to a fibrin clot; fibrin-bound plasminogen is then activated to plasmin, which dissolves the clot. In physiological amounts, t-PA does not bind to circulating plasminogen. Therefore, it does not produce circulating plasmin, which would induce systemic fibrinolysis or fibrinogenolysis. Nor are circulating inhibitors of plasmin, particularly α_2-antiplasmin, depleted by the clot-selective action of t-PA. Indeed, it seems as though the plasmin that is generated locally by t-PA is protected from circulating α_2-antiplasmin by the thrombus and its environment.

Streptokinase and urokinase are *exogenous* systemic activators of the thrombolytic system (Fig. 66-16). Through different mechanisms, these agents convert circulating plasminogen to plasmin. Therefore, doses of streptokinase and urokinase sufficient to cause fibrinolysis of thrombi also generate circulating free plasmin that overwhelms and depletes α_2-antiplasmin and other plasma inhibitors. As a result, systemic hemostasis is impaired because of degradation of circulating fibrinogen and other coagulation proteins and because of an increase in fibrin degradation products. Although these exogenous agents do dissolve clots, they also anticoagulate the patient systemically engendering the risk of hemorrhage, particularly from previous sites of injury and invasion, such as arterial puncture.

Urokinase and streptokinase   After extensive clinical trials by the National Heart, Lung and Blood Institute, the current consensus is that the use of these agents (followed by heparin) is reserved for patients in whom pulmonary emboli have produced a hemodynamically unstable, life-threatening situation and in whom there is no overt potential for hemorrhage. For most patients with pulmonary emboli, heparin alone is the agent of choice on two accounts: (1) no proof of greater effectiveness of streptokinase or urokinase beyond the first day, and (2) the greater incidence of serious hemorrhage that attends the use of thrombolytic agents.

In patients with deep vein thrombosis of the extremities, streptokinase or urokinase seems to achieve more rapid lysis of clot and better preservation of venous valves and vascular integrity than does heparin. However, the high incidence of serious bleeding may limit the use of systemic thrombolytic therapy.

Tissue-type plasminogen activator   As indicated above, in contrast to thrombolytic agents (streptokinase and urokinase) that induce a systemic thrombolytic state in order to dissolve a local clot, tissue-type plasminogen activator (t-PA) affords the prospect of lysing clots by forming the active protease plasmin (Fig. 66-17). In principle, tissue plasminogen activator, because of its intense affinity for fibrin, should have its lytic effects restricted to fibrin in thrombi. Initially, t-PA was isolated from uterine tissue and later from a cultured line of human melanoma cells. More recently, cloning and expression of the t-PA gene in *Escherichia coli* using recombinant-DNA technology has made available large quantities of rt-PA for clinical trials.

The most extensive trials to date have been in patients with coronary arterial thrombi. Overall, this experience suggests that recombinant t-PA (rt-PA) is a safe and effective thrombolytic agent when administered in proper dosage (Table 66-2). It is also apparently not inherently toxic or allergenic. Its short half-life in the circulation (5 to 7 min) makes possible the prompt restoration of normal hemostasis. Finally, because it causes limited derangement of hemostatic mechanisms, elaborate monitoring of the activity of the fibrinolytic system is unnecessary. Dosage is a critical element in avoiding complications. The administration of 0.50 to 0.75 mg/kg body weight intravenously generally evokes only slight systemic fibrinolysis and degradation of fibrinogen. In clinical trials of the effectiveness of rt-PA in coronary occlusion, rt-PA proved to be almost twice as effective as streptokinase in opening coronary arteries that had thrombosed and led to myocardial infarction.

Although experience with recombinant t-PA in venous thromboembolic disease in humans is limited, it is promising. In a recent report of 36 patients with angiog-

TABLE 66-2

Hemodynamic and Arterial Blood Gases, before and after Administration of 40 mg of Tissue-Type Plasminogen Activator

	Before	After
RA	17 mmHg	6 mmHg
RV	53/16 mmHg	41/7 mmHg
PA	53/26 mmHg	43/18 mmHg
$\overline{PA}$	40 mmHg	27 mmHg
$\overline{PW}$	10 mmHg	7 mmHg
C.O.	4.88 L/min	5.73 L/min
O_2 administered	100% face mask	2 L/min via nasal cannula
pH	7.48	7.39
pO_2	73 mmHg	82 mmHg
pCO_2	30 mmHg	30 mmHg
HCO_3^-	22 meq/L	18 meq/L

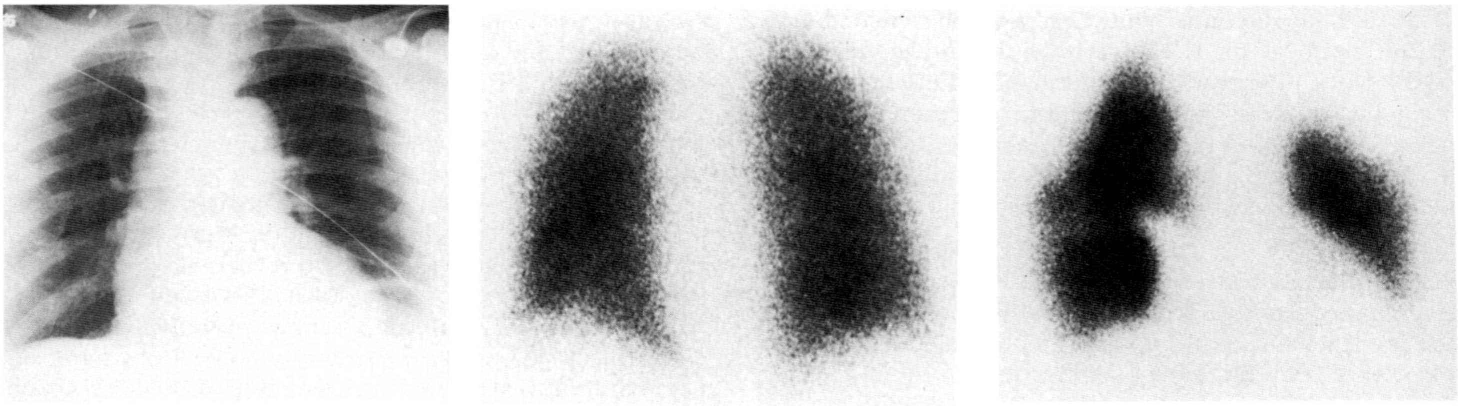

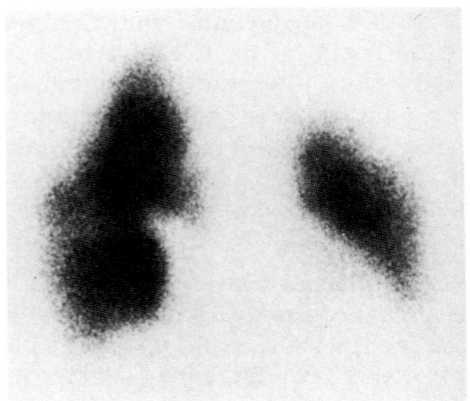

FIGURE 66-17 Tissue-type plasminogen activator (t-PA) in the treatment of acute pulmonary embolism. A 67-year-old male who had undergone an uncomplicated inguinal herniography 2 weeks before presentation. Sudden onset of moderate dyspnea and mild left-sided pleuritic chest pain on day of admission. *A.* Portable chest radiograph. *B* and *C.* Equilibrium phase of the initial ventilation lung scan (*B*) and anterior view of the initial perfusion lung scan (*C*). Ventilation-perfusion scan interpreted as high probability for pulmonary embolism. The patient was heparinized prior to pulmonary angiography. *D.* Pulmonary angiography. Large pulmonary emboli occlude multiple lobar and segmental arteries of the left lung. Clot was also demonstrated in the right lung. The patient received an infusion of 40 mg of recombinant tissue-type plasminogen activator (rt-PA) over 40 min via a peripheral vein. Pulmonary angiography was repeated 90 min after the start of the t-PA infusion. *E.* Post-t-PA pulmonary angiogram. Considerable resolution of the pulmonary emboli. *F* and *G.* Two days after the t-PA infusion. Equilibrium phase of the follow-up ventilation lung scan (*F*) and of the anterior view of the follow-up perfusion lung scan (*G*). Considerable improvement has occurred in the perfusion to both lungs. *(Courtesy of Dr. H. Palevsky.)*

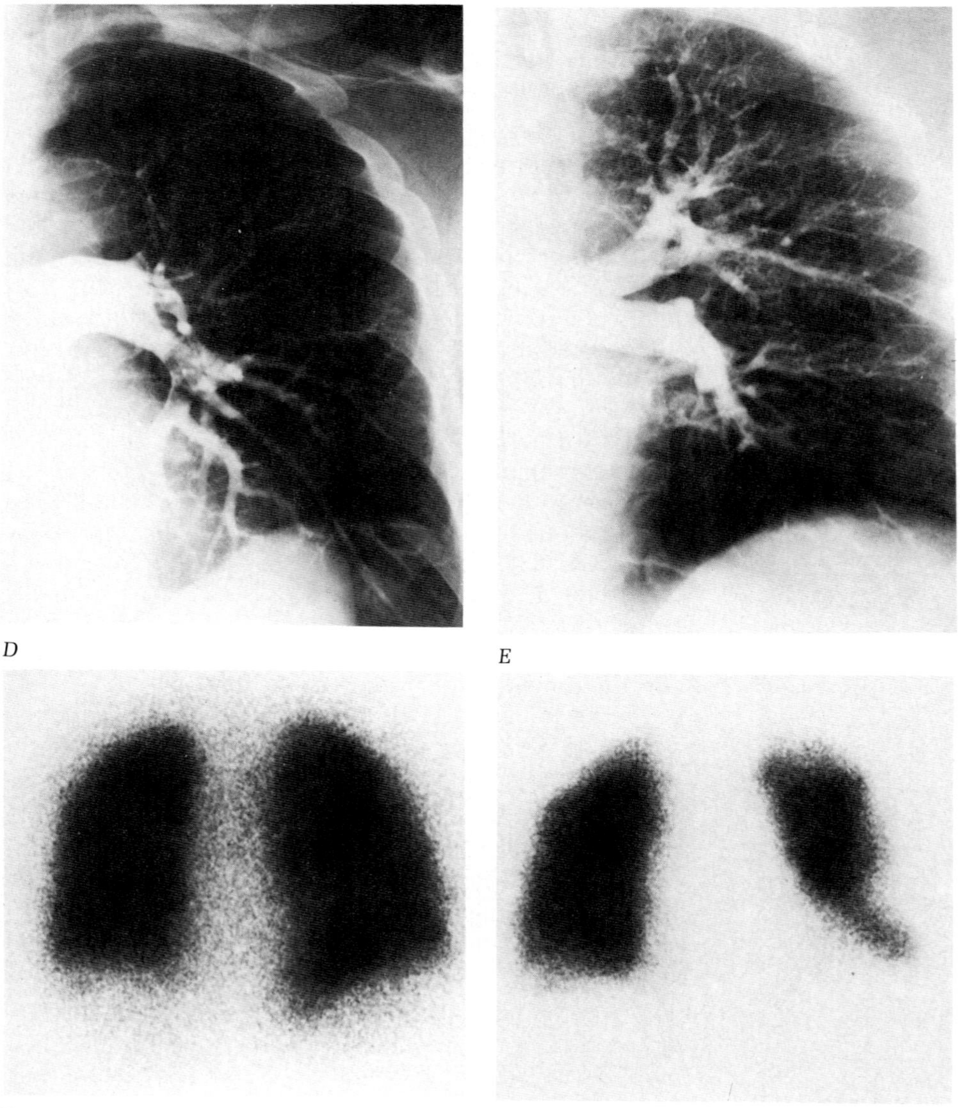

raphically documented pulmonary emboli treated with rt-PA, most patients manifested rapid and marked lysis of the clots. However, in the dosage used (50 mg of rt-PA given intravenously over a 2-h period and then 40 mg over a 4-h period if the initial dosage failed to lyse the clots) systemic complications did occur, ranging from oozing and hematoma at puncture sites (venous and arterial) to more serious bleeding at sites of surgical incision.

Surgical Management

A variety of surgical interventions have been applied in the management of pulmonary emboli. A few have been directed at removing large clots from the pulmonary arteries. But most are designed to deal with peripheral venous thrombosis, e.g., by ligation, plication, or clipping of the inferior vena cava or by placing an umbrella in it (Fig. 66-18). These are considered elsewhere (see Chapter 65).

PROGNOSIS

In acute pulmonary embolism, once therapeutic measures are taken to prevent further formation of thrombi (anticoagulation) or to deny thrombi in the legs access to the lungs (e.g., interruption or blockade of the inferior vena cava), death from embolism is uncommon. Exceptions do occur, even after effective anticoagulation with heparin, particularly if associated disorders persist that predispose to recurrent thrombosis. Also, in some patients who have undergone ligation of the inferior vena cava, emboli recur, presumably either by way of collateral venous channels or from a cul-de-sac above the ligation.

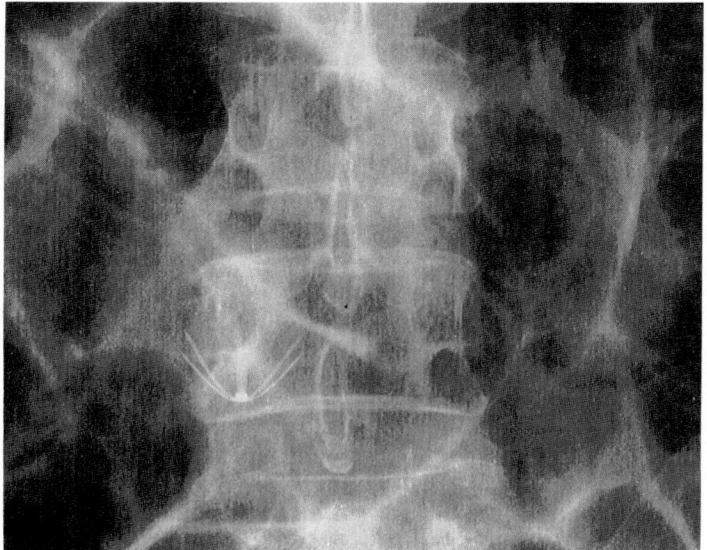

FIGURE 66-18 Umbrella for repeated thromboemboli. A 57-year-old woman with recurrent pulmonary emboli secondary to deep venous thrombosis in the extremities. An umbrella was placed in the inferior vena cava below the renal arteries.

In massive emboli, as clots resolve by fragmentation, dislocation, and fibrinolysis, or are organized and contracted in situ, cardiac output improves, pulmonary artery pressures fall, and right ventricular pressures return to normal. Usually, pulmonary hemodynamics return to original levels in 2 to 8 weeks.

Most surgical patients who are treated at the time of the first embolus recover completely; chronically ill medical patients are more inclined to recurrence because the underlying disorder persists. Exceedingly few treated patients go on to develop chronic cor pulmonale. Instead, chronic cor pulmonale is generally a sequel of unrecognized and untreated pulmonary emboli, underscoring the importance of recognizing pulmonary emboli and dealing with them promptly and effectively.

Deep Venous Thrombosis

About two-thirds of venous thrombi are silent and escape clinical detection. Conversely, only about half of the patients who have signs and symptoms attributed to venous thrombosis prove to have the disease. Accurate diagnosis is essential before starting anticoagulant therapy since the agents have a morbidity and mortality of their own. Pulmonary emboli usually originate as clots in the deep veins of the lower extremities that propagate proximally to femoral and popliteal veins before migrating to the lungs. Therefore, one reasonable approach to establishing the diagnosis of pulmonary embolism is to seek evidence of clot in peripheral veins, bearing in mind that clots in the legs are less likely to be the source of major emboli than those in the thighs and pelvis. Although the search for deep venous thrombosis often does succeed in revealing a venous clot, in nearly one-third of patients with angiographically proven pulmonary embolism the venogram is normal, i.e., a normal peripheral venogram does not exclude the diagnosis of pulmonary embolism.

The frequency of fatal thromboembolism underscores the need to find and deal with sources before embolic material is released. However, the wide array of diagnostic measures is generally nonspecific, costly, and troublesome, often forcing the physician to choose between phlebography, radioisotopes, blood tests, plethysmography, and ultrasound.

CONTRAST VENOGRAPHY (PHLEBOGRAPHY)

Phlebography has become the "gold standard." However, the procedure is not undertaken lightly: it is often painful, sometimes causes hemodynamic upsets because of either the large volume of contrast material that is needed to fill the superficial, deep, and muscular veins or because of sensitivity to the injected dye; occasionally, it aggravates a phlebitis or precipitates local thrombosis. Moreover, it is both expensive and unsuitable for repeated testing.

NONINVASIVE METHODS

The knee is a dividing line for choice of noninvasive methods; impedance plethysmography and venous Doppler tests are most useful for detecting deep venous thrombosis at, or above, the knee, whereas radioactive fibrinogen is best reserved for thrombosis below the knee.

Impedance Plethysmography

This technique is often used in conjunction with the Doppler test to detect proximal venous thrombosis. The method is simple and easy to use in the ambulatory setting. It is currently the most accurate of the noninvasive tests, entailing the use of electronic or mechanical instrumentation to access the sufficiency of venous blood flow from the knee to the right atrium. A pressure cuff placed around the thigh is inflated to just above normal venous pressure, thereby allowing arterial inflow to the limb to continue while venous return is arrested. The resultant increase in venous volume is measured either mechanically (as a change in the circumference of the calf) or electronically (as a change in electrical impedance). Release of the occlusive cuff on the thigh restores venous blood flow causing a uniform decrease in the diameter of the calf veins. The rate of this decrease corresponds to the adequacy of venous flow from the popliteal fossa to the right heart. An obstruction or compromise of venous return is reflected in an abnormal study. This approach can detect virtually all occlusive thrombi in, or proximal to, the popliteal vein. However, it is useless for thrombi in the calf, and it can fail to disclose nonocclusive thrombi in the thigh. When confounding conditions such as right-sided congestive heart failure, external venous compression, and lymphatic obstruction are excluded, the impedence plethysmogram is approximately 90 percent as accurate as contrast venography for detecting proximal deep vein thrombosis. In symptomatic patients, the combination of plethysmography and radioisotopic fibrinogen provides a sensitivity and specificity greater than 90 percent.

Doppler Ultrasound

Doppler ultrasound is best suited for serial studies. It depends on changes in the acoustic characteristics of venous flow arising from different types of venous obstruction. The test correlates well with venography but is technically more difficult to apply than impedance plethysmography. It is also subject to greater interobserver variability in interpretation.

Radioactive Fibrinogen

Fibrinogen, radioactively labeled with ^{125}I, has been extensively applied to detect fresh clots in the deep veins of the legs. The radioactive fibrinogen is injected systemically, and both legs are scanned over successive days for evidence of incorporation of this fibrinogen into new clot. Unfortunately, because of soft tissue absorption of radioactivity and of competing background activity from fibrinogen in fresh wounds, e.g., as from hip surgery, the technique is relatively insensitive for clot above the knee. Furthermore, if there is no active clot formation at the time of fibrinogen injection, the test is apt to be falsely negative.

The test has proved to be most valuable in postoperative patients with propagating clots in leg veins that have led to pulmonary emboli; it is useless in detecting thrombi in the iliac and pelvic veins. Although the radioactive fibrinogen scan has been important in the prophylaxis and treatment of deep vein thrombosis, particularly in surgical patients, it is now only marginally useful in dealing with pulmonary embolism since simpler noninvasive studies can provide more accurate diagnostic information.

OTHER VARIETIES OF EMBOLIC DISEASE

Fat Emboli

The term *fat embolism* refers to a clinical syndrome of neurologic and respiratory abnormalities that occurs within 12 to 24 h after skeletal trauma, particularly as it entails multiple fractures. This syndrome occurs in about 5 percent of patients who have experienced severe and multiple orthopedic injuries: the patient develops fever, unexplained respiratory distress, mental confusion, and often a petechial rash over the body. This syndrome may be mild or progress to respiratory failure and coma. In this syndrome, the lungs are the seat of noncardiac pulmonary edema, considerable intrapulmonary shunting, and a low compliance similar to that seen in the adult respiratory distress syndrome. The neurologic findings sometimes progress to stupor and coma without focal neurologic defects. At autopsy, the patients have fat deposits in many organs, particularly in the pulmonary arteries and the cerebral circulation.

Despite its name, the pathogenesis of fat embolism has not been proven to be the embolization of fat throughout the venous circulation. One suggested explanation is that fractures of the long bones disrupt intramedullary adipose tissue, which then extrudes into the venous circulation. A second preferred alternative is that the trauma induces intravascular biochemical changes that cause circulating chylomicrons to aggregate into fat droplets which, in turn, lodge in the terminal vasculature of various organs. Although there is evidence to support both alternatives, neither has been proven.

PATHOPHYSIOLOGY

Understanding of the end-organ damage caused by fat embolism is incomplete. In the lungs, deposition of the fatty aggregates in the small muscular arteries and arterioles can increase pulmonary arterial pressures sufficiently to evoke cor pulmonale. A capillary leak syn-

drome occurs in fat embolism, presumably due to lysis of the fatty aggregates by lung lipases to form free fatty acids. Thrombocytopenia and the resultant petechiae occur in the fat embolism syndrome, possibly secondary to platelet aggregation by the circulating fat.

CLINICAL FEATURES

The diagnosis of fat embolism syndrome is considered in any patient who, after severe trauma of orthopedic surgery, develops respiratory distress, mental confusion, or petechiae within 3 days of injury. The rash is usually found in the upper part of the body including axillae, chest, flanks, conjunctivae and, at other times, the soft palate. Fever and tachycardia are common. Occasionally, fat can be seen in the retinal vessels.

The hematologic picture is nonspecific. Although increased levels of serum lipase and lipiduria are common in the fat embolism syndrome, these abnormalities are nondiagnostic since they may occur after any trauma. The chest radiograph is generally normal in the early stages of disease but may progress to the picture of noncardiac pulmonary edema. The arterial blood gases are often abnormal (low P_{O_2}, low P_{CO_2}) despite a normal chest radiograph.

DIAGNOSIS

No single clinical feature or laboratory test establishes the diagnosis of the fat embolism syndrome. However, certain diagnostic hints are useful. The fat embolism syndrome rarely occurs beyond the third day after boney trauma. Arterial hypoxemia, although nonspecific, occurs almost invariably in the fat embolism syndrome. Petechial rash described above strongly suggests the disorder. Although high concentrations of lipase in serum are not diagnostic, they may be useful as confirmatory evidence.

TREATMENT

Until recently, treatment of the fat embolism syndrome was largely supportive, directed at ensuring proper hydration, managing respiratory manifestations, and dealing with the underlying trauma. None of these measures had any bearing on *preventing* fat embolism. However, in a recent prospective study, corticosteroids, given to high-risk patients within 12 h of skeletal trauma, proved effective in reducing the incidence of fat embolism syndrome. Anecdotal reports also suggest that corticosteroids may be beneficial even after the fat embolism syndrome has developed.

Prevention of the fat embolism syndrome may be possible during orthopedic surgery, particularly involving the hip. One approach is by venting of the intramedullary canal during the insertion of a total hip prosthesis.

Air Embolism

Air embolism is a potentially life-threatening disorder in which a large bolus of air introduced into the venous circulation travels to the pulmonary circulation. When severe, air embolism can result in total pulmonary arterial obstruction, circulatory collapse, and sudden death. Occasionally, air makes its way into the systemic circulation either through the lungs or a patent foramen ovale, causing infarction in a systemic end-organ, particularly in the central nervous system.

Air embolism may complicate a variety of clinical disorders, including chest injury, instrumentation of central veins, surgery, and hemodialysis. Both the volume and the rate of air introduction are important in producing acute circulatory collapse: a smaller volume injected rapidly into circulation as a bolus may cause as much damage as a larger volume that is introduced slowly. In some patients, the air embolism syndrome is accompanied by noncardiac pulmonary edema and disseminated intravascular coagulation.

The diagnosis of air embolism should be suspected whenever air is accidentally introduced into the venous circulation, particularly when the patient suddenly experiences circulatory collapse. Immediate efforts at resuscitation are directed toward minimizing the volume of the air in the pulmonary circulation: the patient is immediately turned on his or her left side so that the air bubble remains within the right heart. A central venous catheter may prove useful in aspirating air from the right side of the circulation. If these efforts and immediate resuscitation prove fruitless, direct open cardiac massage may be successful in restoring the circulation.

More problematic is the continued presence of small air bubbles within the venous and arterial circulations after air embolization. To dissolve these bubbles, the patient is placed immediately on 100% oxygen and, if possible, moved to a hyperbaric facility. Under hyperbaric conditions, the bubble size can be rapidly reduced. To be effective, hyperbaric therapy must be promptly instituted.

SICKLE CELL DISEASE

Sickle cell disease affects the lungs by causing local thrombosis and occasionally by embolization of marrow elements. Small pulmonary arteries, arterioles, and capillaries are generally affected. Thrombosis in the pulmonary circulation is part of the general proclivity of red blood cells containing S hemoglobin to sickle under appropriate circumstances, particularly hypoxia, stagnation, and clotting follow sickling. In some instances, the thrombus organizes, the vascular lumen is obliterated, and perivascular fibrosis occurs in adjacent lung; in others, recanalization occurs. On occasion, infarction occurs.

Of the factors that predispose in thrombosis in the lungs in sickle cell disease, most important is the low P_{O_2} of mixed venous blood. Not only is the mixed venous P_{O_2} inordinately low, but the O_2 dissociation curve is shifted to the right, thereby handicapping O_2 uptake in the lungs.

Any pulmonary disease that causes alveolar hypoventilation or hypoxemia of blood in the lungs favors sickling and thrombosis. Since patients with sickle cell disease are prone to intercurrent pulmonary infections, particularly pneumonia and tuberculosis, they are predisposed to local areas of alveolar hypoventilation and hypoxia. Patients with severe sickle cell anemia and large fractions of S hemoglobin in their red blood cells are particularly susceptible to intense sickling and thrombosis anywhere, including the lungs, but the vulnerability is not restricted to states of SS hemoglobin. In some heterozygous sickle states, i.e., SC, S thalassemia, and SA hemoglobin, enough S hemoglobin is present to cause extensive thrombosis and infarction during an episode of severe hypoxemia, during acidosis, or during septicemia associated with fever and leukocytosis.

The clinical picture of pulmonary infarction in patients with sickle cell disease can mimic or coexist with bronchopneumonia. The latter may promote local hypoxia which leads to in situ pulmonary thrombosis. An episode often begins with poorly defined or pleuritic chest pain, fever, and sputum that is blood-streaked but fails to disclose any specific bacterial cause. A fleeting episode of breathlessness is usually overlooked. Cyanosis is rare because of the severe anemia. The subsequent course is characterized by an unconvincing response to antibiotics and slow clearing; often a linear scar in the lungs remains as a residue of the infarction. Suspicion of infarction should be high in any black person with S hemoglobin and in white persons of Greek or Italian descent with S thalassemia.

Rarely is occlusive disease sufficiently extensive to cause pulmonary hypertension and cor pulmonale. For this sequence to evolve, many severe episodes of sickling are required. The cor pulmonale that results is unusual because of its association with a high cardiac output and intrinsic myocardial damage that generally complicates sickle cell disease.

Management

Management of the patient with pulmonary thrombosis and infarction in sickle cell disease relies heavily on previous experience with the disease. Few specific measures can be advocated other than conventional supportive treatment. Distinguishing between in situ thrombosis and thromboembolism can be difficult clinically and even by invasive procedures such as angiography or venography. Moreover, because radiographic contrast materials may promote sickling, they have to be used cautiously. To complicate matters, some patients with sickle cell disease are also at increased risk of thromboemboli because of predisposing factors, such as bed rest, congestive heart failure, and dehydration.

Anticoagulants are generally not used in sickle cell disease since there are no data to substantiate their effectiveness.

BIBLIOGRAPHY

Alderson PO, Rujanavech W, Secker-Walker RH, McKnight RC: The role of Xe-133 ventilation studies in scintigraphic detection of pulmonary embolism. Radiology 120:633–640, 1976.
  Based on retrospective data, the overall accuracy of the lung scan compared to pulmonary angiography varies from 5 to 15 percent.

Barrett-Connor E. Pneumonia and pulmonary infarction in sickle cell anemia. JAMA 224:997–1000, 1973.
  Distinguishing pneumonia from sickle cell infarction can be difficult, and empiric therapy may be necessary.

Biello DR, Matter AG, McKnight RC, Siegal BA: Ventilation-perfusion studies in suspected pulmonary embolism. AJR 133:1033–1037, 1979.
  This study outlines commonly used criteria for interpreting ventilation-perfusion lung scans.

Bounameaux H, Vermylen J, Collen D: Thrombolytic treatment with recombinant tissue-type plasminogen activator in a patient with massive pulmonary embolism. Ann Intern Med 103:64–65, 1985.
  The first report of successful clot-selective thrombolysis in a patient with massive pulmonary embolism using recombinant human tissue-type plasminogen activator (rt-PA).

Bynum LJ, Wilson JE: Radiographic features of pleural effusions in pulmonary embolism. Am Rev Respir Dis 117:829–834, 1978.
  Pleural effusion infiltrates and/or atelectasis are the most common radiographic manifestations of pulmonary embolism.

Cines DB: Heparin: Do we understand its antithrombotic activity? Chest 89:420–426, 1986.
A review of mechanisms by which heparin exerts its antithrombotic effects.

Cohen M, Edwards WD, Fuster V: Regression in thromboembolic type of primary pulmonary hypertension during 2½ years of antithrombotic therapy. J Am Coll Cardiol 7:172–175, 1986.
A case report that supports a role for antithrombotic therapy in treating pulmonary hypertension due to "multiple pulmonary emboli" (widespread pulmonary microvascular thrombosis).

Collins FS, Orringer EP: Pulmonary hypertension and cor pulmonale in the sickle hemoglobinopathies. Am J Med 73:814–821, 1982.
Patients had multiple episodes of respiratory distress, chronic syncope or dyspnea, and cor pulmonale which could only be confirmed by right heart catheterization.

Dalen JE, Alpert JS: Natural history of pulmonary embolism. Prog Cardiovasc Dis 17:259–270, 1975.
A description of the epidemiology, pathogenesis, and physiology of pulmonary embolism.

Fareed J: Heparin, its fractions, fragments and derivatives. Sem Thromb Hemost 11:1–9, 1985.
The development of low molecular weight fractions of heparin has brought fresh horizons to the management of thromboembolic diseases.

Goldhaber SZ, Markis JE, Meyerovitz MF, Kim DS, Dawley DS, Sasahara A, Vaughan DE, Selwyn AP, Loscalzo J, Kessler CM, Sharma GVRK, Grossbard EB, Braunwald E: Acute pulmonary embolism treated with tissue plasminogen activator. Lancet 2:886–889, 1986.
In 36 patients with angiographically documented pulmonary embolism, rt-PA was safe and efficacious in rapidly lysing pulmonary emboli.

Haupt HM, Moore GW, Bauer TW, Hutchins GM: The lung in sickle cell disease. Chest 81:332–337, 1982.
In this large autopsy series, alveolar wall necrosis and pulmonary embolization of necrotic marrow often complicated sickle cell disease.

Havig GO: Source of pulmonary emboli. Acta Chir Scand (suppl) 42:1–20, 1977.
This prospective autopsy study documented pulmonary embolism as a significant contributor to inpatient mortality with most clots arising from large capacitance vessels of the lower extremities.

Huisman MV, Buller HR, ten Cate JW, Vreeken J: Serial impedance plethysmography for suspected deep venous thrombosis in outpatients. N Engl J Med 314:823–828, 1986.
This study concluded that the diagnostic accuracy of repeated impedance plethysmography compares favorably with that of venography and that the technique is a safe and effective noninvasive approach to the diagnosis and care of outpatients clinically suspected of acute deep venous thrombosis.

Hull RD, Hirsh J, Carter CJ, Jay RM, Dodd PE, Ockelford PA, Coates G, Gill GJ, Turpie AG, Doyle DJ, Buller HR, Raskob GE: Pulmonary angiography, ventilation lung scanning and venography for clinically suspected pulmonary embolism with abnormal perfusion lung scan. Ann Intern Med 98:891–899, 1983.
This study suggests that there is a large overlap between the results of lung scanning, pulmonary angiography, and venography in the diagnosis of thromboembolism.

Hull RD, Hirsh J, Carter CJ, Jay RM, Ockelford PA, Buller HR, Turpie HG, Powers P, Kinch D, Dodd PE, et al: Diagnostic efficacy of impedance plethysmography for clinially suspected deep-vein thrombosis. Ann Intern Med 102:21–28, 1985.
A randomized trial supporting the high efficacy of impedance plethysmography as a noninvasive test for deep vein thrombosis.

Hyers TM (ed): Pulmonary embolism and hypertension. Clin Chest Med 5(3):1984.
Entire volume devoted to physiology and therapy of thromboembolic disease.

Kakkar VV, Adams PC: Preventive and therapeutic approach to venous thromboembolic disease and pulmonary embolism—can death from pulmonary embolism be prevented? J Am Coll Cardiol 8:146B–158B, 1986.
A practical therapeutic approach emphasizing prevention.

Kelley MA: Thromboembolic disease and fat embolism in the surgical patient, in Goldmann DR, Brown FH, Levy WK, Slap GB, Sussman EJ (eds), *Medical Care of the Surgical Patient*. Philadelphia, Lippincott, 1982, pp. 401–421.
General review of diagnostic and therapeutic approach to both disorders with special emphasis on the high-risk surgical patient.

Kipper MS, Moser KM, Kortman KE, Ashburn WL: Long-term follow-up of patients with suspected embolism and normal lung scan. Perfusion scans in embolic suspects. Chest 82:411–415, 1982.
  A normal perfusion lung scan excludes clinically important pulmonary embolism.

Moser KM, Daily PO, Peterson K, Dembitsky W, Vapnek JM: Shure, D, Utley J, Archibald C: Thromboendarterectomy for chronic, major-vessel thromboembolic pulmonary hypertension. Immediate and long-term results in 42 patients. Ann Intern Med 107:560–565, 1987.
  Forty-two patients with pulmonary hypertension due to chronic, thromboembolic obstruction of the major pulmonary arteries underwent pulmonary thromboendarterectomy. Thromboendarterectomy is feasible, even in patients with severe and protracted hemodynamic compromise. A paper by the same group in the same issue of the journal shows that pulmonary angiography in these patients is safe.

Moser KM, Lemoine JR: Is embolic risk continued by location of deep venous thrombosis? Ann Intern Med 94:439–444, 1981.
  Patients with deep vein thrombosis below the knee rarely had abnormal lung scans, implying that risk of pulmonary embolism was associated with proximal deep vein thrombosis.

Moser KM, Spragg RG, Utley J, Daily PO: Chronic thrombotic obstruction of major pulmonary arteries. Ann Intern Med 99:299–305, 1983.
  Thirteen of fifteen patients in whom pulmonary hypertension was associated with pulmonary hypertension were improved 8 to 144 months after pulmonary thromboendarterectomy.

Murphy BP, Harford FJ, Cramer FS: Cerebral air embolism resulting from invasive medical procedures—Treatment with hyperbaric oxygen. Ann Surg 201:242–245, 1985.
  Systemic embolization from the introduction of venous air is not uncommon, and hyperbaric treatment may be lifesaving.

Novelline RA, Blatarwich OH, Athanasoulis CA, Waltman AC, Greenfield AJ, McKusick KA: The clinical course of patients with suspected pulmonary embolism and a negative pulmonary arteriogram. Radiology 176:561–567, 1976.
  Patients with negative pulmonary angiograms had no significant incidence of pulmonary embolism on subsequent follow-up.

Oh WH, Mital MA: Fat embolism: Current concepts of pathogenesis, diagnosis, and treatment. Orthop Clin North Am 9:769–779, 1978.
  This comprehensive review outlines the biology and clinical aspects of fat embolism syndrome.

O'Quin RJ, Lakshminarayan S: Venous air embolism. Arch Intern Med 142:2173–2176, 1982.
  This review details the clinical aspects and pathophysiology of air embolism syndrome.

Rosebrough SF, Kudryk B, Grossman ZD, McAfee JG, Subramanian G, Ritter-Hrncirik CA, Witanowski LS, Tillapaugh-Fay G: Radioimmune imaging of venous thrombi using iodine-131 monoclonal antibody. Radiology 156:515–517, 1985.
  A description of a new imaging technique which uses antifibrin antibody to document intravascular clot.

Schonfeld SA, Ploysongsang Y, Dilisio R, Crissman JD, Miller E, Hammerschmidt DE, Jacob HS: Fat embolism prophylaxis with corticosteroids. A prospective study in high-risk patients. Ann Intern Med 99:438–443, 1983.
  Prophylactic use of corticosteroids in patients at high risk for fat embolism syndrome reduces the incidence of this complication.

Sharma GV: Historical overview of antithrombotic and thrombolytic therapy. Am J Med 83:2–5, 1987.
  A long view for perspective.

Sharma GV, McIntyre KM, Sharma S, Sasahara AA: Clinical and hemodynamic correlates in pulmonary embolism. Clin Chest Med 5:421–437, 1984.
  The clinical presentation of pulmonary embolism may be dominated by manifestations of pulmonary infarction or by the signs and symptoms of an acute hemodynamic disturbance including shock, tachycardia, or cardiac output.

Shattil SJ: Diagnoses and treatment of recurrent venous thromboembolism. Med Clin North Am 68:577–600, 1984.
  This review discusses the multiple etiology of venous thrombosis and addresses the clinical approach to the patient with recurrent disease.

Sprengers ED, Kluft C: Plasminogen activator inhibitors. Blood 69:381–387, 1987.
  An up-to-date consideration of the role played by plasminogen activator inhibitors in thrombolytic therapy. Much remains to be learned about how they work.

Stein PD, Dalen JE, McIntyre KM, Sasahara AA, Wenger NK, Willis PW III: The electrocardiogram in acute pulmonary embolism. Prog Cardiovasc Dis 17:247–257, 1975.
The electrocardiogram most often shows nonspecific ST- and T-wave abnormalities, whereas ECG manifestations of right heart strain are uncommon.

Turpie AGG, Levine MN, Hirsh J, Carter CJ, Jay RM, Powers PJ, Andrew M, Hull RD, Gent M: A randomized controlled trial of a low-molecular-weight heparin (enoxaparin) to prevent deep-vein thrombosis in patients undergoing elective hip surgery. N Engl J Med 315:925–929, 1986.
A double-blind, randomized trial comparing PK10169 low-molecular-weight heparin with placebo for the prevention of venous thrombosis in patients undergoing elective hip surgery. The authors conclude that prophylaxis with fixed-dose PK10169 heparin is effective and safe for patients undergoing elective hip replacement.

Watson-Williams EJ: Respiratory pharmacology. Antithrombotic and fibrinolytic therapy. Clin Chest Med 7:469–480, 1986.
A survey of the proper use of antithrombotic therapy. However, the proper use of fibrinolytic therapy is still evolving, awaiting the results of ongoing clinical trials.

Weimar W, Stibbe J, van Seyen A, Billian A, DeSomer P, Collen D: Specific lysis of an iliofemoral thrombus by administration of extrinsic (tissue-type) plasminogen activator. Lancet 2:1018–1020, 1981.
Intravenous administration of human tissue-type plasminogen activator (7.5 mg in a 24-h period) induced complete lysis of a 6-week-old renal and iliofemoral thrombosis in a renal-allograft recipient. Thrombolysis was achieved without systemic fibrinolytic activation, hemostatic breakdown, or bleeding.

Williams DO, Borer J, Braunwald E, Chesebro JH, Cohen LS, Dalen J, Dodge HT, Francis CK, Knatterud G, Ludbrook P, et al: Intravenous recombinant tissue-type plasminogen activator in patients with acute myocardial infarction: A report from the NHLBI thrombolysis in myocardial infarction trial. Circulation 73:338–355, 1986.
A multicenter trial of the efficacy and safety of an intravenous infusion of 80 mg of recombinant t-PA over a 3-h period in 47 patients with acute myocardial infarction. The intravenous infusion of rt-PA was generally well tolerated, but this dosage did induce some systemic fibrinogenolysis.

Wilson JE, Pierce AK, Johnson RL, Winga ER, Harrell WR, Curry GC, Mullins CB: Hypoxemia in pulmonary embolism: A clinical study. J Clin Invest 50:481–491, 1971.
At least 10 percent of patients with pulmonary embolism have normal arterial blood gases.

Chapter 67

Cardiac Problems in the Pulmonary Patient

Peter M. Yurchak

Few distinct organ systems are as intimately related functionally as the heart and lungs, together serving to assimilate oxygen into the body and distribute it to each cell of the organism. It is entirely logical that disease or disorder of one system should affect the other. The impact of pulmonary disease on the right heart is considered in Chapter 64, as is the impact of elevated left heart filling pressure (Chapter 60). Mechanisms of dyspnea and the distinction between dyspnea of pulmonary and cardiac disease are discussed in Chapter 68.

CORONARY ARTERY DISEASE

The commonest form of heart disease today is that due to coronary arteriosclerosis. Narrowing of the coronary vessels may lead to reversible ischemia, causing angina pectoris. Obstruction of narrowed vessels results in myocardial infarction, with left ventricular dysfunction, arrhythmias, and death. Considering the length of time that coronary disease has been recognized as an entity, surprisingly little study of its coexistence with chronic lung disease has taken place.

In 1958, Thomas presented the first analysis of coronary disease in 69 patients with coal miner's pneumoconiosis. He found clinical or autopsy evidence of coronary disease in 32 (45 percent). He commented on the need to distinguish the pain of myocardial ischemia from pleuropulmonary pain in reaching a correct diagnosis. The electrocardiogram was seldom of help unless it showed the pattern of clear-cut myocardial infarction. Nonspecific abnormalities were common. The presence of left ventricular hypertrophy on the electrocardiogram or chest radiograph called for a search for coexistent heart disease—coronary, hypertensive, or valvular. Because dyspnea limited the subject's ability to attain the threshold of myocardial ischemia, exercise testing proved to be of limited value in diagnosis. This observation still holds. However, sensitivity of treadmill stress testing has since been refined by combining it with thallium 201 myocardial scintigraphy. It has also become clear that coexistent covert coronary disease may become evident only under the stress of acute respiratory failure and be manifested as either coronary insufficiency, frank myocardial infarction, or serious arrhythmias.

In 212 coal miners with chest disease, Rees et al. found coronary disease in 24 percent, pulmonary heart disease in 48 percent, and *both* in 16 percent. On the basis of a list of criteria for electrocardiographic diagnosis, they detected coronary disease, either alone, or in combination with pulmonary disease, in 70 percent of the miners. However, "false positives did occur."

Subsequent studies of the association between heart and lung disease focused on the seeming infrequency of acute myocardial infarction in subjects with emphysema. In the absence of a more plausible explanation, the apparently protective effect of pulmonary disease was attributed by some to a hypoxia-mediated increase in coronary collateral circulation. However, others have failed to confirm the mutual exclusiveness of acute myocardial infarction and emphysema. Indeed, one report calls attention to a high incidence of "silent" myocardial infarction in individuals with emphysema. Moreover, abnormalities in pulmonary function are quite common (53 percent) in patients undergoing coronary arteriography, presumably due to heavy cigarette smoking, which is a shared risk factor in coronary and pulmonary disease. The possibility has also been raised that the incidence of systemic hypertension is higher in individuals with pulmonary disease than in the population at large.

Pulmonary Function in Acute Myocardial Infarction

Abnormalities in pulmonary function are common in patients with acute myocardial infarction. Two major disorders are responsible for these abnormalities: (1) interstitial pulmonary edema secondary to myocardial dysfunction and (2) chronic obstructive airways disease,

as a rule attributable to cigarette smoking. The observation that the individual experiencing the first myocardial infarction is apt to have a low vital capacity is probably attributable to interstitial pulmonary edema since the vital capacity returns to normal as the patient recovers. Few observations have been made on the management of patients with chronic pulmonary disease who have experienced an acute myocardial infarction.

Electrocardiographic Problems

The electrocardiographic pattern in some individuals with obstructive airways disease may simulate coronary artery disease (see Chapter 34). Because of the hyperinflated lungs and the low diaphragm, the pattern of QRS complexes in the precordial leads is altered, so that there is an overall reduction in the anterior forces; poor R-wave progression is seen in the right and mid-precordial leads. The same pattern can be a legacy of a previous anterior wall myocardial infarction. Other less common causes of the pattern include left ventricular hypertrophy, mitral valve prolapse, and a "normal variant" phenomenon. A stepwise approach to distinguishing among the various possibilities is outlined in Fig. 67-1.

The patient with an acute left-sided penumothorax may also manifest the electrocardiographic pattern of poor R-wave progression: the collection of air in the left hemithorax damps transmission of the electrical potential to the chest surface. The association of chest pain and electrocardiographic changes occasionally leads to the erroneous diagnosis of myocardial infarction.

Therapeutic agents used in the management of both cardiac and pulmonary disease can make their imprints on the electrocardiogram. These are considered subsequently.

LEFT VENTRICULAR FAILURE

Because cardiac and pulmonary disease are so common, an occasional patient is encountered in whom left ventricular failure and chronic obstructive airways disease coexist. The complaint of dyspnea is common to both conditions. Despite the features discussed in Chapter 68 that are helpful in distinguishing between cardiac and pulmonary dyspnea, uncertainties often remain: wheezing and rales occur in either condition, and the noisy respirations of obstructive airways disease sometimes obscure a telltale

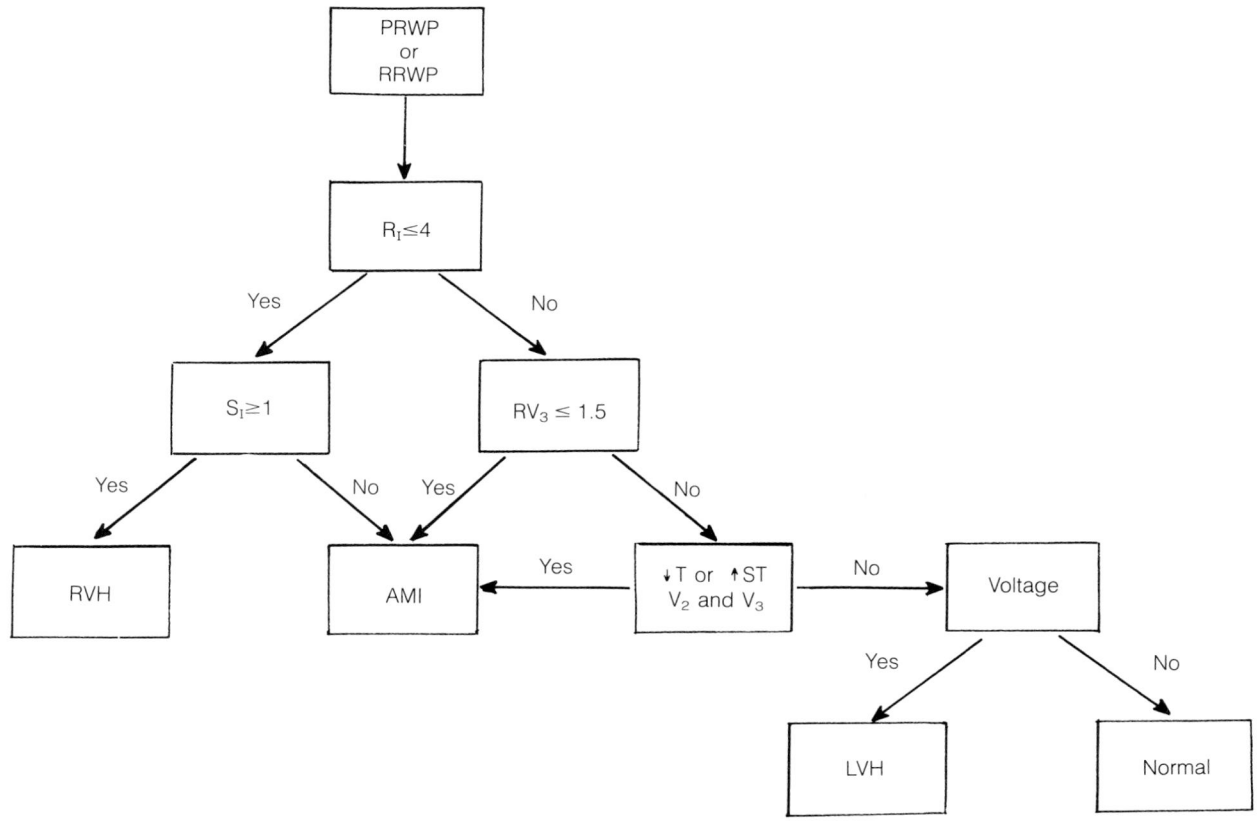

FIGURE 67-1 Approach to the ECG showing poor R-wave progression (PRWP) or reversed R-wave progression (RRWP). R_I, S_I = R, S waves in lead I; RV_3 = R wave in lead V_3; RVH = right ventricular hypertrophy; LVH = left ventricular hypertrophy; AMI = anterior myocardial infarction. (From Zema and Kligfield, 1982, with permission.)

ventricular gallop sound. In the individual with chronic pulmonary disease and chronic dyspnea, worsening of the breathlessness raises the question of whether a superimposed pulmonary process or the onset of left ventricular failure is responsible.

Bass has pointed out that interstitial pulmonary edema improves transmission of sound from hyperinflated regions, thereby imparting a spuriously normal intensity to breath sounds and confusing interpretation of the physical findings. When interstitial pulmonary edema and hyperinflation coexist, the total lung capacity is generally reduced rather than increased; this reduction is attributable largely to a decrease in both the expiratory reserve volume and the residual volume. Also in patients with both disorders, in contrast to those in heart failure, who undergo an increase in the vital capacity as the heart failure is relieved, the reduced vital capacity fails to improve as heart failure clears.

The appearance of the chest radiograph in individuals with both left ventricular or combined heart failure and obstructive airways disease is strongly influenced by the distribution of the pulmonary pathology. For example, basilar emphysema and a low-lying diaphragm may be obscured by pleural effusions and parenchymal congestion; these abnormalities become evident when cardiac failure is relieved (Fig. 67-2). The expected "cephalization" of the pulmonary blood flow that generally accompanies left ventricular failure does not occur in emphysema of the upper lobes because of obliteration of the pulmonary vascular bed at the apices by the pulmonary

disease. This radiographic paradox signals the coexistence of cardiac and pulmonary disease.

Serial chest radiographs and serial determinations of the total and the 1-s forced vital capacities are helpful in identifying the coexistence of the two conditions; when heart failure coexists with obstructive airways disease, the 1-s forced vital capacity, initially near normal, decreases as the heart failure is relieved. As Bass admonishes, "One must remember that, with improvement in cardiac function in a patient who has a coexistent chronic obstructive lung disease, most indices of lung function deviate further away from the predicted normal value."

THE LEFT VENTRICLE IN CHRONIC LUNG DISEASE

The issue of hypertrophy and/or dysfunction of the left ventricle in patients with chronic obstructive disease of the airways was first joined by pathologic studies which reported unexplained left ventricular hypertrophy in from 17.5 to 86 percent of autopsy specimens. However, implication of these findings, i.e., that a mysterious left ventricular abnormality can be a direct consequence of obstructive airways disease, has been challenged over the years on several grounds: the lack of uniformity in the pathologic criteria used to quantify the left ventricular abnormalities, the possibility that systemic hypertension during life had been overlooked, and the likelihood that associated coronary atherosclerosis could have contrib-

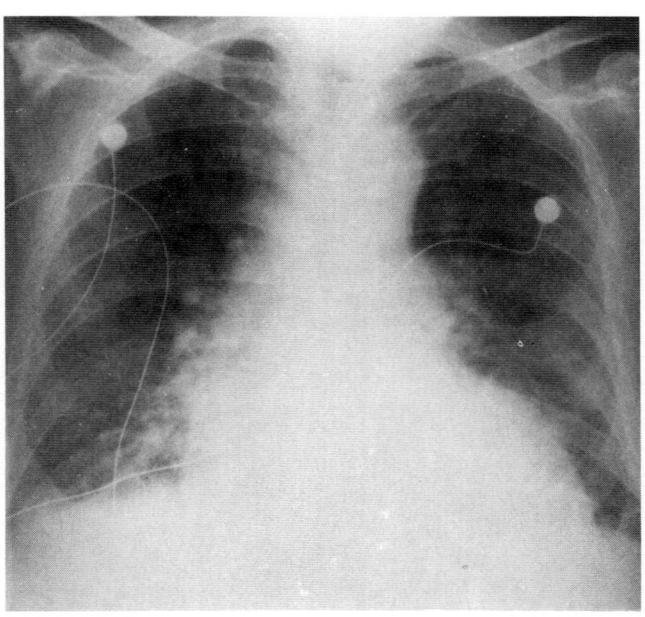

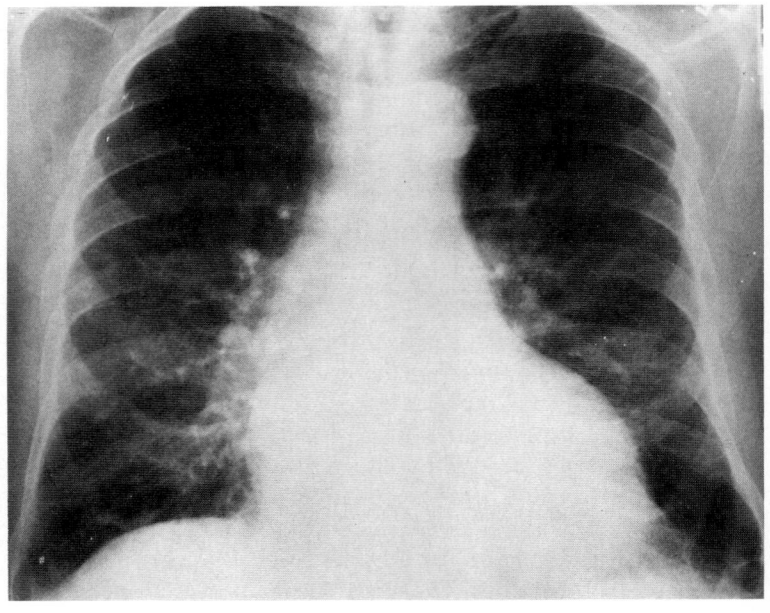

A   B

FIGURE 67-2 Left ventricular failure and obstructive airways disease. *A.* During heart failure, the presence of obstructive airways disease is obscured by pulmonary vascular congestion and pleural effusions. The diaphragm is high, rather than low-lying. *B.* After treatment of the heart failure, hyperinflation, blebs, and a low-lying diaphragm are clearly seen.

uted to left ventricular abnormalities. To this list of caveats can be added the additional qualification that some subjects with undisputed left ventricular hypertrophy may represent a *forme fruste* of early hypertrophic cardiomyopathy for which there is still no generally accepted "marker."

Currently, hypotheses concerning possible mechanisms that might account for otherwise unexplained left ventricular hypertrophy include: hypoxia, hypercarbia, high cardiac output, and bronchopulmonary shunts in the lungs. Anatomically minded writers often implicate the continuous spiral bands of myocardial syncytium that make up the ventricles; i.e., overload of one chamber might cause abnormality of the other because of continuous and shared muscle.

Hemodynamic studies since then have failed to resolve the problem: the same set of data has been interpreted differently by different observers; the validity of pulmonary capillary wedge pressure measurement in the presence of lung disease has been debated; certain criteria such as "systolic time intervals" have proved unreliable in patients with obstructive airways disease. Recently, radionuclide ventriculography and M-mode and two-dimensional echocardiography have failed to settle the issue. At present, the most popular explanation for left ventricular dysfunction in obstructive airways disease (assuming that the two are related) seems to be "ventricular interdependence," i.e., that in patients with right ventricular enlargement, the ventricular septum bulges into the left ventricular cavity. Although anatomic displacement of the septum has been documented in patients with right ventricular overload, its functional significance remains unclear. One problem in obtaining consistent results and interpretations is that the various clinics deal with widely disparate patient populations. Another is that the role of coexistent coronary disease and/or alcohol abuse—either of which might compromise left ventricular function—has not been taken into full account.

VALVULAR HEART DISEASE

Respiratory symptoms are a predominant feature of severe mitral stenosis. About one-third of patients with mitral stenosis experience attacks of "winter bronchitis" that are attributable to their heart disease. As Cortese has noted, "These . . . together with abnormalities on pulmonary function testing, may lead the clinician to make an erroneous diagnosis of primary pulmonary disease. . . . " Indeed, unless chronic pulmonary disease is known to antecede signs of mitral stenosis, it is often difficult to prove that independent pulmonary, as well as cardiac, disease is present. Thus, the entire respiratory syndrome exhibited by a patient with chronic mitral stenosis can arise from the so-called mitral lung.

Derangements in pulmonary function produced by mitral stenosis have been explored for 30 years. Abnormalities of the pulmonary parenchyma, interstitium, blood vessels, and lymphatics contribute to the abnormalities. Although the vital capacity is generally normal, the maximal breathing capacity and maximal mid-expiratory flow rate are generally low; airway resistance is high, and the diffusing capacity is low. Blood flow and ventilation are preferentially shifted to the upper zones of the lungs. Minute ventilation, at rest and during exercise, is abnormally high. In patients with long-standing and severe mitral stenosis, these anatomic changes may preclude a satisfactory result from surgery.

Occasionally, obstructive airways disease obscures the physical findings of valvular heart disease: the overinflated lungs and barrel chest render difficult or impossible the perception and assessment of heart murmurs. For example, the murmur of significant aortic stenosis may be rendered faint and unimpressive. This oversight is potentiated by the fact that many elderly subjects exhibit faint basal systolic murmurs that are caused by ejection of

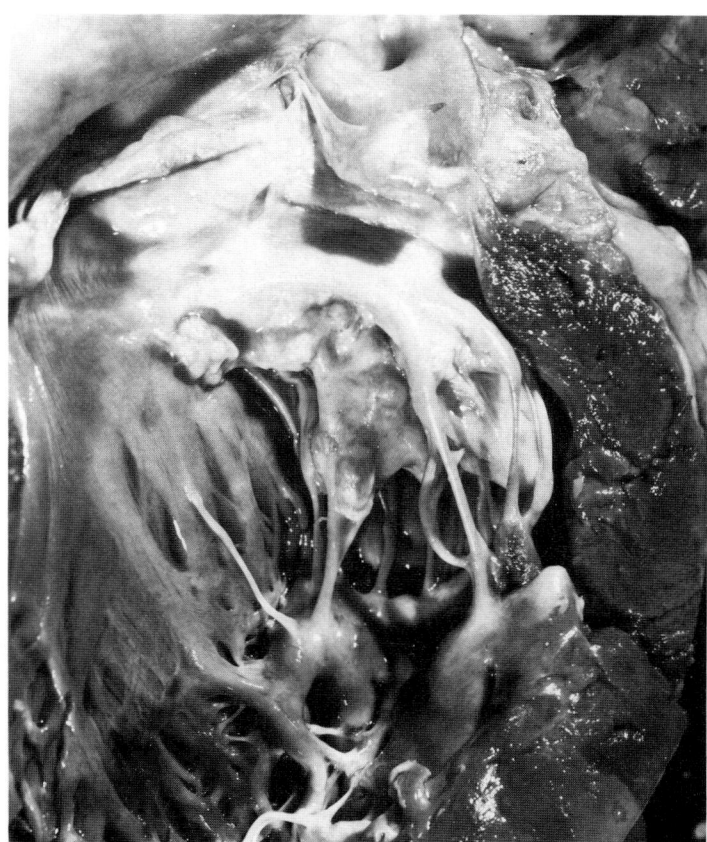

FIGURE 67-3 "Silent" mitral stenosis in long-standing obstructive airways disease. Ventricular aspect of a heavily calcified and stenotic mitral valve that produced no audible signs of its presence in life. This 66-year-old man died of respiratory failure following abdominal surgery.

blood through stiff, albeit nonobstructed, leaflets of the aortic valve. This stiffening, part of the normal aging process, and the murmur that it produces are usually rightly discounted by the examiner as "a few grey hairs on the heart valve." Conversely, symptoms of dyspnea and fatigue are sometimes ascribed to overt lung disease because of the failure to recognize underlying mitral valve disease.

The diastolic rumble of mitral stenosis, often difficult to detect even under ideal circumstances, may also be obscured by the hyperinflated lungs and barrel chest that often accompany chronic obstructive airways disease; posterior displacement of the heart by an enlarged right ventricle adds to the concealment (Fig. 67-3). The development of two-dimensional echocardiography has made it possible to detect these silent lesions without resorting to cardiac catheterization. Magnetic resonance imaging holds promise of being helpful in patients with "silent" mitral stenosis in whom a technically satisfactory echocardiogram cannot be obtained because of changes in the lungs and thorax produced by pulmonary disease.

CARDIAC ARRHYTHMIAS

Disturbances in cardiac rhythm are common in most types of heart disease. But, cardiac arrhythmias often occur in patients with obstructive disease of the airways, even though heart disease is not clinically manifest. Many factors can lead to the development of arrhythmias in acutely ill patients with pulmonary disease (Table 67-1). Successful management hinges on correction of as many of the underlying abnormalities as possible (Table 67-2). Treatment is sometimes handicapped by the inability to with-

draw the initiating medications that are required to manage the pulmonary disorder. When this occurs, it is tempting to administer antiarrhythmic agents. But the roles of these agents in the patients with blood-gas abnormalities and respiratory acidosis who are receiving sympathomimetic agents can create distinctive problems of their own.

At one time, arrhythmias were considered to be uncommon in chronic cor pulmonale. This error was first appreciated in 1958 by Corazza and Pastor, who, in a retrospective electrocardiographic study of 122 subjects hospitalized for treatment of acute exacerbations of chronic lung disease, discovered arrhythmias in 31 percent: about one-third of the arrhythmias were either atrial or ventricular premature beats; sustained arrhythmias were also seen. Supraventricular mechanisms predominated.

TABLE 67-1
Factors Implicated in Cardiac Arrhythmias in Subjects with Chronic Lung Disease

Hypoxia
Hypercarbia
Respiratory acidosis
Stretch reflexes
    Lungs and airway
    Pulmonary vasculature
    Venae cavae
Right atrial distension
Infection, with bronchial irritation
Vagal reflexes (coughing, tracheal suction)
Coronary disease, with myocardial ischemia
Sympathomimetic drugs
Methylxanthines
Digitalis
Metabolic alkalosis (diuretics)
Hypokalemia

TABLE 67-2
Management of Arrhythmias in Patients with Obstructive Disease of the Airways

Diagnostic measures
  Blood-gas values
  Hematocrit, WBC
  Blood chemistry tests
    Potassium
    Magnesium
    Cardiac enzymes
    Digoxin level
    Theophylline level
  Chest radiograph
  Seek signs of infection
  ?Insert Swan-Ganz catheter
  ?Pulmonary arteriography (for suspected pulmonary embolism)
Supportive measures
  Oxygen, if not contraindicated
  Stop sympathomimetics and bronchodilators, if possible
  Intubate for respiratory acidosis or profuse secretions
  Pressors for hypotension
  Volume repletion if pulmonary wedge pressure is low
  Packed blood cells for anemia
  ?Cover possible infection with antibiotics
  ?Heparin for suspected or proven pulmonary embolism
Specific measures
  Atrial fibrillation: digoxin; verapamil
  Atrial flutter: verapamil; cardioversion or rapid atrial pacing
  Supraventricular tachycardia: verapamil; digoxin; rapid atrial pacing
  Multifocal atrial tachycardia: treat the underlying disorder(s)
  Ventricular tachycardia: lidocaine; cardioversion
  Digitalis-induced arrhythmias: phenytoin; potassium repletion

NOTE: WBC = white blood cell count.

Over the next 15 years, only a trickle of studies appeared on the subject. But the advent of intensive-care units, with continuous monitoring of the electrocardiogram, led to the realization that arrhythmias occurred in over three-quarters of patients in whom acute respiratory failure complicated chronic pulmonary disease. This observation was subsequently reinforced by the advent of ambulatory electrocardiographic monitoring that enabled the electrical activity of the heart to be recorded during the entire 24 h.

The incidence of arrhythmias proved to be higher in individuals with combined pulmonary disease and coronary arterial disease than with either disease alone. Moreover, Holter monitoring provided a higher yield of arrhythmias than did either the 12-lead electrocardiogram taken on admission or even continuous monitoring in which the detection of arrhythmias depended on chance observation of the monitor screen.

In general, atrial arrhythmias are commoner than ventricular, and isolated premature beats of either kind are commoner than sustained disturbances in rhythm. Since a sustained tachyarrhythmia could lead to the cascade of consequences depicted in Fig. 67-4, prompt correction of the arrhythmia may be critical for the survival of a seriously ill patient. In patients with a bout of acute respiratory failure that complicates chronic obstructive airways disease, the occurrence of sustained *ventricular* arrhythmias was found to be associated with a mortality of 100 percent. It is not known to what extent associated coronary disease contributed to this dire outcome.

In some patients with stable chronic pulmonary disease, Holter monitoring has shown presence of frequent, or multiform, ventricular ectopic activity. Whether these arrhythmias are ominous is not clear. Although it is widely held that such ectopic activity in a patient with a recent myocardial infarction carries an appreciable risk of death by arrhythmia, this supposition is not supported by the list of causes of death in individuals with chronic pulmonary disease. For example, sudden, unexpected death occurred in only 8 percent of the patients reviewed by Diener and Burrows. Also, most patients with obstructive disease of the airways die in respiratory failure rather than from an arrhythmia. Although it seems likely that the occurrence of ventricular arrhythmias in patients with chronic pulmonary disease implies the coexistence of coronary arterial disease, this hypothesis is still conjectural. Nonetheless, the onset of a ventricular arrhythmia should prompt an urgent search for its cause. Also, the more troublesome the arrhythmia, the more vigorous the treatment: as a rule, lidocaine is given intravenously, whether or not standard antiarrhythmic agents are administered orally.

Multifocal Atrial Tachycardia

All types of supraventricular arrhythmia may be encountered in the acutely ill patient with lung disease. Of these, multifocal atrial tachycardia (MAT) deserves special comment.

MAT was first described as an entity in 1968. It is marked by well-formed and discrete, but multiform, atrial

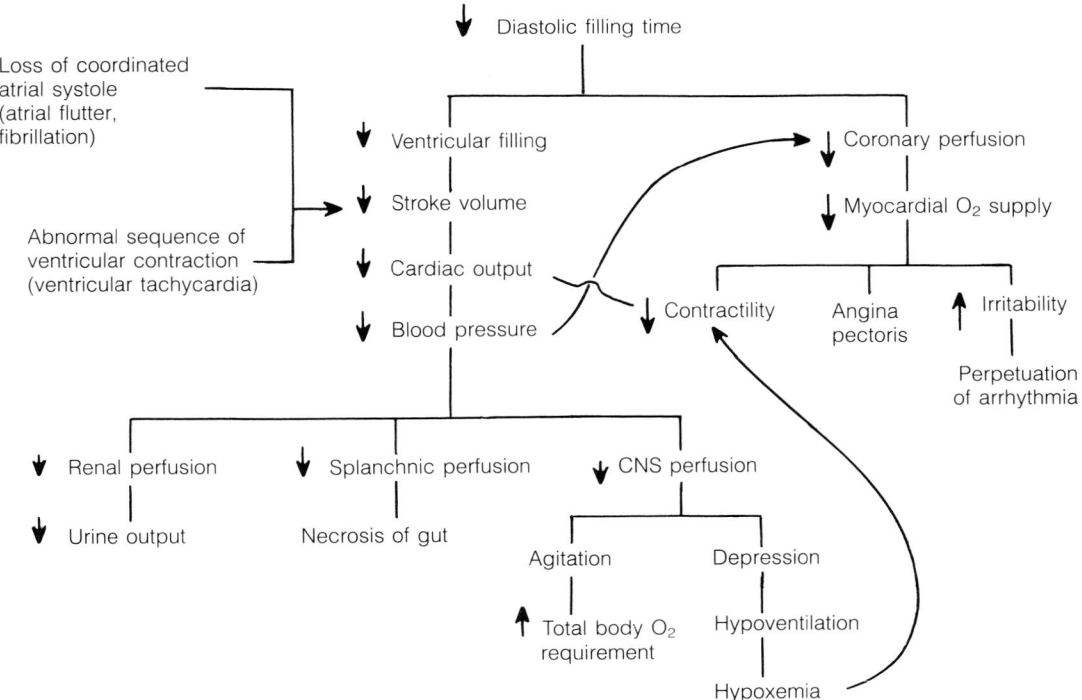

FIGURE 67-4 Cardiovascular effects of tachyarrhythmias.

deflections, at rates of 100 per minute or more. Not only are the deflections multiform, but they are irregular in spacing, resulting in a rapid and irregular *ventricular* response. The usual rate is 120 to 140 per minute, but rates of 200 per minute have been encountered (Fig. 67-5). In that it is an irregular atrial tachyarrhythmia, it resembles atrial fibrillation. However, distinction between the two is critical (Table 67-3, Fig. 67-6). MAT is a so-called secondary arrhythmia, a reflection of some dire underlying problem. It responds to correction of that problem without the use of medications. Digitalis or antiarrhythmic agents are destined to be ineffective unless they improve the underlying problem. Moreover, if digitalis is given, it is often toxic, at times causing death. Conversely, atrial fibrilla-

tion is an isolated, or "primary," arrhythmia that responds to digitalis or verapamil. It is worth emphasizing that mistaking MAT for atrial fibrillation—so that attention is directed solely to the treatment of the arrhythmia—can be disastrous.

Acute respiratory failure complicating chronic bronchitis and emphysema (COPD) is one of the commonest entities associated with MAT; the arrhythmia occurs in about one-third of these patients. Mortality associated with this arrhythmia is extraordinarily high in these patients, i.e., about 80 percent, and increases further with digitalis toxicity.

Toxicity from the injudicious use of digitalis in MAT can be manifested in one of four ways: (1) atrioventricular

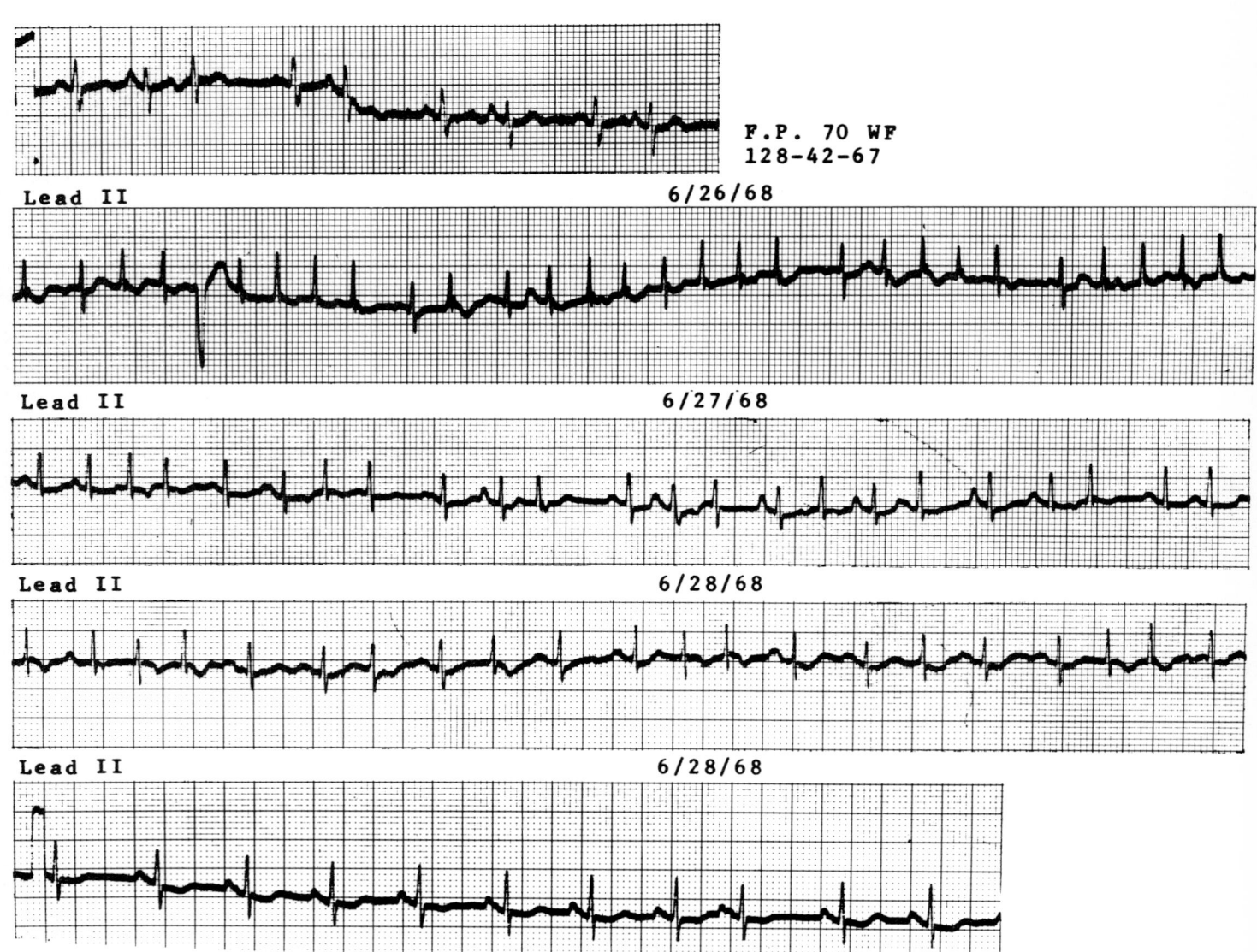

FIGURE 67-5 Multifocal atrial tachycardia (MAT) at rates of 200 per minute in a seriously ill patient with ventilatory failure that required intubation. Even at this very rapid rate, P waves are clearly seen. Note slowing of the rate and eventual reversion to sinus rhythm in the lower strips, coincident with clinical improvement.

TABLE 67-3

Distinction between Multifocal Atrial Tachycardia (MAT) and Atrial Fibrillation (AF)

	MAT	AF
Atrial rate	100–140/min, rarely up to 200/min	300/min or more
Atrial morphology	Multiform, discrete P waves	Multiform, closely spaced fibrillatory waves
Baseline of ECG	Isoelectric between P waves	Continuously undulating
Ventricular-to-atrial response (VR)	1:1	Less than 1:1; ventricular rate 140–160/min
Aberrant ventricular conduction	Rare, even at very rapid atrial rates	May be seen at any ventricular response
Response to carotid sinus pressure, if any	Slowing of VR, transient "smoothing-out" of multi-focality	Slowing of VR, exposing undulating baseline and very rapid fibrillatory waves

NOTE: VR = ventricular rate.

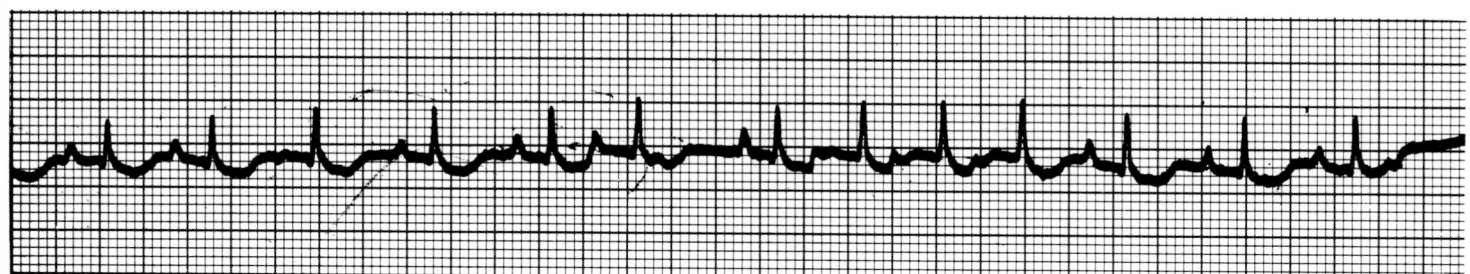

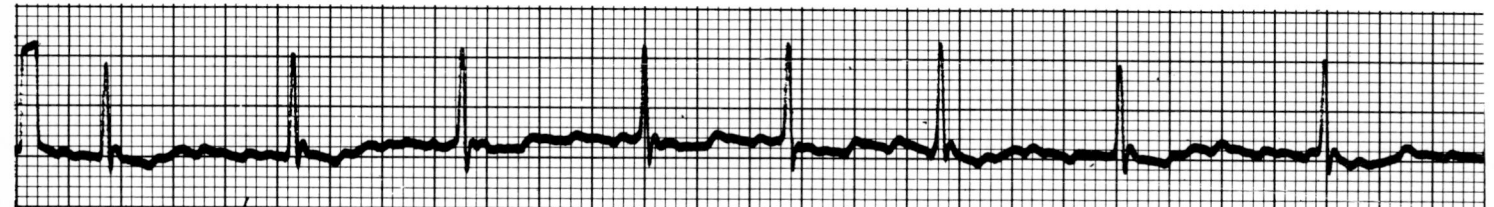

FIGURE 67-6 Comparison of MAT *(above)* and AF (atrial fibrillation) *(below)*. Note the well-formed, discrete P waves and isoelectric baseline in MAT, in contrast to indistinct, low-amplitude fibrillatory waves and undulating baseline in AF.

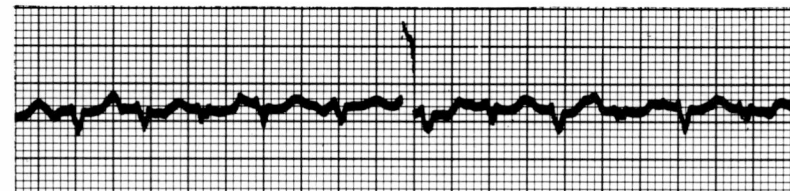

Lead II   Admission

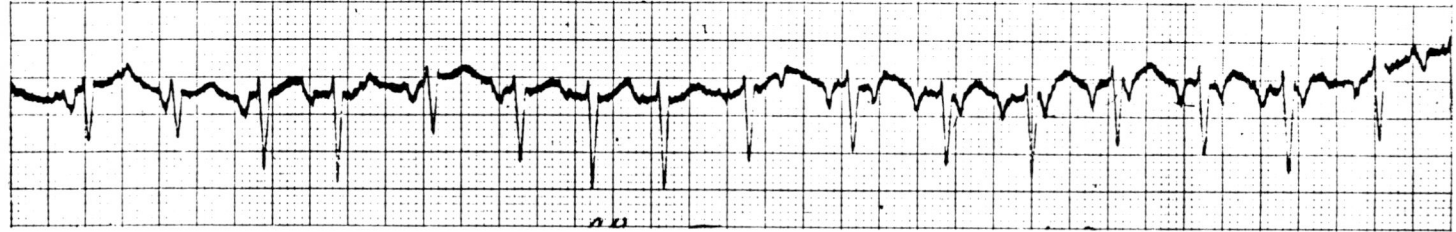

Lead II   Double Std.   Digoxin, 1.0 mg IV, 0.25 mg PO

FIGURE 67-7   MAT with AV block. Upper strip shows MAT on admission. Lower strip shows emergence of periods of 2:1 AV block, with loss of multifocality. This rhythm is highly suggestive of digitalis toxicity.

block, i.e., not every atrial impulse is conducted to the ventricle (Fig. 67-7); (2) decreased multifocality of atrial activity so that the arrhythmia resembles atrial tachycardia with atrioventricular block (see "Atrial Tachycardia with AV Block," below) (an arrhythmia that has long been recognized to be a manifestation of digitalis toxicity); (3) accelerated atrioventricular junctional rhythm, with atrioventricular dissociation; and (4) ventricular ectopic activity.

A variety of antiarrhythmic agents have been used to treat MAT, usually with uncertain or no benefit. Cardioversion appears to be ineffectual. Recently, verapamil, a calcium-channel blocking agent, has proved effective in abolishing the arrhythmia and slowing the heart rate. But it is unclear if there is any other benefit to the patient than the reduction in heart rate. Also, verapamil has potential side effects, e.g., negative inotropism, some of which are serious. The most important consideration in dealing with MAT is detection of the underlying medical problems and correcting them vigorously.

Other Atrial Arrhythmias

Classic paroxysmal supraventricular tachycardia (PAT) is seen almost as frequently as MAT and responds to time-honored measures. Verapamil, given intravenously, has proven highly effective in terminating this arrhythmia. Atrial flutter and atrial fibrillation occur less often than PAT. Several varieties of supraventricular arrhythmias can occur in the same acutely ill patient during a single hospitalization.

Atrial Tachycardia with AV Block

Atrial tachycardia with atrioventricular (AV) block is not uncommon in acute respiratory failure that complicates chronic bronchitis and emphysema. This disorder is char-

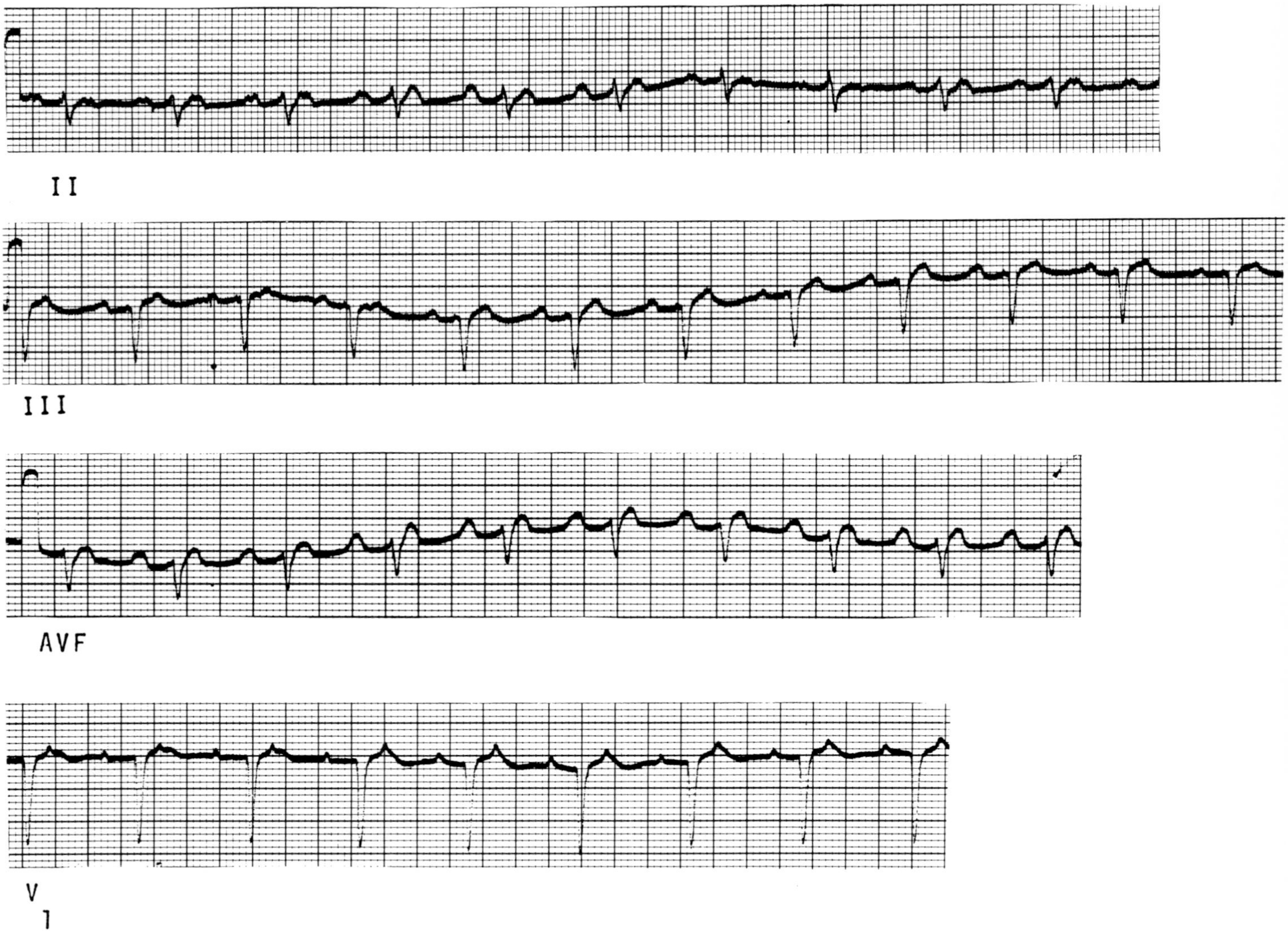

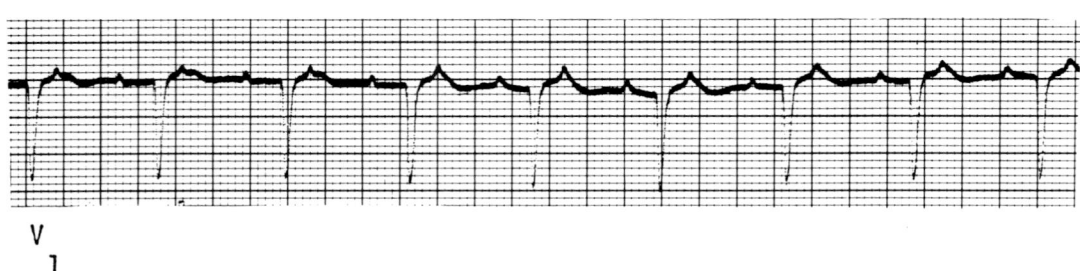

FIGURE 67-8 Atrial tachycardia with 2:1 AV block. The blocked P waves are seen deforming the T waves. (Respirophasic changes in P-wave amplitude are seen in leads II and III.)

acterized by: (1) regular or near-regular, uniform atrial activity, at rates of 120 to 240 per minute; (2) small, upright P waves in the limb leads; and (3) some impairment of AV conduction, usually in the form of 2:1 AV block (Fig. 67-8). If nonconducted P waves nestling in the ST segment are overlooked, the arrhythmia is apt to escape recognition; the arrhythmia is then discounted as a sinus tachycardia instead of being identified as an important arrhythmia. If digitalis toxicity—which is the cause in 90 percent of patients with this arrhythmia—is not recognized, the administration of more digitalis can cause a fatal arrhythmia.

In addition to the 2:1 type of AV block, second degree block can be of the Wenckebach type (Fig. 67-9). This type is also deceptive; the slowly lengthening AV intervals, with sporadic pauses in ventricular rhythm (due to nonconduction of the last atrial impulse of the Wenckebach), are easily missed on casual inspection.

Less common than second degree AV block is 1:1 AV conduction; the arrhythmia then resembles classic paroxysmal supraventricular tachycardia. However, the response of atrial tachycardia with AV block to carotid sinus pressure (or other vagal-potentiating maneuvers) is different: in 1:1 AV block, the block is enhanced without disturbing the atrial mechanism (Fig. 67-10), whereas carotid sinus pressure in classic supraventricular tachycardia either causes it to revert to sinus rhythm or leaves it unaffected.

Emphasis on this arrhythmia is warranted because of its prevalence in patients with obstructive airways disease

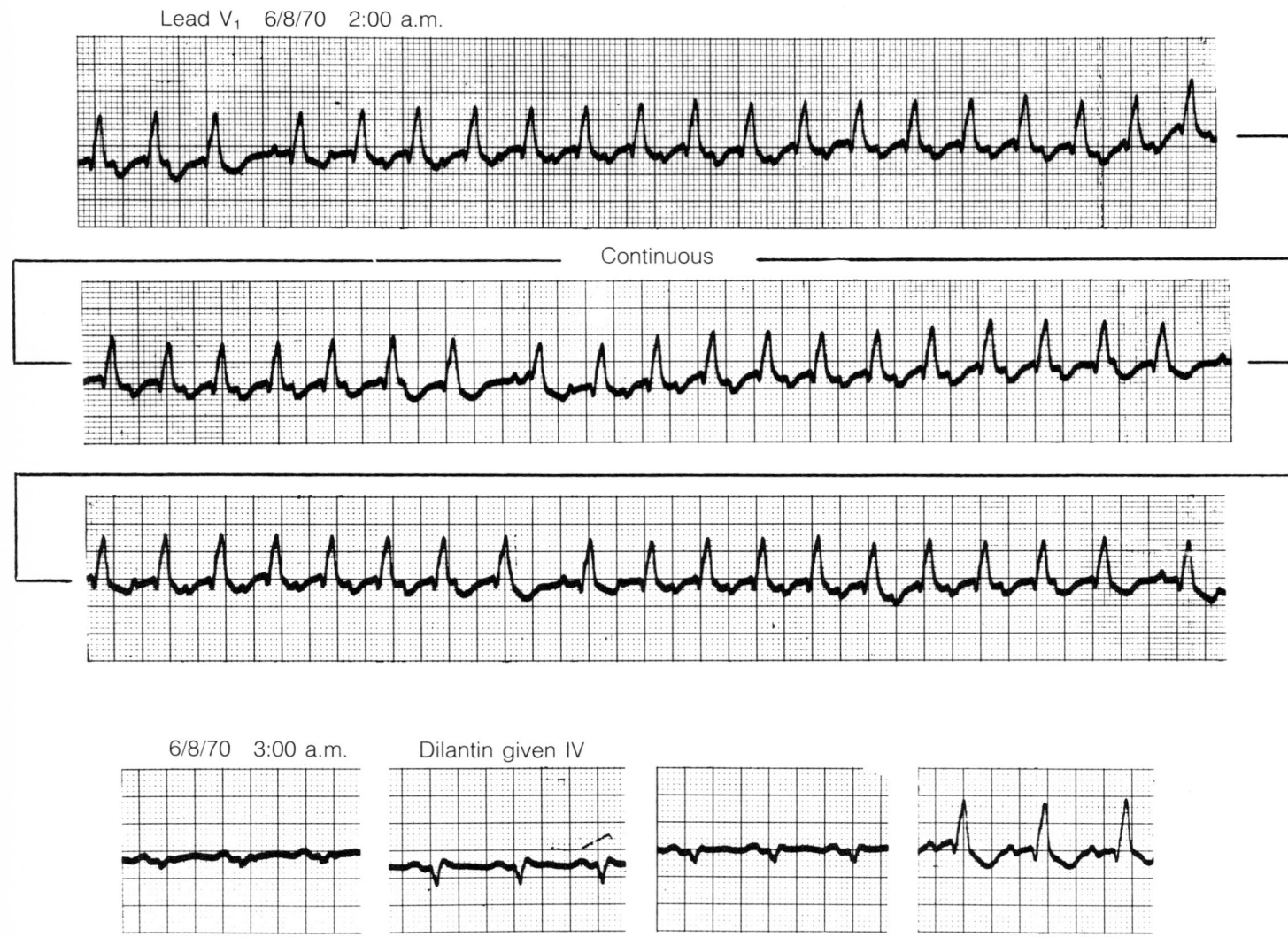

Lead V₁ 6/8/70 2:00 a.m.

Continuous

6/8/70 3:00 a.m.   Dilantin given IV

II   III   AVF   V₁

FIGURE 67-9   Atrial tachycardia with Wenckebach AV block. The three upper strips are a continuous record showing long Wenckebach periods. The P wave (different from the sinus P wave shown below) is seen in the ST segments, with slow lengthening of the PR interval until a pause occurs.

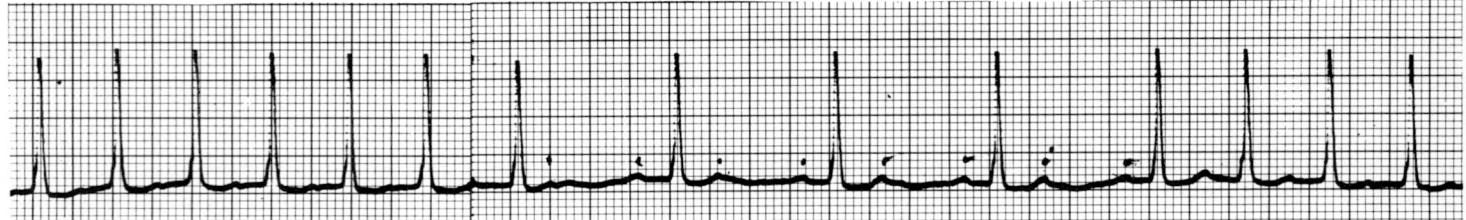

FIGURE 67-10 Carotid sinus pressure in atrial tachycardia with AV block, 1:1 AV ratio. The application of carotid sinus pressure induces 2:1 AV block, exposing P waves (marked with dots) at the same rate as the ventricles.

and the difficulty that is often encountered in detecting it: a patient with a regular 2:1 AV ratio has a regular pulse that simulates a sinus-controlled heart rate at the bedside. Treatment of the arrhythmia consists of withholding digitalis and of correcting potassium depletion if it is present. Phenytoin given intravenously (250 mg over a 5-min period) often restores sinus rhythm without abolishing the digitalis toxicity. On rare occasions, this arrhythmia is not due to digitalis but to underlying heart disease. The determination of serum concentrations of digitalis (digoxin) is a useful strategy for determining if high levels of digitalis are causing the arrhythmia or for excluding digitalis as the causative agent.

Management

The principle underlying the management of arrhythmias in patients with chronic pulmonary disease is that, as a rule, they are "secondary" phenomena. As a corollary, the "primary" underlying derangements must be uncovered and corrected. Digitalis and antiarrhythmic agents can only be viewed as *adjunctive* measures. Table 67-2 outlines a reasonable approach to management.

ADVERSE DRUG EFFECTS IN COMBINED DISEASES

One aspect of the interaction between the heart and lungs (see Chapter 68) is the occurrence of adverse effects on one organ by agents used to treat disorders in the other. For example, β-blocking drugs used to treat angina pectoris and hypertension can induce incapacitating bronchospasm. Oppositely, sympathomimetic amines and methylxanthines that are used as bronchodilators sometimes induce angina and arrhythmias in individuals with coronary arterial disease. As a rule, these untoward side effects occur in individuals in whom cardiac and pulmonary diseases coexist. However, arrhythmias can also be induced in patients who have normal hearts but are seriously ill.

Before considering the effects of drugs on the heart and lungs, consideration of the concept of *adrenergic receptors* is in order.

Adrenergic Receptors: Principles

Long before the 1940s, it had been appreciated that stimulation of the sympathetic nervous system or the administration of certain catecholamines exerted effects on various tissues and organs that seemed to be paradoxical: the effects of a single agent were stimulatory at some sites and inhibitory in others. In 1948, Ahlquist formulated the concept that two different adrenergic receptors, α and β, existed in any structure that is affected by sympathetic activity. For example, α receptors have been shown to be stimulated by both epinephrine and norepinephrine and less so by isoproterenol, and to be responsible for such effects as vasoconstriction and contraction of sphincters in the intestinal and urinary tracts. In contrast, stimulation of β receptors causes vasodilatation, bronchodilatation, and certain distinctive cardiac effects: an increase in heart rate, in contractility, and in conduction velocity, and shortening of the refractory period of the AV node. β receptors are maximally stimulated by isoproterenol and to a lesser extent by epinephrine and norepinephrine.

Propranolol was the first practical example of an agent that could block one type of receptor or the other. It benefited patients with angina pectoris by slowing heart rate and depressing contractility, thereby reducing myocardial requirements for oxygen. However, in susceptible individuals, by blocking β receptors in the airways, it also provoked bronchoconstriction. Currently, it is held to be contraindicated in patients with obstructive airways disease in which a bronchospastic element is present.

In 1967, Lands et al. subdivided β receptors into β_1 and β_2 varieties: β_1 receptors are located only in the heart; β_2 receptors are located in blood vessels and in the airways, where they mediate bronchodilatation. From the outset, a premium was set on developing a specific β_1 blocker. But, as yet, despite intensive search, no agent has yet been devised that is solely a β_1 blocker; all can elicit bronchospasm in susceptible individuals. Acebutolol and metoprolol are among those least likely to do so.

A search also began for agents that might *enhance* β_2-receptor activity (agonists), thereby relieving bronchospasm. Although a variety of β_2 agonists is now available, e.g., terbutaline, metaproterenol, and albuterol, once

again, specificity is incomplete and these agents can stimulate β_1 receptors in the heart, provoking arrhythmias or angina pectoris in susceptible individuals. Although terbutaline is an effective bronchodilator, it is more likely than the others to induce ventricular arrhythmias; albuterol seems to have the least cardiostimulatory effect of this group.

The subjective response of the patient to the start of treatment of angina pectoris with a β-blocking agent is an important guide to the proper choice of agent. If dyspnea intensifies after the medication is taken, the FEV_1 is determined and the determination is repeated after the medication has been temporarily discontinued; if bronchospasm attributable to the agent is manifested, another agent is tried or a different therapeutic approach is undertaken. Calcium-channel blocking agents often provide effective alternatives to β blockers for the treatment of angina pectoris and arrhythmias. These agents do not appear to affect the airways adversely. Indeed, they are probably a wise first choice for the patient with both angina pectoris and obstructive disease of the airways.

At present, it is impossible to predict which patient will experience adverse reaction to β agonists. Should the patient complain of palpitations, an electrocardiogram is indicated to uncover the nature of the arrhythmia.

Methylxanthines and Cardiac Arrhythmias

On occasion, methylxanthines (theophylline and aminophylline) administered intravenously have been reported to be arrhythmogenic. However, the arrhythmogenic effects of theophylline, given intravenously, appear to correlate with large doses and high blood levels. There is as yet no evidence that theophylline given orally has important arrhythmogenic effects, even though the frequency of preexistent ventricular ectopic beats may increase; sustained arrhythmias have not been reported when theophylline has been given by mouth. In contrast, large doses of aminophylline given intravenously have caused sudden death.

Since the metabolism of theophylline is slowed in individuals with chronic liver disease, maintenance dosages may require adjustment in patients who have diseases of both the lungs and liver. Careful monitoring of blood theophylline levels will serve to avoid serious problems.

Pulmonary Effects of Nitroglycerin

Nitroglycerin is widely used in treatment of acute and chronic coronary arterial disease. It is administered either sublingually, topically, or intravenously. Caution is indicated in administering it to individuals in whom coexistent pulmonary disease has caused ventilation-perfusion abnormalities. In these individuals, a decrease in arterial oxygenation occasionally follows the sublingual administration of nitroglycerin, presumably due to aggravation of the ventilation-perfusion mismatch, i.e., the vasodilating effects of nitroglycerin-increased blood flow to relatively hypoventilated regions. Nitroglycerin may also decrease cardiac output. Either the decrease in cardiac output or in oxygenation or both can reduce oxygen delivery to the tissues. Careful monitoring of arterial blood oxygenation is advisable when nitroglycerin is administered to individuals in whom cardiac and pulmonary disease coexist.

BIBLIOGRAPHY

Agarwal BL, Agarwal BV: Digitalis-induced paroxysmal atrial tachycardia with AV block. Br Heart J 34:330–335, 1972.
The incidence of PAT with block is high in individuals with chronic pulmonary disease.

Ahlquist RP: The study of adrenotropic receptors. Am J Physiol 153:586–600, 1948.
Conception and delineation of α- and β-adrenergic receptors, a lucid and impelling 15-page paper.

Alexander S: Cardiac function and arrhythmias in patients with lung disease. Geriatrics 31:42–43, 1976.
This introductory article, as well as the others in a five-part symposium, contains considerable practical information about this subject.

Arsura EL, Solar M, Lefkin AS, Scher DL, Tessler S: Metoprolol in the treatment of multifocal atrial tachycardia. Crit Care Med 15:591–594, 1987.
Metoprolol is effective in the acute and chronic treatment of MAT and may be given to patients with MAT and respiratory failure without serious adverse effects.

Ayres SM, Grace WJ: Inappropriate ventilation and hypoxemia as causes of cardiac arrhythmias: The control of arrhythmias without antiarrhythmic drugs. Am J Med 46:495–505, 1969.
A landmark report that describes arrhythmias induced by over- or underventilation of patients requiring ventilator support.

Badke FR: Left ventricular dimensions and function during exercise in dogs with chronic right ventricular pressure overload. Am J Cardiol 53:1187–1193, 1984.
A recent experimental study in dogs that supports the concept of septum-mediated ventricular interdependence. It is based on hemodynamic techniques and entails measurement of chamber dimensions using ultrasonic crystals implanted on the chamber.

Banner AS, Sunderrajan EV, Agarwal MK, Addington WW: Arrhythmogenic effects of orally administered bronchodilators. Arch Intern Med 139:434–437, 1979.
A clinical study of 20 subjects, using double-blind crossover protocol that tested the effect on chronic ventricular premature beats of ephedrine, aminophylline, terbutaline, and placebo. Terbutaline was found to have considerable arrhythmogenic properties.

Bass H: Lung function in chronic obstructive lung disease: Coexistent left heart failure. Am J Med 48:413–415, 1970.
A succinct summary is provided of the often confusing picture presented by this combination of conditions.

Biggs FD, Lefrak SS, Kleiger RE, Senior RM, Oliver GC: Disturbances of rhythm in chronic lung disease. Heart Lung 6:256–261, 1977.
A review that is unique with respect to the detail provided about the treatment of arrhythmias.

Bove AA, Santamore WP: Ventricular interdependence. Prog Cardiovasc Dis XXIII:365–388, 1981.
A comprehensive overview of the subject, listing 105 references. Experimental and clinical studies are considered in detail.

Brashear RE: Arrhythmias in patients with chronic obstructive pulmonary disease. Med Clin North Am 68:969–981, 1984.
A critical review of the occurrence of arrhythmias in chronic obstructive airways disease and of drug-induced arrhythmias.

Corazza LJ, Pastor BH: Cardiac arrhythmias in chronic cor pulmonale. N Engl J Med 259:862–865, 1958.
The first clinical study calling attention to the importance of this association, emphasizing infection or digitalis toxicity as important etiologic factors.

Cortese DA: Pulmonary function in mitral stenosis. Mayo Clin Proc 53:321–326, 1978.
A detailed examination of pulmonary function in mitral stenosis.

Dean PJ, Groshart KD, Porterfield JG, Iansmith DH, Golden EB Jr: Amiodarone-associated pulmonary toxicity. A clinical and pathologic study of eleven cases. Am J Clin Pathol 87:7–13, 1987.
Pulmonary toxicity developed in 11 of 171 patients undergoing amiodarone therapy. The drug-induced phospholipidosis was reversible clinically in all patients.

DeSilva RA, Graboys TB, Podrid PJ, Lown B: Cardioversion and defibrillation. Am Heart J 100:881–895, 1980.
The group that has pioneered in the use of cardioversion in treating arrhythmias examines its proper application.

Diener CF, Burrows B: Further observations on the course and prognosis of chronic obstructive lung disease. Am Rev Respir Dis 111:719–725, 1975.
A 14-year prospective study of 200 patients with chronic obstructive lung disease, the best such study yet to appear.

Dutt AK, DeSoyza ND, Au WY, Hargis JL, Tuck RL: The effect of aminophylline on cardiac rhythm in advanced chronic obstructive pulmonary disease: Correlation with serum theophylline levels. Eur J Respir Dis 64:264–270, 1983.
Theophylline, in doses that produce therapeutic blood levels, failed to induce ventricular irritability in previously arrhythmia-free subjects, but it did elicit variable effects on preexisting ventricular ectopy. Theophylline was administered intravenously. Holter monitoring was used to detect disturbances in cardiac rhythm.

Eiriksson CE Jr, Writer SL, Vestal RE: Theophylline-induced alterations in cardiac electrophysiology in patients with chronic obstructive pulmonary disease. Am Rev Respir Dis 135:322–326, 1987.
Electrophysiologic testing was performed before and during aminophylline (theophylline ethylenediamine) infusions in 10 male patients with stable obstructive airways disease. Although no arrhythmias were induced, 5 patients had symptoms (3 presyncope and 2 chest pain) with rapid atrial pacing during, but not prior to, the aminophylline infusion.

Friedman GD, Klatsky AL, Siegelaub AB: Lung function and risk of myocardial infarction and sudden cardiac death. N Engl J Med 294:1071–1075, 1976.
> *A prospective study of 464 subjects enrolled in the Kaiser-Permanente Medical Care Program suggests a possible link between lung disease and coronary artery disease.*

Hales CA, Kazemi H: Clinical significance of pulmonary function tests: Pulmonary function after uncomplicated myocardial infarction. Chest 72:350–358, 1977.
> *The effects of uncomplicated myocardial infarction on pulmonary performance is critically analyzed.*

Hazard PB, Burnett CR: Treatment of multifocal atrial tachycardia with metoprolol. Crit Care Med 15:20–25, 1987.
> *In 25 patients with multifocal atrial tachycardia, which was complicating severe cardiopulmonary illness, metoprolol proved effective in the management of multifocal atrial tachycardia.*

Hazard PB, Burnett CR: Verapamil in multifocal atrial tachycardia. Hemodynamic and respiratory changes. Chest 91:68–70, 1987.
> *Verapamil is generally beneficial in the treatment of MAT, but its utility may be limited in many patients by its tendency to aggravate preexisting arterial hypoxemia.*

Henthorn R, Roberts WS, Kelly K, Leier CV: Conversion of atrial flutter: Rapid atrial pacing as a bedside technique. Pace 3:202–206, 1980.
> *The proper use of rapid atrial pacing in treating atrial flutter.*

Holford FD, Mithoefer JC: Cardiac arrhythmias in hospitalized patients with chronic obstructive pulmonary disease. Am Rev Respir Dis 108:879–885, 1973.
> *The first report of the use of Holter monitoring to record continuously the cardiac rhythm. Eighty-nine percent of patients exhibited arrhythmias. The lower incidence of arrhythmias previously reported underscores the unreliability of random electrocardiograms as a basis for determining the frequency of cardiac arrhythmias in this type of patient.*

Hudson LD, Kurt TL, Petty TL, Genton E: Arrhythmias associated with acute respiratory failure in patients with chronic airway obstruction. Chest 63:661–665, 1973.
> *In a large series of patients in acute respiratory failure, ventricular arrhythmias had dire consequences. (Most arrhythmias seen in subjects with lung disease are supraventricular in type.) Unfortunately, no information is given about the incidence of coronary artery disease in this population.*

Jardin F, Gueret P, Prost JF, Farcot JC, Ozier Y, Bourdarias JP: Two-dimensional echocardiographic assessment of left ventricular function in chronic obstructive pulmonary disease. Am Rev Respir Dis 129:135–142, 1984.
> *This report of two-dimensional echocardiography in a small series of patients supports the concept of septum-mediated ventricular interdependence.*

Josephson GW: Dysrhythmogenesis associated with the treatment of acute reversible airway obstruction. Ann Emerg Med 11:425–428, 1982.
> *A recent review of drug-induced arrhythmias in individuals with pulmonary disease.*

Kachel RG: Left ventricular function in chronic obstructive pulmonary disease. Chest 74:286–290, 1978.
> *An even-handed, comprehensive, and critical review of this controversial subject.*

Kleiger RE, Senior RM: Long-term electrocardiographic monitoring of ambulatory patients with chronic airway obstruction. Chest 65:483–487, 1974.
> *To date, this is one of only three studies of Holter monitoring of subjects with chronic pulmonary disease. It emphasizes the findings of the study of Holford and Mithoefer and points up the need for more investigations of this type.*

Kligfield P: Clinical applications of ambulatory electrocardiography. Cardiology 71:69–99, 1984.
> *The emphasis of this review is on the evaluation of arrhythmias in ambulatory patients with coronary disease.*

Krowka MJ, Pairolero PC, Trastek VF, Payne WS, Bernatz PE: Cardiac dysrhythmia following pneumonectomy. Clinical correlates and prognostic significance. Chest 91:490–495, 1987.
> *Cardiac tachydysrhythmias occurred in 53 (22 percent) of 236 consecutive patients undergoing pneumonectomy. Tachydysrhythmias after pneumonectomy occur more frequently following intrapericardial dissection and in patients who develop postoperative interstitial pulmonary edema or perihilar pulmonary edema.*

Lands AM, Luduena FP, Buzzo HJ: Differentiation of receptors responsive to isoproterenol. Life Sci 6:2241–2249, 1967.
  This is a refinement of Ahlquist's adrenergic receptor classification, subdividing β receptors into types 1 and 2. This in turn stimulated search for type-specific therapeutic agents.

Levine JH, Michael JR, Guarnieri T: Treatment of multifocal atrial tachycardia with verapamil. N Engl J Med 312:21–25, 1985.
  Verapamil administered intravenously slowed the atrial rate in subjects with multifocal atrial tachycardia by an average of 30 beats per minute. Whether another benefit also occurred is not indicated. Evidence is provided that this arrhythmia is due to triggered automaticity.

Matthay RA, Berger HJ: Noninvasive assessment of right and left ventricular function in acute and chronic respiratory failure. Crit Care Med 11:329–338, 1983.
  This review provides excellent coverage of studies using radionuclide imaging and echocardiography.

Matthay RA, Depew CC: Obstructive airway disease: Rational therapy with theophylline agents. Geriatrics 35:65–77, 1980.
  This report suggests proper dosages for the intravenous and oral use of these preparations.

Mehrotra PP, Weaver YJ, Higginbotham EA: Myocardial perfusion defect on thallium-201 imaging in patients with chronic obstructive pulmonary disease. JACC 2:233–239, 1983.
  False-positive myocardial scintigraphy using thallium 201 is described in six subjects who were shown to have normal coronary arteries upon study.

Nalos PC, Kass RM, Gang ES, Fishbein MC, Mandel WJ, Peter T: Life-threatening postoperative pulmonary complications in patients with previous amiodarone pulmonary toxicity undergoing cardiothoracic operations. J Thorac Cardiovasc Surg 93:904–912, 1987.
  In four patients with previously diagnosed amiodarone pulmonary toxicity, the adult respiratory distress syndrome developed after cardiothoracic operations for malignant ventricular arrhythmias. Three patients underwent endocardial resection (two died); the fourth had implantation of an automatic defibrillator unit.

Patel AK, Skatrud JB, Thomsen JH: Cardiac arrhythmias due to oral aminophylline in patients with chronic obstructive pulmonary disease. Chest 80:661–665, 1981.
  Aminophylline administered orally to 15 patients with obstructive airways disease increased the incidence of heightened ventricular irritability but not enough to change the grade of the arrhythmia.

Rao BS, Cohn KE, Eldridge FL, Hancock EW: Left ventricular failure secondary to chronic pulmonary disease. Am J Med 45:229–241, 1968.
  An early clinical study of eight patients that includes data obtained by both cardiac catheterization and autopsy. The left ventricular failure in this group seemed to reflect the coexistence of congestive cardiomyopathy and chronic lung disease.

Rees HA, Thomas AJ, Rossiter C: The recognition of coronary heart disease in the presence of pulmonary disease. Br Heart J 26:233–240, 1964.
  Further refinement of criteria of Thomas in clinical and electrocardiographic diagnosis of coronary disease, with autopsy control.

Shine KI, Kastor JA, Yurchak PM: Multifocal atrial tachycardia: Clinical and electrocardiographic features in 32 patients. N Engl J Med 279:344–349, 1968.
  The first delineation of MAT as a clinical-electrocardiographic entity.

Thomas AJ: Coronary heart disease in the presence of pulmonary disease. Br Heart J 20:83–91, 1958.
  The first clinicopathologic study of this association, emphasizing helpful clues to the often elusive diagnosis of coronary disease.

Wadler S, Chahinian P, Slater W, Goldman M, Mendelson D, Holland JF: Cardiac abnormalities in patients with diffuse malignant pleural mesothelioma. Cancer 58:2744–2750, 1986.
  Clinical cardiac abnormalities and cardiac invasion by tumor occur in the great majority of patients with malignant pleural mesothelioma.

Walston A, Brewer DL, Kitchens CS, Krook JE: The electrocardiographic manifestations of spontaneous left pneumothorax. Ann Intern Med 80:375–379, 1974.
  A report that also summarizes the previous literature concerning the electrocardiographic changes in left pneumothorax that mimic anterior myocardial infarction.

Wang K, Goldfarb BL, Gobel FL, Richman HG: Multifocal atrial tachycardia: A clinical analysis in 41 cases. Arch Intern Med 137:161–164, 1977.

A recent study and review of the literature that corroborates the 1968 report of Shine et al.

Weber KT, Janicki JS: Pulmonary hypertension, in Weber KT, Janicki JS (eds), *Cardiopulmonary Exercise Testing.* Philadelphia, Saunders, 1986, pp 222–234.

This chapter on pulmonary hypertension describes the responses to exercise of patients with pulmonary hypertension.

Weisse AB: Contralateral effects of cardiac disease affecting primarily either the left or right chambers of the heart. Am Heart J 87:654–660, 1974.

The first comprehensive review of ventricular interdependence.

Zema MJ, Kligfield P: ECG poor R-wave progression: Review and synthesis. Arch Intern Med 142:1145–1148, 1982.

A summary of the authors' clinicopathologic studies of this subject that includes a review of relevant literature. A stepwise plan for analyzing the electrocardiogram is presented.

Chapter **68**

Pulmonary Disorders Produced by Cardiac Disease

David M. F. Murphy / *Alfred P. Fishman*

Left Ventricular Failure
 Dyspnea
 Signs
 Radiology
 Pleural Effusion
 Pulmonary Function
 Gas Exchange
 Carbon Dioxide Retention
 Distribution of Inspired Air
 Regional Function Studies
 Cardiac Asthma
 Treatment of Pulmonary Edema

Ischemic Heart Disease
 Angina Pectoris (Acute Pulmonary Effects)
 Myocardial Infarction (Subacute Pulmonary Effects)
 Congestive Heart Failure (Chronic Pulmonary Effects)
 Rheumatic Pneumonitis

Valvular Heart Disease
 Mitral Valvular Disease
 Aortic Valvular Disease

Congenital Heart Disease
 Left-to-Right Shunts
 Right-to-Left Shunts

Cardiac Drugs
 β-Adrenergic Antagonists
 Vasodilators
 Amiodarone

Mechanical Ventilation

Cardiac Surgery
 Mitral Valvular Disease
 Coronary Artery Revascularization
 Transplantation

Heart-Lung Interactions
 The Combined Cardiopulmonary System

Ventricular Interdependence
 Systolic Ventricular Interaction
 Diastolic Ventricular Interaction
 Pericardial Effects

Intrathoracic Pressure Effects
Clinical Significance of Ventricular Interdependence
Right Ventricular Pressure Overload
Chronic Pulmonary Disease

Arrhythmias in Cor Pulmonale

Systemic Disease

The Bronchial Circulation
 Bronchopulmonary Anastomoses
 Clinical Importance of the Bronchial Circulation
 Hemoptysis
 Shunts
 Bronchial Hyperreactivity and Cardiac Asthma

The heart, lungs, and blood are traditionally viewed together as a cardiopulmonary apparatus that has evolved in mammals for the sake of external gas exchange (Fig. 68-1). Not only are the heart and lungs coupled mechanically, but they are housed together within the confines of the chest which acts as a bellows, driven by regulatory mechanisms from without. Because of their proximity and interdependence, a disturbance in either the heart or lungs can profoundly affect the performance of the other, thereby threatening the mechanism for external gas exchange. Similarly, an abnormality in the chest bellows or in its regulating mechanisms can compromise the efficient operation of the cardiorespiratory apparatus.

This chapter deals with pulmonary disorders that are secondary to heart disease; almost invariably, it is the left side of the heart—myocardium or valves—that is primarily affected. The converse, cor pulmonale due to respiratory diseases and disorders, is considered elsewhere in this book (see Chapter 64). In Europe, by analogy with *cardiopulmonary* disorders, the disorders considered in this chapter are sometimes designated as *pulmonocardiac disorders*.

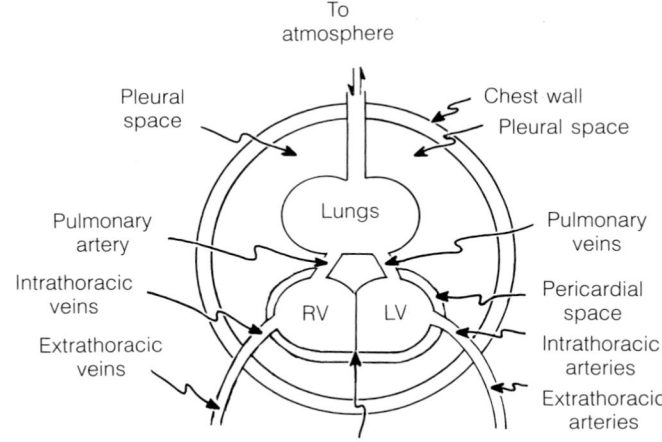

FIGURE 68-1 Schematic representation of the integrated cardiopulmonary system.

LEFT VENTRICULAR FAILURE

A detailed description of the factors that control the formation and distribution of excess fluid in the lungs is provided in Chapter 60. Here it is worth underscoring that the first manifestation of left ventricular failure is dyspnea on effort due to excess water in the lungs. In time, dyspnea present only on exertion is succeeded by dyspnea at rest. The mechanism responsible for the dyspnea is mechanical ("hemodynamic"): an increase in the filling pressures of the left ventricle is reflected in an increase in pulmonary venous pressure and in filtration pressures in the pulmonary microcirculation.

Dyspnea

Dyspnea is a sensation that is easier for patients to describe than for physicians to quantify. Its subjective nature complicates its use as a basis for the functional assessment of heart failure or pulmonary disease. Generally, the term implies not only shortness of breath but also a sense of discomfort; it implies that "breathing is no longer unconsciously or effortlessly performed." A key problem in assessing dyspnea is that it is multidimensional, with sensory, affective, and cognitive components; another is that it covers a multitude of respiratory sensations, ranging from the distressing "tightness of the chest" experienced by asthmatics to the euphoric gulping of air that accompanies winning the 100-yard dash.

MECHANISMS

The early studies of dyspnea focused on the "breathing reserve," i.e., the difference between the maximum breathing capacity (determined as the MVV) and the actual minute ventilation. Cournand and Richards pictured the intensity of dyspnea ("breathlessness") as increasing along with the fraction of the maximum respiratory-force generating capacity utilized in breathing. This useful concept was pushed to the background by developments in assessing the mechanics of breathing. Clearly, patients with pulmonary edema work harder and expend more energy in breathing than do normal individuals: the work and oxygen cost of breathing proved to be high in pulmonary edema. The elastic and resistive components of the work of breathing were shown to be increased; so was the oxygen cost of breathing. The respiratory pattern of high frequency and small tidal volumes was considered to be an automatic adaptation that operated to minimize the work and energy cost of breathing (Fig. 68-2).

A fresh approach to the sensation of dyspnea was heralded by the concept of *length-tension inappropriateness*. According to this theory, perception of dyspnea arises from the disordered relationship between the tension (pressure) generated by the respiratory muscles and the change in length (tidal volume) that results. As part of this

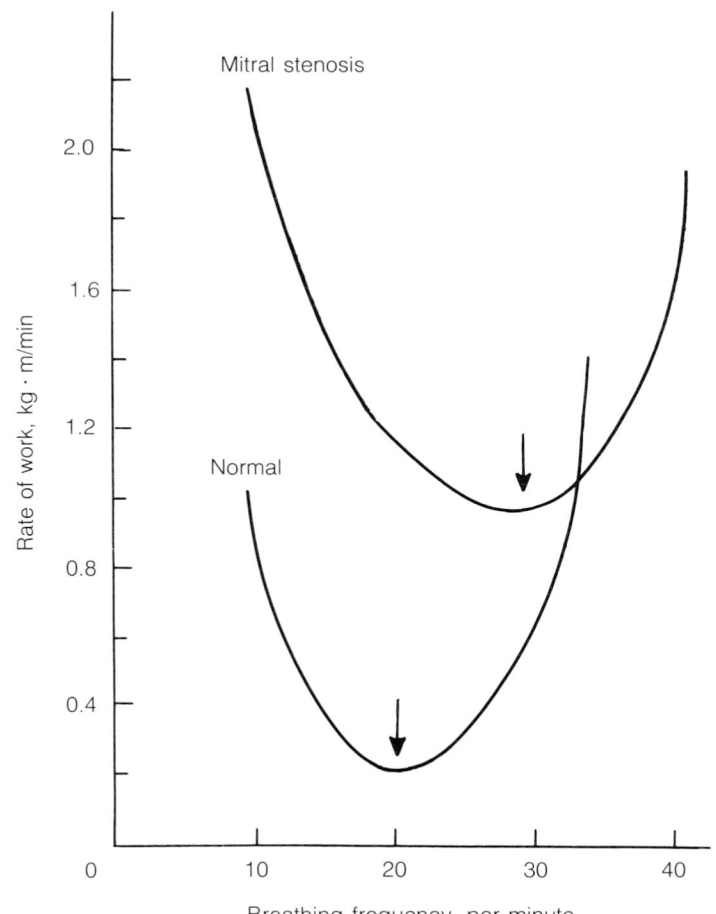

FIGURE 68-2 Mechanical work of breathing at different respiratory frequencies in a normal individual and in a patient with mitral stenosis. As indicated by the arrows, the minimal (optimal) frequency is higher in mitral stenosis than in normals.

concept, it was postulated that a disparity between muscle tension and change in length leads to misalignment of fibers in the muscle spindles; from these spindles, signals are transmitted to higher centers that bring the act of breathing to a conscious level.

More recently, attention has been directed at the psychological and neurophysiological bases for the sensation of dyspnea, and attempts have been made to quantify the sensation using the concepts of psychophysics. The sensation of muscle force seems to arise from receptors in the respiratory muscles which signal changes in muscle tension. The *perceived* magnitude of the load handled by the respiratory muscles seems to be directly dependent on the forces that the muscles generate during loaded breaths rather than the *actual* physical magnitudes of the loads. Also, the intensity of the sensation can be described as a power function of the peak pressure generated by the contracting respiratory muscles and the duration that the contraction is sustained.

If, or how, fatigue of the respiratory muscles contributes to the sensation of dyspnea is unclear. Quantification of the two sensations, i.e., dyspnea and fatigue, for the sake of comparison is a major hurdle in dealing with these subjective phenomena.

DISTINGUISHING BETWEEN CARDIAC AND PULMONARY DYSPNEA

As a rule, there is no problem in identifying if the heart or lungs is the cause of dyspnea. Conventional signs, symptoms, tests, and responses to treatment (e.g., digitalis and diuretics versus bronchodilators) pinpoint etiology and pathogenesis. For example, in the typical case of mitral stenosis or insufficiency, it is generally not difficult to relate shortness of breath, at rest or during exercise, to the valvular abnormality. The same is true of the heavy smoker who is known to have chronic bronchitis. However, the situation does become more complicated in the prototypic overweight, out-of-shape, middle-aged smoker who has both chronic bronchitis and hypertension. The differential diagnosis can also be difficult in the older population in whom cardiovascular disease and chronic obstructive airways disease often coexist. A third troublesome group is that in which asthma begins in later life without apparent cause. However, certain common denominators are useful in sorting out the two groups: (1) *cardiac dyspnea*, almost invariably, pulmonary venous hypertension and a subnormal cardiac output signal left ventricular failure; and (2) *pulmonary dyspnea*, the work of breathing is abnormally high, whereas the breathing reserve (MVV − $\dot{V}_E$) is subnormal.

Certain types of dyspnea have been advocated as more suggestive of disorders of the heart than the lungs or vice versa. Orthopnea (intolerable respiratory distress while lying flat) is a fairly reliable symptom of left ventricular failure, particularly if the sense of urgency to sit upright is a criterion for orthopnea. However, some patients with extracardiac disorders, such as obstructive airways disease, pericardial disease, or bilateral diaphragmatic paralysis, become exceedingly uncomfortable in the supine position. Even more telltale than orthopnea is *paroxysmal nocturnal dyspnea*. Two other patterns of breathlessness were once thought to be distinctive, but they have not worn well: *platypnea* (breathlessness in the upright position that is relieved by the supine position), once thought to be distinctive for severe chronic obstructive airways disease, has also been encountered both in cyanotic, congenital heart disease and in combined heart and lung disease; *trepopnea* (breathlessness limited to one lateral decubitus position), once attributed to heart disease, has also been elicited in patients with pulmonary disease.

Exercise has been widely adopted as a basis for making the distinction between cardiac and pulmonary dyspnea (see Chapters 18 and 164). It affords three different kinds of information: (1) tests of *overall performance* of the cardiorespiratory apparatus, the maximum aerobic capacity ($\dot{V}_{O_2max}$), and the anaerobic threshold (maximum $\dot{V}_{O_2}$ that can be performed without developing metabolic acidosis); (2) tests of *cardiac performance*, such as the electrocardiogram, heart rate, minute ventilation as $\dot{V}_{O_2}$ increases, and radionuclide imaging (e.g., thallium 201); and (3) tests of *pulmonary performance* such as V_D/V_T, $P(A-a)_{O_2}$, arterial oxygenation, and end-tidal P_{CO_2}. However, in practice, exercise testing is used more as a measure for quantifying physical capability and disability on the one hand and of assessing the adequacy of the coronary circulation on the other than for distinguishing between cardiac and pulmonary bases for dyspnea.

Signs

Excess fluid in the lungs is difficult to detect before the stage of severe pulmonary edema. One early manifestation of interstitial edema is an increase in the frequency of breathing. This sign is often overlooked. Presumably, the typical pattern of rapid, shallow breathing that accompanies stiffening of the lungs by excess fluid is due largely to receptors (*juxtacapillary*, or J, receptors) that sense distortions of alveolar and bronchiolar interstitial spaces. Inspiratory rales are late manifestations reflecting free fluid in terminal airways. Pink sputum, often frothy, is even further along and is generally attributed to the leakage of blood from few minute vessels with only a minor contribution from diapedesis through alveolar walls. Surfactant carried into tracheal fluid causes small bubbles.

Radiology

The radiographic findings in acute and chronic pulmonary edema are considered elsewhere (see Chapter 60). In *acute* pulmonary edema, vessels at the top of the lungs are recruited by the expanded pulmonary blood volume. In *chronic* pulmonary edema, cephalization occurs, so that the vasculature of the upper zones is more prominent than that at the lung bases, presumably because of perivascular edema and fibrosis in the dependent part of the lungs.

As pulmonary venous pressure increases acutely, radiographic evidences of interstitial edema appear. The chest radiograph is a sensitive technique for detecting interstitial edema. In the past, it was felt that since chest radiographic interpretation is highly subjective, quantitation would be imprecise. But recent studies have shown that radiographic interpretation can be quantitative and that it correlates well with indicator-dilution measurements made during life and with postmortem determinations of pulmonary extravascular water. The radiographic criteria used for identification of interstitial edema include assessments of hilar size, density, and blunting of outline, and the presence of Kerley lines A, B, and C (Fig. 68-3). Other findings include the presence of widened fis-

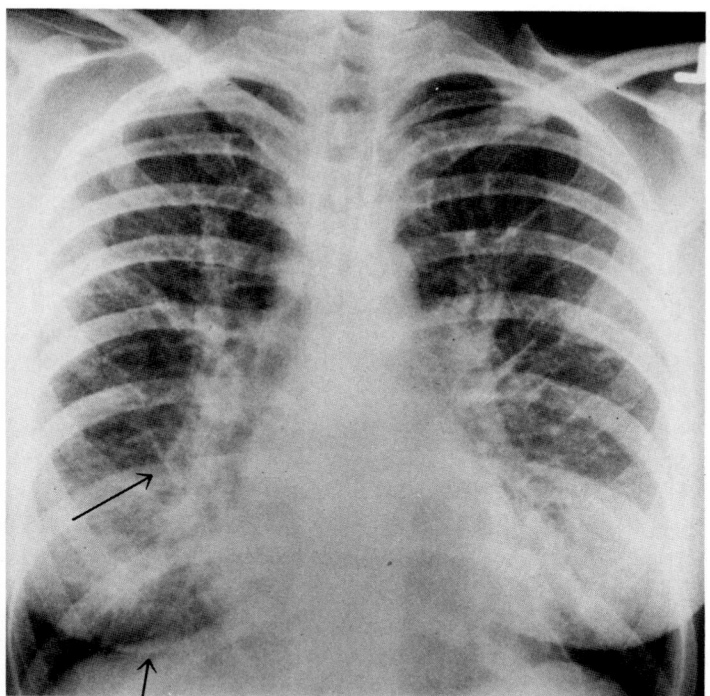

FIGURE 68-3 Mitral stenosis showing interstitial edema. The sharp linear densities (arrows) represent septal edema (Kerley lines).

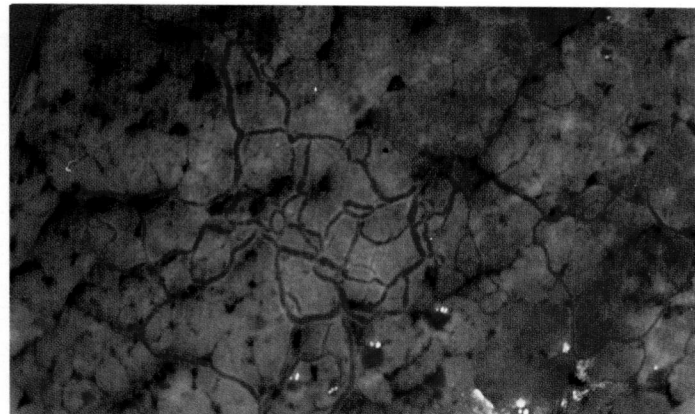

FIGURE 68-4 Lymphatic channels on the surface of the lungs outlined by blood after an episode of hemoptysis.

sures, peribronchial and perivascular cuffs and perihilar haze, subpleural effusion, and diffuse increase in density of the chest radiograph.

In cardiogenic pulmonary edema, the radiographic findings of pulmonary vascular congestion and edema correlate well with determinations of pulmonary venous pressure. Nevertheless, discrepancies exist, including the "posttherapeutic phase lag." This refers to instances where a decline in pulmonary wedge pressure is not associated with corresponding clearing of the radiographic signs of pulmonary edema. This lag is probably attributable to the slow removal of excess extravascular lung water to which the limited capacity of the lymphatic system of the lung probably contributes (Fig. 68-4).

Other radiographic findings which reflect central venous pressures are the size of the azygous vein and of the "vascular pedicle" (Fig. 68-5). The size of the azygous vein correlates well with the right atrial pressure and total blood volume; the width of the "vascular pedicle" reflects the size of the total blood volume. The left border of the pedicle is formed by the relatively rigid subclavian artery, whereas the right border is formed by the compliant right bracheocephalic vein above and the superior vena cava below; increased blood volume expands the right border. The width of the vascular pedicle in normal subjects has been reported to be 48 ± 5 mm. When the width equals or exceeds 62 mm, neck vein distension is usually present. The maximum diameter of the azygous vein in the standard upright chest radiograph is 7 mm. During pregnancy, the arch may dilate to a maximum of 15 mm.

Radiographic appearances often do not permit the clean separation of cardiogenic from noncardiogenic pulmonary edema. Whether recent technological developments, such as nuclear magnetic resonance, density imaging by computed transmission tomography, and Compton scatter tomography, will help in this regard is unclear.

Pleural Effusion

Ten percent of all pleural effusions are due to congestive heart failure. Approximately one-quarter of patients with congestive heart failure and pulmonary edema have pleural effusions. These effusions are usually transudates. For unknown reasons, in patients with congestive heart failure, pleural effusions occur more often, and in large quantities, on the right side than on the left.

A pleural effusion acts as a space-occupying mass: it produces dyspnea as it compresses adjacent lung. Atelectasis is most marked in its vicinity, with a reduction in lung volumes; accompanying these changes are abnormalities in pulmonary mechanics and gas exchange.

Pulmonary Function

In patients with left ventricular failure, the pattern is that of a restrictive ventilatory defect upon which is superimposed an obstructive component of varying degree. In chronic left ventricular failure, the higher the pulmonary venous pressure, the more profound the congestion and edema and the more striking the abnormalities. For convenience, three stages in the evolution of pulmonary edema can be pictured: congestion, interstitial pulmonary edema, and alveolar edema (Fig. 68-6).

PULMONARY CONGESTION

When left ventricular end-diastolic pressure increases, pressure throughout the pulmonary circulation also increases; pulmonary arterial pressure increases somewhat disproportionately, suggesting that reflex, rather than

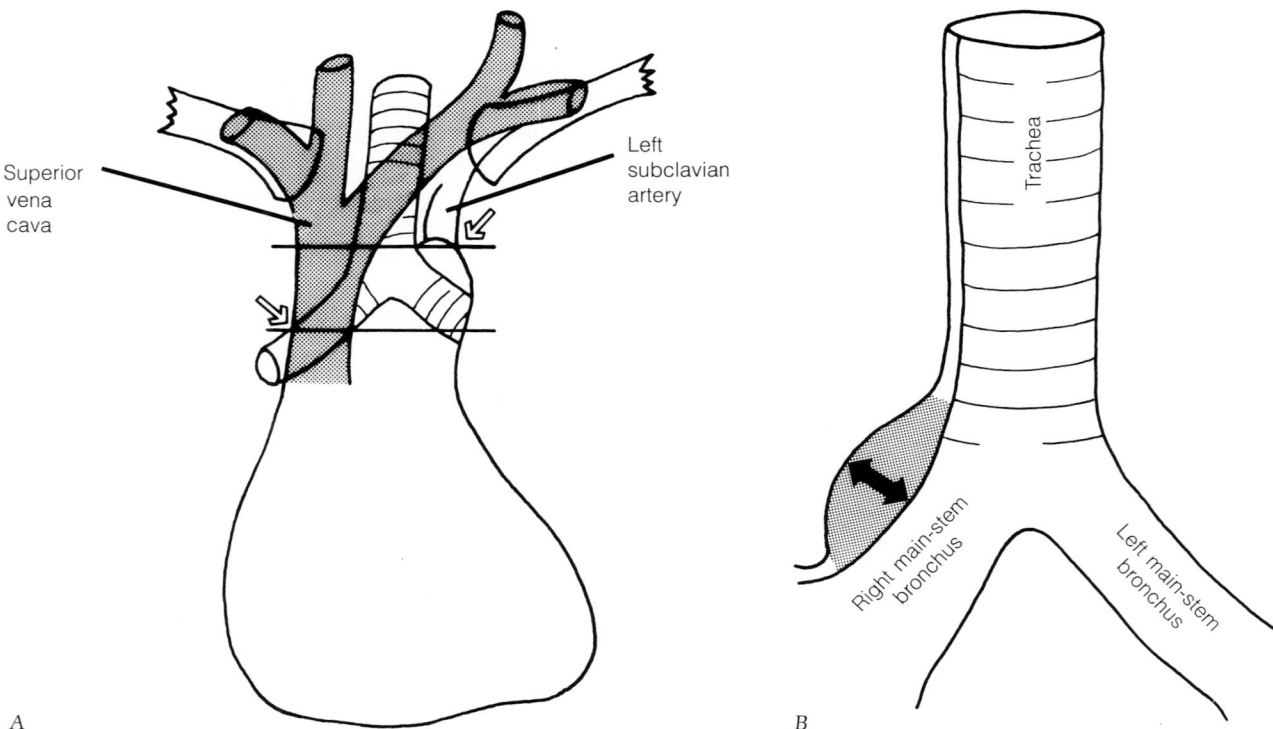

FIGURE 68-5 Radiographic indices of expanded blood volume and increased central venous pressures. A. The distended azygous vein. The upper limit of normal diameter in the conventional upright radiograph is 7 mm. B. The width of the vascular pedicle. The left border of the pedicle is formed by the relatively indistensible subclavian artery. The right border of the pedicle is formed by the more compliant right bracheocephalic vein *above* and the superior vena cava *below*. The landmarks on which the measurements are made are indicated by the two arrows. The upper limit of normal for the width of the vascular pedicle is 53 mm.

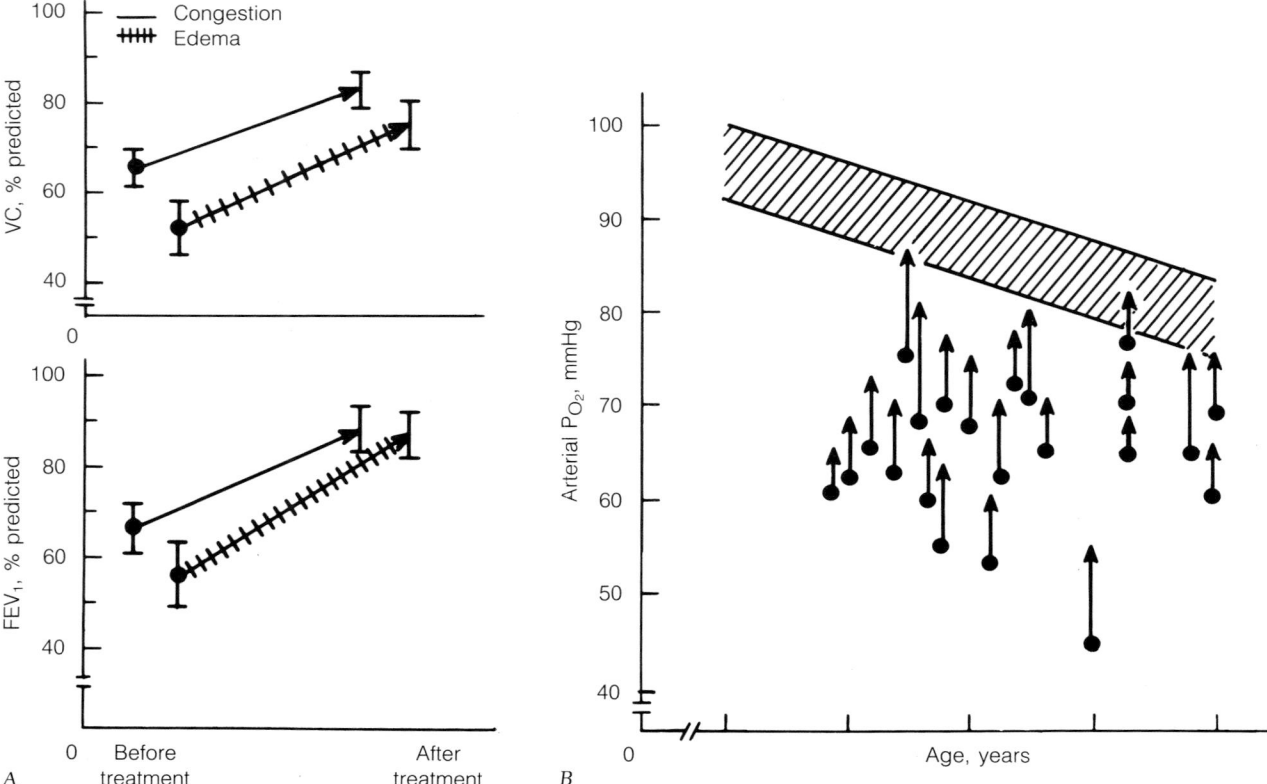

FIGURE 68-6 Schematic representation of changes in some pulmonary function tests in the evolution from pulmonary congestion to pulmonary edema. A. Vital capacity and FEV_1, before and after treatment. B. Changes in lung volumes and arterial P_{O_2} in response to treatment. The progression from congestion to interstitial edema is associated with more profound abnormalities that reverse toward normal after treatment. (*Modified after Sorbini et al. in Giuntini and Pannucio, 1979.*)

simply mechanical factors, are involved. At first, the increment in pressure caused by the increase in pulmonary blood volume leads to the recruitment of unopened vessels. But, if pulmonary venous pressure should increase further, distention succeeds recruitment. The increase in pulmonary capillary blood volume may be reflected in a rise in diffusing capacity. Since the recruitment and distention improves the matching of alveolar ventilation and blood flow, gas exchange improves and arterial oxygen tension increases. Although the compliance of the lungs decreases because of the distended, stiffer blood vessels, elastic recoil pressure decreases at low lung volumes. The resultant change in the shape of the pressure-volume curve is known as the "Von Basch effect" after the German physiologist who first described it in 1887 (Fig. 68-7).

Factors other than increased stiffness contribute to the decrease in pulmonary compliance. Among these are a decrease in lung volumes and a decrease in the compliance of the airways themselves. The congested lung also tends to hold airways open at reduced lung volumes.

INTERSTITIAL EDEMA

The development of interstitial edema is associated with a reduction in all the subdivisions of the total lung capacity (TLC) with relative sparing of the residual volume (RV). As a result, the RV/TLC ratio is high. Closing volumes are also high. In contrast to the inconstant evidence for obstruction of large airways, resistance to airflow through

small airways is consistently high, and specific compliance is both decreased and frequency-dependent.

The common denominator in virtually all these abnormalities is peribronchiolar cuffing that compresses terminal bronchioles, closing peripheral airways at higher lung volumes. The distribution of premature closure of peripheral airways is uneven, and the time constants vary from one part of the lung to another, resulting in uneven distribution of air. This uneven distribution is reflected in the increased slope of phase III of the single-breath oxygen curve (Fig. 68-8).

ALVEOLAR EDEMA

With the onset of alveolar edema, the mechanical functions of the lungs become markedly impaired. At first, peripheral airway resistance increases further, inhomogenicity of airflow becomes more marked, and tests of the function of small airways become increasingly abnormal. When alveolar flooding sets in, ventilation to the flooded airspaces decreases and ventilation-perfusion mismatch becomes evident. Increases in residual volume, accompanied by reductions in diffusing capacity, vital capacity, and the other lung volumes, follow. Vital capac-

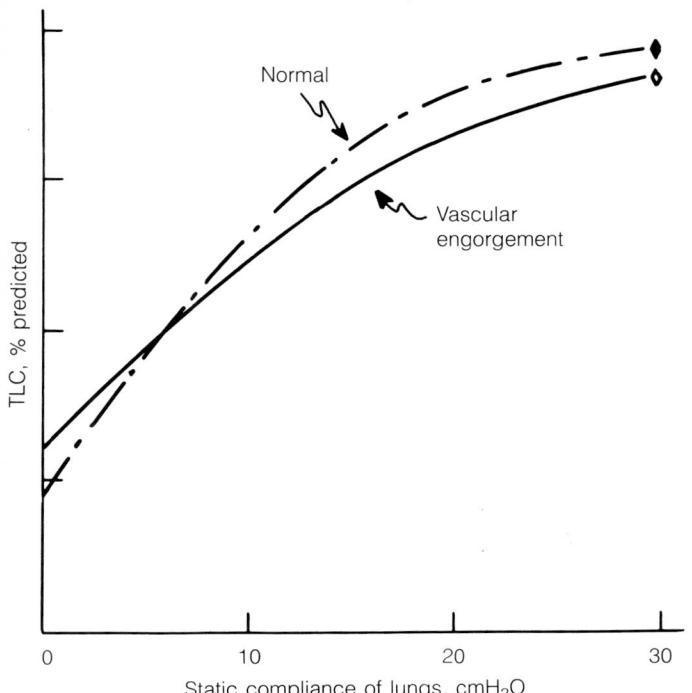

FIGURE 68-7   The Von Basch effect. The pressure-volume relationships of normal lungs are compared with those of engorged lungs.

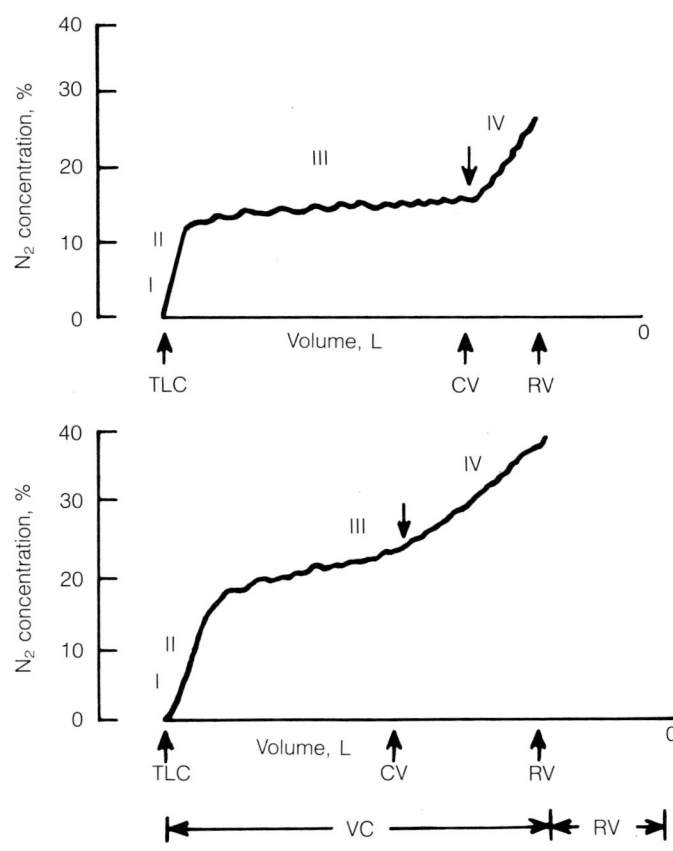

FIGURE 68-8   Schematic representation of closing volumes showing premature closure of the small airways. *Upper,* normal. *Lower,* pulmonary edema.

ity is a simple measurement which correlates well with changes in extravascular lung water: it has been used successfully to monitor the course of patients with congestive heart failure since the 1800s.

Other mechanical changes in the lungs include a decrease in static lung compliance and the appearance of marked static hysteresis of the pressure-volume curve; these changes are attributed to alterations in pulmonary surfactant and to a decrease in lung volume.

Gas Exchange

The alteration in arterial blood gases that occurs with the progressive development of cardiogenic pulmonary edema reflects different physiological changes: hyperventilation, when present, results in reduced arterial P_{CO_2} and respiratory alkalosis; reduction in arterial P_{O_2} reflects ventilation-perfusion mismatch. As a rule, values for arterial O_2 saturation in patients with stable congestive heart failure are of the order of 93 percent; alveolar-arterial differences in P_{O_2} range around 23 mmHg. The physiological dead space increases moderately.

Carbon Dioxide Retention

About 20 percent of patients with congestive heart failure develop progressive CO_2 retention; the resulting increase in arterial P_{CO_2} and respiratory acidosis are not due to coexistent chronic obstructive airways disease. Instead, they are believed to be secondary to marked peribronchial cuffing with fluid or obstruction of the airway lumen by foamy edema fluid (Fig. 68-9). Because this group of patients is not easily recognized, determination of arterial blood-gas composition is mandatory in all patients with pulmonary edema. Metabolic acidosis associated with increased levels of lactate and pyruvate in the blood sometimes occurs, presumably because of poor peripheral and/or hepatic perfusion. Combined respiratory and metabolic acidosis has been reported to occur in 25 to 40 percent of patients with cardiogenic pulmonary edema: increased CO_2 production and increased work of breathing that causes fatigue of the respiratory muscles are largely responsible for the alveolar hypoventilation that underlies the combined respiratory and metabolic acidosis; impaired O_2 delivery to the muscles underlies the concomitant metabolic acidosis.

Distribution of Inspired Air

Obstruction of peripheral airways and abnormal distensibility of different parts of the lung result in maldistribution of inspired air. This inhomogeneity in the distribution of the ventilation can be demonstrated by the 7-min nitrogen washout and the single-breath oxygen test. However, phase III of the single-breath test usually does not become grossly abnormal until interstitial edema is marked.

Regional Function Studies

Determinations of regional blood flow using radioisotopes indicate that increased pulmonary venous pressure is associated with reversal of the normal, gravity-dependent distribution of blood flow. Regional distribution of ventilation is virtually normal in left heart failure. As noted above, ventilation-perfusion relationships are well balanced—often even better than in normal lungs—thereby accounting for the high arterial oxygenation in many patients with chronic pulmonary congestion.

Cardiac Asthma

Reflex bronchoconstriction of the airways ("hyperirritable airways") is often seen in congestive heart failure. When severe, the reduction in airflow accompanied by wheez-

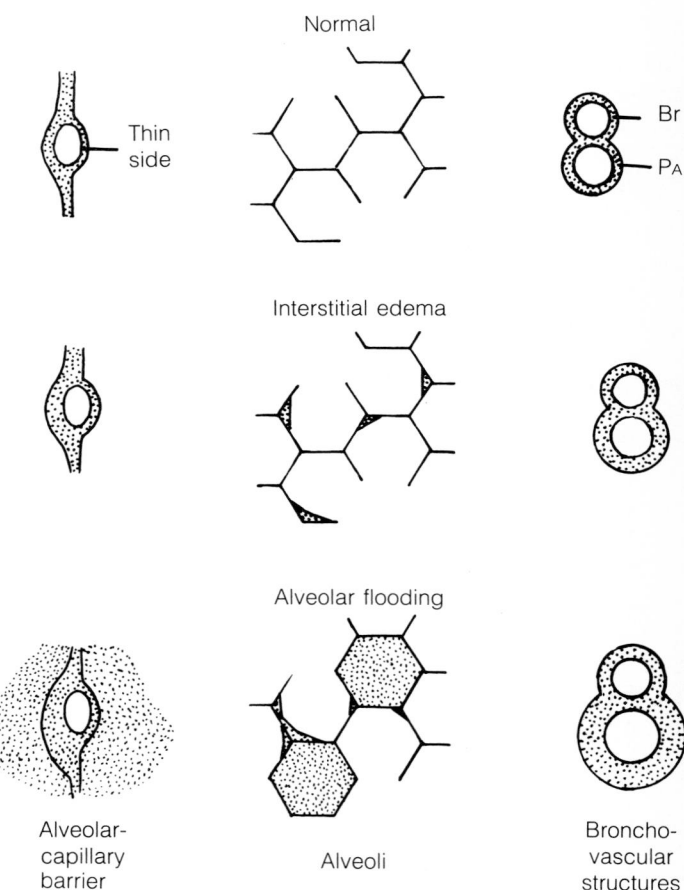

FIGURE 68-9   Progression from interstitial to alveolar edema associated with peribronchial (and perivascular) cuffing. *Upper*. Normal lung. The alveolar-capillary septum incorporates the capillary eccentrically to form a thick and thin side. The alveoli are free of fluid. The peribronchovascular interstitial space is normal. *Middle*. Interstitial pulmonary edema. The thick side of the alveolar-capillary septum is widened. A few alveoli show crescentric filling. The peribronchovascular interstitial space is thickened by excess fluid. *Lower*. Fluid has escaped from the alveolar interstitium into the alveoli. Alveolar flooding is not uniform. There is marked peribronchovascular edema.

ing can cause *cardiac asthma.* Agents such as albuterol and atropine are often effective as bronchodilators in this state, improving the forced vital capacity, the forced expiratory volume delivered in 1 s, and the closing volume; all lung volumes but the total lung capacity increase after these agents are inhaled. The decrements in airway resistance and closing volume that occur after inhalation of atropine are not augmented further by inhalation of albuterol, suggesting a vagal reflex component.

Wheezing in cardiac asthma has generally been attributed to airway narrowing secondary to peribronchiolar cuffing. However, in addition to bronchoconstriction, the mucosa of the airways is edematous, possibly due to interference with bronchial venous drainage. Bronchodilators are apparently less effective in the acute interstitial edema that follows myocardial infarction than in chronic congestive heart failure.

Treatment of Pulmonary Edema

The intravenous administration of powerful diuretics such as furosemide often causes dramatic improvement by reducing left ventricular filling pressure, apparently not only by promoting diuresis but also by increasing venous capacitance. The presence of arterial hypoxemia calls for supplemental oxygen which, in most instances, can be given without concern for the threat of progressive hypercapnia since values for arterial P_{CO_2} are subnormal.

Historically, the administration of morphine has been the mainstay of treatment. Morphine acts by decreasing left atrial, systemic arterial, and central venous pressures, thereby promoting reversal of the pulmonary edema.

The application of occlusive venous cuffs to the limbs, once popular in treating the pulmonary edema of left ventricular failure, is now out of favor. Digitalization of patients in heart failure is most apt to be effective if the patient also has rapid atrial fibrillation. It runs the risk of precipitating a life-threatening arrhythmia if the patient is hypoxemic, acidemic, or hypokalemic. Aminophylline is useful as adjunctive therapy because of its effect on the heart, and because it promotes diuresis and bronchodilation. It also can be helpful if fatigue of the respiratory muscles should supervene, since it strengthens the contraction of the diaphragm.

Vasodilators now feature prominently in the treatment of acute left ventricular failure. They act by improving cardiac ejection via a decrease in peripheral resistance. The increase in cardiac output and the concomitant decrease in left ventricular filling pressure greatly relieve hemodynamic pulmonary edema.

ISCHEMIC HEART DISEASE

Angina Pectoris (Acute Pulmonary Effects)

An acute effect of cardiac dysfunction on pulmonary performance ("pulmocordis") often occurs during an episode of angina pectoris. The onset of angina, e.g., as induced by atrial pacing in susceptible individuals, is associated with an increase in both left ventricular end-diastolic pressure and airway resistance and a decrease in pulmonary compliance. At the end of the attack, the pulmonary and cardiac changes revert to normal.

Myocardial Infarction (Subacute Pulmonary Effects)

In acute myocardial infarction, pulmonary vascular pressures usually remain high for less than a week. Unless gross pulmonary edema supervenes, the major cardiopulmonary abnormalities are a widening of the alveolar-arterial difference in P_{O_2}, arterial hypoxemia, and acute respiratory alkalosis. The physiological dead space/tidal volume ratio also increases. When the venous admixture is large in conjunction with a low cardiac output, the resultant low P_{O_2} of blood contributes to arterial hypoxemia.

Levels of arterial P_{O_2} are inversely related to the increase in left atrial (pulmonary wedge) pressure; abnormal values for arterial P_{O_2} can persist for up to 2 weeks. Elaborate attempts have been made to identify characteristic pulmonary abnormalities after myocardial infarction (presumably due to interstitial pulmonary edema). No measurements have as yet proved more reliable and consistent than repeated determinations of the vital capacity. Not only the vital capacity, but also the residual volume, functional residual capacity, and total lung capacity are decreased.

Regional ventilation and perfusion studies after acute myocardial infarction have shown that ventilation at the lung bases is decreased more than blood flow, presumably due to closure of small airways.

Three to five months after transmural myocardial infarction, some patients still manifest abnormalities in left ventricular function. In about half of these, pulmonary abnormalities (presumably secondary to interstitial pulmonary edema) also persist: hypercapnia, hypoxemia, a widened alveolar-arterial difference in P_{O_2}, and a large arterial dead space/tidal volume ratio.

Congestive Heart Failure (Chronic Pulmonary Effects)

The changes in pulmonary function that occur in chronic congestive heart failure secondary to ischemic heart disease are considered elsewhere (see "Mitral Valvular Disease," below, and Chapter 60) as sequelae of increased pulmonary venous pressure, pulmonary congestion, interstitial edema, and alveolar edema.

Rheumatic Pneumonitis

In addition to changes in the lungs caused by pulmonary edema, the lungs of children dying of rheumatic fever show changes in pulmonary arteries and capillaries, interstitial infiltrates, and alveolar exudates attributable to rheumatic pneumonitis. The lungs generally show intra-

alveolar exudates in association with proliferation of mononuclear cells within alveolar walls that renders the alveolar capillaries bloodless. Vascular changes have also been identified with acute rheumatic fever. Among these are hyaline thrombi in the smaller pulmonary arteries and fibrinoid necrosis of pulmonary arterial walls that often allows red cells to escape. The changes in the pulmonary arteries and capillaries have been attributed to a hypersensitivity vasculitis. Healing of the inflammatory lesions sometimes causes interstitial fibrosis.

One of the sequelae of recurrent bouts of rheumatic pneumonitis is the white or "anemic" lung. At autopsy, large segments of the basal portions of the affected lobes appear blanched and scarred (Fig. 68-10); usually, the lower lobes are most affected.

VALVULAR HEART DISEASE

Valvular heart disease usually affects the lungs by way of pulmonary venous hypertension resulting from a lesion of the left side of the heart. As a rule, since pulmonary venous hypertension is the common denominator, the effects on the lungs are those of cardiogenic pulmonary edema (Table 68-1).

Mitral Valvular Disease

The pulmonary manifestations of chronic left ventricular failure and of chronic stenosis or insufficiency of the mitral valve are virtually identical.

PATHOLOGY

Pulmonary vascular congestion, edema, and their sequelae are regular features of severe mitral stenosis and/or regurgitation (Fig. 68-11). In time, the pulmonary vasculature shows evidence of sustained pulmonary hypertension (thickening of the media of small pulmonary arteries and arterioles; intimal proliferation), whereas the frame-

work of the lungs is thickened as a consequence of chronic interstitial edema. Lymphatics are dilated and tortuous. Hemosiderin in macrophages ("heart failure cells") marks bleeding and lysis of red cells. Occasionally, the organization of the exudate leaves calcifications as its residue. Chronic congestion also leaves its mark on the pulmonary veins, primarily in the form of intimal thickening. The bronchial (systemic) veins are prominent, and some form submucosal varices that give rise to tracheobronchial hemorrhage. Because of the widespread changes in the framework and parenchyma, the lungs become less compliant.

PATHOPHYSIOLOGY

As in chronic left ventricular failure, tight mitral stenosis is accompanied by increases in pulmonary venous and capillary pressures causing pulmonary congestion, interstitial edema, and finally, frank alveolar edema.

PULMONARY FUNCTION

Impairment of pulmonary function in chronic mitral stenosis depends on the functional stage (as defined by the New York Heart Association Classification) and on the duration of chronic passive congestion and edema. In general, as the functional classification worsens beyond stage I, pulmonary function becomes increasingly compromised: vital capacity, forced expiratory flow rates and volumes, maximum breathing capacity, diffusing capacity, and arterial P_{O_2} all decrease. As a rule, the reductions in the inspiratory and total lung capacities suggest a restrictive pattern but are distinctive in that the functional residual capacity remains normal. Reduction in these parameters generally parallels the increase in pulmonary arterial pressure and vascular resistance. However, there are many exceptions to this generalization, pulmonary performance remaining remarkably well preserved despite considerable pulmonary hypertension. Should the ventilatory capacity be inordinately low for the level of pulmonary vascular resistance, a concomitant condition such as chronic bronchitis generally coexists.

Even in those patients in whom the lung volumes are reduced, the usual tests of the distribution of inspired air may be virtually normal. For example, the 7-min nitrogen washout and the helium mixing index often fail to uncover any abnormality; the stiff lungs appear to be emptying normally but from reduced lung volumes (low VC and TLC). This conclusion is in keeping with the normal ratios of FEV_1/FVC. However, in these individuals, the slope of phase III of the single-breath oxygen test is usually abnormally steep.

The vital capacity is a traditional measure for following the course of pulmonary edema in a particular patient. It has also been identified in the Framingham study as a "risk factor" for developing congestive heart failure: a

TABLE 68-1

Serial Vital Capacity and Arterial Blood-Gas Measurements in a Male Who Developed Recurrent Cardiogenic Pulmonary Edema following Insertion of a Prosthetic Heart Valve to Correct Mitral Stenosis

Date	SVC, L	pH	P_{CO_2}, mmHg	P_{O_2}, mmHg	S_{O_2}, %	HCO_3, meq/L
9/20/83	2.49	7.42	44	63	93	27.8
5/23/85	2.48	7.46	47	59	87	33.5
12/27/85	2.31	7.42	45	48	84	29.1
2/17/86	2.64	7.43	41	53	86	27.5

NOTE: SVC = slow vital capacity.

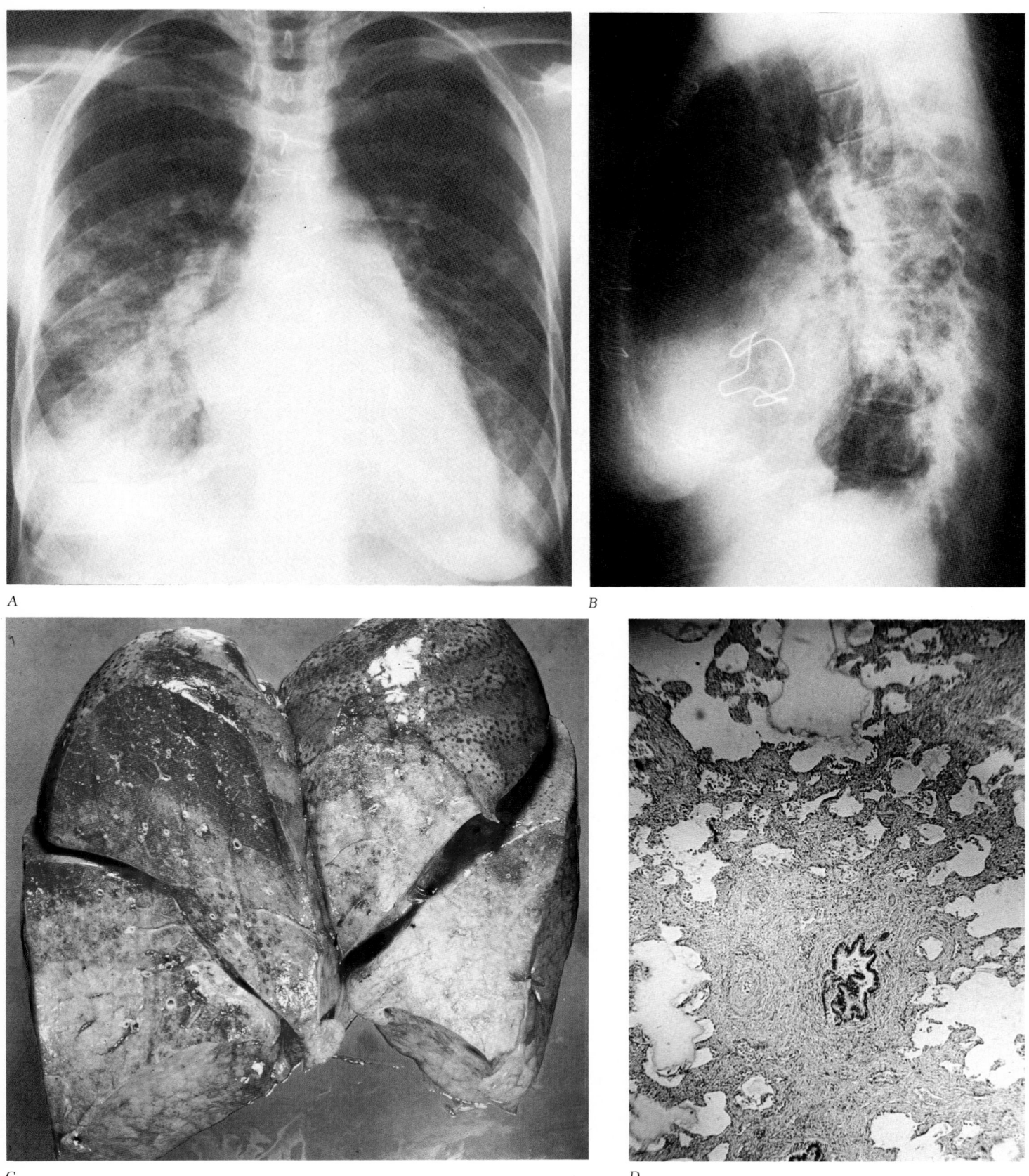

A

B

C

D

FIGURE 68-10 Pulmonary fibrosis after rheumatic pneumonitis "white lung." A and B. Posteroanterior and lateral views of patient with mitral stenosis after mitral valve replacement. C. Sagittal section of whole lungs showing dense fibrosis. D. Histologic appearance of white lung. (*Courtesy of Dr. S. Moolten.*)

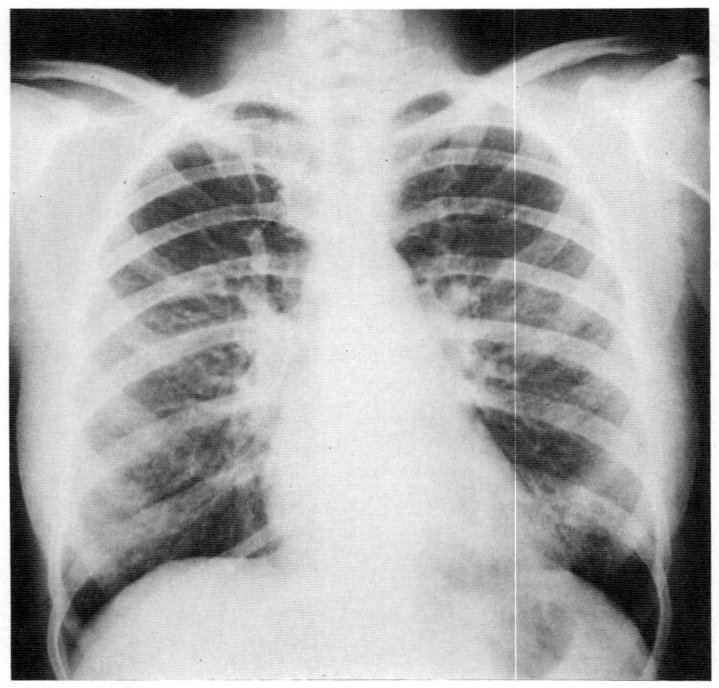
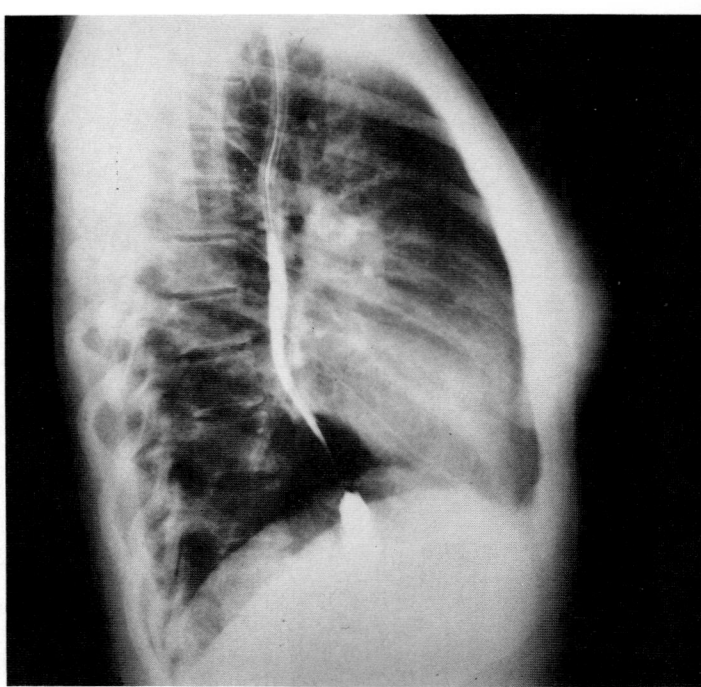

A   B

FIGURE 68-11 Rheumatic heart disease, chronic mitral stenosis. The characteristic changes in the cardiac silhouette are associated with evidence of chronic interstitial edema and fibrosis. *A*. Posteroanterior view. *B*. Lateral view after barium swallow.

recent decrease or a persistent reduction in vital capacity was associated with increased risk of developing congestive heart failure, particularly in individuals known to have either ischemic heart disease or hypertension or rheumatic heart disease.

PULMONARY MECHANICS

As in the case of chronic left ventricular failure, the lungs in mitral stenosis are stiff and the static compliance is decreased. These changes in the elastic work of breathing, coupled with an increase in airway resistance, increase the work of breathing. The respiratory rate is automatically adjusted to minimize the work of breathing; the typical breathing pattern is one of high frequency and small tidal volumes (Fig. 68-2). The shape of the pressure-volume curve is similar to that seen in pulmonary congestion and edema (Fig. 68-7), i.e., static elastic recoil is increased at high lung volumes and reduced at low lung volumes; capillary engorgement is presumably responsible for the decreased elastic recoil pressure at low lung volumes, whereas pulmonary fibrosis, due to long-standing interstitial edema, causes the increased elastic recoil pressure at high lung volumes. The dynamic compliance decreases progressively with increasing severity of mitral stenosis but frequency-dependent decrements in compliance do not often occur.

GAS EXCHANGE

The arterial P_{O_2} and P_{CO_2} at rest are usually normal or only slightly low. The diffusing capacity, no matter how it is determined, is usually decreased.

Although the capillary blood volume (Vc) component of the single-breath diffusing capacity is usually increased in the early stages of mitral stenosis, the membrane component (Dm) is decreased. In the advanced stages of the disease, both components are markedly decreased.

REGIONAL LUNG FUNCTION

Based on studies using radioisotopes, perfusion of the upper zones of the lungs is increased in chronic mitral stenosis, whereas that of the lower zones is decreased. The extent of this reversal in the normal pattern is proportional to the level of unremitting increase in left atrial and pulmonary wedge pressures. Oxygen breathing or infusion of acetylcholine into the pulmonary artery has little effect on this abnormal pattern of distribution of blood flow; it represents mechanical compression and distortions rather than reflex pulmonary vasoconstriction.

Ventilation of the lower lobes is similarly reduced, and ventilation shifts progressively to the upper zones, as both the pulmonary artery and wedge pressure increase. Overall, ventilation-perfusion matching is either un-

changed or even improved. Peribronchiolar edema or scarring may be responsible for the decrease in ventilation to the lower lobes. In keeping with this postulate, closing volumes are increased in patients with severe mitral stenosis.

PULMONARY CIRCULATION

As with other physiological measurements, the hemodynamic consequences of mitral valvular disease depend on

the severity and duration of the valvular abnormalities. Pulmonary arterial and pulmonary capillary pressures, as well as pulmonary venous pressures, are increased in chronic mitral stenosis. Often the increment in pulmonary arterial pressure is disproportionate to the increase in pulmonary venous pressure, suggesting active pulmonary arterial constriction superimposed on the anatomic changes in the intima and media. The cardiac index, often normal at rest, usually fails to increase normally during

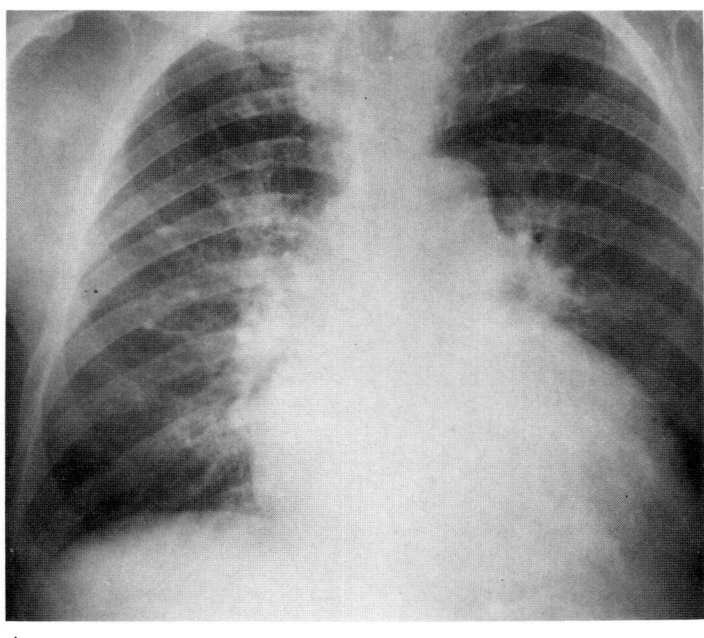

A

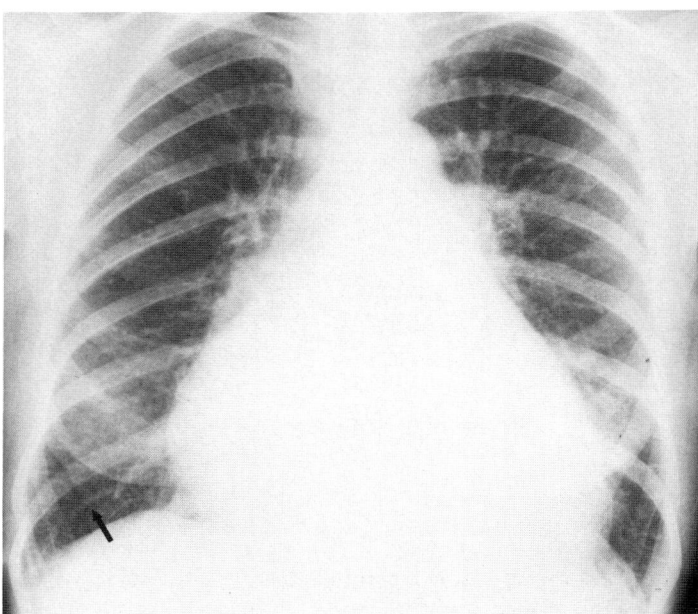

B

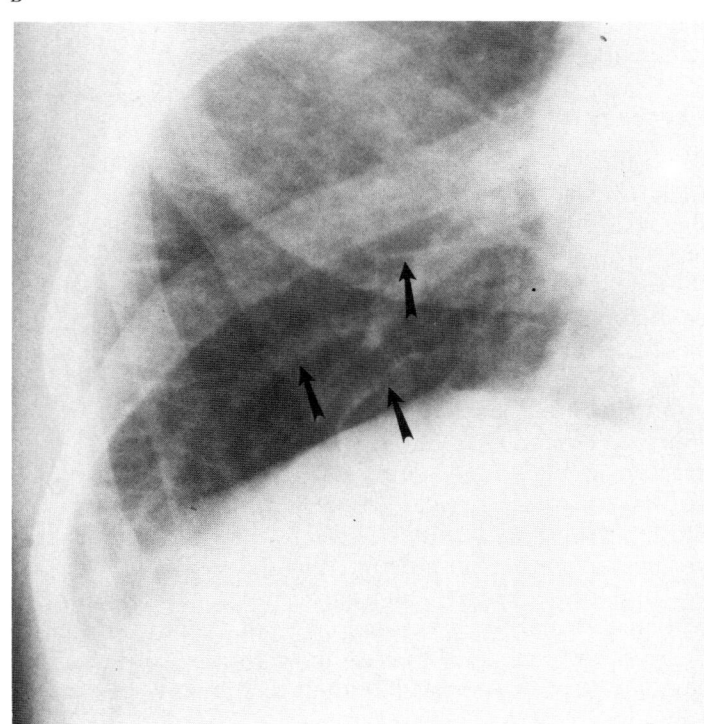

C

FIGURE 68-12 Aortic valvular disease. *A.* Aortic stenosis and left ventricular failure. *B.* Aortic insufficiency; mitral stenosis and mitral insufficiency. Arrow indicates Kerley B line. *C.* Distended lymphatics and increased interstitial markings (arrows). Kerley B lines are seen in the costovertebral angle as linear streaks parallel to the diaphragm.

exercise or decreases; pulmonary blood volume may be increased up to 200 percent in patients with moderate mitral stenosis.

Although enlargement of the main pulmonary arteries on the chest radiograph indicates that pulmonary hypertension is present, it does not necessarily reflect the degree of hypertension. On the whole, pulmonary function correlates poorly with the structural changes in mitral valvular disease. One useful correlate in this group of patients is that patients with low diffusing capacity tend to have hypertensive pulmonary vascular disease.

Aortic Valvular Disease

The effects of aortic valvular disease on pulmonary performance depend, as in the case of mitral valvular disease or myocardial disease, on the degree to which pulmonary venous pressure increases (Fig. 68-12). If interstitial and alveolar edema ensue, the changes in lung volumes, mechanical properties, distribution, and diffusion are the same as those described elsewhere (see Chapter 60) for cardiogenic pulmonary edema.

CONGENITAL HEART DISEASE

The interplay of the heart and lungs in congenital heart disease is primarily by way of the pulmonary circulation. In normal fetal development, arteries and airways develop together. The prealveolar distribution of these structures is usually complete by the 16th month of uterine life; intra-alveolar arteries and alveoli continue to develop after birth during the first 3 years of life. The pulmonary venous and arterial systems develop synchronously.

Congenital cardiac defects affect the prenatal development of the pulmonary circulation. For example, obstruction to pulmonary outflow reduces pulmonary blood flow and pressure, thereby impeding pulmonary arterial growth. Conversely, inordinate pulmonary blood flow also influences growth and development, leading to the appearance of muscle cells within intra-alveolar vessels that ordinarily are nonmuscular. In older patients, pulmonary hypertension alters both the development and the growth of the pulmonary circulation.

As might be expected, different types of abnormalities in pulmonary function are apt to occur in different kinds of intracardiac shunts.

Left-to-Right Shunts

These conditions, typified by atrial septal and ventricular septal defects, are characterized by an increase in pulmonary blood volume and pulmonary blood flow. As a rule, the vital capacity and total lung capacity are minimally reduced, whereas the residual volume is unaffected. The reason for this restrictive pattern is not clear. Also, the

maximum voluntary ventilation, inert gas distribution, and arterial blood-gas composition are normal. In ventricular septal defect, the capillary blood volume component of the single-breath diffusing capacity has been reported to increase.

Right-to-Left Shunts

In patients with cyanotic congenital heart disease, the ventilatory response to hypoxia is blunted and gradually returns to normal after the congenital anomaly is repaired and arterial oxygenation improves (Fig. 68-13). Oxygen delivery in this group of disorders is facilitated by the development of secondary polycythemia and a right shift in the oxygen dissociation curve. Blood lactate levels are usually not elevated, indicating that oxygen delivery to the tissues is adequate.

During exercise, as arterial oxygenation and the abnormal heart fail to ensure adequate O_2 delivery to the tissues, work levels are reduced. O_2 supplementation fails to improve exercise tolerance.

CARDIAC DRUGS

Agents used to treat cardiac disturbances can adversely influence the lungs. Particularly notorious in this regard

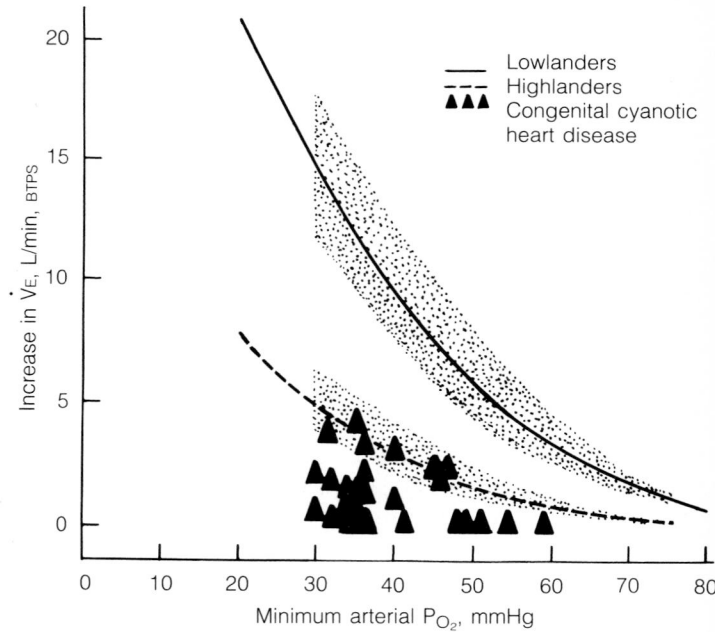

FIGURE 68-13 The ventilatory response to hypoxia in congenital heart disease. Compared are the ventilatory responses to transient hypoxia of normal individuals at sea level (lowlanders), native residents at high altitude (highlanders), and patients with congenital cyanotic heart disease. The shaded envelopes indicate the spread of average responses at rest of 33 lowlanders and five highlanders. Like the highlanders, the congenital cyanotics show a blunted response to the transient hypoxia. *(Modified after Lahiri, Edelman, Cherniack, Fishman, 1969.)*

are the β-adrenergic antagonists administered to patients with obstructive airways disease or hyperreactive airways. Other commonly used agents are vasodilators and amiodarone.

β-Adrenergic Antagonists

β-Adrenergic antagonists used in the treatment of hypertension and angina pectoris engender the risk of inducing bronchospasm and precipitating an attack of asthma. Even β_1 blockers that are reputed to be "cardioselective" can induce bronchospasm in susceptible individuals. In patients with chronic obstructive airways disease, especially asthma, β-adrenergic antagonists should be prescribed carefully for fear of aggravating airway obstruction. In patients with ischemic heart disease and hyperreactive airway disease, calcium channel blockers may be better choices for treating the patient with ischemic heart disease and either chronic bronchitis or other forms of obstructive airways disease.

Vasodilators

Certain vasodilators, such as nitroglycerin, hydralazine, and sodium nitroprusside, run the risk of decreasing systemic arterial oxygen tension by increasing blood flow through hypoventilated areas, thereby promoting ventilation-perfusion mismatch. As a rule, the decrease in arterial oxygenation is mild.

Vasodilators directed at relieving pulmonary hypertension can cause systemic hypotension since they also affect the systemic resistance vessels. Their net effect is a balance between promoting flow through obstructed pulmonary arteries and arterioles without undue dilation of the corresponding systemic vessels. For this reason, they are usually tested for proper dosage by right heart catheterization to see if pulmonary hypertension can be relieved without the undesirable side effect of systemic hypotension.

Amiodarone

Amiodarone, effective in controlling refractory supraventricular and ventricular arrhythmias, has been associated with severe pulmonary toxicity in up to 6 percent of treated patients. Withdrawal of the drug coupled with the administration of corticosteroids generally leads to resolution of the toxic manifestations. The symptoms of amiodarone toxicity include exertional dyspnea, nonproductive cough, weight loss, and occasional low-grade fever. Pleuritic pain is common; physical signs include rales or diminished breath sounds, occasionally with a pleuritic friction rub.

The radiographic findings include bilateral interstitial changes and diffuse or patchy infiltrates. The radiographic changes have to be distinguished from those of pulmonary tuberculosis, pulmonary edema, or pneumonitis. Laboratory studies reveal a high sedimentation rate; white blood cell counts vary from normal to marked leukocytosis. Eosinophilia is not a feature. The concentration of lactic dehydrogenase in serum is often mildly increased.

Under the electron microscope, osmophilic lamellar and granular inclusion bodies are found within the distended lysozymes of macrophages, type II pneumocytes, and interstitial and endothelial cells. These changes resemble those that occur in the dermal histiocytes and pericytes of patients with amiodarone-induced cutaneous lesions.

There seems to be an upper limit (about 400 mg per day) to the maintenance dose of the drug below which pulmonary toxicity is uncommon. Whether the severity of underlying cardiac disease or the coexistence of congestive heart failure contribute to susceptibility is unclear, but most patients who have died from the condition have had severe cardiac dysfunction. Other factors relating to toxicity include the extremely long half-life of amiodarone (up to 45 days) and the higher concentrations of amiodarone in the lungs than in the blood. Although some patients are believed to have a true hypersensitivity reaction, the bulk of the evidence indicates that toxicity is dose-related. Pulmonary angiography should be done with great circumspection in any patient with amiodarone toxicity since there are reports of acute respiratory failure and death following this investigation in these patients.

Pulmonary function tests usually show a restrictive pattern, a reduction in diffusing capacity, and arterial hypoxemia. However, no correlation has been found between the cumulative dose of amiodarone and changes in $FEV_1/FVC\%$, total lung capacity, or diffusing capacity. Patients receiving amiodarone should probably be monitored by serial pulmonary function tests even though it is not clear at this time whether these tests have predictive value in identifying patients at risk.

Treatment includes withdrawal of the agent, with or without administration of corticosteroids. Low-dose corticosteroids may also be useful in patients who have manifested susceptibility to the pulmonary toxic effects of amiodarone but in whom the agent is needed for the control of arrhythmias.

MECHANICAL VENTILATION

As indicated in another chapter (see Chapter 155), another important limit to the use of mechanical ventilation for the treatment of pulmonary disease is imposed by the effects of increased airway pressures on the circulation. In this chapter, the use of positive pressure ventilation in the

treatment of pulmonary edema warrants brief consideration.

The primary reason for resorting to mechanical ventilation is severe pulmonary edema that results in hypercapnia (as well as severe arterial hypoxemia). Mechanical ventilation (after intubation) with positive end-expiratory pressure can be counted on to produce several effects: (1) open closed alveoli and small airways, (2) promote the movement of fluid from alveoli to the peribronchovascular regions as lung volumes are increased, (3) enhance lymphatic drainage, and (4) affect pleural and pericardial pressures and, therefore, venous return and cardiac output—less when the lungs are full of fluid than in normal lungs. In essence, the use of positive end-expiratory pressure (PEEP) strikes a balance between the effects on the one hand of improving gas exchange and promoting the removal of excess water from the lungs and on the other of decreasing the cardiac output. Although reflex mechanisms have been proposed to account for the decrease in cardiac output in experimental animals, the relevance of these studies for the human situation is uncertain. It is even more unclear if the phenomenon of ventricular interdependence (with bulging of the ventricular septum into the left ventricle) is related to the decrease in cardiac output.

CARDIAC SURGERY

Mitral Valvular Disease

Following mitral valve surgery, left atrial pressure, pulmonary vascular resistance, and pulmonary artery pressure tend to return toward normal levels. Preoperatively, patients with mitral stenosis often show mild reductions in vital capacity and diffusing capacity. During the 3- to 5-month interval after thoracotomy, pulmonary function first deteriorates but then returns to normal at 6 to 11 months. By 12 to 24 months, the only abnormality noted is a decrease in diffusing capacity.

Radioisotope studies of regional pulmonary blood flow have revealed that after mitral valve surgery pulmonary blood flow promptly redistributes *toward* normal. During the next 2 years, the distribution of pulmonary blood flow normalizes further. However, the preoperative minor disturbances in regional ventilation persist.

The incidence of postoperative pulmonary complications is higher in patients undergoing mitral valve surgery than after other types of cardiac surgery. Preoperative spirometry is valuable in identifying patients who may have difficult postoperative courses. The presence of considerable preoperative pulmonary dysfunction doubles both the mortality risk for valvular replacement and the frequency of postoperative complications. In smokers, the frequency of pulmonary complications is triple that of nonsmokers.

Coronary Artery Revascularization

Surprisingly, pulmonary dysfunction as identified by spirometry is not associated with an increased mortality after coronary artery revascularization surgery. But advanced age or arterial hypercapnia does increase the risk of postoperative pulmonary complications. Patients with impaired pulmonary function also have about a 10 percent incidence of perioperative myocardial infarction.

After median sternotomy, pulmonary function tests including expiratory flow rates, lung volumes, and arterial oxygenation decrease; they return to within 10 percent of preoperative values by 3 months after surgery.

Transplantation

At present, there are certain pulmonary diseases, such as emphysema, interstitial fibrosis, and cystic fibrosis, which are virtually untreatable when they reach an advanced stage. The only hope for this type of patient is the development of safe and effective organ transplantation. With recent developments in immunosuppressive therapy, advances in this field have been encouraging.

HEART-LUNG TRANSPLANTATION

The first combined heart and lung transplant was performed in 1968 in a 2-month-old baby. Although the infant died 14 h after the operation, it was noted that despite denervation spontaneous respiration returned. From this initial finding, progress in heart-lung transplantation has resulted in some remarkable successes.

There are certain advantages of the combined transplant over a unilateral lung transplantation. These include the fact that all diseased pulmonary tissue is removed, thereby preventing recurrent infections and disordered pulmonary function from affecting the remaining lung. Because of its better blood supply, the tracheal anastomosis used in heart-lung transplantation is more likely to heal than is a bronchial anastomosis.

Among the patients successfully treated to date by heart-lung transplantation are those with primary pulmonary hypertension, Eisenmenger's complex, eosinophilic pneumonia, and sarcoidosis. Donor selection requires a close match of the size of the donor's lungs to the recipient's chest cage, absence of pulmonary infection, and a normal chest radiograph. The donor has to be brought to the recipient, and surgical removal of the donor lungs and heart is carried out in an adjoining surgical theater without trauma to phrenic, vagus, or recurrent laryngeal nerves. Immunosuppression is usually begun in the recipient preoperatively and is continued postoperatively; combinations of cyclosporine and azathioprine have been most successful. Weekly transvenous endomyocardial biopsies are usually performed to identify early rejection,

and if identified, treatment with methylprednisolone is initiated.

When heart-lung transplantation was first tried, it was felt that serial cardiac biopsies could be used to identify pulmonary rejection since heart and lung rejection seemed to occur simultaneously. But, recent studies indicate that this may not be true. Most rejection episodes seem to occur within the first 2 months of transplantation. The major early postoperative complications include cyclosporine toxicity and the reimplantation response.

THE REIMPLANTATION RESPONSE

The reimplantation response is defined as a transient and reversible defect in pulmonary gas exchange, compliance, and vascular resistance, which coincides with the radiographic appearance of pulmonary edema in the postoperative period. It is obviously very important to differentiate this condition from pulmonary infection or the rejection response (Fig. 68-14).

Mortality from heart-lung transplantation is about 17 percent. However, in the 40 percent of patients who survive more than 1 year, cardiac function, pulmonary vascular resistance, and pulmonary function are normal. After heart-lung transplantation for primary pulmonary hypertension, symptoms are remarkably alleviated and arterial oxygenation improves. In the posttransplant period, lung volumes decrease markedly in a restrictive pattern; subsequently, they improve progressively.

One unexpected sequel to heart-lung transplantation has been the development, in about one-third of the patients, of obliterative bronchiolitis in the transplanted lungs. Several months after the transplantation, bronchitic symptoms of cough and mucopurulent sputum develop, signaling recurrent pulmonary infections. Within months of the onset of the bronchitic symptoms, dyspnea develops. The clinical course that follows is similar to that of chronic obstructive airways disease, only developing over months rather than years. Chest radiographs show peribronchial and interstitial infiltrates with variable pleural thickening. Pulmonary function tests reveal an obstructive pattern which improves very little after bronchodilators; a coexisting restrictive pattern is also often present. When reduction in expiratory flow rates becomes severe, arterial hypoxemia develops; hypocapnia, rather than hypercapnia, is characteristic.

In the vulnerable group of patients, abnormalities in pulmonary function often occur within a few months and are usually fully developed within a couple of years after transplantation. The pathologic appearances are those of severe but patchy bronchiolitis obliterans. The disease is progressive, and there has been no sign of spontaneous improvement. Although the pathogenesis of this form of bronchiolitis is uncertain, it is noteworthy that in some patients a chronic graft-versus-host reaction has been reported to produce obstructive airways disease within 2 years following bone marrow transplantation. Other pulmonary complications that have followed heart-lung transplantation include recurrent pulmonary infections, pleural fibrosis, and bronchiectasis.

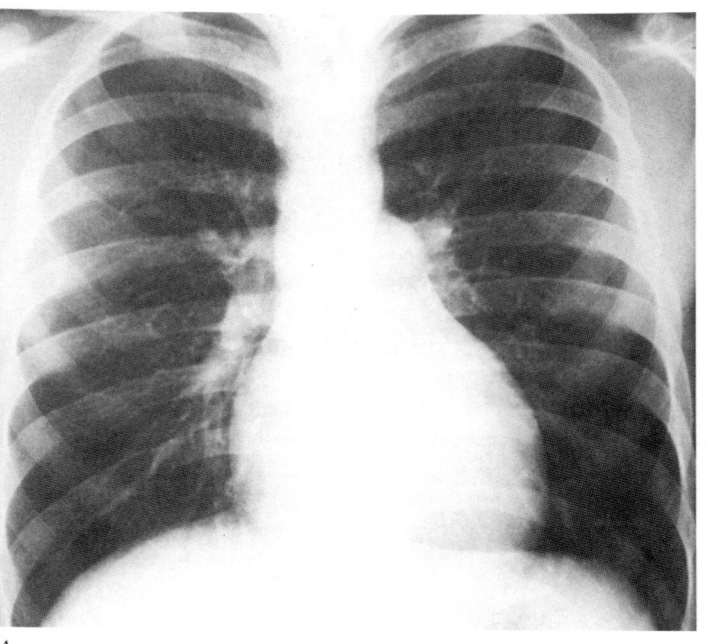

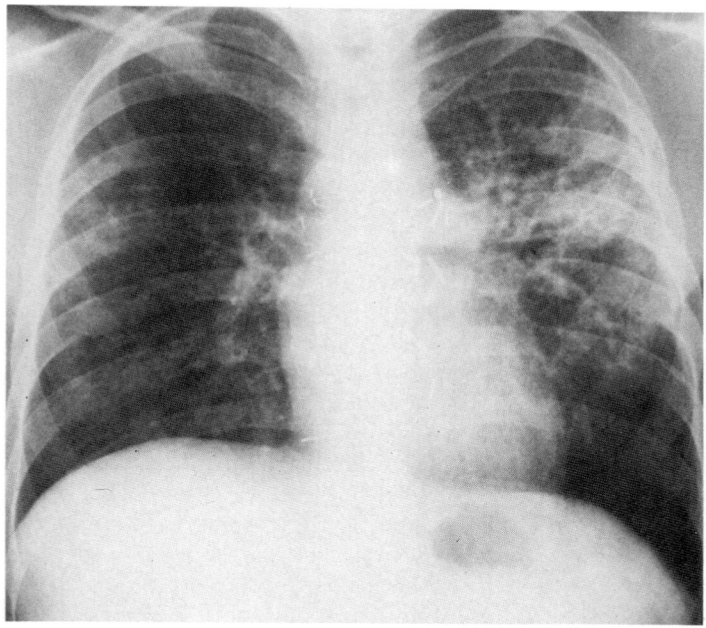

A

B

FIGURE 68-14   Heart-lung transplantation.   *A.* Before transplantation.   *B.* After transplantation showing marked infiltrates on the left. At autopsy, cytomegaloinclusion virus was found. *(Courtesy of Dr. J. Eldredge.)*

UNILATERAL LUNG TRANSPLANTATION

The first unilateral lung transplantation was performed in 1963. This was followed by more than 40 attempts, none of which achieved lasting success. However, recent reports of long-term survivors after unilateral lung transplantation for patients with progressive pulmonary fibrosis are encouraging. One of the problems associated with unilateral lung transplantation was bronchial dehiscence. But the use of cyclosporine instead of corticosteroids and wrapping the bronchial anastomosis with an omental pedicle have provided protection against this serious complication.

Criteria for selecting patients for unilateral lung transplantation include progressive pulmonary fibrosis, unresponsive to corticosteroids, with a life expectancy of 1 year or less. Right ventricular function must be satisfactory. Patients should be weanable from corticosteroids and should not be ventilator-dependent. Patients with bilateral pulmonary sepsis are unsuitable because of the risk of spreading infection to the transplanted lungs. Patients with emphysema may also be unsuitable since loss of elastic recoil in the native lung may cause progressive air trapping and shift the mediastinum toward the transplanted side.

The identification of pulmonary rejection is difficult and requires analysis of clinical, radiographic, and laboratory findings. Sequential lung perfusion scanning can assist in monitoring lung rejection. If an episode of rejection should occur, pulsed doses of methylprednisolone have both diagnostic and therapeutic roles since radiographic and functional improvement tend to occur within hours after intravenous injection.

An important factor favoring unilateral lung transplantation over heart-lung transplantation is the severe scarcity of donors. Whereas heart-lung transplantation requires the lungs and heart of one donor, unilateral lung transplantation permits the separate use of each donor lung and the heart. In other words, three transplants can be served by one donor.

CARDIAC TRANSPLANTATION

The use of immunosuppressive agents to control rejection is not infrequently complicated by nosocomial infection. A wide variety of different infectious agents may be involved. Most commonly reported in order of frequency are bacterial, viral, fungal, protozoal, and nocardial infections.

HEART-LUNG INTERACTIONS

The Combined Cardiopulmonary System

The efficiency of the heart and lungs in respiratory gas exchange depends on their coordinated interactions (Fig. 68-1). An increase in body metabolism automatically adjusts the ventilation, cardiac output, and synchrony between the two sides of the heart so that systemic O_2 delivery increases without flooding the lungs. Disease or disorder of any component draws on reserve mechanisms and imposes a burden on the other components of the system. Malfunctioning in the mechanisms governing the automatic interplay is generally manifested when O_2 requirements are increased. This is the basis for exercise testing that can be used to stress the heart, lungs, or coordinated interplay of the entire cardiorespiratory system.

VENTRICULAR INTERDEPENDENCE

The right and left sides of the heart are arranged as two pumps in series: the right operating as a low pressure-volume pump and the left as a high pressure-volume pump. Several factors affect the performance of this interdependent system, including the dimensions of the ventricles, the interventricular septum, the pericardium, and the intrathoracic pressure.

At the beginning of the twentieth century, Bernheim postulated that left ventricular hypertrophy or dilation could bulge into the right ventricle and compromise its function to produce a state of congestive heart failure. This concept of ventricular interaction prompted Henderson and Prince in 1914 to explore the interdependence of the ventricles of an isolated beating cat's heart. They observed that the volume of fluid ejected by one ventricle decreased as the filling pressure of the other ventricle increased. They proposed that displacement of the interventricular septum might be involved in this phenomenon. In 1943, Starr and his co-workers cauterized the external wall of the right ventricle until it became noncontractile. However, this procedure failed to increase systemic venous pressure, presumably as a consequence of the intact ventricular septum; i.e., the right ventricular function was maintained by the contraction of the left ventricle. Recently, interest has rekindled in the concept of ventricular interdependence, and the phenomenon is believed to be operative during systole and diastole and influenced by the presence or absence of the pericardium.

Systolic Ventricular Interaction

The importance of an intact free wall of the left ventricle in generating right ventricular systolic pressure was demonstrated by cutting the left ventricular free wall. This procedure prevents the left ventricle from generating a considerable increase in systolic pressure. Similarly, changes in right ventricular function can be shown to affect the left ventricle: an increase in right ventricular volume causes an increase in left ventricular pressure.

Diastolic Ventricular Interaction

An increase in diastolic ventricular dimension alters the shape and compliance of the contralateral ventricle. Small increments in right ventricular volume have only minimal effects on the left ventricle. But, as the volume of the right ventricle increases further, left ventricular diastolic pressures increase appreciably. The mechanism underlying this diastolic interdependence seems to be an alteration in ventricular configuration during diastole produced by changes in the volume of the contralateral ventricle. Increasing right ventricular volume deviates the interventricular septum toward the left ventricular free wall, thereby decreasing left ventricular dimensions. Clinical studies have confirmed that acute changes in the volume of one ventricle also alter the diastolic compliance of the contralateral ventricle.

Pericardial Effects

Because the pericardium encases only the heart, intrapericardial pressure is exerted only on the cardiac chambers. In the normal individual, the pericardium is not a restraining influence on cardiac filling or behavior. However, if the heart increases in size acutely, the pericardium becomes constraining. Similarly, if intrapericardial pressure should increase, as in pericardial tamponade, both transmural ventricular pressure and ventricular filling will decrease. In contrast, a slow increase in pericardial pressure, as in the case of a gradually increasing pericardial effusion, will have little effect because the pericardium gradually stretches as the fluid accumulates. The increase in left ventricular diastolic pressure that occurs as right ventricular pressure increases is more marked when the pericardium is present than when it is absent.

Intrathoracic Pressure Effects

During acute bronchospasm, when inspiratory effort is markedly increased in order to promote inspiratory airflow, pleural pressure falls dramatically. The resultant increase in right ventricular filling leads to a leftward shift of the interventricular septum. Left ventricular transmural pressure also increases, leading to a reduced ventricular output and a marked fall in systemic arterial blood pressure—the *pulsus paradoxus* of acute asthma.

A decrease in left ventricular transmural pressure occurs whenever pleural pressure becomes more positive, e.g., during the Valsalva maneuver, pneumothorax, or mechanical ventilation; the decrease in transmural pressure leads to decreased filling of the left ventricle.

Clinical Significance of Ventricular Interdependence

The most common cause of right ventricular failure is left ventricular failure. This effect is exerted predominantly via the shared muscle of the heart and only to a lesser extent by hemodynamic overloading of the right ventricle as a consequence of failure of the left ventricle.

A "reverse Bernheim" syndrome was first proposed in 1956 as cause of the left ventricular dysfunction in patients with atrial septal defect who develop left ventricular failure. In conditions such as tricuspid valvular insufficiency, pulmonary valvular insufficiency, or atrial septal defect in which the right ventricle is subjected to volume overload, left ventricular end-diastolic volume, stroke volume, and stroke work may all decrease. However, despite these changes, left ventricular failure does not usually occur until the right ventricle itself actually fails.

Cross-sectional echocardiography has suggested that the mechanism underlying the left ventricular dysfunction in right ventricular overload is probably a change in the diastolic configuration of the left ventricle produced by changes in the configuration of the interventricular septum; the changes range from slight flattening of the normal curvature to total reversal of the normal concavity. Even though the left ventricle tends to resume its normal circular shape during systole, the movement of the interventricular septum—from a flattened, or inverted, position in diastole to its usual position during systole—assists right ventricular ejection. As a result, right ventricular ejection remains normal when left ventricular function is associated with right ventricular volume overload.

Right Ventricular Pressure Overload

Massive pulmonary embolism or pulmonary stenosis, by causing right ventricular pressure overload, may reduce cardiac output, left ventricular ejection fraction, and both left ventricular end-diastolic and systolic volumes. These hemodynamic consequences have been attributed to distortion of the left ventricle at end-diastole, with failure of the left ventricle to resume its normal shape during systole.

Chronic Pulmonary Disease

In principle, chronic pulmonary disease should adversely affect only the right ventricle; changes in left ventricular function should be secondary to right ventricular overload. This postulate is supported by the pathology of the heart in autopsies of native residents of high altitude. However, it is still unsettled whether left ventricular function is affected by the right ventricular overload of chronic lung disease. Factors complicating interpretation generally include the possibility of coronary artery disease, hypertension, or valvular heart disease. However, in one study of young people with cystic fibrosis, whose average age was 13 years and where other causes for cardiac involvement were unlikely, left ventricular ejection fraction was abnormal in a third of the patients.

ARRHYTHMIAS IN COR PULMONALE

This topic is considered extensively elsewhere in this book (see Chapter 67). Here it will suffice to underscore the importance of round-the-clock monitoring of the cardiac rhythm if the incidence of arrhythmias is to be accurately assessed. Mortality increases in patients with severe advanced obstructive airways disease who develop cardiac arrhythmias. One contributing factor undoubtedly is the presence of left ventricular disease since many of the patients are elderly. Abnormal blood gases, electrolyte disturbances, theophylline, β_2 antagonists, diuretics, and digitalis are important predisposing factors to arrhythmias in these patients. In addition, manipulation of the airways, e.g., tracheal suction, and right ventricular dilation have been implicated in the triggering of bouts of complex premature ventricular contractions and ventricular tachycardia.

Although the use of theophyllines, β_2 antagonists, and digitalis is usually safe in stable patients with chronic obstructive airways disease, this may not be so in the case of the acutely ill patient with respiratory failure. It is particularly important to avoid toxic levels of these agents in the acutely ill, hypoxemic hypercapnic individual who is being vigorously treated. Ventricular arrhythmias in the acutely ill respiratory patient are associated with a high mortality rate, and the incidence of sudden death may be as high as 21 percent.

SYSTEMIC DISEASE

Cardiac involvement, especially in interstitial lung diseases, may be part of a systemic disease or a secondary effect of the disease on the lungs. For example, interstitial fibrosis that develops in diseases such as sarcoidosis, rheumatoid interstitial fibrosis, systemic lupus erythematosus, and progressive systemic sclerosis leads to secondary pulmonary hypertension and right ventricular pressure overload. The systemic disease may also directly involve the heart leading to failure of both ventricles: sarcoidosis sometimes causes conduction defects and cardiomyopathy; progressive systemic sclerosis sometimes causes pericarditis and pericardial effusions. In the vasculitides, e.g., Wegener's granulomatosis or the Churg-Strauss syndrome, the heart and lungs are often involved.

THE BRONCHIAL CIRCULATION

Our knowledge of the bronchial circulation dates back to Leonardo da Vinci's remarkable drawings of his own anatomic dissections during the seventeenth century. Not only did he identify the bronchial circulation's origin from the aorta, but he also illustrated an expanded bron-

chial circulation to a cavity within the lung. The bronchial circulation is now appreciated to be the nutrient circulation of the lungs, supplying the trachea, bronchi, intra- and extrapulmonary airways, bronchovascular bundles and nerves, regional lymph nodes, visceral pleurae, and supporting structures of the lung. In humans, the bronchial circulation arises from at least three main bronchial arteries: as a rule, two supply the left lung and one the right. In most circumstances one bronchial artery, most often the right, arises from an intercostal artery, whereas more than 80 percent of left bronchial arteries arise from the aorta (Fig. 68-15).

Each artery enters the lung at the hilus and divides, to follow the various segments of the bronchial tree. Two or more branches wrap around any given bronchus, penetrating its walls, and extending distally to the terminal bronchiole as a plexus that occupies the peribronchial space. Small arterioles that arise from these two branches pass through the muscle of the bronchial wall to reach the bronchial submucosa, where they give rise to a second submucosal plexus. Thus, both a submucosal and a peribronchial plexus are incorporated into the walls of the bronchial tree extending distally to the terminal bronchioles. Bronchial arteries also supply the walls of both the pulmonary arteries and veins.

The bronchial veins that drain the extrapulmonary airways empty into the right side of the heart via the azygous and hemiazygous veins, whereas those from intrapulmonary airways and parenchyma empty into the left side of the heart via the pulmonary veins. Ample communications exist between bronchial veins so that an increase in atrial pressure on one side of the heart redirects bronchial venous drainage to the opposite side.

In patients in whom the pulmonary circulation is interrupted or sparse, as in certain congenital cardiac defects or unilateral obliteration of one pulmonary artery, the bronchial circulation can proliferate and assume the gas-exchange function of the affected part of the lungs. Evidence is also mounting that the bronchial circulation, by way of its peribronchial plexus, features prominently in the humidification of inspired air and in temperature control. Sites of localized infection in the lungs often show remarkable proliferation of the bronchial circulation in their vicinity. Primary carcinomas of the lung receive their blood supply from bronchial arteries. A large research effort currently under way is exploring the roles of the bronchial circulation in maintaining fluid balance and airway defenses. Knowledge of its role is still incomplete.

Bronchopulmonary Anastomoses

The normal lung is replete with anastomotic channels that link, or can open to link, the bronchial and pulmonary circulations. Among these are: (1) bronchopulmonary arteries which connect small bronchial and pulmonary ar-

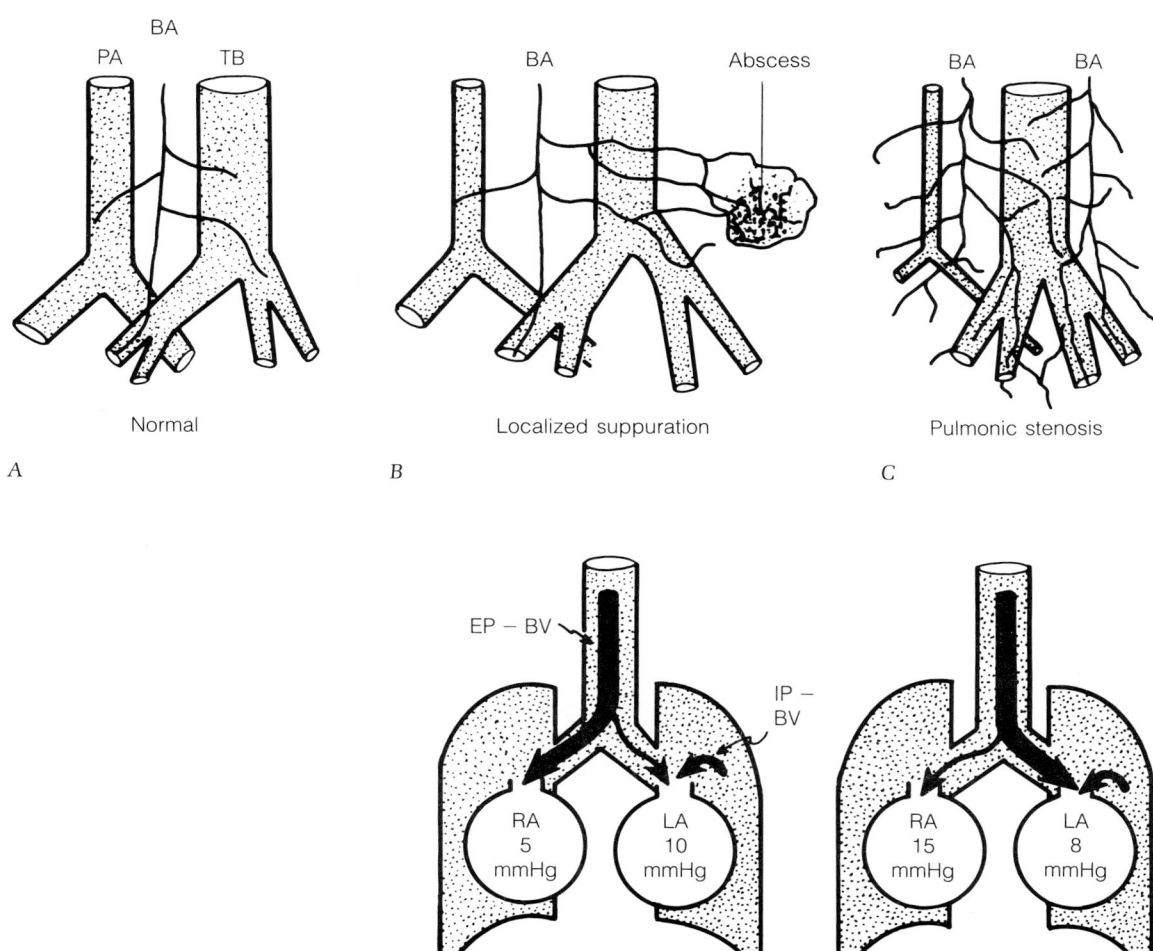

FIGURE 68-15 Schematic representation of the bronchial arterial and venous circulations. *A. Normal bronchial arterial circulation.* These vessels serve a nutrient function. They originate from the aorta or intercostal arteries and supply mediastinal structures, the airways, the supporting structures of the lungs, and the pulmonary vasculature. Distal at the terminal bronchioles, the bronchial and pulmonary microcirculations anastomose by a variety of connections. *B. Local suppuration* (as in bronchiectasis) or *necrosis* (as in infarction) stimulates proliferation of bronchial arteries. Expansion may be enormous, imposing a hemodynamic burden equivalent to a left-to-right shunt. *C. Pulmonic stenosis or atresia.* The expanded bronchial circulation, carrying oxygen-poor blood as in congenital cyanotic heart disease, may perfuse the gas-exchanging surfaces of the lungs, thereby performing a respiratory function essential for life. *D. Normal bronchial venous drainage.* Drainage from *extrapulmonary airways* (trachea and large bronchi) and the supporting structures is predominantly by way of the azygous-hemiazygous system to the right atrium. Drainage from *intrapulmonary* structures is predominantly by way of microanastomoses that lead by way of the pulmonary capillaries to the pulmonary veins and right atrium. *E. Right ventricular failure.* As right atrial pressure increases to exceed left atrial pressure, bronchial venous drainage via the microanastomoses is rearranged in accord with the reversed pressure gradients so that most of the drainage is to the left atrium, thereby constituting venous admixture and contributing to systemic arterial hypoxemia. BA = bronchial artery; BV = bronchial vein; PA = pulmonary artery; TB = tracheobronchial tree; EP-BV = extrapulmonary bronchial vein; IP-BV = intrapulmonary bronchial vein; RA = right atrium; LA = left atrium.

teries, (2) anastomoses between branches of the bronchial arteries and the pulmonary veins, (3) fine communications at the level of the pulmonary lobule and beyond which connect the bronchial and pulmonary microvasculatures, and (4) communications between the bronchial venous plexus and neighboring alveolar capillaries. Under normal conditions, these anastomoses have little functional role aside from a nutrient function. However, hemodynamic imbalances or reactions of the lungs to injury may increase their size and importance. In patients with a lung "destroyed" by suppurative disease, the expanded bronchial circulation can constitute a large hemodynamic burden, equivalent to a large left-to-right shunt.

Clinical Importance of the Bronchial Circulation

Under certain conditions, the bronchial circulation becomes clinically important. Among these are hemoptysis and bronchial hyperreactivity. One intriguing clinical observation is the frequent association of an expanded bronchial circulation, e.g., bronchiectasis, lung abscess, and pulmonary artery stenosis, with clubbing of the digits.

Hemoptysis

Most instances of hemoptysis originate in an expanded bronchial ("collateral") circulation. At times, as in the tetralogy of Fallot or Eisenmenger's complex, bronchial arterial bleeding may be so severe as to result in exsanguination. Occasionally, an expanded bronchial arterial flow can be manifested clinically by a soft, high-pitched murmur under the clavicles, along the borders of the sternum or over the paravertebral distribution (from T-2 to T-5).

In chronic *pulmonary* venous hypertension, e.g., as in mitral stenosis, submucosal bronchial veins often enlarge as the high pulmonary venous pressure diverts blood from the bronchial venous plexus to the azygos vein. Rupture of these submucosal veins may lead to repeated episodes of hemoptysis.

As noted above, inflammatory disease of the lungs, e.g., tuberculosis, bronchiectasis, lung abscess, fungal disease, and bronchitis, is usually associated with an enlarged bronchial circulation. Hemoptysis from a ruptured bronchial arterial branch is not uncommon in these disorders. The same is true of cancer of the lungs.

Although chest radiography is occasionally helpful with respect to the etiology of hemoptysis, particularly in patients with congenital heart disease, arteriography is more definitive. By passing a catheter via the femoral artery to the aorta, the bronchial artery can be identified by injecting radiopaque dye and visualizing its distribution. If bronchial arteriography succeeds in demonstrating the source of bleeding, a Gelfoam compound can be injected to seal the bleeding vessel. This procedure engenders the risk of a complicating transverse myelitis, caused either by spasm of the spinal arteries or inadvertent embolism of these vessels. Nevertheless, the procedure may be lifesaving in patients who are not candidates for resectional surgery. Bronchial arterial angiography is also occasionally valuable for defining vascular anatomy in patients in whom surgical anastomosis is contemplated for pulmonary arterial stenosis.

Shunts

Mention has been made above of the expanded bronchial arterial circulation in the "destroyed lung" and its potential for acting as a left-to-right shunt. In patients with chronic bronchitis and emphysema, the bronchial venous circulation sometimes undergoes considerable proliferation. Should right atrial pressures increase, e.g., as in cor pulmonale and right ventricular failure, a large right-to-left shunt can ensue, contributing to the increase in systemic venous pressure. The right-to-left shunt stems from reversal of bronchial venous drainage from the azygous vein to the pulmonary veins.

Bronchial Hyperreactivity and Cardiac Asthma

Patients in heart failure often manifest bronchial hyperreactivity, and some develop overt wheezing and respiratory distress that resemble asthma from other causes. The bronchial circulation is believed to be importantly involved in the pathogenesis of the obstructive breathing pattern, by way of both mucosal edema and hyperreactivity of bronchial smooth muscles.

Because of the numerous open and potential anastomotic channels between the bronchial and pulmonary circulations, an increase in pulmonary venous pressure is reflected in the bronchial microcirculation, thereby promoting bronchial edema. Moreover, the bronchial venules are exceedingly sensitive to biologically active substances, notably bradykinin and histamine, increasing their permeability markedly when exposed to these agents. Although the last word is not yet in concerning the contributions of the bronchial circulation to bronchial hyperreactivity (or to heat and water exchange in the airways, or increased airway secretions, or mucosal edema, or the transport of mediators to airway walls), the consensus seems to be that the bronchial circulation is importantly involved.

BIBLIOGRAPHY

Aberman A, Fulop M: The metabolic and respiratory acidosis of acute pulmonary edema. Ann Intern Med 762:173–184, 1972.
Eighty-three percent of patients with acute pulmonary edema due to left ventricular failure had acidemia; 24 percent had hypercapnia.

Alexander JK: The cardiomyopathy of obesity. Prog Cardiovasc Dis 27:325–333, 1985.
Hemodynamic derangements in obesity reflect the metabolic demands of a hypermetabolic state, the consequence of pressure overloading of the two ventricles and intrinsic myocardial disorders.

Bernheim PI: De l'asystolie veineuse dans l'hypertrophie du coeur gauche par stenose concomitante du ventricule droit. Rev Med 39:785–794, 1910.
The first account to suggest the importance of ventricular interaction adversely affecting right ventricular performance.

Bove AA, Santamore WP: Ventricular interdependence. Prog Cardiovasc Dis 23:365–388, 1981.
A detailed review of the experimental evidence and clinical significance of ventricular interplay.

Burke CM, Theodore J, Dawkins KD, Yousem SA, Blank N, Billingham ME, Van Kessel A, Jamieson SW, Oyer PE, Baldwin JC et al: Post-transplant obliterative bronchiolitis and other late lung sequelae in human heart-lung transplantation. Chest 86:824–829, 1984.
Serious complications of heart-lung transplantation are described.

Chipps BE, Alderson PO, Roland JM, Yang S, Van Aswegen A, Martinez CR, Rosenstein BJ: Noninvasive evaluation of ventricular function in cystic fibrosis. J Pediatr 95:379–384, 1979.
Seven of twenty-one patients with cystic fibrosis had evidence of abnormal left ventricular function.

Cortese DA: Pulmonary function in mitral stenosis. Mayo Clinic Proc 53:321–326, 1978.
Excellent review of the results of pulmonary function testing in patients with mitral stenosis.

Deffebach ME, Charan NB, Lakshminarayan S, Butler J: The bronchial circulation. Small, but a vital attribute of the lung. Am Rev Respir Dis 135:463–481, 1987.
A comprehensive update of many aspects of the bronchial circulation.

Dexter L: Atrial septal defect. Br Heart J 18:209–225, 1956.
A "reverse Bernheim" syndrome is postulated to explain left ventricular failure in atrial septal defect.

Edelman NH, Lahiri S, Braudo L, Cherniack NS, Fishman AP: The blunted ventilatory response to hypoxia in cyanotic congenital heart disease. N Engl J Med 282:405–411, 1970.
The ventilatory responses to hypoxia in cyanotic congenital heart disease is less than normal. A direct relationship exists between the degree of chronic hypoxemia and the decrease in the ventilatory response.

Estenne M, Yernault JC: The mechanism of CO_2 retention in cardiac pulmonary edema. Chest 86:936–938, 1984.
Studies in a single patient suggest that CO_2 retention is due to increased CO_2 production, physiological dead space, and mechanical impairment.

Fishman AP: Cor pulmonale, in Braunwald E, Isselbacher KJ, Petersdorf RG, Wilson JD, Martin JB, Fauci AS (eds), *Harrison's Principles of Internal Medicine.* New York McGraw-Hill, 1987, pp 993–998.
Includes a consideration of secondary pulmonary hypertension and of evolving experience with the use of pulmonary vasodilators. As a general rule, therapy is directed at treating the underlying disease and vasodilators are reserved for urgent situations to bide time.

Fluck DC, Chandrasekar RG, Gardner FV: Left ventricular hypertrophy in chronic bronchitis. Br Heart J 28:92–97, 1966.
At autopsy, one quarter of 84 patients with chronic bronchitis had left ventricular hypertrophy.

Gallagher CG, Younes M: Breathing pattern during and after maximal exercise in patients with chronic obstructive lung disease, interstitial lung disease, and cardiac disease, and in normal subjects. Am Rev Respir Dis 133:581–586, 1986.
In patients with cardiac disease, the breathing pattern during recovery after maximal incremental exercise was rapid and shallow and differed from that of patients with either obstructive airways disease or interstitial disease, possibly due to the development of pulmonary edema in the cardiac patients during maximal exercise.

Giuntini G, Panuccio P (eds): *Proceedings of the International Congress on Cardiac Lung.* Padova, Italy, Piccin Editore, 1979.
  A large work on the effect of heart disease on the lungs.

Henderson Y, Prince AL: The relative systolic discharges of the right and left ventricles and their bearing on pulmonary congestion and depletion. Heart 5:217–226, 1914.
  Direct experimental evidence of ventricular interaction.

Henning RJ: Effects of positive end-expiratory pressure on the right ventricle. J Appl Physiol 61:819–826, 1986.
  Positive-pressure ventilation with 20 cmH₂O PEEP decreases right ventricular function.

Hertz CW: The effect of heart disease on pulmonary function. Postgrad Med J 52:209–217, 1976.
  Dyspnea in pulmonary congestion is due to an increase in elastic and viscous work.

Hogg JC, Agarawal JB, Gardiner AJS, Palmer WH, Macklem PT: Distribution of airway resistance with developing pulmonary edema in dogs. J Appl Physiol 32:20–24, 1972.
  Peripheral airway resistance increased as left atrial pressure was raised. Above a left atrial pressure of 15 mmHg, increases in resistance were not reversible.

Holford FD, Mithoefer JC: Cardiac arrhythmias in hospitalized patients with chronic obstructive pulmonary disease. Am Rev Respir Dis 108:879–885, 1973.
  Thirty-five patients, 16 of whom had acute respiratory failure and 17 cor pulmonale, were monitored for 72 h. Fifty-four supraventricular tachycardias were detected.

Hudson LD, Kurt TL, Petty TL, Genton E: Arrhythmias associated with acute respiratory failure in patients with chronic airway obstruction. Chest 63:661–665, 1973.
  A 6 percent incidence of second degree atrioventricular block or greater was recorded.

Keats TE, Lipscomb GE, Betts CS III: Mensuration of the area of the azygous vein and its application to the study of cardiopulmonary disease. Radiology 90:990–994, 1968.
  Normal values are reported based on 200 standard chest radiographs.

Lahiri S, Edelman NH, Cherniack NS, Fishman AP: Blunted hypoxic drive to ventilation in subjects with lifelong hypoxemia. Fed Proc 28:1289–1295, 1969.
  The ventilatory response to transient inhalation of nitrogen was significantly less in the congenital cyanotics than in native residents at sea level.

Leblanc P, Bowie DM, Summers E, Jones NL, Killian KJ: Breathlessness and exercise in patients with cardiorespiratory disease. Am Rev Respir Dis 133:21–25, 1986.
  Experimental support for the hypothesis that breathlessness is the perception of respiratory muscle effort and is present when the tension developed by muscles increases, when the muscles are weak, or when both conditions are present simultaneously.

McHugh TJ, Forrester JS, Adler L, Zion D, Swan HJ: Pulmonary vascular congestion in acute myocardial infarction: Hemodynamic and radiologic correlation. Ann Intern Med 76:29–33, 1972.
  Radiologic criteria when related to capillary wedge pressure provide a basis for rational therapy of left ventricular failure due to myocardial infarction.

Mellins RB, Levine OR, Fishman AP: Effect of systemic and pulmonary venous hypertension on pleural and pericardial fluid accumulation. J Appl Physiol 29:564–569, 1970.
  Significantly larger amounts of pleural fluid accumulate after systemic venous hypertension than after pulmonary venous hypertension.

Milic Emili J, Ruff F: Effects of pulmonary congestion and edema on the small airways. Bull Physiopathol Respir 7:1181–1196, 1971.
  Pulmonary congestion and edema cause profound changes in small airways including increased flow resistance and premature airway closure.

Moolten SE: Pulmonary fibrosis in rheumatic heart disease. Am J Med 3:421–441, 1962.
  Description of a distinctive type of interstitial fibrosis seen with rheumatic heart disease.

Murata K, Itoh H, Todo G, Itoh T, Kanaoka M, Furuta M, Torizuka K: Bronchial venous plexus and its communication with pulmonary circulation. Invest Radiol 21:24–30, 1986.
  Radiographic techniques, including bronchiolar arteriography, microradiography, and serial histologic sections, revealed numerous bronchial venous plexuses around the airways and blood vessels into which the bronchial capillaries drain. Frequent communications were shown between the bronchial venous plexuses, the pulmonary veins, and the neighboring alveolar capillaries.

Murphy ML, Adamson J, Hutcheson F: Left ventricular hypertrophy in patients with chronic bronchitis and emphysema. Ann Intern Med 8:307–313, 1974.
At autopsy, 28 percent of patients with chronic bronchitis and emphysema had left ventricular hypertrophy. In 11 percent, no etiology was demonstrable.

Murray JF: The lungs and heart failure. Hosp Pract 20:55–68, 1985.
Excellent review including a section on the measurement of lung water.

Palmer WH, Gree JL, Mills FC, Burke DV: Disturbances of pulmonary function in mitral valve disease. Can Med Assoc J 89:744–750, 1963.
Pulmonary capillary blood volume was increased in patients with moderate mitral stenosis but was consistently decreased in the more seriously ill.

Pepine CJ, Wiener L: Relationship of anginal symptoms to lung mechanics during myocardial ischemia. Circulation 46:863–869, 1972.
Pacing in patients with angina produced changes in the mechanical properties of the lungs.

Pistolesi M, Milne EN, Miniati M, Giuntini C: The vascular pedicle of the heart and the vena azygos. Part II: Acquired heart disease. Radiology 152:9–17, 1984.
Measurement of the vascular pedicle correlated well with total blood volume and mean right atrial pressure.

Snapper JR: Lung mechanics in pulmonary edema. Clin Chest Med 6:393–412, 1985.
Distinguishes among the different patterns of mechanical changes that accompany vascular congestion, interstitial edema, and alveolar edema.

Snashall PD: Pulmonary edema. Br J Dis Chest 74:2–22, 1980.
Excellent review of pulmonary edema, including treatment.

Starr I, Jeffers WA, Meade RH: The absence of conspicuous increments of venous pressure after severe damage to the right ventricle of the dog. Am Heart J 3:291–302, 1943.
Catastrophic damage to the right ventricle had little effect on systemic venous pressure.

Steele P, Ellis JH Jr, Van Dyke D, Sutton F, Creagh E, Davies H: Left ventricular ejection fraction in severe chronic obstructive airways disease. Am J Med 59:21–28, 1975.
A series of 120 patients with severe chronic obstructive airways disease in whom left ventricular function was studied using radionuclides. Left ventricular ejection fraction was subnormal in 32 with acute respiratory failure.

Toronto Lung Transplant Group: Unilateral lung transplantation for pulmonary fibrosis. N Engl J Med 314:1140–1145, 1986.
Reports of two successful unilateral lung transplants.

Turino GM, Fishman AP: The congested lung. J Chron Dis 9:510–524, 1959.
The performance of the congested lung is considered in terms of its anatomic and physiological abnormalities.

Von Basch S: Ueber eine Function des Capillardruckes in den Lungenalveolem. Wien Med Blater 10:465–475, 1887.
Early description of the effect of pulmonary congestion on the pressure-volume relationships of the lung.

Weber KT, Janicki JS (eds): Cardiopulmonary Exercise Testing: Physiologic Principles and Clinical Applications. Philadelphia, Saunders, 1986.
A concise account of the interplay between the heart and lungs and its relationship to gas transport at rest and exercise.

Weber KI, Janicki JS, Shroff SG, Fishman AP: Contractile mechanics and interaction of the right and left ventricles. Am J Cardiol 47:686–695, 1981.
A consideration of cardiac interaction and the role of the septum based on the architecture of the heart and ventricles.

Wood TE, McLeod P, Anthonisen NR, Macklem PT: Mechanics of breathing in mitral stenosis. Am Rev Respir Dis 104:52–60, 1971.
Pressure-volume relationships in mitral stenosis are altered in a similar manner to that seen in vascular engorgement. Airway resistance was doubled, and expiratory flow rates decreased at all lung volumes.

Chapter 69

Pulmonary Vasculitis

Lotte Strauss† / Kenneth V. Lieberman / Jacob Churg

The classic description of necrotizing systemic vasculitis (periarteritis or polyarteritis nodosa) by Kussmaul and Maier is over a century old. Reports by subsequent investigators documented involvement of almost every organ in the body, including the lungs. However, it was apparent from the beginning that pulmonary vasculitis is much rarer than that of the vessels of systemic circulation. Rose and Spencer reviewed 111 patients with polyarteritis nodosa and found pulmonary involvement in less than one-third. Most of their patients in that group had associated granulomatous lesions, falling into the categories of Wegener's granulomatosis and allergic granulomatosis. By now it is well established that these two syndromes account for the majority of cases of pulmonary vasculitis (Table 69-1), whereas the classic polyarteritis nodosa hardly ever involves the lungs.

Although the entity of polyarteritis nodosa was identified by Kussmaul and Maier on the basis of gross exami-

TABLE 69-1
Classification of Pulmonary Vasculitis

1. Wegener's granulomatosis
   a. Lymphomatoid granulomatosis
   b. Midline granuloma
2. Allergic granulomatosis and angiitis (Churg-Strauss syndrome)
   a. Vasculitis in eosinophilic pneumonia due to drugs, to parasites, and to fungi
3. Sarcoidal angiitis (nodular sarcoidosis, necrotizing sarcoid granulomatosis)
4. Takayasu's arteritis and giant cell arteritis
5. Small vessel vasculitis (hypersensitivity angiitis): leukocytoclastic vasculitis and mononuclear vasculitis
6. Other vasculitides: Henoch-Schönlein purpura, cryoglobulinemic vasculitis, Behçet's disease
7. Vasculitis in pulmonary diseases: tuberculosis, fungal infections, extrinsic alveolitis due to organic dusts
8. Vasculitis in pulmonary hypertension
9. Vasculitis in systemic diseases
   a. Collagen diseases: systemic lupus erythematosus, rheumatoid arthritis, progressive systemic sclerosis
   b. Miscellaneous: ulcerative colitis, ankylosing spondylitis, liver cirrhosis, Goodpasture's syndrome, hypocomplementemic vasculitis, malignant tumors, drugs, toxins

†Deceased.

nation at autopsy, the name of the disease was derived from the microscopic appearance of the lesions. Subsequent studies demonstrated that not only medium-size muscular arteries but also small arteries and arterioles were involved. In the instances when the disease was limited to the smaller blood vessels, the entity was designated as *microscopic polyarteritis nodosa*. A clinical distinction was also drawn between the classic polyarteritis nodosa of Kussmaul and Maier for which the etiology is largely unknown and a vasculitis that followed sensitization to foreign proteins or drugs and was designated by Zeek as *hypersensitivity angiitis*. Originally, hypersensitivity angiitis was believed to be the same as microscopic polyarteritis nodosa. However, the current view holds that hypersensitivity angiitis involves mainly venules and capillaries and, to a much lesser extent, the arterioles. In addition to the hypersensitivity states, similar or identical vascular changes were also found in a variety of other diseases (Table 69-1). At present, the noncommital term *small vessel vasculitis* is preferentially applied to this group. Although small vessel vasculitis is most often seen, or perhaps most often recognized, in the skin biopsied because of cutaneous eruption, it also occurs in the internal organs, including the lungs.

WEGENER'S GRANULOMATOSIS

This rare syndrome generally occurs in the fourth and fifth decades of life with a slight male preponderance.

History

Wegener's granulomatosis is a necrotizing, granulomatous vasculitis that classically involves the clinicopathologic triad of upper and lower respiratory tracts and the kidney. Although the first case was described by Klinger, the syndrome was defined by Wegener in 1936. Clinical and pathologic descriptions of the full systemic entity were detailed as well as the recognition of a limited form, without renal involvement. An early report described a high untreated mortality; however, modern therapeutic regimens, including steroids and cyclophosphamide, have dramatically improved the prognosis of these patients with a high percentage of apparent cures.

Pathogenesis

Early investigators hypothesized that the etiology of Wegener's granulomatosis was an exaggerated immunologic response to an inhaled environmental antigen, because of the usual dominance of respiratory tract symptoms in the clinical presentation. No specific antigen, exogenous or endogenous, has been identified. The frequent observation in Wegener's patients of circulating immune complexes (by numerous methodologies), the

correlation of disease activity with circulating immune complexes titer, the presence of circulating rheumatoid factor and cryoglobulins, and polyclonal B-cell activation have led Fauci to suggest that immune complexes may be centrally involved in the pathogenesis of this disease. This would be analogous to the classical Arthus' (type III, hypersensitivity) reaction in which local antigenic rechallenge in an animal previously actively (or passively) immunized results in local immune complex-mediated lesions of necrotizing vasculitis. The tissue immune complexes may be formed in situ (fixed antigenic sites) or may be the result of deposition of circulating immune complexes. This mechanism casts the humoral arm of the immune system in a central role.

There are two sets of observations that cast doubt on the above hypothesis. Firstly, serum complement components (C3, C4) have generally been found to be normal in Wegener's cases. Pathogenic immune complexes would be expected to bind and, therefore, deplete serum complement. The recent report detailing frequent elevation of a circulating C3 breakdown product, however, suggests the presence of complement consumption in Wegener's granulomatosis.

Secondly, the demonstration of immunoglobulin deposits by immunofluorescence microscopy has occurred with much less frequency than would have been expected. Although some investigators have reported granular immunoglobulin deposits in pulmonary alveolar walls, most have reported the striking rarity or absence of deposits in bronchial, paranasal, nasopharyngeal, or cutaneous (extravascular) sites. Immunofluorescence staining has been conspicuously negative in vessel walls. Deposits have also only rarely been demonstrated in renal biopsy material by either immunofluorescence or electron microscopy. However, it must be noted that studies in animal models of Arthus' reaction demonstrated the rapid (within 48 h) loss of antigen and immune complexes from the lesions largely due to digestion by polymorphonuclear leukocytes.

An alternative hypothesis, emphasizing the role of cell-mediated (classically type IV, delayed-type hypersensitivity) immune mechanisms in the genesis of granulomatous vasculitis, has been proposed by Fauci. Sensitized lymphocytes, reacting with antigen, release various lymphokines including macrophage migration inhibition factor. This factor has been demonstrated in lung granuloma extracts from patients with Wegener's granulomatosis.

It then recruits circulating monocytes to the developing lesions where they are transformed to activated macrophages that can release lysosomal enzymes and cause local tissue injury. Immunoperoxidase staining of vascular pulmonary lymphoid infiltrates utilizing monoclonal antibodies has demonstrated that cells of monocyte lineage (OKM1 positive) are the most numerous; T cells (more helper than suppressor-cytotoxic) are also present. The

activated macrophages can then become epithelioid cells, forming multinucleated giant cells, hence creating the mature granulomatous lesion usually recognized in this disorder.

Clinical

The vast majority of patients present with upper respiratory tract complaints: otitis, epistaxis, rhinorrhea, and sinusitis. The characteristic organ involvement is shown in Table 69-2.

CONSTITUTIONAL SYMPTOMS

Systemic manifestations including headache, malaise, weight loss, anorexia, weakness, and fevers are almost invariably present (Table 69-3). In addition, arthralgias (symmetric, polyarticular, small and large joints) are frequent. True arthritis (involving large joints) is less frequent but has been reported as a mode of presentation. Hepatitis, orchitis, and small intestine involvement causing a perforation have each been reported once. Thromboembolic phenomena have been reported. (We have observed a case of deep vein thrombosis complicated by pulmonary emboli.)

RESPIRATORY TRACT

Pulmonary involvement can be expected in virtually all patients. Cough (occasionally with sputum production), dyspnea, chest pain, and hemoptysis can occur. Radiologically, single, or more commonly multiple, unilateral, or more commonly bilateral, nodular solid or cavitary infiltrates are seen (Fig. 69-1). Less commonly, endobronchial lesions can result in airway obstruction even causing atelectasis. Spontaneous pneumothorax with bronchopleural fistula and pleuritis with pleural effusions also occur.

Sinusitis is common (most frequently involving the maxillary, followed by the sphenoid, then the ethmoid sinuses), with mucosal thickening (Fig. 69-2), air-fluid levels, and rarely total sinus obliteration. Superimposed bacterial sinusitis, particularly *Staphylococcus aureus*, especially occurring during treatment with immunosup-

TABLE 69-2
Characteristic Features of Organ System Involvement in Wegener's Granulomatosis

Organ System	Approximate Frequency, %	Typical Features
Nasopharynx	75	Necrotizing granuloma with mucosal ulceration; saddle nose deformity
Paranasal sinuses	90	Pansinusitis; necrotizing granuloma; secondary bacterial infection
Eyes	60	Keratoconjunctivitis; granulomatous sclerouveitis
Ears	35	Serous otitis media; secondary bacterial infection
Lungs	95	Multiple nodular cavitary infiltrates; necrotizing granulomatous vasculitis
Kidneys	85	Focal and segmental glomerulitis; necrotizing glomerulonephritis later in course
Heart	15	Coronary vasculitis; pericarditis
Nervous system	20	Mononeuritis multiplex; cranial neuritis
Skin	40	Dermal vasculitis with secondary ulcerations
Joints	50	Polyarthralgias

SOURCE: From Fauci et al., 1978.

TABLE 69-3
Presenting Signs and Symptoms in Wegener's Granulomatosis

Signs or Symptoms	Patients No.	%
Constitutional		
Joint	37	44
Fever	29	34
Weight loss	14	16
Anorexia or malaise	7	8
Respiratory		
Pulmonary infiltrates	60	71
Sinusitis	57	67
Cough	29	34
Rhinitis or nasal symptoms	19	22
Hemoptysis	15	18
Epistaxis	9	11
Chest discomfort	7	8
Shortness of breath or dyspnea	6	7
Pleuritis or effusion	5	6
Urinary Tract		
Renal failure	9	11
Ocular		
Ocular inflammation (conjunctivitis, uveitis, episcleritis, and scleritis)	14	16
Proptosis	6	7
Cutaneous		
Skin rash	11	13
Nervous system		
Headache	5	6
Aural		
Otitis	21	25
Hearing loss	5	6
Oral		
Oral ulcers	5	6

SOURCE: Fauci et al., 1983.

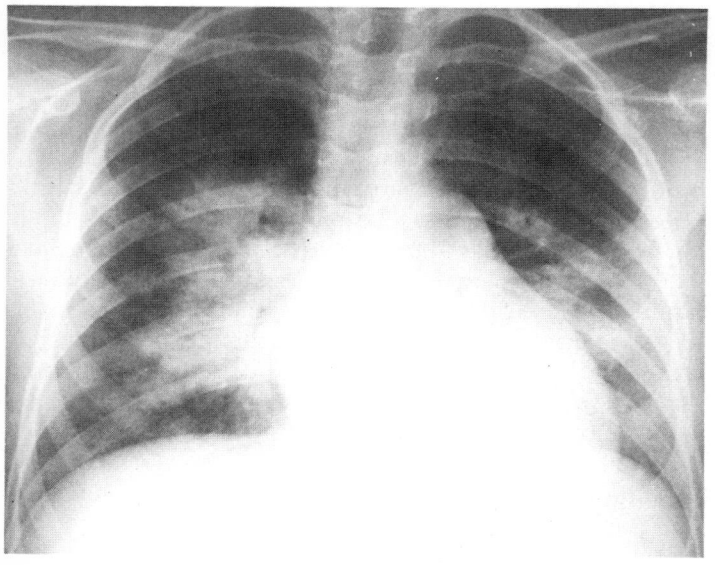

A

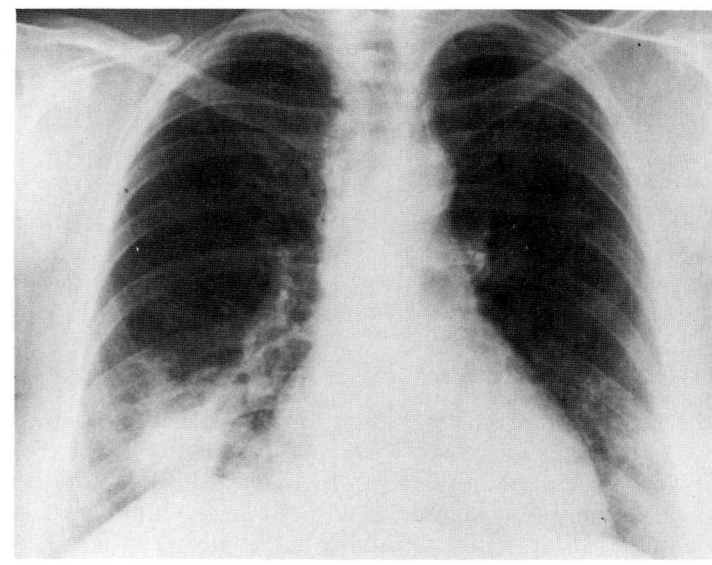

B

C

FIGURE 69-1 Wegener's granulomatosis. Diverse radiographic appearances when first seen by physician. A. Multiple bilateral, poorly defined perihilar densities with early cavitation. B. Bibasal infiltrates with large mass at right lung base. C. Dense opacification of both lung fields more marked on the left. Nodular opacities bilaterally.

pressive agents when other disease manifestations are quiescent, can be confused with Wegener's activity.

Nasal involvement is characterized by rhinitis, rhinorrhea, and epistaxis. Nasal obstruction and shallow mucosal ulcers also occur. Destruction of the cartilagenous nasal septal support of the nasal bridge causes the characteristic "saddle nose" deformity. Otitis media occurs as a result of eustachian tube obstruction (this can be the presenting sign), causing otalgia, otorrhea, and hearing loss. Chronic otitis can lead to cholesteatoma.

Granulomatous inflammation can occur anywhere in the mouth, pharynx, larynx, or trachea, causing pseudotumors (mass lesions) or ulceration. Symptoms can include mouth pain, gingivitis, sore throat, hoarseness, and stri-

dor. Severe subglottic stenosis can necessitate a tracheostomy.

URINARY TRACT

Clinical signs of renal disease are present in the majority of patients with Wegener's granulomatosis. The findings are those of the acute nephritic syndrome. Hypertension and signs of fluid overload (edema, congestive heart failure) are often present. Renal function on presentation can range from normal to mildly impaired to complete renal shutdown with uremia requiring dialysis. Without prompt treatment, mild renal involvement can progress rapidly to severe renal failure. Rarely, Wegener's granulo-

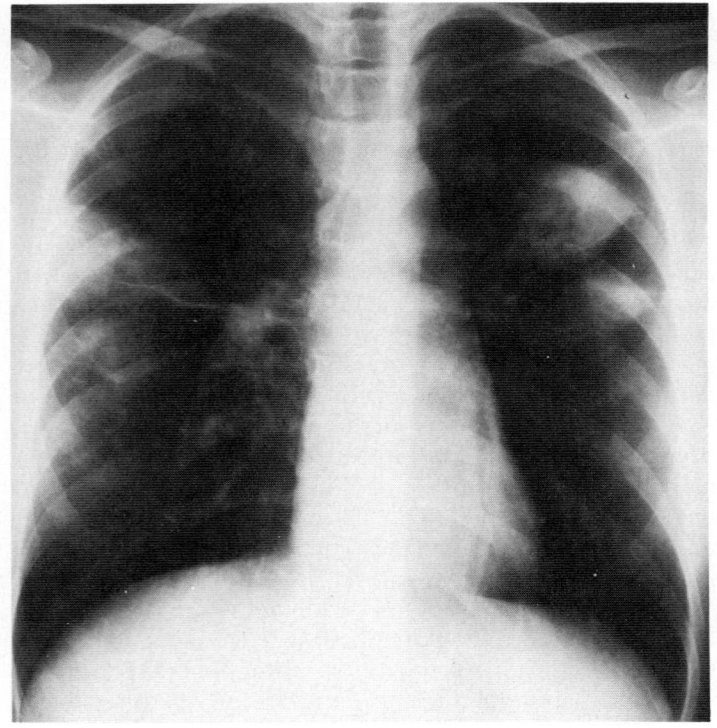

A

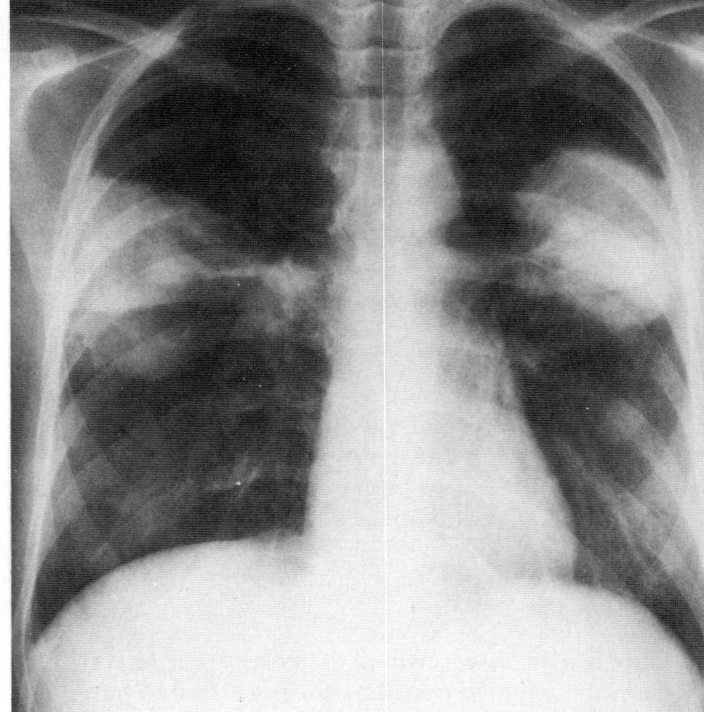

B

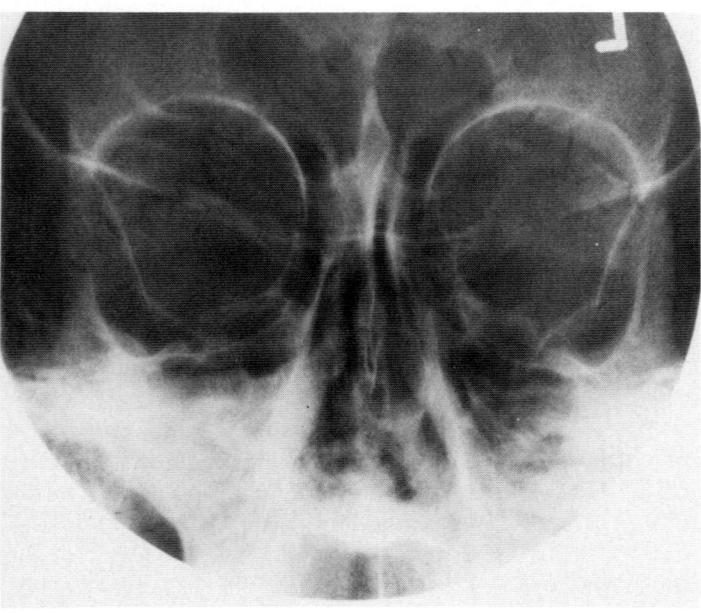

C

FIGURE 69-2 Wegener's granulomatosis. Radiographs of chest and paranasal sinuses. *A.* Bilateral dense masses. *B.* One month later. Considerable growth and confluence of the large masses accompanied by new nodules. *C.* Paranasal sinuses. Bilateral thickening of the mucosal surfaces of both maxillary sinuses with dense opacification particularly on the right.

matosis can present as glomerulonephritis, with the classic respiratory tract involvement developing later in the course.

Although the typical urinary manifestations of Wegener's granulomatosis are usually due to a glomerulonephritis, involvement of many of the elements of the urinary tract have been reported (albeit rarely). Descriptions of the following have appeared in the literature: perinephric hematoma, papillary necrosis, renal artery aneurysms,

necrotizing urethritis, and hydronephrosis secondary to ureteral stenosis caused by a transmural granulomatous inflammation.

OCULAR

Ocular involvement may present with eye pain, disturbances of vision (i.e., decrease or blurriness), chemosis, or proptosis. Proptosis is the result of an inflammatory

retroorbital mass lesion (pseudotumor). Conjunctivitis, episcleritis, scleritis, corneoscleral ulceration, keratitis, optic nerve vasculitis, retinal artery occlusion, uveitis, nasolacrimal duct obstruction, orbital cellulitis, retinal detachment, and retinal hemorrhage have all been seen.

CUTANEOUS

Rarely Wegener's granulomatosis can present with skin lesions, i.e., pyoderma grangrenosum. Other dermatologic manifestations include painful subcutaneous nodules, papules, ulcers, vesicles, petechiae, and palpable purpura.

Pancarditis can occur in Wegener's granulomatosis, as well as limited cardiac involvement: pericarditis, myocarditis, endocarditis-valvulitis, and coronary arteritis. Complete heart block secondary to granulomatous inflammation of the conducting system with nodal arteritis has also been reported.

NERVOUS SYSTEM

Nervous system involvement is usually peripheral with polyneuritis or mononeuritis multiplex due to vasculitis of the vasa nervorum. Centrally, expanding necrotizing granulomatous vasculitic lesions can cause cranial nerve abnormalities. Cortical vein thrombosis or central nervous system vasculitis with hemorrhage can occur. Pituitary involvement manifesting as central diabetes insipidus has been described.

LIMITED WEGENER'S

A limited form of Wegener's granulomatosis without renal involvement has been recognized. This syndrome has also been noted to generally follow a clinically more benign, less fulminating course. Fauci underscored the existence of subclinical renal disease in Wegener's patients. Patients classified as having the limited form (by virtue of the absence of apparent clinical renal disease, i.e., no urinary sediment abnormalities) with abnormal renal biopsies have been described. Further complicating the problem of clinical recognition is the very slow evolution of disease manifestations in some patients: a 16-year period between the first evidence of upper respiratory involvement and the appearance of renal abnormalities has been reported.

The occurrence of Wegener's granulomatosis during pregnancy does not imply a bad outcome. A woman presenting with Wegener's during her first pregnancy was started on prednisone and cyclophosphamide and after the induction of labor, prematurely (because of spontaneous, early rupture of membranes) delivered a small for gestational age infant who did well. Another pregnancy in a woman with Wegener's in remission, still on prednisone and azathioprine, ended successfully with a normal term infant.

Laboratory

Although there are no pathognomonic laboratory tests for Wegener's granulomatosis, the following findings on routine laboratory evaluation are typical: increased erythrocyte sedimentation rate, leukocytosis, thrombocytosis, and anemia. With renal involvement, abnormalities of the urinary sediment can be expected: hematuria, sterile pyuria, and red blood cell casts, along with proteinuria. The serum creatinine may be elevated, reflecting a decrease in creatinine clearance. Characteristically, serum immunoglobulins are elevated, usually IgG and IgA, occasionally IgM, and rarely IgE. The presence of circulating immune complexes has been demonstrated by commonly positive rheumatoid factor, occasionally positive cryoprecipitates, frequently positive Clq binding assay, and positive Raji cell assay. Normal levels of Clq, C3, C4, and CH_{50} have been reported, but C3d (a C3 breakdown product) has been reported to be elevated. The following are characteristically negative: ANA, anti-ds DNA antibodies, LE prep, VDRL, ASLO, and HBsAg. The acute phase reactant C-reactive protein (CRP) is increased. (We have found the CRP to parallel disease activity—unpublished.) A recent report describes the finding of anti-Ro (SSA) antibodies in four out of four tested Wegener's patients. Other recent reports speak of anticytoplasmic autoantibodies against polymorphonuclear neutrophils and monocytes, demonstrable in a high proportion of patients with Wegener's granulomatosis. These antibodies are believed to be of diagnostic significance and may also serve as markers of disease activity. They disappear with remission, but persist despite treatment in incomplete remission and often presage a recurrence. Prior to beginning of immunosuppressive therapy, patients have been found to have normal delayed-type hypersensitivity response by skin test, normal lymphocyte proliferative response to phytohemagglutinin (PHA), and normal numbers of circulating T and B lymphocytes. Studies of the human histocompatibility antigens have demonstrated increased incidence of HLA-B8 (known to have increased frequency in association with other "autoimmune" diseases), increased incidence of HLA-DR2, and increased incidence of the combination of HLA-B7, DR2 (as in systemic lupus erythematosus).

Pathology

The characteristic lesions of Wegener's granulomatosis are necrotizing granulomas and vasculitis. Necrotizing granulomatous lesions typically occur in the upper respiratory tract (nose, paranasal sinuses, nasopharynx, glottis, or adjacent regions), as well as in the lower respiratory tract (trachea, bronchi, lungs) (Figs. 69-3 to 69-5). Generalized, focal necrotizing vasculitis involving both arteries and veins is seen to a varying extent, but almost always in the lungs. The typical renal finding is a glomerulitis characterized by necrosis (and thrombosis) of capillary loops

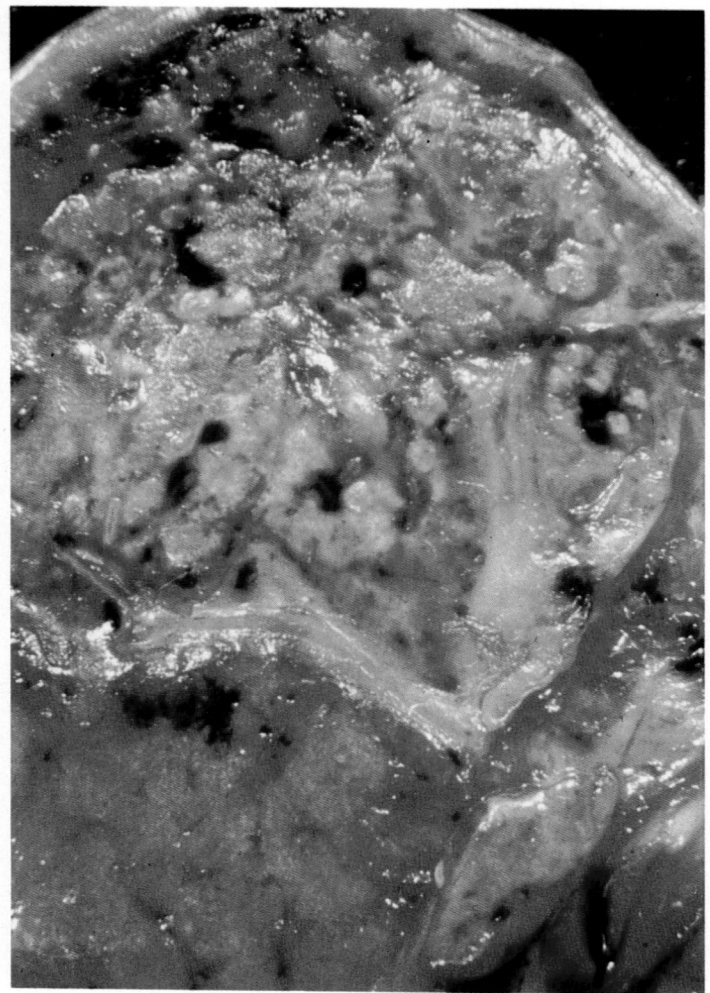
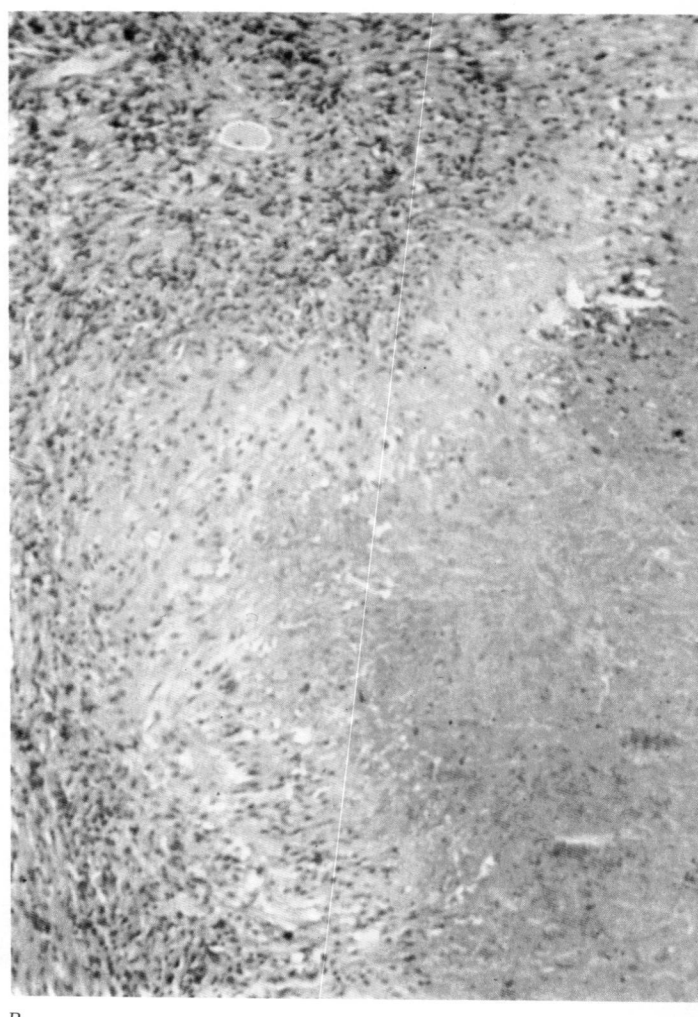

A *B*

FIGURE 69-3 Wegener's granulomatosis. Necrotic lesions. *A.* Large necrotic cavity with a zone of necrosis *(left upper pole)* and adjacent granulomatous inflammation. *B.* Same patient. Edge of the cavity showing a zone of necrosis *(right lower)* and adjacent granulomatous inflammation. H&E, ×25.

or lobules with capsular adhesions and occasional evolution to granulomatous lesions. Virtually any organ system can be involved, with occasional vascular and granulomatous lesions found in the spleen, liver, prostate, epididymis, lymph nodes, and heart.

The variability of the renal findings has been stressed. Most commonly a nonspecific focal and segmental glomerulonephritis is seen on light microscopy. With rapidly progressive disease, a diffuse proliferative or crescentic glomerulonephritis can occur. Granulomatous lesions and vasculitis are only rarely demonstrated. In remission only the sclerosis of glomerular obsolescence is seen. On electron microscopy occasional subepithelial deposits have been reported. Immunofluorescence studies reveal immunoglobulin deposits in only a minority of cases.

Biopsies obtained from the upper respiratory tract often reveal only nonspecific inflammation. Skin biopsies frequently demonstrate only the nonspecific lesion of leukocytoclastic vasculitis. Renal biopsies typically show nonspecific focal and segmental glomerulonephritis and sometimes crescents. The tissue most likely to demonstrate the characteristic lesion of Wegener's granulomatosis is lung; therefore, an open lung biopsy is the preferred technique to rapidly establish a histopathologic diagnosis in a suspected patient.

Differential Diagnosis

A careful clinical evaluation including radiologic evaluation (e.g., sinus films to demonstrate occult sinus disease), serologic studies (to rule out other collagen-vascular diseases), and appropriate biopsies should establish the diagnosis of Wegener's granulomatosis.

The other major pulmonary-renal syndrome, Goodpasture's syndrome, is characterized by circulating anti-

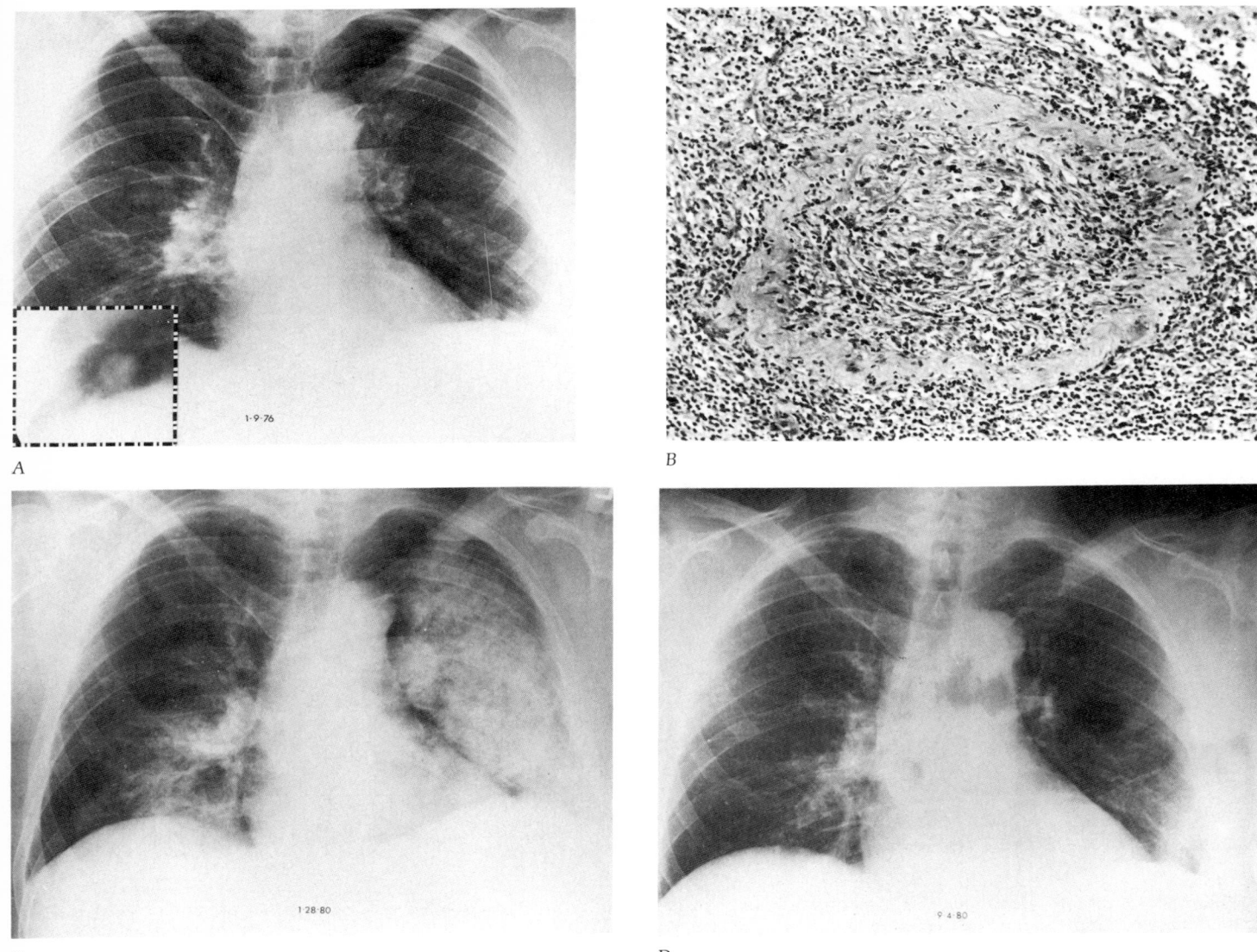

FIGURE 69-4 Wegener's granulomatosis. Resolution of lesions. Fifty-four-year-old man with cough, fever, sweats, and arthralgia. *A*. Multiple pulmonary nodules resembling metastases. *B*. Photomicrograph of lung biopsy showing typical necrotizing granuloma. *C*. Four years after *A*. The left lung is consolidated and there is an infiltrate of the right lung. *Hemophilus influenzae* in sputum. No response to ampicillin. *D*. Nine months after *C*. The lungs cleared while the patient was receiving cyclophosphamide, 100 mg daily. Progressive renal failure. One year later maintained on renal dialysis and cyclophosphamide, 25 mg daily. *(From Israel, 1982)*.

GBM antibodies and linear immunofluorescence staining of basement membranes in lung and kidney. Neoplastic disease may be suggested by the clinical presentation; a biopsy usually establishes the diagnosis. Lymphomatoid granulomatosis is a lymphoproliferative disease that can present as a primarily pulmonary syndrome with systemic symptoms. The primary vasculitic syndromes, systemic lupus erythematosus, Henoch-Schönlein purpura, Sjögren's syndrome, hypersensitivity vasculitis, and polyarteritis nodosa, may need to be considered. Allergic granulomatosis and angiitis can present clinically very similar to Wegener's granulomatosis; however, blood and tissue eosinophilia in addition to an allergic history are charac-

teristic of this syndrome. The purely granulomatous syndromes, sarcoidosis and midline granuloma (Fig. 69-6), must also be excluded.

Treatment

Although Wegener's granulomatosis can exist in an indolent form, with greater than 4-year survival without any specific therapy, the disease is generally considered to have a high untreated mortality rate. Steroids were demonstrated to improve prognosis somewhat; however, the introduction of cytotoxic therapy significantly decreased morbidity and mortality. A number of case reports de-

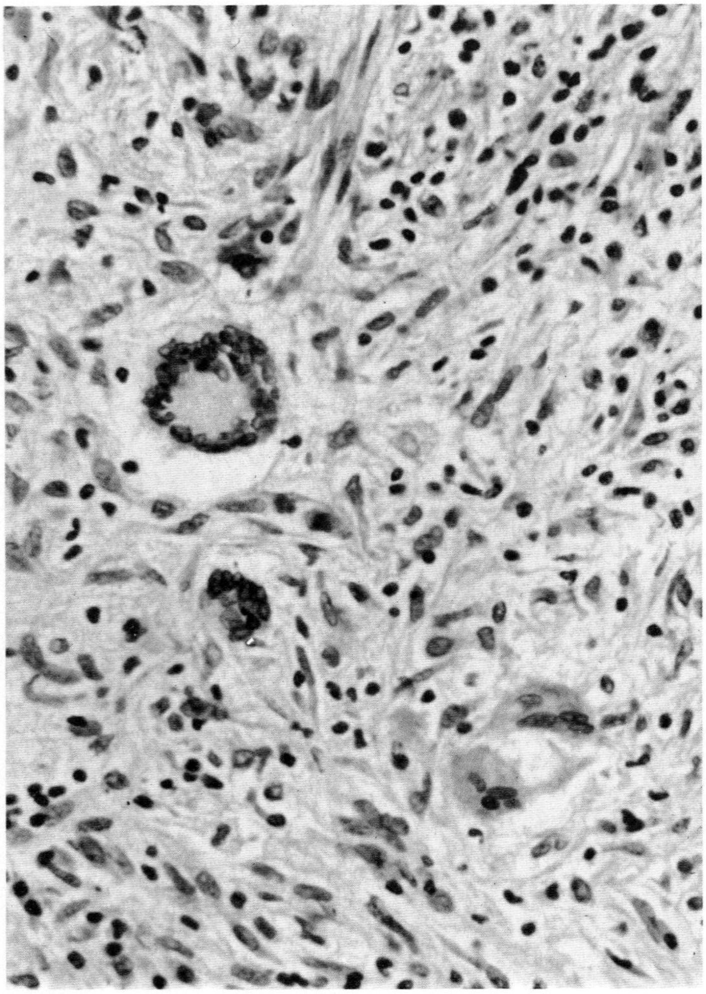

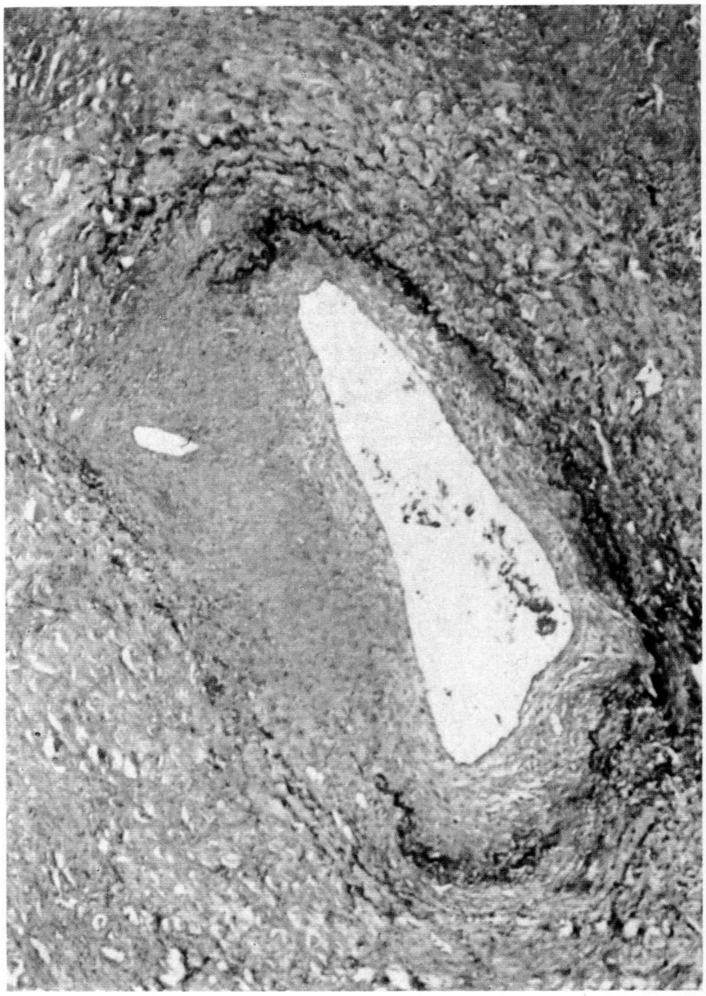

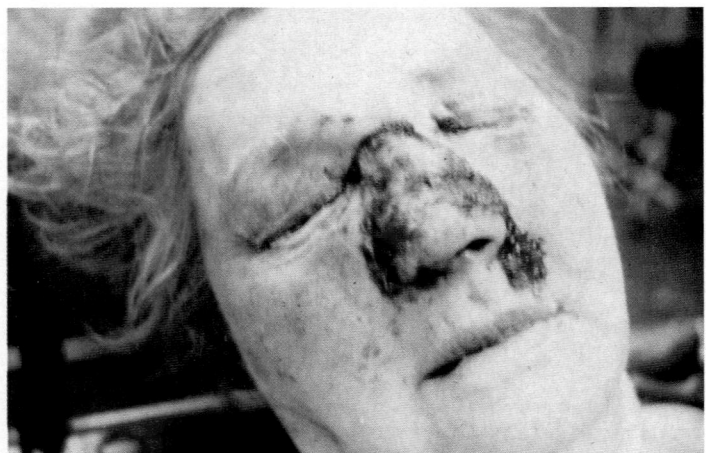

A   B

FIGURE 69-5 Healing in Wegener's granulomatosis. *A.* Later stage showing a healing granuloma with fibroblastic proliferation and scattered multinucleated giant cells. H&E, ×108. *B.* Healing arteritis. The vascular wall is partially destroyed: the elastic lamina has disappeared, and normal elements have been replaced. Elastic van Gieson's stain, ×17.3. *(Courtesy of Dr. Deborah Kay.)*

FIGURE 69-6 Midline granuloma, lymphomatoid (pleomorphic reticulosis) type. Appearance of the face postmortem.

scribed improvement in upper respiratory tract manifestations with steroids alone, development of renal involvement while on steroids, followed by entry into global remission only with the addition of cyclophosphamide (or occasionally azathioprine). Other patients failed to respond to steroids alone and then remitted with the addition of cyclophosphamide. Steroids have been of particular value for ocular manifestations. Incomplete remission induction with prednisone plus azathioprine followed by complete remission when switched to prednisone plus cyclophosphamide has been reported. Although the successful treatment of limited Wegener's with steroids alone has been reported, a similar patient ultimately dying of progressive respiratory failure has also been described. One group has expressed the opinion that, although steroids may suffice for only extrarenal disease, cyclophosphamide is probably mandatory in the presence of renal

involvement (although they also noted rapid pulmonary improvement with the combination of prednisone and cyclophosphamide).

Fauci and others have concluded that the combination of prednisone and cyclophosphamide is the initial treatment of choice for Wegener's granulomatosis. A recommended treatment protocol is as follows. Initial therapy consists of prednisone 1 mg/kg orally daily in divided doses with cyclophosphamide 2 mg/kg orally daily. After 2 to 4 weeks, the prednisone is slowly converted to an alternate day regimen. Depending on the individual patient's course, the prednisone is gradually tapered over the next 6 months to 1 year. After the patient has been in complete remission for at least 1 year, the cyclophosphamide is slowly tapered. Total white blood cell counts need to be carefully monitored and not allowed to drop below 3000 to 3500 per cubic millimeter. Disease reactivation may necessitate remission reinduction with another course of the initial regimen.

Patients with fulminant disease can receive higher doses of cyclophosphamide (4 to 5 mg/kg daily) along with prednisone 2 mg/kg daily, initially. Alternatively, very high dose "pulse" intravenous methylprednisolone (10 to 30 mg/kg daily for 3 to 5 days) has been administered as initial steroid therapy. Two reports have described the use of plasmapheresis in the initial treatment regimen. In one series, steroid plus cyclophosphamide plus plasmapheresis was felt to provide the best control of fulminant disease; it was acknowledged, however, that little clinical improvement occurred with steroids plus plasmapheresis. High dose steroids plus cyclophosphamide have not been directly compared with steroids plus cyclophosphamide plus plasmapheresis.

Recently improvement or control of Wegener's granulomatosis was achieved by adding an antimicrobial agent (trimethoprim-sulfamethoxazole) to the standard cyclophosphamide and steroids regimen, or even using this agent alone. Confirmatory studies have not yet appeared.

LYMPHOMATOID GRANULOMATOSIS

In the past this disease had been confused with Wegener's granulomatosis, but now it is considered to be a distinct entity.

Lymphomatoid granulomatosis is a primarily pulmonary granulomatosis vasculitis that can present a spectrum of disease from benign lymphocytic angiitis and granulomatosis to typical lymphomatoid granulomatosis to a lymphoproliferative malignancy. First described in 1972, lymphomatoid granulomatosis usually presents during the fourth decade of life with a slight male preponderance. Although patients with the benign variant generally do well, many with typical lymphomatoid granulomatosis undergo malignant transformation and, despite

aggressive chemotherapy, have a very poor prognosis. The diffuse pulmonary infiltrates consisting of lymphocytes, histiocytes, and lymphocytoid or plasmacytoid cells with foci of malignant-appearing larger lymphocytes have made difficult the classification of this disease as a collagen-vascular disorder. It is in all probability a neoplastic process.

Clinical

The presenting complaints of patients with lymphomatoid granulomatosis typically include fever, cough, malaise, weight loss, shortness of breath, and chest pain. In addition, cutaneous involvement (erythematous macules or nodules and occasionally ulcerations) (Fig. 69-7), neurologic symptoms (CNS dysfunction, cranial and peripheral neuropathies), arthralgias, myalgias, and gastrointes-

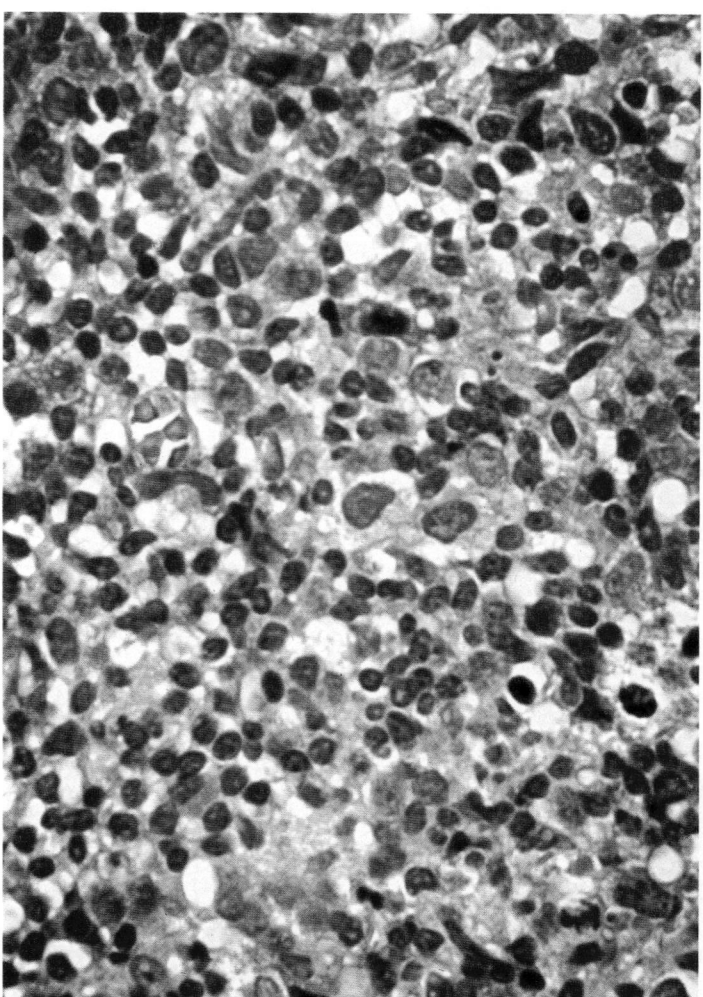

FIGURE 69-7 Lymphomatoid granulomatosis. Nasal biopsy. The nasal mucosa is infiltrated by pleomorphic mononuclear cells. The lungs were involved by an identical process. H&E, ×108. (*Courtesy of Dr. Irving Weiss.*)

tinal complaints are common. Less common findings are splenomegaly, hepatomegaly, lymphadenopathy, and heart, adrenal, or renal involvement.

Laboratory

There are no distinctive laboratory findings. Elevated, normal, and depressed leukocyte counts with lymphocytosis or lymphopenia can be present. Serum immunoglobulin levels are either normal or demonstrate mild, nonspecific polyclonal increases. Anergy is frequently seen. The chest radiograph is characterized by bilateral nodular densities occasionally with cavitation. Diffuse, fluffy alveolar and diffuse reticulonodular infiltrates as well as pleural effusions and rarely hilar adenopathy have been reported.

Pathology

Histologically an angiocentric, angiodestructive inflammatory infiltrate of atypical lymphoreticular cells involving both arteries and veins of lung (100 percent incidence), kidney, liver, brain, spleen, adrenal gland, heart, and lymph nodes (lymphoma) is seen. Distinct granuloma

formation and fibrinoid necrosis are characteristically absent. Malignant lymphoma (histiocytic, immunoblastic sarcoma) is demonstrated during life or at autopsy in possibly as many as 50 percent of patients.

Course

Lymphomatoid granulomatosis is generally a rapidly progressive, lethal disorder. Recently a more favorable outcome has been reported after the early initiation of therapy with corticosteroids and cyclophosphamide. Benign lymphocytic angiitis and granulomatosis is probably a variant characterized by a less aggressive course, paucity of extrapulmonary manifestations, benign histopathologic appearance, and generally favorable response to treatment (chlorambucil or steroids and cyclophosphamide).

BENIGN LYMPHOCYTIC ANGIITIS AND GRANULOMATOSIS

Some clinics distinguish between lymphomatoid granulomatosis and benign lymphocytic angiitis and granulomatosis (Fig. 69-8). Others believe that the two are related,

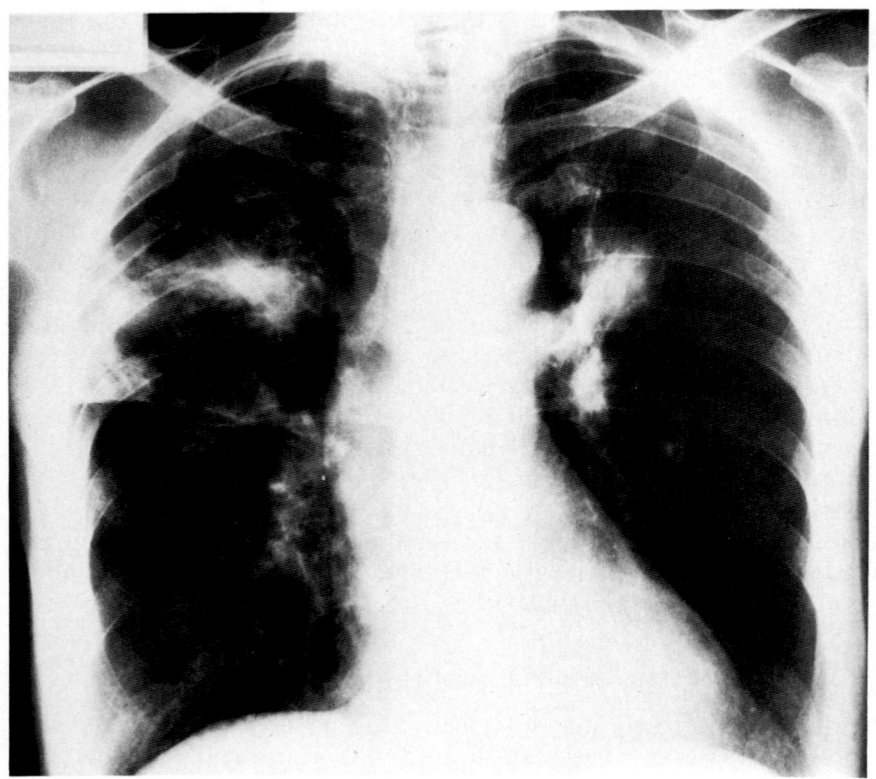
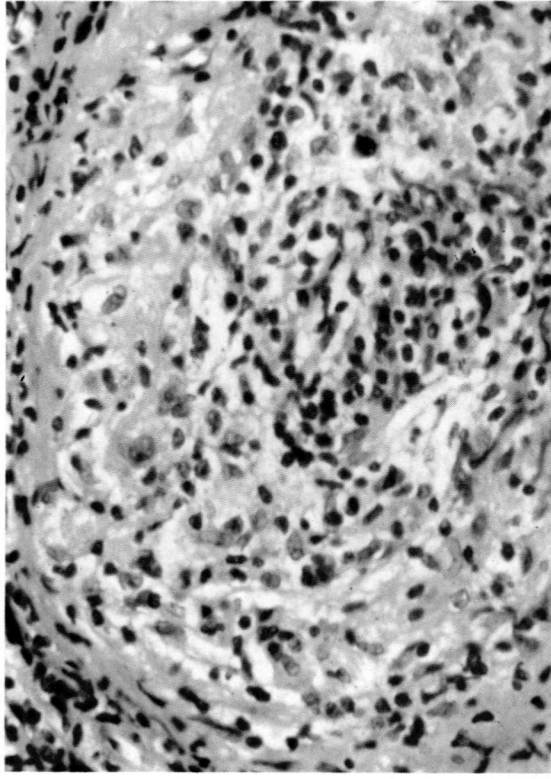

A   *B*

FIGURE 69-8 Lymphocytic angiitis and granulomatosis. *A*. This 70-year-old woman recovered after 6 months of chlorambucil. However, breast cancer developed 3 years later, and she died of metastatic carcinoma of the breast 5 years after this chest radiograph. *B*. Histologic appearance of vascular involvement. The intima of the affected vessel is markedly thickened by an infiltrate of mononuclear cells in which lymphocytes predominate and by beginning fibrosis. The lumen is barely visible. H&E, ×84.5.

the benign lymphocytic angiitis and granulomatosis representing an early form of lymphomatoid granulomatosis. Those who separate the two entities characterize benign lymphocytic angiitis by several criteria: (1) high levels of serum immunoglobulins, particularly of IgE; (2) few extrathoracic manifestations; and (3) responsiveness to a cytotoxic drug, particularly chlorambucil. As a rule, one course of treatment for 6 months has sufficed; occasionally, second courses have been needed.

Although the disorder may resemble pseudolymphoma and angioimmune lymphadenopathy clinically, none of the patients diagnosed as having benign lymphocytic angiitis and granulomatosis have developed a lymphoma. Pathologically, the histologic appearance of lymphomatoid granulomatosis and benign lymphocytic angiitis and granulomatosis are often quite similar. Indeed, the characteristic appearance of each may be visible on the same slide. The clinical findings often tilt the diagnostic balance: in favor of lymphomatoid granulomatosis are cutaneous nodules, neuropathies, and cutaneous anergy; more for benign lymphocytic angiitis and granulomatosis are high levels of immunoglobulins in serum.

MIDLINE GRANULOMA

Midline granuloma is a destructive inflammatory process of upper airways and face. It usually begins in the nose or paranasal sinuses, sometimes in the mouth and rarely in the orbit, and tends to spread through those areas, destroying soft tissues and bone (Fig. 69-6). The disease runs an acute or a chronic course, but is invariably progressive if untreated, and leads to death due to secondary infection, erosion of blood vessels, or involvement of the central nervous system.

Tissue examination shows two or perhaps three patterns. In one, there is intense inflammation and tissue necrosis. Granulomas, sometimes with giant cells, are characteristic, but not always present. Inflammation and thrombosis of blood vessels may be noted. It is usually secondary to the process in the surrounding tissue, but on occasion it represents primary vasculitis. The histologic picture is similar to that of Wegener's granulomatosis and, in some instances, midline granuloma represents an early or a localized form of Wegener's disease. In favor of this interpretation are occasional cases where upper respiratory involvement is associated with crescentic glomerulonephritis, but without evidence of pulmonary disease or systemic vasculitis. Other authors believe that midline granuloma is a distinct entity, a strictly local process. Therapeutically, it responds to high doses of radiation, but rather poorly to steroids and cytotoxic agents. However, the response of upper respiratory lesions of Wegener's granulomatosis to high doses of radiation has not been adequately evaluated.

The second tissue pattern is similar to that of lymphomatoid granulomatosis. This process is often called *polymorphous reticulosis*. The basic disease may be obscured by severe inflammation due to necrosis and secondary infection. If lymphomatoid granulomatosis is simultaneously present in the lung, the diagnosis of the upper respiratory disease becomes easier, but in any biopsy of suspected midline granuloma careful search should be made for malignant looking cells. Some authors sharply separate polymorphous reticulosis from midline granuloma, but the clinical behavior and response of treatment is often similar. Polymorphous reticulosis and lymphomatoid granulomatosis not infrequently progress to a frank malignant lymphoma, which may constitute the third tissue pattern of midline granuloma.

ALLERGIC GRANULOMATOSIS AND ANGIITIS (CHURG-STRAUSS SYNDROME)

Allergic granulomatosis and angiitis is characterized by severe allergy, blood eosinophilia, and multisystemic symptoms, and pathologically by a combination of necrotizing vasculitis and extravascular granulomas. As in Wegener's granulomatosis, the primary site of allergic granulomatosis is the upper and lower respiratory tract. However, unlike Wegener's which usually arises in previously healthy individuals, allergic granulomatosis is almost invariably preceded by asthma and allergic rhinitis, or rarely by sensitization to a drug.

The clinical picture of allergic granulomatosis has been reviewed in detail by Lanham et al. The disease usually begins between the ages of 20 and 40 years, but it also occurs in children and in older persons. Male-to-female ratio is about 1:1. Fever is a common presenting symptom, but it also may be due to eosinophilic pneumonitis which does not necessarily progress to vasculitis. Weight loss, malaise, and weakness are frequent nonspecific manifestations and may be the first indicators of the underlying disease. Splenomegaly, hepatomegaly, and generalized, but usually mild lymphadenopathy are not uncommon.

As in other forms of vasculitis, nearly every organ supplied by systemic circulation may be affected by allergic granulomatosis.

Etiology and Pathogenesis

Asthma and allergic rhinitis usually precede by many years, sometimes 30 or more, but in some patients they appear shortly before or simultaneously with the onset of vasculitis. Asthma begins relatively late in life, around the age of 20 or later, and in individuals who seldom have a family history of allergy. Skin testing reveals sensitivity to various antigens in some but not in all cases. The specific

cause of allergy is generally unknown, although it is sometimes ascribed to infection ("infective asthma"). Some patients are diagnosed as "chronic bronchitis" rather than asthma. In patients who develop allergic granulomatosis, asthma becomes progressively worse with increasing frequency and severity of attacks up to the status asthmaticus. However, surprisingly, in a considerable proportion asthma abates with the onset of vasculitis, only to reappear when vasculitis has been successfully treated.

Allergic granulomatosis occurs only in allergic individuals and, therefore, is presumably due to an antigen-antibody reaction. As is well known, asthma can be induced by a variety of antigens, although the specific offending agent is usually difficult to identify. Increased antibody production may be assumed from the elevation of immunoglobulin levels in the serum, particularly those of IgG and IgE. How an antigen-antibody reaction causes tissue damage is uncertain. One such mechanism may be deposition of immune complexes. Such complexes, containing IgE, were recently demonstrated in the sera but not in the blood vessel walls in five cases of allergic granulomatosis. As an alternative, one may propose a local reaction between the antigen and antibody. Lesions similar to those of allergic granuloma are seen in the tissues around invading parasites such as larva migrans or strongyloides.

Whatever the nature of the immune process, it obviously produces chemotactic substances that attract eosinophils. It is quite possible that eosinophils also contribute to the tissue injury. Fragmentation and necrosis of the eosinophils is accompanied by swelling and eventual destruction of collagen fibers and by development of palisading epithelioid and giant cell granulomas around the necrotic centers. Evidence in support of this concept is provided by cases of Hodgkin's disease where similar palisading granulomas develop in lymph nodes rich in eosinophils.

Although tissue changes in asthma, in eosinophilic inflammation, in granuloma formation, and in necrotizing angiitis are quite different morphologically, they are likely to represent progressive steps of the same process or a combination of processes, that is, antigen-antibody reaction, release of inflammatory mediators, and disintegration of eosinophils. The particular tissue changes express the severity of the underlying immune process and its sequelae, and angiitis is its most striking and most dangerous manifestation.

Clinical

RESPIRATORY TRACT

Pulmonary Manifestations

In addition to asthma, patients with allergic granulomatosis frequently show pulmonary infiltrates accompanied by blood eosinophilia. Such infiltrates wax and wane,

particularly in patients treated with steroids. They precede the onset of vasculitis in at least 75 percent of patients. Radiographically, they are transient and migratory, resembling Loeffler's pneumonia, or persistent, as in chronic eosinophilic pneumonia (Fig. 69-9). Most of the time they are patchy and irregularly distributed, but may be symmetric and peripheral, or on the contrary radiating from the hili. Diffuse infiltrates and miliary or nodular densities also occur. The latter may become confluent and exceptionally break down to form cavities. Hilar lymphadenopathy is sometimes present. Pleural effusion with many eosinophils occurs in perhaps one-third of the cases, but "dry" pleurisy with chest pain or pleural rub is seen on occasion.

Upper Respiratory Tract

Allergic rhinitis accompanies and often precedes asthma in most of the cases. On rare occasions, it is the sole precursor of vasculitis. Nasal obstruction, multiple polyps, and sinusitis are the usual symptoms. Obstruction may be severe enough to require surgical intervention. Radiographic involvement of sinuses can be demonstrated in nearly 90 percent of cases. Before the age of antibiotics, sinus infection by a variety of microorganisms was common; it is seen occasionally even nowadays. A rare patient will have pain and blood discharge and show ulceration of the mucosa and even perforation of the septum, similar to that seen in Wegener's granulomatosis.

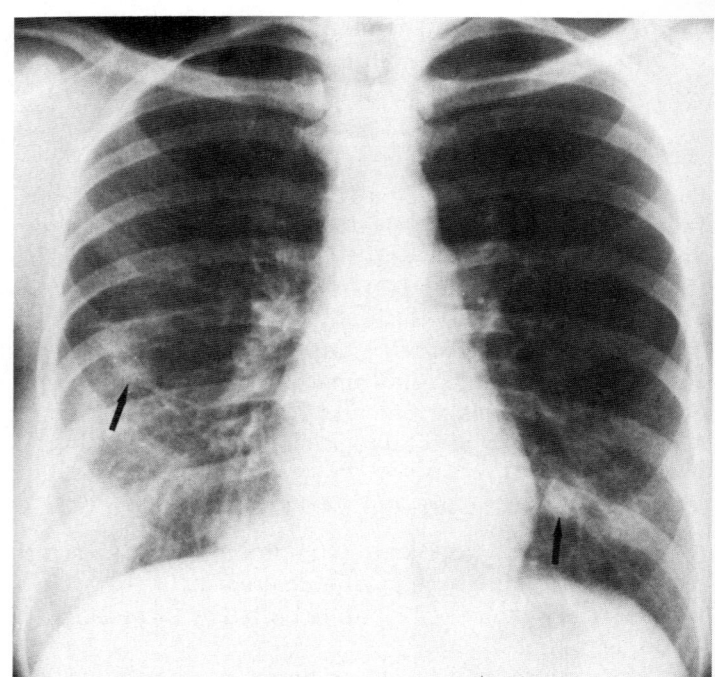

FIGURE 69-9 Churg-Strauss syndrome. Chest radiograph of a 35-year-old woman with recent onset of variegated skin lesions, fever, and arthralgias. Arrows indicate areas of infiltration. Diagnosis established by lung biopsy. (*Courtesy of Dr. W. T. Miller.*)

CARDIOVASCULAR SYSTEM

Involvement of the cardiovascular system is very common and is responsible for serious clinical manifestations. Electrocardiographic abnormalities are found in the majority, and cardiac failure is seen in a considerable proportion of patients. Pericarditis is also common. If left untreated, the congestive failure may become irreversible. Myocardial infarction is a frequent complication of coronary vasculitis. Prognosis is further aggravated by the development of hypertension.

GENITOURINARY SYSTEM

Hematuria, gross or microscopic, and proteinuria are frequent but generally slight or moderate in degree. Nephrotic syndrome is rare and renal failure relatively uncommon. Flank pain usually denotes infarction due to renal vasculitis. Small arterial aneurysms can be demonstrated by angiography of the kidneys and other parenchymal organs (liver, spleen). Vasculitis may contribute to renal failure and also be responsible for the development of hypertension. These manifestations sometimes persist into the postvasculitic phase when most other symptoms have abated. Lower urinary tract involvement, particularly of the ureters and the prostate, occasionally leads to obstruction.

GASTROINTESTINAL TRACT

Involvement of the gastrointestinal tract causes abdominal pain, diarrhea, and hemorrhage. Peritoneal effusion with many eosinophils also occurs. A serious complication is perforation of the bowel with diffuse peritonitis.

NERVOUS SYSTEM

Peripheral neuropathy, mostly mononeuritis simplex, but sometimes symmetric neuritis with sensory and motor disturbances, is a common and diagnostically valuable sign of systemic vasculitis. Cranial nerves, especially the optic nerve, may also be involved. Cerebral manifestations are less common. They vary from nonspecific disorientation, convulsions, or coma to cerebrovascular accidents with paralysis and death, and are caused either by cerebral vasculitis or by hypertension.

JOINTS, MUSCLES, AND CUTANEOUS MANIFESTATIONS

Arthralgias and myalgias are often migratory. True arthritis is rare; it may simulate rheumatoid arthritis. Muscle pain is caused by myositis or more often by local ischemia secondary to vasculitis.

Skin eruptions are very common, ranging from nonspecific macular or papular erythema to urticaria and to palpable purpura; they usually signify involvement of small cutaneous vessels. Deep cutaneous or subcutaneous nodules are less frequent but more diagnostic, since they usually consist of granulomas. The nodules often ulcerate, but ulceration also may be due to skin infarction.

Laboratory

A characteristic feature of allergic granulomatosis is leukocytosis with striking eosinophilia. The eosinophils constitute at least 20 percent of the differential count and sometimes well over 80 percent. In absolute figures, eosinophils exceed 1500 per cubic milliliter and sometimes reach 20,000 or more. However, a single count may miss the peak because of spontaneous wide fluctuations and because of the effect of steroid therapy. Multiple differential counts are essential in such cases. Although in general there is good parallelism between blood eosinophils and the severity of the disease, particularly of eosinophilic pneumonia, granulomas, and vasculitis, exceptions to this rule are not uncommon.

Anemia and high sedimentation rate are frequent, particularly during the vasculitis phase. Serum immunoglobulins IgG and IgE are significantly increased, again during the vasculitis phase, but this phenomenon is nonspecific and is also observed in polyarteritis nodosa and in Wegener's granulomatosis. Immune complexes in the serum and hypocomplementemia are found only occasionally, but rheumatoid factor is moderately elevated in a number of patients.

Pathology

RESPIRATORY TRACT

Lungs
Changes in the lungs precede the development of vasculitis. They are similar to those seen in the asthmatic population and are not necessarily more severe. Characteristically, there is plugging of bronchi by mucus, thickening of bronchial basement membranes, and mucosal inflammation with many eosinophils. Sometimes this inflammation extends into the bronchial wall. Bronchiectases are occasionally seen.

Foci of pneumonitis have a very characteristic structure. The alveoli are filled with and the septa are infiltrated by inflammatory cells, predominantly eosinophils ("eosinophilic pneumonia") (Fig. 69-10). Multinucleated giant cells may be noted in the exudate, and sometimes they are quite numerous. These infiltrates often resolve,

FIGURE 69-10 Allergic granulomatosis and angiitis (Churg-Strauss syndrome). *A.* Eosinophilic pneumonia with foci of early necrosis of the exudate. H&E, ×27. *B.* Edge of a typical granuloma showing necrosis of eosinophils in the center and palisading histiocytes along the periphery *(on left).* H&E, ×90. *C.* Branch of intestinal artery showing fibrinoid necrosis of the wall, surrounded by granulomatous reaction. H&E, ×90. *D.* Branch of pulmonary artery showing fibrinoid necrosis of the wall *(on bottom)*, scanty inflammatory infiltrate with many eosinophils and narrowing of the lumen. H&E, ×90.

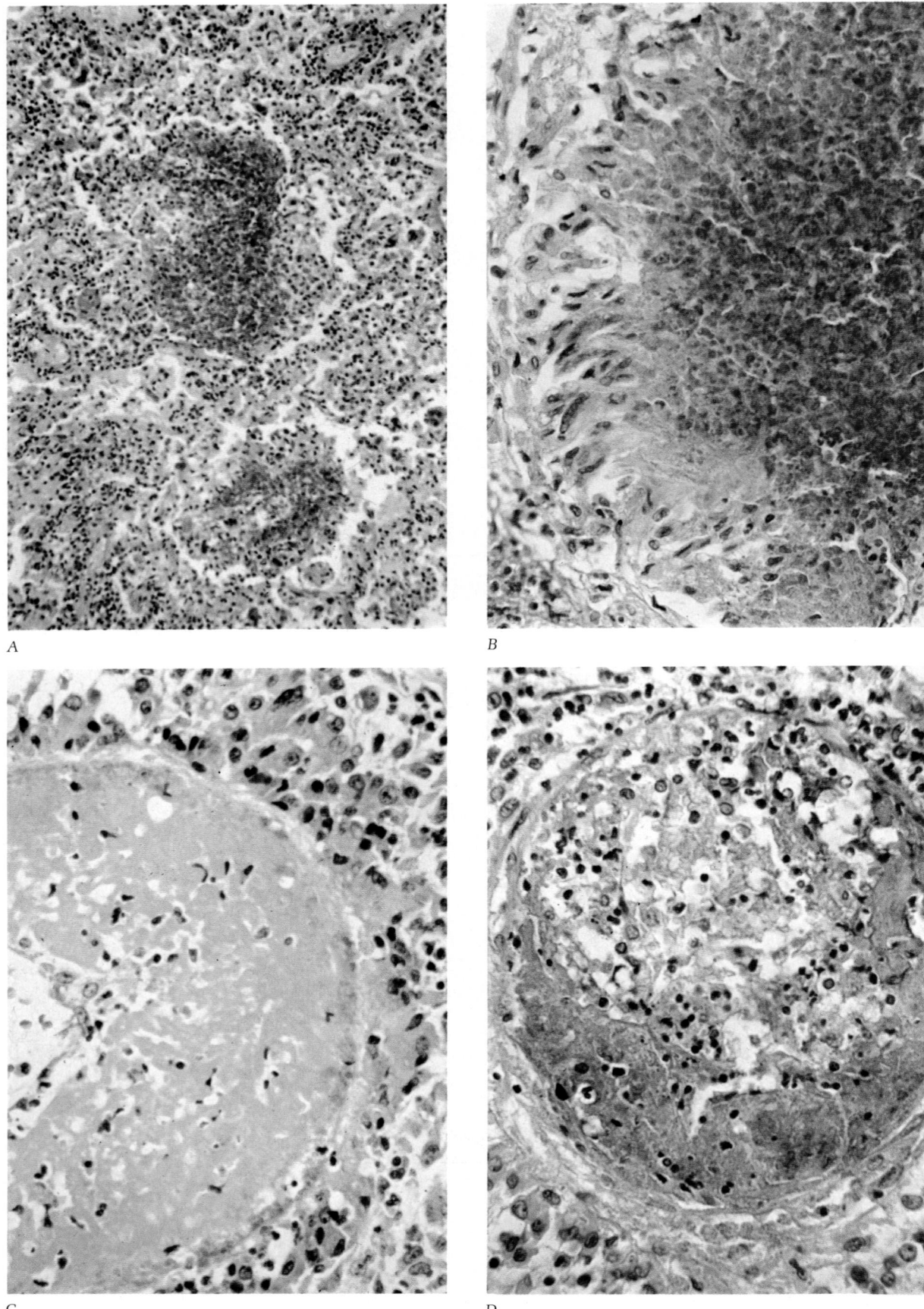

A

B

C

D

but they may persist and progress to granuloma formation. The densely packed eosinophils undergo necrosis with scattering of their granules. The necrosis also involves the parenchymal tissue and leads to disintegration of collagen. Macrophages and giant cells aggregate around the eosinophilic necrotic center and form a palisading layer, one or several cells thick (Fig. 69-10B). The granulomas usually remain small; they evolve, first by clearing of the center of the eosinophilic debris, and occasionally by deposition of calcium, and later by gradual conversion of the cellular periphery into fibrous tissue. Eventually, a nonspecific scar remains, and only the presence of calcification may indicate previous necrosis. Occasionally, active granulomas fuse and form grossly visible nodules. Large aggregates may undergo liquefaction necrosis with formation of cavities, similar to those in Wegener's granulomatosis, but this development is unusual.

Vasculitis may or may not accompany granuloma formation. Vascular lesions are of two types: in the first, granulomas develop in the walls of arteries (Fig. 69-10C) and veins, and lead to local destruction of tissue and necrosis, to narrowing of the lumina or, on the contrary, to aneurysms. Thrombosis is a common complication. The second type of vasculitis resembles polyarteritis nodosa (Fig. 69-10D) showing fibrinoid necrosis and severe inflammation of the wall. The inflammatory exudate usually contains many eosinophils.

Healing of arteritis leads to distortion of the lumina and scarring of the wall with local replacement of the elastic tissue by collagen. Thrombi may or may not recanalize. Healed arteritis can usually be distinguished from arteriosclerosis by the residual defects of the elastic laminae and by their segmental distribution. In most cases of some duration, both active and healing or healed lesions are present simultaneously.

Upper Respiratory Tract

Allergic rhinitis and sinusitis are characterized by edema of the mucosa and loose infiltrates of inflammatory cells with predominance of eosinophils. This is accompanied by the growth of large mucosal "allergic" polyps which consist of markedly edematous connective tissue lined by a single layer of epithelium and containing scattered inflammatory cells, again mostly eosinophils. In a rare case mucosal inflammation, usually granulomatous, is very severe, leading to local ulceration and exceptionally to the destruction of the underlying bone and cartilage of the septum. Vasculitis is seldom seen. Also rare is widespread inflammation of the skin of the nose. Purulent inflammation usually indicates superimposed infection.

NERVOUS SYSTEM

Peripheral neuropathy is usually due to inflammation of the nutrient vessels. Cerebral involvement is also due to vasculitis, which leads to nonspecific symptoms or to psychosis, but may also cause cerebral hemorrhage and

infarction. In other patients, these cerebral accidents are secondary to hypertension. Arthralgias and myalgias usually signify eosinophilic infiltrates or granulomas. Arteritis can occasionally be demonstrated in muscle biopsies. *Cutaneous* arteritis usually involves deeper vessels, but superficial small vessel vasculitis is a common accompaniment of skin eruptions. Cutaneous and subcutaneous nodules represent confluent granulomas.

OTHER ORGANS

Eosinophilic infiltrates, granulomas, and vasculitis can be found in practically every organ system. The heart is often seriously affected by both eosinophilic and granulomatous myocarditis and by coronary arteritis with myocardial infarction. Endocarditis with mural thrombosis is occasionally seen. *Renal* arteritis may lead to infarction and also to hypertension. Small arterial aneurysms are fairly common but are no different from those in other forms of vasculitis. Interstitial granulomas are infrequent, but glomerulonephritis is common. This is usually focal and mild, but on occasion diffuse. Renal failure is uncommon. The *lower urinary tract*, from the renal pelvis to the prostate, is rather frequently affected by eosinophilic inflammation and by granulomas. The diagnosis of allergic granulomatosis can sometimes be established by prostatic biopsy. Eosinophilic infiltrates, granulomas, and vasculitis occur in the gastrointestinal tract, from the stomach to the large intestine. Inflammation may be limited to the mucosa, but more often it involves the entire thickness of the wall. Submucosal infiltrates can produce obstructing masses. Eosinophilic granulomatous appendicitis is a rare complication of allergic granulomatosis. Subserosal infiltrates of the bowel lead to eosinophilic peritonitis. Severe vasculitis causes infarction with perforation and purulent peritonitis.

Therapy and Prognosis

Prior to the introduction of steroids, allergic granulomatosis and angiitis was almost invariably fatal. The leading cause of death was heart disease, followed by cerebral hemorrhage, renal failure, gastrointestinal hemorrhage or perforation, and status asthmaticus. Steroids proved to be remarkably effective, and nowadays survival is the rule rather than an exception.

Essentially, allergic granulomatosis and angiitis is a self-limited process. Cases where the disease "burns itself out" were known in the presteroid era, but the residual damage was usually so severe that the patient's demise followed. Steroids administered early in the course markedly ameliorate the symptoms and the pathologic changes. Therapy should be given in high doses (prednisone 40 to 60 mg per day) for several weeks, until improvement is noted clinically in the cardiac and renal function, peripheral neuropathy, and laboratory indicators (sedimentation rate, white cell count, eosinophilia).

Steroids can be then tapered off gradually, but if symptoms persist or recur, therapy should be extended for a number of months. In a small percentage of cases where steroids prove insufficient, immunosuppressants (cyclophosphamide or azathioprine) should be added, usually with good results. When vasculitis enters the inactive phase (on the average in about 1 year from onset), therapy can be reduced or discontinued, provided no relapses develop. A few patients will run a relapsing course and require retreatment. Asthma and hypertension are the serious residues in the postvasculitic phase and need careful management.

DRUGS, PARASITES, AND FUNGI

A variety of drugs have been associated with the development of eosinophilic pneumonia, among them antibiotics, sulfonamides, hydralazine, and many others. Pulmonary vasculitis seldom develops. Sarcoidlike nodules, necrosis of lung tissue, and fibrinoid necrosis of arteries and arterioles were reported in a patient treated with sulfa drugs, but this patient also had ulcerative colitis (Table 69-1).

Parasites are a fairly frequent cause of eosinophilic pneumonia, particularly in the areas of the world where infestation is frequent and heavy. Larvae of roundworms such as *Ascaris, Ancylostoma, Strongyloides*, and *Toxocara* spend part of their life cycle in the lungs. Pneumonic infiltrates are usually transient, but persistent granulomas similar to allergic granuloma may be seen around the dead larvae (Fig. 69-11A), and pulmonary arteritis is encountered on occasion.

Fungi usually cause nonspecific or granulomatous inflammation, but some noninvasive species, notably *Aspergillus fumigatus* and perhaps also *Candida albicans*, produce an allergic reaction known as allergic pulmonary aspergillosis. The process begins with thick mucous plugs in small bronchi containing fungal hyphae. Eosinophilic infiltrates develop in the surrounding lung tissue and are occasionally accompanied by small granulomas with necrotic, eosinophilic center and peripherally arranged histiocytes (allergic granuloma). Rarely, acute nonnecrotizing vasculitis develops. In very severe cases, the disease progresses to destruction of bronchial wall with spread of intense granulomatous inflammation into the surrounding parenchyma (so-called bronchocentric granuloma) (Fig. 69-11B). Nearby vessels may be involved by direct extension of necrosis and inflammation.

SARCOIDAL ANGIITIS (NODULAR SARCOIDOSIS, NECROTIZING SARCOID GRANULOMATOSIS)

The exact nature of this disease has not been established, but it appears to be related to the more usual forms of sarcoidosis. The presentation is most often with nonspecific pulmonary symptoms, such as cough, chest pain, or shortness of breath, sometimes also fever and weight loss. A fair proportion is asymptomatic, demonstrating only the radiologic findings of nodular lesions, predominantly in the lower lung fields. The nodules occasionally cavitate. Hilar lymphadenopathy is found in the minority of patients, but some have extrapulmonary manifestations such as uveitis. The disease is commonly seen in adults, but occasionally also in children. Women predominate over men by the ratio of 4:1.

Histologically, the nodules consist of conglomerates of sarcoidlike granulomas, which may show necrosis or hyalinization. Individual sarcoid nodules may be seen near the periphery of the conglomerate lesion. Bronchiolar walls are often involved. Arteries and veins are invariably affected by inflammation. Granulomatous nodules (Fig. 69-11C) lie in the adventitia or the media and sometimes extend into the intima, leading to intimal thickening and narrowing or obliteration of the lumina. It should be noted that vascular involvement is also seen in the usual form of sarcoidosis. Nodular granulomatous sarcoidosis responds well to steroid therapy or, if localized, to surgical excision. Prognosis is generally very good.

TAKAYASU'S ARTERITIS

Takayasu's arteritis is a disease of large- and medium-size arteries, such as the aorta and its branches and the pulmonary arteries. Only occasionally does it involve smaller arteries and capillaries.

Clinical

Most of the patients are young women of oriental but also other origins. In more than half the cases, the symptoms appear before the age of 20 years, usually with constitutional acute or chronic manifestations: fever, night sweats, weakness, weight loss, myalgias, and arthralgias. This initial phase may be absent, and the patient is seen in the second phase, referrable to the underlying vascular disease and manifested by decreased arterial blood flow in various regions of the body. This includes blurring of vision or blindness, headaches, fainting, intermittent claudication of arms or legs, absence of pulses, bruit or pain over specific arteries, and Raynaud's phenomenon. Several of these symptoms occur in a specific configuration known as *aortic arch syndrome*. Weakening of the arterial walls predisposes to aneurysms. Hypertension is common and is usually due to renal artery stenosis, to coarctation of aorta, or to loss of elasticity of the arterial walls. Stenosis of pulmonary arteries causes pulmonary hypertension, generally of moderate degree and without pulmonary symptoms, but often with radiologic and electrocardiographic evidence of right heart strain. Cardiac manifestations are mainly due to hypertension, either systemic or

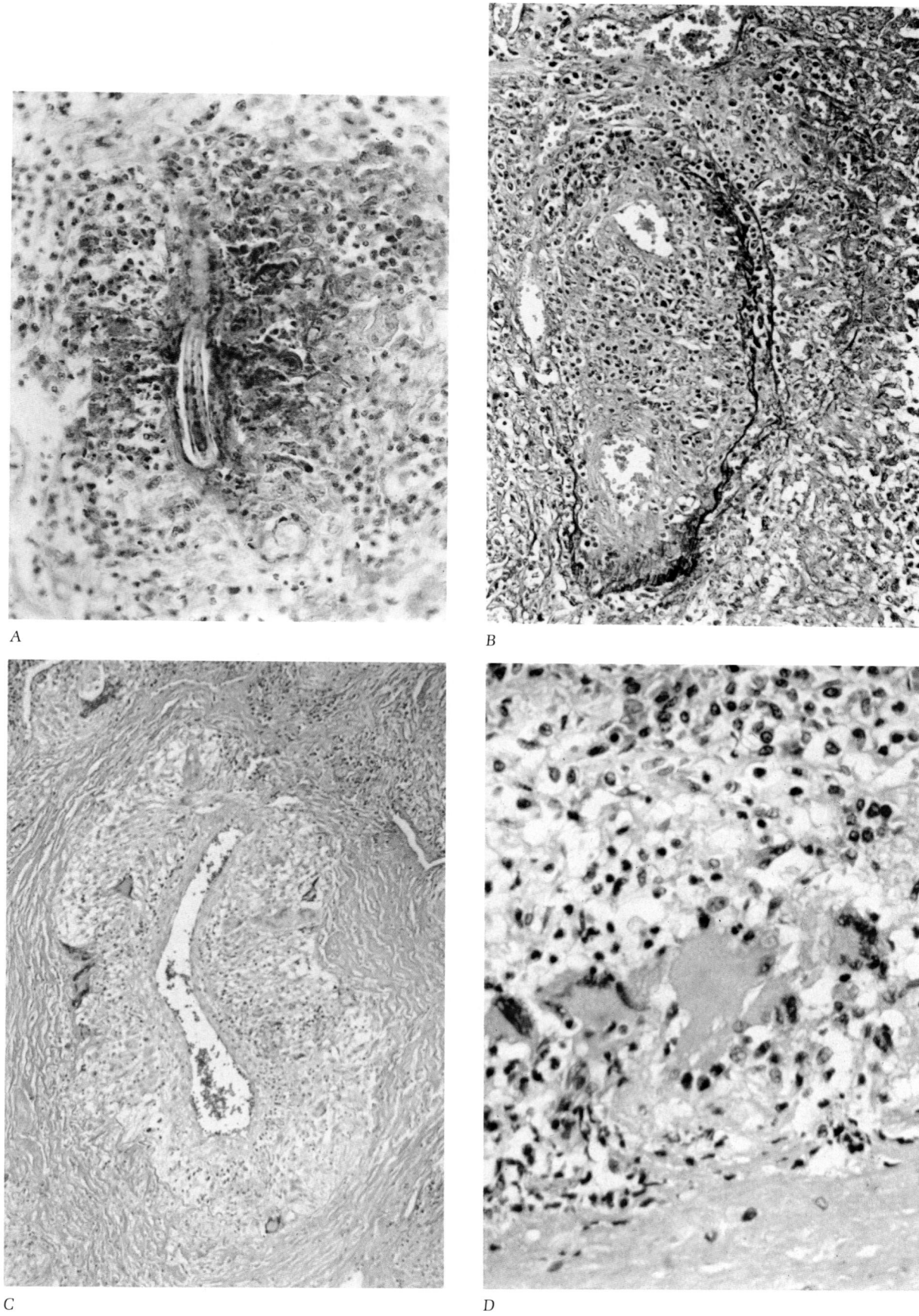

A

B

C

D

pulmonary, leading to left- or right-sided failure. Coronary arteritis with myocardial infarction also occurs. There are suggestions in the literature that Takayasu's arteritis is an autoimmune process, but definite proof is lacking.

Pathology

The characteristic lesion is inflammation of the walls of large arteries. This begins either in the adventitia or in the intima and spreads to involve all three layers. The infiltrate consists of mononuclear cells, lymphocytes, and macrophages, with variable admixture of multinucleated giant cells. Inflammation is succeeded by fibrosis and marked thickening of the intima with progressive narrowing of the lumen and not infrequent thrombosis. Medial involvement leads to fragmentation of the elastics, loss of smooth-muscle fibers, and development of aneurysms. Pathologic changes in small vessels are of a different type, resembling necrotizing arteritis or arteriolitis. Renal glomeruli sometimes show mesangial proliferation or necrotizing inflammation with crescent formation. Mesangiolysis and segmental mesangial sclerosis have also been reported.

Therapy and Prognosis

The inflammatory stage of Takayasu's arteritis apparently responds to steroids in doses of about 30 mg per day, followed by maintenance therapy of 5 to 10 mg per day. Whether this therapy prevents the development of vascular stenosis and other complications is uncertain. More severe and more advanced cases do poorly with or without therapy. Hypertension requires appropriate medication. Vascular surgery, i.e., bypass of the affected arteries, is possible in some cases, e.g., in the coronary circulation where it has been used with some success. On the other hand, bypass of the narrowed renal arteries has been ineffective. The mortality in untreated patients is believed to be on the order of 10 percent, but long-term follow-ups are scanty. The cause of death is most often congestive heart failure, myocardial infarction, renal failure, and cerebrovascular accident. In some cases, the cause of death could not be ascertained even at autopsy.

◄ FIGURE 69-11 Granulomatous inflammatory responses in the lungs. *A.* Allergic type around a larva of *Toxocara.* H&E, ×47. *B.* Bronchocentric granuloma. Severe inflammation of a bronchial wall involving the adjacent small artery which shows partial destruction of the elastic laminae and infiltration of the intima with narrowing of the lumen. Elastica stain, ×32. (*Courtesy of Dr. Andrew Churg.*) *C.* Nodular sarcoidosis. Perivascular sarcoid granuloma involving the vascular wall. H&E, ×21. *D.* Giant cell arteritis. Chronic inflammation with many giant cells in the wall of the aorta. H&E, ×81. (*Courtesy of the Armed Forces Institute of Pathology.*)

GIANT CELL ARTERITIS

Giant cell arteritis is similar to Takayasu's arteritis in certain histologic and clinical aspects but, nevertheless, represents a totally different disease. Giant cell arteritis occurs almost exclusively in elderly individuals, 95 percent of patients being over 65 years of age. Children and young adults are affected very rarely and probably by a separate variant, called juvenile temporal arteritis. There is only slight female predominance.

Clinical

Constitutional symptoms often precede or accompany the development of giant cell arteritis, including fever, night sweats, weakness, anorexia, and fatigue. Sedimentation rate is high. Perhaps half the patients also have polymyalgia rheumatica, characterized by morning stiffness, myalgias, and arthralgias.

The disease affects large arteries, that is the aorta and its branches, rarely the pulmonary arteries, and occasionally also small visceral arteries and capillaries such as glomerular capillaries. Cranial arteries are involved in 50 to 75 percent of cases, causing headaches, blurred vision, and sometimes sudden and generally irrevocable blindness. Tender nodules may be felt along the course of the temporal arteries, or there may be diffuse scalp tenderness, hair loss, erythema, and skin necrosis. Temporal artery pulses are absent. Involvement of the aorta produces the aortic arch syndrome. Pulmonary arteritis seldom gives rise to symptoms. Systemic vasculitis causes myocardial ischemia, gastrointestinal and renal symptoms, and neurologic manifestations which, in severe cases, may simulate polyarteritis nodosa.

Pathology

The typical lesion is granulomatous inflammation with multinucleated giant cells (Fig. 69-11*D*) located in the vascular intima and media, and causing disruption of the elastic membranes, especially the inner elastic lever. The lumen is often thrombosed. In other cases, only nonspecific inflammation is present. Healing leads to bland fibrosis obliterating the lumen. Because the inflammatory lesions are focal in distribution, they may be missed by the biopsy. Visceral arteritis may be of the giant cell type or resemble polyarteritis nodosa. Occasionally, extravascular granulomatous nodules with giant cells are found in the lung and other organs.

Therapy and Prognosis

Giant cell arteritis responds very well to steroid therapy. This should be given as soon as possible in moderately large doses (prednisolone 40 to 50 mg per day) and gradually reduced over a period of weeks or months, depending on the clinical response. Extravascular granulomas also respond. The prognosis is generally good.

SMALL VESSEL VASCULITIS

Small vessel vasculitis is a pathologically defined reaction pattern that has also been termed hypersensitivity vasculitis, leukocytoclastic venulitis, hypersensitivity angiitis, microscopic periarteritis nodosa, allergic angiitis, urticarial vasculitis, and cutaneous vasculitis. This lesion can be the pathologic manifestation of many entities (Table 69-4). Although the hallmark of these syndromes is cutaneous involvement, all have been reported to cause systemic disease.

In 1948 Zeek recognized that the vasculitic syndrome occasionally resulting from the administration of certain drugs or heterologous serum was distinct from the broader clinical entity of periarteritis nodosa described by Kussmaul and Maier in 1866. She termed this syndrome hypersensitivity angiitis. More recently, a classification schema of the vasculitic syndromes was presented by Fauci, including subgroups of hypersensitivity vasculitis. The histopathologic similarities of the clinical syndromes in this large and heterogenous group was emphasized.

Pathogenesis

The lesions of small vessel vasculitis probably result from the host inflammatory response to the local deposition of circulating immune complexes. Various endogenous and exogenous antigens can trigger the host immunologic response. This syndrome is felt to represent the clinical analog of the classic type III hypersensitivity response (immune complex-mediated in the presence of antigen excess, i.e., serum sickness). The acute presentation of a large quantity of antigen, with tissue fixation of antigen,

followed by host antibody production could also lead to localized inflammatory lesions (Arthus' reaction). The presence of circulating immune complexes (by CIq binding, Raji cell, and cryoglobulinemia), hypergammaglobulinemia, and complement consumption, as well as the direct demonstration of complement, immunoglobulin, and occasionally antigen (e.g., hepatitis B surface antigen) in the vascular lesion by immunofluorescence microscopy provides strong evidence for the above hypothesis. The local intradermal injection of histamine in patients with active vasculitis produces a vasculitic lesion at the injection site indistinguishable histologically from the patient's natural lesions. Sequentially biopsying these lesions reveals the very early deposition of immunoglobulins and complement in vessel walls, followed by cellular infiltration. This finding implies the need for a vascular permeability factor, in addition to circulating immune complexes, for the full expression of the clinical syndrome.

In the case of the subgroup of "true" hypersensitivity syndromes (Table 69-4), there is a specific temporal-causal relationship of known antigen exposure and the initiation of vasculitis. The vasculitis in the connective tissue subgroup may be the result of exposure to certain endogenous antigens (e.g., ds DNA, Ro, La, RNP). Malignancies could cause vasculitis by releasing soluble tumor

TABLE 69-4
Small Vessel Vasculitis

"True" hypersensitivity vasculitis
  Classic serum sickness: foreign protein
  Drug reaction: Table 69-5
  Infectious agents: subacute bacterial endocarditis, hepatitis B, rickettsiae, fungi, bacteria (*Streptococcus, Pseudomonas*)
  Chemicals: insecticides, herbicides, petroleum products Foods
Henoch-Schönlein purpura
Mixed cryoglobulinemia: essential, exogenous
Connective tissue disease: rheumatoid arthritis, systemic lupus erythematosus, dermatomyositis, Sjögren's syndrome
Malignancy: lymphoreticular (leukemia, lymphoma, multiple myeloma, carcinoma)
Hypocomplementemia: familial, acquired
Miscellaneous: inflammatory bowel disease, intestinal bypass surgery, primary biliary cirrhosis, chronic active hepatitis (non-B), retroperitoneal fibrosis, Goodpasture's syndrome, α_1-antitrypsin deficiency

TABLE 69-5
Drugs Reported to Cause Small Vessel Vasculitis

Acebutolol	Griseofulvin
Allopurinol	Hydralazine
Ampicillin	Indium
Arsenic	Indomethicin
Aspirin	Isoniazid
Bismuth	Methyldopa
Bromide	Metolazone
Busulfan	Nembutol
Butazolidin	Oxyphenbutazone
Carbamazepine	Paracetamol
Casein	Penicillin
Chloramphenicol	Phenacetin
Chlortetracycline	Phenothiazine
Chlorthalidone	Phenylbutazone
Chlorthiazide	Potassium iodine
Cimetidine	Procainamide
Clindamycin	Propylthiouracil
Coumadin	Quinidine
Cromolyn sodium	Spironolactone
Colchicine	Streptomycin
Dextran	Sulfapyridine
Diphenhydramine	Sulfonamide
Diphenylhydantoin	Tetracycline
Gold	Trimethadione

antigens into the circulation. The etiology of some of the other entities in Table 69-4 is even less clear.

Clinical

The major clinical manifestation of small vessel vasculitis is cutaneous, classically palpable purpura. Other skin lesions include urticaria, vesicles-bullae, papules-petechiae, necrotic ulcerations, subcutaneous nodules, livedo reticularis, and erythema multiforme. Fever, eosinophilia and an elevated sedimentation rate may accompany the lesions. Many patients may manifest only the above findings. A second patient group will manifest the systemic involvement of a generalized vasculitis. These patients usually have involvement of joints, heart, liver, gastrointestinal tract, nervous system, and skeletal muscle. Renal involvement is particularly common in the systemic group, usually with asymptomatic hematuria-proteinuria; however, renal failure can occur. Patients with only cutaneous lesions do not usually progress to systemic involvement. Any of the triggering agents can cause either cutaneous (localized) or systemic (generalized) vasculitis.

Generally, lung involvement is uncommon, consisting of transient diffuse, patchy or nodular infiltrates, pneumonia, and pleural effusions. However, interstitial pneumonitis appears to be common in essential mixed cryoglobulinemia (especially in hepatitis B virus antibody-negative patients). Presenting pulmonary symptoms include asthma, hemoptysis, and pleurisy. Pulmonary function tests and nuclide scans will frequently reveal subtle abnormalities.

Pathology

Vascular lesions involving small arteries, arterioles, capillaries, and especially venules are characteristic. Large and medium vessels are spared. All three vessel layers are involved by a polymorphonuclear leukocytic infiltrate causing leukocytoclasis (presence of nuclear debris), variably accompanied by endothelial swelling and fibrinoid necrosis. A pattern of mononuclear cell infiltration can also be seen, which sometimes represents the end of a spectrum from acute to chronic vasculitis. In addition, a hemorrhagic alveolitis has been described in limited lung biopsy material. Renal involvement can consist of focal or diffuse proliferative or crescentic glomerulonephritis, mesangiocapillary glomerulonephritis, glomerulosclerosis, or focal necrosis.

Therapy and Prognosis

In the cases of "true" hypersensitivity vasculitis, withdrawal of the offending agent, if possible, is the first therapeutic step. Antihistamines or nonsteroidal anti-inflammatory drugs usually control the symptomatology of cutaneous or mild systemic reactions. More severe cuta-

neous manifestations or systemic involvement, especially with renal disease, generally necessitates steroid therapy. Cytotoxic agents and plasmapheresis have been utilized in fulminant cases. Generally, the prognosis of hypersensitivity vasculitis is good, especially those cases limited to cutaneous manifestations; renal involvement has been cited as a more ominous prognostic sign, and pulmonary involvement may also carry serious implications.

OTHER VASCULITIDES

Henoch-Schönlein Purpura

Henoch-Schönlein purpura is characterized by disseminated small vessel vasculitis of leukocytoclastic type, involving most often the skin, kidneys, and gastrointestinal tract. Fibrinoid necrosis of the vascular wall and thrombosis are frequent. Pulmonary involvement is relatively rare, on the order of 5 percent of patients, mainly adults.

The disease often follows upper respiratory infection. A specific microorganism has not been definitely identified, although β-hemolytic *Streptococcus* has been suspected in the past. Skin lesions consist of "palpable" purpura, but platelet counts are normal. Similar lesions probably occur in the gastrointestinal tract leading to melena. Renal manifestations are due to focal or diffuse glomerulonephritis with hematuria and proteinuria. A characteristic feature is glomerular deposits of IgA immunoglobulin and complement (C3) in the mesangium and sometimes also along the capillary walls; other immunoglobulins (IgG, IgM) may be present in lesser amounts. Pulmonary involvement causes hemoptysis and pleuritic pain and ill-defined infiltrates on radiographs. Most of the symptoms resolve spontaneously, but glomerulonephritis may end in chronic renal failure.

Cryoglobulinemic Vasculitis

Cryoglobulinemia refers to the presence in the serum of immune globulins which precipitate in the cold. This property is sometimes associated also with other types of blood proteins, normal, e.g., fibrinogen (cryofibrinogen), or abnormal, e.g., cold precipitable light chains. Cryoglobulins are divided into several classes: monoclonal (type I), polyclonal (type III), or mixed (type II).

The most common combination is that of monoclonal IgM with rheumatoid factor activity and polyclonal IgG, which behaves like antibody to the monoclonal protein. The latter may be IgA or IgG instead of IgM. Vasculitis is most often seen in cases of mixed cryoglobulinemia, either essential or associated with hepatitis B, and perhaps also with other diseases.

The usual clinical presentation of cryoglobulinemia is purpuric rash, especially on the lower extremities, arthralgias, lymphadenopathy, hepatosplenomegaly, and

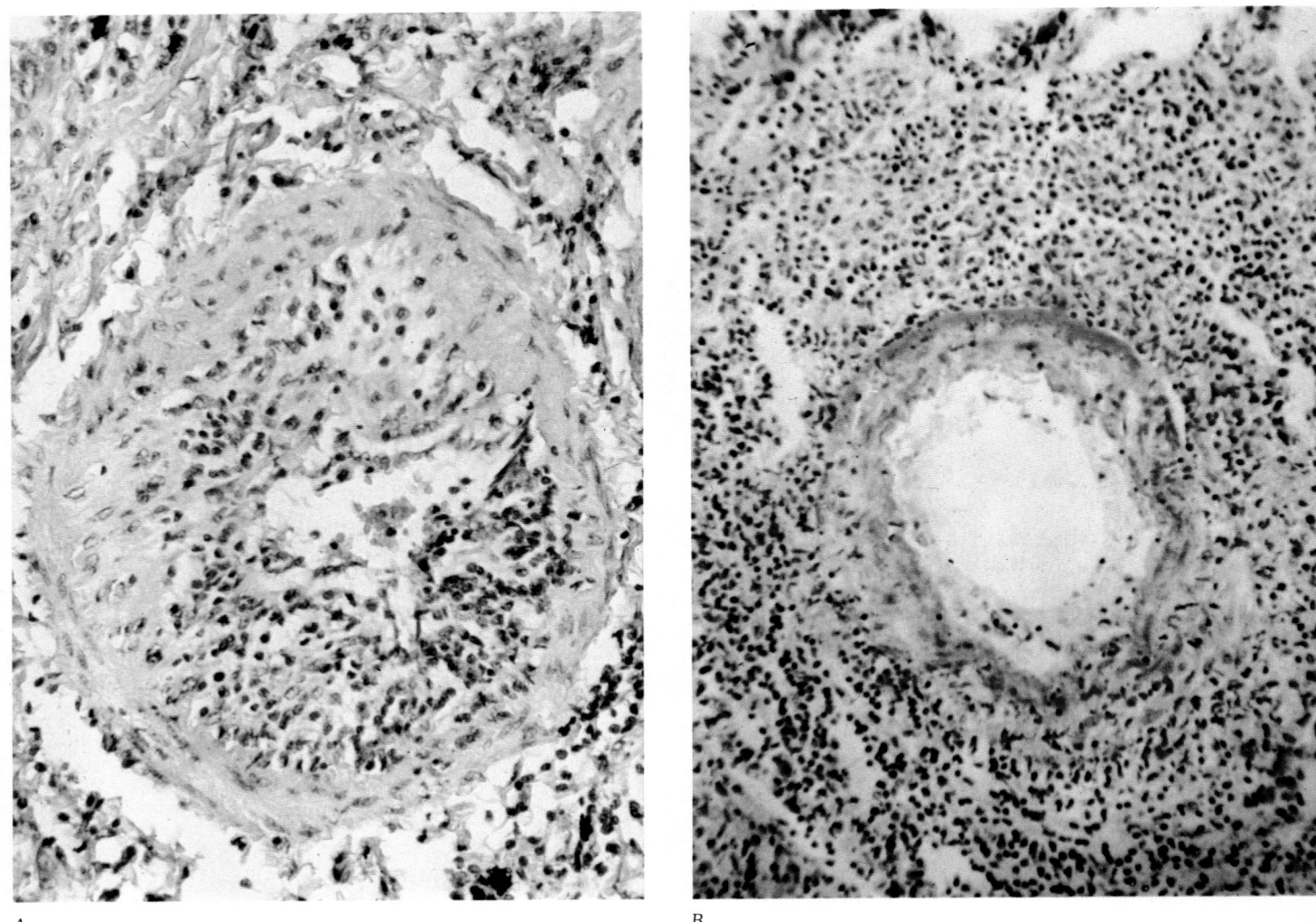

A   B

FIGURE 69-12 Vasculitis in pulmonary disease. A. Pulmonary tuberculosis. A small artery showing chronic inflammation of the intima with narrowing of the lumen. H&E, ×46. *(Courtesy of Dr. Andrew Churg).* B. Pulmonary hypertension. A streak of fibrinoid necrosis in the wall of a small pulmonary artery *(top)*. H&E, ×29.

little or no inflammation. Disruption of such a vessel can cause a massive hemorrhage, although such hemorrhage may also be caused by capillaritis. Treatment includes corticosteroids and cytotoxic agents, with variable success. Diffuse interstitial disease with restrictive findings on pulmonary function testing has also been reported. In some cases, it is caused by healed vasculitis or by progressive intimal sclerosis.

Patients with rheumatoid arthritis who have pleuropulmonary involvement generally have significantly positive tests for rheumatoid factor and evidence of systemic disease; occasionally, other clinical manifestations of rheumatoid arthritis may be absent. Although frequently asymptomatic, the most common lung manifestation of rheumatoid arthritis is pleurisy with or without effusion. Pulmonary nodules, occasionally cavitating, are fre-

quently accompanied by subcutaneous nodules. Diffuse interstitial lung disease (Fig. 69-13) causes pulmonary function abnormalities in approximately one-third of patients with rheumatoid arthritis, although about one-half of those patients have normal chest radiographs. Pulmonary hypertension with or without other pulmonary manifestations has also been reported. This is usually caused by vasculitis, especially of small- and medium-size arteries (Fig. 69-13B). In the acute phase, this arteritis resembles polyarteritis nodosa; in the chronic phase, inflammation is replaced by fibrosis, but occasionally there is a suggestion of a granulomatous process. Corticosteroids and cytotoxic agents may be of benefit in the treatment of pulmonary manifestations.

Pulmonary involvement in progressive systemic sclerosis is virtually universal, and its severity is one of the

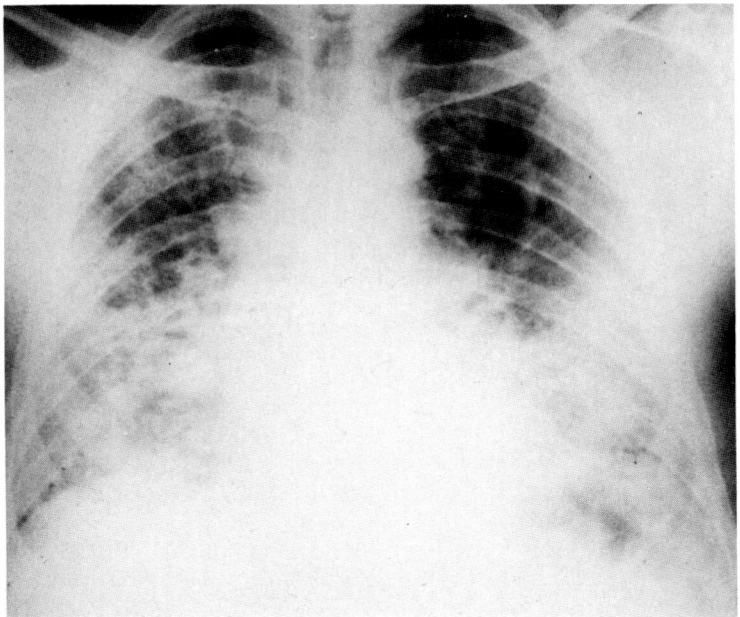

A

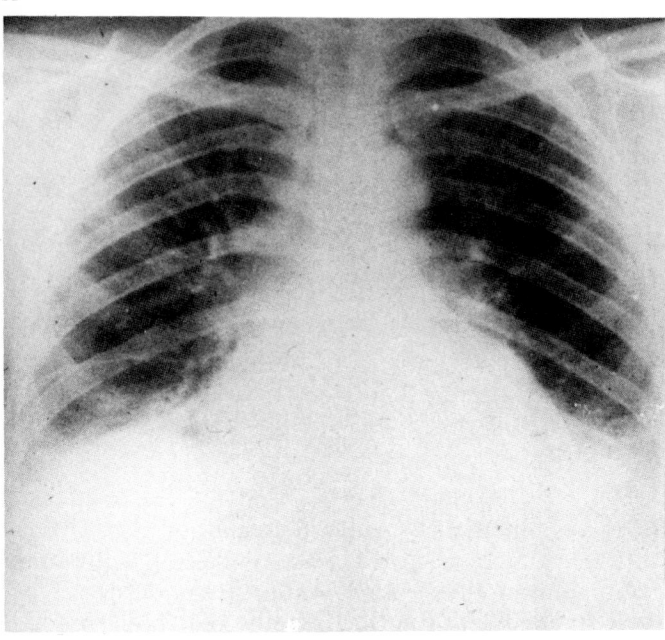

C

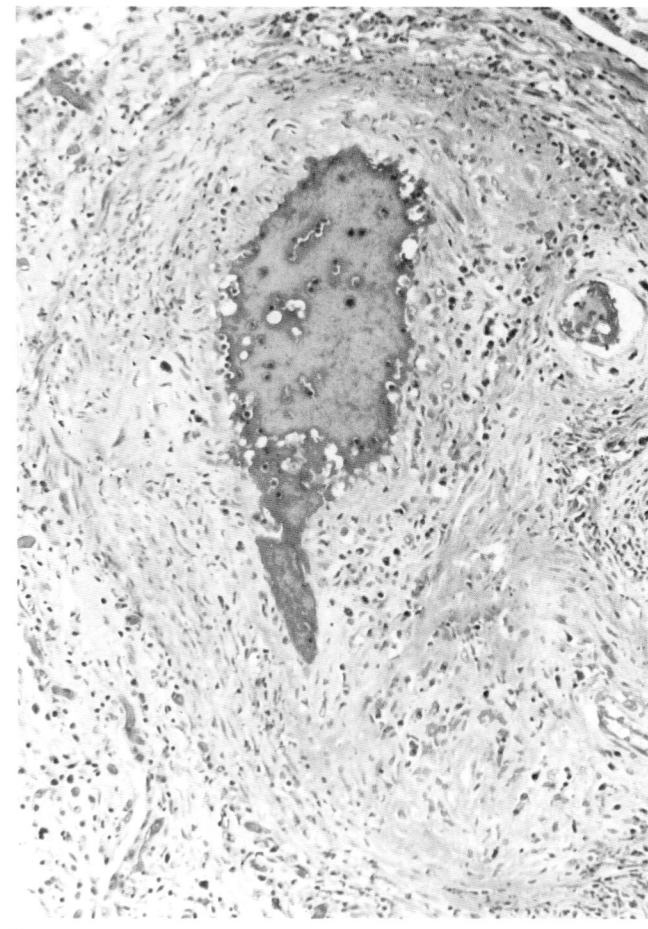

B

FIGURE 69-13 Vasculitis in connective tissue disease. A. Rheumatoid arthritis. Bilateral confluent densities, largely confined to the lower lung fields. There are also rounded nodular densities in the right paracardiac region, right infraclavicular region, and left mid-lung. *(Courtesy of Dr. Alvin S. Teirstein)* B. Rheumatoid arthritis. Small pulmonary artery with chronic inflammation, mainly involving the intima. H&E, ×40. *(Courtesy of Dr. Andrew Churg.)* C. Progressive systemic sclerosis. Bilateral interstitial infiltrates confined to the lower lung fields. Bilateral small pleural effusions. Enlarged cardiac transverse diameter. *(Courtesy of Dr. Alvin S. Teirstein.)*

chief determinants of survival. Diffusion impairment and restrictive lung disease are typical findings. Right ventricular failure can occur secondary to pulmonary hypertension. Chest radiographs may be normal or demonstrate a diffuse reticulonodular interstitial pattern (Fig. 69-13C). Diffuse interstitial fibrosis along with small vessel sclerosis and intimal proliferation are characteristic, but occasionally fibrinoid necrosis is found in the vascular wall. There is no proven effective therapy.

Interstitial lung disease has been described in patients with polymyositis-dermatomyositis, Sjögren's syndrome, and mixed connective tissue disease. In addition, lymphoid interstitial disease presenting a spectrum from benign to malignant lymphoproliferation can be rarely seen in patients with Sjögren's syndrome. Pulmonary hypertension has been noted on occasion in mixed connective tissue disease.

BIBLIOGRAPHY

Albelda SM, Gefter WB, Epstein DM, Miller WT: Diffuse pulmonary hemorrhage: A review and classification. Radiology 154:289–297, 1985.
  A review of the clinical and radiographic features of diffuse pulmonary hemorrhage accompanied by a classification of diseases known to be complicated by pulmonary hemorrhage.

Case records of the Massachusetts General Hospital, Case 31—1986: N Engl J Med 315:378–386, 1986.
  An up-to-date approach to the therapy of Wegener's granulomatosis.

Cupps TR, Fauci AS: The Vasculitides. Philadelphia, Saunders, 1981.
  Comprehensive monograph that is an expansion of the article by Fauci et al., 1978, exploring all aspects of the postulated pathophysiology, classification, characteristics, and treatment of the systemic necrotizing vasculitides.

Fauci AS, Haynes BF, Katz P: The spectrum of vasculitis: Clinical, pathologic, immunologic, and therapeutic considerations. Ann Intern Med 89:660–676, 1978.
  Review of the pathophysiology and immunologic mechanisms of the vasculitides, presentation of a classification schema, and description of recent treatment advances.

Leatherman JW, Davies SF, Hoidal JR: Alveolar hemorrhage syndromes: Diffuse microvascular lung hemorrhage in immune and idiopathic disorders. Medicine 63:343–361, 1984.
  A view of pulmonary vasculitis from the perspective of the various causes of pulmonary hemorrhage.

Leavitt RY, Fauci AS: Pulmonary vasculitis. Am Rev Respir Dis 134:149–166, 1986.
  A review of the immunopathogenic, clinical, and therapeutic features of the pulmonary vasculitides. Combination therapy using cyclophosphamide and corticosteroids is generally effective with a 5-year survival rate of about 90 percent.

McCluskey RT, Fienberg R: Vasculitis in primary vasculitides, granulomatoses, and connective tissue diseases. Hum Pathol 14:305–315, 1983.
  Reviews the problems with the classification and diagnosis of the vasculitides, discussing the pathogenetic importance of immune complexes. Despite the rare identification of the causative antigens (e.g., hepatitis B), in most cases the etiology is unknown.

Rankin JA, Matthay A: Pulmonary renal syndromes. II. Etiology and pathogenesis. Yale J Biol Med 55:11–26, 1982.
  Reviews the classic mechanisms of immune hypersensitivity reactions in relation to pulmonary vasculitides, concluding that the available evidence favors an immune complex and/or cell-mediated etiology.

Rose GA, Spencer H: Polyarteritis nodosa. Q J Med 26:43–81, 1957.
  A large review drawing an important distinction between polyarteritis nodosa with and without pulmonary involvement.

Zeek PM: Periarteritis nodosa: A critical review. Am J Clin Pathol 22:777–790, 1952.
  Historical review of the concept of periarteritis nodosa and a proposal for classification of the various forms of necrotizing angiitis (vasculitis). Includes "hypersensitivity angiitis" resulting from the administration of certain drugs or heterologous serum and characterized by lesions of small vessels only.

Wegener's Granulomatosis

Amin R: Endobronchial involvement in Wegener's granulomatosis. Postgrad Med J 59:452–454, 1983.
  Description of endobronchial involvement with Wegener's granulomatosis presenting with atelectasis and lobar collapse.

Appel GB, Gee B, Kashgarian M, Hayslett JP: Wegener's granulomatosis—Clinical-pathologic correlations and long-term course. Am J Kidney Dis 1:27–37, 1981.
  Presentation of clinical experience emphasizing renal involvement. Renal biopsy findings mostly confirmatory but not specific for Wegener's granulomatosis. Two thirds of lung biopsies were pathognomonic.

Bullen CL, Liesegang TJ, McDonald TJ, DeRemee RA: Ocular complications of Wegener's granulomatosis. Ophthalmology 90:279–290, 1983.
  Description of the ocular manifestations of Wegener's granulomatosis, most commonly orbital inflammation.

Carrington CB, Liebow A: Limited forms of angiitis and granulomatosis of Wegener's type. Am J Med 41:497–527, 1966.
Defines the specific syndrome of limited Wegener's granulomatosis, i.e., no renal involvement. Generally good prognosis with steroid therapy.

De Remee RA, McDonald TJ, Weiland LH: Wegener's granulomatosis: Observations on treatment with antimicrobial agents. Mayo Clin Proc 60:27–32, 1985.
Report on the beneficial effect of antimicrobial agents, chiefly trimethoprim-sulfamethoxazole, in 11 out of 12 cases of Wegener's granulomatosis. In two of the cases the disease was arrested with these agents alone.

Fahey JL, Leonard E, Churg J, Godman G: Wegener's granulomatosis. Am J Med 17:168–179, 1954.
Defines the clinical features of Wegener's granulomatosis—upper and lower respiratory tract and renal involvement, and systemic manifestations.

Fauci AS, Haynes BF, Katz P, Wolff SM: Wegener's granulomatosis: Prospective clinical and therapeutic experience with 85 patients for 21 years. Ann Intern Med 98:76–85, 1983.
Analysis of an extensive patient experience with long-term follow-up. Emphasizes the more recent improved prognosis with steroid-cyclophosphamide therapy.

Gephardt GN, Ahmad M, Tubbs RR: Pulmonary vasculitis (Wegener's granulomatosis). Immunohistochemical study of T and B cell markers. Am J Med 74:700–704, 1983.
Immunoperoxidase staining of the vascular lymphoid infiltrates from lung biopsies of patients with Wegener's granulomatosis demonstrating predominantly T cells and monocytes without identification of immunoglobulin or complement deposition. Provides evidence in favor of a cellular immune mechanism for the disease.

Godman GC, Churg J: Wegener's granulomatosis. Pathology and review of the literature. Arch Pathol 58:533–553, 1954.
Defines the pathologic features of Wegener's granulomatosis—necrotizing granulomatous lesions of the upper and lower respiratory tract, necrotizing systemic vasculitis, and necrotizing glomerulitis.

Haynes BF, Fishman ML, Fauci AS, Wolff SM: The ocular manifestations of Wegener's granulomatosis. Fifteen years experience and review of the literature. Am J Med 63:131–141, 1977.
Description of ocular involvement with Wegener's granulomatosis demonstrating the efficacy of steroid therapy.

Hellmann D, Laing T, Petri M, Jacobs D, Crumley R, Stulbarg M: Wegener's granulomatosis: isolated involvement of the trachea and larynx. Ann Rheum Dis 46:628–631, 1987.
A 26-year-old man with subacute hoarseness and stridor was shown to have Wegener's granulomatosis confined to the trachea and larynx.

Hu CH, O'Loughlin S, Winkelman RK: Cutaneous manifestations of Wegener's granulomatosis. Arch Dermatol 113:175–182, 1977.
Description of the dermatologic manifestations of Wegener's granulomatosis, typically purpuric lesions occasionally with ulceration.

Hui AN, Ehresmann GR, Quismorio FP Jr, Boylen CT, Mayberg H, Koss MN: Wegener's granulomatosis. Electron microscopic and immunofluorescent studies. Chest 80:753–756, 1981.
Describes the presence of granular immunoglobulin deposits in some alveolar walls, although no deposits were seen in electron micrographs.

Jordan JM, Rowe WT, Allen NB: Wegener's granulomatosis involving the breast. Report of three cases and review of the literature. Am J Med 83:159–164, 1987.
Three cases of Wegener's granulomatosis involving the breast are described. In each, the presumed diagnosis was localized or metastatic carcinoma.

Kornblut AD, Wolff SM, Fauci AS: Ear disease in patients with Wegener's granulomatosis. Laryngoscope 92:713–717, 1982.
Describes the otologic manifestations of Wegener's granulomatosis, which is mostly recurrent, or persistent serous otitis media.

Lockwood CM, Bakes D, Jones S, Whitaker KB, Moss DW, Savage CO: Association of alkaline phosphatase with an autoantigen recognised by antibodies in systemic vasculitis. Lancet 1:716–720, 1987.
Confirms the significance of autoantibodies against neutrophils and monocytes in systemic vasculitis, including Wegener's granulomatosis.

Macfarlane DG, Bourne JT, Dieppe PA, Easty DL: Indolent Wegener's granulomatosis. Ann Rheum Dis 42:398–407, 1983.
 Emphasizes the occasional indolent nature of Wegener's granulomatosis with many patients surviving more than 4 years without specific therapy.

Maguire R, Fauci AS, Doppman JL, Wolff SM: Unusual radiographic features of Wegener's granulomatosis. AJR 130:233–238, 1978.
 Catalogs a number of unusual respiratory tract manifestations of Wegener's granulomatosis and redescribes the typical multiple pulmonary nodular infiltrates with a tendency toward cavitation.

McDonald TJ, DeRemee RA, Kern EB, Harrison EG Jr: Nasal manifestations of Wegener's granulomatosis. Laryngoscope 84:2101–2112, 1974.
 Presentation of rhinologic involvement with Wegener's granulomatosis describing the characteristic "saddle nose" deformity.

Ronco P, Verroust P, Mignon F, Lourilsky O, Vanhille P, Meyrier A, Mery JP, Morel-Maroger L: Immunopathological studies of polyarteritis nodosa and Wegener's granulomatosis: A report of 43 patients with 51 renal biopsies. Q J Med 52:212–223, 1983.
 Presentation of immunologic parameters in polyarteritis nodosa and Wegener's granulomatosis including circulating immune complexes, immunofluorescence findings on renal biopsy, complement profile, and hepatitis B status. Notable is the general paucity of specific immunologic abnormalities.

Shasby DM, Schwarz MI, Forstot JZ, Theofilopoulos AN, Kassan SS: Pulmonary immune complex deposition in Wegener's granulomatosis. Chest 81:338–340, 1982.
 Describes immunofluorescence findings suggesting the presence of immune complexes in the pulmonary lesions of Wegener's granulomatosis.

Van Der Woude FJ, Rasmussen N, Lobatto S, Wiik A, Permin H, Van Es LA, Van Der Giessen M, Van Der Hem GK, The TH: Autoantibodies against neutrophils and monocytes: Tool for diagnosis and marker of disease activity in Wegener's granulomatosis. Lancet 1:425–429, 1985.
 Describes the occurrence and the nature of anticytoplasmic autoantibodies against neutrophils and monocytes and details their diagnostic and prognostic value.

Woodworth TG, Abuelo JG, Austin HA III, Esparza A: Severe glomerulonephritis with late emergence of classic Wegener's granulomatosis. Report of 4 cases and review of the literature. Medicine (Baltimore) 66:181–191, 1987.
 A review of an unusual group of 19 patients (15 previously reported) with Wegener's granulomatosis, who presented with severe glomerulonephritis and developed diagnostic respiratory lesions only after 4 to 78 months.

Yoshikawa U, Watanabe T: Pulmonary lesions in Wegener's granulomatosis: A clinicopathologic study of 22 autopsy cases. Hum Pathol 17:401–410, 1986.
 Divides pulmonary lesions into four types: (1) fulminant, with very poor prognosis; (2) classic granulomatous; (3) fibrous scar-type scarring or partial healing; and (4) mixed type. The pulmonary changes in type (1) and type (3) correlate well with similar changes in the systemic circulation and in the renal glomeruli.

Lymphomatoid Granulomatosis and Midline Granulomatosis

Cooke CT, Matz LR, Armstrong JA, Pinerua RF: Asbestos related interstitial pneumonitis associated with glomerulonephritis and lymphomatoid granulomatosis. Pathology 18:352–356, 1986.
 A report of a patient with pulmonary asbestosis who also developed glomerulonephritis and lymphomatoid granulomatosis.

Costa J, Delacretaz F: The midline granuloma syndrome. Pathol Annu 21:159–171, 1986.
 The authors propose a classification (and terminology) that divides the entities previously grouped under "midline granuloma" into four main categories: Wegener's granulomatosis, idiopathic midline destructive disease, lymphomatoid granulomatosis, and angiocentric lymphoma.

DeRemee RA, Weiland LH, McDonald TL: Polymorphic reticulosis, lymphomatoid granulomatosis. Two diseases or one? Mayo Clin Proc 53:634–643, 1978.
 Discussion of two forms of midline granuloma.

Israel HL: Pulmonary angiitis and granulomatosis, in Fishman AP (ed), *Update: Pulmonary Diseases and Disorders.* New York, McGraw-Hill, 1982, pp 243–255.
 A personal perspective by a seasoned expert on distinctions within this category of diseases.

Israel HL, Patchefsky AS, Saldana MJ: Wegener's granulomatosis, lymphomatoid granulomatosis, and benign lymphocytic angiitis and granulomatosis of lung. Recognition and treatment. Ann Intern Med 87:691–699, 1977.
  Utilizing clinical and immunologic assessment, the three syndromes of pulmonary angiitis and granulomatosis are distinguished. Treatment regimens are presented.

Koss MN, Hochholzer L, Langloss JM, Wehunt WD, Lazarus AA, Nichols PW: Lymphomatoid granulomatosis: a clinicopathologic study of 42 patients. Pathology 18:283–288, 1986.
  A study of the histological and clinicopathological findings in 42 patients who had lymphomatoid granulomatosis (LYG).

Liebow AA, Carrington CB, Friedman PJ: Lymphomatoid granulomatosis. Hum Pathol 3:457–558, 1972.
  Description of the distinct lymphoproliferative disease, lymphomatoid granulomatosis. Although patients are improved with steroids, the general prognosis is poor.

Tsokos M, Fauci AS, Costa J: Idiopathic midline destructive disease (IMDD). A subgroup of patients with the "midline granuloma syndrome." Am J Clin Pathol 77:162–168, 1982.
  A proposal to separate idiopathic midlife granuloma from Wegener's granulomatosis.

Allergic Granulomatosis and Angiitis (Churg-Strauss Syndrome)

Brill R, Churg J, Beaver DC: Allergic granulomatosis associated with visceral larva migrans. Am J Clin Pathol 23:1208–1215, 1953.
  Case report of allergic granulomas around parasitic larvae in the lung.

Case records of the Massachusetts General Hospital, Case 30—1986: N Engl J Med 315:308–314, 1986.
  The discussion illustrates the difficulties in distinguishing between "allergic granulomatosis" described by Churg and Strauss and other vasculitides.

Churg J, Strauss L: Allergic granulomatosis, allergic angiitis and periarteritis nodosa. Am J Pathol 27:277–302, 1951.
  Original description of allergic granulomatosis and angiitis.

Clutterbuck EJ, Pusey CD: Severe alveolar haemorrhage in Churg-Strauss syndrome. Eur J Respir Dis 71:158–163, 1987.
  A report of two patients with Churg-Strauss syndrome who presented with life-threatening alveolar hemorrhage as the major manifestation of their disease. One improved on high doses of steroids and cyclophosphamide; the other deteriorated on prednisolone alone, but responded rapidly to the addition of cyclophosphamide and plasma exchange.

Gaffey CM, Chun B, Harvey JC, Manz HJ: Phenytoin-induced systemic granulomatous vasculitis. Arch Pathol Lab Med 110:131–135, 1986.
  Case report of allergic granulomalike lesions induced by sensitization to a drug.

Lanham JG, Elkon KB, Pusey CD, Hughes GR: Systemic vasculitis with asthma and eosinophilia: A clinical approach to the Churg-Strauss syndrome. Medicine (Baltimore) 63:65–81, 1984.
  Extensive review of the clinical features of allergic granulomatosis.

MacFadyen R, Tron V, Keshmiri M, Road JD: Allergic angiitis of Churg and Strauss syndrome. Response to pulse methylprednisolone. Chest 91:629–631, 1987.
  Report of a dramatic improvement in a steroid-dependent asthma patient with biopsy-proven allergic pulmonary angiitis in response to pulsed injections of methylprednisolone intravenously.

Manger BJ, Kraph FE, Gramatzki M, Nusslein HG, Burmester GR, Krauledat PB, Kalden JR: IgE-containing circulating immune complexes in Churg-Strauss vasculitis. Scand J Immunol 21:369–373, 1985.
  Immune complexes of small molecular size and containing IgE were present in the sera of five patients with allergic granulomatosis. Sera in several other types of allergic diseases contained no immune complexes despite a high level of IgE.

Olsen KD, Neel HB, DeRemee RA, Weiland LH: Nasal manifestations of allergic granulomatosis and angiitis (Churg-Strauss syndrome). Otolaryngol Head Neck Surg 88:85–89, 1980.
  Study of upper respiratory disease in allergic granulomatosis.

Strauss L, Churg J, Zak FG: Cutaneous lesions of allergic granulomatosis. J Invest Dermatol 17:349–359, 1951.
  Detailed study of cutaneous lesions in allergic granulomatosis and of their diagnostic significance. Includes a case where allergic granulomatosis followed drug sensitization rather than asthma.

Vasculitis in Eosinophilic Pneumonia

Katzenstein A-L, Liębow AA, Friedman PJ: Bronchocentric granulomatosis, mucoid impaction, and hypersensitivity reactions to fungi. Am Rev Respir Dis 111:497–537, 1975.
  Detailed review.

Liebow AA, Carrington CB: The eosinophilic pneumonias. Medicine 48:251–285, 1969.
  A thorough, by now classic review of eosinophilic pneumonias and their relation to pulmonary allergic reactions.

Sarcoidal Angiitis

Churg A: Pulmonary angiitis and granulomatosis revisited. Hum Pathol 14:868–883, 1983.
  Update of the article by Liebow and reconsideration of the specific identity of granulomatous and vascular diseases.

Liebow AA: Pulmonary angiitis and granulomatosis. Am Rev Respir Dis 108:1–18, 1973.
  Review of several pulmonary diseases characterized by noninfectious granulomatous inflammation and necrotizing vasculitis.

Takayasu's Arteritis and Giant Cell Arteritis

Bradley JD, Pinals RS, Blumenfeld HB, Poston WM: Giant cell arteritis with pulmonary nodules. Am J Med 77:135–140, 1984.
  Case report of giant cell (temporal) arteritis and simultaneous granulomatous giant cell inflammation in the lung.

Halon DA, Turgeman Y, Merdler A, Hardoff R, Sharir T: Coronary artery to bronchial artery anastomosis in Takayasu's arteritis. Cardiology 74:387–391, 1987.
  In a 27-year-old woman with Takayasu's arteritis, angiography demonstrated both pulmonary and systemic vascular involvment. Complete occlusion of the pulmonary arterial branch to the right upper lobe was associated with a large systemic-pulmonary arterial collateral.

Lie JT: Disseminated visceral giant cell arteritis. Am J Clin Pathol 69:299–305, 1978.
  Brief review of giant cell arteritis and description of a disseminated form.

Lupi E, Sanchez G, Horwitz S, Gutierrez E: Pulmonary artery involvement in Takayasu's arteritis. Chest 67:69–74, 1975.
  Demonstration of frequent pulmonary involvement in Takayasu's arteritis.

Rose AG, Halper J, Factor SM: Primary arteriopathy in Takayasu's disease. Arch Pathol Lab Med 108:644–648, 1984.
  Description of pulmonary vascular changes in Takayasu's arteritis.

Yamato M, Lecky JW, Hiramatsu K, Kohda E: Takayasu arteritis: radiographic and angiographic findings in 59 patients. Radiology 161:329–334, 1986.
  A review of 59 patients (57 females, two males) with Takayasu arteritis. Total aortography and pulmonary arteriography are necessary to diagnose and evaluate the extent of the disease.

Small Vessel Vasculitis (Hypersensitivity Angiitis)

Calabrese LH, Clough JD: Hypersensitivity vasculitis group (HVG). A case-oriented review of a continuing clinical spectrum. Cleve Clin Q 49:17–42, 1982.
  A critical review of the spectrum of hypersensitivity vasculitides. Emphasizes the subgroup of "true" hypersensitivity syndromes in which a specific antigen can be incriminated.

Cupps TR, Springer RM, Fauci AS: Chronic, recurrent small-vessel cutaneous vasculitis. Clinical experience in 13 patients. JAMA 247:1994–1998, 1982.
  Describes the clinicopathologic spectrum of small vessel vasculitis. Patients with solely cutaneous disease usually do not develop systemic manifestations and, therefore, have a good prognosis.

Mark EJ, Ramirez JF: Pulmonary capillaritis and hemorrhage in patients with systemic vasculitis. Arch Pathol Lab Med 109:413–418, 1985.
  Review of 13 cases of small vessel vasculitis in the lung accompanying systemic vasculitis. Cases of pulmonary small vessel vasculitis, apparently unrelated to systemic vasculitis, are also mentioned.

Mullick FG, McAllister HA Jr, Wagner BM, Fenoglio JJ Jr: Drug related vasculitis. Clinicopathologic correlations in 30 patients. Hum Pathol 10:313–325, 1979.

> Presents the characteristics of allergic (hypersensitivity) angiitis secondary to drug administration, including a listing of incriminated drugs. Cutaneous vasculitis responds simply to drug withdrawal, while systemic vasculitis may necessitate treatment with steroids.

Sams WM Jr, Thorne EG, Small P, Mass MF, McIntosh RM, Stanford RE: Leukocytoclastic vasculitis. Arch Dermatol 112:219–226, 1976.

> Reviews the causes of small vessel vasculitis including drugs, infections, foreign protein, and chemicals. Presents evidence to support the hypothesis of immune complex mediation.

Other Vasculitides

Bombardieri S, Paoletti P, Ferri C, DiMunno O, Fornai E, Guintini C: Lung involvement in essential mixed cryoglobulinemia. Am J Med 66:748–756, 1979.

> Clinical study of pulmonary manifestations in cryoglobulinemia.

Dreisin RB: Pulmonary vasculitis. Clin Chest Med 3:607–618, 1982.

> A good review of the subject.

Dunnill MS: Pulmonary Pathology. New York, Churchill-Livingstone, 1982.

> Includes brief review of pulmonary hypertensive vasculitis.

Fulmer JD, Kaltreider HB: The pulmonary vasculitides. Chest 82:615–624, 1982.

> A very good review of the subject.

Gamble CN, Wiesner KB, Shapiro RF, Boyer WJ: The immune complex pathogenesis of glomerulonephritis and pulmonary vasculitis in Behçet's disease. Am J Med 66:1031–1039, 1979.

> Case study of Behçet's disease with demonstration of immunoglobulin and complement deposits in the lung and kidney biopsies.

Hunninghake GW, Fauci AS: Pulmonary involvement in the collagen vascular disease. Am Rev Respir Dis 119:471–503, 1979.

> Extensive in-depth review of pulmonary manifestations in collagen diseases and in disseminated vasculitis.

Jones MB, Osterholm RK, Wilson RB, Martin FH, Commers JR, Bachmayer JD: Fatal pulmonary hypertension and resolving immune-complex glomerulonephritis in mixed connective tissue disease. Am J Med 65:855–863, 1978.

> Case report of pulmonary hypertension in mixed connective tissue disease, caused by thromboembolic involvement of small pulmonary arteries.

Lakhanpal S, Tani K, Lie JT, Katoh K, Ishigatsubo Y, Ohokubo T: Pathologic features of Behçet's syndrome: A review of Japanese autopsy registry data. Hum Pathol 16:790–795, 1985.

> A detailed study of the pathology of Behçet's syndrome based on 170 autopsy cases.

Sams WM Jr: Necrotizing vasculitis. J Am Acad Dermatol 3:1–13, 1980.

> Review of various forms of vasculitis with special emphasis on the cutaneous and pulmonary involvement.

Ulbright TM, Katzenstein A-LA: Solitary necrotizing granulomas of the lung: Differentiating features and etiology. Am J Surg Pathol 4:13–28, 1980.

> Review of infectious and noninfectious pulmonary granulomas and demonstration of the frequent occurrence of vasculitis.

Obstructive Disease of the Airways

Chapter 70

The Spectrum of Chronic Obstructive Disease of the Airways

Alfred P. Fishman

Terminology
   Chronic Obstructive Airways Disease
   Chronic Obstructive Pulmonary Disease (COPD),
      or Chronic Obstructive Lung Disease (COLD)
   Chronic Bronchitis
   Emphysema
   Chronic Bronchitis and Emphysema
   Small Airways Disease

Testing for Expiratory Obstruction

Chronic (Obstructive) Bronchitis

Emphysema

Chronic Bronchitis and Emphysema

Small Airways Disease

Hypothetical Natural History of Chronic Bronchitis
and Emphysema
   Predominantly Chronic Bronchitis
   Predominantly Emphysema

Terminology has been a continuing barrier to easy communication about chronic obstructive diseases of the airways. For example, three decades ago, *chronic bronchitis* meant one thing in England and another in the United States. Gradually, *chronic bronchitis and emphysema* was adopted on both sides of the water to mean either chronic bronchitis or emphysema or, more often, a combination of the two. For the last decade or so, *chronic obstructive lung disease* (COLD) or *chronic obstructive pulmonary disease* (COPD) have come into vogue as synonyms for *chronic bronchitis and emphysema.* Clearly, terminology concerning chronic obstructive airways disease has been the product of "lumpers" rather than of "splitters."

One major reason for the lingering ambiguity in terminology has been the engrossment of chest physicians, ever since Laennec, with structural-functional relation-

ships. Although pragmatists have been disinclined to pursue sharper definitions because the broad terms in common use generally suffice for managing individual patients, the needs of epidemiology and preventive medicine have not been satisfied by this solution. Moreover, attempts to bring lessons from the autopsy table to the bedside have met with only limited success so that *chronic bronchitis* continues to be defined in clinical terms, i.e., by persistent cough and sputum, whereas the diagnosis of *emphysema* is generally relegated to the prosector.

Over the years, it became evident that the diagnosis of *chronic bronchitis* needed greater precision, since individuals with persistent cough and sputum differed in their natural histories depending on the presence or absence of airways obstruction. Even the diagnosis of *asthma* has proved to have fuzzy borders. In some instances, the disorder is unmistakable. But, time and time again, the cliché has been reaffirmed that "all is not asthma that wheezes." Indeed, the same clinical syndrome may reflect a variety of etiologies, different pathogenetic mechanisms, and diverse anatomic lesions.

TERMINOLOGY

Although there is still no acknowledged consensus among experts about the terminology of chronic obstructive disease of the airways, the following definitions are consistent with current practice. They would be viewed in the context of a spectrum that consists of primary disorders that blur at their margins (Figs. 70-1 and 70-2). At the left end of the spectrum are the obstructive diseases (cystic fibrosis, asthma) in which intrinsic disease of the airways is the overriding mechanism; at the opposite extremity are the emphysematous disorders in which obstruction to expiration arises from rarefaction of parenchyma secondary to destruction of alveolar walls. Two aspects of the spectrum warrant special mention: (1) "pure" forms of individual diseases, e.g., emphysema, are less common than mixtures, e.g., chronic bronchitis and emphysema; and (2) in chronic bronchitis and emphysema, the most prevalent disorder, the degree and clinical significance of the *bronchitis* and *emphysema* can vary considerably from patient to patient.

Chronic Obstructive Airways Disease

This is a sweeping term that covers the full range of disorders illustrated in Fig. 70-2. The common denominator for this spectrum is increased airway resistance to expiration. Although the span shown in Fig. 70-2 includes *asthma* and *cystic fibrosis,* in practice these two entities usually stand on their own. As a result, *chronic obstructive airways disease* generally has the same encompassing

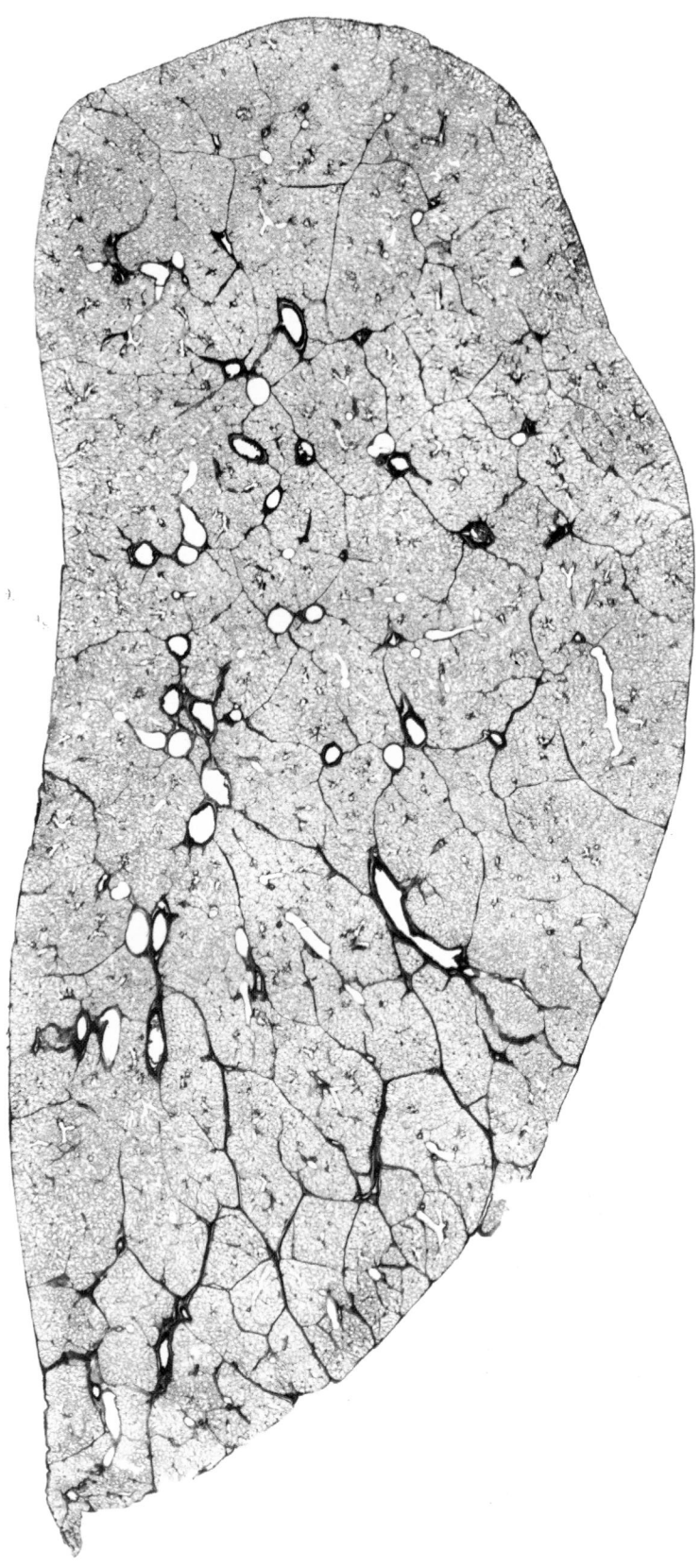

FIGURE 70-1 Normal lung. Sagittal section. For comparison with sections of abnormal lungs in Fig. 70-2. Elastic Van Gieson's stain. *(Courtesy of Dr. S. Moolten.)*

meaning as chronic obstructive pulmonary disease (COPD), chronic obstructive lung disease (COLD), or even *chronic bronchitis and emphysema.*

Chronic Obstructive Pulmonary Disease (COPD), or Chronic Obstructive Lung Disease (COLD)

These two terms are widely used as synonyms for the combination of *chronic bronchitis and emphysema.* The clinical hallmarks of this group are chronic cough, wheezing, expectoration, and dyspnea during a mild exertion if not at rest. Characteristically, airflow is reduced, e.g., the FEV_1 is abnormally low. Bronchodilators do little or nothing to relieve the obstructive breathing. Not only is the airways obstruction irreversible, but it is also progressive. At autopsy, chronic inflammatory changes in the airways are accompanied by irregular enlargement of alveoli and destruction of alveolar walls (Fig. 70-2C). The emphysema is usually pictured as secondary to the bronchitis.

Chronic Bronchitis

The clinical picture is dominated by a chronic productive cough, sputum, and recurrent chest infections. The critical element in this syndrome is airways obstruction during expiration (see Chapter 77). The anatomic correlate is enlargement of the tracheobronchial mucous glands. Persistent cough and expectoration without airways obstruction has a benign course and outlook and does not qualify for inclusion in this entity. *Chronic (obstructive) bronchitis* is distinguished from *asthmatic bronchitis* by its irreversibility, lack of bronchial hyperreactivity, lack of responsiveness to bronchodilators, and distinctive abnormalities in ventilation-perfusion relationships. In Great Britain, *chronic bronchitis* is widely used as a synonym for *chronic bronchitis and emphysema.*

Emphysema

Emphysema continues to be defined primarily in anatomic terms even though radiologic techniques are being increasingly applied for its detection during life. It is caused by enlargement of the airspaces distal to the terminal nonrespiratory bronchiole, accompanied by destructive changes of the alveolar walls. Functional abnormalities result from these anatomic changes. They include loss of lung recoil, excessive collapse of airways on exhalation, and chronic airflow obstruction. Conventional epidemiologic screening tests are not designed to distinguish between the airways on the one hand and the parenchyma on the other in the pathogenesis of airways obstruction.

Chronic Bronchitis and Emphysema

Because of the prevalence of cigarette smoking, a combination of bronchitis and emphysema is much more com-

mon than either *chronic bronchitis* or *emphysema* alone. Usually the description *chronic obstructive pulmonary disease* (COPD) is a synonym for *chronic bronchitis and emphysema.* As a rule, the clinical picture of *chronic bronchitis and emphysema* is seen in heavy smokers and takes 30 years or more to materialize. The full-blown, clinical picture of predominant emphysema can often be distinguished from that of predominant bronchitis. The distinctions have been turned to practical advantage by separating "pink puffers" from "blue bloaters" (Figs. 70-3 and 70-4).

Small Airways Disease

This term is used to describe characteristic abnormalities in pulmonary function that are associated with inflammatory and obliterative changes in the small airways, particularly the bronchioles. The inflammatory process is initiated by irritants, generally inhaled. In addition to respiratory bronchiolitis and hypersecretion in small airways, chronic small airways disease may be associated with a variety of lesions in the small airways: fibrosis, ulceration, metaplasia, and increased muscularization. It is widely held that, despite the characteristic hyperplasia of the mucous glands and the mucous hypersecretion, the functional changes of chronic bronchitis and emphysema are more a consequence of coexisting *small airways disease* than of the *chronic bronchitis.* It is also believed that the syndrome of *chronic bronchitis and emphysema,* particularly *in cigarette smokers,* generally begins as a bronchiolitis. However, much more is known about the natural history of the disorder *after* it becomes clinically evident than about its origins.

TESTING FOR EXPIRATORY OBSTRUCTION

The degree of expiratory difficulty is generally assessed using tests of airflow during expiration. Two broad principles underlie these tests: (1) that an increase in force (measured as pressure) is required to produce a given level of airflow when airway resistance is increased by bronchial narrowing, and (2) that emptying of the lungs is slowed during a maximal forced expiration. In practice, application of the first principle has led to determinations of airway resistance during quiet breathing; applications of the second are typified by the FEV_1 (forced expiratory volume delivered in 1 s). Since the tests differ enormously in complexity and in popularity, determinations of airway resistance are reserved for special pulmonary function laboratories, whereas the FEV_1 has become routine for screening.

In applying these tests, an important caveat must be kept in mind: they only assess obstruction to airflow during expiration in fairly large airways, i.e., from bronchi to

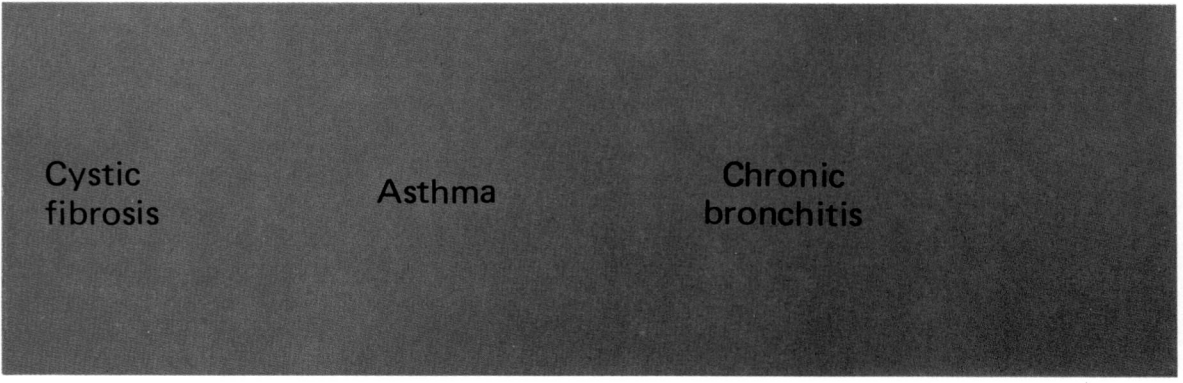

Cystic fibrosis   Asthma   Chronic bronchitis

A

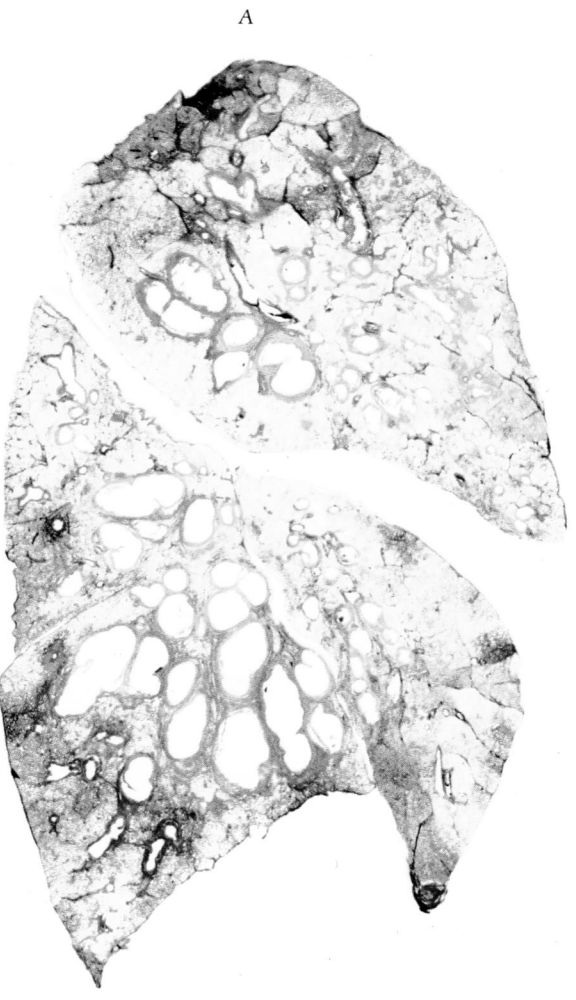

B

FIGURE 70-2 The spectrum of obstructive diseases of the airways. Pictured below the spectrum (A) are sagittal sections of whole lungs illustrating the two poles and middle of the spectrum: predominant airways disease (cystic fibrosis, B), widespread panacinar emphysema (C), and chronic bronchitis and emphysema (D). The cystic fibrosis lung shows remarkable dilatation of the large airways while the intervening pulmonary parenchyma is well preserved. The sagittal section of the rarefied emphysematous lung (C) was difficult to fix and mount because of the widespread destruction and loss of parenchyma. (Courtesy of Dr. S. Moolten.)

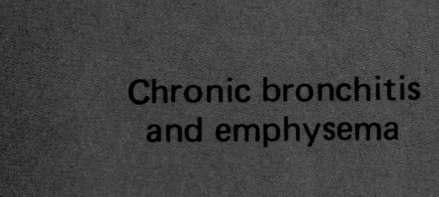

Chronic bronchitis and emphysema   Emphysema

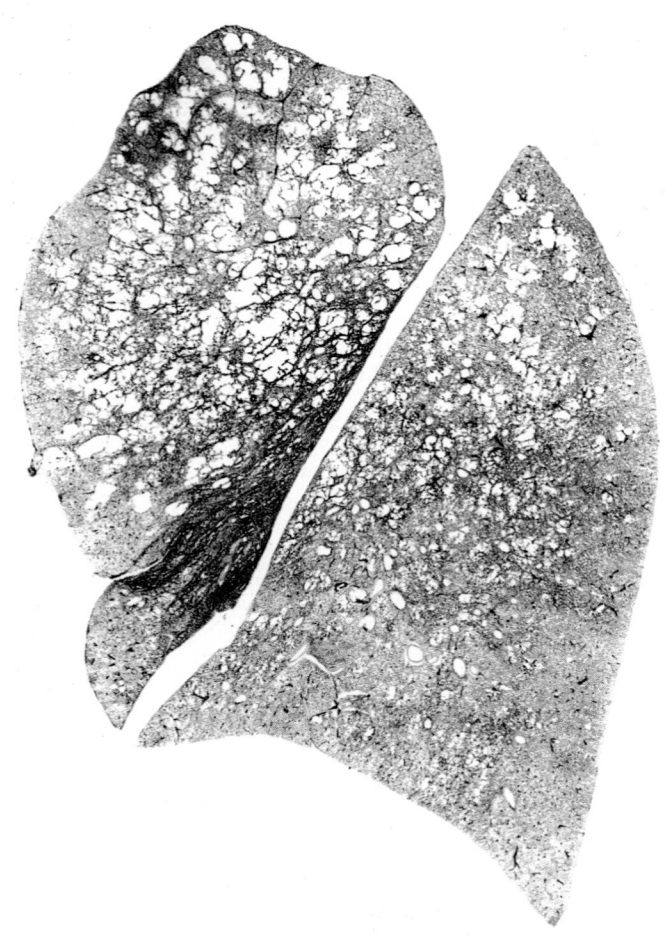

C

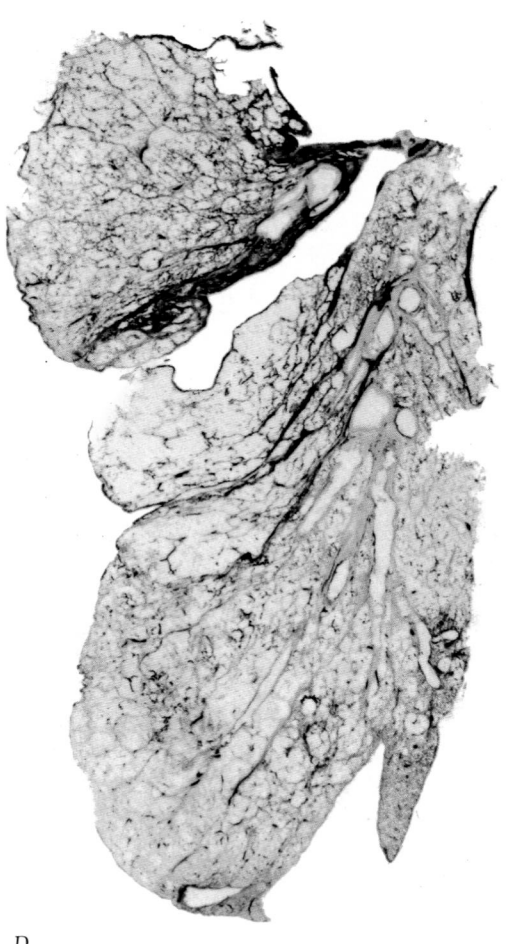

D

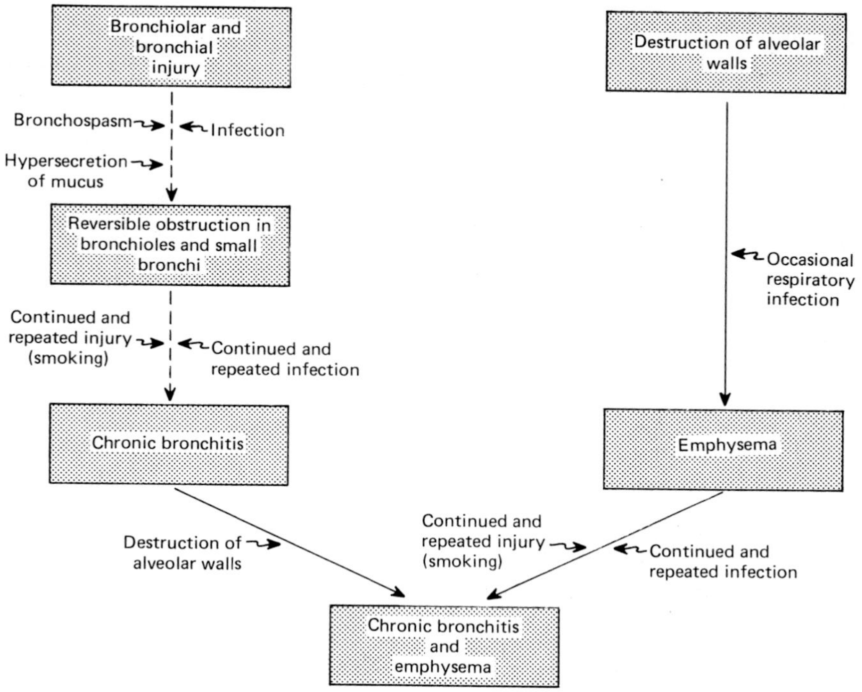

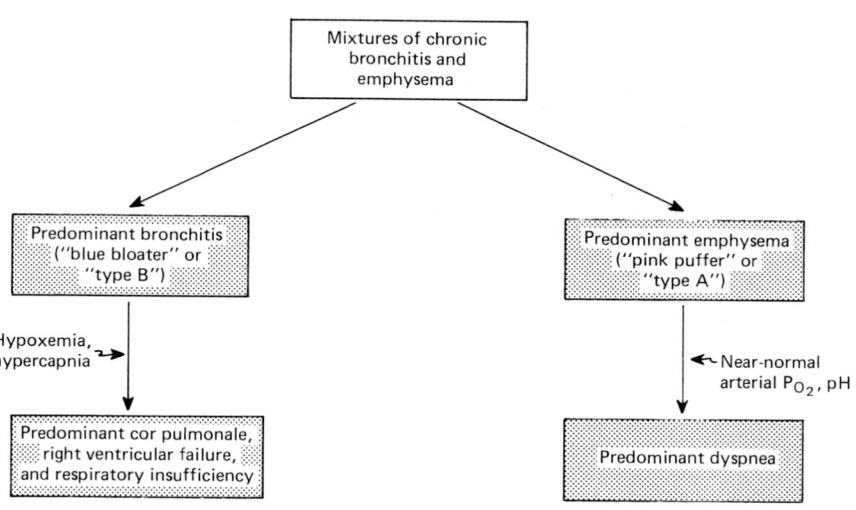

FIGURE 70-3 Schematic representation of the evolution of chronic bronchitis *(left)* and of emphysema *(right)*. Although both can culminate in chronic bronchitis and emphysema, the pathways are different, and either one or the other may predominate. The dashed arrows on the left reflect uncertainty about the origins of chronic bronchitis in small airways disease (bronchiolar inflammation and obstruction).

FIGURE 70-4 The role of arterial hypoxemia and hypercapnia in the evolution of the *blue bloater (left)* or *pink puffer (right)* categories of *chronic bronchitis and emphysema.*

bronchioles greater than 2 mm in diameter. This reservation is important on two accounts: (1) considerable damage to peripheral airways may be present without producing abnormality in tests of airway resistance or of rates of airflow during forced expiration, and (2) in the early stages of airways disease, both tests of airway resistance and of maximum expiratory flow may be within normal limits.

Three different factors can cause airway resistance to increase and FEV_1 to decrease: (1) the intrinsic size of

bronchial lumina, (2) the collapsibility of bronchial walls, and (3) the elastic recoil of the lungs. In a given patient, it may be difficult to sort the relative contributions of each of these factors. Indeed, as a general rule, all three contribute; the practical problem is to sort their relative roles. Of the three, collapsibility of bronchial walls is the most difficult to quantify.

When the diseases pictured on the left of Fig. 70-2 are full-blown, histologic changes can be seen along the entire length of the tracheobronchial tree. One common histo-

logic denomination is a hypersecretory state of the submucosal glands. Mucus-secreting tissue increases at all levels: the volume of glands in the trachea and bronchi is abnormally great; goblet cells appear in parts of the bronchial tree in which they are not normally present. Several different irritants, including smoke and infection, seem to be capable of initiating the same glandular response. Once excessive mucus is produced, the stage appears to be set for bacterial population of the bronchial tree, predisposing to further irritation and damage.

In emphysema (Fig. 70-2D), obstruction to airflow during expiration stems predominantly from a decrease in the elastic recoil of the lungs and, to a lesser extent, from increased compressibility of airways. As a rule, the degree of obstruction is less severe in emphysema than in the intrinsic diseases of the airways shown on the left of Fig. 70-2.

Until recent years, obstruction in the distal airways (bronchioles less than 2 mm in diameter) was beyond the reach of pulmonary function tests. Currently, although the methods are still too troublesome for routine use, they have succeeded in identifying obstructive disease in the terminal bronchioles while resistance of the large airways was still unaltered.

CHRONIC (OBSTRUCTIVE) BRONCHITIS

In Fig. 70-2, the designation *chronic bronchitis* actually signifies *chronic obstructive bronchitis*, which includes two elements: (1) a chronic productive cough for which no specific cardiopulmonary basis can be identified, and (2) obstruction to airflow during expiration. During life, the predominant features are consequences of ventilation-blood flow abnormalities in the lungs (Tables 70-1 and 70-2). At autopsy, the architecture is generally well preserved except for widely disseminated, centrilobular emphysema. Histologic examination of the airways reaffirms that enlargement of the tracheobronchial mucous glands is importantly involved in the pathogenesis of the disorder (see Chapter 77).

However, disturbances elsewhere than in the large airways must also be involved, as suggested by histologic evidence indicating that a similar hypersecretory state also occurs in persons who do not progress to obstructive disease of the airways, e.g., some cigarette smokers. For this reason, some other abnormality of the airways, such as bronchiolar obstruction or obliteration, or emphysema, or both, probably add to the obstructive component during expiration.

TABLE 70-1
Clinical Hallmarks: Predominant Bronchitis versus Predominant Emphysema

	Predominant Bronchitis	Predominant Emphysema
General appearance	Mesomorphic; overweight; dusky with suffused conjunctivae; warm extremities	Thin, often emaciated; pursed-lip breathing; anxious, prominent use of accessory muscles; normal or cool extremities
Age, years	40–55	50–75
Onset	Cough	Dyspnea
Cyanosis	Marked	Slight to none
Cough	More evident than dyspnea	Less evident than dyspnea
Sputum	Copious	Scanty
Upper respiratory infections	Common	Occasional
Breath sounds	Moderately diminished	Markedly diminished
Cor pulmonale and right-sided heart failure	Common	Only during bout of respiratory infection, and terminally
Radiograph	Normal diaphragm position; cardiomegaly; lungs normal or with increased bronchovascular markings	Small, pendulous heart; low, flat diaphragms; areas of increased radiolucency
Course	Ambulatory but constantly on verge of right-sided heart failure and coma	Incapacitating breathlessness punctuated by life-threatening bouts of upper respiratory infections; prolonged course, culminating in right-sided heart failure and coma

TABLE 70-2

Functional Hallmarks: Predominant Bronchitis versus Predominant Emphysema

	Predominant Bronchitis	Predominant Emphysema
FEV_1/VC	Reduced	Reduced
FRC	Mildly increased	Markedly increased
TLC	Normal or slightly increased	Considerably increased
RV	Moderately increased	Markedly increased
Lung compliance	Normal or low	Normal or low
Recoil pressure	Normal or high	Low
MVV	Moderately decreased	Markedly decreased
Airway resistance	Increased	Normal or slightly increased
Dco	Normal or low	Low
Arterial P_{O_2}	Moderately to severely reduced	Slightly to moderately reduced
Arterial hypercapnia	Chronic	Only during acute respiratory infection
Hematocrit	Generally high, may reach 70%	Normal or slightly high, uncommon to exceed 55%
Pulmonary arterial pressure	Generally increased	Normal or slightly increased

NOTE: TLC = total lung capacity; RV = residual volume; D_{CO} = diffusing capacity of carbon monoxide.

Figure 70-3 (left) illustrates the prevalent idea of the evolution of chronic bronchitis. The dashed line reflects uncertainty about how small airways disease and upper airways disease interrelate in the pathogenesis of chronic bronchitis.

EMPHYSEMA

As indicated above, the usual morphologic definition of emphysema includes two components: abnormal and permanent dilatation of the terminal airspaces of the lungs and destruction of their walls. Most, but not all, pathologists emphasize destruction. The definition is useful conceptually, since it separates a state of simple overinflation in which alveolar walls are intact from a morbid state in which dysfunction is secondary to loss of parenchymal substance and rearrangement of pulmonary architecture. Destruction is often obvious, for even in relatively mild examples of emphysema, alveolar walls are visibly damaged or destroyed.

A milestone in the understanding of the etiology of emphysema was the observation that some families with an unusually high frequency of panlobular emphysema unassociated with chronic bronchitis suffer from a deficiency of α_1-antitrypsin in the serum. Among the physiological features of this disorder (Table 70-2) are a low diffusing capacity and relatively well preserved relationships between alveolar blood flow and ventilation in the remaining parts of the lungs. Even though some degree of obstruction to airflow is a regular feature of severe emphysema, loss of elastic recoil accounts only in part for the

airways obstruction. Generally, chronic bronchitis contributes.

Different types of emphysema cause different degrees of pulmonary dysfunction because of differences in the anatomic sites that are predominantly affected. *Panacinar emphysema* is diffusely scattered throughout the secondary lobule and characteristically destroys the alveolar capillary bed. In *centrilobular emphysema*, rarefaction of the lungs is most marked in the center of the secondary lobule, and the enlarged airspaces are interposed between small bronchi and the alveoli. These differences are also important with respect to the radiographic diagnosis of emphysema during life. The greatest difficulty in the radiologic diagnosis of emphysema probably arises in centrilobular emphysema of mild to moderate extent distributed uniformly throughout the lung; less difficulty is experienced in the diagnosis of panacinar emphysema which tends to be much more severe in some regions than in others (Fig. 70-3, right).

CHRONIC BRONCHITIS AND EMPHYSEMA

Interest remains high in quantifying the relative contributions of bronchitis and emphysema to the clinical picture in individual patients since the natural history of the syndrome depends on which component predominates: the predominantly bronchitic patient has a poorer prognosis for longevity because of inhomogeneities in the balance between alveolar ventilation and blood flow that cause hypoxemia and hypercapnia. In contrast, the emphysematous patient generally lives longer, albeit with greater dis-

ability due to breathlessness, because of the preservation of ventilation-blood flow relationships (Fig. 70-4).

The desirability of sorting out and quantifying chronic bronchitis and emphysema should not obscure the fact that the lumping together of the obstructive diseases of the airways has had its rewards. One important consequence has been reaffirmation of spirometry as an exceedingly valuable tool for uncovering obstructive disease of the airways and for following its course. For example, obstructive disease of the airways can be assumed to be present when the FEV_1 and the peak flows are reduced and forced expiration is slowed. Because the FEV_1 is more compromised than the forced vital capacity, the ratio FEV_1/VC (where VC is vital capacity) has gained widespread acceptance as a screening test for obstructive disease of the airways. Also, without serious reduction in the FEV_1, it is difficult to attribute dyspnea to any form of obstructive airways disease.

SMALL AIRWAYS DISEASE

It is now widely held that early in the natural history of chronic bronchitis, obstruction exists in the small airways long before conventional tests of pulmonary function, such as FEV_1 or MVV (maximum voluntary ventilation), become abnormal. Although insufficient to be detected clinically or by the standard tests, the abnormalities in the small airways are enough to derange alveolar ventilation-blood flow relationships and alveolar-capillary gas exchange. The obstruction at first need not be caused by inflammation of the bronchioles; excess secretions can exert the same effect. Although special tests, such as closing volume and frequency dependence of compliance, can uncover obstruction in the peripheral airways at a time when conventional tests are still normal, two practical considerations limit their adoption for routine use: (1) reproducibility of the tests in the same subject is far from ideal; and (2) improved tests of forced expiration, using gases of different density or emphasizing the tail end of the breath, hold promise of being equally sensitive. It is also worth noting that none of these tests, no matter how sensitive, can shed light on the mechanism that is responsible for the obstruction or help to decide whether the cause is within, or without, the lumen of the small airways. Finally, questions may be raised concerning the preoccupation of conventional tests with forced expiration. It is known that elastic recoil may be decreased appreciably and the lung may become hyperinflated without a decrease in the rate of airflow during forced expiration. Therefore, it seems reasonable to anticipate that there are subtle but quantifiable derangements in pulmonary performance even before tests of small airways disease become abnormal.

HYPOTHETICAL NATURAL HISTORY OF CHRONIC BRONCHITIS AND EMPHYSEMA

The natural history of chronic bronchitis and emphysema depends on whether bronchitis or emphysema is the predominant lesion. The two pathways are generally distinguished by designations such as pink puffer or blue bloater.

Predominantly Chronic Bronchitis

The predominantly chronic bronchitic patient is pictured stereotypically as a chronic cigarette smoker whose normal defense mechanisms are continuously besieged by noxious substances in the inhaled smoke. The damage predisposes to infection, particularly in the lower airways; other air pollutants simply add to the insult. Early in the evolution of chronic bronchitis, the closing and residual volumes are somewhat increased; frequency dependence of compliance is present; airway resistance and conventional pulmonary function tests (e.g., the FEV_1) are normal; the arterial P_{O_2} is at the lower limit of normal or slightly subnormal because of slight inhomogeneities in alveolar ventilation-blood flow relationships. This stage is reversible if cigarette smoking stops, air pollutants are avoided, and the individual escapes upper respiratory infections.

In time, the second stage is reached: continued smoking and recurrent infections cause peripheral airways to become increasingly obstructed; some are amputated. The chronic irritation and march of infection begins to affect the large airways. Mucous glands enlarge in the upper as well as lower airways (Reid index increases); hypersecretion is manifested histologically up and down the airways. The production of sputum increases. Conventional tests of obstructive disease become abnormal: the FEV_1 is low, and the residual volume is large. But elastic recoil is still preserved, and the diffusing capacity is normal. Only a few of these patients develop severe derangement in arterial blood-gas levels which sets the stage for cor pulmonale and respiratory failure.

The third stage is characterized by progressive disturbances in ventilation-blood flow relationships caused by airways obstruction and evidences of emphysema (Fig. 70-5). The usual type affects the ends of the respiratory bronchioles (centrilobular emphysema), thereby exaggerating alveolar ventilation-blood flow imbalances. However, in some patients, the destruction is not confined to the center of the lobule; instead, it is widespread throughout the lung, resulting in panacinar emphysema. Reduction in elastic recoil contributes to an increase in airway resistance. As the patient grows older, age exaggerates the loss in elastic recoil and enhances the prospect for infection and further obstruction in the bronchioles and bronchi.

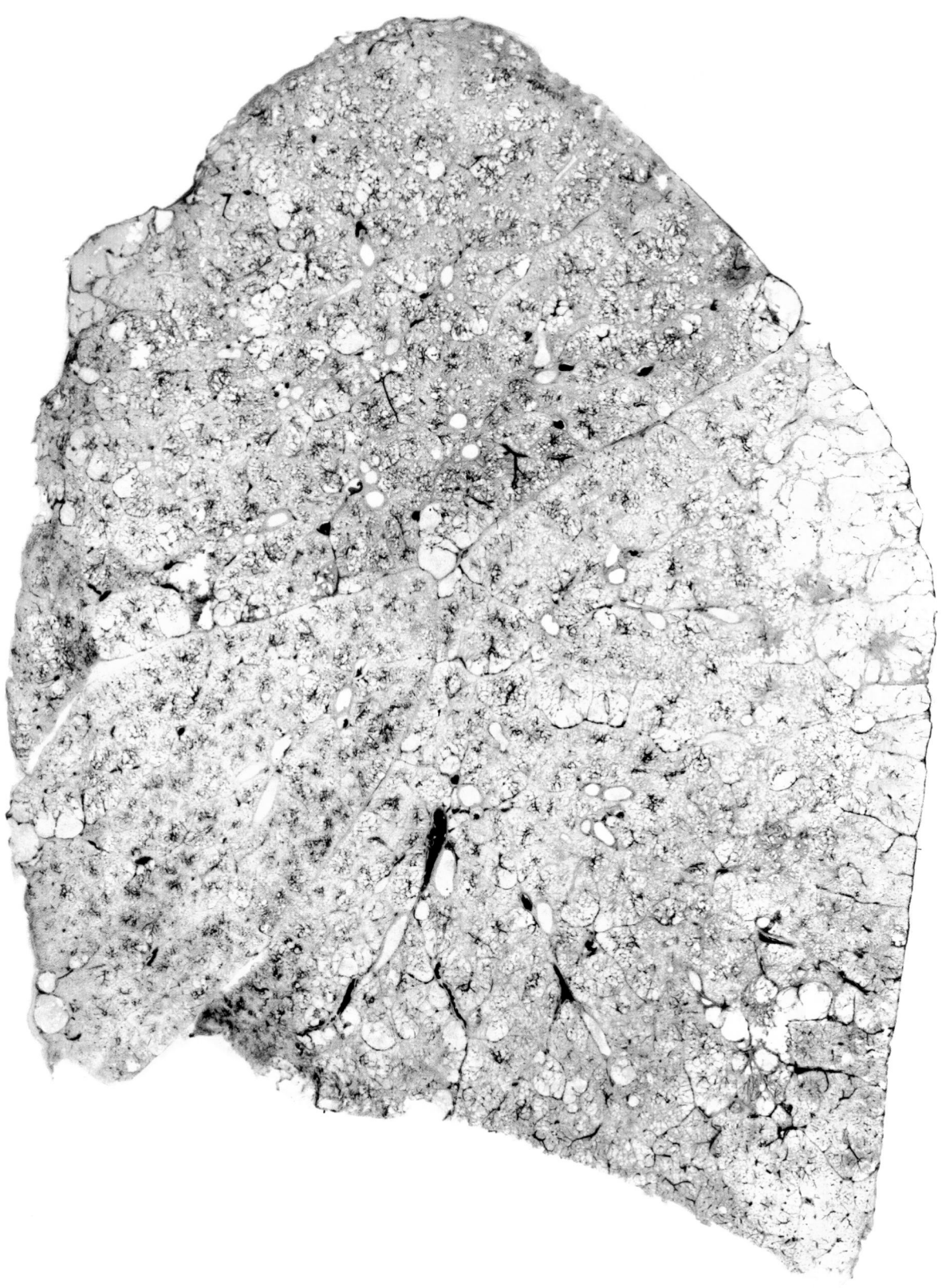

FIGURE 70-5 Sagittal section of the lung from a 45-year-old blue bloater who died in cor pulmonale and respiratory insufficiency.

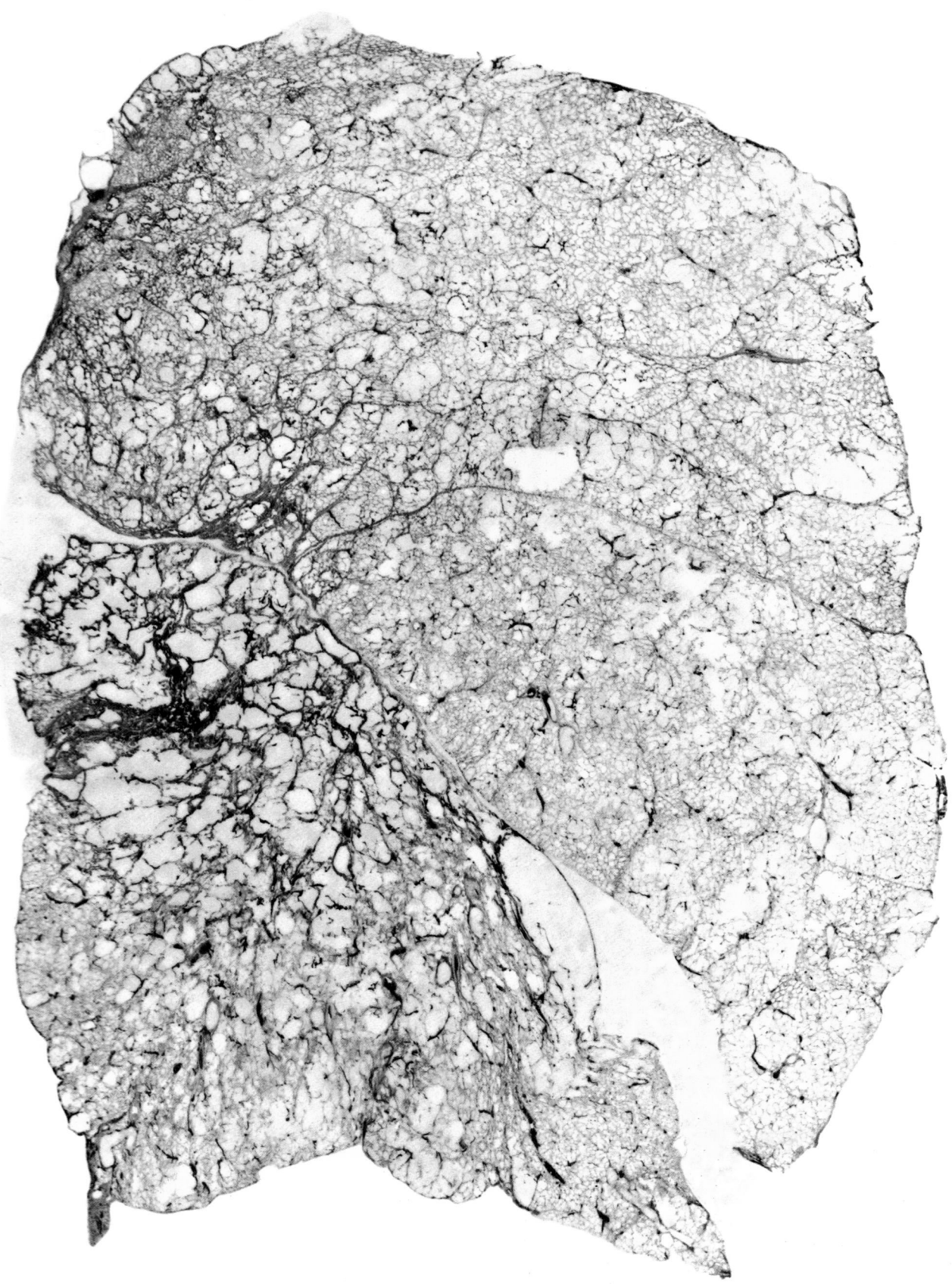

FIGURE 70-6 Sagittal section of the lung from a 67-year-old male pink puffer who died in respiratory insufficiency precipitated by a viral infection. *(Courtesy of Dr. S. Moolten.)*

Although this sequence is plausible, it is linked in spots by tenuous bridges that span gaps of knowledge. For example, little is known about the transition between stage 1 and stage 2 above. Also unknown is why most smokers do not undergo an inevitable progression from obstruction of small airways to disabling chronic bronchitis. Why do a few patients develop alveolar hypoventilation and its consequences, whereas most, with comparable abnormalities in conventional pulmonary function tests, maintain near-normal blood-gas levels except during an acute respiratory infection?

Predominantly Emphysema

Emphysema, even if severe, in the absence of airways obstruction, can remain asymptomatic for a lifetime except for undue breathlessness on exertion. However, most patients with emphysema also have some degree of chronic bronchitis due to cigarette smoking. In contrast with the blue bloater, the emphysematous patient rarely develops cor pulmonale unless hypoxemia becomes sufficiently severe to elicit persistent pulmonary hypertension.

The degree of airflow obstruction in the non-cigarette smoker or coal miner is generally mild. The type of emphysema (panacinar or centrilobular) appears to have little bearing on the degree of airways obstruction. Moderate to severe airways obstruction in emphysema can usually be attributed to an accompanying chronic bronchitis.

Therefore, the natural history of emphysema ranges from breathlessness on exertion for a long lifetime to progressive incapacitating breathlessness at rest as the lungs continue to rarify. Right ventricular overload and cor pulmonale become a problem when arterial hypoxemia supervenes, either acutely in the course of an upper respiratory infection (Fig. 70-6) or chronically because of a concomitant chronic bronchitis. Not infrequently, intercurrent events, such as peptic ulceration, attributable to the indiscriminate use of bronchodilators and corticosteroids, are more life-threatening than the pulmonary disorder.

BIBLIOGRAPHY

Anthonisen NR, Wright EC, Hodgkin JE: Prognosis in chronic obstructive pulmonary disease. Am Rev Respir Dis 133:14–20, 1986.
  Nine hundred and eighty-five patients with chronic obstructive airways disease, but without hypoxemia or other serious disease, were treated in a standard fashion and followed closely for nearly 3 years. Overall mortality was 23% in the 3-year follow-up. Patient age and the initial value of the FEV$_1$ were the most accurate predictors of death.

Bates DV: The fate of the chronic bronchitic: A report of the ten-year follow-up in the Canadian Department of Veteran's Affairs coordinated study of chronic bronchitis. Am Rev Respir Dis 108:1043–1065, 1973.
  The rate of deterioration is much faster in 10 percent of cigarette-smoking men than in the others. The MMEF (maximum mid-expiratory flow rate) and FEV$_1$ are considered to be valuable for the early detection of the members of this small group, thereby allowing institution of prophylactic measures to avoid irreversible changes in pulmonary parenchyma.

Dijkman JH: Morphological aspects, classification and epidemiology of emphysema. Bull Eur Physiopathol Respir 22:241s–243s, 1986.
  Pulmonary function tests, as applied in population studies, do not differentiate between anatomical emphysema and other causes of airflow obstruction. Standard radiology of the thorax provides a morphological approach to the detection of emphysema in advanced disease.

Dodge R, Cline MG, Burrows B: Comparisons of asthma, emphysema, and chronic bronchitis diagnoses in a general population sample. Am Rev Respir Dis 133:981–986, 1986.
  Physician bias may result in labeling male patients as emphysematous and female patients as asthmatic or bronchitic.

Fletcher CM, Peto R, Tinker CM, Speizer FE: The Natural History of Chronic Bronchitis and Emphysema. Oxford, England, Oxford University Press, 1986.
  An important prospective study that assesses the determinants of prognosis in chronic bronchitis. Chronic bronchitis is sharply defined. Only those with measurable abnormalities of expiratory airflow were shown to have a poor prognosis.

Fletcher CM, Price NB: Definitions of emphysema, chronic bronchitis, asthma, and airflow obstruction: 25 years on from the Ciba Symposium. Thorax 39:81–85, 1984.
  A critical review of the report of the Ciba Symposium in 1959 indicates that, even though the original definitions have worn well with respect to distinguishing between chronic bronchitis and emphysema, large gaps remain in the understanding of pathogenesis, that the popular term chronic obstructive bronchitis is inappropriate, and that there is still no sharp definition of asthma.

Greaves IA, Colebatch HJ: Observations on the pathogenesis of chronic airflow obstruction in smokers: implications for the detection of "early" lung disease. Thorax 41:81–87, 1986.
A review of the presumed role of smoking in the evolution of chronic obstructive airways disease.

Keller CA, Shepard JW Jr, Chun DS, Vasquez P, Dolan GF: Pulmonary hypertension in chronic obstructive pulmonary disease. Multivariate analysis. Chest 90:185–192, 1986.
Arterial blood gas criteria were superior to the spirometric and radiographic variables in predicting pulmonary hypertension prior to the development of clinically overt cor pulmonale.

Niewoehner DE, Kleinerman J, Rice DB: Pathologic changes in the peripheral airways of young cigarette smokers. N Engl J Med 291:755–758, 1974.
Based on morphologic studies of young individuals who died out of hospital, respiratory bronchiolitis is postulated to be a precursor of centriacinar emphysema as well as the basis for subtle functional abnormalities found in young smokers.

Petty TL: Definitions, clinical assessment, and risk factors, in Petty TL (ed), *Chronic Obstructive Pulmonary Disease*, 2d ed. New York, Dekker, 1985, pp 1–30.
An attempt, based on a large clinical experience, to formulate acceptable working definitions for the obstructive airways diseases. The approach is that of a "lumper" rather than a "splitter."

Reid LM: The pathology of obstructive and inflammatory airway diseases. Eur J Respir Dis (Suppl)147:26–37, 1986.
Part of a symposium. The diseases included are those commonly called chronic bronchitis, bronchiolitis, bronchiectasis, and asthma. The advocated definitions satisfy the crying need of epidemiologists for sharper categorizations than the popular usage of COPD.

Report of Task Force on Epidemiology of Respiratory Diseases. Division of Lung Diseases, National Heart, Lung and Blood Institute. NIH Publication No. 81-2019, October 1980.
An important attempt to sort chronic bronchitis and emphysema from an epidemiologic point of view.

Sharp JT, Paul O, McKean H, Best WR: A longitudinal study of bronchitic symptoms and spirometry in a middle-aged, male, industrial population. Am Rev Respir Dis 108:1066–1077, 1973.
Challenges the Fletcher definition of chronic bronchitis as being too liberal in that it includes a large number of individuals who will not develop disabling pulmonary disease.

Sparrow D, O'Connor G, Colton T, Barry CL, Weiss ST: The relationship of nonspecific bronchial responsiveness to the occurrence of respiratory symptoms and decreased levels of pulmonary function. The Normative Aging Study. Am Rev Respir Dis 135:1255–1260, 1987.
Increased level of nonspecific responsiveness is significantly associated with wheeze and cough symptoms and decreased levels of pulmonary function in adult men.

Standards for the diagnosis and care of patients with chronic obstructive pulmonary disease (COPD) and asthma. This official statement of the American Thoracic Society was adopted by the ATS Board of Directors, November 1986. Am Rev Respir Dis 136:225–244, 1987.
A statement of a Task Group appointed by the Scientific Assemble of Clinical Problems of the American Thoracic Society.

Tager I, Speizer FE: Role of infection in chronic bronchitis. N Engl J Med 292:563–571, 1975.
A "Medical Progress" review of the epidemiology and natural history of the "cough and phlegm syndromes." It is difficult to pinpoint the role of respiratory infections in adult life in the progressive obstructive airways disease.

Thurlbeck WM: Aspects of chronic airflow obstruction. Chest 72:341–349, 1978.
This report questions several commonly used definitions and commonly accepted concepts. Alternatives are proposed to avoid loose terminology.

Tomashefski JF: Definition, differentiation, and classification of COPD. Postgrad Med 62:88–97, 1977.
COPD is defined as a spectrum of diseases with a common denominator, obstruction to airflow on expiration. Chronic asthma, chronic bronchitis, and pulmonary emphysema are the most prevalent conditions.

Obstructing Lesions of the Larynx and Trachea: Clinical and Pathophysiological Aspects

R. Drew Miller

Obstructing lesions of the larynx and trachea create unique changes that can be differentiated from the more common obstructing disorders of the diffuse lower airways, such as bronchitis, emphysema, and asthma. Because of the noisy respiration associated with many of the lesions, they are commonly misdiagnosed as asthma. However, this misconstruction may be fatal, because the management of obstructive lesions of the major airways is vastly different, and often much more urgent, than that for diffuse airways. Both diagnosis and treatment often require the collaboration of the primary pediatrician or physician, chest physician, otolaryngologist, endoscopist, and surgeon with an interest in head and neck problems and thoracic or pediatric problems.

CHANGING PATTERNS OF FREQUENCY

Obstructing lesions of the larynx and trachea have increased in frequency as part of the accelerated pace of living that has changed lifestyles in industrialized nations. On the one hand, injury to the central airways has become more common as a result of vehicular accidents.

On the other, the introduction of new therapeutic modalities, particularly the combination of cuffed tracheal tubes and controlled ventilation, has introduced a new kind of trauma to the mucosa and cartilaginous rings.

In addition, smoking and air pollution have led to a greater incidence of cancer of the airways, including the larynx and trachea. Why the trachea is less often the site of primary malignancy than the branching airways is not known. It could be that the time of exposure to extrinsic irritants is longer at the bronchial bifurcations, where primary cancer is common, than in the trachea and that the mucociliary escalator operates more rapidly and efficiently in the trachea than in the peripheral airways.

THE COMMON AIRWAY

The trachea is about 11 cm long in the average-sized adult and varies from 17 to 24 mm in diameter. The larynx, even with the cords fully abducted, is somewhat narrower and ovoid. Together with the oral pharynx, the larynx and trachea form the common airway that connects the nose and mouth to the right and left main-stem bronchi. In the young adult, the trachea is mobile in the cervical and mediastinal fascial sheaths. When the neck is extended, one-half of the trachea lies in the neck; when the neck is flexed, the trachea is accommodated almost entirely within the thorax. Aging causes the trachea to become progressively less mobile and predominantly intrathoracic.

Because these central airways account for a large portion of the normal resistance of the airways to airflow, moderate narrowing markedly increases the resistance. If the narrowing is localized, as it is in most obstructing lesions, turbulence is created which exaggerates the pressure drop across the stenotic lumen. The turbulence creates a stridor that is distinctly audible to the unaided ear near the mouth, and that indicates that the airway obstruction is not due to the more common entities of asthma, bronchitis, or emphysema.

Disorders involved in the differential diagnosis of obstruction localized to the central common airway, that is, the trachea, larynx, and hypopharynx, are shown in Table 71-1. In a given situation, many diagnoses can be quickly excluded on the basis of the patient's age and the rarity of the condition in the particular clinical setting. However, other criteria and tests are often needed to clinch the diagnosis.

Innovations in managing lesions of this important central airway in recent years have included resection and primary anastomosis or sleeve resection where surgical removal was thought to be technically impossible in the past. Up to one-half of the tracheal cartilages have been removed and reanastomosed successfully using a laryngeal release surgical procedure to allow better extension

TABLE 71-1

Classification of Potentially Obstructing Diseases of the Trachea and Larynx

I. Developmental—usually seen in infants and children
   A. Vascular anomalies of the aortic arch or its branches; aberrant pulmonary artery
   B. Congenital glottic or subglottic stenosis (web, segment, or diffuse hypoplasia)
   C. Angiomas of the trachea
   D. Sleep apnea in adults with retrognathia

II. Infectious
   A. Infants—usually acute
      1. Croup, epiglottis, and tracheobronchitis with laryngeal edema and spasm
      2. Diphtheria
      3. Sleep apnea from hypertrophied tonsils
   B. Adults
      1. Tuberculosis
      2. Fungi—histoplasmosis, blastomycosis, coccidioidomycosis
      3. Mediastinitis

III. Traumatic
   A. Stricture from therapeutic intubation
   B. Blunt—for example, steering wheel with fracture of trachea
   C. Foreign bodies
   D. Laryngeal and tracheal burns

IV. Neurogenic
   A. Interruption of both recurrent laryngeal nerves
      1. Postoperative
      2. Inflammatory
   B. Obstructive sleep apnea associated with reduced neuromuscular tone in the hypopharynx

V. Neoplastic
   A. Malignant tumors
      1. Squamous cell carcinoma
      2. Cylindroma (adenoid cystic carcinoma)
      3. Mucoepidermoid carcinoma
      4. Adenocarcinoma
      5. Small cell undifferentiated carcinoma
      6. Lymphoma group
      7. Leiomyosarcoma
      8. Chondrosarcoma
      9. Metastatic cancer
     10. Invasive thyroid cancer
     11. Plasmacytoma
   B. Benign
      1. Papillamatosis (childhood and adolescence)
      2. Fibrolipoma
      3. Inflammatory fibrous polyp
      4. Thyroid adenoma

VI. Nutritional
   A. Obesity—that is, hypopharyngeal obstruction

VII. Unknown or uncertain cause
   A. Tracheopathica osteoplastica
   B. Relapsing polychondritis
   C. Tumor-forming amyloid
   D. Tracheomalacia
   E. Sarcoid granuloma of the larynx
   F. Wegener's granuloma of larynx or upper trachea

---

of the tissues. Even more recently neodymium-YAG laser ablation of unresectable tumors has allowed evaporation of the intraluminal part of tumors that have extended into adjacent tissues preventing complete resection. While this is palliative and applicable only to a small proportion of lesions, it offers another dimension in our management armamentarium.

ETIOLOGIC AND PATHOLOGIC CLASSIFICATION OF MAJOR AIRWAY OBSTRUCTION

Developmental Disorders

VASCULAR ANOMALIES

The most common anomalies of the aortic arch compressing the trachea are double aortic arch, right aortic arch with ligamentum arteriosum, and anomalous innominate artery. Less commonly, an anomalous artery has been reported to cause major airway compression. Stridor, wheezing, and episodes of cyanosis occur if secretions are retained. Hyperextension of the neck most often seems to relieve tracheal compression, whereas flexion increases compression. Although these congenital anomalies are present at birth, symptoms become pronounced after several months of growth. Dysphagia is troublesome, and aspiration pneumonitis often confuses the clinical picture. If the constriction is not relieved in the neonatal period, development of the trachea is often permanently impaired, resulting in local stricture and chondromalacia of the involved tracheal rings.

Tracheoesophageal fistulas, which cause respiratory distress, are almost never associated with anomalous stenosis of the trachea. Instead, the respiratory symptoms are secondary to atresia of the esophagus, which causes spillover and aspiration, even if the fistula is small. Thus, the respiratory symptoms in tracheoesophageal fistulas are not due to obstruction of the major airways.

CONGENITAL GLOTTAL AND SUBGLOTTAL STENOSIS

This type of stenosis is not rare. The largest series reported from an endoscopic center exceeds 370 cases. In the infant, about 80 percent of such lesions are confined to the larynx, and the remaining 20 percent occur 2 to 3 mm below the true vocal cords. The mechanism of these le-

sions is probably related to the mesodermal ingrowth laterally on the pharyngeal pouch of the foregut that creates the primordial laryngeal cartilages in the seventh embryonic week. Because of abnormal cartilage found in the stenotic laryngeal lesions, the terms *laryngomalacia* or *congenital laryngeal stridor* have been used.

Mild or moderate stenosis sometimes is clinically silent until acute laryngotracheobronchitis supervenes; edema, with the associated and consequently severe airway obstruction, may be fatal. It has been speculated that failure to examine carefully at autopsy the larynx and upper trachea of children who have died suddenly and of unexplained cause has led to an underestimate of the prevalence of these stenotic lesions.

Conservative management is least hazardous and generally the most successful. Tracheostomy as a temporary bypass is sometimes required in patients who do not respond to humidifying aerosols. With normal growth and medical surveillance for months (or even for as long as 1 year), all but the more severe anomalies are self-correcting.

RETROGNATHISM

Individuals with malformations of the mandible are predisposed to an exaggerated type of snoring associated with an obstructive sleep apnea syndrome. Among the disorders are retrognathia and micrognathia. The retrognathic mandible is displaced posteriorly and retruded with respect to the maxilla; the micrognathic mandible is underdeveloped. A surgical procedure to advance the mandible has been advocated to restore proper skeletal occlusion and to relieve the manifestations of sleep apnea.

ANGIOMAS

Tracheal angiomas are considered congenital because they usually initiate symptoms of dyspnea at approximately 6 months of age. In about one-half of the patients, the tracheal angiomas are associated with angiomas at other sites; they occur twice as frequently in males. Stridor and wheezing vary in intensity and are often associated with cough and cyanosis. Since the angioma is sessile and flat, the upper margin, being just below the vocal cords, is apt to be overlooked at bronchoscopy unless a careful search is made. A biopsy specimen should not be taken, because the lesions are vascular and sometimes contain arteriovenous fistulas. Almost all types of subglottic lesions, especially when sessile, are difficult to detect endoscopically. Sometimes a short fiberoptic laryngoscope or open bronchoscope will allow easier detection. Retrognathia, a variable developmental abnormality, when severe, may allow intermittent upper airway narrowing and, during sleep, total occlusion of the upper airways, leading to the obstructive sleep apnea syndrome.

Infectious Obstruction

INFANTS

Croup is a syndrome associated with epiglottitis, laryngitis, and tracheobronchitis. Inspiratory stridor is the hallmark associated with various degrees of laryngeal obstruction. A virus is presumably responsible for as many as 85 percent of cases; disease of this etiology is often not associated with fever. In the other 15 percent of cases, *Hemophilus influenzae* type B is the chief cause; it is more often associated with fever. *Corynebacterium diphtheriae* is a rare cause of laryngeal obstruction in countries in which immunization is widely practiced.

Viral croup is most common before the age of 3 years, and croup caused by *H. influenzae* is most common in children 3 years or older. Croup of all types is more common in boys than in girls. Some children seem particularly prone to bouts of croup with each respiratory infection, whereas others, with respiratory infections of similar cause, do not develop the croup syndrome. Thus, intrinsic predisposing factors may be present. Laryngeal edema seems to be the key to the development of stridor. Atopic predisposition apparently does not increase the risks of developing croup.

The clinical picture is quite distinctive. The inspiratory stridor associated with severe retraction of the supraclavicular, suprasternal, and subcostal regions in an infant or young child automatically suggests croup.

Management requires a quiet atmosphere containing mist and the administration of supplemental oxygen. When bacterial infection is the cause, appropriate antibiotics are essential. Intermittent positive-pressure breathing and steroids have been advocated, but their value remains unproved. The acute episode of severe inspiratory obstruction often lasts for only a few hours; in some, progressive inspiratory distress has necessitated tracheostomy. In one report, 12 percent of affected children were dead on or soon after arrival at the hospital. Oral intubation of the acutely obstructed infant is widely used to ensure patency of the airway long enough for the acute edema to subside, thus postponing or obviating the need for emergency tracheostomy.

ADULTS

Historically, tuberculosis has commonly involved the larynx. In some parts of the world, where prevalence is still high, this type of involvement persists. In one North American study of a large series of subjects with active tuberculosis, laryngeal lesions were found in 1.5 percent. The lesions were usually not obstructive, even when edema was present. Only 14 percent of subjects with involvement of the larynx had stridor; 10 percent of these underwent tracheostomy. Such patients usually have obvious pulmonary tuberculosis and positive sputum smear

for acid-fast bacilli. Hoarseness is by far the most common presenting symptom of major airway involvement. Cervical adenopathy is usually not present. While tuberculosis has become much less common in North America and Europe, major airway involvement must be considered in new acute or far advanced cases in which the patient's sputum contains tubercle bacilli.

Fungal granulomas, usually in the form of enlarged lymph nodes that compress and invade the trachea, are rare. In an occasional instance, histoplasmosis, blastomycosis, and coccidioidomycosis have been the cause. The obstruction has consistently caused noisy respirations, and the etiology has been confirmed by tracheal tomograms and endoscopic biopsy followed by microbiologic study of the tissue. Appropriate chemotherapy generally affords partial relief of the clinical evidences of airway obstruction.

Ludwig's angina is an acute infection causing upper airway obstruction that occurs predominantly in adults. The initial source of infection may be an abscessed mandibular tooth. It is characterized by brawny induration of the submandibular space and by edema of the floor of the mouth and base of the tongue, sometimes extending into the larynx. The usual causative organism is the *Streptococcus*. This rapidly progressive infection should be treated promptly with penicillin. In advanced disease, wide incision and drainage and tracheostomy may be required as lifesaving measures.

Fibrosing (sclerosing) mediastinitis is most often a consequence to antecedent histoplasmosis mediastinitis. However, it may also be associated with various fibrosing diseases, such as Riedel's struma or retroperitoneal fibrosis. It also has been associated with methysergide therapy for headaches. Regardless of the cause, involvement of the trachea is rarely clinically evident even though the vena cava, esophagus, and pulmonary vessels are frequently compressed.

Trauma

This group of conditions has accounted for the vast majority of major airway obstruction seen in recent years.

THERAPEUTIC INTUBATION

Emergency and intensive care of patients with severe respiratory impairment has not only saved many lives but also has caused iatrogenic problems. Tracheal intubation for 3 to 7 days, using nasal or orotracheal tubes, often causes inflammation and stricture either of the larynx or of the site at which the inflated balloon cuff is exerting pressure. To avoid this complication, when controlled ventilation is in prospect for more than a few days, a tracheostomy is used to introduce a cuffed tube, thereby avoiding the laryngeal or local tracheal trauma. However, this improvement has introduced a new potential site for stricture, i.e., the site of the tracheostomy. The site of stricture strongly influences the dynamics of airway obstruction since the larynx and tracheostomy sites are in the extrathoracic trachea, whereas the cuff site is usually in the intrathoracic trachea.

Many innovations designed to reduce the lateral pressure of the cuff on the tracheal wall, frequent deflation of the cuff seal, and reduction of excessive movement of the tubing by externally connected equipment have reduced the incidence of strictures. However, despite these precautions, the prospect of postintubation stricture should be kept in mind for as long as 2 years after extubation. Of all strictures that produce symptoms, about 80 percent become clinically apparent within 3 months of extubation. Strictures can be dilated by a rigid bronchoscope and by dilators. Bypass tracheostomy is sometimes necessary. At that time, stents can be placed in the strictured area for weeks or months to allow scarring at a larger diameter. Segmental (sleeve) resection of the stricture with end-to-end anastomosis can be done as a last resort since the trachea can be mobilized for anastomosis after resection of a sizable stenotic segment. Dependable tubular prostheses to bridge a large tracheal gap are not currently available.

BLUNT TRAUMA TO CHEST OR NECK

Fracture of the larynx usually results from direct trauma, whereas fracture of the trachea usually follows blunt chest trauma, such as a blow from a steering wheel during an automobile accident; the tracheal fracture is regularly just above the bifurcation. As in the case of blood vessels in the chest, the most vulnerable site for fracture is at the junction of a fixed and free portion of tubing or at a bifurcation where opposing forces cause a sheering effect. Prompt endoscopy is necessary to identify the site of fracture. Usually, surgical intervention is not necessary; on occasion immediate surgical repair is imperative, particularly when major atelectasis has resulted from the tear. Should the fracture result in a persistent and significant stricture of the airway, surgical repair of the stricture becomes necessary.

FOREIGN BODIES

If foreign bodies manage to pass the vocal cords, they usually lodge distal to the bifurcation of the trachea. In children, all sorts of things put in the mouth at play may end up in the major airways. Unless parents or older siblings happen to observe the accident, only cough and wheeze often give a clue to the problem, especially if the object is radiolucent. Obstructive pneumonitis or atelectasis are common complications; but, before this stage, successful bronchoscopic removal of the foreign body, usually with an open, rigid bronchoscope, is one of the most gratifying experiences in the practice of medicine.

Foreign bodies in the airways of adults come from dentures aspirated during accidents or from food during meals, particularly if the presence of a complete upper denture or liberal ingestion of alcohol has dulled the reactivity of the pharynx.

The term *café coronary* has been given to the wedging of a bolus of food, usually steak, in the hypopharynx and upper portion of the larynx. Often it occurs in a restaurant. It is differentiated from a true coronary in that the victim is alert, often participating actively in a conversation across the dinner table, but suddenly cannot talk or breathe. If breathing is judged to be completely obstructed, emergency treatment is directed to produce an "artificial cough." The first and quickest maneuver consists of four blows on the back, with the heel of the hand firmly striking the interscapular spinal column. If breathing does not resume, the second maneuver, consisting of four "manual thrusts," should follow (Fig. 71-1). The rescuer stands behind the victim, embracing the lower part of the chest or upper portion of the abdomen from back to front. After locking the embrace, by grasping one fist with the other hand, the rescuer presses strongly into the victim's chest or upper abdomen with quick backward thrusts. This maneuver causes forceful exhalation, and dislodges the obstructing bolus in at least 60 percent of cases. This second maneuver may be repeated. The third maneuver involves the use of finger probes. The index finger is inserted inside the cheek, deeply into the throat beside the base of the tongue, palpating for the bolus and moving it laterally toward the opposite pharyngeal wall. Care should be taken to avoid pushing the bolus deeper into the larynx. As a result of these three innovative methods, in the past several years pocketknife tracheotomies have rarely been needed.

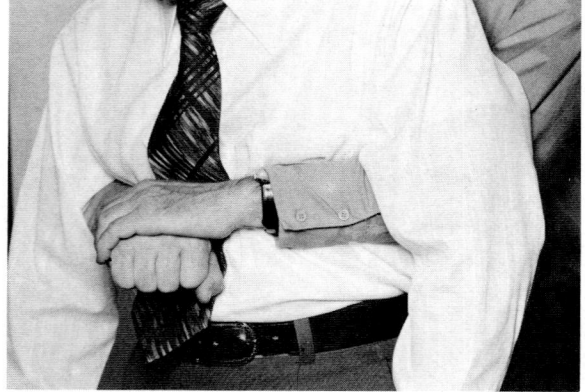

FIGURE 71-1 Arm and fist position over the lower chest and epigastrium for the four "manual thrusts" that are used to dislodge a bolus of food that has been aspirated into the hypopharynx or upper larynx.

INHALATION BURNS

Reports from burn centers reveal that 15 or more percent of patients admitted for special management have significant inhalation burns leading to stenosis of the trachea or larynx. About 20 percent of all patients admitted require laryngotracheal intubation or tracheostomy to maintain life support. Tracheostomy is generally not preferred because the inflammatory response on the internal surface of the trachea predisposes even more to the usual mechanical problems with maintaining a tracheostomy which in turn could enhance further stenosis. With more sophisticated cuffed endotracheal tubes, the longer periods of nasotracheal intubation have been possible without local trauma, and some patients with inhalation burns have been managed for 3 weeks with intubation, avoiding tracheostomy.

Neurogenic Disorders

Impairment of one vocal cord by paralysis of one recurrent laryngeal nerve leads to hoarseness but not to dyspnea, since the other cord can still be abducted. Bilateral paralysis allows good phonation because both cords vibrate similarly, but the chink at the glottis allows ventilation to increase only slightly above resting levels. Most commonly, bilateral paralysis occurs shortly after thyroidectomy so that the nature of the dyspnea and inspiratory stridor is clear. However, sometimes the impairment is delayed or is not immediately evident to the patient. Also, on rare occasions, an obscure neuropathy or diffuse carcinoma of the thyroid gland causes bilateral paralysis. Indirect laryngoscopy identifies the nature of the local laryngeal lesion, but often diagnostic measures are required to identify the underlying cause of nerve paralysis.

Neoplastic Obstruction of Major Airways

Obstruction of the larynx and trachea is caused by both malignant and benign neoplasms.

MALIGNANT TUMORS

Squamous cell cancer of the larynx is very common and usually attracts medical attention because of hoarseness rather than the airway obstruction which occurs later. Prompt attention by a laryngologist offers several modes of treatment, depending on the location and extent of the lesion. Frequently, the larynx can be preserved.

An entirely different problem is posed by squamous cell cancer of the trachea. This, as well as other malignant tumors of the trachea, may mimic diffuse obstructive diseases of the airways and may be mistakenly treated as asthma for a considerable time. The resultant delay complicates the management of a malignant disease that is difficult to treat even under ideal conditions. Sleeve resection and reanastomosis of the major airway is often

especially difficult because of mediastinal nodal involvement and the contiguity of vital structures. When surgical resection is not feasible, radiation therapy affords the prospect for palliation since squamous cell cancers are somewhat responsive to irradiation.

Cylindroma, also called *adenoid cystic carcinoma*, is a low-grade cancer that occurs in the trachea (Fig. 71-2). Fortunately it is uncommon, because it almost never is resectable, and it is resistant to radiotherapy. Some patients have been sustained in their usual way of life by periodic, endoscopic trimming and, more recently, YAG laser evaporation of the tumor; nearly one-half of these have lived comfortably for more than 10 years after the onset of symptoms.

Mucoepidermoid carcinoma is somewhat less malignant (Fig. 71-3) and much less common than the cylindroma. Usually, neither lesion metastasizes, but each is likely to recur locally after partial or attempted complete removal.

Adenocarcinoma in the trachea is usually metastatic, often from the breast, or possibly from a peripheral pri-

mary tumor in the lung. Chemotherapy is occasionally used, the type being dictated by the site of the primary lesion. This tumor is resistant to radiation therapy.

Small cell (oat cell) undifferentiated carcinoma is considered to be inoperable, regardless of its location in the airways. This general rule also applies to the trachea. Tracheal obstruction is usually the result of invasion from mediastinal lymph nodes. Until recently, chemotherapy provided little promise; fewer than 5 percent of patients survived for 2 years after traditional radiation therapy and nitrogen mustard. During the last few years, combined chemotherapy, using three or four anticancer drugs, has improved the outlook considerably for more sustained improvement.

Lymphomas encroach on the trachea by way of diffuse mediastinal lymph node involvement. Although lymphoma is a common neoplasm, it is one of the uncommon causes of significant tracheal narrowing. Encroachment usually results in diffuse, rather than localized, tracheal narrowing. The prognosis is similar to that of the same lymphoma elsewhere in the body. Response to radiation

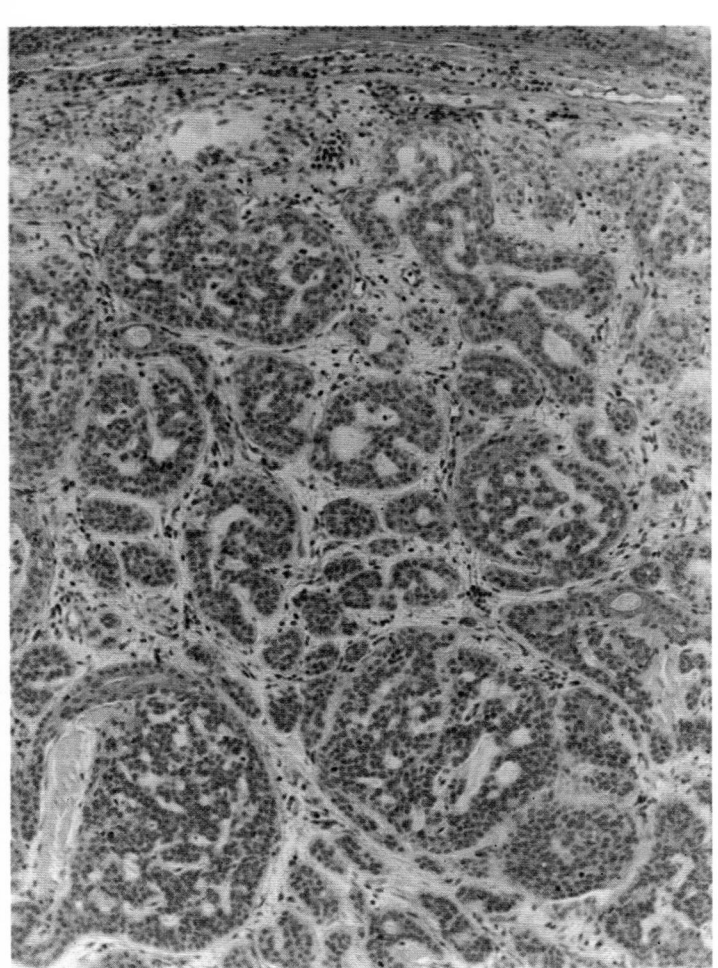

FIGURE 71-2   Adenoid cystic carcinoma (cylindroma) of the trachea. H&E; ×22.

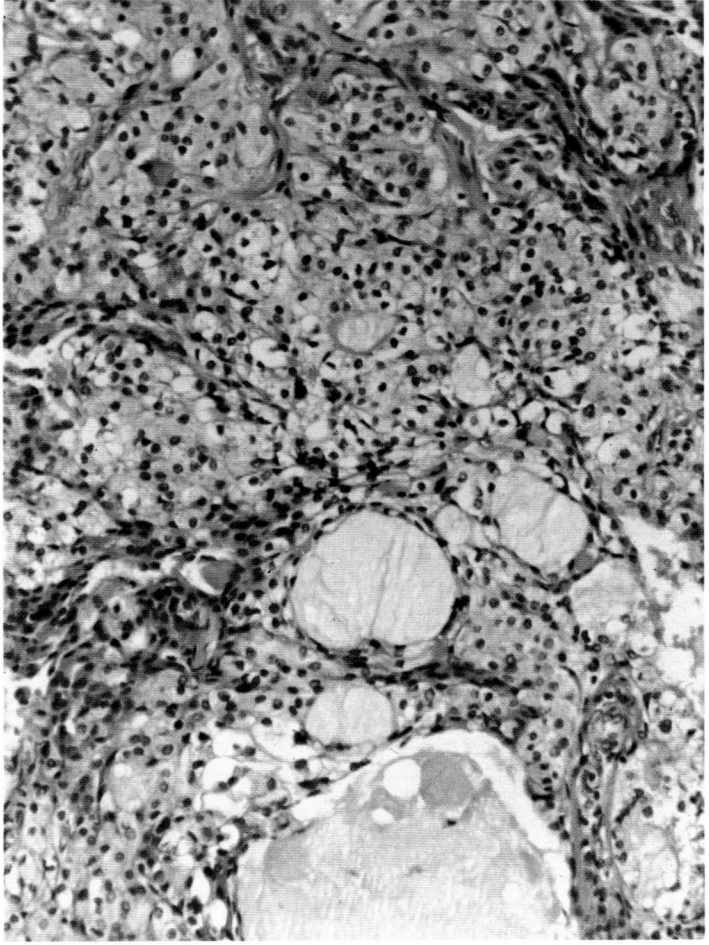

FIGURE 71-3   Mucoepidermoid carcinoma of the trachea showing formation of mucus between areas of epithelioid cells. H&E; ×37.

and chemotherapy usually provides some temporary improvement in airway diameter.

Leiomyosarcoma and chondrosarcoma are very rare tumors in the trachea. If small and low grade, they can be resected; the outcome of surgery is generally a complete recovery.

Invasive thyroid cancer is an uncommon cause of cervical tracheal narrowing. At this late stage the carcinoma is generally beyond cure, but laryngectomy may provide prolonged freedom from airway obstruction.

BENIGN TUMORS

Like malignant tumors, benign tumors of the trachea are much less common than those of the bronchial system. Papillomatosis of the larynx is the most common and distressing of the benign tumors. This usually occurs in children who are less than 6 years old and persists through puberty; occasionally, papillomatosis of the larynx persists into adulthood or may even start in adulthood. The papillomas average 5 mm in diameter (Fig. 71-4A), but they may aggregate to form cauliflowerlike masses (Fig. 71-4B) that extend down into the trachea and occasionally into the bronchi. Even though no viruses have been isolated from the tumors, they are likely to be caused by a tumorigenic, double-stranded DNA-containing virus of the papovavirus or "wart"-producing group. These tumors not only cause severe hoarseness but also impinge on the airway, requiring removal and cautery. An immune deficiency has been suggested by the observation that administration of transfer factor in papillomatosis results in lymphocytic and plasma cell infiltration and sometimes in necrosis in the tumors. Endoscopic removal is still required after administering transfer factor, but less frequently. Individual squamous-covered polyps some-

times occur, particularly in the larynx; they generally do not recur after removal.

Fibrolipomas or lipomas are benign tumors usually found in middle-aged subjects and are rather easily removed endoscopically, usually through a large, rigid bronchoscope.

In contrast to thyroid cancer, thyroid adenomas do not invade the trachea. Even though they may become very large in the thoracic inlet and deviate the trachea considerably, the airway is usually not significantly compromised unless the membranous portion is compressed. If multiple intrathoracic adenomas encompass or compress the trachea from two sides, which is unusual, significant airway narrowing can occur. Most intrathoracic goiters can be removed through a cervical incision.

Obstruction of Upper Airways during Sleep

Obstruction of the hypopharynx and larynx during sleep produces a syndrome of alveolar hypoventilation that is achieving increasing recognition. This topic is considered elsewhere in this book.

Laryngotracheal Disease of Uncertain Cause

TRACHEOPATHICA OSTEOPLASTICA

More than 200 patients with this unusual disease have been reported in the literature. Its cause is obscure. It is characterized by multiple cartilaginous, or even osseous, projections into the tracheal lumen between and overlying cartilages that appear deformed (Fig. 71-5A). Usually, the lower three-fourths of the trachea and the beginning of its bifurcation are affected by lesions that result in considerable rigidity of the walls. The mucosa is usually intact, but it is often thinned, except in the posterior membra-

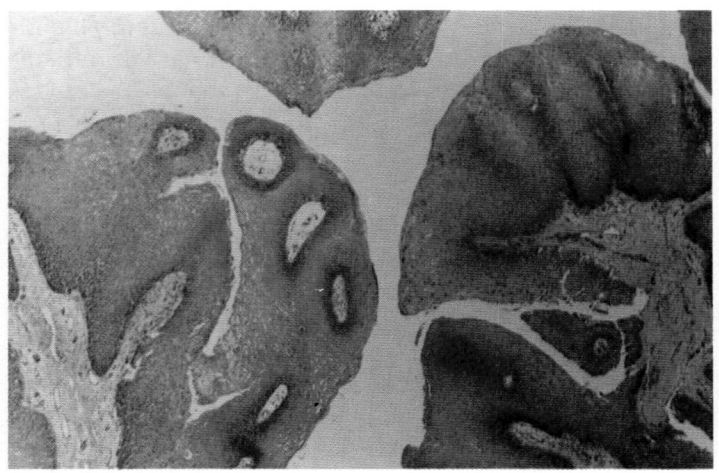

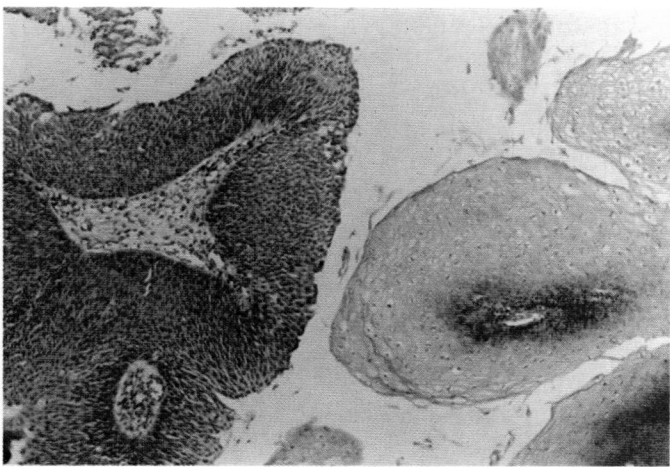

A

B

FIGURE 71-4 Laryngotracheal papillomatosis, usually in children and juveniles, is characterized by many soft wartlike tumors which must be repeatedly removed by cautery until they regress spontaneously. *A.* Simple wartlike formation. H&E; ×6. *B.* Small cauliflowerlike masses. Note cellular atypia of papilloma on left. H&E; ×10.

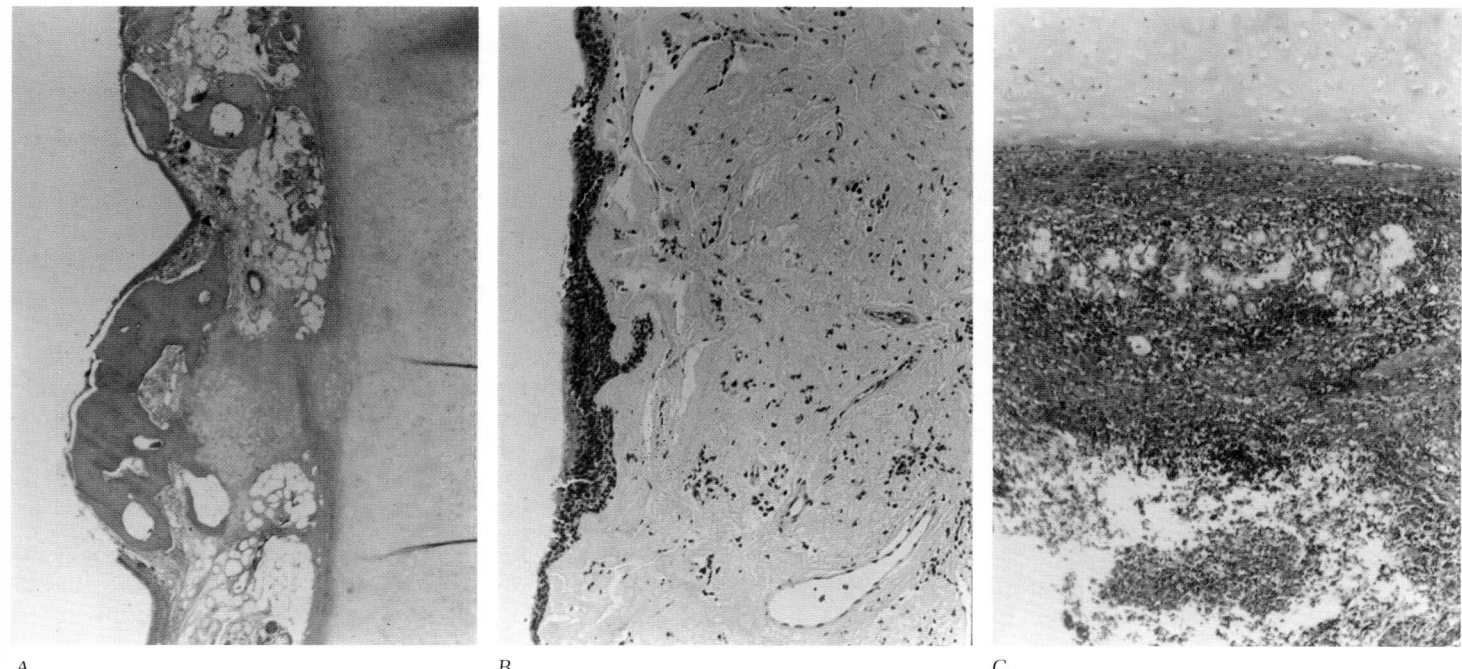

A   B   C

FIGURE 71-5 Laryngotracheal disease of uncertain cause. A. Tracheopathica osteoplastica. Low-power photomicrograph of histologic changes of cartilaginous ring of tracheopathica osteoplastica. Shown is an exuberant growth of cartilaginous rings projecting into the airway lumen covered by respiratory epithelium forming mounds or sharp projection. This not only increases airway resistance by mechanical encroachment but markedly impairs the mucociliary escalator mechanism, leading to retention of secretions in the central airways. H&E; ×4. B. Localized amyloid, left vocal cord. The treatment of tumor-forming amyloid is an endoscopic surgical procedure. Usually lesions are multiple along the tracheobronchial airway and, in these cases, pose a more complex and individualized therapeutic plan. H&E; ×15. C. Wegener's granulomatosis, an increasingly common vasculitis of the upper airways, the lungs, and the genitourinary tract. This biopsy was taken from a laryngeal mass. H&E; ×10.

nous portion, which is conspicuously free of involvement.

Dyspnea or stridor may pose problems. Also, clearing the secretions may be difficult because the mucociliary escalator is impaired at sites of involvement. Endoscopic biopsy is difficult and is usually better accomplished with larger forceps passed through an open, rigid bronchoscope. The condition is seen in about 1 in 2000 bronchoscopies.

RELAPSING POLYCHONDRITIS

This systemic disorder affects cartilage in many sites. It is often associated with rheumatoid arthritis or lupus erythematosus. The "flappy" ears and "saddlenose" deformity cause cosmetic concern, while involvement of the tracheal rings causes severe function impairment because collapsing segments of the trachea or the larynx impair the cough (Fig. 71-6). The disorder occurs at all ages and affects males and females equally. During exacerbations, collapse of the trachea can cause death; on occasion, tracheostomy has been lifesaving.

Painful swelling and redness of various cartilages signal a relapse. Episcleritis, iritis, conjunctivitis, and, later,

cataracts and hearing impairment are part of the disorder. Cardiac valvular and aortic involvement also occur.

Values for excretion of acid mucopolysaccharides in the urine are increased during exacerbations. Histologic study of involved cartilage shows fragmentation and loss of basophilic staining of the matrix, replacement by connective tissue, calcification, and acute-to-chronic inflammation. It has been postulated that lysosomal enzymes cause release of chondroitin sulfate from the cartilage matrix.

TUMOR-FORMING AMYLOID

This is a very rare disease and probably is a subgroup of primary amyloidosis, because it is unrelated to chronic infectious or wasting diseases. The muscle is often involved from submucosa to adventitia, sometimes forming protruding masses that impair airflow in the trachea or major bronchi (Fig. 71-5B). A solitary tumor nodule of the larynx, trachea, or major bronchus is the most common pulmonary form of amyloid. Clinically it first becomes manifest by hoarseness, wheezing, dyspnea, or hemoptysis, depending on the site and intactness of the mucosa. Multiple amyloid masses of the major airways also occur.

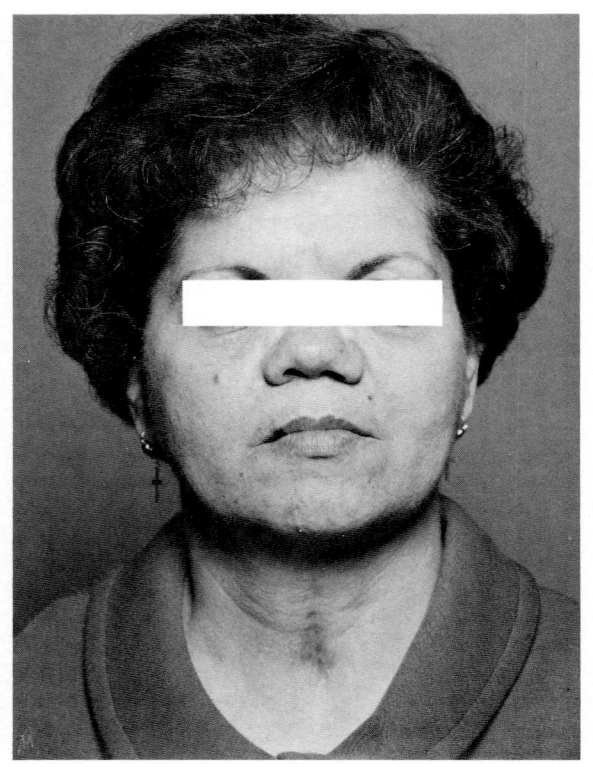

A

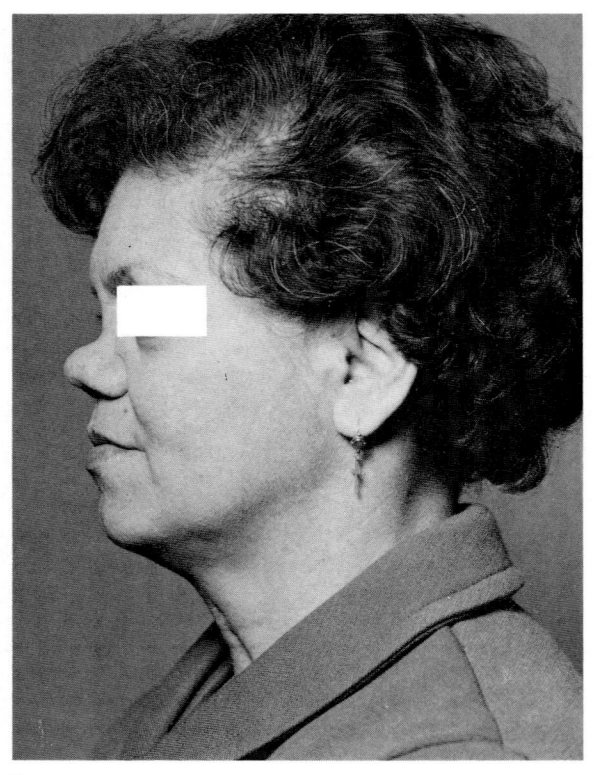

B

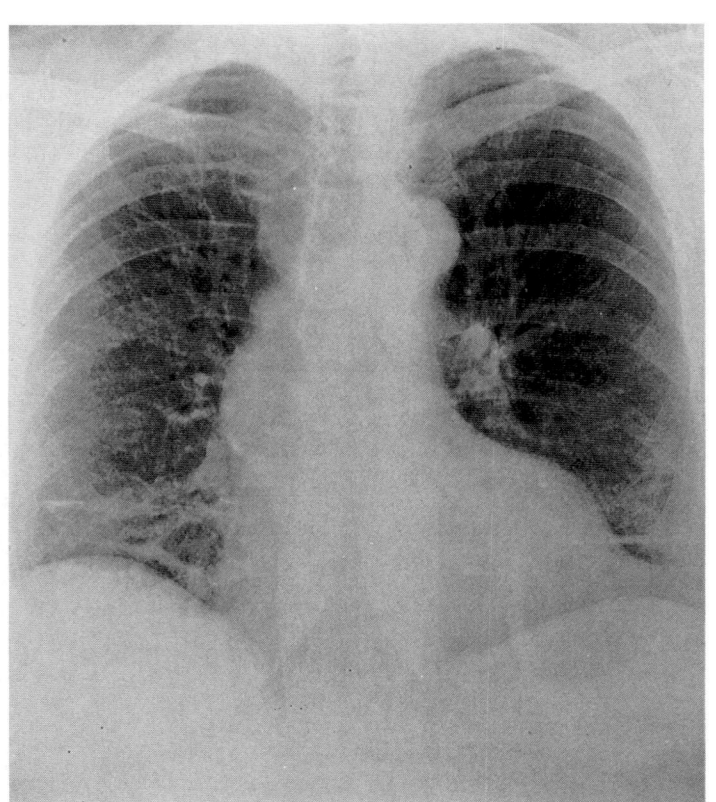

C

FIGURE 71-6 Multicartilaginous changes of relapsing polychondritis. *A.* Front view. Defect from tracheostomy that was necessary to relieve airways obstruction caused by swelling and distortion of cartilages in the trachea and larynx. The helix of each ear was also abnormally pliable. *B.* Profile view. A plastic prosthesis that had been inserted to support the saddle nose was extruded, and the deformity recurred. *C.* Chest radiograph showing numerous areas of linear atelectasis. These were attributed to obstruction of the airways arising from distortion of bronchial cartilages and subsequent inspissation of mucus.

Diagnosis is made by biopsy performed endoscopically, distinction having to be made from tracheopathica osteoplastica. Local lesions can be resected, but the less common diffuse tracheobronchial amyloid is not amenable to treatment.

TRACHEOMALACIA

The condition is so common in newborns that it can be considered a variant of normal. The cartilaginous rings are pliable, or some are congenitally absent, small, or malformed. These abnormalities lead to functional stenosis during an upper respiratory infection. Airway obstruction is usually not evident during quiet breathing. In infants, the diagnosis is made by excluding causes of local secondary tracheomalacia caused by compression by vascular rings, foreign bodies, tracheal web, or mediastinal tumor. Once other causes have been excluded, a program of nonintervention is adopted, because the cartilages can be expected to mature to a normal state, usually by 6 months of age and certainly by 1 year. The aural and other external cartilages are practical guides to maturation since they show concomitant stiffening.

Secondary tracheomalacia in adults is discussed in the earlier section, "Therapeutic Intubation." Continuous compression by cuffed tubes makes secondary tracheomalacia one of the most common causes of major airway obstruction in adults. The key to this problem is prevention during the management of respiratory failure. Fortunately, newer cuffed tubes provide a broader base requiring less focal pressure on the tracheal mucosa. This has led to a decreased incidence of this problem.

SARCOIDOSIS

The larynx is affected in less than 1 percent of patients with sarcoidosis. Hoarseness is virtually a regular feature, and infiltrative and nodular lesions are seen on bronchoscopy. In contrast to the rarity of laryngeal lesions, particularly of involvement of the true vocal cords, endobronchial sarcoidosis is exceedingly common, ranging from 30 to 100 percent, with the highest frequency in stage III sarcoidosis.

WEGENER'S GRANULOMATOSIS

As described in Chapter 69, in Wegener's granulomatosis the respiratory tract is characteristically involved in a granulomatous inflammatory process in which necrosis, ulceration, and necrotizing angiitis are prominent features. Often the process first becomes evident in the nose and sinuses but, in time, laryngeal and pulmonary symptoms develop. Persistent hoarseness is the signal of laryngeal involvement often in conjunction with the lingering symptoms of rhinitis, sinusitis and otitis media. Biopsy of lesions in the nose or larynx reveals the characteristic pathology of Wegener's granulomatosis. By the time of biopsy, clinical evidence of the systemic disorder usually exists in the form of pansinusitis, pulmonary lesions, and glomerulonephritis.

Pathophysiological Aspects

Laryngoscopy and tracheoscopy provide direct access to observation of obstructive lesions, depending on their site. However, not infrequently, pulmonary function tests provide the first clue that the site of obstruction in a dyspneic patient with noisy breathing is in the upper airway.

Spirograms have gradually been replaced by the use of the flow-volume loop during forced vital capacity and forced inspiratory vital capacity maneuvers. This evolution has occurred because the flow-volume loop allows earlier detection and classification of patterns that reflect the dynamic changes in diameter of the trachea and larynx as affected by various lesions. As indicated elsewhere in this book, during forced vital capacity, the normal expiratory maximal flow-volume loop shows early attainment of peak flow, at 6 to 12 L/s, within the first 25 percent of the effort. In the lower three quarters of the vital capacity, airflow during expiration slows progressively because of greater narrowing of all intrathoracic and particularly intrapulmonary airways. The characteristic pattern during normal inspiration and expiration is shown as the outer solid line in Fig. 71-7.

VARIOUS PATTERNS OF FLOW-VOLUME LOOPS

Simulation of major or central airway narrowing can be produced by placing orifices of varied diameters near the mouthpiece in testing a normal subject. Forced expiratory and inspiratory flow-volume loops during vital capacity maneuvers are shown in Fig. 71-7. Obstruction in the major airway reduces flow at the highest point (peak flow) in both the expiratory and the inspiratory loops, resulting in a plateau at the highest flow rates. The diagram in Fig. 71-7 has been redrawn to eliminate the rapid oscillations in the plateau areas of the original records. This "noise" presumably reflects turbulence created by forced flow through local orifices. In the various pathologic states that are described above, three general patterns tend to occur. In "fixed," or rigid, circumferential lesions, such as many cicatricial strictures, the pattern (Fig. 71-8B) looks much like that created by the artificial orifice in the normal subject. Expiratory-inspiratory flows at mid-vital capacity ($FEF_{50\%}/FIF_{50\%}$) are approximately equal, with a ratio near or a little below 1, as in normal subjects. At the lowermost portion of the forced expiration curve, to the right of the plateau in Fig. 71-8B, the loop follows the normal pattern, showing flow limitation by diffuse deflated smaller airways rather than by the orifice of the stricture that limited flow at the higher lung volumes.

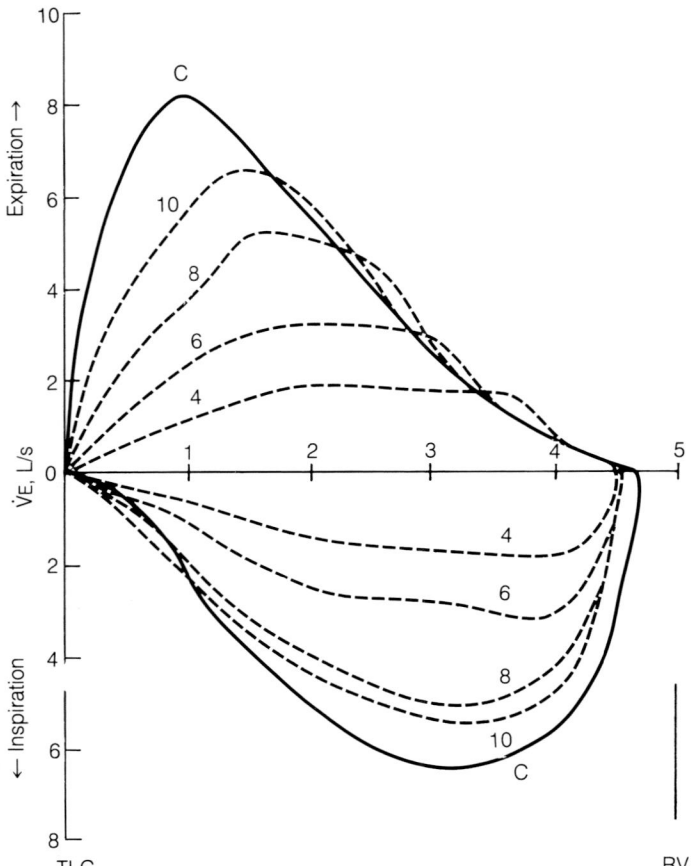

FIGURE 71-7 Family of forced expiratory and inspiratory curves throughout the vital capacity, performed by a normal adult. The greatest difference created by the orifices is at high lung volumes during forced expiration. Solid line shows the pattern without artificial obstruction. Each dashed curve shows the effect of orifices of progressively smaller diameters as labeled. Reduction in expiratory flow by a single obstruction at the opening of the central airways is greatest at the points of peak flow, as contrasted with the diffuse obstruction of smaller airways in which reduction of airflow occurs at lower lung volumes when rates of airflow are lower. The dashed curves resemble those of patients having fixed or rigid pathologic constriction of similar diameter in the tracheal or laryngeal lumen. TLC = total lung capacity. RV = residual volume. *(From Miller and Hyatt, 1969, with permission.)*

Some strictures in the major airway are "variable" and probably not circumferential (Fig. 71-8*C* and 71-8*D*). The physiologically variable lesions show an abnormality on only one portion of the loop, while the other half of the loop is relatively normal as shown. This is in contrast to the fixed lesion where both the inspiratory and expiratory loops are reduced similarly. Each will have a plateau-type deformity. The relative cross-sectional areas during forced expiration and inspiration depend on whether the localized narrowing in the central airway is intrathoracic or extrathoracic. Transmural pressure gradients tend to narrow the variable intrathoracic tracheal lesion during forced expiration, creating an orifice and resulting in a

plateau in the expiratory loop; the smaller the orifice, the lower and broader the plateau (Fig. 71-8*C*). Forced inspiration tends to open the orifice, creating a normal or near-normal inspiratory loop, depending on the resulting cross-sectional area. In contrast, the extrathoracic variable lesion tends to reduce cross-sectional area with forced inspiration because of inward transmural pressure, creating a plateau on the inspiratory loop. The pathologic orifice expands with forced expiration, with a relatively normal expiratory loop.

A variable intrathoracic lesion of the major airway causes expiratory-inspiratory flow ratios at mid-vital capacity ($FEF_{50\%}/FIF_{50\%}$) to be very low (Fig. 71-8*C*, solid line); the ratio resembles that of diffuse obstructive lung disease (Fig. 71-8*A*, dashed line). However, the expiratory loops do have sharply different patterns: the value of $FEF_{50\%}/FIF_{50\%}$ in variable extrathoracic obstruction is usually far above 1, creating a unique pattern and ratio. The so-called fixed lesions are probably not entirely fixed and often show modest changes in orifice diameter during the high transmural pressure changes from forced inspiration to forced expiration.

These distinctions have practical significance. Most fixed lesions (Fig. 71-9) and extrathoracic variable lesions are benign, the latter being most often bilateral vocal cord paralysis. Functionally, variable intrathoracic lesions include a higher proportion of cancers (Fig. 71-10). Elongated narrowing of the trachea, as with diffuse mediastinal adenopathy, causes tracheal narrowing without conforming to any of the three above unusual patterns or to the "scooped out" or concave expiratory flow-volume loop of chronic obstructive pulmonary disease (Fig. 71-8*A*). In diffuse narrowing, the expiratory loop reaches a low peak flow in the upper quarter of the vital capacity and then follows a rather straight diagonal line of uniformly decreasing flow to residual volume. The inspiratory loop also tends not to reach high peak flows but does not contain the characteristic plateau of a localized fixed narrowing. This pattern has been seen in a few cases of lymphoma and has shown dramatic reversion toward normal after irradiation. The airway dynamics in these elongated stenotic lesions are not well understood because too few such cases have been studied.

OTHER ABNORMALITIES IN PULMONARY FUNCTION

If flow-volume loops are not available, certain combinations of spirometric abnormalities may support the clinical diagnosis. The maximal voluntary ventilation is usually reduced more than the 1-s forced expiratory volume (FEV_1), especially if the inspiratory flow is impaired. The 1-s forced inspiratory volume (FIV_1) is often slowed, which is not seen with obstructive bronchitis or emphysema. The relative changes in FEV_1 and peak expiratory flow as compared with FIV_1 and peak inspiratory flow

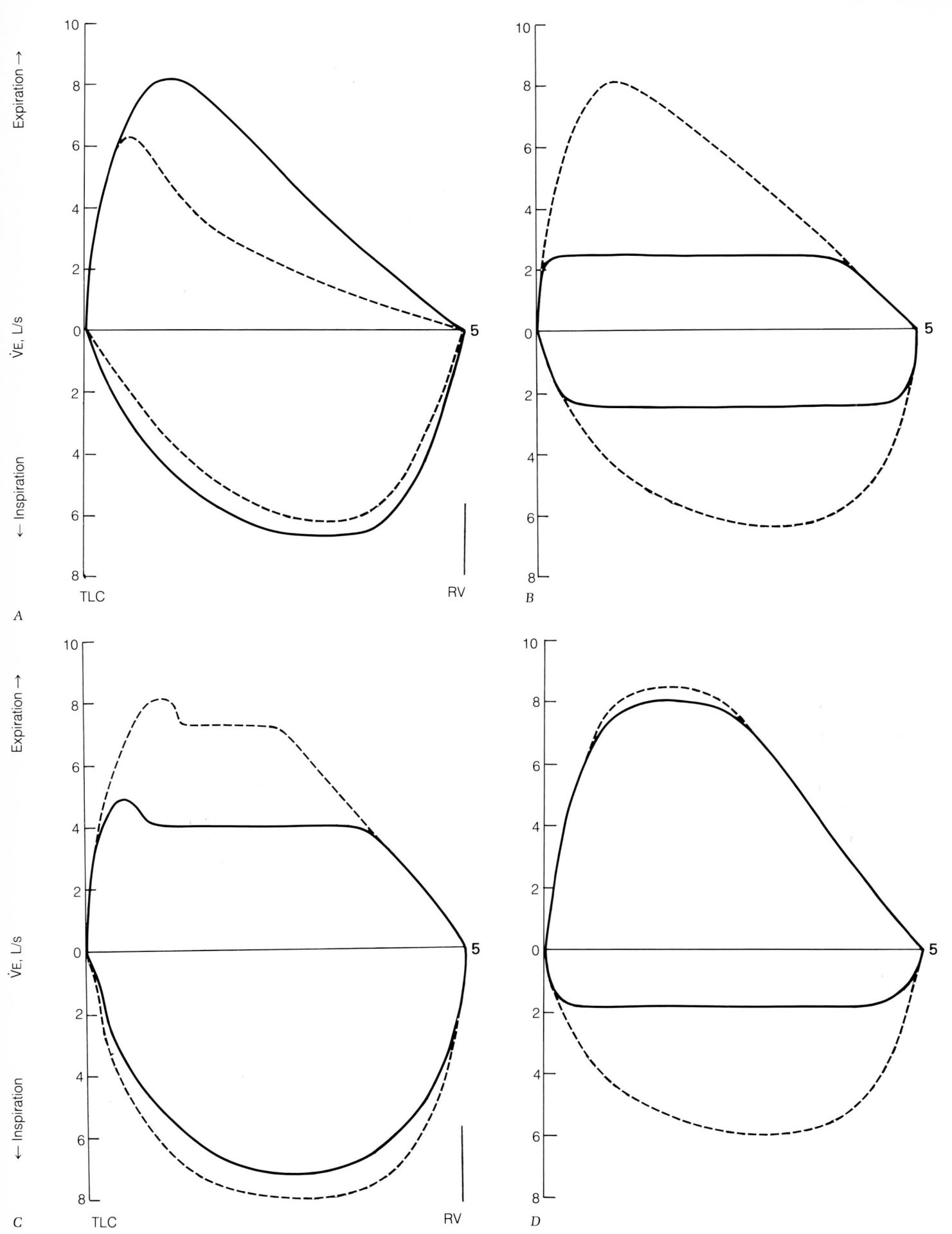

depend on the cross-sectional area at the site of pathologic change during these maneuvers. These changes are not as pronounced or as graphic as those on the flow-volume loop (Fig. 71-8). Airway resistance is usually very high, and indexes of intrapulmonary gas mixing are relatively normal in the absence of bronchitis or retained secretions. Hypoxia occurs during exercise when the lesion produces an orifice of less than 8 mm in diameter.

Clinical Diagnosis

Whenever major airway obstruction is suspected, the patient should be queried about past tracheal intubation, thyroid surgery, and neck or chest injuries. If there is no history of any of these, the occurrence of hemoptysis suggests the possibility of neoplasm. Current or past febrile illness raises the suspicion of nodal compression or infectious invasion of the central airway.

Physical examination should always include listening near the patient's open mouth with the unaided ear during forced inspiration and expiration. Turbulence created in the larynx or trachea is best heard as stridor in this way; it is not heard as well with the stethoscope over the lung fields. Auscultation over the manubrium or neck also may identify the stridor. These findings and a high index of suspicion may lead to a working clinical diagnosis even before pulmonary function tests are done.

CONFIRMATION OF NATURE OF OBSTRUCTION

Laryngoscopy or bronchoscopic examination of the trachea is required for tissue diagnosis of tumors or cicatricial strictures. If the fiber bronchoscope is used, care should be taken not to pass the tip beyond the small opening because of the threat that ventilation will be seriously compromised. The open, rigid bronchoscope has advantages besides providing an adequate airway. Dilatation of a benign stricture often can be carried out, sometimes providing definitive therapy. Prebronchoscopic review of flow-volume loops can guide the choice of the diameter of the rigid bronchoscope used, either for passing easily beyond the stricture or for dilating it, since the plateau of the flow-volume loop provides an estimate of the size of the major airway narrowing (Fig. 71-7). Management is dictated by the nature of the narrowing. Early clinical suspicion of major airway obstruction and appropriate early action can be lifesaving. The remarkable relief of successful diagnosis and correction of a localized obstruction can be equally gratifying to the patient, the physician, and the surgeon.

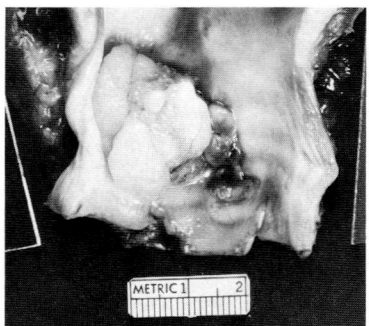

FIGURE 71-10 Variable intrathoracic obstruction. Illustrated is the mucoepidermoid carcinoma (1.6 × 2.1 × 1.0 cm) removed by sleeve resection from the anterolateral wall of the trachea. The patient was a 26-year-old woman who had become cushingoid because of corticosteroid treatment for asthma. Because only one-fourth of the wall was involved, the remainder of the circumference of the wall was free to expand and contract during maximum inspiration, producing a variable loop as in Fig. 71-8C. The expiratory plateau was even lower than the prototype shown in Fig. 71-8C, with flows of only 0.5 L/s.

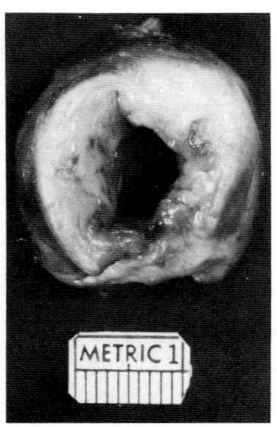

FIGURE 71-9 Tracheal stenosis. Circumferential constriction of the upper trachea followed prolonged cuffed intubation and mechanical ventilation. The strictured segment of trachea affected three cartilaginous rings and produced changes similar to those shown by the solid line in Fig. 71-8B. Postoperatively, the curves resembled those shown by the dashed line in Fig. 71-8B. If these strictures are circumferential and firm, they will result in a fixed orifice-type lesion (Fig. 71-8B). *If the fibrous tissue is loose and somewhat pliable, the loop will be variable as in Fig. 71-8C.*

◄ **FIGURE 71-8** Group of curves illustrating differing patterns resulting from different types of pathologic lesions. *A.* Obstruction of small airways. Solid line displays the normal pattern; dashed line displays the pattern of diffuse obstruction of small airways in which the greatest reduction of flow occurs at the middle and lower thirds of the forced vital capacity (FVC). *B.* Fixed obstruction of cervical or intrathoracic trachea. Solid line shows effect of a structure of the trachea after prolonged controlled ventilation using a cuffed tube for acute respiratory failure. A circumferential cicatricial narrowing occurred at the site of the inflated balloon resulting in a mean diameter of about 7 mm. Resection of the constricted segment, followed by anastomosis of the normal cut edges of the trachea, resulted in the normal loop 12 weeks later (dashed line). *C.* Variable intrathoracic obstruction. Solid line shows curve of variable intrathoracic obstruction resulting from a squamous cell cancer on the lateral wall of the lower part of the trachea. Forced expiration produced a fixed flow because of dynamic compression at the site of the lesion; the dynamic compression uniformly limited airflow until a point about 30 percent from residual volume, where the lowest part of the curve became normal. Forced inspiration is relatively normal. After radiation therapy, flow during expiration improved, but the expiratory pattern remained abnormal (dashed line). *D.* Extrathoracic obstruction. Obstruction outside the thorax (solid line) causes transmural pressure gradients during forced expiration and inspiration to be opposite in direction from those produced by an intrathoracic variable lesion. Bilateral vocal cord paralysis resulted in a slitlike orifice with lateral diameter of 1 to 2 mm and an anteroposterior diameter of approximately 6 to 8 mm during forced expiration, also improving somewhat the anteroposterior diameter. Improvement in flows (dashed curve) followed arytenoidectomy.

BIBLIOGRAPHY

Al-Bazzaz F, Grillo H, Kazemi H: Response to exercise in upper airway obstruction. Am Rev Respir Dis 111:631–640, 1975.
Seven patients with tracheal stenosis demonstrated hypoxemia with exercise. It was corrected after excision or surgical repair of the stenotic lesion. Preoperative fall in Pa$_{O_2}$ averaged 11 mmHg.

American Heart Association, Committee on Emergency Cardiac Care: First aid for foreign body obstruction of the airway (interim recommendations). April 9, 1976.
This is a practical outline of management for acute obstruction by a foreign body in the airways by a group of authorities preparing this consensus statement.

Andrews MJ, Pearson FG: An analysis of 59 cases of tracheal stenosis following tracheostomy with cuffed tube and assisted ventilation, with special reference to diagnosis and treatment. Br J Surg 60:208–212, 1973.
A succinct review of conservative and operative management of benign tracheal strictures and the indications where tracheostomy is required in the management.

Brodovsky DM: Laryngeal tuberculosis in an age of chemotherapy. Can J Otol 4:168–176, 1975.
This concise review shows a prevalence of 1.5 percent of laryngeal tuberculosis among 1383 patients with pulmonary tuberculosis, an interesting observation in this era of successful tuberculosis chemotherapy.

Cramblett HG: Croup (epiglottitis; laryngitis; laryngotracheobronchitis), in Kendig EL Jr (ed), *Pulmonary Diseases*, 2d ed, vol I. *Disorders of the Respiratory Tract in Children.* Philadelphia, Saunders, 1972, pp 209–216.
This report describes the high incidence of epiglottitis, laryngitis, and laryngotracheobronchitis in a pediatric age group, the mechanisms by which the syndrome occurs, the various etiologies, and the generally conservative successful management sometimes requiring more aggressive intervention.

Grillo HC: Obstructive lesions of the trachea. Ann Otol Rhinol Laryngol 82:770–777, 1973.
An extensive review of one of the largest personal experiences in the world of surgical approach to correcting lesions causing severe airflow obstruction in the trachea.

Grillo HC: Management of tracheal tumors. Am J Surg 123:697–700, 1982.
In this series of 110 primary tumors, resection of up to one-half of the trachea was possible. Seventy-three had primary reanastomosis and 17 laryngotracheal resection leading to long-term palliation or cure when complete resection was possible.

Grillo HC, Zannini P: Resectional management of airway invasion by thyroid carcinoma. Ann Thorac Surg 42:287–298, 1986.
Invasion of the trachea by thyroid carcinoma is best managed by resection with airway reconstruction.

Houston HE, Payne WS, Harrison EG Jr, Olsen AM: Primary cancers of the trachea. Arch Surg 99:132–139, 1969.
This review of the literature adds 53 cases of primary cancer of the trachea diagraming location and varieties of surgical approaches.

Hyatt RE: Forced expiration, in Macklem PT, Mead J (eds), *Handbook of Physiology, sect 3: Respiration, vol III: Mechanics of Breathing.* Bethesda, MD, American Physiological Society, 1986, pp 295–314.
A review of the physiological bases for evaluating a forced expiration and of approaches to quantifying the FVC.

Lund T, Goodwin CW, McManus WF, Shirani KZ, Stallings RJ, Mason AD Jr, Pruitt BA Jr: Upper airway sequelae in burn patients requiring endotracheal intubation or tracheostomy. Ann Surg 201:374–382, 1985.
Twenty percent of 217 adult burn patients required endotracheal intubation or tracheostomy. Sixteen percent had significant inhalation injury. Spirometry aided in noninvasive screening and xeroradiograms were helpful in assessing tracheal stenosis.

Mathew OP, Remmers JE: Respiratory function of the upper airway, in Saunders NA, Sullivan CE (eds), *Sleep and Breathing.* New York, Dekker, 1984, pp 163–200.
A consideration of the respiratory functions of the neural, muscular, and mechanical aspects of the upper airway. Other chapters in the book consider the sleep apnea syndromes.

Miller RD, Hyatt RE: Obstructing lesions of the larynx and trachea: Clinical and physiologic characteristics. Mayo Clin Proc 44:145–161, 1969.
   Describes the patterns of flow-volume loops based on the location in the central airways and the dynamic behavior of the obstruction that has come to be the generally accepted classification of major airways obstructing lesions.

Miller RD, Hyatt RE: Evaluation of obstructing lesions of the trachea and larynx by flow-volume loops. Am Rev Respir Dis 108:475–481, 1973.
   Includes a larger series of cases showing variations of the flow-volume loop based on the dynamic behavior of the obstructive lesions.

Parr GV, Unger M, Trout RG, Atkinson WG: One hundred neodymium-YAG laser ablation of obstructing tracheal neoplasms. Ann Thorac Surg 38:374–381, 1984.
   This report describes ablations of nonresectable obstructing tracheal neoplasms in 40 patients, usually requiring more than one treatment.

Powell N, Guilleminault C, Riley R, Smith L: Mandibular advancement and obstructive sleep apnea syndrome. Bull Eur Physiopathol Respir 19:607–610, 1983.
   A case report of an obese patient with retrognathia and obstructive sleep apnea who responded only to advancement of the mandible. This report extends the observations of Lugaresi and Coccagna on heavy snoring and obstructive sleep apnea in micrognathia.

Proctor DF: State of the art, the upper airways. II. The larynx and trachea. Am Rev Respir Dis 115:315–342, 1977.
   This very comprehensive review of the literature and the author's experience is probably the most detailed review of the anatomy, physiology, and pathology of the upper airways.

Proctor DF: Form and function of the upper airways and larynx, in Macklem PT, Mead J (eds), *Handbook of Physiology, sect 3: Respiration, vol III: Mechanics of Breathing.* Bethesda, MD, American Physiological Society, 1986, pp 63–74.
   A well-annotated review of the upper respiratory tract as a conducting airway and the physiological and clinical consequences of obstruction along this path.

Sackner MA, Landa J, Forrest T, Greeneltch D: Periodic sleep apnea: Chronic sleep deprivation related to intermittent upper airway obstruction and central nervous system disturbance. Chest 67:164–171, 1975.
   This report shows graphic sleep studies and the nature of upper airways obstruction as it occurs in various types of sleep apnea.

Widdicombe JG: Role of the parasympathetic cholinergic system in normal and obstructed airways. Respiration 50(Suppl):1–8, 1986.
   The cholinergic motor component of the parasympathetic nervous system supplies several structures which may be important in determining the resistance of normal and diseased airways.

Wolf C, Le Jeune FE Jr, Douglas JR Jr: A technique for intubation of the difficult airway. Otolaryngol Head Neck Surg 96:278–281, 1987.
   A tubular laryngoscope and a hollow wand (or guide) are used to bypass an obstructive friable tumor mass in the hypopharynx for delivery of O_2.

Chapter 72

The Kidney and Acid-Base Disorders in Obstructive Disease of the Airways

George M. Feldman / Zalman S. Agus

The hydrogen ion concentration in bodily fluids is determined by the ratio of the concentrations of carbon dioxide and bicarbonate. Whereas the lungs are responsible for modulating arterial P_{CO_2}, the kidneys are responsible for modulating the concentration of bicarbonate in plasma. In concert, these organs maintain a stable milieu in the extracellular fluid volume that is readily assessed by measuring arterial pH. The role of the kidneys in acid-base homeostasis is to control the metabolic consequence of cellular oxidative metabolism and to respond to other stimuli, such as altered P_{CO_2} resulting from lung disorders.

In addition to their function in acid-base balance, the kidneys maintain circulating arterial blood volume and ionic strength and composition. That is, they respond to varied intake of salt and water and excrete the appropriate quantity of solute and water in the urine to maintain the internal milieu within a tolerable range. In pulmonary disorders and in the treatment of these disorders, this renal role may be compromised.

The normal internal environment is maintained within narrow limits: the arterial blood pH is kept remarkably close to 7.40, whereas virtually all bodily fluids have an osmolality of 285 mosmol/kg body water. In addition, the total water content of the body is maintained at 60 percent of the body weight, compartmentalized into intracellular and extracellular volumes. The extracellular water volume is 25 percent of the total body volume, and the remainder of the water is within cells. The fluid circulating in the vascular system makes up one-third of the extracellular compartment.

Renal maintenance of the internal milieu occurs while large quantities of plasma are being filtered, i.e., 120 ml/min or 170 L per day. This large filtration rate implies that a major function of the kidney is to reabsorb more than 99 percent of the filtered fluid and solute just to maintain circulating volume. This reabsorptive process is remarkably selective in that the reabsorbate is appropriate, both in volume and composition, to maintain the internal environment, whereas noxious substances are duly excreted.

ACID-BASE BALANCE

The normal state of acid-base balance is characterized by arterial blood that has a pH of 7.40 (H^+ concentration of 40 nM), a bicarbonate concentration of 24.5 meq/L, and a P_{CO_2} of 40 mmHg. By convention, discussions of acid-base balance generally focus on acid intake and output rather than base intake and output. However, in biologic systems, the designations *acid* and *base* are complex, because the H^+ or OH^- is often generated from neutral precursors. Outside the body neither ammonium chloride nor sodium lactate is a particularly strong acid or base. However, ingested ammonium chloride is equivalent to ingested hydrochloric acid since the ammonium ion is metabolized to urea and H^+; similarly, ingested sodium lactate is, in effect, converted to bicarbonate.

Normal cellular metabolism generates large quantities of acid daily. By far, most of the metabolic acid is produced in the form of CO_2. In addition, metabolism generates nonvolatile, or "fixed," acid at a daily rate of approximately 1 meq/kg per day. The source of the major portion of these fixed acids is the oxidation of sulfur-containing proteins to sulfuric acid. Although the quantity of acid produced appears small in comparison to exhaled CO_2, if it is not excreted, life-threatening metabolic acidosis ensues. Therefore, for a normal individual, to maintain acid-base balance, 70 meq of fixed acid must be excreted daily. It is the kidneys that are responsible for the excretion of metabolically produced, nonvolatile acid.

Once released from cells, the H^+ ions titrate blood bicarbonate and nonbicarbonate buffers, while the anions, e.g., sulfate, coproduced with the H^+ ions, remain dissociated. In the kidneys, base, in the form of bicarbonate, is actively returned to blood, to replenish the previously consumed blood buffer base. The process of renal regeneration of buffer base depends on the urinary excretion of H^+ ions. That is, for every H^+ ion excreted, a bicarbonate is returned to the body. Although acid excretion by the kidneys is an active cellular process, excretion of the co-

produced anions, such as sulfate, depends entirely on filtration.

In addition to the generation of bicarbonate that titrates or neutralizes acid produced metabolically, the kidneys must also reabsorb the large filtered load of bicarbonate in order to hold constant the bicarbonate content of the body. Assuming a filtration rate of 120 ml/min, 4300 meq of bicarbonate is filtered daily, an amount that is 60-fold greater than that lost metabolically each day. Since excretion and loss into the urine of even a small fraction of this bicarbonate would rapidly result in severe, life-threatening metabolic acidosis, maintenance of acid-base balance requires that the kidney perform two functions: (1) all the filtered bicarbonate must be reabsorbed and returned to the body; this process takes place in the proximal tubule; and (2) buffer base consumed by metabolism must be generated in the process of urinary acid excretion; this takes place in the distal portions of the nephron, the distal convoluted tubule, and the collecting ducts.

Renal Acid-Base Handling

The role of the kidneys in acid-base balance entails a variety of interrelated processes including the reclamation of bicarbonate and the regeneration of buffer base as well as the excretion of acid.

RENAL ACID EXCRETION

In the intercalated cells of the distal nephron, bicarbonate regeneration occurs by the active secretion of hydrogen ions into the lumen, where they are trapped for elimination in the urine, and the simultaneous entry of bicarbonate into the blood (Fig. 72-1). In these cells the generation of acid to be excreted results from the dissociation of carbonic acid into hydrogen ion and bicarbonate. The return of bicarbonate to the blood restores the bicarbonate and nonbicarbonate buffer concentrations to normal.

The intracellular generation of hydrogen ions and their subsequent secretion are predominantly influenced by the arterial P_{CO_2}: the higher the P_{CO_2}, the more rapid the secretory rate. This intracellular response to P_{CO_2} is the basis of the renal compensatory mechanism for respiratory acid-base disorders, i.e., for hypercapnia and hypocapnia. Hydrogen ion secretion by the distal tubules is also stimulated by aldosterone.

This hormone accelerates secretion of H^+ by increasing the cellular production of specific proteins. Intracellular calcium also modulates H^+ secretion, but the factors which regulate cytosolic calcium and the clinical importance of this potential control system have not yet been elucidated.

In addition to the factors above, there are physiological influences that alter the electrochemical gradient that causes H^+ to move out of cells in the distal nephron. The permeability of the collecting duct is such that a minimal

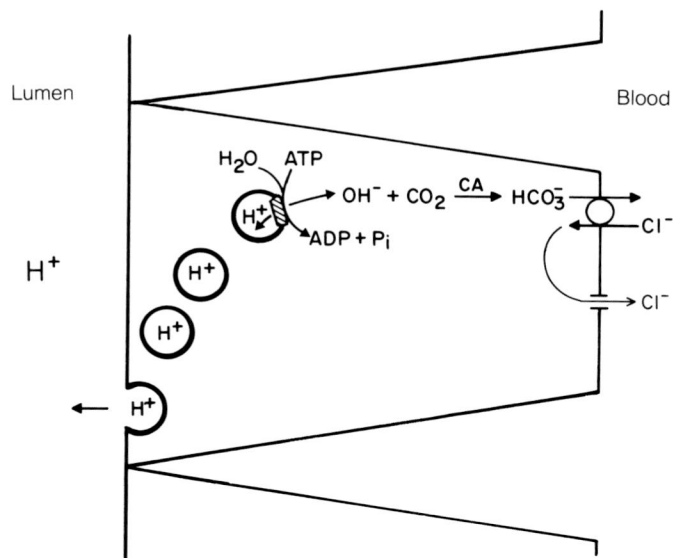

FIGURE 72-1 Schematic representation of distal tubular hydrogen ion secretion. H^+ (from water) is pumped (Koepren and Steinmetz, 1983) into a vesicle and the vesicle empties into the lumen. (Gluck et al., 1982.) CO_2 reacts with OH^- (from water) and with the aid of carbonic anhydrase, CA, bicarbonate is generated. The bicarbonate exits the basolateral side of the cell in exchange for chloride.

pH of approximately 4.5 to 5 can be attained in the urine. At a lower pH (or at a correspondingly higher H^+ concentration), H^+ leaks back into the cell. In addition, as implied by the term electrochemical gradient, the transepithelial voltage also influences cellular H^+ secretion: increasing the concentration of poorly reabsorbed anions enhances luminal electronegativity and accelerates H^+ secretion. Examples of poorly absorbed anions are sulfate, phosphate, and penicillin and its derivatives.

Although the maximal gradient in pH from blood to urine approaches 3 pH units (representing a 1000-fold increase in H^+ concentration), the quantity of acid excreted as free H^+ is trivial in comparison with the metabolic rate of acid production. For example, a pH of 5 represents a H^+ concentration of 10^{-5} eq/L or 10^{-2} meq/L. Daily excretion of 2 L of urine at pH 5 would result in excretion of only 0.02 meq of dissociated H^+ ions in contrast to 70 meq of H^+ that is generated metabolically. To maintain acid-base balance by excreting free H^+ in the urine would, in fact, require excretion of urine at a pH of 1 to 2. Obviously, this would damage the epithelium lining the urinary tract. The problem is resolved by the presence of buffers in the urine which carry more than 99 percent of the excreted H^+. About 40 percent of the excreted H^+ is titrated by urinary buffers, such as phosphate, while the remaining 60 percent is titrated by ammonia produced by the kidneys. Therefore, to maintain acid-base balance the system requires an intact H^+ secretory mechanism, urine low in pH (to permit titration of urinary buffers), and an adequate supply of buffer.

Except in the rare situation of extreme phosphate depletion, the availability of urinary phosphate is not rate-limiting for the renal maintenance of acid-base balance. In contrast, the role of urinary ammonium is of major importance. It is produced in cells of the proximal tubule by the enzymatic breakdown of glutamine into ammonia and glutamate: glutamate is metabolized in the liver, whereas the base, ammonia, is lipid-soluble and diffuses into urinary spaces where it is trapped as ionic ammonium. The greatest concentration of ammonium occurs in the collecting ducts, i.e., at the site where urine pH is kept low by active H^+ secretion. In addition to its systemic effects on acid-base balance, the concentration of potassium in the serum appears to modulate renal ammonia production: hypokalemia stimulates the generation of ammonia, whereas hyperkalemia inhibits generation.

BICARBONATE RECLAMATION

Complete reclamation of filtered bicarbonate is essential for maintenance of a stable concentration of bicarbonate in the plasma. The reclamation process occurs in the proximal portion of the nephron where H^+ ions are secreted into the lumen, thereby converting filtered bicarbonate to carbonic acid (Fig. 72-2). Carbonic anhydrase, situated on the apical membrane of the proximal tubule, promotes the rapid dehydration of carbonic acid into CO_2, which readily diffuses out of the lumen. By the end of the proximal segment of the nephron, approximately 90 percent of the filtered load of bicarbonate has been reabsorbed. Several factors modulate proximal tubule bicarbonate reabsorption: (1) P_{CO_2}, (2) the availability of carbonic anhydrase in the lumen, and (3) the extracellular volume of the patient.

The P_{CO_2} influences the reclamation of bicarbonate in the proximal tubule by way of the intracellular hydration-dehydration reactions of CO_2, which serve as the source of H^+ ions to be secreted: an alteration in intracellular P_{CO_2} immediately alters the supply of hydrogen ions to be secreted into the lumen. Thus, the maintenance of a high bicarbonate concentration in the plasma during respiratory acidosis is, in large part, due to the increased supply of intracellular hydrogen ions. Similarly in respiratory alkalosis, the decrease in P_{CO_2} reduces the supply of intracellular hydrogen ions.

Carbonic anhydrase inhibitors, such as acetazolamide, increase the excretion of bicarbonate by limiting the rate of reabsorption of bicarbonate. In addition to reducing the rate of dehydration of carbonic acid in the lumen, these inhibitors also inhibit the intracellular hydration-dehydration reactions of CO_2 that serve as the source for H^+ ions to be secreted. Carbonic anhydrase inhibitors also seem to interfere with cellular metabolism, thereby limiting the supply of energy needed to move bicarbonate out of the lumen into blood against a prevailing electrochemical gradient.

A third major influence on the reabsorption of bicarbonate in the proximal tubule is the status of the extracellular fluid volume (ECF): in clinical disorders, a decrease in ECF seems to increase the reabsorption of bicarbonate in the proximal tubule; reexpansion of the extracellular fluid volume favors reabsorption of chloride over bicarbonate.

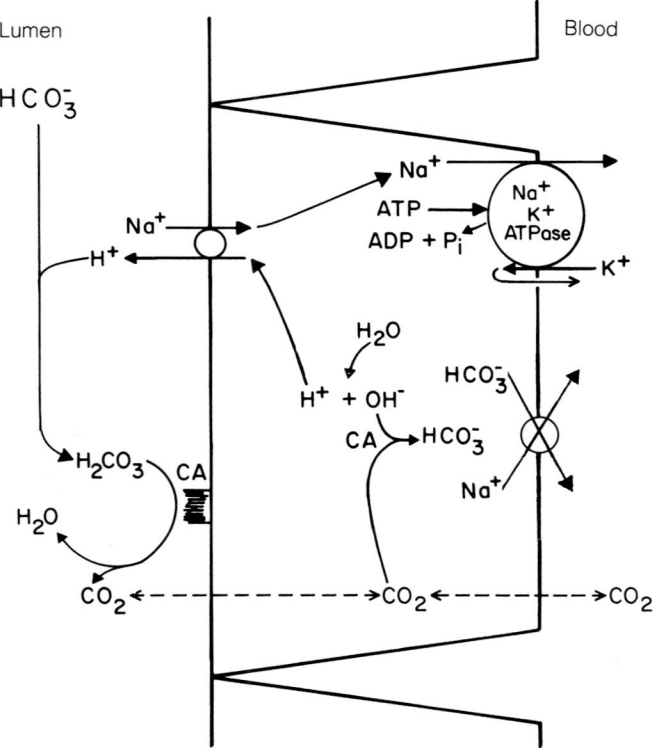

FIGURE 72-2 Schematic representation of proximal tubular reclamation of filtered bicarbonate. In the lumen, filtered bicarbonate reacts with secreted H^+, generating carbonic acid, which is dehydrated by carbonic anhydrase, CA, located on the brush border. The cell secretes H^+ by a process that exchanges H^+ for filtered Na^+. The source of secreted H^+ is water, which in turn generates OH^- and subsequently bicarbonate because of the presence of intracellular CA. Bicarbonate exits the basolateral side of the cell linked in some fashion with Na^+; sodium is also actively pumped out of the cell.

Renal Response to Ventilatory Disorders

Primary disturbances of acid-base balance, either respiratory or metabolic in origin, automatically activate compensatory mechanisms: respiratory disturbances are partly neutralized by the kidneys and metabolic disorders by the lungs. The handling of bicarbonate by the kidneys features prominently in the response of the body to respiratory disorders.

A change in ventilation, that leads to a change in arterial P_{CO_2} and pH, prompts the kidneys to alter bicarbonate reabsorption and acid excretion in such a way as to correct the arterial pH. Although acid-base handling by the

kidneys begins to change immediately after the onset of a disturbance in ventilation, the base content of the body does not reequilibrate for a day or longer: renal compensation for hypocapnia takes more than 1 day to complete; renal compensation for hypercapnia takes more than 3 days to complete.

In response to CO_2 retention, increased secretion of H^+ in the distal nephron and increased excretion of ammonium ion eventually expands the body store of buffer base. In addition to the generating new bicarbonate by the distal nephron, the proximal tubule increases bicarbonate reabsorption, thereby preventing in the urine bicarbonate loss that otherwise would accompany the increased bicarbonate load. Thus, both the proximal and distal nephron play important roles in the metabolic compensation for respiratory acidosis.

Following the onset of hypocapnia, the proximal reabsorption of filtered bicarbonate decreases, thereby causing net urinary loss of base. However, in chronic respiratory alkalosis, the amount of base lost in the urine is inadequate to account for the decrement in total body base content. In fact, Gledhill et al. demonstrated that a large part of the renal response to hypocapnia is a reduction in net acid excretion, thereby retaining metabolically produced hydrogen ions until the new steady state is achieved. It appears that about 50 percent of the compensation to respiratory alkalosis is a consequence of acid retention.

In Vivo Buffering

Even though full renal (metabolic) compensation after the acute onset of a respiratory acid-base disorder is gradual, the concentration of bicarbonate in arterial blood does change immediately. However, instead of reflecting compensation by the kidneys, the immediate changes in bicarbonate concentration reflect the chemical buffering of CO_2 by nonbicarbonate buffers (NBB) that exist throughout the body. Since the stoichiometry of this reaction is such that one bicarbonate is generated (or consumed) for one nonbicarbonate buffer base consumed (or generated), no change occurs in the total buffer base of the body (the sum of bicarbonate and nonbicarbonate bases), i.e., metabolic compensation has not occurred.

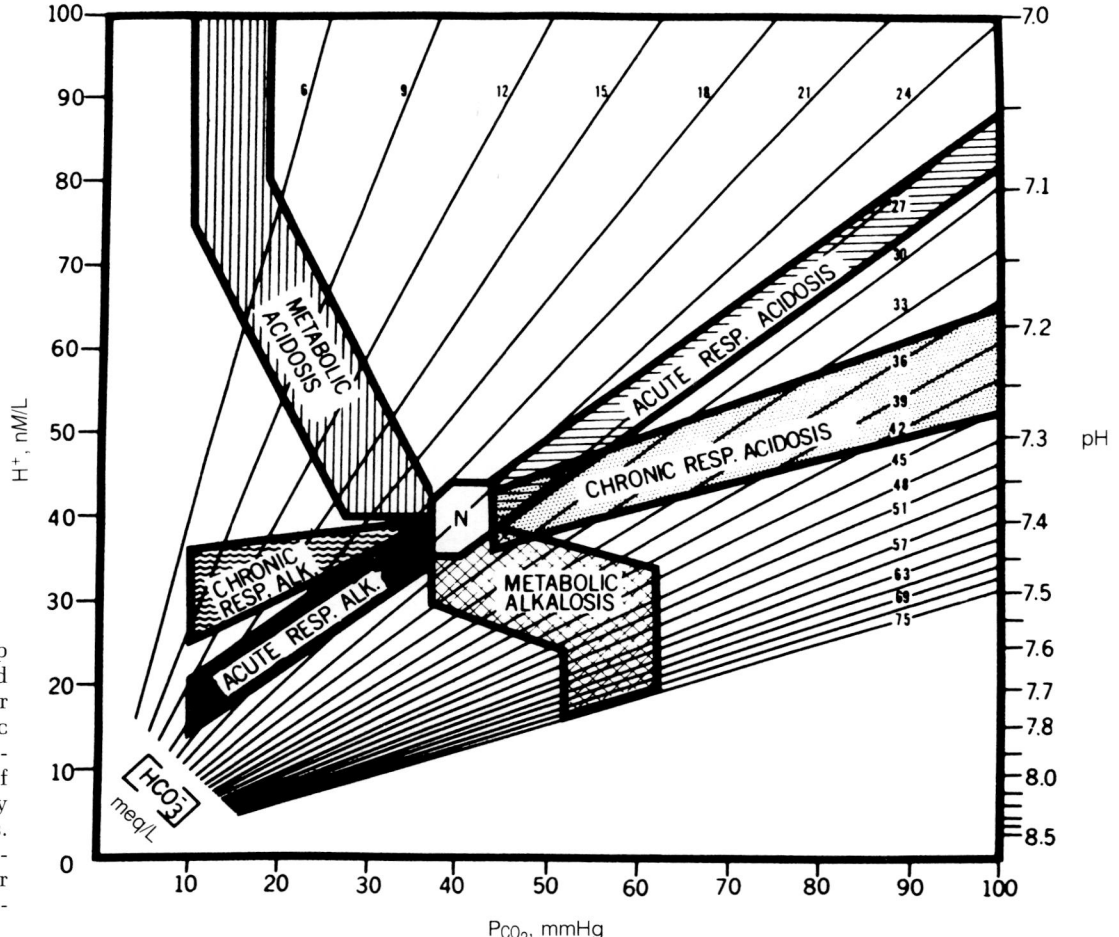

FIGURE 72-3 Acid-base map showing the normal range (N) and the confidence bands for acute or chronic respiratory and metabolic acid-base disturbances. The ordinates are the partial pressure of CO_2 and the hydrogen-ion activity given in nmol/L and pH units. Isopleths for bicarbonate concentration, in milliequivalents per liter, are also shown. (From Goldberg et al., 1973.)

The bands labeled *acute respiratory alkalosis* and *acute respiratory acidosis* on the acid-base map shown in Fig. 72-3 represent the in vivo titration curve of the whole body for CO_2. This confidence band makes it possible to predict the change in bicarbonate concentration that will follow an acute change in P_{CO_2}. Clearly, the increment or decrement in bicarbonate concentration induced by an acute change in P_{CO_2} is not constant; indeed, it varies markedly, depending on the starting point. The factor that controls the amount of bicarbonate generated during CO_2 titration is the initial bicarbonate concentration and not the pH.

Two factors are particularly important in discussing CO_2 titration curves for the entire body: (1) CO_2 titrates nonbicarbonate buffers, not bicarbonate; and (2) the initial bicarbonate concentration is an index of the buffer base content of the entire body, including its nonbicarbonate component. Thus, in patients with compensated metabolic alkalosis and respiratory acidosis in whom bicarbonate concentrations are equivalent, i.e., in whom the buffer base contents are similar, equal changes in P_{CO_2} result in similar degrees of titration of nonbicarbonate buffers and, therefore, produce similar changes in bicarbonate concentration. The results are also similar in patients with metabolic acidosis and respiratory alkalosis. Indeed, the whole body acid-base nomogram developed by Siggaard-Andersen can be used to predict graphically the effect of CO_2 titration on any individual, including those who do not fall into the acute respiratory acidosis-alkalosis confidence band.

In addition to whole-body buffering CO_2, nonbicarbonate buffers also titrate bicarbonate that is infused for therapeutic reasons. Bicarbonate infusion increases the total body content of base, but only a fraction of the added base remains in the form of bicarbonate. The apparent volume of distribution of infused bicarbonate is easily calculated and is referred to as the *bicarbonate space*. The bicarbonate space can vary several-fold, being much larger in metabolic acidosis than in metabolic alkalosis. For many years, the large bicarbonate space in metabolic acidosis was interpreted to mean that the excess H^+ ions on nonbicarbonate buffers titrated the infused bicarbonate. However, the bicarbonate space does not vary with arterial pH. Moreover, in both respiratory and metabolic acid-base disorders, the bicarbonate space varies inversely with the plasma bicarbonate concentration, i.e., it is larger when the bicarbonate concentration is low and less when the bicarbonate concentration is high. The explanation for this phenomenon is based on the buffering ability of bicarbonate as compared to that of the nonbicarbonate buffers: as bicarbonate concentration increases, its ability to buffer also increases, whereas the buffering ability of the nonbicarbonate buffer system remains constant. Thus, as the concentration of bicarbonate in plasma increases, less of added bicarbonate is buffered by nonbicarbonate buffers, more of the added bicarbonate will remain as bicarbonate, and the calculated bicarbonate space decreases.

Diagnostic Approach to Acid-Base Changes

As indicated above, the body buffers and the kidneys respond in a predictable fashion to a change in P_{CO_2}. Also, the resulting changes in bicarbonate and pH are time-dependent so that a larger change occurs in several days than in the first hours. The confidence bands shown in Fig. 72-3 represent the usual pattern of response to an acute change in P_{CO_2}; any deviation can be interpreted as a reflection of processes other than a compensatory response. For example, in a patient with chronic obstructive airways disease, other factors affecting the acid-base status are the concentration of potassium in the plasma, the size of extracellular fluid volume, chloride depletion, diuretics, renal hypoperfusion and coexisting renal disease. The special case of posthypercapnic alkalosis is discussed in the next section.

In evaluating an acid-base disorder, the history and physical examination are invaluable in focusing attention on potential pathologic processes. The composition of blood, with respect to serum electrolytes and blood gases, is then examined for consistency with the clinical impressions. However, in using the acid-base map (Fig. 72-3), it must be kept in mind that the map is based on data from individuals who had a single disorder. Therefore, it does not take into account the possibility of multiple disorders. For example, in a patient with chronic obstructive airways disease whose sputum has turned purulent and who develops nausea and vomiting, the possibility arises of coexistent metabolic alkalosis and acute respiratory acidosis. However, ill-advised application of the arterial blood-gas values from this patient (e.g., pH = 7.25 and P_{CO_2} = 75 mmHg) to the acid-base map would lead to the erroneous conclusion that a chronic respiratory acidosis is present.

Posthypercapnic Alkalosis

In the setting of chronic obstructive lung disease and CO_2 retention, renal compensation increases the concentration of bicarbonate in plasma. The normal renal response to proper treatment of the underlying lung disease and subsequent correction of hypercapnia is correction of the concentration of bicarbonate in the plasma. Occasionally normal renal compensation fails to occur, resulting in the entity of posthypercapnic alkalosis. Appropriate treatment of this condition requires an understanding of the pathophysiology.

Posthypercapnic alkalosis is a subset of the general problem of metabolic alkalosis. Two separate processes are involved in metabolic alkalosis: (1) an excess load of base that is generated either endogenously or exogenously, and (2) maintenance of an abnormally high con-

centration of bicarbonate in the plasma. During hypercapnia, the load of base is the result of renal compensation and de novo bicarbonate generation; in posthypercapnic alkalosis, the key abnormality is maintaining the bicarbonate level in plasma at inordinately high levels.

Maintenance of metabolic alkalosis requires an increase in the reabsorption of bicarbonate by the proximal tubule. As noted above, a reduction in extracellular fluid volume is a major stimulus for increasing the proximal reabsorption of bicarbonate. The occurrence of posthypercapnic alkalosis relates to the tenuous state of the extracellular fluid volume in the hypercapnic individual. In response to hypercapnia, the increased excretion of hydrogen ion in the urine and the increased bicarbonate generated by the secretory process increases concentration of bicarbonate in the plasma. In order to maintain electroneutrality both in the body and the urine, an anion exchange—bicarbonate for chloride—occurs, i.e., the urine is relatively enriched in chloride, while the body becomes depleted of chloride.

During this process, the total sodium content of the body remains stable as does the extracellular fluid volume (unless there is a separate reason for a volume abnormality, e.g., right ventricular failure and the use of diuretics). Correction of metabolic alkalosis requires that the kidneys excrete bicarbonate. This process is also electroneutral. Therefore, a cation, i.e., sodium, must be excreted with bicarbonate. If correction of hypercapnia occurs without simultaneous replacement of sodium chloride, the urinary loss of sodium bicarbonate depletes the extracellular fluid volume, leading to a reduction in renal blood flow and to an increase in the reabsorption of solute, including sodium bicarbonate, by the proximal tubule. In essence, the increased concentration of bicarbonate in the plasma is maintained despite alkalosis for the sake of an adequate circulating volume.

The above discussion emphasizes the role of sodium chloride depletion in maintaining metabolic alkalosis and the requirement that sodium chloride be provided to correct a primary metabolic alkalosis or to prevent a posthypercapnic metabolic alkalosis. However, this recommendation must be reconciled with the clinical observation that a favorable response to potassium chloride therapy alone often occurs in posthypercapnic alkalosis. In part, this is because potassium therapy remedies the total body deficit of potassium that frequently complicates the use of diuretics, a deficit that is partially masked by the substitution of extracellular sodium for intracellular potassium. Potassium chloride therapy enables potassium to reaccumulate inside cells in exchange for sodium while releasing intracellular stores of sodium for return to the extracellular fluid. The net effects of potassium therapy are the same as those of sodium chloride administration, i.e., an increase in extracellular fluid volume and a decrease in the proximal tubular reabsorption of bicarbonate. In addition to the volume reexpansion that occurs with potassium chloride therapy, provision of potassium to a potassium-depleted individual may directly reduce the bicarbonate concentration in plasma: marked potassium deficiency, per se, directly stimulates the secretion of hydrogen ions and the generation of bicarbonate.

DISORDERS OF SODIUM AND WATER HOMEOSTASIS

In addition to selective alterations in acid-base balance, obstructive airways disease alters other aspects of renal function and specifically affects homeostasis of the body fluids. These alterations are manifest as a reduction in the circulating arterial volume, changes in renal hemodynamics, sodium and water retention, edema, and hyponatremia.

Sodium Balance

The amount of sodium in the body determines the extracellular fluid volume. The normal individual controls the daily balance of sodium, and thereby the size of the ECF volume, by excreting in the urine an amount of sodium equal to that taken in by diet. This is achieved by reabsorbing more than 99 percent of the glomerular filtrate. Approximately 24,000 meq of sodium is filtered each day into the proximal tubule, whereas 100 to 200 meq is excreted into the urine. The proximal nephron reabsorbs approximately 70 percent of the filtered load, whereas the remainder is reabsorbed in the more distal portion of the nephron. In response to the changes in the ECF induced by altered sodium intake, the balance between intake and output is accomplished by alterations in transport processes along the entire nephron. Thus, a sudden increase in sodium intake expands the ECF volume and triggers hemodynamic changes which affect sodium transport in the proximal tubule and evoke hormonal changes which modulate changes in the transport of sodium in the distal nephron. Although transport mechanisms differ along the nephron, they do have certain characteristics in common. All depend on the active extrusion of sodium by the sodium pump (Na^+,K^+-ATPase) across the basolateral (serosal or blood) side of the cell. The subsequent lowering of the concentration of sodium in the cytosole creates the gradient by which sodium enters the cell from the lumen. The pathway for the entry of sodium differs along the length of the nephron as does the permeability to water. Although sodium transport throughout the nephron can be inhibited by inhibiting the sodium pump, the differing entry pathways and water permeabilities allow selective modulation by hormonal, hemodynamic, and pharmacologic agents.

PROXIMAL TUBULE

Approximately 70 percent of the filtrate is reabsorbed along the length of the proximal tubule. The permeability of this epithelium is high so that water moves freely between cells and lumen in response to hydrostatic and osmotic pressure gradients. As sodium moves through the cell, from the luminal to the blood side, an osmotic gradient is created that causes water to move out of the tubule into the interstitium; the net effect is the removal of isotonic fluid from the lumen. In addition to sodium, the reabsorbed fluid contains bicarbonate, glucose, amino acids, and phosphate.

Passage of reabsorbed filtrate from the interstitium to the circulating blood is accomplished by the Starling forces (hydrostatic and oncotic pressures) acting across the extensive capillary network that surrounds the proximal tubule. The hydrostatic pressure in the capillary network is low, whereas the oncotic pressure is higher than that of the protein-free filtrate in the tubular lumen. One unique feature of this capillary network is the existence of a postcapillary (glomerular) plexus. The blood entering the capillary bed has undergone filtration in the glomerulus so that its protein concentration is greater than in afferent blood. Since approximately 20 percent of the renal blood flow is filtered at the glomerulus, i.e., the filtration fraction, the protein concentration in the postglomerular arterioles is 20 percent higher than that in the blood both in the preglomerular capillaries and in capillaries elsewhere in the body. The net effect of these events is that the driving forces for fluid movement at the capillary level normally favor uptake into the capillary. The other important consequence of this system is its susceptibility to variation by hemodynamic influences which may alter the filtration fraction and, thereby, the oncotic pressure in the peritubular capillaries.

In most circumstances, changes in ECF volume are accompanied by parallel changes in renal blood flow. In contrast, the glomerular filtration rate usually remains virtually constant, leading to changes in the filtration fraction and in proximal tubular reabsorption (Fig. 72-4). Thus, a decrease in renal blood flow, as occurs during ECF volume depletion, is associated with an increase in filtration fraction and in reabsorption in the proximal tubule. Conversely, expansion of the ECF volume, as occurs when the dietary intake of sodium is high, results in a decrease in the filtration fraction, a decrease in pericapillary oncotic pressure, and a decrease in the uptake of fluid by the capillaries; the net effect is a reduction in proximal tubular reabsorption. This hemodynamic mechanism of volume control is important in obstructive airways disease complicated by right ventricular failure.

DISTAL NEPHRON

Approximately 30 percent of the filtered volume reaches the thick, ascending portion of the loop of Henle. This segment of the nephron is relatively impermeable to water and, as a consequence of active sodium chloride absorption, the luminal fluid becomes hypotonic with respect to plasma. For the entry of sodium chloride into the cell, chloride, sodium, and potassium ions must be present in the lumen. These ions cross the luminal membrane of the cell by attaching to a carrier; this transport pathway is sensitive to diuretics, such as furosemide, bumetamide, and ethacrynic acid, which operate by competitively binding to the cell membrane carrier. Under normal conditions, approximately 20 percent of the filtered sodium load is reabsorbed in this segment.

In the distal convoluted segment, sodium is also actively removed from the urine. Indeed, urine osmolality reaches its minimum (50 mosmol/kg) at this site. The mechanism of sodium reabsorption differs from that in the thick ascending limb of the loop of Henle since sodium enters the cell alone unaccompanied by other ions. The entry of Na^+ generates large voltage gradients across the luminal membrane and across the epithelial cell layer, providing a favorable electrical gradient for the movement of K^+ and H^+ into the tubular lumen. The diuretic, amiloride, by blocking sodium entry into cells through apical channels, eliminates the transepithelial voltage and minimizes the loss of K^+ in the urine.

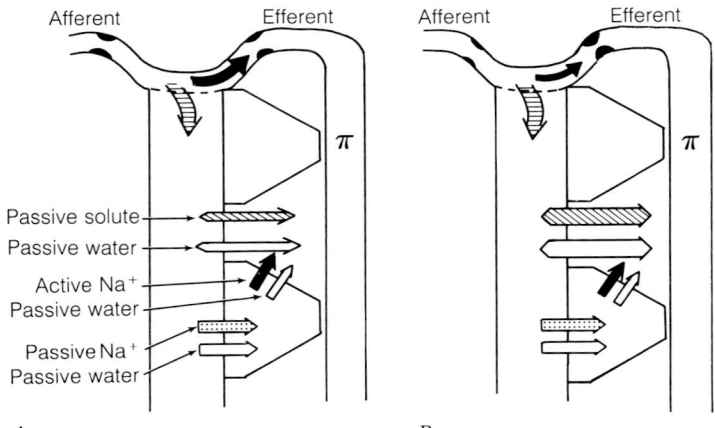

A *B*

FIGURE 72-4 Schematic representations of the influence of decreased renal blood flow on proximal tubule solute and water reabsorption *(B)* and of the normal pattern of proximal tubular reabsorption *(A)*. Glomerular filtration is maintained in the face of decreasing renal blood flow by a reduction in afferent arteriolar resistance and an increase in efferent arteriolar resistance. Consequently, filtration fraction (glomerular filtration rate/renal plasma flow) increases, and hemoconcentration of the efferent arteriolar blood occurs. The rise in peritubular capillary oncotic force, π, increases the net rate of passive solute and water reabsorption between cells. The rates of active solute (Na^+, HCO_3^-, etc.) and passive water transport through cells are unchanged.

Sodium transport into the distal tubular cell is also influenced by aldosterone, which is secreted by the adrenal glands and increases sodium transport by inducing the cellular production of proteins. While enhancing sodium reabsorption, aldosterone also increases the transepithelial voltage, thereby promoting the loss of K^+ and H^+ into the urine. Finally, aldosterone also stimulates directly the secretion of H^+.

Two major stimuli for the secretion of aldosterone by the adrenal glands are angiotensin II and hyperkalemia. In turn, angiotensin II is a product of the action of converting enzyme on angiotensin I; the production of angiotensin I from renin substrate is a function of the circulating level of plasma renin. Since the release of renin from the kidney varies inversely with the renal blood flow and ECF volume, aldosterone serves an important role in the distal nephron in regulating sodium transport in response to changes in ECF volume.

Water Balance

The sodium concentration in body fluids affords a useful measure of the effective osmolality of the plasma; in addition to the renal control mechanisms for handling sodium reabsorption and secretion, the concentration in body fluids is modulated by control of water intake and excretion: the hypothalamus and pituitary gland sense alterations in extracellular fluid osmolality and regulate the effective osmolality (tonicity) by controlling thirst and releasing antidiuretic hormone (ADH).

ADH exerts its effects on the collecting ducts by altering their permeability to water. The driving force for the flow of water across the collecting ducts is hypertonicity of the renal medulla established by high concentrations of sodium chloride and urea. The mechanism that leads to accumulation of these substances in the renal medulla is the same as that which extracts sodium chloride and dilutes urine in the thick ascending limb of the loop of Henle. It is important to emphasize that the renal control of water excretion depends on the delivery of solutes to the loop of Henle and distal nephron, because without this delivery neither dilute nor concentrated urine could be generated.

Disordered Volume Homeostasis

In patients with chronic obstructive airways disease, three disorders, i.e., arterial hypoxemia, hypercapnia, and a decrease in cardiac output when right ventricular failure supervenes, can affect the renal handling of salt and water, each contributing in its own way to the pathogenesis of peripheral edema and ascites.

DECREASED CARDIAC OUTPUT

A decrease in cardiac output, regardless of etiology, is associated with a decrease in renal blood flow and an in-

crease in filtration fraction. The kidney responds to the reduction in renal blood flow by increasing sodium reabsorption in the proximal and distal tubules without regard to the state of total body sodium and water. Because of the right ventricular failure, cardiac output cannot improve; the accompanying reduction in renal blood flow promotes the renal retention of salt and water and the formation of edema and ascites.

During renal hypoperfusion, local production of prostaglandins helps to maintain renal blood flow and glomerular filtration rate. Also, the prostaglandins blunt the vasoconstricting effect of hormones, such as angiotensin II. Inhibition of the cyclooxygenase pathway by nonsteroidal anti-inflammatory agents decreases the production of prostaglandins, thereby reducing renal blood flow and glomerular filtration rate, and aggravating salt and water retention and the formation of edema.

In addition to sodium retention and edema, a decrease in cardiac output can produce hyponatremia, hyperkalemia, and metabolic acidosis. As the filtration fraction and proximal reabsorption increase, a greater proportion of the filtered isotonic fluid is returned to the body and, more importantly, a smaller volume is delivered to the distal sites. Hyponatremia occurs partly because the inadequate delivery of fluid to the distal nephron minimizes the renal capability for excreting water unaccompanied by solute. Retention of water also occurs in some patients because of an increase in ADH levels. The capability for secreting potassium is also decreased by the decrease of fluid flow into the distal nephron, even though aldosterone levels are high. Finally, the reduced rate of flow also minimizes the secretion of hydrogen ions, leading to acid retention and metabolic acidosis.

Renal function is often indirectly affected by the therapeutic use of mechanical ventilation. By increasing intrathoracic pressure, mechanical ventilation can reduce the cardiac output, thereby promoting salt and water retention by the kidneys and leading to edema and hyponatremia. In addition to increasing intrathoracic pressure, mechanical ventilation can contribute to the development of hyponatremia by interfering with the daily insensible loss of water (about 0.5 L) from the airways. This effect is due to the fact that ventilators generally provide for the humidification of inspired air. Although the volume of water eliminated by the lungs is small compared to that of normal kidneys (e.g., capability of about 15 L per day), this small volume may contribute to hyponatremia, particularly if water is being administered or if renal disease impairs the excretion of water.

HYPOXEMIA

Arterial hypoxemia elicits systemic vasodilatation in which the renal circulation shares. Moreover, arterial hypoxemia elicits pulmonary vasoconstriction that may culminate in right ventricular failure, particularly if the

pulmonary hypertension is aggravated by concomitant hypercapnia and acidosis; the impact of a drop in cardiac output on renal function has been considered above. Finally, severe arterial hypoxemia that compromises oxygen delivery can damage renal cells. The segment of the nephron most vulnerable to compromise of oxygen supply is the thick ascending limb of the loop of Henle, possibly because the metabolic demands of sodium chloride transport are large; cellular damage occurs if the oxygen supply is withdrawn for more than a few minutes. Pharmacologic interference with salt transport, using agents such as furosemide, reduces oxygen demand in this region and prolongs its ability to tolerate poor oxygen delivery. However, clinical exploitation of this approach is hampered by the fact that it is only preventive and that it is not effective after the hypoxic insult has occurred.

Less severe hypoxemia may also affect the hormonal state. Without affecting extracellular fluid volume, glomerular filtration rate, plasma volume, or plasma protein concentration in normal individuals, acute hypoxemia does reduce the concentration of aldosterone in plasma. Also, in patients with chronic obstructive airways disease, acute hypoxemia reduces urinary sodium excretion without changing cardiac output or the concentration of vasopressin in plasma.

HYPERCAPNIA

Carbon dioxide also appears to affect renal function. For example, in patients with hypercapnia without hypoxemia, the filtration fraction increases and sodium retention is enhanced, presumably due, in part, to altered intrarenal hemodynamics and increased reabsorption of solutes in the proximal tubule. In addition, an increase in P_{CO_2} may directly increase sodium reabsorption. Thus, active reclamation of sodium and water during hypercapnia may participate in the formation of edema associated with chronic obstructive airways disease.

Carbon dioxide also appears to affect water metabolism by influencing the effect of ADH on the kidneys. For example, pregnant women are hypocapnic and tend to be hyponatremic. Hypocapnia in dogs exaggerates the effect of vasopressin and markedly enhances hyponatremia, whereas hypercapnia effectively blunts the renal response to the same dose of vasopressin. Indeed, this effect of hypercapnia may partially explain the mild hypernatremia (an average increase in the sodium concentration in the plasma of approximately 2 to 4 meq/L) that occurs in patients with chronic obstructive airways disease; in patients with chronic obstructive airways disease who develop acute respiratory failure, hypercapnia may also contribute to the mild hypernatremia that occurs in the face of high levels of ADH and increased sensitivity of the pituitary-hypothalamic axis for releasing ADH.

Clearly, the pathogenesis of the salt and water retention that occurs in some patients with chronic obstructive airways disease is multifactorial. Many factors remain unexplored. For example, the respective roles of atrial natriuretic factor, renin-angiotensin-aldosterone, prostaglandins, and vasopressin in chronic obstructive airways disease await clarification.

DIURETICS

From the preceding discussion it is clear that primary pulmonary pathology can lead to altered renal function with resulting acid-base disturbances, extracellular fluid overload, and electrolyte disorders. Treatment of the lung disease often corrects the renal manifestations. However, if the underlying pulmonary pathology is not reversible, treatment can be directed at the renal disturbances. The therapeutic approach utilizes diuretic agents that function at different segments of the nephron so that they exert different effects on renal function, acid-base balance, and electrolyte balance, and extracellular fluid volume and composition.

Five classes of diuretics have proved useful in treating patients with pulmonary disease: (1) carbonic anhydrase inhibitors, (2) inhibitors of neutral sodium chloride entry into cells, (3) inhibitors of chloride absorption (linked to sodium and potassium) in the thick ascending limb of the loop of Henle, (4) inhibitors of the entry of sodium into apical cells, and (5) inhibitors of aldosterone action. A sixth type of diuretic, i.e, osmotic agents, is of no value in treating these patients. Two new classes of diuretics are under development, i.e., atrial natriuretic hormone and its derivatives, and inhibitors of vasopressin.

Of particular interest in treating hypercapnic states is the carbonic anhydrase inhibitor, acetazolamide. This agent functions primarily in the proximal tubule where, by delaying the dehydration of carbonic acid at the apical membrane, it inhibits the reabsorption of filtered sodium and bicarbonate. The clinical utility of this agent depends on the physiological setting; it is probably most useful when metabolic alkalosis and expansion of the ECF volume occur simultaneously. The potential danger with carbonic anhydrase inhibitors is the induction of metabolic acidosis in a patient who cannot increase ventilation. However, judicious use of acetazolamide may be of benefit by causing a mild metabolic acidosis that stimulates ventilation. Clearly, this form of therapy requires careful and frequent monitoring.

Thiazide diuretics inhibit the entry of neutral sodium chloride into renal tubular cells; they exert their predominant effects in the distal convoluted tubule. Although they induce natriuresis, they are not as potent as the "loop"-active diuretics, such as furosemide, ethacrynic acid, and bumetamide, which inhibit the entry of chloride

into the cells that line the thick ascending limb of the loop of Henle. At this site, chloride reabsorption requires the presence of both sodium and potassium in the luminal fluid. Both classes of diuretics, i.e., the thiazide and loop-active diuretics, are useful in reducing extracellular volume. Side effects are hypokalemia and metabolic alkalosis. In patients with cor pulmonale and right ventricular failure, a decrease in extracellular fluid volume may decrease cardiac preload and evoke systemic hypotension.

Amiloride and triamterene act by blocking the entry of sodium into apical cells in the distal nephron, but the quantity of sodium reabsorbed by this mechanism is small. However, inhibition of sodium transport at this site diminishes the electrical driving force for potassium entry into the lumen, thereby decreasing the secretion of potassium. Consequently, these agents are referred to as *potassium-sparing*. Since these agents are not particularly natriuretic when used alone, they are best used in conjunction with thiazides or loop-active diuretics for their potassium-sparing effect. The most serious side effect of these diuretics is hyperkalemia. Therefore, they should not be used in conjunction with potassium supplementation.

The last group of agents consists of those specific for the aldosterone-dependent reabsorption of sodium and potassium excretion. Aldosterone, a steroid hormone, binds to specific nuclear receptors and, by genetic derepression, stimulates the production of proteins that promote the transport of sodium in the distal portion of the nephron. Spironolactone is a clinically useful agent that competitively inhibits the binding of aldosterone to receptors. Although spironolactone, per se, is not a powerful natriuretic agent, it is an effective antikaliuretic agent; as such, it is often used in conjunction with thiazides or loop-active diuretics. Spironolactone can induce hyperkalemia and reduce the renal generation of hydrogen ions, thereby blunting the renal compensatory response to respiratory acidosis.

BIBLIOGRAPHY

Adrogue HJ, Brensilver J, Cohen JJ, Madias NE: Influence of steady-state alterations in acid-base equilibrium on the fate of administered bicarbonate in the dog. J Clin Invest 71:867–883, 1983.
  This study demonstrates that the bicarbonate volume of distribution varies as a function of the initial bicarbonate concentration and not the initial pH.

Adrogue HJ, Madias NE: Influence of chronic respiratory acid-base disorders on acute CO_2 titration curve. J Appl Physiol 58:1231–1238, 1985.
  A demonstration that whole-body buffering is different after adaptation to altered CO_2 tensions. Along with its companion paper (Madias and Adrogue, 1983) these studies validate the usefulness of the approach of Siggaard-Andersen (1974) to describe acid-base disturbances in terms of buffer base and base excess and plotting whole-body buffering on pH and log P_{CO_2} axes.

Babini R, du Souich P: Furosemide pharmacodynamics: effect of respiratory and acid-base disturbances. J Pharmacol Exp Ther 237:623–628, 1986.
  Only hypercapnia and respiratory acidosis combined with hypoxemia decrease the natriuretic and diuretic effect of furosemide.

Boron WF: Intracellular pH regulation in epithelial cells. Annu Rev Physiol 48:377–388, 1986.
  One of a cluster of papers dealing with intracellular pH and its effects on biologic processes.

Brezis M, Rosen S, Silva P, Epstein FH: Selective vulnerability of the thick ascending limb to anoxia in the isolated perfused kidney. J Clin Invest 73:182–189, 1984.
  Demonstration of effect of anoxia on renal cell survival.

Brezis M, Rosen S, Spokes K, Silva P, Epstein FH: Transport-dependent anoxic cell injury in the isolated perfused rat kidney. Am J Pathol 116:327–341, 1984.
  Demonstration that inhibition of ion transport enhances renal cell survival after exposure to anoxia.

Brezis M, Shanley M, Silva P, Spokes K, Lear S, Epstein FH, Rosen S: Disparate mechanism for hypoxic cell injury in different nephron segments. Studies in the isolated perfused nephron. J Clin Invest 76:1796–1806, 1985.
  Shows that the thick ascending limb responds differently from the proximal tubule.

Claybaugh JR, Wade CE, Sato AK, Cucinell SA, Lane JC, Maher JT: Antidiuretic hormone responses to eucapnic and hypocapnic hypoxia in humans. J Appl Physiol 53:815–823, 1982.
  Demonstrates that humans decrease plasma aldosterone concentrations with acute induction of hypoxemia.

Cohen JJ, Madias NE: Respiratory alkalosis and acidosis, in Seldin DW, Giebisch G (eds), *The Kidney: Physiology and Pathophysiology*. New York, Raven, pp 1641–1661, 1985.
   A current review of the renal response to altered P_{CO_2}.

Coulson RA, Herbert JD: A role for carbonic anhydrase in intermediary metabolism. Ann NY Acad Sci 249:505–515, 1984.
   This study, along with several others in the symposium, suggests that another role for carbonic anhydrase exists; namely, it is a participant in cellular metabolism. This role may link cellular oxidative energy generation to the disposal of the resulting metabolic product, CO_2, in an aqueous environment.

Farber MO, Roberts LR, Weinberger MH, Roberts GL, Fineberg NS, Manfredi F: Abnormalities of sodium and water handling in chronic obstructive lung disease. Arch Intern Med 142:1326–1330, 1982.
   This study of patients with obstructive airways disease and acute respiratory failure documents the reduction in glomerular filtration rate, increase in filtration fraction, and decrease in urinary excretion of sodium. In addition, a variety of hormonal abnormalities were observed.

Farber MO, Weinberger MH, Robertson GL, Fineberg NS, Manfredi G: Hormonal abnormalities affecting sodium and water balance in acute respiratory failure due to chronic obstructive lung disease. Chest 85:49–54, 1984.
   This study extends the observations of hormonal abnormalities previously observed in patients with acute respiratory failure; increased aldosterone concentrations and ADH levels were identified.

Feldman GM, Charney AN: Effect of acute respiratory alkalosis and acidosis on rat intestinal electrolyte transport in vivo. Am J Physiol 242:G486–G492, 1982.
   Demonstrates that P_{CO_2} influences epithelial Na^+ and HCO_3^- fluxes in vivo.

Galla JH, Bonduris DN, Luke RG: The correction of acute chloride-depletion alkalosis in the rat without volume expansion. Am J Physiol 244:F217–F221, 1983.
   The relative importance of chloride depletion, as compared to volume reduction, was assessed by replenishing depleted chloride using salt choline chloride.

Gledhill N, Beirne GJ, Dempsey JA: Renal response to short-term hypocapnia in man. Kidney Int 8:376–386, 1975.
   A human study showing the renal response to one day of hypocapnia.

Gluck S, Cannon C, Al-Awqati Q: Exocytosis regulates urinary acidification in turtle bladder by rapid insertion of H^+ pumps into luminal membrane. Proc Natl Acad Sci USA 79:4327–4331, 1982.
   A study utilizing optical techniques that demonstrated the quantum release of H^+ ions at the luminal membrane.

Goldberg M, Green SB, Moss ML, Marbach CB, Garfinkel D: Computer-based instruction and diagnosis of acid-base disorders. A systematic approach. JAMA 223:269–275, 1973.
   The source of one of many acid-base maps.

Good DW, Knepper MA: Ammonia transport in the mammalian kidney. Am J Physiol 248:F459–F471, 1985.
   An updated review of renal ammonia chemistry and transport.

Heinemann HO: Right-sided failure and the use of diuretics. Am J Med 64:367–370, 1978.
   Gives a valuable perspective to the generic use of diuretics in patients with edema and lung disease.

Hutler HN, Ilnicki LP, Harbottle JA, Sebastian A: Impaired renal H^+ secretion and NH_3 production in mineralocorticoid-deficient glucocorticoid-replete dogs. Am J Physiol 326:F136–F146, 1977.
   The role of mineralocorticoids in renal H^+ secretion and ammonia excretion is demonstrated. This study is particularly pertinent to patients with type IV renal tubular acidosis, i.e., the development of metabolic acidosis due to the failure of adequate renal ammonia generation.

Kaehny WD, Gougoux A, Cohen JJ: Influence of steady-state Pa_{CO_2} on escape from ADH-induced water retention in the dog. Am J Physiol 234:F291–F296, 1978.
   Demonstrates the modulating role of P_{CO_2} on water metabolism and function of ADH.

Kassirer JP, Berkman PM, Lawrenz DR, Schwartz WB: The critical role of chloride in the correction of hypokalemic alkalosis in man. Am J Med 38:172–189, 1965.
   An early clinical study that demonstrates the relevance of potassium chloride therapy for metabolic alkalosis and the importance of KCl as a volume expander.

Koeppen BM, Steinmetz PR: Basic mechanisms of urinary acidification. Med Clin North Am 67:753–770, 1983.
   A review of the cellular mechanisms of H^+ secretion.

Lim VS, Katz AI, Lindheimer MD: Acid-base regulation in pregnancy. Am J Physiol 231:1764–1770, 1976.
Demonstration of coincidence of respiratory alkalosis and hyponatremia in pregnant women.

Madias NE, Adrogue HJ: Influence of chronic metabolic acid-base disorders on the acute CO_2 titration curve. J Appl Physiol 55:1187–1195, 1983.
A demonstration that whole-body buffering is different after adaptation to altered intake of fixed acid. Along with its companion paper (Adrogue et al., 1983) these studies validate the usefulness of the approach of Siggaard-Andersen (1974) to describe acid-base disturbances in terms of buffer base and base excess and to plot whole body buffering on pH and log P_{CO_2} axes.

Maresh CM, Noble BJ, Robertson KL, Seip RL: Adrenocortical responses to maximal exercise in moderate-altitude natives at 447 torr. J Appl Physiol 56:482–488, 1984.
At simulated altitude, hypoxemia reduces plasma aldosterone and K^+ concentrations.

McCurdy DK: Mixed metabolic and respiratory acid-base disturbances: Diagnosis and treatment. Chest 62:35S–44S, 1972.
An effective guide on the diagnostic approach to acid-base disturbances.

Miles DS, Bransford DR, Howath SM: Hypoxia effects on plasma volume shifts at rest, work, and recovery in supine posture. J Appl Physiol 51:148–153, 1981.
Demonstration that hypoxemia does not alter measured blood volume or glomerular filtration rate.

Nattie EE: Gas exchange in acid-base disturbances, in Farhi LE, Tenney SM (eds), *Handbook of Physiology, sect 3: Respiration, vol IV: Gas Exchange*. Bethesda, MD, American Physiological Society, 1987, pp 421–438.
A step-by-step review of the effects of acid-base imbalance on the delivery of O_2 to cell oxidative sites.

Pitts RF: Production and excretion of ammonia in relation to acid-base balance, in Orloff J, Berliner RW (eds), *Handbook of Physiology, sec 8*. Washington, DC, American Physiological Society, pp 455–496, 1973.
A review of the generation and transport of ammonia by the kidneys that puts major emphasis on the role of the permeation of nonionic ammonia across the epithelia of the nephron.

Reihman DH, Farber MO, Weinberger MH, Henry DP, Fineberg NS, Dowdeswell IRG, Burt RW, Manfredi F: Effect of hypoxemia on sodium and water excretion in chronic obstructive lung disease. Am J Med 78:87–94, 1985.
Acute hypoxemia did not alter renal blood flow, systemic concentrations of aldosterone or vasopressin, and the fractional excretion of sodium. Since glomerular filtration rate and Na^+ excretion decreased, it was suggested that hypoxemia alters intrarenal hemodynamics.

Relman AS, Etsten B, Schwartz WB: The regulation of renal bicarbonate reabsorption by plasma carbon dioxide tension. J Clin Invest 32:972, 1953.
A clear demonstration that P_{CO_2} regulates renal bicarbonate transport in vivo.

Schwartz WB, Cohen JJ: The nature of the renal response to chronic disorders of acid-base equilibrium. Am J Med 64:417–428, 1978.
A review that underscores the importance of extracellular fluid volume in acid-base balance. Although overstated, this is an excellent synthesis.

Schwartz WB, Hays RM, Polak A, Haynie GD: Effects of chronic hypercapnia on electrolyte and acid-base equilibrium. II. Recovery, with special reference to the influence of chloride intake. J Clin Invest 40:1238–1249, 1961.
Puts emphasis on extracellular volume as playing a crucial role in posthypercapnic metabolic alkalosis.

Siggaard-Andersen O: *The Acid-Base Status of the Blood*, 4th ed, Baltimore, Williams and Wilkins, 1974.
A textbook that describes blood acid-base chemistry and compares different ways of presenting this information in graphical form. The author uses a physicochemical approach.

Singer RB, Hastings AB: An improved clinical method for the estimation of disturbances of the acid-base balance of human blood. Medicine 27:223–242, 1948.
Presents the first clinically useful nonogram to describe acid-base chemistry utilizing the conceptual term buffer base.

Trivedi B, Tannen RL: Effect of respiratory acidosis on intracellular pH of the proximal tubule. Am J Physiol 250:F1039–F1045, 1986.
Acute acidosis of either respiratory or metabolic origin lowers the intracellular pH of the proximal tubule. However, in the chronic phase, proximal tubular intracellular pH remains low during metabolic acidosis but returns to normal values during respiratory acidosis.

Chapter 73

The Pulmonary Fibroelastic Skeleton: A Functional Perspective

Jerome O. Cantor / Gerard M. Turino

The fibroelastic skeleton of the lung consists of a series of interrelated structures with distinct characteristics. As the tracheobronchial tree and surrounding tissue branch out into the lung, fibers which form the connective tissue network become finer and eventually spread out as individual fibrils in the interstitium, merging with the cellular microenvironment. At each level, this fibrous continuum performs specialized functions which require varied morphologic structure and chemical composition. In this chapter, the fibroelastic skeleton of the lung is considered from several standpoints, including (1) characteristics of connective tissue components, (2) specialized structures, (3) lung development, and (4) changes occurring in disease.

COMPONENTS OF THE FIBROELASTIC SKELETON

Collagen

Collagen is the major constituent of the pulmonary fibroelastic skeleton, accounting for approximately two-thirds of its total mass. The basic subunit of this complex protein consists of three polypeptides wrapped tightly in the form of a triple helix. Fibers result from the spontaneous linkage of large numbers of these strands in the extracellular matrix. The winding and cross-linking of the peptide chains make collagen extremely resistant to stretching. Furthermore, the regularity of these structural features produces a characteristic banding pattern with histologic staining.

Collagen fibers surround airways and blood vessels in a spiral arrangement, imparting a springiness to these structures while preventing their overdistention. As the fibers wind downward into the alveoli, they spread apart. Those with the largest diameter act as struts, providing mechanical support for the alveolar wall. Smaller, more serpiginous fibers are closely associated with capillary walls and serve to regulate the compliance of the microvasculature. Still finer fibers form a meshwork which can insert directly into endothelial and epithelial basement membranes (Fig. 73-1). This distribution of collagen fibers maintains physiological function in the face of mechanical forces which are constantly stretching and twisting the lung tissue during both normal breathing and the extremes of inspiratory and expiratory pressure.

Improvement of techniques to study collagen has resulted in the identification of more than a half-dozen chemically distinct variants of this connective tissue constituent. The mechanical properties of a tissue are related to the relative abundance of these different types of collagen. The tensile strength of tendons, for example, is due to the predominance of thick fibers of type I collagen. The

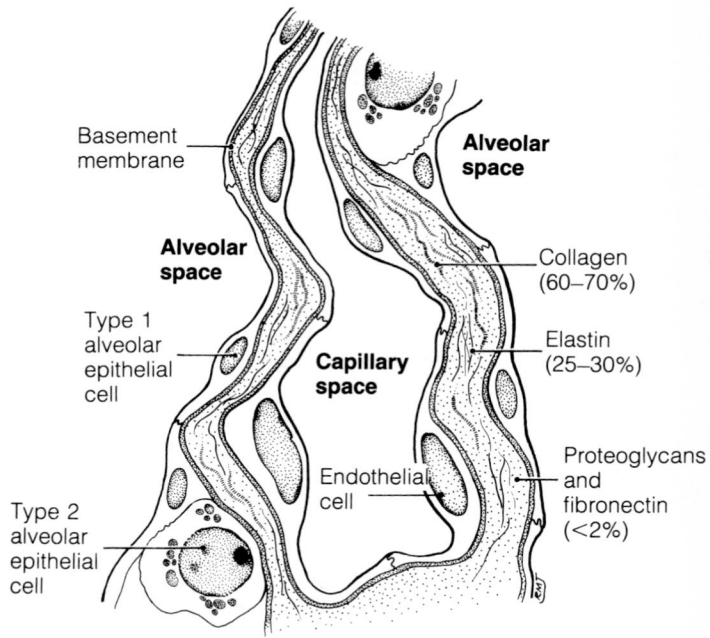

FIGURE 73-1 Representation of the interalveolar septum depicting several of the structures present and indicating the relative abundance of each component of the fibroelastic skeleton.

distensibility of intestinal wall, in contrast, is dependent on the presence of relatively large amounts of type III collagen. Basement membrane, which functions as a semipermeable barrier, contains loosely aggregated type IV collagen. As might be expected, types I and III collagen are important components of lung parenchyma, imparting both strength and flexibility to the tissue. Interstitial fibrosis results in an increase in the ratio of type I to type III collagen, reflected by a loss of lung compliance.

Elastin

While collagen provides support and tethers lung expansion, it does not impart the tissue recoil characteristics necessary for energy efficient movement of air during ventilation. Lung elasticity is primarily the result of highly specialized fibers composed of elastin. This protein is less abundant than collagen, constituting about one quarter of the mass of the pulmonary fibroelastic skeleton. In contrast to collagen, it has an amorphous appearance under the electron microscope.

Elastin readily accommodates a severalfold linear distension, yet returns to its original form when the stretching force is removed. The special properties of elastin are related to its unusual structure, involving long-chain peptides with both coiled and fibrillar regions. Elasticity is believed to result from decreasing entropy as the randomly oriented long-chain peptides become more ordered upon stretching. Release of the distending force allows the protein to resume a more disordered, coiled configuration.

The role of elastin in pulmonary mechanics is demonstrated by pressure-volume measurements of lungs treated with elastase. The plot of this relationship is shifted to the left due to a loss of tissue recoil (Fig. 73-2). At high lung volumes, the restraining action of collagen is manifest by a flattening of the curve. This effect is mitigated by incubation of the lung with collagenase.

Like collagen, assembly of elastin occurs extracellularly (Fig. 73-3). Lysyl residues undergo oxidation and condensation to form cross-links between precursory polypeptides known as tropoelastin, each of which has a molecular weight of about 68,000. Alignment and cross-linking of these nascent elastin chains may be regulated by neighboring glycoprotein moieties, collectively referred to as the microfibrillar component, though their role in this process has not been firmly established.

As a result of cross-linking, the mature elastin molecule is insoluble even in hot alkali. This resistance to chemical breakdown makes elastin a very stable protein with an extremely low rate of turnover. It is therefore an ideal component in tissue systems, such as the lung, which are subjected to continual extreme mechanical force.

Glycosaminoglycans and Fibronectin

While collagen and elastin are the main constituents of the pulmonary fibroelastic skeleton, other less abundant

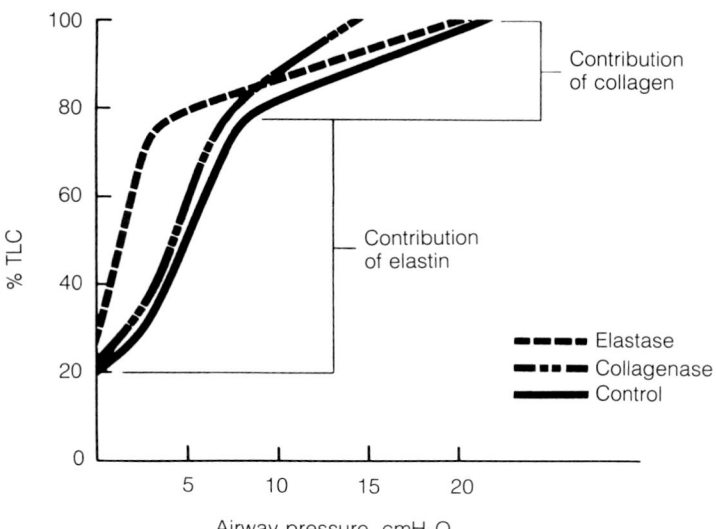

FIGURE 73-2   Graph showing the effects of elastase and collagenase treatment of lungs on the pressure-volume relationship. Following elastase administration, the plot is shifted to the left, indicating a loss of tissue recoil. Collagenase treatment, in contrast, alters the curve at high lung volumes due to a reduction in tissue restraint. *(Reprinted from Turino, 1985.)*

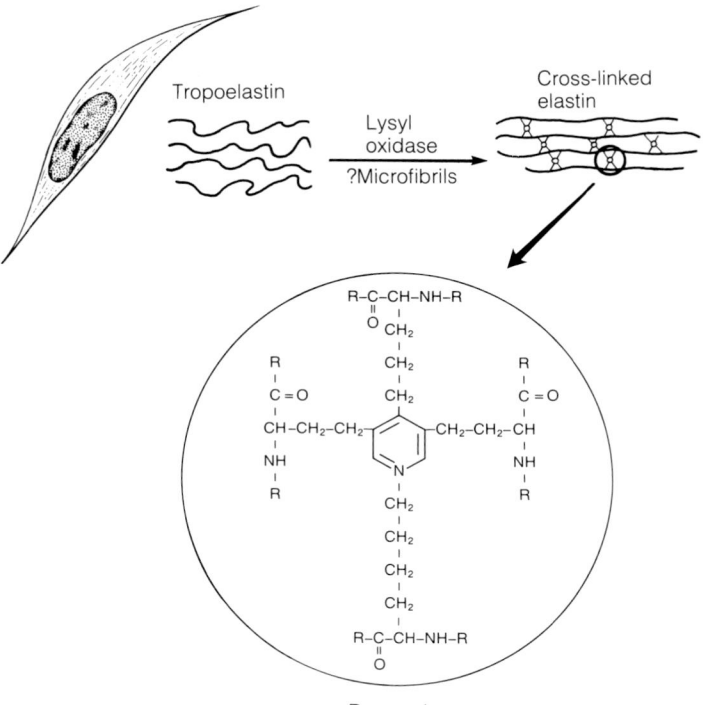

FIGURE 73-3   Depiction of the conversion of tropoelastin to cross-linked elastin. The chemical structure of the major elastin cross-link, demosine, is also shown.

components also play an important role in maintaining lung homeostasis. In particular, proteoglycans and fibronectin stabilize the extracellular matrix and help regulate cellular function. Though each of these molecular species comprises only a very small percentage of the connective tissue mass of the lung, they are nevertheless ubiquitous in the cellular microenvironment.

Proteoglycans consist of a protein core surrounded by covalently linked polysaccharide chains called *glycosaminoglycans*. A number of subtypes of glycosaminoglycans have been identified, including chondroitin sulfate, dermatan sulfate, heparin, heparan sulfate, keratan sulfate, and hyaluronate. With the exception of the last, the polysaccharides all contain sulfate groups which impart electronegativity and facilitate binding to cationic substances in the extracellular matrix. Since a single proteoglycan may contain up to 100 glycosaminoglycans, each composed of an average of 100 sulfated saccharides, it is possible to have 10,000 negatively charged groups per molecule.

Glycosaminoglycans not only surround cells, but are juxtaposed with collagen and elastin, suggesting a functional role for these polysaccharides in the organization of other connective tissue components in the matrix. Studies of salivary gland morphogenesis and amphibian limb regeneration have shown that glycosaminoglycans may also help regulate tissue differentiation.

Fibronectin consists of a group of high molecular weight glycoproteins that can assemble into fibrils which promote cell attachments to one another and to basement membranes. A great deal of interest in fibronectin has been generated as a result of the observation that it is absent on the surface of neoplastic cells, thus facilitating their growth and metastasis. Fibronectin may likewise influence cell movement and proliferation during lung development and repair. Furthermore, it may act to stabilize the extracellular matrix by virtue of its ability to bind to collagen.

In addition to fibronectin, several other adhesive glycoproteins have been identified in the matrix. One of these, laminin, is predominantly associated with basement membrane and is believed to play a role in the attachment of epithelial cells to this structure.

SPECIALIZED CONNECTIVE TISSUE STRUCTURES

Basement Membrane

While the fibroelastic skeleton of the lung provides support and cohesion for airways, blood vessels, and alveoli, it also acts as a scaffold for the cells which line these structures. Pulmonary epithelium and endothelium are attached to a layer of connective tissue called the *basement membrane*. This structure, which may be considered a specialized form of the pulmonary matrix, consists of an amorphous mixture of type IV collagen, proteoglycans, and various glycoproteins, including fibronectin and laminin. The functional relationship between cells and their underlying basement membranes is poorly understood, but it has been postulated that such attachments anchor the intracellular actin filaments that influence cell shape and differentiation. Reestablishment of cellular contact with basement membranes may be a critical component in the repair of lung injuries involving initial destruction and subsequent proliferation of cells.

Pleura

The visceral pleura is a complex structure consisting of an outermost layer of mesothelial cells that rest on a fibrillar network of connective tissue composed primarily of collagen. Beneath this structure is a continuous array of elastic fibers which attach to subjacent alveolar tissue. These elements impart both tensile strength and elasticity to the pleura. The precise relationship between the pleura and lung mechanics needs further investigation, but the large amount of collagen in the pleura suggests that it functions as a restraint. Consequently, a change in the amount or composition of pleural connective tissue, as seen with chronic inflammation of this membrane, can diminish lung compliance, restricting lung inflation.

THE FIBROELASTIC SKELETON IN LUNG DEVELOPMENT

The development of the lung in utero begins with the ingrowth of mesenchyme at the distal end of the embryonic tracheal bud. Bronchi arise from this growth plate and continue to branch off into bronchial tubes which become epithelialized. Throughout much of this early period of lung differentiation, little collagen and elastin is seen in the mesenchyme. The extracellular matrix is composed primarily of amorphous ground substance. As lung development in the human fetus progresses, collagen and later elastin become readily visible. Significant proliferation of elastin occurs in the lung interstitium postnatally, perhaps in response to the mechanical load imposed by ventilation and perfusion.

Biochemical measurements reflect what is seen morphologically. Animal experiments indicate that a very marked upsurge in collagen synthesis is seen late in fetal development. This most likely occurs as a result of rapid lung growth. A similar response can be observed during lung hyperplasia induced by experimental pneumonectomy. Though the rate of collagen synthesis decreases as the lung matures, continual turnover of this protein is maintained even in adult tissue.

Elastin synthesis in the lung, in contrast, is more restricted, remaining dormant throughout early embryogenesis, rising during late fetal development, then returning

to quiescence following maturation. Rapid reexpression of the elastin phenotype can however occur following experimentally induced degradation of this component.

Glycosaminoglycan and fibronectin synthesis is seen at an early stage of embryogenesis. Hyaluronate is especially abundant in the embryonic matrix and may serve to facilitate cell motility and proliferation since this glycosaminoglycan can coat cells and reduce their adhesion to one another. During maturation, the percentage of heparan sulfate in the lung rises, probably due to an increase in basement membrane which contains substantial amounts of this constituent.

That the connective tissue matrix influences cell growth and differentiation is apparent from a number of experimental observations. Disruption of the matrix has been shown, for example, to inhibit normal branching of lung buds during embryogenesis. Conversely, addition of matrix components to lung cell cultures can enhance differentiation. Insight into these types of interactions may be relevant to the repair process as well, since studies suggest its similarity to ontogeny.

THE FIBROELASTIC SKELETON IN DISEASE

Pulmonary Emphysema

The composition of the pulmonary fibroelastic skeleton reflects an equilibrium between synthesis of its constituents and their degradation. There are over 40 types of cells in the lung, many of which are capable of synthesizing one or more connective tissue constituents. There are also a number of cells which contain enzymes that degrade these components. An increase in either synthesis or degradation of pulmonary connective tissue will alter the characteristics of the fibroelastic skeleton. If these changes are of sufficient magnitude, the breathing process will be affected by altered mechanical behavior of the lung.

Pulmonary emphysema is an excellent example of a disease process that involves increased degradation of pulmonary connective tissue. In this case, the main component targeted for destruction is elastin. Loss of this material increases distensibility of the lung and reduces its ability to recoil during expiration. Alveoli become overdistended, and their walls eventually rupture. In patients with emphysema, this process may take years to produce clinical symptoms because of the large functional reserve of the lung. In animal experiments involving insufflation of the lung with a great excess of neutrophil or pancreatic elastase, however, severe emphysema may occur within weeks.

Emphysema is now thought to result from an imbalance between elastase and α_1-antiproteinase, which is synthesized in the liver and binds to the enzyme, preventing it from digesting elastin. Among the factors which may increase the load of elastase in the lung is cigarette smoking. There is evidence that elements in the smoke attract inflammatory cells to the lung. Neutrophils and, to a lesser extent, macrophages then deposit enough elastase locally to overcome its inhibition and permit degradation of elastin. The importance of the neutrophil in this process is confirmed by studies of experimentally induced endotoxin lung injury, in which aggregation of these cells in the interstitium leads to disruption of elastin.

Lung damage may also result from a genetically induced loss of elastase inhibitory capacity. Persons with the rare ZZ phenotype, who markedly lack antiproteinase activity, frequently develop severe emphysema. Much more prevalent is a partial deficiency, seen, for example, in individuals with the ZM phenotype. With the exception of cigarette smokers, the incidence of emphysema in this group does not differ greatly from that of the general population, suggesting that the amount of antiproteinase normally present in the lung is at least twice what is needed to prevent elastin degradation.

In situ inactivation of the antiproteinase may also occur. Oxidation of a methionine residue of the protein, for example, decreases its ability to bind neutrophil elastase. Though this reaction may be reversible, it has nevertheless been postulated to play a role in the development of emphysema in cigarette smokers.

While much research has focused on the mechanism of elastin degradation in the lung, less attention has been paid to the factors which control elastin resynthesis. The importance of elastin resynthesis in emphysema was brought to light by animal experiments which indicate that an upsurge in the synthesis of this protein occurs very shortly after insufflation of the lung with elastase (Fig. 73-4). The enzyme which catalyzes the cross-linking of elastin, lysyl oxidase, undergoes a concomitant steep rise in activity. Recent animal studies indicate that cigarette

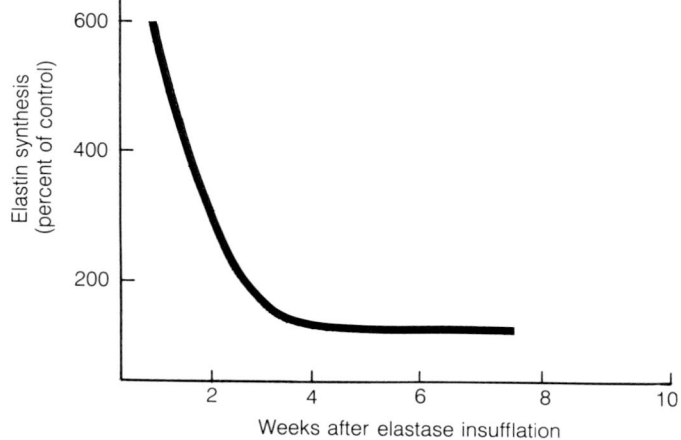

FIGURE 73-4 Graph of the relationship between lung elastin synthesis and the length of time following intratracheal insufflation of elastase into hamsters. Injury to lung elastin results in rapid resynthesis of this connective tissue component.

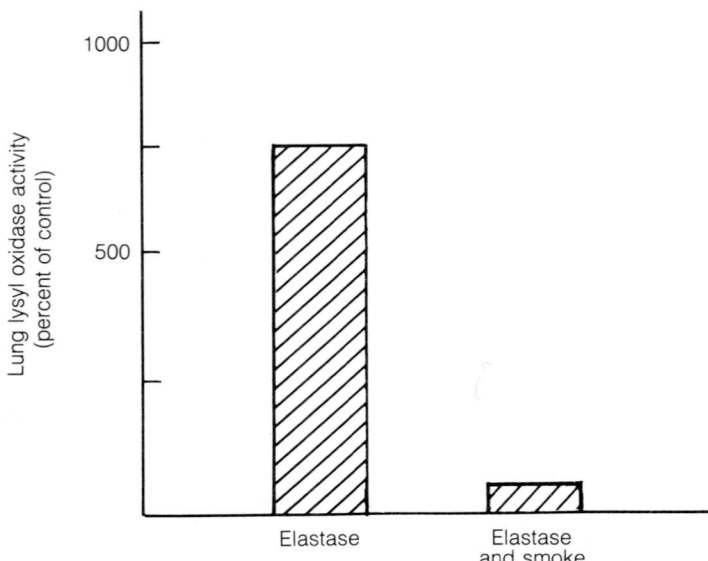

FIGURE 73-5 Graph of the inhibitory effect of repeated exposure to cigarette smoke on lung lysyl oxidase activity, 1 week following intratracheal insufflation of elastase into hamsters.

smoke can markedly decrease cross-linking of newly synthesized elastin following exposure of the lung to elastase. In these experiments, the activity of lysyl oxidase is dramatically reduced, suggesting that elements in cigarette smoke may be directed against this enzyme (Fig. 73-5). The effect of tobacco smoke on elastin cross-linking has likewise been demonstrated in vitro.

Impairment of elastin resynthesis may also occur by interfering with the assembly of the protein in the extracellular environment. Experimentally induced damage to the microfibrillar component shortly after instillation of elastase into the lung significantly impairs formation of new elastin. This finding reinforces the idea that microfibrils are important in elastin synthesis and further suggests that their degradation may be an additional component of the mechanism responsible for the development of emphysema.

Interstitial Pulmonary Fibrosis

In contrast to emphysema, interstitial pulmonary fibrosis involves marked proliferation of connective tissue in the lung. While many chemical and physical substances can initiate the disease, a common early event occurring with a number of these agents is necrosis of type 1 alveolar lining cells. Denudation of the underlying basement membrane results with subsequent rapid proliferation of type 2 cells and abnormal deposition of connective tissue constituents, including collagen, elastin, glycosaminoglycans, and fibronectin. Alterations in the content and distribution of these components may lead to constriction and obliteration of small blood vessels and terminal airways, causing uneven ventilation and perfusion.

At the cellular level, changes in the connective tissue matrix of the lung may have equally adverse effects. Disturbances in glycosaminoglycans or fibronectin can alter the structure and function of cells by interfering with their attachment to basement membranes. Failure of cells to reestablish normal chemical and mechanical relationships following injury may undermine the repair process and lead to scar formation.

Studies of animal models of pulmonary fibrosis indicate that glycosaminoglycans undergo marked proliferation shortly after initiation of lung injury. Deposition of collagen and elastin occurs later and is accompanied by a selective synthesis of dermatan sulfate. Increases in dermatan sulfate have been observed not only in interstitial pulmonary fibrosis but in other forms of injury as well, suggesting that this glycosaminoglycan may be involved in the organization of collagen and elastin in the extracellular matrix.

To date, the molecular sequence of lung repair remains obscure. Nevertheless, a number of studies have shown that inactivation of specific components of the inflammatory reaction can reduce the magnitude of the subsequent fibrotic response. Depletion of serum complement or inhibition of prostaglandin synthesis, for example, has been shown to diminish collagen deposition in experimental pulmonary fibrosis. Instead of affecting collagen synthesis directly, however, these mediators may act through a series of intermediate steps.

With regard to the role of inflammatory cells in causing the fibrotic response, chemical induction of interstitial lung injury in neutropenic animals does not result in diminished connective tissue synthesis. T cells, however, have been shown to modulate the severity of pulmonary fibrosis, perhaps in conjunction with macrophages which secrete factors that regulate collagen synthesis by fibroblasts. Inflammatory cells may further influence fibrosis by releasing enzymes which degrade collagen or other matrix components.

Pulmonary fibrosis may also be ameliorated by direct blockage of connective tissue synthesis. Use of the proline analogue, L-3, 4-dehydroproline, reduces collagen deposition in experimental interstitial injury and also results in an increase in both lung compliance and vital capacity. Another study has shown that administration of an inhibitor of cross-link formation, penicillamine, decreases the amounts of collagen and elastin deposited following experimental interstitial lung injury. A reduction in glycosaminoglycans is likewise observed, though penicillamine is not known to directly affect this component. This finding suggests an interdependence between the synthesis of glycosaminoglycans and that of collagen and/or elastin.

Perhaps the most interesting of these types of studies involves the administration of another cross-link inhibitor, β-aminopropionitrile, to animals with cadmium chlo-

ride-induced lung injury. Those animals treated with the agent developed emphysema, while those left untreated formed lesions more consistent with interstitial fibrosis. These results emphasize the fundamental importance of connective tissue synthesis in determining the form of lung disease which develops after tissue injury.

Acute Lung Injury

Studies of experimentally induced endotoxin lung injury indicate a rapid proliferation of glycosaminoglycans, with preferential synthesis of dermatan sulfate and chondroitin-4-sulfate. Though the precise mechanism underlying this response is unknown, it may be triggered by release of degradative enzymes from neutrophils which migrate to the lung in large quantities after exposure to endotoxin. Though elastin breakdown is observed in this model, the resultant emphysema is generally of a mild nature. If galactosamine is administered to reduce α_1-antiproteinase production by the liver, however, a more severe form of emphysema results, again illustrating the importance of the proteinase inhibitor in preventing marked destruction of elastin (Fig. 73-6).

As in endotoxin injury, a specific increase in the synthesis of dermatan sulfate and chondroitin-4-sulfate is observed at an early stage of hyperoxic lung damage. Again, this may be related to mass migration of neutro-

phils to the lung. One study has shown that after exposing the lung to 100% oxygen for 3 days, neutrophils entering the interstitium disintegrate and disperse their contents throughout the parenchyma. With regard to damage of elastin, α_1-antiproteinase activity may be reduced by oxidation and by saturation of available binding sites with excess elastase. Nevertheless, the marked parenchymal remodeling seen in hyperoxic injury is not primarily due to release of neutrophil enzymes since it may also occur in neutropenic animals. Most of the tissue injury may rather be caused by disruption of alveolar lining epithelium and capillary endothelium by highly reactive oxygen radicals. Necrosis of one or both of these cell types may be an important factor in the progression of acute inflammation to chronic interstitial lung disease.

CONCLUSIONS

Further investigation of the microarchitecture of the fibroelastic skeleton is needed. A number of connective tissue processes, such as cross-linking, occur extracellularly and depend on specific molecular alignments to form chemical bonds. New arrangements resulting from altered connective tissue deposition may produce a structurally abnormal matrix in disease. Such irregularities may additionally interfere with normal degradative mechanisms, causing excessive buildup of connective tissue.

Only a small amount of information is presently available concerning the chemical and structural relationships between components of the extracellular matrix under normal circumstances and in disease. One study involving ligamentum nuchae fibroblasts indicates that cross-linking of elastin occurs only when the cells are grown on dead fetal ligament. Such interactions between matrix components may help explain the ability of different cell types to organize connective tissue in accordance with the requirements of a given tissue.

With regard to treating interstitial fibrosis, insight into changes in the extracellular matrix will be especially important. Most cases of the disease become clinically apparent well after initial inflammatory events have subsided, when the pulmonary parenchyma may already be programmed to undergo fibrosis by virtue of basic changes in matrix relationships. Effective therapy may therefore depend on modifying the extracellular environment. To do so will require a much greater knowledge of the disturbances which have occurred in the matrix and how they may perpetuate altered synthesis and degradation of connective tissue components. Ultimately, a deeper understanding of the intermediate steps in collagen, elastin, and glycosaminoglycan neosynthesis in different forms of injury may allow control and modulation of the process to preserve normal lung architecture and limit alveolar destruction or interstitial proliferation.

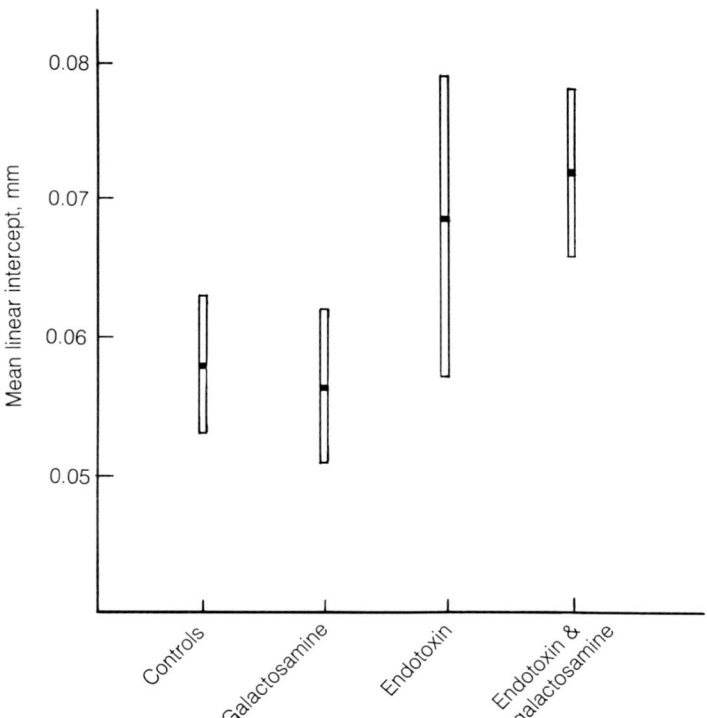

FIGURE 73-6   Graph depicting the increase in severity of lung emphysema, as measured by the width of the alveoli, following reduction of α_1-antiproteinase activity by galactosamine in endotoxin-treated rats.

BIBLIOGRAPHY

Bray BA, Osman M, Ashtyani H, Mandl I, Turino GM: The fibronectin content of canine lungs is increased in bleomycin-induced fibrosis. Exp Mol Pathol 44:353–363, 1986.
   Lungs from beagles in which fibrosis had been induced with bleomycin contained 0.99% Fn, more than a twofold increase over normal.

Clark JG, Greenberg J: Modulation of the effects of alveolar macrophages on lung fibroblast collagen production rate. Am Rev Respir Dis 135:52–56, 1987.
   Alveolar macrophages (AM) can either stimulate or inhibit lung fibroblast collagen production.

Clark JG, Kuhn C III, McDonald JA, Mecham RP: Lung connective tissue. Int Rev Conn Tissue Res 10:249–331, 1983.
   Well-referenced, comprehensive review of pulmonary connective tissue.

Crouch EC, Moxley MA, Longmore W: Synthesis of collagenous proteins by pulmonary type II epithelial cells. Am Rev Respir Dis 135:1118–1123, 1987.
   Interactions between pneumocyte-derived fibronectin and type IV procollagen contribute to the formation of the epithelial basement membrane and to the attachment of these cells in normal or injured lung.

Crouch E, Quinones F, Chang D: Synthesis of type IV procollagen in lung explants. Am Rev Respir Dis 133:618–625, 1986.
   A study of the synthesis of type IV procollagen, the major collagenous component of basement membranes, in slices of adult rat lung.

Doherty JB, Ashe BM, Argenbright LW, Barker PL, Bonney RJ, Chandler GO, Gahlgren ME, Dorn CP Jr, Finke PE, Firestone RA et al: Cephalosporin antibiotics can be modified to inhibit human leuko- cyte elastase. Nature 322:192–194, 1986.
   Certain low relative molecular mass inhibitors of mammalian serine proteases, including modi- fied cephalosporin antibiotics, can inhibit human leukocyte elastase (HLE, EC 3.4.21.37), an enzyme whose degradative activity on lung elastin has been implicated as a major causative factor in the induction of pulmonary emphysema.

Freeman BA, Tanswell AK: Biochemical and cellular aspects of pulmonary oxygen toxicity. Adv Free Rad Biol Med 1:133–164, 1985.
   Discussion of the mechanisms of oxygen radical-mediated lung damage.

Gosline J, Rosenbloom J: Elastin, in Piez KA, Reddi AD (eds), Extracellular Matrix Biochemistry. New York, Elsevier, 1985, pp. 191–227.
   The biochemistry and physical chemistry of elastin.

Hance AJ, Crystal RG: Collagen, in Crystal RG (ed), The Biochemical Base of Pulmonary Function, vol 2, in Lenfant C (ed), Lung Biology in Health and Disease. New York, Dekker, 1976, pp 213–257.
   Detailed information about collagen structure and function.

Ivaska K: Effect of extracellular glycosaminoglycans on the synthesis of collagen and proteoglycans by granulation tissue cells. Acta Physiol Scand [Suppl] 494:1–53, 1981.
   Role of glycosaminoglycans in extracellular matrix organization.

Janoff A: Elastases and emphysema. Am Rev Respir Dis 132:417–433, 1985.
   Current concepts regarding the pathogenesis of emphysema.

Kerr JS, Chae CU, Nagase H, Berg RA, Riley DJ: Degradation of collagen in lung tissue slices ex- posed to hyperoxia. Am Rev Respir Dis 135:1334–1349, 1987.
   Exposure of animals to oxidant gases produces a mild emphysema. Proteolytic enzymes are involved in hyperoxiamediated degradation of lung collagen.

Kirk JM, Da Costa PE, Turner-Warwick M, Littleton RJ, Laurent GJ: Biochemical evidence for an increased and progressive deposition of collagen in lungs of patients with pulmonary fibrosis. Clin Sci 70:39–45, 1986.
   The results demonstrate an increased deposition of lung collagen in patients with cryptogenic fibrosing alveolitis (idiopathic pulmonary fibrosis).

Last JA, Reiser KM: Effects of silica on lung collagen. Ciba Found Symp 121:180–193, 1986.
   The consecutive changes in collagen are described after a single intratracheal injection of 50 mg crystalline silica (quartz) into rats.

Laurent GJ: Lung collagen: more than scaffolding. Thorax 41:418–428, 1986.
   A review of the structure and function of lung collagen in health and disease.

Lemaire I, Beaudoin H, Dubois C: Cytokine regulation of lung fibroblast proliferation. Pulmonary and systemic changes in asbestos-induced pulmonary fibrosis. Am Rev Respir Dis 134:653–658, 1986.
> A study of the production of fibroblast growth factors derived from alveolar macrophages (AM) and peripheral blood mononuclear leukocytes (PBML) during the development of asbestos-induced fibrosis.

Mechanic GL, Farb RM, Henmi M, Ranga V, Bromberg PA, Yamauchi M: Structural crosslinking of lung connective tissue collagen in the blotchy mouse. Exp Lung Res 12:109–117, 1987.
> Male mice with the sex-linked mutation Blotchy (Blo) have a defect in copper metabolism, which results in deficient activity of a number of copper-containing enzymes. Inbred Blo/y mice spontaneously develop lung abnormalities which resemble emphysema and often die of ruptured aortic aneurysm.

Quinones F, Crouch E: Biosynthesis of interstitial and basement membrane collagens in pulmonary fibrosis. Am Rev Respir Dis 134:1163–1171, 1986.
> Maximal collagen synthetic activity that occurs 1 to 2 weeks after bleomycin administration is associated with a selective increase in the synthesis and accumulation of interstitial collagens.

Reiser KM, Tyler WS, Hennessy SM, Dominguez JJ, Last JA: Long-term consequences of exposure to ozone. II. Structural alterations in lung collagen of monkeys. Toxicol Appl Pharmacol 89:314–322, 1987.
> Long-term exposure to relatively low levels of ozone (0.61 ppm, 8 h/day for 1 year) may cause irreversible changes in lung collagen structure.

Riley DJ, Kramer MJ, Kerr JS, Chae CU, Yu SY, Berg RA: Damage and repair of lung connective tissue in rats exposed to toxic levels of oxygen. Am Rev Respir Dis 135:441–447, 1987.
> Lung collagen is degraded, and an emphysematous lesion is produced in rats after exposure to 98% O_2 for 60 h.

Rosenquist TH: Organization of collagen in the human pulmonary alveolar wall. Anat Rec 200:447–459, 1981.
> Definitive ultrastructural study of lung collagen.

Sandberg LB, Soskel NT, Leslie JG: Elastin structure, biosynthesis and relation to disease states. N Engl J Med 304:566–579, 1981.
> Excellent introduction to elastin structure and function.

Schellenberg JC, Liggins GC: Elastin and collagen in the fetal sheep lung. I. Ontogenesis. Pediatr Res 22:335–338, 1987.
> The ontogenesis of elastin (desmosine), collagen (hydroxyproline), and DNA concentrations and their rates of increase were studied in fetal sheep lungs from day 60 until term.

Spencer H: Pathology of the Lung. Oxford, Pergamon, 1977, pp 1–13.
> Morphologic description of lung development in utero.

Turino GM: The lung parenchyma—a dynamic matrix. Am Rev Respir Dis 132:1324–1334, 1985.
> Glycosaminoglycans and elastin in lung injury and repair.

Chapter 74

The Pathogenesis of Emphysema

Robert M. Senior / Charles Kuhn III

The Protease-Antiprotease Hypothesis

Emphysema Associated with α_1-Antitrypsin Deficiency
   α_1-Antitrypsin
   α_1-Antitrypsin Deficiency, PiZ

Emphysema in Smokers
   Lung Injury Produced by Inflammatory Cells
   Decreased Function of Intrapulmonary Elastase Inhibitors
   Decreased Repair of Injured Pulmonary Extracellular Matrix

Conclusions

For more than two decades the definition of emphysema has been "a condition of the lungs characterized by enlargement of airspaces distal to the terminal bronchioles accompanied by destruction of their walls." This definition was amended recently to exclude lungs in which enlargement and destruction of peripheral airspaces are associated with diffuse pulmonary fibrosis.

Symptoms and signs of chronic obstructive lung disease are usually present in patients with severe emphysema, but clinical features, radiographic findings, and even pulmonary function tests have all proved to be insensitive and imprecise methods for detecting and quantifying emphysema. Recent studies suggest that computed tomography may be a reliable method; however direct inspection of lung tissue emphysema is the only certain method. As might be expected, the requirement for lung tissue has hampered studies of the pathogenesis of emphysema in humans.

Cigarette smoking is the overwhelming factor associated with emphysema. Many studies attest to a rough dose-response relationship between smoking and emphysema and to the rarity of more than minimal emphysema among those who have never smoked. Other factors that have been associated with emphysema include environmental air pollution, hereditary deficiency of α_1-antitrypsin (α_1-AT), and hereditary abnormalities of extracellular matrix synthesis such as cutis laxa.

THE PROTEASE-ANTIPROTEASE HYPOTHESIS

From the time of Laennec, in the early nineteenth century, through the 1950s, mechanical explanations of airspace enlargement and destruction dominated thinking about the pathogenesis of emphysema. In 1963 Laurell and Eriksson reported an association of chronic airflow obstruction with deficiency of serum α_1-AT, and in 1964 Gross and associates described the first reproducible model of emphysema in experimental animals by injecting the lungs with the plant protease papain. These two observations indicated that emphysema could be induced by proteolytic injury to the lung extracellular matrix, and they eventually led to the protease-antiprotease hypothesis of emphysema that has been the prevailing concept of the pathogenesis of emphysema in recent years.

According to this hypothesis, there is a steady or episodic release of proteolytic enzymes into the lungs, primarily from phagocytic cells. Plasma protease inhibitors, especially α_1-AT, permeate lung tissue and prevent the proteolytic enzymes from digesting structural proteins of the lungs. Other protease inhibitors are synthesized locally in the lungs. Emphysema may result from an augmentation of protease release, a reduction in the pulmonary antiprotease defense, or a combination of both increased protease burden and decreased protease inhibitory capacity.

A number of proteases have been examined in experimental animals for the ability to produce emphysema following intratracheal instillation. The capacity to degrade elastin has proved to be the essential requirement. Proteases that are inactive against elastin fail to produce emphysema even though some, such as bacterial collagenase, cleave other extracellular matrix components. These studies have led to acceptance of the idea that degradation of lung elastin is central to the pathogenesis of emphysema.

EMPHYSEMA ASSOCIATED WITH α_1-ANTITRYPSIN DEFICIENCY

The clearest example of the association of protease-antiprotease imbalance and emphysema in humans is inherited deficiency of α_1-AT. Although the number of people with this deficiency is small, the pathogenic mechanisms seem to have implications for the far-commoner emphysema that occurs in smokers.

α_1-Antitrypsin

Human plasma contains at least six proteins that function as protease inhibitors. Together they make up about 10 percent of the total plasma protein. At a concentration of approximately 150 mg/dl, α_1-AT has the highest concentration of the plasma protease inhibitors. α_1-AT is also

present in other body fluids and can be recovered from the lungs by bronchoalveolar lavage. α_1-AT belongs to a family of inhibitors against serine proteases called the *serpins* (*serine protease inhibitors*); these have considerable sequence homology, particularly around their reactive sites. The serpins are important for homeostasis, since they exert some control over such major proteolytic cascades as the complement system and coagulation.

α_1-AT is a glycoprotein of molecular weight 52,000 that is synthesized primarily by the liver. It is a single polypeptide chain of 394 amino acids without internal disulfide bonds. There are three carbohydrate side chains that account for 12 percent of the molecular weight. The normal α_1-AT gene has been cloned and sequenced and the complete amino acid sequence of the protein deduced by that means, confirming the sequence that was obtained by direct protein sequencing. α_1-AT inhibits many serine proteases and does so on a 1:1 molar basis. Its capacity to inhibit serine proteases besides trypsin has led some authors to prefer the terms α_1-*proteinase inhibitor* or α_1-*antiprotease*.

Protease inhibition by α_1-AT involves proteolytic cleavage of the α_1-AT followed by formation of a complex between the attacking protease and the modified α_1-AT. The complex renders the protease inactive, and because the complex is quite stable, inactivation is essentially permanent. Serine proteases attack α_1-AT at the methionine residue at position 358 and produce proteolytic cleavage at the peptide bond between this methionine and the adjacent serine at position 359.

α_1-AT associates with neutrophil elastase much faster than with trypsin or other serine proteases. Indeed, the association rate with neutrophil elastase is so fast in comparison with other proteases that inhibition of neutrophil elastase appears to be the primary role of α_1-AT. Elastase is a major constituent of neutrophil azurophil granules. It is released from neutrophils during phagocytosis and is capable of digesting bacterial components, suggesting that one function is to help dispose of microorganisms. As its name clearly indicates, neutrophil elastase is active against elastin; however, its activity extends to many other proteins encompassing other components of the extracellular matrix including fibronectin and basement membrane (type IV) collagen. With this broad spectrum of activity the enzyme may assist in removing tissue debris and may help neutrophils penetrate tissues to sites where they are needed for the inflammatory process. Neutrophil elastase is one of the proteases that has been shown to produce emphysema in experimental animals. Thus, chronic unrestrained activity of this enzyme in the lungs because of an intrapulmonary deficiency of functional α_1-AT might be expected to result in the development of emphysema.

The genetic aspects of α_1-AT have been elucidated in detail. α_1-AT is specified by the proteinase inhibitor (Pi) locus on chromosome 14 and is transmitted co-dominantly. Thus, the gene product from each parent is expressed in the offspring. There is extraordinary polymorphism of α_1-AT. More than 80 phenotypes have been identified. A nomenclature for Pi polymorphism uses letters to specify the individual types. The original letters were chosen to reflect electrophoretic mobility: F = fast; M = medium; S = slow; and Z = ultraslow. The normal phenotype, PiM, exists in greater than 90 percent of the population.

α_1-Antitrypsin Deficiency, PiZ

Several α_1-AT phenotypes are associated with low plasma concentrations of α_1-AT and emphysema. Of these, the PiZ phenotype is by far the most common. Affected individuals have about 15 percent of the normal concentration of α_1-AT in the plasma. The prevalence of the PiZ allele (genotype) in the United States is about .012. Thus, the classic deficiency occurs once in 6000 people. In Sweden, where the deficiency was first detected, the gene frequency is .03, and the deficiency occurs once in every 1000 people.

Most individuals (80 to 90 percent) with PiZ eventually become symptomatic with chronic obstructive lung disease. In many, the rate of deterioration of lung function (measured by the annual decline in FEV_1) is nearly twice the average rate for persons with chronic obstructive lung disease who have normal α_1-AT phenotypes, but considerable variability is observed, and some persons reach advanced age with minimal respiratory symptoms. Smoking has a marked effect on the age at which shortness of breath appears. On the average, PiZ smokers have symptoms by age 40, about 15 years earlier than PiZ nonsmokers. The basis for the chronic obstructive lung disease is panacinar emphysema (Fig. 74-1A) that is often worst in the basal parts of the lungs.

The PiZ phenotype also predisposes to liver disease. An increased risk of hepatitis and cirrhosis exists in children. Among adults, chronic liver disease and hepatoma are found with increased frequency. Cirrhosis is found in 10 to 20 percent of those over the age of 50.

The diagnosis of PiZ can be made in clinical laboratories by standard serum protein electrophoresis. The electrophoretogram shows a low, flat baseline in the α_1-globulin region instead of the normal peak (Fig. 74-2A). It should be noted that the densitometric tracing itself must be inspected for the absence of an α_1 peak rather than relying upon the quantity of α_1-globulin calculated from the tracing. The reason is that the quantity of α_1-globulin is usually reported as normal because traces of albumin trail into the α_1-globulin region offsetting the baseline. For confirmation of PiZ, as well for determination of other Pi phenotypes, isoelectric focusing is currently the procedure most widely used (Fig. 74-2B).

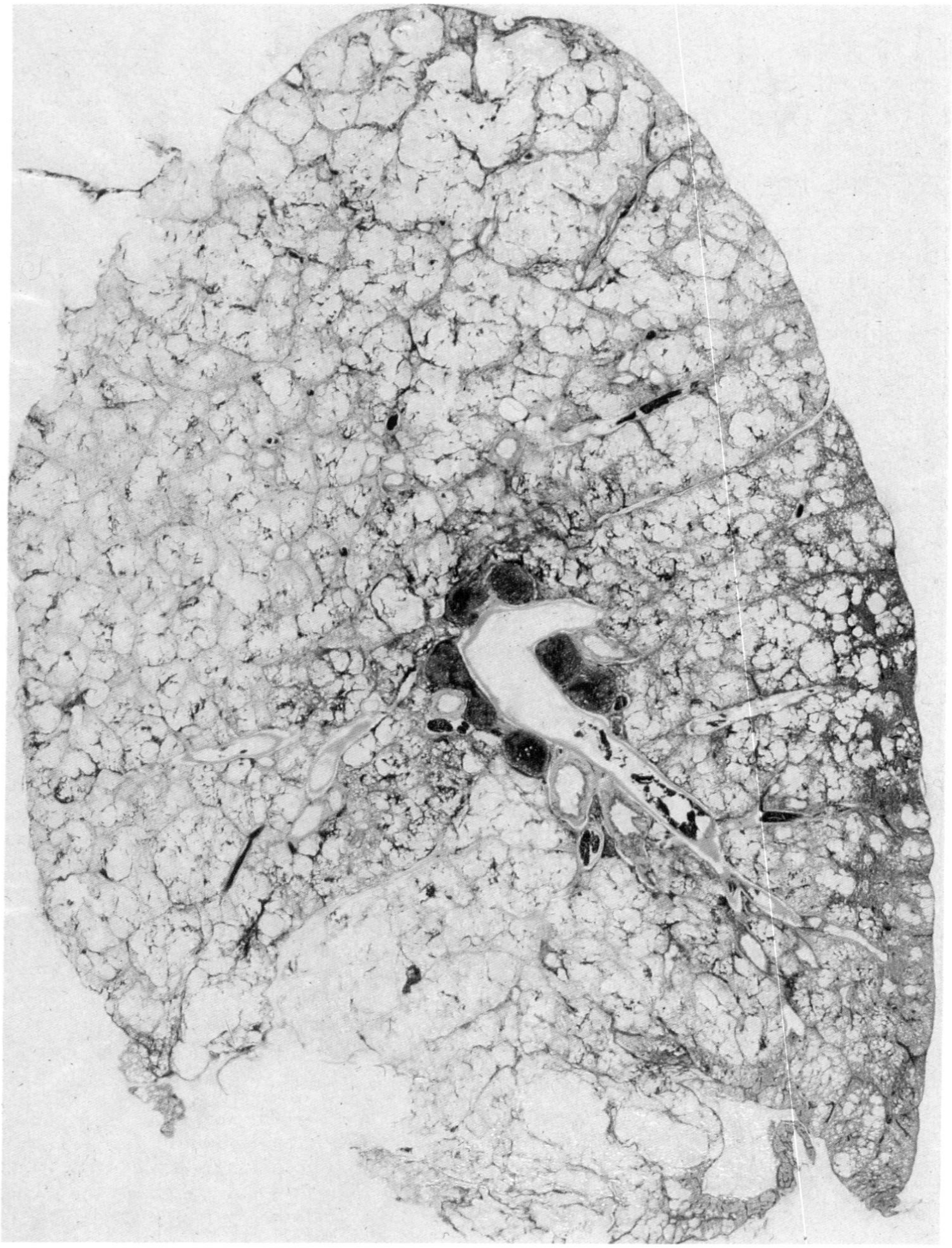

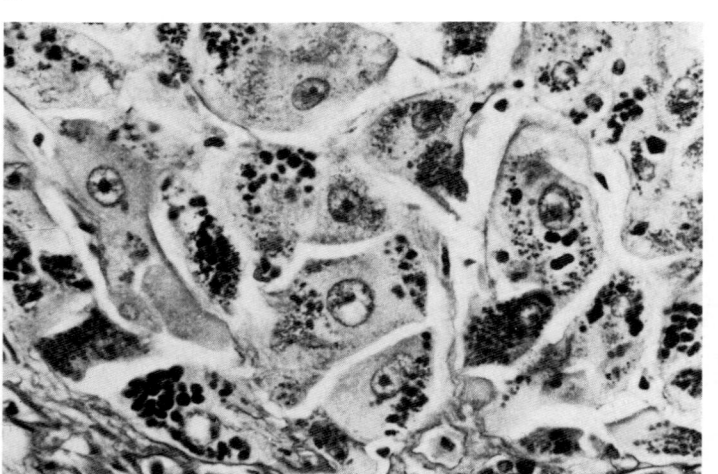

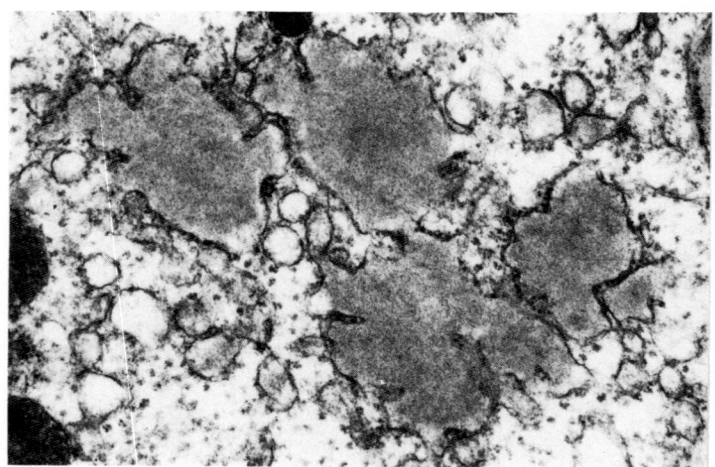

FIGURE 74-1 The pathology of PiZ type α_1-AT deficiency. A. Panacinar emphysema. Paper-mounted whole lung section. B. Globular cytoplasmic inclusions in hepatocytes. Periodic acid-Schiff stain after diastase digestion (×1250). C. Electron micrograph showing dilated cisterns of endoplasmic reticulum containing α_1-AT in a hepatocyte. These correspond to the globular inclusions in B (×25,000).

A

B

C

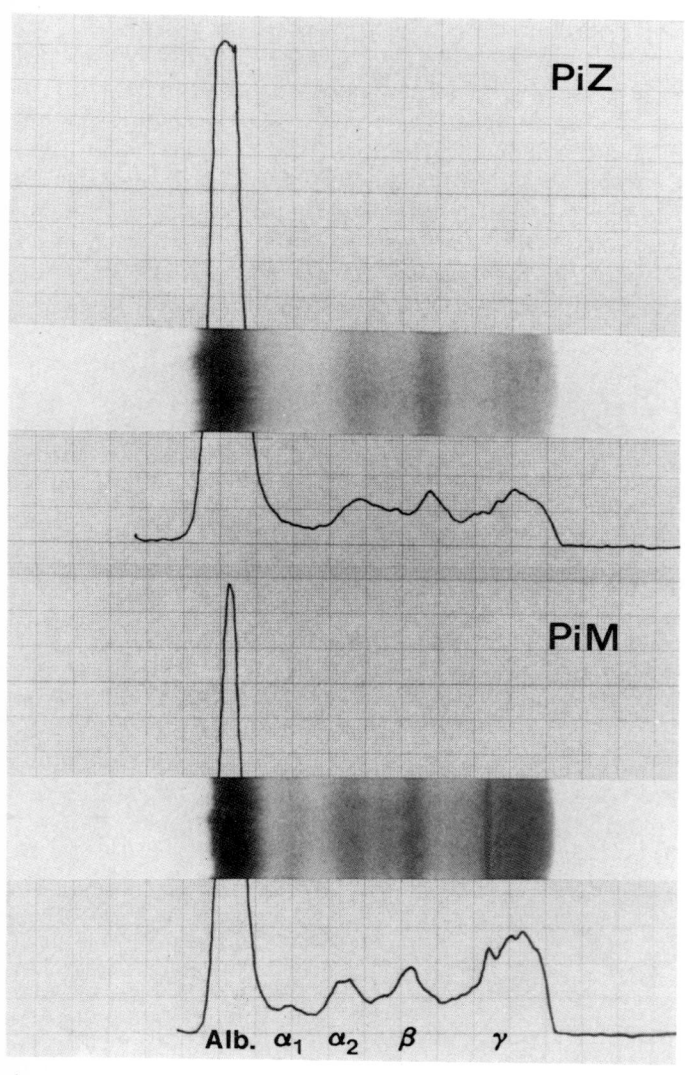

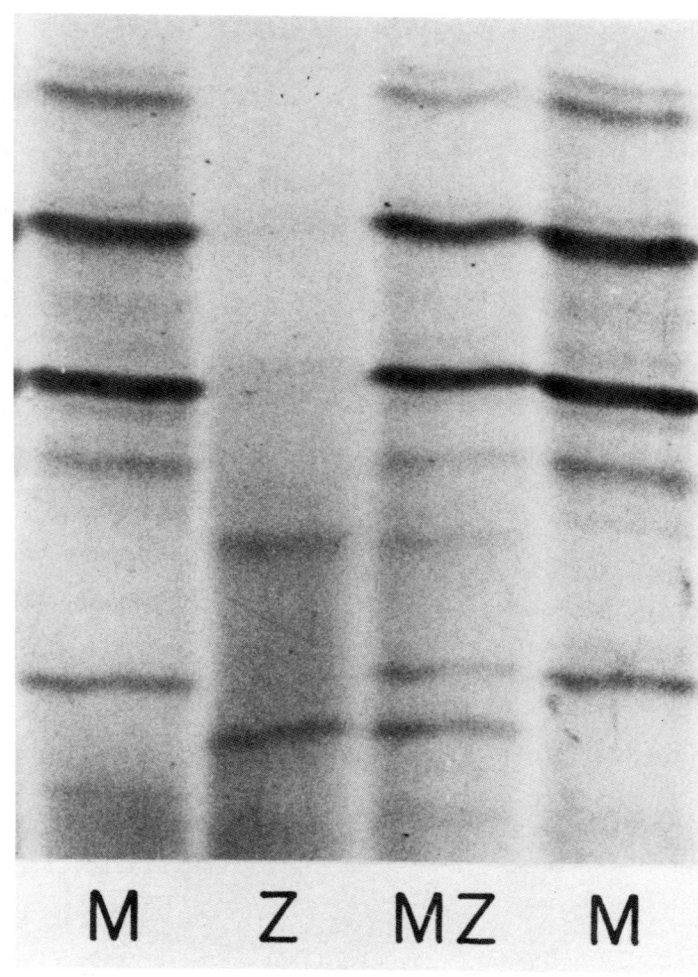

FIGURE 74-2   A. Serum protein electrophoresis in PiZ and PiM showing the absence of the normal peak in the α_1-globulin region in PiZ. B. Patterns of PiM, Z, and MZ on isoelectric focus. By this analysis, α_1-AT has microheterogeneity and thus appears as multiple bands. From above, in the M lane, the major bands visible are numbers M4 and M6; the minor bands visible are M2, M7, and M8. From above, the Z lane shows only bands Z4 and Z6. From above, the MZ lane shows bands M2, M4, M6, M7, Z4, M8, and Z6. *(Provided by John A. Pierce, M.D.)*

The abnormality leading to the PiZ type α_1-AT is a point mutation at position 342 with coding for lysine instead of glutamic acid. The resulting change in amino acid composition and charge of the molecule do not affect the ability of the mutant α_1-AT to function as an inhibitor; mole for mole the Z protein is as effective as the M protein in inhibiting elastase. Moreover, transcription of the α_1-AT gene in the liver is not affected. The levels of messenger RNA for α_1-AT are equal in liver cells from individuals with PiZ and PiM, and the messenger RNAs translate α_1-AT equally well in cell-free systems. The abnormality does, however, affect the processing of the protein in the hepatocyte. Instead of being transported through the endoplasmic reticulum and Golgi apparatus, becoming gly-

cosylated and then secreted, most of the abnormal protein accumulates in the endoplasmic reticulum of the hepatocyte where it can be detected in liver biopsies as periodic acid-Schiff (PAS)-positive globular inclusions in the cytoplasm of the hepatocyte (Fig. 74-1B and C). Thus, low levels of α_1-AT in body fluids and in bronchoalveolar lavage fluid in PiZ result from failure of hepatic secretion of the protein. In the near future, treatment for α_1-AT deficiency due to PiZ may include chronic replacement therapy with α_1-AT that has been isolated from normal human plasma or produced by recombinant DNA technology.

Individuals who are heterozygous for the Z gene (PiMZ) make up 2 to 3 percent of the U.S. population. These persons have approximately 60 percent of the nor-

mal plasma α_1-AT concentration. Although some controversy still exists, this common phenotype does not appear to lead to an increased risk of chronic obstructive lung disease.

EMPHYSEMA IN SMOKERS

Unchecked intrapulmonary elastase activity is generally accepted now as the predominant mechanism for emphysema in smokers. Proof is still lacking, however, that smokers who develop emphysema have an excess of intrapulmonary elastase activity, or an intrapulmonary deficiency of elastase inhibition, or both, because it is difficult to obtain biochemical and morphologic data in the same individuals. Thus, compelling biochemical findings reported by some investigators, such as decreased antielastase activity in bronchoalveolar lavage fluid from smokers and increased elastin fragments in plasma from smokers with chronic obstructive lung disease, are not backed by documentation of coexisting emphysema. Among the most suggestive evidence for elastolytic injury as a pathogenic factor in emphysema due to smoking is the immunohistochemical, in which antibody to neutrophil elastase has localized neutrophil elastase in smokers' lungs specifically in the emphysematous areas.

Although elastases from inflammatory cells are central in current thinking about emphysema in smokers, it is likely that the pathogenesis of emphysema in smokers is more complex than simply excessive intrapulmonary elastase (Fig. 74-3). Tobacco smoke not only causes pulmonary inflammation that burdens the lungs with increased elastase, but it also inactivates pulmonary defenses against elastase activity and blunts repair of injured pulmonary extracellular matrix. The contribution each of these effects of smoking makes to causing emphysema is unknown. It would not be surprising if their relative importance differed between individual smokers who develop emphysema.

Lung Injury Produced by Inflammatory Cells

Low-level, chronic pulmonary inflammation is a consistent feature of smoking and may be a major mechanism for the development of emphysema associated with smoking. That smokers have chronic inflammation has been demonstrated in a number of ways. By bronchoalveolar lavage, smokers yield 5 to 20 times the number of cells recovered from nonsmokers. Most of the increased cellularity in the lavage fluid is due to alveolar macrophages, but there are also more neutrophils than normal. Minces of lung tissue from smokers contain more neutrophils than are retrieved from that of nonsmokers and, by direct count, smokers' lungs have about twice as many neutrophils in alveolar walls as are found in the alveolar walls of nonsmokers. A distinctive finding in smokers is macrophage collections in the respiratory bronchioles. These are already present in young adults who smoke. The alveolar macrophage

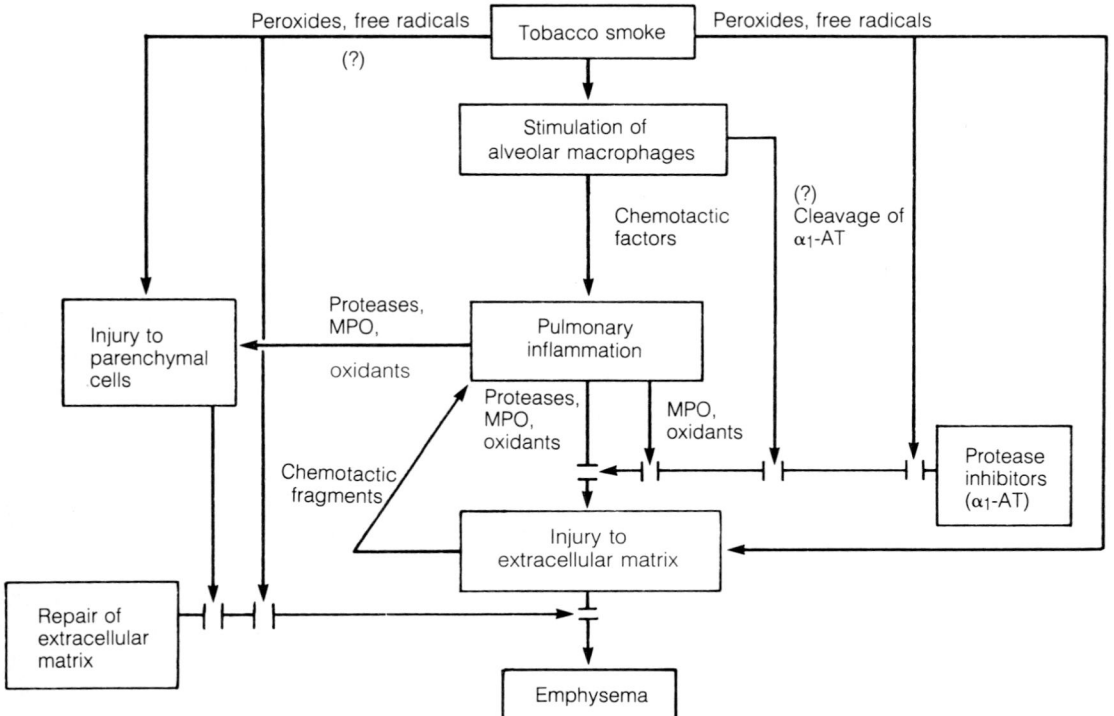

FIGURE 74-3 Schematic summary of current concepts of the pathogenesis of emphysema due to smoking. Smoking causes pulmonary inflammation that leads to increased intrapulmonary release of proteases, myeloperoxidase (MPO), and oxidants. Proteases injure the lung extracellular matrix, whereas MPO and oxidants lead to injury of pulmonary parenchymal cells and the lung extracellular matrix and to inactivation of intrapulmonary protease inhibitors. Peroxides and free radicals associated with tobacco smoke directly inactivate intrapulmonary protease inhibitors, damage the lung extracellular matrix, and blunt repair of the lung extracellular matrix by injuring the cells responsible for matrix synthesis and by disturbing normal extracellular processing of matrix macromolecules.

accumulations in respiratory bronchioles and the increased numbers of neutrophils in alveolar walls present in smokers' lungs have been replicated in experimental animals exposed to tobacco smoke.

Animal studies point to particulates as the ingredients in tobacco smoke that provoke the accumulation of macrophages and neutrophils in smokers' lungs. It seems most likely that the particulates act indirectly, by stimulating production of endogenous chemotactic factors that recruit inflammatory cells to the lungs, rather than by directly attracting neutrophils and monocytes from the circulation. Alveolar macrophages are apt to be a predominant source of chemotactic factors provoked by smoking, as these cells take up tobacco smoke particulates and are known to release chemotactic activity for inflammatory cells. Some evidence suggests that tobacco smoke boosts the output of neutrophil chemotactic activity by alveolar macrophages. It is possible that smoking leads to other sources of intrapulmonary chemotactic activity as, for example, from airway epithelial cells that can produce chemotactic leukotrienes. Peptides released by proteolytic enzymes from collagen, elastin, and other components of the extracellular matrix are also chemotactic, raising the possibility that breakdown of the lung extracellular matrix by inflammatory cell proteases may be a mechanism for perpetuating pulmonary inflammation.

Both neutrophils and macrophages may be involved in the breakdown of lung elastin in smokers. Many investigators have attempted to prove the importance of one or the other cell type, if only because therapeutic strategies would be much simpler if only a single cell and single enzyme were causative. The elastolytic activities of neutrophils are much better understood than are those of alveolar macrophages. This has occurred because neutrophils contain large amounts of a serine elastase that has allowed for isolation and characterization, whereas human macrophages have little associated elastase activity that can be collected for study.

NEUTROPHILS

Emphysema has been produced in animals by intratracheal injection of human neutrophil homogenates. Neutrophil elastase seems to be the most important constituent of these preparations as this enzyme alone is sufficient to cause the lesions. In vivo, however, other neutrophil constituents and nonproteolytic reactions generated by neutrophils may act together with elastase to injure the lungs.

Normally, neutrophils are only a small percentage of the inflammatory cells in the lung tissue at any time, but their life span is only a few hours, indicating a substantial turnover of these cells within the lungs. It has been estimated that approximately a half-billion neutrophils enter the pulmonary parenchyma daily in adults, and that over the period of a year these cells might release at least 8 mg of elastase into the lungs. This quantity of neutrophil elastase is far more than that needed to produce emphysema acutely in dogs. Thus, even under normal circumstances substantial amounts of neutrophil elastase need to be disposed of in the lungs. If smoking increases the neutrophil flux through the lungs, one might expect that substantially more neutrophil elastase permeates the lung tissue than normal and that there is a corresponding increased risk of damage to the lung's elastic fiber network.

ALVEOLAR MACROPHAGES

Although an increased pool of macrophages is present in the lungs of smokers, and macrophages predominate at the sites of earliest smoke-induced lung injury, a direct role for the alveolar macrophage in causing emphysema has not been established. In contrast to neutrophils, intratracheal injection of homogenates of macrophages does not produce emphysema. Some animal alveolar macrophages, when placed in cell culture, secrete easily measured amounts of a metalloproteinase type of elastase not inhibited by α_1-AT, but in the same kinds of studies human alveolar macrophages release amounts of elastase activity that are barely at the limits of detection by current methods. In recent efforts, however, in which cells are put into direct contact with extracellular-matrix-containing elastin, human alveolar macrophages have been reported to degrade elastin and to be even more effective than neutrophils when serum is present in the test systems.

The biochemical characteristics of human alveolar macrophage elastase are not certain. Different laboratories have found activity belonging to different biochemical classes of proteases. To complicate the situation further, human monocytes have elastase activity resembling neutrophil elastase that they lose as they mature into macrophages. Also, human alveolar macrophages can internalize neutrophil elastase by specific receptors and later release it in a still active form.

As summarized in Table 74-1, alveolar macrophages might affect intrapulmonary elastase balance in a number of ways. Alveolar macrophages might promote elastase activity by releasing several types of elastases, by inactivating α_1-AT, and by recruiting neutrophils to the lungs and stimulating them to release elastase. On the other hand, alveolar macrophages may limit intrapulmonary elastase activity by secreting elastase inhibitors and by removing elastases by receptor-mediated endocytosis. At this time the relative importance of these diverse macrophage functions is not known, nor is it known how smoking affects these activities or how macrophages of different individuals compare.

A concluding comment should be made about mechanisms that may exist in vivo to account for proteolytically

TABLE 74-1
Effects of Alveolar Macrophages on Elastase-Antielastase Balance

Increased elastase activity
  Release of elastase activity
    Metalloelastase
    Cysteinyl elastase
    Serine (neutrophil) elastase
  Inactivation of α_1-AT
    Oxidation by activated oxygen species
    Proteolysis by metalloelastase
  Recruitment of neutrophils
    Secretion of chemoattractants
  Stimulation of elastase release from neutrophils
    Secretion of neutrophil secretagogue activity
Decreased elastase activity
  Release of elastase inhibitors
    α_1-AT
    α_2-Macroglobulin
    Tissue inhibitor of metalloproteinases (TIMP)
  Receptor-mediated endocytosis of elastases
    Neutrophil elastase
    Elastase-α_2-macroglobulin complexes

SOURCE: Adapted from Janoff, 1985.

induced injury to extracellular matrix. Studies of degradation of extracellular matrix by alveolar macrophages and neutrophils have revealed that, under some circumstances, even high concentrations of protease inhibitors may not protect the matrix from proteolytic activity released by these cells. Lack of protection seems to occur because (1) inflammatory cells can adhere tightly to the matrix, excluding the inhibitor-containing fluid from the interface between the cell and the matrix, and (2) inflammatory cells generate oxidants that inactivate protease inhibitors in the immediate vicinity of the cells.

Decreased Function of Intrapulmonary Elastase Inhibitors

When α_1-AT is exposed to oxidants, its active-site methionine residue becomes converted to methionine sulfoxide. This change in the α_1-AT molecule decreases markedly the rate at which it associates with neutrophil elastase and, for practical purposes, means that it is no longer an inhibitor of neutrophil elastase. Oxidation has the same effect on another intrapulmonary neutrophil elastase inhibitor, the low-molecular-weight bronchial mucus inhibitor, also known as *antileukoprotease*, which is produced by serous secretory cells of mucous glands and probably by nonciliated secretory (Clara) cells of the bronchioles.

Tobacco smoke and oxidizing radicals released by neutrophils and monocytes, particularly in the presence of myeloperoxidase and chloride ion, can oxidize α_1-AT. Accordingly, it has been suggested that one mechanism by which smoking predisposes to emphysema is inactivation of intrapulmonary elastase inhibitors. Support for this idea has been developed in animals in which it has been found that repeated administration of oxidants, with corresponding decreases of both circulating and intrapulmonary elastase inhibitory capacity, leads to pulmonary emphysema.

Attractive as this idea is, however, it has proved to be difficult to obtain agreement as to whether smokers actually oxidize their intrapulmonary elastase inhibitors. In some studies, α_1-AT recovered by lavage has been less active in inhibiting elastase than would be expected from the amount of the protein present. Other studies of bronchoalveolar lavage fluid, however, have failed to observe differences between smokers and nonsmokers in either the amount of functional α_1-AT or the proportion of the total α_1-AT that is functional. Moreover, reductions in lavage fluid elastase inhibitory capacity have not been observed immediately after smoking.

Whether intrapulmonary oxidation of α_1-AT and other protease inhibitors will turn out to be an important mechanism in the pathogenesis of emphysema associated with smoking cannot be stated at the time of this writing. What does seem clear is that looking for differences between most smokers and nonsmokers may not be revealing since most smokers do not develop emphysema. One might predict that intrapulmonary oxidation is kept in check in most smokers by means of scavenger molecules such as ceruloplasmin, as well as by reduction pathways, as for example by the enzyme methionine sulfoxide-peptide reductase that can restore the functional activity of oxidized α_1-AT. An interesting direction of research in this area has been to devise changes in the α_1-AT molecule to make it more resistant to oxidation. Already, recombinant DNA technology has produced an α_1-AT molecule in which valine is substituted for methionine at position 358. The recombinant α_1-AT retains its elastase inhibitory capacity upon exposure to oxidants.

Decreased Repair of Injured Pulmonary Extracellular Matrix

Normally in adult tissue the turnover of elastin is extremely slow and its rate of biosynthesis low. After an intratracheal injection of elastase into an experimental animal, however, there is acute depletion of lung elastin followed by a burst of synthesis of extracellular matrix so that over a few weeks the elastin content of the lungs returns to normal, although the lungs develop emphysema. Restoration of lung elastin content in this model of emphysema matches most analyses of emphysematous human lungs which have shown a normal elastin content. A further point of similarity between the experimental

lesion and human emphysema is that the newly synthesized lung elastin in the animal model is disorganized. Disorganized elastic fibers in emphysematous human lungs have been recognized for over a century.

Studies of the biosynthesis of lung elastin after elastase-induced injury have shown that the accelerated synthesis of extracellular matrix plays an important role in minimizing the extent of damage to the architecture of the lungs. If this "repair" phase is disturbed, for example by chemically blocking the synthesis of normal elastin, the experimental animals develop far more severe emphysema, complicated by bullae and cor pulmonale.

Several types of information indicate that smoking may have deleterious effects upon lung elastin synthesis. Tobacco smoke inhibits lysyl oxidase, the enzyme that performs the first step in the formation of lysine-derived cross-links between elastin molecules during the formation of elastic fibers, and in experimental animals with lung injury produced by intratracheal elastase, the addition of tobacco smoke inhalation (1) enhances the effect of small doses of elastase on lung compliance and alveolar size, (2) blunts the reaccumulation of lung elastin, and (3) decreases the incorporation of labeled lysine into cross-

links of the lung elastin. Considering these findings, it is plausible that smoking suppresses lung elastin synthesis in people and thereby accentuates the effects of an increased load of elastase-producing inflammatory cells in the lungs and a decreased intrapulmonary elastase inhibitory activity that may also be consequences of smoking.

CONCLUSIONS

Emphysema is thought to result from disruption of the network of elastic fibers in the lung due to an intrapulmonary imbalance between elastases and their inhibitors. In α_1-AT deficiency the imbalance arises from a primary deficiency of the main circulating inhibitor of neutrophil elastase. Smoking, by far the dominant cause of emphysema, has multiple effects known to injure the elastic network of the lung that include (1) causing pulmonary inflammation which increases the pulmonary burden of elastases, (2) inactivating intrapulmonary elastase inhibitors, and (3) reducing biosynthetic repair of pulmonary elastic tissue.

BIBLIOGRAPHY

Abboud RT, Fera T, Richter A, Tabona MZ, Johal S: Acute effect of smoking on the functional activity of α_1-protease inhibitor in bronchoalveolar lavage fluid. Am Rev Respir Dis 131:79–85, 1985.

The α_1-AT in bronchoalveolar lavage fluid from smokers who had not smoked for 8 h was almost fully functional. A minor degree of inactivation of α_1-AT was found 1 h after smoking two to four cigarettes.

Albin RJ, Senior RM, Welgus HG, Connolly NL, Campbell EJ: Human alveolar macrophages secrete an inhibitor of metalloproteinase elastase. Am Rev Respir Dis 135:1281–1285, 1987.

Elastase activity directed against lung extracellular matrix is currently believed to be important in the pathogenesis of pulmonary emphysema. However, experimental proof of this hypothesis is complicated by the influence of assay conditions for the detection of metalloproteinase activity.

Banda MJ, Clark EJ, Werb Z: Regulation of alpha$_1$ proteinase inhibitor function by rabbit alveolar macrophages: Evidence for proteolytic rather than oxidative inactivation. J Clin Invest 75:1758–1762, 1985.

Rabbit alveolar macrophages inactivated α_1-AT by elastolytic proteases under conditions where oxidative activity was prevented, suggesting that oxidation is not necessarily the only mechanism for loss of functional α_1-AT within the lungs of smokers.

Becklake MR, Irwig L, Kielkowski D, Webster I, de Beer M, Landau S: The predictors of emphysema in South African gold miners. Am Rev Respir Dis 135:1234–1241, 1987.

A case control study showed that in gold miners shifts worked in high dust, smoking, and age were all shown to be strong and independent predictors of emphysema at autopsy. Prediction, however, was not improved by addition of any of the clinical features examined. These findings agree with previous cross-sectional studies in South African gold miners, showing an exposure response relationship between mining service and airflow limitation measured by lung function tests in life.

Bergin C, Muller N, Nichols DM, Lillington G, Hogg JC, Mullen B, Grymaloski MR, Osborne S, Pare PD: The diagnosis of emphysema: A computed tomographic-pathologic correlation. Am Rev Respir Dis 133:541–546, 1986.

In 32 patients undergoing resectional lung surgery for tumors, preoperative computed tomography yielded an accurate estimate of emphysema as determined by direct inspection of the surgical specimen.

Bruce RM, Cohen BH, Diamond EL, Fallat RJ, Knudson RJ, Lebowitz MD, Mittman C, Patterson CD, Tockman MS: Collaborative study to assess risk of lung disease in PiMZ phenotype subjects. Am Rev Respir Dis 130:386–390, 1984.
Analysis of lung function in adults with PiMZ, including smokers, did not show differences compared with carefully matched adults with PiM.

Buist AS, Burrows B, Eriksson S, Mittman C, Wu M: The natural history of air-flow obstruction in PiZ emphysema: Report of an NHLBI workshop. Am Rev Respir Dis 127:S43–S45, 1983.
A survey of adults with PiZ showed large variability in the rate of decline of FEV$_1$.

Campbell EJ, Senior RM, Welgus, HG: Extracellular matrix injury during lung inflammation. Chest 92:161–167, 1987.
A review of mechanisms by which inflammatory cell proteolytic enzymes can degrade lung matrix despite the presence of protease inhibitors.

Campbell EJ, Wald MS: Hypoxic injury to human alveolar macrophages accelerates release of previously bound neutrophil elastase: Implications for lung connective tissue injury including pulmonary emphysema. Am Rev Respir Dis 127:631–635, 1983.
Human alveolar macrophages can accumulate neutrophil elastase and later release it, suggesting that macrophages may participate in the pathogenesis of emphysema by serving as vectors for neutrophil elastase.

Carrell RW: α_1-Antitrypsin: Molecular pathology, leukocytes, and tissue damage. J Clin Invest 78:1427–1431, 1986.
Reviews many current concepts about the function of α_1-antitrypsin.

Chapman HA Jr, Stone OL: Comparison of live human neutrophil and alveolar macrophage elastolytic activity in vitro: Relative resistance of macrophage elastolytic activity to serum and alveolar proteinase inhibitors. J Clin Invest 74:1693–1700, 1984.
Human alveolar macrophages degraded more elastin than did neutrophils when both cell types were incubated with elastin in the presence of serum. Macrophage elastolytic activity was due to more than a single enzyme.

Cohen AB, Rossi M: Neutrophils in normal lungs. Am Rev Respir Dis 127:S3–S9, 1983.
A review of neutrophil traffic in the lungs with estimates of the elastase load that may be released into the tissues and discussion of factors that may be involved in triggering elastase release from neutrophils.

Damiano VV, Tsang A, Kucich U, Abrams WR, Rosenbloom J, Kimbel P, Fallahnejad M, Weinbaum G: Immunolocalization of elastase in human emphysematous lungs. J Clin Invest 78:482–493, 1986.
By immunohistology, neutrophil elastase was found in emphysematous regions of smokers' lungs.

Eriksson S, Carlson J, Velez, R: Risk of cirrhosis and primary liver cancer in alpha$_1$-antitrypsin deficiency. N Engl J Med 314:736–739, 1986.
In a retrospective autopsy survey the PiZ phenotype carried a statistically increased risk for cirrhosis and primary liver cancer in adult males.

Flenley DC: Pathogenesis of pulmonary emphysema. Q J Med 61:901–909, 1986.
A survey of current understanding of the pathogenesis of pulmonary emphysema.

George PM, Travis J, Vissers MCM, Winterbourn CC, Carrell RW: A genetically engineered mutant of α_1-antitrypsin protects connective tissue from neutrophil damage and may be useful in lung disease. Lancet 2:1426–1428, 1984.
Recombinant DNA technology was used to produce an α_1-AT molecule resistant to oxidants but effective as an inhibitor of neutrophil proteases.

Hoidal JR, Niewoehner DE: Cigarette smoke inhalation potentiates elastase-induced emphysema in hamsters. Am Rev Respir Dis 127:478–481, 1983.
In hamsters, neither smoking nor low-dose intratracheal elastase separately produced emphysema, but emphysema did develop when elastase and smoking were administered in tandem.

Hubbard RC, Crystal RG: Antiproteases and antioxidants: strategies for the pharmacologic prevention of lung destruction. Respiration 50:56–73, 1986.
Because of the key roles of oxidation and proteolysis in the pathogenesis of emphysema, reasonable strategies to prevent lung destruction in high-risk individuals include such therapeutic interventions as augmentation of lung levels of α_1-antitrypsin and the administration of antioxidants.

Hunninghake GW, Crystal RG: Cigarette smoking and lung destruction: Accumulation of neutrophils in the lungs of cigarette smokers. Am Rev Respir Dis 128:833–838, 1983.
Increased numbers of neutrophils were found in smokers' lungs both by bronchoalveolar lavage

and by extracting lung tissue. In vitro, cigarette smoke stimulated release of neutrophil chemotactic activity from alveolar macrophages.

Janoff A: Elastases and emphysema: Current assessment of the protease-antiprotease hypothesis. Am Rev Respir Dis 132:417–433, 1985.
A comprehensive review of many aspects of the hypothesis that elastolytic activity in the lungs is the cause of emphysema.

Kew, RR, Ghebrehiwet B, Janoff A: The fifth component of complement (C5) is necessary for maximal pulmonary leukocytosis in mice chronically exposed to cigarette smoke. Clin Immunol Immunopathol 43:73–81, 1987.
Recruitment of elastase-containing leukocytes to the alveoli and small airways of cigarette smokers is thought to be a major contributing factor in the pathogenesis of pulmonary emphysema. Cigarette smoke induces an increase in leukocytes in the lungs of mice by mechanisms which are partly dependent on C5, a potent chemoattractant for these cells.

Kucich U, Christner P, Lippmann M, Kimbel P, Williams G, Rosenbloom J, Weinbaum G. Utilization of a peroxidase antiperoxidase complex in an enzyme-linked immunoabsorbent assay of elastin-derived peptides in human plasma. Am Rev Respir Dis 131:709–713, 1985.
An immunoassay for elastin-derived peptides showed elevated serum elastin peptide concentrations in people with chronic obstructive lung disease.

Kuhn C III: The biochemical pathogenesis of chronic obstructive pulmonary diseases: protease-antiprotease imbalance in emphysema and diseases of the airways. J Thorac Imaging 1:1–6, 1986.
A critical appraisal of the role of an imbalance between proteases and their inhibitors not only in the pathogenesis of emphysema, but also of bronchitis and bronchiectasis.

Ludwig PW, Schwartz BA, Hoidal JR, Niewoehner DE: Cigarette smoking causes accumulation of polymorphonuclear leukocytes in alveolar septum. Am Rev Respir Dis 131:828–830, 1985.
Smokers and animals exposed to cigarette smoke showed double to triple the numbers of neutrophils in their alveolar walls compared with alveolar walls of nonsmokers.

Osman M, Cantor JO, Roffman S, Keller S, Turino GM, Mandl I: Cigarette smoke impairs elastin resynthesis in lungs of hamsters with elastase-induced emphysema. Am Rev Respir Dis 132:640–643, 1985.
Smoke exposure impaired the resynthesis of lung elastin after intratracheal elastase in hamsters.

Pedersen JZ, Franck C: Increased serum levels of ceruloplasmin in severe chronic airflow obstruction. Eur J Respir Dis 70:140–144, 1987.
Ceruloplasmin levels were significantly elevated in patients with severe chronic airway obstruction, as compared with smoking and nonsmoking control groups, suggesting that the increased ceruloplasmin in CAO is a measure of antioxidant activity, which may play a part in the pathogenesis of pulmonary emphysema.

Riley DJ, Kerr JS: Oxidant injury of the extracellular matrix: Potential role in the pathogenesis of pulmonary emphysema. Lung 163:1–13, 1985.
A review of evidence that oxidants may have direct effects upon lung extracellular matrix.

Rubin LJ, Windberg P, Taylor W, Heatfield B: Pulmonary vascular structural and functional changes in papain-induced emphysema in dogs. Am Rev Respir Dis 136:704–709, 1987.
Chronic emphysema produced in dogs by aerosol administration of papain results in elevated pulmonary artery pressure, which is characterized pathologically by medial hypertrophy of small pulmonary arteries.

Snider GL, Kleinerman J, Thurlbeck WM, Bengali ZH: The definition of emphysema: Report of a National Heart, Lung and Blood Institute, Division of Lung Diseases Workshop. Am Rev Respir Dis 132:182–185, 1985.
A presentation of the current definition of emphysema.

Weiss SJ, Regiani S: Neutrophils degrade subendothelial matrices in the presence of alpha-1-proteinase inhibitor: Cooperative use of lysosomal proteinases and oxygen metabolites. J Clin Invest 73:1297–1303, 1984.
In an in vitro system, neutrophils degraded the extracellular matrix even in the presence of α_1-AT. Failure of protease inhibition by α_1-AT in this system appeared to be due to inactivation of the α_1-AT by oxidants released from the neutrophils.

Weitz JI, Landman SL, Crowley KA, Birken S, Morgan FJ: Development of an assay for in vivo human neutrophil elastase activity. Increased elastase activity in patients with α_1-proteinase inhibitor deficiency. J Clin Invest 78:155–162, 1986.
A specific fibrinopeptide released from fibrinogen by neutrophil elastase was found increased in the plasma of individuals with antitrypsin deficiency, suggesting unrestrained activity of neutrophil elastase.

Bullous Disease of the Lung

David M. F. Murphy / Alfred P. Fishman

A bulla is a large, air-containing space within the substance of the lungs that results from destruction, dilatation, and confluence of airspaces distal to terminal bronchioles (Fig. 75-1). By definition, it is larger than 1 cm in diameter. Its walls are made up of attenuated and compressed parenchyma. Distinctions are drawn between bullae, blebs, and cysts (Table 75-1).

A bleb is an accumulation of air between the layers of the visceral pleura. The thin covering of a bleb predisposes to rupture and the entry of air into the pleura.

Cysts are epithelial-lined cavities that may resemble bullae on the chest radiograph. Many fall into the category of hamartomas, i.e., developmental anomalies in which are found mixtures of mesenchymal and epithelial components that are normally present in the lung. The pathologic nature of cystic lesions is generally reflected in their names: cystic adenomatoid malformations, peripheral bronchogenic cysts, congenital polycystic disease, atypical bronchopulmonary sequestrations.

Bullous disease refers to multiple bullae in otherwise normal lungs. It is different in etiology and pathogenesis from bullae that occur in conjunction with underlying lung disease, e.g., obstructive airways disease with bullae.

Pathologists are often inclined to view bullous disease as a subset of panacinar emphysema. Hence, *bullous emphysema* is commonly used as a synonym for bullous disease. But this is probably an oversimplification on at least three accounts: (1) panacinar emphysema tends to occur in the lower lobes, whereas bullous disease favors

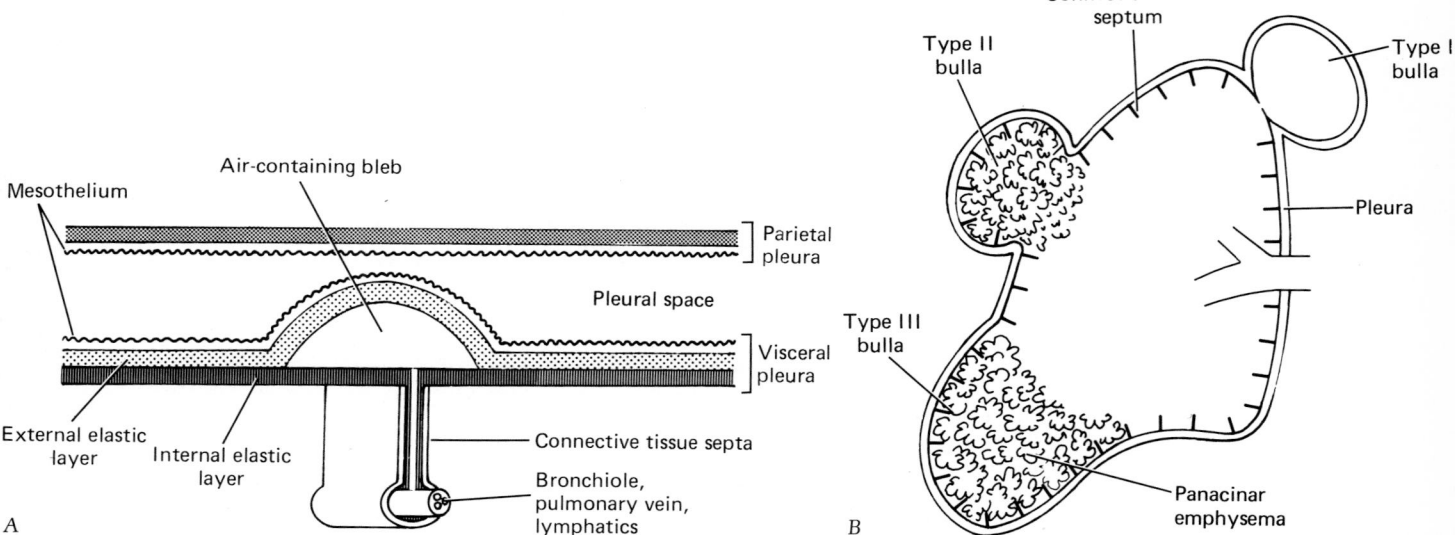

FIGURE 75-1 Blebs and bullae. *A.* Development of a bleb. A bleb is an accumulation of air within the pleura that is not confined by connective tissue septa within the lung. Air that escapes within the substance of the lungs makes its way to the surface, separating the internal from the external elastic layers on the visceral pleura. *B.* Different types of bullae. In contrast to a bleb, a bulla is confined by connective tissue septa of the lung and is deep to the internal elastic layer of the visceral pleura. Three different types of bullae are shown arising from a lung which has been removed from within the chest wall. A type I bulla is shown at the apex, a type II in the middle zone, and type III arising at the base. The short dark lines denote connective tissue septa. Panacinar emphysematous parenchyma is present within the types II and III bullae. *(After Reid, 1967, with permission.)*

TABLE 75-1

Characteristics of Blebs, Bullae, and Cysts

	Bleb	Bulla	Cyst
Site	Within visceral pleura	Arises within secondary lobule	Lung parenchyma or mediastinum
Size	1–2 cm	1 cm to greater than 75% of a lung	2–10 cm
Lining	Elastic laminae of the pleura	Connective tissue septa	Epithelium
Associated condition	Spontaneous pneumothorax		Respiratory infection

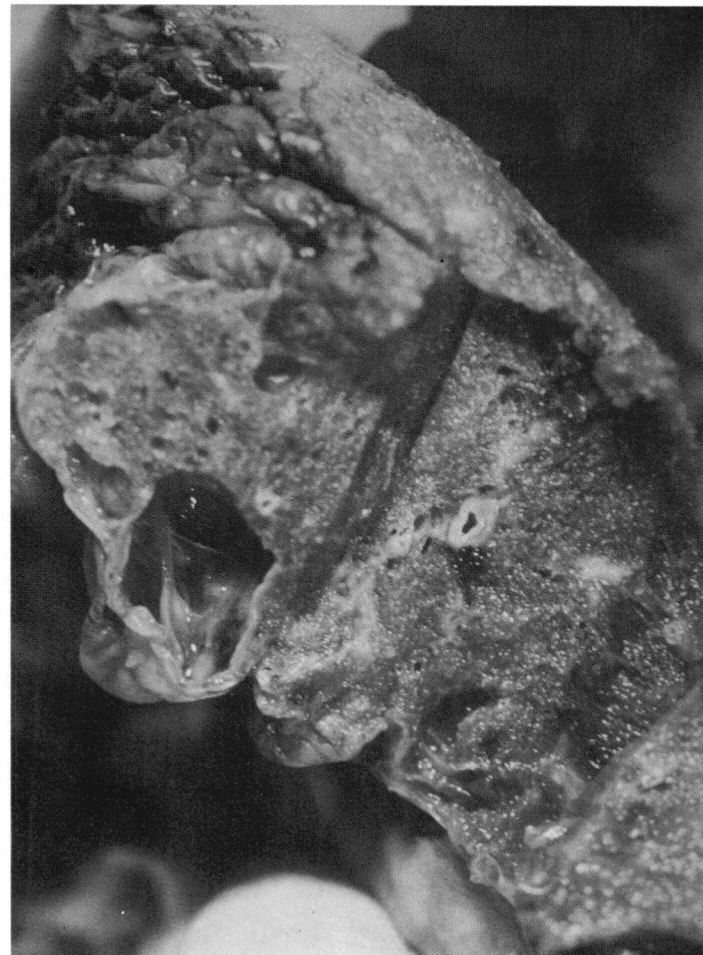

FIGURE 75-2 Bullae projecting from the cut surface of the lung. *(Courtesy of Dr. I. Gordon.)*

the upper lobes; (2) the natural history of the two disorders is quite different; and (3) panacinar emphysema has certain distinctive features not shared by bullous disease, e.g., a "winter-tree" appearance on angiography.

The etiology of bullous disease is unknown. The large areas of rarefaction within the substance that characterize bullae generally begin in the upper lobes. No unusual mechanical stresses, strains, or distorting elements due to intrinsic lung disease of the airways or pulmonary parenchyma have been identified. One form of bullous disease is commonly referred to as *vanishing lung*. Although this is felt to be a degenerative nonobstructive type of pulmonary disease, its etiology and pathogenesis are obscure. Biochemical abnormalities, such as α_1-antitrypsin deficiency, have not been identified in bullous disease.

Bullae within the intact chest are ordinarily relaxed, compressed, or molded to fit adjacent anatomic configurations. However, when the lungs are freed from these constraints by removal from the thoracic cavity, bullae project like bubbles from the lung surface (Fig. 75-2). Large bullae sometimes expand sufficiently to extend across the midline or up into the neck and cause compression of adjacent pulmonary parenchyma.

PATHOGENESIS

How bullous disease develops is still unclear. Several hypotheses have been tendered over the years, but none have been proven. However, the speculations do illustrate possible mechanisms. Among these are the following: (1) that weakness of the alveolar walls predisposes to the formation of bullae, particularly at the apices of the lungs where pleural pressures are most negative; this' theory underscores the proclivity of bullae for the upper lobes and stresses the influence of mechanical forces acting upon flawed tissue; (2) that inflammatory disease of a bronchiole leads to progressive air trapping and "tension airspaces"; (3) that some form of disordered collateral ventilation is responsible; (4) that the same mechanisms

as those responsible for generalized emphysema underlie the formation of bullae; and (5) that underlying paraseptal emphysema is the etiology.

Of all the hypotheses, that of underlying paraseptal emphysema is the more popular. It envisages destruction of alveoli adjacent to connective tissue septa or the pleura (Fig. 75-3); small "bubbles" develop along the edges of the lung when the pleura is involved. Occasionally, the bubbles become visible on the chest radiograph. As a rule, small bubbles and bullae produce neither symptoms, signs, nor discernible alteration in pulmonary function. But, should one or more rupture, spontaneous pneumothorax ensues. Recurrent pneumothoraxes secondary to paraseptal emphysema and small bullae is an indication for surgical resection of the affected area.

One reasonable basis for panacinar emphysema, bubbles, and bullae is an underlying fault in connective tissue. Support for this view is provided by the occurrence of bullae in Marfan's syndrome, a heritable disorder of

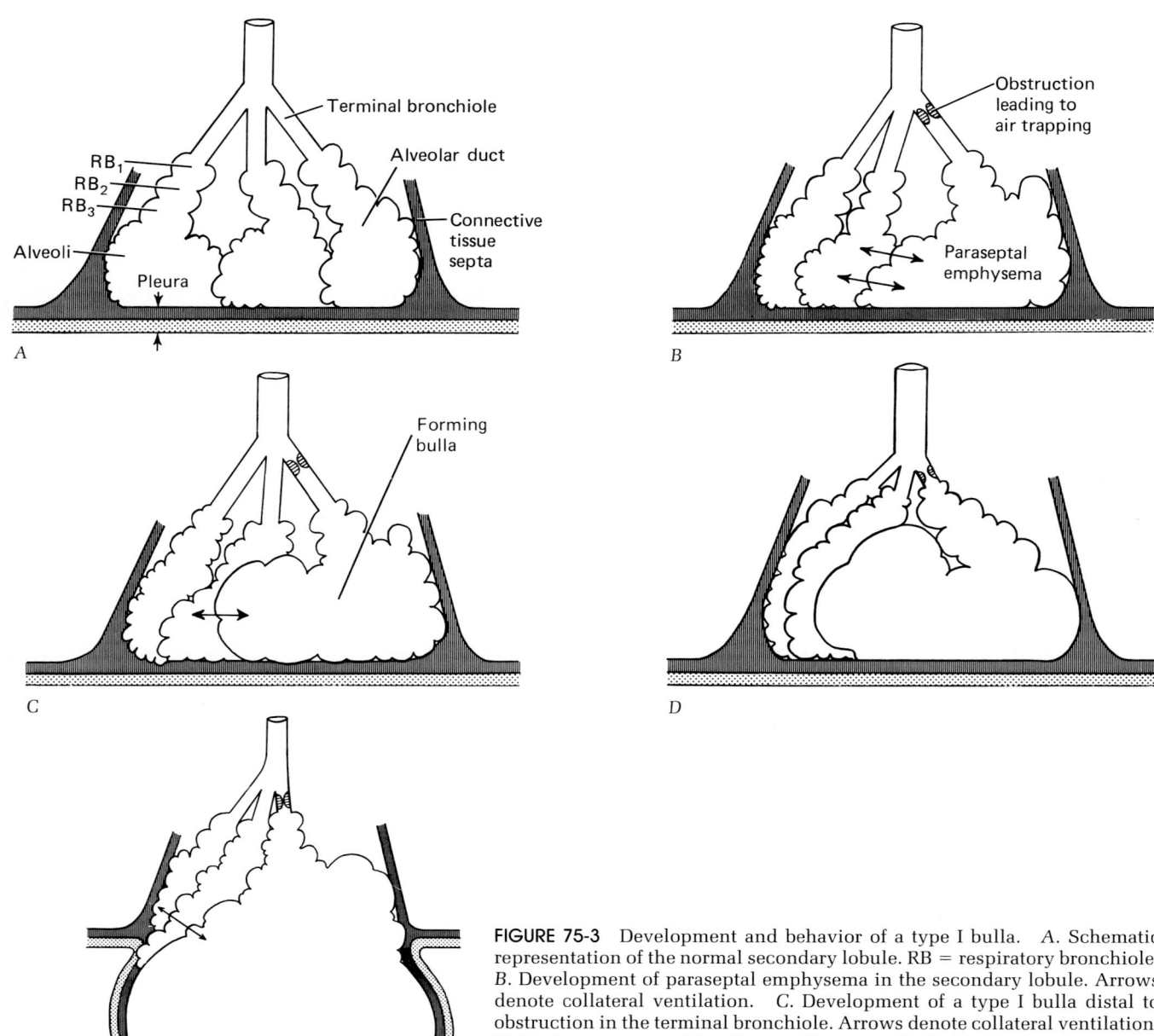

FIGURE 75-3 Development and behavior of a type I bulla. *A.* Schematic representation of the normal secondary lobule. RB = respiratory bronchiole. *B.* Development of paraseptal emphysema in the secondary lobule. Arrows denote collateral ventilation. *C.* Development of a type I bulla distal to obstruction in the terminal bronchiole. Arrows denote collateral ventilation. *D.* Limitation imposed by chest wall on type I bulla leading to compression of adjacent lung. *E.* Effect on type I bulla when the lung is removed from within the chest wall. *(After Fraser RG, Paré GAP: Diagnosis of Diseases of the Chest, 2d ed, Saunders, Philadelphia, 1977, with permission.)*

connective tissue. As a rule, the bullae are apical in location. Not infrequently they give rise to pneumothoraxes, most of which are recurrent and bilateral; spontaneous pneumothorax vies with aortic dissection as the primary diagnostic consideration in an individual with Marfan's syndrome who develops sudden, severe chest pain. In contrast to bullae that occur in lungs that are otherwise normal anatomically, bullae that arise in diseased lungs seem to form as a consequence of local distortions and nearby scarring.

CLASSIFICATION OF BULLAE

Bullae are classified into three main types (Fig. 75-1*B*).

Type I bullae are characterized by a narrow neck that connects the bulla with pulmonary parenchyma. This type of bulla is presumably caused by overinflation of a volume of lung tissue, as may follow partial obstruction to the lumen of the bronchiole supplying the region. As a result of the partial obstruction, air trapping occurs (Fig. 75-3). In support of this idea is the association of bronchi-

olitis and bullae. The walls of type I bullae are thin, and their interiors are empty. Scanning electron microscopy has disclosed not only that the thin neck is a consistent feature but also that the pleural mesothelial cells on their external surface are either reduced in number or completely absent, revealing bundles of collagen fibers lying naked and separated from each other by small pores or crevices. Type I bullae are usually found at the apices of the lung and along the edges of the lingula and middle lobes. They also occur often in association with paraseptal emphysema.

In contrast, type II bullae arise from the subpleural parenchyma and are characterized by a neck of panacinar emphysematous lung tissue. Also, the interior of these airspaces consists of emphysematous lung in which blood vessels are still present, and in contrast to the type I bulla, the outer wall is formed by pleura covered with intact mesothelial cells. Although connective tissue septa are present within the bullae, they are not found in the wall. Type II bullae may occur anywhere in the lung but are most frequent in the upper lobe, on the anterior surface of the middle lobe, and over the diaphragm.

Type III bullae consist of slightly hyperinflated lung connected to the rest of the lung by an extremely broad base that extends deep into the parenchyma. This type is believed to represent an atrophic form of emphysema.

DISTRIBUTION OF BULLAE

As indicated above, the tendency for bullae to occur in the upper lobes is usually attributed to the greater mechanical stresses imposed on the apices than on the bases of the lungs. Because intrapleural pressures near the apices of the lungs are more negative than at the bases, apical alveoli are subjected to greater expanding stresses than are basal alveoli. Radioactive gas studies and in situ freezing techniques have demonstrated that the alveoli in the upper zones of the lungs are considerably larger than those in the lower zones. As indicated elsewhere in this book, gravity plays a role in this feature of the upright lung, behaving like a coiled spring which when allowed to dangle in the upright position shows larger gaps between coils at its top than at its bottom.

Engineering techniques used to study the distribution of stresses in aircraft have been applied to the analysis of stresses on the lung. They have shown that the larger expanding stresses at the apices are directed primarily in a vertical direction but also, to a lesser extent, laterally. These stresses tend to increase with expansion of the lung but are also manifest when the lung volume decreases below functional residual capacity. The increase in apical stress at low lung volumes has been attributed to an increase in the rigidity of the lungs as the residual volume is approached.

CLINICAL FEATURES

In asymptomatic patients, bullae are usually detected in the course of routine chest radiography. However, in some patients, bullae give rise to progressive dyspnea or chest pain (Fig. 75-4). On occasion, a patient with bullous disease of the lungs develops sudden severe breathlessness due to the development of a spontaneous pneumothorax (Fig. 75-5) or a sudden increase in the size of a bulla due to air trapping. The development of bullae in individuals with obstructive airways disease tends to aggravate breathlessness, presumably as a consequence of reducing expiratory flow rates.

In the individual known to have bullous disease, the onset of fatigue, generally accompanied by an increase in coughing and sputum production, usually heralds the presence of infection in a bulla (Fig. 75-6). Pleuritic chest pain is occasionally part of the syndrome. Fever and leukocytosis are often not prominent and Gram stain of the sputum often shows only a mixed flora without a predominant organism. Radiographically, infection is usually identified by the appearance of an air-fluid level (Fig. 75-6). It is generally held that the mechanism responsible for fluid in a large airspace (bulla) is somewhat akin to that responsible for a parapneumonic pleural effusion. Alternatively, the occurrence of fluid has been attributed to impeded drainage of the contents of the bulla due to obstruction of microscopic communications between the airspace and the pulmonary parenchyma. On occasion, infection of a bulla causes it to disappear completely. More often, the air-fluid level persists for months after the infection has cleared in response to treatment.

The physical findings in a patient with one or more bullae usually reflect the state of the lungs overall or in the immediate vicinity of the bulla. Only infrequently do giant bullae reach a size sufficient to cause the expected localized decrease, or absence, of breath sounds and the expected increase in resonance to percussion over the bulla.

RADIOLOGIC FEATURES

Although routine chest radiography is the most practical method for identifying the presence of bullae, this technique discloses only about 15 percent of bullae. In a given patient, serial radiographs over years are invaluable in tracing the evolution of the disease. The presence of bullous lung disease is suggested by areas of increased radiolucency sharply delineated by fine radiopaque lines that delineate the walls of the bullae. These lines, "hairline shadows," are composed of compressed and fused connective tissue or pleura. Because these hairline shadows appear incomplete on the chest radiograph, they display only segments of the wall of the bulla (Fig. 75-5). It is

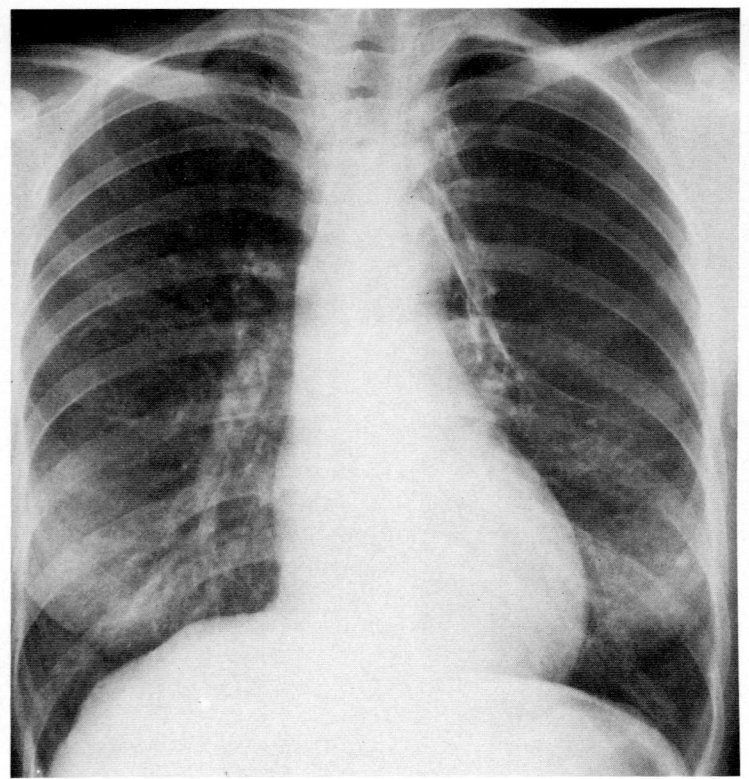

A

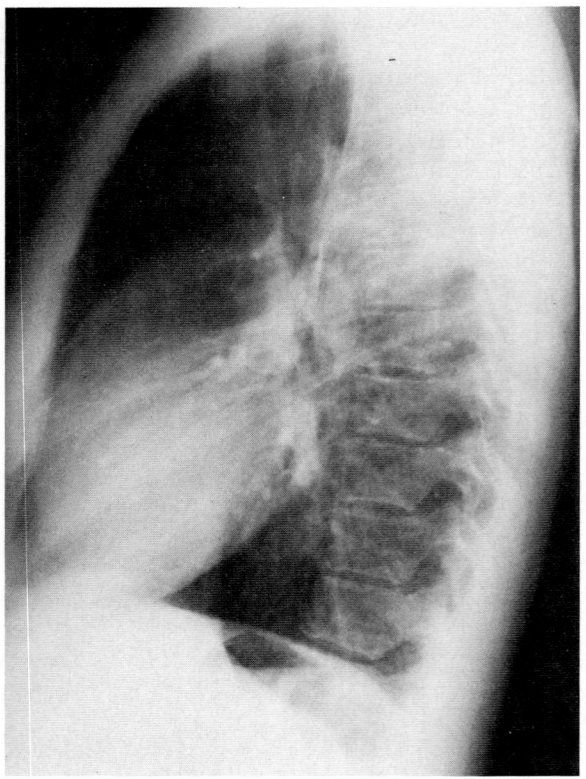

B

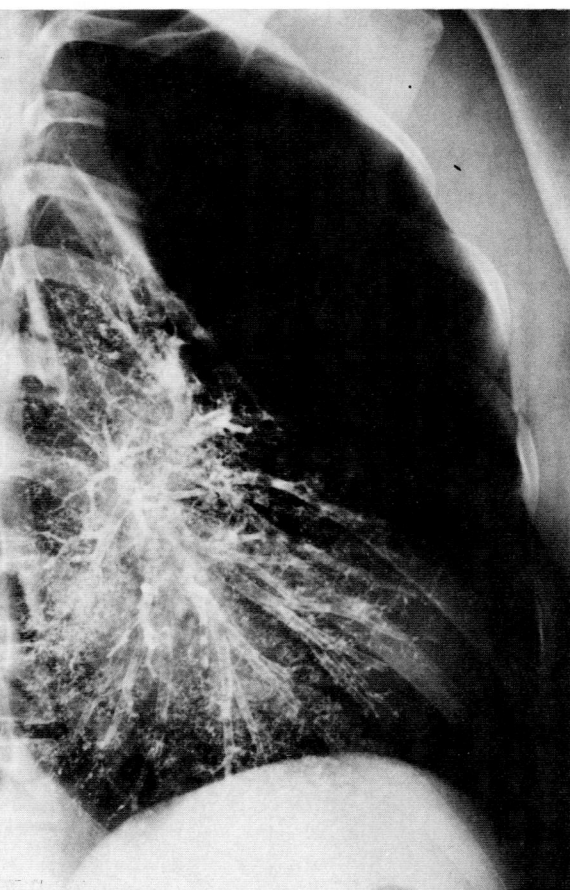

C

FIGURE 75-4 Large bulla in a 35-year-old woman admitted because of chest pain and increasing dyspnea. *A.* Chest radiograph (PA view). A large translucent area in the left upper lung represents a bulla that is causing compression of adjacent lung. *B.* Chest radiograph (lateral view). A hairline shadow outlines a large bulla in the left upper lobe. *C.* Bronchogram of left lung. Compression of the bronchial tree by the large bulla is evident.

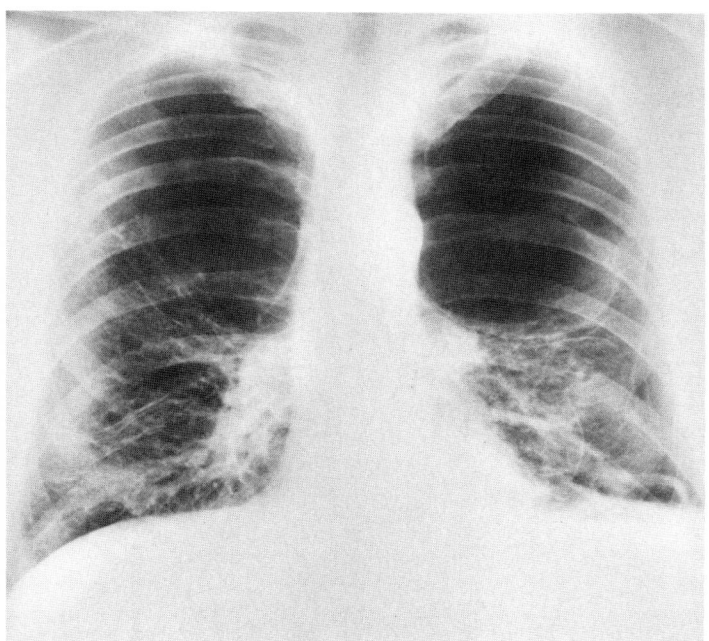

A

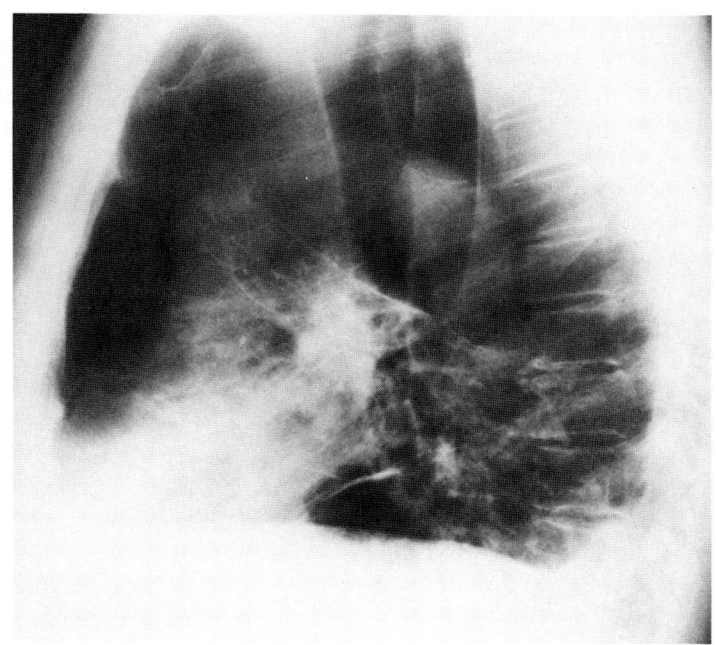

B

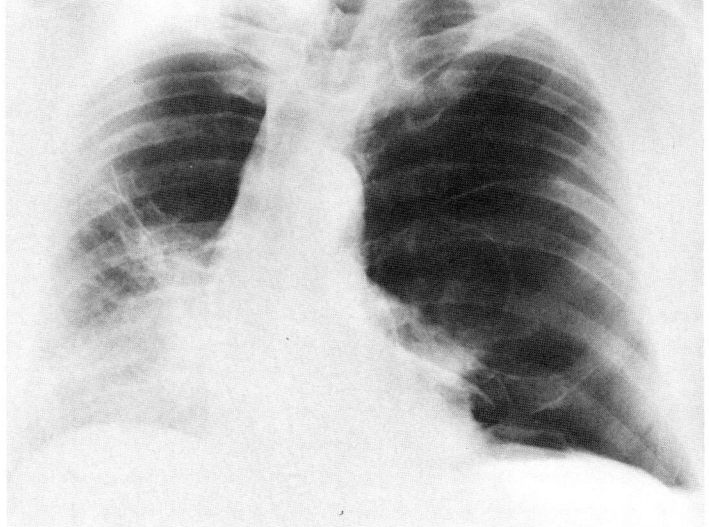

C

FIGURE 75-5   Bullous disease in a 53-year-old male. *A*. Chest radiograph (PA view) showing upper zonal areas of increased radiolucency. *B*. Chest radiograph (lateral view) showing hairline borders of multiple bullae. *C*. Chest radiograph showing a left-sided pneumothorax with residual inflated bullae. *(Courtesy of Dr. S. Flicker.)*

usually not difficult to distinguish the hairline shadows produced by a bulla from the thicker, sometimes irregular, walls of a cavity. More troublesome is the distinction between bullae and cysts. In favor of bullae is the presence of other radiologic signs of emphysema or fibrotic lung disorders. The differential diagnosis of multiple enlarged thin-walled airspaces on the chest radiograph in adults is shown in Table 75-2.

The superimposition of a chronic infiltrate on an existing bulla raises the possibility of a concomitant fungal or tuberculous infection. Also, a localized air-fluid level on the chest radiograph raises the prospect of infection; the differential diagnosis then includes lung abscess, pul-

monary tuberculosis, pulmonary fungal disease, cavitary lung carcinoma, pulmonary hemorrhage within a bulla, congestive heart failure, or carcinoma arising from a bulla (Fig. 75-7).

Fluid in a Bulla

The presence of fluid in a bulla, especially if the bulla is located subpleurally, occasionally prompts the mistaken diagnosis of loculated hydropneumothorax. Computed tomography is helpful in separating these two conditions: when locules within the bulla fill with fluid, the bulla shows characteristic strands or septa sometimes in a "step

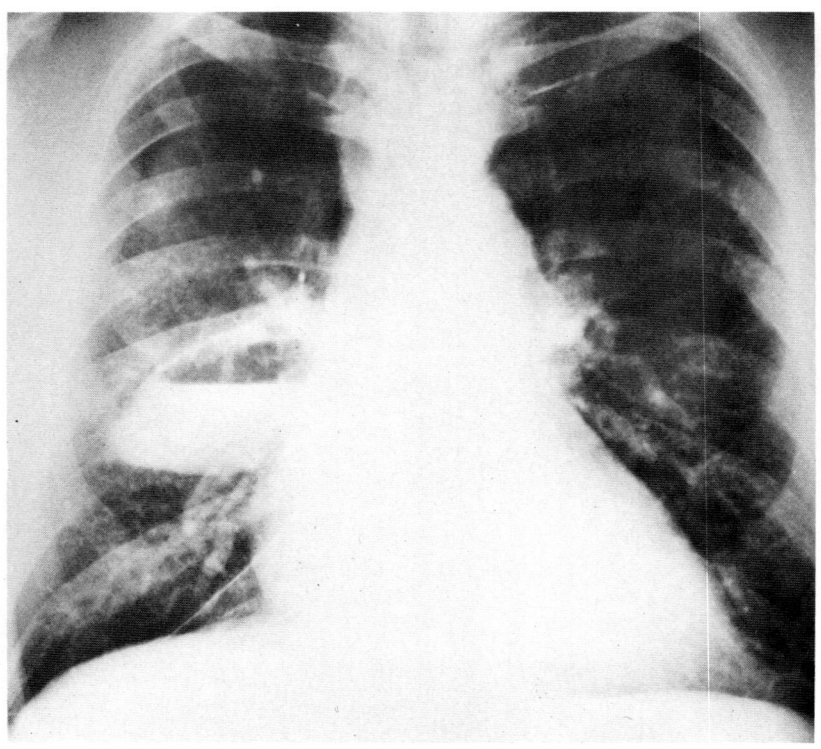
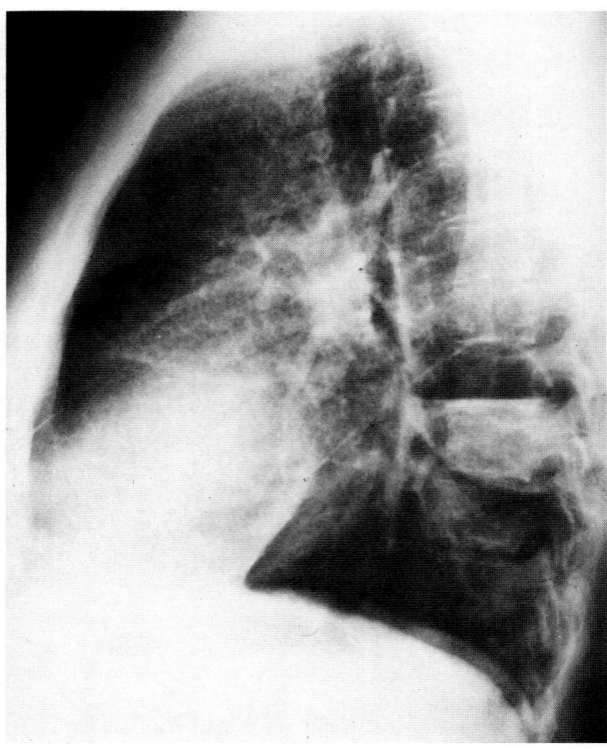

A   B

FIGURE 75-6 An infected bulla in a 44-year-old male with mitral stenosis.   A. Chest radiograph (PA view). A translucent area is visible in the right midzone with a clearly defined air-fluid level.   B. Lateral radiograph.

TABLE 75-2
***The Differential Diagnosis of Thin-Walled
Enlarged Airspaces in the Lungs***

Cystic bronchiectasis
Pneumatoceles
Fungal infections (coccidioidomycosis)
Septic emboli
Parasitic disorders

ladder" configuration; in contrast, a loculated hydrothorax shows no septa.

Special Techniques

A forced expiration is sometimes helpful in demonstrating the presence of bullae either on the chest radiograph or during fluoroscopy: air trapping during the expiration accentuates their outline by preventing them from decreasing in size as the surrounding lung empties. Large bullae sometimes displace the mediastinum contralaterally and compress the opposite lung; sometimes it is difficult to distinguish between a large bulla and a pneumothorax. Conventional tomography, once used for this purpose, has largely been succeeded by computed tomography which provides valuable anatomic information

about the size, number, and relationships of bullae; compression of adjacent lung; and disposition of the pulmonary vasculature.

Angiography provides even more precise information about the state of the pulmonary vasculature (Fig. 75-8). It is particularly valuable in evaluating the compressed lung adjacent to a large bulla. Pulmonary artery pressures can also be obtained at the time of angiography (Table 75-3). In addition to the compressing effect on pulmonary blood vessels caused by air trapping within bullae, relaxation of parenchyma in their vicinity contributes to an increase in pulmonary arterial pressure by decreasing elastic recoil of the perivascular tissues and increasing tissue pressure. A regional bronchogram at the time of bronchoscopy is sometimes helpful in assessing the state of the airways in the region of lung compression (Fig. 75-4).

Useful preoperative information can also be obtained from lung scanning using radioisotopes (Figs. 75-9 and 75-10). A perfusion scan provides a qualitative assessment of the pulmonary vasculature. The results of ventilation scans vary with the technique: a *single*-breath xenon 133 scan often fails to demonstrate ventilation of a bulla, whereas a *continuous* ventilation scan often shows slow filling and emptying of the bulla. Complete lack of communication between the airways and the bulla is reflected in the absence of filling during all phases of the continuous ventilation scan.

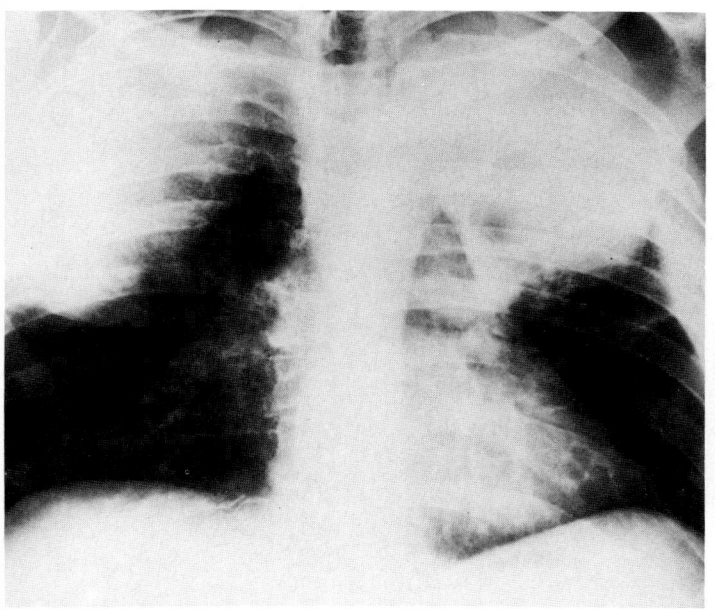

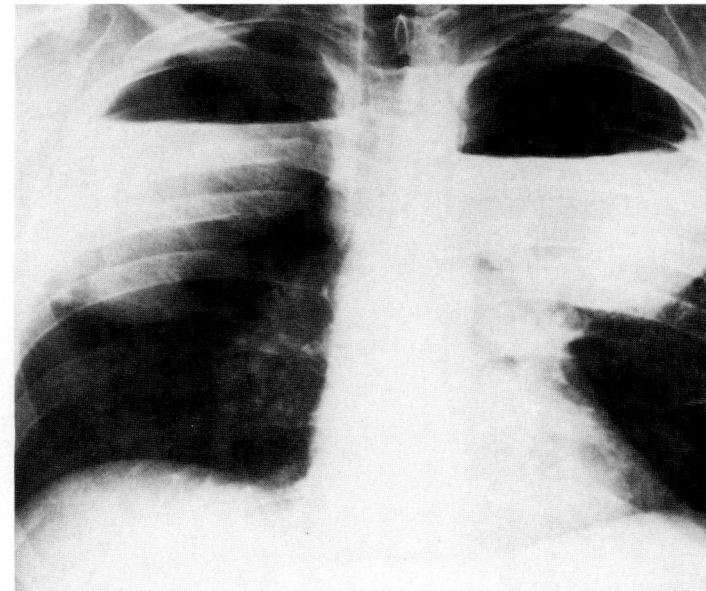

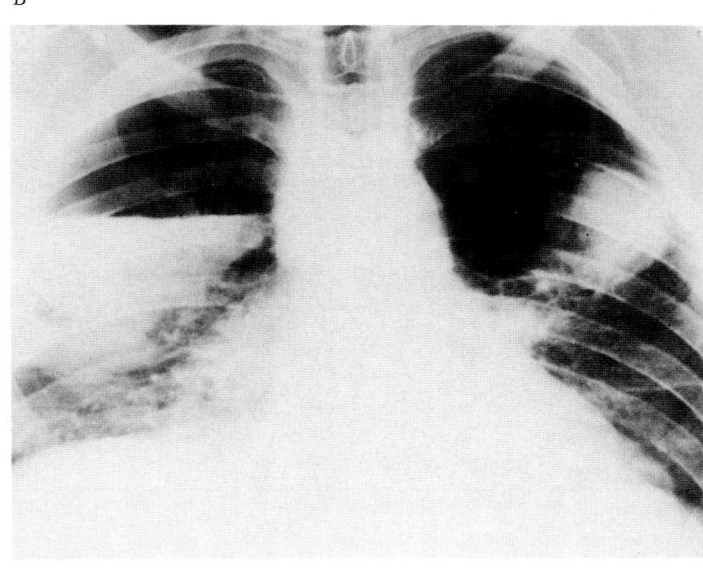

FIGURE 75-7 Infected bullae.   A. Bilateral infected bullae in a 62-year-old male.   B. Fluid levels in both bullae.   C. Clearing of the infection revealed a bronchogenic carcinoma on the left. (Courtesy of Dr. M. Feierstein.)

A

B

C

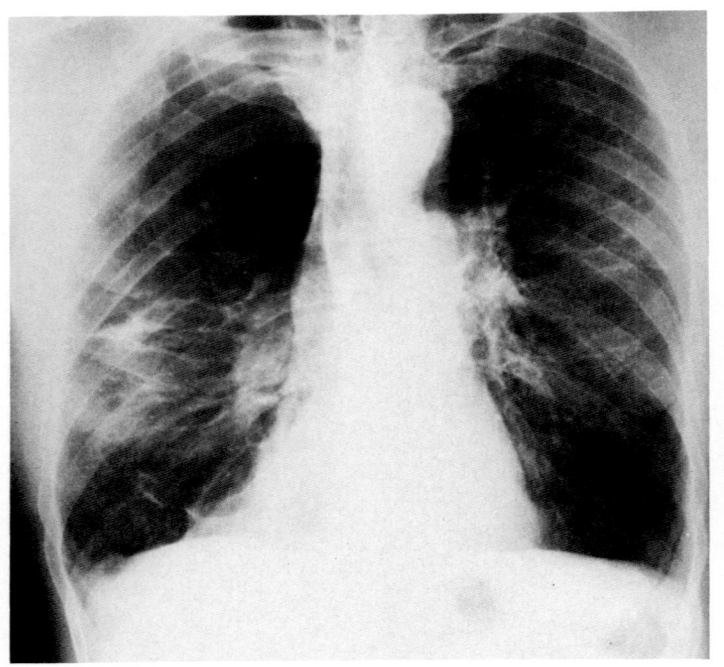

A

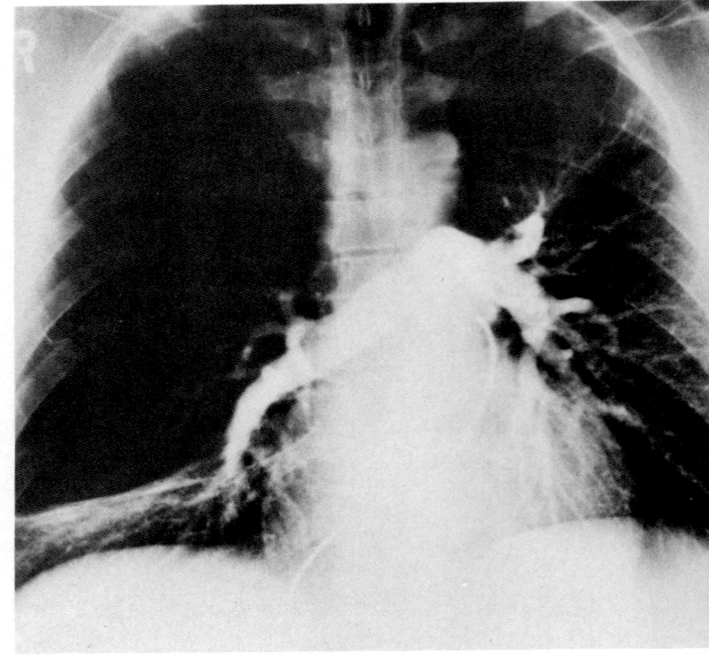

B

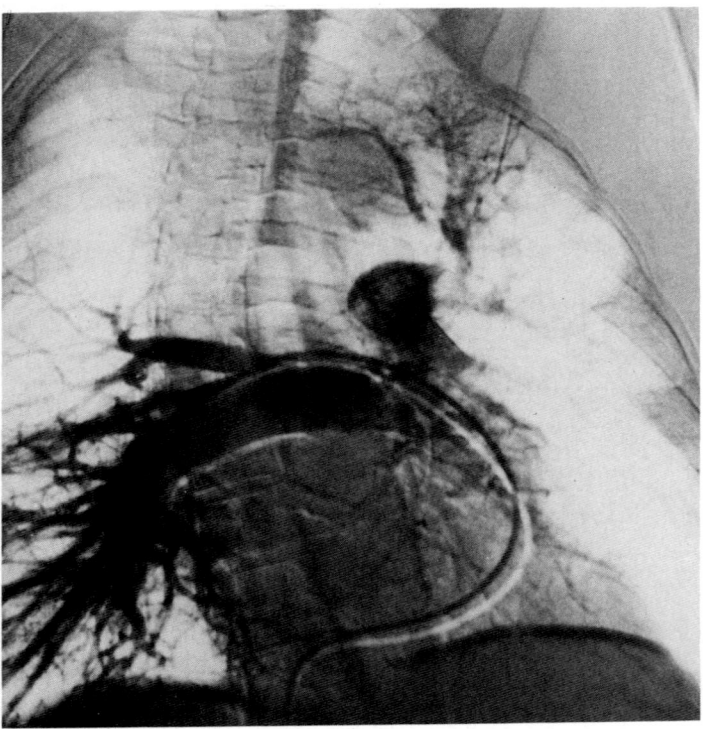

C

FIGURE 75-8 Bullous lung disease in a 65-year-old black male. The patient had progressive unrelenting dyspnea. *A.* Conventional PA chest radiograph revealing bilateral bullae. A large bulla in the right upper lobe has compressed the remaining lung on the right. *B.* Pulmonary arteriogram showing compression of the right lower lobe vasculature. *C.* Pulmonary arteriogram, subtraction technique. (*Courtesy of Dr. H. Naidech.*)

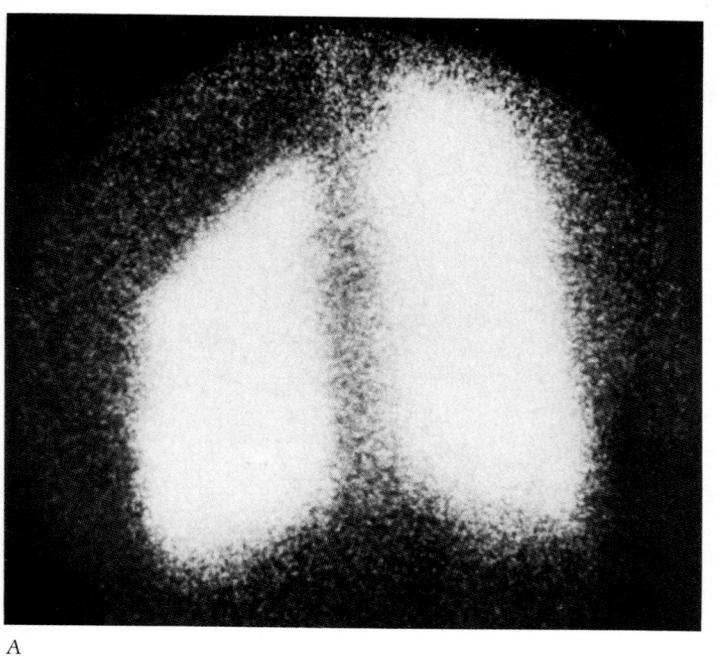 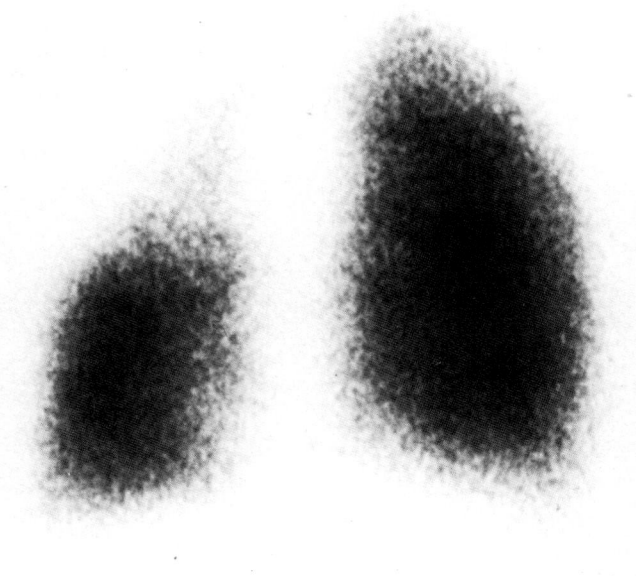

A   B

FIGURE 75-9 Lung scans in the preoperative evaluation of patients for bullectomy. *A*. Preoperative ventilation lung scan (^{133}Xe). Ventilation is absent in the left upper zone. *B*. Preoperative perfusion lung scan using ^{131}I-macroaggregated albumin. Blood flow is absent in the left upper zone while it is maintained at the left base. *(Courtesy of Dr. A. Alavi.)*

TABLE 75-3
Pulmonary Function Tests in a 65-Year-Old Black Male with Bullous Lung Disease

	Prebronchodilator		
Spirometry	Actual	% Pred.	Pred.
FVC, L	1.21	38	3.16
FEV$_1$, L	0.74	30	2.46
FEV$_3$, L	1.03	35	2.94
FEV$_1$/FVC%	61		80
FEV$_3$/FVC%	85		97
FEF$_{25-75}$, L/s	0.34	11	3.21
PEFR, L/s	3.05	46	6.57
FIF$_{25-75}$, L/s	1.30	23	5.67
SVC, L	1.42	38	3.72
IC, L	1.13	48	2.38
ERV, L	0.28	21	1.33
FRC, L	1.60	44	3.59
RV, L	1.31	58	2.26
TLC, L	2.73	47	5.85
RV/TLC%	48.11	123	39.00
D$_{LCO}$, single breath, ml/min/mmHg	10.06	40	25.18
Pulmonary vascular pressures			
Pulmonary artery, mmHg	60/22		30/16
Mean, mmHg	27		20

TABLE 75-4
Pulmonary Function Tests

Test	Bullous Disease	Obstructive Airways Disease and Bullae
TLC, L	N	N ↑
RV, L	N	↑
FRC, L	N	↑
FRC,* L	↑	↑
RV/TLC%	N	↑
FEV$_1$, L	N ↓	↓
FVC, L	N ↓	↓
FEV$_1$/FVC%	N	↓
MVV, L/min	N	↓
D$_{CO}$/V$_A$, (ml/min/mmHg)/L	N	↓
Raw, cmH$_2$O/L/s	N ↑	↑
Cst, exp, L/cmH$_2$O	N ↑	↑
Pst, TLC, cmH$_2$O	N ↓	↓

*FRC determined by body plethysmography.

NOTE: N = normal, ↑ = increased, ↓ = decreased.

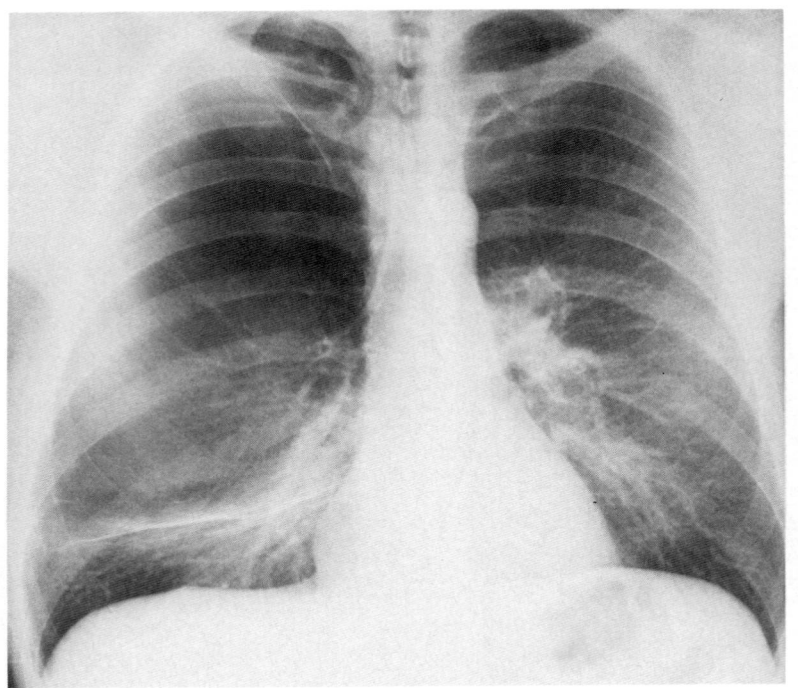
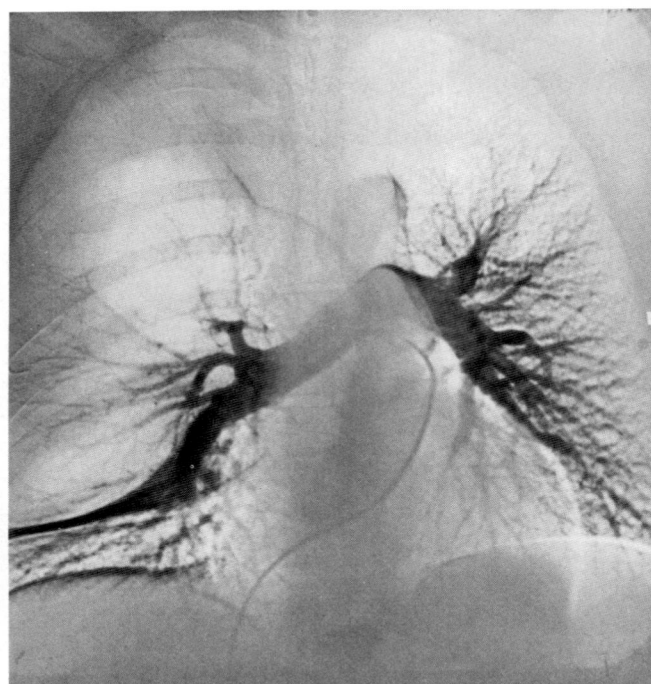

A

B

Isotope	^{99m}Tc Microspheres 3 mCi			^{133}Xe Gas 20 mCi		
Differential lung function						
Ventilation	Right lung			Left lung		
Anterior	52			48		
Posterior	37			63		
Total lung	44			56		
Perfusion						
Anterior	48			52		
Posterior	37			63		
Total lung	42			58		
	Right lung			Left lung		
Ventilation	Upper	Mid	Lower	Upper	Mid	Lower
Anterior	14	18	19	19	19	11
Posterior	12	11	14	19	26	18
Total lung	13	14	17	19	23	14
Perfusion						
Anterior	8	18	22	17	23	12
Posterior	8	15	14	18	26	19
Total lung	8	16	18	18	25	15

C

FIGURE 75-10 Large bulla in a 38-year-old man admitted because of increasing dyspnea. *A.* A chest radiograph (PA view). A large translucent area in the right upper lung represents an enlarging bulla that is causing compression of adjacent lung. *B.* Pulmonary arteriogram, subtraction technique. The pulmonary vasculature is compressed by the large bulla. *C.* Quantitative regional ventilation and perfusion obtained from the lung scans of this patient. Ventilation is markedly reduced in the right upper zone. Perfusion is absent in the right upper zone while it is present at the base. *(A and B. Courtesy of Dr. M. Ora; C. Courtesy of Dr. P. Germon.)*

PULMONARY PATHOPHYSIOLOGY

Pulmonary Function Tests

Pulmonary function tests have considerable practical value in distinguishing patients with localized bullae and normal intervening lungs from those in whom localized bullae are part of obstructive airways disease (Table 75-4). This distinction is important since those with obstructive airways disease are generally poor surgical candidates because of impaired pulmonary function.

In individuals with bullous disease, the volume of air in the lungs can be estimated either by radiograph, by body plethysmography, or by closed circuit methods (helium dilution) and nitrogen washout. Using the radiographic method, pulmonary function tests in bullous disease are generally normal as long as the bullae occupy one-third or less of the volume of the lung. Expansion of a large bulla that compresses intervening normal lung produces a restrictive pattern.

The volume of air trapped in bullae can be determined as the difference between the functional residual

TABLE 75-5
Pulmonary Function Tests in a 44-Year-Old Male with a Large Noninfected Bulla and Mitral Stenosis

| | Prebronchodilator | | |
Spirometry	Actual	% Pred.	Pred.
FVC, L	2.67	57	4.70
FEV_1, L	1.57	42	3.76
FEV_3, L	2.31	52	4.47
$FEV_1/FVC\%$	59		
$FEV_3/FVC\%$	87		
FEV_{25-75}, L/s	0.76	16	4.69
PEFR, L/s	3.86	43	9.50
FIF_{25-75}, L/s	2.41	34	7.03
MVV, L/min	59	43	137
SVC, L	2.89	62	4.70
IC, L	2.27	65	3.47
ERV, L	0.62	51	1.23
FRC, L	2.86	87	3.29
TGV*	4.71		3.29
RV, L	2.24	109	2.06
TLC, L	5.13	76	6.71
RV/TLC%	43.63	137	31.79
DL_{CO}, single breath, ml/min/mmHg	17.65	60	29.45
Gaw/VL, cmH_2O/s	0.07		0.13–0.34

*Measured by body plethysmography.

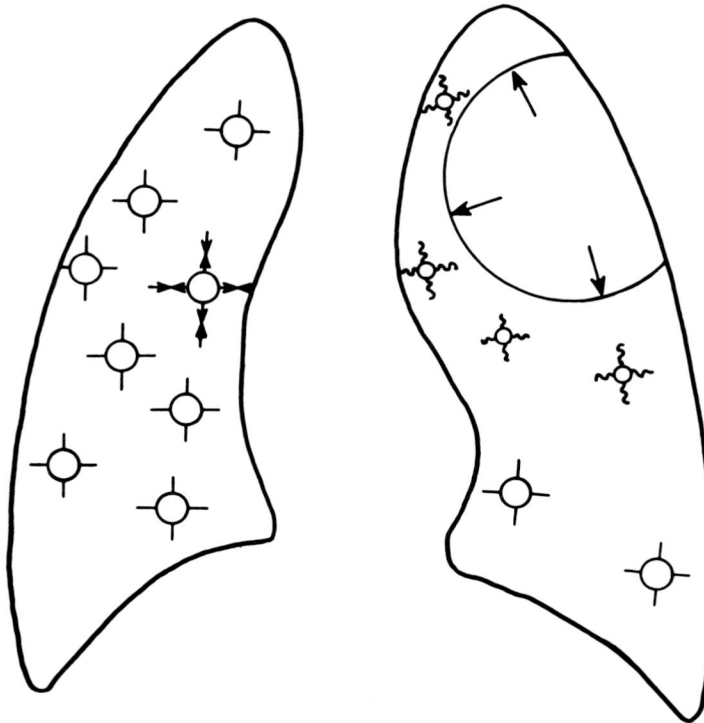

FIGURE 75-11 The effects of an enlarging airspace on radial traction exerted by elastic tissue on the airways. The reduction in lumen diameter is associated with an increase in airway resistance.

capacities determined plethysmographically and by using a closed circuit method (helium dilution) (Table 75-5); the difference is due to the inability of the inert gas used in the closed circuit method to enter the bullae. However, although the nitrogen washout curve is usually normal, the concentration of N_2 in alveolar gas at the close of 7 min of breathing 100% O_2 is often abnormal.

Pulmonary Mechanics

As large bullae expand, acting as growing space-occupying lesions, they first relax and then they compress adjacent lung tissue. Relaxation of the surrounding pulmonary parenchyma decreases radial traction on the airways, thereby increasing resistance to airflow (Fig. 75-11). The effects of bullectomy on mechanics are inconsistent: in some patients, removal of a large bulla increases the static recoil pressure of the lungs and decreases both airways and upstream resistances (Fig. 75-12); in others, bullectomy decreases the elastic recoil pressure.

Distinction between widespread emphysema on the one hand and bullae on the other has practical significance since resection of an emphysematous lung offers a less certain therapeutic response than does resection of large bullae. However, since each reduces the static elastic recoil pressure of the lungs on its own, the diffusing ca-

pacity is usually determined to aid in the distinction. The basis for determining the diffusing capacity is that it correlates better with morphologic estimates of emphysema than do most other tests. However, although a combination of a decrease in diffusing capacity and in static elastic recoil does favor the diagnosis of emphysema (and would discourage attempts at surgical bullectomy), it must be kept in mind that both the elastic recoil and the diffusing capacity can be decreased by bullae that compress the lungs.

Exercise

Both progressive and steady-state exercise testing have been used to determine if the tracheobronchial tree and the lung tissue between bullae are normal or abnormal. Exercise is invariably used as part of a constellation of tests to determine the state of the airways and parenchyma, keeping in mind the distortions introduced by the space-occupying bullae.

In patients with a few circumscribed bullae but otherwise normal lungs, exercise reveals that the alveolar-arterial difference in P_{O_2}, the VD/VT ratio, the DL_{CO}, and the arterial oxygenation remain normal or near normal.

Patients in whom bullae are associated with panacinar emphysema differ in that the alveolar-arterial difference in P_{O_2} is widened, both at rest and during exer-

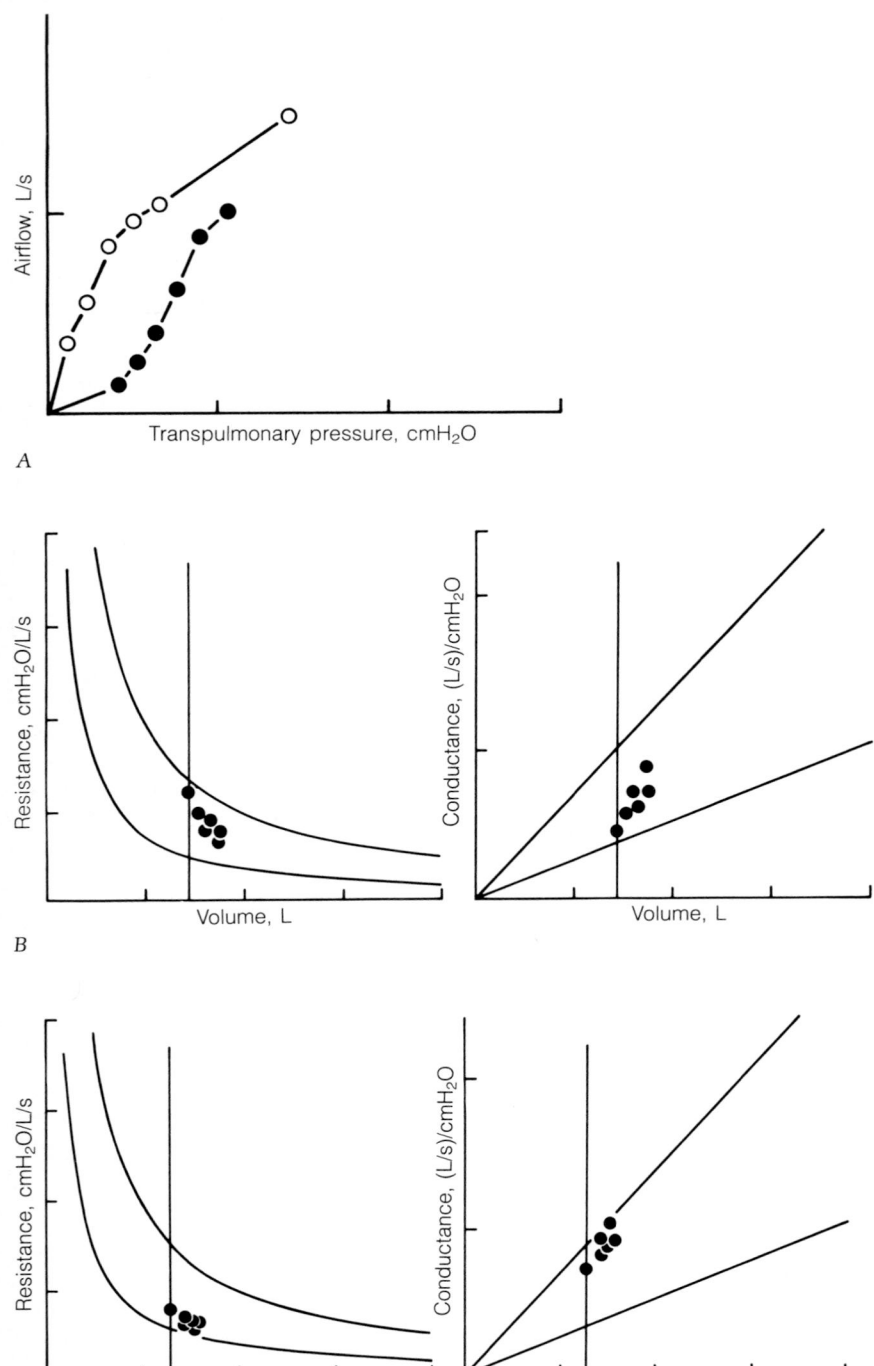

FIGURE 75-12 Airway resistances, pre- and postoperative. *A.* Pre- and postoperative maximum flow static recoil pressure curves. After operation, upstream resistance decreased. ● = preoperative; ○ = postoperative. *B.* Preoperative airway resistance and conductance. *C.* Postoperative airway resistance and conductance. After bullectomy, airway resistance decreased and conductance increased.

cise, and they develop arterial hypoxemia during exercise. The arterial Pa_{CO_2} tends to hover around the upper limits of normal at rest and during exercise; the V_D/V_T ratio is higher in this group than in the group with normal intervening lung; also, steady-state diffusing capacities are reduced in this group and fail to increase normally during exercise. In many of these patients, the $D_{L_{CO}}$ is

reduced at rest and arterial hypoxemia develops during exercise.

Patients in whom bullae are associated with chronic bronchitis show a widened alveolar-arterial difference in P_{O_2} and an increased V_D/V_T ratio at rest. However, the decrease in arterial P_{O_2} during exercise is only modest even though arterial Pa_{CO_2} at rest is abnormally high and

increases further during exercise, indicating progressive alveolar hypoventilation.

Pulmonary Circulation

As a rule, pulmonary arterial pressures and blood flow are within normal limits in patients with bullous disease at rest, i.e., the bullae act like amputated segments of lung, limiting the volume of the vascular bed available for recruitment as cardiac output increases. However, in patients in whom the extent of the pulmonary vascular bed has been severely curtailed by widespread bullous disease, the pulmonary arterial pressures tend to rise, both at rest and during exercise, in a few instances reaching levels of pulmonary hypertension that lead to cor pulmonale. Exercise in patients with bullous disease is generally associated with abnormally high increments in pulmonary arterial pressure as the normal increases in pulmonary blood flow are accommodated in the restricted vascular bed. Underlying pulmonary disease exaggerates the increments in pulmonary arterial pressure during exercise.

COMPLICATIONS

The major complications of bullous lung disease are infection of the bulla, massive hemorrhage, and spontaneous pneumothorax. Recurrent spontaneous pneumothorax may be a complication of paraseptal emphysema.

TREATMENT

Many patients with bullous disease of the lungs can be managed medically. Because the natural history of a bulla is unpredictable, the patient with bullous disease should be monitored by chest radiography at regular intervals to ensure that the situation is stable. Bullae occasionally enlarge suddenly and rapidly for no apparent reason.

Medical

The finding of a bulla in an asymptomatic patient calls for reassurance, a recommendation for annual chest radiography, advice to stop smoking, and an alert to the need for a prompt visit to a physician should symptoms develop. Activities that promote rupture of bullae, e.g., contact sports and scuba diving, should be proscribed. Chronic bronchitis, asthma, or emphysema associated with bullae require treatment in their own right.

Infection of a bulla requires sputum specimens for culture and Gram stain. Fiberoptic bronchoscopy is usually done if sputum studies fail to disclose the nature of the infection; sterile sheathed catheters are sometimes helpful in obtaining noncontaminated respiratory tract secretions for culture. Direct sampling of fluid from

within the bulla is rarely useful in making the diagnosis. Once the diagnosis of an infected bulla has been established, treatment is begun using chest physiotherapy and antibiotics. The choice of antibiotic depends on the Gram stain and sputum cultures. Treatment is prolonged since poor drainage of the bulla inevitably slows resolution of the disease process. The course of the infection is followed by repeated chest radiographs (Fig. 75-7). Most infections of bullae eventually respond to medical therapy. Large infected bullae that are slow to respond may require surgical intervention because of the possibility that an infected bulla may empty into the contralateral lung.

Surgical

In certain patients, surgical intervention provides symptomatic relief and improved exercise tolerance. However, the surgical outcome depends on the size and number of bullae, the condition of the intervening lung, and the occurrence of postoperative complications.

LOCALIZED BULLAE WITH NORMAL INTERVENING LUNG

Surgical removal of large bullae brings about remarkable symptomatic improvement in some of these patients (Table 75-6). There are certain definite indications for surgical intervention. For example, certain complications of

TABLE 75-6

*Preoperative and Postoperative Pulmonary Function Tests in Bullous Disease**

Spirometry	Preoperative Actual	% Pred.	Pred.	Postoperative Actual
FVC, L	3.97	77	5.15	4.64
FEV$_1$, L	2.72	66	4.14	3.36
FEV$_3$, L	3.60	73	4.93	4.25
PEFR, L/s	6.05	63	9.60	7.07
FEV$_{25-75}$, L/s	1.68	33	5.08	2.41
FEV$_1$/FVC%	69		83	72
FEV$_3$/FVC%	91		97	91
FIF$_{25-75}$, L/s	5.67	74	7.61	5.92
MVV, L/min	98	76	128	129
SVC, L	4.28	83	5.15	4.73
IC, L	2.88	91	3.16	3.36
ERV, L	1.29	65	1.99	1.37
RV, L	0.81	39	2.04	1.90
TLC, L	5.08	71	7.17	6.63
RV/TLC%	16		29	28.63
FRC, L	2.10	52	4.03	3.27
DL$_{CO}$, single breath, ml/min/mmHg	21.04	64	32.93	26.43

* Thirty-eight-year-old man who underwent successful bullectomy. Second study done 20 months postoperatively.

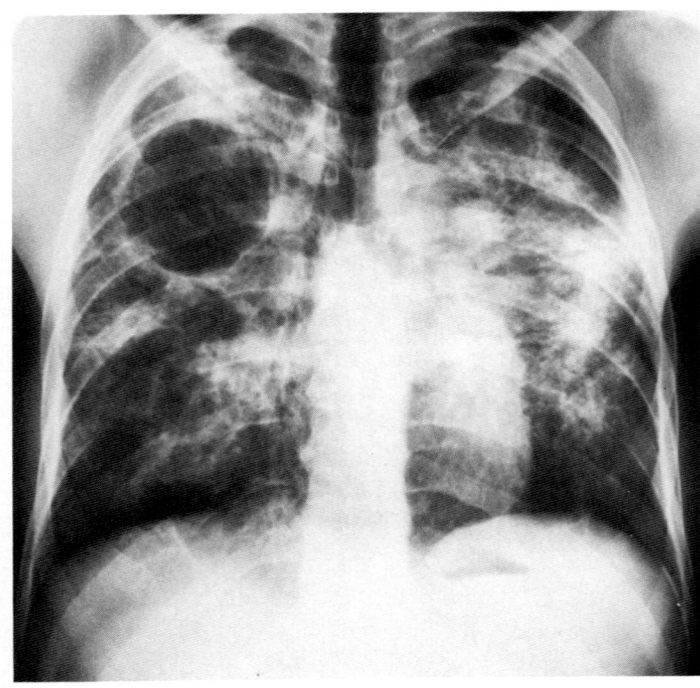

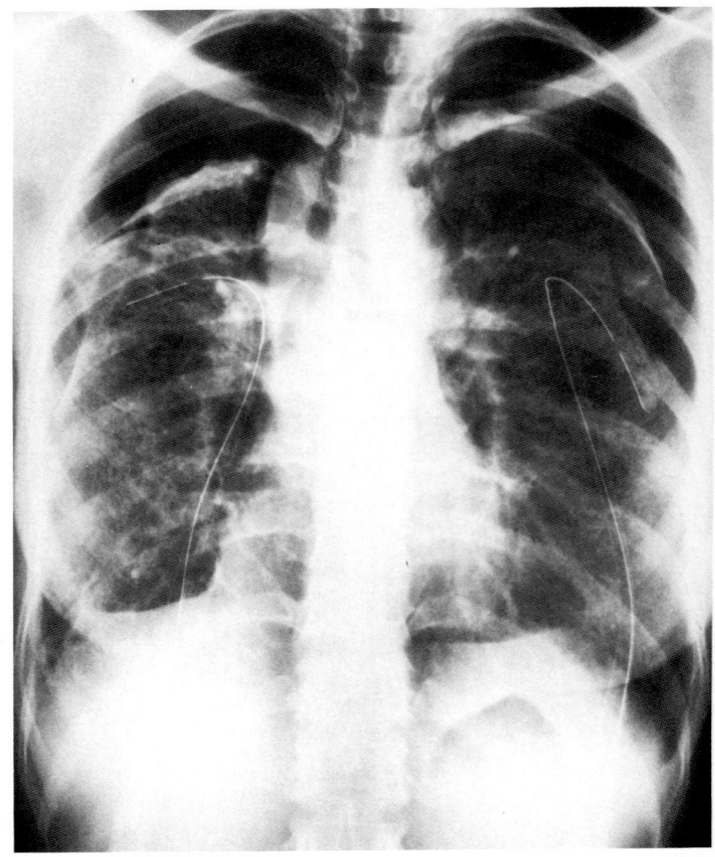

FIGURE 75-13 Bullae in sarcoidosis. *A*. A bulla in a 27-year-old male with sarcoidosis. *B*. Bilateral pneumothorax in a 26-year-old woman with sarcoidosis. A large bulla was found at the right apex.

bullous disease, i.e., spontaneous pneumothorax or massive hemorrhage, demand urgent surgical intervention even though the bullae may be small. In less urgent circumstances, the indications for operating on bullae that coexist with relatively normal surrounding parenchyma are as follows: (1) bullae that have reached such size as to cause dyspnea; (2) bullae that are increasing in size or have attained such a size as to compress surrounding lung tissue; (3) bullae that are responsible for recurrent pneumothoraxes; (4) infected bullae that fail to respond to medical treatment; (5) acute respiratory insufficiency attributable to the bullae; (6) acute distension of a bulla; and (7) severe chest pain attributable to a change in a bulla, e.g., distention.

As a rule, small-wedge excisions or plications of large bullae have brought about larger increments in expiratory flow rates than has lobectomy. This is not surprising since removal of more lung tissue is unlikely to improve a disorder characterized by the loss of lung tissue. The overall mortality in this type of surgery is about 1.5 percent. Median sternotomy has less postoperative morbidity than does a standard thoracotomy.

The size of the bulla is a principal factor in determining the outcome of surgery: the best functional improvement occurs where the bulla comprises 70 to 100 percent

of the hemithorax (Fig. 75-12); postoperative increments in FEV_1 range from 50 to 200 percent. Good results can also be anticipated when the involved lung contributes little to overall ventilation. Another good prognostic sign is the finding of large volumes of trapped air in the lung.

The most common causes of mortality are infection and respiratory failure, but the sudden development of a contralateral pneumothorax or herniation of a bulla across the mediastinum is an occasional cause of death. Postoperative complication rates tend to be high, i.e., between 14 and 44 percent. Not surprisingly, persistent air leaks and pleuropulmonary infections have been the major cause.

LOCALIZED BULLAE WITH ABNORMAL INTERVENING LUNG

Bullae can complicate both fibrotic and obstructive pulmonary disease. As a rule, there is no reason for surgical intervention unless a life-threatening complication should suddenly arise (Fig. 75-13).

When bullae occur in association with widespread panacinar emphysema (demonstrated by a marked reduction in DL_{CO} and a "winter tree" appearance of the pulmonary vessels on angiography), little improvement can be expected from bullectomy. This is particularly true if the FEV_1 is less than 30 percent of predicted. Elderly indi-

viduals in whom the bullae are associated with widespread emphysema have a high surgical mortality, i.e., about 9 percent. In chronic bronchitis associated with bullae, surgical removal of the bullae is sometimes followed by improvement, especially when large bullae are removed. However, this improvement is generally short-lived and not sustained for more than 6 months. Two signs auger a poor prognosis: (1) a prolonged productive cough, and (2) secondary pulmonary hypertension. The outlook after surgery is better for those who stop smoking than for those who do not.

MONALDI PROCEDURE

One older surgical procedure that is still occasionally useful in patients with large bullae and poor respiratory function is the Monaldi procedure. Originally this procedure entailed two stages, but recently a one-stage procedure has been substituted. The procedure entails surgical resection of a small piece of a rib that overlies the bulla. A purse string suture is then inserted into the parietal pleura, picking up the wall of the bulla and the visceral pleura. The bulla is then opened through the purse string, and a catheter with retaining balloon is inserted. The purse string is tightened, the balloon is inflated, and a continuous drainage using an underwater seal is applied. Symptomatic improvement occurs in 90 percent of the survivors, but the mortality of the procedure is high, i.e., up to 6 percent.

BIBLIOGRAPHY

Carr DH, Pride NB: Computed tomography in pre-operative assessment of bullous emphysema. Clin Radiol 35:43–45, 1984.
  Discusses the role of computed tomography in the assessment of bullae for surgery.

CIBA Guest Symposium: Terminology, definitions and classifications of chronic pulmonary emphysema and related conditions. Thorax 14:286–299, 1959.
  Standard definitions in pulmonary emphysema.

Current status of the surgical treatment of pulmonary emphysema and asthma. A statement by the Committee on Therapy, American Thoracic Society. Am Rev Respir Dis 97:486–488, 1968.
  Committee statement on the indications for surgical treatment of emphysema.

Fitzgerald MX, Keelan PJ, Cugell DW, Gaensler EA: Long-term results of surgery for bullous emphysema. J Thorac Cardiovasc Surg 68:566–568, 1974.
  Excellent analysis of the results of surgery in a series of 84 patients with bullous emphysema.

Gaensler EA, Cugell DW, Knudson RJ, Fitzgerald MX: Surgical management of emphysema. Clin Chest Med 4:443–463, 1983.
  Recent review with historical perspective.

Gelb AF, Gold WM, Nadel JA: Mechanisms limiting airflow in bullous lung disease. Am Rev Respir Dis 107:571–578, 1973.
  Discussion of the mechanical factors that affect expiratory flow rate in bullous emphysema.

Godwin JD, Webb WR, Savoca CJ, Gamsu C, Goodman PC: Multiple thin-walled cystic lesions of the lung. AJR 135:593–604, 1980.
  Excellent discussion of the radiologic differential diagnosis of cystic lung lesions.

Goldstein DS, Karpel JP, Appel D, Henry Williams M: Bullous pulmonary damage in users of intravenous drugs. Chest 89:266–269, 1986.
  The incidence of bullous lung disease was found to be 2 percent in a large group of intravenous drug abusers.

Harris J: Severe bullous emphysema. Successful surgical management despite poor preoperative blood gas levels and marked pulmonary hypertension. Chest 70:658–660, 1976.
  Describes the successful surgical outcome in a hypoxemic hypercapnic patient with pulmonary hypertension.

Holden WE, Mulkey DD, Kessler S: Multiple peripheral lung cysts and hemoptysis in an otherwise asymptomatic adult. Am Rev Respir Dis 126:930–932, 1982.
  An unusual example of pulmonary cysts lined by benign epithelium and primitive mesenchyme.

Hughes JA, MacArthur AM, Hutchison DCS, Hugh-Jones P: Long-term changes in lung function after surgical treatment of bullous emphysema in smokers and ex-smokers. Thorax 39:140–142, 1984.
  After operation, lung function declined faster in those who continued to smoke.

Jensen KM, Miscall L, Steinberg I: Angiography in bullous emphysema: Its role in selections of the case suitable for surgery. Am J Roentgenol 85:229–245, 1961.
Discusses the value of angiography in preoperative assessment.

Laurenzi GA, Turino GM, Fishman AP: Bullous disease of the lung. Am J Med 32:361–377, 1962.
The measurement of diffusing capacity during exercise may separate those patients with diffuse emphysema and bullae from those with localized bullae.

Law JW, Heard BE: Emphysema and the chest film: A retrospective radiological and pathological study. Br J Radiol 35:750–761, 1962.
Radiologic and pathologic correlation.

Lee M, Prisco DL, Berger HW, Lajain F: One stage surgery for bilateral bullous emphysema via median sternotomy: Report of three cases. Mt Sinai J Med 50:522–526, 1983.
One of several recent articles describing the use of median sternotomy for severe bilateral bullous emphysema and resulting lower morbidity.

MacArthur AM, Fountain SW: Intracavitary suction and drainage in the treatment of emphysematous bullae. Thorax 32:668–672, 1977.
A recent application of the older Monaldi procedure—mortality was 6.5 percent.

Mahler DA, D'Esopo ND: Periemphysematous lung infection. Clin Chest Med 4:51–57, 1981.
Review of the clinical and radiologic manifestations and the management of the infected bullae.

Morgan MD, Denison DM, Strickland B: Value of computed tomography for selecting patients with bullous lung disease for surgery. Thorax 41:855–862, 1986.
Concludes that computed tomography alone can be used to identify bullae that are amenable to surgery and can measure their volume and ventilation. The surgical removal of such clearly identified bullae is safe and associated with symptomatic and functional improvement.

Ohata M, Suzuki H: Pathogenesis of spontaneous pneumothorax with special reference to the ultrastructure of emphysematous bullae. Chest 77:771–776, 1980.
Scanning electron microscopy studies in paraseptal bullae.

Peters JI, Kubitschek KR, Gotlieb MS, Awe RJ: Lung bullae with air-fluid levels. Am J Med 82:759–763, 1987.
Fourteen patients in whom air-fluid levels developed in preexisting emphysematous bullae were treated either with oral penicillin or oral tetracycline. Complete resolution of symptoms and air-fluid levels occurred in all patients over two to 32 weeks (mean, 12).

Pride NB, Barter CE, Hugh-Jones P: The ventilation of bullae and the effect of their removal on thoracic gas volumes and tests of overall pulmonary function. Am Rev Respir Dis 107:83–98, 1973.
The most consistent changes in pulmonary function in 18 patients treated surgically were an increase in arterial oxygenation and a decrease in functional residual capacity.

Reid L: The Pathology of Emphysema. Chicago, Year Book, 1967.
Classification of bullae into three main types.

Richards DW: The aging lung. Bull NY Acad Med 32:407–416, 1956.
Identifies a form of bullous emphysema sometimes referred to as "vanishing lung" as a chronic degenerative nonobstructive lung disease.

Tenholder MF, Jones PA, Matthews JI, Hooper RG: Bullous emphysema. Progressive incremental exercise testing to evaluate candidates for bullectomy. Chest 77:801–803, 1980.
Another dimension in the selection of patients with bullous emphysema for surgery.

West JB: Distribution of mechanical stress in the lung, a possible factor in localization of pulmonary disease. Lancet 1:839–841, 1971.
Interesting paper on the role of mechanical stress in the distribution of pulmonary disorders— the higher frequency of bullae at the apices is explained by the higher negative pressures generated around the upper lobes and the greater expanding stresses.

Witz JP, Roeslin N: La chirurgie de l'emphyseme bulleux chez l'adulte: Ses résultats éloignes: Rev Fr Mal Respir 8:121–131, 1980.
Results and analysis of a large French series.

Wood JR, Bellamy D, Child AH, Citron KM: Pulmonary disease in patients with Marfan's syndrome. Thorax 39:780–784, 1984.
In a review of 100 patients, eleven were found to have had one or more episodes of pneumothorax, five had bullae evident on the chest radiograph, and four had pulmonary fibrosis.

Chapter 76

Epidemiology of Bronchitis and Emphysema

Ian T. T. Higgins

The earliest descriptions of emphysema date from the latter half of the seventeenth century. There are sporadic references to the disease during the eighteenth century, and by the 1820s it had been well defined, clearly described, and recognized to be common. Enlargement of airspaces, trapping of air, and rupture of alveolar walls were described first by morbid anatomists. Clinicians subsequently confirmed their findings and also noted the association between productive cough and emphysema. The diagnosis of chronic bronchitis was first applied by Badham in 1805 to patients with chronic cough, breathlessness, and recurrent exacerbations during the winter months. Badham attributed this syndrome to the emphysema which he subsequently observed at autopsy. There are many references to these diseases during the nineteenth century. Climate, weather, exposure to cold or damp, changes in temperature, and long-standing local irritation from dust or overdried air were believed to be the important causative factors. There was also much speculation on the mechanism of production of emphysema. During the first half of the twentieth century, these diseases evoked little interest, but since then, stimulated very much by the London fog of December 1952, which evoked considerable concern in Britain, and the progressive rise in mortality from emphysema in this country, there has been widespread and increasing recognition of their importance.

SIZE OF THE PROBLEM

In 1983, there were 62,000 deaths attributed to chronic bronchitis, emphysema, and chronic obstructive pulmonary disease (COPD). This is 3 percent of all deaths and makes the group the fifth highest specific cause of death in the United States. These diseases are cited on death certificates as contributory causes of death about one and one-half times as often as underlying causes. Thus, there are probably about 150,000 deaths from or with chronic bronchitis, emphysema, or COPD each year in the United States. As the underlying cause of death, these diseases have nearly doubled since 1970, and there has been an increasing proportion of deaths among females. The male-female sex ratio was 4.3:1 in 1970 and 2.36:1 in 1983 (Table 76-1).

Estimates from the National Health Survey indicate that nearly 8 million people in the United States have chronic bronchitis, 2 million have emphysema, and 7 million have asthma. The total number of persons affected by these diseases is however unknown because an unknown number of persons have more than one disease. Moreover, these figures are believed to be underestimates because they include only reported cases. Many surveys have reported a prevalence of 10 to 40 percent, depending on age, sex, and definition of disease that is used. These diseases cause serious disability. The frequency of limitation of activity exceeds that reported for any other major disease category. Over 50 percent of patients report limitation of activity and over 25 percent bed disability.

The economic cost of these diseases has been rising steadily and is now believed to be about $6.5 billion, $2.3 million due to direct costs for health care and the rest for indirect costs of morbidity, loss of earnings, and premature death.

DEFINITIONS

The term *chronic obstructive lung diseases* has become increasingly used to cover the diagnoses *chronic bronchitis, emphysema,* and sometimes *asthma*. This is unfortunate, since it has led to confusion of meaning and confounded temporal and geographic comparisons. The

TABLE 76-1

Number of and Ratio of Male-to-Female Chronic Obstructive Lung Disease (COLD) Deaths for Three Time Periods, United States

Cause of death	1970		1975		1980	
	Men	Women	Men	Women	Men	Women
Chronic bronchitis	4,282	1,564	3,260	1,452	2,380	1,348
Emphysema	18,901	3,820	14,849	3,946	10,133	3,744
COLD and allied conditions	3,601	848	13,411	4,182	24,820	10,734
Total COLD deaths	26,784	6,232	31,520	9,580	37,333	15,826
M/F ratio	4.30		3.29		2.36	

SOURCE: National Center for Health Statistics, 1982, and unpublished mortality data. From Chronic Obstructive Lung Disease: A Report of the Surgeon General, 1984. Dept. H.H.S. PHS Office on Smoking and Health, Rockville, MD.

situation has been potentially exacerbated in the ninth revision of the International Classification of Causes of Death by the use of the rubric "Chronic Obstructive Pulmonary Disease and Allied Conditions," which includes bronchitis, emphysema, asthma, bronchiectasis, and extrinsic allergic alveolitis.

Studies relying on information from certificates have to use the diagnoses specified on those certificates. Studies in which data are collected by questionnaire, lung function testing, and other tests are amenable to much greater diagnostic precision. Epidemiologists have tried to add precision to the diseases they study by clear definitions. Thus, carefully specified answers to well-standardized questions and precisely defined indices of functional level have gone some way to permitting valid comparisons between observations made by different observers and by the same observer in different places. Although there is still controversy, the presence of productive cough for 3 months in the year for two consecutive years is widely accepted as a minimal requirement for the diagnosis of chronic bronchitis. While there is probably less agreement on what constitutes minimal obstructive airways, a 1-s forced expiratory volume ($FEV_{1.0}$) of less than 65 percent of prediction and a 1-s forced expiratory volume to forced vital capacity ratio ($FEV_{1.0}/FVC$) of less than 80 percent has proved useful. Emphysema is generally regarded as a pathologic diagnosis which cannot be made reliably during life. It has, therefore, seldom been used in epidemiologic studies except those which analyze available data. Agreed definitions of allergy and of bronchial hyperreactivity are still needed for epidemiologic studies.

DISTRIBUTION OF DISEASE

Time Trends

At the turn of the century the reported death rate from chronic bronchitis and emphysema in the states for which mortality data were published by the federal government—

The National Death Registration Area—was 20 per 100,000 population. The rates declined steadily and fairly uniformly to a low of 1 or 2 per 100,000 in the late 1940s. Then the death rates for emphysema began a steady rise, and 10 years later a more modest increase occurred in the rates for chronic bronchitis. The increase in rates has been noted in all states and also in certain cities. It has affected men and women, whites and nonwhites. Since 1968 an increasing number of deaths have been certified as due to COPD. The result has been an apparent decline in the annual death rates from chronic bronchitis, emphysema, and asthma. When these COPD deaths are added to those due to bronchitis, emphysema, and asthma, the rates are still increasing (Fig. 76-1). Figure 76-1 shows that the rates have flattened in men but are rising steadily in women.

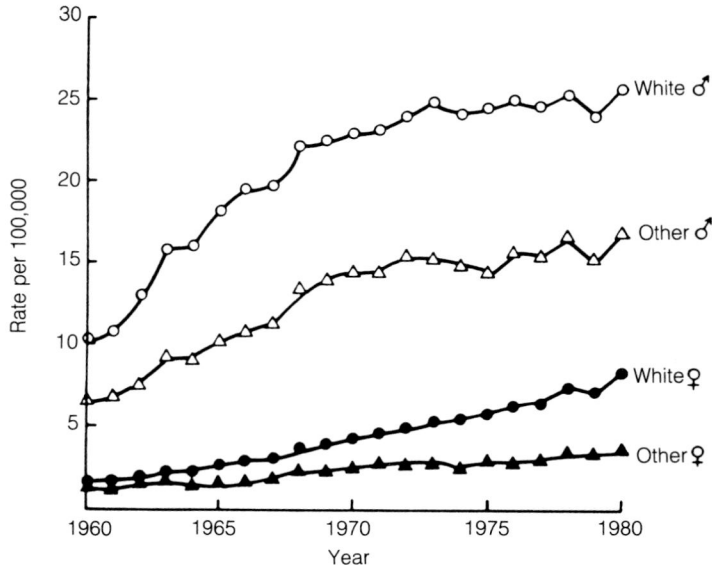

FIGURE 76-1 Age-adjusted mortality from chronic obstructive lung disease (COLD) for whites and nonwhites in the United States, 1960 to 1980. (*Source: National Center for Health Statistics, 1982, and unpublished data. From Chronic Obstructive Lung Disease. A Report of the Surgeon General.*)

There is a fairly pronounced seasonal variation in mortality and morbidity from these diseases. In the United States, approximately one-third of the total deaths in a year from these chronic respiratory diseases occur in December, January, or February and the smallest number of deaths occurs in August and September.

Geographic Comparisons

There are large differences between different countries in the reported death rates from chronic bronchitis and emphysema. Some of these are due to differences in diagnosis, terminology, classification, or coding of causes of death in different countries, but when these are allowed for, differences still remain. Comparisons of respiratory symptom prevalence and lung function values found in special surveys provide support for these conclusions based on mortality. Comparable chronic respiratory disease is prevalent in certain underdeveloped communities, notably in rural New Guinea and Egypt and among Malaysian and Australian aborigines.

Mortality rates from bronchitis and emphysema often vary in different places within countries. In the United States, there is a three- to four-fold variation between the states with the highest and the lowest rates. Certain states (Arizona, Wyoming, Montana, Nevada) have exceptionally high rates. Differences in age distribution can explain some of the variation, but climate, pollution, and migration presumably contribute. In the United Kingdom there is a clear association between bronchitis death rates and density of population. Rates for men and women of comparable age are twice as high in the most densely populated areas as in the rural areas. Urban and rural differences are much less apparent in the United States.

PERSONAL CHARACTERISTICS: AGE, SEX, RACE, AND SOCIOECONOMIC CIRCUMSTANCES

Mortality and morbidity rates increase with age in both sexes. Most aspects of lung function, but especially ventilatory lung function, also decline with age. Age-adjusted and age-specific mortality rates are higher in men than in women. In the United States the rates are consistently higher in whites than in nonwhites.

In England and Wales for at least 50 years bronchitis mortality rates have been approximately six times as high in the lowest as in the highest social class. More recently a comparable gradient of morbidity has also been noted. In the United States mortality rates are twice as high among semiskilled workers and laborers as among professional workers. A higher prevalence of respiratory symptoms and lower ventilatory lung function have been reported in the less well educated. Smoking has been shown to be strongly related to socioeconomic circumstances, the less well educated smoking more and more heavily than the better educated. Smoking, therefore, is likely to be an important factor in the social class gradient. Occupation is also important in the etiology of these diseases, but occupational exposures to respiratory irritants cannot explain the socioeconomic gradient, since this is also seen in married women. Other suggested explanations include poor housing, overcrowding in the home with resulting increased cross-infection, too early return to manual work after a respiratory infection, residence of poor people in more polluted parts of cities, and social drift whereby those with chronic respiratory disease tend to decline in social standing.

ETIOLOGIC FACTORS

Smoking

Cigarette smoking is the most consistently important determinant of chronic bronchitis and emphysema. Cigarette smokers have about 10 times the risk of nonsmokers of dying from chronic bronchitis and emphysema. Pipe or cigar smokers have a much smaller risk—between one and one-half and three times that of nonsmokers. Among cigarette smokers, the risk of dying from bronchitis and emphysema increases with increasing numbers of cigarettes smoked. The reduction in mortality from giving up smoking appears to be less for bronchitis and emphysema than for respiratory cancer.

Persistent, productive cough is much more prevalent among cigarette smokers than among nonsmokers or ex-smokers: the prevalence increases with the number of cigarettes smoked. Other respiratory symptoms such as wheezing, breathlessness, and recurrent chest illnesses, while more frequent in smokers than in nonsmokers, are less closely related to the amount smoked. Pipe and cigar smokers have usually been found to have a lower prevalence of symptoms than cigarette smokers. The prevalence of chronic bronchitis is higher in inhalers than in noninhalers. It is more prevalent among persons who extinguish and relight their cigarettes and in those who leave the cigarette constantly in the mouth. The rate of development of symptoms is higher, and of remission of symptoms is lower, in smokers than in nonsmokers.

Ventilatory lung function is almost invariably lower on the average among cigarette smokers than among nonsmokers or ex-smokers. Pipe and cigar smokers have intermediate values. Lung function declines more rapidly among cigarette smokers than among nonsmokers, ex-smokers, or smokers of pipes or cigars. These changes in morbidity and lung function are compatible with the histologic changes which have been shown to be related to smoking.

Although cigarette smoking is well established as the most important cause of chronic obstructive airways dis-

ease, only a minority of even heavy smokers develop the disease. Much research is being directed to determining the degree to which the disease is caused by aspects of smoking that have been up to now inadequately specified, such as tar content of cigarettes, puff volume, depth of inhalation, and the frequency of personal characteristics, such as allergy or atopy and bronchial hyperreactivity. Apart from understanding the mechanisms whereby such factors result in respiratory disability and decline in lung function, better identification of susceptible subjects would provide a powerful impetus toward prevention.

Cigarettes smoked today differ substantially from those smoked 25 years ago. Tar and nicotine contents are now less than half of what they used to be, filters are almost universal, and there have been considerable changes in the manufacture and use of new synthetic products. How these changes have affected smokers' health is imperfectly known. Evidence suggests that, while reduced cigarette tar may have reduced cough and mucous hypersecretion, it may not have reduced breathlessness and obstructive airways disease. Further studies are needed to assess the effect of smoking cigarettes with very low tar and nicotine. It is fairly well established that smokers who switch to low-yield cigarettes compensate for the reduction in nicotine (and possibly also for the reduction in tar) by altering the pattern of their smoking. The number of puffs per cigarette and the volume of smoke inhaled are usually increased while the number of cigarettes smoked per day and depth of inhalation may be increased in some groups of smokers but not in others.

Passive Smoking

Recent interest has focused on the effects of inhalation of the smoke of others by nonsmokers. The prevalence of respiratory symptoms, particularly coughing and wheezing, tend to be higher and the level of ventilatory lung function lower in the nonsmoking wives of smoking husbands as well as among the nonsmoking children of smoking parents. The effect, even if small, is important because of the frequency of the exposure and also its involuntary nature.

Air Pollution

The classic episodes of severe pollution that occurred in the Meuse Valley, Donora, London, New York, and other cities showed conclusively that fogs could kill and make people ill. Much of the mortality and morbidity was due to respiratory disease. Those with preexisting chronic disease, particularly of the lungs or heart, were recognized to be especially vulnerable, but the occasional onset of symptoms in young children and in animals, as well as the recurrence of symptoms in patients who had become asymptomatic, suggested that fog could initiate as well as exacerbate respiratory disease.

Apart from these episodes, adverse effects of pollution on the respiratory tract have often been demonstrated. Thus, temporal and spatial variations in mortality, morbidity, respiratory symptom prevalence, lung function levels, and sickness absence have been shown to correlate with various measures of air pollution in different populations and in different segments of the population. Studies have been conducted in patients with respiratory disease, in infants and young children, in representative samples of the general population, and in a number of occupational groups, notably those which are widely distributed yet socially and economically fairly uniform, such as telephone and transport workers.

Uncertainty remains about the levels of the various pollutants that produce the untoward respiratory effects. Current federal primary ambient air quality standards are shown in Table 76-2. There is not universal agreement on the adequacy of these standards, particularly the 24-h levels. Moreover, the particulate standard takes no cognizance of the type or size distribution of the particles. Recommended changes including the incorporation of size distributions of particles and consideration of 1- and 3-h standard for SO_2 are now under consideration by the Environmental Protection Agency's administrator.

Interaction between pollutants with resulting synergism may be important, but it is difficult to carry out epidemiologic studies to explore it successfully. Controlled laboratory studies are more likely to illuminate this aspect of air pollution. However, interaction between pollution and smoking has been suggested in several epidemiologic studies.

Indoor Pollution

Recognition that people spend 80 percent or more of their time indoors, coupled with the increasing tendency to hermitically seal houses, has concentrated concern on indoor pollution. It has been found that certain pollutants are likely to be higher indoors than outside. Particles, mainly resulting from smoking, and NO_2 arising from indoor heating and cooking, particularly when stoves are poorly vented, have been found to be dominated by indoor sources. A number of studies have indicated that the occurrence of respiratory illnesses may be more frequent, the prevalence of respiratory symptoms higher, and the level of ventilatory lung function lower in persons who live in homes using gas for heating and/or cooking than in persons living in homes using electricity. This difference has been attributed to the differences in NO_2 concentrations between such homes. In considering adverse responses to low levels of air pollutant, it is, therefore, important to realize that apparent biologic responses to very low levels of ambient outdoor pollutant concentrations may really be due to responses to appreciably higher indoor concentrations.

TABLE 76-2
Current National Ambient Air Quality Standards

Pollutant	Concentration	Comments
Sulfur dioxide (SO$_2$)	80 μg/m^3 (0.03 ppm) 365 μg/m^3 (0.14 ppm)	Annual arithmetic mean Maximum 24-h concentration not to be exceeded more than once per year
Total suspended particulates (TSP)	75 μg/m^3 260 μg/m^3	Annual geometric mean Maximum 24-h concentration not to be exceeded more than once per year
Carbon monoxide (CO)	10 mg/m^3 (9 ppm)	Maximum 8-h concentration not to be exceeded more than once per year
	40 mg/m^3 (35 ppm)	Maximum 1-h concentration not to be exceeded more than once per year
Ozone (O$_3$)	235 μg/m^3 (0.12 ppm)	Not more than 1 day per calendar year with maximum hourly average concentration above 235 μg/m^3
Nitrogen dioxide (NO$_2$)	100 μg/m^3 (0.05 ppm)	Annual arithmetic mean (generally monitored continuously)
Lead	1.5 μg/m^3	Maximum arithmetic mean averaged over a calendar quarter (frequently monitored weekly)

SOURCE: Reprinted from Code of Federal Regulations, Title 40, Part 50, 1984.

Occupational Exposures

Since the time of Ramazzini, dust exposure at work has been considered an important etiologic factor of respiratory disease. During the nineteenth century much of the disease that was described was no doubt silicosis, other pneumoconiosis, or tuberculosis, but some of it must certainly have been bronchitis and/or emphysema. The development of chest radiography improved diagnosis and facilitated differentiation of these diseases with the result that Collis in 1931 could refer confidently to bronchitis as the first of the dust diseases. Type of dust was clearly important, with the high death rates among sandstone workers, tin and copper miners, and cotton strippers and grinders being striking. In contrast, death rates from bronchitis among coal miners were only moderately high, and there was considerable variation from place to place. Since 1900, although death rates among all coal miners in England and Wales have been roughly 40 percent higher than the corresponding rates for other men, the rates have varied in different coal mining areas from below the national average to about twice the average. In Britain high bronchitis mortality rates are also reported among foundry workers (especially molders and core makers), furnace workers, cotton textile workers, and unskilled laborers, while high morbidity rates have been noted among miners, furnace, forge, foundry, gas, coke, glass, and chemical workers. In the United States national information on occupational mortality is limited but suggests high death rates from chronic bronchitis and emphysema among miners, metal molders, and unskilled laborers.

Special surveys comparing persons occupationally exposed to dust with comparable controls have supported the view that exposure to a wide variety of dusts contributes to the development of chronic bronchitis and emphysema. Thus, coal, gold, and fluorspar miners and foundry, furnace, cotton, and flax workers have been found to have a higher prevalence of respiratory symptoms and chronic bronchitis and lower average ventilatory function than persons of the same age living in the same area but with no occupational dust exposure. The quantitative relationship between lifetime dust dosage and respiratory disease and disability has been most thoroughly investigated in coal miners. In them, chronic bronchitis and emphysema has not usually been found to be closely related to dose. In Britain, the prevalence of bronchitis was found to increase with increasing dust dosage in persons aged 25 to 44 but not in older persons.

Lifetime dust dosage may be more closely related to disease and disability in occupations involving exposure

to dusts other than coal. Thus, among metal miners in the United States the prevalence of symptoms and bronchitis has been reported to be higher in those with silicosis than in those without and to increase with increasing duration of mining. An increasing prevalence of respiratory symptoms with increasing dust exposure has also been found among asbestos miners and millers, and there are a few reports of increased respiratory disease among talc and cement workers. Exposure to dusts of vegetable origin appears more likely to cause chronic bronchitis than exposure to most mineral dusts. Thus, apart from byssinosis, a specific occupational disease, workers with cotton, flax, and hemp also experience an increased prevalence of bronchitis. A high prevalance of respiratory symptoms has also been reported among grain handlers. Allergic sensitization to various fungi appears to play a dominant role, though nonspecific irritation from various parts of the grain may also contribute.

Exposure to fumes and gases at work has received much less epidemiologic study than exposure to dusts. Oxides of nitrogen have been incriminated as a cause of obliterative bronchitis in silo fillers and following blasting in enclosed spaces in the course of underground mining. Respiratory impairment and reduced lung function have followed exposure to chlorine gas. Emphysema is generally recognized as a sequel to cadmium fume inhalation, whereas asthma and an inordinate rate of decline of ventilatory lung function can follow exposure to toluene di-isocyanate.

Heredity

Heredity was considered to be etiologically important by clinicians in the nineteenth century. Several recent lines of evidence have reinforced this idea: (1) relatives of bronchitic subjects have a higher prevalence of bronchitis than do the relatives of controls; (2) siblings of bronchitic subjects occasionally have a higher frequency of bronchitis than their spouses; (3) the FEV_1 correlates more closely among family members than among spouses; and (4) concordance rates are higher among monozygotic than dizygotic twins.

The observation that deficiency of the serum protein α_1-antitrypsin could lead to the early development of emphysema indicated clearly the occasional importance of single gene substitutions as a cause of emphysema, but since the homozygous deficiency is found in fewer than 2 percent of all cases of severe emphysema, it can hardly be a major determinant of the disease. The possibility of increased susceptibility to respiratory irritants among carriers who are heterozygous for the gene has been suggested but is as yet unproved. In cystic fibrosis, another genetically determined disease associated with an increased risk of chronic bronchitis and emphysema, heterozygous carriers do not share this increased risk.

Infection

Persons with chronic bronchitis usually have a higher frequency of pneumonia, pleurisy, and acute bronchitis than other persons. They also report a higher mean annual number of colds and a much higher frequency for colds to "go down on the chest." This susceptibility appears to date from childhood. Much current research is directed at elucidating the role of childhood respiratory illnesses in relation to subsequent development of chronic bronchitis and airway obstruction.

The role of infectious agents in the recurrent exacerbations which are so characteristic of chronic bronchitis and emphysema is still uncertain.

Miscellaneous Factors

A high prevalence of chronic bronchitis has been reported among persons who were gassed in World War I. More recently, a high frequency of bronchitis and lung cancer and reduced expiratory flow rates have been found in workers employed in a Japanese poison gas factory. Whether infection of the teeth and paranasal sinuses are important etiologic factors in chronic bronchitis is uncertain.

FOLLOW-UP STUDIES OF CHRONIC RESPIRATORY DISEASE

The mortality of patients with chronic bronchitis exceeds that expected for men of the same age. Indeed, death rates are approximately four times those expected for men of the same age in the general population. Prognosis becomes worse as the degree of airway obstruction increases. Prognosis is grave in patients with chronic O_2 desaturation, CO_2 retention, radiographic evidence of generalized emphysema, and cor pulmonale.

Mortality has also been determined in representative samples of the population after varying numbers of years from the initial examination. This has confirmed the overwhelming influence of smoking on the occurrence of mortality from bronchitis and emphysema (COPD). In one study that followed up the mortality of a number of British populations after 20 to 25 years, no death out of 104 attributed to COPD occurred in a nonsmoker. Those men with an $FEV_{1.0}$ of more than two standard deviations below the mean had a mortality rate from COPD which was 50 times that of those with an FEV that was above average. The study showed, in addition, that simple bronchitis (or mucous hypersecretion) in the absence of airflow obstruction had little effect on mortality.

TABLE 76-3
Points for Risk Factors (Tecumseh Index of Risk)*

Age	Points	Cigarettes/day	Points	FEV$_1$ % Predicted	Points	Change in Cigarettes/day	Points	Risk of OAD† Total Points	Risk (cases/100)
				Men					
25	0	0	0	121	−14	−60	−9	≤7	Low risk
27	1	10	2	118	−12	−50	−7	8–14	1
29	2	20	5	115	−10	−40	−6	8–17	2
31	3	30	7	112	−8	−30	−4	8–19	3
33	4	40	9	109	−6	−20	−3	20	4
35	5	50	11	106	−4	−10	−1	21	5
37	6	60	13	103	−2	0	0	22	6
39	7			100	0	10	1	23	7
41	8			97	2	20	3	24	8
43	9			94	4	30	4	25	9
45	10			91	6	40	6	26	11
47	11			88	8	50	7	27	13
49	12			85	10	60	9	28	15
51	13			82	12			29	18
53	14			79	14			30	20
55	15			76	16			31	23
57	16			73	18			≥32	High risk
59	17			70	20				
61	18								
63	19								
65	20								
				Women					
25	0	0	0	121	−16	−60	−17	≤10	Low risk
27	1	10	4	118	−14	−50	−14	11–17	1
29	2	20	9	115	−11	−40	−11	18–20	2
31	3	30	13	112	−9	−30	−8	21–23	3
33	4	40	18	109	−7	−20	−6	24	4
35	5	50	22	106	−5	−10	−3	25	5
37	6	60	27	103	−2	0	0	26	5
39	7			100	0	10	3	27	6
41	8			97	2	20	6	28	7
43	9			94	5	30	8	29	8
45	10			91	7	40	11	30	10
47	11			88	9	50	14	31	11
49	12			85	11	60	17	32	13
51	13			82	14			33	14
53	14			79	16			34	17
55	15			76	18			35	19
57	16			73	21			36	21
59	17			70	23			≥37	High risk
61	18								
63	19								
65	20								

*This point system is based on the number of cases (per 100 population) of obstructive airways disease expected within 10 years.

†OAD = obstructive airways disease.

Prediction of Obstructive Airways Disease

During the past 5 years, interest has been directed to predicting obstructive airways disease from knowledge of a relatively small number of characteristics which can be simply measured. A number of models, depending on the risk factors included, have been developed from the Tecumseh study, an ongoing longitudinal study of cardiorespiratory and other diseases in Tecumseh, Michigan, to specify the proportion of the population that will develop obstructive airways disease in 10 or in 15 years. The simplest of these models has been tested in a number of other communities and has been found to predict disease in those populations. The factors included in the model are: age, sex, level of 1-s forced expiratory volume, number of cigarettes smoked per day, and whether or not cigarette smoking continues, changes, or is discontinued during the 10 or 15 years of follow-up. In order to facilitate the use of the model by clinicians, a scoring system has been developed. Points are allocated for each risk factor, and a total score is calculated. This score provides an estimate of the individual's risk of developing obstructive airways disease in either 10 or 15 years. Table 76-3 gives the points allocated for each of the factors included in the model. Figure 76-2 presents estimates of the probabilities of developing obstructive airways disease for a 45-year-old man, depending on whether he continues to smoke or gives up smoking. Thus, if his $FEV_{1.0}$ is 75 percent of predicted and he smokes 40 cigarettes per day, his chance of developing obstructive airways disease is about 40 in 100. On the other hand, were he to quit smoking after his initial examination, his risk would be reduced by more than half to about 16 per 100. Such a clear demonstration of the benefits of giving up smoking should provide a strong stimulus to quitting, though at present this still needs to be proved.

LESSONS FROM EPIDEMIOLOGY FOR PREVENTION

Epidemiologic studies have shown the overwhelming importance of cigarette smoking as a cause of chronic bronchitis and emphysema. Apart from the direct effect of smoking on the respiratory tract, interactions between smoking and occupational exposures or smoking and air pollution suggest that smoking may also act indirectly to modify the effects produced by these other determinants. Clearly the major emphasis in any program of prevention must be on smoking. The main objectives should be to discourage young people from taking up smoking, to reduce the number of people now smoking, and to develop less hazardous cigarettes for those unable to quit. Continuing smokers should be advised not to inhale and to use filter cigarettes. The use of low tar and low nicotine cigarettes should be recommended because of the reduction in mucous hypersecretion that is anticipated and because such cigarettes may also reduce the risk of lung cancer. Advice that cigarette smokers should switch to cigars or even a pipe is unwise unless they are also discouraged from inhaling cigar or pipe smoke as they used to inhale cigarette smoke.

Prompt and adequate treatment of acute respiratory diseases and of exacerbations of chronic bronchitis will reduce time lost from work, but that such treatment has apparently little influence on the natural history of chronic bronchitis indicates that prevention, rather than early detection or treatment, is likely to be the only effective approach.

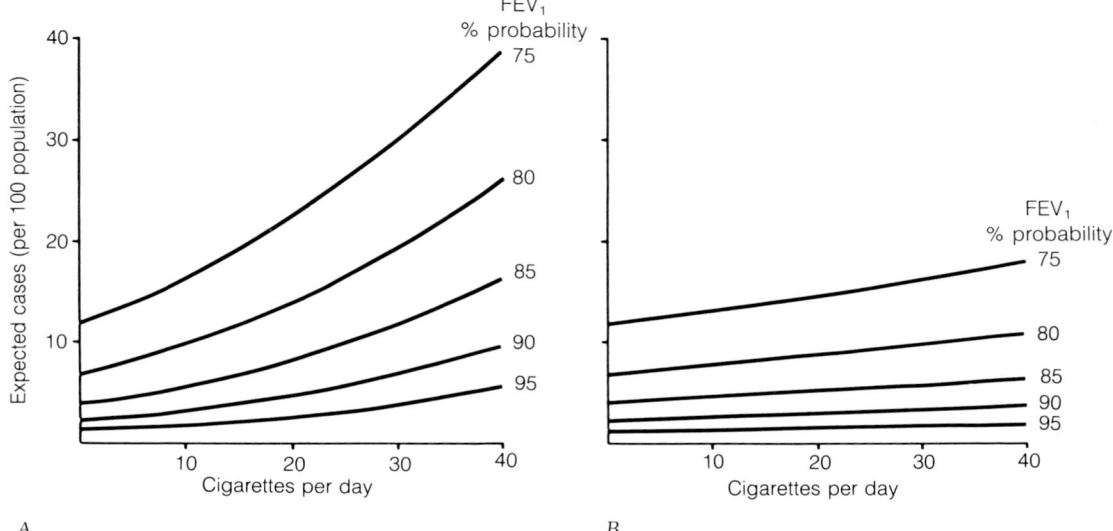

FIGURE 76-2 Risks of developing obstructive airways disease within 10 years for a 45-year-old man. *A.* Continues smoking. *B.* Stops smoking. *(From Higgins et al., 1982.)*

BIBLIOGRAPHY

Anderson HR, Bland JM, Patel S, Peckham C: The natural history of asthma in childhood. J Epidemiol Community Health 40:121–129, 1986.
  The incidence and prognosis of childhood asthma and wheezing illness was studied using data obtained at ages 7, 11, and 16 from a national cohort of 8806 children born in 1958.

Badley EM, Lee J, Wood PH: Impairment, disability, and the ICIDH (International Classification of Impairments, Disabilities, and Handicaps) model. II: The nature of the underlying condition and patterns of impairment. Int Rehabil Med 8:118–124, 1987.
  This paper presents a further exploration of the conceptual scheme proposed in the International Classification of Impairments, Disabilities, and Handicaps, which links underlying condition, impairment, and disability.

Baillie M (1793): *Morbid Anatomy of Some of the Most Important Parts of the Human Body.* London, Bulmer, 1912.
  An atlas of morbid anatomy largely from specimens in the museum of his uncle, Dr. William Hunter. The specimen illustrating emphysema was the lung of Dr. Samuel Johnson.

Burchfiel CM, Higgins MW, Keller JB, Howatt WF, Butler WJ, Higgins IT: Passive smoking in childhood. Respiratory conditions and pulmonary function in Tecumseh, Michigan. Am Rev Respir Dis 133:966–973, 1986.
  The relationship of passive smoking to respiratory conditions and pulmonary function was assessed using a cross-sectional design in the defined population of Tecumseh, Michigan.

Carstensen JM, Pershagaen G, Eklund G: Mortality in relation to cigarette and pipe smoking: 16 years' observation of 25,000 Swedish men. J Epidemiol Community Health 41:166–172, 1987.
  In 25,129 Swedish men, there were clear covariations (p < .001) between the amount of tobacco smoked and the risk of death due to cancer of the oral cavity and larynx, esophagus, liver, pancreas, lung, and bladder as well as due to bronchitis and emphysema, ischemic heart disease, aortic aneurysm, and peptic ulcer. Pipe smokers showed similar risk levels to cigarette smokers.

Crofton JW, Douglas A: *Respiratory Diseases,* 2d ed. Oxford, Blackwell, 1975, pp 320–359.
  Reliable general account of the group of diseases.

Ferris BG Jr: Epidemiology standardization project. Am Rev Respir Dis 118:1–120, 1978.
  Recommended methods for use in epidemiologic studies.

Ferris BG Jr, Speizer FE, Spengler JD, Dockery D, Bishop YM, Wolfson M, Humble C: Effects of sulfur oxides and respiratory particles on human health. Methodology and demography of populations in the study. Am Rev Respir Dis 120:767–779, 1979.
  Description of the Harvard six cities study of air pollution. Study with some initial results on pollution levels and respiratory effects.

Higgins MW, Keller JB: Estimating your patient's risk of COPD. J Respir Dis 4:97–108, 1983.
  Presentation of the Tecumseh index of risk and how to measure it in patients and other individuals.

Higgins MW, Keller JB, Becker M, Howatt W, Landis JR, Rotman H, Weg JG, Higgins I: An index of risk for obstructive airways disease. Am Rev Respir Dis 125:144–151, 1982.
  Based on the Tecumseh Community Health study over a period of 15 years, predictors of obstructive airways disease are identified. The risk factors indentified included age, sex, cigarette smoking, respiratory symptoms, chronic bronchitis, asthma, respiratory tract infections, reduced lung function, and familial chronic bronchitis.

Laennec RTH: *A Treatise on the diseases of the Chest and on Mediate Auscultation,* Forbes J (transl). New York, Samuel Wood & Sons, 1830.
  Chapter 3 "Of Emphysema of the Lungs" describes the clinical characteristics of the disease, including a recognizable account of the blue bloater.

Morgan WKC, Seaton A: *Occupational Lung Diseases.* Philadelphia, Saunders, 1975, pp 265–273.
  Standard text on occupational lung diseases.

NAS-NRC Committee on the Epidemiology of Air Pollutants. Epidemiology and air pollution. Washington, DC, National Academy Press, 1985.
  A report for EPA administrators. The committee established a common base of state-of-the-art knowledge through the circulation and discussion of background papers assembled by experts.

Rosenblatt MB: Emphysema. Geriatrics 18:517–527, 1963.
  A good review of the history of these diseases.

The Health Consequences of Smoking. Chronic Obstructive Lung Disease. A Report of the Surgeon General, 1984. Dept H.H.S. PHS Office on Smoking and Health, Rockville, MD.
  A useful review of chronic obstructive pulmonary disease, emphasizing its relationship to smoking but also presenting other risk factors.

Chronic Obstructive Pulmonary Diseases

Lynne M. Reid

Chronic obstructive diseases of the lungs include four conditions that are very different though all of them cause airways obstruction: bronchiolitis, chronic bronchitis, emphysema, and asthma. Even the way they produce airways obstruction is different. Since each can be separately identified and has different implications for prevention, treatment, and management, the umbrella terms *chronic obstructive lung disease* and *chronic obstructive pulmonary disease,* with their catchy abbreviations of COLD and COPD, have no place in medical use.

Bronchiolitis is discussed first, since it focuses attention on acute changes in small peripheral airways; it is caused most commonly by infection and less often by noxious chemicals. It is important in infant, child, and adult.

Chronic bronchitis is the response to chronic irritation. Early in the disorder, changes are confined to bronchi, i.e., to the large airways; at this time, airways obstruction is uncommon; in the later stages, the bronchioli or small airways are also involved, and airways obstruction is a regular occurrence. Tobacco smoking is the commonest cause: occupational factors come a long way behind.

Asthma arises from acute, and readily reversible, constriction of bronchial muscle. It affects airways of all sizes, from terminal bronchioli to the hilus, so obstruction really affects large and small airways, sometimes selectively at a particular level. In some patients with asthma, the changes are only functional; in others, structural changes are also present.

These three conditions (bronchiolitis, chronic bronchitis, and asthma) are commonly associated with a normal alveolar region of the lung.

Emphysema includes a variety of anatomic types; some varieties of this alveolar disease change the lungs' compliance or distensibility and are associated with severe airways obstruction. In the type of emphysema that causes airways obstruction, the alveolar region is abnormally compliant, thereby producing a secondary or functional effect on the airways: loss of elasticity causes the airways to collapse prematurely during expiration, probably the small ones first and later the large.

Although more than one of these four conditions often affects a patient at the same time, each is sometimes present alone. In this chapter, bronchiolitis, chronic bronchitis, and cor pulmonale are considered separately to identify features peculiar to the definition, diagnosis, pathogenesis, and prognosis of each; asthma is considered elsewhere (Chapters 79 and 80). By understanding the effects of a condition when it occurs alone, it is possible to

analyze better the effect of a combination of these diseases.

Whether obstruction is in large, medium, or small airways, ventilation to the affected region is reduced. Regardless of the level at which the obstruction to airways starts or ends, if it is widespread enough, blood-gas tensions are deranged.

Certain misleading generalizations, which have doubtless arisen from a desire to simplify, are current about these four diseases. This group of diseases, emphysema in particular, has been ill-served by the attempt to "lump" and simplify. The following true, but somewhat paradoxical, generalizations make it clear why it is difficult to relate structure to function or disability in a simple way.

1. Chronic bronchitis is often crippling and fatal without any emphysema being present.
2. Some forms of emphysema are crippling and fatal without there being any chronic bronchitis.
3. Other types of emphysema are widespread and structurally severe but lead to no incapacity for the patient.
4. Emphysema is not a single entity. It is currently described in structural terms, and on this basis several varieties can be identified. Even if these are regrouped on a functional, radiographic, or pathogenic basis, the term *emphysema* still includes a variety of conditions.

To understand these diseases in a clinical setting, we rely heavily on the results of radiographic techniques and functional testing. The use of function tests is to diagnose the presence of airways obstruction and to assess its severity and its reversibility. The radiograph makes it possible to detect whether certain types of emphysema are present and of sufficient severity to explain disability.

A simple schema of the important bases for obstruction in these various diseases is shown in Table 77-1. This table provides a practical checklist that can be applied in considering the management and treatment of a particular patient.

TABLE 77-1
Causes of Airways Obstruction

Block of lumen
  Mucus
  Pus
Changes in wall
  Epithelial height
  Edema
  Inflammatory-cell infiltration
  Muscle hypertrophy
  Muscle constriction
  Fibrosis (including stenosis and obliteration of lumen)
  Change in mechanical properties

DEFINITIONS

In the last decades, definitions have gradually evolved that have been accepted internationally and have improved communication and diagnosis. They offer a framework within which the various unsolved problems can be identified and described. Although each definition has a different basis, i.e., clinical, physiological, or pathologic, largely reflecting the striking characteristic of the given disease, the definitions as a group have the advantage of practicality. *Asthma* is defined in terms of deranged function as reversible airways obstruction, *emphysema* in terms of structure as abnormally large airspaces, and *chronic bronchitis* by the presence of a symptom, sputum production. *Bronchiolitis* has not been so succinctly defined, but we may do it etymologically as inflammatory changes of the distal airways, the bronchioli.

Recently developed function tests have encouraged physiologists to hope that obstruction in small airways can be detected earlier than was previously possible. These "sensitive" pulmonary function tests have led to the concept of small-airways disease, a noninfective obstructive state arising *only* in small airways. As yet, it is unclear whether this concept will be edifying in more than a few patients. Disease in bronchioli is, of course, part of the picture associated with chronic bronchitis.

In this account bronchi are taken to be large airways and bronchioli small airways. Although by reference to the definitions given later a sharp anatomic junction between the two can be identified, functionally there is probably no such sharp division, and the small bronchi probably often behave like bronchioli.

Even newer methods of measuring function in the small airways do not satisfactorily distinguish the two main causes of small-airways obstruction—mechanical obstruction and a secondary functional effect from loss of elastic recoil. It seems that when the results of common tests of ventilatory capacity are normal, "sensitive tests" (e.g., the flow-volume curve and the single-breath N_2 test) will detect evidence of both early closure of small airways and a minor increase in uneven ventilation. Obstruction within small airways can also be discovered by the responses to gases that are less dense than air. Thus, if the large airways are patent and there is obstruction in small airways, the use of a $He-O_2$ mixture will cause a smaller change in the flow-volume curve in patients than in normal subjects. However, it is not possible to be sure whether the premature closure of small airways is due to a disease of adjacent alveoli, producing a secondary functional effect on the small airways, or to changes in the small airways themselves.

Some smokers with normal ventilatory capacity show premature closing of the small airways. From the point of view of correlation between structure and function, it is not possible to say whether this finding reflects changes

in small airways *themselves* or in the alveolar region. Tobacco smoke probably causes both. Clearly it is necessary to follow up groups of early smokers to analyze whether this finding is of help in predicting those subjects who will later develop disability.

ANATOMIC BACKGROUND AND UNITS OF LUNG STRUCTURE

Cartilage is important for the support of the airway wall and for its relation to muscle insertion. Constriction of smooth muscle in the airways contributes to airways obstruction in several of these disorders and is of special significance, as it is treatable.

Cartilage is found as C-shaped plates in the anterior and lateral walls of main bronchi (Fig. 77-1). Muscle is located posteriorly as bundles which insert into the posterior ends of the cartilage plates. Mucous glands are numerous in the intervals between the plates of cartilage and especially in the posterior wall external to the muscle coat. The gland ducts penetrate the muscle. As the airways enter the lung, plates of cartilage come to surround the whole circumference. This point of transition in the arrangement of the cartilage is associated with an important change in the arrangement of the muscle. In the airway within the lung, the muscle surrounds the entire lumen and is not attached to the cartilage. Within the lung, muscle contraction can cause complete occlusion of the lumen, as occurs in asthma. In contrast, the airways

outside the lung are not exposed to sphincteric action of the muscle.

Earlier, in Chapter 2, an idealized system of airway anatomy is given, of the sort used in studies of lung clearance or respiratory function tests. In the paragraphs that follow, the facts of airway branching are described as seen in radiographic, including bronchographic, examination and as applicable to pathologic specimens and to computed tomography (CT).

In the walls of the intrapulmonary airways the cartilage is arranged in a series of plates which distally become sparse (Fig. 77-2). Bronchi, by definition, are those airways which are proximal to the last plate of cartilage; bronchioli are those distal. Two classes of bronchi can be distinguished—the *large bronchi*, where cartilage is so abundant that any section of the airway includes cartilage in its wall, and the *small bronchi*, where a chance histologic section may not include cartilage. Mucous glands and cartilage are coterminous, i.e., all bronchi as just defined have submucosal glands. A difference in behavior of large and small bronchi is seen in massive collapse or airlessness of a lobe, a difference that is important in analyzing the bronchographic appearances in bronchiectasis.

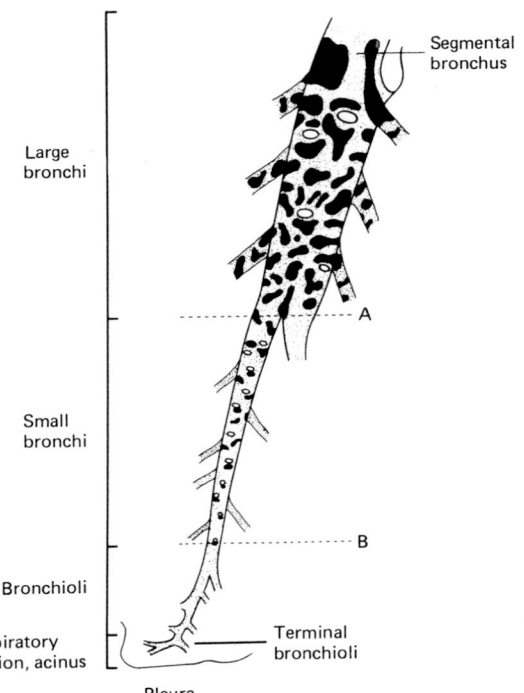

FIGURE 77-2 Diagrammatic representation of arrangement of cartilage (black plates) in the wall of an axial bronchus of the posterior basal bronchopulmonary segment. The bronchus has been opened longitudinally and flattened. Proximally to level A, the cartilage (black) supports the entire circumference of the bronchial wall continuously along its length (large bronchi). Distal to the last plate of cartilage at B are bronchioli. Between A and B are small bronchi: in some respects the small bronchi resemble the large; in others they may behave like bronchioli.

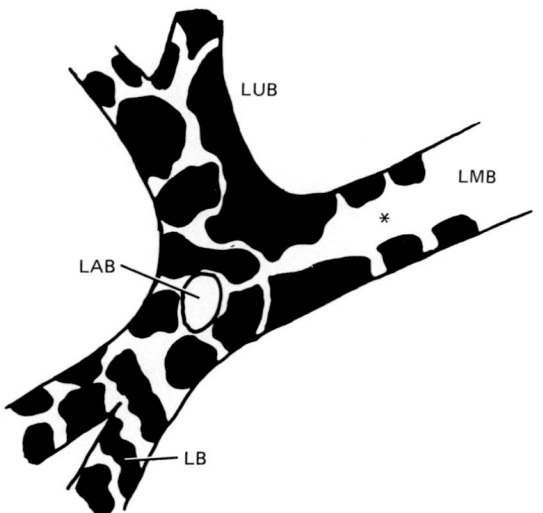

FIGURE 77-1 Diagrammatic representation of arrangement of cartilage (black plates) in large bronchi—posterior view. The disposition of cartilage (black) is shown at the end of the left main bronchus (LMB) and around the origin of the bronchus to the left upper lobe (LUB) and the apical branch (LAB) of the lower lobe (LB). In the main bronchus the cartilage is arranged in rings, open posteriorly, and separated by the membranous portion (*).

Thus, the large intrapulmonary bronchi have such inherent rigidity that their lumen stays patent, whereas the small bronchi behave as bronchioli or alveoli in that their walls appose. Broadly speaking, two sorts of intrasegmental pathways can be recognized for airways. One is an *axial pathway* which runs the longest possible course within a bronchopulmonary segment and passes directly from the hilus of the lung to the distal pleural surface. The other is a lateral pathway, the type that supplies regions between the hilus and the distal pleural surface.

An axial pathway to the posterior basal segment gives rise to 25 or more branches between the segmental bronchus and a terminal bronchiolus close to the pleura. If a generation is taken as the length of bronchus between two branches, then we can describe any airway in terms of its number of generations of branching. The length of an axial pathway and the number of its generations varies with the size and shape of the segments: the shorter segments have fewer branches.

Along lateral pathways there are fewer generations, and alveoli are reached in about five generations along the first lateral airway in a segment. To compare segments it is convenient to count the segmental bronchus as the first generation. The older method of counting the trachea as the first has the disadvantage that segmental bronchi within the various lobes have a different count. It is better, for radiographic and pathologic studies, to compare airways by generation than by size because the latter will vary with functional state, in disease and with age and size of the individual.

At the distal end of any airway, be it axial or lateral, a *respiratory bronchiolus* is reached which, while having the structure of a bronchiolus in part of its wall, elsewhere has alveoli opening into its lumen.

A *terminal bronchiolus* is the airway immediately before a respiratory bronchiolus and is the most distal bronchiolus with a complete epithelial lining.

Three units have practical application in clinical and radiographic description. Each reflects the features of branching of the bronchial tree.

First, the *bronchopulmonary segment* is the essential topographic unit. A lung contains 9 or 10 segments. The variation in the pattern of branching of the bronchi at the hilus is so great that the segments cannot be satisfactorily described by reference only to the position of the supplying bronchus. The critical feature is the position of the segment in the lung (see Chapter 35).

Second, the respiratory unit is the *acinus* (Fig. 77-3). It includes all lung distal to a terminal bronchiolus, that is, it includes several generations of respiratory bronchioli, alveolar ducts, and alveoli. Acini vary in size and shape as do the segments. The diameter of an acinus is between 0.5 and 1.0 cm.

Third, the *lobule* includes the cluster of three to five acini at the end of any airway (Fig. 77-4). Neither an aci-

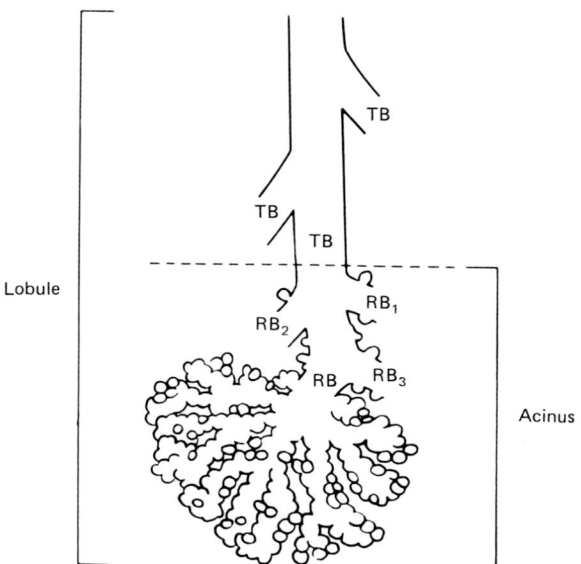

FIGURE 77-3 Diagrammatic representation of an acinus, i.e., the respiratory unit supplied by a terminal bronchiolus (TB). This is the airway immediately proximal to a respiratory bronchiolus (RB), which has alveoli opening into its lumen. Several generations of RB occur before alveolar ducts and alveoli are reached. The acinus is 0.5 to 1 cm in diameter.

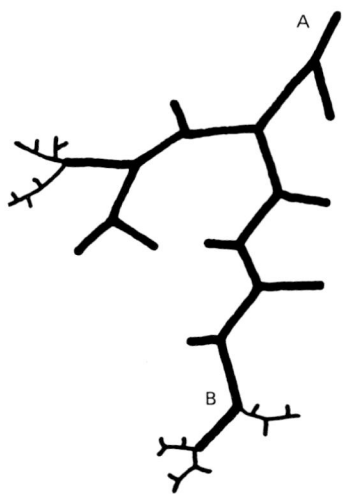

FIGURE 77-4 Diagram showing patterns of branching of the small airways at the end of a bronchial pathway. These include small bronchi and bronchioli. At first, branches arise at intervals of approximately 0.5 to 1 cm, "the *centimeter* pattern" (A). Beyond B, branches arise at intervals of about 2 mm, "the *millimeter* pattern." At the end of each pathway, three to five branches (terminal bronchioli), each 2 mm or so long, make up the region of the millimeter pattern. Terminal bronchioli fill in a bronchogram; the acini beyond do not.

nus, a lobule, nor a segment is surrounded by connective tissue septa, although part of their circumference is sometimes demarcated in this way.

Collateral Ventilation

No unit within a lobe is isolated from its neighbor. Only the pleura isolates. In only one lung in two is the oblique fissure complete, meaning that often not even a lobe is an end unit. The incompleteness of the septa in human beings is essential to *collateral airdrift,* the term used by van Allen and colleagues to describe the phenomenon of air drifting across alveolar walls. This capability means that air can pass from acinus to acinus, lobule to lobule, and segment to segment without using airways. Its effects are essential to understanding what may happen with airway obstruction. Block, even obliteration, of airways is not necessarily associated with airlessness; the lung may be well aerated and normal to naked-eye examination although its supplying airways are no longer patent. Even if alveoli appear normal, it does not follow that the supplying airway is normal. Collateral air drift to some extent renders airways and alveoli independent of each other.

Collateral air drift operates in the infant and child as well as the adult, but it is less efficient in the infant. In the normal lung, it operates through small openings such as the pores of Kohn. In severe panacinar emphysema the "holes" are so much larger that impediment to its operation is much less. Regional variation in the concentration of septa renders air drift less effective in some parts of the lung, such as the lingula or the medial segment of the middle lobe. The resultant relative isolation of parts of the lung makes them more prone both to collapse and to the development of bullae.

In this chapter, bronchiolitis, chronic bronchitis, and emphysema are considered, as well as cor pulmonale, a common complication of these disorders. Asthma is discussed in detail elsewhere.

BRONCHIOLITIS

Bronchiolitis may be acute or chronic. The acute is more common since acute bronchiolitis, caused by infection, is a frequent and serious childhood disease. Chronic bronchiolitis is not often made as a separate diagnosis, although it is not uncommon pathologically. Since it is a feature of chronic bronchitis, it is usually comprehended within the term referring to the larger airways. In the adult, in an otherwise healthy person, acute bronchiolitis arises from infection or from the inhalation of noxious gases.

With acute bronchiolitis—whether in infant, child, or adult—conventional pulmonary function tests of the sort that are discussed for chronic bronchitis are not usually considered. In the patient sick with an acute bronchiolitis, it is the magnitude of the disturbance in blood-gas levels that determines the seriousness of the disease and offers a guide to management.

In the adult, acute infective tracheitis and bronchitis are usually present without much airways obstruction. In acute bronchiolitis in childhood the large airways are also affected, but it is the suffocative nature of the obstructive inflammatory lesions in the bronchioli that dominates the clinical picture since the lesions impair oxygenation of arterial blood and promote retention of CO_2. In these patients, autopsy examination of fatal cases has shown that mechanical obstruction of small airways occurs from secretion in the lumen as well as from swelling of the airway wall by edema and inflammatory cell exudate and by obliterative changes.

Mechanical obstruction of the bronchioli leads to severe disturbance of lung function. In adult chronic bronchitis, it is the changes in the bronchioli that are functionally most significant.

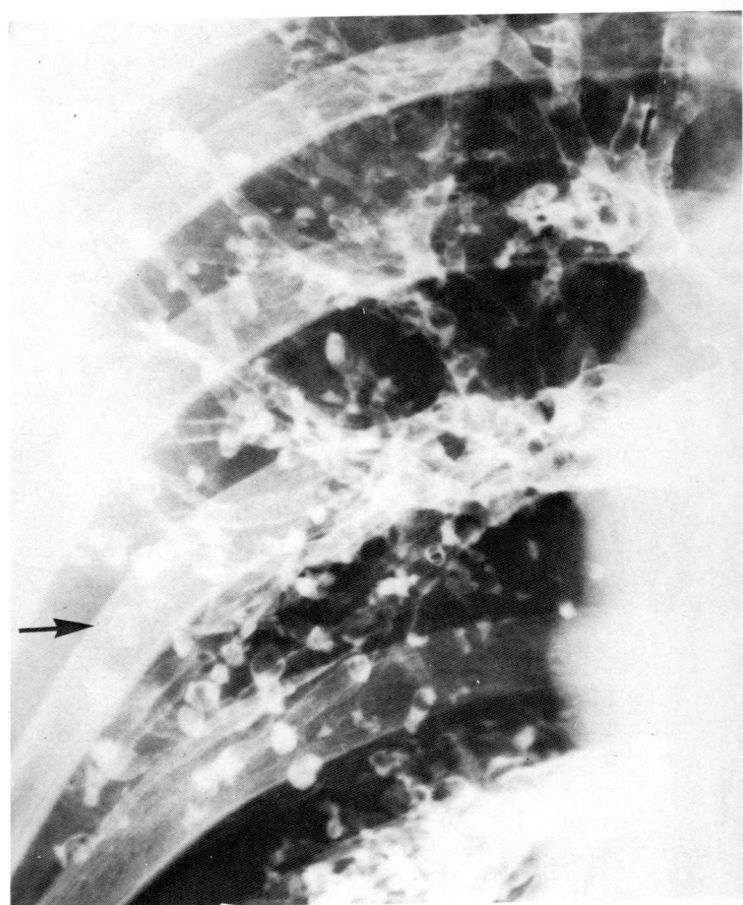

FIGURE 77-5 Bronchographic demonstration of bronchiolectasis in right apical region (arrow). The dilated regions are proximal to sites of bronchiolitis obliterans, demonstrated by the distal regions of nonfilling.

Inflammation of large airways can cause reflex constriction of peripheral small airways. Such a reflex effect arises from the upper respiratory tract, as when the nose is the site where an attack of asthma is triggered or when a cold produces constriction of intrapulmonary airways.

An acute incident of bronchiolitis, if in a previously healthy lung, usually resolves without sequelae. In a child or adult, acute bronchiolitis caused by infection or noxious gases is sometimes followed by impairment, even loss, of small-airway patency (Fig. 77-5). The inflammatory exudate of acute bronchiolitis is followed by fibrosis of small- and medium-size airways, i.e., of anatomic bronchioli and small bronchi. If this obliteration and stenosis is patchy through a large unit of lung, such as a lobe, it sometimes leads to residual hyperlucency on the radiograph. Particularly in a child, the hyperlucency is often unilateral, and this is a radiographic feature of Macleod's (Swyer-James) syndrome.

CHRONIC BRONCHITIS: MUCOUS HYPERSECRETION WITH OR WITHOUT INFECTION

An important step in the study and understanding of chronic bronchitis was the acceptance that sputum production arising from mucous hypersecretion is an early preclinical stage of chronic bronchitis. A smoker's cough was recognized as potentially serious. Severe chronic bronchitis is a common crippling disease that is characterized by cough, sputum production, airways obstruction, and recurrent "infections." In some patients, mucous hypersecretion seems to lead inevitably and incurably to disability. It is not yet possible to predict which individuals are at risk. One working hypothesis is that bronchiolar involvement is the critical factor.

Soon after World War II, when infectious diseases were largely controlled by antibiotics, when in affluent societies smoking was increasing, and when, most importantly, because of better control of disease the population was aging, it became apparent that this condition is one of the major diseases in the community as judged either by sick leave from work or by human disability and suffering. The earlier stages became increasingly important not just to epidemiologic studies but to patient management. It is apparent that with all the advances of modern medicine, treatment of the late stages of the disease is unsatisfactory. At this time it cannot be cured, although there is much that can be done to support the patient.

The role of inflammatory mediators in the persistence and progression of symptoms is being explored as is the interaction between airways obstruction, mucous hypersecretion, and airway hyperreactivity to constrictor drugs. In most patients, each contributes to the pathologic and clinical features of the disease at some stage. Taking animal studies together with the clinical, there is dissociation between these features. The simple interpretation of mucous hypersecretion being associated with hyperreactivity and each then, by mechanical or functional means respectively, contributing to airways obstruction is not the whole story.

Definition

Simple chronic bronchitis is defined as hypersecretion of mucus sufficient to cause cough and expectoration on most days, for at least 3 months of the year, over two successive years. Description of the condition is further qualified by whether the sputum is purulent, indicating infection, and whether the patient has airways obstruction. For example, a particular patient who produces nonpurulent sputum and is not obstructed at one time would, at other times, be a sufferer from purulent obstructive bronchitis. The disease seems to start in large airways and only later to spread to small. Recent studies have shown that in mucous hypersecretion the constituents of the bronchial liquid are different from the normal. Not only is total content increased, but there are changes in the nature of the glycoconjugate and lipid constituents.

Hypersecretion of mucus is the hallmark of chronic bronchitis and is its earliest clinical feature (Fig. 77-6). The hypersecretion starts in large airways and is not usually associated with airways obstruction. The airways of the normal lung are sterile, and mucous hypersecretion can develop without infection. On occasion, bacteria can be cultured from the airways although there is no pus in the secretion. The airways are colonized by bacteria, but whether this should be regarded as infection is debatable. Certainly there is no evidence of invasive infection.

As the chronic bronchitis persists and progresses, excessive mucus is produced also in small airways (Fig. 77-7)—i.e., medium-sized bronchi and bronchioli—and obstruction develops; obstructive bronchitis occurs while sputum is still nonpurulent.

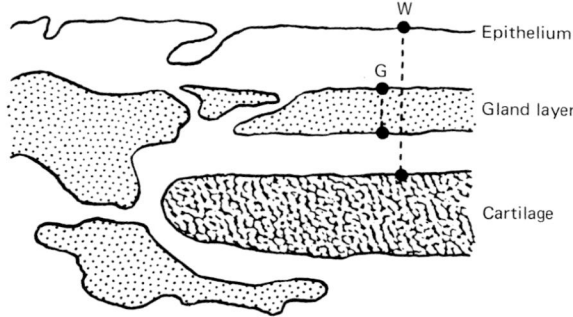

FIGURE 77-6 Diagrammatic representation of gland-to-wall (G/W) ratio. At a site where epithelium is parallel to cartilage, gland thickness (G) is measured; at the same point, the wall thickness, i.e., the distance from epithelium to perichondrium (W), is also measured.

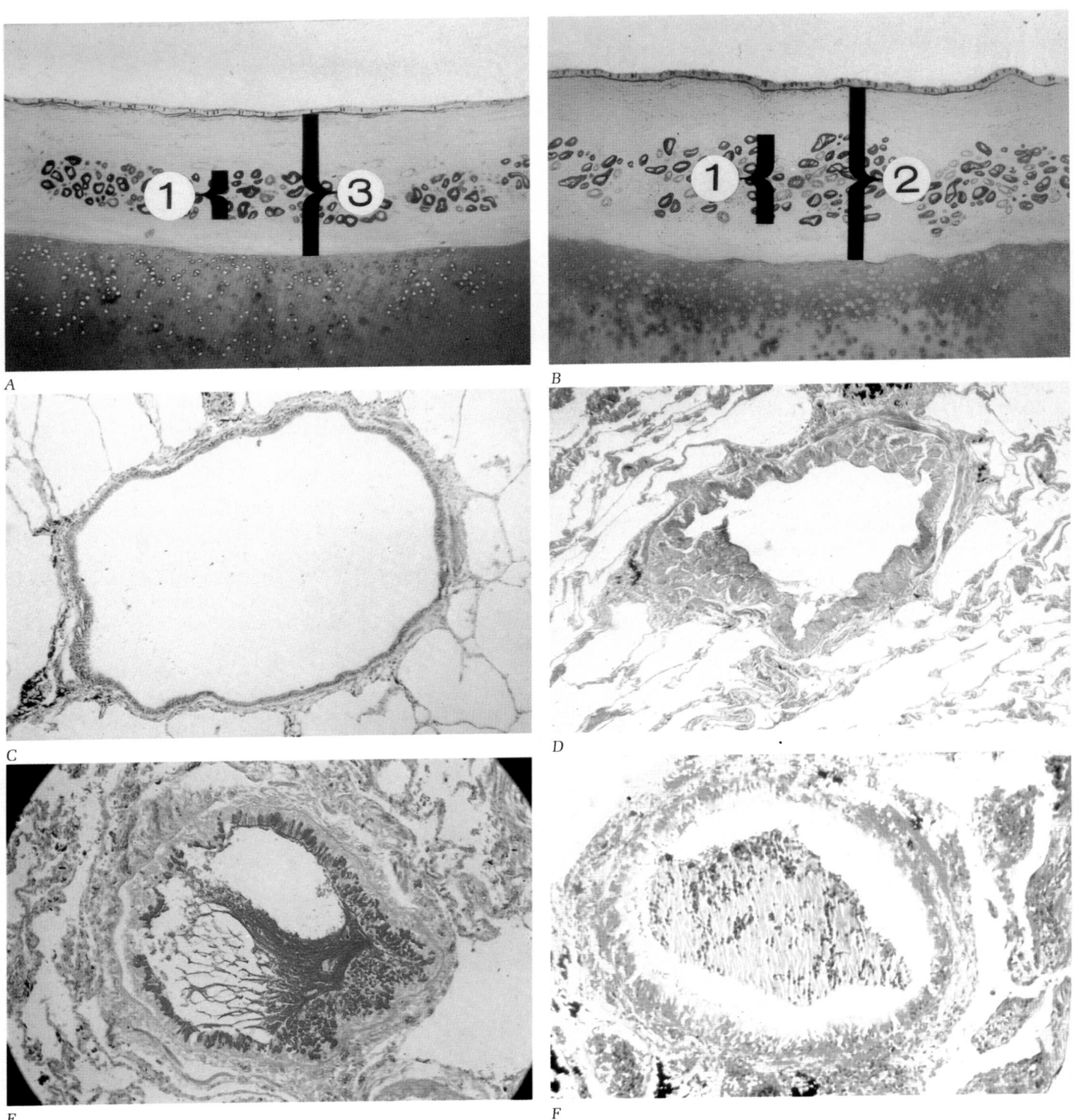

FIGURE 77-7 Changes in the airways produced by chronic bronchitis. *A.* Submucosal gland from normal main bronchus showing gland-wall ratio of 1:3. *B.* Submucosal gland from bronchus of patient with chronic bronchitis showing gland-wall ratio of 1:2. *C.* Normal bronchiolus with few mucous cells. *D.* Bronchiolus of patient with chronic bronchitis showing a large number of mucous cells. *E.* As in *D,* showing lumen partly blocked by mucus. *F.* As in *E,* with pus and mucus in lumen. *A* and *B* show mucus glycoprotein blue; *C* to *F* show mucus red.

For practical purposes, sputum volume can be assumed to reflect changes in large airways, whereas obstruction indicates changes in bronchioli or small airways. It is the changes in the large airways that are present at the onset of the disease and in its milder forms. With progression in severity the bronchioli are also affected, and it is then that obstruction develops.

Bronchial Secretion and Sputum

Mucous secretion is a function of the normal bronchial tree but not in amounts sufficient to produce sputum. Submucosal glands are found in the walls of normal bronchi and mucus-secreting cells in the surface epithelium of the airways, particularly of the bronchi. Normally, mucus-secreting cells are sparse in bronchioli. In the normal subject, the volume of the glands beneath the surface is about 40 times that of the mucus-secreting cells of the mucosal surface.

Normal airway mucus does not contain typical glycoprotein. Recent studies of normal human volunteers have revealed new facts about normal airway mucus. Bronchial aspirate from normal human volunteers gives very little macromolecular yield. It does not contain a component of buoyant density typical of an epithelial glycoprotein: it contains a glycoconjugate of higher buoyant density with sugars typical of an epithelial glycoprotein and some that are typical of a proteoglycan. Cholesterol and neutral lipids are also important constituents by weight. In organ culture human airway yields a similar glycoconjugate: only if stimulated by methacholine is a typical epithelial glycoprotein produced, indicating the potential for its synthesis by normal airway. In the normal human volunteers who smoked, albeit mildly, dry weight yield was not increased, but a small amount of glycoprotein of buoyant density typical of epithelial glycoprotein had appeared together with glycolipid. In chronic bronchitis when sputum is present typical epithelial glycoprotein and glycolipid is found in the greatly increased macromolecular yield from any bronchial lavage or aspirate.

Sputum includes the special mucous secretion of the airway epithelium as well as tissue fluid or serum components (Fig. 77-8). The secretions of the epithelium contain large acid glycoproteins, i.e., up to molecular weights of 7×10^6. Although they vary in weight, they are similar in chemical structure. Glycoproteins consist of polypeptide chains with oligosaccharide side chains. In bronchial glycoprotein, threonine and leucine are the main amino acids, but also there is a handful of disulfide bonds. The oligosaccharide side chains include galactosamine, glucosamine, fucose, and also acid residues—sialic acid and sulfate as an ester. The sialic acid groups are probably linked terminally. In purulent sputum a much higher concentration of serum components is found.

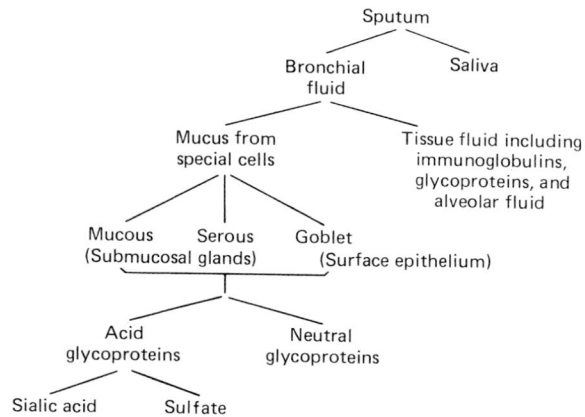

FIGURE 77-8 The diverse components of sputum. Not only is sputum a mixture of saliva and bronchial fluid, but the bronchial fluid that contributes to it is also a conglomerate.

It is the mucous glycoprotein and lipid that confers on sputum its special viscoelastic properties. Serum yields five times the macromolecular dry weight of non-purulent sputum, but the latter is 10 times more viscid. Sputum can be separated into a sol and a gel phase by centrifugation. The same acid glycoprotein is found in both but in lower concentration in the sol. Clearance of airways is achieved by the mucociliary escalator. Cilia are present to the distal end of the epithelium of respiratory bronchioli. The cilia operate in a liquid layer, probably similar to the sol phase of sputum. Thick secretions, bacteria, or particulate matter are shifted up on the surface of this liquid layer.

Mucous Hypersecretion

Persistent mucous production is associated with hypertrophy of submucosal glands in the trachea and large and small bronchi. A quick and simple method of gauging gland hypertrophy is by measuring the gland and wall thickness of an airway and expressing these as a ratio (Fig. 77-6). The main, or lobar, bronchi are most suitable for these measurements since glands are distributed more or less evenly around their walls, and points are numerous at which the surface of cartilage plates is parallel to the epithelium. In the normal person, the ratio of gland thickness to thickness of the wall between epithelium and cartilage is less than 0.3. The ratio has the advantage that this normal value is the same for various airways in the same lung, for airways from large and small lungs, from male and female, and from child and adult. One qualification to this generalization is that under the age of 4 years the normal gland-wall ratio is slightly higher.

In chronic bronchitis, the mucous glands hypertrophy. In patients who produce sputum regularly for 5 years or more, the ratio is above 1:3, sometimes as high as 4:5; there is no overlap with the normal. Patients who produce only a trace of sputum or who have a smoker's early morning cough fall midway between normal and those with well-established sputum production.

It is not known what degree of gland hypertrophy or of mucous production is necessary before sputum is produced. Doubtless the sputum threshold is different in different individuals (Fig. 77-9). Some individuals who have a degree of gland hypertrophy insufficient to lead to sputum production under basal conditions probably will quickly achieve the levels of gland hypertrophy associated with sputum production when stimulated by irritants such as tobacco smoke or infection.

The gland-wall thickness ratio is sometimes supplemented by other measurements such as those concerned with acinar size. These are useful in assessing gland size in bronchial biopsy tissue.

Secretory Cell Increase

Secretory cells are more numerous in large than in small airways. Their distribution is patchy: although only 1 in 20 or 30 cells is a secretory one, these tend to be clumped. Cross section of most bronchioli in a normal lung includes at most only a couple of secretory cells.

In chronic bronchitis, it is usually the glands in the bronchi that hypertrophy first; the increase in goblet-cell number, and particularly their appearance peripherally,

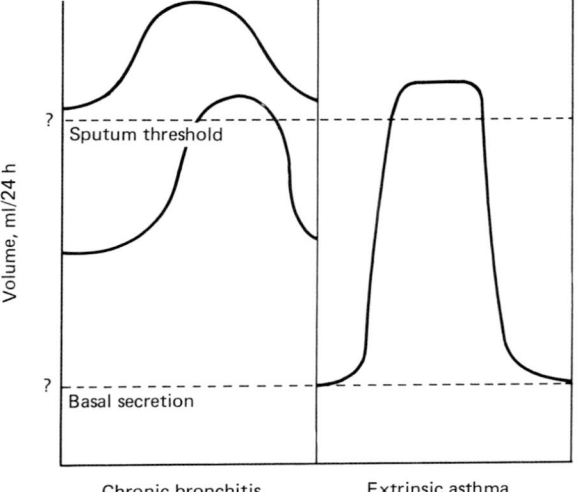

FIGURE 77-9 Sputum threshold. The amount of fluid produced by a normal bronchial tree is not known, nor is the increase necessary for a patient to reach sputum threshold; hence, the question marks. On stopping smoking a subject may fall below this level (upper dashed line) but still be hypersecreting; some may revert to normal. A subject may temporarily and reversibly produce sputum.

occurs later. Bronchiolar involvement is an important feature of the disease labeled *chronic bronchitis*. The degree to which the bronchioli are affected is probably the most significant feature in determining disability. In general, it can be said that hypertrophy of the submucosal glands is associated with increase in the number of goblet cells in bronchioli, and the greater the degree of gland hypertrophy, the more severe and uniform is the increase in the bronchioli. The changes in the bronchioli tend to be patchy: in a single microscopic section the size of a postage stamp, of 5 to 12 small airways, 1 or 2 can be virtually without goblet cells, whereas the others show an obvious increase.

Although gland hypertrophy in bronchi and the increase in secretory cells in bronchioli usually occur together and to a similar degree, this is not necessarily so; gland hypertrophy is sometimes striking when bronchiolar secretory-cell increase is minimal; the number of bronchiolar goblet cells is sometimes impressive when gland hypertrophy is not. The volume of mucous glands in a normal adult is roughly 4 ml; of goblet cells it is 0.1 ml. A threefold increase in gland thickness means 27-fold increase in volume. Although it is doubtless that the glands contribute more to the sputum than do the surface epithelial secretory cells (goblet cells), it is the surface cells that are more related to disability since they are responsible for mucous secretion in small airways that normally are free of it. Because of the small size of their lumen, the peripheral airways are more easily blocked than the larger airways. The possible dissociation between the two aspects of mucous hypersecretion is important to the understanding of certain clinical features and probably explains why no consistent correlation has emerged between the amount or duration of sputum production and a patient's disability. Some severely disabled patients have only a short history of sputum production. Others suffer no great disability and yet have produced sputum for 30 years or more.

Obstruction

A variety of structural changes lead to encroachment on lumen of small and large airways (Table 77-1). Gland hypertrophy is associated with an absolute increase in wall thickness, and this thickening encroaches on the lumen. The epithelium that has an increased number of goblet cells is higher than normal, and there is probably some degree of edema as well as of muscle hypertrophy. These features have different rates of reversal.

Etiologic Factors

From epidemiologic studies it seems that the most common association with chronic bronchitis, i.e., with chronic sputum production, is the habit of tobacco

smoking—particularly of cigarettes. It is likely that the response by the airway epithelium of mucous hypersecretion is a nonspecific response to an irritant. In view of the differences in the types of intracellular glycoprotein, differences in the nature of mucus could arise from different causes of chronic bronchitis or according to the speed with which these changes develop.

Animal Models

Taking the stigmata of chronic bronchitis to be an increase in submucosal gland size and in surface epithelial secretory cell number, helpful information has been obtained from animal models of chronic bronchitis. These changes have been produced in a variety of ways and in a variety of species.

First it was important to produce these changes without infections being present, since the early stages of the human disease are not associated with infection. With SO_2 and with tobacco smoke these changes have been produced both with and without ulceration of the surface epithelium. Recent studies have shown that nonsecretory cells present within the surface epithelium can develop secretory granules within 24 h of starting exposure to an irritant. And secretory cells that contain a few discrete granules quickly come to have many granules with characteristics of a typical mucus-secreting cell or goblet cell—a cell stuffed with numerous confluent granules containing acid glycoprotein.

At first the changes are only in trachea and large intrapulmonary bronchi, but gradually the same changes are found also in small peripheral airways, the bronchioli. The increase in goblet cell number is dose-related, and with higher doses the changes appear more quickly at the periphery. The epithelium becomes higher, and the concentration of secretory cells per unit area of epithelium also increases. Ciliated cells and basal cells, as well as the secretory cells, are more numerous.

A variety of types of glycoprotein are secreted by the epithelial cells and glands. Speaking generally, no abnormal type of glycoprotein is found in chronic bronchitis, but an increasing proportion of cells come to secrete an acid, rather than a neutral, glycoprotein; of the acid radicals, it is a resistant sialic acid and sulfate that particularly increase. This pattern is similar to that found in human disease. Experimentally, anti-inflammatory agents have been shown to modify this behavior. Phenylmethyloxadiazole, for example, "protects" against the increase in secretory cell number but does not prevent the change in glycoprotein types.

Isoproterenol also produces an increase in secretory cell number and in gland size in the living animal. Pilocarpine produces a similar effect, but there are sufficient differences in the histochemical features of the glycoprotein and in the morphology of the new cells to suggest that the mechanisms by which these drugs act are different.

Recovery from these changes has also been shown experimentally, and although the distribution of glycoprotein types returns to normal in weeks, the time necessary for secretory cell number and gland size to revert must be measured in months.

Infection also causes gland hypertrophy. Experimental *Mycoplasma* pneumonia in a lobe of the piglet's lung evokes, within a couple of weeks, a gland-wall ratio of 0.5 in the trachea and large airways, representing a statistically significant hypertrophy, since the gland-wall ratio for the pig is similar to the human. There is no evidence of infection of the glands, suggesting that perhaps the hypertrophy is mediated through a nervous reflex stimulated by the changes at the lung periphery. It could be important in understanding the onset of chronic bronchitis in certain diseases, particularly cystic fibrosis, when peripheral infection is probably the first event, and gland hypertrophy and goblet-cell increase are secondary to it. The airway secretions also contain antiproteases.

It is difficult in the human to follow the transition from the normal to the hypersecretory state that carries the diagnosis of chronic bronchitis. This is being done in the canine model of bronchitis produced by inhalation of SO_2 gas. The findings before SO_2 exposure are similar to those described for the normal human airway. With exposure to SO_2, aspirate increased in volume as did its dry weight yield: in some dogs typical epithelial glycoprotein appeared that is similar to that recovered from the sputum of human chronic bronchitis. The dogs were studied during many months exposure to SO_2, either 50 or 200 ppm (parts per million), and during as many months of recovery. From these studies the following generalizations can be made. Individual variation and susceptibility was apparent: three of four dogs exposed to 100 parts even after 10 months exposure to SO_2 dry weight yield and constituents were no different from the normal pre-SO_2 levels. When mucous hypersecretion is present, the constituents of bronchial mucus are abnormal. But which comes first, increase in amount of secretion or abnormal constituents? It seems abnormal constituents are observed before increase in amount of secretion is apparent clinically. Change in the glycoconjugate molecule secreted is an early finding, as is the appearance of glycolipid. The significance of these findings for early diagnosis or airway irritation and their implication for management have still to be explored.

Clinical Course of Chronic Bronchitis

The earliest stage of chronic bronchitis is the production of nonpurulent sputum, with no evidence of airways obstruction; the sputum is sterile on culture. The next stage is associated with the evidence of infection. It is to detect the early stages of peripheral airways obstruction that some recently described tests of respiratory function, e.g., closing volume, have special application (see Chapter

163). These stages are important for two reasons—to detect the presence of impairment to function and to predict the patient who is at risk of worsening function. Because the reasons for clinical deterioration are so poorly understood, such analysis is essential to improved understanding of pathogenesis. Only then will it be possible to choose the appropriate treatment.

In the normal lung, the airways are sterile and often remain so even in chronic bronchitis with disability. Although the word *infection* is usually applied if bacteria can be recovered from the airway secretions, it is probably useful to think of their presence as a stage of colonization of the airways by bacteria since the secretions usually do not contain pus cells. The airways now resemble the upper respiratory tract or gut, where it is normal to find bacteria on the epithelial surface and in the lumen. This colonization is not, of course, the normal state for the airways. It may be that the presence of particulate matter, such as bacteria, contributes to continuing secretion of mucus. Many patients produce purulent sputum, either continuously or intermittently, which is not associated with systemic signs of infection.

In the early stages of the disease, a patient often presents to the doctor for the first time because a cold has "settled in the chest." In the disabled patient, "exacerbations" of chronic bronchitis cause the patient to consult the physician: the patient's symptoms usually worsen; shortness of breath becomes more severe; blood-gas tensions either become abnormal or, if so already, worsen. Sputum sometimes decreases during these exacerbations. The patient rarely has a temperature or an increased white blood cell count. These incidents often arise when atmospheric pollution is worse or with the onset of a cold or flu. It seems that initially the trouble is retention of secretions so that obstruction increases. After some days more definitive evidence of infection may become apparent. It is presumed that bacteria have multiplied within the retained secretions. The use of antibiotics in the management of chronic bronchitis contributed to this interpretation of the changes. Antibiotics given prophylactically do not seem to affect the number of such incidents that a patient suffers, but they have been reported to shorten the duration and severity as judged by absence from work.

Pathologic Findings

In the airways the main findings are a high gland-wall ratio and an increase in the number of secretory cells in the surface epithelium. In the bronchioli the number of secretory cells is increased. These changes have been described above with the discussion of mucous hypersecretion, the main feature of chronic bronchitis.

When obstruction develops and causes disability, it is the small bronchi and bronchioli that are implicated. A bronchogram reveals the effect on regional lung function. Peripheral filling is severely impaired, and irregularities

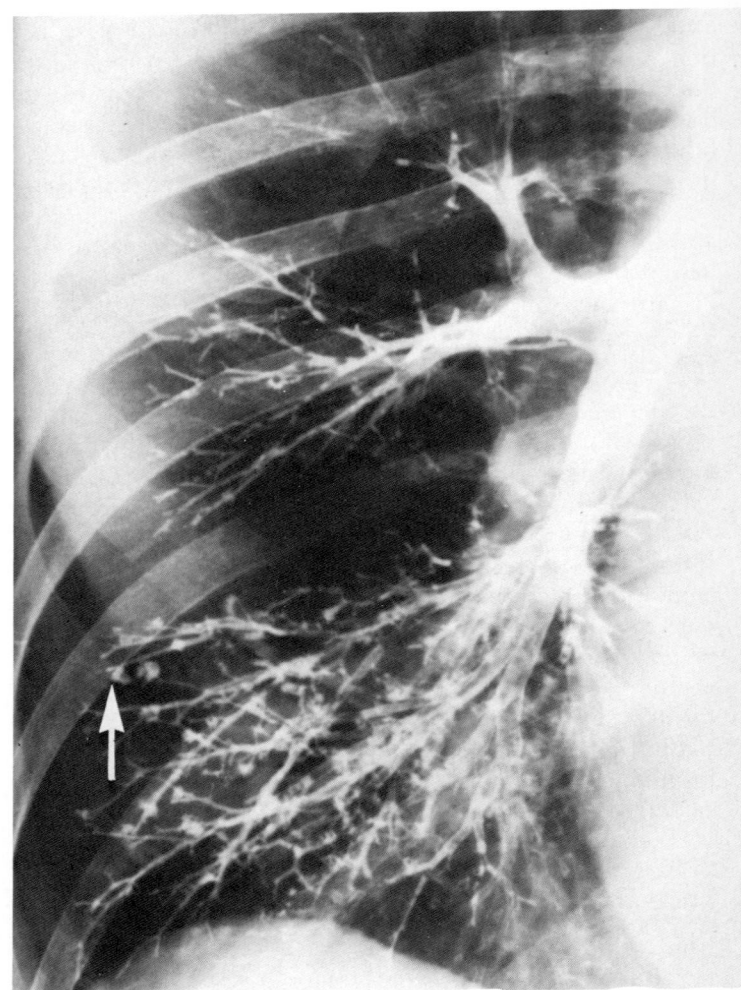

FIGURE 77-10 The small airways in chronic bronchitis. Bronchogram in chronic bronchitis showing poor peripheral filling in lower lobe and regions of bronchiolectasis (arrow).

in the lumen of the filled airways are apparent (Fig. 77-10). Acute and chronic changes coexist: the walls of the small airways show thickening because of edema or inflammatory cell infiltrate; chronic changes have distorted the airways. The wall is thickened by an increase in muscle and connective tissues and in the height of the epithelium. The lumina are irregular because of dilatation and narrowing. Bronchiolitis sometimes produces ulceration which is almost invariably associated with fibrosis. Fibrosis gives rise to stenosis or even bronchiolitis obliterans.

Part of these changes is due to the acute damage produced by infection. Less clear is the role of continuing mucous hypersecretion and colonization by bacteria in producing chronic inflammatory changes in the walls of the small airways. The acute clinical exacerbations have raised the possibility that deterioration in a patient's respiratory reserve is caused by episodic damage to peripheral small airways and that each incident produces its

quota of irreversible structural damage. However, a patient's deterioration is usually gradual and not related to the intermittent bouts of infection. Instead, it seems likely that hypersecretion of mucus and the presence of secretion within the airway lumen—whether or not it is colonized by bacteria—are in some way linked to the deterioration in airway functions. The possibility of amplification of injury by mediators of inflammation released from inflammatory cells into the tissue or airway lumen needs also to be considered.

Clinical Stages and Reversibility

By the time that the patient with chronic bronchitis first presents to the physician, respiratory function is usually already impaired, often severely. Gregg has recognized an earlier stage of mucous hypersecretion than sputum production, namely, early morning throat clearing. It is of interest that even at this stage many individuals—this symptom would hardly be thought to justify calling the subject a "patient"—have respiratory reserve reduced below normal values. Almost all patients who had presented with respiratory problems due to chronic bronchitis had serious impairment of lung function. When the patient has mild impairment of respiratory function, the bronchogram usually shows damaged airways; in those patients whose activities are curtailed, bronchograms always show widespread and severe damage.

Radiographic and Bronchographic Findings

The chronic changes in the airways do not show in a radiograph. Even though the plain radiograph of a chronic bronchitic patient is usually normal, a bronchogram often reveals a variety of changes. A bronchogram can be considered a respiratory function test that in some ways resembles an intravenous pyelogram: it tests the ability of airways to conduct the test substance to the periphery. The use of a radiopaque medium identifies those airways that do conduct, and how far. In chronic bronchitis, the obliterated airways are bronchioli or small bronchi.

The bronchographic appearance of airways supplying regions of nonfilling offers clues to the nature of the airway changes. In the earliest stages of chronic bronchitis the bronchogram is either normal or, if there is patchy nonfilling, those airways that do fill appear normal. If the endings of the filled airways look squared off, either secretion or more distal disease is preventing filling while the airways are normal up to the point where the filling ends. In the later stages, in addition to regions of nonfilling, small peripheral airways show irregularities, stenosis, and dilatations (Fig. 77-10).

The terms *bronchiectasis* and *bronchiolectasis* are again coming into use. In addition to giving an anatomic message, the terms point to a different sort of injury. The dilatation of airways, large or small, enshrined in the term

is often of little consequence compared to the other structural features. Bronchitis obliterans and bronchiolitis obliterans are two synonyms for bronchiectasis or bronchiolectasis that point to more significant structural features than dilatation. Obliteration of bronchi or bronchioli is associated with nonfilling of distal airways with grave functional implication: frequently the bronchi that have filled have an irregular shape and outline pointing to distortion and scarring. Collateral ventilation often results in a lobe or lung that appears normally aerated in a straight radiograph: only a bronchogram reveals that this is largely achieved by collateral ventilation since so many airways are obliterated. These injuries are commonly the result of infection—typically one incident of pneumonia for example, with or without associated airlessness or collapse, has left severe scarring and distortion of airways. If the infection resolved, this may be all that is wrong—"dry" bronchiectasis. If the cavities and patent proximal airways continue to hypersecrete because they are the site of chronic infection, then sputum production often continues—"wet" bronchiectasis. The symptoms are indistinguishable from purulent chronic bronchitis.

Correlations have been made between the bronchographic and histologic appearances of specimens. The dilatations that appear as small "pools" of radiopaque material, of the order of 3 to 5 mm in diameter, represent dilated bronchioli, usually proximal to the site of bronchiolitis obliterans. Bronchiolar lesions are often so numerous that filling, particularly in the basal segments, is poor.

Sometimes a dense collection of radiopaque medium, up to 1 cm in diameter with an irregular outline, is seen. This collection represents the rare occasion when radiopaque medium reaches the alveolar region and localizes in a region of panacinar emphysema. Contrast medium has not been demonstrated within a region of centriacinar emphysema.

Cystic Fibrosis

Although features of cystic fibrosis resemble those seen in chronic bronchitis, their pathogenesis is probably different. In the adult chronic bronchitic, mucous hypersecretion develops in response to irritation, with infection following (Fig. 77-11). The child with cystic fibrosis has increased susceptibility to lower pulmonary airway infection, the reason for which is not known, but which is associated with bronchiolitis. It is the infection that leads to mucous hypersecretion, probably by a nervous reflex producing submucosal mucous gland hypertrophy in larger airways. The presence of mucus in the airways predisposes to colonization by bacteria and offers a nidus in which bacteria can multiply. The possibility that in this disease the cells and mediators of inflammation lead to persistence and amplification of injury opens new fields for investigation and perhaps therapy.

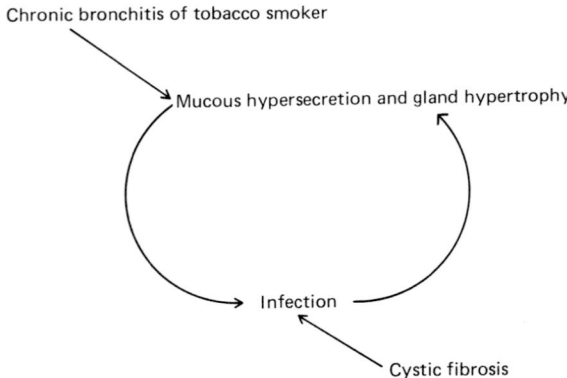

FIGURE 77-11 Mucous hypersecretion in chronic bronchitis and in cystic fibrosis. Mucous hypersecretion is a nonspecific response to irritation and is ultimately associated with infection. Cystic fibrosis produces the changes of mucous gland hypertrophy because of susceptibility to infection.

No abnormality in the lungs of the newborn with cystic fibrosis can be detected by any one of the methods currently available. In particular, submucosal gland size, goblet cell number, and type of intracellular acid glycoprotein are normal. This has far-reaching implications for treatment and prognosis in these patients. If infection can be prevented or acute infection completely eradicated, the changes of chronic bronchitis can be prevented. If infection develops in the child with cystic fibrosis, mucous gland hypertrophy, goblet cell increase, and extension to the periphery soon follow. In chronic bronchitis, as in the common forms of bronchiectasis, the lesions are more common and more severe basally. In cystic fibrosis even the early lesions are diffuse and commonly in the upper as well as the lower lobes, emphasizing that, even if it is not yet identified, there is an intrinsic abnormality of lung tissue or its secretions in this disease.

"EMPHYSEMATA"

This somewhat pedantic Greek plural is used to emphasize that no matter how we consider emphysema it includes a variety of types.

Definition

Emphysema is a condition of the lung characterized by increase beyond the normal in the size of the airspaces distal to the terminal bronchiolus, i.e., within the acinus.

The structural definition has the advantage that it leads to recognition of several anatomic types that have different clinical, radiographic, and functional significance. This definition is shorn of any references to dilatation or destruction. Previous inclusion of *dilatation* or *destruction* in the definition was intended to differentiate the benign from the more serious forms of the disease. It

was once believed possible to encompass all types of emphysema within these two mechanisms. Since it soon became apparent that this approach was too simple, it seems best to drop reference to mechanisms in the definition.

General Comments

Emphysema is sometimes a crippling and fatal disease, even though there is no chronic bronchitis or structural distortion of the airways. In these instances, airways obstruction is a secondary feature caused by the effects of alveolar disease on the airways.

Certain types of emphysema that are striking pathologically are not associated with disability. Thus, size of the emphysematous holes does not correlate well with presence of disability or the degree of airways obstruction. This discrepancy explains some of the disappointing results obtained in early attempts to correlate disability with structural emphysema that was assessed in terms of tissue-air ratio. The answer was nonsense: some of the highest emphysema counts were found in subjects who had never experienced any impairment of respiratory function.

It is doubtful whether airways obstruction due to chronic bronchitis can be reliably separated from airways obstruction due to emphysema. Respiratory function tests are particularly useful in identifying that airways obstruction is present, in quantifying its severity, and in judging its reversibility. The radiograph is important in diagnosis and in the management of the patient. Although the radiograph cannot diagnose certain types of emphysema, the type of emphysema and its severity that can be diagnosed from the radiograph are important in assessing disability and prognosis. The severe grades of panacinar emphysema can be diagnosed from the chest radiograph.

Anatomic Types

Several anatomic types of emphysema can be recognized by a characteristic distribution of large airspaces within the acinus (Fig. 77-12).

PANACINAR

In panacinar emphysema, all alveoli within the acinus are affected and to roughly the same degree. The change may be so severe that virtually the whole of the acinus has disappeared; if many acini disappear, a "spider web" or "candy floss" appearance results. This anatomic type is seen in primary emphysema as associated with α_1-antitrypsin deficiency, in compensatory over-inflation, and in types of emphysema representing hypoplasia.

CENTRIACINAR OR CENTRILOBULAR

The alveoli arising from respiratory bronchioli are mainly affected. This type of emphysema is found in widespread and severe form in subjects who have no respiratory disa-

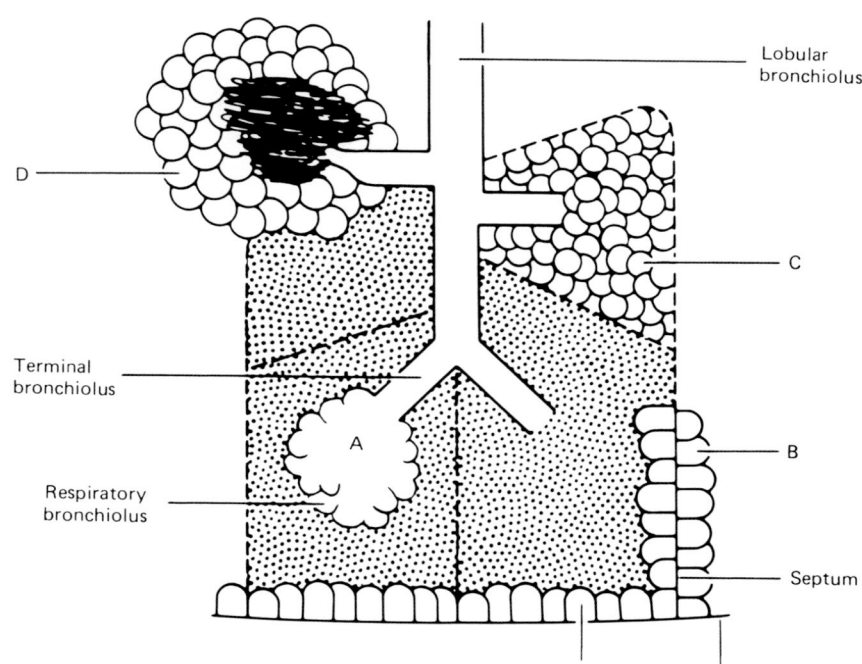

FIGURE 77-12 Anatomic varieties of emphysema. A = centriacinar (centrilobular); B = periacinar or paraseptal; C = panacinar; D = irregular (scar). The dashed lines mark the edge of an acinus. Usually the edge is not demarcated by a connective tissue septum, and so collateral airdrift can occur.

bility and for whom we do not therefore have respiratory function tests in life.

PERIACINAR OR PARASEPTAL

The enlarged airspaces are under the pleura or along connective tissue septa and are thus at the periphery of the acinus. Since it is only when the periphery of the acinus is bordered by connective tissue that the periacinar region is affected, the term *paraseptal* is a useful synonym.

IRREGULAR

Irregular emphysema is the term used to describe large airspaces with no uniform or particular anatomic distribution within the acinus. It includes the enlarged airspaces that sometimes occur in the vicinity of a scar.

Although there has been widespread agreement and acceptance of these terms, inconsistency in their use has contributed to the confusion that still surrounds the emphysemas. These are anatomic terms and should be used to describe anatomic features, e.g., *not* to imply cause or pathogenesis. The unit of reference is the acinus, and so the term should be used with reference to a single acinus and not to a region, e.g., a localized region of panacinar has been erroneously called centriacinar emphysema because of local intensity of the change. These types are sometimes found in the same lung and, if so, should be separately identified. Centriacinar and panacinar considered just as anatomic types have different distribution within the whole lung. Centriacinar is commonly found

in upper lobes, panacinar as often in the lower as the upper. Centriacinar does not commonly develop into panacinar emphysema.

Pathogenesis of Emphysema: Mechanisms

The large airspaces of emphysema arise in one of the following four ways: hypoplasia, atrophy, overinflation, and destruction.

HYPOPLASIA

Hypoplasia creates a paradoxical sort of emphysema in that the large airspaces represent underdevelopment of the lung or a failure of growth. In the normal lung, alveoli multiply after birth to produce the adult number of about 300×10^6 alveoli by the age of 8 (Fig. 77-13). Congenital or acquired lesions interfere with this multiplication. The result is a panacinar type of emphysema, severe and often evident in the radiograph. Examples are Macleod's syndrome, atresia of a bronchus, lobar emphysema of childhood, and some forms of adult bullous disease.

ATROPHY

After normal development has been completed, in some subjects alveoli atrophy and enlarge (i.e., become emphysematous); the process occurs in the aged lung—*senile emphysema*. The process is characterized by loss of total alveolar surface area and of alveolar number.

Certain types of primary or unexplained emphysema are still in this pigeonhole, but this group is a catchall.

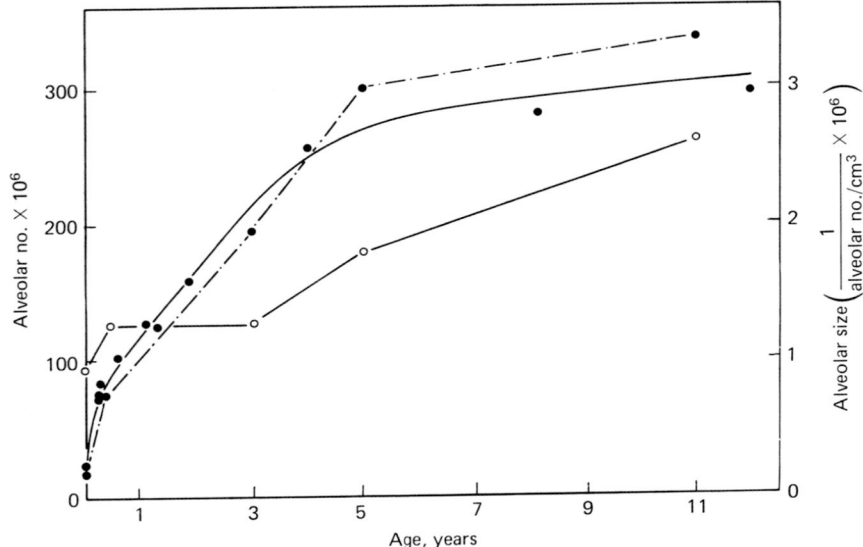

FIGURE 77-13 The normal increase in alveolar size and number with age. At birth the alveoli are represented by a total of 20×10^6 primitive sacs; by 8 years of age the adult number of 300×10^6 has developed. Lung disease in childhood can interfere with this growth and lead to emphysema. ●——●, alveolar number (Dunnell MS: *Postnatal growth of the lung. Thorax 17:329–333, 1962.*); ●—·—●, alveolar number (Davies G, Reid LM: *Growth of the alveoli and pulmonary arteries in childhood. Thorax 25:669–681, 1970.*); ○——○, alveolar size (Davies G, Reid LM: *Growth of the alveoli and pulmonary arteries in childhood. Thorax 25:669–681, 1970*).

α_1-Antitrypsin deficiency, in which enzymes seem to destroy the alveolar wall, was once in this group but can be reassigned to the destruction group.

OVERINFLATION

The alveoli are increased in size beyond the normal expansion that occurs in maximum inspiration. Examples are emphysema with check-valve obstruction or emphysema with distension of a lobe compensatory to excision or collapse, *compensatory emphysema.* Compensatory growth does not seem to include increase in alveolar units above the normal total, but an increase of lung volume above normal before alveolar multiplication is complete causes this process to occur faster than is normal.

DESTRUCTION

In this type, alveolar walls that were once present are damaged with complete or partial destruction or ulceration of alveolar walls. This destruction characterizes post-inflammatory states in which airspaces enlarge, but alveolar architecture is still recognizable. An example is healed sarcoidosis.

One of the uses of this quartet of mechanisms is to help refine analysis of the way in which a given type of emphysema develops. For example, patients with inherited deficiency of α_1-antitrypsin are prone to develop widespread severe panacinar emphysema. This implies that the lung developed normally and that then there was regression. On the other hand, it has been claimed that emphysema is found in children with α_1-antitrypsin deficiency. If this is so, then it implies that childhood multiplication and development of alveoli was abnormal and that this type of emphysema is a form of hypoplasia. In

fact, it is not yet answered whether the lungs in these patients had developed normally. The factors contributing to the development of emphysema in the absence of this antiprotease are considered in detail in Chapter 74. The bullous region associated with atresia of a bronchus probably arises in part from hypoplasia—a failure of alveoli to multiply normally in the affected region—and in part from overinflation—increase in volume inappropriate to the alveolar growth—because it is ventilated by collateral ventilation, which favors an inspiratory volume and air trapping.

Classification of Types of Emphysema

The point of departure for the classification that follows is that, although emphysema is defined in anatomic terms, large airspaces do not correlate with disability, whereas airways obstruction does (Fig. 77-14). The classification that follows combines anatomic observations with evidence of airways obstruction. Since intrinsic airways disease often coexists with emphysema, the final interpretation of the role of the emphysema in the airways obstruction also requires appraisal of the extent and type of the associated disease of the airways.

Emphysema without Airways Obstruction ("Benign" Emphysema)

Among these benign types of emphysema, each anatomic variety is represented.

AGED LUNG

A mild form of panacinar emphysema is seen in about one-half the lungs of people over 70 years of age. It is not

apparent on the radiograph, although the "aged chest" can often be detected by the striking reduction in rib calcification which makes the vascular pattern surprisingly obvious and the lung fields appear clear. This condition is not associated with disability.

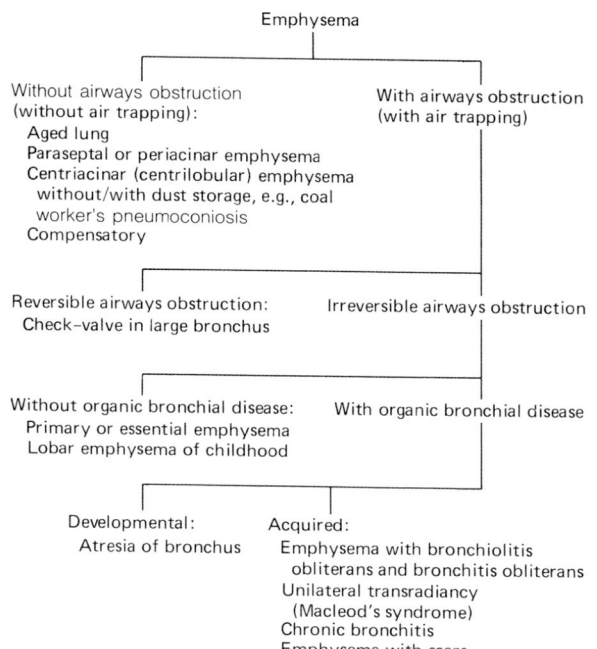

FIGURE 77-14 Classification of emphysema according to the presence, or absence, of appreciable airways obstruction.

When inflated in the laboratory the lungs are normal in size or small, and when the inflating pressure is released, the lungs deflate normally but rather more slowly than does a young lung. The alveolar number is reduced, and alveolar diameters are enlarged. When the enlargement is only twofold, alveolar volume is enlarged eight times, and alveolar surface area is considerably reduced (Fig. 77-15). Although the arteriogram shows a reduction in background haze, it is nowhere as severe as in the more severe grades of panacinar emphysema that are associated with airways obstruction.

PERIACINAR OR PARASEPTAL EMPHYSEMA

This type of emphysema does not cause airways obstruction, although it may be detected on the radiograph or in the tomogram (Fig. 77-16). It may be the start of a large bulla or give rise to a pneumothorax.

COMPENSATORY EMPHYSEMA AND EMPHYSEMA WITH CHECK-VALVE OBSTRUCTION

In each of these conditions there is an increase above the normal in volume of the lobe or lobes affected. Little is known of the effect on structure of compensatory emphysema that persists for years, but if the lung was normal before it was overexpanded, its function remains good. Radiographically the blood vessels are spread out, and so the concentration of vessels is often less than normal, but the background density or grayness is normal. In overinflation associated with a check valve, e.g., from a foreign body or tumor in the airway lumen, the background density is reduced. The region is hyperlucent, presumably

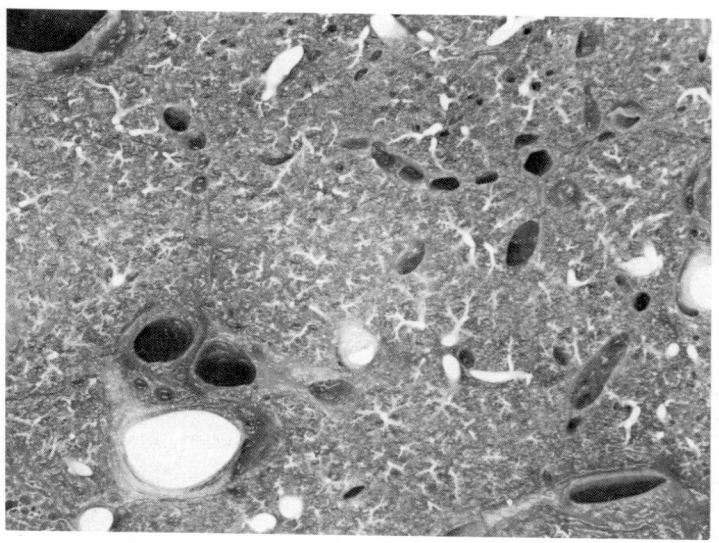

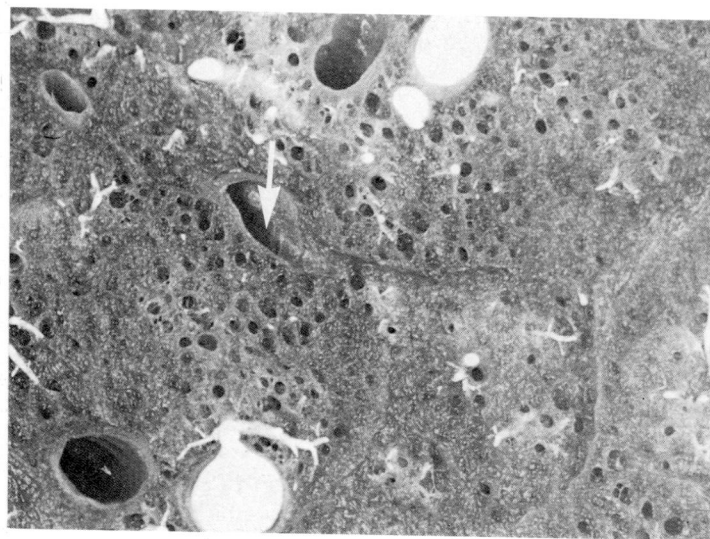

A   B

FIGURE 77-15 Close-ups of thick lung sections. Normal young (A) and aged (B) lung. The lungs were fixed in inflation, and the pulmonary artery was injected with white medium. In B, large spaces stretch from the central artery (containing the white injection medium) to the peripheral unfilled vein (arrow), changes characteristic of panacinar emphysema.

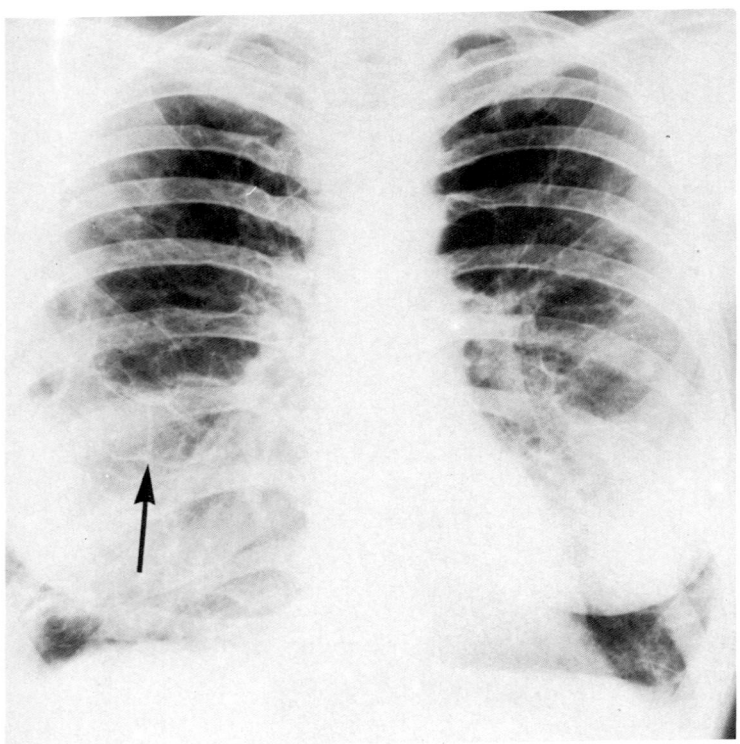

FIGURE 77-16 Radiograph of a patient with widespread periacinar or paraseptal emphysema. The intersecting line shadows (as at arrow) represent walls of small bullae, found mainly peripherally.

because the air trapping, characteristic of this sort of emphysema, is associated with decreased blood flow to the region.

CENTRIACINAR (CENTRILOBULAR) EMPHYSEMA

Autopsy studies of people who die with no history of lung disease and who had normal radiographs in life reveal that in about one-quarter of such subjects centriacinar emphysema is present. This type of emphysema is often widespread and severe, but since the chest radiograph is normal, it is not possible to diagnose its presence during life.

Centriacinar emphysema is found particularly in the upper or apical parts of the lung or of a lobe; for example, in the lower lobe it is mainly the apical segment that is affected. It is more common in males than females. These features are different from panacinar emphysema, which, either as in the aged lung or in primary emphysema, affects the base certainly as much as the apex and probably more; moreover, it has no predilection for the male lung. Centriacinar emphysema is rare before the age of 40. The distribution of centriacinar emphysema corresponds with the regions of maximum strain exerted by gravity. The stresses produced by gravity are greater the larger the lung, and centriacinar emphysema appears to be more common in large lungs. However, multifactorial influences contribute to the pathogenesis of centriacinar emphysema since smoking and very dusty occupations increase slightly the incidence of this form of emphysema.

Although these lesions often are striking if etched by dust, whether from an occupational source or from urban pollution (Fig. 77-17), dust storage is not the cause of centriacinar emphysema. The clinical significance of centriacinar emphysema is uncertain. There is no evidence to suggest that it causes disability. It has also been proposed that centriacinar emphysema contributes to disability in patients who have another pulmonary disease, such as chronic bronchitis. Patients with centriacinar emphysema who develop cor pulmonale invariably have associated chronic bronchitis which, because of hypoxemia, is the cause of the pulmonary hypertension.

Emphysema with Airways Obstruction ("Malignant," or Disabling, Emphysema)

PRIMARY OR ESSENTIAL EMPHYSEMA (IDIOPATHIC, CRYPTOGENIC).

Of the types of emphysema associated with airways obstruction, primary, or essential, emphysema is of utmost importance. Clinically, this type of emphysema is associated with airways obstruction, but there is no structural lesion of the airways. The functional effect is secondary to alveolar disease, which is panacinar emphysema of a severe degree (Fig. 77-18). Only for this type of emphysema is there proof that emphysema can cause airways obstruction, because it occurs in the presence of normal airways.

Clinical Presentation

Patients with this type of emphysema present clinically with shortness of breath but with virtually no sputum production. The condition occurs in relatively young adults and in women as often as in men. About one in five patients is deficient in α_1-antitrypsin (see Chapter 74). Airways obstruction is severe, and the diffusing capacity is low.

Pathologic Features

The lungs show severe panacinar emphysema that usually affects the whole lung, although the severity often varies locally. The lower lobes are sometimes worst affected. In spite of the severe airways obstruction functionally, even at autopsy the bronchi are usually empty of secretions, and it is possible with a pair of scissors to follow patent airways right to the lung periphery.

The panacinar emphysema is at least grade III (airspaces 2 to 5 mm) and often grade IV (airspaces more than 5 mm) (Fig. 77-18). This severity represents a great loss in alveolar surface area and in pulmonary vascular bed. If enough of a lobe or of the lung is affected, this type and grade of emphysema is detectable on the radiograph.

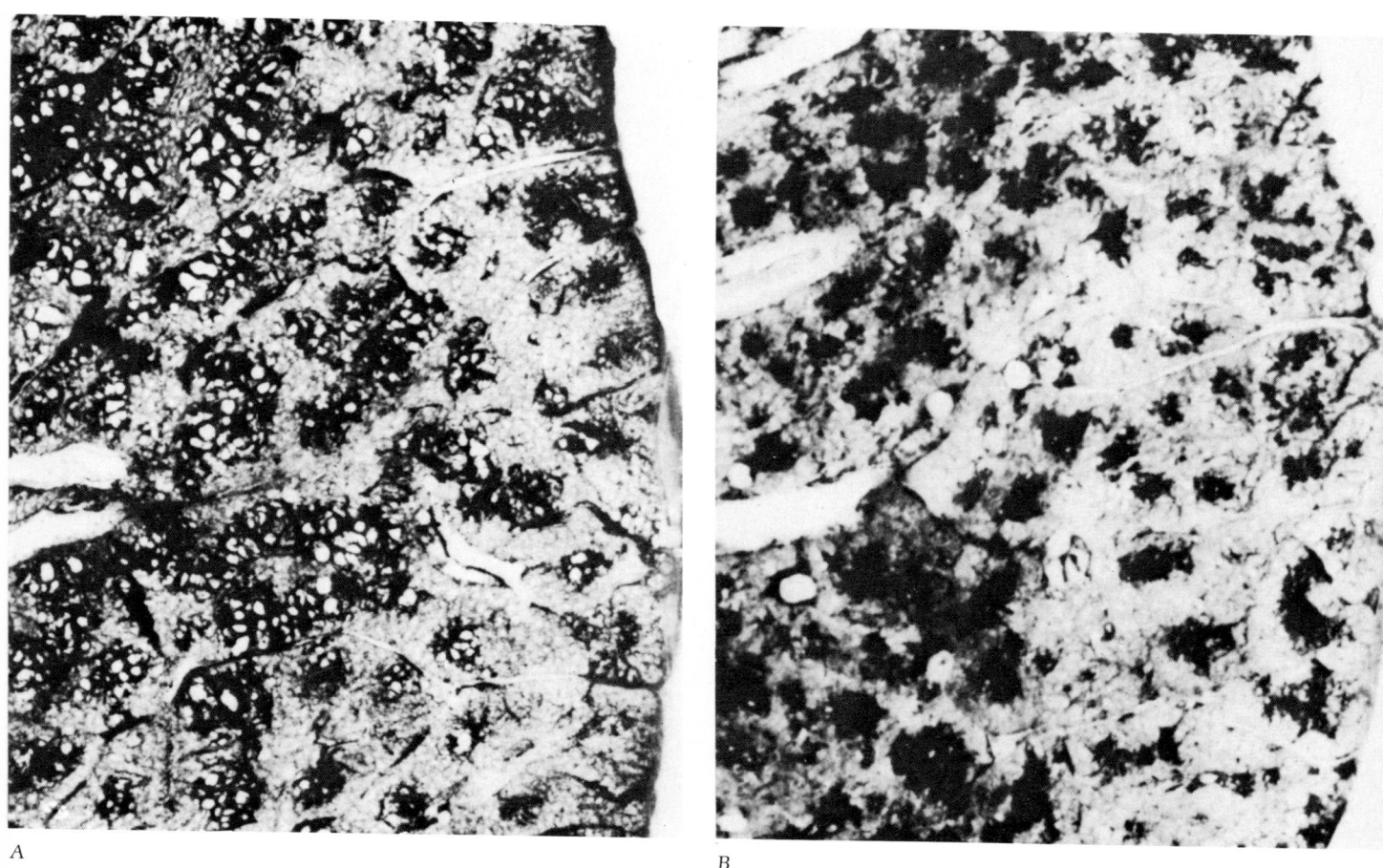

FIGURE 77-17 Centriacinar (centrilobular) emphysema. Sagittal sections of lung. A. City dweller. Enlarged airspaces predominantly alveoli from respiratory alveoli, containing collections of town dust. B. Coal miner. Centriacinar storage of dust with no emphysema.

Correlation of Radiographic and Pathologic Findings

In chronic bronchitis, even if fatal, and in asthma, the radiograph is usually normal. The same is true of emphysema with a few important exceptions. Only panacinar emphysema is apparent in the radiograph (Fig. 77-19), and for this type to be evident, it must be at least grade III in severity, and at least two-thirds of the lungs must be affected to produce the criteria for the radiologic diagnosis of widespread severe panacinar emphysema listed in Table 77-2. This generalization means that centriacinar emphysema is not detectable on the chest radiograph and that panacinar of grade II severity, as occurs in the aged lung, will not be detected even if it affects the whole of both lungs.

In the severe panacinar emphysema (as associated with α_1-antitrypsin deficiency) the radiographic features reflect the functional changes. Excess air is present in the lung (Table 77-2). Whereas the arteries in a patient with asthma are of normal size, in a patient with severe panacinar emphysema they are narrower than normal. Injection studies show that these vessels dilate to normal size if injected with radiopaque material postmortem. The narrow vessels in life are in regions with most loss of peripheral vascular bed and presumably reflect local reduction in blood flow. To increase objectivity in assessing arterial size, Simon advocated the use of the largest vessels as "marker" vessels for size. When narrow vessels are found in at least four of the six zones, the patient has widespread severe panacinar emphysema. Grade III or IV panacinar emphysema causes the affected region to appear avascular on the chest radiograph, sometimes demarcated by a line. A localized bulla shows up in this way even if the rest of the lung is normal.

If the changes under items 1 and 2 in Table 77-2 are found in four or more of the six lung zones, severe panacinar emphysema will be found through at least two-thirds of the lung.

Bullae against the diaphragm may produce a low and flat diaphragm but not the other criteria of widespread emphysema.

Using the above criteria, the only condition that commonly causes difficulty with the radiographic diagnosis of severe *panacinar* emphysema is left ventricular failure.

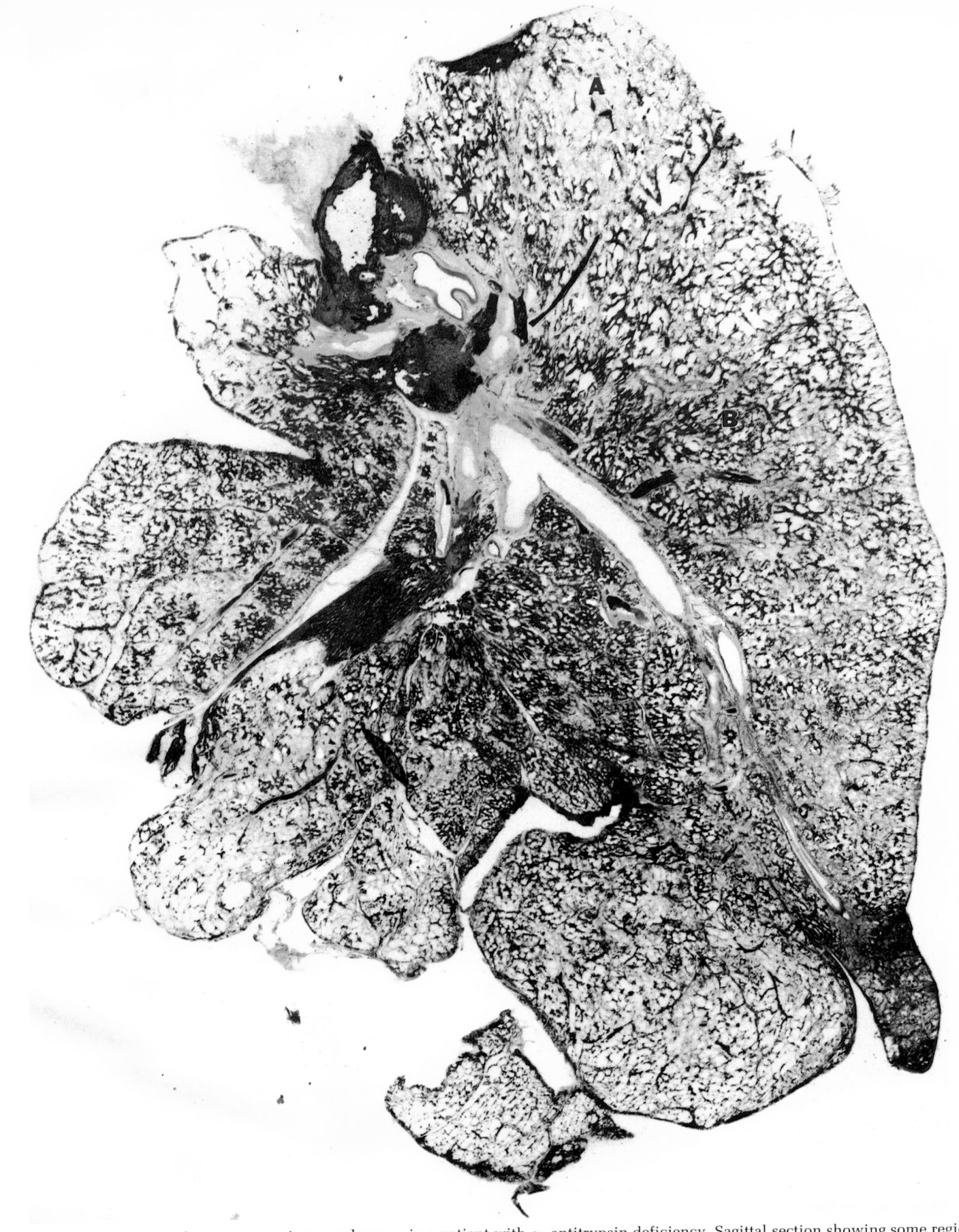

FIGURE 77-18 Widespread, severe panacinar emphysema in a patient with α_1-antitrypsin deficiency. Sagittal section showing some regions of grade III panacinar emphysema (airspaces up to 5 mm); and some of grade IV (airspaces larger than 5 mm). *(Courtesy of J. C. Wagner.)*

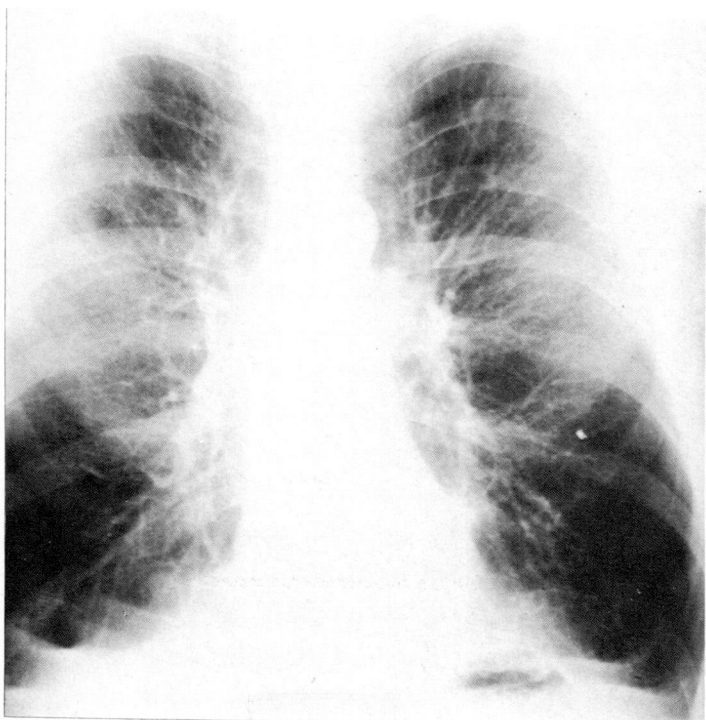

FIGURE 77-19 Radiograph of widespread severe panacinar emphysema. (See Table 77-2.)

TABLE 77-2

Criteria for Radiographic Diagnosis of Widespread Severe Panacinar Emphysema (Grade III)*

1. Signs of excess air in the lungs
   a. Low, flat diaphragms
   b. Large retrosternal translucent area
2. Cardiovascular changes
   a. Narrow vertical heart
   b. Sometimes a prominent pulmonary trunk
   c. Hilar vessels normal or large
   d. Overall lung vessels small (compared to marker vessels)
3. Signs of local vessel loss (sometimes)
   a. Bulla: demarcated by a line
   b. Bullous area: not demarcated by a line

*If more than four of the six zones are affected, emphysema is *widespread*; if fewer than four of the six zones are affected, it is local.

When the left ventricle fails, the diaphragm returns to normal level and the blood vessels increase in diameter and appear uniform. The reason for reversal of radiographic changes is not clear but seems related to pulmonary congestion. When the heart failure is corrected, the radiography again shows emphysema.

Some patients with chronic bronchitis also have severe panacinar emphysema. In this group prognosis is related to the presence of this radiographic appearance. A group of patients with chronic bronchitis (cough and sputum production) were followed over 10 years and divided into those with a normal radiograph, those who showed bullous or localized emphysema on the radiograph, and those who showed the features of widespread severe panacinar emphysema. In the first two groups, 20 percent mortality occurred at the end of 5 years, mostly for reasons unrelated to the lung; the results for the second 5-year period were similar. In those who showed evidence of widespread, severe panacinar emphysema, the mortality was 50 percent, mostly from respiratory or cardiac causes, and there were few survivors at 10 years. The signs we have reported are those that are found with the severe panacinar emphysema associated with deficiency of α_1-antitrypsin.

α_1-Antitrypsin Deficiency

This condition is dealt with in detail elsewhere in this book so that only certain points will be mentioned here.

In a previous section emphasis was placed on the need for separate assessment of emphysema from airways disease. The person with α_1-antitrypsin deficiency, whether a homozygote or heterozygote, illustrates this need since airways obstruction often develops from airways disease and not from emphysema. Not all homozygotes with this deficiency develop emphysema; certainly not all heterozygotes do. During life, radiographic evidence is necessary to prove that emphysema is indeed present.

More and more people with this antitrypsin defect are being reported as instances of emphysema on the basis of airways obstruction; at least some of these individuals probably have chronic bronchitis rather than emphysema as the basis for the airways obstruction. The habit of tobacco smoking seems to increase the risk of developing emphysema, particularly in the homozygote. Although heterozygotes may also be prone to develop chronic bronchitis, this is a different issue and should be addressed separately from that of emphysema.

A predilection for the lower lobes either exclusively or at first in the patient with emphysema and α_1-antitrypsin deficiency has been contrasted with the predisposition of severe bullous emphysema for the upper lobes. However, the emphysema of α_1-antitrypsin deficiency often affects the upper, or apical, zones as well as the lower lobes, or basal regions.

Careful clinical follow-up of these patients should help answer a number of critical questions as to the evolution of this disease. Rarely in a patient is a normal chest radiograph succeeded by one of fully developed emphysema. However, the emphysema of α_1-antitrypsin deficiency will probably prove an exception to this generalization. Moreover, it seems reasonable that these patients lose alveolar surface area and experience impairment of diffusion before lung compliance increases enough to pro-

duce the radiographic appearance of widespread severe panacinar emphysema. In essence, tests of diffusion, ventilation, and mechanics of breathing would be expected to be abnormal before radiographic evidence of emphysema appears.

Lobar Emphysema of Childhood

Lobar emphysema of childhood presents as an acute emergency when the volume of the affected lobe increases sufficiently to displace mediastinal structures. Treatment is then by surgical resection of the affected lobe. This clinical picture arises from a variety of pathologic conditions (Table 77-3). Sometimes the presentation is less acute, surgical treatment is not necessary, and the children continue to adult life with an emphysematous lobe or lobes. In any series of bullae treated surgically in adult life, some examples will be found that suggest that they have been present since early childhood.

Table 77-3 gives a list of types of emphysema that have been found in a lobe or lung removed surgically. For completeness, compensatory emphysema has been included, although this does not cause a clinical emergency.

TABLE 77-3
Childhood Lobar Emphysema

Type	Number of Airways	Alveoli Number	Alveoli Size
Polyalveolar lobe	N	↑ *	N or ↑
Overinflation	N	N*	↑
Hypoplastic emphysema	↓	↓	↑
Atresia of bronchus	N	N*	↑
Compensatory emphysema	N	N	↑

* After birth alveolar multiplication is so rapid that this type may come to have too few alveoli for age if postnatal multiplication is impaired.

NOTE: N = normal; ↑ = increased; ↓ = decreased.

Acquired Hypoplastic Emphysema of Childhood (e.g., Macleod's Syndrome)

Swyer and James first described this entity in 1953 in a single patient. The next year Macleod described the syndrome in a series of adult patients. It is characterized by unilateral hyperlucency associated with air trapping during expiration in the hyperlucent lung so that mediastinal

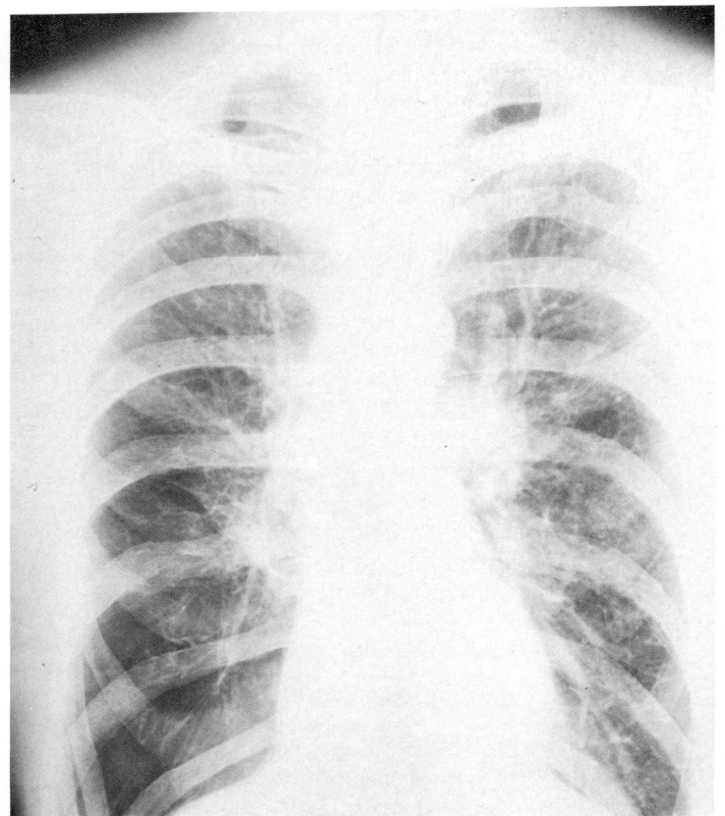

A

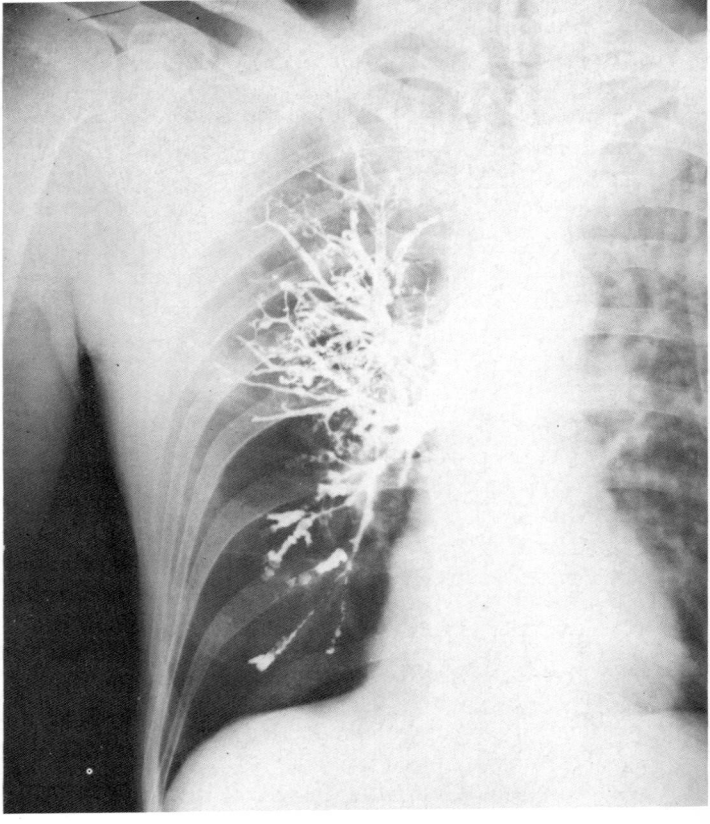

B

FIGURE 77-20 Macleod's (Swyer-James) syndrome. *A.* Unilateral hyperlucency of the right lung, showing small hilar and intrapulmonary arteries. *B.* Bronchogram of the right lung, showing no normal peripheral filling but more severe changes in the lower than in the upper half of lung.

structures shift away from the affected side. The pulmonary artery to the affected lung is small (Fig. 77-20). This condition is a consequence of patchy bronchiolitis obliterans through the lung, acquired during childhood from an incident of infection. This condition sometimes affects a lobe, or part of a lobe, as well as a lung; about one-third of the patients have evidence of airway damage in some part of the contralateral lung. That patchy bronchiolitis obliterans is the cause is suggested by the likelihood that the patient would probably not have survived diffuse disease of both lungs and that if too many small airways had been blocked, the affected lobes would have become airless, and collateral ventilation would not have sufficed to maintain aeration. The affected regions show panacinar emphysema with relatively few but large airspaces, but, paradoxically, the volume of the lobe, or lung, is greater or smaller than normal, or is normal. The conclusion is that the lung is underdeveloped and that the alveoli have not been multiplied normally. The basis for this failure in development is probably the reduced blood flow associated with aeration by collateral ventilation which holds the lung in an expanded position but reduces ventilatory movement. This conclusion is consistent with the idea that growth can be considered, in part, as work hypertrophy.

The bronchiolitis results from bacterial infections, including tuberculosis, or from viral infections. Instances have occurred in which the lung is known to have been normal radiographically before the bout of infection. The small pulmonary artery that is seen on the radiograph and by angiography reflects reduced flow since in those instances where the lobe, or lung, has been resected surgically, the artery has proved to be only slightly smaller than normal. The reduced pulmonary arterial size and hypoplasia of cartilage seem to represent a general failure to grow rather than the cause of emphysema.

COR PULMONALE

Chronic lung disease affects the heart in a variety of ways. Heart failure may develop with or without preexisting right ventricular hypertrophy (RVH); RVH need not be associated with right ventricular failure (see Chapter 64). The use of the term *cor pulmonale* in different ways by different authorities has led to confusion. Elsewhere in this book, it is defined as enlargement of the right ventricle without distinguishing between hypertrophy and dilatation. However, an expert committee of the World Health Organization has recommended that the term cor pulmonale be confined to those cases where RVH has been demonstrated. It *is* desirable that hypertrophy and dilatation should be assessed separately. Dilatation can be detected on the radiograph; hypertrophy cannot.

To diagnose RVH reliably and to assess its severity it is necessary to weigh the ventricles. The septum (S) is included with the left ventricle (LV). To separate the muscle of the two ventricles, fat, coronary vessels, and valves are excised. Then the free wall of the right ventricle (RV) is cut from the septum, save that the right-sided chordae tendineae are shaved off to be included in the right ventricular mass. Wall thickness is an unreliable estimate since dilatation may completely mask hypertrophy. On the other hand, if the wall of the right ventricle is above 3 mm, it indicates hypertrophy.

Right ventricular hypertrophy can then be assessed on the basis of weight and also of the ratio between LV + S, and RV. In the normal, the ratio (LV + S)/RV lies between 2.3:1 and 3.3:1, and the RV weighs 60 g or less. Right ventricular hypertrophy is established by a weight of 80 g or more or a ratio of less than 2:1. If left ventricular hypertrophy is also present, the ratio may be within normal levels or raised. The advantage of using the ratio, as well as the absolute weights, is that these figures can be used throughout childhood, and in a small heart the ratio may indicate RVH when the absolute weight does not.

The electrocardiogram in cor pulmonale is considered in Chapter 34 in considerable detail. However, it is instructive to review certain results and conclusions of Millard, who applied the method described above for assessing right ventricular hypertrophy at autopsy and compared these findings with vectorcardiographic features during life.

He found that the most reliable evidence of RVH is a frontal plane mean QRS axis between and including +91°. and ±180°. This criterion did not give any false positives and enabled the diagnosis to be made in 85 percent of cases where hypertrophy was confined to the right ventricle. It therefore seems to be the most reliable single sign and also more reliable than any group of signs that has been suggested for diagnosis. However, he concluded that the *degree* of RVH cannot be assessed with certainty by this or any other method of interpretation of the ECG. The presence of left ventricular hypertrophy or of ischemic disease—common in elderly bronchitic patients—masks the signs of RVH and limits the usefulness of the electrocardiogram in diagnosing RVH. Finally, the presence of emphysema in the overlying lung seems to have little effect on these signs.

Cor Pulmonale and Emphysema

Some years ago Dornhorst described the clinical paradox that patients with equally severe airways obstruction associated with chronic bronchitis showed wide variation in certain clinical features. At one extreme were patients "pink and puffing" while at the other extreme were some who, with the same degree of airways obstruction, were

"blue and bloated." He considered that this difference might arise from difference in the drive of their respiratory center—i.e., the pink puffers working hard to maintain oxygenation of their blood but conscious of breathlessness; the blue bloaters failing to respond to their abnormal blood-gas levels and so developing edema but, at rest, anyway, seemingly comfortable. Most patients fall somewhere between these extremes (see Chapter 70).

The pathologic findings in the lungs and heart of these patients increase the paradox. It is the pink and puffing who tend to have severe panacinar emphysema. The blue and bloated often have no emphysema; some have mild panacinar; some have centriacinar. In the group with severe panacinar emphysema, with great loss of peripheral blood vessels, RVH is rare, and when it is present, it is mild. In the blue and bloated group with intact lung periphery there is often RVH, and it is usually severe. This group with the seemingly intact lung is the one with pulmonary hypertension.

How to explain this paradox? In the group with an intact lung periphery there is some loss of distal arteries and arterioles up to 40 μm in diameter, but the muscular resistance arteries of the lung, which are just proximal, are still present, and these respond to hypoxia with increase in wall thickness. In the partially muscular and nonmuscular arteries that are precapillary in position, muscle appears by differentiation from precursor cells. In widespread severe panacinar emphysema, much larger arteries, including the muscular ones, are missing, and although there is a greater drop in the volume of the circulation, the muscular arteries are greatly reduced. Pulmonary artery arcades open up, that offer a "run off."

The reason for the dyspnea in the pink and puffing group is not clear, but it may depend on the Hering-Breuer reflex, a stretch reflex from the lung which stops inspiration and leads to expiration when the lung is appropriately stretched. This stimulus to expiration may develop more rapidly in widespread panacinar emphysema because the lung is so compliant that, on inspiration, it quickly reaches a level to stimulate expiration.

BIBLIOGRAPHY

Aubier M, Murciano D, Viires N, Lebargy F, Curran Y, Seta JP, Pariente R: Effects of digoxin on diaphragmatic strength generation in patients with chronic obstructive pulmonary disease during acute respiratory failure. Am Rev Respir Dis 135:544–548, 1987.
  Digoxin has a potent effect on diaphragmatic strength generation that may be beneficial in patients with chronic obstructive pulmonary disease during acute respiratory failure.

Bhaskar KR, O'Sullivan DD, Opaskar-Hincman H, Reid LM, Coles SJ: Density gradient analysis of secretions produced in vitro by human and canine airway mucosa; identification of lipids and proteoglycans in such secretion. Exp Lung Res 10:401–422, 1986.
  Describes the production of glycoconjugates and lipid by normal human and canine airway under basal and stimulated conditions. Typical epithelial glycoprotein is not normally present in airway mucus.

Bhaskar KR, O'Sullivan DD, Seltzer J, Rossing TH, Drazen JM, Reid LM: Density gradient study of bronchial mucus aspirates from healthy volunteers (smokers and nonsmokers) and from patients with tracheostomy. Exp Lung Res 9:298–308, 1985.
  Describes the constituents of mucus aspirated from airways of normal human volunteers. It demonstrates that typical epithelial glycoprotein is not present in a detectable amount.

Brooks SM, Zipp T, Barber M, Carson A: Measurements of maximal expiratory flow rates in cigarette smokers and nonsmokers using gases of high and low densities. Am Rev Respir Dis 118:75–81, 1978.
  In smokers and nonsmokers maximal respiratory flow was measured at various lung volumes using air and gas mixtures of different densities. This strategy demonstrated the presence of reduced ventilation not shown by air breathing, indicating previously undetected degrees of peripheral airways obstruction in smokers.

Burrows B, Knudson RJ, Camilli AE, Lyle SK, Lebowitz MD: "Horseracing effect" and predicting decline in FEV from screening spirometry. Am Rev Respir Dis 135:788–799, 1987.
  In men with chronic bronchitis who continue to smoke FEV_1/FVC is the best predictive test of rapid decline in function. In other types of patients with chronic bronchitis such prediction is not effective.

Cropp A, DiMarco AF: Effects of intermittent negative pressure ventilation on respiratory muscle function in patients with severe chronic obstructive pulmonary disease. Am Rev Respir Dis 135:1056–1061, 1987.

The reduced respiratory muscle strength and increased work of breathing in patients with severe chronic obstructive pulmonary disease (COPD) may predispose these patients to the development of respiratory muscle fatigue and consequent respiratory failure.

Dantzker DR, D'Alonzo GE: The effect of exercise on pulmonary gas exchange in patients with severe chronic obstructive pulmonary disease. Am Rev Respir Dis 134:1135–1139, 1986.
The worsening hypoxemia during exercise in patients with severe chronic obstructive airways disease is due to an inadequate ventilatory response and the effect of a decreased mixed venous PO₂ on the end-capillary PO₂ of low VA/Q lung units and shunt.

Davies P, McBride J, Murray GF, Wilcox BR, Shallal JA, Reid LM: Structural changes in the canine lung and pulmonary arteries after pneumonectomy. J Appl Physiol 53:859–864, 1982.
While compensatory overinflation growth after resection in the adult dog increases weight and surface area of the residual lung, it does not increase alveolar number. If resection is carried out before alveolar multiplication is completed, this occurs faster but does not increase the final alveolar number.

Dornhorst AC: Respiratory insufficiency. Lancet 1:1185–1187, 1955.
This article first described the paradox of the "pink and puffing" and "blue and bloated" chronic bronchitic patient.

Edelman NH, Rucker RB, Peavy HH: NIH workshop summary: Nutrition and the respiratory system. Chronic obstructive pulmonary disease (COPD). Am Rev Respir Dis 134:347–352, 1986.
An overview of nutrition as it relates to the management of patients with severe chronic obstructive airways disease.

Fletcher C, Peto R, Tinker C, Speizer FE: *The Natural History of Chronic Bronchitis and Emphysema*, an eight year study of early chronic obstructive lung disease in working men in London. Oxford, Oxford University Press, 1976.
An analysis of epidemiologic studies of chronic bronchitis that cover the decades since World War II. It is over this time that "chronic bronchitis" was recognized as a significant problem and its features analyzed.

Gilmartin JJ, Gibson GJ: Mechanisms of paradoxical rib cage motion in patients with chronic obstructive pulmonary disease. Am Rev Respir Dis 134:683–687, 1986.
An investigation of the nature of paradoxical motion of the rib cage in patients with chronic obstructive pulmonary disease.

Gregg I: Proceedings of 11th Aspen Emphysema Conference. Department of Health, Education and Welfare, U.S. Government Printing Office, Arlington, Va, 1969, p 235.
An important study of early detection and reversibility of chronic bronchitis. The role of infection in onset and deterioration is also considered.

Gregg I, Trapnell D: The bronchographic appearances of early chronic bronchitis. Br J Radiol 142:132–139, 1969.
Bronchography demonstrates the presence of distorted and scarred airways, even in early cases of chronic bronchitis. Infective incidents are probably not as benign as some epidemiologic studies suggest.

Hislop A, Reid LM: Growth and development of the respiratory system, in Davis JA, Dobbing J (eds), *Scientific Foundations of Paediatrics*, 2d ed. London, Heinemann, 1981, pp 390–431.
This chapter describes normal lung growth and development and how childhood disease can disturb it and cause emphysema. It also describes developmental varieties of childhood lobar emphysema.

Korn RJ, Dockery DW, Speizer FE, Ware JH, Ferris BG Jr: Occupational exposures and chronic respiratory symptoms. A population-based study. Am Rev Respir Dis 136:298–304, 1987.
Data from a random sample of 8515 white adults residing in six cities in the eastern and midwestern United States were used to examine the relationships between occupational exposures to dust or to gases and fumes and chronic respiratory symptoms. Chronic respiratory symptoms and disease can be independently associated with occupational exposures.

Lopez-Vidriero MT, Reid LM: Bronchial mucus in asthma, in Weiss EB, Segal MS, Stein M (eds), *Bronchial Asthma: Mechanisms and Therapeutics*, 2d ed. Boston, Little Brown, 1985, pp 218–235.
Includes more detail on the biochemical nature of secretion in the various hypersecretory airway conditions.

McHardy VU, Inglis JM, Calder MA, Crofton JW, Gregg I, Ryland DA, Taylor P, Chadwick M, Coombs D, Riddell RW: A study of infection and other factors in exacerbations of chronic bronchitis. Br J Dis Chest 74:228–238, 1980.

A carefully controlled analysis of the features associated with exacerbation of chronic bronchitis, including viral infection and sputum eosinophils, in two patient groups from Edinburgh and London. The results are compared with a similar study made 20 years ago.

Millard FJC: The electrocardiogram in chronic lung disease. Br Heart J 29:43–50, 1967.
To my knowledge this is still the only electrocardiographic interpretation of right ventricular hypertrophy based on weights of cardiac ventricles.

O'Donnell DE, Sanii R, Anthonisen NR, Younes M: Effect of dynamic airway compression on breathing pattern and respiratory sensation in severe chronic obstructive pulmonary disease. Am Rev Respir Dis 135:912–918, 1987.
In patients with severe obstructive airways disease, application of negative pressure at the mouth while expiratory flow was at its maximum caused a highly significant increase in the sense of breathing effort.

Reid LM: The Pathology of Emphysema. London, Lloyd-Luke, 1967.
The analysis of emphysema and chronic bronchitis in this chapter is based on the approach reported more fully in this monograph.

Reid LM: Anatomic and pathophysiologic factors in infections of the airways and pulmonary parenchyma in infants and children: Anatomic factors. Pediatr Res 11:210–215, 1977.
A symposium that considered facts known and unknown about the common disease of bronchiolitis in the infant—still the age most at risk for acute bronchiolitis.

Reid LM, Jones RC: Experimental chronic bronchitis. Internat Rev Exp Pathol 24:335–382, 1983.
A review of experimental studies in which the structural changes of chronic bronchitis have been produced in animal models.

Sassoon CS, Hassell KT, Mahutte CK: Hyperoxic-induced hypercapnia in stable chronic obstructive pulmonary disease. Am Rev Respir Dis 135:907–911, 1987.
Hyperoxic-induced hypercapnia is primarily due to impairment in gas exchange rather than to depression of ventilation.

Sassoon CS, Te TT, Mahutte CK, Light RW: Airway occlusion pressure. An important indicator for successful weaning in patients with chronic obstructive pulmonary disease. Am Rev Respir Dis 135:107–113, 1987.
Airway occlusion pressure is a useful predictor for successful weaning during discontinuation of assisted ventilation (AV) in patients with chronic obstructive pulmonary disease (COPD).

Selinger SR, Kennedy TP, Buescher P, Terry P, Parham W, Gofreed D, Medinger A, Spagnolo SV, Michael JR: Effects of removing oxygen from patients with chronic obstructive pulmonary disease. Am Rev Respir Dis 136:85–91, 1987.
A study of the acute physiological effects of removing oxygen from patients with chronic obstructive pulmonary disease receiving long-term oxygen therapy. Removing oxygen caused an increase in pulmonary vascular resistance.

Seltzer J, Scanlon PD, Drazen JM, Ingram RH, Reid LM: Morphologic correlation of physiologic changes caused by SO_2-induced bronchitis in dogs: The role of inflammation. Am Rev Respir Dis 129:790–797, 1984.
The correlation of functional disturbance with structural changes is described in a canine model of chronic bronchitis produced by SO_2.

Simon G: Principles of Chest X-Ray Diagnosis, 4th ed. London, Butterworth, 1978.
This author relates radiographic appearance to the proved pathologic lesions. He understands that different structural types of emphysema have a different functional significance and that only panacinar emphysema can be reliably diagnosed in the radiograph.

Snider G, Lucey E, Sonte P: State of the art: Animal models of emphysema. Am Rev Respir Dis 133:149–169, 1986.
An up-to-date review of animal studies of varieties of lung injury that cause emphysema, i.e., enlargement of airspaces in the alveolar region of the lung.

Sparrow D, O'Connor G, Colton T, Barry CL, Weiss ST: The relationship of nonspecific bronchial responsiveness to the occurrence of respiratory symptoms and decreased levels of pulmonary function. The Normative Aging Study. Am Rev Respir Dis 135:1255–1260, 1987.
Nonspecific bronchial responsiveness was assessed by an abbreviated methacholine challenge test in 458 male participants of the Normative Aging Study. Increased level of nonspecific responsiveness is significantly associated with wheeze and cough symptoms and decreased levels of pulmonary function in adult men.

Standards for the diagnosis and care of patients with chronic obstructive pulmonary disease (COPD) and asthma. This official statement of the American Thoracic Society was adopted by the ATS Board of Directors, November 1986. Am Rev Respir Dis 136:225–244, 1987.
This statement represents the combined efforts of a Task Group appointed by the Scientific Assemble of Clinical Problems of the American Thoracic Society.

Stoller JK, Gerbarg ZB, Feinstein AR: Corticosteroids in stable chronic obstructive pulmonary disease: Reappraisal of efficacy. J Gen Intern Med 2:29–35, 1987.
The 14 available randomized clinical trials were evaluated according to a methodologic "review of systems" and an examination of the statistical precision of the outcome results.

Theodore AC, Beer DJ: Pharmacotherapy of chronic obstructive pulmonary disease. Clin Chest Med 7:657–671, 1986.
One of a series of papers in the same volume dealing with different aspects of treating patients with chronic obstructive airways disease.

van Allen CM, Lindskog GE, Richter HG: Collateral respiration. Transfer of air collaterally between pulmonary lobules. J Clin Invest 10:559–590, 1931.
A function of lung critical to understanding the pathophysiological and radiologic features of airway diseases in which lung tissue continues to be aerated although supplying airways are obstructed, even obliterated.

West JB: Distribution of mechanical stress in the lung, a possible factor in localisation of pulmonary disease. Lancet 1:839–841, 1971.
The stress pattern can explain the development of centriacinar emphysema in normal adults over the age of 40. This type is not caused by the storage of dust, whether occupational or urban.

World Health Organization: Report of an Expert Committee on Chronic Cor Pulmonale. WHO Techn Rep ser no 213, 1961.
The definition of chronic cor pulmonale in terms of right ventricular hypertrophy was and is a real advance, as it emphasizes the need for separate analysis of right ventricular failure and hypertrophy.

Chapter **78**
Cystic Fibrosis

Thomas F. Scanlin

Cystic fibrosis is one of the most common, recessively inherited disorders and the most common lethal genetic disease in the white population. It is a generalized dis- order of exocrine glands. Symptoms involving the lungs and pancreas usually dominate the clinical picture. Two aspects of the disease make it particularly difficult to diag- nose and manage: (1) there is tremendous variability in the degree and type of involvement of different organs in different individuals and (2) the basic defect in cystic fi- brosis is not known.

GENETICS

Cystic fibrosis has an autosomal recessive pattern of in- heritance. The incidence of the disease in whites in the United States is estimated to be about 1 in 2000 live births (Table 78-1); although rare in Asians and in African blacks, the estimated incidence in blacks in the United States is about 1 in 17,000. It also has a remarkable gene frequency: about 1 in 20 whites are heterozygous carriers of the cystic fibrosis gene.

It has not been proved that cystic fibrosis represents either a single disease entity or a single gene defect. How- ever, evidence is mounting that a single locus is involved. Genetic counseling has been handicapped by the lack of a reliable test to detect carriers and a reliable means of pre- natal diagnosis. Current practice is to advise parents of a child diagnosed as having cystic fibrosis that they are het- erozygous carriers and that all their children will have a 1 in 4 chance of being homozygous for cystic fibrosis; also, that their children who do not have cystic fibrosis have a 2 in 3 chance of being heterozygous carriers of the cystic fibrosis gene. It is important to provide genetic counseling for siblings and cystic fibrosis patients when they reach adolescence.

TABLE 78-1
Calculated Risk for Each Pregnancy to Yield a Cystic Fibrosis Progeny

Parents	Estimated Risk
Both are from general white population*	1/2000
Both are known carriers of the cystic fibrosis gene†	1/4
One is an aunt or uncle of an individual with cystic fibrosis	1/160 to
Other has no family history of cystic fibrosis	1/120
One is an unaffected sibling of a cystic fibrosis individual	1/120
Other has no family history of cystic fibrosis	
One is a known carrier of cystic fibrosis	1/80
Other has no family history of cystic fibrosis	
One is an individual with cystic fibrosis	1/40
Other has no family history of cystic fibrosis	

*Based on estimated carrier frequency of 1/20.

†Parent of a child with cystic fibrosis—presumed obligate heterozygote.

Because of the lack of a test for carriers, in 1985 close relatives of cystic fibrosis patients could be informed only about the likelihood that they are carriers: they were told that a spouse unrelated to an individual with cystic fibrosis has a 1 in 20 chance of being a heterozygous carrier.

However, the understanding of the genetic basis of cystic fibrosis took a long leap forward in the closing months of 1985 when it was shown that the cystic fibrosis gene was closely linked with other genetic markers, e.g., with the PON gene for the enzyme paraoxonase, suggesting that the two genes are located on the same chromosome. The directions to be pursued in localizing the cystic fibrosis gene were immediately apparent: for example, the marker, e.g., the PON gene, could be cloned to determine the chromosome and band where both the cystic fibrosis gene and the marker gene are located; then, by screening chromosome-specific libraries for the closely linked probes, the chromosomal locus of the cystic fibrosis gene could be explored.

Using this approach, evidence has mounted that the gene for cystic fibrosis is located on the long arm of chromosome 7 (Fig. 78-1). Although the precise nature and location of the cystic fibrosis gene in the chromosome is not yet known, it is already possible to use the available information as a basis for the genetic counseling of some families who have a child with cystic fibrosis. In these families, analysis of DNA, obtained from a sample of either the chorionic villus or of the amniotic fluid from the pregnant parent, makes it possible to identify, with greater than 95 percent confidence, the cystic fibrosis phenotype of the fetus. The prospect has also been raised that the accuracy of these tests can be improved even further by combining the DNA analysis with determinations of the concentration of intestinal villi enzymes in samples of amniotic fluid obtained during the 15th to 18th week of pregnancy.

It seems inevitable that new probes, with tighter linkages to the locus of the cystic fibrosis gene, will soon be identified. For the present, there can be no doubt that localization of the cystic fibrosis gene to the long arm of chromosome 7 heralds a new era for both genetic counseling and for basic research in cystic fibrosis. However, until the precise molecular defect is defined, the descriptive approach to the pathogenesis of cystic fibrosis must prevail.

PATHOGENESIS AND PATHOPHYSIOLOGY

Since the basic defect in cystic fibrosis has not yet been elucidated, it is not possible to describe precisely the pathogenesis of this complex disorder of *all* the exocrine glands. The hypotheses that have been proposed to explain the pathogenesis of cystic fibrosis include an abnormal glycosylation of glycoproteins, altered autonomic regulation, abnormal ion transport, and unique cystic fibrosis factors.

Every exocrine gland seems to be primarily affected, albeit to different degrees, in cystic fibrosis. Because the exocrine glands perform highly specialized functions in a variety of organs, i.e., in the skin, respiratory tract, gastrointestinal tract, and reproductive system, the list of possible symptoms and complications in cystic fibrosis is impressive. In Table 78-2 the complications and symptoms are listed according to the age group in which they occur most often. Obstruction of exocrine ducts by viscous secretions seems to play a cardinal role in the pathogenesis of almost all manifestations of the disease. In 10 to 20 percent of cystic fibrosis patients, the first manifestation of the disease is often *meconium ileus*, i.e., obstruction of the intestines by thick, viscous meconium stool; chronic pulmonary disease, pancreatic insufficiency, and focal biliary cirrhosis progress gradually throughout the course of the disease, albeit at different rates in different patients. Progressive obstruction of exocrine ducts is a regular feature of the disease, except in sweat glands where obstruction of ducts does not seem to be implicated in the pathogenesis of the exocrine disorder.

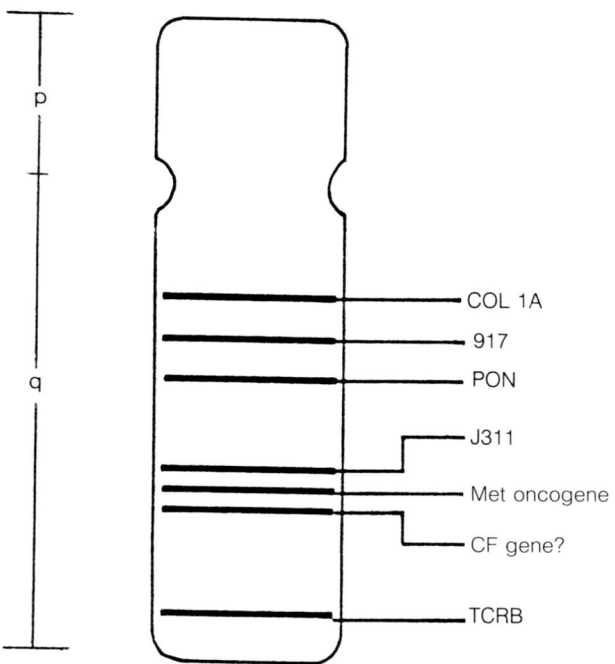

FIGURE 78-1 Partial genetic map of human chromosome 7 showing the approximate location of the cystic fibrosis (CF) gene locus in relationship to other genetic markers. 917 and J311 are "anonymous" DNA probes which were demonstrated to have a linkage to cystic fibrosis and were subsequently mapped to the long arm of chromosome 7. PON is the serum protein paraoxonase, and COL 1A, TCRB, and Met Oncogene represent gene loci for collagen, the T-cell receptor β chain, and the human met oncogene, respectively. The map summarizes the data available in January 1986. See Newmark (1985) for a discussion and the original references.

TABLE 78-2

Complications and Presenting Symptoms of Cystic Fibrosis by Age Group

Infancy	Childhood	Adolescence/Adult
Meconium ileus	Pulmonary infections with staphylococcus & pseudomonas	Chronic bronchitis
Obstructive jaundice	Malnutrition with steatorrhea and pancreatic insufficiency	Pansinusitis
Edema with hypoproteinemia, anemia, and hypoprothrombinemia	Heat prostration with hypoelectrolytemia and metabolic alkalosis	Hemoptysis
Failure to thrive	"Atypical asthma" with clubbing and/or bronchiectasis	Chronic abdominal pain
Intussusception	Esophageal varices	Delayed sexual development
Volvulus	Hypersplenism	Obstructive aspermia
Rectal prolapse	Nasal polyps	
Recurrent pneumonia/bronchiolitis		

Respiratory Tract

In the lungs, hypersecretion of viscid mucus and of chronic bacterial infection combine to produce a progressive and distinctive type of chronic obstructive airways disease that eventually leads to diffuse, severe bronchiectasis. Whether the viscid secretions are primary or are secondary to chronic bacterial infections remains unsettled. In favor of a primary disturbance is the demonstration of hyperplasia of the mucus-secreting cells in the airways of neonates with cystic fibrosis who have not yet developed any evidence of bacterial infection or chronic colonization of the airways. Using sophisticated culture methods, bacterial pathogens can almost invariably be isolated from the respiratory tract of cystic fibrosis patients. The most common pathogens isolated from sputum cultures are *Staphylococcus aureus* and *Pseudomonas aeruginosa*; less commonly found are mucoid *Escherichia coli*, *Klebsiella*, and *Hemophilus influenzae*. In later stages of the disease, *Pseudomonas* usually predominates.

A variety of alterations in the immune system occur in cystic fibrosis. Most appear to be secondary to the chronic pulmonary infection, and a specific deficiency in defense mechanisms has not been identified in cystic fibrosis to account for the persistence of these pathogens in the respiratory tract of these patients.

Typically, respiratory secretions increase when a cystic fibrosis patient, already chronically colonized with *Pseudomonas*, develops a viral respiratory tract infection. In turn, the increase in secretions leads to a gradual increase in cough and sputum and then to an exacerbation of the pulmonary disease usually manifested by increase in respiratory rate, retraction of the chest during inspiration, and diffuse, coarse inspiratory rales. Fever and leukocytosis are common. On the chest radiograph, the degree of hyperinflation increases, and both peribronchial thickening and nodular/cystic densities are more marked than usual. Pulmonary function tests become more abnormal than at baseline; usually RV (residual volume) increases, VC (vital capacity) decreases, and the $FEF_{25-75\%}$ (forced expiratory flow) also decreases. Effective treatment using anti-*Pseudomonas* antibiotics and chest physiotherapy generally succeeds in restoring most indices of pulmonary function to, or almost to, baseline. However, *Pseudomonas* persists in sputum culture.

The most attractive hypothesis to account for this pattern of response to treatment is that treatment has reduced the number, and possibly the virulence, of organisms. However, despite the virtual return to baseline after a particular exacerbation, the cumulative effect of repeated episodes is a progressive bronchiectasis or atelectasis, or a combination of the two accompanied by a gradual and irreversible decrease in pulmonary function. The striking degree of airway destruction and the relative sparing of pulmonary parenchyma at autopsy are shown in Fig. 78-2. A simplified scheme to illustrate the evolution of the process is shown in Fig. 78-3.

Gastrointestinal Tract

Although pancreatic function may be either normal or abnormal at birth, it gradually becomes increasingly abnormal as the ducts become progressively obstructed by a thick viscous secretion from the exocrine portion of the pancreas; pancreatic enzymes that are trapped in the ducts lead to autodestruction of the pancreas. A cycle of destruction and obliteration of the ducts is set into motion leading to cystic dilatation of ducts proximal to sites of obstruction and fibrosis of the body of the pancreas. In advanced stages of the disease, the fibrotic process in the pancreas sometimes causes obliteration of the islets of Langerhans and diabetes.

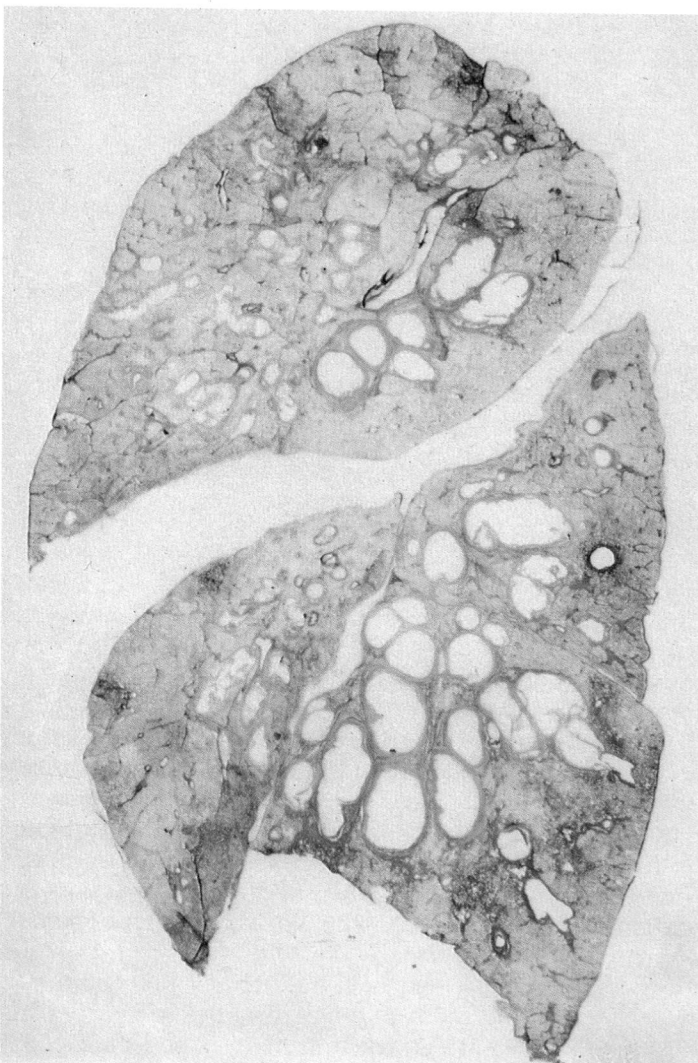

FIGURE 78-2 Section of lung from autopsy of a patient with cystic fibrosis demonstrating remarkable dilatation of large airways with preservation of intervening pulmonary parenchyma. *(Courtesy of Dr. S. Moolten.)*

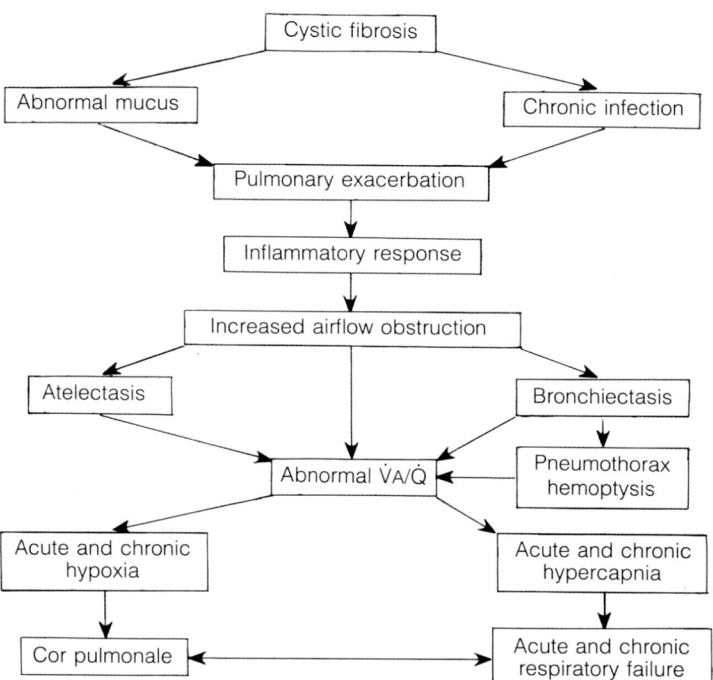

FIGURE 78-3 Simplified scheme for pathogenesis and progression of pulmonary disease in cystic fibrosis.

The liver and biliary tract are also involved in cystic fibrosis. Here too, the primary mechanism appears to be obstruction of ducts by abnormally viscid secretions. The earliest pathologic change is focal biliary cirrhosis, that may be present in early infancy. In some patients, the focal cirrhosis progresses to diffuse cirrhosis and portal hypertension. Some newborn infants with cystic fibrosis develop the *inspissated bile syndrome* characterized by prolonged obstructive jaundice starting at 2 to 8 weeks of age; the jaundice often clears without therapy. In approximately 20 to 30 percent of cystic fibrosis patients the gallbladder is small, presumably because of underdevelopment secondary to obstruction by viscid secretions.

The most striking pathologic change in the intestines is hyperplasia of the mucous glands and goblet cells. Biochemical abnormalities in intestinal mucins may contrib-

ute to malabsorption of specific nutrients and bile acids. Much of the malabsorption in cystic fibrosis can be corrected by administering pancreatic enzymes. However, the abnormal mucins may lead to a slowing of intestinal transit time; the slowing, combined with maldigestion of food substances, sometimes causes fecal impaction in the terminal ileum and ileocecal area, a condition referred to as *meconium ileus equivalent*. The fecal impaction, in turn, occasionally causes volvulus or intussusception of the bowel.

Reproductive Organs

Except for an increase in viscosity and an abnormal midcycle ferning pattern in cervical mucus, no consistent pathologic changes occur in the female reproductive tract. However, in the male reproductive tract, the vas deferens is either atretic or absent from birth. Although the pathogenesis of this lesion is not certain, it is possible that viscous secretions may contribute to obstruction in utero followed by failure of development of the vas deferens. Spermatogenesis and testicular development is otherwise normal. Because of either partial or complete obstruction of the vas deferens, approximately 98 percent of males with cystic fibrosis are aspermic.

Sweat Glands

The sweat glands manifest no distinctive histologic changes. Nonetheless, their function is abnormal, and the characteristic abnormalities feature prominently in vari-

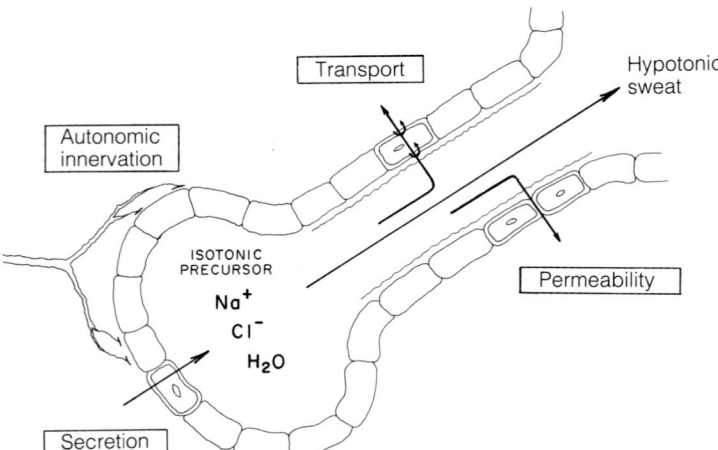

FIGURE 78-4 Schematic representation of a sweat gland illustrating normal function and the altered mechanisms which have been proposed to explain the elevated sweat electrolytes in cystic fibrosis.

ous theories proposed to explain the pathogenesis of cystic fibrosis (Fig. 78-4). Micropuncture has shown that the precursor solution secreted by the sweat glands is isotonic to plasma, both in individuals with cystic fibrosis and in normals (Fig. 78-4). In normal individuals, as the sweat flows along the duct of the gland, sodium and chloride are reabsorbed so that by the time that the opening at the skin surface is reached, sweat is hypotonic to plasma with respect to both sodium and chloride concentrations. Because the isotonic precursor solution is the same in both cystic fibrosis and non-cystic fibrosis individuals, it is unlikely that a defect in the secretion of either water or electrolytes is the primary abnormality of the sweat glands in cystic fibrosis. Likewise, since the amount and rate of sweat produced by the sweat glands in individuals with cystic fibrosis are the same as in non-cystic fibrosis individuals, it is unlikely that a disturbance in the autonomic control of secretion is a primary factor. However, these observations do not exclude the possibility that autonomic control of the secretion of other substances, or that the effects of autonomic stimulation on membrane reabsorption, could be involved in the pathogenesis of the sweat gland defect in cystic fibrosis.

Although several abnormalities identified with cystic fibrosis can influence either sodium reabsorption or Na^+,K^+-ATPase activity, a primary defect in sodium transport has not been found. For example, the abnormality in membrane Ca^{2+}-ATPase activity that has been reported to occur in erythrocytes of patients with cystic fibrosis probably stems from an abnormal lipid composition of the erythrocyte membranes, which in turn, is secondary to the malabsorption of lipids in cystic fibrosis patients. Also, the hypotheses that relate either the regulation of calcium secretion or the coupling of ion fluxes to mucous secretion to the basic defect in cystic fibrosis require further testing.

In contrast to the lack of evidence for a primary defect in sodium transport is the mounting evidence that epithelial cells in patients with cystic fibrosis are poorly permeable to chloride ions. The relative impermeability to chloride ions is held to be responsible for the characteristic increase in potential differences across isolated perfused sweat glands and epithelial cells from the respiratory tract in cystic fibrosis.

The decreased permeability of epithelial cells to chloride ions features prominently in several theories concerning the pathogenesis of cystic fibrosis. For example, either abnormal glycosylation or sulfation of the glycoproteins of the extracellular matrix or of the chloride channel proteins, or an abnormal response of the chloride channel to sympathetic agonists or to a "second messenger," such as calcium, has been invoked as an explanation for the defect in chloride permeability. Although the recent demonstrations that chloride fluxes are decreased in cells cultured from sweat glands, respiratory tract epithelia, and skin fibroblasts of patients with cystic fibrosis do suggest that the defect in chloride permeability is intrinsic to the cystic fibrosis cell, a discrete chloride channel has been neither isolated nor characterized. A large research effort is currently under way to identify the nature of the chloride defect and to discover the basic abnormality that is responsible for it.

The red cell membrane contains a band 3 glycoprotein that is involved in its chloride exchange. This glycoprotein apparently functions normally in cystic fibrosis. Nonetheless, the possibility remains that a similar glycoprotein operates as the hypothetical chloride channel in epithelial cells and that an abnormality in the structure or function of this channel could relate closely to the basic defect in cystic fibrosis. The recent localization of a gene for a nonerythroid band 3 protein to the long arm of chromosome 7 will permit this hypothesis to be thoroughly tested.

The defect of the sweat glands in cystic fibrosis and the search for underlying mechanisms have prompted extrapolations to the function of other epithelial cells in cystic fibrosis, i.e., of the lungs, pancreas, intestines, liver, and reproductive glands. However, it would still be premature to advocate a unifying hypothesis that would interrelate the multiple abnormalities in the organs, glands, and cells of patients with cystic fibrosis.

DIAGNOSIS

The diagnosis of cystic fibrosis requires the demonstration of abnormally high levels of sodium and chloride in the sweat of an individual who has the characteristic history and symptoms of cystic fibrosis. The most prominent clinical features of cystic fibrosis are chronic pulmonary disease and pancreatic insufficiency, and the strongest family history in favor of cystic fibrosis in a particular

individual is cystic fibrosis in a sibling. If the clinical picture and/or the family history support the diagnosis, and if two sweat tests using the quantitative pilocarpine iontophoresis method are clearly positive, the diagnosis of cystic fibrosis can be made with assurance. However, because cystic fibrosis is a complex clinical syndrome (Table 78-2), because clinical manifestations are sometimes subtle, and because family history is not always straightforward, a high index of suspicion, coupled with a battery of clinical tests, is sometimes required to establish the diagnosis, especially in the adolescent or young adult.

Since cystic fibrosis occurs with a high frequency in the general population, it should be considered often in the differential diagnosis of a large number of symptoms. Although Table 78-2 categorizes the symptoms according to the age at which they occur most often, these symptoms at any age should prompt the consideration of the diagnosis of cystic fibrosis.

The most consistent feature of cystic fibrosis is the abnormally high concentration of sodium and chloride in sweat. The only reliable sweat test entails quantitative iontophoresis of pilocarpine. This method depends on the determination of the concentration of both sodium and chloride in an adequate, measured volume of sweat. One hundred milligrams of sweat is the minimum acceptable amount. When a preweighed, measured pad is used, this amount ensures that an adequate sweat flow rate (1 g/m^2 per minute) has been achieved and that the sample is large enough for the determination of sodium by flame photometry and of chloride by titration. In children, concentrations of less than 50 meq/L are usually regarded as normal. However, the average of values for sodium and chloride concentrations is about 20 meq/L for normal individuals and 95 meq/L for individuals with cystic fibrosis. In children, values between 45 and 60 meq/L are borderline elevated; such values call for repetition of the sweat test until

a clear pattern emerges. The concentration of sodium and chloride in sweat increases gradually with age. An age-corrected scale of normal, abnormal, and borderline values of the concentration of sodium in sweat is available (Fig. 78-5). Conditions other than cystic fibrosis in which the concentration of sodium and chloride in sweat are abnormally high include malnutrition, adrenal insufficiency, hereditary nephrogenic diabetes insipidus, ectodermal dysplasia, and fucosidosis. Except in some instances of malnutrition, these conditions are readily distinguished from cystic fibrosis.

The finding of abnormal concentrations of sodium and chloride in sweat automatically prompts evaluation of the patient to determine if, and to what extent, other organs are affected.

EVALUATION

Chest Radiography

Rarely is the chest radiograph completely normal in cystic fibrosis. In the individual with minor pulmonary symptoms, the manifestations may be questionable, i.e., mild hyperinflation and minimal peribronchial thickening. However, radiographic findings become more distinctly abnormal as the disease increases in severity. Peribronchial thickening, which is often most prominent in the upper lobes of the lungs early in the course of the disease, usually progresses to involve all lobes. In the advanced stage of pulmonary involvement, ring shadows, cystic lesions, and nodular densities become increasingly apparent, and areas of bronchiectasis and atelectasis become increasingly evident. The central pulmonary artery often begins to enlarge in middle stages of the disease, but the cardiac silhouette remains within normal limits until the disease is far advanced. The variability in the chest radiographs is illustrated in Fig. 78-6 for three siblings with cystic fibrosis when each was 17 years old.

Pulmonary Performance

In cystic fibrosis the lungs are usually morphologically and functionally normal at birth. Over the years, the abnormal tracheobronchial secretions and infections progressively impair pulmonary function in almost all patients with cystic fibrosis. When the stage of full-blown pulmonary disease is reached, all the pulmonary function abnormalities that are seen in chronic bronchitis and emphysema and in asthma can occur. However, there is also one complicating regular feature of cystic fibrosis, i.e., bronchiectasis, that modifies pulmonary performance in these patients: chronic, local infection and damage to the airways increases the compliance of the bronchiectatic airways and causes them to collapse during rapid expirations or cough.

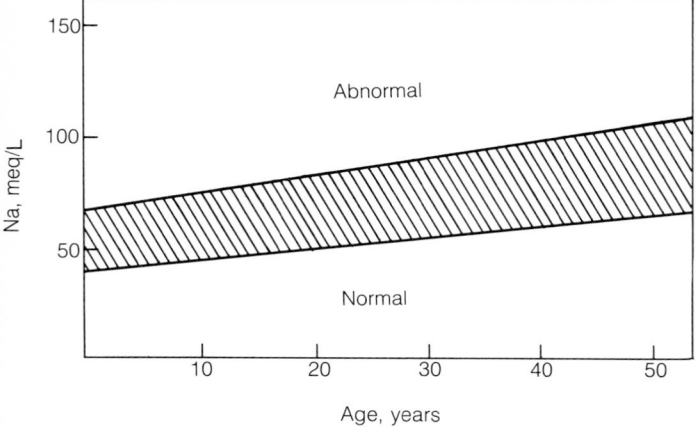

FIGURE 78-5 Graph of sweat test results versus age; normal, elevated and borderline (stippled). (*Modified after Jones, Steige, and Logan, 1970.*)

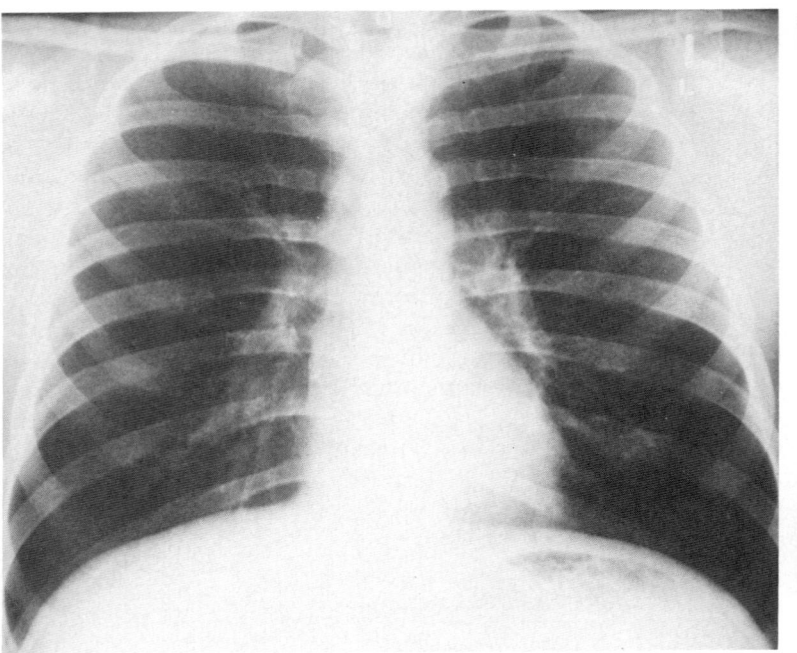

A

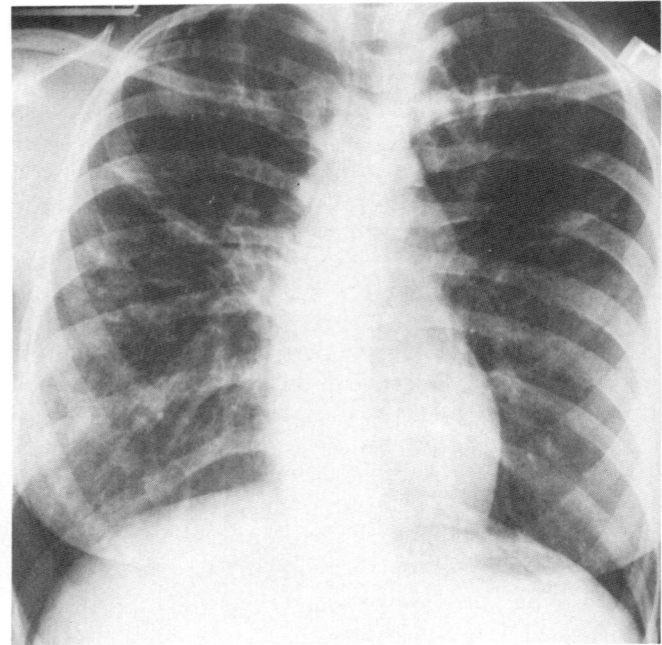

B

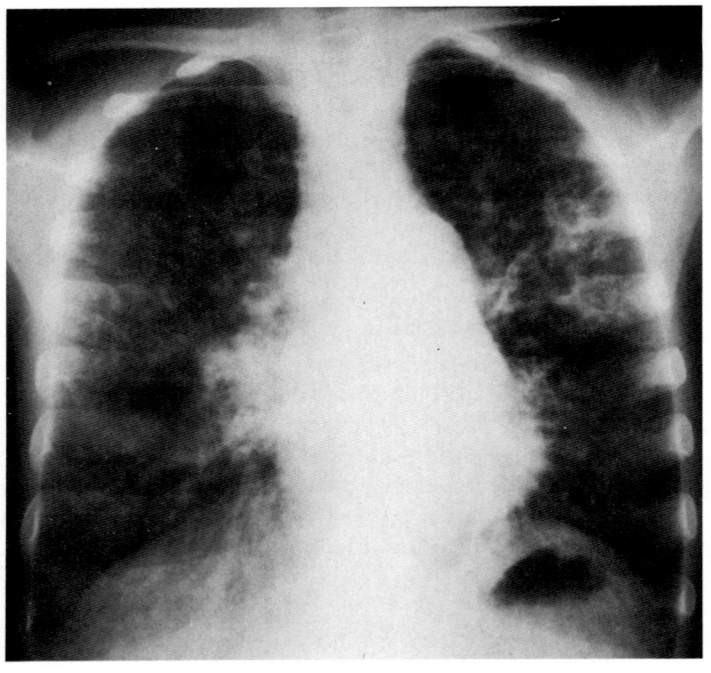

C

FIGURE 78-6   Chest radiographs of three siblings with cystic fibrosis taken when they were 17 years of age.   A. Mild hyperinflation; otherwise normal. Patient is now 21 years of age and was hospitalized once for treatment of electrolyte depletion. He works full-time. B. Diffuse peribronchial thickening, mild hyperinflation, and cystic changes in both upper lobes. Patient is now 24 years of age and has been hospitalized three times for exacerbation of pulmonary infections and once for hemoptysis. She is married and works full-time. C. Severe hyperinflation, diffuse peribronchial thickening, multiple infiltrations, and increased pulmonary vascular markings and heart size. The patient died 1 month later from respiratory failure complicated by congestive heart failure.

The usefulness of pulmonary function testing in cystic fibrosis falls into two categories: (1) tracing the natural history of the disease and (2) assessing the value of therapeutic interventions. However, the earlier stages of the pulmonary disorder are the most difficult to quantify. In *infants*, tests are constrained almost entirely to those that do not depend on the understanding and cooperation of the patient. Notable among these are body plethysmography to determine the functional residual capacity and the

esophageal balloon technique to determine airway resistances; and more recently, occlusion of expiration on three successive breaths (expiratory volume clamping) has been used to assess passive respiratory mechanics in infants.

In some infants, even though their lungs are clinically and radiographically normal, both the residual volume and the airway resistances are abnormally high and the dynamic compliance is abnormally low. An intercurrent pulmonary infection augments the abnormalities in the

three tests; subsidence of the infection restores them toward normal. It is noteworthy that because of the uncertainties that attend pulmonary function testing in infancy, the variations in the time and severity of onset, and the variable impacts of the recurrent pulmonary infections, the early stages in the evolution of pulmonary abnormalities in cystic fibrosis are poorly documented.

Until age 6, determination of arterial blood-gas composition is generally used as a measure of overall pulmonary function, both in the stable state of the pulmonary disorder and during an intercurrent infection. However, this test is neither easy to perform nor to interpret in the early years of life because of the ventilatory and metabolic upsets that often accompany anxiety and crying.

After age 6, pulmonary function tests originally designed for adults can be done quite readily on children. In terms of pulmonary performance, this is the part of the natural history that can be described with most confidence in cystic fibrosis.

OBSTRUCTION IN SMALL AIRWAYS

The small airways, i.e., the bronchioles, are vulnerable to obstruction early in the course of cystic fibrosis. At this stage, as in cigarette smokers, tests for small airways disease are apt to be abnormal, while tests for obstruction of large airways are still normal. Three factors interact in causing this obstruction: (1) intrinsic disease of the smaller airways, often in association with bronchiectasis in the proximal larger airways; (2) viscid secretions, impaired ciliary action, and impaired cough; and (3) progressive decrease in elastic recoil.

The progressive reduction in elastic recoil in cystic fibrosis is predominantly a function of overinflation due to the intrinsic airways disease rather than to a loss of pulmonary parenchyma. This mechanism differs from that of bronchitis and emphysema, in which the combined effects of parenchymal destruction as well as overinflation are responsible for the decrease in elastic recoil. It is noteworthy (Fig. 78-2) that emphysema is not a regular feature of cystic fibrosis and that in some patients it only occurs late in the course of the disease.

The tone of muscle in the airways increases only slightly in cystic fibrosis. Exercise elicits bronchodilation that is followed shortly by bronchoconstriction. Both the bronchodilation and bronchoconstriction are far less impressive in cystic fibrosis than in asthma. Indeed, exaggerated bronchomotor responses in cystic fibrosis raise the possibility of superimposed asthma. In distinguishing between the contributions of intrinsic airways disease caused by cystic fibrosis from that due to asthma, maximal expiration-flow curves are sometimes helpful: in severe cystic fibrosis, the record is curvilinear because of a high rate of airflow at the start of expiration followed by an abrupt decrease in slope, a pattern consistent with

early emptying of the fast components followed by the emptying of the slower regions; in asthma, the initial increase is less striking and the falloff is relatively linear.

A useful test for detecting small airways disease is the relative decrease in $\dot{V}_{max}$ when an inspired mixture of He–20% O_2 (HeO$_2$) is substituted for air. An abnormal density dependence of $\dot{V}_{max}$ signifies small airways obstruction. Another manifestation of obstruction of small airways is the superimposition of the two curves at higher lung volumes than in normal individuals. Because of the bronchiolar locus of the early lesions in cystic fibrosis, abnormalities in frequency-dependent tests (e.g., dynamic compliance at various breathing frequencies), in volume-dependent tests (e.g., closing volume), and in maximal expiratory flow ($\dot{V}_{Emax}$) at low lung volume are demonstrable even though tests of large airways disease [e.g., forced expiratory volume in 1 s (FEV$_1$) and airways resistance] are still normal.

LUNG VOLUME ABNORMALITIES

The lung volumes change in cystic fibrosis as expected in chronic obstructive airways disease. As in the case of chronic bronchitis and emphysema, and of asthma, the residual volume increases, followed by an increase in functional residual capacity and, sometimes, by an increase in total lung capacity. The increase both in the residual volume and in functional residual capacity are due, as indicated above, to a combination of an increase in obstructive airways disease and a decrease in elastic recoil.

Abnormalities in Gas Exchange

Early in evolution of the pulmonary abnormalities in cystic fibrosis, i.e., when tests of small airways disease are needed to uncover that a pulmonary disorder is present, ventilation-perfusion abnormalities usually widen the alveolar-arterial ΔP_{O_2} and increase the ratio of the dead space to tidal volume. These abnormalities portend increasing inhomogeneities in alveolar ventilation and blood flow as the child grows to adulthood. The diffusing capacity for carbon monoxide is low at rest and does not increase normally during exercise. This observation is difficult to reconcile with the preservation of the gas-exchanging surfaces of the lungs, without emphysema, until late in the course of the disease (Fig. 78-2).

As the obstructive disease of the airways progresses and exaggerates the imbalances between alveolar ventilation and blood flow, arterial hypoxemia ensues; this is followed, in time, by pulmonary hypertension, cor pulmonale, and right ventricular failure. Late in the course of the disease, hypercapnia and respiratory acidosis contribute to the final picture of respiratory failure. At this juncture, the ventilatory response to inhaled CO_2 is depressed, evidences of acute CO_2 retention supervene, and respiratory depression by oxygen breathing or sedatives may

bring the patient closer to the brink of respiratory depression and coma. Bouts of infection punctuate the course of the illness; in each episode pulmonary function deteriorates but almost invariably returns toward baseline, except in the preterminal stages of the disorder.

Sputum Culture

The unique respiratory flora obtained from cultures of the sputum from cystic fibrosis patients serves as an aid in establishing the diagnosis of cystic fibrosis and in guiding the antimicrobial therapy of exacerbations of the disease. *Pseudomonas aeruginosa* and *Staphylococcus aureus* are found alone, or in combination, in sputum cultures from many patients with cystic fibrosis. Once present, these organisms, especially *Pseudomonas*, are rarely eradicated from cultures despite the use of either intermittent, intravenous, or continuous antibiotics administered by mouth or by nebulizer. Although these organisms are sometimes found in sputum cultures from patients with pulmonary diseases other than cystic fibrosis, their association with cystic fibrosis is so consistent that a dedicated attempt to obtain a sputum culture is an integral part of the evaluation of all patients, including infants and young children suspected of having cystic fibrosis.

Pancreatic Function

The evaluation of pancreatic function is an important part of establishing the diagnosis of cystic fibrosis since 80 to 90 percent of patients with cystic fibrosis have pancreatic insufficiency. In infants with pancreatic insufficiency, the most striking feature of the history and physical examination is often failure to thrive; the record of bowel movements may disclose only loose or frequent stools. In the older child, whose diet includes more fat and protein, a history of bulky, foul, malodorous stools is often easier to elicit. The best way to document malabsorption is to collect stools for 72 h and test for fat content while the patient is ingesting a known quantity of fat (approximately 100 g per day). A coefficient of malabsorption greater than 7 percent is usually considered to be abnormal; in patients with cystic fibrosis, the coefficient of malabsorption often is of the order of 20 to 30 percent.

In infants and young children, the determination of trypsin or chymotrypsin activity in a properly collected stool specimen is an accurate way to determine the content of pancreatic enzymes. However, in older patients, the trypsin or chymotrypsin activity in a stool sample may be artificially low because of a delayed transit time that causes partial inactivation of the enzyme. In some instances, a secretin stimulation test may be helpful in demonstrating pancreatic insufficiency. For this purpose a triple-lumen tube is introduced into the duodenum. The response to secretin is usually abnormal: the volume of secretion is small, the fluid is viscid, and the bicarbonate

ion concentration is low. This test is not often used in children because it is cumbersome to perform.

For infants, the serum immunoreactive assay for trypsin is used in some clinics as a screening test. As a rule, serum levels of trypsin are abnormally high, usually reflecting the continuing destruction of the pancreas. However, the assay does not provide an accurate measure of pancreatic function. Another approach is the use of certain compounds, such as N-benzyl-L-tyrosyl-p-aminobenzoic acid, that are ingested orally and subsequently hydrolyzed by pancreatic enzymes. The amount of hydrolysis is quantified by determining the amount of aminobenzoic acid that is present in serum or excreted in the urine. This test, still in the developmental stage, affords the prospect of a useful test for the assessment of pancreatic function in cystic fibrosis.

Liver Function

Evaluation of liver function is an important part of the work-up in cystic fibrosis. In infants and children, the concentrations of bilirubin and transaminases in serum sometimes increase transiently. However, concentrations of these substances are usually normal, even in patients with mild to moderate amounts of focal biliary cirrhosis. The prothrombin time is sometimes prolonged in cystic fibrosis due to a combination of malabsorption and decreased synthesis by the liver. An occasional patient presents with bleeding esophageal varices from advanced cirrhosis; endoscopy and upper gastrointestinal contrast studies are then often helpful in demonstrating the varices.

Semen Analysis

Occasionally, an adult male, found to have aspermia in the course of an evaluation for infertility, is subsequently found to have cystic fibrosis. A complete semen analysis is part of the evaluation of an adult male with cystic fibrosis. Azoospermia is found in more than 97 percent of males with cystic fibrosis.

TREATMENT

The intensive, comprehensive treatment programs that were designed to deal with particular symptoms, to correct deficiencies, and to prevent the progression and complications of cystic fibrosis have led to a dramatic increase in the median age of survival (Fig. 78-7). Although the value of this comprehensive treatment is beyond cavil, far less certain is the rationale for each type of treatment and how much of each treatment is necessary in a given patient. At present, the best approach still seems to be the determination of the type and degree of abnormality present for each patient separately and the designing of a treat-

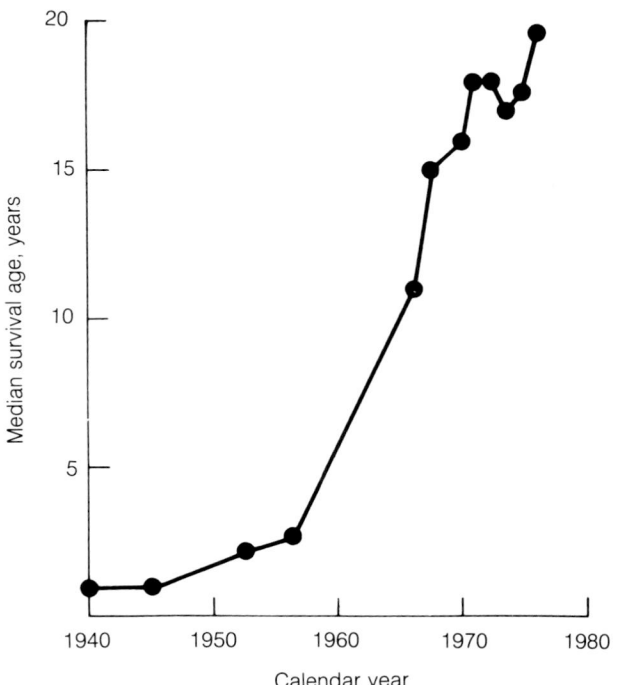

FIGURE 78-7 Survival of patients with cystic fibrosis. Median survival age was obtained from estimates in the literature before 1968 and from the Data Registry of the Cystic Fibrosis Foundation after 1968. [From Mischler EH, after Davis PB (ed), Seminars in Respiratory Medicine 6:271, 1985.]

ment program that will improve, or maintain, function of the organ systems that are involved.

To ensure that the treatment regimen meets the needs of the individual patient, that necessary treatment is not omitted, or that side effects of prescribed treatments do not go unnoticed, it is often desirable to have the patient admitted to the hospital during the process of diagnosis and evaluation. Hospitalization also provides an excellent opportunity to counsel the patient, the parents, and the family about the diverse aspects of the diagnosis, treatment, prognosis, and inheritance pattern of cystic fibrosis. It provides the opportunity to monitor the response of individual patients to each component of the individual therapeutic program.

An important aspect of the care of cystic fibrosis patients has been the establishment and organization of a network of over 100 cystic fibrosis centers throughout the United States and an even larger network throughout the world. Most of the larger cystic fibrosis centers use a team approach to the care of cystic fibrosis patients. A cystic fibrosis care team usually includes physicians, nurses, respiratory and/or physical therapists, nutritionists, and social workers.

Management of the Pulmonary Disease

More than 98 percent of patients with cystic fibrosis die from either respiratory failure or pulmonary complica-

tions. The goals of treating the pulmonary disorder in cystic fibrosis are to prevent and to treat the complications of obstruction and infection in the airways. Although management of the pulmonary disorder consists of multiple components that are applied in combination, the individual components of the therapy are discussed separately below.

Chest Physiotherapy

Almost all treatment programs for cystic fibrosis include a strategy that is intended to clear the pulmonary secretions in order to prevent the complications arising from plugging of the airways by the viscous mucous secretions. Chest physiotherapy, i.e., "percussion and postural drainage," performed regularly, is the most widely prescribed of these tactics. In young infants and children, chest physiotherapy is generally done routinely twice a day. In older patients, the manual chest physiotherapy is often replaced by either vibrators and mechanical percussors, or a combination of exercise and either forced expirations or forced coughing maneuvers. Although it is reasonable, and widely held, that this type of program does improve clearance of mucous secretions and maintain pulmonary function, objective proof is not available. However, it has been shown that in patients with *moderate* pulmonary disease who do no chest physiotherapy for a period of 3 weeks, pulmonary function deteriorates; in these patients, reinstitution of percussion and postural drainage for a 3-week period restores pulmonary function to baseline levels. At present, most cystic fibrosis centers recommend that all patients with cystic fibrosis clear pulmonary secretions with some method that is applied regularly, twice daily. They also recommend that chest physiotherapy be applied more often during an exacerbation of the pulmonary infection. Unfortunately, the recommendation of chest physiotherapy—a time-consuming and often arduous form of treatment—on a regular basis is difficult to implement without considerable support and encouragement by family and health professionals.

Antibiotics

In the treatment of cystic fibrosis during the past few decades, antibiotics have been the key element responsible for increased survival. However, antibiotic regimens are not standardized: at one extreme are the clinics that treat all patients with cystic fibrosis with antistaphylococcal antibiotics uninterruptedly, from the time of diagnosis; during an exacerbation, additional antibiotics are administered by mouth or intravenously. At the opposite end are the clinics that reserve the use of antibiotics solely for severe exacerbations of the pulmonary infection because of concern about the prospect of promoting the emergence of newer and more resistant strains of *Pseudomonas*.

A reasonable compromise seems to be an intermediate position that balances the dangers of overzealous ad-

ministration of antibiotics against the progressive damage to airways and the bronchiectasis that result from untreated pulmonary infection. This position entails culture of the sputum of patients at the time of diagnosis and at regular intervals thereafter. When signs and symptoms herald an increase in pulmonary infection—i.e., either increased cough and/or sputum production, or fresh abnormalities on the physical examination, the chest radiograph, or the pulmonary function tests—the use of percussion and postural drainage is increased and the appropriate antibiotic is given orally.

Currently, the most useful agents for treating staphylococcal infections are dicloxacillin, cephalexin, the newer cephalosporins, and chloramphenicol. Early in the course of the pulmonary disease, a small fraction of *Pseudomonas* organisms may be sensitive to tetracycline, trimethoprim-sulfamethoxazole or chloramphenicol. Occasionally, even *Pseudomonas* organisms that are resistant according to laboratory tests apparently respond to these antibiotics. But, if the signs and symptoms do not improve, if they become too severe to manage on an ambulatory basis, or if the bacteria are resistant to those antibiotics that can be given by mouth, the patient is admitted to the hospital, usually for a 2-week course of intravenous antibiotics.

For the treatment of a pulmonary exacerbation of cystic fibrosis caused by a *Pseudomonas* organism, a combination of an aminoglycoside given intravenously and a semisynthetic penicillin is generally used. This combination of antibiotics is presumed to act synergistically on *Pseudomonas*, and the *Pseudomonas* is less likely to become resistant to either antibiotic.

Most popular of the antibiotic combinations currently in use are gentamicin and carbenicillin and more recently, tobramycin and ticarcillin. In order to achieve high levels of the antibiotic in the airways and secretions, the aminoglycoside is generally administered in higher doses and more often than usual. For example, gentamicin, 7.5 mg/kg per day in four divided doses, is given instead of 5 mg/kg per day in three divided doses. The resulting concentrations in serum are monitored: instead of the usual therapeutic serum levels for gentamicin and tobramycin of 4 to 8 μg/ml, the usual goal in cystic fibrosis is a serum level of 8 to 10 μg/ml; some clinics advocate even higher levels. Serum concentrations of antibiotic, renal function, and hearing are monitored to avoid toxic reactions. The higher levels of 8 to 10 μg/ml do not seem to elicit greater toxicity than the usual levels. No advantage has been demonstrated for further increments in dosage.

Some of the newer antibiotics, e.g., piperacillin, azlocillin, and ceftazidime are also quite effective against *Pseudomonas*. Although they may be effective at first when given alone, resistance often develops quickly. Usually, these agents are used in combination with an aminoglycoside. Because the sensitivity and resistance patterns of the *Pseudomonas* organisms often change, different combinations are tried at different times, relying empirically on the combination which appears to be most effective for the particular strain of *Pseudomonas*.

Pseudomonas, once found in the sputum, are rarely eradicated. However, most other manifestations of an exacerbation of pulmonary disease improve during a 2-week course of antibiotics administered intravenously, i.e., the densities seen on the chest radiograph decrease, the white blood cell count decreases, fever and respiratory rate decrease, and pulmonary function tests, which often deteriorate at the start of an exacerbation, return to their previous baseline. Although many patients will begin to show improvement after 5 to 7 days, most cystic fibrosis clinics continue antibiotics intravenously for at least 2 weeks in order to decrease the relapse rate and to avoid a decrease in the interval between exacerbations. Indeed, some clinics routinely recommend a 3- to 4-week course of antibiotics given intravenously to treat an exacerbation of a pulmonary infection in cystic fibrosis.

In the occasional patient in the hospital who experiences a relapse, or manifests an increase in symptoms shortly after the intravenous administration of antibiotics is stopped, long-term, intravenous administration of aminoglycoside can be continued using a heparin lock. This technique may be useful in allowing the patient to return home while still receiving effective doses of aminoglycosides. Another approach that has been advocated is the administration of antibiotics by inhalation in order to increase concentrations in airways that are infected by *Pseudomonas*. Although it has been argued that inhalation will not deliver effective concentrations to diseased portions of the lungs because of the interference with ventilation by local airway obstruction, in some instances inhaled antibiotics seem to be helpful. Gentamicin or tobramycin, 20 to 40 mg/ml, given in 1 to 2 ml of inhaled solution two or three times per day are often used. As a rule, inhalation of antibiotics is reserved for those patients who have been hospitalized repeatedly for exacerbations of pulmonary symptoms that recur at increasing frequency and after shorter intervals between exacerbations. Often if inhalation therapy is started after completing a course of intravenous antibiotics, the interval before the next exacerbation occurs is prolonged. It should be emphasized that all the above practices with respect to antibiotics—continuously by mouth, long-term intravenously, and inhalation—are based more on the individual experiences of different cystic fibrosis clinics than on controlled clinical trials.

Recent reports from several large cystic fibrosis clinics have indicated an increasing incidence and prevalence of infections with *P. cepacia* in cystic fibrosis patients. Many of these organisms have proved to be resistant to most antibiotics; in some of the patients colonized with these organisms, pulmonary function and clinical condition have deteriorated rapidly. This problem and the best approach to management are currently under study.

Mist and Mucolytics

Mist therapy, delivered either by sleeping in a mist tent or by the intermittent inhalation of an aerosol, was a common form of treatment several decades ago. The goal was to "liquefy" the cystic fibrosis secretions. However, this treatment could not be shown to be helpful to cystic fibrosis patients, and the use of mist tents has largely been discontinued. Intermittent aerosols are still used to deliver bronchodilators and mucolytics.

A number of mucolytic agents have been tried over the years. Of these, one that has endured is N-acetylcysteine. In the test tube, this agent is quite effective in dissolving the mucin components and in decreasing the viscosity of cystic fibrosis sputum. Although some clinics have found it to be a useful adjunct to therapy in cystic fibrosis patients, others have encountered an inordinate frequency of bronchospasm or tracheitis. Some difficulties in the past can now be attributed to the use of a 20% (almost undiluted) solution of N-acetylcysteine, which can be irritating because of its extremely high osmolarity. The incidence of side effects can be decreased greatly by using a 5% solution of N-acetylcysteine for inhalation and by greater discrimination in its use; during an exacerbation, when cough and sputum production increase, the 5% solution is inhaled two to three times per day, before chest physiotherapy. Should the patient develop bronchospasm, demonstrated by physical examination or by pulmonary function testing, a bronchodilator is tried to reverse the bronchospasm. If successful, the bronchodilator and the N-acetylcysteine are administered jointly by inhalation. However, should the bronchospasm persist in face of the bronchodilator, N-acetylcysteine is not given to that individual patient.

Bronchodilators

Bronchodilators are often used in treating the pulmonary manifestations of cystic fibrosis. This use is individualized on several accounts for each patient. For example, in many patients, bronchospasm that is reversible by bronchodilators at one point in the course of their illness will prove refractory a short time later. Some cystic fibrosis patients undergo deterioration in pulmonary function after the use of bronchodilators, probably from the collapse of airways secondary to a decrease in the tone induced in tracheobronchial smooth muscle. In young infants who are audibly wheezing, a bronchodilator can be tried and continued if bronchospasm is relieved. In older patients, pulmonary function testing proves a more objective and quantitative measure of effectiveness.

Corticosteroids have been used with good results in infants with severe obstructive airways disease that does not respond to antibiotics and bronchodilators, and in cystic fibrosis patients in whom the pulmonary disease is complicated by either severe asthma or allergic broncho-

pulmonary aspergillosis. Preliminary observations suggest that cystic fibrosis patients may benefit from the long-term administration of corticosteroids on alternate days. Presumably, the effect of the corticosteroids is to decrease the inflammatory response of the airways; this treatment regimen is currently being evaluated in a multicenter trial.

Nutritional Support

Patients with cystic fibrosis require careful evaluation to determine if partial or complete pancreatic insufficiency is present and to design a nutritional program to correct any deficiency. The mainstay in managing the pancreatic insufficiency is the pancreatic enzyme preparations that are now available in the form of enteric-coated capsules containing coated microspheres. These pancreatic enzymes are ingested along with any food that contains protein, fat, or complex carbohydrates. The dosage of these enzymes is adjusted to ensure a relatively normal bowel pattern, adequate weight gain or maintenance of ideal weight for height, and a decrease in bowel symptoms, such as cramping and flatulence.

However, despite enzyme replacement, the correction of pancreatic insufficiency is incomplete so that the patients require more than 100 percent of recommended caloric intake. In some, an even greater caloric intake is required because of the increased energy expenditure due to an increased work of breathing secondary to chronic pulmonary infection. Aggressive nutritional supplementation, using either oral supplements or nocturnal nasogastric feeding of hydrolyzed formulas, has been helpful in the short run in promoting weight gain at this stage of disease. Hyperalimentation is used less often except in infants with meconium ileus.

As a rule, patients with cystic fibrosis are advised to take each day a double dose of a multivitamin preparation and a supplement of vitamin E. Infants, those in whom prothrombin time is prolonged, and those who take antibiotics uninterruptedly, require supplemental vitamin K. Supplemental salt is needed by cystic fibrosis patients to prevent electrolyte depletion, metabolic alkalosis, and heat prostration: for infants, 1 to 2 g of salt per day are added to their feeding formulas; children and adults are encouraged to salt their foods liberally and to take salt-containing liquids and snacks during hot weather.

NATURAL HISTORY AND PROGNOSIS

The comprehensive treatment program of cystic fibrosis has unequivocally improved the overall survival of patients with cystic fibrosis: 30 years ago the median survival was only a few years of age; now it is about 24 years of age (Fig. 78-7). However, because cystic fibrosis is a complex clinical disorder that affects different organs to

different degrees, it is difficult to depict a paradigm of the patient with cystic fibrosis: some patients die in childhood or early adolescence, others are alive and more than 30 years old.

The individual variability in the natural history of cystic fibrosis is clearly shown by comparing the serial chest radiographs from two individuals with cystic fibrosis shown in Figs. 78-8 and 78-9, respectively. Radiographs in the early life of a patient with cystic fibrosis are likely to show persistent pneumonia and/or atelectasis (Fig. 78-8A and B). With appropriate management, the pulmonary parenchyma generally clears dramatically (Fig. 78-8C), but hyperinflation and peribronchial streaking become manifest (Fig. 78-8D). Patches of infiltration, atelectasis, and enlargement of hilar and mediastinal nodes are seen as the disease progresses (Fig. 78-8E). Further developments include lobar atelectasis, cyst and abscess formation, and increasing lung densities due to retention of secretions and pneumonia (Fig. 78-8F). Late complications include bronchiectasis, pneumothorax, and cor pulmonale (Fig. 78-8F).

Figure 78-9 documents the condition of the chest in a patient with a milder expression of the disease. At the time of diagnosis, pneumonia was present (Fig. 78-9A). Antibiotic therapy produced some resolution (Fig. 78-9B), and ultimately lung aeration appeared almost normal (Fig. 78-9C). In adult life this patient developed some parenchymal streaks from retained secretions and fibrotic scarring (Fig. 78-9D and E) but maintains an active and productive life at 28½ years of age.

An important determinant of the natural history in cystic fibrosis is the severity of the pulmonary disease and the rate at which it progresses. Although most patients improve in response to therapy, skillful management does less to influence the course of the severely affected patient than of the mildly affected patient (Fig. 78-10).

A variety of scoring systems have been devised for cystic fibrosis patients. The clinical scoring system devised by Shwachman and Kulczyclci, and the chest radiograph scoring system devised by Brasfield and associates, are widely used. However, although these and more elaborate scoring systems are useful in categorizing patients according to the severity of their disease, none has proved useful in prognosticating the future course of a particular patient.

Because cystic fibrosis is a genetic disease, the question of a familial pattern of severity is often raised. Figure 78-6 shows chest radiographs of three siblings with cystic fibrosis demonstrating the occurrence of mild, moderate, and severely affected individuals in the same family. The capsule histories, which are included in the legend to Fig. 78-6, also illustrate the variability in courses experienced by these individuals.

Patients with cystic fibrosis can be categorized not only with respect to severity of illness but also with respect to survival. For example, more than one-half of cystic fibrosis patients who had undergone surgery for meconium ileus before 1965 died in the first 2 months of life. Although this situation had improved markedly by 1976, the survival rate for meconium ileus patients was still not as good as for all other cystic fibrosis patients. Also, the survival rate was much lower for females than for males, especially in the adolescent age group. Because of improvements in the collection of mortality statistics, comparisons of current data with those of previous years may be somewhat misleading. However, the age for 50 percent survival has not been increasing as rapidly in recent years as in the 1970s (Fig. 78-7). Indeed, it seems that the average duration of life for cystic fibrosis patients is approaching a plateau.

COMPLICATIONS

The course of cystic fibrosis is often characterized by a gradual decrease in pulmonary function punctuated by further abrupt declines during exacerbations. Malnutrition, when present despite therapy, usually correlates best with the severity of the pulmonary disease. However, the course of cystic fibrosis can be suddenly changed by certain complications of the disease.

Hypoelectrolytemia and Metabolic Alkalosis

Hypoelectrolytemia and metabolic alkalosis are serious complications that are especially apt to occur during periods of hot weather when losses of sodium and chloride in patients with cystic fibrosis increase. Electrolyte depletion may be life-threatening, especially in infants and young children (Table 78-3). Prompt fluid replacement with isotonic saline is critical in these situations.

Intestinal Obstruction

Acute or chronic crampy abdominal pain attributable to some degree of intestinal obstruction, is common in patients with cystic fibrosis. If the obstruction is incomplete and manifested solely by a tender right lower quadrant mass, medical therapy, using oral mineral oil and N-acetylcysteine, in conjunction with hyperosmolar enemas containing an agent such as diaztrizoate methylglucamine

TABLE 78-3
Hypoelectrolytemia and Metabolic Alkalosis in Two Cystic Fibrosis Patients

Patient	Serum Electrolytes, meq/L				Serum pH
	Na	K	Cl	CO_2	
No. 1	123	2.2	49	48	7.60
No. 2	125	2.4	55	41	7.63

SOURCE: Modified from Scanlin, 1983 (with permission).

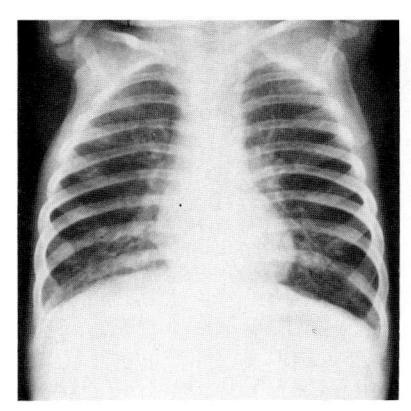

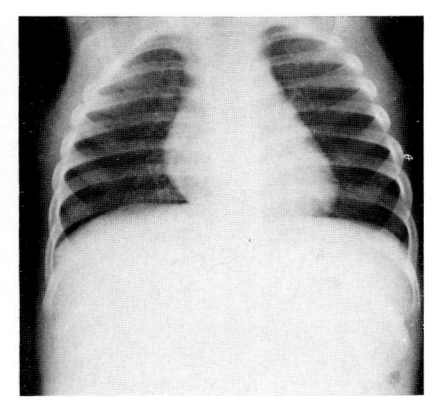

A

B

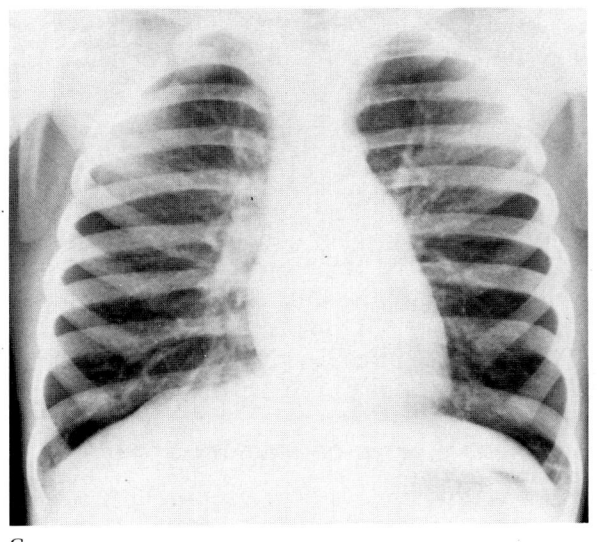

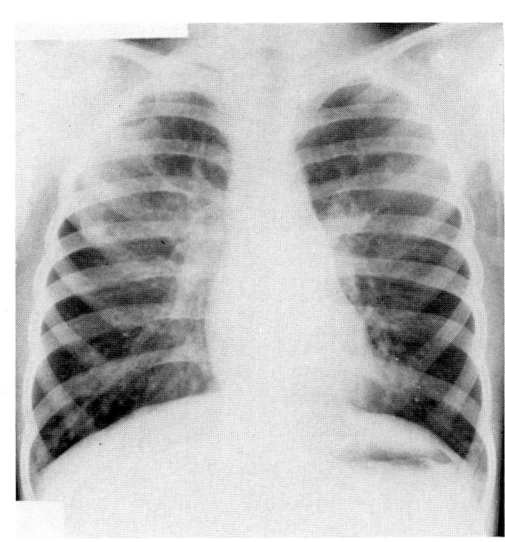

C

D

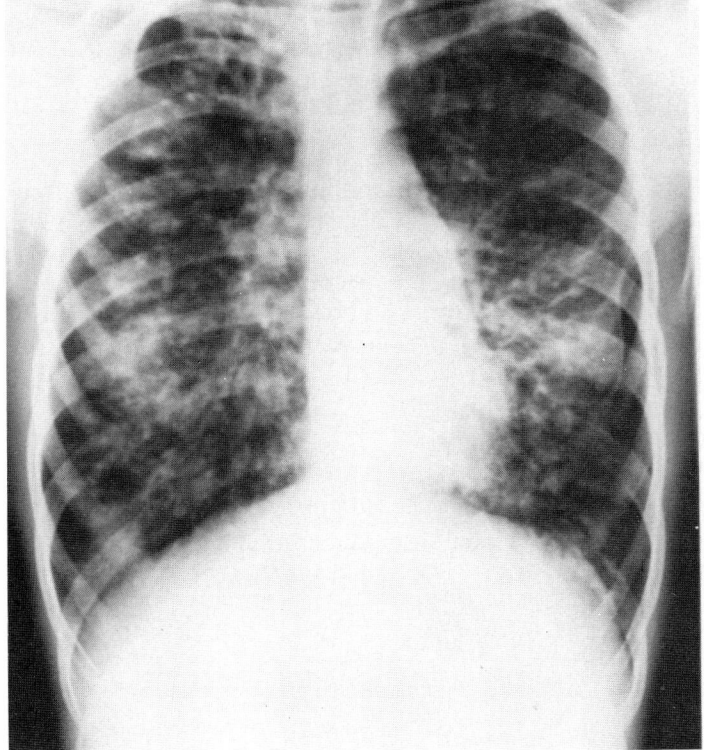

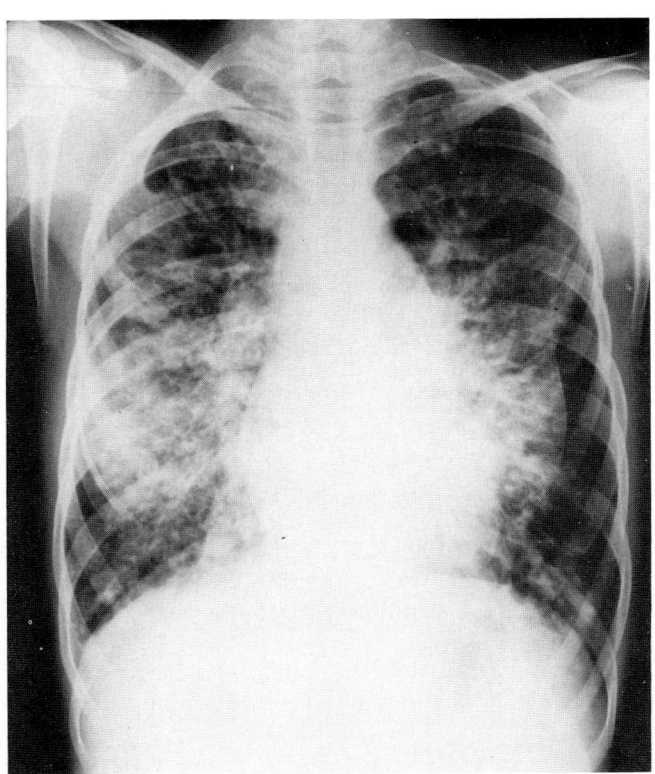

E

F

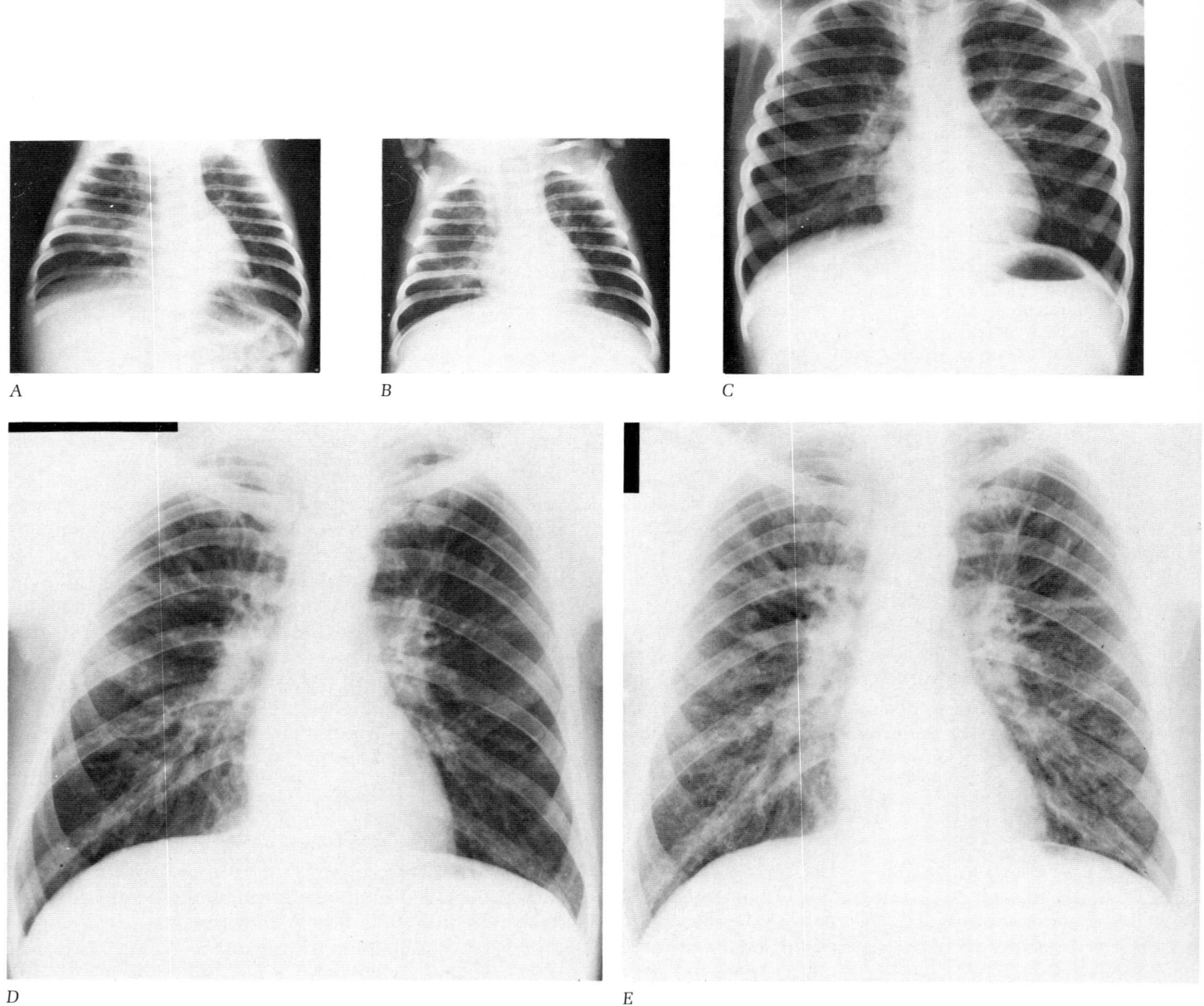

A

B

C

D

E

FIGURE 78-9 A 28-year course of cystic fibrosis in a white male. *A.* First admission in 1949 as a 2½-month-old infant with a chronic cough and failure to thrive. Areas of blotchy pulmonary infiltration. *B.* One week later, after treatment with antibiotics, the chest radiograph shows considerable clearing. The diagnosis of cystic fibrosis was made at 3 years 6 months of age. *C.* Age 3 years 9 months. Diffuse, mild streaking of the pulmonary parenchyma. During the ensuing 20 years the patient was generally well except for episodes of cough, emphysema, and pulmonary infection with staphylococci, *Haemophilus influenzae* and, since age 19, *Pseudomonas.* *D.* Age 23 years. Irregular streaks from retained secretions. At 27 years the patient was treated with antibiotics for recurrent hemoptysis. *E.* Age 28 years, 6 months. Minimal progression of pulmonary streaks. The patient's heart remains normal. He is currently doing well. *(From Matthews, Dearborn, and Tucker, 1980.)*

◄ **FIGURE 78-8** The 20-year course of cystic fibrosis in a white female. The diagnosis of cystic fibrosis was made at 4 months. *A.* First admission at 9 months, with severe pulmonary obstruction. *B.* Age 15 months. Improvement to antibiotic therapy only after cortisone was added. *C.* Age 5 years. Continued improvement. Lungs virtually normal. *D.* Age 8 years. A radiating pattern of fibrosis. *E.* Age 17 years. Chronic parenchymal disease with bronchiectasis in the upper lobes. *F.* Age 20 years. Recurrent hemoptysis, dyspnea, chest pain, and loss of weight. Over a period of 1 month the patient's condition deteriorated. The infiltrates are more confluent and the heart is enlarged due to cor pulmonale. The patient died. *(From Matthews, Dearborn, and Tucker, 1980.)*

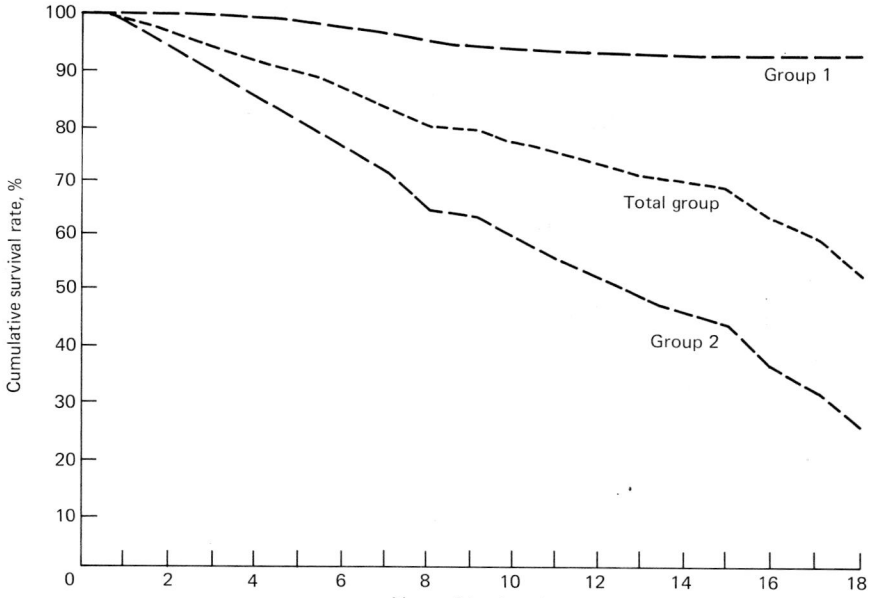

FIGURE 78-10 Correlation between chest radiograph scores and the cumulative survival rate. Scoring is based on chest radiography during the first year after diagnosis at the start of a comprehensive treatment program; chest radiograph in group 1 is much more normal than in group 2. Total of both groups consists of 535 patients. In group 1, consisting of 280 patients, there were 267 survivors; in group 2, consisting of 255 patients, there were 149 survivors. *(From Matthews, Dearborn, and Tucker, 1980.)*

(Gastrografin) may remove the fecal mass. Patients with a past history of crampy abdominal pain and previous incomplete obstruction are occasionally seen with radiographic evidence of intestinal obstruction manifested by bowel and air-fluid levels. After the neonatal period, intestinal obstruction is referred to as *meconium ileus equivalent.* An impacted fecal mass may serve as the leading edge for a volvulus or intussusception. Surgery is generally performed whenever necessary in cystic fibrosis. But, careful pre- and postoperative management is essential to avoid deterioration in pulmonary function that may follow the use of anesthesia.

Atelectasis

Atelectasis of a segment or lobe of the lung sometimes occurs in cystic fibrosis. Acute atelectasis is generally associated with few symptoms (Fig. 78-11A). However, if untreated, the end result of atelectasis will be a severely bronchiectatic segment, or lobe, of the lung (Fig. 78-11B). Vigorous chest physiotherapy, in conjunction with antibiotic therapy, is often successful in reexpanding the affected segment or lobe. Bronchoscopy is occasionally helpful. However, as a rule, it is not more effective than medical therapy. Resection of a persistently atelectatic or bronchiectatic lobe is undertaken only when the remaining areas of the lung are in relatively good condition, when overall pulmonary function is good, and if the evidence is convincing that the affected segment is responsible for intolerable symptoms, notably fever, cough, or sputum production.

Pneumothorax

Recurrent pneumothorax is exceedingly common in cystic fibrosis, particularly in older patients (Fig. 78-11C).

Tension pneumothorax occurs in up to 30 percent of these patients. Tube thoracostomy is indicated when the pneumothorax occupies more than 10 percent of the area of the hemithorax. Because the frequency of recurrence is high, attempts are made often at the time of the initial pneumothorax to obliterate the ipsilateral pleural space by instilling a solution of a sclerosing agent such as quinacrine or tetracycline. This type of preventive measure is advocated especially for those patients in whom pulmonary function is sufficiently compromised to make them poor candidates for surgery.

Hemoptysis

Expectoration of a small amount of blood-streaked sputum is a fairly common occurrence in cystic fibrosis. It is generally managed by intensifying home therapy for pulmonary infection. In contrast, hemoptysis (the expectoration of at least 30 to 60 ml of fresh blood) requires hospitalization even though the chest radiograph remains virtually unchanged (Fig. 78-11D). The probable mechanism for the hemoptysis is erosion of an area of localized infection into a bronchial vessel. Massive hemoptysis (blood loss from 300 to 2500 ml) is uncommon. But, when it does occur, it is a life-threatening situation. Bronchoscopy, and sometimes thoracic surgery, may be required to control the hemorrhage. Bronchial artery embolization has been used successfully in cystic fibrosis patients. But, experience with this technique in cystic fibrosis is limited.

Esophageal Varices

Although less common, some patients with cystic fibrosis do bleed from esophageal varices that are secondary to hepatic cirrhosis and portal hypertension. Once the

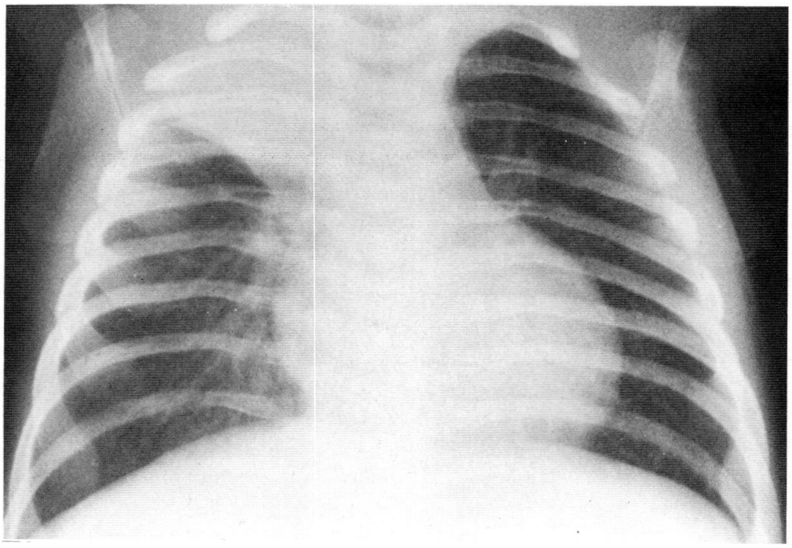

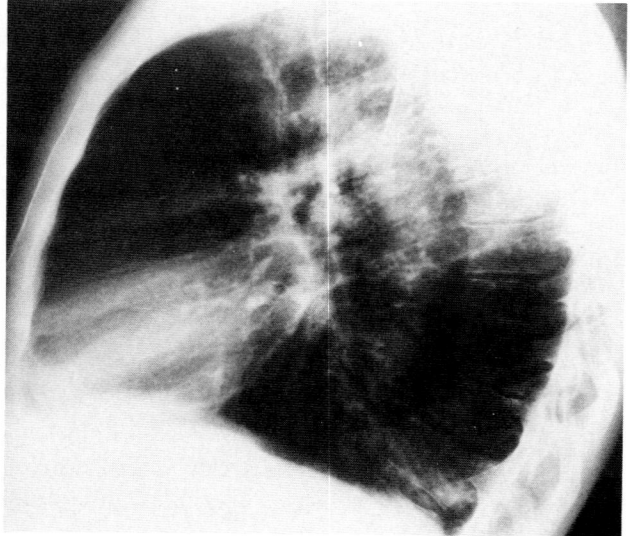

FIGURE 78-11 Chest radiographs of patients with pulmonary complications of cystic fibrosis. *A.* Atelectasis of the right upper lobe in a 4-month-old male. The atelectasis resolved with antibiotics and chest physiotherapy. *B.* The same patient at 9 years of age with mild hyperinflation, central bronchiectasis, resolving right upper lobe infiltrate. The diagnosis of allergic bronchopulmonary aspergillosis was made, and the patient improved after treatment with prednisone. *C.* Pneumothorax of the right lung (arrows) in a 13-year-old male. The pneumothorax resolved after tube thoracostomy and tetracycline sclerosis. The patient died 3 years later from respiratory failure with congestive heart failure. There were no recurrences of the pneumothorax. *D* and *E.* A 34-year-old male showing hyperinflation and diffuse peribronchial thickening. The radiograph was taken during an episode of significant hemoptysis, and no acute changes were seen on the radiograph. He works full-time and has not had another episode of hemoptysis in the last 3 years.

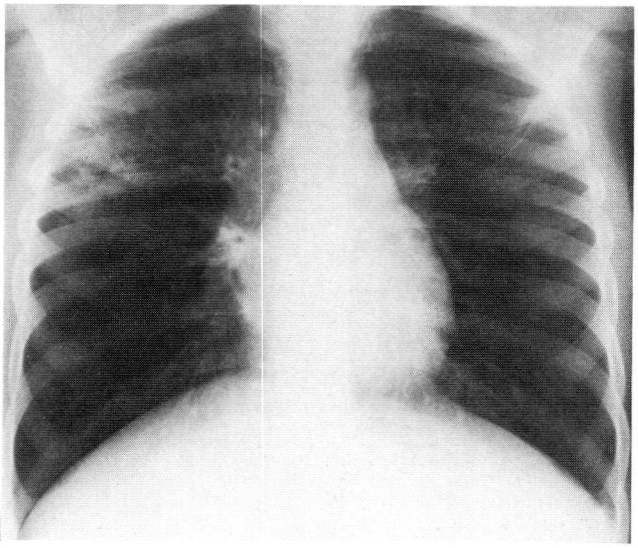

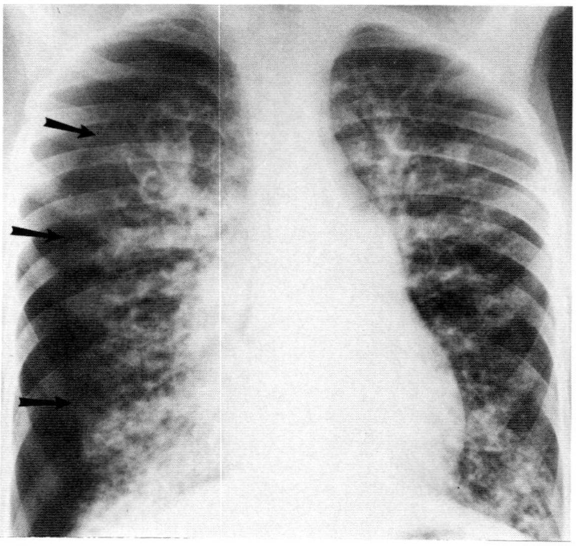

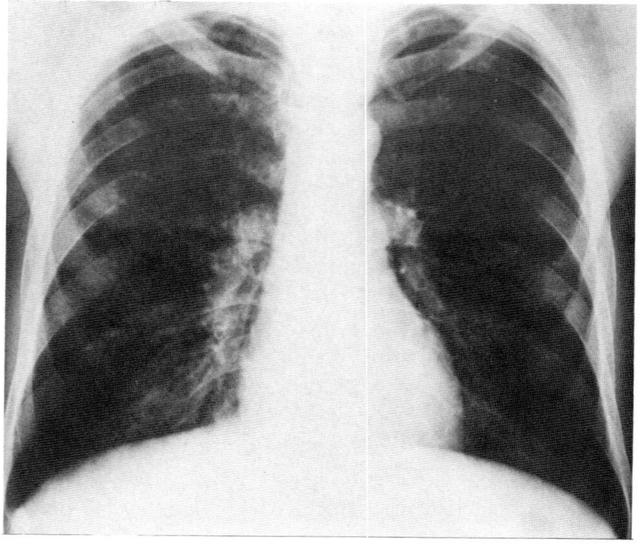

source of bleeding has been identified as varices rather than hemoptysis, endoscopy is undertaken to sclerose the varices. Although portacaval shunts have been successfully done in cystic fibrosis, the outcome has not been uniformly good.

Cor Pulmonale

As the pulmonary disease progresses and the degree of hypoxia increases, patients with cystic fibrosis eventually develop pulmonary hypertension and cor pulmonale. An increase in hypoxia during exacerbation of the pulmonary disease often precipitates overt right ventricular failure. During the acute episode antibiotic treatment for the underlying pulmonary disorder is intensified, and a cardiotonic program consisting of oxygen and diuretics is added. Digitalis and pulmonary vasodilators have not been of proven benefit in cystic fibrosis. Whether the use of nocturnal oxygen—as has proved successful in patients with chronic obstructive airways disease who develop serious hypoxemia during sleep—will work equally well in cystic fibrosis to minimize the degree of pulmonary hypertension is currently under study.

Respiratory Failure

With the advent of respiratory failure in cystic fibrosis, i.e., hypercarbia ($Pa_{CO_2} \geq 55$ mmHg) in addition to arterial hypoxemia, management becomes extremely difficult. As a rule, cystic fibrosis patients do not respond as well to mechanical ventilation, and have more complications from mechanical ventilation, than do patients with other forms of chronic obstructive airways disease.

Mechanical ventilation is generally instituted when an acute episode, such as viral pneumonia or status asthmaticus, throws the patient into respiratory failure. This approach is particularly indicated in the patient who has had good pulmonary function before the episode. Mechanical ventilation is less apt to be successful if the patient has previously experienced a bout of respiratory failure, i.e., acute hypercapnia coupled with the chronic arterial hypoxemia. When respiratory failure marks the end of a chronic course of progressive pulmonary insufficiency despite adequate medical therapy, mechanical ventilation is usually of no avail. However, none of the indications or contraindications for mechanical ventilation are absolute, and a great deal of the outcome depends on the availability of a dedicated and skilled intensive-care team skilled in the handling of patients with cystic fibrosis.

Pregnancy

Pregnancy can complicate the course of cystic fibrosis. A national survey in 1975 identified 129 pregnancies in 100 women with cystic fibrosis; since then, the number has increased. Although the frequency of still births and neonatal deaths is greater than in the general population, there is no excess of congenital malformations.

During the final trimester of pregnancy, pulmonary function deteriorates and pulmonary symptoms increase. However, in those women in whom pulmonary function and nutritional status were good before pregnancy, pulmonary function returned to the pregravid level after delivery; the patients also continued to do well afterward. However, those women who had severe pulmonary disease and poor nutritional status did not return to their pregravid status; indeed, pulmonary function continued to deteriorate after pregnancy.

PSYCHOSOCIAL ISSUES

Careful attention to the emotional, social, and financial well-being of the patient with cystic fibrosis, and of the family, has considerable value in favorably influencing the course of the disease. At the time of diagnosis, it is important to strike an optimistic note while educating the patient about the illness and its management. As part of the early encounter with the patient, it is important to identify and reinforce the emotional and financial strengths of the family as well as weaknesses that will need buttressing. Medical care for cystic fibrosis is costly, especially if hospital admissions are required. Many states have crippled children's programs that provide support for patients and families who do not have adequate resources. Several states have also established special programs for adults with cystic fibrosis.

As the disease runs it course, counseling and feedback about the progression of the disease is essential. As the patient and the family go about setting educational, career, and family goals, they will need guidance in realistic planning. It is vital that the physician develop and maintain a positive attitude. The patient who gives up hope is a candidate for rapid deterioration. Conversely, even patients with severe pulmonary disease can continue to function well and to be productive. However, at the stage when medical therapy can be of no further avail, patient and family will require considerable emotional support to accept the inevitable. In recent years, many cystic fibrosis clinics allow patients to die at home rather than in the hospital. The family will require specific instructions about how to provide physical and emotional comfort for the patient in the home. Usually home visits by some members of the cystic fibrosis team are required. Not all families have the strength or the resources to care for the dying cystic fibrosis patient at home.

FUTURE DIRECTIONS

Since most patients with cystic fibrosis eventually die of respiratory failure at a relatively young age, consideration

must be given to the possibility of heart-lung transplantations for these patients. To date, only a few heart and lung transplants have been attempted in cystic fibrosis. In the first attempt in this country, the patient survived for almost 2 months but died from complications of the immune suppression. Recently, there have been several apparent successes.

Infection with *Pseudomonas* organisms is a critical aspect of cystic fibrosis that has attracted a great deal of attention. To date, *Pseudomonas* organisms have demonstrated a remarkable capacity to change expression of phenotype and to develop resistance to new antibiotics. The newer quinoline antibiotics, taken orally, are currently undergoing clinical trials. If these prove to be effective, they could reduce the cost and the morbidity of treatment for cystic fibrosis.

There is a concern that the marked improvement in survival which occurred over the last two decades is approaching a plateau. For another upsurge to occur in the mean survival curve, physicians must look to new directions from basic research. Two immediate problems to be solved are the detection of heterozygotes and improvement in prenatal diagnosis. As indicated above, during the past year, spectacular progress in applying molecular genetics and recombinant DNA technology has localized the cystic fibrosis gene to chromosome 7. Although there is still much work to be done before the cystic fibrosis gene is identified and the function of its product is described, enough has already been accomplished to warrant a realistic expectation that major breakthroughs will soon occur in the diagnosis and treatment of cystic fibrosis.

BIBLIOGRAPHY

Blumer JL, Stern RC, Yamashita TS, Myers CM, Reed MD: Cephalosporin therapeutics in cystic fibrosis. J Pediatr 108:854–860, 1986.
  Cefsulodin and ceftazidime have been evaluated extensively in the treatment of acute pulmonary exacerbation in cystic fibrosis, and both have been found to be safe and effective.

Brasfield D, Hicks G, Soong S, Tiller RE: The chest roentgenogram in cystic fibrosis: A new scoring system. Pediatrics 63:24–29, 1979.
  Description of a widely used scoring system which has been correlated with a clinical scoring system and with pulmonary function.

Cropp GJ, Pullano TP, Cerny FJ, Nathanson IT: Exercise tolerance and cardiorespiratory adjustments at peak work capacity in cystic fibrosis. Am Rev Respir Dis 126:211–216, 1982.
  Demonstration of abnormal physiological adaptations to exercise in cystic fibrosis patients with advanced lung disease.

Davis PB (ed): Cystic fibrosis. Semin Resp Med 6:243–333, 1985.
  A collection of timely articles describing the current state of the art in the clinical management of cystic fibrosis and the prospects for the immediate future. The tone of this collection is upbeat, in large measure due to the excitement about the likelihood of locating the chromosomal site of the cystic fibrosis gene and its practical applications.

Davis PB, di Sant'Agnese PA: Assisted ventilation for patients with cystic fibrosis. J Am Med Assoc 239:1851–1854, 1978.
  Retrospective summary of experience with mechanical ventilation with cystic fibrosis patients.

Desmond KJ, Schwenk WF, Thomas E, Beaudry PH, Coates AL: Immediate and long-term effects of chest physiotherapy in patients with cystic fibrosis. J Pediatr 103:538–542, 1983.
  Controlled study demonstrating that chest physiotherapy maintains pulmonary function in cystic fibrosis.

Fellows K, Khaw KT, Schuster S, Shwachman H: Bronchial artery embolization in cystic fibrosis. Technique and long-term results. J Pediatr 95:959–963, 1979.
  First report of the use of this technique in cystic fibrosis.

Fick RB Jr, Olchowski J, Squier SU, Merrill WW, Reynolds HY: Immunoglobulin-G subclasses in cystic fibrosis. IgG2 response to Pseudomonas aeruginosa lipopolysaccharide. Am Rev Respir Dis 133:418–422, 1986.
  An investigation into why pulmonary macrophage phagocytosis of Pseudomonas aeruginosa is defective when this pathogen is opsonized with IgG antibodies isolated from serum samples from patients with cystic fibrosis (CF).

Fox WW, Bureau MA, Taussig LA, Martin RR, Beaudry PH: Helium flow-volume curves in the detection of early small airway disease. Pediatrics 54:293–299, 1974.
  Describes the application of a sensitive test for detection of small airways disease in cystic fibrosis.

Ingram RH Jr, McFadden ER Jr: Pulmonary performance in cystic fibrosis, in Fishman AP (ed), *Pulmonary Diseases and Disorders.* New York, McGraw-Hill, 1980, pp 614–617.
   Overview of pulmonary functions in cystic fibrosis.

Isles A, Maclusky I, Corey M, Gold R, Prober C, Fleming P, Levison H: *Pseudomonas cepacia* infection in cystic fibrosis. An emerging problem. J Pediatr 104:206–210, 1984.
   Highly resistant forms of this organism are now of great concern for cystic fibrosis populations.

Jones JD, Steige H, Logan GB: Variations of sweat sodium values in children and adults with cystic fibrosis and other diseases. Mayo Clinic Proc 45:768–773, 1970.
   Demonstrates the increase in sweat electrolytes with age.

Kaliner M, Shelhamer JH, Borson B, Nadel J, Patow C, Marom Z: Human respiratory mucus. Am Rev Respir Dis 134:612–621, 1986.
   A review of respiratory secretions with particular reference to the mucous glycoproteins.

Katz JN, Horwitz RI, Dolan TF, Shapiro ED: Clinical features as predictors of functional status in children with cystic fibrosis. J Pediatr 108:352–358, 1986.
   Clinical features apparent at diagnosis are valuable prognostic indicators in children with cystic fibrosis.

Lamarre A, Reilly BJ, Bryan AC, Levison H: Early detection of pulmonary function abnormalities in cystic fibrosis. Pediatrics 50:291–298, 1972.
   Demonstrates that hypoxemia may precede changes in other parameters of pulmonary function.

Landau LI, Phelan PD: The variable effect of a bronchodilating agent on pulmonary function in cystic fibrosis. Pediatr Pharm Therapeut 82:863–868, 1973.
   Demonstrates decreased airflow in some patients with cystic fibrosis following administration of bronchodilators.

Laufer P, Fink J, Bruns T, Unger G, Klabfleisch J, Greenberger PA, Patterson R: Allergic bronchopulmonary aspergillosis in cystic fibrosis. J Allergy Clin Immunol 73:44–48, 1984.
   Good description of this complication of cystic fibrosis which is common in the United Kingdom and in some parts of the United States.

Lawson D (ed): *Cystic Fibrosis: Horizons,* Proceedings of the 9th International Cystic Fibrosis Congress. Brighton, England, Wiley, 1984.
   Contains review articles of several major areas of research in cystic fibrosis and new abstracts through June 1984.

Marks J, Pasterkamp H, Tal A, Leahy F: Relationship between respiratory muscle strength, nutritional status, and lung volume in cystic fibrosis and asthma. Am Rev Respir Dis 133:414–417, 1986.
   Respiratory muscle strength is not related to nutritional status in patients with cystic fibrosis and asthma.

Matthews LW, Dearborn DG, Tucker AS: Cystic fibrosis, in Fishman AP (ed), *Pulmonary Diseases and Disorders.* New York, McGraw-Hill, 1980, pp 600–613.
   Excellent presentations of the natural history of cystic fibrosis and the correlation of severity of changes on chest radiographs with survival curves.

McLaughlin FJ, Matthews WJ, Strieder DJ, Khaw KT, Schuster S, Shwachman H: Pneumothorax in cystic fibrosis: Management and outcome. J Pediatr 100:863–869, 1982.
   Emphasizes need for chemical or surgical treatment to prevent recurrences of pneumothorax in cystic fibrosis.

Mellins RB, Levine OR, Ingram RH Jr, Fishman AP: Obstructive disease of the airways in cystic fibrosis. Pediatrics 41:560–573, 1968.
   Classic description of the pulmonary function abnormalities in cystic fibrosis.

Mullins RE, Lampasona V, Conn RB: Monitoring aminoglycoside therapy. Clin Lab Med 7:513–529, 1987.
   Monitoring of serum aminoglycoside concentrations is essential in patients with cystic fibrosis in order to avoid their toxic effects.

Newmark P: Testing for cystic fibrosis. Nature 318:309, 1985.
   Editorial discussing advances in molecular genetics of cystic fibrosis.

Olsen MM, Gauderer MW, Girz MK, Izant RJ Jr: Surgery in patients with cystic fibrosis. J Pediatr Surg 22:613–618, 1987.
   A 15-year review of Children's Hospital patients with cystic fibrosis (CF) who underwent surgery disclosed 578 instances in 210 patients (mean 2.7 per patient).

Orenstein DM, Franklin BA, Doershuk CF, Hellerstein HK, Germann KJ, Horowitz JG, Stern RD: Exercise conditioning and cardiopulmonary fitness in cystic fibrosis. Chest 80:392–397, 1981.
> *Presents evidence that a supervised exercise program can improve exercise tolerance in cystic fibrosis patients.*

Palmer J. Dillon-Baker C, Tecklin JS, Wolfson B, Rosenberg B, Burroughs B, Holsclaw DS, Scanlin TF, Huang NN, Sewell EM: Pregnancy in patients with cystic fibrosis. Ann Intern Med 99:596–600, 1983.
> *Detailed analysis of pregravid and postpartum courses in a group of women with cystic fibrosis.*

Palumbo AP, Isobe M, Huebner K, Shane S, Rovera G, Demuth D, Curtis PJ, Ballantine M, Croce CM, Showe LC: Chromosomal localization of a human band 3-like gene to 7q35–7q36. Am J Hum Genet 39:307–316, 1986.
> *Localization of a gene candidate for the epithelial chloride transport.*

Redding GJ, Restuccia R, Cotton EK, Brooks JG: Serial changes in pulmonary functions in children hospitalized with cystic fibrosis. Am Rev Respir Dis 126:31–36, 1982.
> *Detailed documentation of response to standard therapy for exacerbation of cystic fibrosis pulmonary infection.*

Richardson VF, Robertson CF, Mowat AP, Howard ER, Price JF: Deterioration in lung function after general anaesthesia in patients with cystic fibrosis. Acta Paediatr Scand 73:75–79, 1984.
> *Well controlled study documenting change in lung function with general compared to local anesthesia.*

Rosenstein BJ, Langbaum TS: Misdiagnosis of cystic fibrosis. Need for continuing follow-up and reevaluation. Clin Pediatr (Phila) 26:78–82, 1987.
> *Eight of 271 patients evaluated over a 15-year period in whom the diagnosis of cystic fibrosis was made on the basis of a compatible clinical picture and at least two positive quantitative pilocarpine iontophoresis sweat tests were subsequently shown to have normal sweat electrolyte concentrations.*

Scanlin TF: Cystic fibrosis, in Fleisher G, Ludwig S (eds), *Textbook of Emergency Pediatrics.* Baltimore, Williams & Wilkins, 1983, pp 532–556.
> *Practical details of emergency management of complications of cystic fibrosis.*

Scanlin TF, Wang YM, Glick MC: Altered fucosylation of membrane glycoproteins from cystic fibrosis fibroblasts. Pediatr Res 19:368–374, 1985.
> *Includes references describing the glycoprotein alterations in cystic fibrosis.*

Sobonya RE, Taussig LM: Quantitative aspects of lung pathology in cystic fibrosis. Am Rev Respir Dis 134:290–295, 1986.
> *The lungs of nine patients with cystic fibrosis were studied by morphometric techniques to determine the amount of bronchiectasis, emphysema, pneumonia, bronchial gland enlargement, and small airways narrowing and density.*

Stern RC, Boat TF, Orenstein DM, Wood RE, Matthews LW, Doershuk CF: Treatment and prognosis of lobar and segmental atelectasis in cystic fibrosis. Am Rev Respir Dis 118:821–826, 1978.
> *Retrospective review of medical and surgical management of atelectasis in a larger cystic fibrosis center.*

Talamo RC, Rosenstein BI, Berninger RW: Cystic fibrosis, in Stanbury JA, Wyngaarden JB, Frederickson DS, Goldstein JL, Brown MS (eds), *The Metabolic Basis of Inherited Disease,* 5th ed. New York, McGraw-Hill, 1983, pp 1889–1917.
> *Comprehensive review of cystic fibrosis literature through 1980 (533 references). Thorough discussion of cystic fibrosis factors.*

Taussig LM: *Cystic Fibrosis.* New York, Theime-Stratton, 1984.
> *Comprehensive reviews of topics in cystic fibrosis.*

Tepper RS, Hiatt PW, Eigen H, Smith J: Total respiratory system compliance in asymptomatic infants with cystic fibrosis. Am Rev Respir Dis 135:1075–1079, 1987.
> *The determination of total respiration system compliance is a useful noninvasive method for detecting early pulmonary function abnormalities in CF infants.*

Thomassen MJ, Demko CA, Doershuk CF, Stern RC, Klinger JD: Pseudomonas cepacia: decrease in colonization in patients with cystic fibrosis. Am Rev Respir Dis 134:669–671, 1986.
> *P. cepacia infections have been associated with shorter survival in some patients with cystic fibrosis. The results suggest that infection is via patient-to-patient transmission. Segregation measures decrease colonization with this organism.*

Tomashefski JF Jr, Bruce M, Goldberg HI, Dearborn DG: Regional distribution of macroscopic lung disease in cystic fibrosis. Am Rev Respir Dis 133:535–540, 1986.
  Macroscopic morphometry applied to lungs obtained at autopsy confirmed that in cystic fibrosis the lung disease and remodeling are unevenly distributed in favor of the upper lobes.

Welsh MJ, Widdicombe JH: Research on cystic fibrosis: Step 3? J Appl Physiol 59:1999–2001, 1985.
  Editorial review of meeting at National Institutes of Health to discuss recent research strategies in cystic fibrosis. Focus on chloride defect.

Chapter 79

Asthma: General Features, Pathogenesis, and Pathophysiology

E. R. McFadden, Jr.

Asthma is a disease of the airways that is characterized by increased responsiveness of the tracheobronchial tree to a multiplicity of stimuli. Functionally, the hallmark of this illness is widespread narrowing of the airways that changes in severity either spontaneously or as a result of therapy. Clinically, the disorder is manifested by paroxysms of cough, dyspnea, and wheezing which generally occur together. However, an occasional patient presents with only cough or dyspnea.

GENERAL FEATURES

Prevalence and Natural History

Asthma is a chronic disease that is episodic in nature and in which acute exacerbations are interspersed with symptom-free periods of variable duration. It is a common malady that affects both children and adults; it has been suggested that approximately 4 percent of the population in the United States has the disorder. Asthma can begin at any age, but about one-half of the affected individuals develop the disease before age 10 and another one-third before age 40. Long periods of remission are not uncommon.

Typically, acute exacerbations tend to be episodic and short-lived, and to be followed by complete recovery. However, sometimes there is a phase in which the patient experiences some degree of airway obstruction daily. This phase can be mild, sometimes punctuated by bouts of severe obstruction persisting for days to weeks, i.e., *status asthmaticus.*

The mortality of asthma is low, averaging approximately 0.3 deaths per 10,000 persons. Typically, 2000 to 3000 people die of the disease per year, and the deaths tend to occur in the very young and in the elderly. The death rate from asthma may be increasing: data from 1983 and 1984 indicate an excess death rate of 200 cases per year. The reasons for this purported increase are not clear. Some consider it to be artifactual, a consequence of a recent change in reporting practices.

Although asthma has a low mortality, its morbidity is staggering and its socioeconomic consequences are awesome. It is estimated that asthma results in over 27 million patient visits, 6 million lost work days and 90.5 million days of restricted activity per year. In addition, asthma is believed to account for approximately 134,000 admissions per annum to hospital, the average stay being 8.3 days. Families with asthmatic members may spend as much as 18 percent of their total income on treatment; according to the pharmaceutical industry, $292 million was spent in 1975 for medications to treat airway diseases. The cost of medications has risen sharply since then.

Asthma differs from other forms of chronic obstructive airways disease in that its course is not relentlessly progressive and pulmonary dysfunction is rarely permanent. Clinical expression of the disease varies greatly not only among asthmatics but from time to time in the same patient: at a particular time, an individual with asthma may be normal by functional and clinical criteria; asymptomatic, with functional defects of varying degree; symptomatic, with varying severity of obstruction; or in a state of status asthmaticus, with or without respiratory failure. The factors that determine this behavior have not been completely elucidated. One of them, however, is the degree of lability of the tracheobronchial tree.

Airway Reactivity

The airways are not rigid tubes. Instead, they are dynamic structures that change diameter in response to a variety of stimuli. For example, when the need arises for large volumes of air to be moved, as during exercise, bronchodilation occurs. Conversely, when it is important to limit or decrease the volume of air inspired, such as upon expo-

sure to irritant gases, the lung defends itself by cough and bronchoconstriction. This ability of the airways to alter their size in response to endogenous and exogenous stimuli has been designated *airway reactivity*. This term tends to be used synonymously with smooth-muscle contraction. However, more than one pathologic process can result in airway narrowing. For example, mucosal edema with or without inflammatory cellular infiltrate, increased mucous secretion with or without changes in clearance, alterations in parenchymal elasticity, the loss of stability of distal bronchioles, and changes in airway vasculature can all contribute to a reduction in the caliber of the airway lumen. The predominant response depends on such variables as the nature of the offending agent, its distribution within the tracheobronchial tree, the duration and intensity of the exposure, and the responsivity of the host.

In asthmatic individuals, responsivity of the airways is markedly increased. Patients with asthma develop more intense bronchoconstriction to milder stimuli than do healthy individuals. Increased airway reactivity is the cardinal feature of asthma and is believed by many to be the primary predisposing influence in the advent of the disease. Heightened airway responsiveness also occurs in the first-degree relatives of asthmatics and in some patients with allergic rhinitis, cystic fibrosis, and chronic bronchitis. Heightened airway reactivity may also be transiently acquired by normal individuals after viral infections of the upper respiratory tract or after acute exposure to certain air pollutants.

In asthma, airway reactivity increases on repeated exposure to inciting stimuli and decreases when they are avoided. As exposure increases, the airways become more responsive to nonspecific stimuli. This endogenous hyperresponsiveness of the tracheobronchial tree accounts for much of the morbidity associated with the disease, and it correlates with many clinical features of the illness, such as severity, symptom intensity, quantity of medications required, and the degree of diurnal fluctuation in pulmonary function. Therefore, the phenomenon of heightened airway reactivity of asthmatics is an important feature of the disease that can be used in clinical practice not only to diagnose the presence of asthma but also to help assess its severity and to anticipate the requirements for treatment.

In general, three classes of stimuli have been used to measure bronchial reactivity: (1) pharmacologic and immunologic aerosols, e.g., methacholine, histamine, propranolol, prostaglandin $F_{2\alpha}$, and leukotrienes; (2) physical chemical agents, e.g., ozone, sulfur dioxide, distilled water, and hypertonic solutions; and (3) thermal stimuli, e.g., exercise and voluntary hyperventilation of cold air. The methods for each have been standardized. There seems to be little to choose from among such diverse tests as methacholine, histamine, exercise, and the hyperventilation of frigid air.

The distribution of airway responsiveness in the population at large is unknown. However, instead of constituting a unique group, asthmatics may represent the extreme end of a normal distribution. If this is the case, it is conceivable that normal individuals could develop changes in the airway reactivity that could move them into the asthmatic range; conversely, asthmatics might undergo reduction in airway reactivity toward normal. This type of distribution is consistent with clinical observations and makes a strong case for developing methods by which airway reactivity can be reduced.

Despite its importance in asthma, little is known about the mechanism(s) by which airway hyperreactivity develops and the factors that sustain it. Three types of factors have been invoked: (1) an increase in the inherent reactivity of the airway smooth muscle, (2) an abnormality in autonomic nervous control, and (3) a breakdown in airway defenses secondary to inflammatory processes. Unfortunately, none of these is entirely satisfying, per se. Indeed, the likelihood is strong that multiple influences, including an interplay among the diverse inflammatory mediators released by the various cells involved in the inflammatory process, are involved. Particularly appealing as a common denominator are the metabolites of arachidonic acid: the prostaglandins and leukotrienes generated by the metabolism of arachidonic acid in the plasma membrane of the resident and inflammatory cells can reproduce most of the physiological effects seen in acute and chronic airway disease.

Airway Reactivity and Circadian Changes

One major clinical manifestation of increased airway reactivity is a marked circadian variation in pulmonary function. Asthmatic patients often manifest an increase in respiratory symptoms during the night and early morning. Nocturnal asthma is a common and troubling symptom. It occurs in 70 to 80 percent of patients and is often difficult to manage. The marked swings in pulmonary function during the night have been implicated in causing respiratory arrest and sudden death in asthmatic patients (Fig. 79-1). For example, eight of the nine respiratory arrests in asthmatics treated at the Brompton Hospital occurred between midnight and 6 A.M. In this group, large diurnal swings in flow rates occurred during the 24 h before the respiratory arrests; peak flow rates in the morning were less than 50 percent of the highest daily reading.

Numerous etiologic factors have been proposed to explain this phenomenon: exposure to allergens in the bedding, late phase reactions to antigen exposure early in the day, supine posture with secondary airway changes, fluctuations in airway caliber during REM sleep, timing of bronchodilator administration, gastroesophageal reflux, impaired mucociliary clearance, and airway cooling. Although many of these external factors may contribute to

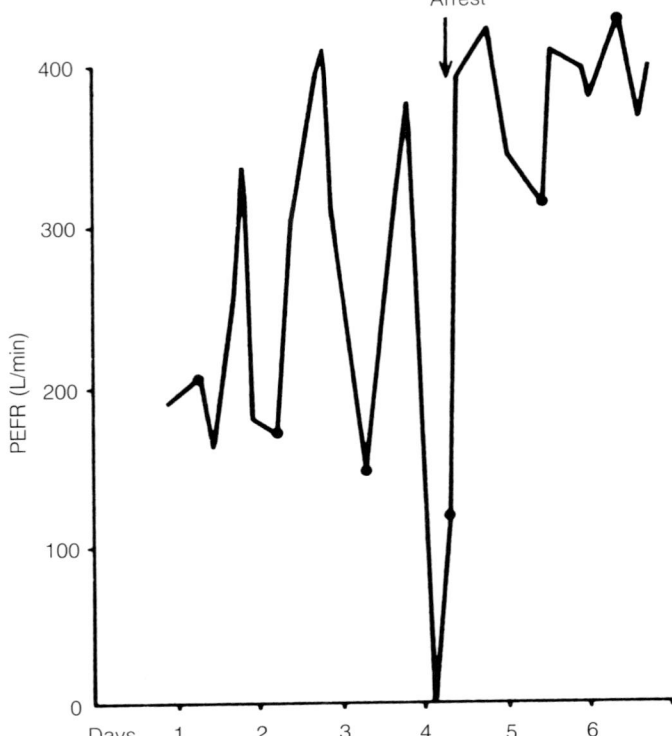

FIGURE 79-1 Daily, four hourly recordings of peak expiratory flow rate (PEFR) in a 52-year-old male patient. Note: recurrent morning falls in PEFR of greater than 50 percent preceded the respiratory arrest on the fifth day. *(From Hetzel, Clark, Branthwaite, 1977.)*

bronchospasm at night in individual patients, they do not provide a universal explanation for nocturnal asthma. Many biologic functions show variability over a 24-h period, and airway function is no exception. One reasonable explanation for nocturnal asthma is that it results from a complex interaction of several coincident circadian rhythms which in normal subjects cause only small changes in airway caliber but in asthmatics cause bronchospasm severe enough to rouse the patient.

PATHOGENESIS

With respect to etiology, asthma is a heterogeneous disease and it has proved useful to classify the forms of this illness by the principal stimuli that incite, or are associated with, acute episodes. However, distinction between various types of asthma is artificial, and the response of any given subclassification may be initiated by more than one type of stimulus. Seven major types of stimuli can provoke acute episodes of asthma: allergens, exercise, infections, and occupational, environmental, pharmacologic, and emotional stress.

Allergens

The role played by immunologic host factors in the pathogenesis of asthma is unclear. Most experts believe that a suspected or proven allergic component can be found in up to 35 to 55 percent of asthmatic patients. Most of the allergens that provoke asthma are airborne, and in order to induce a state of sensitivity, they must be reasonably abundant in the environment for considerable periods of time. However, once sensitization has occurred, minute amounts of the offending agent can produce exacerbations of the disease.

The process of sensitization is believed to be initiated by the interaction of an environmental antigen with peripheral lymphoid tissue. In the presence of participating regulatory T cells, the antigen causes mature B cells to proliferate and to differentiate into B cells that secrete IgE and plasma cells. The IgE then circulates until a part of its epsilon chain combines with a high-affinity receptor located on the membrane of mast cells and basophils. Once coated with antibody, these cells are primed to release their mediators on subsequent exposure. In the lungs, most mast cells are located in peripheral airways, in the submucosa of the airways close to capillaries and smooth muscle. In the large central airways, mast cells interdigitate with surface epithelial cells. Basophils circulate freely in the blood.

When an antigen bridges two adjacent molecules of membrane-bound IgE, a chain reaction is initiated that culminates in exocytosis of the cell granules and the release of the potent biologic mediators of the immediate hypersensitivity reaction that they contain (Fig. 79-2A). Some of the compounds released, such as histamine, platelet activating factor, leukotrienes, and prostaglandins, have direct effects on airway smooth muscle and pulmonary capillary permeability. Others, such as the eosinophil chemotactic factor of anaphylaxis, high-molecular-weight neutrophil chemotactic factor of anaphylaxis, lymphocytic chemotactic factor, and leukotriene B_4, are chemotactic and recruit polymorphonuclear cells, lymphocytes, and platelets to the site of release.

These events in the plasma membrane also activate phospholipase A_2 resulting in the formation of arachidonic acid, which is the precursor of a number of potent, biologically active agents (Fig. 79-2B). The mediators derived from arachidonic acid are a diverse group of highly active pharmacologic materials that together possess all the functions necessary for fully expressed immediate and long-term inflammatory reactions. Arachidonic acid is metabolized by two distinct pathways, the lipoxygenase and cyclooxygenase pathways. The products of the lipoxygenase pathway are the hydroxyeicosatetraenoic acids (HETEs) which are further metabolized to the leukotrienes (LTB_4, LTC_4, LTD_4, and LTE_4). The latter three are the constituents of slow-reacting substance of anaphylaxis. LTB_4

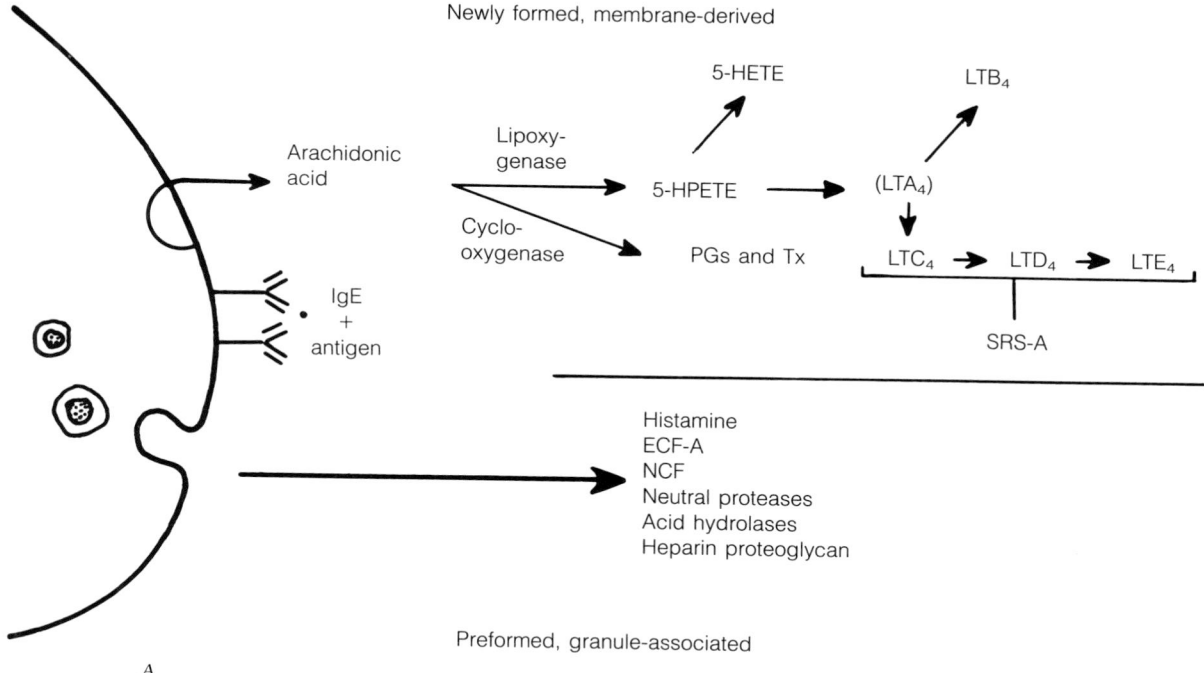

Newly formed, membrane-derived

Preformed, granule-associated

A

FIGURE 79-2　*A*. Antigen-antibody reaction at the surface of the mast cell with the elaboration of preformed granual associated mediators and newly formed membrane-derived mediators.　*B (opposite)*. Membrane events associated with the release of arachidonic acid. ECF-A = eosinophil chemotactic factor of anaphylaxis; NCF = neutrophil chemotactic factor of anaphylaxis; 5-HETE = 5-hydroxyeicosatetraenoic acid; 5-HPETE = 5-hydroperoxy-eicosatetraenoic acid; LT = leukotriene; PG = prostaglandin; SRS-A = slow reacting substance of anaphylaxis; Tx = thromboxane. *(From Barnes and Costello, 1984.)*

and the HETEs are powerful chemotactic agents, whereas LTC_4, LTD_4, and LTE_4 are among the most potent and long-acting bronchoconstricting agents that have been studied in humans. These agents also increase vascular permeability and mucus release from human airways and decrease its clearance.

The products of the cyclooxygenase pathway are prostaglandins, prostacyclin, and thromboxane. These compounds can be characterized as potent bronchoconstrictors, chemotactic factors, and substances that both generate mucus and inhibit its removal. The chemotactic factors can recruit the enzymatic contents of eosinophils and neutrophils into the reaction.

As a group, these products are responsible for the physiological and pathologic changes of the allergic asthmatic attack by acting on bronchial smooth muscle to cause bronchoconstriction, on ciliated epithelium to reduce mucociliary clearance, on bronchial glands to cause mucous secretion, and on blood vessels to cause vasodilation and increased permeability.

After inhaling an antigen, the usual response in a sensitized individual is the prompt development of airway obstruction. Typically, the airflow limitation occurs within minutes and regresses spontaneously during the next 30 to 60 min. In a considerable number of patients (between 15 to 50 percent depending upon the study), this initial reaction is followed in several hours by a second wave of obstruction, the so-called late reaction. Frequently, the late reaction is more severe than the first initial obstructive response and tends to be resistant to sympathomimetics. In some situations, particularly when the antigen load is high, a single exposure may produce recurrent bouts of airflow limitation over the course of several days.

The immediate reaction is presumed to be chiefly the result of the elaboration of the mediators of immediate hypersensitivity that act directly on bronchial and vascular smooth muscle to cause bronchoconstriction, vasoconstriction, and edema. The late reaction probably represents an infiltrative phase that results from the chemotactic mediators that were initially elaborated and the secondary effector cells that they recruit. One cell that seems to play a central role in the inflammation of the late phase is the eosinophil. Eosinophils are prominent in the airways of asthmatics, and the eosinophilic protein, a major basic protein, is known to kill ciliated respiratory epithelium. In fact, it is now recognized that during severe episodes of asthma the sputum contains quantities of

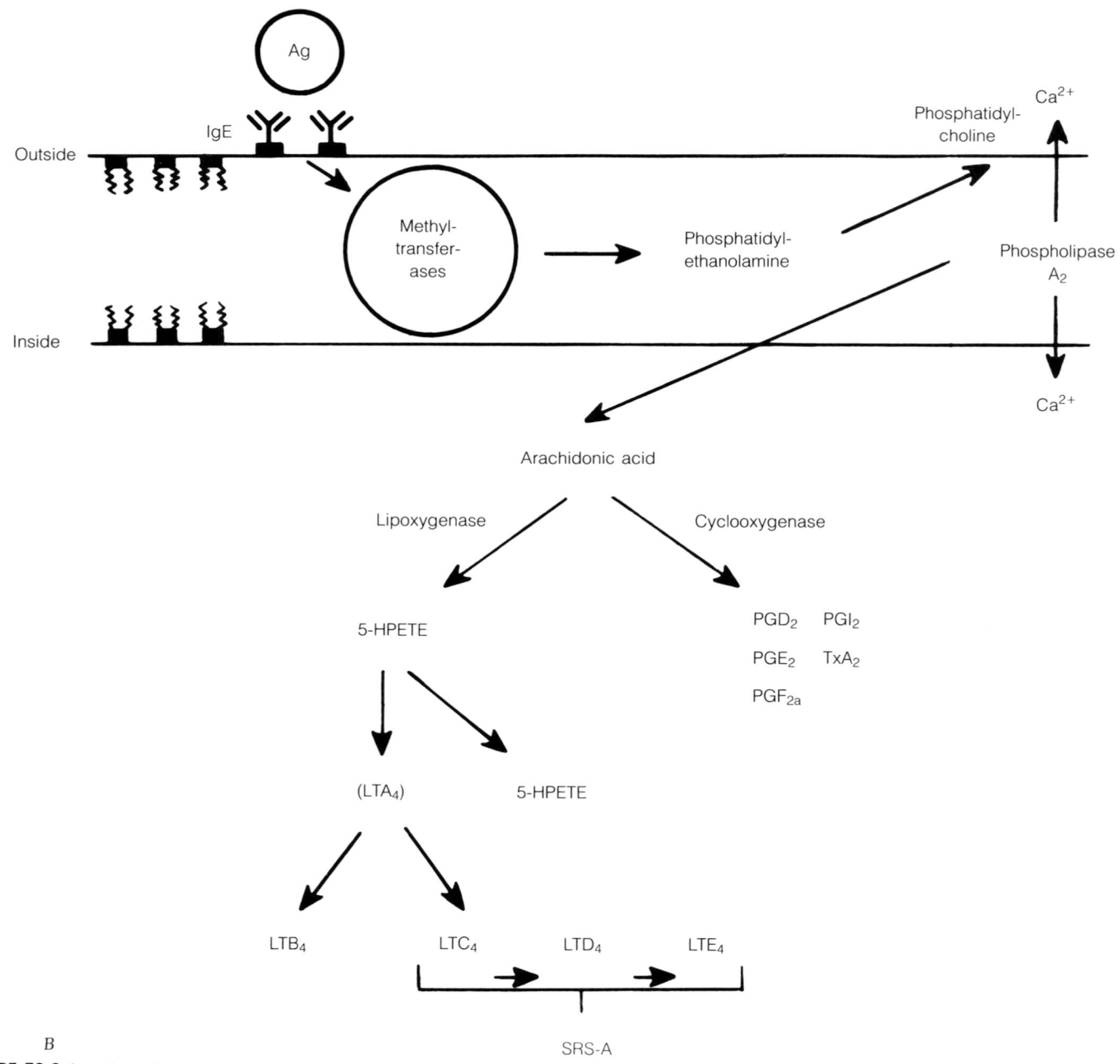

B

FIGURE 79-2 *(continued)*

major basic protein that are toxic to respiratory epithelium in vitro. High concentrations of major basic protein are also found in the bronchial walls and areas of denuded epithelium.

Physical Exertion

Asthma can be exacerbated by physical exertion. This phenomenon has been designated as *exercise-induced asthma*. It is a particularly troublesome feature of the asthmatic diathesis in children and young adults because of their high level of physical activity. However, it can also be observed in the elderly and probably operates to some extent in every asthmatic patient. As a rule, the patient with exercise-induced asthma develops cough, wheezing, and/or dyspnea at the end of the period of exercise, not during its performance. Usually the induced attack is short-lived and regresses spontaneously. Although exercise can occasionally be the only stimulus that evokes acute episodes of asthma, more often it is only one of the many nonimmunologic triggers for this release.

The magnitude of postexertional airway obstruction

is strongly influenced by the environment in which exercise is performed. For example, inhalation of cold air during physical exertion markedly augments the severity of the airway obstruction; conversely, warm humid air blunts or abolishes it. Consequently, activities such as ice hockey, skiing, or ice skating present more difficulty to an affected individual than does swimming in an indoor heated pool.

Although the airflow limitation in exercise-induced asthma is somehow related to thermal changes within the intrathoracic airways during hyperpnea, the mechanism by which this occurs is unknown. Large minute ventilations and/or low temperatures decrease the water content of inspired air and increase the thermal load of the airways. As a result, greater movement is required of heat and water from the mucosal surface to warm the inspired air to body temperature and humidity. The more heat and water to be transferred, the larger the subsequent obstructive response. Conversely, low ventilation and high inspired temperatures and humidity minimize the transfers, thereby decreasing the magnitude of the response. If there is no movement of heat and water from the respiratory tract during hyperpnea, airway obstruction tends not to develop.

The importance of the water content of the inspired air during periods of hyperpnea in determining the severity of airflow limitation in asthmatics has been well documented. The vapor pressure of the inspired air is a critical determinant of the severity of an upcoming attack of asthma. This is because, under all circumstances but the most extreme, 60 to 80 percent of the total heat lost from the mucosa comes from the evaporation of water. The higher the vapor pressure in the incoming air, the less water has to be vaporized and the smaller the thermal consequences. It has been proposed that vaporization of water from the mucosa during inspiration causes an increase in surface osmolarity, and it is the increase in osmolarity and not the cooling of the airways that provokes exercise-induced asthma. Since the evaporation of water causes both cooling of the airways and changes in osmolarity to develop simultaneously, it is not possible to separate physiologically the effects of these two processes. However, it has not yet been proved that changes in the osmolarity of the airway surface fluid do occur; not only is water evaporated during inspiration recovered during expiration, but any net water loss could be replaced by mechanisms involved in the epithelial transport of water.

The level of ventilation operating primarily via airway cooling has been shown to be the major determinant of bronchospasm in exercise-induced asthma. A variety of mechanisms have been proposed to explain how airway cooling elicits exercise-induced asthma. Among those that have been discounted are the following: (1) thermally sensitive neural receptors in the respiratory tract as reflex mediators of the response to airway cooling, (2) choliner-

gic mechanisms, and (3) mast cell degranulation with release of mediators. Currently being investigated is the possibility that the bronchovascular congestion and hyperemia play an important role in eliciting exercise-induced asthma.

Respiratory Infections

Upper respiratory tract infections are among the most common of the stimuli that evoke acute exacerbations of asthma. Like exercise, provocation of bronchospasm by infection is probably somewhat operative in every asthmatic patient. The role of bacterial infection in inducing acute exacerbations of asthma appears to be minimal; viruses, not bacteria, are the major etiologic agents. Therefore, the use of antibiotics in treating acute exacerbations of asthma has no basis. Neither does the use of vaccines directed against bacterial flora.

In children under the age of 2 years, respiratory syncytial virus plays a major etiologic role. With increasing age, rhinoviruses become increasingly more important as pathogens along with influenza, parainfluenza, and *Mycoplasma*. In adults, the rhinoviruses and influenza virus type A seem to be major precipitants of infection-induced wheezing. Simple colonization of the tracheobronchial tree is insufficient to evoke acute episodes of bronchospasm; active infection appears to be required. The incidence of viral infection is substantially higher in children than in adults: as many as 40 percent of wheezing episodes in children during the fall and winter months may be viral-related.

Asthmatic individuals are neither more susceptible to upper respiratory tract infection than nonasthmatics nor do they have an immunologic defect that predisposes them to respiratory illnesses. Nor do asthmatics who are taking corticosteroids in usual doses, either orally or by inhalation, appear to be at increased risk of viral or bacterial infections. Finally, although asthmatics do have more symptomatic episodes of nasal congestion, sore throat, cough, and hoarseness than do nonasthmatics, fewer of these episodes can be proved, either by isolation of an etiologic agent or by an increase in antibody titers, to be related to infection.

The mechanisms by which viral respiratory tract infections evoke wheezing are unknown. Infection, which increases the responsiveness of the tracheobronchial tree in both normal individuals and asthmatics, may play a role by increasing reactivity to nonspecific stimuli. The increase in responsivity can last for 2 to 8 weeks after the onset of the illness. The primary mechanism responsible for these changes is probably viral replication in the respiratory epithelium, which causes cellular damage and the release of arachidonic acid metabolites; these metabolites plus the involvement of polymorphonucleocytes could elicit both acute and chronic inflammatory changes. It is

uncertain whether uncovering of irritant sensory receptors in the epithelium, leading to an increase in their sensitivity, is also involved.

Occupational Stimuli

Since asthma affects approximately 4 to 5 percent of the population at large and about one-third of the cases develop in adult life, asthma can be expected to develop by coincidence in 1 to 2 percent of all workers during their working lives. When the incidence of asthma in a particular occupational environment is several times the normal level, the cause is more likely to be occupational than coincidental. In the cotton industry, 25 to 29 percent of workers exposed to the carding process and 10 to 29 percent of those involved in spinning develop airway obstruction. About 6 percent of animal handlers become clinically sensitive to animal proteins, and perhaps 5 to 10 percent of workers using isocyanates develop respiratory problems. Occupational asthma is not uncommon in bakers exposed to cereal, flours, or insect contaminants, or in the platinum refining industries.

Although a wide variety of occupations can be associated with asthma, in general, bronchoconstriction in industry results from exposure to six different types of agents: metal salts, wood and vegetable dusts, pharmaceutical agents, industrial chemicals and plastics, biologic enzymes, and animal, bird, fish, and insect proteins. In a given industry, a worker may be exposed to more than one agent. At least three mechanisms, immunologic, pharmacologic, and inflammatory, contribute to the development of airway obstruction. For example, repeated exposure to some environmental substances can bring about IgE-mediated immunologic reactions in animal handlers, metal dust workers, and pharmaceutical industry workers. In byssinosis, pharmacologically induced bronchoconstriction is believed to occur as the result of a histamine-releasing substance in the cotton bract. Other examples of pharmacologically induced bronchoconstriction are organic phosphorus insecticides that act as anticholinesterases and substances with a β-adrenergic agonist action used in manufacturing plastics. Acute inflammatory bronchoconstriction most often follows exposure to irritant gases and vapors, such as hydrochloric acid, sulfur dioxide, hydrogen sulfite, ammonia, and fumes from heated plastics. In these circumstances, low environmental concentrations tend to affect primarily those individuals who have increased bronchial hyperreactivity; in high concentration, even normal persons can develop an acute chemical bronchitis.

Occupational lung disease related to metal salts was first described in photographic workers. It can be found in any industry using metal salts. Although this phenomenon typically occurs in individuals working with complex salts of platinum, chromium, and nickel, it also oc-

curs following exposure to salts of other metals in the saline chemical grouping. The reaction is believed to be IgE-mediated. Metallic dusts, per se, are innocuous.

A number of wood and vegetable sources cause asthma. The list includes castor bean oil; colophony (pine resin which is used as a flux in tin or lead soldering); cotton; flax and hemp; grain flours such as barley, corn, oats, rye, and wheat; green coffee beans; gums such as acacia and arabic, which are used in the printing industry; mushrooms; soy bean oil; soy flour; tea; tobacco; and woods such as western red cedar and oak. Exposure can come about through working with these materials in industries as diverse as farming, food processing, vegetable oil manufacturing, baking, grain handling, and meat wrapping. Other occupations that entail this risk are textile working, dock working, electrical working, carpentry, and printing. Many of the proteins listed above are potent immunologic sensitizers because they have multivalent antigenic determinants. As a result, immunologic and/or pharmacologic mechanisms dominate.

The pharmaceutical agents which have been shown to produce airways disease are cimetidine, penicillins, phenylglycine acid chloride, piperazine, sulfasalazine, tetracycline, and spiramycin. Pharmacists, nurses, physicians, and factory workers who handle these agents are at risk of developing asthma by inhaling these materials.

Industrial chemicals and plastics, such as toluene diisocyanate (TDI), phthalic acid anhydride, trimellitic anhydride (TMA), persulfates, ethylenediamine, paraphenylenediamine, and other dyes are sometimes important causes of occupational asthma. These products are widely used in industry so that exposure to them, in one form or another, is quite common. For example, TDI is an important component in the production of polyurethane (which is used in the paint, varnish, and plastic industries), of coating for wires in the electronic industry, and of foam packaging for insulation. In addition to workers who are directly exposed, TDI sensitivity occasionally is manifested clinically by clerical personnel of factories that use or make TDI and by people who live near a factory that uses it. TDI can cause disease on either an immunologic or a pharmacologic basis.

Another widely used industrial compound is trimellitic anhydride (TMA). Exposure to TMA can produce three distinct syndromes: (1) a typical asthmatic reaction (cough and wheezing) after a latent, or sensitization, interval; (2) an asthmatic attack accompanied by systemic manifestations, i.e., arthralgia, myalgia, and fever—the so-called TMA flu, a syndrome readily recognized by people who work with the compound; and (3) epistasis, rhinorrhea, cough, dyspnea, and wheezing after heavy exposure for brief periods, i.e., high dosages.

One of the most widely publicized forms of occupational asthma in recent times involved biologic enzymes incorporated into laundry detergents. In some industries,

enzymes of *Bacillus subtilis* were added to laundry detergents to facilitate biodegradation of the product. Allergic reactions rapidly developed, and an outbreak of asthmalike symptoms occurred in industrial workers and consumers alike. In addition to bacterial enzymes, medicinal enzymes used for replacement therapy, such as pancreatic enzymes and pituitary preparations as well as pepsin and trypsin, have all produced respiratory symptoms in workers who prepare the compounds. The mechanism appears to be immunologic in nature.

Exposure to organic proteins in the sera, secretions, and/or dust from birds, insects, mammals, and fish is another major cause of occupational asthma. This form of asthma is most frequently seen in veterinary practice and in medical research. But, it also occurs in occupations as diverse as seafood processing, pesticide research, beekeeping, grain handling, and silkworm cutting. Insect dyes, such as carmine, can also produce occupational asthma in clothing manufacture, largely because of the development of IgE-reagenic sensitivity.

The diagnosis of occupational asthma is made on the basis of a careful and complete history, both of the patient's type of work and the work environment, including the materials used. It is also important to bear in mind that exposure to sensitizing chemicals, such as those in plastics, can occur in leisure or other non-work-related activity. A good clue to the diagnosis is the pattern of the patient's symptoms. For all but the immunologic reactions, the characteristic pattern is that the patient consistently develops wheezing, chest tightness, or cough, with or without sputum production or rhinitis, toward the end of the work shift. These manifestations tend to worsen during the night and then either improve, or resolve completely, by morning. Absence from work during weekends or vacation periods generally brings about a remission. The presence of similar patterns of symptoms in other employees is also helpful diagnostically.

The diagnosis of occupationally related asthma is readily confirmed by monitoring pulmonary function in the work environment. Identifying the responsible agent can occasionally be quite difficult. Frequently, some form of inhalational challenge test involving the suspected specific inducing agent may be needed.

Environment and Air Pollution

It is quite common for asthmatic subjects to volunteer that changes in the weather worsen their symptoms. The most frequent complaints about changes are cold and dampness. Although the effects of cold air on pulmonary function have been extensively studied, the role that cold air plays in nonexercise, weather-related exacerbations of asthma is unknown. In the main, the evidence linking weather and asthma is associative. For example, increases in hospital admission rates for asthmatic patients have been reported in the Netherlands and New York to coincide temporally with cold fronts or with sudden changes in ambient temperature. In Melbourne, Australia, and Birmingham, England, outbreaks of asthma have been associated with severe thunderstorms. The reasons for these epidemics are unknown, and although a number of causes have been suggested, few of them have been critically assessed.

Asthma can also be exacerbated by extremely high levels of air pollution. Levels of particulates or sulfur dioxide that exceed 100 μg/m^3 have been associated with an increase in both mortality and morbidity in patients with pulmonary disease. This degree of air pollution is encountered in heavy industrial, densely populated, urban areas. Often it is associated with thermal inversions or other causes of stagnant air masses. In this circumstance, although the general population often develops respiratory symptoms, patients with asthma and other respiratory diseases tend to be very severely affected. The most notable examples of this phenomenon are the killer smogs that occurred in the Meuse Valley in Belgium in 1930; Donora, Pennsylvania, in 1948; and London, England, in 1952. Epidemics of asthma also occurred in the Tokyo-Yokohama Basin in Japan in the late 1960s. Since the development and enforcement of clean air standards, such epidemics have all but disappeared.

The more important pollutants seem to be sulfur dioxide, ozone, and nitrogen dioxide. These compounds derive from either the incomplete combustion of fossil fuels from industrial or other sources leading to the formation of an SO_2-particulate complex or to photochemical reactions involving ultraviolet radiation from sunlight acting on atmospheric hydrocarbons or nitrogen oxides from automobile emissions to produce high-energy oxidants. The two processes are not mutually exclusive, and both can be operative in the same area. The components of the SO_2-particulate complex are di- and trioxides of sulfur, sulfuric acid, nitrogen dioxide, carbon monoxide, and particulates. This type of pollution is usually found in large industrial areas, particularly near smelters or factories that burn high-sulfur oil or coal. The major pollutant produced as the result of atmospheric photochemical reactions is ozone, but nitric oxide and other oxidants are also present. Typically, the type of atmospheric condition conducive to photochemical reactions is encountered in areas with a sunny climate and a heavy concentration of automobiles; the result is the usual Los Angeles smog.

Sulfur oxides and particulates are the most common form of air pollution. Sulfur dioxide is a highly irritating gas. As a rule, atmospheric concentrations range between 0.01 and 0.1 ppm; in times of major pollution, peak concentrations may reach 1 to 1.5 ppm. Respiratory disturbances do not typically occur in normal individuals unless the ambient concentration is substantially above 1 ppm by volume. Although concentrations of this magnitude are

uncommon in most urban areas, as indicated above they do occur in some industrial environments. Asthmatics appear to be far more reactive to SO_2 than are healthy people. However, the results of epidemiologic studies concerning sulfur dioxide as a major aggravating stimuli for asthma have been inconclusive.

The physiological effects of SO_2 can be reduced by resorting to nasal breathing. The gas is highly soluble, and passage through the nose can scrub a considerable fraction of it. The combination of breathing cold air and low doses of SO_2 causes more airway obstruction than does either stimulus alone. The mechanism by which sulfur dioxide produces bronchoconstriction is unknown. The possibility of mast cell involvement has been suggested by studies indicating that pretreatment with large doses of disodium cromoglycate attenuates the airway effects of subsequent exposure to sulfur dioxide.

Ozone is another fairly common form of outdoor pollution, particularly in the western and southwestern regions of the United States. Unlike sulfur dioxide, ozone affects healthy people almost as severely as it does asthmatics. The consequences of ozone exposure are slower to develop than those of sulfur dioxide, and they persist longer. In severe pollution, the concentration can reach 1.0 ppm. Single exposures at higher concentrations for 2 to 3 h induce mild degrees of bronchoconstriction that may last for 24 h. Ozone also increases nonspecific bronchial reactivity in atopic and nonatopic individuals. Adaptation and desensitization to ozone do occur. Typically, the adaptation is short-lived, so that it cannot be relied on for protection against the injurious effects of this agent. Recent observations in animals indicate that ozone has the capability of causing the airway epithelium of a number of animal species to produce prostaglandins and leukotriene precursors, raising the possibility that its effects may be mediated through inflammatory mechanisms.

Two of the most important indoor air pollutants are carbon monoxide and nitrogen dioxide. Indoors, these gases are emitted by gas- and woodburning stoves and space heaters. Elevated concentrations in ambient air occur when air exchange rates are low. Carbon monoxide is by far the most lethal of the two but has no special untoward effects in asthmatics. Nitrogen dioxide is an oxidant like ozone and can readily form acids such as SO_2. However, the effect of this gas on pulmonary function is unclear.

Pharmacologic Stimuli

The pharmacologic agents most commonly associated with the induction of acute episodes of asthma are aspirin, drug additives such as tartrazine, and food preservatives such as metabisulfite. The typical aspirin-sensitive respiratory syndrome usually begins with perennial vasomotor rhinitis that is followed by hyperplastic rhinosinusitis and nasal polyps. Progressive asthma then appears. On exposure to aspirin, affected individuals typically develop ocular and nasal congestion and acute, often severe, episodes of airway obstruction. The reaction usually occurs within $\frac{1}{2}$ to 3 h after ingestion of standard doses of aspirin and can last for many hours thereafter. The prevalence of aspirin sensitivity in asthmatic subjects varies from report to report: values from 3 to 19 percent have been reported in the literature with an average of 10 percent. This disease is primarily seen in adults, but also occurs in children. In addition to aspirin, there is a great deal of cross reactivity with other nonsteroidal anti-inflammatory compounds including indomethacin (Indocin), fenoprofen (Nalfon), naproxen (Naprosyn), zomepirac (Zomax), ibuprofen (Motrin), mefenamic acid (Ponstel), and phenylbutazone (Butazolidin). Acetaminophen sodium salicylate, choline salicylate, salicylamide, and propoxyphene seem to be well tolerated.

Patients with aspirin sensitivity can be desensitized and made refractory to the adverse effects of aspirin by the daily administration of the drug. The mechanism responsible for the desensitization is not understood. The loss of response can last from 2 to 5 days, but aspirin sensitivity recurs if the daily administration of aspirin is discontinued. Desensitization to aspirin or indomethacin also produces cross tolerance to other nonsteroidal anti-inflammatory agents.

Asthmatics with aspirin sensitivity may also cross-react to various types of dyes used in food coloring and industry. The most common dye known to have this effect is tartrazine, or yellow dye no. 5. The exact frequency of tartrazine sensitivity is unsettled: reports varying from less than 10 up to 80 percent have appeared in the literature. Sensitivity to tartrazine and other dyes seems never to occur alone but always as a complication of aspirin-sensitive asthma. Tartrazine and other potentially troublesome additives are present in many medications used to treat airway and nasal diseases and may be unwittingly administered to sensitive individuals.

The mechanism by which aspirin and dyes produce bronchospasm is unknown. One popular theory holds that the inhibition of the cyclooxygenase pathway of arachidonic acid by aspirin and other nonsteroidal anti-inflammatory drugs leads to a decrease in prostaglandin production and a concomitantly greater production of leukotrienes. This hypothesis is unlikely to be the sole explanation since it does not explain why cyclooxygenase inhibition affects only some asthmatic subjects but not all.

Another insidious form of drug-induced bronchospasm is caused by sulfite ingestion. Sulfites are widely used as sanitizing and preservative agents, and the compounds commonly employed for this purpose include potassium metabisulfite, potassium bisulfite, sodium bisulfite, sodium sulfite, and sulfur dioxide. These chemicals are extensively used in the fast-food and restaurant

industry and can be found in a wide variety of food substances as preservatives including salads, fresh fruits, potatoes, wine, and shellfish. Sulfiting agents are also widely employed in the pharmaceutical industry so that sulfites are contained in some intravenous solutions, analgesics, cardiovascular drugs, cyclotropic agents, and solutions of bronchodilators administered via aerosol nebulization. The mechanism by which sulfiting agents produce asthma is unknown.

In the last several years, a number of asthmatic- and anaphylacticlike reactions have been documented after exposure to sulfites. Most often, these reactions have occurred in restaurants featuring salad bars, where sulfites were used on the ingredients to keep them fresh. However, these reactions are not confined to restaurants. For example, severe bronchospastic episodes have been observed in patients using parenteral medications, aerosolized bronchodilators, and ophthalmologic topical solutions containing metabisulfite. A cardinal diagnostic feature for sulfite-induced bronchospasm is the onset of respiratory symptoms soon after a meal or after the consumption of beer or wine. The diagnosis can be confirmed in the laboratory by determining pulmonary function before and after a controlled exposure to the offending agent.

Asthma can also be aggravated by β-blocking drugs. Nonselective β blockers, such as propranolol, readily produce airway obstruction not only in asthmatics but also in their first-degree relatives and in some patients with hay fever. To avoid this complication, β_1-selective blockers have been developed. Although these agents generally do not elicit respiratory complaints when they are used in low dosage, adverse responses still occur when the dose is increased or when these agents are given to extremely sensitive patients. In some patients, minute exposures, such as the topical use of ophthalmologic solutions containing the selective β_1 drug, timolol, have sufficed to precipitate an attack of asthma.

Psychological Factors

The role played by psychological factors in the induction of acute airway obstruction in susceptible individuals has been recognized since the early seventeenth century when van Helmont described an episode of asthma following a period of emotional turmoil:*

> A citizen being by a Peer openly disgraced and injured, unto him he might not utter a Word without the fear of the utmost Ruine; in silence dissembles and bears the reproach, but straight away after an Asthma arises.

In fact, the notion that asthma was a psychological disease gained such wide acceptance that by the late nine-

* van Helmont JB: *Oriatrike or Physick Refined.* London, Lodowick Lloyd, 1662.

teenth and early twentieth centuries William Osler wrote in his textbook of medicine that asthma was primarily of psychological origin.

Abundant data now exist to show that psychological factors can interact with the asthmatic diathesis to worsen, or ameliorate, the disease process in perhaps 50 percent of the patients. However, it is extremely unusual for psychological factors to be the sole trigger. Psychological stimuli appear to exert their effects via vagal efferent activity. Suggestion seems to be an important influence in some asthmatics. Given the right suggestion, reactive individuals increase or decrease appropriately the pharmacologic effects of adrenergic or cholinergic stimuli on the airways. The extent to which psychological factors participate in the induction or the continuation of any given exacerbation of asthma is unknown. Undoubtedly, it varies from patient to patient and in the same patient from episode to episode.

PATHOPHYSIOLOGY

No matter which of the above stimuli incites an acute episode of asthma, once the attack begins characteristic changes occur in the pulmonary mechanical and gas-exchanging properties of the lungs; virtually all aspects of pulmonary function are affected. Asthma alters pulmonary flow-resistance properties, pressure-volume relationships, pulmonary elasticity, chest wall mechanics, distribution of ventilation, and ventilation-perfusion relationships.

Pulmonary Mechanics

During an acute episode of asthma, airway resistance increases markedly. The increase in airway resistance is caused by contraction of bronchial smooth muscle and by luminal narrowing produced by a combination of mucosal edema and retention of secretions. The pathophysiological expression of these pathologic changes is a prolongation of forced expiratory time, a low vital capacity, a marked depression of forced expiratory volumes and flow rates, and hyperinflation that is accompanied by derangements in chest wall geometry and respiratory muscle activity. The degree of abnormality present in each of these measurements is quite variable and depends on the severity of the attack. However, on the average, the best preserved index is the forced vital capacity (FVC). Next in decreasing order are the 1-s forced expiratory volume (FEV_1), flow rates determined high in the vital capacity, and then flow rates low in the vital capacity (Fig. 79-3). When a patient presents for treatment, the FVC can be expected to be about 50 percent of predicted, the FEV_1 to average between 30 and 35 percent of predicted, and the flow rates to be 20 percent or less. In absolute terms, the

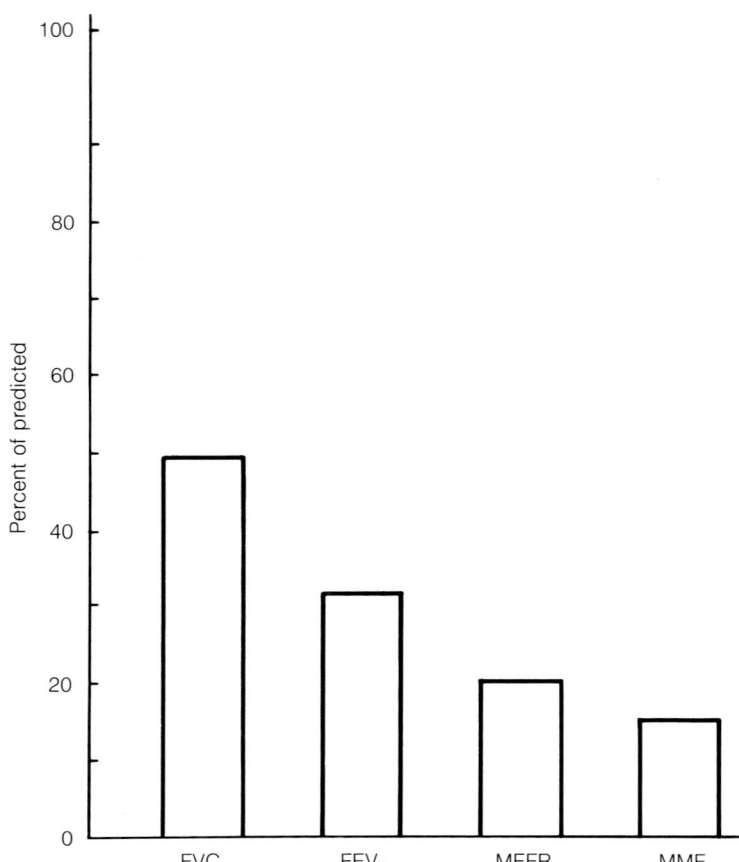

FIGURE 79-3 Pattern of spirographic abnormalities associated with acute episodes of asthma. MEFR = maximum expiratory flow rate; MMF = maximum mid-expiratory flow. *(From McFadden, 1983.)*

FEV_1 tends to be around 1 L and the peak flow about 2.5 L/s.

In addition to intraluminal obstruction during an acute attack of asthma, the airways seem to become unstable and dynamic airway collapse is accentuated, causing distal airways to close at higher volumes and lower transmural pressures than normal and at points closer to the alveoli. In some individuals, airway closure may occur even during tidal breathing, and during very severe episodes, the airflows that the patients manage to accomplish during quiet respiration may actually equal the maximum flow rates that they can achieve.

Marked alterations in lung volumes often accompany the changes in the flow-resistive properties. While the symptoms are acute, the residual volume (RV) and the functional residual capacity (FRC) tend to be markedly increased whereas the total lung capacity (TLC) remains normal or nearly so. In patients presenting for urgent treatment in the emergency room, the average values for FRC and RV are of the order of 200 and 400 percent of predicted, respectively.

Speaking teleologically, the increase in lung volumes in acute asthma, and the concomitant enlargement of the airway calibers, can be regarded as a mechanism for offsetting the intrinsic obstruction of the airways. However, there is a limit to this sort of gain in that the more the lungs are inflated, the more difficult it becomes to inflate them further: as the resistive work of breathing decreases on one hand, the elastic work increases on the other.

The mechanisms responsible for hyperinflation in asthma are unknown. Part of the increase in RV is undoubtedly due to premature airway closure. More difficult to explain are the changes in FRC. Since there is often a decrease in elastic recoil in asthma and a change in chest wall configuration, the increase in FRC might be explained simply on a mechanical basis. Thus, because the lungs are viscoelastic, they are readily deformed. However, as they are stretched more and more, it becomes increasingly difficult to inflate them further. Therefore, simply conducting respiration at higher lung volumes would increase the elastic work of breathing. To offset this, some asthmatics have the ability to change reversibly the elastic properties of the lung so that the pressure-volume characteristics shift upward and to the left. As a result, for any given volume the elastic pressures necessary to effect respiration decrease. Originally, this phenomenon was thought to be the result of stress relaxation, presumably related to prolonged overdistention of terminal alveoli. However, these changes in elasticity have since been shown to occur acutely after various types of provocation. The mechanism responsible for the reversible change in elastic properties remains enigmatic.

In the past, dynamic factors have also come under suspicion. Since expiration is prolonged because of the increased resistance to flow, the time for expelling a normal amount of air may be insufficient so that the FRC would increase until a new balance was struck between the frequency of respiration and the degree of obstruction. Although dynamic forces may play a role, it now seems that their contribution is minor.

Another factor contributing to the increase in FRC is persistence of inspiratory intercostal and accessory muscle activity during expiration. Normally these muscles are activated only during inspiration when they work together with the diaphragm to generate the pleural pressures necessary for air to flow into the thorax. During acute asthma, the chest wall is held in the inspiratory position by the active use of inspiratory muscles, thereby maximizing patency of the airways while minimizing resistive work. This increased load may contribute to the sensation of dyspnea and place affected individuals at increased risk of developing respiratory muscle fatigue and respiratory failure.

Pulmonary Gas Exchange

In the normal lungs, the distribution of incoming air is heavily influenced by the distribution of time constants,

i.e., by the product of the resistance of a particular airway and the compliance of alveoli that it subtends. In normal lungs, the distribution of the time constants within the lungs is about the same everywhere so that virtually all alveoli tend to fill and empty synchronously. During an attack of asthma, obstruction to airflow is nonuniformly scattered throughout the lungs, causing the time constants to become widely disparate. If the increased airflow resistance in asthma were uniformly distributed throughout the tracheobronchial tree, the alveoli would continue to fill and empty synchronously although on a slower time base. This is not the case.

Both in acute episodes of asthma and during recovery, maldistribution of inspired air is such that large segments of the lungs receive a very small fraction of each incoming breath while small segments receive most of the air. The overall result is that a relatively small number of alveolar units are *hyperventilated* with respect to their perfusion, giving rise to hypocapnia and a large physiological dead space while a very large number of alveoli are being *hypoventilated* with respect to their perfusion, giving rise to hypoxemia and widening of the alveolar-pulmonary venous difference in Pa_{O_2}. The net effect on the oxygenation of systemic arterial blood depends upon the algebraic sum of the O_2 contents of pulmonary venous blood leaving the hypo- and hyperventilating areas of the lungs (see Chapter 13).

The most common pattern of arterial blood-gas abnormalities in acute asthma is a combination of hypoxemia, hypocapnia, and respiratory alkalosis. Virtually all asthmatic patients develop arterial hypoxemia during acute exacerbations. As a rule and within limits, the more se-

vere the obstruction, the lower the arterial Pa_{O_2} (Fig. 79-4). For example, in patients at sea level, it is extremely unusual for the arterial Pa_{O_2} to fall below 50 mmHg during an uncomplicated attack of asthma. However, when arterial hypoxemia is more marked, airflow limitation is apt to be exceedingly severe. In most acute exacerbations, the oxyhemoglobin saturation remains normal, or near normal, because of a shift in the oxyhemoglobin dissociation curve induced by alkalosis.

Seventy to seventy-five percent of asthmatics who visit an emergency room have hypocarbia and respiratory alkalosis (Fig. 79-5). Usually the degree of hypocarbia is not severe and the arterial Pa_{CO_2} is in the low 30s. When airway obstruction is severe ($FEV_1 = 0.5$ L, or 15 to 20 percent of predicted), arterial Pa_{CO_2} tends to normalize; should the obstruction progress (FEV_1 less than 15 percent of predicted), hypercapnia begins to occur. Typically, the hypercarbia is modest, with values for Pa_{CO_2} ranging between 50 and 55 mmHg. In the emergency room, normocarbia is found in about 20 percent of the patients, whereas hypercarbia and respiratory acidosis are found in about 10 percent or fewer.

A metabolic acidosis sometimes occurs in asthma, usually when the disease is very severe. It is more common in children than adults. It is caused by lactic acidosis secondary to impaired O_2 delivery or utilization in peripheral tissues. Metabolic acidosis can also be caused by excessive use of sympathomimetics to treat the acute episode.

The abnormalities in gas exchange in very severe episodes of acute asthma are substantially less than those observed in the respiratory failure of other forms of

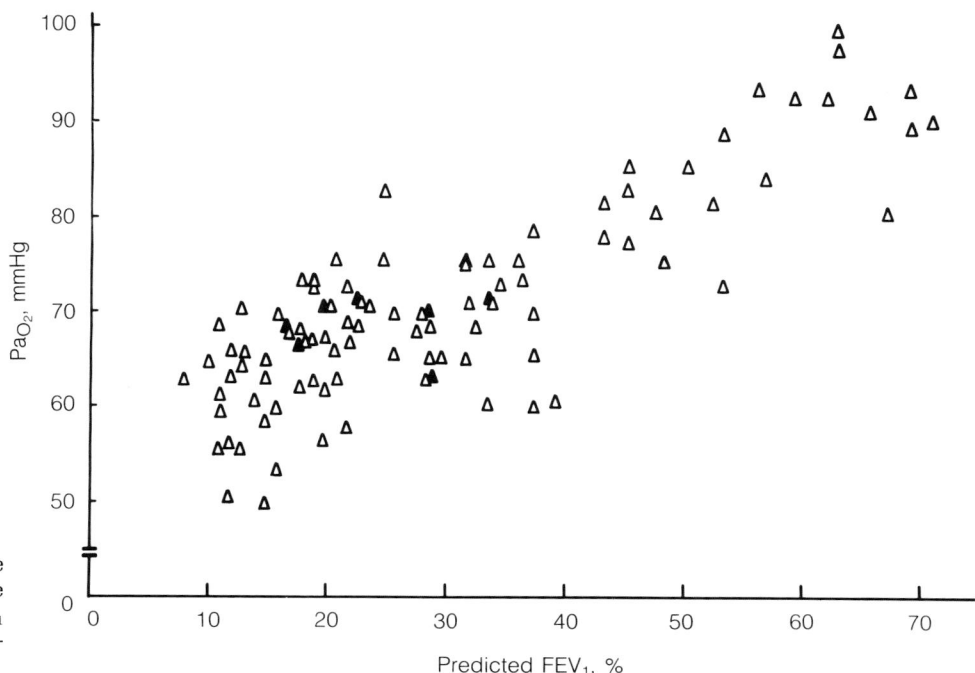

FIGURE 79-4 The relationship between the arterial oxygen tension (Pa_{O_2}) and the degree of airway obstruction as measured by FEV_1 during acute episodes of asthma. *(From McFadden and Lyons, 1968.)*

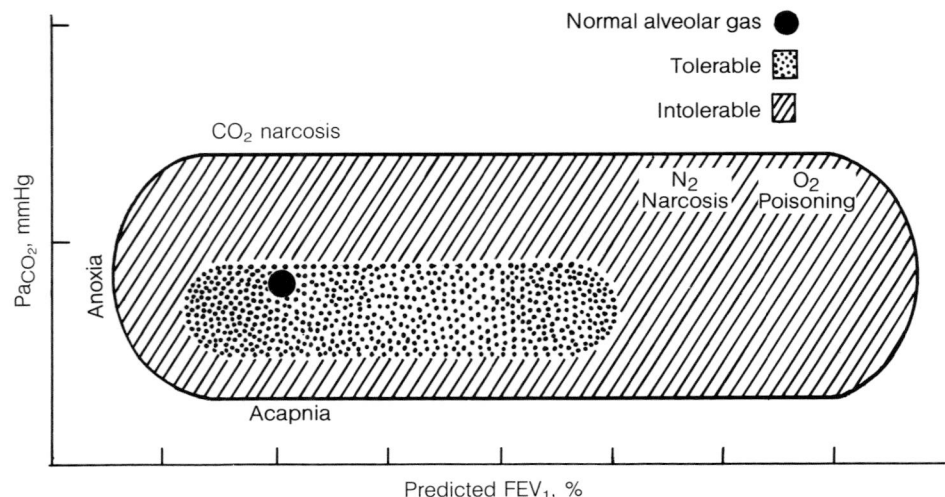

FIGURE 79-5 The relationship between arterial carbon dioxide tension (Pa_{CO_2}) and the degree of airway obstruction as measured by FEV_1 during acute episodes of asthma. *(From McFadden and Lyons, 1968.)*

chronic obstructive airways disease: whereas values for Pa_{O_2} of between 40 to 50 mmHg and for Pa_{CO_2} greater than 55 mmHg are unusual even in status asthmaticus, values for Pa_{O_2} less than 30 mmHg and for Pa_{CO_2} greater than 60 mmHg are the rule in patients with chronic respiratory failure. However, although usually modest, the changes in Pa_{O_2} in asthma respond slowly to treatment: arterial hypoxemia and widened alveolar-arterial differences in Pa_{O_2} often continue for several weeks following a single episode of the disease.

Cardiac Function

In addition to altering the mechanical and gas-exchanging properties of the lung, the acute airways obstruction of asthma can also compromise cardiac function. A number of reversible electrocardiographic abnormalities can occur, including sinus tachycardia, premature ventricular contractions, P pulmonale, right axis deviation, right bundle branch block, clockwise rotation, and right ventricular strain patterns; nonspecific ST-T changes have also been observed. In general, the more severe the airways obstruction and the more abnormal the blood gases and electrolytes, the more likely is the patient to have one or more of these electrocardiographic abnormalities.

Severe episodes of asthma are often accompanied by pulsus paradoxus, i.e., widening of the respiratory variations in blood pressure. As a rule, the decrease in blood pressure with respiration is small, averaging about 8 to 10 mmHg; a decrease in blood pressure greater than 15 mmHg occurs in fewer than 20 percent of the patients. Typically, the greater the airways obstruction, the greater the pulsus paradoxus. The development of pulsus paradoxus during acute exacerbations of asthma is attributable to marked swings in intrathoracic pressure. These swings in intrathoracic pressure induce cyclic changes in stroke volume by altering left ventricular preload. Other contrib-

utory factors may be a reduction in the size of the left ventricular cavity by a subtle shift of the ventricular septum into the left ventricle during inspiration and an increase in left ventricular afterload secondary to an increase in transmural left ventricular pressures (see Chapter 68).

Clinical-Physiological Correlates

The physical signs associated with acute airways obstruction are tachycardia, tachypnea, wheezing, increases in the anterior-posterior diameter of the thorax, the use of the accessory muscles of respiration, pulsus paradoxus, and diaphoresis. The last three signs are particularly useful manifestations of severe airways obstruction. Nonetheless, the absence of either accessory muscle use or pulsus paradoxus does not rule out the presence of major airflow limitation. To be evident clinically, these signs require the development of large negative swings in intrathoracic pressure during respiration. Consequently, if a person is breathing rapidly and shallowly, the pressure swings may not suffice to elicit these signs. Because they share a common pathogenesis, pulsus paradoxus and the use of the accessory muscles of respiration usually coexist.

In the patient requesting emergency therapy for asthma, the pulse rate is usually of the order of 100 beats per minute and the respiratory frequency between 25 to 28 breaths per minute. However, heart rates in excess of 120 per minute and breathing frequencies greater than 30 per minute are not uncommon.

In response to appropriate therapy administered aggressively, acutely ill individuals tend to cease rapidly to complain of breathlessness and wheezing. The use of the accessory muscles and the pulsus paradoxus also tend to remit quickly. However, other signs of asthma, such as rhonchi and wheezing, tend to linger without a constant relationship to the patients' symptoms. In fact, in many

patients who consider themselves to be asymptomatic, physical examination reveals that they are still wheezing.

Most signs and symptoms in the asthmatic patient cannot be counted on to parallel the changes in pulmonary function. For example, at a time when the patient believes that the asthmatic attack is over, even though pulmonary mechanics will be significantly better than before treatment, they will still be quite abnormal. At this juncture, the FEV_1 typically averages 50 percent of predicted, whereas the RV is approximately 200 percent. When the signs of asthma have dissipated, and the patient has clear lungs to auscultation, forced expiratory volumes, flow volumes, and residual volume will still be grossly abnormal. Under these circumstances, the FEV_1 tends to be between 60 and 70 percent of predicted and the RV 150 to 160 percent of predicted. Flow rates in the mid-vital capacity will usually be only 30 to 40 percent of normal; this abnormality often persists for a long time in the face of aggressive therapy.

These data indicate that one cannot rely on the loss of subjective complaints, or even the sign of wheezing, as indicating that the lungs have returned to functional normalcy. Also, the end of a clinical episode of asthma is typically associated with a large residuum of obstructive airways disease. Since the residual obstruction encroaches on the patient's pulmonary reserve, the patient will tolerate poorly any further reductions in pulmonary function and be predisposed to an increase in the frequency and severity of attacks of asthma. For this reason, many clinics urge that treatment of each acute episode of asthma be continued until the patient has become functionally normal.

BIBLIOGRAPHY

Adelroth E, Morris MM, Hargreave FE, O'Byrne PM: Airway responsiveness to leukotrienes C4 and D4 and to methacholine in patients with asthma and normal controls. N Engl J Med 315:480–484, 1986.
Leukotrienes C4 and D4 appear to be unique bronchoconstrictors with a possible role in the pathogenesis of asthma.

Barnes NC, Costello JF: Mast-cell-derived mediators in asthma. Arachidonic acid metabolites. Postgrad Med 76:140–151, 1984.
A review of the potential role of the cell membrane-related, lipid-derived mediators of immediate hypersensitivity in asthma.

Befus D: The role of the mast cell in allergic bronchospasm. Can J Physiol Pharmacol 65:435–441, 1987.
The role of mast cells in bronchoconstriction is complex and entails complex interactions with other cells of the airways.

Bernstein IL: Occupational asthma. Clin Chest Med 2:255–272, 1981.
An overview of occupational asthma from pathophysiological, etiologic, diagnostic, and therapeutic standpoints.

Cade JF, Woolcock AJ, Rebuck AS, Pain MC: Lung mechanics during provocation of asthma. Clin Sci 40:381–391, 1971.
A description of the alterations that develop in the pressure flow and volume characteristics of the lungs and airways during the development of, and recovery from, acute episodes of asthma.

Cuss FM, Barnes PJ: Airway smooth muscle and disease workshop: epithelial mediators. Am Rev Respir Dis 136:S32–S35, 1987.
A review of the various epithelial abnormalities observed in asthma that may lead, via different mechanisms, to increased bronchial hyperresponsiveness, a fundamental feature of asthma. The same issue of the journal contains other related review articles, e.g., inflammatory mediators.

Drazen JM, Boushey HA, Holgate ST, Kaliner M, O'Byrne P, Valentine M, Widdicombe JH, Woolcock A: The pathogenesis of severe asthma: a consensus report from the Workshop on Pathogenesis. J Allergy Clin Immunol 80:428–437, 1987.
A review of the mechanisms involved in causing severe asthma.

Ellis EF: Role of infection in asthma. Adv Asthma Allergy Pulmon Dis 4:28–33, 1977.
A consideration of the role of viral infections as exacerbating factors in asthma.

Fick RB Jr, Metzger WJ, Richerson HB, Zavala DC, Moseley PL, Schoderbek WE, Hunninghake GW: Increased bronchovascular permeability after allergen exposure in sensitive asthmatics. J Appl Physiol 63:1147–1155, 1987.
Based on bronchoalveolar lavage in humans, it is concluded that allergen exposure in sensitive asthmatics causes an acute increase in bronchovascular permeability to serum proteins.

Freedman S, Tattersfield AE, Pride NB: Changes in lung mechanics during asthma induced by exercise. J Appl Physiol 38:974–982, 1975.
> *This paper, together with that of McFadden and Lyons (1969) and Cade et al. (1971), provides a comprehensive overview of the changes in the pressure, flow, and volume characteristics of the lungs and airways during the development of, and recovery from, acute episodes of asthma.*

Frigas E, Gleich GJ: The eosinophil and the pathophysiology of asthma. J Allergy Clin Immunol 77:527–537, 1986.
> *The hypothesis is advanced that the eosinophil mediates damage to the respiratory epithelium and is the prime effector cell in the pathophysiology of asthma.*

Gilbert IA, Fouke JM, McFadden ER Jr: Intra-airway thermodynamics during exercise and hyperventilation in asthmatics. J Appl Physiol (in press).
> *Exercise and hyperventilation produce identical thermal profiles within the airways of asthmatics. Therefore, these stimuli can be used interchangeably to study exercise-induced asthma.*

Godfrey S: Controversies in the pathogenesis of exercise-induced asthma. Eur J Respir Dis 68:81–88, 1986.
> *Exercise-induced asthma is considered in terms of the stimulus, the intermediary pathway, and the response. Various controversies about each of these components are discussed.*

Greenberger PA, Patterson R: Allergic bronchopulmonary aspergillosis. Model of bronchopulmonary disease with defined serologic, radiologic, pathologic and clinical findings from asthma to fatal destructive lung disease. Chest 91:165S–171S, 1987.
> *A review of allergic bronchopulmonary aspergillosis, a complication of asthma, that results in immunologic lung destruction.*

Haltom JR, Strunk RC: Pathogenesis of exercise-induced asthma: Implications for treatment. Ann Rev Med 37:143–148, 1986.
> *Current concepts of the pathogenetic mechanisms of exercise-induced asthma are reviewed along with implications for treatment of this condition.*

Hargreave FE, Ryan G, Thomson NC, O'Byrne PM, Latimer K, Juniper EF, Dolovich J: Bronchial responsiveness to histamine or methacholine in asthma: Measurement and clinical significance. J Allergy Clin Immunol 68:348–355, 1981.
> *A review of the authors' experience with the measurement of nonspecific airway reactivity. The article describes methodology, interpretation of data, interrelationships among tests, and how changes in airway responsiveness correlate with fluctuations in the clinical features of asthma.*

Hetzel MR, Clark TJ, Branthwaite MA: Asthma: Analysis of sudden deaths and ventilatory arrests in hospital. Br Med J 1:808–811, 1977.
> *The incidence of episodes of unexpected ventilatory arrest, some of which led to sudden death, was studied in 1169 consecutive hospital admissions for asthma.*

International symposium on special problems and management of allergic athletes. J Allergy Clin Immunol 73(Suppl):629–748, 1984.
> *A compendium of papers that deals with airway reactivity and exercise-induced asthma. Many of the current areas of controversy are highlighted.*

Knowles GK, Clark TJH: Pulsus paradoxus as a valuable sign indicating severity of asthma. Lancet 2:1356–1359, 1973.
> *The presence of pulsus paradoxus during acute episodes of asthma heralds severe airway obstruction.*

Martin J, Powell E, Shore S, Emrich J, Engel LA: The role of respiratory muscles in the hyperinflation of bronchial asthma. Am Rev Respir Dis 121:441–447, 1980.
> *Describes the effect of persistent inspiratory intercostal and accessory muscle activity during expiration on lung volumes in asthma.*

Mathison DA, Stevenson DD: Aspirin sensitivity in rhinosinusitis and asthma. Immunol Allergy Pract 5:17–26, 1983.
> *An overview of aspirin sensitivity.*

McFadden ER Jr: Asthma: Airway dynamics, cardiac function, and clinical correlates, in Middleton E, Reed CE, Ellis EF (eds), *Allergy Principles and Practice.* St. Louis, Mosby, 1983, pp 845–862.
> *The interplay between the heart and lungs and its clinical implications.*

McFadden ER Jr, Kiser R, DeGroot WJ: Acute bronchial asthma: Relations between clinical and physiologic manifestations. N Engl J Med 288:221–225, 1973.
> *Explores the manner and extent to which the symptoms of acute airway obstruction reflect the alterations in physiology.*

McFadden ER Jr, Lenner KA, Strohl KP: Postexertional airway rewarming and thermally induced asthma. New insights into pathophysiology and possible pathogenesis. J Clin Invest 78:18–25, 1986.
> *The severity of exercised-induced asthma depends not only on airway cooling but also on the rapidity and magnitude of airway rewarming immediately thereafter.*

McFadden ER Jr, Lyons HA: Arterial blood gas tensions in asthma. N Engl J Med 278:1027–1032, 1968.
> *A description of the changes that occur in arterial blood-gas tensions in adults and children during acute episodes of asthma.*

McFadden ER Jr, Lyons HA: Serial studies of factors influencing airway dynamics during recovery from acute asthma attacks. J Appl Physiol 27:452–459, 1969.
> *An account of the alterations that develop in the pressure flow and volume characteristics of the lungs and airways during the development of, and recovery from, acute episodes of asthma.*

Rebuck AS, Read J: Assessment and management of severe asthma. Am J Med 51:788–798, 1971.
> *The electrocardiographic and cardiac manifestations associated with acute episodes of asthma are described.*

Schwartz HJ: Observation on the uses and effects of sulfiting agents in foods and drugs. Immunol Allergy Pract 6:31–34, 1984.
> *A state-of-the-art review on the role of food preservatives as asthmogenic stimuli in asthmatics.*

Spykerboer JE, Donnelly WJ, Thong YH: Soc Sci Med 22:553–558, 1986. Parental knowledge and misconceptions about asthma: A controlled study.
> *The parents of 128 asthmatic children were interviewed about their knowledge and misconceptions of asthma. Two-thirds or more gave correct responses to questions about etiology and pathogenesis, pathophysiology, symptomatology, precipitants, and outcome of asthma.*

Weng TR, Langer HM, Featherby EA, Levison H: Arterial blood gas tensions and acid-base balance in symptomatic and asymptomatic asthma in childhood. Am Rev Respir Dis 101:274–282, 1970.
> *This paper, and that of McFadden and Lyons (1968), deals with the changes in arterial blood-gas tensions that occur in adults and children, respectively, during acute episodes of asthma.*

Chapter 80

Asthma: Acute and Chronic Therapy

E. R. McFadden, Jr.

How to best relieve and/or prevent the acute impediments to breathing induced by episodes of asthma has been debated since antiquity. Over the centuries, a number of remedies have materialized, each with a champion and each advocated as a panacea. Some, like the inhalation of fish oil or silver nitrate, quickly proved disappointing and disappeared. Others, such as the anticholinergic alkaloids and the forerunners of the adrenergic agonists, have not only withstood the test of time but have also prompted a search for new formulations or congeners with more ideal properties. Meanwhile, the continuing search for better and more selective therapeutic modalities has produced a bewildering array of nostrums. Only recently have the available medications begun to be evaluated critically and their relative effectiveness compared scientifically.

TREATMENT: GENERAL ASPECTS

The therapeutic aim in the treatment of acute asthma is threefold: relief of bronchospasm, mobilization of secretions, and maintenance of alveolar ventilation. The three goals are interdependent. They can also be readily satisfied by proper use of current medications.

Acute asthma calls for bronchodilators. Both the β-adrenergic agonists and the methylxanthines not only serve this purpose well, but they also increase ciliary transport by increasing the frequency of the ciliary beat, increase the amount of the protein in the secreted mucus, and increase the fluid on the surfaces of the airways. The old idea that adult asthmatics need fluid replacement to offset increased respiratory water losses or decreased mucous viscosity has not been backed by scientific data. It now seems that controlling the airways obstruction by administering appropriate therapy controls the problems in the mucociliary escalator.

In *chronic asthma*, airway responsiveness can be controlled by agents that presumably reduce airway inflammation.

Clinical Pharmacology

Five classes of drugs are useful in the treatment of asthma. Three of them, i.e., the adrenergic agonists and the methylxanthines noted above and the anticholinergics, are bronchodilators; these are used to relieve the symptoms of acute airways obstruction. The other two classes, the glucocorticoids and cromones, do not dilate the airways. Instead, they exert their effects by modulating the various components of acute and subacute inflammation.

Adrenergic Agonists

The adrenergic agonists, or sympathomimetics, are a group of compounds that mimic the effects of the adrenal medullary hormones and neurotransmitters of the sympathetic nervous system. Their chemical structure (catecholamines) is simple. They exert their effects at a biochemical level through the formation of cyclic adenosine monophosphate (cAMP). Because the interplay of cAMP and intracellular calcium flux is the natural modulator of the tone of airway smooth muscle, these agents are uniquely effective as bronchodilators.

The physiological effects of the adrenergic agonists are mediated by activation of α- and β-adrenergic receptors at cell surfaces. The α effect is thought to be of little therapeutic importance. The β effect can be subdivided into two components: β_1 and β_2; only the latter, with its increase in high-energy phosphate compounds in respiratory smooth muscle, is of major therapeutic use in relieving airway constriction. The β_1 effect is cardiac via a positive inotropic effect. Therefore, agents with only selective β_2 activity are ideal for dealing with acute bronchoconstriction.

Four classes of sympathomimetic agents are currently available for clinical use in the United States: the catecholamines, the resorcinols, the saligenins, and a new

form of "pro-drug" which is metabolized in vivo to its active state.

CATECHOLAMINES

The native catecholamines consist of dopamine, norepinephrine, and epinephrine. They are the neurotransmitters of the sympathetic nervous system. Each has profound effects on multiple organs, including the lungs. However, only epinephrine, which has mixed α, β_1, and β_2 effects, has proven to be efficacious clinically in the treatment of reversible airways obstruction. Synthetic derivatives of epinephrine have been formulated to be more selective in their actions. Among these are isoproterenol, isoetharine, rimiterol, and hexoprenaline (Fig. 80-1). Since isoproterenol has only β activity, it lacks some of the undesirable effects of epinephrine. But since it still has equal activity of β_1 and β_2 receptors and although it is quite effective as a bronchodilator, it is also a potent cardiac stimulant.

Isoetharine is a derivative of isoproterenol that has primarily β_2 activity. It is a far less potent bronchodilator but much more selective in its action. Rimiterol and hexoprenaline have similar pharmacologies to isoetharine but are unavailable in the United States. All drugs in this class have in common a 3,4-hydroxybenzene ring and an ethylamino side chain with a hydroxy group on the second carbon. They differ from each other mainly in the size of the terminal amino substitution. Because of their molecular configuration, the catechols are rapidly metabolized (on first pass) both intracellularly and in the gastrointestinal tract by nonspecific enzymes. Therefore, they have short half-lives and are not effective when given by mouth. As a group, the catecholamines are rapid-acting, potent bronchodilators, and isoproterenol is the standard to which other agents are compared with respect to their airway and cardiac effects. The chief disadvantages of these drugs are their short durations of action and their absolute, or relative, lack of β_2 selectivity.

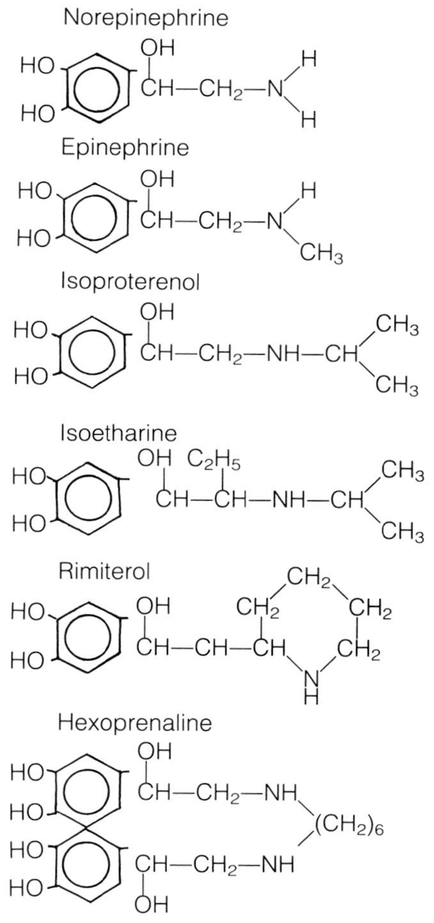

RESORCINOLS

In the search for longer-acting agents that have fewer cardiac side effects, the catechol nucleus has been replaced with a 3,5-hydroxybenzene ring (resorcinol) (Fig. 80-2), or substituted into at the 3-hydroxy position (saligenin) (Fig. 80-3); the bulk of the terminal amino substitution has also been increased. These structural modifications circumvent the metabolic pathways involved in the degradation of the catecholamines and have given rise to the long-acting drugs that have a high degree of airway selectivity and are effective by all routes of administration. The resorcinols in common use are metaproterenol, terbutaline, and fenoterol.

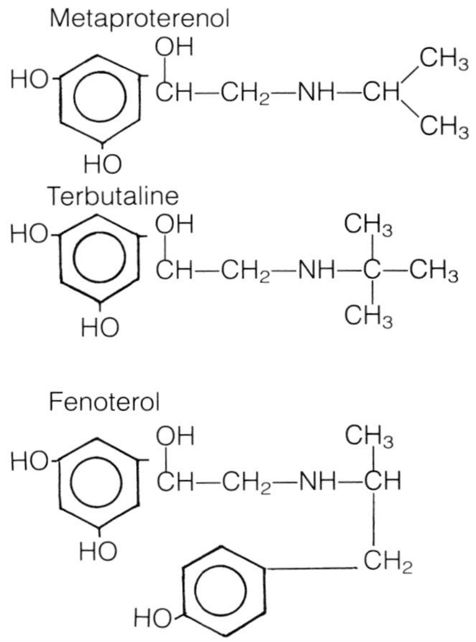

FIGURE 80-1 Chemical structures of the catecholamine bronchodilators. (From McFadden, 1981.)

FIGURE 80-2 Chemical structures of the resorcinol bronchodilators. (From McFadden, 1981.)

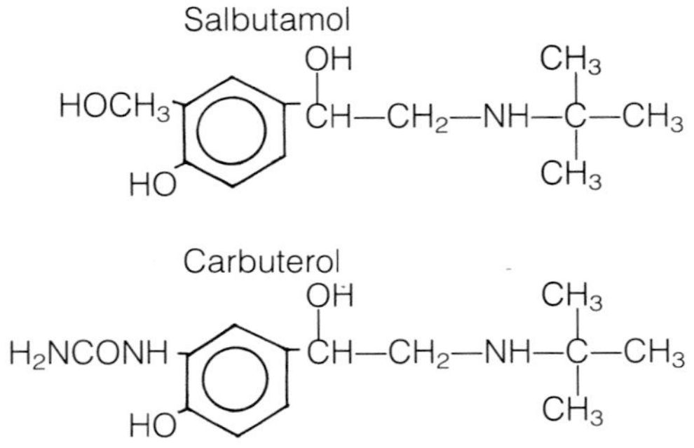

FIGURE 80-3 Chemical structures of the saligenin bronchodilators. *(From McFadden, 1981.)*

SALIGENIN

The only saligenin available in the United States as a relatively selective β_2 bronchodilator is albuterol. In most patients, its bronchodilating effects last longer than do those of isoproterenol, and it is less apt to elicit a serious tachycardia.

PRO-DRUGS

A fresh approach to sympathomimetic therapy has been the recent development of pro-drugs that remain inactive until they are metabolized. One example is bitolterol. This compound is a diester sympathomimetic that is cleaved to release the active catecholamine, colterol (Fig. 80-4). Because the level of esterase is greater in the lungs than in the heart, bitolterol is an effective bronchodilator without significant cardiac side effects.

CHOICE OF ADRENERGIC AGONIST

In practice, the choice of adrenergic agonist depends on the desired effect. The catecholamines achieve peak bronchodilatation within 5 min of inhalation but, depending on the dose, their effects are spent in 1 to 2 h. The noncatecholamines are somewhat slower in onset and achieve near maximum bronchodilatation within 10 to 15 min. However, their half-lives are quite long, varying from 3 to 6 h, again dose-dependent. Although the drugs differ distinctly, in experimental studies in animals with respect to their relative cardiostimulatory and bronchodilator effects, the results of human studies are less clear-cut. From a practical clinical standpoint, albuterol, terbutaline, and

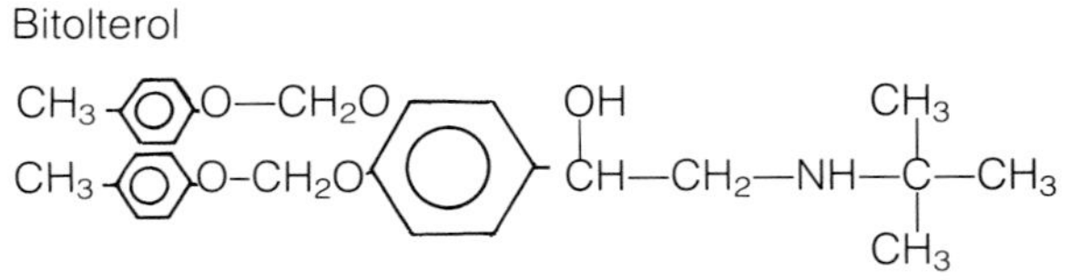

FIGURE 80-4 Chemical structure of bitolterol. *(From McFadden, 1986.)*

fenoterol are probably as potent as isoproterenol in relieving bronchospasm; bitolterol, metaproterenol, and the catecholamines are somewhat less effective. In terms of cardiac effects, isoproterenol is the most active, whereas isoetharine, rimiterol, and hexoprenaline (in therapeutic doses) tend not to cause obvious cardiovascular problems. Of the saligenins and resorcinols, metaproterenol has the greatest β_1 effects; fenoterol is next.

Terbutaline and albuterol are similar in their effects but somewhat more cardioselective than the others. The major side effects to their use as bronchodilators are tremors and palpitations and, to a lesser extent, metabolic disturbances. The development of a tremor is a specific β_2 effect. Its frequency is directly proportional to the dose of drug and, therefore, to amount of drug delivered to the skeletal muscles.

Although they are highly β_2-selective, none of the newer adrenergic agonists are totally devoid of cardiac stimulant properties. Like tremor, heart rate increases as the plasma levels of the drug increase. Therefore, large doses and oral routes of administration increase the incidence of cardiac side effects. Usually these drugs are well tolerated and the cardiac response, when present, is confined to a mild tachycardia. However, arrhythmias have been reported with terbutaline and albuterol, particularly in patients who have preexisting tendencies to cardiac irregularities.

Like the native catecholamines, the synthetic sympathomimetics can produce an increase in the blood concentrations of glucose, insulin, nonesterified free fatty acids, lactate, pyruvate, and ketones, and a decrease in serum potassium, phosphate, calcium, and magnesium. Typically, these metabolic effects are small and do not become manifest clinically. However, a metabolic acidosis can be induced by the excessive administration of these agents parenterally. Moreover, ketoacidosis has occasionally occurred in diabetic patients receiving these agents.

In general, the adverse effects of β-adrenergic agonists result from excessive sympathetic stimulation and disappear when the drugs are discontinued. Unlike the nonselective drugs of the past, the newer β_2 agents are quite safe. Deliberate or accidental ingestion of large quantities of albuterol or terbutaline, i.e., 20 to 30 times the usual daily oral dose, has occurred without fatality.

Methylxanthines

In one form or another, the methylxanthines, caffeine, theophylline, and theobromine, have been in continuous use in the treatment of airways obstruction for approximately 150 years. Theophylline is the most widely used. Its major pharmacologic action is to relax bronchial smooth muscle. This effect is most marked when the muscles are constricted. Like the β agonists, theophylline also improves contractility of the diaphragm, rendering it less suscepti-

ble to fatigue; it also accelerates mucociliary transport. Finally, by antagonizing the effects of adenosine on mast cells, it reduces mediator release.

THEOPHYLLINE

This is a medium potency drug, the bronchodilating activity of which is proportional, over the range of 3 to 25 μg/ml, to the logarithm of the serum concentration. The degree of improvement in lung function is small, at levels less than 10 μg/ml; the incidence of serious side effects increases at levels above 25. Therefore, the therapeutic range is usually taken to be 10 to 20 μg/ml.

The mechanism responsible for the bronchodilator effect of theophylline is unknown. Although it has been assumed that theophylline increases the intracellular levels of cyclic adenosine monophosphate by inhibiting phosphodiesterase, this hypothesis is now being contested: phosphodiesterase activity is not reduced at concentrations of theophylline that are achieved with the usual therapeutic doses; also, other phosphodiesterase inhibitors are not bronchodilators.

Until recently, it was generally held that the absorption of theophylline from the gastrointestinal tract was erratic owing to its poor solubility in water. However, the advent of reliable serum assays has shown that the drug is rapidly and completely absorbed from both liquid and plain, uncoated tablet preparation. Indeed, enteric coating, intended to promote uniform absorption from the gastrointestinal tract, decreases the dissolution of tablets and can cause serum levels to vary erratically. Absorption is slowed but still complete when sustained release formulations are used. Absorption may be slower at night so that predose levels in the morning are higher than those at night. This effect is most marked when sustained release formulations are used but does occur with other formulations as well. However, the importance of this phenomenon clinically is not yet established.

There is considerable intra- and intersubject variability in the absorption and clearance of theophylline. In adult volunteers and in moderately ill asthmatics, plasma half-lives for theophylline vary between 2 and 11.5 h (Fig. 80-5). Variations of similar magnitude also occur in children. In general, the "rapid eliminators" require larger doses and more frequent administration of the agent to achieve the desired therapeutic effect.

In addition to the intrinsic variability described above, theophylline clearance is decreased importantly in a variety of circumstances and populations: neonates, the elderly, those with acute and chronic hepatic dysfunction, and those undergoing congestive heart failure. Clearance also decreases during febrile illnesses. Conversely, theophylline clearance increases in children, cigarette smokers, users of marijuana, and those ingesting a high carbohydrate-low protein diet. In each of the situations

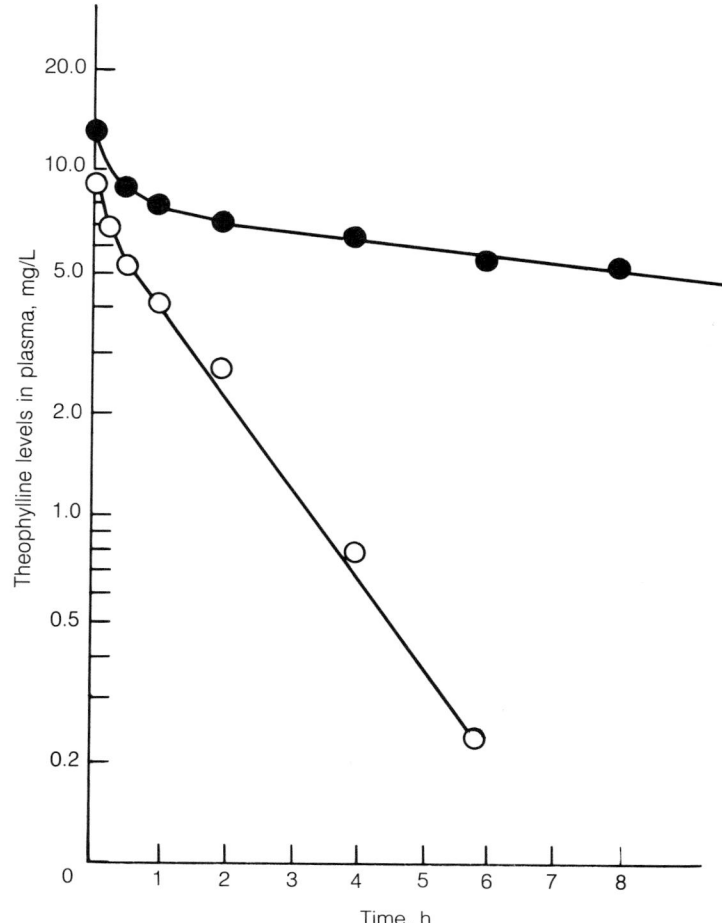

FIGURE 80-5 Examples of extremes of theophylline kinetics. ● = child, 8 years old, 38.8 kg; $t_{\frac{1}{2}} \cong 10$ h. ○ = child, 7 years old, 21.4 kg; $t_{\frac{1}{2}} \cong 1.6$ h. *(Based on data in Ellis, Koysooko, Levy, 1976.)*

noted above, dosage requirements fall and rise in accord with the changes in theophylline clearance. Concurrent medications also influence elimination: clearance is decreased by the macrolide antibiotics (erythromycin and troleandomycin), allopurinol, cimetidine, and propranolol. It increases with phenobarbital and phenytoin, or any other agents that induce the formation of hepatic enzyme.

PREPARATIONS

For the long-term management of reversible airways obstruction, both rapid and sustained release formulations of theophylline are available. The choice of product depends on the therapeutic goal. To treat acute symptoms, a rapidly absorbed preparation, such as uncoated tablets or liquids, is recommended. However, for chronic prophylaxis, the use of these formulations would entail unduly wide fluctuations in, and the need for, unacceptably short dosing intervals. For example, in individuals in whom elimination kinetics are rapid, it is often exceedingly diffi-

cult to maintain blood concentrations of the agent at therapeutic levels even when intervals between doses are as
short as 6 h; moreover, in keeping with the swings in
blood levels, the patients often manifest cyclic symptoms
of over- and underdosage. To overcome this problem, a
number of sustained release formulations have been developed for chronic prophylaxis. These compounds improve time-concentration profiles and diminish the variation between peak and trough serum levels, thereby
enabling longer intervals between doses. In the last several years, dosage schedules have been reduced progressively from every 6 to 8 to 12 h to once per 24 h. The
obvious advantage of the sustained release compounds is
improved patient compliance and, thereby, better control
of symptoms.

In using sustained release preparations, the dose of
medication is adjusted according to the patient's clinical
response and the blood levels of theophylline. Since a
minimum of three to four half-lives is required for a
steady state to be reached, theophylline levels are determined only after 3 to 4 days of therapy and then only in
order to ensure proper timing of the dose. As a rule, random samples do not give very useful information. When
twice a day compounds are used, bloods are drawn 4 to
6 h postdose to determine the peak level and 10 to 12 h
postdose to determine the nadir. Based on this information, dosage adjustment is easily accomplished. Thereafter, if the patient fares well, periodic monitoring of the
trough level is all that is required.

The side effects of theophylline are nervousness, nausea, vomiting, anorexia, abdominal discomfort, and headache. Increasing plasma levels tend to be associated with
increasing clinical manifestations. Approximately 1 percent of children and 4 percent of adults are unable to tolerate the drug even at very low plasma levels. The risk of
serious toxic effects such as seizures and cardiac arrhythmias increases when the plasma levels exceed 30 μg/ml.
Theophylline also increases the secretion of gastric acid.

Anticholinergics

The anticholinergic drugs, atropine sulfate, atropine
methylnitrate, and ipratropium bromide, constitute one of
the oldest forms of therapy for airways disease. These
agents are administered only by inhalation. All are effective bronchodilators that act by overriding the constrictor
effects on bronchial smooth muscle and the secretory effects on bronchial mucosa exerted by the release of the
parasympathetic nervous transmitter. Until the 1940s,
when isoproterenol was introduced, atropine was the
only form of aerosol therapy available to treat respiratory
disease.

In the last quarter century, the use of anticholinergic
therapy has fallen into disfavor. The drugs in this class
have a slow onset of action, and their peak bronchodilator

activity may not be reached for 30 to 60 min. Thus, their
use has been superseded by more rapidly acting agents. In
addition, atropine sulfate is rapidly absorbed from the airway mucosa, and its systemic effects can be troublesome
because of its actions on the smooth muscle or neurologic
pathways of multiple organ systems. Moreover, in high
doses, atropine sulfate can interfere with mucociliary
transport by increasing the viscosity of the sputum and
decreasing ciliary motility. The quaternary compounds
(atropine methylnitrate and ipratropium bromides) represent a major advance in this form of treatment since they
are devoid of these side effects because of their very high
degree of local activity within the airways when administered by inhalation.

The anticholinergics are medium-potency bronchodilators, and whether they afford a first-line therapy for
asthma is currently an open question. Because of the relatively slow onset of action, other agents are generally preferable in emergency situations. However, there is a group
of patients that does respond favorably to the antimus-
carinics. Unfortunately, there is no good way of determining the responders prospectively. Consequently, in dealing with acute asthma, anticholinergics are usually
reserved as second-line therapy in patients who are severely ill and unresponsive to β agonists and methylxanthines. Anticholinergics do interact synergistically with
the sympathomimetics and methylxanthines. In nonur-
gent situations, anticholinergic agents are often useful in
treating the paroxysmal cough associated with irritated
airways. They are also quite effective in reducing the volume of sputum.

Cromoglycate

Disodium cromoglycate (cromolyn sodium; cromolyn)
was introduced into clinical practice in 1967 as a mast
cell stabilizing agent in the treatment of allergic asthma.
Although early trials in Great Britain had shown cromolyn to be highly effective, it was far less successful when
introduced into the United States in 1973. The discrepancy finally proved to be due largely to the different populations in which it was used: in the United States, cromolyn was used only in patients who could not be controlled
with β agonists or theophylline, or as a steroid-sparing
agent in patients who had become glucocorticoid-depend-
ent. Subsequent clinical trials have demonstrated this
approach to be inappropriate, and cromolyn has since
emerged as a first-line agent in the treatment of reversible
airways disease.

Cromolyn sodium is effective only by inhalation. It is
supplied as a powder, as a solution, and in metered-dose
inhalers. In each of its formulations, cromolyn is extremely safe: the incidence of adverse reactions is around
2 percent, and when such reactions do develop, they are
usually minimal in nature and cease when the drug is

withdrawn. Irritation of the throat, cough, occasional minor bronchospasm, and transient skin rashes are the most common side effects. The throat irritation and cough are seen most frequently when cromolyn is administered as a powder; they do not occur when given in solution or via a pressurized inhaler. More serious problems such as generalized dermatitis, myositis, and other hypersensitivity reactions do occur but are exceedingly rare. Cromolyn has no significant smooth-muscle relaxant properties. The major action of the drug appears to be the stabilization of mast cell membranes, thereby inhibiting the release of the mediators of immediate hypersensitivity. It does not inhibit the pharmacologic activity of the mediators of immediate hypersensitivity, nor does it affect the fixation of reagenic antibody to mast cells or the interaction between antigen and antibody. Many clinical trials of cromolyn have been conducted. In the main, success rates range from 60 to 90 percent. The composite data make it clear that cromolyn has broad uses, is effective in both adults and children, works in patients without an allergic history, and compares quite favorably to theophylline as first-line therapy for asthma.

Cromolyn is quite versatile and has been reported to block, or attenuate, the bronchoconstriction that follows exposure to antigen, exercise, cold air, sulfur dioxide, ultrasonic aerosols, toluene di-isocyanate, western red cedar, propranolol, and colophony. Although protective effects against histamine and methacholine have also been reported, this has not been a universal finding. Since the mechanisms of action of each of the above provocations differ, it is clear that cromolyn has a complex pharmacology.

In the case of antigen, cromolyn suppresses both the immediate and late onset reactions that follow exposure to a variety of aeroallergens (Fig. 80-6). It also prevents impairment of mucociliary transport. From a clinical standpoint, these therapeutic activities are extremely important and allow the drug to be used quite effectively to achieve acute and chronic prophylaxis. For these purposes, the drug need not be given chronically or around the clock. A single administration of cromolyn prior to the unavoidable exposure to known allergens can keep the patient symptom-free and prevent the development of both the immediate and late phases. This approach is best suited for short-term, intermittent exposures such as cutting grass, visiting homes in which there are pets, working occasionally with laboratory animals, and cleaning dusty or moldy areas. In these circumstances, the protective effect of the drug lasts for 3 to 4 h. Chronic or perennial exposure to antigen requires both more intense and prolonged therapy.

Cromolyn also provides effective prophylaxis for exercise-induced asthma. Here, too, the drug need not be given on a chronic basis; a single dose, a few minutes before exercise, is all that is needed. However, unlike the

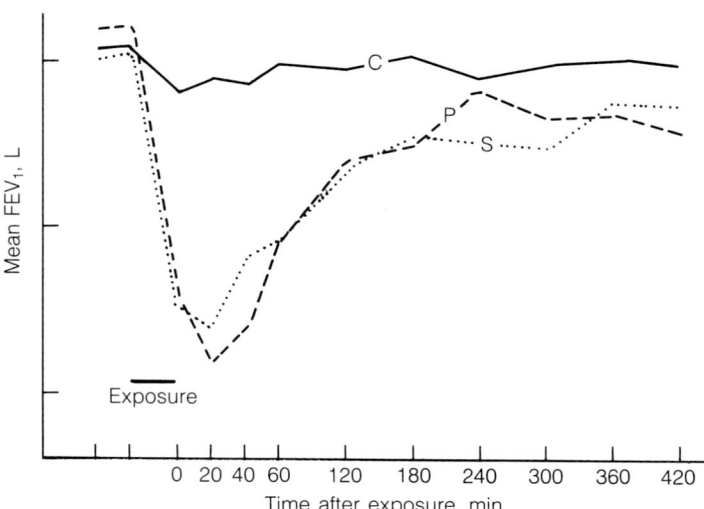

FIGURE 80-6 The effects of cromolyn sodium on the immediate response to antigen exposure. Mean FEV_1 before and after exposure to laboratory animals in 10 subjects with LAA (laboratory animal allergy) on three exposure days. S = screening day (day 1); P = placebo day; C = cromolyn day. *(From Gross, 1980.)*

situation with antigen, cromolyn does not totally block the response: airways obstruction still develops after cromolyn, but it is attenuated and the patient's symptoms are ameliorated. The protective effect lasts for 2 to 3 h.

In addition to its acute protective effects, cromolyn can also be used prophylactically to reduce bronchial reactivity: the long-term administration of cromolyn to asthmatics during their allergy season substantially reduces the responsivity of their airways to specific and nonspecific stimuli; after cromolyn, the patients have more symptom-free days and require less medication than without the drug. Stopping cromolyn causes airway hyperresponsivity to recur. For cromolyn to be used prophylactically in reducing bronchial reactivity, it must be given while the airways are being exposed to repetitive or chronic stimuli. Also, it must be administered for more than 2 weeks. When given out of season, or for short periods, cromolyn has little or no effect.

Glucocorticoids

Glucocorticoids were first used in the treatment of asthma in 1950. These agents are widely held to be a cornerstone in the management of patients with severe disease. Although all agree about the efficacy of the glucocorticoids in asthma, few data are available to settle when they should be used and what are the optimum dosage and schedule of administration.

The mechanisms by which steroids produce their effects are unknown. One hypothesis is that glucocorticoids bind to cytosol receptors, thereby initiating a membrane

phenomenon that culminates in a decrease in the availability of arachidonic acid and its metabolites. Another possibility includes the synthesis of new β-adrenergic receptors. Steroids also reduce cellular infiltration with polymorphonuclear cells, particularly eosinophils.

Regardless of mechanism, the effects of glucocorticoids are not immediate: as a rule, 6 to 12 h are required for their effects to become evident. Therefore, when corticosteroids are given to treat acute asthma, the other forms of therapy are continued aggressively until the corticosteroids take effect. Reliance on the corticosteroids alone in treating asthma is unwarranted.

Prevailing dose schedules for dealing with acute severe asthma are largely empirical. Currently, high dosages are in vogue. Some clinics use initial doses of corticosteroids that range from 100 to 1000 μg of hydrocortisone or its equivalent followed by similar doses every 2 to 4 h. In a recent study in our clinic, based on asthmatics who had proved to be refractory to 8 h of conventional treatment, those who received corticosteroids (2 mg/kg bolus followed by 0.5 mg/kg/h) had significantly greater resolution of airways obstruction after 24 h than those given placebo (Fig. 80-7). An initial delay of at least 6 h preceded remission of airways obstruction; thereafter, subjective and objective improvement continued. By 12 h, the mean increase in FEV_1 became statistically significant. The amount of hydrocortisone administered (approximately 1 g per 13 h for a person weighing 70 kg) succeeded in maintaining serum levels of cortisol equal to, or greater than, 150 μg/dl. Whether similar results can be accomplished using a smaller dose remains to be established.

Glucocorticoids are also quite helpful in the outpatient treatment of acute exacerbation of asthma that cannot be controlled by increasing the dosage of standard bronchodilators. Once again, treatment is empirical. However, as a rule, treatment is begun using dosages equivalent to 40 to 60 mg of prednisone per day. The dose is tapered by 5 to 10 mg every third to fourth day until an amount equivalent to 15 mg of prednisone is being administered. Tapering is then continued more gradually until corticosteroids are completely discontinued. In practice, a 12- to 20-day treatment period has no substantial effect on the hypothalamic-pituitary-adrenal axis.

Long-term glucocorticoid therapy should be undertaken only in patients in whom beneficial effect can be demonstrated using objective pulmonary function tests. If long-term treatment is necessary, an alternate day schedule, using a medium-duration preparation such as prednisone, minimizes side effects. Doses of prednisone as high as 30 to 40 mg are well tolerated. However, calcium loss from bone may pose a problem. Long-acting preparations should not be used in long-term therapy since they defeat the purpose of the alternate day regimen.

An alternative approach to the oral administration of glucocorticoids is the inhalation of a high-potency glucocorticoid that undergoes minimal systemic absorption, e.g., beclomethasone, triamcinolone, or funisolide. When used as recommended, these drugs are free of systemic side effects and, at least in adults, are not associated with clinical features of hypercorticism or disturbances in the hypothalamic-pituitary-adrenal axis. Because of the high local concentrations that are achieved in the mouth and pharynx, these compounds are associated in about 10 percent of patients with symptomatic candidiasis and/or dysphonia. The frequency of these complications can be decreased by proper timing of the inhalations.

The use of inhaled steroids facilitates the withdrawal of oral glucocorticoids in steroid-dependent patients. It may also decrease bronchial reactivity, particularly in patients with seasonal asthma. The usual daily dose of the inhaled drugs can be taken to be equivalent to 10 to 15 mg of prednisone. Hence, inhalation will have little effect if these agents are given to patients who require a larger oral dosage. Typically, corticosteroids by inhalation are begun when the oral dose of prednisone decreases to 15 to 20 mg daily. To reduce airway lability, the administration of glucocorticoids by inhalation should start at the onset of seasonal antigen exposure and be continued for the duration. There are no data to support a role for inhaled steroids in treating acute exacerbations of asthma.

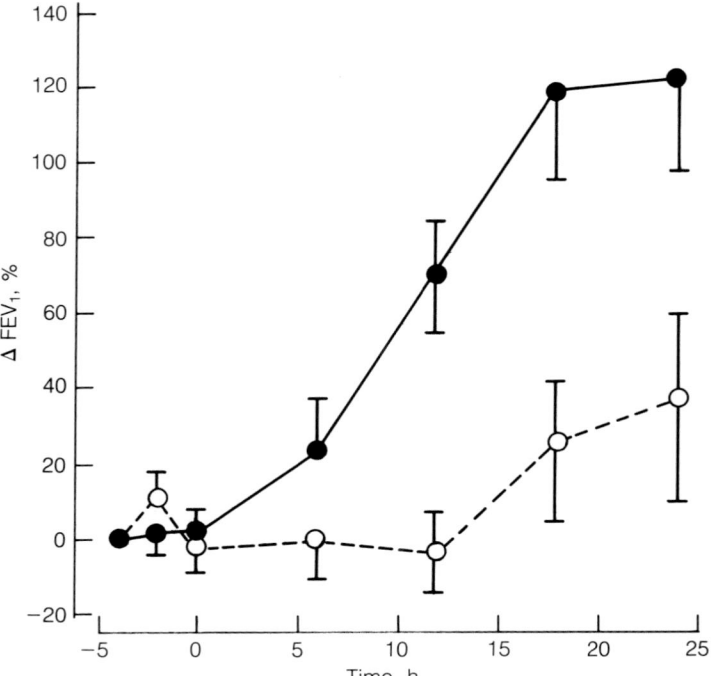

FIGURE 80-7   Effects (average ± 1 SEM) of treatment with hydrocortisone on pulmonary mechanics (ΔFEV_1) in acute asthma. Airways obstruction decreased progressively in the glucocorticoid-treated patients so that, by 12 h, the difference between the two groups was statistically significant. Test infusions were begun at time zero. ● = steroids; ○ = placebo. *(From Fanta, Rossing, McFadden, 1983.)*

TREATMENT: THE ACUTE EXACERBATION

The goal in treating acute asthma is to eliminate the patient's symptoms and improve pulmonary function as quickly as possible with a minimum of side effects. In principle, a variety of drugs can be used to achieve this goal. However, until recently, few objective data have been available concerning either their relative effectiveness or their toxic-therapeutic ratios in an emergency setting. Therefore, until recently, empiricism has predominated in the choice of bronchodilators.

β-Adrenergic Agonists

There now seems to be a consensus that the β-adrenergic agonists should be the first-line therapy for acute episodes of asthma. The administration of agents such as epinephrine and isoproterenol in emergency situations increases FEV_1 or peak flow rates by 50 to 60 percent over their pretreatment values. Of the two, isoproterenol is the more potent. Salbutamol, terbutaline, metaproterenol, and fenoterol also have similar effects in symptomatic patients. Therefore, the results are not drug-specific. The degree of bronchodilatation obtained by administering β_2 selective agents (nebulized terbutaline, salbutamol, metaproterenol, and fenoterol) to acutely ill asthmatics is equal to, or only slightly better than, that obtained using the catecholamines (injected epinephrine, inhaled isoproterenol, or isoetharine).

The experience with acute asthma in young patients indicates that very large doses of both non-β_2- and β_2-selective drugs are well tolerated, thereby dispelling fears of the potential arrhythmogenic hazards of sympathomimetics, especially in patients with preexisting tachycardia. This is in contrast to the propensity for arrhythmias manifested by patients with chronic obstructive airways disease in whom serious disturbances also exist in blood-gas composition and in electrolyte balance (see Chapter 67). Even when treated with high doses of agents such as epinephrine and isoproterenol, which have marked inotropic and chronotropic activity, the pulse rates and blood pressures of acutely ill asthmatics fall as airways obstruction dissipates. It is also likely that acute airways obstruction in older subjects could be treated with adrenergic agonists but, because of the higher risk of concurrent heart disease, a β_2-selective agent should be used.

In the past, ineffectiveness reported by the patient of large doses of sympathomimetics self-administered before presenting for urgent treatment had been regarded as prima facie evidence of drug resistance. However, the report by the patient that self-administered β agonists have failed to terminate an acute exacerbation of asthma *outside the hospital* does not predict the response to this class of drugs in the emergency room. Nor does it imply acquired tolerance: no significant differences have been found between either the degree of bronchodilatation or the incidence of adverse effects in those who take sympathomimetic agents as outpatients and those who do not.

The inhaled route should be the first form of therapy used to relieve airways obstruction and the patient's symptoms. Administration by inhalation delivers the drug directly to the airways so that only small quantities of medication are required to achieve the desired therapeutic effect; unwanted systemic action, or side effects, are minimized. In addition, the onset of action is substantially quicker with aerosols than with the oral route, as is the time to peak response. As in the case of arrhythmias, fears about the potential limitations of inhaled therapy in acutely ill patients have not been substantiated.

Aminophylline

As indicated above, the methylxanthines are only medium potency compounds. In contrast to the adrenergic agonists, the intravenous administration of the usually recommended doses of aminophylline tends to produce only a 15 to 25 percent increase in pulmonary function over the first few hours of treatment. Part of the reason for this modest response is that the dose-effect curve for this drug is linear and not sigmoidal as is the case for the sympathomimetics. Therefore, a large increase in blood levels is needed to achieve significant effects on the airways. This phenomenon can pose a substantial problem for individuals who have been taking the medication on a regular basis: elimination of the loading dose in these individuals in order to prevent toxicity frequently precludes the achievement of the high blood levels required for immediate effects.

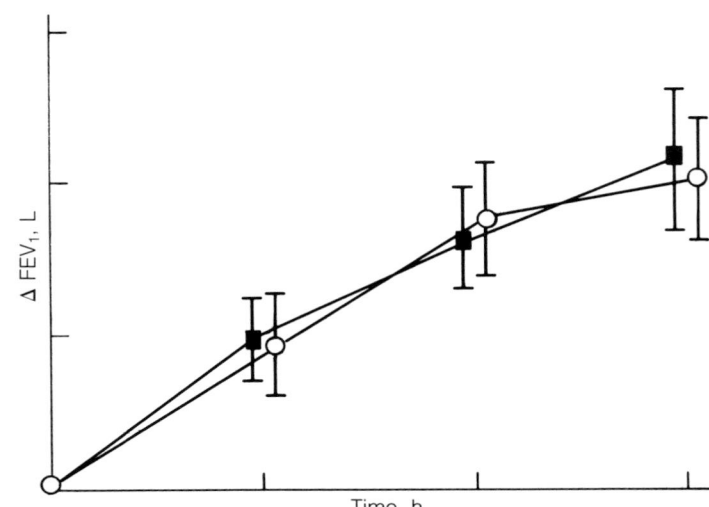

FIGURE 80-8 Comparison of the effects on pulmonary mechanics (FEV_1) of inhaled metaproterenol (■) and of metaproterenol in combination with intravenous aminophylline (○) on the resolution of airways obstruction in an acute attack of asthma. (*From Siegel, Sheppard, Gelb, Weinberg, 1985.*)

Whether or when to use aminophylline in combination with a β-adrenergic agonist has not yet been settled (Fig. 80-8). As a rule, combined therapy of a β agonist with methylxanthine is reserved for the more severely ill, i.e., those patients who have very *severe* airways obstruction and who will require long-term therapy.

Anticholinergic Agents

These drugs are not used as first-line agents to treat acute asthma. Like the methylxanthines, atropine, in all its formulations, is a medium-potency bronchodilator with a slow time course of action; both of these features limit its usefulness in emergency situations. Although anticholinergics combined with sympathomimetics have been reported to produce additive bronchodilatory effects, the results have been inconsistent except for an increase in the duration of bronchodilatation.

Nonresponders in the Emergency Room

Approximately 25 percent of patients with acute asthma require prolonged therapy before remission can be induced; in one-half of this group, hospitalization becomes necessary. Although, as a rule, all asthmatics improve somewhat within the first hour of treatment, those with the most severe airflow obstruction tend to respond least well. The typical individual who is ultimately admitted enters the emergency room with severe impairment and does not improve sufficiently to increase the FEV_1 above 40 percent of predicted. This type of individual behaves as though maximum bronchodilatation is achieved quickly and the subsequent persistent obstruction to airflow is due to airway inflammation and impaired mucociliary transport. As soon as this type of individual is identified, corticosteroids are probably in order. Experience has taught that unless the inflammatory component of their disease is brought under control by glucocorticoids, individuals who do not respond quickly in the emergency room are not apt to show much improvement during the next 24 h in hospital despite continued intensive therapy.

STATUS ASTHMATICUS

As indicated above, perhaps 10 to 15 percent of patients who present for therapy will require admission to the hospital for control of symptoms. In some, the disease can be life-threatening; these are said to be experiencing *status asthmaticus.*

Status asthmaticus differs only quantitatively from more usual asthma attacks, and it is completely reversible with prolonged aggressive therapy. Typically, status asthmaticus does not develop quickly. Instead, it tends to occur in a patient who has been experiencing persistent

asthma for several days. Five historical and clinical features of asthma help in recognizing those at risk of developing status asthmaticus: recurrent serious episodes of airways obstruction in the immediate past despite adequate treatment; short-lived relief of symptoms following aggressive therapy in the emergency room; a history of severe episodes of asthma with the need for repeated hospitalizations or large amounts of corticosteroids; failure of the signs and symptoms of severe airways obstruction, particularly the use of accessory muscles and pulsus paradoxus, to resolve; and a low FEV_1 or PEFR that does not exceed 40 percent of predicted within an hour of administering sympathomimetics in large doses. Any one of these findings should alert the physician to the likelihood that the present exacerbation is severe and requires more than routine therapy.

Once the candidate for status asthmaticus has been identified, arterial blood gases and pulmonary mechanics are monitored. The intuitive expectation that such patients would have severe hypoxemia and hypercapnia proves not to be so. Unlike the patient with respiratory insufficiency due to chronic bronchitis, the respiratory insufficiency of asthma is infrequently associated with frank respiratory failure: values for arterial $Pa_{O_2} < 45$ mmHg at sea level or $Pa_{CO_2} > 60$ mmHg are rare. When they do occur, they commonly represent therapeutic misadventures on the part of the treating physician. When present on admission to the emergency room, mild hypercapnia frequently resolves in response to aggressive therapy.

The hospital course of a patient with severe asthma follows a fairly predictable pattern. Nationwide, the average stay is 8.3 days; in approximately one-half of the admissions, a viral infection of the respiratory tract proves to be responsible for the episode. In a large series of 127 patients reported by Bond and Williams, the PEFR in each patient was less than 100 L/min. In 27 of the 127 patients, the Pa_{CO_2} was high on admission, averaging 54 mmHg; of these, 23 were treated successfully without intubation. Only four required ventilatory support; the average Pa_{CO_2} in this group was 75 mmHg. Patients with hypercapnia who were treated without intubation improved at the same rate as did those without hypercapnia. Overall, 5 to 6 days of aggressive treatment were required before the patients felt well enough to be considered for discharge. Hypercapnia did not develop in any patient in whom pulmonary mechanics were improving.

Therapy of status asthmaticus differs little from that of any other acute episode, save that the time scale is prolonged. As indicated above, without glucocorticoids little improvement in pulmonary function is apt to occur in 24 to 36 h. Therefore, the early use of these drugs is advisable. Routine monitoring of pulmonary function is mandatory. If PEFR or FEV_1 is improving, gas exchange cannot be deteriorating unless the patient's ability to ventilate

has been compromised, e.g., as by sedatives. If pulmonary mechanics are poor but stable, and the patient is eucapnic or hypocapnic, current therapeutic measures can be safely continued. If, however, mechanics are deteriorating or if the patient is hypercapnic, careful and continuous monitoring of arterial blood gases is mandatory. If Pa_{CO_2} is increasing, intubation may be necessary. In adults, ancillary measures such as anesthesia, bronchoscopy with lavage, and the intravenous administration of sympathomimetics are unnecesary.

CHRONIC THERAPY

The aims of this phase of the therapy of asthma are to control symptoms, decrease morbidity, and prevent acute episodes from developing. These goals can be achieved either by reducing airway reactivity or by chronic administration of bronchodilators, or both. Pharmacologic modulation of bronchial hyperreactivity can be achieved by the regular use of inhaled steroids or cromolyn sodium. Bronchodilators, per se, although they can afford protection against many acute stimuli, do not reduce airway responsivity; therefore, they produce only short-lived symptomatic relief. For the treatment of chronic asthma, cromolyn sodium and perhaps aerosolized corticosteroids should be kept in mind as first-line drugs that should be employed early in the treatment program.

With respect to achieving bronchodilatation, in chronic asthma as in acute asthma, aerosolized sympathomimetics are the drugs and route of choice. As noted above, inhalation provides the most effective treatment with the fewest side effects. For example, with respect to the resorcinols and saligenins, depending on the compound, the amount of drug released from a metered-dose inhaler is usually one-tenth to one-twentieth of the smallest effective dose that is marketed for oral use. Moreover, of this small quantity, only 10 to 15 percent is deposited in the airways. Therefore, the use of metered-dose inhalers is associated with low concentrations of the drug in the systemic circulation and few systemic side effects. Moreover, as has been repeatedly shown for β-adrenergic drugs, the small quantity of drug delivered to the airways by aerosol is at least as potent, and as long-acting, as conventional doses of medication taken by mouth.

Two major problems encountered in the use of inhalation therapy are the inability of some patients to master the technique required for proper usage of metered-dose inhalers and the inexpertness of the physicians instructing them: it has been estimated that perhaps 40 to 50 percent of patients using metered-dose nebulizers are unable to coordinate activation of the device with inhalation despite careful instruction and that up to 60 percent of general internists do not know how to either demonstrate the proper procedures or detect and correct improper proce-

dures. To overcome these difficulties, several approaches have been taken. Some pharmaceutical companies have begun to market powdered aerosols in which an active agent is micronized and released into a moving airstream by special devices, e.g., Spinhalers and Rotohalers. Since these insufflators are triggered by the patient's inhalation, they can readily be employed by anyone, even children and the elderly, who cannot synchronize the activities required for proper use of a propellant-driven nebulizer. These devices are quite effective, and no significant differences have been found between the bronchodilating ability of a given drug contained in a powder or in a pressurized aerosol.

Another approach designed to maximize aerosol deposition in the airways, currently popular in Europe and catching on in the United States, is the incorporation of a *spacer* between the delivery system and the patient's mouth. This approach is directed at eliminating the need for coordination of activation of the canister with the patient's inspiration and thereby decreasing the undesirable deposition of the aerosol in the patient's oropharynx: because of the spacer, the aerosol remains suspended sufficiently long for the patient to inhale deliberately at a slow inspiratory rate.

Another approach to chronic therapy that has become quite popular, particularly in the United States, is the use of long-acting theophyllines. The rationale is that a reasonably constant serum level of theophylline will protect the patient from developing acute symptoms. The approach works particularly well in treating patients with nocturnal, and early morning, attacks of asthma.

SPECIAL THERAPEUTIC CIRCUMSTANCES

Three clinical situations will suffice to illustrate special problems that complicate the management of a patient with asthma: pregnancy, advancing age, and cardiac disease.

Pregnancy

Pregnancy and asthma frequently coexist. Intuitively, an argument can be made that the two conditions could interact either to the detriment or advantage of the patient. In fact, in about half of the patients, the combined effect is neutral, i.e., no substantial change occurs in the asthma, in about 30 percent the asthma gets better, and in about 20 percent it gets worse. It is the last category that commands the attention of physicians.

The treatment of acute airways obstruction in pregnancy is frequently complicated by fears of both the expectant mother and the physician about untoward effects of the medication on the fetus. In reality, these fears tend to be groundless so that the care of a pregnant woman differs little from that of other asthmatics.

Although double-blind, controlled studies do not exist, worldwide experience indicates that sympathomimetics, methylxanthines, cromones, and glucocorticoids can be used safely. However, prudence does dictate that medications be withdrawn, if possible, particularly during the first trimester. If this is not possible, one should use whatever medication is required to stabilize the patient. Improving the mother, or keeping her symptom-free, is the best protection that the fetus can obtain. The medications in common use, such as the β agonists and methylxanthines, do cross the placenta and can be found in the fetal circulation at the time of delivery. They also cross into breast milk. Because these transfers are concentration-dependent, they can be minimized by keeping maternal blood levels low. Since the amounts transferred are exceedingly small, and since accumulation does not seem to occur in fetuses or infants, therapy with either a β agonist or a methylxanthine need not be interrupted during pregnancy or while breast feeding.

Elderly Patients

The elderly present special treatment problems such as hypersensitivity to stimulating drugs and confounding concurrent diseases, especially cardiac disease (see below). In this population, it is frequently quite helpful to start the patient on very low doses of medications and then gradually increase the amount to achieve the desired therapeutic effect. Inhaled sympathomimetics, with spacers if necessary, frequently work quite well as do long-acting methylxanthines. This approach minimizes the possibility of amplifying preexisting tremors and increasing rate-related cardiac problems, such as arrhythmias and/or angina.

Coexistent Cardiac and Airways Disease

The coexistence of cardiac disease and asthma can be particularly difficult to treat because of the competing therapeutic rationales and overlapping symptoms (see Chapters 67 and 68). Before the advent of β_2 agonists delivered by aerosol, because of their combined bronchodilator and diuretic activities, methylxanthines were favored in treating patients with primary airways disease and concomitant congestive heart failure and/or ischemic heart disease. However, since theophylline produces both inotropic and chronotropic activity, it can evoke undesirable cardiac effects. Therefore, striking a balance between beneficial and adverse consequences by adjusting dose was often difficult to accomplish.

With the advent of the β_2-adrenergic agonists that can be delivered by aerosol, some of the problems have become easier to control. Although there is as yet no pure β_2-receptor agonist, and even though β_1 effects do begin to appear as the dosage of available β_2 agonists is increased, cardiac arrhythmias or aggravation of angina are unusual. Indeed, terbutaline and salbutamol, when given by aerosol to patients with congestive heart failure, increase cardiac output and stroke volume, without changing heart rate; concomitantly, peripheral vascular resistance decreases, and left and right ventricular ejection fractions increase while the ventricular diastolic volume decreases. These changes occur within 10 min of inhalation and disappear after 30 min. This improvement in myocardial performance is achieved without an increase in myocardial oxygen consumption. In contrast, nonspecific agents such as epinephrine and/or isoproterenol increase myocardial oxygen consumption, thus making the heart work harder instead of more efficiently. Because they act to decrease peripheral vascular resistance, thereby decreasing the cardiac afterload, the β_2 agonists also tend to be safer. Indeed, the intravenous administration of salbutamol and terbutaline have been helpful in treating various cardiac and circulatory disorders, including acute myocardial infarction (with and without cardiogenic shock), coronary arterial disease accompanied by heart failure, and other types of congestive cardiomyopathies.

BIBLIOGRAPHY

Bergman B, Bokstrom H, Borga O, Enk L, Hedner T, Wangberg B: Transfer of terbutaline across the human placenta in late pregnancy. Eur J Respir Dis 65(Suppl):81–86, 1984.
  A presentation of data on placental and breast transfer of terbutaline.

Bernstein IL: Cromolyn sodium in the treatment of asthma: Coming of age in the United States. J Allergy Clin Immunol 76:381–388, 1985.
  A review of cromolyn as a treatment for asthma, with emphasis on mechanisms of action, and comparisons with alternative therapies.

Bondi E, Williams MH Jr: Severe asthma. Course and treatment in hospital. NY State J Med 77:350–353, 1977.
  Evaluation of the presenting features and hospital course of patients with severe asthma.

Bowler SD, Mitchell CA, Armstrong JG, Scicchitano R: Nebulized fenoterol and i.v. aminophylline in acute severe asthma. Eur J Respir Dis 70:280–283, 1987.
For the majority of patients presenting with acute severe asthma, it is likely that high doses of nebulized β₂ agonist alone will produce near maximal bronchodilation in the short term.

Chan-Yeung M, Lam S: Occupational asthma. Am Rev Respir Dis 133:686–703, 1986.
A state of the art review ranging from historical perspective to diagnostic treatment and prevention.

Chervinsky P: Concomitant bronchodilator therapy and ipratropium bromide. A clinical review. Am J Med 81:67–73, 1986.
A review of the use of ipratropium bromide concomitantly with other bronchodilators, with a focus on its use in patients with asthma. Overall, the combination of ipratropium with other agents appears to offer promise in therapy for asthma.

Dawson JR, Poole-Wilson PA, Sutton GC: Salbutamol in cardiogenic shock complicating acute myocardial infarction. Br Heart J 43:523–526, 1980.
An examination of the effects of salbutamol and terbutaline in patients with severe heart disease.

Ellis EF, Koysooko R, Levy G: Pharmacokinetics of theophylline in children with asthma. Pediatrics 58:542–547, 1976.
The pharmacokinetics of theophylline following intravenous injection of aminophylline, 4 mg/kg of body weight, were determined in 30 children with asthma and in six normal adult volunteers. Children eliminate theophylline more rapidly on the average than do adults and show pronounced interindividual differences in the elimination of the drug.

Falliers CJ, Tinkelman DG: Alternative drug therapy for asthma. Clin Chest Med 7:383–391, 1986.
This article reviews experimental and clinical data on the efficacy, safety, mode of action, and therapeutic indications for cromolyn and related inhalational compounds; ketotifen; α-adrenergic blockers; calcium-channel blockers; nonsteroidal anti-inflammatory drugs; and such diverse agents as immunosuppressive drugs, ether, alcohol, ascorbic acid, and other nutritional substances.

Fanta CH, Rossing TH, McFadden ER Jr: Emergency room treatment of asthma: Relationships among therapeutic combinations, severity of obstruction and time course of response. Am J Med 72:416–422, 1982.
An evaluation of the factors influencing the response of asthmatics to treatment in an emergency setting.

Fanta CH, Rossing TH, McFadden ER Jr: Glucocorticoids in acute asthma. A critical controlled trial. Am J Med 74:845–851, 1983.
A controlled trial of the time course of action of glucocorticoids in acute asthma in patients known to be resistant to standard therapy.

Greenberger PA, Patterson R: Management of asthma during pregnancy. N Engl J Med 312:897–902, 1985.
A review of the therapeutic considerations of asthma and pregnancy.

Gross NJ: Allergy to laboratory animals: Epidemiologic, clinical, and physiologic aspects, and a trial of cromolyn in its management. J Allergy Clin Immunol 66:158–165, 1980.
A double-blind controlled trial in 10 subjects with laboratory animal-induced bronchospasm showed that prior use of cromolyn offered considerable or complete protection against both immediate and late bronchospasm in all subjects but one.

Gross NJ, Skorodin MS: Anticholinergic, antimuscarinic bronchodilators. Am Rev Respir Dis 129:856–870, 1984.
A review of the pharmacology and clinical application of atropine and congeners in the treatment of airways disease.

Hendeles L, Weinberger M: Theophylline. A state-of-the-art review. Pharmacotherapy 3:2–44, 1983.
A review of the pharmacology and clinical utility of theophylline preparations.

Joad JP, Ahrens RC, Lindgren SD, Weinberger MM: Relative efficacy of maintenance therapy with theophylline, inhaled albuterol, and the combination for chronic asthma. J Allergy Clin Immunol 79:78–85, 1987.
Theophylline and combination regimens were associated with significantly fewer days with symptoms (52% and 55%) than albuterol (72%). The transient duration of effect from inhaled albuterol appears to limit its usefulness as maintenance therapy.

Kaliner MA, Barnes PJ: *The Airways.* New York, Dekker, 1987.
  A comprehensive review of neural mechanisms that may be important in diseases of the airways, such as asthma.

Lindberg C, Boreus LO, DeChateau P, Lindstrom B, Lonnerholm G, Nyberg L: Transfer of terbutaline into breast milk. Eur J Respir Dis 65(Suppl):87–91, 1984.
  A presentation of data on placental and breast transfer of terbutaline.

Lulich KM, Goldie RG, Ryan G, Paterson JW: Adverse reactions to beta 2-agonist bronchodilators. Med Toxicol 1:286–299, 1986.
  A review of side effects of β_2 agonists and how to circumvent toxicity.

McFadden ER Jr: Beta 2 receptor agonists: Metabolism and pharmacology. J Allergy Clin Immunol 68:82–93, 1981.
  A review of the structure-function relationships and pharmacology of adrenergic agonists.

McFadden ER Jr: *Inhaled Aerosol Bronchodilators.* Baltimore, Williams & Wilkins, 1986.
  Monograph on aerosol therapy for lung diseases including pharmacokinetics and pharmacodynamics of inhaled substances (bronchodilators).

Miech RP, Stein M: Respiratory pharmacology. Methylxanthines. Clin Chest Med 7:331–340, 1986.
  A review of the changes in the last decade with respect to theophylline: its analogs, its mode of action, and its pharmacokinetics.

Murphy S, Kelly HW: Cromolyn sodium: A review of mechanisms and clinical use in asthma. Drug Intell Clin Pharm 21:22–35, 1987.
  The cellular and clinical pharmacology of cromolyn sodium are reviewed.

Popa V: Respiratory pharmacology. Beta-adrenergic drugs. Clin Chest Med 7:313–329, 1986.
  A review of the large literature on beta agonists, emphasizing three aspects: the structural, pharmacokinetic, pharmacodynamic, and toxicologic properties; the relative advantages and disadvantages of various routes of administration; and the pharmacologic factors that may limit further development of these compounds for therapy.

Rebuck AS: Asthma: non-responsiveness to conventional therapy. Eur J Respir Dis 147:105–109, 1986.
  A review of the management of asthma that is refractory to conventional therapy, including strategies to deal with poor responsiveness to corticosteroids.

Rebuck AS, Chapman KR: Asthma: 2. Trends in pharmacologic therapy. Can Med Assoc J 136:483–488, 1987.
  A review of approaches to managing asthma of different severity.

Townley RG, Suliaman F: The mechanism of corticosteroids in treating asthma. Ann Allergy 58:1–6, 1987.
  The diverse effects of corticosteroids are reviewed with reference to managing difficult cases of asthma.

Tukiainen P, Lahdensuo A: Effect of inhaled budesonide on severe steroid-dependent asthma. Eur J Respir Dis 70:239–244, 1987.
  High-dose budesonide treatment (1600 µg/day) improves the clinical status of patients with severe steroid-dependent asthma more than does a low-dose therapy (400 µg/day), without causing systemic side effects.

Wang RYC, Lee PK, Yu DYC, Tse TF, Chow MS: Myocardial metabolic effects of intravenous terbutaline in patients with severe heart failure due to coronary artery disease. J Clin Pharmacol 23:362–368, 1983.
  An examination of the effects of salbutamol and terbutaline in patients with severe heart disease.

Woolcock AJ: Therapies to control the airway inflammation of asthma. Eur J Respir Dis 147:166–174, 1986.
  The natural history of the development of airway inflammation in asthma is reviewed together with the known histopathologic changes, measurable effects, and symptoms.

Chapter *81*

Pulmonary Rehabilitation

Andrew L. Ries

Comprehensive rehabilitation programs for patients with chronic pulmonary diseases are typically administered by a medical–allied health professional team. They provide an integrated approach directed toward stabilizing disease and improving exercise tolerance and functional capacity for these patients.

The primary goal of these programs is to restore the patient to the highest possible level of independent function. This goal may be accomplished by helping patients become more knowledgeable about their disease, more actively involved in their own health care, and more independent in performing daily care activities and, therefore, less dependent on family, friends, health professionals, and expensive medical resources. Rather than focusing solely on reversing a chronic, progressive disease process, rehabilitation programs attempt to reverse the patient's disability from the disease.

In 1974, the American College of Chest Physicians' Committee on Pulmonary Rehabilitation adopted the following definition:

> Pulmonary rehabilitation may be defined as an art of medical practice wherein an individually tailored, multidisciplinary program is formulated which through accurate diagnosis, therapy, emotional support, and education, stabilizes or reverses both the physio- and psychopathology of pulmonary diseases and attempts to return the patient to the highest possible functional capacity allowed by his pulmonary handicap and overall life situation.

This definition focuses on three important features of successful rehabilitation programs:

1. *Individual.* Patients with disabling obstructive disease of the airways require individual assessment of their needs, individual attention, and a program designed to meet realistic individual goals.
2. *Multidisciplinary.* Pulmonary rehabilitation programs provide access to information from a variety of health care disciplines which is integrated by an experienced staff into a comprehensive, cohesive program tailored to the needs of each patient.
3. *Attention to Physio- and Psychopathology.* To be successful, pulmonary rehabilitation programs must pay attention to psychological and emotional problems as well as help to optimize medical therapy to improve lung function.

Within this general framework, successful pulmonary rehabilitation programs have been established in various places, ranging from inpatient or outpatient hospital settings to physicians' offices and utilizing different health professionals. The key to a successful program is a dedicated, enthusiastic, and motivated staff (often with at least one full-time member) who can coordinate program activities, relate well to patients, and be given the medical and administrative support necessary. In addition, the goals of these programs as preventive health measures must be understood by patients, referring physicians, administrators, and third-party payers.

Although pulmonary rehabilitation programs have been developed primarily for patients with chronic obstructive airways disease (e.g., emphysema, chronic bronchitis, and chronic asthma), selected portions of these programs may be useful for patients with other chronic pulmonary disorders.

COMPONENTS OF A PULMONARY REHABILITATION PROGRAM (TABLE 81-1)

Patient Selection

Any patient with symptomatic obstructive airways disease is eligible for a pulmonary rehabilitation program.

TABLE 81-1
Components of a Pulmonary Rehabilitation Program

Patient evaluation
Medical evaluation
Physiological tests—pulmonary function, exercise, arterial blood gases
Psychosocial evaluation
Goal setting
Program content
Education
Chest physiotherapy instruction
Exercise training
Psychosocial support

The appropriate patient recognizes that he or she has obstructive airways disease, perceives some limitation or disability related to that disease, is motivated to do something to improve his or her health status, and has some pulmonary reserve. Patients with very mild disease may not perceive their problem as severe enough to warrant a comprehensive care program, and patients with very severe disease may be too limited to benefit appreciably. Therefore, these programs are best suited for patients with moderate to moderately severe disease.

Other factors also condition the success of the rehabilitation process. Pulmonary rehabilitation is not a primary mode of therapy for obstructive airways disease. Therefore, patients should be stabilized on standard medical therapy before beginning a program. Assessment and the treatment plan can then be based on the patient's optimal baseline level of function. Patients should not have other disabling or unstable conditions which would limit their ability to participate fully and to concentrate on rehabilitation activities. These include, but are not limited to, unstable heart disease, psychiatric illness, or concurrent evaluation for a potentially severe health problem.

The ideal patient for pulmonary rehabilitation, then, is one with moderate to moderately severe disease, stable on standard medical therapy, not distracted or limited by other serious or unstable medical conditions, willing and able to learn about his or her disease, and motivated to devote the time and effort necessary to benefit from a comprehensive care program.

Patient Evaluation

The initial step in the rehabilitation process is the assessment of the patient's medical history, clinical state, physiological stage of disease, and psychosocial state. This initial appraisal makes it possible to set individual goals that are compatible with both the patient's needs and expectations and the program's objectives.

MEDICAL EVALUATION

Review of the patient's medical history and past records, coupled with a thorough physical examination, enables the staff to characterize the patient's lung disease and to assess its severity. Other medical problems that might preclude or delay participation in the program are identified. The chest radiographs and electrocardiogram help to complete the clinical picture. Available pulmonary function tests, exercise tests, and arterial blood gases, drawn at rest and during exercise, provide objective indexes of functional status. If necessary at this juncture, additional information can be gathered and further therapeutic measures initiated before the patient begins the rehabilitation program. At the time that the program is begun, the patient's condition should be stable.

DIAGNOSTIC TESTING

The testing procedures depend on the individual patient and the facilities available. Spirometry and determination of lung volumes are useful for staging the patient's disease. More sophisticated tests, such as diffusing capacity or airway resistance, are not generally required.

Exercise testing as a preliminary to a rehabilitation program serves two purposes: (1) to assess the patient's exercise tolerance and blood gases (for hypoxemia or hypercapnia), and (2) as a basis for a safe and appropriate prescription for subsequent training.

The maximum exercise tolerance of patients with obstructive airways disease is limited largely by the maximum minute ventilation ($\dot{V}_{E_{max}}$) reached during exercise. $\dot{V}_{E_{max}}$ can be approximated from the resting maximal voluntary ventilation (MVV) which, in turn, can be estimated from the $FEV_{1.0}$ (e.g., MVV = $35 \times FEV_{1.0}$). Although spirometric measurements ($FEV_{1.0}$) can be used to estimate a patient's maximum work capacity ($\dot{V}_{O_2max}$), the exercise tolerance of patients with obstructive airways disease will depend considerably on an individual patient's perception and tolerance of the subjective symptom of dyspnea. Many patients are physically inactive and deconditioned due to their limited lung function and fear of dyspnea. Therefore, it is important to exercise each patient to determine the current level of function and the tolerance for dyspnea. It is easiest to perform this test using the form of exercise to be used for training (e.g., treadmill for walking program); however, the results from one type of exercise (e.g., cycle ergometer) can be translated to similar forms of exercise (e.g., walking). During testing, the work load, heart rate, electrocardiogram, and arterial oxygenation are monitored. These measurements represent the minimum. Clinics with special interests include others (e.g., $\dot{V}_E$, $\dot{V}_{O_2}$).

The determination of arterial blood-gas composition, at rest and during exercise, is important because of the possibility of exercise-induced hypoxemia. The sampling of arterial blood during exercise complicates testing. Therefore, increasing reliance is now placed on cutaneous oximetry to provide estimates of arterial oxygen saturation (Sa_{O_2}). Although this noninvasive technique is useful for continuous monitoring and for approximate values of blood oxygenation, it is not entirely accurate (95 percent confidence limits for Sa_{O_2} = ±4 to 5 percent).

PSYCHOSOCIAL ASSESSMENT

Successful rehabilitation requires attention not only to physical problems but also to psychological, emotional, and social ones. Patients with chronic illness, such as chronic obstructive airways disease, develop psychosocial problems as they struggle to deal with symptoms that

they often understand poorly. They become depressed, frightened, anxious, and increasingly dependent on others to care for their needs. Progressive dyspnea frightens some patients, causing a vicious "fear-dyspnea" cycle: in the patient with progressive disease, less exertion results in more dyspnea that evokes more fear and anxiety that, in turn, produce more dyspnea. Ultimately, the patient avoids physical activity that is associated with these unpleasant symptoms. In the extreme, some patients set up a stationary "command post" from which they rarely venture forth except to seek relief in physician offices and hospitals.

In anticipation of these problems, the initial evaluation includes an assessment of the patient's psychological state (e.g., depression or other psychological tests). Close attention is paid to psychosocial clues gained during the screening interviews (e.g., information about family and social support, living arrangement, activities of daily living, hobbies, employment potential). Spouses, family members, and close friends may provide valuable insights and are included in the screening process (and program).

SETTING GOALS

After evaluating a patient's medical, physiological, and psychosocial state, specific goals are set. These must be compatible with the individual patient's disease, needs, and expectations and realistic with respect to the goals of the rehabilitation program. Patients and family members are included in this process so that all understand what can, and cannot, be expected.

Program Content

EDUCATION

It is essential that the patient (and family members) understand the patient's disease and that instruction be directed toward coping with the specific problems of the individual. Although instruction can be given individually or in small groups, it must be adapted to the different learning abilities and needs of the individual patient. The educational program may consist of classroom, individual, and audiovisual formats. Among the topics covered can be: how normal lungs work, what is COPD, medications, nutrition, travel, stress reduction and relaxation, when to call your doctor, and planning a daily schedule. Individual instruction and coaching may be provided on the use of respiratory therapy equipment and oxygen, breathing techniques, bronchial drainage, chest percussion, energy-saving techniques, and self-care tips. The general philosophy of the program should be to encourage patients to assume responsibility for and to become active participants and partners in taking care of themselves.

CHEST PHYSIOTHERAPY

Many patients with obstructive airways disease use, abuse, and are confused about techniques for respiratory and chest physiotherapy. Rehabilitation programs must assess each patient's needs and provide instruction in proper techniques. Good bronchial hygiene is important for all patients, especially those who produce excess mucus. The patient should be taught appropriate techniques for coughing and postural drainage. Instruction in pursed-lip and diaphragmatic breathing helps to improve ventilatory pattern (e.g., slow respiratory rate) and gas exchange. It also helps the patient to gain control over the symptom of dyspnea; relaxation training also helps in this regard. Patients who use respiratory therapy equipment are instructed in its proper use, care, and cleaning. For those who require O_2-enriched air, available methods for oxygen delivery should be reviewed to help select the best system and application for their needs (e.g., continuous versus ambulatory therapy).

EXERCISE

Exercise conditioning should be considered for all patients. Benefits are both physiological and psychological. This is an ideal opportunity for patients to learn their capacity for physical work and to use and practice methods (e.g., breathing and relaxation techniques) for controlling dyspnea.

The exercise program needs to be safe and appropriate for each patient's interest, environment, and level of function; it is based on the results of the initial exercise testing. Training utilizes methods easily adapted to the home setting. Walking programs are used extensively and have the advantage of encouraging patients to expand their social horizons. In inclement weather, patients can frequently walk indoors (e.g., shopping malls). Other types of exercise (e.g., cycling, swimming) are also effective. Patients should be encouraged to incorporate regular exercise into other activities they enjoy (e.g., golf, gardening). Since many patients with obstructive disease of the airways have limited exercise tolerance, emphasis during training should be placed on increasing endurance. Greater endurance will enable them to become more functional within their physical limits. An increase in the level of exercise often ensues as the patients gain experience with the exercise and confidence in their ability to perform without harm.

Exercise Prescription

After the initial exercise test to assess a patient's maximal exercise tolerance, training begins at a level that the patient can sustain for several minutes. This is an adequate starting point for a training program designed to increase endurance as well as level.

It must be remembered that principles of exercise testing and training derived from normal populations are seldom applicable to pulmonary patients who are limited by ventilation and dyspnea. For instance, most patients with clinically significant, chronic pulmonary disease can be trained at higher percentages of their maximum exercise tolerance than can normal individuals because the patients can sustain their ventilation at high percentages of their MVV. Therefore, training levels often approach (or even exceed) the maximal level determined by the exercise tolerance test. Patients with milder disease can be trained at submaximal levels that are higher than the usual 60 or 70 percent of maximum expected in normal individuals. In addition, these patients will usually not reach maximum predicted heart rates, so it is important not to set a standard heart rate. The level of exercise is titrated to that which pushes the patient toward his or her maximum and is adjusted according to the patient's perception and tolerance for dyspnea. Ratings of perceived symptoms (e.g., breathlessness) help in teaching patients to exercise to "target" levels for breathing discomfort.

A major problem in planning a safe exercise program for the patient with obstructive airways disease is the possibility of exercise-induced hypoxemia. Changes in arterial oxygenation cannot be predicted reliably from measurements of pulmonary function or gas exchange made at rest. Normal individuals do not develop hypoxemia with exercise. In patients with *mild* obstructive disease of the airways, the Pa_{O_2} may remain unchanged or increase during exercise. However, in patients with moderate to severe obstructive airways disease, the Pa_{O_2} during exercise may increase, decrease, or remain unchanged. Therefore, it is important to determine if appreciable hypoxemia does occur during exercise so that proper oxygen concentrations can be delivered during exercise for safe training. Because of the availability of convenient, portable systems for delivering oxygen to the ambulatory patient, arterial hypoxemia is no longer an obstacle to exercise training.

Other Forms of Exercise

Exercise programs for patients with obstructive airways disease generally focus on the lower extremities (e.g., walking). Other types of exercise may also be beneficial for these physically limited individuals.

The role of respiratory muscle fatigue in patients with obstructive airways disease as a potential cause of respiratory failure and of limitation to ventilation has stimulated efforts to train the ventilatory muscles. Either isocapnic hyperventilation or inspiratory resistive loading has been used and shown to improve function of these muscles. However, exercise performance after ventilatory muscle training alone has not consistently improved. To explain the inconsistencies, Pardy and coworkers have reported that the benefits of ventilatory muscle training are most

evident in the subset of patients with obstructive airways disease who develop electromyographic evidence of diaphragmatic fatigue during exercise. However, at present, there is no simple expedient for selecting the patients most apt to benefit from this type of exercise training.

Exercise training of the upper extremities is associated with a higher ventilatory demand (for a given level of oxygen consumption) than is lower-extremity exercise. Some patients with obstructive airways disease who are handicapped in performing daily activities that draw heavily on the arms (e.g., dressing, bathing, shopping, carrying) seem to benefit from upper-extremity training exercise. However, too few studies along this line have yet been done to draw conclusions about the efficacy of this approach.

PSYCHOSOCIAL SUPPORT

This is the final important component of a comprehensive pulmonary rehabilitation program. From the realization that their disease is chronic and incurable, patients with obstructive airways disease develop a variety of psychosocial symptoms that reflect their progressive feelings of hopelessness and inability to cope with their disease. Depression and anxiety (particularly fear of dyspnea) are common. Patients show symptoms of denial, anger, and isolation and become sedentary and dependent on family members, friends, and medical services to provide for their needs. Overconcern with other physical problems and psychosomatic symptoms develop. Sexual dysfunction and fear of sexual activities is a common, often unspoken, consequence contributing to personal and family difficulties. These patients often have evidence of cognitive and neuropsychological dysfunction, possibly related to, or exacerbated by, the effects of arterial hypoxemia on the brain.

Successful pulmonary rehabilitation programs must attend not only to physical problems but also to psychosocial ones. This is provided best by enthusiastic and supportive staffers who are able to communicate effectively with patients and devote the time and effort necessary to understand and motivate them. Close family members and friends are included in the program so that they can understand and cope better with the patient's disease. Support groups and group therapy sessions are very effective. Patients with severe psychological disorders may benefit from individual counseling and psychotherapy. Psychotropic drugs should generally be reserved for patients with severe levels of dysfunction.

RESULTS OF PULMONARY REHABILITATION

Comprehensive pulmonary rehabilitation programs for patients with obstructive airways disease have proved to

TABLE 81-2
Benefits of Pulmonary Rehabilitation

Decreased hospitalization needs
Improved quality of life
Decrease in respiratory symptoms (e.g., dyspnea)
Decrease in psychological symptoms (e.g., fear, depression)
More independence
Increased physical activity—ability to perform activities of daily living
Increased exercise capacity and endurance
Increased knowledge about disease
Return to work possible
? Prolonged survival

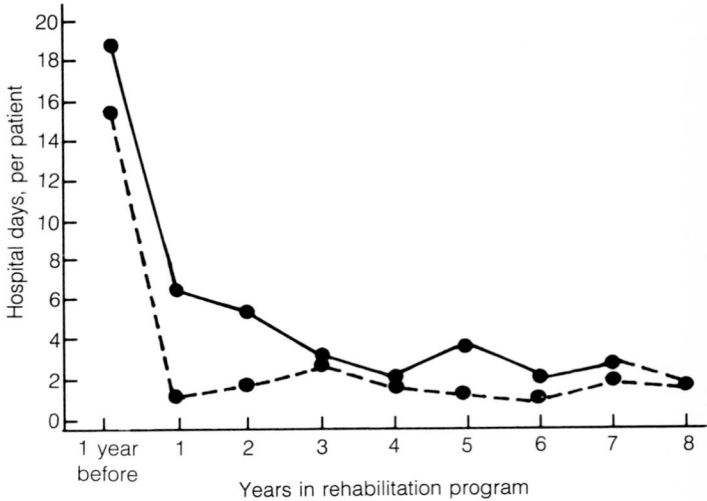

FIGURE 81-1 Hospitalization requirements before and during 8 years of follow-up after pulmonary rehabilitation. The solid line represents data for all patients; the dashed line represents data only for those patients who survived in the program for 8 years. *(Modified after Hodgkin, Zorn, Connors, 1984.)*

be cost-effective (Table 81-2). One tangible benefit has been a decrease in the number of days of hospitalization and in the use of medical resources (Fig. 81-1). Another outcome has been improvement in the quality of life, manifested by a reduction in respiratory symptoms, an increase in exercise tolerance and level of physical activity, greater independence and increased ability to perform the activities of daily life, and an improvement in psychological function with less anxiety and depression and increased feelings of hope, control, and self-esteem. Even those patients with severe disease have benefited from rehabilitation because of an improved understanding of their disease, increased levels of activity, and improved exercise tolerance.

Overall, pulmonary rehabilitation programs have neither improved pulmonary function in patients with obstructive airways disease nor slowed the expected deterioration in pulmonary function. Nor has it been shown convincingly that survival is increased after pulmonary rehabilitation. However, some patients with moderate disease have been able to return to work and to increase their ability to perform in vocational and recreational activities. In those severely disabled by their disease, vocational benefits have generally been difficult to demonstrate. The success of vocational rehabilitation also depends on factors other than the degree of respiratory impairment, including the patient's motivation, level of education, capability for retraining, physical demands of a particular job, and support and understanding from an employer.

FUTURE OF PULMONARY REHABILITATION

Chronic obstructive disease of the airways (COPD) is a chronic, progressive, and largely irreversible disease which develops insidiously over many years and is generally moderate to severe when recognized. The goals of medical therapy are: (1) to slow the expected decline in lung function and (2) if possible, to improve lung func-

tion. Once the patient has been stabilized using standard medical therapy, it is unlikely that much additional improvement in pulmonary function can be expected. Therefore, to demonstrate improvement as the result of a rehabilitation program requires a controlled study of patients with chronic obstructive airways disease whose function would be expected to decline over time. Such a study has not yet been done.

In addition, the benefits of pulmonary rehabilitation are most evident as changes in the quality of life, changes that although difficult to measure, may be critical in understanding the benefits and cost effectiveness of these programs. Recently, approaches for measuring the quality of life have been developed and used to assess the cost-benefit ratio of clinical interventions. Clinical trials that examine the benefits of pulmonary rehabilitation are needed.

In addition to assessing the overall benefits of comprehensive pulmonary rehabilitation programs in patients with obstructive airways disease, a better understanding of specific components would be helpful. Much needs to be learned about the optimal methods for performing exercise testing and training in pulmonary patients. Standard approaches are needed for detecting and managing exercise-induced hypoxemia. The best type of exercise training for patients with obstructive airways disease remains to be established. Finally, since the multidisciplinary, individualized program entailed in rehabilitation calls for a considerable and concerted effort from both patients and staff, improved methods are needed for the selection of those patients who are apt to complete and to benefit from the program.

BIBLIOGRAPHY

American Thoracic Society: Pulmonary rehabilitation. Am Rev Respir Dis 124:663–666, 1981.
Position statement defining pulmonary rehabilitation and describing components and benefits of such programs.

Belman MJ, Wasserman K: Exercise training and testing in patients with chronic obstructive pulmonary disease. Basics of RD 10:1–6, 1981.
Succinct review of exercise testing and training for patients with obstructive disease of the airways emphasizing differences from normal individuals.

Casaburi R, Wasserman K: Exercise training in pulmonary rehabilitation. N Engl J Med 314:1509–1511, 1986.
A perspective, based on physiological principles, of the application of exercise training in pulmonary rehabilitation.

Derenne J-PH, Macklem PT, Roussos CH: The respiratory muscles: Mechanics, control, and pathophysiology. Am Rev Respir Dis 118:119–133; 373–390; 581–601, 1978.
Review of respiratory muscle function and possible relationships of dysfunction to pulmonary disorders.

Dudley DL, Glaser EM, Jorgenson BN, Logan DL: Psychosocial concomitants to rehabilitation in chronic obstructive disease: Part 1. Psychosocial and psychological considerations; Part 2. Psychosocial treatment; Part 3. Dealing with psychiatric disease (as distinguished from psychosocial or psychophysiologic problems). Chest 77:413–420; 544–551; 677–684, 1980.
Three-part series reviewing psychosocial problems in obstructive airways disease and their management.

Haas A, Cardon H: Rehabilitation in chronic obstructive pulmonary disease. Med Clin North Am 53:593–606, 1969.
Five-year follow-up of 252 patients with obstructive airways disease treated with rehabilitation versus 50 patients treated without. Twenty-five percent of rehabilitation group returned to work compared with 3 percent of controls. Mortality rates: 22 percent in experimental versus 42 percent in control group.

Hodgkin JE, Zorn EG, Connors GL (eds): Pulmonary Rehabilitation—Guidelines to Success. Boston, Butterworth, 1984.
A comprehensive reference source for pulmonary rehabilitation—rationale, methods, and results.

Hudson LD, Tyler ML, Petty TL: Hospitalization needs during an outpatient rehabilitation program for severe chronic airway obstruction. Chest 70:606–610, 1976.
Four-year follow-up of hospitalizations before and after pulmonary rehabilitation. In 64 patients, hospital days were reduced 51 percent at 1 year. In 44 patients alive at 4 years, there was a 57 percent average yearly reduction.

Hughes RL, Davison R: Limitations of exercise reconditioning in COLD. Chest 83:241–249, 1983.
Review of current status of exercise training in chronic obstructive airways disease.

Kaplan RM, Atkins CJ, Timms R: Validity of a quality of well-being scale as an outcome measure in chronic obstructive pulmonary disease. J Chron Dis 37:85–95, 1984.
Description and example of a quality-of-life instrument used to evaluate outcomes of an intervention for patients with chronic obstructive disease of the airways.

Lertzman MM, Cherniack RM: Rehabilitation of patients with chronic obstructive pulmonary disease. Am Rev Respir Dis 114:1145–1165, 1976.
Comprehensive state-of-the-art review of pulmonary rehabilitation.

Make BJ: Pulmonary rehabilitation: myth or reality? Clin Chest Med 7:519–540, 1986.
One of a series of papers in the same volume dealing with the diverse aspects of pulmonary rehabilitation.

Moser KM, Archibald C, Hansen P, Ellis B, Whelan D: Shortness of Breath—A Guide to Better Living and Breathing, 3d ed. St. Louis, Mosby, 1983.
Excellent book for patient education.

Moser KM, Bokinsky GE, Savage RT, Archibald CJ, Hansen PR: Results of a comprehensive rehabilitation program: Physiologic and functional effects on patterns with chronic obstructive pulmonary disease. Arch Intern Med 140:1596–1601, 1980.
Description and results of a comprehensive pulmonary rehabilitation program. Emphasizes safety, feasibility, and benefits of exercise training for patients with chronic obstructive disease of the airways.

Paine R, Make BJ: Pulmonary rehabilitation for the elderly. Clin Geriatr Med 2:313–335, 1986.
  The individual practitioner can successfully incorporate many of the elements of pulmonary rehabilitation in dealing with patients with chronic obstructive airways disease.

Pardy RL, Rivington RN, Despas PJ, Macklem PT: The effects of inspiratory muscle training on exercise performance in chronic airflow limitation. Am Rev Respir Dis 123:426–433, 1981.
  Inspiratory muscle training in 12 patients with obstructive disease of the airways improved muscle endurance without changing muscle strength. Exercise performance increased in seven patients, six of whom had electromyographic evidence of inspiratory muscle fatigue during pretraining exercise. The five patients without inspiratory muscle fatigue showed no improvement in exercise performance.

Ries AL: The role of exercise testing in pulmonary diagnosis. Clin Chest Med 8:81–89, 1987.
  General description of principles of exercise testing and their application to patients with pulmonary disease.

Ries AL, Farrow JT, Clausen JL: Accuracy of two ear oximeters at rest and during exercise in pulmonary patients. Am Rev Respir Dis 132:685–689, 1985.
  Accuracy of ear oximetry compared to arterial blood measurements. Ninety-five percent confidence limits ±4 to 5 percent for Sa_{O_2} and ±2.5 to 3.5 percent for change in Sa_{O_2} from a previous value.

Ries AL, Farrow JT, Clausen JL: Pulmonary function tests cannot predict exercise induced hypoxemia in chronic obstructive pulmonary disease. Accepted for publication, Chest, 1987.
  With exercise, patients with chronic obstructive airways disease undergo a variable change in Pa_{O_2} (increase, no change, decrease); the change cannot be predicted from pulmonary function tests at rest.

Ries AL, Moser KM: Comparison of isocapnic hyperventilation and walking exercise training at home in pulmonary rehabilitation. Chest 90:285–289, 1986.
  Isocapnic hyperventilation exercise training can be performed successfully by patients with obstructive airways disease in an unsupervised home setting. In contrast, walking exercise training did not improve ventilatory muscle endurance.

Tiep BL, Lewis MI: Oxygen conservation and oxygen-conserving devices in chronic lung disease. A review. Chest 92:263–272, 1987.
  The cost of oxygen can be substantially reduced while increasing the portability and range of home oxygen therapy.

Hypoventilation Syndromes and Sleep Disorders

Chapter 82

Disorders of Alveolar Ventilation

Richard P. Millman / Alfred P. Fishman

General Alveolar Hypoventilation according to Etiology
    Inadequate Ventilatory Drive
    Mechanical Impairment of the Breathing Apparatus

Treatment of Chronic Alveolar Hypoventilation
    Assisted Ventilation
    Medical Management

Clinical instances of alveolar hypoventilation are usually sorted into two major groups according to whether the lungs are normal or abnormal (Table 82-1). The telltale feature of both groups is an abnormally high arterial P_{CO_2}. Although a decrease in arterial P_{O_2} invariably accompanies the hypercapnia, arterial P_{O_2} has proved less useful than P_{CO_2} as a hallmark of alveolar hypoventilation. In the patient with normal lungs, either the drive from the respiratory neurons is at fault, or the chest bellows is operating ineffectively (Fig. 82-1). In contrast, in the patient with abnormal lungs—as is discussed in considerable detail in the sections on chronic obstructive airways disease—abnormal blood-gas tensions result from widespread imbalances between alveolar ventilation and perfusion. Sleep exaggerates the degree of hypoventilation no matter what its etiology.

In the patient with general alveolar hypoventilation and normal lungs, both lungs share globally in the hypoventilation, some parts being affected more than others because of regional differences in their mechanical properties. Early in the disease, i.e., before unrelated parenchymal disease can add ventilation-perfusion abnormalities, the decrease in arterial P_{O_2} corresponds, millimeter of mercury for millimeter of mercury, to the increase in arterial P_{CO_2}. Later on, particularly in cigarette smokers, the ravages of obstructive airways disease often add a component of ventilation-perfusion abnormalities that exaggerate the drop in alveolar P_{O_2}.

Hypoventilation may occur both acutely and chronically. The acute forms of alveolar hypoventilation may occur as complications of drug overdose or as a consequence of neuromuscular diseases such as bulbar poliomyelitis, myasthenia gravis and the Guillain-Barré syndrome. They usually present as clinical crises. The acute

TABLE 82-1
Pathogenesis of Chronic Alveolar Hypoventilation

Chronic alveolar hypoventilation with normal lungs (general)
  Inadequate ventilatory drive
    1. Functional depression of ventilatory drive:
      Sleep
      Hypercapnia
      Metabolic alkalosis
      Drugs (narcotics, sedatives)
      Myxedema
    2. Anatomic damage to respiratory neurons:
      Bulbar poliomyelitis
      Encephalitis
      Brain-stem infarction
      Brain-stem neoplasm
      Bilateral cervical cordotomy
    3. Idiopathic alveolar hypoventilation
    4. Organic depression of motor pathways (Ondine's curse)
  Mechanical impairment of the breathing apparatus
    1. Peripheral neuromuscular disorders:
      Poliomyelitis
      Guillain-Barré syndrome
      Myasthenia gravis
      Muscular dystrophy
      Polymyositis
      Bilateral diaphragmatic paralysis
    2. Disorders of the chest cage:
      Kyphoscoliosis
      Obesity-hypoventilation syndromes
    3. Obstruction to the upper airways:
      Tracheal stenosis
      Obstructive sleep apnea
Chronic alveolar hypoventilation with abnormal lungs (net)
  Obstructive disease of the airways

syndromes are considered elsewhere in this book as instances of acute respiratory failure.

The chronic forms of general alveolar ventilation are usually more difficult to recognize. They are apt to be overlooked on two accounts: (1) since the patient generally is free of pulmonary complaints, the physician fails to consider inadequate ventilation as a possible cause (Fig. 82-2); and (2) a normal total ventilation under the emotional stress of the physical examination may obscure an alveolar ventilation that is inadequate when the patient is alone and unobserved. Even when alveolar hypoventilation is suspected, the act of observing the patient's breathing, or of introducing an arterial needle, often evokes sufficient hyperventilation to restore the arterial gas tensions to normal. Indeed, unless attention is paid to the possibility that an inexplicably high value for serum bicarbonate represents renal compensation for chronic respiratory acidosis, the prospect of chronic hypercapnia due to chronic alveolar hypoventilation often fails to be taken into proper account. Not infrequently, the existence of chronic alveolar hypoventilation is first suspected when an inordinate depression of the ventilation—or even coma—follows the

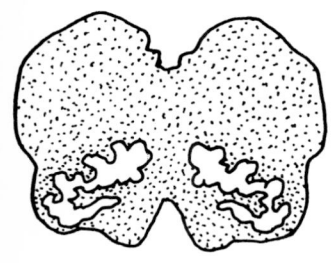

Drugs
Anatomical lesions
Metabolic alkalosis
Hypothyroidism
Idiopathic

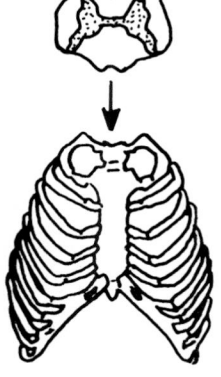

Myasthenia gravis
Guillain—Barré syndrome
Amyotrophic lateral sclerosis
Injury to cervical spine
Poliomyelitis

Kyphoscoliosis (severe)
Polymyositis
Obesity
Diaphragmatic fatigue
Hypokalemia, hypophosphatemia

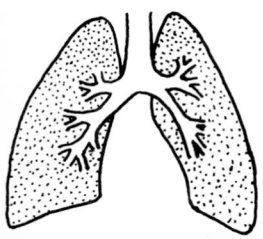

Obstructive airways disease
Pulmonary edema (severe)
Pulmonary interstitial disease
    (end-stage)

FIGURE 82-1   Causes of chronic alveolar hypoventilation. The upper two parts represent extrapulmonary causes of alveolar hypoventilation; the lower third lists causes of alveolar hypoventilation secondary to intrinsic pulmonary disease.

administration of a usual dose of a sedative or when signs of CO_2 intoxication occur during the breathing of O_2-enriched air.

The clinical consequences of alveolar hypoventilation are directly attributable to the hypoxemia, hypercapnia, and acidosis. The abnormal blood-gas levels exert their predominant effects in distinctive ways: hypoxia, acute or chronic, causes pulmonary hypertension by inducing pulmonary (arterial and arteriolar) vasoconstriction. In contrast, hypercapnia exerts its effects primarily on the central nervous system, and the consequence depends largely on the acuity of exposure: acute hypercapnia and the associated acidosis produce cerebral vasodilatation, increased cerebrospinal fluid pressure, and neurologic disturbances that range in their manifestations from weakness, irritability, lassitude, and cloudy senso-

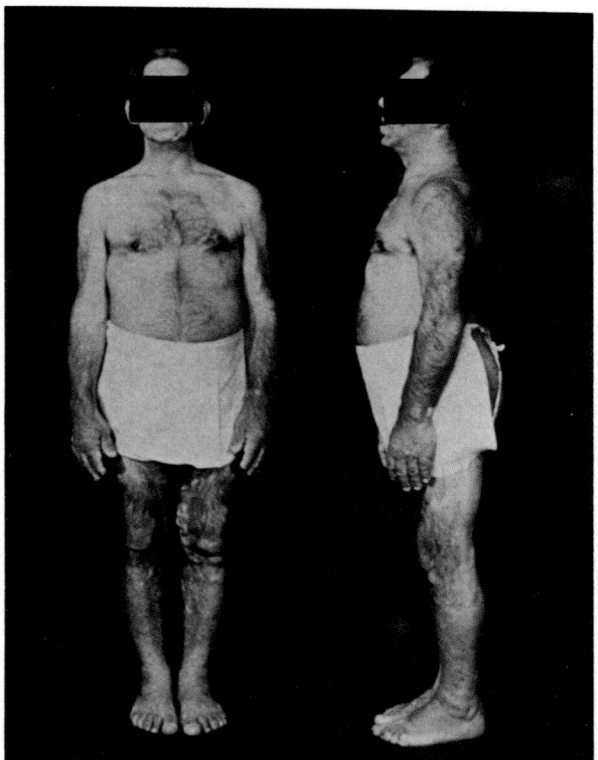

A

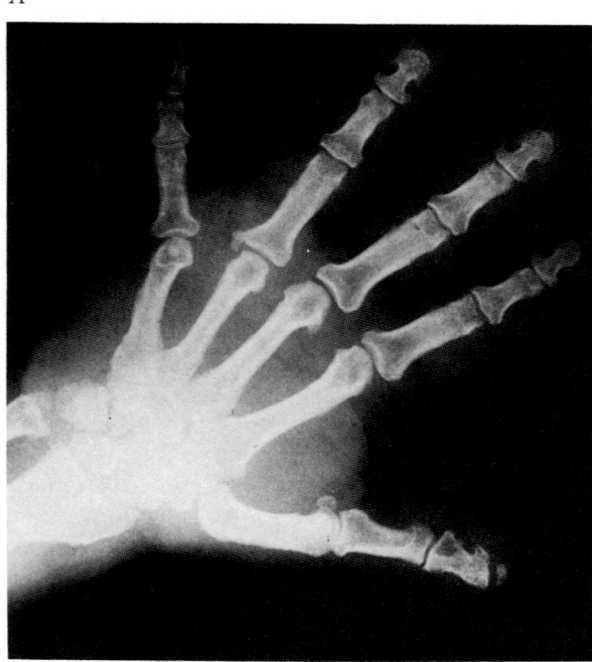

B

FIGURE 82-2   Chronic alveolar hypoventilation that escaped detection for many years. Fifty-year-old man with acromegaly who had received irradiation to the region of the pituitary for visual disturbances. Normal lungs but severe hypoxemia and hypercapnia. Characteristic acromegalic appearance with muscular habitus. Radiographic changes in the fingertips (and in the skull) were consistent with the diagnosis of acromegaly.

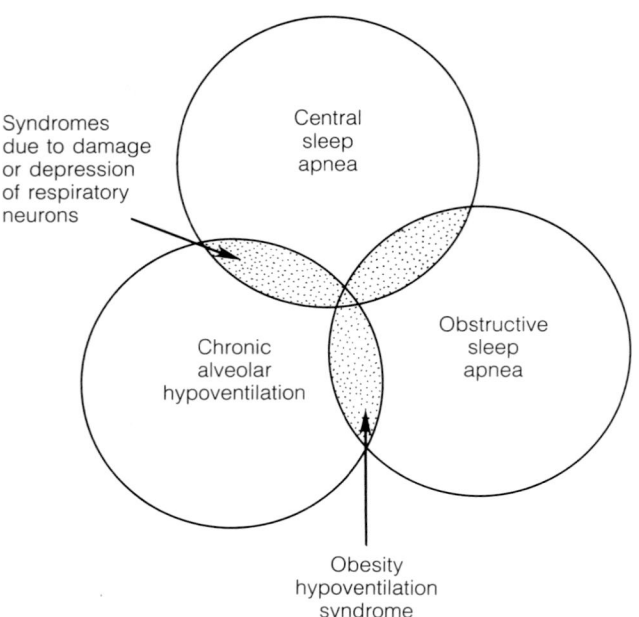

FIGURE 82-3 Overlap of the syndromes of chronic alveolar hypoventilation and sleep apnea.

rium to somnolence, confusion, and narcosis. In contrast, chronic (compensated) hypercapnia may have little more to show for it than dilated conjunctival vessels and watery eyes.

The respiratory acidosis that accompanies alveolar hypoventilation generally acts to exaggerate the pulmonary hypertension induced by hypoxia. The deleterious effects of acidosis on the circulation are counterbalanced by its contribution to the ventilatory drive: acidosis is part of the chemical stimulus to breathing during alveolar hypoventilation; relief of acidosis, as by the infusion of amine buffers, depresses total and alveolar ventilation.

GENERAL ALVEOLAR HYPOVENTILATION ACCORDING TO ETIOLOGY

In this section some of the familiar syndromes of chronic alveolar hypoventilation categorized in Table 82-1 are highlighted. As indicated in a separate chapter, chronic alveolar hypoventilation sometimes complicates the sleep apnea syndromes (Fig. 82-3).

Inadequate Ventilatory Drive

The disorders in this category elicit chronic alveolar hypoventilation even though the lungs are normal. The cause is an abnormally low ventilatory drive from the res-

piratory neurons to the respiratory muscles because of either anatomic damage or functional depression.

FUNCTIONAL DEPRESSION OF THE VENTILATORY DRIVE

Alveolar hypoventilation is a regular feature of sleep, both in normal people and patients with disorders of the lungs and respiratory apparatus. In normal people, arterial P_{CO_2} usually does not increase by more than 5 to 6 mmHg; in patients with obstructive disease of the airways and hypercapnia, the increments in P_{CO_2} are often greater. The span of CO_2 retention during sleep, from normal individuals, through heavy snorers, and up to individuals with the sleep apnea syndromes is considered in Chapter 83.

Metabolic alkalosis can cause functional depression of respiratory neurons. Often it occurs in a complicated setting in which hypoxia, severe derangements in acid-base balance, hypokalemia, and dehydration coexist. In metabolic alkalosis that is associated with hypochloremia and intracellular alkalosis, functional depression of respiratory neurons may be quite striking (Fig. 82-4). For example, furosemide, which is quite popular as a diuretic, promotes chloride excretion by the kidney and causes intracellular depletion of hydrogen ions. When used to excess, it may depress ventilation, an undesirable side effect when diuretics are used to treat the heart failure that complicates cor pulmonale and alveolar hypoventilation. Hypochloremia, another common side effect of vigorous diuretic therapy, interferes with lasting correction of hypercapnia.

Another common type of functional depression of central respiratory neurons is produced by narcotics. Some heroin addicts who are on methadone maintenance

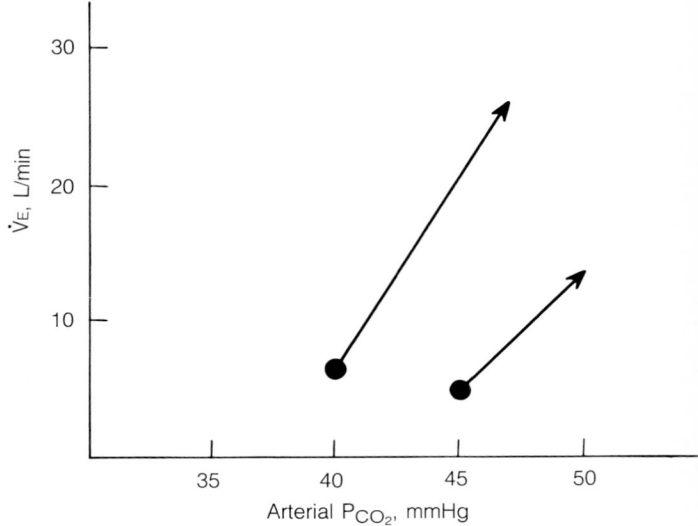

FIGURE 82-4 Graph of the effect of certain types of induced metabolic alkalosis on the ventilatory response to breathing 5% CO_2 in air. The pattern of response illustrated can be produced by administration of a diuretic such as furosemide or sodium bicarbonate. The response curve is shifted to the right with a reduction in slope.

programs develop alveolar hypoventilation and manifest blunted ventilatory responses to both acute hypoxia and hypercapnia as part of overall depression of the central nervous system.

Severe myxedema has been associated with marked central respiratory depression and chronic hypoventilation. Even in mild to moderate hypothyroidism chemosensitivity is depressed, but it returns to normal upon replacing thyroid hormone.

ANATOMIC DAMAGE TO RESPIRATORY NEURONS

Anatomic damage to respiratory neurons is an occasional sequel to an overt inflammatory process, e.g., diffuse encephalitis or bulbar poliomyelitis; occasionally it complicates cerebrovascular thrombosis. Usually the onset is flagrant, and respiratory damage is unmistakable. Often widespread damage to the central nervous system causes chronic alveolar hypoventilation without any clinical evidence that acute injury has occurred. The damage is manifested only long after the undetected acute episode has subsided, and its nature is revealed at autopsy. These patients occasionally exhibit normal ventilation during the day, but either hypoventilate while asleep or manifest central sleep apnea.

IDIOPATHIC ALVEOLAR HYPOVENTILATION

In some individuals, chronic alveolar hypoventilation develops without apparent cause (Fig. 82-5). Once suspicion is aroused, tests reveal that respiratory neurons in the brain are unresponsive to stimulation and that although the respiratory apparatus is intact, it fails to receive adequate drive. Because the cause of the inadequate ventilatory drive cannot be identified during life, these individuals have been designated as victims of "primary" or "idiopathic" alveolar hypoventilation. At autopsy, some show evidence of old, diffuse, unsuspected inflammatory disease of the brain. In others, the brain appears normal. Because of the inadequate ventilatory drive, despite a perfectly adequate chest bellows and capacity to breathe, these individuals develop arterial hypoxemia, respiratory acidosis, cor pulmonale, and right ventricular failure. They show no evidence of apnea during nighttime sleep recording.

A continuing trickle of individuals with this syndrome is still being reported. The disorder is detected primarily in persons who are in the third to fifth decades of life. Clinical manifestations are mild and arise principally from chronic hypoxemia (cyanosis, severe polycythemia of unknown cause). Until the nature of the disorder is elucidated, patients can be suspected for years of having congenital cyanotic heart disease. Minor, nonspecific neurologic manifestations are also common. Arterial blood-gas levels reveal severe hypoxemia and hypercapnia, usually with a near-normal pH. Irregular breathing patterns are

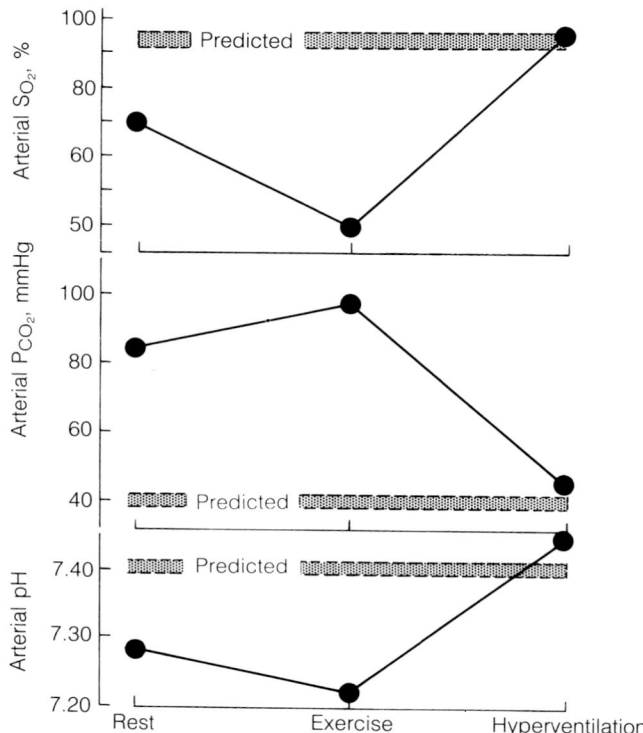

FIGURE 82-5 Blood-gas levels in a thin 53-year-old man with idiopathic alveolar hypoventilation. Arterial hypoxemia and respiratory acidosis were present at rest. During exercise the increase in ventilation was inadequate for the metabolism; the blood-gas levels became more abnormal. However, deliberate hyperventilation at rest restored blood-gas levels to normal.

common. The ventilatory responses to acute hypercapnia, to acute hypoxia, and to exercise are subnormal. Hypoventilation persists night and day but is exaggerated at night. Most of these patients develop severe polycythemia and die of cor pulmonale and right ventricular failure.

ORGANIC DEPRESSION OF MOTOR PATHWAYS (ONDINE'S CURSE)

Some infants develop marked alveolar hypoventilation during sleep despite normal blood-gas levels while awake. The disease of these infants has been designated as *Ondine's curse:*

> Since you left me, Ondine, all of the things my body once did by itself, it does now only by special order. . . . It is an exhausting piece of management I've undertaken. I have to supervise five senses, two hundred bones, a thousand muscles. A single moment of inattention, and I forget to breathe. He died, they will say, because it was a nuisance to breathe.

The defect in Ondine's curse seems to be in the automatic or metabolic pathway, which is under involuntary con-

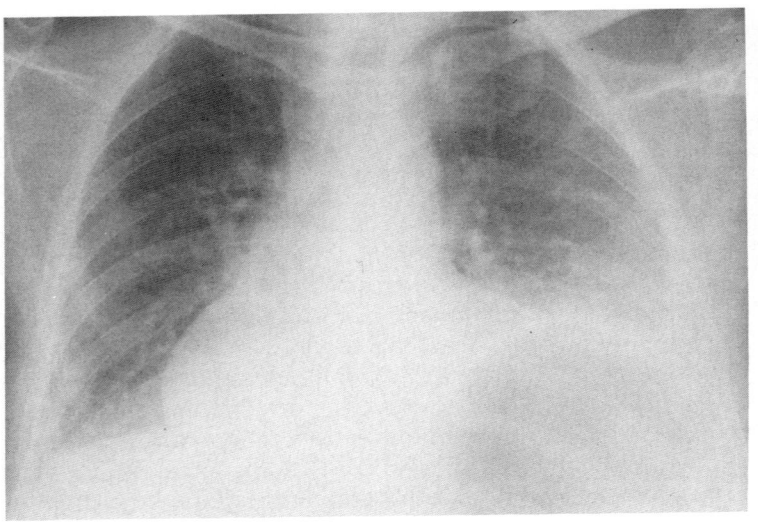
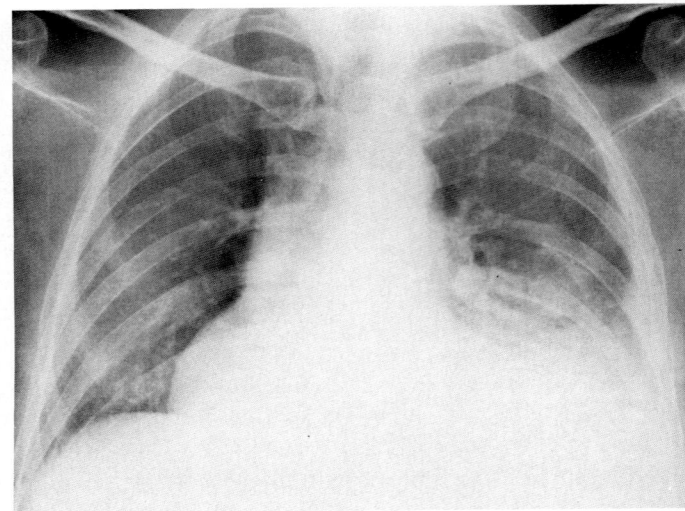

A   B

FIGURE 82-6 Diaphragmatic paralysis in a 38-year-old man who had paralytic poliomyelitis in childhood. Diaphragmatic paralysis was unsuspected until acute respiratory failure was precipitated by an acute respiratory infection. The left diaphragm is paralyzed; the right is weak. *A.* Chest radiograph on admission at maximum inspiration. There is haziness over the left lung obscuring the outline of the diaphragm. *B.* One week later. The diaphragm is clearly outlined.

trol; the behavior pathway is intact. Automatic control can be selectively impaired, and Ondine's curse reproduced, by lesions at the cervicomedullary junction or by destruction of the tegmentum of the pons or medulla below the trigeminal outflow. The syndrome is also caused by surgical procedures that aim to relieve intractable pain by severing the spinothalamic tract via a ventrolateral incision into the second cervical segment.

Mechanical Impairment of the Breathing Apparatus

PERIPHERAL NEUROMUSCULAR DISORDERS

Various kinds of neuromuscular disorders lead to alveolar hypoventilation. These include the Guillain-Barré syndrome, amyotrophic lateral sclerosis, poliomyelitis, myasthenia gravis, muscular dystrophy, polymyositis, and bilateral diaphragmatic paralysis.

Paralysis of the diaphragm is a common denominator for alveolar hypoventilation in a variety of neuromuscular diseases. The patients often complain of disturbed sleep, morning headaches, daytime fatigue and somnolence, and breathlessness while supine. Sleep and the supine position enhance the likelihood of clinical alveolar hypoventilation. Not infrequently the first evidence of respiratory impairment in patients with bilateral diaphragmatic paralysis is a bout of acute respiratory failure that may be precipitated by infection (Fig. 82-6).

It is often difficult to diagnose diaphragmatic paralysis, weakness, or fatigue. An important clue is the inward ("paradoxical") movement of the abdominal wall during inspiration. When standing, both the chest and the abdomen move in the same direction. However, while supine,

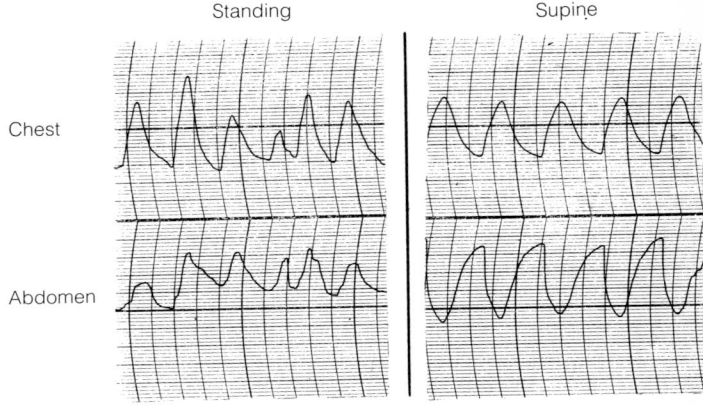

FIGURE 82-7 Thirty-three-year-old male with idiopathic diaphragmatic paralysis that caused shortness of breath while lying flat. Chest and abdominal movement in both the standing and supine positions monitored by a respiratory inductive plethysmograph. In the supine position, the chest and abdomen move oppositely. Pulmonary function studies in the sitting and supine positions are shown in Table 82-2.

the chest moves inward during inspiration and the abdomen moves out (Fig. 82-7 and Table 82-2). Moreover, diagnosis of bilateral diaphragmatic paralysis is reinforced by the further decrease in vital capacity when the supine position is assumed.

Although fluoroscopy of individuals with unilateral paralysis of the diaphragm often reveals impaired descent of the affected diaphragm during inspiration and paradoxical upward movement during a sniff test, paradoxical

1339

TABLE 82-2

Pulmonary Function Tests in Sitting and Supine Positions (Same Patient as in Fig. 82-7)

	Sitting	Supine
VC, L	2.74	1.26
FEV_1/FVC, %	77	70
FEF_{25-75}, L/s	1.43	0.60
FIF_{25-75}, L/s	4.18	2.11
MVV, L/min	96	43
PI_{max}, mmHg	45	30
PE_{max}, mmHg	118	80

NOTE: PI_{max} = maximum inspiratory pressure; PE_{max} = maximum expiratory pressure.

movement is often not as evident in bilateral paralysis. For this reason, measurement of transdiaphragmatic pressures has·been advocated: in normal individuals, a maximum inspiration causes the transdiaphragmatic difference in pressure to exceed 25 cmH₂O; in individuals in whom the diaphragm is paralyzed, transdiaphragmatic pressure does not change during either a quiet, or a maximal, inspiration.

KYPHOSCOLIOSIS

Severe deformity and dwarfing predispose to alveolar hypoventilation. Because of the severely deformed, stiff chest and the small lungs, the mechanics of breathing are abnormal (Fig. 82-8); the abnormal elastic resistance of the chest wall somehow sets a ventilatory pattern of rapid shallow breathing, one in which alveolar ventilation is sacrificed for dead-space ventilation. In this way, the deformity not only sets the stage for chronic alveolar hypoventilation but also has other indirect consequences: (1) the alveolar ventilation of a childlike lung is obliged to satisfy the metabolic requirements of an adult; (2) the deformed, stiff chest limits the ventilation during exercise; and (3) any additional impairment of ventilation or gas exchange, as by a bronchitis or pneumonia, may further compromise the critically limited lung and elicit the clini-

cal manifestations of respiratory and cardiac failure. Moreover, once CO_2 retention is established, any further depression of the ventilation, as by sedatives or O_2, may have lethal consequences.

OBESITY-HYPOVENTILATION SYNDROME

In 1810 Wadd noted the relationship between massive obesity, periodic breathing, and daytime somnolence. In 1918 Osler coined the designation *Pickwickian*. The association of cardiocirculatory disorders and massive obesity was described by Kerr and Logan in 1936; 20 years later, Burwell and associates revived the designation Pickwickian syndrome and spelled out the clinical features of marked obesity, somnolence, twitching, cyanosis, secondary polycythemia, periodic respiration, cor pulmonale, and right ventricular failure. Subsequent investigators demonstrated blunting of the ventilatory responses to acute hypercapnia and hypoxia. In 1966 Gastaut demonstrated using polysomnography that the obesity hypoventilation syndrome could result from repetitive episodes of obstructive apnea during sleep.

Obstructive sleep apnea is now the most common cause of the obesity-hypoventilation syndrome. However, there remains a subgroup of obese hypoventilators who fail to develop any evidence of apneas on all-night polysomnography—even though they do develop appreciable arterial hypoxemia while asleep. It is not understood why obese patients without obstructive sleep apnea develop alveolar hypoventilation. Nor is it clear why other obese individuals, many much more obese, remain eucapnic and without apneas during sleep.

Attempts to invoke a universal mechanical explanation that would, per se, account for the development of alveolar hypoventilation in obese patients without apnea have consistently been unconvincing (Fig. 82-9): since the work and energy cost of breathing are increased in all extremely obese individuals, whereas only a few develop the obesity-hypoventilation syndrome, some factor(s) other than the mechanical load of obesity has to be invoked to account for the alveolar hypoventilation.

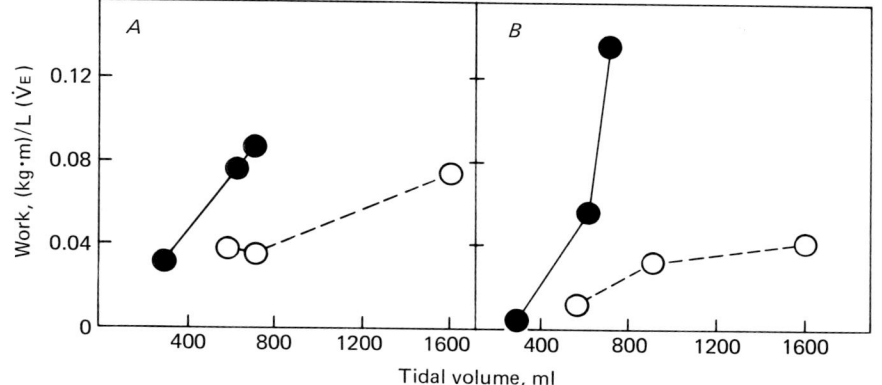

FIGURE 82-8 The work of breathing on the lungs (A) and on the chest (B) in kyphoscoliosis. The kyphoscoliotic subject (●) breathes at smaller tidal volumes than does the normal subject (○). Compared with the normal subject, the kyphoscoliotic patient demonstrates inordinate increases in the work of moving both the chest wall and the lung. (*Modified after Bergofsky, Turino, Fishman, 1959.*)

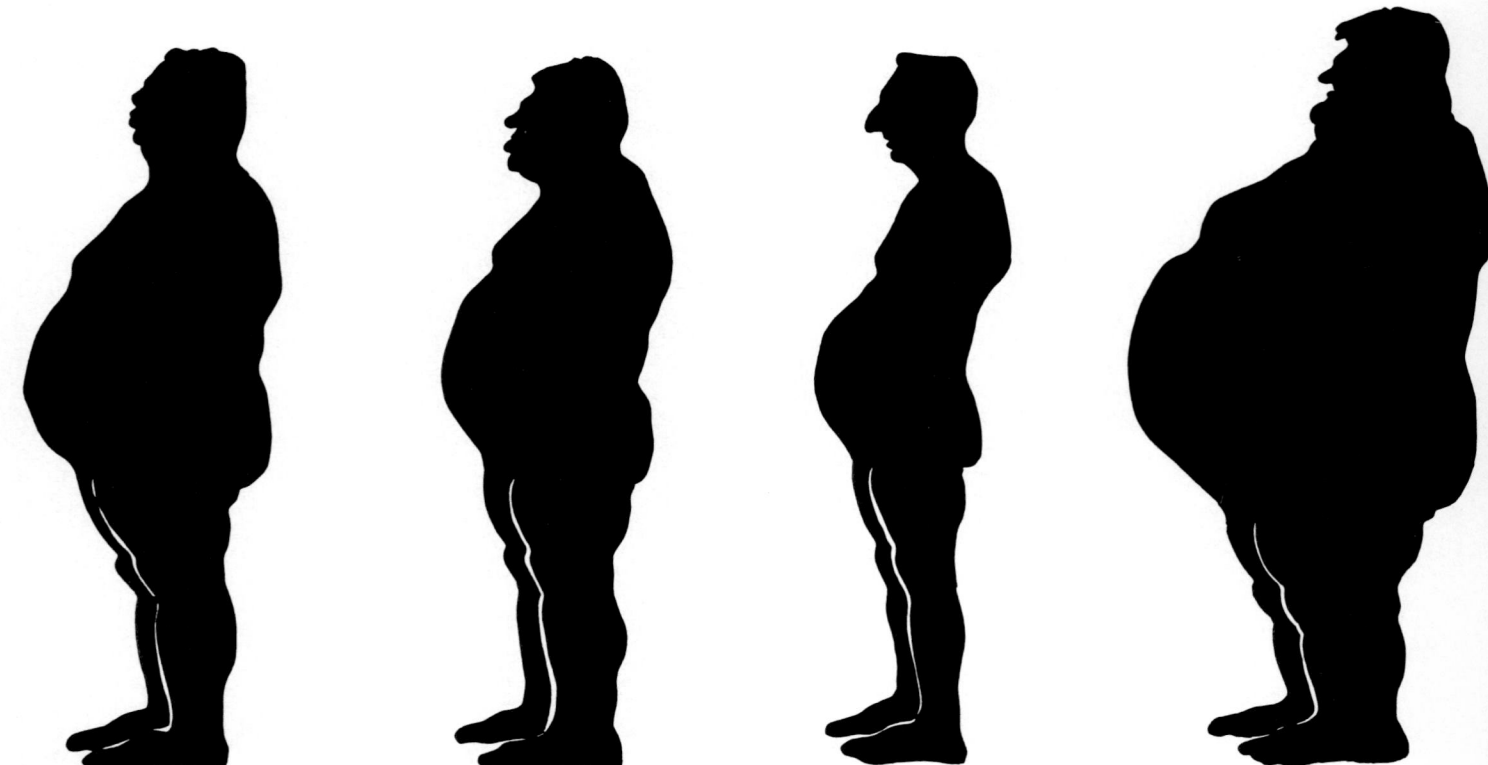

FIGURE 82-9 Silhouettes of four obese men. The three on the left had severe chronic alveolar hypoventilation. The most obese (right) weighed 750 lb and had normal blood gases and no evidence of obstructive sleep apnea.

Several mechanisms have seemed to tip the balance in favor of alveolar hypoventilation in certain patients: (1) a congenitally poor ventilatory response to CO_2 and/or hypoxia, (2) idiopathic (primary) alveolar hypoventilation that is not directly related to obesity, (3) a lesion in the brain that is responsible for both obesity and blunted chemosensitivity (encephalitis), and (4) acquired damage to the respiratory apparatus.

One curious aspect of the alveolar hypoventilation that occurs in patients who are extremely obese is enlargement of the left ventricle as well as the right ventricle (Fig. 82-10). The right ventricular enlargement (cor pulmonale) is easy to attribute to the hypoxia and acidosis of alveolar hypoventilation. However, the reason for left ventricular enlargement is much more subtle. Generally, it is attributed to the inevitable expansion of the circulating blood volume in obesity, along with left ventricular overloading due to increased cardiac output (in keeping with the high metabolic rate of obesity) and the frequent occurrence of systemic hypertension in extreme obesity.

TREATMENT OF CHRONIC ALVEOLAR HYPOVENTILATION

The guiding principle in treating alveolar hypoventilation is to improve alveolar ventilation to the point of restoring the arterial blood-gas levels either to normal or, more often, to tolerable levels of abnormality. The particular method used to improve the aeration of the blood varies according to the degree of abnormality, the initiating mechanism, the age of onset, and the clinical urgency. A few other general principles of treatment also warrant brief mention: (1) systematic management involves repeated measurements of arterial blood-gas levels as a guide to the use of mechanical ventilators and O_2 therapy; (2) acute life-threatening episodes of alveolar hypoventilation are usually precipitated by reversible factors, such as infection, oversedation, the administration of high concentrations of O_2, and acute bronchospasm; (3) patients with chronic alveolar hypoventilation may be asymptomatic even though the arterial blood-gas levels are distinctly abnormal; in such patients, in whom an acute upper respiratory infection or respiratory depressants may precipitously drive the blood gases to intolerable levels, the aim of treatment is to restore a tolerable degree of chronic alveolar hypoventilation.

Assisted Ventilation

In the 1950s, the use of iron lung negative pressure ventilators was instrumental not only in saving the lives of many victims of paralytic poliomyelitis, but also in paving the way for many other types of mechanical ventila-

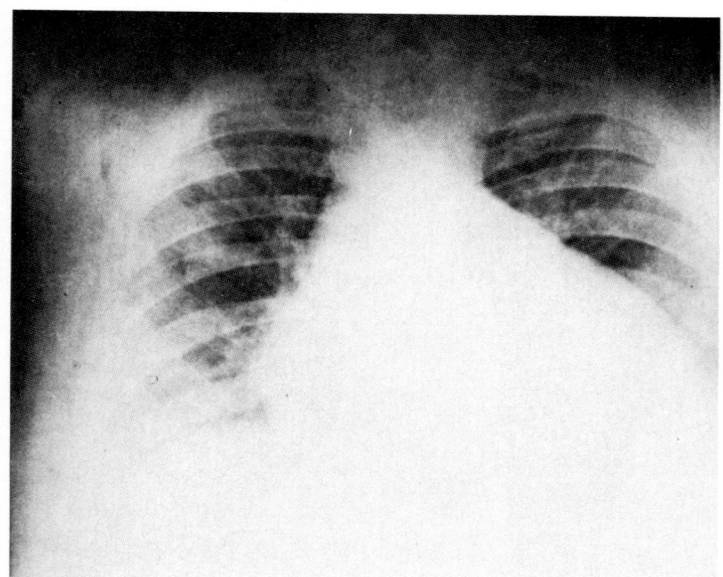

A

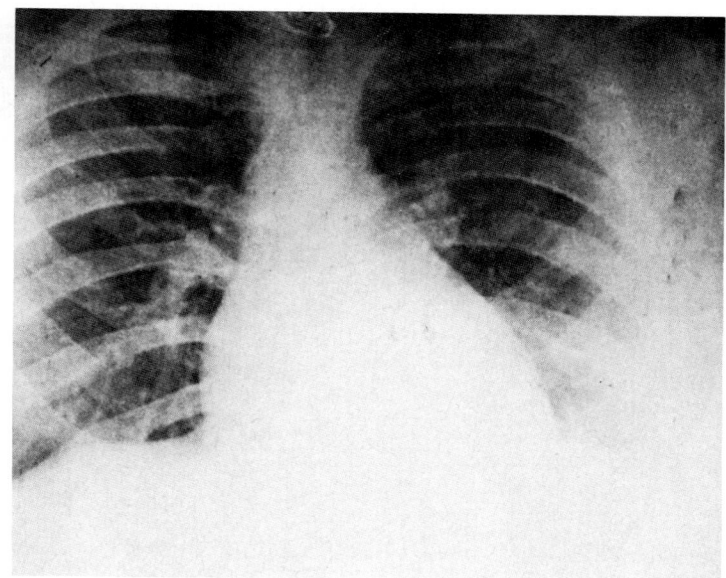

B

		Normal		During heart failure		After heart failure	
P_PA, mmHg	60 / 40 / 20						
P_wedge, mmHg	25 / 15 / 5						
End diastolic RV, mmHg	25 / 15 / 5						
C.O., L/min	15 / 10 / 5						
Sa_O2, %	100 / 80 / 60						
ΔC.O. / Δ O2 consumption, ml/100 ml	700 / 500 / 300						
		Rest	Exer.	Rest	Exer.	Rest	Exer.

C

FIGURE 82-10 The pulmonary circulation in the obesity-hypoventilation syndrome. Radiographic appearance of the heart during heart failure (A) and after recovery (B). Hemodynamic changes at rest and during exercise compared to normal (C). During exercise a slight increase in cardiac output (C.O.) and in filling pressure accompanies a further increase in pulmonary artery pressure.

tors for use in patients with alveolar hypoventilation of all sorts. Since then, the "TANK" respirator has been succeeded by other forms of assisted ventilation: the rocking bed to produce passive diaphragmatic movement; cuirass, or "tortoise shell," respirators which apply negative pressure only to the anterior chest wall; positive pressure ventilators; and constant volume respirators usually used in conjunction with tracheostomy. Recently, a positive pressure ventilator linked to the patient by a nasal mask has been used to effect continuous positive airway pressure ventilation (nasal CPAP). The more recent equipment has made assisted ventilation, either continuous or nocturnal, much more comfortable and less complicated while providing ready access to the patient.

Electrophrenic respiration has been tried repeatedly during the past two decades and continues to have strong advocates in certain clinics. The technique of radiofrequency electrophrenic pacing is currently being tried to

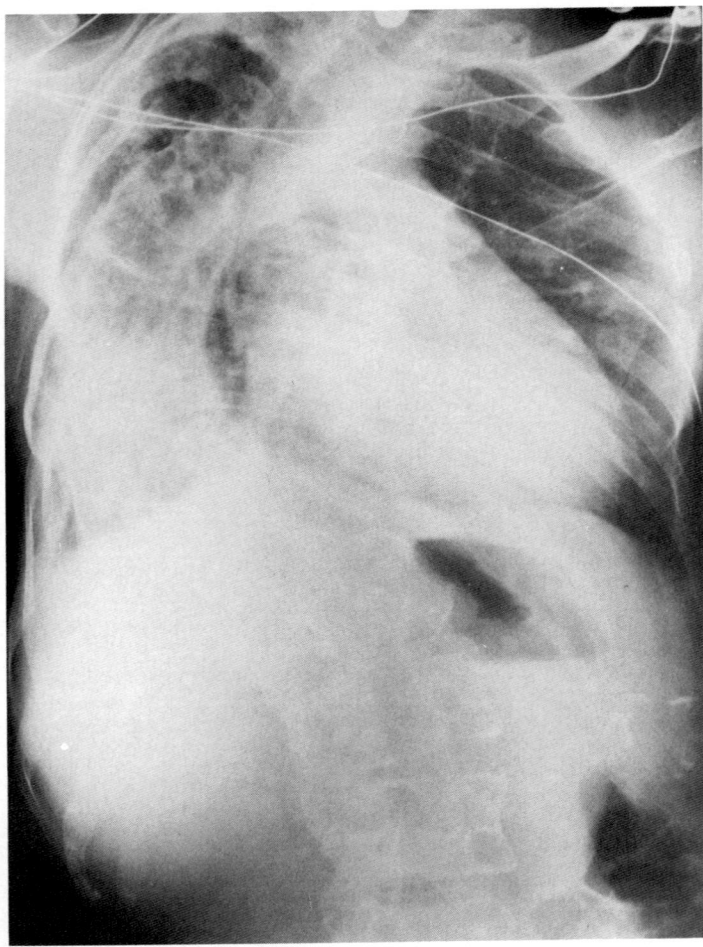

FIGURE 82-11 Chest radiograph from a 27-year-old white female with severe kyphoscoliosis from childhood polio. Her pulmonary function deteriorated after placement of a Harrington rod. After repetitive admissions to the medical intensive-care unit for acute exacerbations of her chronic respiratory failure, she was placed in a tent-type cuirass ventilator at night. Application of negative inflating pressures to both the patient's rib cage and her abdomen allowed her to have effective ventilation at night for the first time. After 10 days, there was a 20-mmHg fall in her P$_{CO_2}$ and improved daytime functioning.

pulse to subcutaneously implanted receivers, which then pace the diaphragm. The desired tidal volume and frequency are determined empirically. Although the technique appears to be well tolerated for prolonged periods of time, to date only few patients have been treated in this fashion.

It is worth stressing that nocturnal assisted ventilation is sometimes helpful in breaking the cycle involving pulmonary hypertension and the retention of salt, water, and bicarbonate during sleep, a sequence that further worsens lung mechanics and blunts respiratory chemosensitivity; the quality of daytime lifestyle subsequently improves (Fig. 82-11). Also, sleep-associated alveolar hypoventilation in patients with normal lungs (or chronic obstructive airways disease) is sometimes exaggerated by diaphragmatic or generalized neuromuscular weakness. In these patients, the use of nocturnal assisted ventilation not only improves the quality of daily life but also avoids the serious complications of sleep-aggravated alveolar hypoventilation.

Medical Management

The medical management of patients with inadequate ventilatory drive has included drugs that increase the ventilatory responsiveness to acute hypercapnia. For example, medroxyprogesterone acetate has sometimes been successful in improving CO_2 responsiveness and the arterial blood-gas tensions in resting patients with the obesity-hypoventilation syndrome. The use of this agent is based on the observation that, during the latter portion of the menstrual cycle or during pregnancy, the CO_2 response is heightened, and the resting arterial P$_{CO_2}$ is low. Progesterone has been shown to be responsible for this phenomenon; it acts by decreasing the threshold, and increasing the slope, of the CO_2 response curve by directly stimulating the medullary chemoreceptor.

Because of the depressant effects of high bicarbonate levels on the ventilation, one cornerstone of medical management is reducing bicarbonate levels in blood to normal. Acetazolamide, a carbonic anhydrase inhibitor, is commonly used for this purpose. Administration of chloride salts to combat hypochloremia is also helpful by producing a bicarbonate diuresis. The disadvantage of overzealous administration of potent diuretics that promote metabolic alkalosis accompanied by the loss of hydrogen ion from cells, including the respiratory neurons, has been noted above.

improve ventilation in patients who have a general hypoventilation syndrome as well as in patients with high cervical spinal cord transection. Indwelling phrenic electrodes are placed on the cervical portion of both phrenic nerves, and external radio transmitters transmit the im-

BIBLIOGRAPHY

Bergofsky EH: Respiratory failure in disorders of the thoracic cage. Am Rev Respir Dis 119:643–669, 1979.
  Up-to-date review of the topic.

Bergofsky EH, Turino GM, Fishman AP: Cardiorespiratory failure in kyphoscoliosis. Medicine 38:263–317, 1959.
  Classic description of respiratory function in kyphoscoliosis.

Bradley TD, Rutherford R, Lue F, Moldofsky H, Grossman RF, Zamel N, Phillipson EA: Role of diffuse airway obstruction in the hypercapnia of obstructive sleep apnea. Am Rev Respir Dis 134:920–924, 1986.
  The presence of diffuse airway obstruction is an important predisposing factor to the development of chronic CO_2 retention in obstructive sleep apnea.

Brouillette RT, Hunt CE, Gallemore GE: Respiratory dysrhythmia. A new cause of central alveolar hypoventilation. Am Rev Respir Dis 134:609–611, 1986.
  In an infant who developed chronic respiratory failure after aseptic meningoencephalitis at 5 months of age, the subsequent course indicated that disorganized as well as diminished output from the central respiratory pattern generator can result in central alveolar hypoventilation.

Davis JN, Goldman M, Loh L, Casson M: Diaphragm function and alveolar hypoventilation. Q J Med 45:87–100, 1976.
  Diaphragm paralysis can lead to chronic alveolar hypoventilation.

DeBacker WA, Heyrman RM, Wittesaele WM, Van Waeleghem JP, Vermiere PA, DeBroe ME: Ventilation and breathing patterns during hemodialysis-induced carbon dioxide unloading. Am Rev Respir Dis 136:406–410, 1987.
  Carbon dioxide unloading during hemodialysis with acetate-buffered dialysate is accompanied by alveolar hypoventilation.

Ellis ER, McCauley VB, Mellis C, Sullivan CE: Treatment of alveolar hypoventilation in a six-year-old girl with intermittent positive pressure ventilation through a nose mask. Am Rev Respir Dis 136:188–191, 1987.
  When all else failed, the use of IPPV with 5 cmH_2O of PEEP administered through a nose mask during sleep maintained both oxygen saturation and transcutaneous CO_2 levels within the normal range.

Fishman AP, Goldring RM, Turino GM: General alveolar hypoventilation. A syndrome of respiratory and cardiac failure in patients with normal lungs. Q J Med 35:261–274, 1966.
  Classic description of chronic alveolar hypoventilation syndromes.

Gibson GJ, Pride NB, Davis JN, Loh LC: Pulmonary mechanics in patients with respiratory muscle weakness. Am Rev Respir Dis 115:389–395, 1977.
  Evaluation of lung function in patients with weakness of the respiratory musculature.

Glenn WL, Gee JBL, Cole DR, Farmer WC, Shaw RK, Beckman CB: Combined central alveolar hypoventilation and upper airway obstruction. Treatment by tracheostomy and diaphragm pacing. Am J Med 64:50–60, 1978.
  Diaphragm pacing may be an effective means of testing central alveolar hypoventilation but may precipitate obstructive sleep apnea in susceptible patients.

Goldstein RS, Molotiu N, Skrastins R, Long S, de Rosie J, Contreras M, Popkin J, Rutherford R, Phillipson EA: Reversal of sleep-induced hypoventilation and chronic respiratory failure by nocturnal negative pressure ventilation in patients with restrictive ventilation impairment. Am Rev Respir Dis 135:1049–1055, 1987.
  Nocturnal negative pressure ventilation is effective in preventing sleep-induced reductions in alveolar ventilation.

Hoeppner VH, Cockcroft DW, Dosman JA, Cotton DJ: Nighttime ventilation improves respiratory failure in secondary kyphoscoliosis. Am Rev Respir Dis 129:240–243, 1984.
  Nighttime ventilation through a permanent tracheostomy proved to be an effective alternative for long-term treatment of the cardiorespiratory failure caused by severe kyphoscoliosis.

Kerby GR, Mayer LS, Pingleton SK: Nocturnal positive pressure ventilation via nasal mask. Am Rev Respir Dis 135:738–740, 1987.
  A continuous positive airway pressure mask, originally developed for patients with obstructive apnea, was connected to a portable positive-pressure volume respirator in five patients with neuromuscular disease. In five of the six, blood gases improved considerably during the 6 months of use.

Lavie CJ, Crocker EF Jr, Key KJ, Ferguson TG: Marked hypochloremic metabolic alkalosis with severe compensatory hypoventilation. South Med J 79:1296–1299, 1986.
  An uncommon, but not extraordinary patient with alveolar hypoventilation secondary to metabolic alkalosis. A larger perspective can be found in report by Fishman, Goldring, and Turino, 1966.

Loh L, Goldman M, Newsom Davis J: The assessment of diaphragm function. Medicine 56:165–169, 1977.
Transdiaphragmatic pressure is the most useful tool for assessing bilateral diaphragmatic paralysis or weakness.

Marks CE, Goldring RM: Chronic hypercapnia during methadone maintenance. Am Rev Respir Dis 108:1088–1093, 1973.
Methadone can blunt the ventilatory response to CO_2 and lead to the development of chronic hypercapnia.

Mellins RB, Balfour HH Jr, Turino GM, Winters RW: Failure of autonomic control of ventilation (Ondine's curse). Medicine 49:487–504, 1976.
Classic description of Ondine's curse.

Olgiati R, Levine D, Smith JP, Briscoe WA, King TKC: Diffusing capacity in idiopathic scoliosis and its interpretation regarding alveolar development. Am Rev Respir Dis 126:229–234, 1982.
Diffusion in idiopathic scoliosis is reduced purely by the reduced lung volumes. There is a partial failure of alveolar enlargement as a result of the thoracic deformity rather than an atrophy of the alveoli or pulmonary vasculature.

Riley DJ, Santiago TV, Daniele RP, Schall B, Edelman NH: Blunted respiratory drive in congenital myopathy. Am J Med 63:459–466, 1977.
Central depression of ventilation can occur frequently in the setting of congenital myopathies. The resulting chronic respiratory failure can effectively be managed by assisted ventilation at night.

Sandham JD, Shaw DT, Guenter CA: Acute supine respiratory failure due to bilateral diaphragmatic paralysis. Chest 72:96–98, 1977.
The supine position increases the degree of alveolar hypoventilation that occurs with diaphragmatic paralysis.

Sinha R, Bergofsky EH: Prolonged alteration of lung mechanics in kyphoscoliosis by positive pressure hyperventilation. Am Rev Respir Dis 106:47–56, 1972.
Intermittent positive pressure breathing increases lung compliance in kyphoscoliotic patients and decreases the work of breathing.

Sivak ED, Ahmad M, Hanson MR, Mitsumoto H, Wilbourn AJ: Respiratory insufficiency in adult-onset acid maltase deficiency. South Med J 80:205–208, 1987.
This article describes four patients with respiratory muscle weakness associated with signs of cor pulmonale and symptoms of alveolar hypoventilation.

Smith PEM, Calverly PMA, Edwards RHT, Evans GA, Campbell EJM: Practical problems in the respiratory care of patients with muscular dystrophy. N Engl J Med 316:1197–1205, 1987.
Drawing on their special experience gained from the respiratory core of patients with Duchenne's muscular dystrophy, the authors indicate the implications for other conditions involving chronic weakness of the inspiratory muscles.

Sutton FD, Zwillich CW, Creagh CE, Pierson DJ, Weil JV: Progesterone for outpatient treatment of the Pickwickian syndrome. Ann Intern Med 83:476–479, 1979.
Progesterone by stimulating ventilation has some benefit in the treatment of chronic alveolar hypoventilation.

Yasuma F, Nomura H, Sotobata I, Ishihara H, Saito H, Yasuura K, Okamoto H, Hirose S, Abe T, Seki A: Congenital central alveolar hypoventilation (Ondine's curse): a case report and review of the literature. Eur J Pediatr 146:81–83, 1987.
In an infant with congenital central alveolar hypoventilation ("Ondine's curse"), diaphragmatic pacing resulted in remarkable improvement.

Zwillich CW, Natalino MR, Sutton FD, Weil JV. Effects of progesterone on chemosensitivity in normal man. J Lab Clin Med 92:262–269, 1978.
Progesterone administration increases ventilatory responsiveness to hypercapnia and hypoxia.

Zwillich CW, Pierson DJ, Hofeldt FD, Lifkin EG, Weil JV: Ventilatory control in myxedema and hypothyroidism. N Engl J Med 292:662–667, 1975.
Mild hypothyroidism and myxedema are associated with blunted ventilatory responses to chemical stimuli.

Chapter *83*

Sleep Apnea Syndromes

Richard P. Millman / Alfred P. Fishman

Obstructive Sleep Apnea Syndromes
    Pathogenesis
    Clinical Features
    Diagnosis
    Treatment

Central Sleep Apnea Syndromes
    Pathogenesis
    Clinical Features
    Diagnosis
    Treatment

Relationship between Central and Obstructive Apnea

Apnea during Sleep in the Elderly

Effect of Sleep on Respiration in Pulmonary Disease
    Chronic Obstructive Airways Disease
    Asthma

In 1966, Gastaut and co-workers called attention to repetitive pauses in breathing that occurred in some patients during sleep. Since then, considerable attention has been paid to the behavior of respiration during sleep, not only in individuals suspected of sleep apnea, but also in patients who have underlying pulmonary disorders, notably chronic obstructive airways disease, i.e., chronic bronchitis and emphysema (COPD) and asthma. Pursuit of this interest has relied heavily on the polysomnograph in conjunction with the simultaneous monitoring of the stage of sleep, airflow at the nose and mouth, respiratory effort, arterial oxygen saturation, and heart rate as diagnostic tools.

As experience has grown, old terms have taken on more precise meanings: *apnea* is now defined as a cessation of airflow for 10 s or longer. There is less of a consensus about the definition of *hypopnea*: some clinics define hypopnea as a 50 percent reduction in airflow associated with a 4 percent fall in oxygen saturation. However, this definition is not entirely satisfying when applied to relatively healthy adults and children who fail to develop appreciable O_2 desaturation (despite a drop in arterial P_{O_2}) because of the shape of the oxyhemoglobin dissociation curve.

Based on all-night polysomnographic evaluation of normal subjects, *sleep apnea* has been defined as greater than five apneas per hour or more than 30 apneas per night. Because of the unexpected finding that subjects older than 65 years have a high incidence (35 to 40 percent) of recurrent apneas, some of which are asymptomatic and others symptomatic, this definition of sleep apnea has been seriously challenged. From a clinical standpoint, the designation "sleep apnea syndrome" should be applied to those individuals who not only experience frequent apneas and hypopneas during sleep but who also manifest symptoms (e.g., hypersomnolence, cor pulmonale, polycythemia) due to recurrent fragmentation of sleep and arterial hypoxemia.

Two distinct clinical syndromes of sleep apnea have been identified based on pathophysiological mechanisms: *obstructive and central*. The syndrome of *obstructive sleep apnea* is characterized by episodes of either *obstructive apnea*, during which respiratory effort continues despite pharyngeal obstruction to airflow (Fig. 83-1), or of *mixed apnea*, during which respiratory effort is absent at the start of the apnea but then starts again before airflow resumes.

By definition, the syndrome of *central sleep apnea* entails a cessation of both respiratory effort and airflow. This kind of "pure" central apnea is responsible for less than 5 percent of instances of sleep apnea. As a rule, the designation *central sleep apnea syndrome* is reserved for patients who have repetitive episodes of apnea that are solely central in type. However, some clinics are more lax than others in this regard and categorize patients as having the syndrome of central sleep apnea when the central apnea pattern predominates—even though up to 45 percent of the apneic events may be clearly obstructive in nature.

OBSTRUCTIVE SLEEP APNEA SYNDROMES

The obstructive sleep apnea syndrome can be regarded as a continuum that begins with snoring (mild to severe) and extends through the more significant disturbances of hypersomnolence and frequent nocturnal arousals to the severe derangements of obstructive sleep apnea (the classic Pickwickian syndrome).

Snoring is a sound produced by vibration of the soft palate and posterior faucial pillars when air is inspired through the mouth into a partially narrowed upper airway; the frequency of the sound ranges from 40 to 60 cycles per second. In an individual who snores tolerably and is otherwise normal, snoring accompanies each breath and has a harmonic quality.

In contrast with normal snoring, the typical snore associated with the sleep apnea syndrome is loud and intermittent rather than continuous. It marks the start of

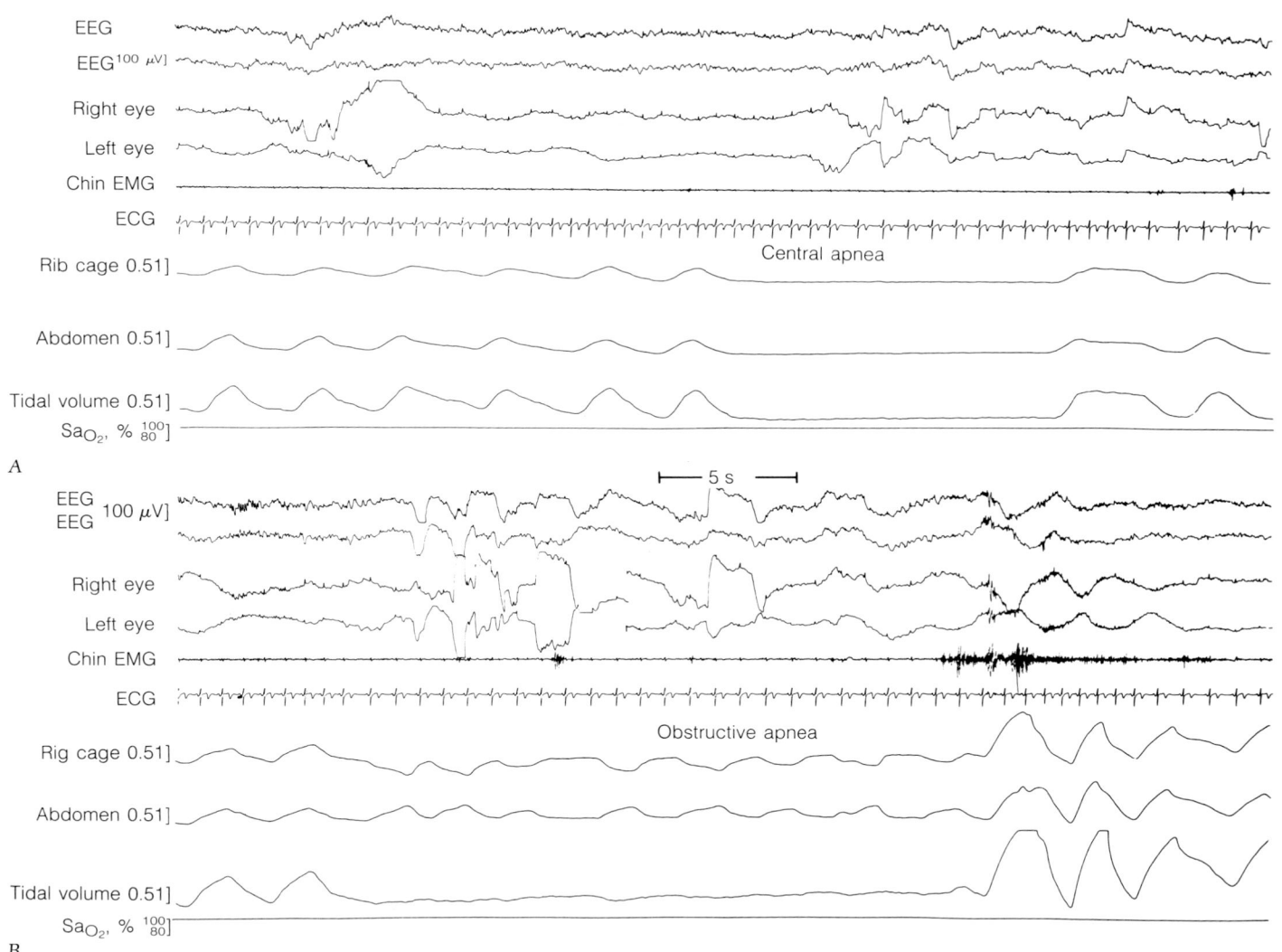

FIGURE 83-1 Records illustrating distinctions between central and obstructive apneas. Respiratory inductive plethysmography in a 40-year-old man. Upper and lower panels are part of a continuous record during REM sleep. *A*. In *central apnea*, the absence of deflections associated with the tidal volume (cessation of breathing) was associated with an absence of both rib cage and abdominal movements. *B*. In *obstructive apnea*, the movements of the rib cage and abdomen are paradoxical. EEG = electroencephalogram; Chin EMG = submental electromyogram; ECG = electrocardiogram; Sa_{O_2} = arterial O_2 saturation determined by ear oximetry. (*From Phillipson and Bowes, 1982.*)

breathing after a bout of complete airway closure and heralds the inrush of air through a narrow pharyngeal orifice. In most cases, the complete closure is brought about by movement of the tongue and soft palate posteriorly to occlude both the oropharynx and nasopharynx (Fig. 83-2). Occlusion occurs when the force tending to collapse the airway, i.e., negative pharyngeal pressure, exceeds opposing forces generated by contraction of the upper airway muscles. The occlusion persists as long as continued diaphragmatic contraction sustains the negative hypopharyngeal pressure; arousal activates the musculature of the upper airways, thereby undoing the obstruction. In moderate to severe obstructive apnea, the episodes of apnea occur periodically, separated by several breaths (Fig. 83-2). In this way, recurrent cycles of sleep and apnea alternate with arousal and breathing.

Pathogenesis

The pathogenesis of upper airway obstruction during sleep is not entirely clear. However, three major factors appear to be involved, to different degrees, from patient to patient: the configuration of the upper airway, neural control of the respiratory muscles, and hormonal balance.

CONFIGURATION OF THE UPPER AIRWAY

It seems evident that the narrower the caliber of the airway, the easier it is for closure to occur. Indeed, computed tomography has shown that the prototypical, middle-aged obese patient with obstructive sleep apnea has a narrow upper airway. However, many patients with sleep apnea do have a normal body habitus. In some, airways are narrowed by structural derangements such as adenotonsillar

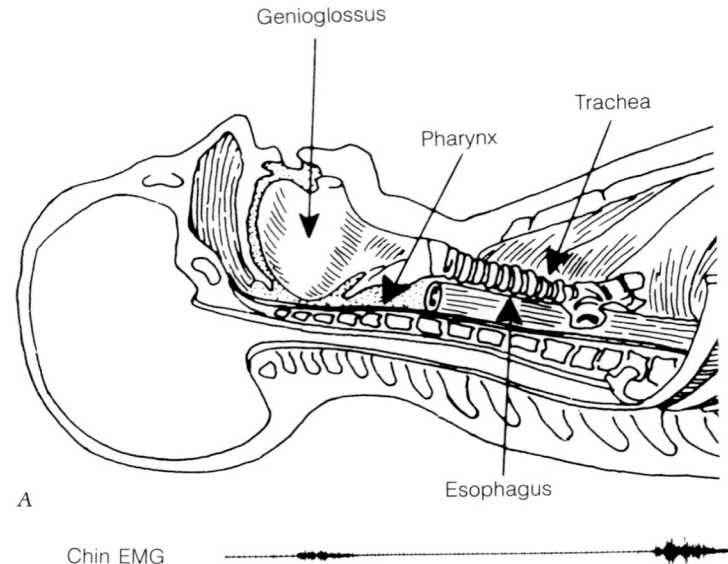

Genioglossus

Pharynx

Trachea

Esophagus

A

FIGURE 83-2 Obstructive sleep apnea. *A.* Sagittal section showing architecture in vicinity of the tongue predisposing to upper airway obstruction. *(See also Frontispiece.) B.* Severe obstructive sleep apnea syndrome. Polysomnographic tracings in a 51-year-old man demonstrating the typical cyclical pattern of apnea, profound arterial O_2 unsaturation, and bradycardia, alternating with activation of upper airway muscles and large tidal volumes. Pes = esophageal pressure as a measure of respiratory effort; Chin EMG = submental electromyogram; ECG = electrocardiogram; Sa_{O_2} = arterial O_2 saturation determined by ear oximetry. *(From Phillipson and Bowes, 1982.)*

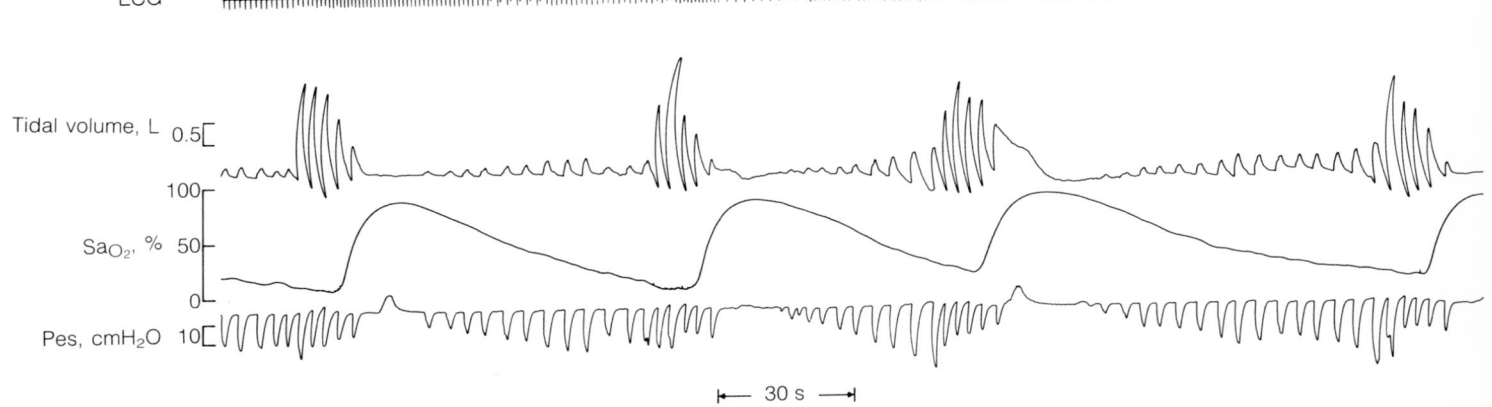

Chin EMG

ECG

Tidal volume, L 0.5

100

Sa_{O_2}, % 50

0

Pes, cmH_2O 10

|← 30 s →|

B

hypertrophy (Fig. 83-3), macroglossia (hypothyroidism, acromegaly), retrognathia, and micrognathia. In others, who by inspection have no evident narrowing of the upper airway, sophisticated diagnostic tools, such as acoustic reflection methods and cephalometric radiography, have disclosed narrow airways that are unusually collapsible.

Narrowing of the nasopharynx by deviation of the nasal septum, or enlargement of the nasal adenoids or by allergic rhinitis, increases the negativity of hypopharyngeal pressure during inspiration, thereby contributing further to the collapse of the oro- and nasopharynx.

NEURAL CONTROL OF THE RESPIRATORY MUSCLES

The respiratory system is dramatically affected by the stage of sleep. Since mechanical features operate continuously regardless of state, and since apneas are intermittent events, nonmechanical influences must be involved in the pathogenesis of sleep apnea. Among these are neural influences which, in conjunction with the intrinsic caliber

of the upper airway, determine its degree of patency. The neural influences exert their effects by way of the coordinated function of *all* respiratory muscles—not only those of the upper airway (Fig. 83-4) but also those of the chest wall and the diaphragm. The upper airway does not collapse during wakefulness because muscle tone of the multiple muscle groups in the airway work is high. During non-rapid eye movement (NREM) sleep, neural activity to these muscles decreases, causing the airway to narrow somewhat. During rapid eye movement (REM) sleep, the respiratory motor neurons are inhibited, causing the upper airway to become atonic.

In NREM sleep, obstructive and central apneas occur intercurrently. One explanation attributes this intercurrence to instability in the ventilatory control system, just as in Cheyne-Stokes breathing (see Chapter 25). According to this concept, *central* apnea ensues during NREM sleep when the arterial P_{CO_2} falls below the apneic threshold, thereby turning off respiratory drive (see Chapter 9); ventilation resumes as arterial hypoxemia and hypercapnia develop and restore the ventilatory drive. Instability of

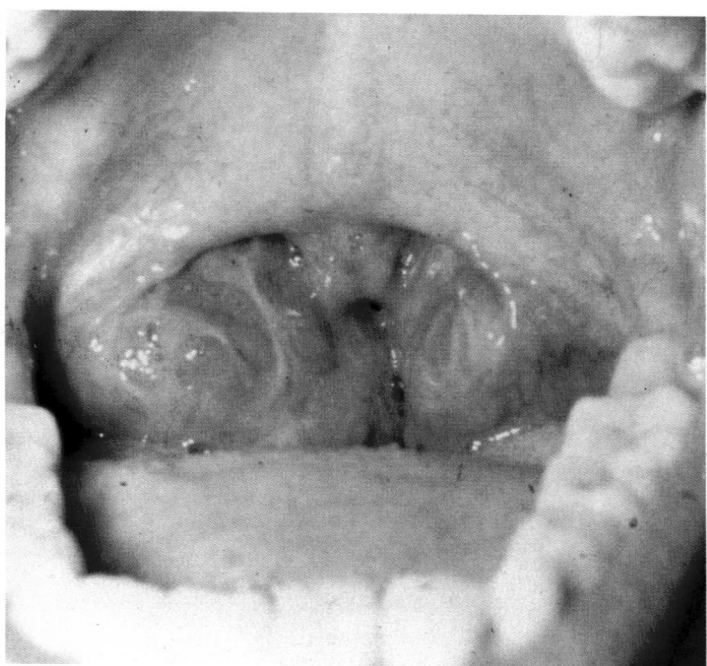

FIGURE 83-3 Marked airway narrowing secondary to tonsillitis in a 10-year-old child. His parents observed the acute onset of intermittent loud snoring and obstructive apneic episodes.

the ventilatory control system operates differently in *obstructive* apnea. Respiratory neural activity never stops completely. In this instance, neural efferent activity to the diaphragm is presumably unlinked from that to the muscles of the upper airway, possibly due to the differences in their intrinsic responsiveness to hypoxia and hypercapnia. Should the diaphragm receive a greater neural input than the upper airway muscles, the pharynx would collapse. However, mitigating against the concept of different intrinsic responsiveness is the normal ventilatory response of the total respiratory system to hypoxic and hypercapnic stimuli in the awake state. Moreover, even though individuals who are hypoxic or hypercapnic during the day generally have reduced ventilatory responses to hypoxia and hypercapnia, respectively, it is not clear whether the blunted responsiveness is the cause, or the result, of the abnormal arterial blood gases.

During REM sleep, both obstructive and central apneas may result from episodic inhibition of neural efferent activity to the diaphragm and muscles of the upper airway. Asynchronies are prone to develop during phasic events, such as eye movements and muscle twitches. For example, during these movements, inspiratory activity of the diaphragm is intermittently inhibited. Similarly, the inspiratory activity of the upper airway musculature is largely absent or diminished throughout REM sleep. As in the case of the postural muscles, the accessory and intercostal muscles also become atonic during REM sleep. Therefore, episodic and asynchronous inhibition of the diaphragm and upper airway muscles probably contribute to the pathogenesis of apneas. In keeping with this concept, most apneas do occur at the time of phasic events.

HORMONAL BALANCE

The role of hormonal balance in the pathogenesis of sleep apnea is uncertain. Premenopausal women seem to be protected against developing obstructive sleep apnea presumably because circulating progesterone is a respiratory stimulant. Oppositely, at least in some instances, administration of testosterone has triggered the onset of apnea. Hypothyroidism can cause obstructive sleep apnea not only by way of macroglossia that narrows the upper airway but also by disturbance of ventilatory control.

Clinical Features

The clinical features of the obstructive sleep apnea syndrome (Table 83-1) appear to be a direct consequence of the multiple episodes of hypoxemia and sleep fragmentation that occur each night. During the apneic period, hypoxia, hypercapnia, and acidosis develop and intensify until an arousal occurs and breathing resumes. Hypoxemia and acidemia produce transient increases in systemic and pulmonary arterial pressures during the night; in most instances, the blood pressures return to normal levels upon awakening. However, persistent systemic hypertension is not uncommon. Indeed, it has recently been proposed that obstructive sleep apnea is an important cause of "essential hypertension" in middle-aged men. In some patients, sustained pulmonary hypertension is sufficiently severe to elicit cor pulmonale and right ventricular failure.

During each apnea, alveolar hypoventilation develops. But, as a rule, the breaths interposed between the apneic episodes suffice to restore alveolar ventilation to normal, i.e., no net CO_2 retention occurs during the night.

TABLE 83-1
Clinical Features of the Obstructive Sleep Apnea Syndrome

Excessive daytime sleepiness
Frequent nocturnal awakening
Insomnia
Loud snoring
Morning headaches
Intellectual deterioration
Personality changes, irritability
Impotence
Systemic hypertension
Arrhythmias
Pulmonary hypertension, cor pulmonale
Polycythemia

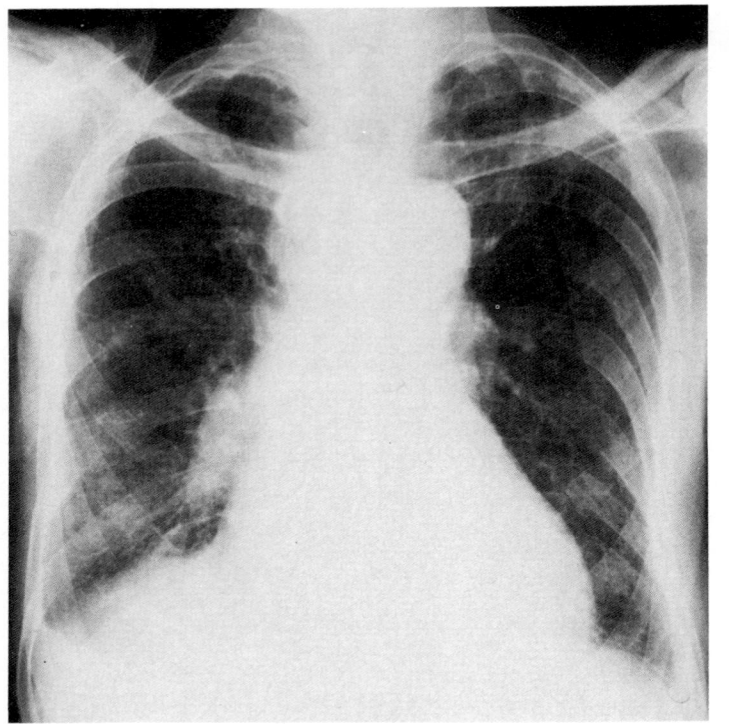

A

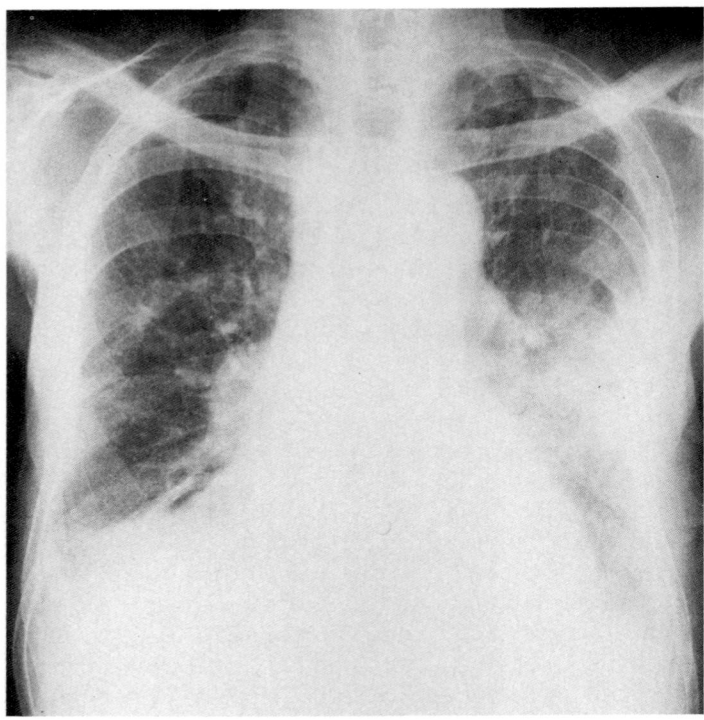

B

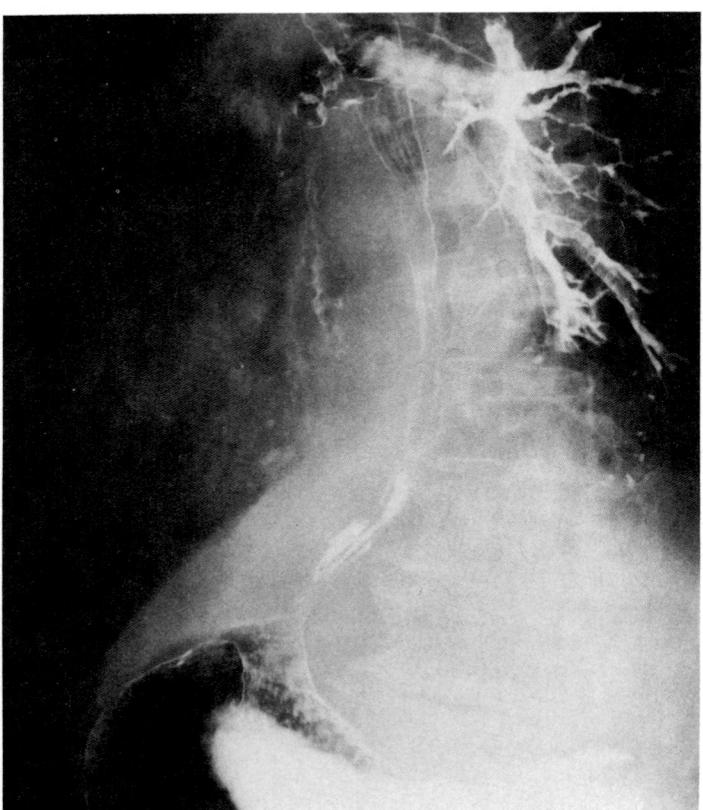

C

FIGURE 83-4 Cricopharyngeal motor dysfunction in a 99-year-old man, leading to insufficiency rather than to obstruction of the upper airway. *A*. Before hospitalization. Patient in good health. *B*. Aspiration pneumonia. *C*. Barium swallow showing aspiration of barium into both lung fields.

One clinical clue to persistent hypercapnia is the occurrence of morning headaches, which subside as the day progresses. The headaches probably result from hypercapnia-induced cerebral vasodilatation. It is not clear why a small proportion of those with obstructive sleep apnea develop the chronic hypoventilation and the persistent daytime hypercapnia that occurs in the Pickwickian syndrome. It is possible that the net increase in P_{CO_2} that occurs in some patients at night leads to an increase in renal bicarbonate reabsorption, thereby enabling the patient to tolerate higher levels of P_{CO_2} without developing severe acidosis. It is also possible that these patients are predisposed to developing CO_2 retention because of a lower ventilatory response to CO_2. However, blunting of the hypercapnic ventilatory response may result from, rather than lead to, chronic hypercapnia.

During the apneic episodes, arterial hypoxemia, in conjunction with repetitive respiratory efforts against a closed upper airway, increases vagal tone, thereby causing bradycardia, occasionally with sinus arrest. Alternating episodes of bradycardia and tachycardia that correspond respectively to the apneic and breathing periods are common. Although cardiac ischemia may increase ventricular irritability and promote ectopy, significant ventricular arrhythmias occur primarily if the arterial oxygen saturation falls below 60 percent. Nocturnal sudden death, presumably due to an arrhythmia, has occurred in patients with the Pickwickian syndrome. Whether nocturnal sudden death due to arrhythmia also occurs in patients with less severe forms of obstructive sleep apnea is unknown.

Multiple arousals fragment the sleep of patients with obstructive sleep apnea. Although some patients do complain of frequent nocturnal awakening and in some instances of frank insomnia, most arousals go unrecognized. Occasionally, a patient is awakened by the sense of not breathing. Unless the patient panics, the discomfort generally resolves rapidly. It is not clear whether it is the recurrent hypoxemia or the sleep fragmentation that causes the patient to experience excessive daytime sleepiness and to doze off inappropriately, i.e., while reading, watching television, conversing, or even while driving an automobile. The sleep-deprived individual may undergo changes in personality, become irritable, and undergo intellectual deterioration. Impotence is a common complaint.

Diagnosis

The most reliable diagnostic test is still the overnight evaluation using polysomnography. However, in patients with a severe sleep apnea syndrome, a daytime study can reveal not only the diagnosis but also the severity of the apnea. Typical variables monitored during these studies are outlined in Table 83-2; the essentials are the determi-

TABLE 83-2

Variables Measured during Polysomnography

Sleep staging
  Electroencephalogram (EEG)
  Electrooculogram (EOG)
  Submental electromyogram (EMG)
Ventilation
  Nasal and oral thermistors
  Tracheal breath sounds
  Respiratory inductive plethysmography
Respiratory effort
  Abdominal-thoracic strain gauges
  Respiratory inductive plethysmography
  Esophageal pressure
  Diaphragmatic and intercostal EMG activity
Gas exchange
  Ear oximetry
  Transcutaneous CO_2 electrode
  Indwelling arterial catheter
Heart rate

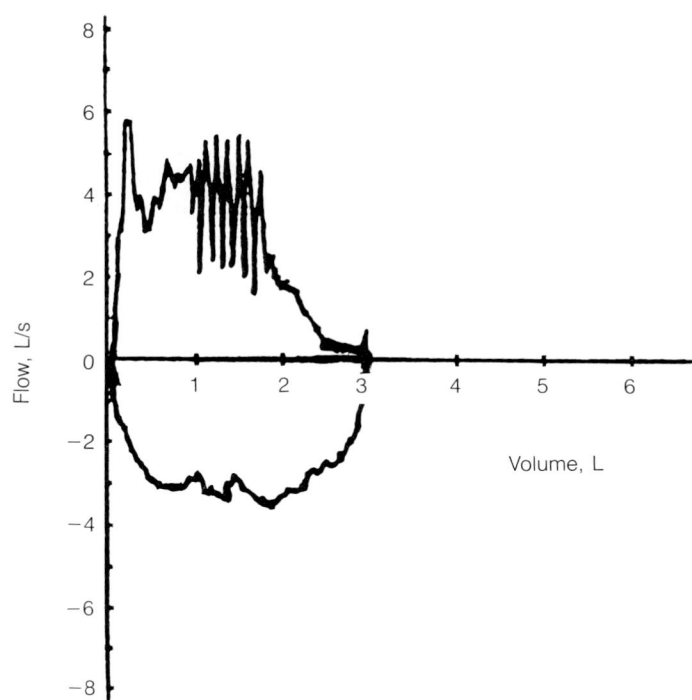

FIGURE 83-5 Flow-volume loop in obstructive sleep apnea. The inspiratory limb is flattened and a saw-toothed pattern is evident in the expiratory limb. Once popular as a screening test for obstructive sleep apnea, it has been succeeded by the all-night polysomnogram.

nation of the stage of sleep, airflow, respiratory effort, oxygen saturation of arterial blood, and heart rate.

At present, there is no adequate screening test for obstructive sleep apnea. The initial popularity of the flow-volume loop as a screening test has waned considerably in light of recent observations that have invalidated reliance

of certain patterns (Fig. 83-5) as reliable indicators of the syndrome.

Once a diagnosis of obstructive sleep apnea is made on the basis of polysomnography, the determination of the patient's hematocrit to detect hypoxia-induced polycythemia and the sampling of arterial blood to determine the level of oxygenation and the P_{CO_2} are useful in defining the severity of the disease. Occasionally, thyroid function studies reveal unexpected hypothyroidism as an underlying cause of obstructive sleep apnea. Examination of the upper airway by an experienced otorhinolaryngologist is essential in identifying surgically treatable causes of the apnea.

Treatment

Successful treatment requires that therapy be individualized according to the patient's needs. Unfortunately, the correlation between symptoms and polysomnographic findings is often poor. Moreover, it is often difficult to justify treatment in relatively asymptomatic individuals who have positive polysomnographic findings, especially the elderly, since little is known about the natural history of the disorder if left untreated. Therefore, therapy should be directed not only at normalizing the sleep disturbance but, more importantly, at abolishing symptoms.

Despite these caveats, certain principles of therapy can be applied to most patients with obstructive sleep apnea (Table 83-3): weight loss is often helpful in decreasing the severity of the illness. The consumption of alcohol and/or sedatives in the evening should be avoided since these agents exacerbate apnea during sleep; not only does alcohol reduce upper airway muscle (genioglossus) activity in humans (leaving diaphragmatic activity unaffected), but it also impairs responses to arousal stimuli.

TABLE 83-3
Treatment of Obstructive Sleep Apnea

General measures
  Weight loss
  Avoidance of alcohol and sedatives
Medications
  Medroxyprogesterone
  Protriptyline
  Nasal decongestants
Surgery
  Tracheostomy
  Tonsillectomy
  Uvulopalatopharyngoplasty
  Nasal septal repair
Mechanical approaches
  Nasal CPAP
  Tongue retaining device
  Nasopharyngeal airway

Medical management is often disappointing in obstructive sleep apnea. Medroxyprogesterone, which is effective in alveolar hypoventilation syndromes, is of little value in obstructive sleep apnea. Protriptyline, a nonsedating tricyclic antidepressant, has proved useful in decreasing daytime hypersomnolence and the frequency of nocturnal apneas. Its mechanism of action is unclear. However, protriptyline does decrease the duration of REM sleep where the worst apneas tend to occur. In animal studies the drug has been shown to increase the tonic activity of the upper airway muscles. In practice, the use of protriptyline is often hampered by its anticholinergic effects, particularly urinary retention; also, tachyphylaxis develops during prolonged usage. Antihistamines and inhaled nasal steroids are sometimes effective in patients in whom allergic rhinitis and reversible nasal obstruction contribute to upper airway collapse.

It has long been recognized that the administration of oxygen entails the risk of prolonging obstructive apnea. Originally, prolongation of the apnea was attributed to the abolition of hypoxia which was regarded as a potent arousal stimulus. However, hypoxia has proved to be a rather weak arousal stimulus. Indeed, long-term oxygen therapy is currently being tried as a mode of therapy in obstructive sleep apnea.

Tracheostomy has been the traditional mainstay of therapy for obstructive sleep apnea because the tracheostomy site lies below the level of the obstruction. However, with the advent of newer surgical procedures and nasal positive airway pressure (CPAP), fewer tracheostomies are being done. As a rule, the procedure is now reserved for the most severe cases, specifically those with the Pickwickian syndrome (Fig. 83-6). In some individuals, even though tracheostomy relieves the symptoms and abolishes the apneas, chronic alveolar hypoventilation and hypercapnia persist.

Less severely affected individuals are treated by tonsillectomy or a uvulopalatopharyngoplasty (UPP). The UPP entails surgical excision of the tonsils, the uvula, and the posterior portion of the soft palate with tightening of the posterior pharyngeal wall. The procedure alleviates symptoms of snoring in 90 to 95 percent of the patients, but only decreases apneas and excessive daytime hypersomnolence in about 50 percent. Unfortunately, unless gross anatomic deformity is present, it does not yet seem possible to identify which patient will benefit from the procedure. The results appear to be directly related to the excisional technique employed and the skill of the surgeon as well as to the anatomy of the pharynx. Other surgical procedures, such as nasal septal repair, mandibular advancement and mandibular osteotomy, and expansion hyoidoplasty are helpful in selected patients.

Not all patients are willing to undergo surgery or are candidates for surgery. Certain alternatives are available. For example, mechanical devices, such as the nasopha-

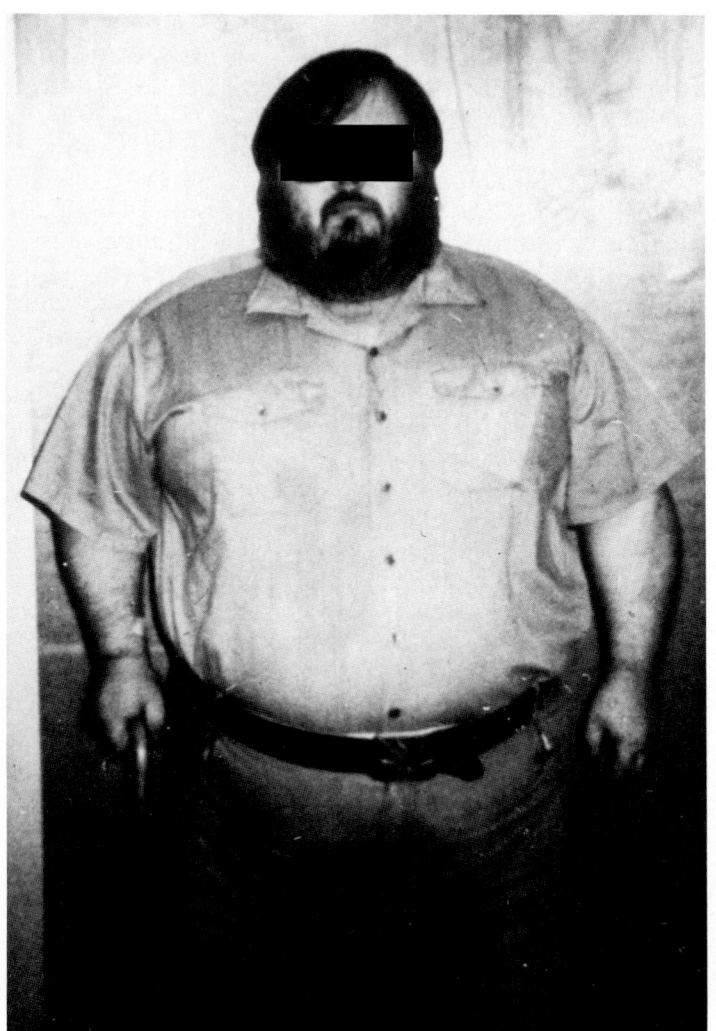
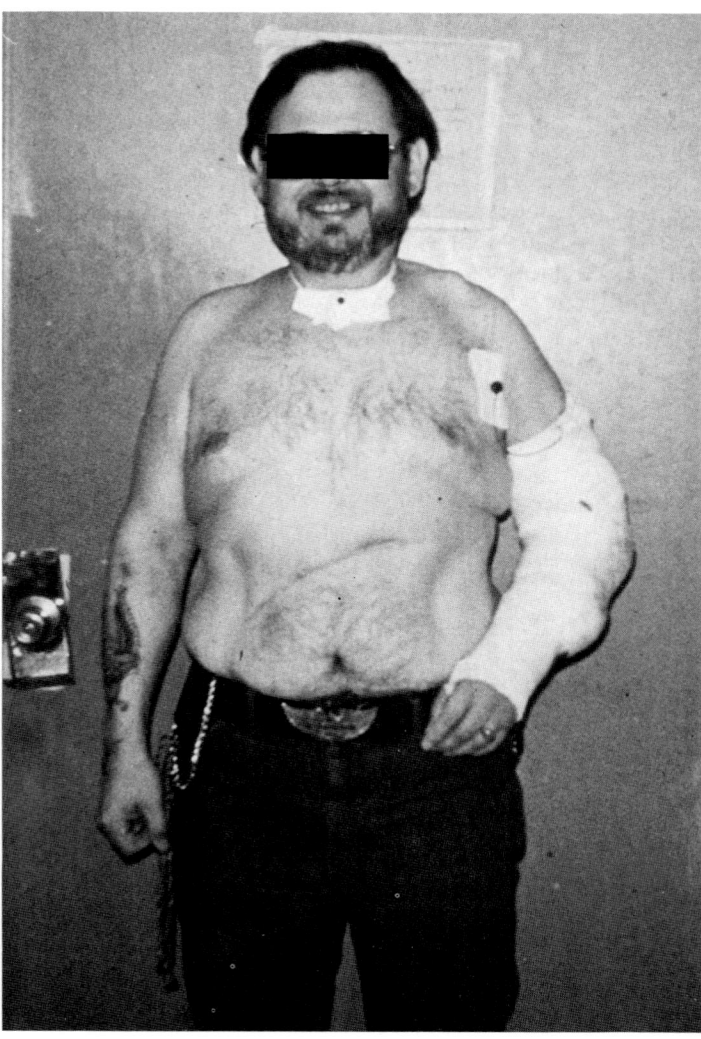

A   B

FIGURE 83-6 Obstructive sleep apnea in a morbidly obese individual. *A.* Before weight loss. Polysomnography revealed repetitive episodes of obstructive apnea with arterial O_2 unsaturation to 60 percent. He was treated with a tracheostomy and a gastric stapling procedure. *B.* One and one-half years later. The patient then weighed 180 pounds. Repeat polysomnography with the tracheostomy plugged revealed rare apneas. After closure of the tracheostomy, the patient remained asymptomatic.

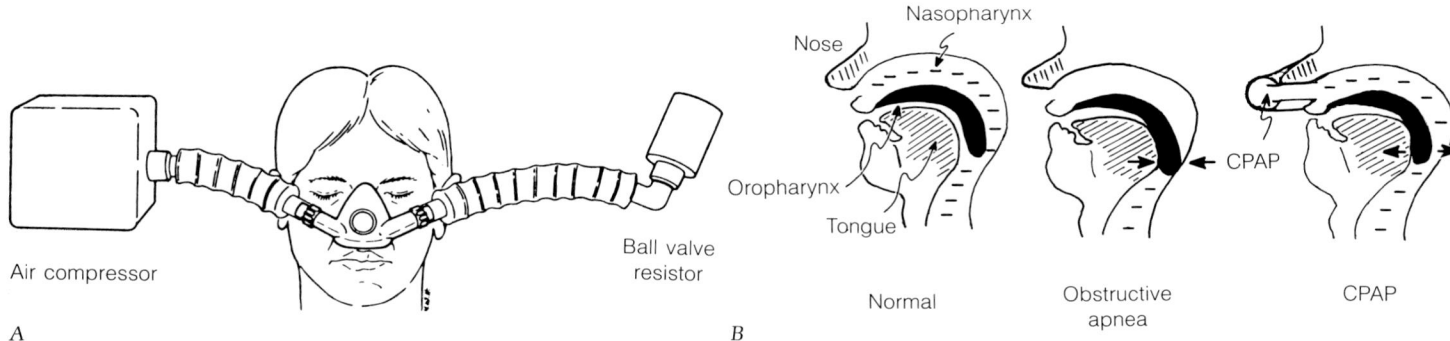

A   B

FIGURE 83-7 Nasal CPAP in treating obstructive sleep apnea. *A.* Schematic representation of the system used for CPAP: an air compressor, a tight-fitting nose mask, and a ball value resistor to adjust pressure. *(From Sanders, 1984.)* *B.* The operation of the CPAP. By creating a positive pressure in the oropharynx and nasopharynx, the negative pressure developed in the hypopharynx during inspiration is overcome. *(From Sullivan, Issa, Berthon-Jones, Eves, 1981.)*

ryngeal airway or the tongue-retaining device, have proved to be helpful in some instances, but the devices are cumbersome and often uncomfortable. Excellent results have recently been obtained using nasal CPAP or by delivering continuous airflow to the nose (Fig. 83-7).

CENTRAL SLEEP APNEA SYNDROMES

Pathogenesis

Central apnea has traditionally been regarded as a separate entity from obstructive and mixed apneas. Many neurologic diseases that damage respiratory neurons and are known to produce chronic alveolar hypoventilation also produce central apnea (Table 83-4). Among these are bulbar poliomyelitis, encephalitis, brain-stem neoplasm, brain-stem infarction, spinal cord surgery, and cervical cordotomy. In fact, these patients usually have coexistent hypoventilation during the daytime, which is exacerbated with sleep.

However, there are other causes of central apnea that are not associated with neurologic disease and alveolar hypoventilation. Periodic central apneas occur during NREM sleep in most new arrivals to high altitude; they are related to hypoxic stimulation of the carotid body. In these individuals, alveolar hyperventilation, rather than hypoventilation, underlies the development of apnea: the hyperventilation that occurs between apneic episodes lowers the P_{CO_2} below the apneic threshold, thereby triggering the onset of apnea; while there is a decrease in P_{O_2} and an increase in P_{CO_2} during the apnea, the carotid body is stimulated, ventilation resumes, and the cycle is repeated. In REM sleep, concurrent inhibition of the diaphragm and upper airway can cause central apnea. Hypothyroidism, by functionally depressing ventilatory drive, can also cause central apnea. In elderly individuals, central apnea frequently occurs without obvious neurologic dysfunction.

TABLE 83-4
Pathogenesis of Central Sleep Apnea

Anatomic damage to respiratory neurons:
  Bulbar poliomyelitis
  Encephalitis
  Brain-stem infarction
  Brain-stem neoplasm
  Spinal cord surgery
  Bilateral cervical cordotomy
Functional alteration of ventilatory drive:
  Hypothyroidism
  High altitude
Uncertain—aging

Clinical Features

The clinical features of central sleep apnea caused by neurologic damage are essentially those produced by alveolar hypoventilation: the patients are either asymptomatic or show signs and symptoms of chronic hypoxemia and hypercapnia. In addition, they may have symptoms consistent with sleep fragmentation, including frequent awakenings and daytime sleepiness. Some authors have reported troublesome snoring and daytime hypersomnolence. However, these manifestations may be related to the inclusion in their series of up to 45 percent *obstructive* apneas and hypopneas.

Diagnosis

Diagnosis is best made, as in the case of obstructive sleep apnea, by all-night polysomnography. To confirm pure, or predominantly, central apnea, the absence of respiratory effort during an apneic event can be best confirmed using an esophageal balloon or a carefully calibrated respiratory inductive plethysmograph.

Treatment

The treatment of central sleep apnea that accompanies neurologic disease is essentially that of chronic alveolar hypoventilation. Ventilatory support, primarily at night, can be provided by a rocking bed, an iron lung, a cuirass body shell, or positive pressure ventilation either via a tracheostomy, a lip-seal ventilator, or a nasal CPAP mask. Phrenic nerve pacing has been useful in some patients with normal chest bellows and lungs.

Ventilatory stimulation, using either medroxyprogesterone acetate or acetazolamide (that causes a metabolic acidosis), is occasionally successful in reversing central sleep apnea but seems to be more effective in dealing with the central apnea of high altitude. Supplemental oxygen, by abolishing hypoxia-induced stimulation of the carotid body, can prevent the development of central apnea at high altitude. Sometimes nasal CPAP is also effective in abolishing central apnea.

RELATIONSHIP BETWEEN CENTRAL AND OBSTRUCTIVE APNEA

There is now reason to believe that central and obstructive apneas need not be a consequence of different pathophysiological mechanisms. Occasionally, the administration of acetazolamide or the breathing of O_2-enriched mixtures has converted central to obstructive apnea (Fig. 83-8). Phrenic nerve pacing has also been reported to convert central to obstructive apnea. Moreover, mild hypothyroidism, as noted above, can produce either obstructive or central apnea.

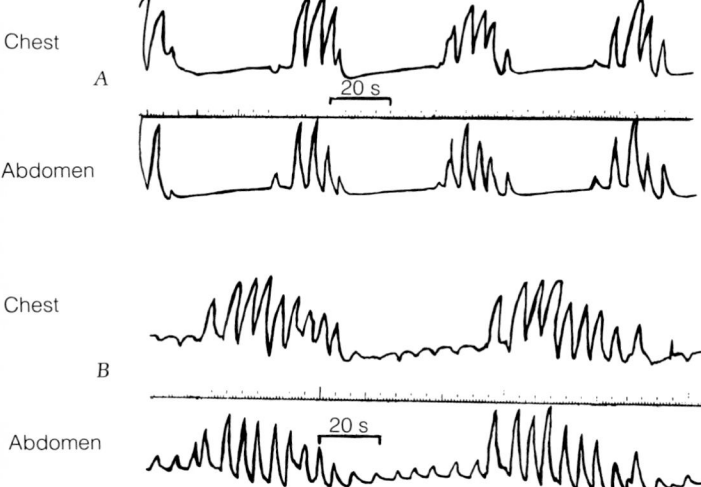

FIGURE 83-8 Periodic breathing in the elderly. *A.* Stages 1 to 2 sleep. Chest and abdominal movements recorded by a respiratory inductive plethysmograph reveals recurrent central apneas. *B.* Administration of O₂. Obstructive apneas develop with paradoxical motion of the chest and abdomen during the apneic periods.

One possible common denominator in the pathogenesis of the two types of apnea is the unlinking of the respiratory muscles, specifically the diaphragm, intercostal muscles, and upper airway muscles during the various stages of sleep. As indicated previously, during NREM sleep, these muscle groups probably have different activation thresholds and response slopes to hypercapnia and hypoxia. During REM sleep, depending on whether the inhibition of the diaphragm and muscles of the upper airway are asynchronous or synchronous, either obstructive or central apnea can result.

In keeping with the concept of unlinking, the metabolic acidosis produced by acetazolamide could act like phrenic nerve pacing by selectively stimulating the diaphragm more than the muscles of the upper airway; the resulting negative pharyngeal pressure would predispose the upper airway to collapse.

APNEA DURING SLEEP IN THE ELDERLY

Several studies have demonstrated recently that up to 40 percent of healthy elderly subjects without sleep complaints experience a sufficient number of episodes of either central or obstructive apnea during sleep to be categorized as having sleep apnea. However, even though there is general agreement that apnea is quite common in the elderly, there is no consensus about the clinical significance of frequent apneas in the asymptomatic elderly individual. There are several reasons for the uncertainty: (1) since individuals older than 60 years were not used in originally defining the sleep apnea syndrome, the standard definition may not apply to the elderly; (2) the inci-

dence of frequent apneas during sleep is the same as in those who complain of disrupted sleep; and (3) arousals from light sleep to awakening occur as frequently in the elderly without apnea as in those with apnea. Therefore, it may be erroneous to assume that sleep disruption in the elderly is caused necessarily by periodic apneas. Other processes such as nocturnal myoclonus may be as important, or more important.

It is widely held, but not well substantiated, that the elderly are more sleepy during the daytime and that they tend to doze off quite easily. Unfortunately, subjective assessment of daytime sleepiness is often imprecise. One test is the Multiple Sleep Latency Test which simply involves determining how long it takes a patient to fall asleep four to five times a day at 2-h intervals. When the tendency to fall asleep is measured in asymptomatic elderly individuals with apnea using the Multiple Sleep Latency Test, they do have a greater tendency to doze off during the daytime. However, it is difficult to translate this index of increased daytime sleepiness to performance capabilities. Although some elderly individuals with proven apneas and definite complaints of disrupted sleep have performed poorly on intellectual and cognitive function testing, it is not clear that the run-of-the-mill asymptomatic elderly person with apnea has any deficits in cognitive capabilities. This is an important area for clinical research since the results may strongly influence decisions about treatment.

From the cardiovascular standpoint, it is clear that elderly individuals may experience considerable hemodynamic stress during sleep. However, the natural history of the elderly with apnea but without evidence of systemic or pulmonary hypertension while awake is uncertain, particularly with respect to developing cardiac complications if the apneas are left untreated. Nor is it clear whether apneas during sleep contribute to death during the night that often occurs in the older age groups. Should the apneas be implicated, the common use of hypnotics and sedatives in the elderly would have to be reassessed with respect to the risk of nocturnal sudden death.

Little is also known about the treatment of sleep apnea in the elderly. There is little experience with any of the conventional therapeutic modalities that are being used to alleviate apnea and snoring in the middle-aged individuals. The lack of information is compounded by a general lack of knowledge about the clinical significance and natural history of apnea if left untreated in an asymptomatic elderly patient who is found to have apnea on polysomnographic testing.

EFFECT OF SLEEP ON RESPIRATION IN PULMONARY DISEASE

Polysomnography has also been applied to patients with cardiopulmonary disorders who do not have sleep apnea.

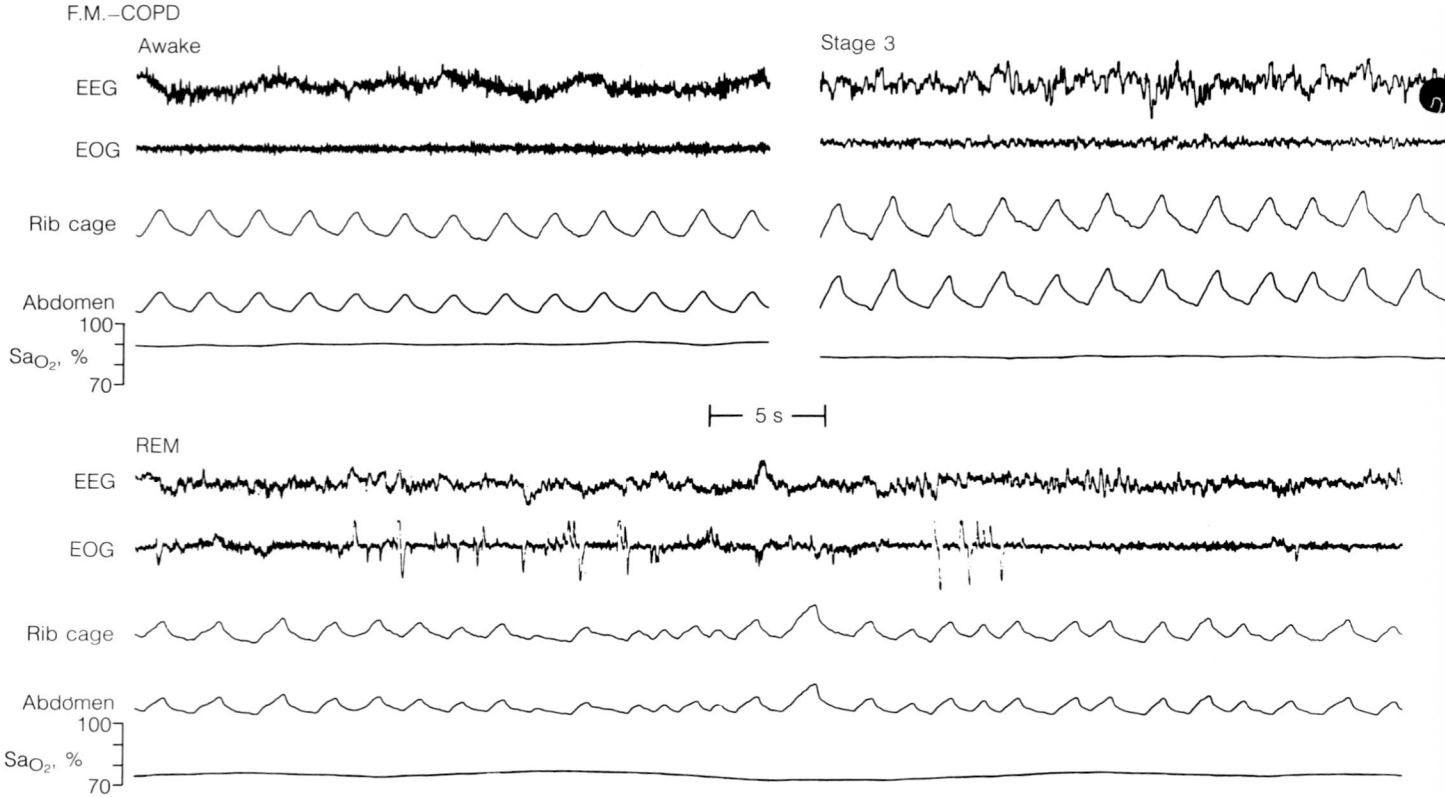

FIGURE 83-9 Sleep recording from a 58-year-old man with chronic bronchitis and emphysema demonstrating the effect of sleep on arterial O_2 saturation. The channels from top to bottom show electroencephalogram, electrooculogram, rib cage and abdominal movement, and oxygen saturation. The most profound desaturation occurs during REM sleep with loss of intercostal muscle tone. *(From Phillipson, Bowes, 1982.)*

The bulk of the information available is about chronic obstructive airways disease (COAD), i.e., chronic obstructive lung disease (or COLD, usually used as a synonym for chronic bronchitis and emphysema) and asthma. Observations have also been made on patients with chronic interstitial lung disease. Arterial hypoxemia often becomes more marked in both groups during REM sleep, but the mechanisms appear to be different. However, neither routine pulmonary function tests nor exercise testing has succeeded in identifying the patient with obstructive airways disease or interstitial lung disease at risk for arterial O_2 unsaturation during REM sleep: instead, in obstructive airways disease, the best predictor for exaggerated arterial hypoxemia during sleep is the level of hemoglobin during wakefulness; for interstitial lung disease, the best predictor is the arterial O_2 saturation in the supine patient. (Unpublished observations of Kline LR, Goldszmidt AJ, Laufe MD, and Pack AI.)

Chronic Obstructive Airways Disease

Patients categorized as having chronic obstructive pulmonary disease, presumably chronic bronchitis and emphysema, undergo a considerable drop in arterial oxygenation during sleep; the drop is unrelated to apneic events. The greatest degree of oxygen unsaturation occurs during REM sleep (Fig. 83-9), when intercostal muscle activity decreases markedly, thereby minimizing the contribution of the rib cage to ventilation. In patients with chronic bronchitis and emphysema, the lungs are hyperinflated and the shortened diaphragms function with reduced mechanical efficiency. The loss of intercostal muscle activity during REM sleep decreases the functional residual capacity (FRC), resulting in closure of small airways and microatelectasis. Arterial hypoxemia is then a consequence of two possible mechanisms: ventilation-perfusion mismatching or alveolar hypoventilation.

Another factor that may contribute to arterial hypoxemia is a sleep-related reduction in the clearance of pulmonary secretions. Patients with large quantities of mucous secretion are particularly vulnerable to obstruction of small airways, with subsequent mismatching of alveolar ventilation and blood flow.

The end-state chronic bronchitic ("blue bloater") tends to develop more arterial hypoxemia during sleep than does the patient with pure emphysema ("pink puffer"). The blue bloater has a greater degree of daytime

hypoxemia. Therefore, a reduction in oxygen tension during sleep is associated with a greater fall in oxygen saturation because of the shape of the oxyhemoglobin dissociation curve. Furthermore, in these patients, the degree of sleep-related hypoxemia is inversely related to their ventilatory responsiveness to hypercapnia while awake. These disturbances in the arterial blood gases and their blunting effects on the chemical control of ventilation may contribute to the severe nocturnal hypoxemia that sometimes occurs in blue bloaters.

Moderate to severe arterial hypoxemia, particularly if severe, sometimes causes sustained pulmonary hypertension and cor pulmonale. The best therapeutic approach is nocturnal supplemental oxygen: by preventing the nocturnal exaggeration of arterial hypoxemia, the supplemental oxygen reduces pulmonary artery pressures, improves right ventricular function, decreases nocturnal cardiac arrhythmias, and prolongs survival.

Asthma

Symptoms of asthma often become manifest during sleep. The descriptive term *morning dipper* has been applied to those patients in whom asthma worsens in the early morning hours. The mechanisms for this phenomenon are not well understood. One possibility is that the exacerbations are related to circadian decreases in plasma epinephrine levels while histamine levels are increasing. Whether gastroesophageal reflux, airway cooling, or reduced clearance of airway secretions plays a role is unclear.

Attacks of asthma can occur during both NREM and REM sleep. They are associated with audible wheezing, increased activity of the diaphragm and intercostal and sternocleidomastoid muscles, and asynchronous movement of the abdomen and chest wall. Apneic events are not observed unless the patient has coexistent sleep apnea, nor is arterial hypoxemia a common occurrence.

BIBLIOGRAPHY

Ancoli-Israel S, Kripke DF, Mason W, Messin S: Sleep apnea and nocturnal myoclonus in a senior population. Sleep 4:349–358, 1981.
  Elderly subjects with symptoms of disrupted sleep frequently have sleep apnea or nocturnal myoclonus.

Anthonisen NR: Long-term oxygen therapy. Ann Intern Med 99:519–527, 1983.
  Oxygen decreases pulmonary vascular resistance and improves survival in COPD patients.

Berssenbrugge A, Dempsey J, Iber C, Skatrud J, Wilson P: Mechanism of hypoxia-induced periodic breathing during sleep in humans. J Physiol 343:507–524, 1983.
  Periodic apnea induced by hypoxia results from oscillations in CO_2 about a CO_2-apnea threshold.

Berthon-Jones M, Sullivan CE: Ventilatory and arousal responses to hypoxia in sleeping humans. Am Rev Respir Dis 125:632–639, 1982.
  At normal alveolar P_{CO_2}, hypoxia is a poor arousal stimulus in humans.

Block AJ, Faulkner JA, Hughes RL, Remmers JE, Thach B: Factors influencing upper airway closure. Chest 86:114–122, 1984.
  State-of-the-art review of mechanisms leading to the development of obstructive apnea.

Block AJ, Wynne JW, Boysen PG: Sleep-disordered breathing and nocturnal oxygen desaturation in postmenopausal women. Am J Med 69:75–79, 1980.
  Postmenopausal women, unlike premenopausal women, may have episodes of apnea, hypopnea, and oxygen desaturation during sleep.

Bonora M, St John WM, Bledsoe TA: Differential elevation by protriptyline and depression by diazepam of upper airway respiratory motor activity. Am Rev Respir Dis 131:41–45, 1985.
  Protriptyline's efficacy in the treatment of obstructive sleep apnea may be related to a selective augmentation of upper airway muscle activity.

Bradley TD, Brown IG, Zamel N, Phillipson EA, Hoffstein V: Differences in pharyngeal properties between snorers with predominantly central sleep apnea and those without sleep apnea. Am Rev Respir Dis 135:387–391, 1987.
  Patients with idiopathic central sleep apnea may have abnormalities of upper airway mechanics that might contribute to the pathogenesis of central apneas.

Bradley TD, McNicholas WT, Rutherford R, Popkin J, Zamel N, Phillipson EA: Clinical and physiologic heterogeneity of the central sleep apnea syndrome. Am Rev Respir Dis 134:217–221, 1986.
  Central sleep apnea is a heterogeneous disorder associated with alveolar hypoventilation as well as intact alveolar ventilation.

Carskadon MA, Brown ED, Dement WC: Sleep fragmentation in the elderly: Relationship to day-time sleep tendency. Neurobiol Aging 3:321–327, 1982.
Elderly patients with sleep apnea have a greater tendency for daytime sleepiness.

Carskadon MA, Dement WC: Respiration during sleep in the aged human. J Gerontol 36:420–423, 1981.
There is approximately a 40 percent incidence of sleep apnea in healthy elderly subjects.

Catterall JR, Douglas NJ, Calverley PMA, Shapiro CM, Brezinova V, Brash HM, Flenley DC: Transient hypoxemia during sleep in chronic obstructive pulmonary disease is not a sleep apnea syndrome. Am Rev Respir Dis 128:24–29, 1983.
Hypoxemia during sleep occurs in nonobese COPD patients in the absence of apneas.

Cherniack NS: Sleep apnea and its causes. J Clin Invest 73:1501–1506, 1984.
Sleep apnea may result from instability of the ventilatory control system.

DeMarco FJ, Wynne JW, Block AJ, Boysen PG, Taasan VC: Oxygen desaturation during sleep as a determinant of the "blue and bloated" syndrome. Chest 79:621–625, 1981.
Blue bloaters demonstrated the greatest reductions in oxygen saturation during sleep.

Espinoza H, Antic R, Thornton AT, McEvoy RD: The effects of aminophylline on sleep and sleep-disordered breathing in patients with obstructive sleep apnea syndrome. Am Rev Respir Dis 136:80–84, 1987.
Aminophylline reduces central apnea and the central component of mixed apneas but has no effect on obstructive apnea.

Fleetham JA, Mezon B, West P, Bradley CA, Anthonisen NR, Kryger MH: Chemical control of ventilation and sleep arterial oxygen desaturation in patients with COPD. Am Rev Respir Dis 122:583–589, 1980.
Awake ventilatory response to hypercapnia inversely correlated with the degree of nocturnal oxygen desaturation.

Fletcher EC, DeBehnke RD, Lovoi MS, Gorin AB: Undiagnosed sleep apnea in patients with essential hypertension. Ann Intern Med 103:190–195, 1985.
Thirty percent of middle- and older-aged men with "essential hypertension" were found to have obstructive sleep apnea syndrome. Their data raise the question of whether sleep apnea syndrome could be the cause of this hypertension.

Garay SM, Rapoport D, Sorkin B, Epstein H, Feinberg I, Goldring RM: Regulation of ventilation in the obstructive sleep apnea syndrome. Am Rev Respir Dis 124:451–457, 1981.
Awake ventilatory responses do not relate to the severity of the sleep apnea phenomenon.

Gastaut H, Tassinari C, Duron B: Polygraphic study of the episodic diurnal and nocturnal (hypnic and respiratory) manifestations of the Pickwick Syndrome. Brain Res 2:167–186, 1966.
A landmark paper that prompted many of the subsequent papers on the control of breathing during sleep.

Guilleminault C (ed): Sleep and Its Disorders in Children. New York, Raven, 1987.
An important start at collecting information on sleep disorders in children.

Guilleminault C, Connolly S, Winkle R, Melvin K, Tilkian A: Cyclical variation of the heart rate in sleep apnoea syndrome. Lancet 1:126–131, 1984.
Sinus bradycardia alternating with tachycardia, corresponding to periods of apnea and breathing, respectively, is frequently seen in obstructive sleep apnea.

Haponik EF, Smith PL, Bohlman ME, Allen RP, Goldman SM, Bleecker ER: Computerized tomography in obstructive sleep apnea. Correlation of airway size with physiology during sleep and wakefulness. Am Rev Respir Dis 127:221–226, 1983.
Airways are narrowed in obese patients with obstructive sleep apnea.

Hudgel DW, Chapman KR, Faulks C, Hendricks C: Changes in inspiratory muscle electrical activity and upper airway resistance during periodic breathing induced by hypoxia during sleep. Am Rev Respir Dis 135:899–906, 1987.
The latest in a series of papers dealing with the sites of airway obstruction during periodic breathing in sleep.

Issa FG, Sullivan CE: Respiratory muscle activity and thoracoabdominal motion during acute episodes of asthma during sleep. Am Rev Respir Dis 132:999–1004, 1985.
Asthma attacks during sleep were characterized by audible wheezing, augmentation of respiratory muscle activity, and asynchronous rib cage and abdominal movement.

Kales A, Vela-Bueno A, Kales JD: Sleep disorders: sleep apnea and narcolepsy. Ann Intern Med 106:434–443, 1987.
A review of the differential diagnoses of narcolepsy versus sleep apnea syndromes.

Kimmelman CP, Levine SB, Shore ET, Millman RP: Uvulopalatopharyngoplasty: A comparison of two techniques. Laryngoscope 95:1488–1490, 1985.
> *The specific surgical technique employed can affect the results of the uvulopalatopharyngoplasty (UPP).*

Knight H, Millman RP, Gur RC, Saykin AJ, Doherty JU, Pack AI: Clinical significance of sleep apnea in the elderly. Am Rev Respir Dis 136:845–850, 1987.
> *Although apnea during sleep in the elderly may be associated with an increase in daytime sleepiness, it need not cause other physiological or neuropsychological consequences.*

Lahiri S, Maret K, Sherpa MG: Dependence of high altitude sleep apnea on ventilatory sensitivity to hypoxia. Resp Physiol 52:281–301, 1983.
> *Recurrent central apnea during sleep at high altitude results from hypoxic stimulation of the carotid body.*

Leiter JC, Knuth SL, Bartlett D: The effect of sleep deprivation on activity of the genioglossus muscle. Am Rev Respir Dis 132:1242–1245, 1985.
> *Sleep deprivation in normal subjects leads to a selective decrease in genioglossus electromyographic activity during hypercapnic rebreathing.*

Lugaresi E, Coccagna G: Sleep, snoring and sleep-apnea syndromes, in Fishman AP (ed), *Pulmonary Diseases and Disorders.* New York, McGraw-Hill, 1980, pp 445–451.
> *A summary of an early European study linking heavy snoring to sleep apnea and alveolar hypoventilation with records of the ventilatory and circulatory disturbances.*

Martin RJ, Sanders MH, Gray BA, Pennock BE: Acute and long-term ventilatory effects of hyperoxia in the adult sleep apnea syndrome. Am Rev Respir Dis 125:175–180, 1982.
> *Long-term nasal oxygen can be used to treat obstructive sleep apnea.*

McNicholas WT, Tarlo S, Cole P, Zamel N, Rutherford R, Griffin D, Phillipson EA: Obstructive apneas during sleep in patients with seasonal allergic rhinitis. Am Rev Respir Dis 126:625–628, 1982.
> *Obstruction of the nose increases the negative pressure in the hypopharynx and leads to upper airway collapse during sleep.*

Miller A, Granada M: In-hospital mortality in the Pickwickian syndrome. Am J Med 56:144–150, 1974.
> *The Pickwickian syndrome is associated with nocturnal sudden death.*

Miller WP: Cardiac arrhythmias and conduction disturbances in the sleep apnea syndrome. Prevalence and significance. Am J Med 73:317–321, 1982.
> *The prevalence of serious ventricular arrhythmias and conduction disturbances in patients with obstructive sleep apnea syndrome is lower than previously reported.*

Millman RP, Bevilacqua J, Peterson DD, Pack AI: Central sleep apnea in hypothyroidism. Am Rev Respir Dis 127:504–507, 1983.
> *Central sleep apnea may occur in mild hypothyroidism associated with significant depression of hypoxic and hypercapnic ventilatory responses.*

Millman RP, Kimmel P, Shore ET, Wasserstein AG: Sleep apnea in hemodialysis patients: The lack of testosterone effect on its pathogenesis. Nephron 40:407–410, 1985.
> *Testosterone therapy had no effect on the severity of obstructive sleep apnea in chronic hemodialysis patients.*

Montplaisir J, Walsh J, Malo JL: Nocturnal asthma: Features of attacks, sleep and breathing patterns. Am Rev Respir Dis 125:18–22, 1982.
> *The duration and frequency of apneas were no more frequent in asthmatics compared to normal controls. Attacks did not occur in stages 3 to 4 sleep.*

Orr WC, Imes NK, Martin RJ: Progesterone therapy in obese patients with sleep apnea. Arch Intern Med 139:109–111, 1979.
> *Progesterone did not appear to work in men with obstructive sleep apnea.*

Phillipson EA, Bowes G: Sleep disorders, in Fishman AP (ed), *Update: Pulmonary Diseases and Disorders.* New York, McGraw-Hill, 1982, pp 256–273.
> *A comprehensive review of the pathophysiology of sleep disorders and the influence of sleep on intrinsic pulmonary disease.*

Phillipson EA, Bowes G: Control of breathing during sleep, in Cherniack NS, Widdicombe JH (eds), *Handbook of Physiology, sect 3: The Respiratory System, vol II: Control of Breathing*. Bethesda, MD, American Physiological Society, 1986, pp 649–689.
> *A comprehensive review, in typical handbook style, of the physiology of the different stages of sleep followed by a full consideration of the ventilatory and arousal responses to respiratory stimuli.*

Remmers JE: Obstructive sleep apnea. A common disorder exacerbated by alcohol. Am Rev Respir Dis 130:153–155, 1984.
> *Alcohol exacerbates obstructive sleep apnea by depressing upper airway muscle activity and depressing arousal responses.*

Remmers JE, deGroot WJ, Sauerland EK, Anch AM: Pathogenesis of upper airway occlusion during sleep. J Appl Physiol 44:931–938, 1978.
> *Upper airway occlusion results from the interaction between upper airway muscle activity and the negative hypopharyngeal pressure that develops with contraction of the diaphragm.*

Rivlin J, Hoffstein V, Kalbfleisch J, McNicholas W, Zamel N, Bryan AC: Upper airway morphology in patients with idiopathic obstructive sleep apnea. Am Rev Respir Dis 129:355–360, 1984.
> *Even in nonobese patients with sleep apnea, the upper airway has a smaller cross-sectional diameter than seen in normal individuals.*

Sandblom RE, Matsumoto AM, Schoene RB, Lee KA, Giblin EC, Bremmer WJ, Pierson DJ: Obstructive sleep apnea syndrome induced by testosterone administration. N Engl J Med 308:508–510, 1983.
> *Case report of reversible obstructive sleep apnea precipitated by the administration of testosterone for hypogonadism.*

Sanders MH: Nasal CPAP effect on patterns of sleep apnea. Chest 86:839–844, 1984.
> *Nasal CPAP is an effective mode of treatment of obstructive sleep apnea.*

Shepard JW, Garrison MW, Grither BS, Dolan GF: Relationship of ventricular ectopy to oxyhemoglobin desaturation in patients with obstructive apnea. Chest 88:335–340, 1985.
> *Ventricular arrhythmias can occur when the oxygen saturation falls below 60 percent.*

Shore ET, Millman RP: Abnormalities in the flow-volume loop in obstructive sleep apnoea sitting and supine. Thorax 39:775–779, 1984.
> *The flow-volume loop is a poor screening test for obstructive sleep apnea.*

Shore ET, Millman RP, Silage DA, Chung DC, Pack AI: Ventilatory and arousal patterns during sleep in normal young and elderly subjects. J Appl Physiol 59:1607–1615, 1985.
> *Mean ventilation did not differ between young and elderly subjects in different stages of sleep; periodic apneas occurred more frequently in the elderly during light sleep.*

Simmons FB, Guilleminault C, Miles LE: The palatopharyngoplasty operation for snoring and sleep apnea: An interim report. Otolaryngol Head Neck Surg 92:375–380, 1984.
> *The UPP is often a safe treatment modality in obstructive sleep apnea.*

Skatrud J, Iber C, Ewart R, Thomas G, Rasmussen H, Schultz B: Disordered breathing during sleep in hypothyroidism. Am Rev Respir Dis 124:325–329, 1981.
> *Mild hypothyroidism without macroglossia can cause obstructive sleep apnea.*

Smith PL, Haponik EF, Allen RP, Bleecker ER. The effects of protriptyline in sleep-disordered breathing. Am Rev Respir Dis 127:8–13, 1983.
> *Protriptyline works in obstructive sleep apnea apparently by decreasing REM sleep, a period where the most severe apneas are observed.*

Strohl KP, Redline S: Nasal CPAP therapy, upper airway muscle activation, and obstructive sleep apnea. Am Rev Respir Dis 134:555–558, 1986.
> *Nasal CPAP works in obstructive sleep apnea primarily as a pneumatic splint.*

Sullivan CE, Issa FG, Berthon-Jones M, Eves L: Reversal of obstructive sleep apnoea by continuous positive airway pressure applied through the nares. Lancet 1:862–865, 1981.
> *Five patients with severe obstructive sleep apnea were treated with continuous positive airway pressure (CPAP) applied via a comfortable nose mask through the nares. Low levels of pressure (range 4.5 to 10 cmH$_2$O) completely prevented upper airway occlusion during sleep in each patient and allowed an entire night of uninterrupted sleep.*

Suratt PM, Wilhoit SC, Cooper K: Induction of airway collapse with subatmospheric pressure in awake patients with sleep apnea. J Appl Physiol 57:140–146, 1984.
  Patients with obstructive sleep apnea have upper airways which are more collapsible.

Tilkian AG, Guilleminault C, Schroeder JS, Lehrman KL, Simmons FB, Dement WC: Hemodynamics in sleep-induced apnea. Studies during wakefulness and sleep. Ann Intern Med 85:714–719, 1976.
  Pulmonary and systemic arterial pressures rise transiently during obstructive apneas.

Weil JV, Cherniack NS, Dempsey JA, Edelman NH, Phillipson EA, Remmers JE, Kiley JP: NHLBI workshop summary. Respiratory disorders of sleep. Pathophysiology, clinical implications, and therapeutic approaches. Am Rev Respir Dis 136:755–761, 1987.
  This report focuses on unanswered questions on the interplay between breathing and sleep.

Weil JV, Kryger MH, Scoggin CH: Sleep and breathing at high altitude, in Guilleminault C, Dement W (eds), *Sleep Apnea Syndromes.* New York, Liss, 1978, pp 119–136.
  Medroxyprogesterone and acetazolamide can be used to treat high altitude central sleep apnea by stimulating ventilation.

White DP, Zwillich CW, Pickett CK, Douglas NJ, Findley LJ, Weil JV: Central sleep apnea. Improvement with acetazolamide therapy. Arch Intern Med 142:1816–1819, 1982.
  Acetazolamide is an effective mode of therapy for central apnea.

Wilhoit SC, Brown ED, Suratt PM: Treatment of obstructive sleep apnea with continuous nasal airflow delivered through nasal prongs. Chest 85:170–173, 1984.
  Continuous nasal airflow prevents collapse of the upper airway in patients with obstructive apnea.

Yesavage J, Bliwise D, Guilleminault C, Carskadon M, Dement W: Preliminary communication: Intellectual deficit and sleep-related respiratory disturbance in the elderly. Sleep 8:30–33, 1985.
  Symptomatic elderly men with sleep apnea performed poorly on cognitive function testing.

Zwillich CW, Natalino MR, Sutton FD, Weil JV. Effects of progesterone on chemosensitivity in normal man. J Lab Clin Med 92:262–269, 1978.
  Progesterone administration increases ventilatory responsiveness to hypercapnia and hypoxia.

Chapter *84*

Control of Breathing in the Neonate and the Sudden Infant Death Syndrome

Henrique Rigatto

One remarkable feature about breathing in the neonatal period and early infancy is its tendency to become periodic with frequent apneas. The phenomenon of periodic breathing has been recognized since the beginning of medicine. Hippocrates (460–370 B.C.) referred to it in his patient Philliscus: "His respiration was rare and large, like a person who forgot for a time the need of breathing and then suddenly remembered." Yet, after more than 2000 years, the mechanism responsible for this respiration remains poorly understood. Apnea and periodic breathing not only affect preterm infants, but also term infants.

Because evidence is mounting that apnea causes brain damage and may predispose to the sudden infant death syndrome (SIDS), its treatment and prevention are important. SIDS occurs in one to three infants per 1000, and it is the most frequent cause of mortality between the neonatal period and the end of the first year (Table 84-1). In this chapter the concept is developed that periodic breathing, apnea, and SIDS are likely to have a common pathophysiological mechanism involving the control of breathing.

TERMINOLOGY

Periodic breathing is defined as pauses in respiratory movements that last for 10 to 15 s alternating with breathing.

Apnea is defined as a longer arrest of respiratory movements, i.e., longer than 20 s.

Bradycardia is defined as a heart rate of fewer than 80 beats per minute.

Although the duration used to distinguish between periodicity and apnea are empirical, they have proved useful and have been widely adopted. Periodic breathing is common and is regarded as benign because the respiratory pause is short. In contrast, apnea is a serious condition. It is usually accompanied by a decrease in heart rate to fewer than 80 beats per minute, whereas in periodic breathing the heart rate decreases only slightly, if at all (Fig. 84-1).

Sudden infant death syndrome is defined as "the sudden death of any infant or young child, which is unexpected by history and in which a thorough postmortem examination fails to demonstrate an adequate cause of death." Fundamental to this definition is the concept of "adequate cause," which has led to considerable controversy and difference of opinion.

Near-SIDS is a term used to define a high-risk state that is characterized by the sudden onset of apnea with cyanosis or pallor, prompting resuscitative efforts by parents. Near-SIDS is believed to have the same etiology as SIDS, and it is widely used as a human model.

CLASSIFICATION OF APNEA

Apneas in the neonate can be classified either according to the absence or presence of underlying disease (Table 84-2) or according to the absence or presence of breathing efforts during the period of no airflow (Fig. 84-2). The classification based on respiratory efforts as related to airflow is as follows:

Central apneas: no flow and no observable efforts to breathe.

Obstructive apneas: no flow despite breathing efforts.

Mixed apneas: begin as central apnea and end as obstructive apnea.

Breath-holding apneas: flow stops at mid-expiration and an expiration occurs just before breathing starts again.

Figure 84-3 shows the frequency distribution of these types of apneas in healthy neonates.

CLINICAL FEATURES AND PATHOGENESIS

About 40 to 50 percent of preterm infants breathe periodically during the neonatal period. The incidence of peri-

TABLE 84-1
Morbidity and Mortality from Disorders in the Control of Breathing

Disease (ICD/9 Code)	Hospitalization 1983*			Physician Office Visits 1980 + 1981 (000)	Deaths under 1 Year 1981
	First Listed (000)	Second Listed (000)	Length of Stay (days)		
SIDS (798.0)	1	1	5.0	—	5295
Apnea (770.8)	11	23	10.2	—	1675
Total	12	24	9.8	†	6970

* Under age 15.

† Not available.

NOTE:— — = Virtually no visits. Fewer than 350,000 visits are statistically unreliable. These estimates have a standard error of 30 percent or more. ICD = International Classification of Diseases.

SOURCES: Hospital Discharge Survey, National Center for Health Statistics (NCHS); Ambulatory Medical Care Survey, NCHS; and Vital Statistics of the NCHS.

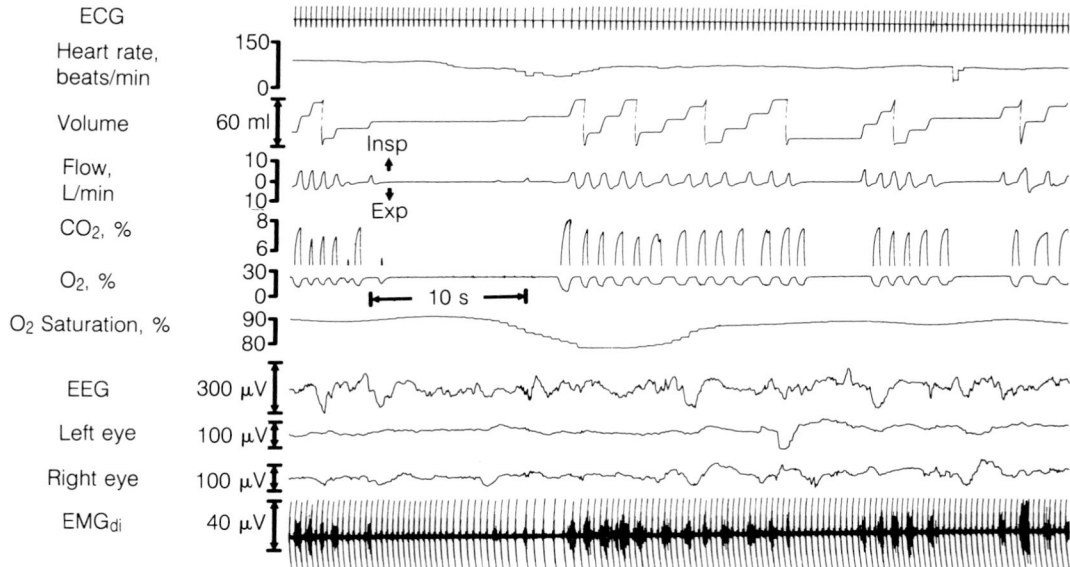

FIGURE 84-1 Apnea followed by periodic breathing in a preterm infant at 33 weeks of gestation, 12 days old. A pronounced decrease in heart rate accompanies arterial hypoxemia during apnea. The heart rate does not change during periodic breathing. EMG$_{di}$ = diaphragmatic electromyogram.

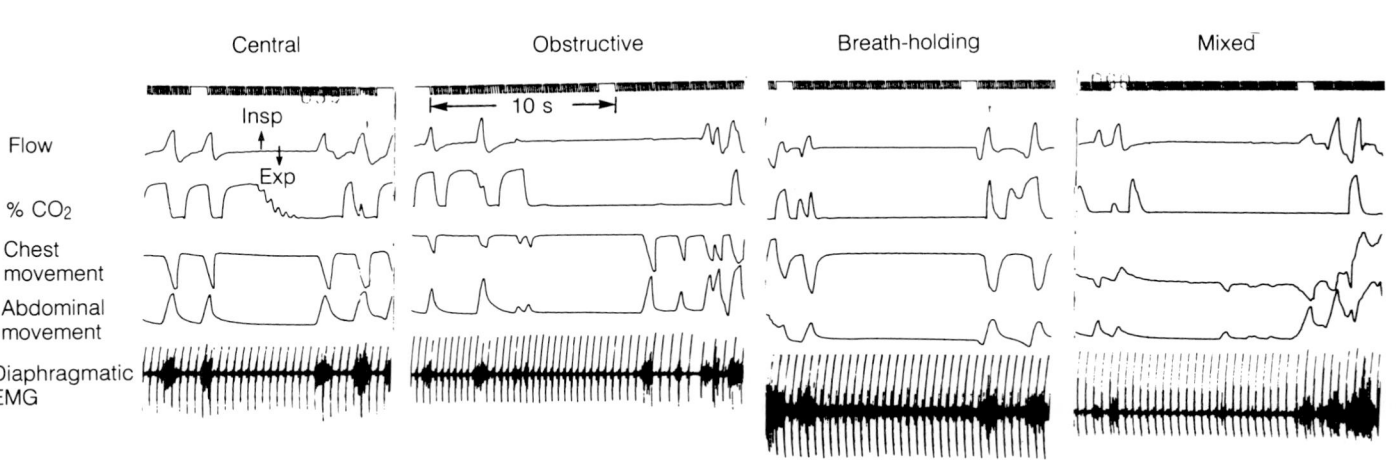

FIGURE 84-2 Types of apnea. Apneas are categorized according to whether airflow is present and to the absence ("central" type) or presence ("obstructive" type) of diaphragmatic activity (and of corresponding chest and abdominal movements). Mixed apneas showed features of both central and obstructive types. In the breath-holding type, flow stops at mid-expiration, and an expiration occurs just before the next inspiration.

TABLE 84-2

Apnea and Related Clinical Problems in Infants in a Neonatal Intensive Care Unit: 1-Year Review (September 1985 to September 1986)*

Related Causes	Number of Infants with Apnea	Percent of Infants
Not associated with obvious disease	11	19
Associated with obvious disease		
Mucus in the larynx	16	26
Bronchopulmonary dysplasia	11	19
Respiratory distress syndrome	11	19
Pneumonia or sepsis	3	5
Seizures	2	3
Intracranial bleeding	1	2
Patent ductus arteriosus	1	2
Congenital heart disease	1	2
Other†	2	3
Total	59	100

* Based on data from the Children's Hospital, University of Manitoba, Winnipeg, Canada.

†Include one patient with gastroesophageal reflux and one with apnea induced by gavage feeding.

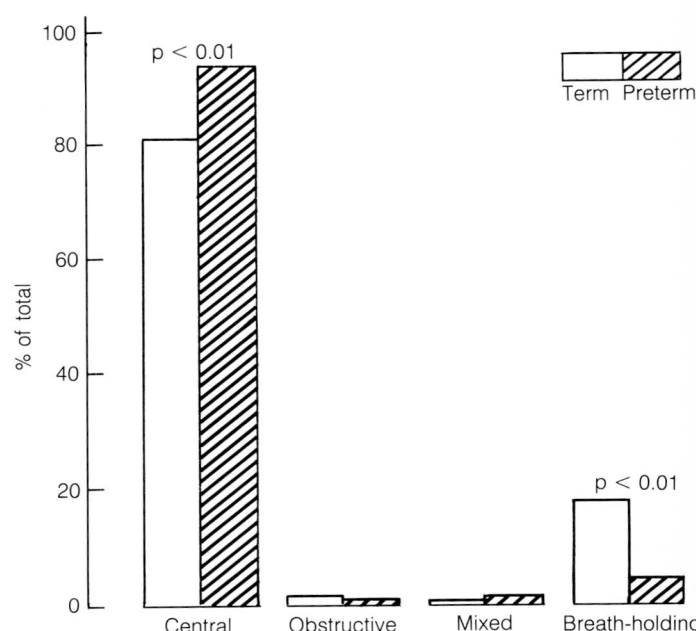

FIGURE 84-3 Frequency distribution of the various types of apneas in healthy preterm and term infants. Central apneas were predominant. The frequency of breath-holding apneas was greater in term than in preterm infants. Obstructive and mixed types of apneas were rare.

odic breathing increases remarkably with prematurity; it is 90 percent at 28 to 29 weeks of gestation. Approximately half of the infants with periodic breathing develop apnea at one time or another.

Periodic breathing unaccompanied by other clinical disturbances is occasionally encountered during the routine clinical examination; as noted above, in this benign form, there is no significant decrease in heart rate. However, apnea can appear unexpectedly in infants breathing periodically; frequently, the apnea is associated with a pronounced decrease in heart rate, cyanosis or pallor, and poor peripheral perfusion. The onset of apnea in these infants is usually heralded by alarms designed to detect apnea and to monitor heart rate. Once recovered in response to either manual stimulation or to oxygen delivered by bag, the infant seems well and usually remains in good clinical condition.

Apnea in Infants without Underlying Disease

As indicated above, apnea without underlying disease affects primarily preterm infants. The pronounced increase in the frequency of apnea with prematurity is probably related to immaturity of anatomic structures and of physiological mechanisms. Arborization of dendrites at 30 weeks of gestation is meager, and neuroconduction and synaptic relay are impaired. Delays in the traffic of neuromessages make the system oscillate. Unfortunately, the degree of immaturity in structure has not yet been

quantified. Nor is it clear how much this immaturity is responsible for impaired neurophysiological traffic.

Periodic breathing and apnea probably have common physiopathologic roots; apnea is probably only a severe manifestation of the disturbance that induces periodic breathing. The unsettled question is where these disturbances occur along the negative feedback loop that controls respiration. It seems likely that more than one factor is involved in producing apnea.

In infants who breathe periodically and develop apnea, the ventilatory system is depressed as reflected in the high $P_{A_{CO_2}}$ and a low minute ventilation; compared to that in infants who breathe uninterruptedly, the CO_2 response curve is shifted to the right and the slope is slightly decreased. This physiological configuration predisposes the system to oscillate. Compared to those in infants who breathe continuously, the peripheral chemoreceptors of infants with periodic breathing and apnea seem quite active, as reflected by the longer apneic periods and the more pronounced decrease in ventilation that the periodic breathers manifest while breathing high-oxygen mixtures. Hypoxia can be a contributing factor, since inhalation of a low-oxygen mixture easily induces periodic breathing and apnea in these infants. In response to a hypoxic inspired mixture, small infants manifest a transient increase in ventilation followed by a decrease (Fig. 84-4); apnea usually appears during the late response. The initial increase in ventilation reflects peripheral chemoreceptor activity; the mechanism responsible for the late

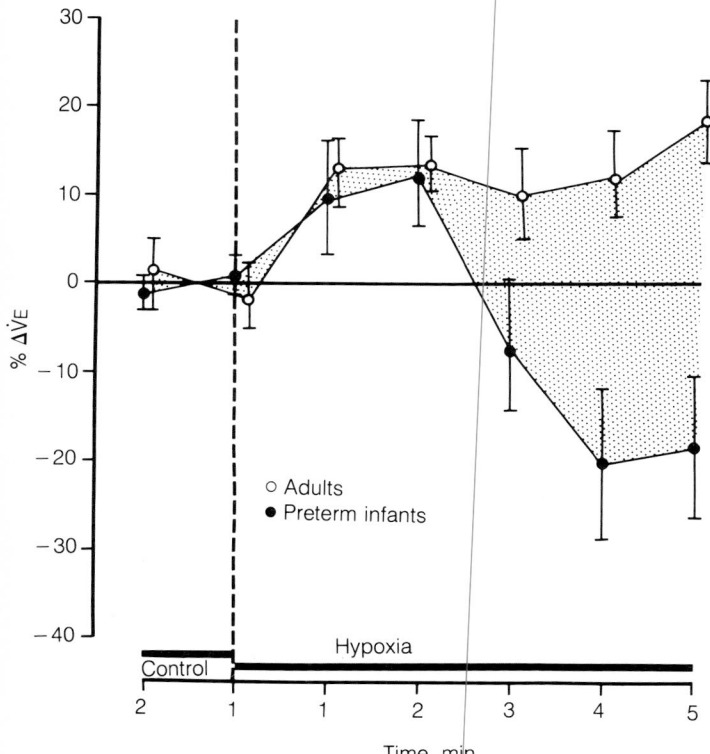

FIGURE 84-4 Percent change in ventilation when 15% O_2 was substituted for 21% O_2 in preterm infants (closed circles) and 12% O_2 substituted for 15% O_2 in adult subjects (open circles). Hyperventilation is sustained in adults but not in preterm infants.

response is controversial. In kittens, the late decrease in ventilation is probably due to mechanical failure, possibly the result of an increase in pulmonary impedance caused by hypoxia-related bronchoconstriction (Fig. 84-5). The same mechanism may also explain why the ventilatory response to CO_2 in neonates is less under hypoxic than hyperoxic conditions.

The sleep state appears to be a contributing factor, since periodic breathing and apnea are more frequent during rapid eye movement (REM) sleep than during quiet sleep. The neonate sleeps almost uninterruptedly, continuously alternating between REM sleep and quiet sleep. This pattern increases instability in the respiratory control system. Indeed, minor alterations during sleep, such as a startle or a sigh, produce apnea in these infants. The almost continuous change in the baseline ventilation during sleep is what Haldane called "the hunting of the respiratory centre."

Although sleep modulates breathing, it does not cause apnea; apnea also occurs during wakefulness. The high prevalence of apnea during REM sleep may be related to muscle activity in this stage: during REM sleep, the tone of the intercostal muscles is abolished in conjunction with a decrease in diaphragmatic activity and in the tone of the adductor muscles of the upper airway—a

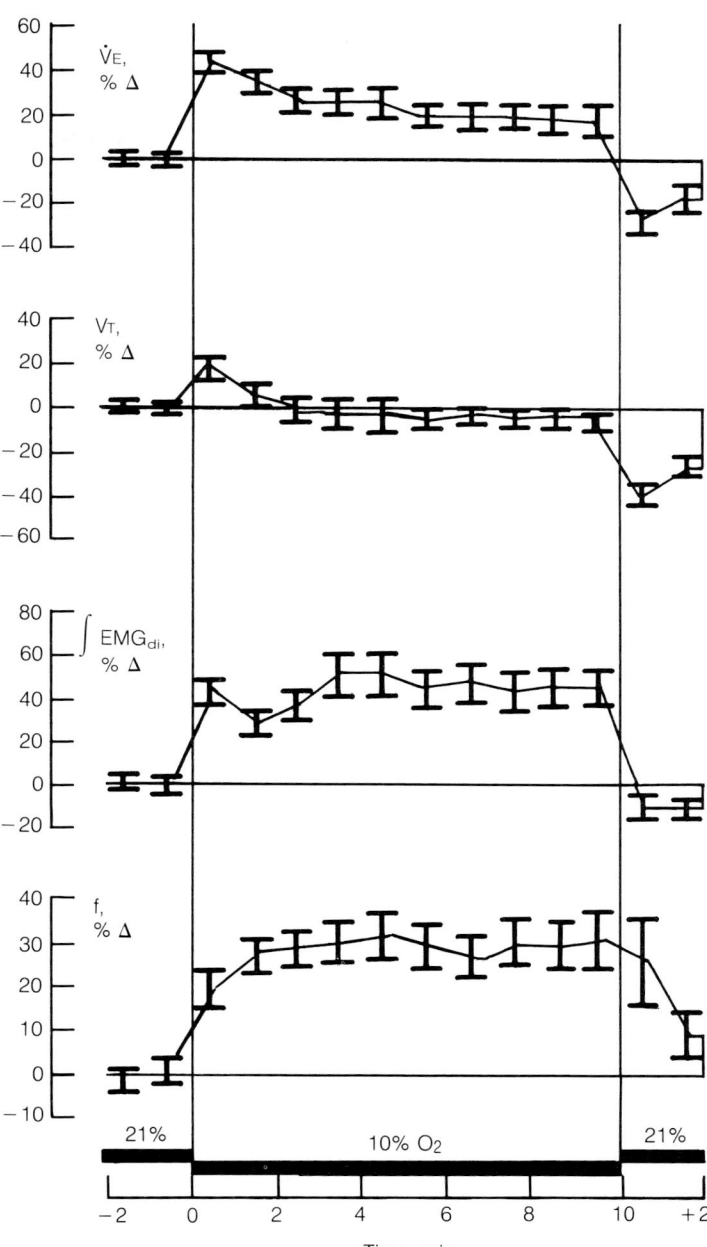

FIGURE 84-5 The ventilatory response to hypoxia in newborn kittens. An immediate increase in ventilation is followed by a decrease. The late decrease is primarily related to a decrease in tidal volume; the diaphragmatic activity and the frequency remain high during hypoxia. This pattern suggests that the late decrease in ventilation during hypoxia is primarily peripheral rather than central in origin, possibly related to bronchoconstriction and to either increased pulmonary impedance or uncoupling of diaphragm and lungs.

combination of factors likely to induce chest distortion, impairment of the braking mechanism during expiration, pulmonary collapse, and apnea (Fig. 84-6). During chest distortion, which is further enhanced by an unusually compliant chest wall, diaphragmatic work increases by

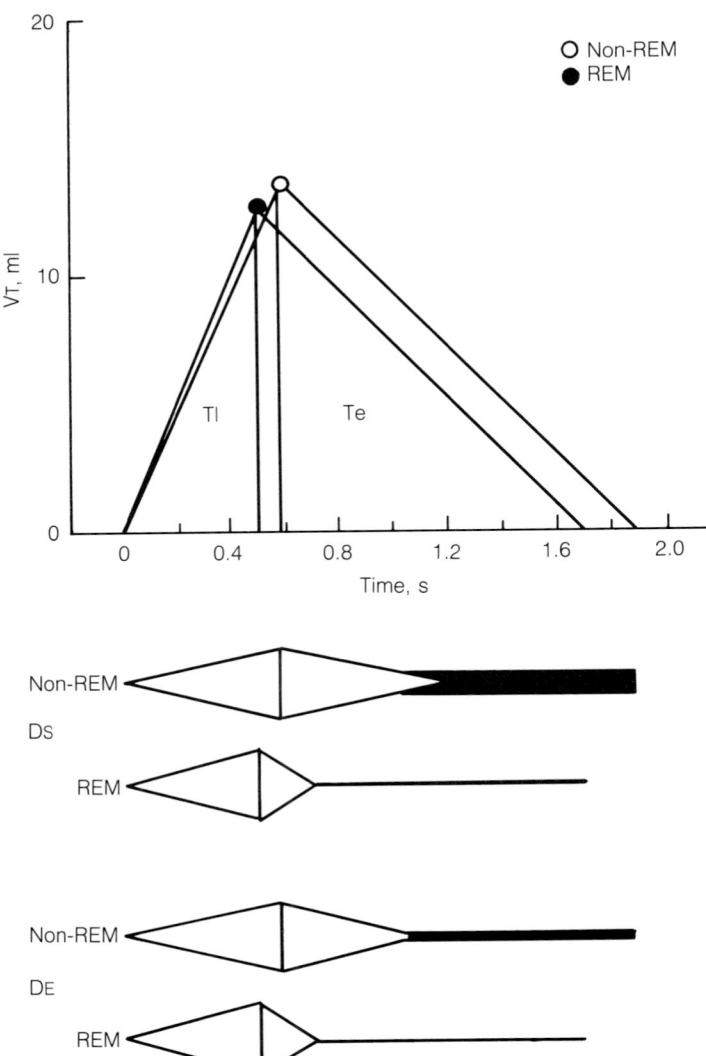

FIGURE 84-6 Schematic representation of changes in tidal volume, "timing," and diaphragmatic EMG in non-REM (quiet) and REM (active) sleep. Total phasic activity is greater in non-REM sleep than in REM sleep. Also, in both sleep states it is shorter in the esophageal EMG (DE) than in the surface EMG (DS). Expiratory phase activity as a proportion of total phasic activity decreases significantly from non-REM to REM sleep. Ti = inspiratory time; Te = expiratory time.

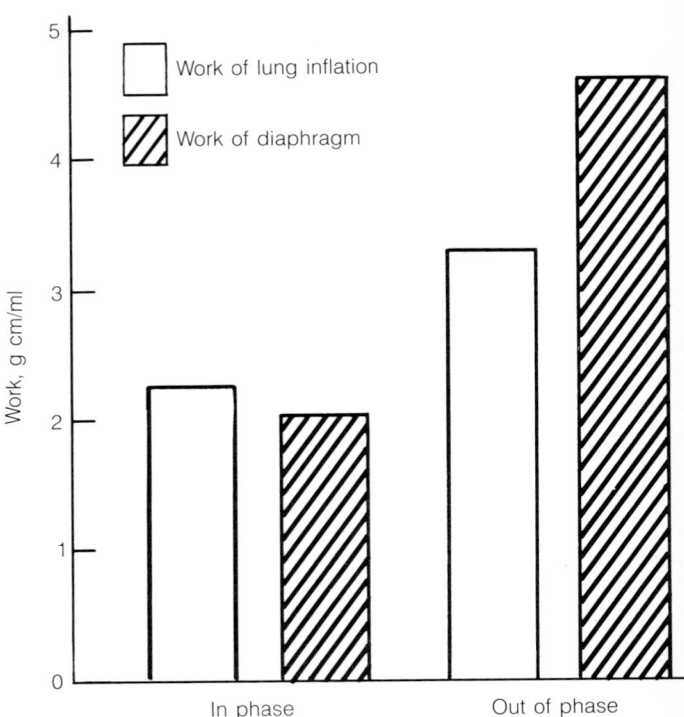

FIGURE 84-7 Work done in inflating the lungs and work done by the diaphragm when breathing is in phase or out of phase. The work of lung inflation is not significantly different when the breathing is in phase or out of phase. However, the work of the diaphragm is approximately 40 percent greater when the breath is out of phase than when it is in phase.

about 40 percent, adding to the mechanical impairment (Fig. 84-7). This observation is compatible with the finding that the application of nasal continuous positive airway pressure (nasal CPAP) or of continuous negative pressure around the chest tends to abolish apnea.

In summary, periodic breathing and apnea are highly prevalent in neonates, probably owing to immaturity of the anatomic structures at this age. Superimposed on this immaturity is the almost continuous change in resting ventilation during sleep produced by chemical and nonchemical mechanisms, thereby providing the "coup de mort" to respiratory stability. Apnea then results.

All infants who weigh less than 1800 g, and larger babies who are sick, should be on apnea and heart rate monitors. Since most apneas of prematurity are idiopathic, a likely cause cannot be found. In infants without obvious underlying disease, most apneas are central (more than 85 percent) or of the breath-holding type; obstructive and mixed apneas are rare (Fig. 84-3), except in infants with bronchopulmonary dysplasia who are recovering from the respiratory distress syndrome, i.e., with some residual disease; in these infants, the prevalence of mixed and obstructive apneas is high, at times accounting for 40 to 50 percent of apneas.

Apnea in Infants with Underlying Disease

Underlying disease can be identified in most infants who develop apnea that is of clinical concern during the neonatal period. Among the underlying diseases are the following:

1. *Bronchopulmonary dysplasia.* These infants are recovering from hyaline membrane disease; usually they are also receiving 23 to 35 percent supplemental oxygen. They are on the verge of hypoxia, their respiratory pump is still compromised by abnormally high pulmonary im-

pedance, and bronchoreactivity is high as the result of the underlying disease. In these infants, the onset of apnea depends on the occurrence of hypoxia and, to a lesser extent, to airways obstruction. The incidence of mixed apnea and the risk of SIDS is high. The transcutaneous P_{O_2} is invariably low, i.e., almost 45 to 48 mmHg.

2. *Patent ductus arteriosus,* in preterm infants who are not being mechanically ventilated. The clinical findings usually include tachypnea, mild intercostal retraction, prominent arterial pulses, and a heart murmur. The decrease in pulmonary vascular resistance after birth leads to an increase in the left-to-right shunt through the patent ductus arteriosus; pulmonary edema develops, and apnea becomes prominent. Accompanying the pulmonary edema is an increase in Pa_{CO_2}, a decrease in Pa_{CO_2}, and a slight decrease in pulmonary compliance. Closure of the ductus is associated with a return to normal values and a decrease in the incidence of apnea.

The diagnosis of patent ductus arteriosus (PDA) is made by clinical findings and ultrasound. The clinical constellation includes heart murmur, tachypnea, prominent or bounding pulses, slight increase in liver size (the liver is rarely more than two finger breadths below the right costal margin), and increased Pa_{CO_2}. Increased Pa_{CO_2} may be an early sign of pulmonary edema, which may or may not be apparent radiographically. Diagnosis using ultrasound is based on direct visualization of the ductus and an abnormally high ratio of left-atrial-to-aortic diameters. At times, ultrasound findings can be disappointing despite a clinically significant PDA. In intubated infants, the presence of PDA may delay extubation because of the increased ventilatory support that is required.

3. *Intracranial bleeding,* in the immediate neonatal period, usually in infants who are receiving ventilatory assistance. In these infants, apnea occurs primarily from the second day of life, whereas idiopathic apneas are more prevalent after the fifth day. If the bleeding is severe, the infant is likely to develop circulatory collapse and die, often after cyanosis and seizures. Should the intracranial hemorrhage be mild and occur in an infant who is not receiving ventilatory assistance, prolonged apnea and cyanosis may ensue; both may be refractory to stimulation. Although the cause of the apnea seems to be a lack of central drive, the precise nature of the neurodisturbance is unclear. Since bleeding in these infants usually does not occur in the midbrain, apnea must be related to injury of neural structures elsewhere in the brain.

The diagnosis of intracranial hemorrhage changed dramatically with the advent of ultrasonography. Major intracranial bleeding, intraventricular and intraparenchymal (grades III and IV of Papille), is associated with cyanosis, shock, metabolic acidosis, seizures, bloody cerebrospinal fluid, and decrease in the serum hemoglobin concentration. The prognosis for patients in grades III and IV

of Papille is poor, but if the hemorrhage is less severe (grades I to II of Papille), the prognosis is much better.

4. *Pneumonia or sepsis.* In infants between 2 and 6 weeks of age who are brought to the hospital because of an apneic episode associated with limpness and need for resuscitative measures, a useful rule of thumb is to consider them as having a pneumonia with possible sepsis, probably viral. The clinical picture generally includes cyanosis or pallor, poor peripheral perfusion, mottling, poor feeding, poor tonus, and sometimes seizures. Pneumonia or sepsis causes apnea because of the individual, or combined, effects of hypoxia, sensitization of pulmonary reflexes, and central depression.

The diagnosis of pneumonia, with or without sepsis, is often difficult unless the pneumonia is severe. Therefore, suspicion of pneumonia must be high if the radiographic signs are to be appreciated. Apnea is a striking feature of pneumonia in large babies, whereas systemic involvement dominates the scene in preterm infants.

5. *Respiratory distress syndrome.* The cause is either a lack of surfactant (type 1) or pulmonary aspiration or fluid retention (type 2). The infants are tachypneic; the sudden respiratory arrest occurs while they are receiving supplemental oxygen. The apnea may occur during its acute phase or, more often, during the recovery phase of the underlying disease.

The respiratory distress syndrome presumably causes apnea because the respiratory muscles fatigue while performing the inordinate work of moving the stiff lungs and distorted chest wall. In some instances, arterial hypoxemia may contribute to the apnea.

6. *Congenital heart disease,* cyanotic or acyanotic; in term infants, attacks of apnea may occur at the beginning of extrauterine life. Apnea is the result primarily of arterial hypoxemia and secondarily of pulmonary edema.

Other types of apnea or periodic breathing are rare. *Seizures* may present as isolated, "dusky" spells. Usually there is a history of asphyxia. The mechanism for the apnea is probably transient hyperventilation that lowers Pa_{CO_2} to levels below threshold values required to stimulate breathing. Anticonvulsants generally eliminate the apnea. *Hypoglycemia* may be associated with apnea in infants of diabetic mothers and also in small-for-date infants; presumably impaired muscular performance is responsible for the apnea. *Hypocalcemia* may also cause apnea in small-for-date infants. Both hypoglycemia and hypocalcemia are now rarely associated with apnea because of the prophylactic administration of glucose and of calcium gluconate to small infants.

Gavage feedings are frequently associated with apnea and bradycardia, probably vagal in origin. The same mechanism is involved in apnea accompanying *mucus in the larynx* during the immediate neonatal period; this is quite common in term infants with some degree of as-

phyxia (Table 84-2). Infants who experience dusky spells in the first 24 h of life that seem inclined to continue should be investigated for the presence of *H-type esophageal fistula. Gastroesophageal reflux* may also cause apnea, primarily after feeding. *Maternal oversedation* leading to respiratory depression predisposes infants to apnea shortly after delivery. Finally, *increase in incubator temperature* has been associated with apnea. In all these later types of apneas the baseline clinical condition is generally good.

SIDS AND NEAR-SIDS

Clinical and Epidemiologic Features

The two most striking features about SIDS and near-SIDS are the absence of warning signs and their occurrence during sleep. Because there are no warning signs preceding death, characterization of SIDS is best made through its epidemiologic framework.

SIDS occurs mostly during winter months, at ages ranging from 1 to 4 months, and it occurs most commonly in malnourished infants of poor socioeconomic background. Males are more often affected than females, and some ethnic groups have the highest risk, e.g., American Indians (5.93 per 1000), Alaskan natives (4.5 per 1000), and blacks of low socioeconomic status (5.04 per 1000). Preterm infants or infants that are of low birth weight for their gestational age are most often affected. Infants with bronchopulmonary dysplasia, of mothers addicted to barbiturates or who smoke during pregnancy, are at increased risk. Low Apgar scores and a history of resuscitative efforts are common in infants who die of SIDS. Siblings of SIDS families are at high risk (20 per 1000), and the same seems to be true for near-SIDS. Infants who die of SIDS tend to have mild respiratory symptoms in the preceding week, occasionally requiring hospitalization between the time of birth and death. SIDS occurs most often during sleep, the greatest number of deaths occurring between 12 a.m. and 9 a.m. Whether infants who experience frequent apnea during the neonatal period are more apt to die of SIDS is unsettled.

The epidemiologic background of near-SIDS mimics that of SIDS. This is why it has been used as a model for SIDS. Like SIDS, near-SIDS also occurs more frequently during sleep. Although infants who present with near-SIDS seem to be at higher risk for SIDS, the relationship between the two is not clear.

Diagnosis

The diagnosis of SIDS is based on the history and the pathologic findings, integral parts of the definition of SIDS. In contrast, the diagnosis of near-SIDS is highly speculative and based on history alone. Most near-SIDS infants, once admitted to hospital, have a normal physical examination and behave unremarkably. Prolonged studies during sleep of these infants have given contradictory results, some investigators finding the ventilatory response to CO_2 decreased, others not. Our laboratory has been unable to identify disturbances that would compromise survival in infants with near-SIDS. This raises the question of whether near-SIDS is a good model of SIDS or, alternatively, if the normal findings in near-SIDS upon hospitalization bear upon events during an acute crisis. Because of the lack of warning signs and of positive laboratory results in near-SIDS, attempts to use near-SIDS to define the events surrounding death in SIDS have failed.

Pathogenesis

The profusion of etiologic mechanisms offered in explanation of SIDS led Collins and Piper to refer to the SIDS as "a disease of theories." However, the notion that SIDS is a disturbance of the respiratory control system that occurs during sleep—a time when the cardiorespiratory control system is known to be more vulnerable than while awake—is a major working concept. The hypothesis is that in some infants vulnerability in the respiratory control system during sleep leads to apnea which, in conjunction with viral-induced upper airway obstruction and hypoxemia, is irreversible because of failure to arouse. The attractiveness of this hypothesis is that it inherently relates sleep, viral infection (common cold), and death.

The problem with the hypothesis is that, even though the pathologic findings of medial hypertrophy in the pulmonary arteries and arterioles of infants who die of SIDS is consistent with the hypoxemic theory, there is as yet no direct evidence that arterial hypoxemia occurs. Furthermore, REM sleep could predispose to SIDS by preventing arousal at the end of apnea. Impaired arousal may occur if the lung collapses because of a lack of intercostal tone, a lack of postinspiratory diaphragmatic activity, and a lack of adductor tone of the muscles of the larynx. Once again, there is no direct evidence that this occurs.

Finally, some investigators have implicated a disturbance in the chemical control of breathing in the pathogenesis of near-SIDS, i.e., a decrease in ventilatory response to CO_2 and an increase in susceptibility to mild hypoxia; but these findings have not been corroborated by others. Our laboratory is currently exploring the hypothesis that the cardiorespiratory control system does fail during sleep in SIDS and that some of the difficulty to arouse at the end of a sleep apnea may be related to the presence in some neonates of the same chemical mediator that hinders arousal in utero.

In summary, the unpredictability of SIDS has made the understanding of its pathogenesis difficult. Because this disease has no warning signs, its elucidation is likely to be slow. Because SIDS may be a sleep apnea in which

arousal does not occur, it will perhaps be solved when there is a physiological and neurochemical understanding of why infants become apneic during sleep. It seems important, therefore, to clarify the mechanisms for cardiorespiratory control during sleep using experimental fetuses and neonates. Although the near-SIDS model may still turn out to be more useful than it presently seems to be, it is unlikely, in the end, to explain the pathogenesis of SIDS.

TREATMENT

Apnea

The first consideration in managing apnea is whether the apnea is severe enough to warrant treatment. More than five apneas per 24 h, accompanied by occasional change in the infant's color, signifies that the apnea is serious and that theophylline should be administered. The first dose of theophylline is given intravenously (85% anhydrous theophylline) over a 5-min period; subsequent doses are given orally in an alcoholic solution (5.3 mg/ml). Serum theophylline levels are monitored twice weekly. In some instances, the maintenance dose has to be decreased to 1.5 mg/kg per dose to avoid toxicity. Experience with this drug has been gratifying. Theophylline abolishes, or reduces, apnea by increasing alveolar ventilation by way of central nervous stimulation. The half-life of the drug is longer during the neonatal period than during later life, and serum levels that would be considered toxic in older children are usually tolerated in infants. Side effects are few in infants; usually a slight increase in heart rate is seen; although hematemesis, jitteriness, seizures, or albuminuria are possible, they are extraordinarily rare. Doxapram, a central nervous system stimulant, has recently been used in infants in whom theophylline has failed. The agent is administered intravenously (1 mg/kg per hour). Although the oral administration of doxapram promises to be clinically effective, extensive studies of pharmacokinetics and effectiveness using the oral route are not yet available.

Arterial hypoxemia, when present, is treated by increasing the fraction of O_2 inspired air (FI_{O_2}) in steps of about 5 percent. Whenever FI_{O_2} is increased, arterial P_{O_2} must be monitored closely to minimize the risk of retrolental fibroplasia. In infants recovering from the respiratory distress syndrome, arterial oxygenation is usually monitored by an ear oximeter. The baseline saturation is kept at 94 percent: higher values are unnecessary since the goal is to wean the infant from supplemental oxygen; lower values tend to produce apnea and bradycardia.

Other useful therapeutic measures include nursing the infant in the prone position and using water beds. Much more equivocal as therapeutic measures are interventions designed to keep the baby's temperature within normal range, the use of "rocker" beds, and tactile and auditory stimulation.

Treatment for apnea related to specific diseases is primarily directed at the underlying disease using ventilatory support as needed for the apnea. Except for ventilatory support, there is little to offer in dealing with intracranial hemorrhage. Although sedation of the neonate has been advocated as a measure that is helpful in preventing intracranial bleeding, its value has not been confirmed. Patency of the ductus arteriosus is treated with indomethacin, 0.2 mg/kg every 24 h, for three doses; if this approach should fail, surgical closure is indicated. Pneumonia or sepsis is treated with antibiotic coverage, blood, and ventilatory support. Apnea related to congenital heart defects requires assisted ventilation and the appropriate cardiac surgery. Apnea associated with seizures is treated with anticonvulsants, phenobarbital and diphenylhydantoin (Dilantin). Apnea caused by maternal narcotics usually responds well to naloxone 0.005 mg/kg. The bradycardia associated with gavage feeding usually resolves without use of atropine. The H type of esophageal fistula is treated surgically. Gastroesophageal reflux is treated by positioning the infant head up and by thickening the formula.

In resorting to ventilatory support, it must be kept in mind that the lungs of these infants are usually normally compliant so that low ventilatory pressures must be used to avoid lung damage and hyperventilation. The required duration of ventilatory support depends on the cause of apnea, but is usually short.

SIDS

Since SIDS is a disease of unknown etiology and pathogenesis, a standard therapeutic approach has not been established. Currently, infants presenting with a diagnosis of near-SIDS are often admitted to the hospital for respiratory studies. Because of frequent apneas and poor ventilatory response to chemical stimuli, some of these infants are sent home with monitors on the assumption that the home use of monitors may prevent SIDS. However, the value of home monitors in preventing SIDS is still not known; its benefit-risk ratio has not been settled. Although it has been proposed that respiratory stimulants such as theophylline or caffeine may help prevent SIDS, there are no data to support this proposition. At present, SIDS does not seem to be preventable.

BIBLIOGRAPHY

Barrington KJ, Finer NN, Peters KL, Barton J: Physiologic effects of doxapram in idiopathic apnea of prematurity. J Pediatr 108:124–129, 1986.
 Doxapram abolishes apnea by increasing minute ventilation.

Davi MJ, Sankaran K, Simons KJ, Simons FE, Seshia MM, Rigatto H: Physiologic changes induced by theophylline in the treatment of apnea in preterm infants. J Pediatr 92:91–95, 1978.
 Theophylline reduces apnea by central ventilatory stimulation as reflected by an increase in $\dot{V}_E$ and in the ventilatory response to inhaled CO_2.

Haddad GG, Leistner HL, Lai TL, Mellins TB: Ventilation and ventilatory pattern during sleep in aborted sudden infant death syndrome. Pediatr Res 15:879–883, 1981.
 The ventilatory response to CO_2 was not decreased in near-SIDS infants as compared to that in controls.

Harding R, Johnson P, McClelland ME: Respiratory function of the larynx in developing sheep and the influence of sleep state. Resp Physiol 40:165–179, 1980.
 The activity of the thyroarytenoid muscle, an important adductor of the larynx, is abolished in REM sleep, thereby decreasing end-expiratory pressure.

Hayakawa F, Kakanda S, Kuno K, Nakashima T, Miyachi Y: Doxapram in the treatment of idiopathic apnea of prematurity: Desirable dosage and serum concentration. J Pediatr 1:138–140, 1986.
 Doxapram is effective in the treatment of prematurity in patients in whom theophylline has failed.

Henderson-Smart DJ, Read DJC: Reduced lung volume during behavioral active sleep in the newborn. J Appl Physiol 46:1081–1085, 1979.
 Loss of intercostal tonus during REM sleep produces a decrease of 30 percent in functional residual capacity.

Hoffman HJ, Hunter JC, Damus K, Pakter J, Peterson DR, van Belle G, Hasselmeyer EG: Diphtheria-tetanus-pertussis immunization and sudden infant death: Results of the National Institute of Child Health and Human Development Cooperative Epidemiological Study of Sudden Infant Death Syndrome risk factors. Pediatrics 79:598–611, 1987.
 Diphtheria-pertussis-tetanus immunization is not a significant factor in the occurrence of SIDS.

Hunt CE, Brouillette RT: Sudden infant death syndrome: 1987 perspective. J Pediatr 100:669–678, 1987.
 A summary of current knowledge regarding SIDS, apnea, pneumograms, and home monitors. The cause(s) of SIDS remains unknown.

Kahn A, Van de Merckt C, Dramaix M, Magrez P, Blum D, Rebuffat E, Montauk L: Transepidermal water loss during sleep in infants at risk for sudden death. Pediatrics 80:245–250, 1987.
 Infants with an apparently life-threatening event had significantly higher evaporation rate values during NREM sleep than did control and sibling infants.

Kelly DH, Shannon DC: Periodic breathing in infants with near-miss sudden infant death syndrome. Pediatrics 63:355–360, 1979.
 Periodic apnea is more frequent in near-SIDS patients who later had SIDS.

Kitterman JA: Arachidonic acid metabolites and control of breathing in the fetus and newborn. Semin Perinatol 11:43–52, 1987.
 Prostaglandins participate in the control of breathing in the fetus during parturition and at birth.

Lee DS, Caces R, Kwiatkowski K, Cates D, Rigatto H: A developmental study on types and frequency distribution of short apneas (3 to 15 seconds) in term and preterm infants. Pediatr Res 22:344–349, 1987.
 The effect of sleep on the frequency distribution of various types of apneas during the first 4 months of age suggests that central apneas are predominant in preterm and term infants; obstructive and mixed apneas are rare.

Luz J, Winter A, Cates D, Moore M, Rigatto H: Effect of chest and abdomen uncoupling on ventilation and work of breathing in the newborn during sleep. Pediatr Res 16:296A, 1982.
 The work of the diaphragm during chest distortion is increased by 40 percent.

Naeye RL: Pulmonary arterial abnormalities in sudden infant death syndrome. N Engl J Med 289:1167–1170, 1973.
 Thickening of the medium smooth-muscle layer in the small pulmonary arteries is suggestive of chronic hypoxemia in SIDS victims.

Perrin DG, Becker LE, Madapallimatum A, Cutz E, Bryan AC, Sole MJ: Sudden Infant Death Syndrome: Increased carotid body dopamine and noradrenaline content. Lancet 2:535–537, 1984.
> Victims of SIDS have a 10-fold increase in dopamine concentration in the carotid body. This may be the mechanism preventing arousal in SIDS.

Purpura DP: Dendritic differentiation in human cerebral cortex: Normal and aberrant development patterns, in Kreutzberg GW (ed), *Advances in Neurology*. New York, Raven, 1975, pp 91–116.
> Dendritic differentiation in the 30-week preterm infant is poor.

Rigatto H: Apnea, in Thiebeault DW, Gregbry GA (eds). *Neonatal Pulmonary Care*, 2d ed. Norwalk, CT, Appleton-Century-Crofts, 1986, pp 641–655.
> Comprehensive review of pathogenesis of apnea and treatment.

Rigatto H, Brady JP: Periodic breathing and apnea in preterm infants. I. Evidence for hypoventilation possibly due to central respiratory depression. Pediatrics 50:202–218, 1972.
> Neonates with periodic breathing and apnea have a depressed respiratory system with a high Pa_{CO_2} and a decreased ventilatory response to CO_2.

Rigatto H, Brady JP: Periodic breathing and apnea in preterm infants. I. Evidence for hypoventilation possibly due to central respiratory depression. Pediatrics 50:202–218, 1972.
> Neonates with periodic breathing and apnea have a depressed respiratory system with a high Pa_{CO_2} and a decreased ventilatory response to CO_2.

Rigatto H, Brady JP: Periodic breathing and apnea in preterm infants. II. Hypoxia as a primary event. Pediatrics 50:219–228, 1972.
> Hypoxia induces periodic breathing and apnea in preterm infants.

Rigatto H, de la Torre Verduzco R, Cates DB: Effects of O_2 on the ventilatory response to CO_2 in preterm infants. J Appl Physiol 39:896–899, 1975.
> The ventilatory response to CO_2 in the preterm infant is the opposite of that in adult subjects; i.e., it is greater the higher the background concentration of O_2.

Shannon DC, Kelly DH: SIDS and near-SIDS. N Engl J Med 306:959–1028, 1982.
> Comprehensive review of theories developed to explain the course of SIDS.

Nontuberculous Infections of the Lungs: General Aspects

Approach to the Patient with Pulmonary Infections

Morton N. Swartz

The clinical scenario of a pulmonary infection characteristically involves a patient with fever, pulmonary symptoms such as cough (with or without sputum production) or shortness of breath, and a pulmonary lesion on radiographic examination. Delineation of the infecting agent requires a sequence of steps. Since the pulmonary process in this patient may be noninfectious in nature, an *early step* is the consideration of the categories and clinical features of any possible "mimics" of pulmonary infection that might be relevant. On finding no clues for a noninfectious process, the *next step* is to define the gross pathologic and pathogenetic features of the pulmonary infection: frank pneumonia, focal infiltrate, lung abscess, chronic cavitary lesion, bronchiectasis, miliary lesions. As a corollary, since pulmonary infections are generated occasionally by the hematogenous rather than by the bronchogenic route, possible initiating pathogenetic factors in the pathogenesis of the pulmonary infection should be weighed.

The *third step* takes into account likely etiologic agents on the basis of frequency statistics. To assist in this appraisal, it is helpful to resort to clinically meaningful groupings. For example, pneumonia can be divided into three major groupings: (1) *community-acquired,* (2) *nosocomial,* and (3) *in the immunocompromised patient.* Each, in turn, would be considered either as *typical,* i.e., direct sputum examination or culture provides the diagnosis; this subset would include primarily the common bacterial pneumonias; or *atypical,* i.e., sputum examination and culture fail to provide a diagnosis; this subset would consist primarily of viral or mycoplasmal pneumonia.

The *fourth step* in defining the etiologic agent involves the careful search for clinical clues. This is particularly important in the patient with atypical pneumonia. Epidemiologic information may be extremely important. For example, coccidioidomycosis becomes a consideration in a patient who develops atypical pneumonia in the San Joaquin Valley of California but not in a patient with atypical pneumonia who has spent his or her whole life in New York City.

Other sources of clinical clues may be provided by the patient's symptomatology. A desultory onset of symptoms over a week or 10 days and a prominent headache might suggest *Mycoplasma pneumoniae* pneumonia. On the other hand, an abrupt onset of illness with recurrent (over several days) shaking chills after a prodromal period

of 24 h or less, particularly if associated with mild diarrhea for 1 or 2 days, might suggest Legionnaires' disease. Further clinical clues may be provided by physical findings. Thus, a relative bradycardia in a patient with the clinical picture of pneumonia might suggest psittacosis or Legionnaires' disease; extensive periodontal disease and an absent gag reflex might indicate the likelihood of aspiration pneumonia; or the occurrence of bullous myringitis might implicate a mycoplasmal etiology.

Other general clinical clues as to etiology of an atypical pneumonia may be provided by examination of the results of initial blood counts, urinalysis, and routine blood chemistries. For example, the presence of mild liver function abnormalities might suggest Q fever, tularemia, miliary tuberculosis, or Legionnaires' disease. A hemolytic anemia with a markedly elevated level of cold agglutinins would direct attention to the possibility of M. pneumoniae pneumonia; or the presence of pigmented casts in the urine and markedly elevated serum levels of creatine phosphokinase might focus attention on the possibilities of influenza virus pneumonia, Legionnaires' disease, or a pulmonary infiltrate associated with intravenous drug abuse.

The *fifth step* involves categorization of the radiographic features. This step is particularly helpful in evaluating the immunocompromised patient where the number of possible etiologies is so extensive. However, it is important to bear in mind that there are no radiographic findings that are specific enough to define the microbial etiology of a given pneumonia or pulmonary infiltrate. The only definitive way to reach a specific etiologic diagnosis is through demonstration of the infecting organism, i.e., by examination of stained smears of sputum and pleural fluid or other biologic materials, or by culture of respiratory secretions and blood, or by demonstrating an increase in antibody titer against the infecting microorganism. Nonetheless, the radiographic picture, taken along with other clinical information, can favor one or several etiologic agents. Accordingly, it is of value to define the radiographic pattern as: (1) lobar or segmental consolidation, (2) patchy bronchopneumonia, (3) nodules (large, small, or miliary), or (4) interstitial process. Multiple large, round pulmonary densities in a renal transplant recipient suggest *Nocardia* infection rather than *Pneumocystis* pneumonia, whereas in a heroin addict with cough, fever, and pleuritic chest pain, such densities suggest acute right-sided endocarditis rather than pneumococcal pneumonia.

The *sixth step*, examination of an appropriately stained smear of sputum or pleural fluid (or occasionally a buffy coat of centrifuged blood), often provides a provisional diagnosis. Although given as the sixth step in progression to an etiologic diagnosis, in practice, examination of an appropriately stained smear of sputum is performed earlier in the evaluation process and can pro-

vide a shortcut to diagnosis if the findings are reasonably definitive. Gram-stained smear provides information not only concerning the morphology and the tinctorial properties of bacteria (and some fungi) but, most importantly, concerning the presence of polymorphonuclear leukocytes and squamous cells, the latter indicating that the specimen originated in the upper, rather than the lower, respiratory tract. On occasion, when clinical features warrant, other special staining methods (e.g., Giemsa for *Pneumocystis carinii* or direct fluorescent antibody for *Legionella pneumophila* or *Legionella micdadei*) may provide a diagnosis. Culture of sputum (and blood) may be required for etiologic diagnosis of some pneumonias when evaluation of a Gram-stained smear has not supplied a provisional diagnosis, either because the infecting agent cannot be distinguished from components of the normal upper respiratory flora incorporated in the specimen or because the particular microorganism is not visible on Gram-stained smear (e.g., *Aspergillus* species or M. pneumoniae). In some patients, an etiologic diagnosis cannot be made on the basis of examination of initial stained smears of sputum and on the results of initial bacteriologic culture. In such circumstances, a definitive diagnosis can sometimes be made only retrospectively, by serologic means, as in psittacosis, Q fever, or adenovirus pneumonia.

The *seventh step* involves selection of initial antimicrobial therapy. If examination of the Gram-stained (or other) smear does not provide the necessary insights as to etiology, then beginning therapy is empiric and based primarily on available clinical clues. Thus, for a community-acquired pneumonia in an otherwise healthy adult, therapy might start with a β-lactam antibiotic, such as penicillin or ampicillin, or a second generation cephalosporin, such as cefamandole or cefuroxime. If, on the other hand, a patient with the AIDS-related complex develops fever, cough, and a bilateral pulmonary infiltrate that is consistent radiologically with *Pneumocystis* infection, then empiric therapy with trimethoprim-sulfamethoxazole would be more appropriate. Clearly, the selection of drug(s) for empiric therapy depends on the clinical setting and on the gravity of the pulmonary process.

The *eighth step* in the approach to the patient with a pulmonary infection entails the performance of an invasive diagnostic procedure to obtain either uncontaminated lower respiratory tract secretions or pulmonary tissue for microbiologic and histologic analysis. This step becomes necessary in those patients in whom the rate of progression of the illness precludes the initiation of a meaningful trial of empiric therapy or requires that such a trial be concluded prematurely. These restrictions apply particularly to the immunosuppressed patient for whom the number of possible etiologies and therapeutic options is large: the rapid progression of the disease does not permit sequential trials of individual antimicrobial agents,

and the hazard of potential side effects precludes the indiscriminate use of multiple drug combinations. At this juncture, only specific etiologic diagnosis can direct meaningful therapeutic efforts.

Among the invasive procedures that are available are: (1) transtracheal aspiration, (2) bronchial brushing, (3) bronchoalveolar lavage, (4) fiberoptic bronchoscopy with transbronchial biopsy, (5) needle biopsy of the lung, and (6) open lung biopsy via limited thoracotomy. The choice of invasive diagnostic procedure should be individualized for each patient. Important considerations in this decision include the type and location of the pulmonary lesion, the ability of the patient to cooperate with the required manipulations, the presence of the coagulopathies, and experience of the particular hospital in performing each of the procedures.

NONINFECTIOUS PROCESSES TO BE CONSIDERED IN THE DIFFERENTIAL DIAGNOSIS OF PULMONARY INFECTIONS

The list of noninfectious disorders that mimic pulmonary infections is extensive (Table 85-1). These are considered briefly in the course of taking the initial history and explored in greater detail should evaluation of the gram-stained smear (and culture) of sputum be unrevealing, or if the initial response to empiric antimicrobial therapy proves unsatisfactory, or if radiographic findings are atypical.

Drug-Induced Pulmonary Disease

Drugs producing pulmonary reactions are conveniently considered in two categories: *noncytotoxic* and *cytotoxic* drugs. Noncytotoxic drugs producing hypersensitivity pneumonitis include antimicrobials, anticonvulsants, diuretics, antiarrhythmics, tranquilizers, and antirheumatic agents (Table 85-2).

NONCYTOTOXIC DRUGS

The commonly used antibacterial drug, nitrofurantoin, can produce two patterns of pulmonary reaction: (1) *acute*, that occurs within 2 weeks of starting therapy and consisting of dyspnea, nonproductive cough, fever, crackles, and diffuse interstitial or patchy infiltrates (often with pleural effusion), and (2) *chronic*, which is less common and occurs after months to years of continuous treatment; the picture of the chronic form is one in which exertional dyspnea and nonproductive cough appear gradually and are unaccompanied by fever; the pattern is not that of a pneumonia.

Sulfasalazine (and other sulfonamides) can produce hypersensitivity lung disease that includes cough, fever, dyspnea, and peripheral hazy acinar or diffuse reticular

TABLE 85-1
Noninfectious Causes of Febrile Pneumonitis Syndrome (Mimics of Pulmonary Infection)

Drug-induced pulmonary disease
  Noncytotoxic drugs
  Cytotoxic drugs

Extrinsic allergic alveolitis

Injury due to inhaled toxic gases

Chronic eosinophilic pneumonia

Interstitial lung disease associated with connective tissue disorders
  Systemic lupus erythematosus
  Polymositis-dermatomyositis
  Mixed connective tissue disease

Interstitial lung disease associated with pulmonary vasculitis
  Wegener's granulomatosis
  Lymphomatoid granulomatosis
  Churg-Strauss syndrome (allergic angiitis and granulomatosis)
  Polyangiitis overlap syndrome

Interstitial lung disease associated with pulmonary airway disease
  Allergic bronchopulmonary aspergillosis
  Bronchocentric granulomatosis
  Bronchiolitis obliterans and bronchiolitis obliterans with organizing pneumonia

Chronic interstitial pneumonias of unknown etiology
  Usual interstitial pneumonia (UIP)
  Lymphocytic interstitial pneumonia (LIP)
  Desquamative interstitial pneumonia (DIP)
  Giant cell interstitial pneumonia (GIP)

Pulmonary neoplasms
  Carcinoma or lymphoma

Sarcoidosis

Pulmonary infarction

Radiation pneumonitis

Adult respiratory distress syndrome (ARDS)
  Associated with extrapulmonary sepsis
  Associated with oxygen toxicity, chemical inhalation or aspiration, or aspiration of gastric contents
  Associated with pancreatitis
  Associated with fat embolization
  Associated with shock of various etiologies
  Associated with drug overdose
  Associated with chest trauma

Pulmonary leukoagglutinin transfusion reactions

Miscellaneous
  Pulmonary alveolar proteinosis
  Plasma cell granuloma
  Histiocytosis X
  Idiopathic pulmonary hemosiderosis
  Goodpasture's syndrome

TABLE 85-2

Noncytotoxic Drugs Capable of Inducing a Picture Resembling Pulmonary Infection

Antimicrobial agents
  Nitrofurantoin
  Sulfasalazine; other sulfonamides
  Amphotericin B (acting with leukocyte transfusions)
Anticonvulsants
  Phenytoin
  Carbamazepine
Diuretics
  Hydrochlorothiazide
Antiarrhythmics
  Amiodarone
Narcotics
  Heroin
  Methadone
  Propoxyphene
Antirheumatic agents
  Gold salts
  Penicillamine
Drugs that can induce a lupus erythematosus-like syndrome
  Hydralazine
  Procainamide
  Isoniazid

TABLE 85-3

Cytotoxic Drugs Capable of Inducing a Picture Resembling Pulmonary Infection

Acute or chronic pneumonitis with pulmonary fibrosis
  Antibiotics
    Bleomycin; mitomycin; neocarzinostatin
  Alkylating agents
    Busulfan; cyclophosphamide; chlorambucil; melphalan; chlorozotocin
  Nitrosoureas
    Carmustine (BCNU); semustine (methyl CCNU); lomustine (CCNU); chlorozotocin
  Antimetabolites
    Methotrexate; azathioprine; mercaptopurine; cytosine arabinoside
  Miscellaneous
    Vinblastine; VM-26; vindescine
Hypersensitivity lung disease
  Antimetabolites
    Methotrexate
  Antibiotics
    Bleomycin
  Miscellaneous
    Procarbazine
Noncardiogenic pulmonary edema
  Antimetabolites
    Methotrexate; cytosine arabinoside
  Alkylating agents
    Cyclophosphamide
  Miscellaneous
    VM-26

infiltrates. Although synergistic pulmonary toxicity between amphotericin B administered intravenously and leukocyte transfusions has been suggested, it has not been confirmed.

Phenytoin can produce hypersensitivity responses in the lung 3 to 6 weeks after initiation of therapy. Fever, cough, and dyspnea are accompanied by radiographic findings of bilateral acinar, nodular, or reticular infiltrates. The presence of a maculopapular skin rash, generalized lymphadenopathy, and peripheral eosinophilia direct attention toward hypersensitivity and away from the diagnosis of pulmonary infection.

Pulmonary reactions occasionally occur with the diuretic hydrochlorothiazide. The sudden onset of cough, dyspnea, fever, chest pain, and crackles after the agent is ingested and after finding radiographic evidence that is suggestive of pulmonary edema raises the prospect of a hypersensitivity mechanism.

Pulmonary side effects occasionally follow 5 to 6 months of therapy with the antiarrhythmic agent amiodarone. Exertional dyspnea, nonproductive cough, malaise, and fever (in about half the patients) are gradual in onset, over weeks to several months. The radiographic findings generally resemble those of chronic eosinophilic pneumonia, tuberculosis, or diffuse interstitial disease, and consist of peripheral areas of consolidation that affect primarily the upper lobes. In some instances, coarse reticular interstitial infiltrates are present. Withdrawal of the medi-

cation coupled with the administration of corticosteroids usually leads to complete resolution.

Patients receiving gold salts as treatment for rheumatoid arthritis occasionally develop a nonproductive cough, fever, and progressive dyspnea over the course of several weeks. The radiographic findings are primarily those of diffuse reticulonodular infiltrates. Hydralazine, procainamide, and isoniazid are capable of inducing a lupuslike syndrome; the clinical picture often includes pleuropulmonary involvement.

CYTOTOXIC DRUGS

Three clinicopathologic patterns characterize cytotoxic drug-induced pulmonary disease: (1) chronic pneumonitis with pulmonary fibrosis, (2) acute hypersensitivity lung disease, and (3) noncardiogenic pulmonary edema (Table 85-3). A variety of predisposing factors may contribute to the development of these reactions. The cumulative dose of certain drugs (e.g., bleomycin, busulfan, and carmustine) appears to be particularly important. Older age seems to be a risk factor for pulmonary toxicity from bleomycin.

Syndrome of Acute or Chronic Pneumonitis with Fibrosis

Essentially all types of cytotoxic drugs capable of inducing pulmonary disease can produce this kind of reaction. The clinical manifestations develop over weeks to months and include nonproductive cough, progressive dyspnea on exertion, fatigue, and malaise. End-inspiratory crackles are audible on examination. The radiographic findings are consistent with those of an interstitial inflammatory process and pulmonary fibrosis. Fever is not intrinsic to this process. An exception is the case of cyclophosphamide-induced pulmonary injury, where over 50 percent of patients exhibit fever. However, since cytotoxic drugs are administered to patients whose underlying disease (or its complications) is often associated with fever, distinguishing between chronic pneumonitis with pulmonary fibrosis and pulmonary infection becomes an important practical issue.

Syndrome of Hypersensitivity Lung Disease

Methotrexate, bleomycin, and procarbazine have each caused an acute syndrome of dyspnea, nonproductive cough, fever, and occasionally pleuritic chest pain. The presence of blood eosinophilia and a skin rash suggest a hypersensitivity reaction. The radiographic findings include a diffuse reticular pattern as well as, in some patients, bilateral acinar infiltrates.

Extrinsic Allergic Alveolitis (Hypersensitivity Pneumonitis)

Inhalation of organic dusts can produce chills, fever, nonproductive cough, dyspnea, and pulmonary crackles a few hours after exposure to an organic dust or vapor to which the sensitive individual is exposed. The chest radiograph usually shows bilateral patchy acinar infiltrates, thus completing a picture suggestive of pulmonary infection. The history of a specific exposure provides the clue to diagnosis, particularly when such episodes have been recurrent. Over two dozen such diseases have been described. Farmer's lung occurs with hypersensitivity to moldy hay containing *Thermoactinomyces* species and *Micropolyspora faeni*. "Air-conditioner" or "humidifier" lung is associated with exposure to similar moldy antigens stemming from occult microbial growth on these air-exchanging systems in offices and homes (Fig. 85-1). In other hypersensitivity pneumonitides, the offending antigens may be of avian origin (pigeon breeder's disease) or from other environmental fungi contaminating natural products in industry (e.g., in maple bark stripper's lung; in moldy sugar cane in bagassosis).

Injury Due to Inhaled Toxic Gases

An acute syndrome mimicking acute bacterial or viral pneumonia clinically and radiologically can follow exposure to nitrogen dioxide in silo-filler's disease.

Chronic Eosinophilic Pneumonia

Chronic eosinophilic pneumonia usually has a course of weeks to months, characterized by fever, night sweats, nonproductive cough, and dyspnea. Pulmonary crackles are variably present. Chest radiographs show a characteristic pattern of peripheral acinar infiltrates that usually involves the upper lobes and resembles the appearance of butterfly pulmonary edema on the photographic negative. In contrast with the usual infectious pneumonias, peripheral blood eosinophilia is common. Occasionally, onset of eosinophilic pneumonia is acute, raising the possibility of drug hypersensitivity.

Interstitial Lung Disease Associated with Connective Tissue Disorders and Pulmonary Vasculitis

A variety of connective tissue disorders and vasculitides may mimic pulmonary infections (Table 85-1). Systemic lupus erythematosus may be associated with transitory infiltrates, interstitial disease, or frank consolidation of a noninfectious nature. Interstitial pneumonitis occurs in 5 to 10 percent of patients with polymyositis and may be mistaken for a pulmonary infection since pulmonary manifestations and fever may precede muscle weakness.

Three types of vasculitis in particular may mimic pulmonary infection. Wegener's granulomatosis involves the lung in approximately 95 percent of cases. The lesions radiologically appear as patchy infiltrates or as sizable nodular lesions, the latter suggesting a lung abscess or cavity due to mycobacterial or mycotic infection (Fig. 85-2). Allergic angiitis and granulomatosis (Churg-Strauss syndrome) occurs in the setting of asthma and peripheral eosinophilia; it characteristically involves the lung, producing pulmonary infiltrates associated with granulomatous and vasculitic lesions. The polyangiitis overlap syndrome combines some of the characteristic features of classic polyarteritis nodosa and of allergic angiitis and granulomatosis, including prominent pulmonary involvement in some instances.

Interstitial Lung Disease Associated with Pulmonary Airway Disease

Allergic bronchopulmonary aspergillosis, characterized by cough, wheezing, fever, and intermittent pulmonary infiltrates, can suggest a pulmonary infection, although an accompanying eosinophilia provides a clue to the true nature of the process. Bronchocentric granulomatosis, a necrotizing process of unknown etiology involving small bronchi, may in some patients produce an acute febrile illness. The pulmonary lesions vary from mucoid impaction to diffuse and nodular infiltrates. Bronchiolitis obliterans, an occasional complication of pulmonary viral infections and inhalation of chemical irritants, can also occur without apparent cause; the latter is often associ-

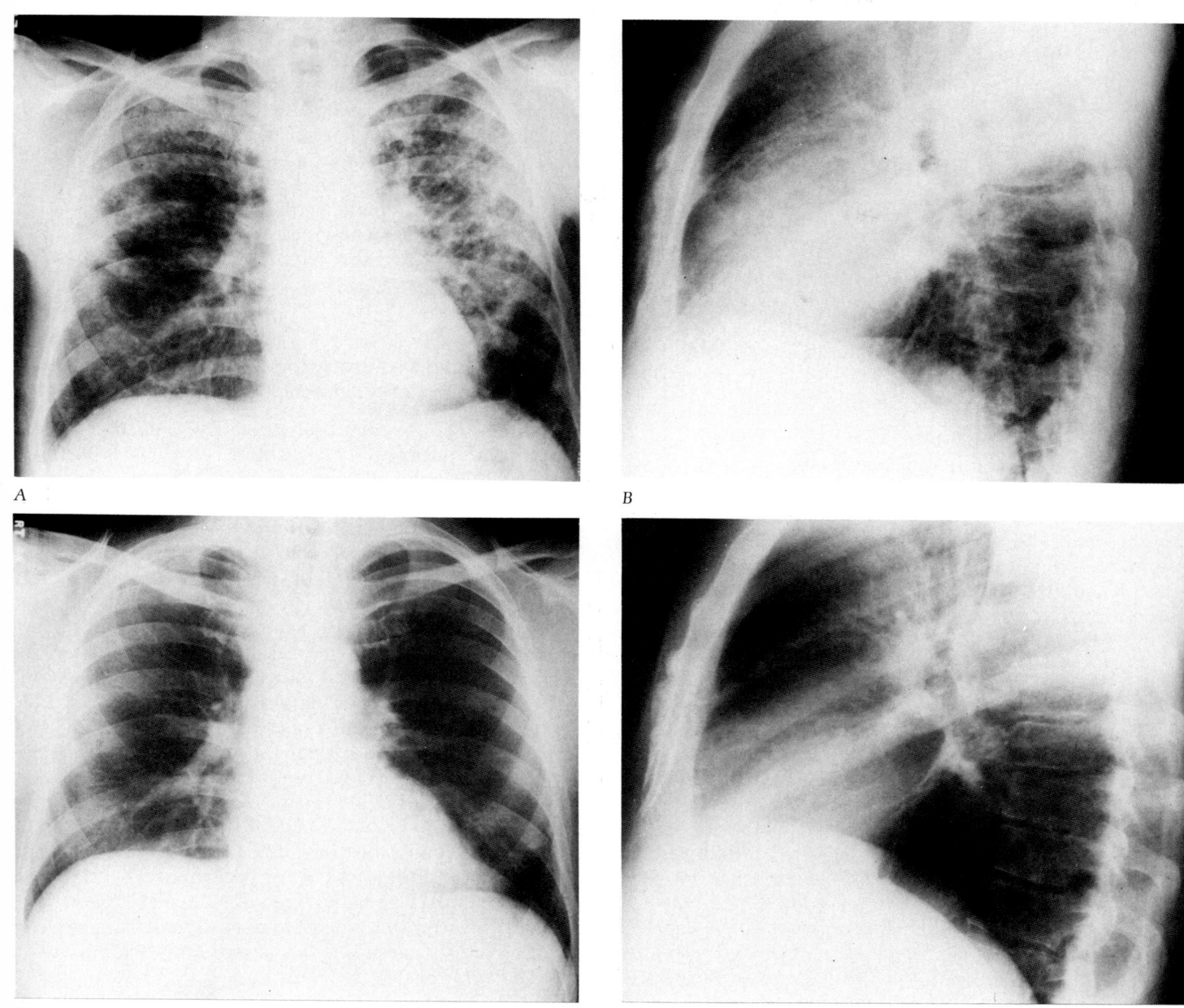

FIGURE 85-1 Hypersensitivity pneumonitis following introduction into home of two humidifiers containing stagnant water. Forty-five-year-old male. PA and lateral views.   *A* and *B*. Dense bilateral infiltrates associated with acute onset of incapacitating dyspnea.   *C* and *D*. Resolution of infiltrates and breathlessness while taking large doses of steroids.

ated with patchy areas of pneumonitis, necrosis of bronchiolar epithelium, and occlusion of terminal airways by granulation tissue.

Chronic Interstitial Pneumonias of Unknown Etiology

A variety of interstitial pneumonias, known as usual interstitial pneumonia (UIP), lymphocytic interstitial pneumonia (LIP), desquamative interstitial pneumonia (DIP), and giant cell interstitial pneumonia (GIP), are conditions of unknown etiology that are defined on histologic

grounds (Fig. 85-1). Most often they present clinically as afebrile subacute or chronic processes characterized by progressive dyspnea, cyanosis, nonproductive cough, pulmonary crackles and a radiographic picture of diffuse reticulonodular infiltrates (more prominent at the lung bases) or a "ground-glass" pattern. Thus, the clinical picture would not suggest a pulmonary infection. However, in a minority of patients, the onset may be rapid, with fever suggesting an acute respiratory infection. A subacute onset in an immunocompromised individual raises the possibility of a *Pneumocystis* infection.

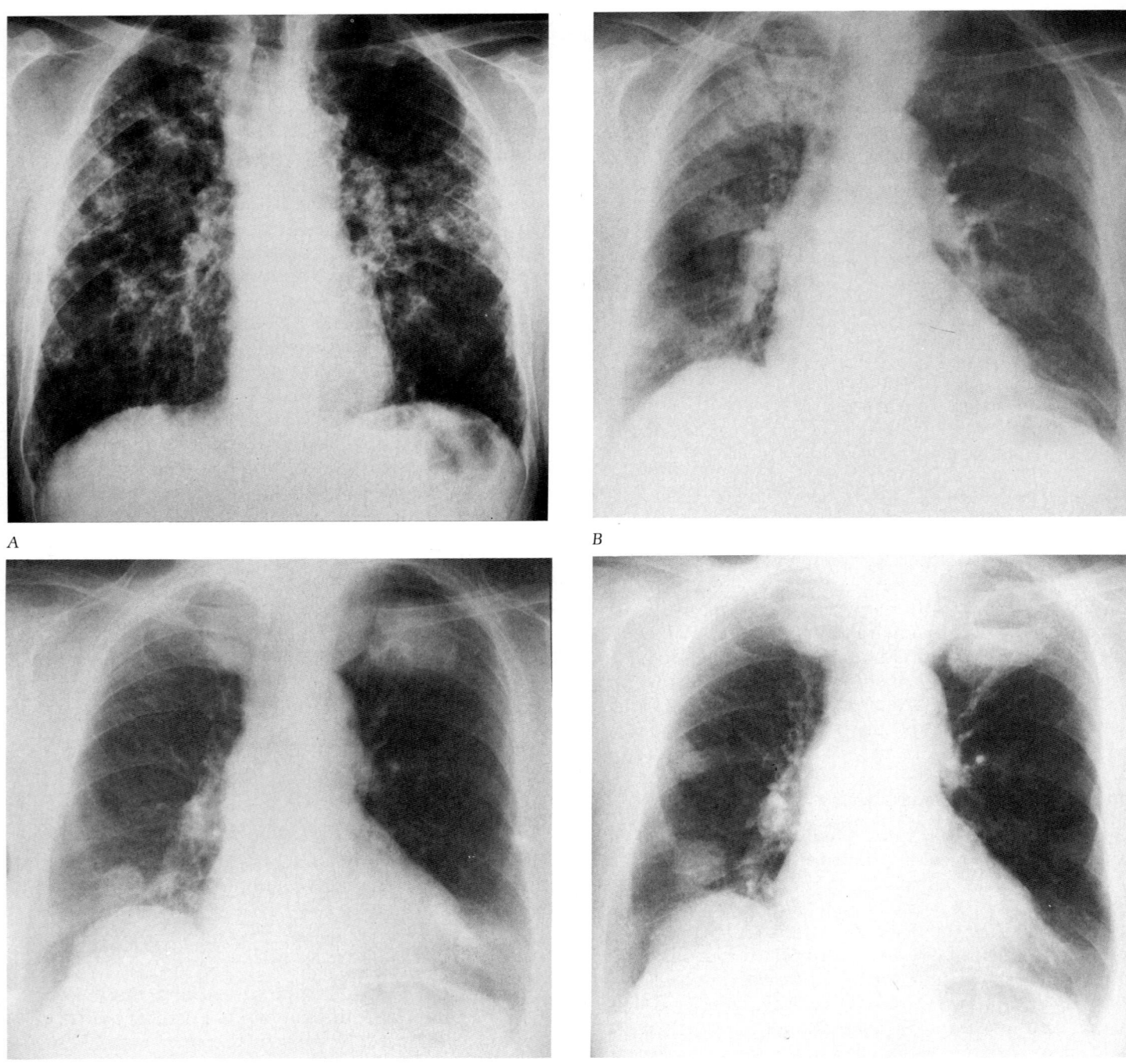

A

B

C

D

FIGURE 85-2 Wegener's granulomatosis. *A.* Onset with chills and fever in 64-year-old male, previously healthy. Lung biopsy interpreted as Wegener's granulomatosis. Partial clearing in response to combined chemotherapy (cyclophosphamide and prednisone). *B.* Onset with malaise, headaches, and fever in 62-year-old female, previously healthy. Bilateral maxillary sinusitis. Widespread, nodular pulmonary infiltrates most marked on right. *C.* Same patient as *B* after 3 years of intermittent combined chemotherapy. Bilateral large masses. *D.* Same patient as *C*, 2 months later. Necrosis within mass in left upper lobe has produced a fluid level.

Pulmonary Neoplasms

Bronchial obstruction by a bronchogenic carcinoma may produce obstructive pneumonia ("drowned lung") or atelectasis. Infection is common as a secondary feature. Recurrent pneumonia in the same portion of the lung should suggest this possibility. Hodgkin's disease and non-Hodgkin's lymphoma may present with fever, cough, dyspnea, and pulmonary lesions suggesting infection. In Hodgkin's disease, a single mass lesion may be present and cavitate, suggesting a lung abscess.

Sarcoidosis

In the patient with sarcoidosis and interstitial lung disease, fever is uncommon unless hilar adenopathy or other features, such as erythema nodosum, are present as well (Fig. 85-3). Thus, this process is usually not mistaken for a primary pulmonary infection.

Pulmonary Infarction

Fever, dyspnea, pleuritic chest pain, leukocytosis, and segmental pleural-based infiltrates (and possibly accompanying pleural effusion) of pulmonary infarction might also suggest the diagnosis of pneumococcal pneumonia. The additional presence of blood-streaked sputum might suggest the possibility of *Streptococcus pyogenes* pneumonia with its hemorrhagic tracheobronchitis. Occasionally, several round lesions in the lung of a febrile, dyspneic patient with pulmonary emboli might suggest aspirational or bacteremic lung abscesses.

Radiation Pneumonitis

The acute phase of radiation pneumonitis usually develops within 3 or 4 months of initiation of radiation therapy. It is characterized by fever, dyspnea, cough, and radiographic changes (infiltrates or ground-glass density) sharply demarcated geometrically to the portal of irradiation rather than to natural pulmonary anatomic divisions. This reaction might be mistaken for a bacterial pneumonia. The late phase of radiation pneumonia, characterized by pulmonary fibrosis, occurs 9 months or later following radiation therapy and is not accompanied by fever.

Adult Respiratory Distress Syndrome

Many unrelated conditions (Table 85-1) involving the lungs primarily or having their initial impact elsewhere have in common the capacity to cause diffuse damage to the alveolar-capillary membrane and produce noncardiogenic pulmonary edema. The process progresses rapidly with inflammatory cell infiltration and pulmonary fibrosis. Extensive pulmonary infiltrates are evident on chest radiographs. Many of the underlying processes producing adult respiratory distress syndrome (ARDS) are associated with fever, and thus fulminant bacterial or viral pneumonia becomes a major diagnostic consideration.

Pulmonary Leukoagglutinin Transfusion Reactions

An acute pulmonary reaction may follow receipt of a blood transfusion with which there has been passive transfer of leukoagglutinins and antibodies cytotoxic to recipient lymphocytes. The clinical picture of an abrupt onset of chills, fever, tachycardia, cough, and dyspnea accompanied by numerous fluffy and nodular perihilar infiltrates on radiograph might easily be mistaken for an acute pulmonary infection.

Miscellaneous Mimics of Pulmonary Infection

Pulmonary alveolar proteinosis usually begins slowly with dyspnea as the principal symptom. Radiographic features are those of a bilateral diffuse predominantly perihilar airspace disease. The radiographic, but not the clinical, manifestations might suggest pulmonary infection. Fever is ordinarily absent. However, since pulmonary alveolar proteinosis may occasionally be associated with hematologic malignancies (e.g., lymphoma and acute leukemias) that themselves cause fever, the mimickry of pulmonary infection might apply. In addition, pulmonary alveolar proteinosis is sometimes complicated by pulmonary infections (e.g., nocardiosis—most frequently, cryptococcosis, aspergillosis, tuberculosis, and histoplasmosis).

Plasma cell granuloma is a postinflammatory pseudotumor of the lung. The combination of cough, fever, and radiologic changes of atelectasis and consolidation suggests the diagnosis of pulmonary infection associated with bronchial obstruction.

Eosinophilic granuloma of the lung (pulmonary histiocytosis X) usually is manifested as a noninfectious interstitial pulmonary process with dyspnea and nonprogressive cough. However, in about 15 percent of patients fever occurs, suggesting the possibility of pulmonary infection. The radiographic findings are those of small nodules and reticulation or honeycombing; these findings in the febrile patient might suggest the diagnosis of miliary tuberculosis, invasive mycotic infection, or viral disease, e.g., varicella-zoster.

PULMONARY INFECTIONS: PATHOLOGIC AND PATHOGENETIC FEATURES

The various pulmonary infections can be categorized according to their distinctive pathologic aspects and pathogenetic features.

Bacterial Pneumonia

Bacterial pneumonia commonly results from bronchogenic spread of infection following microaspiration of secretions. Such particles are able to reach terminal airways and alveoli and there initiate infection, which has the anatomic distribution and radiologic appearance of subsegmental, segmental, or lobar pneumonia. Sometimes, particularly in the elderly or in debilitated patients, pneumonia may be patchy, with a peribronchial and multifocal distribution. Factors that predispose to these patchy pneumonias include aspirated material, preexisting chronic bronchitis, diffuse acute tracheobronchial inflammation (e.g., influenza) and specific infecting microorganisms (e.g., oral anaerobic bacteria).

The progression of a pulmonary infiltrate or lobar consolidation to parenchymal destruction (necrotizing pneumonia or lung abscess) usually is the consequence of

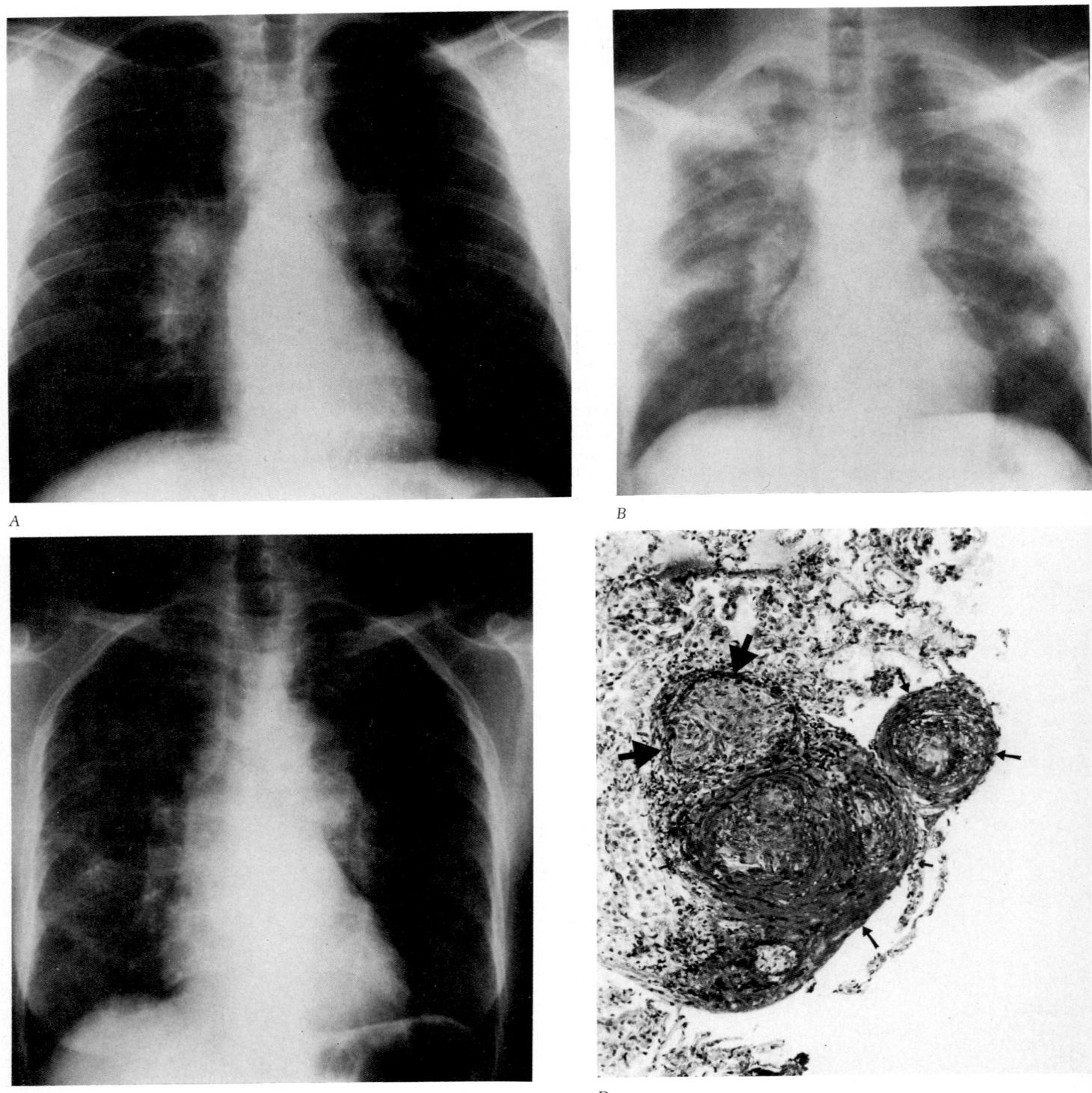

A

B

C

D

FIGURE 85-3   A to C. Chest radiographs illustrating the various stages of sarcoidosis.   A. Stage I, bilateral hilar adenopathy.   B. Stage II, bilateral hilar adenopathy with parenchymal infiltrates.   C. Stage III, parenchymal infiltrates without hilar adenopathy.   D. Transbronchial lung biopsy from a patient with sarcoidosis. Small arrows indicate granuloma with a surrounding rim of collagen (confirmed by positive trichrome staining). The large arrows indicate a granuloma without a surrounding rim of collagen. Original magnification ×10. (*From Rossman and Dauber, 1982*)

one or two factors: (1) the nature of the infecting organism(s), and (2) the presence of bronchial obstruction by tumor or foreign body. Although *Streptococcus pneumoniae* is the most frequent cause of bacterial pneumonia, it almost never produces necrosis of the lung unless there is a complicating factor such as bronchial obstruction, mixed infection, or bacterial superinfection. In contrast, aspirational polymicrobial pneumonia is frequently a necrotizing process. Pleural extension of such anaerobic pulmonary infections often results in putrid empyema. *Klebsiella pneumoniae* not infrequently causes a necrotizing pneumonia with progression to abscess or chronic cavity formation, and in the upper lobe the latter may mimic pulmonary tuberculosis.

Pneumonia may occasionally develop via the bacteremic rather than the bronchogenic route. The clinical setting and the radiographic pattern usually suggest this form of pathogenesis. The intravenous drug abuser with fever, cough, purulent sputum, a murmur of tricuspid insufficiency, numerous irregular infiltrates and rounded densities on chest radiograph, and *Staphylococcus aureus* bacteremia undoubtedly has acute right-sided endocarditis rather than primary *S. aureus* pneumonia. Similarly, an extensively burned patient with secondary infection of involved skin surfaces, with *Pseudomonas aeruginosa* bacteremia and multiple nodular pulmonary densities, is

likely to have bacteremic *Pseudomonas* pneumonia with bacterial invasion of pulmonary arterial walls rather than pneumonia developing via the bronchogenic route. Frankly septic pulmonary emboli, arising from septic thrombosis of the jugular vein as a complication of postanginal sepsis, sometimes produce a clinical and radiographic picture suggestive of multifocal bronchopneumonia. However, on the chest radiograph, the lesions are nodular; histologically, they represent pulmonary infarcts (following emboli) upon which are engrafted pyogenic infection and abscess formation.

Lung Abscess

Lung abscess is an area of pulmonary infection that has gone on to parenchymal necrosis. It is usually solitary but may occur as multiple discrete lesions. Most often it is secondary to aspiration of anaerobic organisms that are components of the normal flora of the upper respiratory tract and are associated with periodontal disease. If the process is subacute, the clinical features may be overlooked initially so that the first evidence of illness appears only after breakdown of tissue has resulted in an abscess cavity. Should there be some degree of ball valve bronchial obstruction, ingress of air may occur while contained pus fails to drain, producing the radiographic pic-

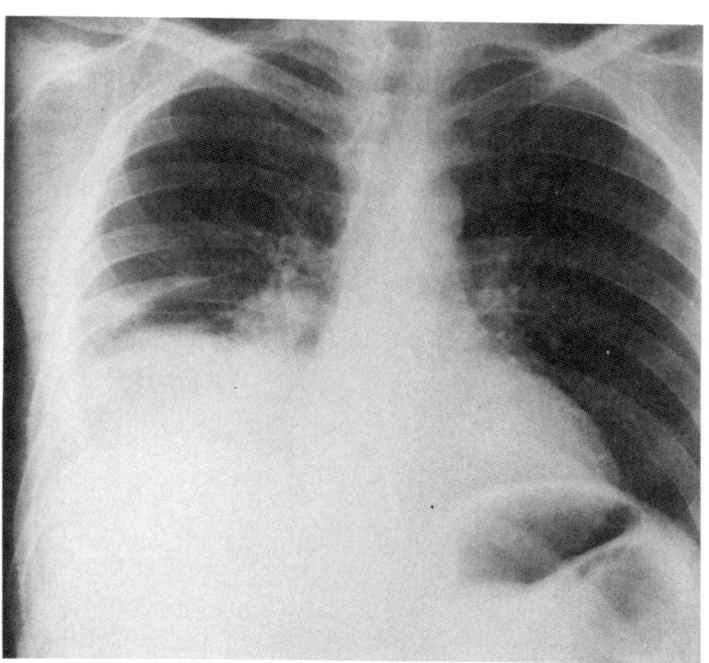
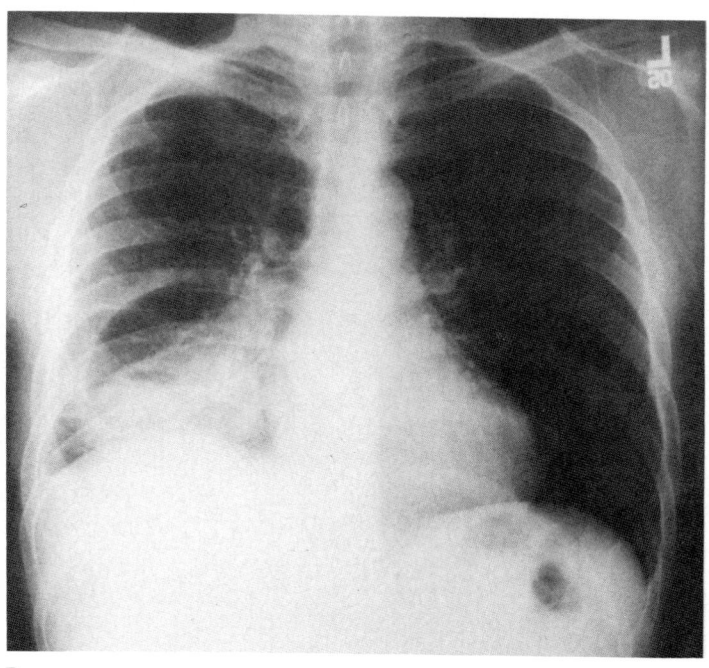

A   *B*

FIGURE 85-4   Necrotizing pneumonia, probably secondary to aspiration. Thirty-nine-year-old male, smoker and drinker, previously healthy. Onset with cough, shortness of breath, fever, and right-sided pleuritic pain. Despite antibiotics, signs and symptoms progressed to include high fevers, night sweats, greenish sputum, leukocytosis, and manifestations of hypertrophic osteoarthropathy.   *A.* On admission. Consolidation of right lower lobe, right hilar mass (or adenopathy), and right pleural effusion. Mediastinoscopy and bronchoscopy revealed no tumor. *B.* Three months later. Process in right lower lobe more circumscribed. Right lower lobectomy revealed extensive necrotizing pneumonia, multiple abscesses, and "reactive" lymph nodes. Postoperatively, free of signs and symptoms including hypertrophic osteoarthropathy.

ture of an air-fluid level. Alternatively, the initial process may be an aspirational (anaerobic) necrotizing pneumonia with extensive microscopic foci of abscess formation; this process may be clinically evident as a severe pneumonia, i.e., "pulmonary gangrene." Progression of this process with confluence of small necrotic foci can either cause one or more lung abscesses or lead to a grossly shrunken and destroyed lobe.

Other causes of lung abscess are: (1) progression of a bronchogenic pneumonia due to a pathogen with necrotizing potential, e.g., *K. pneumoniae*, or *Nocardia asteroides* in an immunocompromised patient, (2) bacteremic spread of infection, and (3) septic pulmonary emboli. Lung abscesses complicating necrotizing pneumonia (Fig. 85-4) should be distinguished from pneumatoceles; the latter are thin-walled, air-filled structures that often develop early in the course of staphylococcal pneumonia, particularly in infants and young children, and that usually disappear over the course of a few months.

Bronchitis and Bronchiectasis

Acute bronchitis is an inflammatory process, usually of viral origin, confined to the bronchi and bronchioles; it does not extend appreciably to surrounding pulmonary parenchyma and is not evident on radiographic examination. Purulent secretion is a common concomitant even though there is no discernible bacterial infection; sometimes purulent secretion represents bacterial superinfection that is evident on examination of Gram-stained smears of sputum and sputum culture. The diagnosis of an acute exacerbation of chronic bronchitis is based solely on clinical grounds; the manifestations are increased cough, dyspnea, and enhanced production of purulent sputum, with or without fever, in a patient with chronic obstructive pulmonary disease. Bacteriologic examination generally reveals large numbers of pneumococci or nontypable *Hemophilus influenzae*, either as infecting organisms or as chronic colonizers of the bronchial tree (which is the site of a newly acquired viral infection).

Bronchiectasis is characterized by destruction of epithelial, elastic, and muscular elements of bronchi resulting in their irreversible dilatation. The major proximate cause is repeated or chronic bacterial infection. However, predisposition to such infections may be a consequence of a variety of factors including certain types of prior infection (pertussis, adenoviral, or rubeola infections, necrotizing pneumonia), bronchial obstruction, immunodeficiencies, congenital anatomic lung disease (e.g., congenital tracheobronchomegaly), and other hereditable disorders such as ciliary dysfunctional states and α_1-antitrypsin deficiency. As a result of repeated infections, stasis of secretions, and peribronchial fibrosis, bronchi are grossly distorted or completely destroyed. Although pneumonia or lung abscess may accompany recurrent acute infections, exacerbations are usually confined to bronchial and peribronchial tissues.

Chronic Cavitary Disease

Chronic cavitary pulmonary tuberculosis commonly begins with a focus of pneumonitis, usually in the subapical posterior portion of an upper lobe (Fig. 85-5). This patch of pneumonitis occurs at a latent site of earlier metastatic infection (Simon focus) produced by lymphohematogenous spread from primary pulmonary tuberculous lesions. Progressive caseation necrosis at this site, followed by drainage of caseous material through the

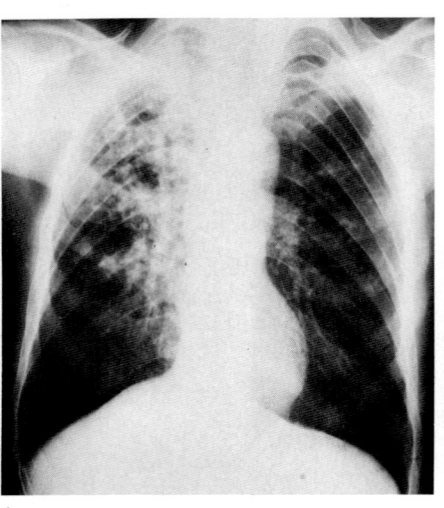 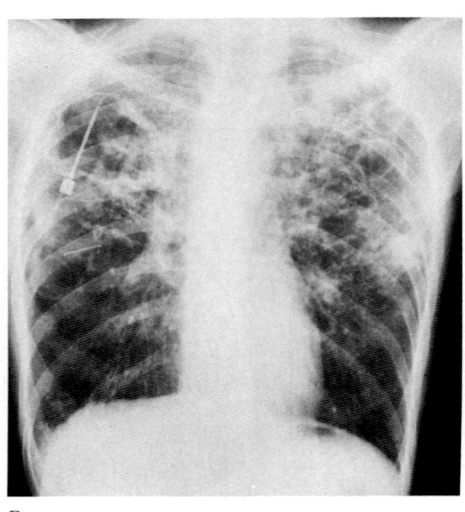 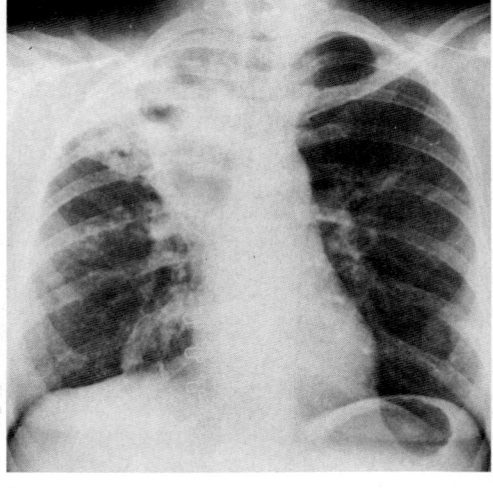

A   *B*   *C*

FIGURE 85-5 Tuberculous cavities. In each instance, the organisms were seen on smear and identified by culture. *A.* Fifty-six-year-old black male. Cavity in midst of consolidation. *B.* Seventy-two-year-old black male. Bilateral, multiple cavities. *C.* Forty-eight-year-old black female. Spread from original involvement of right upper lobe.

bronchial tree, produces a cavity. The cavity is encased in a rigid wall of fibrous tissue.

In addition to pyogenic lung abscess and pulmonary tuberculosis, other pulmonary infections can produce chronic cavities. These include nocardial infections, actinomycosis, and chronic primary pulmonary mycoses (particularly histoplasmosis, occasionally coccidioidomycosis, uncommonly blastomycosis). Sporotrichosis can involve the lung and produce cavities, usually thin-walled. Rare parasitic infestation of the lung (paragonimiasis, echinococcosis) can take the form of cavitary disease as well.

Pulmonary cavities may also occur in noninfectious disorders, e.g., Wegener's granulomatosis, lymphoma or bronchogenic carcinoma, bland pulmonary infarcts, and intrapulmonary nodules of rheumatoid lung disease. Such cavitary lesions, as well as the cystic lesions that occur in chronic pulmonary sarcoidosis and in the markedly dilated bronchi of saccular bronchiectasis, can be sites of growth of "fungus balls." These represent tangled masses of fungal hyphae and debris lying freely within pulmonary cavities as noninvasive saprophytic growths. The mycotic agent involved most commonly is an *Aspergillus* species (usually *A. fumigatus*), and the infection is known as an aspergilloma.

Miliary Lesions

Hematogenous dissemination of tuberculosis can follow initial infection in children or adults (Fig. 85-6). It also can result from breakdown of formerly quiescent sites of pulmonary or extrapulmonary infection. Clinically, unexplained fever is accompanied by miliary lesions (very small and uniform in size and shape) on the chest radiograph; histologically, these lesions are foci of granulomatous reaction. Similar radiographic lesions also occur in the course of hematogenously disseminated mycotic infections such as cryptococcosis and histoplasmosis.

MICROBIAL ETIOLOGIES OF PNEUMONIA

In dealing with a patient with pneumonia it is helpful, while microbiologic data are being gathered, to consider the relative frequencies of various etiologies as an aid in selecting initial antimicrobial therapy. Categorization of pneumonias by clinical settings is a practical first step (Table 85-4).

Community-Acquired Pneumonia

An estimated 2 to 2.5 million cases of pneumonia occur annually in the United States. The largest category con-

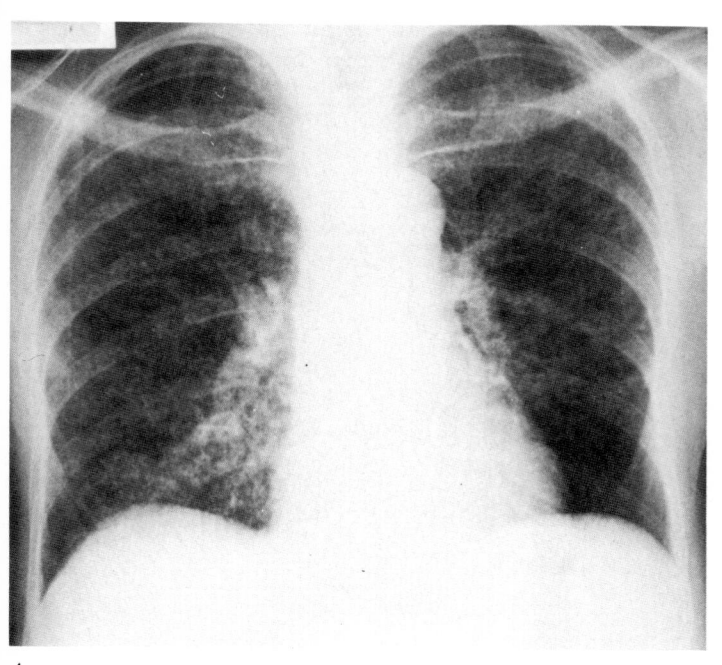
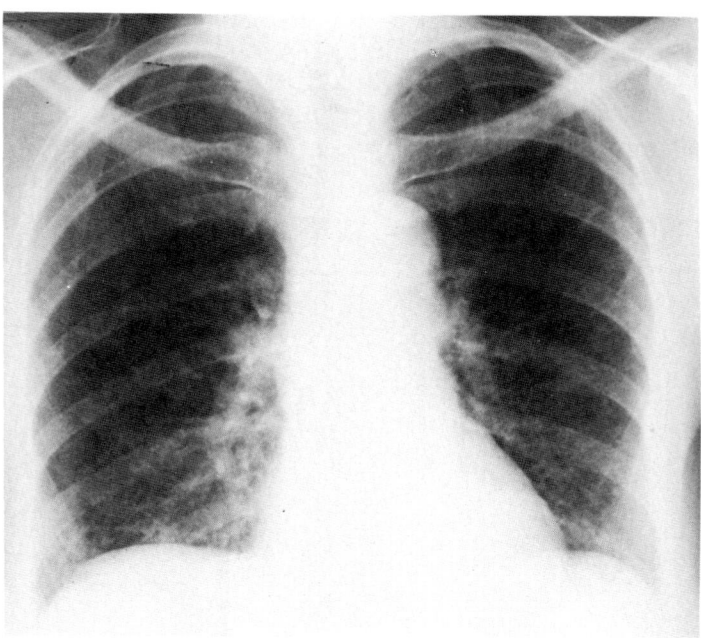

A

B

FIGURE 85-6 Miliary tuberculosis. A 64-year-old black female complaining of urinary frequency and progressive weight loss for 1 year. *A.* On admission. Close inspection reveals fine nodular lesions throughout both lung fields. *B.* Four weeks later. The lesions are larger and many have become confluent, especially on the right. Bronchoscopic washings, biopsy, and culture positive for *M. tuberculosis*. Urine culture strongly positive for *E. coli* but negative for *M. tuberculosis*.

sists of community-acquired pneumonias. A global view of the relative frequencies of the major groupings can be seen in a compilation of data from 11 series reported over the past 20 years (Table 85-5). These cases represent patients with pneumonia of sufficient severity to have warranted hospital admission. Clearly, not all patients with pneumonia require hospitalization. At one institution, as many as 50 percent of patients reporting to an emergency room with pneumonia were believed not to require hospi-

talization. In a Seattle study involving a large medical cooperative, 15 percent of all pneumonias were due to *M. pneumoniae* (Fig. 85-7), but only 2 percent of the patients with *M. pneumoniae* pneumonia were hospitalized. Thus, this etiology is likely to be underrepresented in a compilation such as is shown in Table 85-5.

TABLE 85-4
Practical Categorization of Pneumonia by Clinical Setting

Community-acquired pneumonia
  Typical (i.e., classic) pneumonia
  Atypical pneumonia
  Aspiration pneumonia
Pneumonia in the elderly
  Community-acquired
  In nursing home residents
Nosocomial pneumonia
Pneumonia in immunocompromised hosts
  Pneumonia in patients with immunoglobulin deficiencies
  Pneumonia in patients with granulocyte deficiency
  Pneumonia in patients with cellular immune deficiences
    Pneumonia in patients with neoplastic disease
    Pneumonia in transplant recipients
    Pneumonia in patients with AIDS
    Pneumonia in other immunocompromised patients

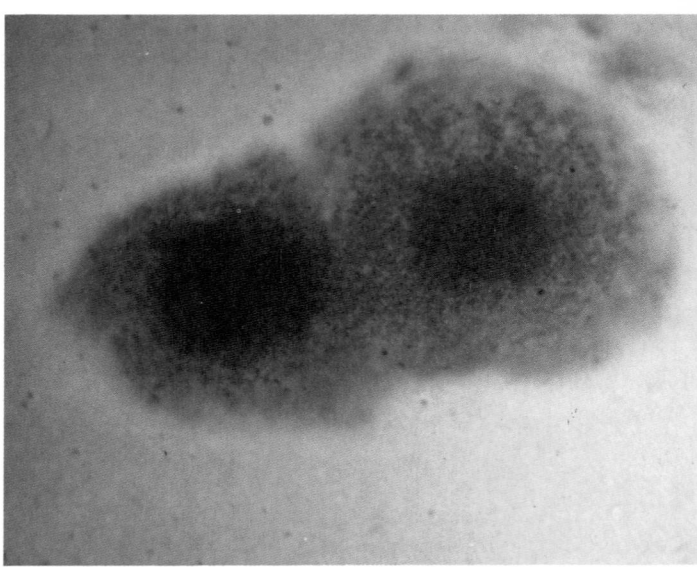

FIGURE 85-7 Subculture on mycoplasma agar of *Mycoplasma* isolated from sputum of a 22-year-old man with atypical pneumonia. The two colonies show the "fried egg" appearance that is more typical of *M. hominis* and other *Mycoplasma* species than of *M. pneumoniae* on primary isolation. ×45; Dienes stain.

TABLE 85-5
Relative Frequencies of Major Categories of Community-Acquired Pneumonia

Year	Author	Total No. Patients	No. with Bact. Etiology	% with Bact. Etiology	No. with Pneumococci	Pneumococcal Etiology: % Total Bacterial	No. Viral (V), Chlamydial (C), Mycoplasmal (M)	% V, C, M of Total	No. Unknown Etiology	% Unknown of Total
1967	Mufson	427	200	47	Most	Most	85	20	142	33
1968	Lepow	98	46	47	Most	Most	11	11	41	42
1969	Fiala	192	128	67	106	83	?	?	64	33
1971	Fekety	100	66	66	62	94	5	5	29	29
1972	Sullivan	292	166	57	103	62	?	?	126	43
1973	Dorff	148	109	74	71	65	13	9	25	17
1980	Ebright	106	56	53	38	68	?	?	50	47
1981	White*	210	43	20	24	56	70	33	107	51
1982	McFarlane†	127	123	97	96	76	?	?	4	3
1985	Berntsson‡	127	58	46	49	84	22	17	27	21
1985	Woodhead	50	38	76	16	42	3	6	9	18
	Totals	1877	1033	55	565	71	209	18	624	33

*Ten patients had more than one infectious agent implicated by isolation or serologic means.

†Percentages difficult to determine because 21 patients were reported with two pathogens, three patients with three pathogens, and one patient with four pathogens.

‡These data fail to add up to 100 percent since an additional 20 patients had two or more pathogens implicated and relative roles of each were not assessed; therefore, not included in this tabulation.

Bacterial etiologies are the most frequent (55 percent) in community-acquired pneumonias. Of the bacterial species involved, *S. pneumoniae* is the predominant, accounting for 71 percent of cases with a bacterial etiology. Eighteen percent of patients have definable nonbacterial etiologies such as *Mycoplasma*, viruses, *Chlamydia*, and *Coxiella burnetii*. In one-third of the cases of community-acquired pneumonia, the etiologic agent cannot be defined by the available methodologies. Some of these cases undoubtedly represent viral and mycoplasmal pneumonias that have not been identified. It is also likely that others represent: (1) patients with pneumococcal pneumonia whose sputum cultures failed to grow this somewhat fastidious microorganism, (2) patients with *Legionella* pneumonia, (3) patients with aspirational pneumonia caused by oral anaerobes, or (4) patients with as yet undescribed etiologic agents.

BACTERIAL PNEUMONIA

S. pneumoniae is the preeminent bacterial etiology of community-acquired pneumonia. *H. influenzae*, usually unencapsulated strains, may produce pneumonia in patients with chronic bronchitis. It also may be the causative agent of pneumonia in the chronic alcoholic. However, apart from *S. pneumoniae*, the most important pathogen in this type of patient, by virtue of its virulence and special antibiotic susceptibilities, is *K. pneumoniae*. During an outbreak of influenza viral infections, bacterial superinfections often occur, usually in the elderly or in individuals with chronic cardiopulmonary disease. Patients with secondary bacterial pneumonia often have a period of up to 4 days of clinical improvement following the initial influenzal illness before the onset of overt pulmonary infection. The superinfecting microorganisms are the potential pathogens that would ordinarily colonize the upper airways but that invade opportunistically a tracheobronchial tree that has been recently damaged. These organisms include *S. pneumoniae*, *H. influenzae*, *S. aureus*, and *K. pneumoniae*. The use of antibiotics at the time of the initial respiratory infection is not only useless against viral influenza but may selectively promote the emergence of a more resistant bacterial flora in the respiratory tract. *S. aureus* is a very uncommon cause of community-acquired pneumonia. Indeed, the occurrence of several cases of *S. aureus* pneumonia in the community during the winter months is usually a good indicator of the presence of an ambient influenza outbreak.

Pneumonia due to *S. pyogenes* is quite uncommon. Usually it occurs as a superinfection in a patient with influenza or as a primary pneumonia in the course of a regional outbreak of group A streptococcal infections (as still occurs from time to time when a new M-antigenic type appears in a community).

ATYPICAL PNEUMONIA SYNDROME

In evaluating patients with community-acquired pneumonia, it is often helpful to consider separately a group of patients whose illness is characterized by little, if any, sputum production and, if sputum is raised, examination on Gram-stained (and Ziehl-Neelsen stained) smears and routine culture fail to reveal a microbial etiology. Often, but not always, the clinical onset of illness is less acute than in the typical bacterial pneumonias, the radiologic picture is more likely to consist of patchy infiltrates or an interstitial pattern rather than a lobar consolidation, and a peripheral leukocytosis is less common. For convenience, this grouping has been designated *atypical pneumonia*.

The entities in the category of atypical pneumonia are highly heterogeneous (Table 85-6), and the syndrome accounts for about 40 to 50 percent of cases of community-acquired pneumonia. *M. pneumoniae* is the etiology in about 30 percent of the cases of atypical pneumonia. Respiratory viruses are responsible for about another 20 percent. However, the predominant etiologic agent varies considerably with the season and the prevalence of influenza A in the community. A viral respiratory illness becomes a major cause of atypical pneumonia during an outbreak of the latter. The newly described TWAR strain of *Chlamydia psittaci*, an infectious agent that causes pneumonia and can be spread from person to person without an avian host, appears to be responsible for 12 to 21 percent of cases of atypical pneumonia. This form of pneumonia typically occurs in young adults as a sporadic mild pneumonia. Occasional outbreaks have occurred.

The epidemiologic and clinical characteristics of certain types of atypical pneumonias may provide a basis for suspecting these etiologies before results of specific labo-

TABLE 85-6
Etiologies of Community-Acquired Atypical Pneumonias

Mycoplasma
   M. pneumoniae
Respiratory tract viruses
   Influenza; adenovirus, respiratory syncytial virus (RSV); parainfluenza virus
Other viral agents
   Varicella-zoster; measles; Epstein-Barr virus (EBV)
Rickettsia
   C. burnetii (Q fever)
Chlamydia
   C. psittaci (psittacosis); *C. psittaci* var TWAR
Bacteria
   Legionella; *F. tularensis*; *Y. pestis*; *B. anthracis*
Fungi
   Histoplasma; *Blastomyces*; *Coccidioides*

ratory tests become available. In adults, *M. pneumoniae* pneumonia, in contrast to bacterial pneumonia, often begins insidiously with malaise, fever, and prominent headache. Sore throat is common, but coryza is minimal or absent. Nonproductive cough develops over the next few days and is the hallmark of this disease. Skin rash (erythema multiforme) and bullous myringitis, usually appearing late in the course of illness, are uncommon findings but, when present, do suggest the diagnosis. Mini-outbreaks of *M. pneumoniae* infection in households are frequently not appreciated because of the long incubation period (3 weeks) and the varied forms that the illness can assume. One characteristic sequence to illustrate the diversity of clinical presentations is as follows: the infection with *M. pneumoniae* is introduced by a grade school child whose illness may be a sore throat and earache; three weeks later a parent develops atypical pneumonia; and several weeks later a second child of high school age develops a troublesome persistent dry cough with minimal fever. Outbreaks have occurred in military camps.

Infections with respiratory viruses occur predominantly in the winter and early spring. Influenza virus is the one agent that may be associated with sizable outbreaks or major epidemics. Primary influenza viral pneumonia usually occurs in the setting of an influenza A outbreak. It occurs especially in patients with underlying heart disease, particularly mitral stenosis. Other risk factors include chronic pulmonary disease and pregnancy. Unlike secondary bacterial pneumonia after influenza—a complication that occurs after a period (1 to 4 days) of improvement following a typical influenzal upper respiratory illness—primary influenza pneumonia immediately follows typical influenza. Very rarely, in the course of systemic infection with viruses whose principal impact is not ordinarily on the respiratory tract, viral pneumonia develops in an otherwise healthy individual. Pulmonary infiltrates occur in 16 percent of young adults with varicella, but only 2 to 4 percent have clinical manifestations suggestive of pneumonia. Pneumonia in children with varicella is more likely to represent bacterial superinfection than primary viral pneumonia. On rare occasions, pulmonary infiltrates develop in patients with clinical infectious mononucleosis; the infiltrates represent atypical pneumonia due to Epstein-Barr virus.

Q fever, due to *C. burnetii*, like many of the other causes of the atypical pneumonia syndrome, is suspected on the basis of epidemiologic clues. Transmission of this disease to humans occurs as a result of inhalation of aerosols from surroundings contaminated by·placental and birth fluids of infected livestock (cattle, sheep, goats) and domestic animals (cats). Veterinarians, ranchers, and medical investigators, such as those who use goats or sheep to produce antibodies, are at particular risk. Since the incubation period of Q fever is approximately 20 days, a source of exposure during foreign travel may easily be overlooked. Although the clinical picture resembles that of *M. pneumoniae* pneumonia, the onset may be more abrupt, with chills and high fever. Liver function abnormalities or clinical hepatitis in a patient with atypical pneumonia is suggestive of Q fever.

Chlamydia trachomatis causes pneumonia in the newborn but has not been proven to be a cause of pneumonia in adults who are otherwise healthy. However, *Chlamydia psittaci*, the causative agent of psittacosis, is spread to humans by avian species. Although psittacine birds (parakeets, parrots) are the major reservoir, human infection can be acquired from pigeons, sparrows, and turkeys. In a patient with atypical pneumonia, the clinical features that raise the possibility of this etiology are relative bradycardia, splenomegaly and hepatomegaly, or hepatic dysfunction. *C. psittaci* var TWAR produces atypical pneumonia without the usual bird-to-human transmission of *C. psittaci* infection. The clinical picture of TWAR-strain infection is indistinguishable from that of *M. pneumoniae* pneumonia.

Legionella infections (due to *L. pneumophila* and other *Legionella* species) account for 2 to 4 percent of cases of atypical pneumonia. Although *Legionella* is an important nosocomial pathogen, it is also responsible for community-based sporadic cases and major outbreaks. The occurrence of summer outbreaks associated with the use of air conditioners and evaporative condensers should call attention to this possible cause of atypical pneumonia. Various extrapulmonary manifestations have been attributed to Legionnaires' disease. Among these are a relative bradycardia, diarrhea for 24 h at the onset of illness, confusion and obtundation, mild renal dysfunction (azotemia, microscopic hematuria, proteinuria), acute rhabdomyolysis, and mild hepatic dysfunction. Although many of these manifestations also occur with other pneumonias, the coincidence of several of these features should raise the possibility of *Legionella* infection. This is particularly important in view of the fact that the antibiotic treatment (erythromycin) for Legionnaires' disease differs from that for the more common bacterial pneumonias and that the mortality of Legionnaires' disease, if inadequately treated, can be as high as 15 percent. Recurrent chills, which occur over several days in Legionnaires' disease, are rare in pneumococcal pneumonia unless septic complications, e.g., endocarditis or pericarditis, develop. Although the initial radiographic picture of *Legionella* pneumonia is often that of an interstitial, segmental, or bronchopneumonic pneumonia, if the disease is untreated, the process progresses to lobar or multilobar consolidation, a picture that mimics pneumococcal or *Klebsiella* pneumonia.

The other noteworthy bacterial types of atypical pneumonia are those due to *Francisella tularensis*

(tularemic pneumonia), *Yersinia pestis* (plague pneumonia), and *Bacillus anthracis* (anthrax pneumonia). These are all singularly uncommon causes of pneumonia, and the principal clues to diagnosis again derive from epidemiologic considerations. Exposure to *F. tularensis* comes through contact with tissues of an infected animal (rabbit), animal (coyote, cat) bites, inhalation of infectious aerosols, tick or deerfly bites, or ingestion of contaminated water or poorly cooked meat from an infected animal. Ulceroglandular tularemia, or the typhoidal form of tularemia, may be complicated by patchy pulmonary infiltrates. Indeed, it is likely that typhoidal tularemia often represents infection initially acquired via the bronchogenic route. Plague is less common than tularemia in the United States and is sharply localized to southwestern United States and California. The diagnosis should be considered in an individual from an endemic area who has a septic illness (septicemic plague) or painful localized lymphadenopathy with fever (bubonic plague) and a history of bites by rodent fleas or of handling tissues of infected animals, such as prairie dogs or coyotes. Pneumonia occurs as a complication in 10 to 15 percent of patients with bubonic or septicemic plague. Primary (inhalation) pneumonic plague is extremely rare and occurs only as a result of exposure to aerosolized particles from an infected animal or following close contact with cases of plague pneumonia. Anthrax pneumonia (inhalation anthrax) is also extremely rare in this country; it is a consequence of the inhalation of anthrax spores during the processing, or use, of goat hair or wool (usually imported from the Middle East, Asia, or Africa).

The principal clues that the cause of atypical pneumonia in a given patient might be a primary pulmonary mycosis are epidemiologic. For example, the principal endemic areas for histoplasmosis in this hemisphere are in midwestern United States and Central America. The organism is present in high concentrations in soil sites where avian, chicken, or bat excrement has accumulated. Movement of soil in such endemic areas by cleaning chicken coops, knocking down old starling roosts, or cleaning out old attics or basements can expose individuals to high concentrations of airborne spores that, when inhaled, produce an acute pneumonia. Atypical pneumonia in an individual with this type of geographic exposure, or in a spelunker, should automatically raise the possibility of histoplasmosis.

Blastomycosis occurs in most states in this country, but the endemic area is principally in the southeastern and south central areas. Rural exposure to soil contaminated with animal excrement appears to be a risk factor. Skin lesions, either verrucous or ulcerative, are the most common extrapulmonary manifestations of blastomycosis and afford a clinical clue to diagnosis.

Coccidioidomycosis is endemic in southwestern United States (California, particularly the San Joaquin Valley; Arizona) and in neighboring portions of Mexico. Infection is usually acquired in these areas by inhaling highly infectious arthrospores. Occasionally, major dust storms carry the arthrospores considerable distances from their soil source and produce unexpected outbreaks of infection. Archeologic digs sometimes cause infection in those living elsewhere who receive an artifact uncovered in the explorations. Erythema nodosum may be associated with any of the primary pulmonary mycoses, but most often with coccidioidomycosis. The coincidence of this hypersensitivity skin lesion and an atypical pneumonia syndrome in an individual from an endemic area suggests the possibility of one of these pulmonary mycoses.

ASPIRATION PNEUMONIA

Community-acquired aspiration pneumonia may occur following an overt episode of aspiration, e.g., of gastric contents, or of bronchial obstruction by a foreign body. More often the predisposing circumstances are less clear-cut, e.g., alcoholism, nocturnal esophageal reflux, pyorrhea, a prolonged session in the dental chair, epilepsy, or chronic sinusitis in a patient with absent gag reflex. In these circumstances, since the pneumonia may develop more insidiously than after overt aspiration, the relationship of the developing pneumonia to the predisposing circumstances may not be appreciated at the time. For this reason, specific questioning regarding such possible pathogenetic factors and evaluation of the gag reflex should be part of the examination of any patient with pneumonia.

If untreated, aspiration pneumonia may progress rapidly to a necrotizing process that is usually due to anaerobic organisms. The process may involve a pulmonary segment, a lobe, or an entire lung with ultimate extension to the pleura ("putrid empyema"); in some patients, the necrotizing pneumonia culminates in lung abscesses. In others, aspiration produces an illness of several weeks duration that is characterized by malaise, productive cough, and low grade fever. If a chest radiograph is first taken after several weeks of untreated illness, it may show little, if any, evidence of pneumonia but will clearly identify a well-formed lung abscess.

In community-acquired aspiration pneumonia, insight into the etiologic agents has been primarily obtained from bacteriologic studies after transtracheal aspiration; these studies have provided a statistical basis for selecting the initial antimicrobial therapy. Anaerobic bacteria are etiologically involved in about 90 percent of community-acquired aspiration pneumonias and lung abscesses. In 40 to 65 percent of these patients, anaerobic organisms are the sole infecting agents; in 40 to 45 percent, the etiology is a mixture of anaerobes and aerobes. The most common anaerobes are the *Bacteroides melaninogenicus-asaccharolyticus* group, *Fusobacterium nucleatum*, peptostreptococci, peptococci, and microaerophilic strepto-

cocci. β-Lactamase-producing *Bacteroides* species and members of the *B. fragilis* group are present in about 15 percent of cases. Members of the *B. melaninogenicus* group may be the most important contributors in such mixed infections. A rare form of anaerobic aspiration pneumonia (actinomycosis) that is community-acquired is that due to *Actinomyces israelii*, part of the normal flora in the gingival crevice (Fig. 85-8). The direct extension of such a necrotizing pneumonia to the pleura *and chest wall* is a characteristic finding that strongly suggests the diagnosis of actinomycosis.

Although anaerobic members of the oropharyngeal flora have a preeminent role in community-acquired aspiration pneumonia and lung abscess, occasionally, gram-negative enteric bacilli such as *K. pneumoniae*, *Escherichia coli*, and *Proteus* species may be the etiology.

Persistence of a necrotizing pneumonia or lung abscess despite antimicrobial therapy that would be expected a priori to be effective raises the possibility of an underlying bronchogenic carcinoma, particularly if the patient is edentulous.

Pneumonia in the Elderly

Community-acquired pneumonia in the elderly primarily involves two groups: one population that lives at home and another that resides in nursing homes. The latter, from the point of view of oropharyngeal flora and extent of exposure to antimicrobial agents, might be regarded as midway between community residents and patients in hospital. S. pneumoniae is responsible for 40 to 50 percent of community-acquired pneumonia in the elderly. H. influenzae, primarily nontypable strains, is the second most common etiology, isolated from 13 to 20 percent of geriatric patients in the community. In similar geriatric patients, other gram-negative bacilli (*Klebsiella, E. coli, Enterobacter, Proteus,* and *Pseudomonas*) have been implicated in 6 to 37 percent of bacterial pneumonias of defined etiology. S. aureus is responsible for from 2 to 10 percent of cases in the same age group. Thus, in the elderly, the two leading bacterial causes of community-acquired pneumonia are S. pneumoniae and H. influenzae as in other adults, but S. pneumoniae is a somewhat less common cause in the older population. Gram-negative bacilli appear to play a somewhat greater relative role in causing community-acquired pneumonia in the elderly than in other adults.

Data concerning the etiologies of pneumonias that develop in the elderly who live in nursing homes are sparse. But, in one study, K. pneumoniae were isolated (blood, sputum, or transtracheal aspirates) from 40 percent of 35 elderly patients in nursing homes and from only 9 percent of 35 similarly aged patients living in the community. In the same comparison, S. pneumoniae was implicated as etiology in 43 percent of the elderly community dwellers and in 26 percent of the nursing-home dwellers. S. aureus was isolated about twice as commonly from the nursing home population as the community-based population. According to this sort of statistical information, in the elderly patient who has acquired pneumonia outside the hospital, S. pneumoniae and H. influenzae should be regarded as the leading etiologic candidates, but gram-negative bacilli (particularly K. pneumoniae) should be kept in mind as possible causative agents—especially in nursing home patients in whom gram-negative bacilli and S. aureus are clearly important.

Nosocomial Pneumonia

Between 150,000 and 200,000 cases of nosocomial pneumonia occur annually in the United States; this is the most common fatal hospital-acquired infection. The strikingly different bacterial etiologies of nosocomial pneumonia from those of community-acquired pneumonia serve to direct the clinician's initial thinking about etiology and therapeutic approach before results of cultures become available.

About 60 percent of hospital-acquired pneumonias are due to aerobic gram-negative bacilli. Of these, most belong to the Enterobacteriaceae (*K. pneumoniae, E. coli, Enterobacter* species, *Proteus,* and *Serratia*). The other gram-negative species involved are primarily *P. aeruginosa* and other nonfermentative bacilli; in respiratory in-

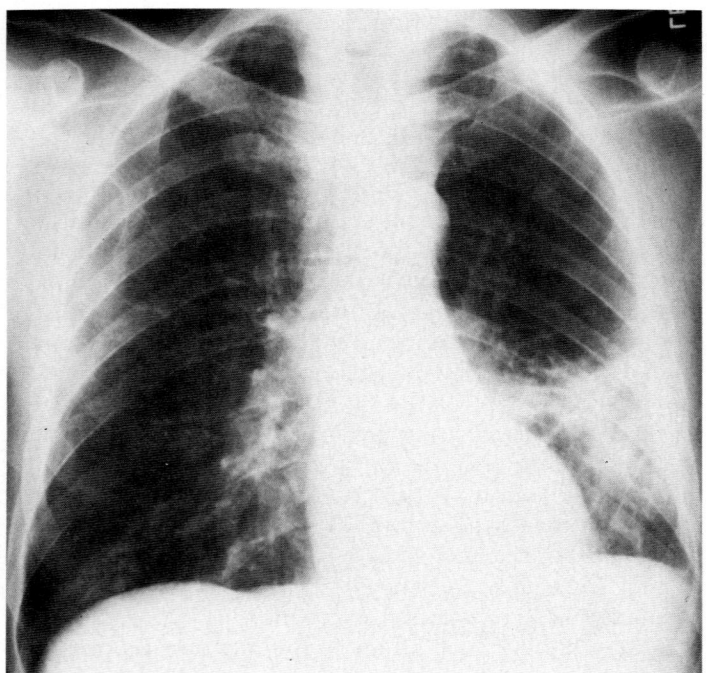

FIGURE 85-8 Actinomyces. Fifty-four-year-old chronic alcoholic male with pyorrheic gums. Admitted with signs of brain tumor. Chest radiograph shows mass in left lower lobe. Computed tomography consistent with brain metastasis. Transthoracic needle aspirate revealed *A. israelii*.

tensive-care units *Acinetobacter* species, *Pseudomonas cepacia*, and *Pseudomonas maltophila* have been implicated in localized outbreaks of nosocomial pneumonia. In one recent study, *P. aeruginosa* was the commonest pathogen isolated from patients with nosocomial pneumonia. *S. aureus* is the cause of 11 to 14 percent of nosocomial pneumonias. In only about 5 percent of patients with hospital-acquired pneumonia is the pneumonia pneumococcal in etiology. Since gram-negative bacilli rapidly colonize the oropharynx of ill hospitalized patients, they are the most common cause of aspiration pneumonias that occur subsequently.

Nosocomial outbreaks of *Legionella* pneumonia have occurred in hospitals secondary to environmental problems related to potable water, air-conditioning systems or water-cooling towers. Although in these circumstances immunocompromised patients have been particularly at risk, patients with alcoholism and chronic obstructive airways disease have also been particularly vulnerable.

In previous years, attention focused on nosocomial pneumonias of bacterial etiology. However, it is now appreciated that hospital-acquired viral pneumonias are also of considerable impact. During major influenza outbreaks, the incidence of nosocomial pneumonias increases and is accompanied by considerable mortality. These pneumonias represent primary influenza viral pneumonia or, more often, bacterial pneumonia complicating influenza.

Statistical information about the etiologies of nosocomial pneumonia does provide some knowledge that is of general predictive value. However, in dealing with the individual patient, more useful information is provided by awareness of the bacterial species that is most often involved in nosocomial pneumonia in the particular hospital and the antimicrobial susceptibilities of sputum isolates from patients in that institution. The hospital epidemiologist or the physicians working in an intensive-care unit often can provide insights into the cause of outbreaks of nosocomial pneumonia either in the hospital or in their specific sector, respectively. With respect to treating a particular patient, examination of sputum (or a tracheal or transtracheal aspirate) after Gram staining is essential as a guide to the selection of initial antimicrobial therapy.

Pneumonia in the Immunocompromised Host

To utilize statistics in assessing the likely etiology of a febrile pneumonitis syndrome in a patient who has an underlying disorder of host defenses, it is helpful to distinguish among several categories of abnormal defense mechanisms. Depending on the underlying defect, the types of pneumonia developing in these settings can differ.

HYPOGAMMAGLOBULINEMIA

Patients who have congenital or acquired deficiencies of the immunoglobulins are particularly susceptible to recurrent pneumonias caused by encapsulated bacterial species, particularly *S. pneumoniae* and *H. influenzae* type B.

GRANULOCYTE DEFICIENCY

This category includes patients who have deficiencies both in granulocyte function and in granulocyte numbers.

Defects in Granulocyte Function
Patients with the hyperimmunoglobulin E syndrome, characterized by chronic eczema, "cold" cutaneous abscesses, and mucocutaneous candidiasis, have a chemotactic defect for polymorphonuclear leukocytes. As a result, they are subject to recurrent skin and sinopulmonary infections. The principal bacteria causing pneumonia in these patients are *S. aureus*, *H. influenzae*, and to a lesser extent, *S. pneumoniae*.

Patients with chronic granulomatous disease (CGD) of childhood suffer from an inherited disorder of oxidative microbicidal activity of polymorphonuclear leukocytes and monocytes. These patients are subject to suppurative lymphadenitis, soft tissue and hepatic abscesses, and sometimes to pneumonia. Pathogens producing infections in this setting are primarily *S. aureus*, Enterobacteriaceae (*K. pneumoniae*, *Serratia*), *Pseudomonas* (often *P. cepacia*), *Nocardia*, *Candida* species, and *Aspergillus* species.

Granulocytopenia
Granulocytopenia (fewer than 500 granulocytes per microliter of blood) is an important risk factor for pulmonary infections, particularly those caused by gram-negative bacilli, *S. aureus*, and fungi such as *Aspergillus* and *Candida* species. The predisposing granulocytopenia usually develops in the course of treating leukemia to induce a remission, during leukemic relapse, aplastic anemia, or cytotoxic drug therapy for neoplastic disease, or in association with organ transplantation. The pulmonary infections that occur in recipients of bone marrow transplants represent a special case because of the combination of profound granulocytopenia, severe combined immunodeficiency, and graft-versus-host disease produced by intense cytotoxic drug or radiation therapy that is used to ablate the bone marrow. As a result, an additional group of infecting agents [cytomegalovirus (CMV) and *P. carinii*] becomes likely on statistical grounds.

Pneumonias that affect granulocytopenic hospitalized patients occur most often via the microaspiration route. Although mixed anaerobic oral commensals may be responsible, gram-negative bacilli (*P. aeruginosa* particularly) are the most frequent etiologies. In about 75 percent

of patients with leukemia who develop gram-negative bacillary pneumonia, the responsible bacterial species has colonized the oropharynx within the preceding 3 days. Bacteremic spread of infection to the lung can also occur from an initiating site of infection in the perineum, intestinal tract, or urinary tract. However, although bacteremia occurs in 30 to 40 percent of patients with gram-negative bacillary pneumonia, the pulmonary infection usually precedes the bacteremia.

CELLULAR IMMUNE DEFICIENCY

The number of immunocompromised patients who have defects primarily in T-cell function and/or numbers has increased markedly in recent years on several accounts: (1) the prolonged survival of patients with neoplastic disease, (2) the increasing number of organ transplantations (and the attendant use of cytotoxic drugs), (3) the increasing number of patients with collagen-vascular disease (that are responsive to drugs such as cyclophosphamide and corticosteroids), and (4) the current annual doubling of the number of patients in the United States with acquired immunodeficiency syndrome (AIDS). These diverse entities share a common clinical picture of fever and a pulmonary infiltrate. The principal immunodeficiency in each of these situations is fundamentally a lack of cell-mediated immunity. However, because the causes of the same clinical picture of fever and a pulmonary infiltrate are so diverse among these entities, it is worthwhile to

TABLE 85-7
Etiology of Syndrome of Fever with Pulmonary Infiltrates in 100 Patients with Neoplastic Disease

Etiology	No. of Patients
Infectious agents (73)	
Conventional bacterial species	26
Viruses	11
Fungi	10
N. asteroides	5
P. carinii	6
M. tuberculosis	1
Mixed infections	14
Noninfectious causes (27)	
Pulmonary emboli	3
Recurrent tumor	8
Radiation pneumonitis	7
Pulmonary edema	1
Drug-induced pneumonitis	5
Leukoagglutinin reaction	2
Pulmonary hemorrhage	1

SOURCE: Data from Rubin and Greene, 1981.

consider each of the groups separately as a basis for approaching diagnosis from a statistical viewpoint.

Pneumonia in Patients with Neoplastic Disease
Although patients with neoplastic diseases are considered as a specific category of patients with deficient cell-mediated immunity for present purposes, the group is far from uniform. Variations in the nature of the neoplastic process (leukemia, lymphoma, carcinoma) and in the duration and type of therapy (cytotoxic drugs, radiation, corticosteroids) may evoke differing patterns of immunosuppression and pulmonary pathology. Until recently, in patients with leukemia and lymphoma, bacterial etiologies have been 2 to 15 times as common as fungal causes of fatal pneumonias. But, in recent years, the percentage of fatal fungal pneumonias appears to be increasing.

The diversity of infectious and noninfectious causes of the febrile pneumonitis syndrome in patients with neoplastic disease is shown in Table 85-7. In patients with neoplastic disease, and in patients who have undergone renal transplantation, important clues to narrow the field of etiologic possibilities are provided by two considerations: (1) the rate of progression of the illness, and (2) the radiologic features of the pulmonary process (see "Radiologic Features of Pneumonia," below). An acute pulmonary process, developing in 24 to 36 h, should suggest either: (1) a bacterial etiology (usual respiratory pathogens, nosocomial gram-negative bacilli, S. aureus, Legionella species), (2) pulmonary emboli, (3) pulmonary edema, (4) pulmonary hemorrhage, or (5) a leukoagglutinin (transfusion) reaction. A *subacute to chronic* process developing over several days to weeks suggests a different set of etiologic considerations: (1) fungal infection (*Aspergillus, Mucor, Cryptococcus, Candida,* etc.), (2) nocardial infection, (3) viral infection (common respiratory viruses causing pneumonia in healthy individuals, CMV, varicella-zoster virus, herpes simplex virus, and adenoviruses), (4) protozoal infection (strongyloidiasis), (5) mycobacterial infection (principally *Mycobacterium tuberculosis* but also atypical mycobacteria), (6) radiation pneumonitis, (7) drug-induced pulmonary toxicity or hypersensitivity reaction, or (8) involvement of the lungs by tumor or leukemia.

Pneumonia in Transplant Recipients
Although the infecting agents that cause pneumonia in transplant recipients are common to the various types of organ transplantation, certain opportunistic infections are more common for certain organs (e.g., bone marrow) than for others (e.g., kidney).

Another clue to the etiology of pneumonia in transplant recipients is the time after transplantation at which the pulmonary process develops. In the renal transplant recipient, pulmonary infections during the first month after organ transfer are almost always due to conventional

bacterial pathogens rather than to fungal, viral, or protozoal agents. Should an opportunistic infection occur during this interval, environmental contamination in the transplant unit becomes a serious consideration. Usually the problem is one of infection with *Legionella* spread via potable water or airflow systems or the airborne spread of *Aspergillus* species, commonly associated with construction and renovation. A single instance of either of these types of infection in the early posttransplant period should prompt an immediate epidemiologic investigation to forestall a nosocomial outbreak in this highly vulnerable population.

In the 1 to 6 months after renal transplantation, serious opportunistic infections pose the greatest risk because of the cumulative effects of continuing immunosuppression, particularly if pulses of antirejection therapy have been administered. Viral pneumonias due to CMV, adenovirus, and herpes simplex can occur during this period. CMV infection, symptomatic and asymptomatic, is particularly noteworthy in transplant recipients because of its frequency and the possible additional element of immunosuppression it may add, per se. From 40 to 90 percent of renal transplant recipients and most cardiac transplant recipients develop evidence of CMV infection after transplantation. In the series reported by Rubin and Greene, CMV was the cause of 15 percent of 54 episodes of pulmonary disease that followed renal transplantation. The clin-

ical and radiographic picture is that of an interstitial pneumonia. The incidence of CMV infection (Fig. 85-9) in bone marrow transplantation (BMT) is considerably greater: about 50 percent of allogeneic BMT patients develop interstitial pneumonitis, and CMV is the etiology in about half of these cases; in the other half, the etiology is unclear.

During the same vulnerable period (1 to 6 months after transplantation) *Aspergillus* and *Nocardia* infections of the lung occur, usually complicating a preceding bacterial pneumonitis or CMV infection. Reactivation of latent pulmonary infection with *Coccidioides immitis, Blastomyces dermatitidis,* and *Histoplasma capsulatum* may also occur during this period of cumulative immunosuppressive effects. In this circumstance, a careful epidemiologic history is of paramount importance.

P. carinii pneumonia occurs during the same 1- to 6-month period of immunosuppression as that in which other opportunistic pulmonary infections usually become manifest. There appears to be a particularly close association between CMV and *Pneumocystis* infections. Fine pulmonary crackles, characteristic of an interstitial process, are common in *Pneumocystis* pneumonia. In one study involving renal transplant recipients, *P. carinii* was identified as the etiology of only 2 percent of pneumonias. Many renal transplant programs now utilize prophylactic trimethoprim-sulfamethoxazole to prevent pyelonephritis in the renal graft and also in patients with symptomatic CMV infection to prevent *Pneumocystis* infection. This practice may further decrease the incidence of *Pneumocystis* infection in the renal transplant population.

Pulmonary infections with *Cryptococcus neoformans* tend to occur later in the posttransplant period (after 4 to 6 months). They may take the form of pneumonitis or miliary disease that may present simultaneously with cryptococcal meningitis.

Pneumonia in Patients with Acquired Immunodeficiency Syndrome

The relative frequencies of the various causes of pulmonary infiltrates in patients with AIDS show prominent differences from those observed in organ transplant recipients and patients with neoplastic disease (Table 85-8): *P. carinii* is clearly the preeminent cause of pneumonia in this setting. Pyogenic bacteria are less common causes of pneumonia in patients with AIDS than in transplant recipients and in patients with hematologic and other malignancies. Pulmonary infections with *Nocardia* and *Aspergillus* are remarkably infrequent among pulmonary infections in patients with AIDS (Table 85-8). About 30 percent of patients with AIDS have two or more coexisting pulmonary infections.

Noninfectious processes must also be considered as possible causes of pulmonary infiltrates in febrile patients with AIDS. Unexplained interstitial pneumonias occur.

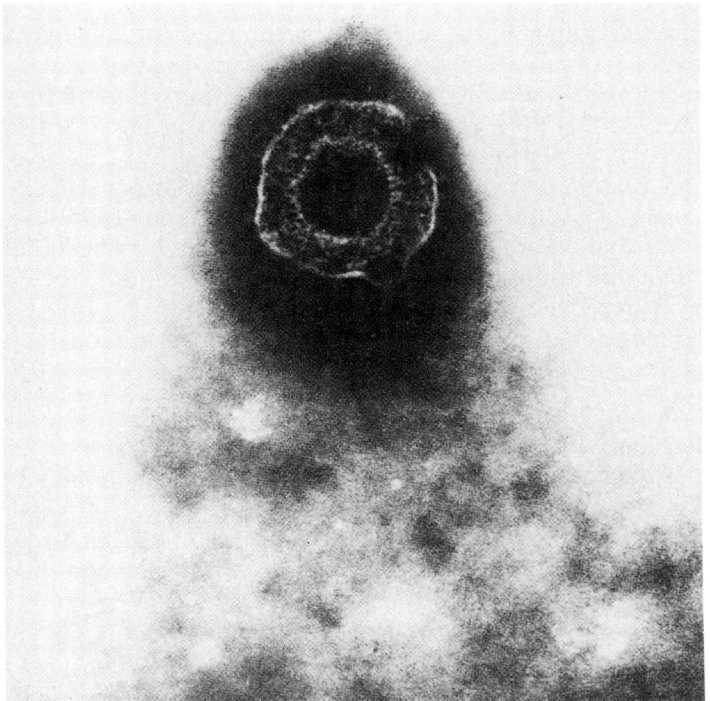

FIGURE 85-9 *Electron micrograph of cytomegalovirus. (Courtesy of Dr. S. Stagno and of the Research Resources Information Center, National Institutes of Health.)*

TABLE 85-8
Etiology of 778 Pulmonary Infections in Patients with AIDS

Infectious Agent	Percent
P. carinii	57
M. avium-intracellulare	14
Cytomegalovirus	13
M. tuberculosis	6
Pyogenic bacteria	3
Legionella species	3
Cryptococcus	2
Other fungi (*Candida, Histoplasma, Aspergillus*)	1
Herpes simplex	0.4
Nocardia	0.1
Toxoplasma	0.1
Miscellaneous other infectious agents	0.4
	100.0

SOURCE: Compilation of data from Murray et al., 1984, and Talavera and Mildvan, 1986.

Lymphocytic interstitial pneumonias of unknown etiology appear to be common in children with AIDS but rare in adults. Antecedent infection with Epstein-Barr virus (EBV) was implicated as the etiology of lymphocytic interstitial pneumonia (LIP) in one child with AIDS. The detection by in situ hybridization of human immunodeficiency virus (HIV) RNA in a relatively high frequency (0.1 percent) of cells in the lung of an infant with AIDS and LIP implicates this virus itself in LIP.

About 8 percent of patients with AIDS and pulmonary processes have Kaposi's sarcoma in the lung.

In addition to the statistical evidence that shows a predominant role for *P. carinii*, certain clinical clues as to the nature of the pulmonary process can be provided by epidemiologic considerations and physical findings. For example, tuberculosis is endemic in Haiti. Among Haitians with AIDS, tuberculosis is an important possible cause of a pulmonary infiltrate. The presence of extensive chorioretinitis (with the "melted cheese and catsup" appearance of the fundus) suggests widespread CMV infection that often also involves the lung. The presence of intra-oral and pharyngeal lesions of Kaposi's sarcoma raises the question of pulmonary involvement by the same process.

RADIOGRAPHIC FEATURES OF PNEUMONIA

The radiographic features of a pneumonia do not provide a specific etiologic diagnosis. This can come only from additional microbiologic information. However, the radiographic pattern combined with clinical and epidemiologic information can narrow the diagnostic considerations while microbiologic data are being obtained; they also aid in the selection of initial antimicrobial therapy. Several radiographic patterns can be helpful in categorizing certain infectious and noninfectious etiologies: (1) airspace or alveolar pneumonia, (2) broncho- or lobular pneumonia, (3) interstitial pneumonia, and (4) nodular infiltrates. Although the chest radiographs of a particular patient may not fit neatly into one or another of these categories, identification of a predominant pattern can be helpful in directing attention to certain etiologies.

Alveolar Pneumonia

This form of consolidation occurs when certain organisms, notably *S. pneumoniae*, induce inflammatory edema in peripheral alveoli. When the extent of the consolidation involves an entire lobe, this is the classic "lobar pneumonia." But, more often, the process is not that extensive, although the pathogenesis is the same. An air bronchogram is characteristic. Loss of volume is absent or minimal during the acute stage of consolidation, but some atelectasis may develop owing to obstruction of bronchi by exudate during resolution of the process.

K. pneumoniae is another bacterial cause of community-acquired pneumonia which, like pneumococcal pneumonia, shows homogeneous parenchymal consolidation containing air bronchograms. Although *K. pneumoniae* pneumonia classically involves the right upper lobe and produces a dense homogeneous lobar consolidation with bulging of the fissure (Fig. 85-10A), these features are not pathognomonic and cannot be relied on for diagnosis without supporting bacteriologic data. The propensity for *K. pneumoniae* to produce tissue destruction and abscess formation (Fig. 85-10B) may, in fact, result in a shrunken, rather than an expanded, lobe. Pneumococcal pneumonia may also cause bulging of the fissure, albeit less commonly and less prominently. Extensive alveolar consolidation may occur with a variety of other bacterial causes of pneumonia including mixed anaerobes of aspiration pneumonia and a variety of gram-negative bacilli involved in nosocomial pneumonias (Fig. 85-11).

Occasionally, an unusual configuration of airspace consolidation, "spherical pneumonia," occurs, particularly in children, with pneumococcal or *H. influenzae* pneumonias. It has also been reported with Q fever.

In the setting of the compromised host, alveolar consolidation on the chest radiograph suggests a variety of etiologies. Among the infectious causes, bacterial agents are a major consideration. If the consolidation is lobar or multilobar, *L. pneumophila* is an important possibility to consider. Other likely infectious agents are fungi (e.g., *Aspergillus*), *Nocardia*, and *M. tuberculosis*. Less often, viruses (e.g., CMV) elicit a predominantly alveolar pattern. Bilateral diffuse involvement with an airspace pattern resembling pulmonary edema is not uncommonly a feature of *P. carinii* pneumonia.

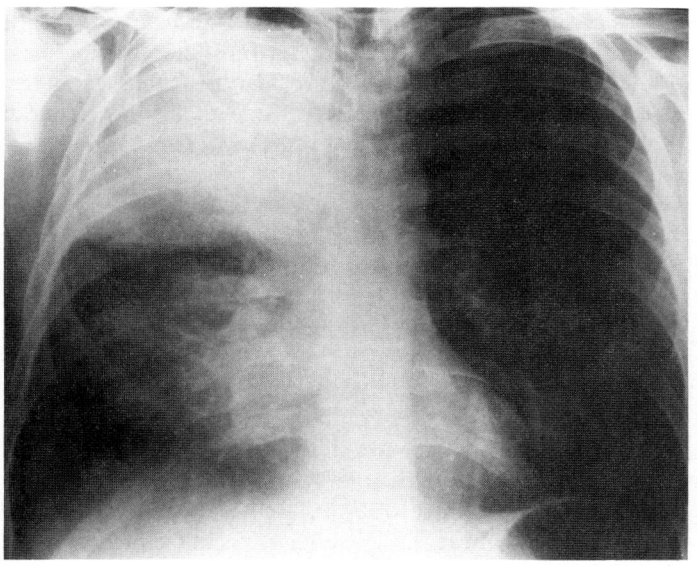

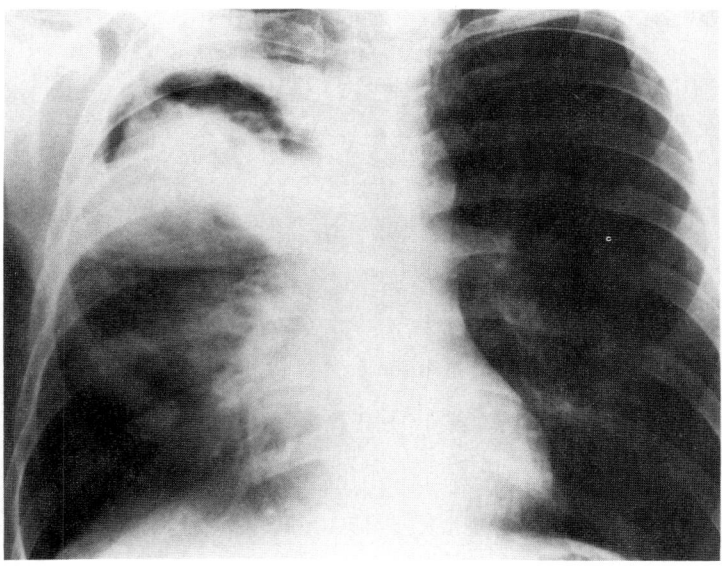

A   *B*

FIGURE 85-10   *A.* Dense lobar consolidation involving right upper lobe in an alcoholic patient with *Klebsiella pneumoniae* pneumonia. The minor fissure is bulging downward. There is also involvement of the right middle lobe. *(Courtesy of Dr. R. Greene.)*   *B.* Same patient as *(A)* but 7 days later. Progression of *K. pneumoniae* pneumonia despite antibiotic therapy to become a necrotic process with formation of multiple abscesses. *(Courtesy of Dr. R. Greene.)*

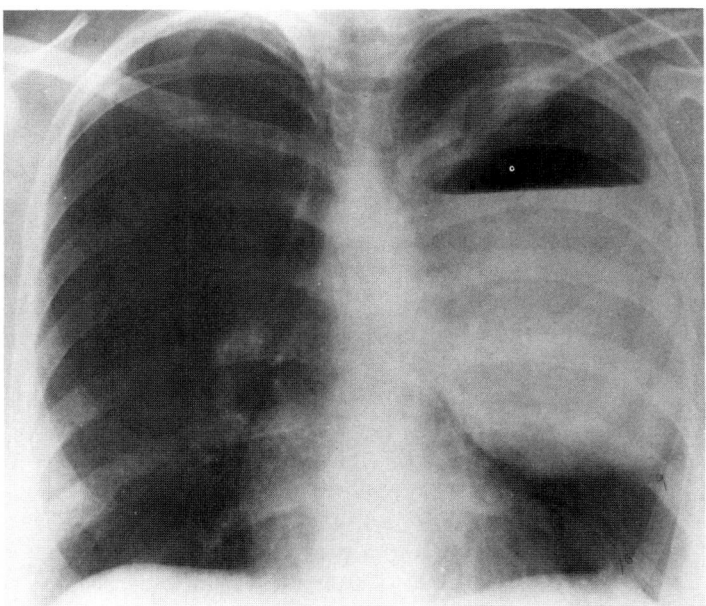

FIGURE 85-11   Left upper lobe pneumonia in a 17-year-old female due to *S. aureus* that has progressed to formation of a huge lung abscess. Note air-fluid level. *(Courtesy of Dr. R. Greene.)*

Bronchopneumonia

In bronchopneumonia the focus of infection and the inflammatory response is in the bronchi and surrounding parenchyma. Consolidation is segmental in distribution, and involvement is patchy; segmental involvement may become confluent to produce a more homogeneous pattern. Bronchopneumonic patterns are commonly observed in pulmonary infections due to *S. aureus* or nonencapsulated *H. influenzae*. With *S. aureus* infections, macro- and microabscess formation may occur rapidly. Also, pneumatoceles occur during the first week of lung involvement in about half the children with *S. aureus* pneumonia. These cystic spaces are believed to be the consequence of a check valve opening between a peribronchial abscess and an adjacent bronchus.

A bronchopneumonic pattern of consolidation is commonly observed when pneumonia is engrafted on underlying bronchiectasis or chronic bronchitis. In such predisposing circumstances, *S. pneumoniae* infection may produce a bronchopneumonic pattern rather than its usual lobar consolidation. In the presence of underlying emphysema, the radiographic pattern of pneumococcal pneumonia may also be altered from its usual homogeneous pattern to one that contains multiple radiolucencies (representing unconsolidated emphysematous areas) that may be misinterpreted for abscesses.

Segmental bronchopneumonia is the radiographic picture in psittacosis pneumonia due to *Chlamydia psittaci* var TWAR and in many viral pneumonias (Fig. 85-12). Any of the bacterial species that cause nosocomial pneumonia can produce a radiographic pattern of bronchopneumonic consolidation.

Interstitial Pneumonia (Peribronchovascular Infiltrate)

A reticular or reticulonodular pattern of infiltration is the radiographic representation of interstitial inflammation,

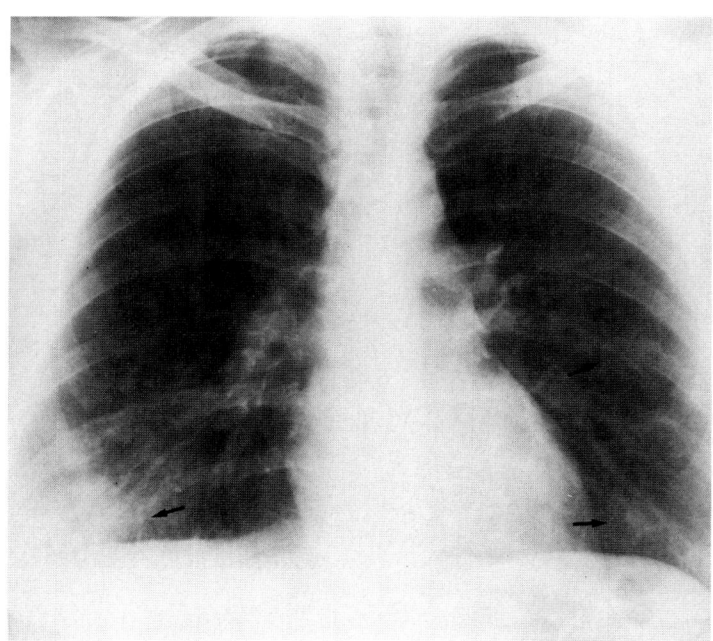

FIGURE 85-12 Multifocal (arrows) pneumonia in a patchy bronchopneumonic pattern in a 36-year-old housewife. Clinical course and laboratory findings were consistent with a viral etiology, but viral isolation was not attempted.

i.e., a peribronchovascular infiltrate. In otherwise healthy individuals, *M. pneumoniae* is high on the list of community-acquired causes of a radiographic pattern of interstitial pneumonia. In some instances, interstitial infiltration progresses to produce patchy consolidation of airspaces, most often in the lower lobes. Pneumonias due to respiratory viruses sometimes have an interstitial pattern that progresses to patchy segmental consolidation or to diffuse airspace disease that resembles pulmonary edema. A variety of noninfectious causes of interstitial lung disease (e.g., hypersensitivity lung disease, collagen-vascular disease, or sarcoidosis) may also produce a reticular pattern on the chest radiograph.

In immunocompromised patients, particularly in those with AIDS, the infectious causes of interstitial pneumonia are broadened to include early *P. carinii* pneumonia and additional opportunistic viral agents (CMV, varicella-zoster, herpes simplex, and probably EBV and possibly HIV). Noninfectious causes of a reticular pattern on chest radiography in an immunocompromised host include drug-induced (bleomycin, methotrexate, etc.) pneumonitis, early radiation pneumonitis, and pulmonary edema.

Nodular Infiltrates

Nodular infiltrates are considered here as large (>1 cm^2 on the chest radiograph), well-defined, rounded focal lesions. Such a lesion may represent an aspirational lung abscess (without telltale air-fluid level), a fungal or tuberculous granuloma, or a lesion of pulmonary nocardiosis. Multiple nodular infiltrates may also represent the necrotic lesions that develop in the lung secondary to the septic vasculitis produced by *P. aeruginosa* bacteremia or the consequences of fungemic spread of candidal infection from an infected intravascular catheter. Infected nodular pulmonary lesions are sometimes caused by septic pulmonary infarcts produced by infected emboli that originate from right-sided bacterial endocarditis, septic thrombophlebitis of pelvic veins, or septic jugular vein phlebitis. On rare occasions, similar nodular lesions are produced by necrotic (but not infected) pulmonary infarctions; primary or metastatic neoplastic lesions may have a similar appearance. Nodular lesions that undergo rapid necrosis with cavity formation can be a feature of Wegener's granulomatosis.

In the immunocompromised patient, nodular infiltrates may be due to bacteremic or fungemic spread of infection, most often as a nosocomial infection caused by an infected intravenous catheter. In this type of patient, nodular lesions should bring to mind the possibilities of pulmonary nocardial infection, aspergillosis, or other fungal infections. Tuberculous granulomas in the lungs may develop or enlarge in the immunosuppressed patient. Metastatic neoplasm or lymphoma sometimes presents a similar radiologic picture.

MILIARY PULMONARY DISEASE

Disseminated miliary lesions of infectious nature suggest miliary tuberculosis, histoplasmosis, or blastomycosis in either the normal or immunosuppressed host (Fig. 85-13). In the immunosuppressed patient, a miliary pattern may also be seen in disseminated cryptococcal infection.

SMALL NODULAR INFILTRATES

Multiple small nodules, larger than miliary lesions but smaller than the gross nodular lesions described above, raise the possibility, in the immunocompromised host, of varicella-zoster or CMV infection of the lung.

NONINVASIVE DIAGNOSTIC STUDIES

Noninvasive studies can provide information indicating the specific microbial cause of a pulmonary infection or can narrow the field of likely etiologic agents.

Direct Examination of the Sputum

This subject is considered in some detail in Chapter 30. Here, certain aspects are reviewed as they relate to the approach to the patient.

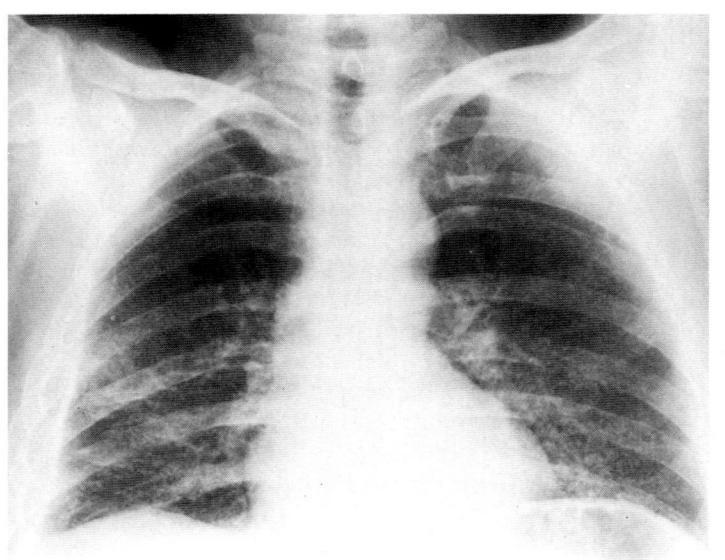
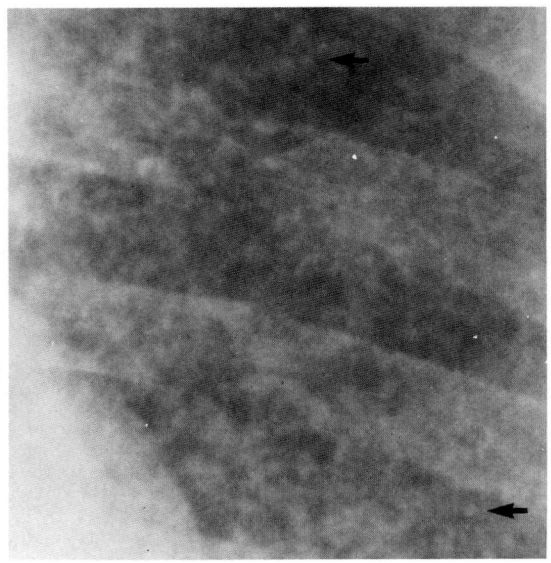

A

B

FIGURE 85-13 Miliary tuberculosis in a 45-year-old immigrant from Portugal with old calcified tuberculous empyema on the right. *A.* Fine nodularity present in both lungs. *B.* Arrows point to individual miliary lesions which are more readily visible with added magnification. *(Courtesy of Dr. R. Greene.)*

CYTOLOGIC EXAMINATION

Examination of Gram-stained sputum smears can be of major value in pinpointing a bacterial etiology of pneumonia and guiding initial therapy. The most valuable bacteriologic information from sputum examination is that in which the results from stained smears and cultures are mutually confirmatory. The quality of a sample of expectorated or induced sputum submitted for examination is the prime determinant of the results that can be expected. Culture of sputum that consists principally of saliva is valueless. What are sought are lower respiratory secretions produced by a cough, not nasopharyngeal secretions. Cytologic examination provides an evaluation of the quality of the sample and its suitability for culture and interpretation of a Gram-stained smear made from it. Scanning of Gram-stained smears or application of specific quantitative criteria is helpful in selecting meaningful specimens for bacteriologic evaluation on smear and in culture. Squamous epithelial cells (normally exfoliated from the oropharynx) when present in numbers over 25 per low-power (×100) magnification field (Fig. 85-14) indicate that the specimen is unsatisfactory; culture of such a specimen correlates poorly with results from culture of a transtracheal aspirate. The presence of numerous polymorphonuclear neutrophils on Gram-stained smear (10 to 25 or more per low-power microscopic field) in the absence of an excessive number of squamous cells (see above) is indicative of a good specimen for bacteriologic evaluation.

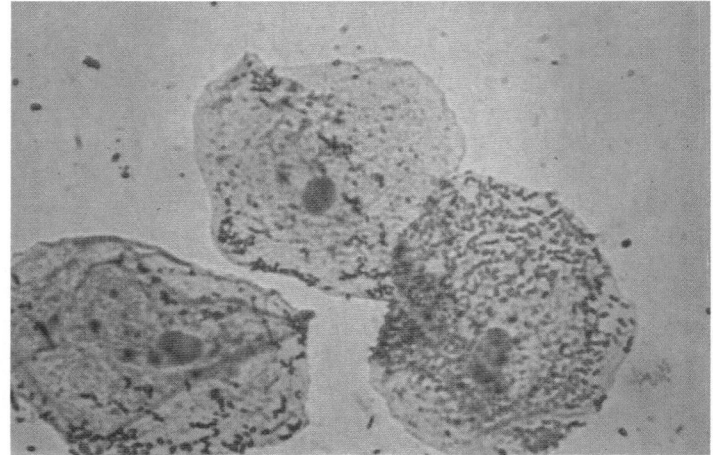

FIGURE 85-14 Three large oropharyngeal epithelial cells from a specimen of "sputum" that is inadequate for Gram-stain analysis and culture because of its origin in the upper respiratory tract. Note the large number of organisms agglutinated on the surface of the squamous epithelial cells. ×400.

EXAMINATION OF GRAM-STAINED SMEARS FOR BACTERIA

The oil immersion fields examined, and the immediately adjacent fields, should not contain any squamous cells; each should also contain at least three or four neutrophils or bronchoalveolar lining cells. The presence of squamous cells not only indicates that the specimen is derived from the upper respiratory tract but may be confusing to the uninitiated because of the large number of bacteria, often gram-positive diplococci, which might be mistaken for S. pneumoniae, adherent to the surface of these cells.

A variety of bacterial respiratory tract pathogens have rather characteristic morphologies and strongly suggest an etiologic role when present in considerable numbers in a suitable specimen of sputum (or in a transtracheal aspirate) that contains the proper numbers of inflammatory cells. Such organisms include S. pneumoniae (gram-positive, oval or lancet-shaped diplococci), H. influenzae (small, pleomorphic gram-negative bacilli), Branhamella catarrhalis (gram-negative, biscuit-shaped diplococci), or the similar appearing Neisseria meningitis, enteric gram-negative bacilli (not distinguishable from one another with respect to species except for large encapsulated rods that are suggestive of Klebsiella), and S. aureus (large gram-positive cocci in small groups or clusters) (Fig. 85-15). Since normal oral flora includes a variety of streptococcal species that are morphologically somewhat similar to S. pneumoniae, sputum smears may be misinterpreted. Thus, a definite predominance of gram-positive diplococci in multiple appropriate oil immersion fields needs to be observed to implicate S. pneumoniae. A quantitative aspect to the evaluation has been suggested: ≥10 gram-positive lancet-shaped diplococci per oil immersion field predicts the isolation of S. pneumoniae from sputum cultures in approximately 90 percent of patients.

Gram-stained smears can be helpful not only in the etiologic diagnosis of community-acquired bacterial pneumonia due to the usual respiratory pathogens, but also in supporting a diagnosis of atypical pneumonia when sputum examinations repeatedly show neither neutrophils nor bacteria. Uncommon bacterial species may be implicated in a pulmonary infection on the basis of unusual morphology on Gram-stained smear: irregularly staining, beaded, delicate gram-positive branching filaments suggest either Nocardia or Actinomyces.

Several organisms, uncommon causes of pulmonary infection, have morphologic characteristics that may mimic other more common respiratory pathogens. Pasteurella multocida and Acinetobacter species, both small

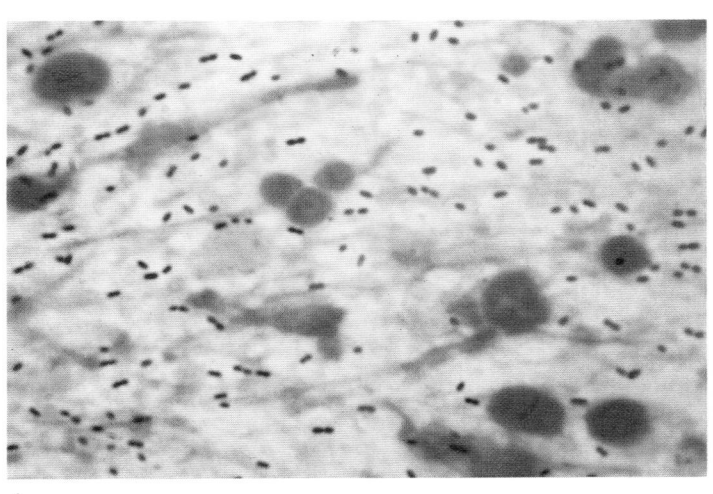

A

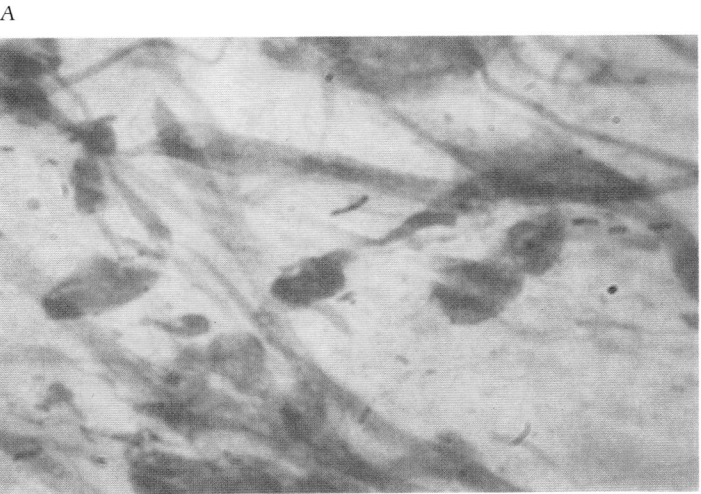

C

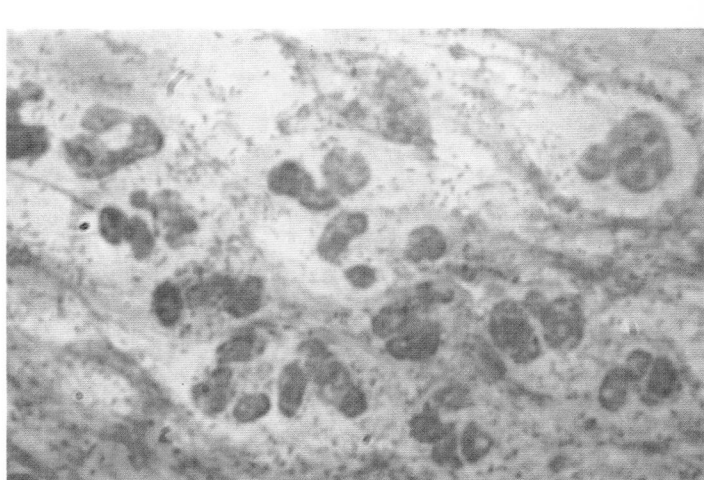

B

FIGURE 85-15 A. Gram-stained smear of sputum from patient with pneumococcal lobar pneumonia. ×1000. In this field there are numerous gram-positive lancet-shaped diplococci and polymorphonuclear leukocytes. B. Gram-stained smear of sputum from patient with bronchopneumonia superimposed on chronic bronchitis. This field (×1000) is teeming with gram-negative coccobacilli. Many polymorphonuclear leukocytes are present. H. influenzae was isolated from sputum as predominant organism. C. Gram-stained smear of sputum from patient with lobar pneumonia due to K. pneumoniae. In this field (×1000) there are moderate numbers of polymorphonuclear leukocytes and large, thick gram-negative bacilli. (A to C Courtesy of H. Provine.)

gram-negative coccobacilli, have each been mistaken in sputum of patients with pulmonary infections for either *H. influenzae* or *B. catarrhalis,* or for a mixture of the two.

Sputum or pleural fluid with foul odor provides evidence of involvement of anaerobic organisms in infective processes such as lung abscess, aspiration pneumonia, empyema or, occasionally, bronchiectasis. In these settings, the findings on Gram-stained smear may corroborate the preliminary diagnosis. Organisms of the *B. melaninogenicus-asaccharolyticus* group are small, gram-negative coccobacilli. *Fusobacterium nucleatum* is a long, tapering pale-staining gram-negative bacillus with irregularly staining gram-positive internal granules. Purulent secretions or pus from such anaerobic infections contain numerous neutrophils and usually a mixture of bacterial species, including anaerobic and microaerophilic streptococci on stained smear.

EXAMINATION OF ZIEHL-NEELSEN SMEARS FOR MYCOBACTERIA

Although the number of new cases of tuberculosis reported annually has been decreasing for the past several decades, this decline appears to have leveled off the past year or two. This plateau appears to be primarily the result of the increased number of individuals in particularly high risk groups, especially immigrants from Southeast Asia and Haiti and individuals with AIDS. Pulmonary tuberculosis in these settings may take the form of chronic cavitary tuberculosis or forms more likely to suggest pyogenic or atypical pneumonia, i.e., progressive primary tuberculosis or tuberculous pneumonia. Acid-fast smears of sputum can provide the very first evidence of this disease. Mycobacteria are seen on smear of about 50 percent of specimens that subsequently prove to contain *M. tuberculosis.* Atypical mycobacteria may be demonstrated on sputum smears of patients, usually older individuals with slowly progressive pulmonary disease. In patients with AIDS, disseminated *Mycobacterium avium-intracellulare* infection is usually diagnosed by isolating the organism from blood culture or by histopathologic diagnosis on biopsy. However, the organism can be demonstrated on acid-fast smears and culture of respiratory secretions even though there may be little radiographic evidence of pulmonary infection directly attributable to its presence.

Modified Ziehl-Neelsen stained smears are helpful in detecting *Nocardia.*

FUNGAL WET MOUNTS (KOH PREPARATIONS)

Fungal wet mounts are employed when epidemiologic considerations suggest community-acquired pulmonary mycoses (coccidioidomycosis and blastomycosis particularly). It should be a routine part of evaluation of respiratory secretions and lung biopsy materials from immunocompromised patients where additional fungal pathogens, e.g., *Aspergillus* or *Mucor,* can be involved.

DIRECT IMMUNOFLUORESCENT MICROSCOPY

The principal current use of the direct fluorescent antibody (DFA) technique is in the diagnosis, using sputum, of Legionnaires' disease or pneumonia due to *L. micdadei.* A monoclonal antibody to an antigen common to the different *L. pneumophila* serogroups is commercially available for use with DFA techniques in diagnosis. A fluorescent antibody against *L. micdadei* has been available from the Centers for Disease Control for similar use in diagnosis. Since patients with Legionnaires' disease often produce little sputum, this approach has limited use. Although the specificity of this test is high (over 90 percent), the sensitivity is low. In patients raising a satisfactory expectorated sputum, DFA can provide the diagnosis. In patients who raise little if any sputum, DFA may allow rapid diagnosis on transtracheal aspirates, needle lung aspirates, specimens from fiberoptic bronchoscopy, or lung biopsy.

GIEMSA AND OTHER SPECIAL STAINED SMEARS FOR DIAGNOSIS OF *PNEUMOCYSTIS* INFECTION

Since *Pneumocystis carinii* pneumonia is an alveolar process, examination of routinely collected sputum for *P. carinii* is generally not regarded as rewarding in immunosuppressed patients with neoplastic disease or transplant recipients. In these patients, fiberoptic bronchoscopy and transbronchial biopsy combined with bronchoalveolar lavage provide the highest diagnostic yield (see below). However, in patients with AIDS, sputum examination for *P. carinii* may be more helpful. In a study of 20 patients with *Pneumocystis* pneumonia at an institution where there was considerable experience in diagnosing AIDS and *P. carinii* pneumonia, microscopy of induced sputum (prepared by cytocentrifugation and stained with Grocott's methenamine silver stain) revealed *P. carinii* in 55 percent. Comparative percentages in the same patients for bronchial washings, bronchial brushings, and transbronchial lung biopsy were about 80 percent, 55 percent, and 90 percent, respectively.

SPECIAL MICROSCOPIC EXAMINATIONS

Occasionally, in the setting of an apparent pulmonary inflammation with features atypical for infection, microscopic examinations using stains other than the Gram stain may be indicated. For example, Wright-stained smears may show the presence of eosinophils in allergic pulmonary aspergillosis or other causes of pulmonary infiltrates that are accompanied by eosinophilia. Cytologic examination of exfoliated sputum using Papanicolaou's stain may reveal a pulmonary neoplasm. Birefringent calcium oxalate crystals (needlelike in rosettes or arranged like sheaves of wheat) in sputum cytologic specimens have been reported as suggesting pulmonary infection with *Aspergillus* (aspergilloma; occasionally, invasive

aspergillosis), a fungus that excretes oxalic acid as a metabolic product.

In the intubated or tracheotomized patient whose tracheobronchial secretions commonly contain neutrophils and often some bacteria on Gram-stained smears, it may be difficult at times to distinguish between colonization and nosocomial pneumonia. The presence on light microscopy ($\times 400$) of characteristic elastin fibers with split ends (in a drop of tracheal aspirate to which a drop of 40% KOH has been added), in the appropriate clinical setting, is a strong indicator of a necrotizing pulmonary infection.

Intense bacteremias sometimes accompany pulmonary infections, and the etiologic agent may be demonstrable on stained smears of the buffy coat of centrifuged blood: pneumococci have been identified in Gram-stained or Wright-Giemsa stained smears of buffy coats of splenectomized patients; occasionally, *M. avium-intracellulare* have been found intracellularly in acid-fast stains of buffy coats from patients with AIDS.

Additional special microscopic examinations may be indicated in immunocompromised patients who have patchy pulmonary infiltrates on the chest radiograph. For example, the presence of the hyperinfection syndrome of strongyloidiasis (often accompanied by *E. coli* bacteremia) can be established by finding filariform larvae in the sputum and in the stool after the latter is suitably prepared by concentration techniques. Although eosinophilia is often present in patients with strongyloidiasis, it may be absent in the hyperinfection syndrome.

SPUTUM CULTURES

In most patients with the common types of community-acquired and nosocomial bacterial pneumonia, the etiologic diagnosis can be made based on the combined results of a Gram-stained smear of sputum and of properly culturing a suitable exudative portion of a freshly obtained sputum specimen. The criteria for a proper sample of sputum have been noted above (cytologic examination of sputum). Culture entails streak dilution on blood agar and McConkey media. Reliance on "routine" sputum specimens of doubtful quality, collected by paramedical personnel and automatically cultured (often after prolonged transit times to the laboratory) without screening for suitability, is responsible for the obsolete conclusion that sputum cultures are of limited value in the diagnosis of pneumococcal pneumonia. Before strict attention began to be paid to the quality of sputum specimens, only about half of the patients with bacteremic pneumococcal pneumonia had positive sputum cultures. However, more recently, a comparative study of cultures of expectorated sputum, of sputum contained at bronchoscopy, and of sputum obtained by transtracheal aspiration, showed that in 16 patients with acute bacterial pneumonia, the pneumonia was due to *S. pneumoniae* in 13 and that in these 13 patients, each of the three types of specimens obtained from each patient yielded almost pure cultures of *S. pneumoniae* (on the third and fourth quadrants of dilution-streaked blood agar plates).

Expectorated sputum should not be cultured anaerobically, since contamination with oral anaerobes is inevitable and the results will be uninterpretable. Because patients with Legionnaires' disease often raise little if any sputum suitable for culture, most attempts to isolate *Legionella* resort to specimens obtained either by transtracheal aspiration, fiberoptic bronchoscopy, or lung biopsy or at thoracentesis. Cultures of such materials are plated on buffered charcoal-yeast extract agar. Occasionally, *Legionella* species can be isolated from sputum by using a semiselective medium that contains cefamandole, polymyxin B, anisomycin, an organic buffer, and α-ketoglutarate.

Cultures for myobacteria are undertaken when clinical circumstances raise the possibility of pulmonary infections due to *M. tuberculosis* or atypical mycobacteria. Similarly, cultures of sputum for primary invasive mycotic agents, e.g., *H. capsulatum*, *B. dermatitidis*, and *C. immitis*, are dictated by clinical and epidemiologic circumstances. In immunosuppressed patients, cultures of sputum are also directed toward a variety of opportunistic fungi, including *Cryptococcus neoformans*, *Aspergillus* species, and Mucoraceae.

Most hospitals do not have facilities for isolating viruses by tissue culture. This lack poses little problem in dealing with most community-acquired viral pneumonias for which viral isolation is not necessary and the cost is prohibitive. However, viral isolation from throat washings is warranted in certain circumstances, e.g., to prove the presence of an outbreak of influenza, to establish that an outbreak among young children is due to respiratory syncytial virus, and to identify a specific viral agent, such as an adenovirus, as the cause of a serious pneumonia that is not responding to antibacterial therapy. In immunosuppressed patients with pneumonia, a variety of opportunistic viral infections (CMV, varicella-zoster virus, herpes simplex) are diagnostic considerations. Because CMV and herpes simplex are frequently present in the oral secretions of immunosuppressed patients, isolation of these viruses is apt to be meaningful only if the materials used for the isolation procedure were obtained either by transtracheal aspiration, lung biopsy, or bronchoalveolar lavage.

BLOOD CULTURES

Blood cultures should always be performed in patients with suspected bacterial pneumonia. Bacteremia occurs in approximately 30 percent of patients with pneumococcal pneumonia. Demonstration of bacteremia in other patients with pneumonia may indicate that the pulmonary

infection is secondary to bacteremia originating from a focus of infection elsewhere, e.g., acute right-sided *S. aureus* endocarditis or *P. aeruginosa* infection of thermal burns. In patients with AIDS and disseminated *M. avium-intracellulare* infection, blood cultures are almost always positive. The lysis centrifugation technique permits ready and rapid isolation of the mycobacterium and quantifies the intensity of the bacteremia.

BACTERIAL ANTIGEN DETECTION IN SPUTUM AND URINE

The quellung reaction was extensively used in the preantibiotic era to identify *S. pneumoniae* in sputum. It entails the use of light microscopy to detect capsular swelling after pneumococcal antiserum is added to a loopful of sputum. The occurrence of the quellung reaction was shown to correlate closely with the presence of *S. pneumoniae* in sputum culture, i.e., in about 90 percent of the patients. In recent years, this procedure has been reserved primarily for the identification of pneumococci in the cerebrospinal fluid of patients with meningitis.

Currently, this approach has been superseded by the use of latex particles coated with polyvalent pneumococcal antibodies. Although pneumococcal antigen has been detected by this approach in the sputum of 80 to 90 percent of patients with pneumococcal pneumonia in whom it has been tried, only a small number of patients have as yet been studied. Pneumococcal antigen can also be detected in sputum by counterimmunoelectrophoresis, but this technique seems to be slightly less sensitive and technically more difficult.

False positives occur with the various methods of antigen detection. For example, antigen is often detected in sputum in patients with chronic bronchitis even though they do not have pneumonia. The diagnostic value of antigen detection is still limited. However, it is not far-fetched to anticipate that antigen detection coupled with semiquantitative microscopically directed culture will prove to be the most valuable approach to diagnosis of community-acquired bacterial pneumonia.

Enzyme-linked immunosorbent assay (ELISA) for *Legionella* antigenuria is both sensitive and specific in the diagnosis of Legionnaires' disease.

RAPID VIRAL DIAGNOSIS BY ANTIGEN DETECTION

The need for methods that can rapidly identify viruses stems from the recent introduction of effective chemotherapy for several viral agents that cause pulmonary infections and from the long time (3 to 10 days) required for viral isolation and identification by tissue culture. Both radioimmunoassay and ELISA tests have been applied successfully to respiratory secretions for the rapid identification of influenza A and B, parainfluenza, and respiratory syncytial virus antigens. Although this approach is still evolving, it does offer considerable promise for rapid

(within 12 h) diagnosis of infections not only due to community-acquired respiratory viruses but also due to other (opportunistic) viruses that otherwise require lung biopsy for identification.

Serologic Tests

Serologic tests are sometimes of considerable help in establishing the etiologies of a number of pulmonary infections where the causative agents are difficult to isolate. However, this approach, requiring the demonstration of a fourfold or greater rise in titer between acute and convalescent samples, neither enables rapid diagnosis nor provides assistance in initial selection of antimicrobial therapy. Complement-fixation tests are of value in the diagnosis of psittacosis. The indirect immunofluorescent antibody test may provide a retrospective diagnosis of Legionnaires' disease, but the antibody rise occasionally may not be demonstrable for 4 to 6 weeks after the clinical onset. Cold agglutinins develop in about half the patients with *M. pneumoniae* pneumonia, but such antibodies occur in other conditions; complement-fixation testing is the preferred diagnostic procedure.

Serologic tests are also helpful in the diagnosis of invasive infection due to the primary pulmonary mycotic pathogens. Serum IgM precipitins (latex agglutination, immunodiffusion) appear with primary coccidioidomycosis. Abnormally high complement-fixation titers ($\geq 1:32$) are present in most patients who have disseminated infection due to *C. immitis*. A fourfold increase in complement-fixation titer to yeast and to mycelial phases of *H. capsulatum* (or possibly a single titer of $1:64$ or higher), and the presence of H and M precipitin bands, strongly suggest histoplasmosis. Complement-fixation tests for blastomycosis lack sensitivity and specificity: titers of $\geq 1:8$ suggest recent or active disease, particularly if precipitins to the A antigen are also present. Cryptococcal antigenemia is detectable by latex particle agglutination in patients with cryptococcal pneumonia or disseminated cryptococcal infection.

Serologic tests (paired acute and convalescent sera) may be helpful for the retrospective diagnosis of infections due to influenza A and B, respiratory syncytial, adenoviruses, and parainfluenza viruses.

Skin Tests of Delayed Hypersensitivity

The tuberculin skin test is of great importance in the evaluation of a pulmonary infection of unknown etiology. The intermediate (5 tuberculin unit) purified protein derivative (IPPD) test should be used if no information is available about previous testing. A positive test does not distinguish between prior and current infection, but, in individuals who are either less than 35 years old or who are members of high-risk groups (usually immigrant), a positive reaction carries considerable diagnostic weight.

A negative second strength PPD skin test in a patient who is not anergic is strong evidence against a tuberculous etiology of a pulmonary process. However, several caveats are noteworthy: (1) since it may take 4 to 6 weeks for the skin test to become positive, the tuberculin skin test may be initially negative in progressive primary pulmonary tuberculosis, and (2) in the patient who was infected long ago, cutaneous hypersensitivity may wane; in the elderly individual, in whom waning has occurred, repeat testing several weeks later may show a positive result (booster effect), whereas the original IPPD skin test was negative.

Fungal skin tests do not distinguish between current and past infection; indeed, active disease is often accompanied by a negative skin test. The coccidioidin skin test is the best of the available tests, but the diagnosis of coccidioidomycosis is not excluded by a negative test. Blastomycin and histoplasmin skin tests are of little value because of frequent false-negative results and cross reactions. Also, the performance of the histoplasmin skin test may falsely elevate antibody levels to the *H. capsulatum* mycelial antigen.

A negative skin test response to a specific antigen must be interpreted in the light of possible anergy related to underlying conditions such as malnutrition, immunosuppressive and corticosteroid therapy, and AIDS. A battery of control antigens (mumps, *Candida*, *Trichophyton*, streptokinase-streptodornase) serves to detect such anergy.

Gallium Scan

Increased gallium 67 uptake by the lungs can be found in patients with *P. carinii* pneumonia and essentially normal chest radiographs. With the greater awareness of the early changes of *P. carinii* pneumonia on the radiographs of patients with AIDS, this radionuclide study is of less value. It can only indicate a pulmonary inflammatory process but cannot define the specific etiology.

INITIAL ANTIMICROBIAL THERAPY

Initial therapy of community-acquired pneumonia is based on the clues provided by clinical, epidemiologic, and radiologic information and by evaluation of stained smears of sputum. In the case of a presumed bacterial pneumonia in which an etiologic agent is identified on the sputum smear, initial treatment is tailored to this organism. But, if the etiologic agent cannot be identified in the sputum smear, initial therapy is directed at the likely causative agents. In adult patients with mild pneumonia, a pneumococcal etiology is most likely and empiric treatment with penicillin is reasonable; ampicillin (or cefuroxime) might be used in the same circumstance for the patient who has a history of chronic bronchitis. Treatment of a child with pneumonia and a nondiagnostic sputum examination might turn to cefuroxime because of the possibility that a β-lactamase producing *H. influenzae* type B is involved. The initial treatment of community-acquired aspiration pneumonia or lung abscess might well be with penicillin G; if the therapeutic response is unsatisfactory, or if the patient had received prolonged penicillin therapy previously, then clindamycin might be preferable.

In the more seriously ill patient who has a community-acquired pneumonia in a special setting, other antibiotics might be used in empiric initial therapy. For example, if in the setting of an influenza outbreak the likelihood of *S. aureus* pneumonia as a superinfection is a serious consideration, nafcillin might be substituted for penicillin G. Also, in the alcoholic patient who has a dense lobar consolidation, a first-generation cephalosporin (cephalothin, cefazolin) plus gentamicin would be appropriate as initial therapy.

In community-acquired atypical pneumonia, *M. pneumoniae* pneumonia and Legionnaire's disease are the important treatable considerations, and erythromycin is the drug of choice for initial therapy. If epidemiologic factors suggest Q fever or psittacosis, tetracycline is in order as initial therapy.

Nosocomial pneumonia which is probably bacterial in nature but in which sputum smears are not diagnostic should be treated for the most likely bacterial etiologies (*S. aureus, Klebsiella, E. coli, Serratia, Enterobacter, P. aeruginosa*). Cognizance should be taken of local epidemiologic data, e.g., in a given intensive-care unit clusters of cases of pneumonia that are due to the less common and difficult-to-treat organisms, such as *Acinetobacter* or *P. cepacia*, and antibiotic susceptibility patterns. Initial presumptive therapy might reasonably consist of a combination of nafcillin (or a first-generation cephalosporin) and an aminoglycoside (gentamicin, tobramycin, or amikacin, depending on known susceptibility patterns in the given institution).

Although third generation cephalosporins are effective against many of the gram-negative species causing nosocomial pneumonia, the possibility of resistant organisms, e.g., *P. aeruginosa*, often makes it desirable to use the third-generation cephalosporins in conjunction with an aminoglycoside in the treatment of serious nosocomial pneumonia, particularly in the immunocompromised or granulopenic host. In the latter circumstance, in life-threatening infection where *Legionella* species may be the etiology, erythromycin is added to the therapeutic program.

In oncology or intensive-care units that are experiencing a high incidence of *P. aeruginosa* infections, initial therapy might consist of a combination of ticarcillin (or piperacillin) and an aminoglycoside. In the febrile granulocytopenic patient who has been treated for 10 days with

a cephalosporin and aminoglycoside for presumed sepsis of unknown etiology, the development of a wedge-shaped pulmonary infiltrate might raise the question of a fungal infection, e.g., *Aspergillus*, that warrants the intravenous administration of amphotericin B.

Extrapulmonary findings sometimes suggest the etiology of a pulmonary process and, thereby, direct initial therapy. Thus, acyclovir given intravenously would be indicated in the immunocompetent or immunosuppressed adult who has varicella-zoster and a diffuse pulmonary infiltrate that consists of small-sized nodules.

The patient with AIDS, who develops on chest radiograph a bilateral interstitial or airspace process that is compatible with *P. carinii* pneumonia, is likely, on statistical grounds, to have *P. carinii* pneumonia. Initial therapy using trimethoprim-sulfamethoxazole is appropriate for the mildly ill patient; invasive diagnostic procedures are undertaken if a favorable response does not materialize in several days. In the patient whose illness is severe when first seen, whose course has progressed rapidly, whose radiographic picture is complex, and whose pulmonary infiltrates may represent multiple etiologies, not only is initial therapy begun using trimethoprim-sulfamethoxazole but an invasive procedure is performed simultaneously in order to obtain a tissue diagnosis.

INVASIVE DIAGNOSTIC PROCEDURES

In certain circumstances, a more aggressive approach is required to uncover the etiology of a pneumonia or other pulmonary infection. This approach entails either the foregoing of the initial empiric trial of antibiotics or the foreshortening of the duration of such a trial and resorting to invasive diagnostic procedures. Such an approach may be required at the outset for the patient who has either a severe, rapidly progressive community-acquired pneumonia or for a life-threatening community-acquired pneumonia that has caused the patient's condition to deteriorate despite empiric antimicrobial therapy. In the immunocompromised patient, early invasive diagnostic approaches are mandated by the large number of etiologic agents that may be responsible, the frequent involvement of multiple infectious or noninfectious etiologies in the pulmonary process, the multiplicity of different antimicrobial choices available for targeting to different organisms, e.g., bacteria, viruses, fungi, protozoa, and chlamydia, and the rapidity with which clinical deterioration may preclude further diagnostic and therapeutic actions.

Transtracheal Aspiration

The use of transtracheal aspiration (TTA) is reserved primarily for the patient in whom bacterial pathogens are highly likely as the etiologic agents, but either the patient cannot expectorate sputum or the specimen is nondiagnostic, and in whom the severity of the illness outweighs the risks either of the procedure or of awaiting the outcome of empiric antimicrobial therapy. Also, TTA may be appropriate in a seriously ill patient in whom pneumonia has not responded to therapy directed at likely pathogens (based on initial sputum examinations) or in a patient in whom pneumonia is under treatment but pulmonary superinfection is suspected. TTA is generally not helpful in patients with chronic obstructive airways disease because their tracheobronchial trees often harbor numerous S. pneumoniae and H. influenzae without concurrent pulmonary infection. Since the differential diagnosis of pulmonary infection in immunosuppressed patients includes a number of viral, fungal, and protozoal pathogens as well as noninfectious etiologies, alternative methods (bronchoscopy, bronchoalveolar lavage, open lung biopsy, transthoracic needle aspiration) that can provide tissue or abundant cells for histopathologic examination are preferable.

Contraindications for TTA include: (1) patient unwillingness or inability to cooperate, (2) prior antibiotic therapy (unless bacterial superinfection is suspected), (3) the presence of abnormalities in coagulation (such as platelet counts under 100,000 per microliter or prothrombin times of under 60 percent of normal), and (4) values for arterial $P_{O_2} < 60$ mmHg (with or without supplemental oxygen).

Specimens obtained by TTA should be examined on smears stained by Gram stain, Ziehl-Neelsen stain, modified acid-fast stain, and DFA for *Legionella*. Cultures should be obtained for aerobic and anaerobic bacteria, *Legionella*, fungi and mycobacteria (if indicated by clinical features). If *Pneumocystis* infection is a possible consideration, a smear stained by Giemsa or methenamine silver stain is indicated.

Flexible Fiberoptic Bronchoscopy with Lung Biopsy

When the seriousness of the pulmonary process and lack of definable etiology by noninvasive measures indicate the necessity for biopsy in order to obtain histopathologic and cultural identification of the cause of the pulmonary lesions, choice has to be made among one of several invasive procedures. The choice depends on the experience and skill with the different procedures at a given hospital. Also important in determining the proper procedure are location and radiographic appearance of the pulmonary lesions.

Fiberoptic bronchoscopy using specialized devices to shield against oropharyngeal contamination is used at some institutions to obtain tracheobronchial secretions for culture and as a substitute for transtracheal aspiration in certain acute bacterial pneumonias. A peripheral nodule or cavity (over 1 cm in diameter) that is readily visualized on conventional (posteroanterior and lateral) radiographs and fluoroscopy, and is in an accessible location, may be aspirated and biopsied by needle percutane-

ously. A nodule that is inaccessible to needle aspiration, or a peripherally placed process where the need for histopathology is not apt to be met by needle aspiration and biopsy, is best approached by open lung biopsy.

Fiberoptic bronchoscopy in conjunction with transbronchial lung biopsy provides an etiologic diagnosis in about 50 percent of immunosuppressed individuals who do not have AIDS and in 60 to 90 percent of individuals who do have AIDS, in whom *P. carinii*, CMV, and *M. avium-intracellulare* infections are common.

Contraindications to transbronchial biopsy include inability of the patient to cooperate, marked hypoxemia, bleeding disorders (particularly those associated with hypoprothrombinemia, thrombocytopenia refractory to platelet transfusion, uremia), and pulmonary hypertension.

Tissue specimens are processed for histopathologic examination (hematoxylin and eosin stain, tissue acid-fast stains, Gomori's methenamine-silver stain, periodic acid-Schiff stain, tissue Gram stain, and Dieterle silver stain). Impression smears from tissues are made using sterile slides which, after appropriate fixation, are stained with Giemsa (for *Pneumocystis)*, Gram, and Ziehl-Neelsen stains. As indicated, DFA staining for *Legionella* is performed on separate impression smears. Appropriate cultures are made using tissue obtained either transbronchially or at open lung biopsy.

BRONCHOALVEOLAR LAVAGE

In patients with AIDS, fiberoptic bronchoscopy coupled with subsegmental bronchoalveolar lavage (BAL) has proved particularly useful, providing a diagnosis in over 95 percent of cases of *Pneumocystis* pneumonia. BAL only, without transbronchial biopsy, is often substituted in patients who are thrombocytopenic, or on mechanical ventilation, or severely hypoxemic. The material obtained by BAL is processed for smear and culture. As indicated elsewhere (see Chapter 104), a variety of stains are available for demonstrating the presence of *Pneumocystis* in the cytocentrifuged material: Giemsa stain is rapid and stains intracystic bodies; toluidine blue stains cyst walls; Gram-Weigert and Gomori's methenamine-silver stains take slightly longer to perform.

Stained cytocentrifuged BAL specimens can also be helpful in establishing other diagnoses: Papanicolaou's stain is useful in detecting neoplastic cells and in identifying viral cytopathic effects in epithelial cells.

In at least two-thirds of immunosuppressed patients with CMV pneumonia, the diagnosis can be made by finding inclusion bodies in cytocentrifuged BAL specimens and by immunofluorescent monoclonal antibody staining. CMV is isolated even more often on culture in these patients, but culture alone is not sufficient to establish the diagnosis, since finding the organism may only represent viral shedding in the presence of pulmonary disease due to other causes.

Percutaneous Transthoracic Needle Lung Biopsy

Percutaneous needle biopsy is often the invasive diagnostic procedure of choice for a sizable (>1.0 cm) pulmonary nodule or cavity that is located peripherally. The use of smaller gauge needles has reduced the frequency of pneumothorax as a complication. Diagnostic yields of 60 to 80 percent have been obtained in immunocompromised individuals with pneumonia. This procedure has also provided the diagnosis in 70 percent of patients in whom the underlying lesion was granulomatous. The small core of tissue and aspirated fluid is examined by stained smear and culture for various infectious agents (see "Flexible Fiberoptic Bronchoscopy with Lung Biopsy"). Cytologic examination should be done for neoplastic cells. However, because of the nature of the specimen, histopathologic examination is generally fruitless.

Open Lung Biopsy

Open lung biopsy provides the most definitive procedure for histopathologic diagnosis in the immunocompromised host. It provides sufficient lung tissue for diagnosis and also makes it possible to sample several different sites. It is particularly suitable for evaluating processes that may not be infectious, e.g., neoplasm such as Kaposi's sarcoma, antineoplastic drug toxicity, drug hypersensitivity, and lymphocytic interstitial pneumonia. Open lung biopsy has provided a specific diagnosis in 60 to 90 percent of immunocompromised patients in whom it has been employed. Its major advantages include the ability to control bleeding, air leaks, and the airway. Its disadvantages relate to the thoracotomy: the need for general anesthesia, the inherent delay in preparing the patient for the surgical procedure, the need for intubation, the usual placement of a chest tube, and postoperative splinting due to incisional pain. The mortality of the procedure is about 1 percent. Bleeding is a complication in about 1 percent of patients and delayed pneumothorax in about 9 percent.

Fiberoptic bronchoscopy combined with transbronchial biopsy and segmental BAL is the usual initial invasive diagnostic procedure in the immunocompromised patient with an undefined diffuse pulmonary process. If this fails to provide a diagnosis, then open lung biopsy is indicated. For the patient in whom the pace of the illness does not allow this sequential approach, open lung biopsy may have to be the first choice. It is also preferred in the patient who is unable to cooperate with fiberoptic bronchoscopy or in whom thrombocytopenia or hypoxemia presents additional problems for transbronchial biopsy.

Processing of lung biopsy specimens should include: special stained imprint smears for *P. carinii*, bacteria, fungi, viral inclusion bodies; cultures for bacteria, viruses, fungi, mycobacteria; tissue sections stained for histology and for various infectious agents (see "Flexible Fiberoptic Bronchoscopy with Lung Biopsy").

BIBLIOGRAPHY

Bartlett JG: Invasive diagnostic techniques in respiratory infections, in Pennington JE (ed), *Respiratory Infections: Diagnosis and Management.* New York, Raven, 1983, pp. 55–77.
  A thorough evaluation of the advantages, disadvantages, indications, and contraindications for each of the invasive pulmonary diagnostic procedures: (1) transtracheal aspiration, (2) fiberoptic bronchoscopy with transbronchial biopsy, (3) transthoracic needle aspiration, and (4) open lung biopsy.

Bartlett JG: The technique of transtracheal aspiration. J Crit Illness 1:43–49, 1986.
  A concise review of the indications, contraindications, and technique of transtracheal aspiration.

Bartlett JG: Diagnosis of bacterial infections of the lung. Clin Chest Med 8:119–134, 1987.
  A review of the basic principles involved in the choice of specimens for the identification of respiratory bacterial pathogens, the major bacterial pathogens, and the various diagnostic techniques.

Bartlett JG, Finegold SM: Anaerobic infections of the lung and pleural space. Am Rev Respir Dis 110:56–77, 1974.
  An important paper defining the predisposing circumstances and prominent role of anaerobic organisms in pleuropulmonary disease.

Bartlett JG, Gorbach SL, Finegold SM: The bacteriology of aspiration pneumonia. Am J Med 56:202–207, 1974.
  The authors define the leading role of anaerobic organisms such as Bacteroides melaninogenicus, Fusobacterium species, and anaerobic streptococci in aspiration pneumonia.

Berntsson E, Blomberg J, Lagergard T, Trollfors B: Etiology of community-acquired pneumonia in patients requiring hospitalization. Eur J Clin Microbiol 4:268–272, 1985.
  A high incidence (16 percent) of mixed infections was noted in this series of 127 patients with pneumonia in Sweden. Fifty-six percent of patients with viral infection and 44 percent of those with mycoplasma infection had simultaneous evidences of pneumococcal infection.

Bodey GP, Elting L, Kassamali H, Lim BP: *Escherichia coli* bacteremia in cancer patients. Am J Med 81:85–95, 1986.
  During a ten-year period, 621 episodes of Escherichia coli bacteremia occurred in 575 cancer patients. The infection was most common in patients with acute leukemia and genitourinary and gastrointestinal malignancies.

Cairns MR, Durack DT: Fungal pneumonia in the immunocompromised host. Semin Respir Infect 1:166–185, 1986.
  A well referenced article that thoroughly reviews the epidemiology, pathogenesis, clinical features, diagnostic procedures, and therapy of all the major mycotic infections of the lung occurring in immunocompromised patients.

Chayt KJ, Harper ME, Marselle LM, Lewin EB, Rose RM, Oleske JM, Epstein LG, Wong-Staal F, Gallo RC: Detection of HTLV-III RNA in lungs of patients with AIDS and pulmonary involvement. JAMA 256:2356–2359, 1986.
  In situ hybridization detected HTLV3 RNA in a relatively high percentage (0.1 percent) of cells in the lung of an infant with lymphocytic interstitial pneumonia but not in the lungs of 10 other patients with AIDS and other pulmonary problems, suggesting a possible etiologic role for HIV in development of lymphocytic interstitial pneumonia in children with AIDS.

Cooper JAD, White DA, Matthay RA: Drug-induced pulmonary disease. Part I: Cytotoxic drugs. Am Rev Respir Dis 133:321–340, 1986.
  This review is the most complete and current summary of the pulmonary injury produced by cytotoxic drugs. Clinical features and pathogenetic mechanisms are considered in detail.

Cooper JAD, White DA, Matthay RA: Drug-induced pulmonary disease. Part 2: Noncytotoxic drugs. Am Rev Respir Dis 133:488–505, 1986.
  This comprehensive review deals with noncytotoxic drugs capable of producing radiologically evident pulmonary disease. It includes consideration of clinical aspects and likely mechanisms of pathogenesis.

Curnutte JT, Boxer LA: Clinically significant phagocytic cell defects, in Remington JS, Swartz MN (eds), *Current Clinical Topics in Infectious Diseases—6.* New York, McGraw-Hill, 1985, pp. 103–105.
  A complete and up-to-date review of the impaired mechanisms and clinical expression of granulocyte defects. Mechanisms by which specific microorganisms deflect normal microbicidal defenses are also considered.

Dorff GJ, Rytel MW, Farmer SG, Scanlon G: Etiologies and characteristic features of pneumonias in a municipal hospital. Am J Med Sci 266:349–358, 1973.
In this series of 148 cases of pneumonia reported from a municipal hospital, 74 percent were of bacterial etiology. The mortality was 17.5 percent for the overall series.

Ebright JR, Rytel MW: Bacterial pneumonia in the elderly. J Am Geriatr Soc 28:220–223, 1980.
The etiologies of 106 cases of community-acquired pneumonia, of which 31 percent occurred in individuals of 65 years of age or older, are reviewed. Laboratory facilities allowed only bacteriologic diagnosis. The frequency of a gram-negative bacillary etiology in the elderly was three times as high as in younger adults.

Epler GR, Colby TV, McLoud TC, Carrington CB, Gaensler EA: Bronchiolitis obliterans organizing pneumonia. N Engl J Med 312:152–158, 1985.
A clinical, radiographic, and pathologic study of 50 patients with bronchiolitis obliterans associated with patchy organizing pneumonia. It is distinguished from bronchiolitis obliterans associated with irreversible bronchial obstruction.

Fekety FR Jr, Caldwell J, Gump D, Johnson JE, Maxson W, Mulholand J, Thoburn R: Bacteria, viruses and mycoplasmas in acute pneumonia in adults. Am Rev Respir Dis 104:499–507, 1971.
One hundred patients with community-acquired pneumonia are reviewed with respect to etiologies. Only 50 percent of patients seen in emergency room with pneumonia required hospitalization.

Fiala M: A study of the combined role of viruses, mycoplasmas and bacteria in adult pneumonia. Am J Med Sci 257:44–51, 1969.
In 192 adults with pneumonia, a bacterial etiology was found in 67 percent. Of the bacterial pneumonias, 83 percent were due to S. pneumoniae.

Fishman JA: Diagnostic approach to pneumonia in the immunocompromised host: Semin Respir Infect 1:133–144, 1986.
A concise, well-organized approach to the diagnosis of pneumonia in the immunocompromised host. Clinical and radiologic clues and noninvasive studies are outlined, as well as various approaches to a histologic diagnosis.

Garb JL, Brown RB, Barb JR, Tuthill RW: Differences in etiology of pneumonias in nursing home and community patients. JAMA 240:2169–2172, 1978.
The best available data comparing in the elderly the etiologies of bacterial pneumonia acquired while living at home in comparison with those acquired among residents of nursing homes.

Grayston JT, Kuo C, Wang S, Altman J: A new *Chlamydia psittaci* strain, TWAR, isolated in acute respiratory tract infections. N Engl J Med 315:161–168, 1986.
The most complete clinical, epidemiologic, and microbiologic report of a new C. psittaci strain (TWAR) which is spread from human to human (unlike conventional C. psittaci) and causes a clinical picture resembling M. pneumoniae pneumonia.

Habermehl K-O: Rapid diagnosis of respiratory virus infections in patients with acute respiratory disease. Diagn Microbial Infect Dis 4:17S–22S, 1986.
A good correlation is shown between tissue culture isolation of influenza A and respiratory syncytial viruses and demonstration of their antigens in respiratory tract mucus by radioimmunoassay and ELISA.

Korvick JA, Yu VL: Legionnaires' disease: an emerging surgical problem. Ann Thorac Surg 43:341–347, 1987.
Legionnaires' disease is an important, although often overlooked, complication in the postoperative patient. Patients undergoing a transplant procedure are at highest risk, but occurrence is common in the surgical patient undergoing general anesthesia, endotracheal intubation, or both.

LaForce MF: Hospital-acquired pneumonia: Epidemiologic summary and clinical approach, in Pennington JE (ed), *Respiratory Infections: Diagnosis and Management*. New York, Raven, 1983, pp 135–142.
A concise overview of the magnitude of the problem, pathogenetic factors, and microbial agents involved in nosocomial pneumonia.

Lee SH, Barnes WG, Schaetzel WP: Pulmonary aspergillosis and the importance of oxalate crystal recognition in cytology specimens. Arch Pathol Lab Med 110:1176–1179, 1986.
In a patient with a large mycetoma-containing cavity complicated by invasive aspergillosis, sputum cytology (and lung at autopsy) showed numerous calcium oxalate crystals. Literature on pulmonary oxalosis with Aspergillus infection of the lung is reviewed.

Lepow ML, Balassanian N, Emmerich J, Roberts RB, Rosenthal MS, Wolinsky E: Interrelationships of viral, mycoplasmal, and bacterial agents in uncomplicated pneumonia. Am Rev Respir Dis 97:533–545, 1968.
> *A review of the etiologies of 98 cases of community-acquired pneumonia. In this study a close relationship was not shown between viral and mycoplasma infections and bacterial pneumonia, but virologic techniques were those of the 1960s.*

McFarlane JT, Ward MJ, Finch RG, Macrea AD: Hospital study of adult community-acquired pneumonia. Lancet 2:255–258, 1982.
> *Bacterial etiologies predominated in this series of 127 patients in Nottingham, England, with community-acquired pneumonias. Seventy-five percent of the pneumonias were pneumococcal. Legionella species were the second commonest etiology (15 percent), a much more frequent cause of pneumonia than reported elsewhere.*

Mufson MA, Chang V, Gill V, Wood SC, Romansky MJ, Chanock RM: The role of viruses, mycoplasmas and bacteria in acute pneumonia in civilian adults. Am J Epidemiol 86:526–544, 1967.
> *Etiologies of over 400 cases of community-acquired pneumonia in adults are described. Viral or mycoplasma etiology is found in 20 percent.*

Murray JF, Felton CP, Garay SM, Gottlieb MS, Hopewell PC, Stover DE, Teirstein AS: Pulmonary complications of the acquired immune deficiency syndrome: Report of a National Heart, Lung, and Blood Institute Workshop. N Engl J Med 310:1682–1688, 1984.
> *This article, based on over 400 patients with AIDS, provides an excellent evaluation of the relative frequencies of the different opportunistic pathogens causing pulmonary disease in this setting.*

Niederman MS, Fein AM: Pneumonia in the elderly. Clin Geriatr Med 2:241–268, 1986.
> *Because recognition of pneumonia may be difficult and therapy is fraught with problems, mortality is high in the elderly. Accordingly, serious attention must be paid to prevention, including the use of pneumococcal and influenza vaccines as well as careful attention to the patient's host defense status.*

Ognibene FP, Shelhamer J, Gill V, Macker AM, Loew D, Parker MM, Gelmann E, Fauci AS, Parrillo JE, Masur H: The diagnosis of *Pneumocystis carinii* pneumonia in patients with acquired immunodeficiency syndrome using subsegmental bronchoalveolar lavage. Am Rev Respir Dis 129:929–932, 1984.
> *Bronchoalveolar lavage provided a diagnosis of Pneumocystis pneumonia in 16 of 18 patients in whom the diagnosis was proven by transbronchial biopsy.*

Pennington JE: Gram-negative bacterial pneumonia in the immunocompromised host. Semin Respir Infect 1:145–150, 1986.
> *A good overview of the incidence, bacteriology, pathogenesis, diagnosis, and treatment of gram-negative bacillary pneumonias in immunosuppressed (particularly granulopenic) patients.*

Pitchenik AE, Ganjei P, Torres A, Evans DA, Rubin E, Baier H: Sputum examination for the diagnosis of *Pneumocystis carinii* pneumonia in the acquired immunodeficiency syndrome. Am Rev Respir Dis 133:226–229, 1986.
> *The values of sputum, bronchial washings, bronchial brushings, and transbronchial lung biopsy in making the diagnosis of Pneumocystis pneumonia in 20 patients with AIDS are compared.*

Popovsky MA, Abel MD, Moore SB: Transfusion-related acute lung injury associated with passive transfer of antileukocyte antibodies. Am Rev Respir Dis 128:185–189, 1983.
> *The clinical and laboratory features of five patients with leukoagglutinin-related transfusion-induced noncardiogenic pulmonary edema are reviewed.*

Ramsey PG, Rubin RR, Tolkoff-Rubin NE, Cosimi AB, Russell RS, Greene R: The renal transplant patient with fever and pulmonary infiltrates: Etiology, clinical manifestations and management. Medicine 59:206–222, 1980.
> *A thorough review of the infectious and noninfectious causes of fever and pulmonary infiltrates in 54 renal transplant recipients. It should be noted that this experience related to the period before widespread use of cyclosporin A for immunosuppression.*

Rossman MD, Dauber JH: Sarcoidosis: Assessment of inflammatory activity, in Fishman AP (ed), *Update: Pulmonary Diseases and Disorders*. New York, McGraw-Hill, 1982, pp 193–204.
> *A comparison of bronchoalveolar lavage, determination of angiotensin-converting enzyme and gallium 67 scanning (three tests) to evaluate the activity of sarcoidosis. The problems with each of these tests as a clinical tool for the management of patients with sarcoidosis are discussed.*

Rubin RH: Pneumonia in the immunocompromised host, in Fishman AP (ed), *Update: Pulmonary Diseases and Disorders.* New York, McGraw Hill, 1982, pp 1–25.
   A comprehensive review of the diverse etiologies responsible for the high incidence of pneumonia in immunocompromised patients.

Rubin RH, Greene R: Etiology and management of the compromised patient with fever and pulmonary infiltrates, in Rubin RH, Young LS (eds), *Clinical Approach to Infection in the Compromised Host.* New York, Plenum, 1981, pp 123–161.
   A thorough and practical consideration of the various causes of fever with pulmonary infiltrates in compromised patients, particularly those with neoplastic disease and those who have undergone renal transplantation. Valuable clues to etiologic considerations are stressed.

Rytel MW, Preheim LC: Antigen detection in the diagnosis and in the prognostic assessment of bacterial pneumonias. Diagn Microbiol Infect Dis 4:35S–46S, 1986.
   A review of the limited data available on the evaluation of methods for detecting pneumococcal antigen in the sputum of patients with pneumococcal pneumonia.

Salata RA, Lederman MM, Shlaes DM, Jacobs MR, Eckstein E, Tweardy D, Toossi Z, Chmielewski R, Marino J, King CH, Graham RC, Ellner JJ: Diagnosis of nosocomial pneumonia in intubated, intensive care unit patients. Am Rev Respir Dis 135:426–432, 1987.
   Emphasis is placed on the finding of elastin fibers in tracheal aspirates of patients with necrotizing nosocomial pneumonias.

Segreti J, Bone RC: Overwhelming pneumonia. Dis Mon 33:1–59, 1987.
   A review of various considerations in dealing with overwhelming pneumonia.

Seidenfeld JJ, Pohl DF, Bell RC, Harris GD, Johanson WG Jr: Incidence, site, and outcome of infections in patients with the adult respiratory distress syndrome. Am Rev Respir Dis 134:12–16, 1986.
   A study of 108 infections in 129 patients with ARDS and evaluation of the organisms responsible, the body sites involved, and the outcomes of therapy.

Shanley JD, Jordan MC: Viral pneumonia in the immunocompromised patient. Semin Respir Infect 1:193–201, 1986.
   A concise review of the roles of CMV, varicella-zoster, herpes simplex, and adenoviruses in causing pneumonia in transplant recipients.

Sliman R, Rehm S, Shlaes DM: Serious infections caused by Bacillus species. Medicine 66:218–223, 1987.
   Thirty-eight patients with serious infections caused by organisms belonging to the genus Bacillus are described. The predisposing role of intravascular devices, trauma, immunosuppression and intravenous drug abuse is emphasized.

Springmeyer SC, Hackman RC, Holle R, Greenberg GM, Weems CE, Myerson D, Meyers JD, Thomas ED: Use of bronchoalveolar lavage to diagnose acute diffuse pneumonia in the immunocompromised host. J Infect Dis 154:604–610, 1986.
   The value of cytotoxic examination of bronchoalveolar lavage in the diagnosis of CMV pneumonia in bone marrow recipients is emphasized. Two-thirds of the patients diagnosed by open lung biopsy could be diagnosed by bronchoalveolar lavage.

Sullivan RJ Jr, Dowdle WR, Marine WM, Hierholzer JC: Adult pneumonia in a general hospital. Arch Intern Med 129:935–942, 1972.
   In this review of the microbial etiologies of 292 patients hospitalized for pneumonia, a bacterial etiology was implicated in 57 percent. Serologic evidence of concomitant viral infection was found in 10 percent of the bacterial pneumonias.

Talavera W, Mildvan D: Pulmonary infections in the acquired immunodeficiency syndrome. Semin Respir Infect 1:202–211, 1986.
   A review of the various infectious agents identified in several hundred pneumonias in patients with AIDS at one large hospital in New York City.

Thorsteinsson SB, Musher DM, Fagan T: The diagnostic value of sputum culture in acute pneumonia. JAMA 233:894–895, 1975.
   A straightforward study showing concordance in cultures for pneumococci in specimens of expectorated sputum and tracheobronchial secretions obtained via transtracheal aspiration and bronchoscopy in 16 patients.

Verghese A, Berk SL: Bacterial pneumonia in the elderly. Medicine 62:271–285, 1983.
   A comprehensive review of the literature of the predisposing factors and etiologies of community-acquired and nosocomial pneumonias in the elderly.

White RJ, Blainey AD, Harrison KJ, Clarke SKR: Causes of pneumonia presenting to a district general hospital. Thorax 36:566–570, 1981.

  In this series of cases of community-acquired pneumonia from England, the combination of viral, mycoplasmal, chlamydial and rickettsial (C. burnetii) etiologies exceeded bacterial by 60 percent.

Woodhead MA, MacFarland JT, Rodgers FG, Laverick A, Pilkington R, Macrae AD: Aetiology and outcome of severe community-acquired pneumonia. J Infect 10:204–210, 1985.

  A study of the etiologies of severe community-acquired pneumonia in Nottingham, England. The mortality was 50 percent, and 88 percent of all cases required ventilatory assistance. The most frequent etiologies were S. pneumoniae (32 percent), Legionella (30 percent), and S. aureus (10 percent).

Chapter *86*

Pulmonary Defense Mechanisms to Microbial Infections

Herbert Y. Reynolds

Overview: Normal Lung Host Defenses

Special Defenses in Certain Areas
   Nose and Oropharynx
   Conducting Airways
   The Alveolar Spaces
   Interplay between Alveolar Macrophages
     and Polymorphonuclear Granulocytes
   Lymphocytes in the Alveolar Spaces

Potential Defects in Host Defenses That Can Be Associated
with Respiratory Infections

OVERVIEW: NORMAL LUNG HOST DEFENSES

The atmosphere we breathe is not simply "air" but represents a complex mixture of gases and particulates. To this ambient air are further added virus- and bacteria-containing droplets, found in respiratory secretions coughed or sneezed by our immediate neighbors, which can be aerosolized into our airways. Moreover, we frequently aspirate secretions from the upper respiratory tract, particularly during sleep. To perform air exchange adequately, the respiratory system must recognize and eliminate these unwanted elements in inspired air. This nonrespiratory activity of purifying inspired air and keeping lung tissues free of infection has been collectively termed *lung host defense.*

Components of the defense system are spaced along the entire respiratory tract from the point of air intake at the nares to the level of oxygen uptake on the alveolar surface. Conducting airways functionally extend from the nose to the respiratory bronchioles. In this segment of the airways, nasal turbinates, the epiglottis, larynx, and other anatomic barriers exist. Dichotomous branching of the respiratory tree causes the airstream to deflect and particles carried in it to impact on the mucosal surface. Entrapment in mucus and other locally derived proteins (such as secretory IgA), ciliary clearance, and coughing serve to remove this particulate material from the respiratory tract.

Distal to the respiratory bronchioles in the air-exchange units, other components of host defense become important (Fig. 86-1). The lining material of the alveoli (surfactant), iron-containing proteins (transferrin), other immunoglobins such as IgG opsonins, or properdin (factor B), which may initiate the alternative pathway of complement activation, all have varying activity against inhaled particles or microorganisms.

Alveolar macrophages are the principal phagocytic cells in the airspaces and scavengers of the alveolar surfaces. What evades these other mechanisms and alights on the alveolar surface is efficiently consumed by roaming macrophages, which may be assisted by other components of the humoral immune system and various lipoproteins and glycoproteins mixed in the alveolar lining fluid. In the event that local phagocytes and alveolar defenses are inadequate, an inflammatory reaction can be initiated, which unleashes the potent polymorphonuclear neutrophils (PMNs), complement factors, and other vasomediators and humoral immune elements from systemic sources. Prior contact with a microbial agent or some sensitizing substance in the airways may induce specific antibody (secretory IgA to prevent mucosal adherence or an IgG opsonin to facilitate phagocytosis) thereby helping the lung to deal more efficiently with it on rechallenge at a future time.

In summary, coordinated function of lung defense mechanisms along the respiratory tract is remarkably ef-

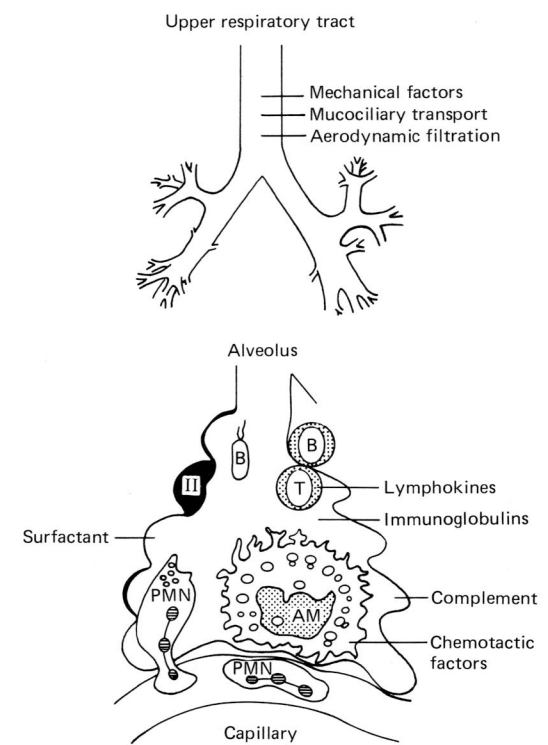

FIGURE 86-1 Schematic representation of the defense mechanisms of the lung.

fective in removing or neutralizing microorganisms, particulates, and noxious gases that are inhaled with respired air or aspirated in nasopharyngeal secretions. Lung infections and overt harm from air pollutants are rare for the healthy human, considering our constant exposure to airborne substances in ambient air or to our own indigenous bacterial flora. Many of the mechanical barriers and reflex actions are concentrated in the nose and oropharynx and along the conducting airways, and the combination of adherence to the mucosal surface, mucociliary clearance, and coughing removes the bulk of debris. These are surveillance mechanisms that either function mechanically, or they may be activated by nonspecific or nonimmunologic stimuli. In addition, several augmenting mechanisms exist that enhance the responsiveness of the defense system and make it flexible and adaptable, but require more time or complexity to activate. One of these is the lung's ability to mount immune responses (humoral and cellular) to various antigenic stimuli. Another is the potential to mount readily an inflammatory response in the pulmonary parenchyma, which allows components in plasma and blood cells to bolster the local resources of the lung.

SPECIAL DEFENSES IN CERTAIN AREAS

Nose and Oropharynx

These areas are the normal channels for inhaled air to reach the glottis and pass into the extrathoracic portion of the trachea before it enters the thorax. With nasal breathing, air is partially conditioned for correct humidity and temperature as it flows over the nasal turbinates and mucosa into the posterior pharynx. Because of nasal obstruction or ventilation requirements for exercise and exertion (usually breathing at more than 20 to 30 L/min), mouth breathing becomes essential, and inhaled air may have to pass well into the trachea before appropriate climatic conditions are obtained. The nasal mucosa is very vascular and has great potential to add copious amounts of fluid to the surface; mucous secretion is plentiful, also. In the mouth, as fluid is basically required to masticate food and to be a lubricant of sorts for the tongue and larynx, its origin is in the parotid and salivary glands, where amylase and sialic acid are provided. Host defense mechanisms in the nose and mouth must filter contaminants in the air and control indigenous bacteria, which are plentiful in both areas.

In the nose, sneezing (or blowing) is the counterpart of coughing and provides a high-velocity ejection from the nares of any pollen or large-sized particle (>10 μm in diameter) that is an irritant or a nuisance there. Course hairs in the nares also facilitate exclusion of gross particles or their entrapment in mucus. For substances that attach to the mucosa, one response of the nose is to exude large quantities of watery secretions to wash off its surface. Mucociliary clearance is operant also. Downspouts leading from the ears and lacrimal glands and from sinus cavities provide multiple points for more fluid to be added to the nasal secretions but also create vulnerable points that can cause the gutters to become clogged. The complex plumbing in the nose works if there is good gravitational flow and the orifices stay open; if not, sinusitis, otitis media, and occluded tear ducts result.

Substances in nasal secretions that control bacteria or viruses have received most attention, and perhaps Dr. Alexander Fleming's characterization of the bacteriolytic enzyme lysozyme initiated research on defense mechanisms in the upper respiratory tract. With the contemporary research effort into the secretory immune system, which began in the early 1960s and focused on the role of immunoglobulins, especially that of secretory IgA (SIgA), the nose was the first portion of the respiratory tract to be investigated (parotid gland secretions are considered part of the digestive tract). Nasal secretions, like those from other external or mucosal surfaces, are rich in IgA, which is synthesized locally by submucosal plasma cells. IgA accounts for about 10 percent of the total protein content in nasal wash. IgG and siderophilin are present in smaller amounts, and IgE probably is not secreted by normal nonatopic people, although its detection in nasal wash has been controversial. As an example, in 10- to 20-ml specimens of normal subjects' nasal washings, which were concentrated fivefold, we measured about 0.5 mg of total protein; this protein consisted of 15% albumin, 15% SIgA, about 1% IgG, and almost no IgE. Free secretory component (SC) can be detected in nasal wash fluid. Of the nasal immunoglobulins, SIgA is the major source of antibody; only in people with allergic rhinitis will IgE antibody be substantial. The usual specificity of IgA antibody is antiviral. After nasal immunization of normal subjects with various viral or mycoplasmal vaccines, appropriate neutralizing IgA antibody can be elicited. Although these antibodies are protective against homologous and live microbial challenge, the duration of protection is often brief and the antibody titers diminish rapidly unless repeated exposure occurs. Certainly this antibody system is a major host defense mechanism in the upper airway, but it is still poorly understood and has proved difficult for investigators to harness and to manipulate in a predictable manner. The dream that a number of good nasal viral vaccines could be used broadly in the population to immunize against common agents, thus reducing one of the greatest causes of minor morbidity and time lost from work, seems to be fading away. Success with certain bacterial vaccines may be more promising.

In the mouth, the sweeping action of the tongue against all surfaces during chewing, swallowing, and expectorating should make it difficult for bacteria to stay in

place and to stick. Yet bacteria adhere to buccal squamous cells, and many accumulate in crevices around teeth and gums. Many kinds are present: aerobes and anaerobes, spirochetes, gram-positive and gram-negative species, and some that specialize in making dental plaque and decaying teeth. A common feature of host defense in the mouth and nose is the plentiful amount of SIgA in secretions that bathe each area. The parotid glands and probably the submandibular salivary glands secrete IgA as their principal humoral immune substance, which accounts for 12 to 15 percent of the total protein content. In this fluid, albumin represents about 10 percent of the protein, but IgG is barely detectable (<1 percent). In parotid fluid IgA is found in monomeric and dimeric forms, and free secretory component can be detected as well. Thus, normal nasal and parotid (or salivary) secretions have about the same composition of immunoglobulins. Crevicular fluid that seeps from the edge of the gum resembles an ultrafiltrate of plasma and has a high total protein content, which is mainly IgG but contains a little IgA. As with the nasal immune system, it has been possible to manipulate SIgA in the mouth and to produce antibodies against certain cariogenic strains of streptococci, that will subsequently prevent bacterial adherence to teeth. Substantial success can be achieved in preventing caries with intrasalivary gland immunization in animal models. As for human host defenses, regular brushing and flossing, coupled with some fluoride in the water supply and moderation of candy or sugar in the diet, may still be the best solution.

Two reasons for including a section on the nose and mouth in a review of respiratory infections are (1) to remind us that there is an upper portion of the respiratory tract that has some features in common with the lower part, particularly the mucosal surface, and (2) to emphasize that infections in the nose, sinuses, ears, and teeth and gums are common and often have ramifications for the diagnosis or successful treatment of illness in the lower respiratory tract. Aspiration of anaerobic bacteria in oral secretions contributes to lung abscess formation, whereas, chronic sinusitis often accompanies such diseases as cystic fibrosis, ciliary dyskinetic syndromes, asthma, and dysgammaglobulinemia. Acute viral infections of the nose may be a prelude to bacterial lung infection, and various allergic diseases can simultaneously cause rhinitis and symptoms of hyperreactive airways (asthma syndrome). Control of asthma symptoms may be very difficult unless an unrecognized sinus infection is discovered and treated. The presence of nasal polyps in an asthmatic may be expected, but their development in a child with recurrent respiratory infections must raise the possibility of cystic fibrosis. Chronic aspiration pneumonias in a neurologic patient with an incompetent larynx may require drastic measures to separate completely the upper and lower tracts by oversewing the vocal cords and then making a tracheostomy.

Conducting Airways

Within this segment of the respiratory tract, situated between the upper airway (nose, oropharynx, and larynx) and the air-exchange area of the terminal bronchioles and alveoli, mucociliary clearance and coughing are the principal means of cleansing the mucosal surface. SIgA and other antibodies probably prevent epithelial attachment of certain bacteria and viruses as well to the ciliated cells. Multiple branching points of the respiratory tree increases impaction of airborne particulates against the mucosa. Because many respired particles ($<5>1\ \mu m$ in size) are filtered out in the conducting airways, host defenses must be efficient. However, this segment is susceptible to many diseases, e.g., epithelial cell infection with viruses and *Mycoplasma*, bronchoconstriction in asthmatic syndromes, bronchitis, bronchiectasis, colonization with bacteria, irritation from noxious gases, and lung cancer.

The respiratory mucosa is coated with viscous fluid which is secreted by bronchial glands, globlet cells, and probably by Clara cells (nonciliated bronchiolar secretory cells found in the terminal bronchioles). Some of this fluid is derived from the intravascular space by diffusion through the blood-air barrier. Special proteins, such as SIgA and SC, can be added locally along airways by immunoglobulin-secreting plasma cells and epithelial cells. The result is a mucosal fluid layer of great complexity, still incompletely characterized, covering the airways. Few attempts have been made in humans to retrieve selectively mucosal secretion from the trachea and along the bronchi for analysis. However, the preliminary results indicate that these portions of the mucosa actively produce IgA and α_1-antichymotrypsin and secrete potassium ion (but other electrolytes are lower in proportion than present in plasma); the mucosa has a low pH of about 6.8 to 6.9.

Beating cilia arising from the epithelial lining cells propel these secretions up the respiratory tract; periodic coughing can assist the process. The combination of an intact mucosal lining and overlying mucous secretions provides a protective layer which can entrap inhaled particles and repel noxious gases or vapors. Thus, little penetrates or sticks to the respiratory surface, and this seems to be an important function in lung host defense. Bacteria and other infectious agents may transiently colonize the airways, but mucociliary clearance effectively removes them. Tight cellular junctions between epithelial cells also prevent passage of macromolecules into the submucosa. However, several circumstances can alter the intactness of this protective barrier, which may make this portion of the respiratory tract vulnerable or susceptible to disease: (1) nutrition may affect the integrity of mucosal epithelial cells and may allow certain bacteria to adhere; (2) cigarette smoke or noxious fumes can disrupt the anatomy of epithelial junctions and enhance the passage of

airway substances into areas usually inaccessible; and (3) some bacteria can elaborate proteolytic enzymes that may break down IgA, thus, promoting their selective coloniza-tion.

Lymphoid tissue is present along the entire respira-tory tract, extending from the nose and oropharynx to the respiratory bronchioles and alveolar ducts. At least three levels of pulmonary lymphoid tissue organization can be defined: true lymph nodes situated at the root of the lung as hilar nodes, lymphoid nodules, and lymphoid aggre-gates. The level of organization within lymphoid struc-tures decreases progressively down the airways.

Lymphoid nodules may occur in the mucosal surface of large- and medium-sized bronchi and are particularly numerous at points of airway bifurcation. They consist anatomically of follicles that contain small- and medium-sized lymphocytes, but lack capsules and germinal cen-ters that are characteristic of true lymph nodes. On the airway side, these submucosal follicles are covered by a single layer of flattened, nonciliated surface epithelium, which is often observed to be infiltrated with lympho-cytes. These bronchial-associated lymphoid tissues (BALT) bear some resemblance to gut-associated lymph-oid tissues (Peyer's patches) and probably serve as a reser-voir for immunocompetent cells in the lungs that eventu-ally migrate into the airspaces. Whereas BALT is easily demonstrated in some rodents and rabbits, subhuman pri-mates and humans have decidedly less obvious amounts of this lymphoid tissue, and it may not be as relevant to airway defenses as initially thought, especially in the adult.

Loosely organized collections of lymphocytes (lymphoid aggregates) are concentrated in the distal air-ways, especially at the bronchoalveolar junctions, the in-terface for ciliated epithelial cells of the terminal bronchi-ole, and the alveolar lining cells. These aggregates provide the opportunity for close interaction between lymphoid cells and inhaled antigens that are deposited in the lower respiratory tract. Also, in the vicinity of the respiratory bronchioles, lymphatic channels begin that might provide these lymphocytes with a route to draining lymph nodes (hilar nodes) where immunologic responses develop.

The Alveolar Spaces

The defenses enumerated above (Fig. 86-1) are not perfect in that they may not quantitatively eliminate all particles inspired into the lungs, but their overall effectiveness is excellent. Airways distal to the major bronchi are proba-bly sterile in normal subjects. However, some particles of small size and certain geometry can elude all the above-named mechanisms and reach the air-exchange surface of the alveolar spaces. When this occurs, another group of

host defense factors must take over. Anatomically, lung structure changes at the level of respiratory bronchioles, and in the terminal units (alveolar ducts and alveoli) cili-ated epithelium and mucus-secreting cells (goblet cells and mucous glands) are no longer present. Therefore, mucociliary clearance does not exist, nor does coughing effectively clear material from the alveoli. Microbial clear-ance and the removal of other antigenic material from al-veoli depend entirely on cellular and humoral factors. These include phospholipid surfactant and proteins (im-munoglobulins and complement factors) in the alveolar lining material and phagocytic cells, i.e., alveolar macro-phages and PMNs.

Inhaled or aspirated bacteria are an appropriate ex-ample. If a bacterium of critical size (0.5 to 3 μm in diame-ter) is deposited in an alveolus, the microbe may encounter at least three substances that conceivably could inactivate it, exclusive of its eventual inactivation by phagocytosis. The actual pathway the aerosolized microbe takes is not certain, but it may have to contact the alveolar wall, roll and tumble along in the alveolar lining fluid picking up a coat of the various soluble lipoprotein substances pres-ent, encounter a patch of IgG or a complement factor (C3b) or possibly some nonimmune opsonin like a fibronectin fragment, dodge around a proteolytic enzyme that is con-tending with an antiprotease, and finally keep squirming away from some phagocyte trying to catch it. Neverthe-less, the chase does not last very long, and an alveolar macrophage captures the bacterium within a few minutes. With experimental murine models in which bacteria are aerosolized into the lungs and lung histology is then ex-amined soon after, bacteria do not remain free on the alve-olar surface but are almost quantitatively ingested by mac-rophages. Mice, when exposed to an aerosol cloud of bacteria (*Staphylococcus aureus* or *Proteus mirabilis*), will respire low numbers of organisms into their alveoli. Within a few minutes, staphylococci are almost all within alveolar phagocytic cells; the ingestion of gram-negative organisms is somewhat slower. Gram-negative bacteria are usually cleared from lungs more slowly.

Of particular importance is the activity and specific-ity of alveolar space opsonins. First, surfactant, secreted by type II pneumocytes, may have antibacterial activity against staphylococci and rough colony strains of some gram-negative rod bacteria. Second, immunoglobulins, principally of the IgG class (may account for 5% total pro-tein in alveolar fluid and subclasses IgG_1 and IgG_3 may be most important) and, in lesser concentration, monomeric and secretory forms of IgA may have specific opsonic anti-body activity for the bacterium. Third, complement com-ponents, especially properdin factor B, might interact with the bacterium and trigger the alternative comple-ment pathway. One or all of these possibilities can pre-pare the bacterium for ingestion by an alveolar macro-

phage, or the active complement sequence can lyse it directly. Although alveolar macrophages avidly phagocytose some inert particles, they may ingest viable bacteria with considerably less enthusiasm. Coating or opsonizing the organisms will enhance phagocytosis approximately tenfold in an in vitro culture system. IgG is capable of selectively enhancing alveolar macrophage phagocytosis, and the complement (C3b fragment) can function in concert with IgG to enhance or amplify the process. The effect of nonimmune opsonins must be considered as well. Certainly surfactant, as mentioned, has a role, as well as fibronectin (large-molecular-weight fragments of 220,000 daltons) and cytophilic or cell-membrane-bound IgG.

Phagocytosis, defined as the ingestion of particulate matter by cells, is a complex process that is divided into two phases: attachment of the particle to the cell surface and internalization. Attachment of the particle to the surface of the phagocytic cell appears to be essential prior to ingestion. This binding may occur at random but is greatly enhanced by opsonization of the particle by antibody (especially IgG) or one component of the complement system, C3b. Opsonin-dependent phagocytosis is mediated by receptors on the cell surface for immunoglobulin or complement. Receptors for the Fc portion of IgG (IgG3 and IgG1 primarily) and for the third component of complement (C3b) have been identified on human monocytes and alveolar macrophages. There is evidence that the number and function of these receptors can be modulated by lymphocyte products, such as γ-interferon, and other mediator substances. Ingestion of membrane-bound particles occurs via a process that is energy-dependent and involves the actin-myosin system of the phagocytic cell. The plasma membrane of the ingesting cell surrounds the bound particle, enclosing it in an endocytic vesicle.

Phagocytic cells have well-developed mechanisms that operate to kill internalized pathogens. Fusion of the vacuole (or phagosome) containing an engulfed organism with lysosomes within the cell follows the actual ingestion of the pathogen. This process exposes the pathogen to hydrolytic enzymes and other bactericidal proteins, as well as myeloperoxidase, an enzyme that in combination with oxygen metabolites is extremely active in killing phagocytosed organisms. However, several organisms are known to interfere with phagosome-lysosome fusion and are able to promote their own intracellular survival. An important factor of the antimicrobial systems in phagocytic cells is their ability to generate reduced oxygen species, such as hydrogen peroxide, superoxide anion, and hydroxyl radicals. In response to a phagocytic stimulus, neutrophils, monocytes, and macrophages undergo a respiratory burst that results in increased oxygen consumption, accelerated utilization of glucose, and activation of the hexose monophosphate shunt, with generation of re-

duced pyridine nucleotide (NADPH) and the production of reduced oxygen metabolites. These have sufficient antimicrobial activity, both independently and in the presence of myeloperoxidase. Myeloperoxidase (MPO) is a lysosomal enzyme present in abundance in neutrophils and to a lesser extent in monocytes. Macrophages contain little or no demonstrable MPO, although they may have some other peroxidase activity. MPO reacts with hydrogen peroxide and a halide (usually chloride) to form highly reactive products (especially hypochlorous acid) with potent antimicrobial activity, probably mediated via halogenation and/or oxidation of the surface of the ingested pathogen. Even though macrophages lack myeloperoxidase, it is likely that toxic oxygen species remain an important microbicidal mechanism for these cells.

Following containment of bacteria, the fate of alveolar macrophages is not certain. They are long-lived tissue cells that can survive at least for several months and presumably are capable of handling repeated bacterial and other microbial challenges (reusable phagocytes). Because they are mobile cells, they can migrate quickly to other areas of the respiratory tract (to the region of the respiratory bronchioles) and get aboard the mucociliary escalator for elimination from the lungs. In addition, macrophages gain entry into lung lymphatics at this same place and can be carried to regional lymph nodes. This exit gives them access to systemic lymphoid tissue and is important in initiating cellular immune responses. Undoubtedly, macrophages are instrumental in degrading antigenic material and presenting it to appropriate T lymphocytes in these nodes. Activated macrophages, as may be found in certain diseases such as sarcoidosis, have enhanced capacity to present antigens to T lymphocytes. Increasingly, attention is being given to the effector immune role of macrophages.

The alveolar macrophage has acquired an interesting dual role in the respiratory tract—as a phagocyte to dispose of debris, to process foreign antigens, and to kill ingested microorganisms and as an effector cell to initiate immune responses and the inflammatory reaction. The secretion of chemotactic factors by alveolar macrophages may be important in generating parenchymal inflammation and attracting PMNs to the lung. Alveolar macrophages can usually inactivate microorganisms and host defense surveillance is successful; clinical disease and pneumonitis rarely develop. However, if a sufficiently large bacterial inoculum reaches the lower respiratory tract, or if particularly virulent microorganisms are inhaled, the macrophage system can be overwhelmed. PMNs are recruited to help out. This situation points out the dual phagocytic protection present in the alveolar spaces and raises the intriguing question of how the influx of other phagocytic cells is initiated and modulated.

Interplay between Alveolar Macrophages and Polymorphonuclear Granulocytes

Alveolar macrophages are the most numerous resident phagocytes present in the alveoli (about one cell per three to four alveoli). They are the bona fide first line of cellular defense on the air side of the lower respiratory tract. A few PMNs (about 1 per 100 alveoli), are present, but primarily they are reserve phagocytic cells held close by in the intra-vascular compartment. A plentiful supply of PMNs resides in the blood of lung capillaries as part of the body's pool of marginated PMNs. Even though PMNs are in close proximity to alveolar spaces, they are nonetheless separated by several planes of tissue: capillary endothelium, interstitial space, and alveolar epithelium. Depending on the species of bacteria that are inhaled into the lungs, alveolar macrophages and/or PMNs are selected to respond to the inoculum. Experimentally in mice, a small dose of aerosolized S. aureus is contained solely by macrophages, whereas Klebsiella and Pseudomonas evoke a PMN exudate in alveoli. To prove that PMNs were needed to defend against gram-negative bacilli, mice have been rendered selectively granulocytopenic and then challenged with aerosolized bacteria. As Klebsiella and Pseudomonas were cleared poorly, such experimental results indicate that circulating PMNs must be available to enter lung tissue and work with macrophages. Gram-negative bacteria seem to require more of a PMN phagocytic cell response for containment or clearance from the lungs than gram-positive species. Perhaps this is related to cell wall products, such as lipopolysaccharide endotoxin, that these gram-negative organisms contain or to the release of unidentified exotoxins. Certainly, patients and animal models that are immunosuppressed to the point that circulating blood PMN levels are low or absent are at significantly increased risk for infection, especially bacterial infection with aerobic gram-negative rods and with certain fungi such as Aspergillus species.

Many factors may govern the kinetics of the macrophage-PMN interchange in the lung. Certainly the species of organism, virulence, and inoculum size are all important for lung clearance in the normal, nonimmune animal or human. As the lung is capable of mounting an extensive inflammatory response, this is a potent mechanism to augment host defenses. The development of inflammatory response and hence pneumonia is a deliberate and controlled reaction in the lungs. When the pulmonary parenchyma mounts an extensive inflammatory response, it may be perceived as clinical illness, and a chest radiograph usually reveals an infiltrate.

Granulocyte movement into the alveoli is an orderly reaction initiated from the alveolar side. This is termed directed migration, or chemotaxis. At least two mechanisms for chemotactic activity that can set in motion the inflammatory response in the alveoli and amplify the PMN response. The first is best illustrated with the example of gram-negative rod bacteria known to contain endotoxins. Some complement components, particularly factor B, are present in small amounts in bronchoalveolar fluids. Bacterial endotoxin can directly activate the alternative complement pathway, leading to the formation of fragments such as C5a that are known to be potent stimulators of PMN chemotaxis. In addition, the inflammatory response may include activation of the kinin system. This could result in generation of kallikrein, which has chemotactic activity, and bradykinin, which is capable of increasing vascular permeability and could account for the accumulation of fluid and other humoral substances in alveoli that accompanies pneumonia. The second mechanism may emanate from the alveolar macrophage itself. Following phagocytosis of opsonized bacteria, or other forms of activation, chemotactic factors are synthesized and secreted that will selectively attract PMNs. Several substances with chemoattractant activity have been found to be produced by human alveolar macrophages. These include two low-molecular-weight proteins (one about 5000 daltons size and another <1000 daltons size) and lipoxygenase pathway metabolites of arachidonic acid, namely leukotrienes. Leukotriene B$_4$ is one of the most important of these.

Lymphocytes in the Alveolar Spaces

When cells are retrieved from the alveolar surface by bronchoalveolar lavage, about 7 to 10 percent of the respiratory cells are lymphocytes; characteristics of these cells are given in Table 86-1A and B. Two major populations of lymphoid cells are recognized, those that depend on the thymus gland for differentiation (T cells) and those that differentiate independently of thymus in the bone marrow (B cells). The T and B lymphocytes are indistinguishable by usual morphologic criteria but can be differentiated by membrane surface markers. The B cells serve as precursors for cells that synthesize immunoglobulins and, hence, antibody molecules that are the basis of humoral immunity. They have easily detectable surface immunoglobulin, a receptor for the third component of complement, and a receptor for the Fc portion of immunoglobulin.

The T lymphocytes perform functions associated with cell-mediated immunity. The characteristic adherence of sheep red blood cells to T cells generally identifies thymus-derived lymphocytes. Subsets of human T cells, as mentioned, can be identified with special mouse monoclonal antisera as T-suppressor-cytotoxic (CD8) cells or T-helper-inducer (CD4) cells. (CD is a cluster of differentiation antigen.) In the presence of specific antigen, immune or sensitized T lymphocytes synthesize and secrete a number of biologically active soluble factors (lymphokines) and, in an immunologically specific manner, can

TABLE 86-1A
T-Lymphocyte Subgroups in Lung Lavage Fluid from Normal Subjects

Fluid	Cell Count, $\times 10^6$	Lymphocytes, %	T Cells, %	T Helper, %	T Suppressor, %
Lung lavage*	$10 \pm 4\dagger$	7 ± 1	73 ± 5	46 (35–55)	25 (18–32)
Blood				48 (40–60)	28 (22–40)

*Cells from 300-ml lavages of six normal nonsmokers.

†Mean $\pm$ SEM, range observed in parentheses.

Source: From Hunninghake and Crystal, 1981.

TABLE 86-1B
Enumeration of Immunoglobulin-Secreting Cells in Lung Lavage from Normal Subjects

Fluid	IgG	IgA	IgM	IgE
Lung lavage*	489 (268–891)	633 (290–1380)	18 (2–144)	13† (2–83)
	175 (102–301)	100 (38–261)	32 (15–67)	0

*Geometric means are given for data from 12 normal volunteers. Numbers expressed per 10^6 lymphocytes; ranges appear in parentheses.

†Detected in only half of the subjects.

SOURCE: From Lawrence EC et al: J Clin Invest 62:832–835, 1978.

lyse cells that carry membrane antigens to which they are immune without the involvement of immunoglobulin or complement (cell-mediated cytotoxicity). The T lymphocytes can be identified by functional tests that measure their proliferative (blastogenic) response to mitogens such as phytohemagglutinins and concanavalin A or by various helper functions (inducing B cells to synthesize IgM) or suppressor activity.

As shown in Table 86-1A, about 70 percent of the lymphocytes in lavage fluid are T cells, and about 5 percent are B cells; the ratio of T to B cells in lavage fluid is roughly that of peripheral blood, although in blood more circulating B cells are identified (about 15 percent). Common to all lung lymphocyte studies is a significant proportion of cells that cannot be identified with the usual immune reagents; these are classified as null cells. Within the null cell group are natural killer lymphocytes (about 5 to 8 percent) that are not especially active in the normal lung. With phenotypic markers, the T cells can be divided into two principal groups, the helper-inducer lymphocytes and suppressor-cytotoxic lymphocytes. In normal individuals there is a greater percentage of T_H cells—about 45 percent of the total T cells versus approximately 25 percent T_S cells. The ratio of these subtypes of T cells is about 1.5 in lung lavage fluid, which is about the same as found among peripheral blood lymphocytes. About 1 to 5

percent of lung lymphocytes seem to be able to release or secrete class-specific immunoglobulin. Enumeration of these cells has found that IgG- and IgA-secreting cells are much more numerous than IgM-producing cells. Representative values are given in Table 86-1B.

As indicated above, alveolar macrophages and lymphocytes have the capacity to produce many cellular mediators that affect each other as well as other inflammatory or immune effector cells. This dynamic but complex interaction is illustrated in Fig. 86-2 which illustrates alveolar macrophage-lymphocyte interactions on the alveolar surface. As may be seen in this figure, monocyte precursors from the blood differentiate into mature macrophages under the influence of vitamin D metabolites and other unknown stimuli to become long-lived aerobic metabolizing phagocytes. Their most important activity is to scavenge the alveolar surface and ingest debris that accumulates there and microbes aerosolized or aspirated into the lungs. However, macrophages have the potential to become "activated" cells and then are capable of producing and secreting an enormous array of enzymes and cellular mediators. These *cytokines* can affect the function of other cells such as lymphocytes or release chemotactic factors that can attract polymorphonuclear neutrophils and lymphocytes in the alveoli. Of particular note as chemotactic agents are LTB_4 and IL-1 (interleukin 1); the latter, when secreted by activated macrophages (especially in active lung forms of sarcoidosis), may attract T lymphocytes to the lungs.

Among the populations of T lymphocytes in the alveoli, most are T-helper-inducer cells and a lesser percentage are T-suppressor-cytoxic lymphocytes; the normal ratio of helper-suppressor T lymphocytes is about 1.5. When activated, T-helper cells are capable of producing regulatory cytokines ("lymphokines") that are important in modulating the function of other immune cells. Interleukin 2 (IL-2) quantitatively seems most important. This substance has many identified functions. IL-2, formerly known as a T-cell growth factor (TCGF), can stimulate other T cells to proliferate and, thereby, expand clones of

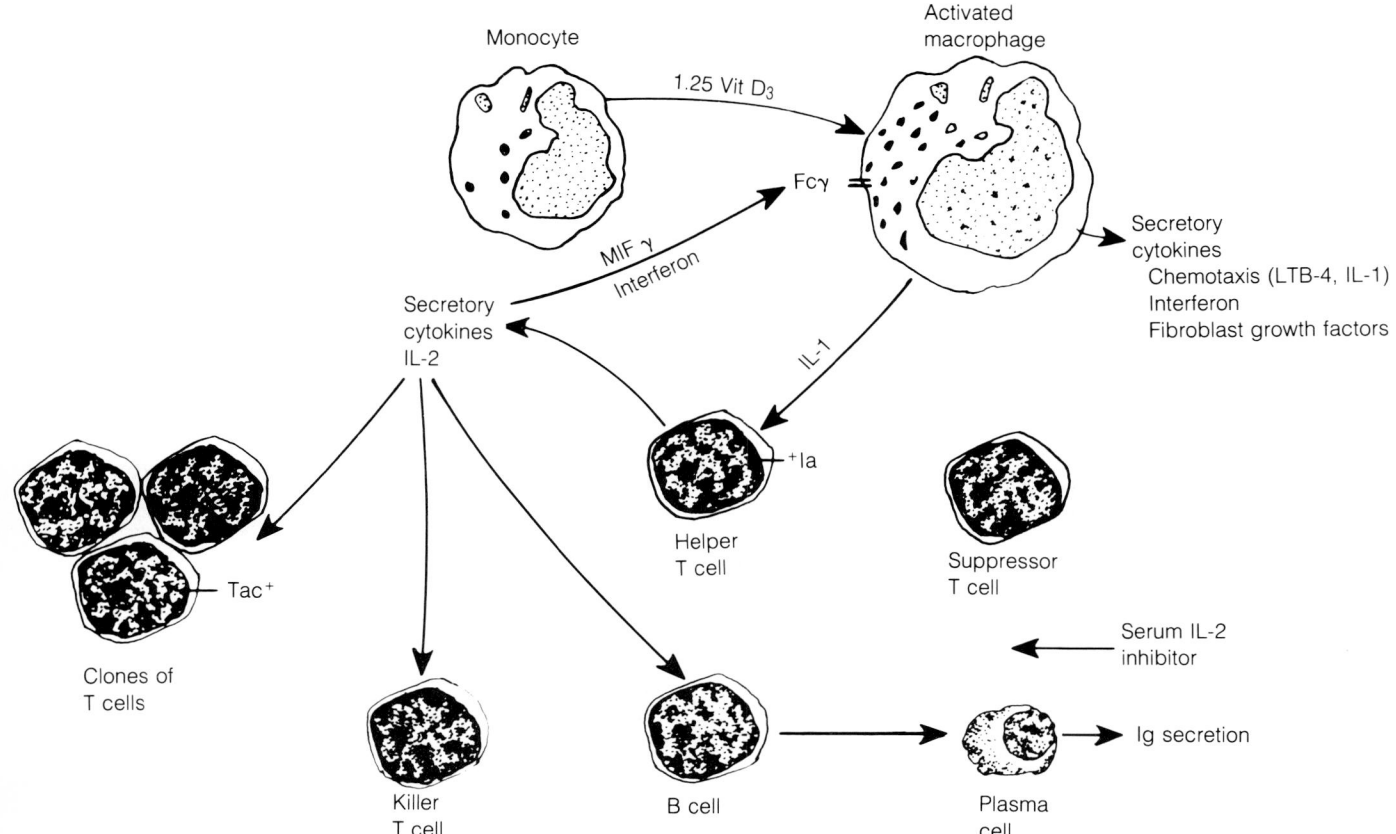

FIGURE 86-2 Immunologic interactions on the alveolar surface involving alveolar macrophages and lymphocytes.

lymphocytes. The receptor cells must have a Tac surface antigen (Tac⁺) to respond properly to IL-2. IL-2 can activate killer T cells. A few killer lymphocytes can be identified among the T-cell population in the alveoli, but these cells seem to be dormant in normal individuals until stimulated. IL-2 can stimulate B lymphocytes to turn into plasma cells that can, in turn, synthesize various classes of immunoglobulins. This is a mechanism by which local production of immunoglobulin (and antibodies) in the lung can occur.

In the other direction, activated T-helper cells can produce several monokines that affect macrophage function. Such a substance is migration inhibition factor (MIF) which may immobilize macrophages engaged in phagocytosis. Of special interest is γ-interferon, which seems to produce more Fc receptors on the macrophage's cell membrane; in turn, the increased number of Fc receptors enhances phagocytic uptake. γ-Interferon may have other functions as well that promote cellular immunity. The role of T-suppressor lymphocytes in these interactions is less clear: an array of specific mediators such as those attributed to T-helper lymphocytes has not been identified for T-suppressor lymphocytes. The scheme shown in Fig. 86-2 may help to explain certain derangements found in a number of lung diseases that have excessive or defi-

cient secretion of cellular monokines and lymphokines or feature changes in the relative proportions of lymphocytes. Examples of such cellular imbalances include sarcoidosis, hypersensitivity pneumonitis, and the acquired immunodeficiency syndrome.

POTENTIAL DEFECTS IN HOST DEFENSES THAT CAN BE ASSOCIATED WITH RESPIRATORY INFECTIONS

Infection can affect any portion of the respiratory tract—upper airways (nose, sinuses, and oropharynx), conducting airways (trachea down to the respiratory bronchioles), or the alveolar area. Exposure to a virulent microorganism or to a large inoculum, if inhaled or aspirated into the lungs, may cause illness in a normal person, but in many of the cases in which recurrent or chronic infection is a problem, the general apparatus at fault can be the pulmonary host defense system. Some malfunctioning or compromised component of this intricate defense system often can be correlated with a propensity for infection (Table 86-2). For example, an endotracheal tube allows direct access to the lung, bypassing the larynx and the other upper airway structures. If ciliary movement and clearance are impaired because viral or mycoplasma res-

1418

TABLE 86-2
Lung Host Defenses for Airway Challenge

Host Mechanism	Potential Defect	Impact and Potential Infection
Conducting Airways		
Mechanical barriers (larynx, pharynx, etc.)	Bypassing barriers with an endotracheal tube or tracheostomy	Aspiration, direct aerosol of microorganisms into airway
Mucociliary clearance (cough)	Intrinsic structural defect in cilia; ciliotoxic infections	Stagnant secretions, coughing, bronchiectasis, sinusitis
Bronchoconstriction	Hyperreactive airways; intrinsic asthma	Poor removal of secretions; excessive secretions
Local immunoglobulin coating— secretory IgA	IgA deficiency; functional deficiency from breakdown by bacterial IgA1 proteases	Sinopulmonary infections; abnormal colonization with bacteria
Iron-containing proteins (transferrin, lactoferrin)	Iron deficiency	May not inhibit certain bacteria (*Pseudomonas, Escherichia coli*)
Alveolar Milieu		
Other immunoglobulin classes (opsonic IgG)	Acquired hypogammaglobulinemia; selective IgG4 and IgG2 deficiency	Sinopulmonary infections; pneumonia with encapsulated bacteria
Alternative complement pathway activation	C3 and C5 deficiency	Trouble with infection but not life-threatening
Surfactant	Decreased synthesis; acute lung injury	Loss of opsonization activity; alveolar collapse (atelectasis)
Alveolar macrophages	Subtle effects from immunosuppression; cannot kill intracellular microbes	Propensity for *Pneumocystis* and *Legionella* infections; poor containment of mycobacterium
Polymorphonuclear granulocytes	Absent because of immunosuppression: intrinsic defects of motility; lack of chemotactic stimulus	Poor inflammatory response, associated with gram-negative bacillary infection and fungi (*Aspergillus*)
Augmenting Mechanisms		
Initiation of immune responses (humoral antibody and cellular immunity)	Immunosuppression	Inadequate SIgA or IgG antibody available (more susceptible to viral, mycoplasmal, and bacterial infections)
Generation of an inflammatory response (influx of PMN granulocytes, eosinophils, lymphocytes, and fluid components)	Generally reflects status and supply of PMN granulocytes; impaired adherence	Same as for PMN granulocytes; C5 deficiency might decrease inflammatory response

piratory infection has occurred—these microorganisms can be ciliotoxic and destroy these organelles or disrupt the epithelial cell—the removal of secretions can be impaired. Coughing is a means of compensating for poor ciliary clearance, however, and this may be one beneficial reason that frequent coughing persists as an aftermath of such infections. In a group of healthy students with minor viral upper respiratory infections, abnormalities in small airway lung function tests could be found up to 2 months after infection, indicating that the effects of even mild infection can be protracted. Moreover, viral particles perhaps contained within the infected airway epithelial cells can be aspirated into the alveoli and ingested by alveolar macrophages. When challenged with a bacterial species, concomitant infection of macrophages with virus can impair the bactericidal activity of macrophages resulting in poor killing of the bacteria. The aftermath of secondary bacterial pneumonia, often caused by staphylococci, fol-

lowing influenza infection, is well recognized. Thus, viruses may potentially damage two components of the host defense apparatus.

Defects in the ultrastructure of cilia located on the apical edge of the airway epithelial lining cells causes dyskinetic motion of cilia; removal of mucus and respiratory secretions is sluggish and ineffective. Occasionally, this will be the cause of bronchiectasis and a constellation of upper respiratory infections that comprise one of the hereditary syndromes of ciliary dyskinesis. Infertility especially in males may be associated, and the evaluation of this problem may bring the respiratory symptoms to the physician's attention. If the postoperative patient, perhaps because of abdominal pain or depressed consciousness, cannot cough well, secretions accumulate in the airways.

In patients with hypogammaglobulinemia or dysgammaglobulinemia, the absence of opsonic antibody can fos-

ter infections with encapsulated bacteria. A number of common bacteria that colonize the airways of patients with chronic bronchitis and chronic obstructive pulmonary disease (COPD) usually associated with cigarette smoking, can elaborate a specific IgA protease directed toward cleaving the α_1 form of the IgA heavy chain in its hinge region adjacent to the Fc portion. These bacteria are *Streptococcus pneumoniae* and *Hemophilus influenzae*; *Neisseria* species can also secrete an IgA1 proteolytic enzyme. This is a potential mechanism by which bacteria could inactivate a substantial portion of secretory IgA coating the conducting airways and perhaps gain better access to the ciliated epithelial cells for attachment. While this mechanism is somewhat theoretical and not quantitative, deficiencies in IgG, especially IgG subclasses IgG2 and IgG4 in combination (often with IgA also) or IgG4 alone, are well correlated with respiratory infections and chronic inflammation contributing to bronchiectasis. Presumably an absence of these subclasses denies phagocytic cells the potential of opsonic antibody which enhances the membrane attachment of opsonized particles or bacteria and promotes ingestion. The process of phagocytosis and dependence on opsonins is now quite complex, and other elements in the alveolar milieu and lining fluid may be essential also. These other factors include certain complement components (C3b), large size fragments of fibronectin, lipoproteins associated with surfactant and cytophilic IgG subclasses that reside in the macrophages' cell membrane. As a practical consideration, it should be remembered that the IgG2 subclass may contain antibodies that are especially helpful in warding off certain infections, for antibodies made to polysaccharide antigens, as found in *Streptococcus* and *Hemophilus* species, and to teichoic acid, as present in staphylococci, exist within the IgG2 subclass. Possibly antibodies to lipopolysaccharides, as contained in the cell walls of gram-negative bacilli such as *Pseudomonas* and *Klebsiella* species, are also of this subclass. The diagnosis, therefore, of an IgG deficiency is quite important for the recent availability of intravenous preparations of IgG make selective replacement therapy a reality for these patients. Cytotoxic antineoplastic chemotherapy and other forms of immunosuppression can produce granulocytopenia, which prevents the mobilization of PMNs and creation of a good inflammatory reaction. All these deficiencies in pulmonary host defense, whether acquired or inherent, are associated with obvious syndromes of respiratory infection. Moreover, the normal person without antecedent lung disease is equally at risk for the development of infection under some of the circumstances just discussed.

In adults, the reason for having a respiratory tract infection is often obvious: chronic bronchitis, aggravated by cigarette smoking, or chronic obstructive lung disease. Occasionally, however, the physician is confronted with a relatively young person who has an unexpected number of respiratory problems which seem inappropriate. The problem may not be an overt lung infection. It may be a cough and excessive sputum, poorly controlled allergic rhinitis, asthma, frequent sinusitis, recurrent nasal polyps, and bouts of otitis media. Because the severity of these respiratory problems may not seem great, they may not readily alert the physician that something unusual is present. But the physician should be prepared to evaluate this type of patient thoroughly. A propensity for infection may not have been obvious in childhood but became apparent in the patient's teens or early 20s. Because genetic defects usually are manifested in infancy, this patient's situation may suggest falsely that the defect is not genetic. That assessment may not be accurate, because subtle or minor forms of host deficiency disease are being recognized increasingly in adults. Diseases such as cystic fibrosis, selective absence of IgG subclass immunoglobulin, structural defects in cilia, and possibly IgA deficiency are the diseases that should be considered in a differential diagnosis. Other very rare problems relating to poor granulocyte motility and a deficiency in the complement cascade may need consideration as well. Recurrent respiratory infections often provide the clue to all these syndromes.

Thus, to summarize, a combination of upper respiratory tract infections and lower airway infections (bronchitis or pneumonia) indicates the possibility of several immunodeficiency syndromes that are not found exclusively in the pediatric age group but can exist in young adults as mild, heterozygous, nonlethal forms of disease. As mentioned, possible diseases include cystic fibrosis, defects in the mucociliary clearance apparatus or dyskinetic ciliary syndromes, acquired hypogammaglobulinemia, and dysfunction of phagocytic cell killing or motility (responsiveness to chemoattractant stimuli). A detailed patient history can immediately provide important information about affected siblings, infertility, or a striking change in respiratory health that makes an acquired abnormality likely. Preliminary screening tests also are indicated and usually include: microbial cultures of respiratory secretions (of particular interest would be the isolation of a mucoid strain of *P. aeruginosa*); analysis of electrolytes contained in a sample of sweat (ionoelectrophoresis method); quantitative serum immunoglobulins, including subclasses of IgG; secretory IgA as sampled in parotid fluid or nasal wash samples; subtyping blood lymphocytes; assessing ciliary clearance with an aerosol, isotopic tracer method; a nasal mucosal biopsy for electron-microscopy views of ciliary cross sections to define ultrastructure; sperm motility in males of appropriate age; and documentation of the extent of bronchiectasis by CT scanning of the chest or possibly fiberoptic bronchoscopy and selective bronchorrhaphy. A thorough evaluation by an ear, nose, and throat specialist is often helpful because of the recurrent sinusitis, otitis media, and nasal polyps that might be present.

In a different context certain forms of pneumonia il-

lustrate possible deficiencies in other lung cells such as alveolar macrophages, lymphocytes, or PMNs. As opsonization of certain encapsulated bacteria is necessary for optimal phagocytosis by macrophages and PMNs, the lack of appropriate IgG antibodies against pneumococci, *Hemophilus* species, and staphylococci may contribute to infections with these common bacteria. However, some other microbial causes of pneumonia may be related to lymphocyte function and cell-mediated immunity. Infection with *Legionella* bacteria will illustrate this point. After an infection with *L. pneumophila,* which causes the majority of lung infections among this genus of bacteria, the host develops specific IgM and IgG serum antibodies. However, subjecting the organisms to a mixture of specific antibody plus complement in vitro does not create a lytic state for the bacteria that is sufficient to kill them. However, the availability of these opsonins does ensure that the *Legionella* organisms can attach and be ingested by various phagocytic cells including PMNs, blood monocytes, and alveolar macrophages, but once inside the phagocytes, *Legionella* multiply without impedence and eventually kill and disrupt the host cells. However, immune lymphocytes can be taken from a subject who has successfully weathered a *Legionella* infection and stimulated to produce lymphokines in their cell culture medium (now identified as γ-interferon). Then the lymphokine mediators can be reacted with virgin phagocytes to energize them, i.e., activate the cells through cellular immunity. Now such stimulated phagocytes after ingesting the *Legionella* inoculum will contain the growth of the bacteria within themselves and thus cope with the infection, although they are not actually able to kill the bacteria. Immunomodulation to create cell-mediated immunity would seem to be an important factor in optimizing lung host defense by macrophages and PMNs and perhaps preventing recurrent infection. These mechanisms are similar in concept to other situations involving facultative intracellular microbes including mycobacterial species.

Another contemporary example is the acquired immunodeficiency syndrome (AIDS) in which the human host is infected with a retrovirus (HIV) that has a propensity to destroy certain subpopulations of T lymphocytes, namely, the T cells belonging to the inducer-helper subset. The patients may have a number of respiratory infections, involving organisms such as viruses (cytomegalovirus or herpes simplex), *Pneumocystis carinii, Mycobacterium tuberculosis* or *avium-intracellulare,* and fungi (*Cryptococcus* species) and much less infrequently with *Toxoplasma gondii* and *Legionella.* Most of these infectious agents have the common requirement to reside in a macrophage or similar cell as a facultatively dependent intracellular organism. Just why the AIDS victim should have such trouble with this group of infections is not certain, but a possible explanation may involve the relative imbalance of lymphocytes found in the alveoli, as sampled by bronchoalveolar lavage of the lung. Normal values for T lymphocytes have been given in Table 86-1. In AIDS patients, the recoverable alveolar lymphocytes reflect a decrease in the T-helper variety from HIV infection; however, there is a surprising increase in the suppressor-cytotoxic specie of T lymphocytes. Thus, the alveolar macrophage may exist in an environment where it cannot be activated sufficiently, i.e., induction of cell-mediated immunity, to contain or kill organisms such as *Pneumocystis* or *Mycobacterium.* A kind of double suppressor effect may exist. Macrophages themselves tend to have suppressive function for they are not especially good cells for producing or sustaining proliferative responses by lymphocytes when co-cultured with them under cell culture conditions. In the situation of AIDS, there is an additional decrease in T-helper lymphocytes that ordinarily might help active macrophages through various monokines (Fig. 86-2) such as γ interferon and migration inhibition factor. This is coupled with a relative increase in T-suppressor lymphocytes that probably dampens further macrophage function. The net effect may be a macrophage that cannot be activated nor respond appropriately to cellular stimuli that are needed to optimize its intracellular antimicrobial processes. AIDS patients suffer chronic and repeated respiratory infections which ultimately are usually quite significant in determining the morbidity and mortality of the syndrome.

BIBLIOGRAPHY

Beck CS, Heiner DC: Selective immunoglobulin G$_4$ deficiency and recurrent infections of the respiratory tract. Am Rev Respir Dis 124:94–96, 1981.
  IgG4 seems quite necessary to prevent respiratory infections.

Brieland JK, Kunkel RG, Fantone JC: Pulmonary alveolar macrophage function during acute inflammatory lung injury. Am Rev Respir Dis 135:1300–1306, 1987.
  Pulmonary alveolar macrophages from injured lungs enhance mechanisms responsible for induction of oxidase activity, and changes in their functional responses may be important in the mediation and resolution of acute inflammatory lung injury.

Clark JG, Greenberg J: Modulation of the effects of alveolar macrophages on lung fibroblast collagen production rate. Am Rev Respir Dis 135:52–56, 1987.
  Alveolar macrophages (AM) may function as effector cells that can either stimulate or inhibit lung fibroblast collagen production.

Czopp JK, McGowan SE, Center DM: Opsonin-independent phagocytosis by human alveolar macrophages: Augmentation by human plasma fibronectin. Am Rev Respir Dis 125:607–609, 1982.
   Optimal phagocytosis requires many factors, some nonimmune, as well as specific antibodies.

Elias JA, Jimenez SA, Freundlich B: Recombinant gamma, alpha, and beta interferon regulation of human lung fibroblast proliferation. Am Rev Respir Dis 135:62–65, 1987.
   A study designed to understand the processes controlling tissue fibrosis by characterizing the effect of recombinant gamma, alpha$_A$, alpha$_D$, and beta interferons on the proliferation of slowly and rapidly proliferating normal human lung fibroblasts.

Etzkorn ET, Lillis PK, McAllister CK: Tuberculosis in Korea. The relationship between prior therapy and drug resistance. Chest 90:247–250, 1986.
   A review of 121 culture-positive cases of pulmonary tuberculosis from 1979 to 1984, including both Korean and American patients, at the major US military hospital in Korea indicated that most antituberculosis drug resistance occurred in patients with a history of previous antituberculosis therapy.

Fick RB Jr, Reynolds HY: Changing spectrum of pneumonia—News media creation or clinical reality? Am J Med 74:1–8, 1983.
   As title implies, new forms of pneumonia in more immunoderanged hosts.

Haslam PL, Dewar A, Butchers P, Primett ZS, Newman-Taylor A, Turner-Warwick M: Mast cells, atypical lymphocytes, and neutrophils in bronchoalveolar lavage in extrinsic allergic alveolitis: Comparison with other interstitial lung diseases. Am Rev Respir Dis 135:35–47, 1987.
   Extrinsic allergic alveolitis (idiopathic pulmonary fibrosis) may provide an example of a human disease in which delayed hypersensitivity disorders involve mast cells as well as lymphocytes.

Hollsing AE, Granstrom M, Vasil ML, Wretlind B, Strandvik B: Prospective study of serum antibodies to *Pseudomonas aeruginosa* exoproteins in cystic fibrosis. J Clin Microbiol 25:1868–1874, 1987.
   Serum immunoglobulin G to four purified antigens from Pseudomonas aeruginosa were determined in 62 patients with cystic fibrosis by enzyme-linked immunosorbent assay. Titers of serum antibody to phospholipase C seem to be a reliable indicator of chronic colonization with P. aeruginosa.

Holter W, Goldman CK, Casabo L, Nelson DL, Greene WC, Waldmann TA: Expression of functional IL 2 receptors by lipopolysaccharide and interferon-gamma stimulated human monocytes. J Immunol 138:2917–2922, 1987.
   The induction of monocytic IL 2 receptors by lipopolysaccharide may point to a functional role for this receptor during monocyte/macrophage responses to microbial infections.

Horwitz MA: Cell-mediated immunity in Legionnaires' disease. J Clin Invest 71:1686–1697, 1983.
   Preliminary review for paper by Nash et al.

Hunninghake GW, Crystal RG: Pulmonary sarcoidosis: A disorder mediated by excess helper T-lymphocyte activity at sites of disease activity. N Engl J Med 305:429–434, 1981.
   Normal values for T-lymphocyte subsets were established.

Jakab GJ: Mechanisms of virus-induced bacterial superinfections of the lung. Clin Chest Med 2:59–66, 1981.
   Review of animal research by a leading contributor to this topic.

Kallenberg CG, Schilizzi BM, Beaumont F, De Leij L, Poppema S, The TH: Expression of class II major histocompatibility complex antigens on alveolar epithelium in interstitial lung disease: relevance to pathogenesis of idiopathic pulmonary fibrosis. J Clin Pathol 40:725–733, 1987.
   Class II antigens are expressed not only on alveolar epithelium that is infiltrated by T8 cells in interstitial pulmonary fibrosis but also in the interstitial pulmonary disease caused by sarcoidosis and microbial infections.

Little JW, Hall WJ, Douglas RG Jr, Mudholkar GS, Speers DM, Patel K: Airway hyperreactivity and peripheral airway dysfunction in influenza A infection. Am Rev Respir Dis 118:295–303, 1978.
   Impact of mild viral disease on the lower respiratory tract lasts longer than expected.

Merrill WW, Naegel GP, Olchowski JJ, Reynolds HY: Immunoglobulin G subclass proteins in serum and lavage fluid of normal subjects: quantitation and comparison with immunoglobulins A and E. Am Rev Respir Dis 131:584–591, 1985.
   IgG subclasses are of increasing interest in lung diseases.

Monick M, Glazier J, Hunninghake GW: Human alveolar macrophages suppress interleukin-1 (IL-1) activity via the secretion of prostaglandin E$_2$. Am Rev Respir Dis 135:72–77, 1987.
   The apparent defect in the release of IL-1 by human alveolar macrophages may be due in part to the release of large amounts of PGE$_2$, which suppresses various lymphocyte functions.

Mulks MH, Kornfeld SW, Plaut AG: Specific proteolysis of human IgA by *Streptococcus pneumoniae* and *Haemophilus influenzae.* J Infect Dis 141:450–456, 1980.
  Specific cleavage of α heavy chain by bacterial proteases.

Naegel GP, Young KR, Reynolds HY: Receptors for human IgG subclasses on human alveolar macrophages. Am Rev Respir Dis 129:413–418, 1984.
  More details about IgG receptors.

Nardell E, McInnis B, Thomas B, Weidhaas S: Exogenous reinfection with tuberculosis in a shelter for the homeless. N Engl J Med 315:1570–1575, 1986.
  An investigation of an outbreak of tuberculosis in a large shelter for the homeless to assess the role of exogenous reinfection as opposed to reactivation of endogenous infection as the cause of secondary tuberculosis in this population. Exogenous reinfection may have been an important factor in this highly susceptible population.

Nash TW, Libby DM, Horwitz MA: Interaction between the Legionnaires' disease bacterium (*Legionella pneumophila*) and human alveolar macrophages. J Clin Invest 74:771–782, 1984.
  Makes case for cellular-mediated immune activation of macrophages to help contain Legionella organisms.

Nathan CF: Secretory products of macrophages. J Clin Invest 79:319–326, 1987.
  A comprehensive review of the role played by the secretions of macrophage in the response to injury.

Peck R: Neuropeptides modulating macrophage function. Ann NY Acad Sci 496:264–270, 1987.
  Neuroendocrine hormones may act either positively or negatively in regulating the activities of the macrophage.

Reynolds HY: Lung host defenses: A status report. Chest 75S:239–242, 1979.
  Author's initial summary on topic.

Reynolds HY: Lung inflammation: Role of endogenous chemotactic factors that attract polymorphonuclear granulocytes. Am Rev Respir Dis 127:516–525, 1983.
  Reviews kinetics of lung inflammatory response.

Reynolds HY: Respiratory infections may reflect deficiencies in host defense mechanisms. Disease-A-Month 31:1–98, 1985.
  More in-depth presentation of the topic.

Reynolds HY: Lung inflammation: Normal host defense or a complication of some diseases? Ann Rev Med 38:295–323, 1987.
  Several examples of diseases that feature inflammation as part of their pathophysiology have been selected for this review, i.e., asthma, chronic bronchitis, interstitial lung diseases, and acute lung injury leading to adult respiratory distress syndrome.

Reynolds HY, Chrétien J: Respiratory tract fluids: Analysis of content and contemporary use in understanding lung diseases. Disease-A-Month 30:1–103, 1984.
  Contains baseline values for cells and proteins in respiratory secretions and the alveoli (sampled by lung lavage).

Reynolds HY, Atkinson JP, Newball HH, Frank M: Receptors for immunoglobulin and complement on human alveolar macrophages. J Immunol 114:1813–1819, 1975.
  Details about macrophage receptors.

Rossman CM, Forrest JB, Lee RM, Newhouse MT: The dyskinetic cilia syndrome: Ciliary motility in immotile cilia syndrome. Chest 78:580–582, 1980.
  Reviews topic and outlines defects.

Seligmann M, Pinching AJ, Rosen FS, Fahey JL, Khaitov RM, Klatzmann D, Koenig S, Luo N, Ngu J, Reithmuller G et al: Immunology of human immunodeficiency virus infection and the acquired immunodeficiency syndrome—an update. Ann Intern Med 107:234–242, 1987.
  Recent advances in the understanding of the pathogenesis of infection with human immunodeficiency virus (HIV) stems from the demonstration that the membrane glycoprotein, CD4, is the cellular receptor for HIV. This glycoprotein is found mainly on the surface of a major subpopulation of T lymphocytes and also on macrophages, natural killer cells, some B lymphocytes, and neuronal cells.

Spurzem JR, Saltini C, Rom W, Winchester RJ, Crystal RG: Mechanisms of macrophage accumulation in the lungs of asbestos-exposed subjects. Am Rev Respir 136:276–280, 1987.
  Both enhanced recruitment of blood monocytes and increased local proliferation of alveolar macrophages contibute to the accumulation of mononuclear phagocytes in the lung of persons with chronic asbestos exposure.

Tomassi TB Jr: Mechanisms of immune regulation at mucosal surfaces. Rev Infect Dis 5:S784–S792, 1983.
  Status of IgA reviewed by person who initially investigated it.

Wallace JM, Barbers RG, Oishi JS, Prince H: Cellular and T-lymphocyte subpopulation profiles in bronchoalveolar lavage fluid from patients with acquired immunodeficiency syndrome and pneumonitis. Am Rev Respir Dis 130:786–790, 1984.
  Immunology of AIDS lung disease presented.

Young KR, Rankin JA, Naegel GP, Paul ES, Reynolds HY: Bronchoalveolar lavage cells and proteins in patients with the acquired immunodeficiency syndrome: An immunologic analysis. Ann Intern Med 103:522–533, 1985.
  Immunology of AIDS lung disease presented.

Chapter 87

Bacterial Colonization of the Respiratory Tract

Waldemar G. Johanson, Jr.

Definitions

The term *colonization* refers to the persistence of microorganisms at a particular site. Some sites within the respiratory tract are normally colonized by certain species of bacteria. Colonization is considered abnormal when bacteria are present which are highly likely to cause disease or when normally sterile regions are colonized. The distinctions between colonization phenomena which are normal and those which are not and between colonization and infection are often difficult to make.

DEFINITIONS

Colonization can be defined as the persistence of bacteria at a body site without evidence of a host response. *Infection* implies either a host response or evidence of injury to host tissues. Presence and persistence of the bacteria are easy to demonstrate. The problem with these definitions lies in the *host response*. For example, normal people may have local and/or circulating antibody against bacteria which have colonized their oropharynx, certainly evidence of a host response. Patients who have been endotracheally intubated for respiratory failure often demonstrate bacteria persistently in tracheal secretions in the presence of neutrophils. Does this indicate infection or merely colonization? Also, the term *persistence* in this context means continual presence over some period of time. What is the period of time? It is known that some individuals may harbor pathogenic strains of *Streptococcus pneumoniae*—especially type 3—in their upper respiratory tracts for years in the absence of infection and that some individuals appear to be lifelong nasal carriers of *Staphylococcus aureus*. On the other hand, acquisition of these organisms and persistence for even a brief time by other individuals may pose a substantial risk of infection. As a practical matter, we are usually concerned with colonization over brief periods in clinical medicine; colonization is considered to have occurred if the same bacterial species are identified at a site in two cultures, or even in a single culture if one can reasonably expect their continual presence if a second culture were obtained a day later.

SITES OF COLONIZATION AND THE NORMAL FLORA

Organisms which infect the lungs often enter the body via the mouth and oropharynx. Therefore, for the purposes of this chapter, the mouth and oropharynx are considered to be part of the upper respiratory tract.

The mouth and oropharynx are heavily colonized by certain species of bacteria. The level of contamination can be easily demonstrated by quantitative cultures of saliva which typically contains 10^8 to 10^9 aerobic bacteria per milliliter and about equal numbers of anaerobic species. The anterior nares and nasal passages are less heavily contaminated but are universally colonized with bacteria. Organisms which are commonly isolated from these sites are listed in Table 87-1.

Despite their contiguity with the nasal passages, the paranasal sinuses are normally sterile. Bacteria are infrequently found distal to the vocal cords in normal people, and the airways and lung distal to the carina are considered to be normally sterile. The mechanisms which maintain the sterility of these regions, despite their proximity to massive bacterial contamination, are known collectively as host defenses and are discussed elsewhere in this text (see Chapter 86). This chapter focuses on the mechanism of bacterial colonization and its significance in the pathogenesis of respiratory infections.

TABLE 87-1

Bacteria Which Colonize the Normal Upper Respiratory Tract

Streptococcus viridans
Streptococcus pyogenes
Streptococcus pneumoniae
Staphylococci, including *S. aureus*
Neisseria species
Branhamella catarrhalis
Hemophilus species, including *H. influenzae*
Lactobacilleae
Corynebacteria
Various obligate anaerobes

The fundamental problem facing those who want to define the bacterial flora of a region of the body is sampling. Certainly in the case of the respiratory tract the possibility for contamination of samples obtained from distal airways or lung by proximal secretions is large since most samples are obtained with instruments which pass through the nose or mouth. Further, since most such instrumentation requires at least topical anesthesia, aspiration of oropharyngeal contents may produce positive cultures from sites which were sterile prior to the sampling procedure.

On the other hand, small numbers of bacteria are present in ambient air and are inhaled into the lung periphery. Oropharyngeal secretions are regularly aspirated into the tracheobronchial tree by healthy persons, at least during sleep. However, lung antibacterial defenses are highly efficient, and viable bacteria which are introduced into the lungs tend to be swiftly inactivated and/or removed so that the number of viable organisms which remain diminishes rapidly. Thus, the results of one sample at one point in time represents the interplay of all these factors: artifacts induced by sampling, ongoing inoculation by inhalation or aspiration, and bacterial clearance processes.

These considerations explain the occasional recovery of bacteria from aseptically resected lung tissue or aseptically sampled distal airways in healthy persons. The bulk of the evidence suggests that these regions are usually sterile in normal individuals; if bacteria are present, they are those of the upper respiratory tract representing recent contamination, and they do not persist.

CHARACTERISTICS OF THE NORMAL FLORA

The initial bacterial flora of the upper respiratory tract is acquired within the first few days of life from the infant's environment, including his or her attendants. Thereafter, the bacterial flora tends to demonstrate the characteristics listed in Table 87-2. Despite the incredible array of bacteria in nature, only a few species are found commonly in the human respiratory tract. Further, while humans show a high degree of similarity among individuals for broad groups of organisms, the exact strains and proportion of various strains which make up the normal flora differ widely among healthy people but tend to remain quite

TABLE 87-2
Characteristics of the Normal Bacterial Flora
Restricted variety of organisms present
Composition resistant to change in an individual
Varies among regions of the upper respiratory tract
Excluded from some contiguous sites, e.g., paranasal sinuses, airways

constant over time for a single individual. Certain organisms, such as *Hemophilus influenzae*, are readily acquired by most members of a family following introduction by one family member. Other organisms, such as β-hemolytic streptococci, are much less likely to be shared while others, such as gram-negative bacilli, are almost never found in other family members when one individual is colonized.

In addition, rather marked differences in bacterial flora exist between geographic regions of the upper respiratory tract in a single individual. For example, *Streptococcus mutans* is regularly present in dental plaque but absent from the dorsum of the tongue, while the reverse pattern is characteristic of *Streptococcus salivarius*.

These observations suggest that maintenance of the normal flora is not a happenstance. Rather, powerful selective processes appear to be operative which determine both the composition of the normal bacterial flora and its geographic extent in the respiratory tract. These are the factors which determine colonization. Further, it is alterations in these factors which cause the abnormal patterns of colonization which are often associated with disease.

DETERMINANTS OF THE NORMAL FLORA

A variety of hypotheses have been advanced in attempts to explain the normal flora. The physiochemical milieu of the oropharynx may certainly explain why a number of bacterial species fail to colonize human hosts. These considerations are of undoubted importance in understanding why anaerobic bacteria flourish in the gingival crevices but fail to colonize exposed mucosal surfaces. They do not, on the other hand, explain why one individual carries *S. aureus* in his nose while another does not, or why certain species of aerobic bacteria persist in one human host while others predominate in a different individual. Physiochemical properties such as pH, redox potential, or availability of certain nutrients explain a small but important fraction of the observations in question.

Bacterial interference refers to the laboratory, and possibly clinical, phenomenon in which one bacterial species inhibits the growth of another. Known mechanisms underlying this observation include the preferential consumption of essential nutrients by one species and elaboration of one of a variety of antibacterial substances by certain species. Even though bacterial interference has been studied in vitro for more than 100 years, its significance in vivo remains largely speculative. Some years ago it was noted that intentional colonization of newborn infants with an avirulent strain of *S. aureus*, 502A, tended to diminish colonization and infection by highly pathogenic strains of *S. aureus*. Attempts to prevent postoperative oropharyngeal colonization with gram-negative bacilli associated with antimicrobial therapy by manipulation of

the normal flora have been reported. Many organisms contained in the normal flora are capable of inhibiting the growth of gram-negative bacilli in vitro, and penicillin therapy markedly reduces the number of these inhibitory organisms and was associated with gram-negative colonization in vivo. Penicillin resistance was induced in the normal flora by administering small doses of this drug preoperatively; these resistant inhibitory organisms persisted despite high doses of penicillin postoperatively, and colonization by gram-negative bacilli was diminished. Neither follow-up nor confirmatory studies of those interesting observations have been reported.

If bacterial interference is important in vivo, one would expect that alteration of the existing flora by antimicrobial therapy would lead to long-lasting changes in the normal flora; such are not observed. It is probable that this phenomenon plays little role in determining the normal flora.

The concept that the normal flora may be regulated by selective adherence of only certain bacteria to regional epithelial cells is relatively recent but is supported by a variety of observations. Members of the normal flora adhere in large numbers to normal oropharyngeal cells during incubation in vitro, whereas other bacteria do not. Further, cells recovered from different regions of the mouth and oropharynx adhere organisms in vitro in similar proportions to that found by culturing the region in vivo. Alterations of the host which cause increased adherence of certain organisms such as gram-negative bacilli in vitro are associated with a markedly increased risk of colonization with the same organisms in vivo. Finally, epithelial cell adherence of bacteria has been extensively studied in the gut and urinary tract. The accumulated evidence strongly suggests that this does represent an important, if not essential, step in the establishment of a new microbial flora.

Unfortunately, bacterial adherence to mammalian epithelial cells appears to occur through a broad variety of binding mechanisms. In general, bacterial binding sites are located on appendages called *fimbriae* in gram-positive organisms and *pili* in gram-negative bacilli, but non-pili-associated binding of the latter has been described as well. However, binding mechanisms differ for most of the species which have been studied and, in some bacteria, multiple mechanisms may coexist. For example, *Escherichia coli* is known to adhere to cells via mannose-sensitive and mannose-resistant ligands on pili and by a third ligand which is not associated with pili. In some situations there appears to be a reciprocal relationship between the adherence of two differing bacterial species in that cells which adhere many of one species will adhere few of the other and vice versa. This appears to be especially true of streptococci and *E. coli*. In that instance, streptococci bind via a lipoteichoic acid ligand to fibronectin on the epithelial surface; *E. coli* does not bind to fibronectin and,

if this protein is on the cell surface, cellular adherence is prevented. If cell-surface fibronectin is absent or diminished, streptococci do not adhere, but *E. coli* is able to bind directly to the cell surface. The widely varying nature of the bacterial cell adherence process in the upper respiratory tract makes it unlikely that manipulation of this mechanism will prove to be clinically useful. In the urinary tract, however, and perhaps at other sites where a limited variety of organisms are important, immunization with bacterial adhesins appears to provide protection against colonization and infection.

Bacterial binding to the various cell types which may be present in the normal upper respiratory tract has received relatively little attention but may prove to be of fundamental importance in understanding these complex interactions. Fibronectin accumulates on the surface of squamous cells as the latter mature and become keratinized. Bacteria which bind to cell surface fibronectin become more numerous as a consequence of cell age, whereas other bacterial species may predominate if epithelial cell turnover is high. *N. meningitides* binds only to nonciliated cells in the nasopharynx, although colonization with these organisms produces a marked toxic effect on ciliated cells as well. In contrast, *Bordetella pertussis* and *Mycoplasma pneumoniae* bind selectively to the cilia of respiratory cells. Observations such as these suggest that the interactions between bacterial adhesins and respiratory cell surface receptors are both highly specific but widely variable among organisms which may inhibit the respiratory tract.

BACTERIAL COLONIZATION AND INFECTION

Bacterial infections of the respiratory tract may follow inoculation by bloodborne or airborne bacteria. In these situations prior colonization of the upper respiratory tract is unimportant, if it occurs at all. However, the great majority of bacterial infections are preceded by colonization by the offending bacterium prior to the onset of invasive disease. Two patterns of colonization are important to consider: (1) colonization of usually contaminated sites in previously healthy individuals by highly virulent organisms, and (2) colonization of persons with underlying disease by any of a variety of organisms, not necessarily those possessing great virulence. In the latter circumstance, the extent of colonization often includes normally sterile sites.

Colonization of Normal Individuals by Highly Virulent Organisms

Several organisms might serve as examples of this interaction: *Neisseria meningitides*, *Streptococcus hemolyticus*, and probably *Streptococcus pneumoniae*. Although long-

term colonization of healthy individuals with each of these organisms is known to occur, outbreaks of acute disease also occur and can be traced to transmission of organisms from person to person. The role of adherence in colonization by such organisms is controversial. Highly virulent respiratory pathogens are typically encapsulated, and the presence of an extracellular capsule markedly diminishes adherence to epithelial cells in vitro. Thus, several investigators have found that avirulent, nonencapsulated mutants adhere more readily to respiratory epithelial cells than do encapsulated strains associated with infections. Further, using labeled antibody against capsular antigens, pneumococci were rarely found on the surface of regional epithelial cells, even in individuals who were demonstrably colonized by usual cultural techniques. These observations have been used to suggest that epithelial cell adherence is not an important factor in colonization by these organisms.

Recent evidence shows that virulent organisms can switch the production of both extracellular appendages and capsular material off and on with incredible rapidity. Loss of the capsule and production of pili or fimbriae would facilitate mucosal adherence. On the other hand, presence of the capsule confers resistance against host defenses, especially phagocytes, and would promote tissue invasion. An interesting series of experiments with *N. meningitides* supports this sequence of events. Although encapsulated strains adhere poorly to nasopharyngeal cells in vitro, organisms incubated with small explants of nasopharyngeal mucosa adhere and penetrate the epithelium.

Colonization of Persons with Underlying Disease

In this situation the properties of the responsible organism are of less importance than the altered state of the host. Abnormal colonization patterns are commonly observed in the presence of either acute or chronic underlying disease and may be manifested by the presence of organisms normally excluded from the respiratory tract or the presence of organisms at sites which are normally sterile.

The propensity of bacterial infections to develop on the background of a respiratory viral infection may be in part related to such phenomena. Infection of cells in tissue culture with influenza A virus markedly increases their adherence of *S. aureus*. Disruption of the airway epithelium by influenza infection in vivo exposes sites to which bacteria adhere readily in contrast to the resistance of the normal epithelium.

Gram-negative enteric bacilli infrequently colonize the upper respiratory tracts of healthy individuals but are found in most individuals with serious, life-threatening illnesses. The frequency of colonization of elderly people parallels their degree of chronic disability. Colonization by gram-negative bacilli correlates well with the degree to which these organisms adhere to respiratory epithelial cells in vitro: cells obtained from colonized individuals adhere large numbers, while cells from noncolonized people do not. Binding sites for gram-negative bacilli appear to be present on normal respiratory squamous cells since enzymatic treatment of such cells in vitro markedly increases bacillary adherence. It appears that fibronectin, a large protein molecule which is normally present on the surface of these cells, protects these binding sites. Cells from colonized individuals are deficient in fibronectin, a finding which may be related to the proteolytic activity of secretions.

Patients with chronic bronchitis may demonstrate a persistent bacterial flora in distal airways, as demonstrated some years ago with meticulous techniques to avoid contamination. The mechanisms underlying this observation have received little attention. It seems likely that adherence of the responsible organisms to sites in distal airways is involved, but this is an unproven hypothesis. Increased adherence could be related to the development of islands of squamous epithelium, loss of ciliary activity, or alterations in secretion. A similar occurrence of chronic colonization of a normally sterile site is often present in individuals with chronic sinusitis. In this situation, as in chronic bronchitis, it is always difficult to distinguish between causes and effect. Chronic inflammation is associated with a number of mucosal changes, one of which is bacterial colonization. These abnormalities lead to impaired mucociliary function, reduced drainage, and retention of secretions, all of which promote bacterial infection.

Clinical Distinctions between Colonization and Infection

The importance of colonization lies in two areas: (1) since it is the initiating pathogenetic step for many infections, colonization represents a significant risk factor in some circumstances, and (2) confusion with infection may lead to inappropriate treatment—failure to treat actual infections on the one hand or antimicrobial treatment of incidental colonization on the other.

Clinical decision making in the first instance involves an analysis of risk versus benefit. The analysis of risk must include the likelihood of infection developing, the severity of illness if it does, and the potential harm associated with prophylactic therapy. Each of these factors varies widely in individual circumstances. For example, asymptomatic nasal colonization with *S. aureus* does not require treatment in most subjects but may be beneficial for a patient with recurrent furunculosis or a surgeon who is experiencing staphylococcal wound infections. Asymptomatic group A streptococcal colonization should usually be treated because of the severity of potential disease and the minimal risk of treatment.

By far the most common problems with colonization

in clinical chest disease involve colonization of the airways in individuals with acute or chronic underlying disease. Gram-negative bacilli appear in tracheobronchial secretions in at least 50 percent of patients who are intubated for ventilatory support. Similarly, colonization of the respiratory tract by new pathogens, usually gram-negative bacilli, occurs in at least 20 percent of patients undergoing treatment for pneumococcal pneumonia or other specific infections. In these circumstances the clinician must decide whether the appearance of new organisms represents a significant superinfection or merely colonization. Well-validated criteria for this decision making are not available. As a general rule, it is wise to remember the axiom that patients, not laboratory results, are being treated, and if the patient is doing well, the new culture findings should not be acted upon. Some clinicians recommend performing serial microscopic examinations of tracheobronchial secretions, believing that an increase in neutrophils, along with increasing numbers of gram-negative bacilli, is a more reliable criterion of superinfection than culture results alone. Others recommend quantitative cultures of secretions; increasing colony counts or absolute values greater than 10^6 per milliliter have been said to identify patients with new infections. Invasive sampling procedures, including transtracheal aspiration, transthoracic needle aspiration, and more recently, fiberoptic bronchoscopy with distal lung samples obtained by a protected specimen brush technique, have been recommended by some. Each of these approaches has advocates and advantages in some circumstances. Each adds substantially to the cost of patient care and none can be recommended as routine procedures. Our approach is to limit our concern to those patients who seem likely to have superinfections on clinical grounds and to investigate those patients by bronchoscopy and selection sampling if the causative organisms are unclear and if specific antimicrobial therapy is likely to make a significant difference in the patient's outcome.

BIBLIOGRAPHY

Beachey ED: Bacterial adherence: Adhesion-receptor interactions mediating the attachment of bacteria to mucosal surfaces. J Infect Dis 143:325–345, 1981.
  Good overview of the interactions between bacteria and mammalian epithelial cells.

Driks MR, Craven DE, Celli BR, Manning M, Burke RA, Garvin GM, Kunches LM, Farber HW, Wedel SA, McCabe WR: Nosocomial pneumonia in intubated patients given sucralfate as compared with antacids or histamine type 2 blockers. The role of gastric colonization. N Engl J Med 317:1376–1382, 1987.
  Retrograde colonization with gram-negative bacteria of the pharynx from the stomach may be more likely when the gastric pH is relatively high. In patients receiving mechanical ventilation, the use of a prophylactic agent against stress-ulcer bleeding that preserves the natural gastric acid barrier against bacterial overgrowth may be preferable to antacids and H2 blockers in avoiding retrograde colonization.

Higuchi JH, Johanson WG: The relationship between adherence of Pseudomonas aeruginosa to upper respiratory cells in vitro and susceptibility to colonization in vivo. J Lab Clin Med 95:698–705, 1980.
  Demonstrations of altered upper respiratory cell adherence by surgical stress and an associated increased susceptibility to colonization in experimental animals.

Irwin RS, Erickson AD, Pratter MR, Corrao WM, Garrity FL, Myers JR, Kaemmerlen JT: Prediction of tracheobronchial colonization in current cigarette smokers with chronic obstructive bronchitis. J Infect Dis 145:234–241, 1982.
  A recent study of tracheobronchial colonization in chronic bronchitis using transtracheal aspiration; previous articles using bronchoscopic techniques are well referenced.

Karam GH, Griffin FM Jr: Invasive pulmonary aspergillosis in nonimmunocompromised, nonneutropenic hosts. Rev Infect Dis 8:357–363, 1986.
  The isolation of Aspergillus from respiratory secretions of normal hosts usually signifies tracheobronchial colonization, not disease. Invasive pulmonary aspergillosis should be considered when Aspergillus is isolated from the respiratory secretions of anyone who has pneumonia, regardless of host defense status.

Mackowiak PA: The normal microbial flora. N Engl J Med 307:83–93, 1982.
  Scholarly review of the normal bacterial flora with a thorough discussion of the factors which determine it.

Neiderman MS, Merrill WW, Ferranti RD, Pagano KM, Palmer LB, Reynolds HY: Nutritional status and bacterial binding in the lower respiratory tract in patients with chronic tracheostomy. Ann Intern Med 100:795–800, 1984.
  Demonstration that colonization of the airways is associated with bacterial adherence to washed cells and that the latter phenomenon may be influenced by host factors.

Palmer LB: Bacterial colonization: pathogenesis and clinical significance. Clin Chest Med 8:455–466, 1987.
A review of bacterial colonization of the respiratory tract as a precursor of serious invasive infection.

Salata RA, Lederman MM, Shlaes DM, Jacobs MR, Eckstein E, Tweardy D, Toossi Z, Chmielewski R, Marino J, King CH, et al: Diagnosis of nosocomial pneumonia in intubated, intensive care unit patients. Am Rev Respir Dis 135:426–432, 1987.
The authors studied 51 intubated, intensive care unit patients prospectively in an attempt to develop criteria for the early detection of pulmonary infection. Patients with infection had new or progressive pulmonary infiltrates plus 1 of the following: positive blood culture results, radiographic evidence of cavitation, or histologic events of pneumonia; or 2 or more of the following: new fever, new leukocytosis, or grossly purulent tracheal aspirates.

Stanislawski L, Simpson WA, Hasty D, Sharon N, Beachey EH, Ofek I: Role of fibronectin in attachment of *Streptococcus pyogenes* and *Escherichia coli* to human cell lines and isolated oral epithelial cells. Infect Immunol 48:257–259, 1985.
A detailed study of the interactions between two different bacterial species and host cells indicating the complexity of these processes.

Stephens DS, Hoffman LH, McGee ZA: Interaction of *Neisseria meningitides* with human nasopharyngeal mucosa: Attachment and entry into columnar epithelial cells. J Infect Dis 148:369–376, 1983.
Fascinating study of the interaction of a pathogenic bacterium with nasopharyngeal explants demonstrating selective adherence to nonciliated cells, uptake, and passage through the cells.

Tuomanen EI, Hendley JO: Adherence of *Bordetella pertussis* to human respiratory epithelial cells. J Infect Dis 148:125–130, 1983.
Demonstration of selective adherence to only ciliated cells of a highly virulent bronchial pathogen.

Vincent JL, Cabolet P, Berre J, Serruys-Schoutens E, Kahn RJ: Bronchopulmonary superinfections in the critically ill. Acta Anaesthesiol Belg 38:117–122, 1987.
The authors review the mechanisms by which bacterial colonization is accomplished and the routes to nosocomial infection.

Woods DE, Straus DC, Johanson WG, Bass JA: Role of salivary protease activity in adherence of gram-negative bacilli to mammalian buccal epithelial cells *in vivo*. J Clin Invest 68:1435–1440, 1981.
Buccal cell adherence of gram-negative bacilli was found to increase postoperatively in patients undergoing coronary artery bypass in association with a reduction in cell-surface fibronectin and an increase in salivary protease activity.

Chapter 88

Nosocomial Pneumonias

George W. Counts / Walter E. Stamm

The acquisition of an infection after admission to an acute care hospital in the United States is estimated to occur at a ratio of 5.7 episodes per 100 admissions. At this rate, approximately 2 million hospital-acquired or nosocomial infections occur annually. By definition, these infections are neither present nor incubating on admission to a hospital. Urinary tract infections represent the most common nosocomial infection, accounting for 42 percent of the total. Surgical wound infections cause 24 percent of nosocomial infections, with pneumonia (10 percent) and bacteremia (5 percent) responsible for smaller numbers of infections. All other types of infections combined are responsible for the remaining 19 percent of nosocomial infections. In addition to the considerable morbidity and mortality resulting from nosocomial infections, hospital charges for care of these patients exceed $1 billion annually in the United States.

A variety of factors unique to the hospital setting make the epidemiology of nosocomial infections complex. These include the close approximation of many susceptible patients, the intimate exposure of these patients to hospital personnel, the increased susceptibility of hospitalized patients (by virtue of their underlying disease or immunosuppressive therapy) to infection, the unusual reservoirs for microorganisms provided by the hospital environment, the presence of pathogens with unique properties (such as antibiotic resistance) often found in the hospital, and invasive hospital procedures that bypass normal epithelial and mucosal defense mechanisms providing microorganisms direct entry to deeper tissues. Pneumonia is the third most common type of nosocomial infection, causing an estimated 200,000 cases per year;

these infections are particularly important because they account for a majority of all deaths from nosocomial infections.

PREDISPOSING FACTORS

Pathophysiology

In most healthy persons, intact pulmonary defense mechanisms keep the lower respiratory tract free from potentially pathogenic bacteria (see Chapter 86). Organisms responsible for nosocomial pneumonia are believed to reach the lung via one of three routes: (1) aspiration of oropharyngeal secretions, (2) hematogenous spread from distant sites of infections, and (3) inhalation of contaminated aerosols. A majority of nosocomial pneumonias result from aspiration of oropharyngeal material. After introduction of microorganisms into the lower respiratory tract, whether pneumonia results is a function of competing factors such as the number of organisms (inoculum size), their virulence, and local and systemic host defense mechanisms (Fig. 88-1).

Host Factors

Pneumonias acquired in the community prior to admission to a hospital are most often caused by organisms such as *Streptococcus pneumoniae* and *Hemophilus influenzae*. After admission, patients are exposed to and become colonized with more resistant gram-negative bacilli. Colonization occurs in the oropharynx, as well as the skin and gastrointestinal and urinary tracts. As a prelude to pneumonia, any factor which increases the potential for aspiration of oropharyngeal contents is a risk factor for the development of nosocomial pneumonia (Figs. 88-2 to 88-4). Increased frequency of aspiration in persons with depressed level of consciousness is not unexpected; one study using a radiolabeled tracer showed that aspiration could be demonstrated in 70 percent of such persons. However, it was further noted that aspiration also occurred during sleep in 45 percent of apparently healthy individuals. Other factors facilitating aspiration are dysphagia, nasogastric intubation, artificial airways, and tracheostomies. The type of bacteria causing pneumonia secondary to aspiration reflects the type of organisms comprising the oropharyngeal flora. Increased throat carriage of gram-negative bacilli accounts for the increased frequency of gram-negative bacilli as a cause of nosocomial pneumonias. Ordinarily these bacteria are uncommon as a component of throat flora, being present in approximately 2 to 18 percent of healthy adults. However, gram-negative bacilli rapidly colonize the throats of seriously ill persons, especially those admitted to an intensive-care unit (ICU).

The composition of the microbial flora on a mucosal surface appears to be determined in part by the ability of

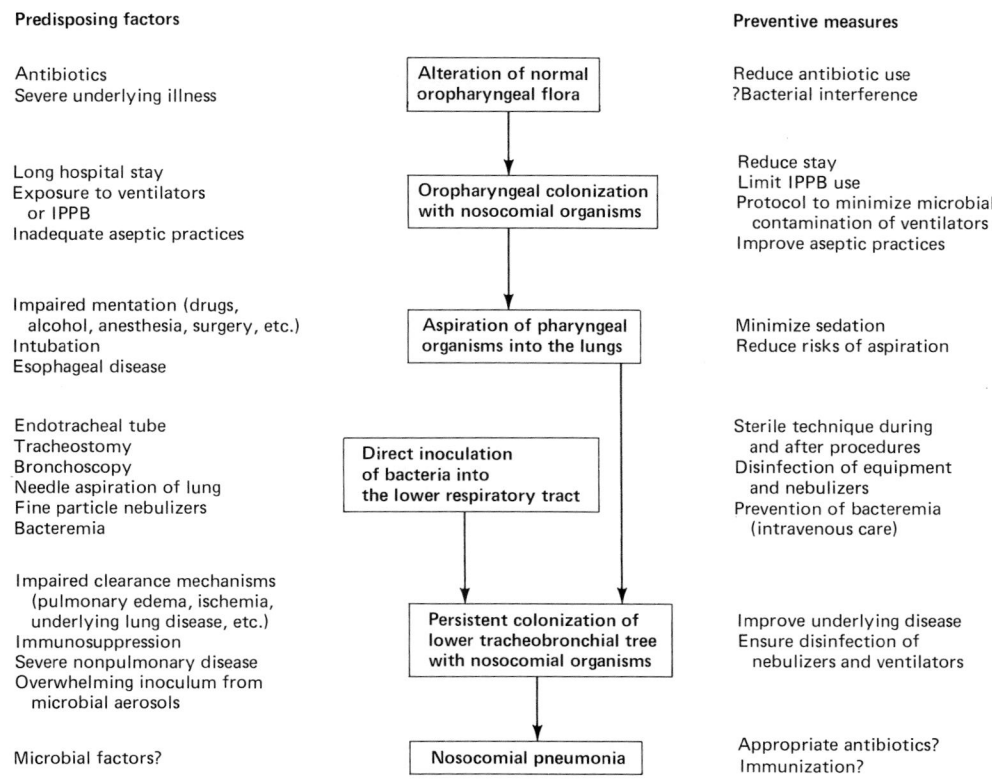

Predisposing factors

Antibiotics
Severe underlying illness

Long hospital stay
Exposure to ventilators
  or IPPB
Inadequate aseptic practices

Impaired mentation (drugs,
  alcohol, anesthesia, surgery, etc.)
Intubation
Esophageal disease

Endotracheal tube
Tracheostomy
Bronchoscopy
Needle aspiration of lung
Fine particle nebulizers
Bacteremia

Impaired clearance mechanisms
  (pulmonary edema, ischemia,
  underlying lung disease, etc.)
Immunosuppression
Severe nonpulmonary disease
Overwhelming inoculum from
  microbial aerosols

Microbial factors?

Preventive measures

Reduce antibiotic use
?Bacterial interference

Reduce stay
Limit IPPB use
Protocol to minimize microbial
  contamination of ventilators
Improve aseptic practices

Minimize sedation
Reduce risks of aspiration

Sterile technique during
  and after procedures
Disinfection of equipment
  and nebulizers
Prevention of bacteremia
  (intravenous care)

Improve underlying disease
Ensure disinfection of
  nebulizers and ventilators

Appropriate antibiotics?
Immunization?

Center flowchart boxes:

Alteration of normal oropharyngeal flora

↓

Oropharyngeal colonization with nosocomial organisms

↓

Aspiration of pharyngeal organisms into the lungs

Direct inoculation of bacteria into the lower respiratory tract

↓

Persistent colonization of lower tracheobronchial tree with nosocomial organisms

↓

Nosocomial pneumonia

FIGURE 88-1 Pathogenesis of nosocomial pneumonias.

bacteria to adhere to specific epithelial cells. Thus, changes in epithelial cell binding characteristics or an increase in binding sites may be responsible for the increased pharyngeal carriage by persons at risk for gram-negative bacillary pneumonia, e.g., persons severely ill, persons admitted to ICUs, alcoholics, and diabetics.

To develop nosocomial pneumonia, a patient must have impaired bacterial clearance mechanisms in addition to aspiration. Tracheostomy, intubation, tracheobronchial suctioning, and bronchoscopy all permit organisms to bypass local nasal and oropharyngeal defense mechanisms—specifically the nasal mucosa, vibrissae, and turbinates; the bacterial trapping and clearance action of the mucociliary epithelium and mucous layer; and the gag and cough reflexes. Local secretory antibodies, phagocytic cells, and nasopharyngeal lymphoid tissues are bypassed as well. Many diseases frequently seen in hospitalized patients, including pulmonary edema, chronic bronchitis, emphysema, and respiratory infections, impair the clearance of bacteria from the lungs. Smokers are also known to have less effective clearance mechanisms than nonsmokers. The relative importance of individual components of the host immune response (alveolar macrophages, secretory and humoral antibodies, complement, lymphoid cells, etc.) in protecting against nosocomial pneumonia remains unclear.

Environmental Factors

Several factors appear to underlie the importance of admission to an ICU as a risk factor for the development of nosocomial pneumonia. The most critically ill persons of greatest susceptibility to infection are concentrated in such units. Other contributing factors include the use of ventilatory support devices, which increase colonization by gram-negative bacilli, and the high intensity of care provided, which facilitates person-to-person transmission via equipment or the hands of personnel. Among ICU patients, differences exist in the risk of nosocomial pneumonia as evidenced by the fact that postoperative patients account for about three-fourths of all cases in adults. Those with upper abdominal and thoracic procedures have higher pneumonia rates than patients having procedures at other sites. Presumably the impairment of effective pulmonary toilette and the inability to clear the airways by coughing and deep breathing are responsible for the increased rates in patients with thoracoabdominal procedures.

Nosocomial pneumonia rates are also considerably higher in patients who use ventilatory devices compared with those who do not; 20-fold differences have been reported in some studies. Two decades ago, the association between respiratory therapy devices that generated aero-

(Text continued on page 1436)

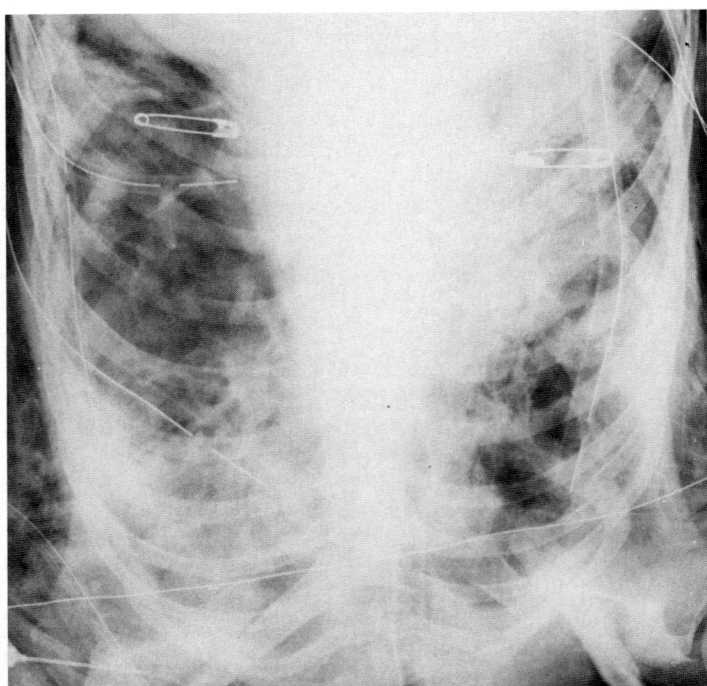

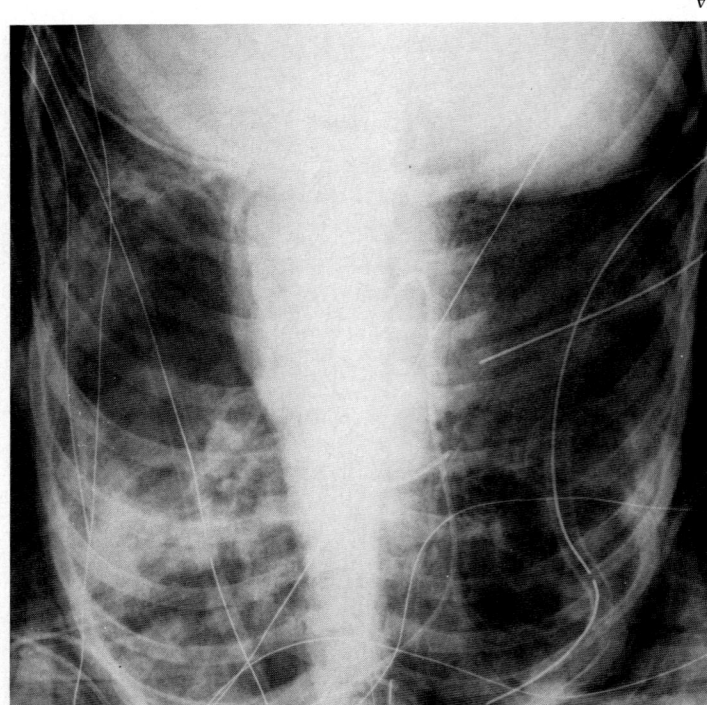

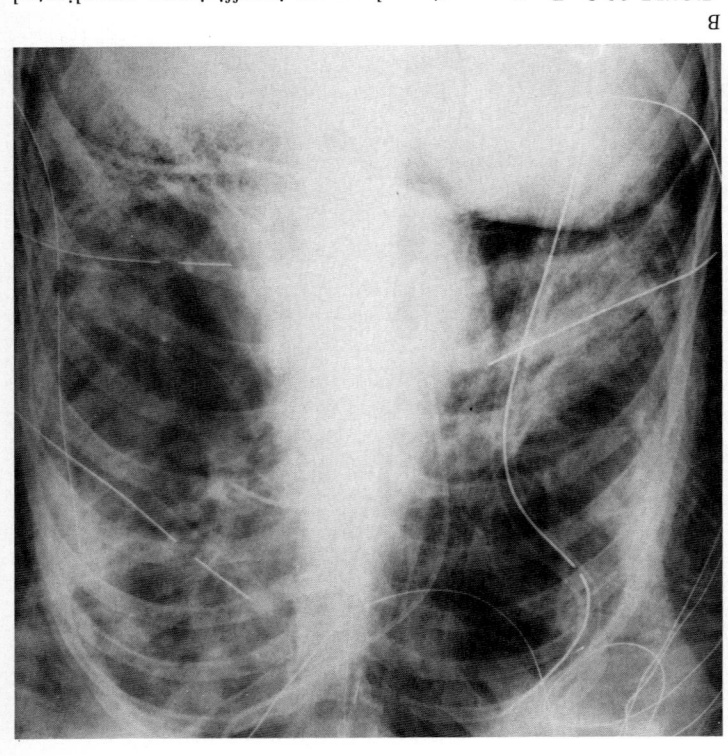

FIGURE 88-2 Posttraumatic pulmonary insufficiency complicated by nosocomial staphylococcal and *Serratia* pneumonia. A 21-year-old male was in excellent health until crush injury to the right side of his chest resulted in a right clavicular fracture, multiple rib fractures, and bilateral pneumothoraxes. An initial chest radiograph after placement of bilateral chest tubes and endotracheal intubation showed no infiltrates. Mechanical ventilation, using 40% O_2 as the inspired mixture, achieved an arterial P_{O_2} of 74 mmHg. *A.* Five days after injury and intubation. Temperature spiked to 103°F. A left upper lobe infiltrate and early pneumatocele are present. Gram stain of specimen obtained via nasotracheal suction showed alveolar macrophages, many white blood cells, and large numbers (++++) of gram-positive cocci. Cultures of sputum and drainage from the left chest tube grew *Staphylococcus aureus*; therapy with intravenous methicillin, 8 g daily, was begun. Continued arterial hypoxemia was treated with positive end-expiratory pressure (15 cmH_2O), high-O_2 inspired gas mixture (70% O_2), frequent suctioning, and constant monitoring of pulmonary wedge pressures. *B.* Seven days after methicillin was started. The left upper lobe infiltrate has improved slightly, but new infiltrates have appeared in the right middle lobe and left lower lobe. A repeat Gram stain of sputum showed plump gram-negative rods and many white blood cells: cultures of sputum, right and left pleural fluid, and blood all grew *Serratia marcescens* resistant to methicillin but sensitive to gentamicin. Intravenous gentamicin, 5 mg/kg per day, and cefotaxime, 2 g every 4 h, were begun. *C.* One week later. Patient remained febrile. Bilateral diffuse infiltrates appeared. Increasing difficulty in maintaining arterial P_{O_2}. Gram stain and cultures of sputum and pleural fluid continued to show *S. marcescens*; the patient expired.

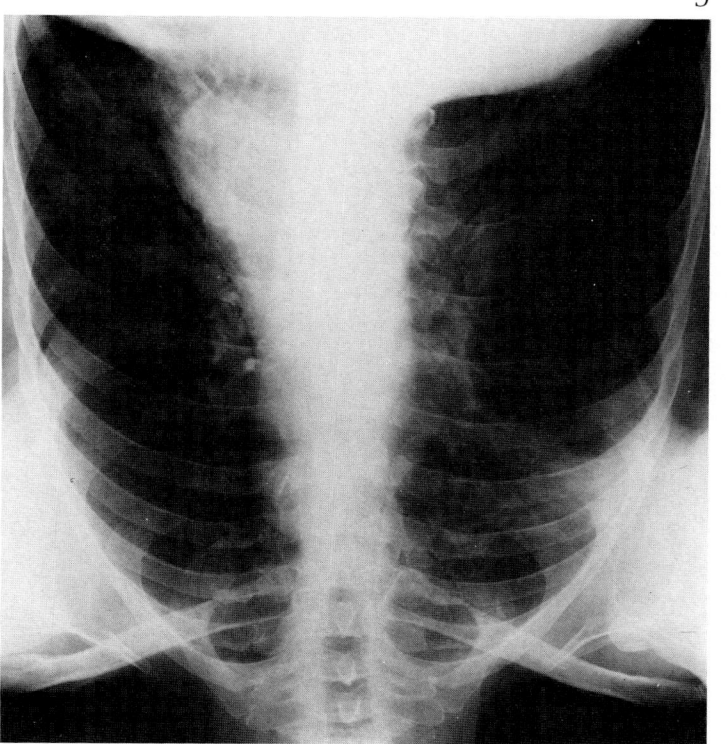

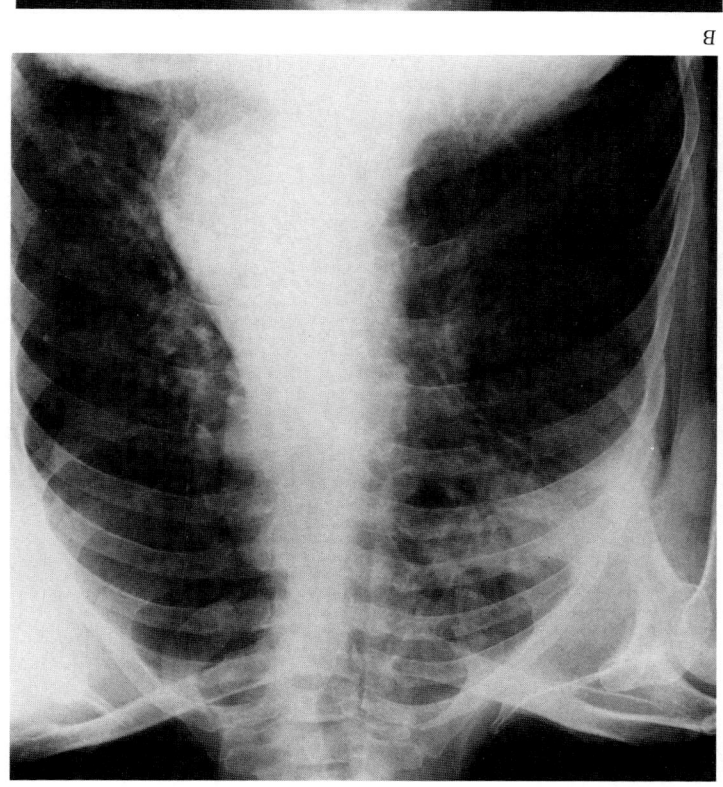

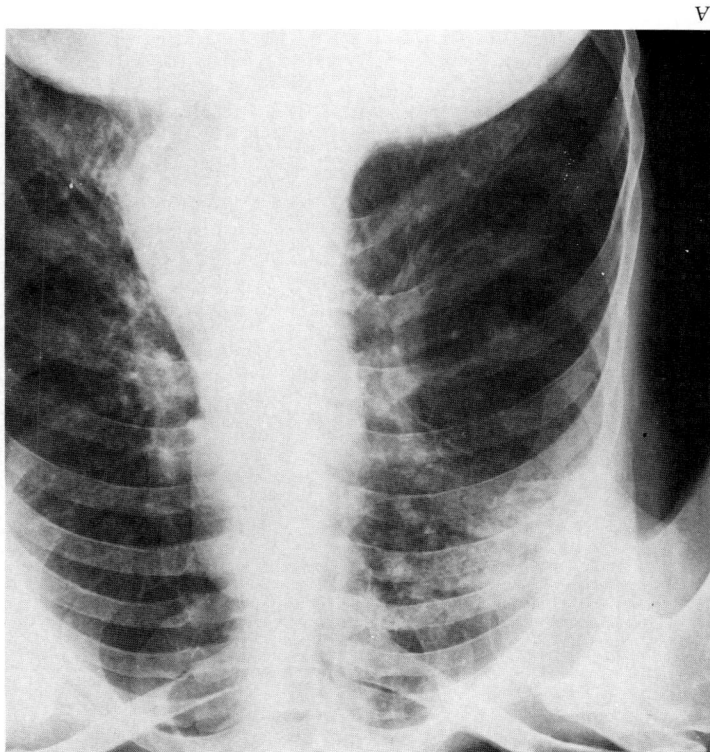

FIGURE 88-3 Postoperative nosocomial pneumonia due to *Klebsiella pneumoniae*. A 52-year-old man with previous history of heavy smoking (85 pack-years) and mild chronic bronchitis and emphysema underwent elective surgical repair of a ventral hernia. He required 1 h of general anesthesia and 2 h of endotracheal intubation in the recovery room. Postoperatively, marked peri-incisional pain necessitated frequent morphine and caused pronounced splinting. Deep-breathing exercises and intermittent positive pressure breathing were administered to prevent atelectasis. On the sixth postoperative day, the temperature spiked to 102°F, and the white blood cell count increased from 10,260 to 18,480 per cubic millimeter. *A.* Right upper lobe infiltrate. Sputum increased in amount and on Gram stain many white cells, a few alveolar macrophages, and many (++++) gram-negative bacilli were seen. Sputum cultures grew *K. pneumoniae*, but blood cultures were sterile. Treatment with intravenous cefotaxime 2 g every 4 h and gentamicin 5 mg/kg was begun. Four days later, the patient became afebrile and his white blood cell count dropped to 8060 per cubic millimeter. Sputum production concomitantly decreased. Gentamicin and cefotaxime were given for a total of 10 days. *B.* Fifteen days after start of therapy. Some clearing of infiltrate. *C.* Thirty days after start of therapy. Clearing continues.

FIGURE 88-4 Nosocomial staphylococcal pneumonia superimposed on cavitary pulmonary tuberculosis. A 54-year-old man was admitted with a 4-month history of cachexia, 40-lb weight loss, progressive cough, and increasing dyspnea. A purified protein derivative skin test had been positive 1 year prior to admission. A. On admission. A large cavitary lesion is present in the right upper lobe in association with smaller cavities in the right lower lobe, and a diffuse infiltrate on the left. Gram stain of sputum showed many white blood cells and many (++++) pleomorphic gram-negative rods; many (++++) acid-fast bacilli were seen on Ziehl-Neelsen stain. The white blood count was 24,000 per cubic millimeter, temperature was 101°F, and P_{O_2} was 38 mmHg while breathing ambient air. The initial diagnosis was widespread cavitary tuberculosis with probable endobronchial spread and possible superimposed bacterial pneumonia; sputum cultures subsequently grew Hemophilus influenzae and Mycobacterium tuberculosis. The patient required intubation, mechanical ventilation, and intensive respiratory therapy to maintain satisfactory oxygenation of arterial blood. Ampicillin was begun intravenously; isoniazid, ethambutol, and rifampin were started by mouth. After 5 days, mechanical ventilation was no longer required, and the patient was extubated. B. One month later. Clearing of the left-sided infiltrate and some improvement in the right lower lobe process. However, nonpulmonary problems (malnutrition, anemia, persistent diarrhea) necessitated further hospitalization. C. Fiftieth hospital day. Increase in cough and sputum production. Temperature spiked to 101°F, and the white blood count increased from 6200 to 14,600 cells per cubic millimeter. A new infiltrate is present in the left lower lobe; sputum Gram stain demonstrated many white blood cells and (++++) gram-positive cocci. Sputum cultures grew Staphylococcus aureus, and intravenous nafcillin was begun. Six days later, the fever and white count returned to normal, and 3 weeks later the chest radiograph returned to baseline (A).

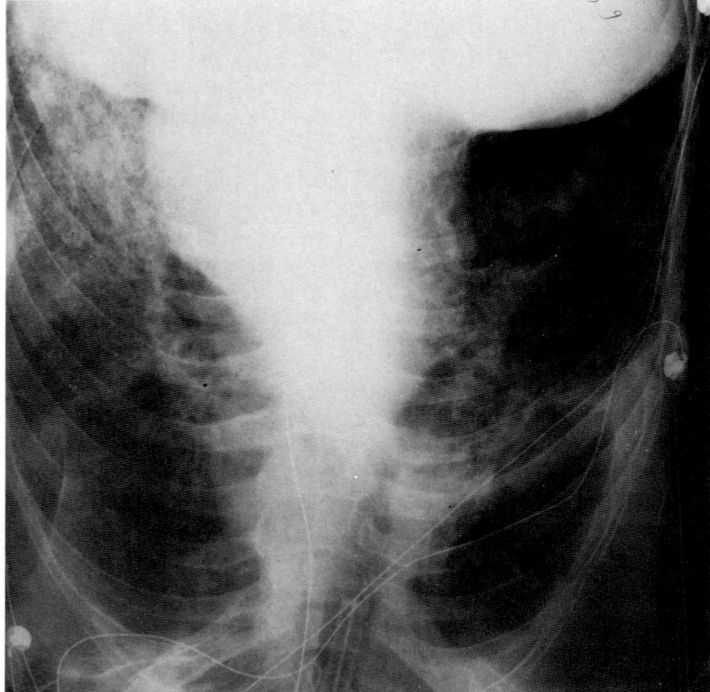

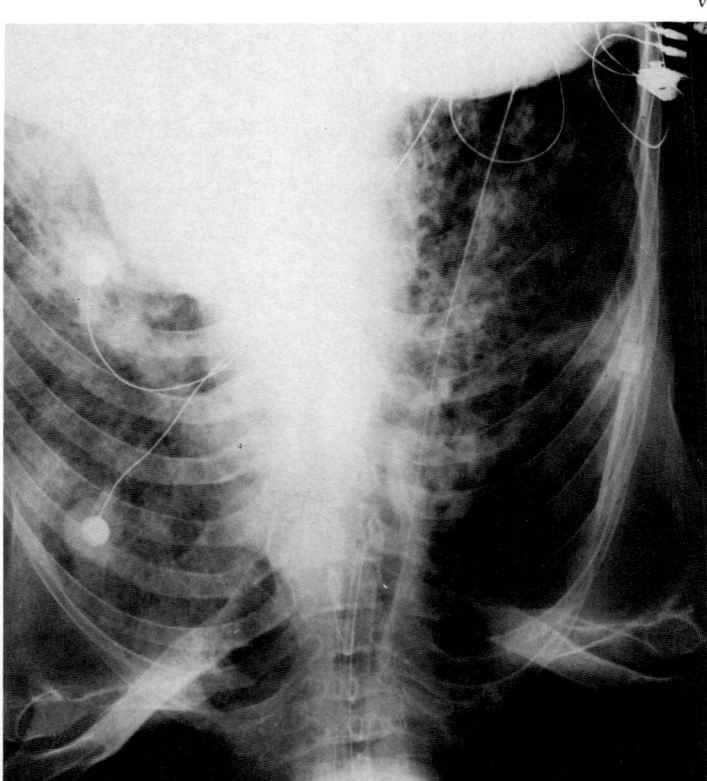

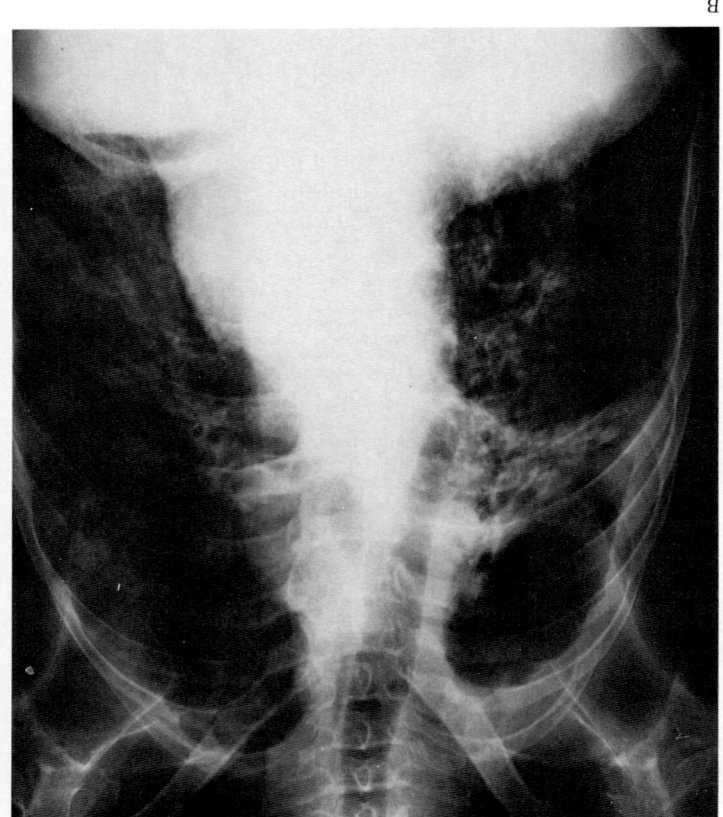

sols contaminated with gram-negative bacilli and nosocomial pneumonia was well described. Many outbreaks of nosocomial pneumonia due to contaminated components of respiratory therapy equipment were reported. As a result of these epidemics, guidelines for the care and decontamination of respiratory therapy equipment were adopted in most hospitals in the 1970s. The number of such outbreaks has since dramatically fallen, and exposure to contaminated respiratory therapy equipment is now considered an uncommon cause of nosocomial pneumonia. Instead of exposure to contaminated equipment, the higher pneumonia rates associated with ventilatory devices may be due to other associated procedures such as tracheal suctioning or bronchoscopy, or to the severity of underlying illness in these patients.

Gram-negative bacilli can be readily recovered from the ICU environment. It has been difficult to determine whether organisms are transferred from the ICU environment to patients, causing subsequent pulmonary infection, or whether they represent shedding into the environment from patients who are colonized or infected. One study of tracheal colonization in 20 ICU patients with prolonged intubation suggested that Enterobacteriaceae (Escherichia coli, Klebsiella, Proteus) originated in the hypopharynx perhaps due to pooling above the endotracheal or tracheostomy tube cuff, with subsequent spillage into the trachea upon deflation. On the other hand, non-Enterobacteriaceae (Pseudomonas and Acinetobacter) appeared to have been directly introduced into the trachea from exogenous sources. These organisms constituted 32 percent of organisms present in the hypopharynx, but represented two-thirds of the gram-negative bacilli acquired in and colonizing the trachea after the first day. These observations suggest a direct role for the environment as a source of gram-negative organisms colonizing and causing nosocomial pneumonia in ICU patients, especially those pneumonias caused by non-Enterobacteriaceae.

ETIOLOGY

Aerobic gram-negative bacilli are responsible for the majority of cases of nosocomial pulmonary infections, with gram-positive cocci and fungi causing smaller numbers of cases (Table 88-1). Standard culture methods, however, would not detect viruses or other "newer" pathogens such as Legionella. One prospective study including both children and adults suggested that up to 20 percent of nosocomial pneumonias were caused by viruses. Influenza, para-influenza, and respiratory syncytial viruses were associated with the majority of cases. The latter two agents, however, generally cause asymptomatic or mild infections in adults. During community outbreaks of influenza, nosocomial acquisition may occur, with the reservoir of infection being other infected patients or the hos-

TABLE 88-1
Etiologic Agents in Nosocomial Pneumonia

Organism	Fraction of Pneumonias Associated with Each Group of Agents, %*				
	CDC‡ (1973)	Graybill (1973)	Klick (1975)	Simmons† (1983)	Craig (1984)
Aerobic gram-negative bacilli	45	55	93	68	67
Aerobic gram-positive cocci	17	30	7	24	11
Fungi				5	—
Uncertain	39	26	—	—	22

* Totals exceed 100 percent because of multiple isolations from individual cases of pneumonia.

† National Nosocomial Infection Study, 1980, including only cases in which a pathogen was recovered.

‡ Data from Centers for Disease Control (CDC) surveillance sources, 1973.

pital staff. Nosocomial influenza B virus infection has also been reported. Symptoms were relatively mild with few serious complications and few instances of actual pneumonitis.

Appreciation of Legionella as a new cause of nosocomial pneumonia is increasing. Legionella appears to be an ubiquitous waterborne organism. Many hospitals have noted outbreaks of nosocomial Legionnaires' disease, often associated with recovery of the organism from water sources in the hospital environment. In one study in which there had been no documented instances of Legionnaires' disease, a prospective study found that Legionella caused 14 percent of cases of nosocomial pneumonia. The authors estimate that 3.8 to 6.6 percent of fatal nosocomial pneumonias may be due to Legionella.

The pathogenic role of anaerobic bacteria in nosocomial pneumonias not complicated by lung abscess or empyema remains uncertain. Normally, anaerobic bacteria vastly outnumber aerobes in the oropharynx, and hence anaerobes should logically be involved in causing pneumonias that follow oropharyngeal aspiration. Careful anaerobic bacteriologic studies have shown that anaerobes were present in the transtracheal aspirates of more than 30 percent of patients with hospital-acquired pneumonia that occurred after observed aspiration. However, facultative gram-negative bacilli were also isolated from most of these patients, and the pathogenic role of each type of organism remains in doubt. Strict anaerobes may require prior infection with facultative gram-negative bacilli to produce tissue necrosis and the anaerobic conditions necessary for their growth. Anaerobes clearly participate as pathogens in suppurative lung abscesses or empyemas that sometimes complicate nosocomial pneumonia.

DIAGNOSIS

Nosocomial pneumonia varies in clinical presentation, and there are no specific characteristics for infection caused by any particular pathogen. The following features are usually present: fever, cough, leukocytosis, and purulent sputum, in association with the development of a new infiltrate on chest radiograph, or an extension of a prior infiltrate. Nosocomial pneumonias usually present as patchy, nonlobar, alveolar infiltrates, without an associated pleural effusion. While any pulmonary segment may be involved, infection most often begins in the lower lobes. Widespread, multilobe involvement rarely occurs. Microabscess formation, cavitation, or empyema may subsequently develop.

Because of nonspecific clinical features, a high index of suspicion must be maintained in order to reliably recognize nosocomial pneumonia. The disease should be strongly considered in certain clinical situations: (1) patients predisposed to aspiration, (2) patients receiving ventilation support or respiratory therapy, (3) patients with recent surgery, especially thoracoabdominal procedures, (4) patients with tracheostomies, (5) patients with preceding pneumonia, and (6) immunocompromised patients.

Ordinarily, diagnosis of nosocomial pneumonia is made on the basis of clinical features plus an evaluation of sputum. Because of contamination by oropharyngeal microorganisms, examining expectorated sputum is of limited value. Multiple types of organisms are usually present, and it is difficult to identify a specific pathogen. The usefulness of examining expectorated sputum can be increased by screening the specimen for suitability. Gram-stained smears which have fewer than 10 squamous epithelial cells per low-power field ($\times$100) are felt to be truly representative of lower respiratory tract secretions and sufficiently free of oropharyngeal contamination. Some authors use the presence of 25 or more polymorphonuclear white blood cells per low-power field as a second criterion for specimen suitability.

Unless specific contraindications exist, transtracheal aspiration (TTA) should be performed on all moderately ill patients with suspected nosocomial pneumonia from whom a suitable expectorated sputum specimen cannot be readily obtained. This technique usually yields the responsible pathogen(s) without contamination of the specimen. Because of the large number of anaerobic organisms normally present in the oropharynx, anaerobes associated with lower respiratory infections can be identified only with a technique such as TTA, which bypasses the oropharynx. In a study of 488 patients undergoing TTA, the incidence of false-negative cultures was 1 percent among persons sampled before administration of antibiotics, and the incidence of false-positive cultures was 21 percent. Experience with this procedure suggests that complica-tions occur at an acceptably low rate, and one should not hesitate to use it to diagnose a disease with 20 to 50 percent associated fatality.

Many patients who develop nosocomial pneumonia are likely to be seriously ill in intensive-care units and already intubated or with tracheostomies. Because of the difficulty in the early recognition of pneumonia in that setting, regular monitoring of the microbial flora of the lower respiratory tract of intubated patients, usually by Gram stain of tracheal aspirates, may be considered. With the development of pneumonia, the stains would show new or increased numbers of white blood cells and a new or predominant organism. Others have advocated periodic culture surveillance of sputum in high-risk patients to identify the predominant gram-negative pathogens present and their antimicrobial susceptibilities. Secondary bacteremia may accompany nosocomial pneumonia, and blood cultures should always be obtained. If present, pleural fluid should also be Gram-stained and cultured.

Since aerobic gram-negative bacilli and gram-positive cocci are responsible for the overwhelming majority of cases of nosocomial pneumonia, more invasive diagnostic tests are rarely required. Most nosocomial pneumonias are associated with sputum production and occur in immunocompetent patients. However, nosocomial pneumonias in immunocompromised patients are more likely to be caused by unusual or opportunistic pathogens, for which an aggressive approach is warranted, including consideration of percutaneous needle aspiration, bronchiolar lavage, transbronchial biopsy and aspiration, or open lung biopsy (see Chapter 109).

Many disease processes may resemble nosocomial pneumonia. In many cases, the patient's underlying disease process dominates the clinical picture, obscuring the diagnosis of newly acquired pneumonia. In hospitalized patients, fever and leukocytosis may arise from a variety of processes (most commonly nonpulmonary infections, neoplasms, inflammatory diseases, and drug fever) or may be absent in the presence of pneumonia in patients with uremia, hematologic malignancy, immunosuppression, or steroid therapy. Noninfectious causes of pulmonary infiltrates (pulmonary edema, pulmonary infarction, atelectasis, aspiration of gastric contents, drug reactions, or vasculitis) not infrequently seen in hospitalized patients may be associated with fever and leukocytosis. Nosocomial bacterial pneumonia may be particularly difficult to diagnose in patients with acute lung injury and respiratory failure [adult respiratory distress syndrome (ARDS)]. Changes in the chest radiograph in such patients may be difficult to differentiate from pneumonia, and fever and leukocytosis may be present in both conditions. However, in most cases, ARDS can be distinguished from nosocomial pneumonia by radiologic features, by the absence of purulent sputum, and by the clinical setting.

TREATMENT

Therapeutic decisions in patients with nosocomial pneumonia are guided by estimations of the likely pathogen based on clinical clues, Gram stain and culture results, surveillance data, and any other diagnostic tests performed. Knowledge of the prevailing causative microorganisms and their antibiotic-resistant patterns in a given hospital or unit can be of great assistance in directing initial antibiotic choices. These patterns vary from hospital to hospital. Seriously ill medical patients or postoperative patients in ICUs, whose sputum Gram stain shows predominantly gram-negative bacilli or mixed flora and for whom no surveillance data are available, should receive empiric combination chemotherapy with a β-lactam drug and an aminoglycoside. Newer cephalosporins (e.g., cefotaxime, cefoperazone, ceftriaxone, ceftizoxime, and ceftazidime) have excellent activity against a broad range of gram-negative bacilli. One of these drugs (dosages of 4 to 12 g per day) could be combined with gentamicin (3 to 5 mg/kg per day). If surveillance data suggest a likelihood of gentamicin-resistant strains, tobramycin or amikacin should be used. For pneumonias known or suspected to be caused by *Pseudomonas aeruginosa*, an extended spectrum penicillin such as ticarcillin, piperacillin, or mezlocillin could be added to the above combination or substituted for the cephalosporin. Cefoperazone and ceftazidime have better activity than older β-lactam drugs against *P. aeruginosa*. However, most authorities believe that at this time these drugs should not be used as monotherapy for *P. aeruginosa* infections in seriously ill patients. Aminoglycosides penetrate poorly into bronchial secretions and should also not be used alone to treat nosocomial pneumonia. The value of the endotracheal administration of aminoglycoside as an adjunct to parenteral therapy in the treatment of pneumonia caused by gram-negative bacilli is controversial. If the initial Gram stain shows only gram-positive cocci or mixed flora, a penicillin such as nafcillin or methicillin (8 to 12 g per day) could be added to the two-drug combination or substituted for the cephalosporin, depending on the clinical assessment.

The necessity of including a drug effective against anaerobes in the antimicrobial regimen used to treat nosocomial pneumonia remains unproven. In the absence of lung abscess, empyema, or a Gram stain suggesting the presence of anaerobes, such specific therapy seems unnecessary.

After 48 h, the initially selected antibiotic regimen should be reassessed. At this time, presumptive results of sputum and blood cultures should be available, as well as knowledge of the clinical, laboratory, and radiographic response to therapy. The duration of antibiotic therapy necessary for successful treatment of nosocomial pneumonia has not been clearly established. Therapy must be individualized for each patient's clinical course, but 10 to 14 days generally suffice. Since sputum colonization with the infecting strain often persists long after clinical improvement has occurred, eradication of the infecting organism from sputum should not be used as a therapeutic end point.

PREVENTION

Figure 88-1 lists general measures important in the prevention of nosocomial pneumonia. The use of antimicrobial agents given either parenterally or by inhalation to prevent pneumonia in hospitalized patients has generally been complicated by the emergence of resistant isolates. It is of interest, however, that small amounts of antibiotics, (i.e., subinhibitory concentrations) appear to alter buccal epithelial binding sites for gram-negative bacilli, thus preventing adherence and colonization. The ultimate utility of this observation has not been determined.

Efforts to enhance host defenses against those pathogens most often responsible for nosocomial pneumonia are still largely investigational. Passive immunization using specific immunoglobulin or monoclonal antibody and active immunization with a vaccine against multiple species of gram-negative bacilli are avenues being explored.

The ultimate goal of infection control programs is the prevention of nosocomial infections of all types. For the specific prevention of pneumonia, measures include the following: (1) the development of guidelines for the prevention of contamination of ventilatory devices and respiratory therapy equipment; (2) policies and procedures for aseptic patient care practices, e.g., tracheal suctioning and care of vascular lines; and (3) surveillance of infections and antibiotic susceptibility patterns of microbial ecology present in high-risk areas. A national study of the efficacy of nosocomial infection control programs seemed to validate this approach as a preventive measure. Programs which had a specially trained physician, a ratio of one infection control nurse per 250 beds, and intensive surveillance reduced nosocomial pneumonia rates by 27 percent in surgical patients and by 13 percent among medical patients.

BIBLIOGRAPHY

Andrews CP, Coalson JJ, Smith JD, Johanson WG: Diagnosis of nosocomial bacterial pneumonia in acute, diffuse lung injury. Chest 80:254–258, 1981.
    Authors analyzed autopsies of patients dying with ARDS and concluded that the diagnosis of bacterial pneumonia in that setting was often erroneous. Overall 29 percent of cases were misdiagnosed.

Bartlett JG, O'Keefe P, Tally FP, Louie TJ, Gorbach SL: Bacteriology of hospital-acquired pneumonia. Arch Intern Med 146:868–871, 1986.
    Study included only patients diagnosed by TTA, blood, or empyema culture. Most common causes were gram-negative bacilli (47 percent), anaerobes (35 percent), Staphylococcus aureus (31 percent), and Streptococcus pneumoniae (26 percent).

Baumgartner JD, Glauser MP, McCutchan JA, Ziegler EJ, Van Melle G, Klauber MR, Vogt M, Muehlen E, Leuthy R, Chiolero R, Geroulanos S: Prevention of gram-negative shock and death in surgical patients by antibody to endotoxin core glycolipid. Lancet 2:59–63, 1985.
    A double-blind prophylactic study using human antiserum to E. coli J5; while there was no difference in the incidence of gram-negative infections, the risk of septic shock was significantly higher in controls than J5 recipients.

Craig CP, Connelly S: Effect of intensive care unit nosocomial pneumonia on duration of stay and mortality. Am J Infect Control 12:233–238, 1984.
    Nosocomial pneumonia was the most common infection acquired by ICU patients and was associated with a threefold prolongation of hospital stay and a fourfold increase in mortality compared to patients developing pneumonia outside an ICU. Effect was not a consequence of ventilatory support or acute respiratory failure.

Dixon RE: Nosocomial respiratory infections. Infect Control 4:376–381, 1983.
    General review of frequency, risk factors, and preventive measures for nosocomial pneumonias.

Graybill JR, Marshall LW, Charache P, Wallace LK, Melvin VB: Nosocomial pneumonia: A continuing major problem. Am Rev Respir Dis 108:1130–1140, 1973.
    Organisms responsible were mainly Pseudomonas and Klebsiella-Enterobacter. Almost 20 percent of the nosocomial pneumonias were attributable to Streptococcus pneumoniae, a figure higher than found in most other studies.

Haley RW, Culver DH, White JW, Morgan WM, Emori TG, Munn VP, Hooton TM: The efficacy of infection surveillance and control programs in preventing nosocomial infections in US hospitals. Am J Epidemiol 121:182–205, 1985.
    Results of the Centers for Disease Control (CDC) Study on the Efficacy of Nosocomial Infection Control, which showed that infection control programs could decrease infection rates; for nosocomial pneumonia, a reduction of 27 percent in postoperative patients and 13 percent in medical patients was seen.

Huxley EJ, Voroslav J, Gray WR, Pierce AK: Pharyngeal aspiration in normal adults and patients with depressed consciousness. Am J Med 64:564–568, 1978.
    An indium tracer study showed that aspiration occurred as expected in 70 percent of persons with altered mental status, but surprisingly also in 45 percent of normal adults while sleeping.

Johanson WG, Higuchi JH, Chaudhuri TR, Woods DE: Bacterial adherence to epithelial cells in bacillary colonization of the respiratory tract. Am Rev Respir Dis 121:55–63, 1980.
    Prospective study of noncolonized surgery patients found that increased adherence of gram-negative bacilli to buccal epithelial cells was associated with increased oropharyngeal colonization by gram-negative bacilli. With increased adherence of Pseudomonas, 11/16 patients became colonized compared to 0/16 patients whose buccal cells did not have increased adherence.

Johanson WG, Pierce AK, Sanford JP: Changing pharyngeal bacterial flora of hospitalized patients: Emergence of gram-negative bacilli. N Engl J Med 281:1137–1140, 1969.
    Throat carriage of gram-negative bacilli was uncommon in healthy persons but increased dramatically in hospitalized sick patients.

Klick JM, duMoulin GL, Hedley-White J, Teres D, Bushnell LS, Feingold DS: Prevention of gram-negative pneumonia using polymyxin aerosol as prophylaxis. II. Effects on the incidence of pneumonia in seriously ill patients. J Clin Invest 55:514–519, 1975.
> *In a study of ICU patients, an overwhelming majority of cases were caused by aerobic gram-negative bacilli. The study showed that polymyxin reduced the incidence of gram-negative pneumonia, but resistant isolates emerged.*

Lowy FD, Carlisle PS, Adams A, Feiner C: The incidence of nosocomial pneumonia following urgent endotracheal intubation. Infect Control 8:245–248, 1987.
> *The risk of nosocomial pneumonia following emergency or urgent endotracheal intubation was studied prospectively. Pneumonia developed in 35 of 78 (45%) patients within 3 days of intubation. Emergency endotracheal intubation appears to contribute to the overall incidence of nosocomial pneumonia.*

Muder RR, Yu VL, McClure JK, Kroboth FJ, Kominos SD, Lumish RM: Nosocomial Legionnaires' disease uncovered in a prospective pneumonia study. JAMA 249:3184–3188, 1983.
> *In a community hospital with no history of Legionnaires' disease, 14 percent of nosocomial pneumonia cases were found to be due to Legionella.*

Podnos SD, Toews GB, Pierce AK: Nosocomial pneumonia in patients in intensive care units. West J Med 143:622–627, 1985.
> *Excellent comprehensive and succinct review paper.*

Reinarz JA, Pierce AK, Mays BB, Sanford JP: The potential role of inhalation therapy equipment in nosocomial pulmonary infection. J Clin Invest 44:831–839, 1965.
> *This study established the connection between contaminated respiratory therapy equipment and nosocomial gram-negative pneumonia.*

Rosenow EC, Wilson WR, Cockerill FR: Pulmonary disease in the immunocompromised host. Mayo Clin Proc 60:473–487, 610–631, 1985.
> *A comprehensive review of all aspects of pulmonary disease in these patients, including infectious and noninfectious causes, community-acquired and nosocomial pneumonias, and therapy strategies.*

Schwartz SN, Dowling JN, Benkovic C, DeQuittner-Buchanan M, Prostko T, Yee RB: Sources of gram-negative bacilli colonizing the tracheae of intubated patients. J Infect Dis 138:227–231, 1978.
> *A prospective study of intubated patients suggested that organisms such as E. coli, Klebsiella, and Proteus colonize the hypopharynx and are then aspirated into the lung upon deflation of the cuff, while non-Enterobacteriaceae such as Pseudomonas and Acinetobacter are introduced into the trachea directly from an environmental source.*

Simmons BP, Wong ES: CDC guidelines for the prevention and control of nosocomial infections. Guidelines for the prevention of nosocomial pneumonia. Am J Infect Control 11:230–239, 1983.
> *CDC National Nosocomial Infection Study of 1980, including only those cases in which an etiology was established; gram-negative bacilli were responsible for two-thirds of cases.*

Stamm WE, Bennett J: Nosocomial Infections, in Top FV, Wehrle PE (eds), *Communicable and Infectious Diseases.* Chicago, Mosby, 1981, pp 444–461.
> *General review of nosocomial infections, including epidemiology.*

Sugarman B, Donta ST: Effect of antibiotics on the adherence of Enterobacteriaceae to human buccal cells. J Infect Dis 140:622–625, 1979.
> *Interesting observation that subinhibitory concentrations of antibiotics interfere with binding sites and decrease attachment of gram-negative bacilli.*

van Uffelen R, Rommes JH, van Saene HK: Preventing lower airway colonization and infection in mechanically ventilated patients. Crit Care Med 15:99–102, 1987.
> *Within three days of application of 2% polymixin E and tobramycin in an adhesive paste to the buccal mucosa of patients undergoing mechanical ventilation, the oral cavity of each patient was free of gram-negative bacilli, and no patient developed tracheal aspirates containing gram-negative bacilli or nosocomial pneumonia.*

Van Voris LP, Belshe RB, Shaffer JL: Nosocomial influenza B virus infections in the elderly. Ann Intern Med 96:153–158, 1982.
> *Hospital-acquired outbreak of influenza B virus infections affecting patients and staff of a Veterans Administration medical center.*

Wong LK, Barry AL, Horgan SM: Comparison of six different criteria for judging the acceptability of sputum specimens. J Clin Microbiol 16:627–631, 1982.
> *Authors concluded that methods based on the number of epithelial cells were quite satisfactory. There was good reproducibility among the various methods.*

Chapter 89
Systemic Infection and the Lungs

Jay A. Fishman

Bacteremia

Microbial Characteristics and the Dissemination of Infection
  Bacterial Adhesion
  Bacterial Products: Exotoxins and Secreted Glycoproteins
  Bacterial Products: The Bacterial Cell Wall (Endotoxins)
  Recently Identified Mediators: Cachectin and Interleukin 1

Septic Shock without Endotoxin
  The Neutrophil

Patterns of Pulmonary Injury in Systemic Infection

Syndromes of Lung Injury
  Intravascular Infections
  Occult Infection: Burns, Sickle Cell Anemia, Alcoholism

Treatment of Systemic Infections Involving the Lungs

The position of the lungs in the circulation and their extensive microvascular network gives them a unique exposure to bloodborne cells, organisms, hormones, toxins, and debris from bodily processes. In the absence of arteriovenous shunting, all venous blood returning from the peripheral vasculature must pass through the pulmonary circulation. The lymphatic drainage from the gastrointestinal tract and liver is also conducted to the lungs, both directly across the diaphragm and more circuitously via the thoracic duct and superior vena cava. As a result, it is not surprising that extrapulmonary infection and/or inflammation is rapidly reflected by changes within the pulmonary parenchyma. To gain access to the circulation, infection and its by-products must first bypass both the specific (immune) and nonspecific (inflammatory) protective responses of the infected tissues themselves. Infection located outside the lungs affects the lungs in four ways: (1) directly, by the embolization of organisms, inflammatory cells, tissue debris, and coagulation products via the blood to the pulmonary vessels; (2) directly, by extension of subdiaphragmatic or pleural processes to the lungs via lymphatics or tissue invasion; (3) indirectly, via the effects of toxins or products made by the infecting organisms; or (4) indirectly, as an effect of some of the

many circulating mediators of inflammation or components of the immune response of the host (Fig. 89-1).

In general, the lung is protected from the effects of toxins or bacteria in the blood by the filtration and metabolic functions of the liver, spleen, and bloodborne phagocytes. Thus, only when these systemic defenses either fail or are overwhelmed are the lungs subjected to direct injury by extrapulmonary processes (Table 89-1). Many metabolic derangements which are part of the host inflammatory response (protein catabolism, acute phase reactant synthesis, leukocytosis, proteinuria) occur both when the infection is localized or has spread systemically. Some of these changes occur acutely (e.g., fever), whereas others persist after the acute symptoms have resolved. Information on the systemic actions of the newly described mediators of inflammation (e.g., cachectin/tumor necrosis factor) coupled with those long known to have systemic vascular effects (e.g., histamine, serotonin) afford prospects for explaining a variety of enigmatic pulmonary syndromes (e.g., the adult respiratory distress syndrome).

BACTEREMIA

Bacterial, viral, and fungal organisms are present in the circulation more often than is generally appreciated. Leakage of organisms into the bloodstream across the colonic mucosae, from tooth brushing, from in-hospital procedures (e.g., bronchoscopy, liver biopsy, sigmoidoscopy), and in the course of localized infections of the urinary tract, lungs, gallbladder, or sinuses is common. Usually this leakage is nonthreatening to the immunologi-

TABLE 89-1
Systemic Infections Affecting the Lungs

Bacteremia, fungemia, viremia (seeding, bleeding, thrombosis)
Septic embolus (+/− infarction)
Septic shock (shock lung, ARDS)
Cardiac failure, myocarditis (Coxsackie virus, leptospirosis, T. gondii, diphtheria)
Pericardial disease (tuberculosis, S. pneumoniae, Candida)
Hemorrhage (toxic shock syndrome, dengue)
Direct extension (hepatic amebiasis, retropharyngeal abscess)
Pulmonary eosinophilia (filariasis, Strongyloides)
Hypotension/volume loss (cholera, pancreatitis)
Vasculitis (rickettsia)
Hemolysis/hypoxemia (clostridia)
Empyema/pleural infection (streptococci, anaerobes)
Immune depression (cytomegalovirus, HIV-AIDS)
Tick-borne disease (tularemia, Rocky Mountain spotted fever, Q fever)
Louse-borne disease (relapsing fever—Borrelia)
Airway obstruction/pharyngitis (diphtheria)
Paralytic disease (tetanus, polio, tick paralysis)

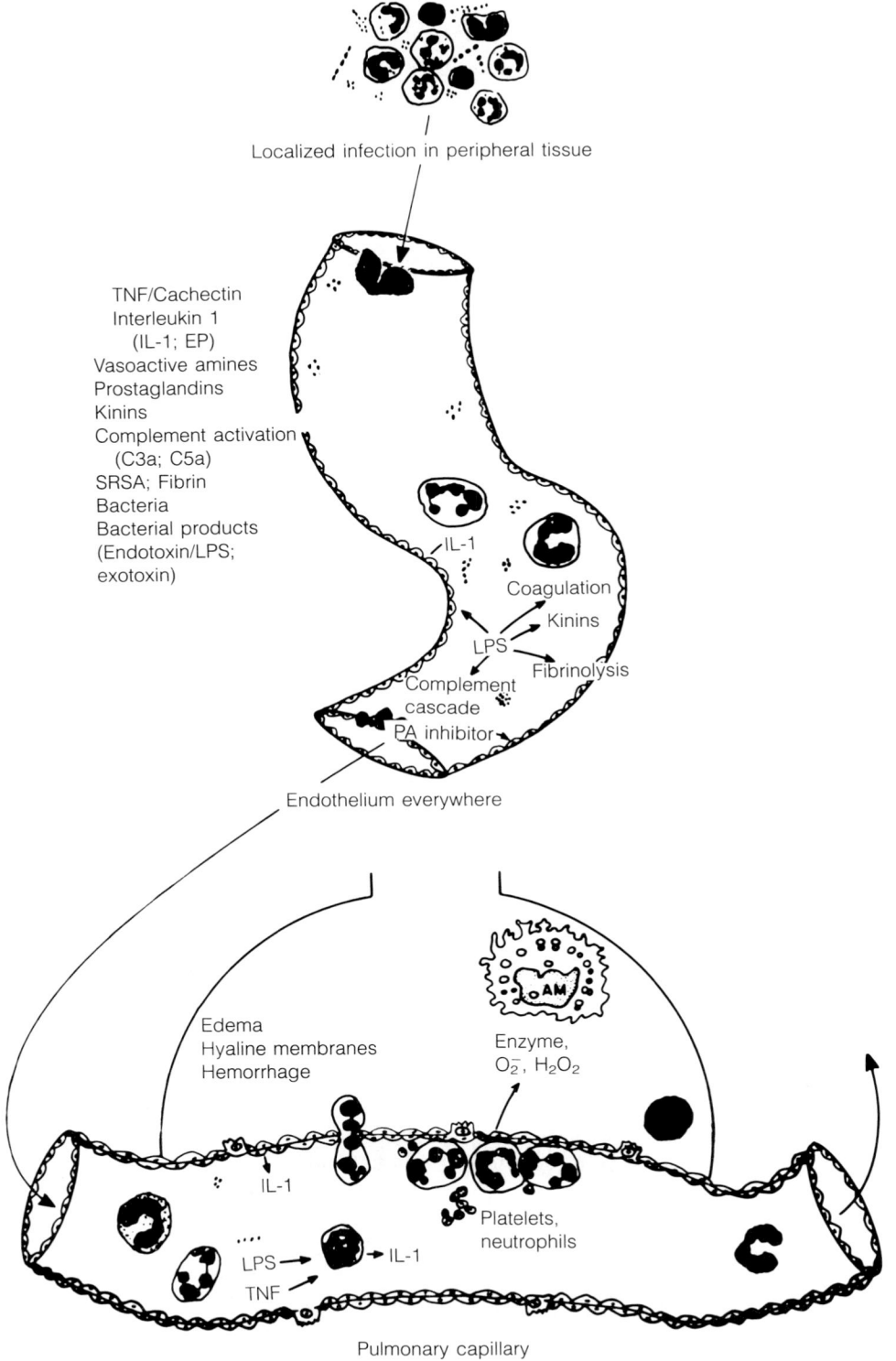

FIGURE 89-1 Systemic infection and inflammation initiates an array of host responses. Bacterial products, host factors, cells, and cellular debris are released locally into the circulation. Distant effects are due to bacteria, bacterial products, inflammatory cells, and a large group of mediators active in the pulmonary circulation and elsewhere in the body.

cally normal host. "High-grade" bacteremia or persistent infection of the blood elicits distinctive systemic effects. A working definition of clinically meaningful infection of the bloodstream is that infection detected by three or more positive blood cultures for the organism(s), collected sterilely and drawn more than 4 h apart. This bacteremia is distinguished from *sepsis*, which is the life-threatening clinical syndrome caused by infection. Popular usage has tended to blur the crispness of these definitions so that these terms are often used interchangeably.

Whether an infection will become high-grade depends on the location of infection, the defense mechanisms of the infected host, and the organism(s) involved. Infection that causes "pus under pressure," e.g., obstruction of drainage from a viscus, the biliary tree, or the urinary tract, or a large or perivascular abscess, is likely to cause leakage of organisms into the bloodstream. Similarly, intravascular infection (e.g., endocarditis), infected vascular grafts, and central venous catheters have immediate access to the circulation. Organisms also differ in their ability to gain access to the circulation, to adhere to vascular endothelium, and to elaborate the factors responsible for many of the systemic effects of infection. The ability of the host's immune system to handle these blood-borne organisms determines the outcome of the infection. The effects of infection on the lungs are both direct, e.g., embolization of cells, bacteria and debris, and indirect, e.g., mediated by hormones, toxins, and intermediate interactions between host and bacteria. Which cells or bacteria are involved is determined by the characteristics of the infection and of the inflammatory/immune response.

Bacteremia is often used to describe the presence of any bacterium, fungus, or parasite in the blood. According to the Centers for Disease Control, these infections account for 4 to 10 out of every 1000 patient discharges, and approximately 7.5 percent of all infections. Of all blood culture isolates at the Massachusetts General Hospital, approximately 35 to 40 percent are aerobic gram-positive species (largely *Staphylococcus* and *Streptococcus*), 35 to 40 percent are aerobic gram-negative species (largely *Escherichia coli*, *Klebsiella*, and *Pseudomonas*), 10 to 15 percent are anaerobic bacteria, and 5 to 10 percent are *Candida* and other fungi. Up to 25 percent of all blood isolates represent duplicate positive cultures, or species of unknown pathogenic importance, including *Propionibacterium*, *Staphylococcus epidermidis*, and diphtheroids. Fungi and mycobacterial species are becoming of greater importance as immunocompromised patients represent an increasing segment of the total population. Bacteremia is detected in up to 6 percent of infections that do not primarily involve the bloodstream. However, this is known to be an underestimate; the true incidence is probably four- to fivefold greater. Mortality from known bacteremia ranges from 20 to 40 percent. Antibiotic therapy has not significantly reduced this mortality, especially in the gram-negative bacteremias.

The organisms responsible for bacteremia are largely those colonizing the gastrointestinal tract, respiratory tract, and skin. Thus, bacteremia arising from the gastrointestinal tract is often due to *E. coli* and to the anaerobic *Bacteroides fragilis*. In burn patients, whose skin is colonized with *Pseudomonas aeruginosa* or *Staphylococcus aureus*, bacteremia involves these pathogens. Patients on assisted ventilation develop bacteremia due to colonization of the equipment, of the humidifying water, and ultimately of their respiratory tracts with the local hospital flora, often *Pseudomonas*, *Serratia*, or *Proteus* species. The organisms change as the patient enters the hospital environment. For example, in intensive-care patients, Johanson et al. demonstrated the role played by debility in the colonization of the respiratory tract by gram-negative bacilli; coma, hypotension, tracheal intubation, acidosis, neutrophilia, and anemia accompany the development of colonization. The use of antibiotics changes both the specific bacteria involved by altering the colonization pattern (e.g., up to a fivefold increase in the fecal carriage of *P. aeruginosa*) and by increasing the proportion of organisms resistant to the antibiotic agents. Clusters of patients with infection due to organisms new to a specific clinical setting should raise suspicion of an increased nosocomial hazard, e.g., carriage of *Staphylococcus* or *Salmonella* by physician or nurse, release of fungi into the hospital by construction or demolition in the vicinity, or colonization of equipment. The recent increase in incidence of fungal and anaerobic bacteremias reflects technological advances in culturing of the blood and, to an even greater extent, the increased survival of immunocompromised patients and the increase in usage of a wide variety of surgical and mechanical interventions by the physician.

MICROBIAL CHARACTERISTICS AND THE DISSEMINATION OF INFECTION

Only those organisms that are suited to the human environment survive to cause significant disease. Thus, the relatively few organisms that cause the majority of the invasive infections have advantageous properties, including digestive enzymes that allow penetration into tissue, "stickiness" or adherence factors, protective membrane glycoproteins, or exotoxins that either interfere with the host's immune function or injure the infected tissues. These are called *virulence factors*, and vary according to both the organism and the preferred sites for establishing a nidus of infection. For example, the small group of organisms that live inside host cells, e.g., *Listeria monocytogenes*, are uniquely protected against the immune surveil-

lance mechanisms of the host. In particular, organisms that infect the lungs and are not directly aspirated through the airways must either adhere to, and cross, the vascular endothelium or cross the pleural surface of the lung to enter the pulmonary parenchyma. Bacteria reaching the lungs must be present in sufficient numbers or with the necessary properties to avoid clearance by the local humoral, phagocytic, and mechanical protective mechanisms of the lungs. As is discussed below, in establishing a pneumonitis, some effects are mediated by the effects of organisms on the endothelial cells or on neutrophils without direct invasion of tissue.

Bacterial Adhesion

Some of the current research focuses on the molecules responsible for adherence to host cells, i.e., *adhesins*. The ability to stick to and to colonize endothelial surfaces allows the successful dissemination of bloodborne infection to other tissues. The organisms most often responsible for metastatic infection (*Staphylococcus aureus*, *Salmonella*, group A streptococci, *Pseudomonas aeruginosa*, *Haemophilus influenzae*) all have specialized surfaces that enable adherence to endothelial or mucosal surfaces. For example, streptococci are covered either by fibrillae or by a fine fuzzy coating of lipotichoic acid (LTA) and proteins, including the M proteins, that serve as intermediaries in the process of binding to a wide range of cell types. Important differences between strains and target tissues allow certain strains to bind preferentially to the pharyngeal epithelium of patients who have rheumatic carditis, whereas others exhibit preferential binding for cutaneous epithelial cells. The amount of binding is determined by the density of receptors for LTA on the cell surfaces. LTA also mediates some of the binding of streptococci to fibronectin, a ubiquitous glycoprotein that is found in serum and attached to cell surfaces, and to glycoproteins, including heparin and collagen. Fibronectin may be the intermediary ("receptor") for streptococcal, and some staphylococcal, binding to cell surfaces; receptors for fibronectin appear to be a family of cell surface glycoproteins that vary in distribution and in their affinity for fibronectin and related molecules. Adherence of most of the Enterobacteriaceae is achieved by way of fimbriae or pili, small tubular surface projections that bind to common cell surface oligosaccharide receptors. The type and amount of fimbriae varies with culture conditions, including the concentration of estrogens. Nonspecific bacterial adherence is proportional to the level of hydrophobicity of the bacterial or fungal surface glycoproteins. Adherence properties are important determinants of the ability of organisms to colonize medical devices: artificial heart valves, catheters, vascular grafts, suture materials. The chemical composition, surface irregularity, and hydrophobicity of the materials determine the incidence of infection of these surfaces. In some cases, the presence of these organelles of adherence on the surfaces of bacteria may predispose to phagocytosis and clearance of the organisms by the host. Noncolonizing strains of bacteria are often isolated from the blood of bacteremic patients. Although some insights have been gained, many determinants of bacterial invasiveness remain to be clarified.

Bacterial Products: Exotoxins and Secreted Glycoproteins

The second characteristic of bacteria and fungi that determines the systemic effects of infection is the group of products synthesized and/or secreted by the infecting organisms. This is a large group of "exotoxins" and enzymes, only few of which have been well described, and a number of which cause tissue injury or metabolic effects. Because of the intricate interactions of the components of the host's response to bacteremia or localized infection, it is difficult to evaluate the role of any one of these factors in pulmonary injury in isolation from any other. For example, in the setting of *P. aeruginosa* bacteremia, it is difficult to separate the effects of the pseudomonal cytotoxin from those of bacterial endotoxin, lipopolysaccharide (LPS), or lipid A from the cell walls of the gram-negative organisms. Many mediators of the responses to these substances are shared, and the physiological actions of these agents in vivo are unclear.

In general, exotoxins are more important in gram-positive infections than in gram-negative. A few exotoxins merit individual mention. S. aureus α toxin mediates the formation of nonphysiological calcium channels in pulmonary endothelium in vitro and the initiation of the arachidonic acid cascade in isolated perfused rabbit lungs. These changes are accompanied by pulmonary hypertension, probably due to thromboxane A_2 release, though the vasodilator prostaglandin, prostacyclin, is also activated; the toxin may also be responsible for direct pulmonary endothelial cell injury. However, the in vivo role of these changes is unclear.

Two additional staphylococcal exotoxins have been implicated in the development of toxic shock syndrome (TSS). This syndrome was recognized in late 1979 and consisted of high fever, a diffuse macular erythroderma accompanied by desquamation that included the palms and soles of the feet, hypotension, and involvement of at least three organ systems from among the following: mucous membranes (hyperemia); gastrointestinal tract (diarrhea or vomiting); muscles (myalgias or twice normal creatine phosphokinase levels); kidneys (pyuria without urinary tract infection or twice normal concentration in serum of creatinine or urea nitrogen); hepatic (twice normal concentration in serum of total bilirubin or transaminases); blood (thrombocytopenia, less than 100,000 per milliliter); central nervous system (altered mental status

without focal neurologic signs when normotensive without fever). These findings usually occur in young menstruating women without microbiologic evidence of infection other than the presence (in 97 percent) of positive cultures for *S. aureus* (10 percent in vaginal cultures). Up to 80 percent of these isolates were of phage types 29 and 52, and more than 93 percent produced staphylococcal exotoxin C or enterotoxin F (as compared with fewer than 15 percent of random isolates). These putative toxins may represent two activities of the same protein. Although TSS has commonly occurred in association with tampon use, 13 percent of cases have occurred in the absence of menstruation (5 percent in men), in the setting of cutaneous or surgical infection, or after childbirth or abortion. The absence of bacteremia in up to 90 percent of TSS suggests a major role for an exotoxin activity. The lungs are often involved in TSS with changes consistent with "shock lung" (Fig. 89-2): pulmonary hemorrhage, edema, atelectasis, hyaline membrane formation, and capillary thrombosis are prominent in the absence of pulmonary infection (Fig. 151-3). TSS is probably not different from pediatric staphylococcal scarlet fever that was epidemic in 1927, and it shares certain features with other exfoliative staphylococcal and streptococcal infections. Staphylococci and streptococci produce in excess of 20 bacterial products, i.e., toxins, enzymes, factors, the in vivo roles of which in the development of infections remain unclear. Among these, the hyaluronidases, lipases, coagulases, hemolysins, streptokinase, and streptolysins are believed to enhance the spread of infection along, or through, tissue planes and may account for the ability of these organisms to cause bacteremic infection. These organisms are also among the most common oropharyngeal colonizers and nosocomial organisms in hospitals, so that the frequency of infection with these agents may also reflect their preponderance in the environment.

The gram-negative organisms also produce a variety of toxins, proteases, and immunologically active factors. Like *S. aureus*, *P. aeruginosa* produces a nonenzymatic protein, *cytotoxin*, that also induces prostacyclin production and creates discrete nonphysiological transmembrane channels in cultured pulmonary artery endothelial cells similar to those described for staphylococcal α toxin. These channels allow the influx of calcium, which may modulate arachidonic acid metabolism in the cell. However, this organism also appears to have some unique characteristics which allow it to cause lung injury. (1) *P. aeruginosa* is frequently associated with the development of the adult respiratory distress syndrome (ARDS) during bacteremia or pneumonia (Fig. 89-3). In this setting, it is associated with microvascular lung injury which appears to be due to the pulmonary vascular sequestration of stimulated blood neutrophils even in the absence of infection of the pulmonary parenchyma. (2) It is also a major pulmonary pathogen that can adhere to pulmonary endothe-

lium, cause capillary thrombosis and inflammation, and invade the pulmonary interstitium (Fig. 89-4). *Pseudomonas* may mimic pulmonary thromboembolism with infarction during high-level bacteremia associated with bacterial invasion of pulmonary vessel walls. (3) In the absence of granulocytes, *Pseudomonas* cytotoxin has been shown to mimic the presentation of ARDS in sheep and pigs. *Pseudomonas* also causes ARDS in the neutropenic patient. This effect is due to a marked and irreversible increase in pulmonary vascular permeability which is distinct from the reversible, prostaglandin-mediated increase in pulmonary vascular resistance described above. This effect is also separable from the effects of bacterial endotoxin (see below), which has an overlapping array of pulmonary manifestations. These multiple manifestations of *Pseudomonas* infection illustrate a variety of mechanisms by which systemic infection may cause significant pulmonary injury.

Bacterial Products: The Bacterial Cell Wall (Endotoxins)

The third feature of infection that will cause systemic manifestations is the presence of the bacterial structural components associated with septic shock. At this juncture, a brief review of the structure of the cell wall of gram-negative bacteria is necessary. Surrounding the bacterial plasma membrane that borders the cytoplasm is the rigid layer made up of peptidoglycans or mucopeptides. This is the site of action of the penicillin and cephalosporin antibiotics which inhibit cell wall synthesis. Outside this membrane is the outer membrane, which consists of polysaccharides, proteins, and lipids. These components give the bacterium its O antigen and are responsible for the major serotypes by which bacteria are compared antigenically. This outer membrane also contains the LPS, or endotoxin moiety. Some strains of bacteria have additional cell layers that contain either organelles of adherence (pili or fimbriae) or of motility (flagella), and capsular or envelope polysaccharide antigens (the K antigen of *Klebsiella* and *E. coli*, the V1 of *Salmonella*). The K antigen appears on the smooth strains of gram-negative bacteria and is antiopsonic and antiphagocytic, thereby contributing to the inability of these organisms to be killed by serum that lacks specific antibodies to the infecting bacterium. In contrast, "rough" strains of bacteria that lack the K antigen have exposed O antigen, bind complement (C3b), and are more readily lysed or phagocytosed. These features may either confer tissue specificity or contribute to the invasiveness of certain organisms.

The syndrome of septic shock is usually associated with a gram-negative bacteremia. The syndrome consists of tissue hypoperfusion, systemic acidemia, hemodynamic instability, and hematologic disorders (Table 89-2). It may also be associated with metastatic infection with abscess formation. However, hypotension and metastatic

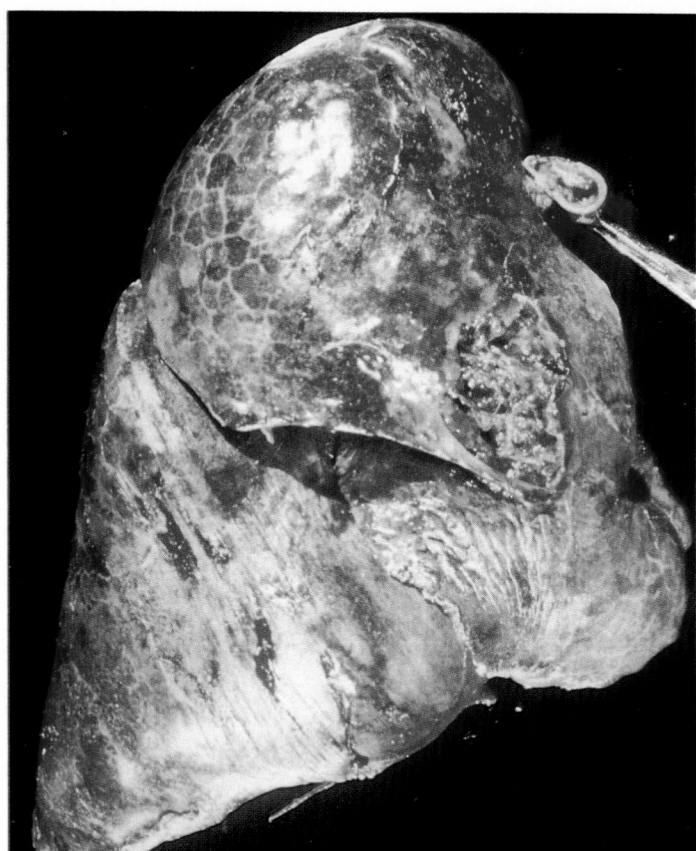

FIGURE 89-2   Toxic shock syndrome due to S. *aureus* bacteremia in a 20-year-old male following knee joint arthroscopy. Pleural hyperemia and inflammation (A) accompanies the parenchymal hemorrhage and consolidation of staphylococcal pneumonitis (B). Cavitation with abscess formation was prominent (C).

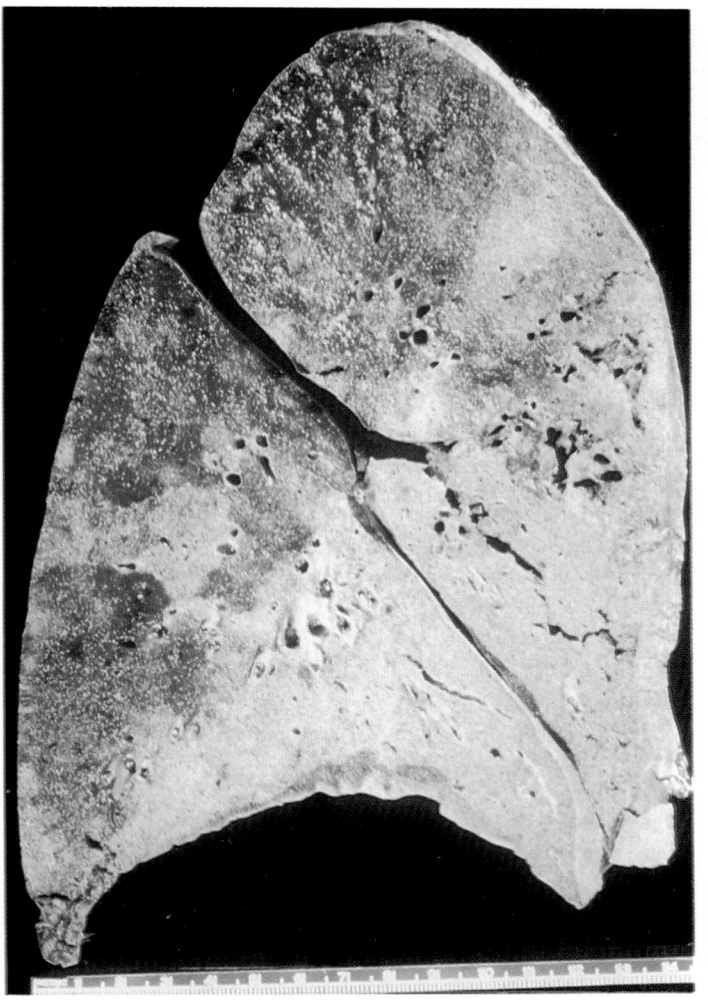

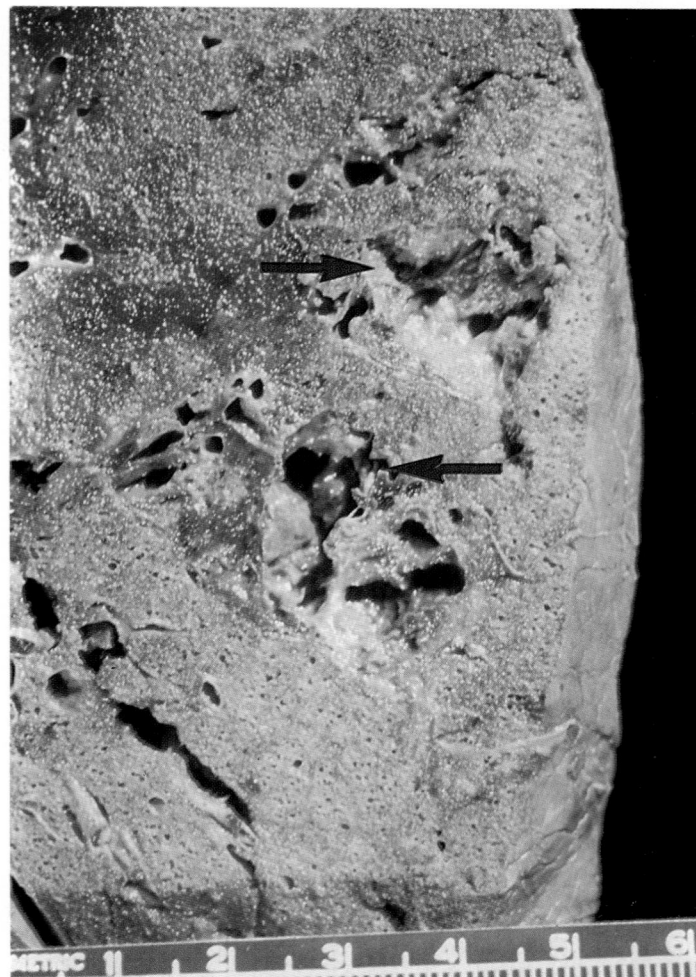

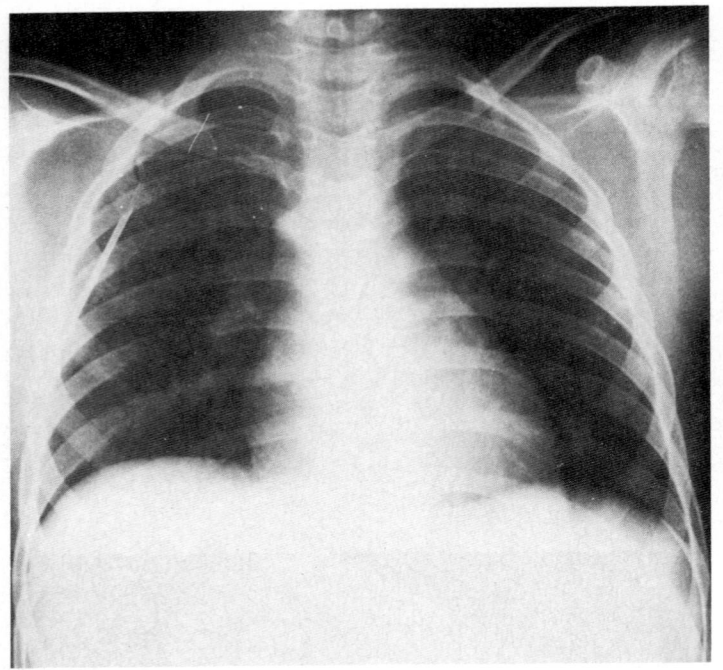

A

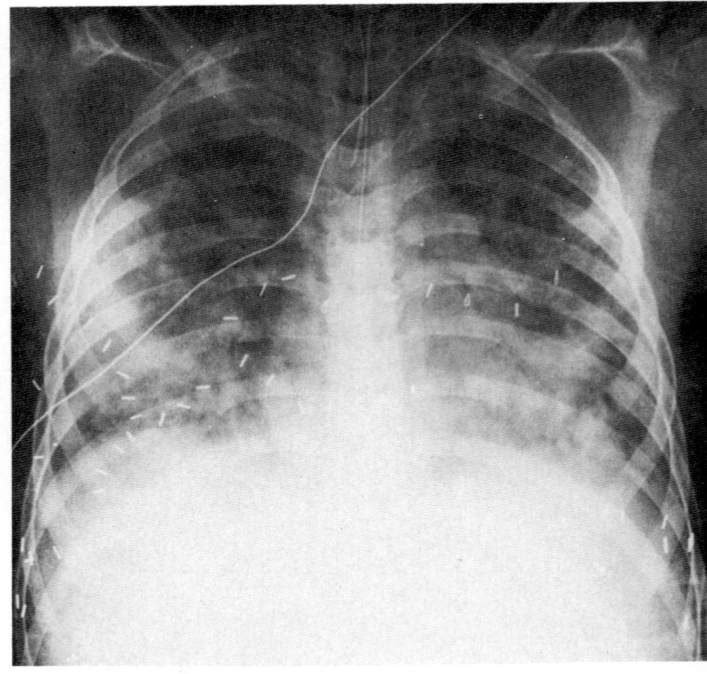

B

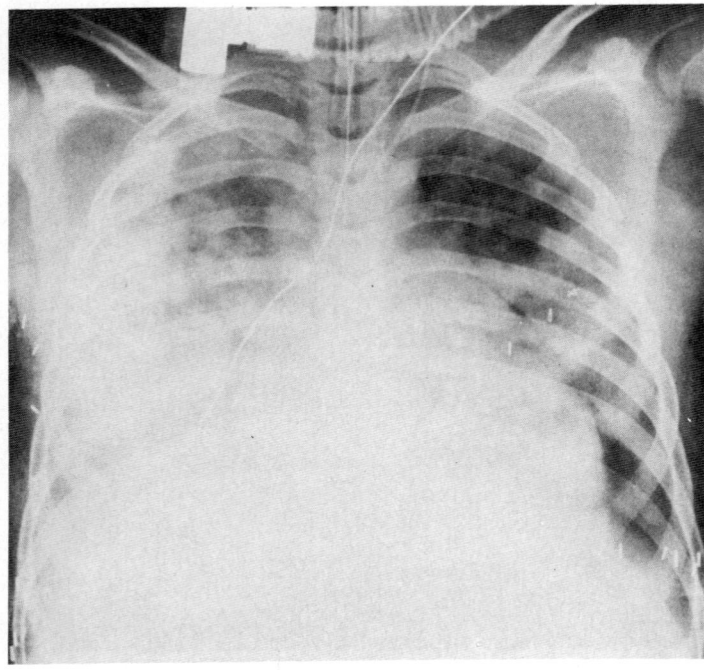

C

FIGURE 89-3 A child was admitted after 55 percent body burns with a clear chest radiograph (A). After 2 weeks and multiple skin grafting procedures, the patient developed a mild cough. Sputum contained no inflammatory cells and contained sheets of gram-negative rods on Gram stained smear. Therapy was initiated for *P. aeruginosa* empirically, despite an unchanged chest radiograph. Forty-eight hours into therapy, bronchopneumonia developed on chest radiograph (B) and progressed rapidly (72 h, C) requiring intubation. The patient survived. Cultures of sputum grew *P. aeruginosa*.

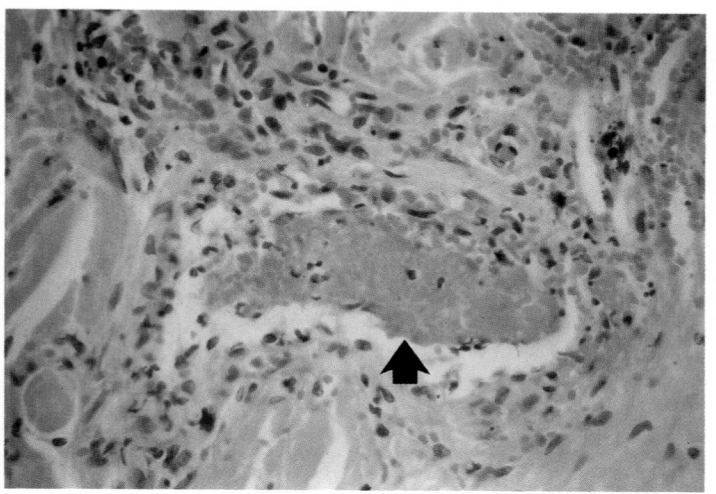

A

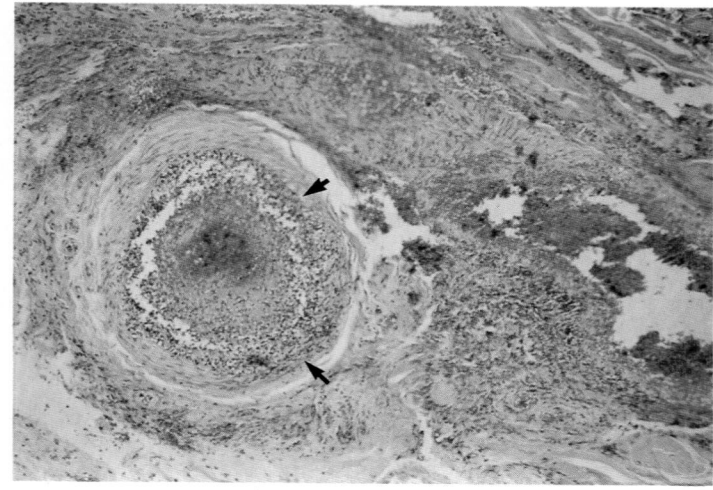

B

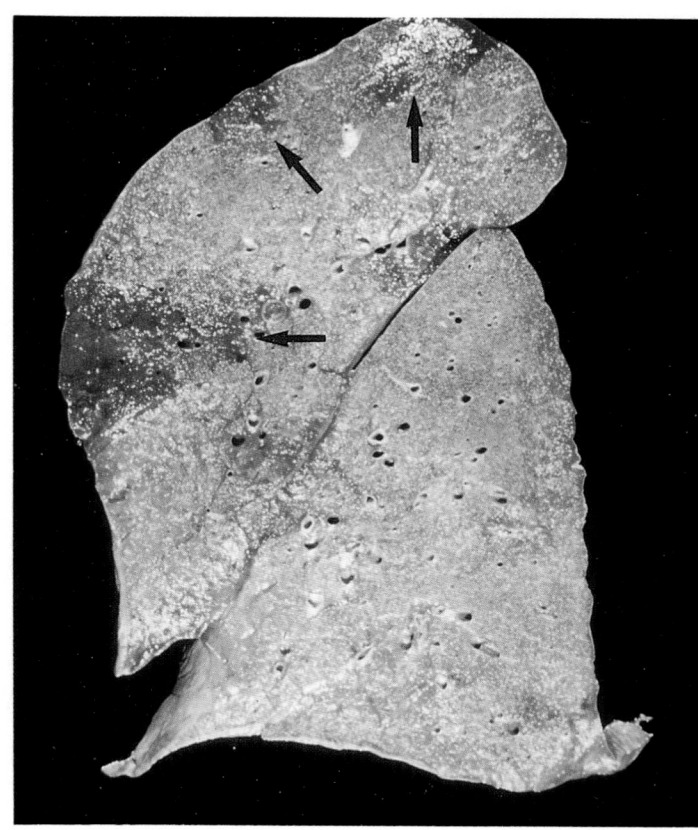

C

FIGURE 89-4   *Pseudomonas aeruginosa* bacteremia from an infected pelvic vein thrombus presented as cutaneous vasculitis (A) with small arteries occluded by fibrin thrombi (arrow) and with bacterial and leukocytic infiltration of the vascular wall (arrows, B). The patient developed multiple septic pulmonary emboli with infarction (arrows, C) with both organisms and leukocytes deep within the emboli. The pattern of microvascular thrombosis due to disseminated intravascular coagulation and ecthyma gangrenosum (arterial vasculitis due to infection) is characteristic of persistent high-grade bacteremia with *Pseudomonas* and other gram-negative bacteria.

infection also occur in association with infections caused by gram-positive, fungal, and viral organisms. It is, therefore, worth trying to distinguish between the physiological changes evoked by endotoxin derived from gram-negative organisms and those produced by bacteremic, or invasive, infection from other causes. Bacterial endotoxins are mixtures of all the components of the bacterial outer membrane including lipids, proteins, and polysac-

charides. Most of the biologic effects of endotoxin are mimicked by the "core glycolipid," which is lipid A (lipoidal acylated glucosamine disaccharide) attached to an acidic heterooligosaccharide. The roles played by the protein and sugar moieties in the in vivo syndrome are poorly defined. It is also unclear whether the active endotoxin is free or bound to intact bacteria. In general, the structure of lipid A is preserved intact among the various

TABLE 89-2
Manifestations of Gram-Negative Rod Bacteremia*

General signs
  Malaise, anxiety
  Fever, chills
  Hypothermia
  Dyspnea, cough
  Hyperventilation
  Altered mental status
  Accelerated angina
  Anorexia
  Nausea, vomiting
Symptoms
  Skin lesions
  Jaundice
  Bleeding
  Cardiac ischemia
  Tachypnea
  Aspiration
  Hemodialysis hypotension
  Hemoptysis
Clinical
  DIC (emboli, bleeding)
  Ecthyma gangrenosum
  Hypotension, shock
  Respiratory alkalosis
  Metabolic acidosis
  Oliguria, anuria
  Hemodynamic instability, congestive heart failure
  Hypoxemia
  Jaundice
  Leukopenia, thrombocytopenia
  Glucose intolerance
  Gastrointestinal ischemia

* Altered in those with underlying immune dysfunction, cardiac or pulmonary disease, extremes of age.

TABLE 89-3
Effects of Bacterial Endotoxins

Activation of complement (C3 and alternative pathway, inflammation)
Hageman factor activation (fibrinolysis)
Plasma thromboplastin antecedent (coagulation)
Interleukin 1 release (fever, catabolic state, leukocyte activation)
Cachectin/TNF synthesis (fever, IL-1, hypotension, cachexia)
Prostaglandin activation (pulmonary hypertension, platelet activation, vasoconstriction, leukocyte activation)
Kinin activation (edema, hypotension)
Endothelial injury (leukocyte margination, TNF, clotting)
Decreased surfactant function

Enterobacteriaceae; minor changes in the structure of lipid A cause considerable changes in the biologic activity of the bacterial endotoxins.

Support for the role of endotoxin in the pathogenesis of sepsis stems from the reproduction of the manifestations of this disorder by administering purified bacterial cell wall extracts to experimental animals. The manifestations include activation of the complement cascades, the coagulation and fibrinolytic systems, the kallikrein and bradykinin systems, and the induction of the physiological alterations associated with gram-negative sepsis in experimental animals given lipid A or endotoxin (Table 89-3). Further evidence comes from the ability of antibodies to core glycolipid to block many of the manifestations of sepsis due to gram-negative organisms. A precursor of lipid A (called lipid X) has also been shown to block certain systemic effects of lipid A, possibly through competition for a receptor that mediates some of the effects of endotoxin. Endotoxin has a variety of local and systemic effects in experimental systems. However, it may well be that many of the manifestations currently attributed to endotoxemia may prove to be related to other bacterial or host factors. Moreover, the ability to block the effects of administered endotoxin using diverse blocking agents, i.e., antibodies to cachectin/tumor necrosis factor, opiate antagonists (e.g., naloxone), prostaglandin or protease inhibitors, and platelet inhibitors, suggests that a variety of mechanisms mediate the effects currently ascribed to endotoxin.

A number of observations about the effects of endotoxin are pertinent. First, acute infusion of endotoxin to animals causes a biphasic physiological response similar to that seen clinically in bacteremic shock. Within 5 min, a stage of hypoperfusion and hypotension develops. This initial phase is not clearly related to the serum level of endotoxin. It appears to entail the pooling of blood in the splanchnic bed and peripherally; cardiac function appears to be unaffected. The initial phase is followed by a progressive fall in arterial blood pressure associated with a loss in vascular tone and an increase in vascular permeability. Endotoxin prompts the release of a broad spectrum of vasoactive substances into the circulation: serotonin, histamine, catecholamines, thromboxane and prostaglandins, endorphins, adrenal corticosteroids, lysozymes, lipases, proteases, and elastases, kallikrein, and bradykinin. Some are released from neutrophils at the site of localized infection; others are parts of the systemic response to infection and to endotoxin. The relative contribution of each of these factors, as with the contributions of the organisms themselves, is controversial.

Second, the depletion of some serum complement components caused by endotoxin is associated with the release of chemotactic factors, notably those of the alternative pathway, via the cleavage of C3. These factors me-

diate the release of kinins and histamine, chemotaxis and activation of neutrophils and monocytes, B-lymphocyte proliferation, bacterial opsonization, and vascular permeability. (Some of these activities are due to the lipid A-associated protein portion of the endotoxin complex rather than to the lipid-sugar alone.) Activation of serum complement is *not* necessary for the development of hypotension in this syndrome, but may account for some of the changes seen in vivo that are duplicated by other mediators. However, the alveolocapillary leakage during endotoxemia appears to be partially mediated by complement activation.

Third, activation of Hageman factor, resulting in the simultaneous initiation of both fibrinolysis and coagulation (owing to the cleavage of pre-plasma-thromboplastin antecedent) may be responsible for the syndrome of DIC (disseminated intravascular coagulation or consumptive coagulopathy with dysfunctional coagulation and bleeding diathesis) in endotoxemia. DIC should be suspected when unexplained bleeding, thrombocytopenia, prolongation of coagulation parameters, fibrin split products, or systemic microemboli occur in the absence of liver disease or other explanation for coagulopathy. DIC will result in the thrombosis of small blood vessels systemically due to the deposition of fibrin at sites of injury to the vascular endothelium (see below) and to trapping of microemboli in small vessels (Fig. 89-4). The syndrome of DIC is not unique to gram-negative bacteria; it is seen in a wide variety of gram-positive, fungal and, occasionally, viral infections, and it is a prominent feature of some carcinomas. DIC is a concern in only 5 to 10 percent of patients with a major infection.

Fourth, endotoxin also causes direct vascular endothelial injury, directly and by way of the systemic activation of neutrophils and monocytes that adhere to the injured cells or are trapped in the pulmonary capillaries. The principal direct actions of endotoxin are on small blood vessels that are innervated by the sympathetic nervous system. One indication of pulmonary endothelial injury is the leakage of endothelial angiotensin converting enzyme into blood flowing through the lungs. The development of pulmonary hemorrhages and/or pulmonary vascular microthrombi, therefore, relate both to the picture of DIC and to derangements in the endothelial surface and its anticoagulant functions by endotoxin. Sludging of blood in areas of increased pulmonary vascular resistance and alveolar capillary leakage also predispose to vascular thrombosis in small vessels. Stagnant anoxia causes vascular shunting around the anoxic areas, thereby interfering with the oxygenation of the blood leaving the lungs.

Endotoxin damages pulmonary microcirculatory endothelium causing an increase in permeability ("leaky vessels"). Adding to this direct effect are injuries arising from substances elaborated in response to infection, damage caused by microthrombi, and activated neutro-phils; in addition, endotoxin exerts powerful vasomotor effects on the pulmonary vascular bed, e.g., it elicits pulmonary vasoconstriction. Local release of prostaglandins further complicates the microcirculatory responses to endotoxin. These mechanisms are considered elsewhere in this book (Chapter 59). Much of the histopathology of shock lung is nonspecific. Pulmonary capillary endothelium remains grossly intact. However, the loss of alveolar epithelial type I cells occurs acutely and is accompanied by hyaline membrane formation, hemorrhagic edema, and type II cell proliferation. Chronic injury causes interstitial fibrosis, which is reflected in disturbances of oxygen exchange. Large leaks across the capillary endothelium are, apparently, rapidly repaired. Leakage of serum proteins into the alveolar spaces affects the concentration, and the surface activity, of pulmonary surfactant, thereby predisposing to the development of atelectasis during bacteremia and shock. Endotoxin also forms complexes with surfactant that alters the morphology, surface charges, and surface tension properties of this material. Complexes of endotoxin with pulmonary surfactant appear to be more toxic in mice than endotoxin alone. Thus, the interaction of bacteria, or bacterial products, with the lungs may increase the toxicity of systemic infection.

Endotoxin is cleared from the circulation in two phases: a rapid hepatic clearance that accounts for more than 50 percent, and a gradual second phase. Less than 5 percent of circulating endotoxin is deposited in the lungs. However, endothelium throughout the body and leukocytes release mediators of inflammation locally; within the lungs the effects of small amounts of endotoxin are greatly amplified. Endotoxin is deactivated by a variety of metabolic mechanisms including deacylation and dephosphorylation. Some of this activity is carried out by circulating leukocytes. The binding of endotoxin to lipoproteins, acute phase reactants, or antibodies also decreases its toxicity.

Recently Identified Mediators: Cachectin and Interleukin 1

Less than nanogram quantities of endotoxin per milliliter can produce injury to monocytes, macrophages, or pulmonary endothelial cell lines in vitro and in vivo. This corresponds to less than 10,000 molecules per cell. The amplification of the effects of bacterial endotoxin are a part of the infected individual's inflammatory response and are relatively nonspecific. A few mediators of endotoxin's systemic effects have been recently identified. Cachectin, or tumor necrosis factor (TNF), is a polypeptide hormone synthesized and secreted by circulating macrophages, fixed reticuloendothelial cells, lymphocytes, and probably other cell types. It is released in milligram quantities within minutes of exposure of macrophages to endotoxin. Its actions are mediated by a relatively specific receptor

on the surface of its target cells; this receptor also binds the related lymphokine, *lymphotoxin*. TNF has a short serum half-life (approximately 6 min); therefore, its systemic effects are due to either its continuous production or to a series of second mediators, e.g., interleukin 1. TNF appears to play a role in the anorexia and the weight loss that accompanies chronic infections, such as that seen in trypanosomiasis or in the acquired immunodeficiency syndrome (AIDS). Administration of TNF induces a syndrome similar to endotoxemia: fever, hypotension, acidosis, and DIC. Antibodies or passive immunization to TNF protects against the lethal effects of administered endotoxin. TNF causes activation of neutrophil adherence, degranulation, and phagocytosis. TNF also suppresses endothelial anticoagulant activity and enhances procoagulant activity, changes that correlate with the tendency to thrombosis during gram-negative bacteremia. TNF is also a pyrogen.

Interleukin 1 (IL-1) is also known as *endogenous pyrogen*, lymphocyte activating factor, or the *leukocytic endogenous mediator*. IL-1 and TNF mediate some of the same inflammatory reactions including fever, neutrophilia, and systemic metabolic changes. Of note, IL-1 production can occur in many cell types such as monocytes (including pulmonary and peripheral blood macrophages), endothelial cells, and epithelial cells. Its synthesis is induced by TNF and by microorganisms, endotoxin, inflammation and trauma, and immune stimulation. IL-1 can also induce endothelial cell procoagulant activity mediated by plasminogen activator inhibitor. Thus, IL-1 and TNF appear to be major mediators of many of the effects of endotoxin. These effects are augmented by many other factors released in the process of the host response to infection, and are themselves amplified by other lymphokines, e.g., γ-interferon and lymphotoxin, and by cellular activities. Of potential therapeutic importance is the synthesis of TNF messenger ribonucleic acid (mRNA), and the translation of this mRNA into TNF protein, which is blocked by corticosteroids. However, this blockage, including the protective effect on alveolar-capillary permeability, has proved effective only if corticosteroids are administered *prior* to the administration of the endotoxin. Similarly, corticosteroids appear to suppress IL-1 release. At present, even though much remains to be learned about how the corticosteroids exert their effects, it appears that there is no therapeutic role for corticosteroids once bacterial sepsis has developed.

SEPTIC SHOCK WITHOUT ENDOTOXIN

Septic shock is not limited to infections with gram-negative organisms; it occurs in association with almost all bacterial, fungal, and viral species. Endotoxin has been isolated from rickettsia, spirochetes, and some fungi (in-

cluding *Candida*). The importance of its association with gram-negative infection is emphasized by the mortality of gram-negative bacteremia (20 to 30 percent), and of gram-negative septic shock (50 percent). In the setting of ARDS, the mortality of gram-negative sepsis may approach 80 to 90 percent. However, in both gram-negative and gram-positive bacteremias, the level of bacteremia is correlated with hypotension and mortality. Although the mechanisms responsible for gram-positive, viral, and fungal shock are more elusive than those considered above for gram-negative shock, it is likely that the same mediators of inflammation, i.e., histamine, complement, TNF, IL-1, neutrophil activation, and locally active exotoxins and enzymes, are important in all infections. The apparent lack of specificity of the hypotensive effects of inflammation are demonstrated by early studies on the equal ability of tissue necrosis, turpentine-induced sterile abscesses, or localized intraoperative infection to produce hypotension in experimental animals. Similarly, in a variety of hosts, DIC occurs in infections due to mycobacteria, fungi, parasites, rickettsia, and viruses. In the absence of endotoxin, the development of septic shock may be a question of the degree, rather than of the uniqueness, of the syndrome seen with gram-negative infections.

Comparison of gram-positive and gram-negative sepsis suggests that the hemodynamic consequences encountered clinically are generally more dramatic with gram-negative bacteremia: the decrease in systemic vascular resistance and the drop in central venous pressure are more rapid and profound than that in gram-positive infection, as are the oliguria and metabolic acidosis. The decrease in blood pressure is also more protracted and refractory to therapy. Cardiac output is normal or high in both types of sepsis even though a myocardial depressant factor appears in the circulation. In time, this "high output" state is succeeded by heart failure. The change to a "low output" state is predictive of high mortality in all infections. Similarly, advancing age, immune compromise, cardiac disease, hepatic dysfunction, fluid loss, renal failure, and the delayed or incorrect choice of the initial antibiotics and supportive therapy correlate with increased mortality.

As noted previously, many of the gram-positive organisms produce exotoxins and enzymes that may injure infected tissues and elicit inflammation. Some, like the pneumococci (*Streptococcus pneumoniae*) and *S. aureus*, can cause a destructive pneumonia or pericardial tamponade. Unique toxins from diphtheria (myocarditis), *Shigella* and cholera (intestinal fluid loss), *anthrax* (systemic edema), and clostridia (hemolysis, edema, myonecrosis) have other mechanisms for inducing hypotension or shock. The appropriate choice of antibiotic therapy should be guided by the isolation of the causative organism *before* therapy is begun because of the broad spectrum of organisms that can cause a syndrome of septic shock.

The Neutrophil

Many of the effects of systemic infection have been attributed to miscellaneous factors that exert systemic effects. Although it is likely that neutrophil activation also plays a primary role in damaging the lungs during infection, like complement, TNF, and endotoxin, neutrophils are *not* essential for lung injury in infection; ARDS and bacteremic pneumonia are frequently seen in the neutropenic-bacteremic patient. During infection, neutrophils accumulate rapidly in the alveolar capillaries. It appears that if these cells are "activated," then pulmonary injury can occur. In the presence of bacteria, viruses, fungi, endotoxin, IL-1, TNF, microemboli, complement activation, or other leukocyte activators, the neutrophils marginate, degranulate, release lymphocyte and monocyte chemoattractants and leukocyte activators, and cause pulmonary injury. The local release of IL-1 and TNF into the pulmonary circulation may augment that released at the site of extrapulmonary infections. In the setting of pneumonia, neutrophil accumulation and activation will persist. Within an hour of the initial insult, pulmonary capillary endothelial injury occurs, with edema and interstitial accumulation of protein and cells. The release of proteolytic enzymes, oxygen free radicals, and arachidonic acid metabolites, which affect permeability and increase vascular tone, will continue to injure the pulmonary parenchyma for as long as the stimulus persists. Pulmonary injury is potentiated by both hypoxia and hyperoxia and by conditions associated with chronic inflammation, such as bronchiectasis, bronchitis, chronic interstitial disease, and radiation or chemotherapy injury.

The major barriers to infection are the intact cutaneous and mucous membranes. Once these physical barriers have been breached, the second line of defense is the ability of the host to neutralize invading organisms by opsonization, complement-mediated lysis, and/or phagocytosis. Blockade of the systemic effects of lipid A by antibodies does not prevent the spread of infection throughout the body. Systemic immunization using intact bacteria, e.g., *P. aeruginosa* and *E. coli*, enhances pulmonary clearance of those bacteria to which antibodies have been raised. Preformed immunoglobulins may appear in pulmonary edema fluids within hours of bacterial seeding, and improve the clearance of bacteria, both from the alveolus and the circulation. Antibodies directed against surface antigens of bacteria, fungi, and viruses may protect the host by blocking the ability of the organism to adhere, penetrate, or move within tissues. When systemic defenses fail, the prevention of pulmonary involvement in disseminated infection depends on the clearance of bacteria by the lung, i.e., by lymph fluid, coughing, local immunoglobulins, and resident phagocytes. The potential for marginating neutrophils to add to pulmonary injury in addition to clearing invasive organisms has been noted above. In some animal models of bacteremia associated with shock, hypoxemia, atelectasis, and pulmonary edema, a reversible decrease occurs in the phagocytosis and killing of bacteria by alveolar macrophages. The mechanisms responsible for this depressed activity are unclear, but this decrease in the function of alveolar macrophages during bacteremias may contribute to the development of pneumonia due to the seeding of the pulmonary parenchyma from the blood or due to aspirated oropharyngeal organisms in the setting of reduced bacterial clearance.

PATTERNS OF PULMONARY INJURY IN SYSTEMIC INFECTION

Three major patterns of pulmonary injury occur in response to infection outside of the lungs. First is the direct extension of infection to the pulmonary parenchyma or pleural space. This often involves the decompression of an intra-abdominal or pharyngeal abscess along tissue planes into the thoracic cavity. These may be catastrophic clinical events, as in the rupture of a subphrenic or a hepatic abscess due to *Entamoeba histolytica* across the diaphragm with the sudden development of amebic pneumonia. A more insidious picture occurs when a peritonsillar abscess (or infections of the parapharyngeal space) or submandibular infection (Ludwig's angina) decompresses into the retropharyngeal space (Table 89-4). This potential space extends down to the level of thoracic vertebrae 1 or 2, and may allow the drainage of pus directly into the mediastinum causing mediastinitis.

The second major pattern of involvement of the lungs is due to embolic spread of infection to the lungs and to the pleura. This may entail only bacteremic or lymphatic spread of organisms to the lungs, or the seeding of the pleura or of pleural fluid causing empyema. It may also be due to septic embolization of an infected thrombus (Fig. 89-4) or to the debris of a distant infection. Bacteremia tends to cause multiple areas of pneumonia throughout the parenchyma. This is a pattern seen in miliary tuberculosis or in staphylococcal bacteremia due to endocarditis (Fig. 89-5). Multiple abscesses develop; they are usually peripheral in location. When pulmonary emboli develop as a complication of septic thrombophlebitis or of tricuspid valvular infective endocarditis, infarction may accompany infection. In this situation, abscess formation is rapid and unimpeded by appropriate host responses as infarcted tissues become necrotic. Rarely do emboli become secondarily infected. However, infarction may accompany pneumonia due to *Aspergillus* or *P. aeruginosa* because of their vascular tropism and to the vasculitis that these organisms cause (Fig. 89-4).

The third pattern of pulmonary injury occurs in both

TABLE 89-4
Extrapulmonary Infectious Disease Emergencies Affecting the Respiratory System

Syndrome	Signs/Symptoms	Organisms	Comments
Gram(−) bacteremia	Ecthyma gangrenosum, hypotension, acidosis	P. aeruginosa, E. coli, Klebsiella	Endotoxic shock, often ARDS, DIC
Meningococcemia	Petechial hemorrhagic rash, hypotension, DIC	Neisseria Meningitidis	Early high-dose penicillin therapy
Toxic shock syndrome	Hypotension, multiorgan dysfunction, DIC, erythema of skin	S. aureus	Late desquamation, men and women, after surgery, childbirth, soft-tissue infections
Erysipelas, scalded skin	Rapidly advancing cutaneous erythema	Staphylococcus, Streptococcus	Often with bacteremia
Infective endocarditis	Congestive heart failure, lung abscess	All	Prior procedures, drug abuse
Sinusitis	Fever of undetermined origin, headache, cavernous sinus thrombosis	Anaerobes, Pneumococcus, nosocomial gram(−) fungus	After nasotracheal intubation, especially immunosuppressed patients
Ludwig's angina, peritonsillar abscess, retropharyngeal abscess	Dysphagia, raised tongue, tonsillitis, pharyngitis, trismus	Oral anaerobes, Staphylococcus, Streptococcus	Early therapy, may need tracheostomy abscess drainage mediastinitis
Epiglottitis	Stridor, obstruction with manipulation, "cherry-red" epiglottis	H. influenzae type B, Streptococcus, Staphylococcus	Early elective intubation in children
Diphtheria	Pustular pharyngitis, pseudomembranes	Corynebacterium diphtheriae	Antitoxin, rule out mononucleosis
Tetanus	Trismus, dysphagia, diplopia, pupil dilatation	Clostridium tetani, C. botulinum	Toxoid, wound debridement, support
Guillain-Barré	Ascending paralysis, neuritis	Mycoplasma pneumoniae Many viruses	After respiratory illness, postimmunization, trauma
Strongyloidiasis	Diarrhea, gram(−) bacteremia, pneumonia, eosinophilia	Strongyloides stercoralis	Immunosuppressed host
Hepatic-bronchopleural fistula	"Anchovy paste" sputum, hepatic abscess	Entamoeba histolytica	Tamponade, "sterile" right pleural effusion
Immunocompromised patient	Dyspnea, cough, fever, tachypnea, acidosis, altered mental status, hematologic or metabolic changes	All	Radiographic changes often absent
Acquired immunodeficiency syndrome (AIDS)	Dyspnea, cough, fever, skin lesions, weight loss, diarrhea, confusion	Human immunodeficiency virus, Cryptococcus neoformans, Toxoplasma gondii	Rule out Pneumocystis and metastatic tumor; look for central nervous system involvement

pulmonary or extrapulmonary infections. The pattern is one of widespread lung injury in association with a significant infection that causes the activation of the complement cascade, neutrophil trapping and activation, production of cachectin/TNF and interleukin 1, and activation of the mediators of inflammation. High on the list of initiating mechanisms are infection with bacteremia, oxygen toxicity, and major nonpulmonary trauma. This picture, at its worst, is ARDS, or shock lung. The presence of bacterial products, i.e., enzymes, endotoxin, and toxins, may promote the development of pulmonary edema, hyaline membranes, interstitial fibrosis, hemorrhage and cellular injury that characterize the histopathol-ogy of these patients' lungs (Chapter 142). As noted previously, some bacteria or bacterial products may cause this syndrome when abscesses decompress into the circulation, when loculated infection maintains a high-grade bacteremia, in the course of intravascular infection, or in gram-negative sepsis. The syndrome should be regarded as the climax to the interplay of a large number of systemic mediators activated by tissue injury and by inflammation. It is clear that the effects of infections on the lungs form overlapping patterns that are often further complicated by the development of pneumonia or other pulmonary disturbances, such as pulmonary edema caused by left ventricular failure.

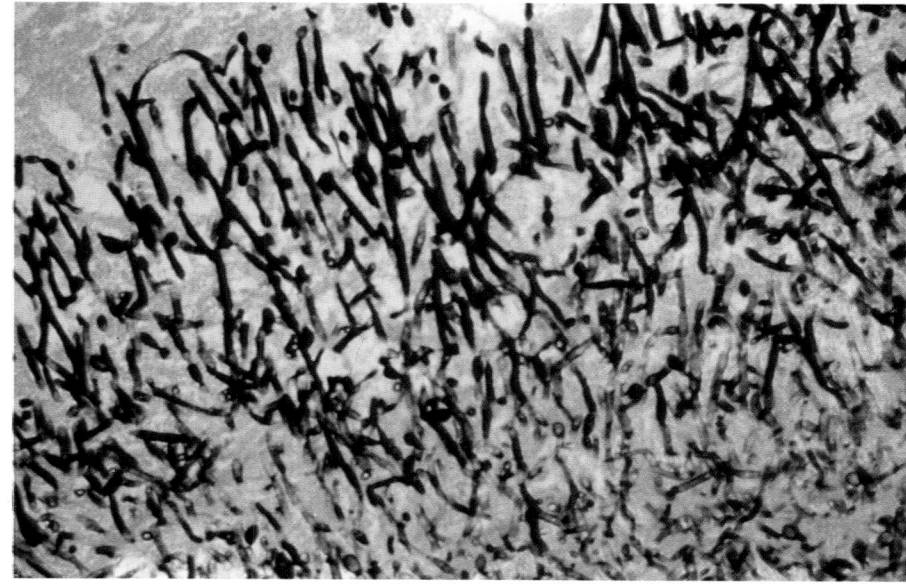

FIGURE 89-5 Fungal right-sided endocarditis (IE) in a patient with 50 percent total body burns resulted in an embolus of *C. albicans* from the infected valve *(A)* to the bifurcation of the pulmonary artery *(B)*. Pleural involvement with fungal seeding of the pleural surface is a common complication of right-sided IE *(C)*.

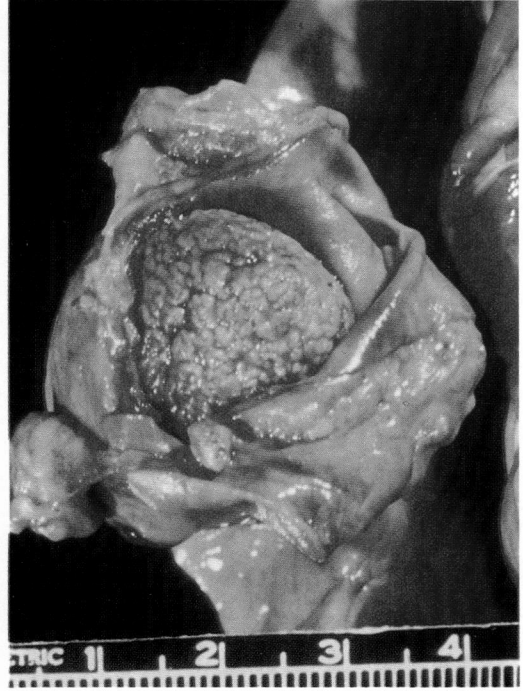

B

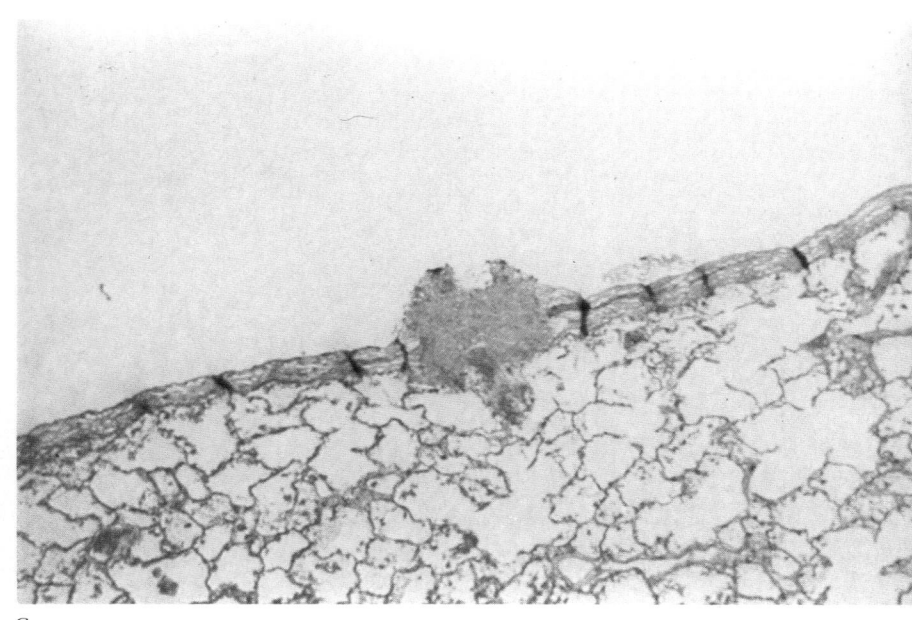

A

C

SYNDROMES OF LUNG INJURY

Intravascular Infections

Disseminated infection and high-grade bacteremias are most often associated with infection in, or adjacent to, the bloodstream. The best described entity of this type is infective endocarditis (IE). The terms *acute* or *subacute endocarditis* were descriptive names applied to heart valve infections in the preantibiotic era; the infections were largely staphylococcal and streptococcal. Most of the criteria for infections that might involve the lungs apply to infective endocarditis (IE). For a given organism to cause IE, it must adhere to a heart valve, replicate, and produce infec-

tion that is relatively resistant to host defenses. In principle, these qualifications should limit the number of species that can produce the syndrome. However, even though streptococci and staphylococci account for more than 80 percent of all instances of IE, the frequency of gram-negative, anaerobic, and fungal infections as the cause of IE is increasing. Many of the latter organisms gain access to the circulation by way of the newer invasive therapies, including central venous catheters and pacemakers; some of the increased incidence is also due to the prolonged survival of patients after severe trauma, e.g., burns, or with immune compromise caused by either cancer or the therapeutic agents used to treat it.

The development of IE depends on the preexistence of an irregular or damaged heart valve or endocardial surface onto which fibrin and/or platelets have been deposited. Turbulence of blood flow or the erosion caused by a cardiac catheter may suffice to cause injury, even though the "classic" disruption is the scarring of the mitral and aortic valves as a result of rheumatic carditis. This nonbacterial, thrombotic endocarditis (NBTE) is then superinfected by a strain of bacteria that can adhere to the fibrin mesh. Transient bacteremia from dental work, surgery, airway manipulation, endoscopy, urologic procedures, and a variety of minor traumas are sufficient to infect the endocardial surface. The ability of the bacteria to secrete enzymes that allow deeper penetration into the fibrin or cardiac tissue renders the infection impervious to host defenses. The growth of the fibrin/platelet/bacterial thrombus on the valve ("vegetation") prevents the penetration of neutrophils to the main nidus of infection.

The systemic effects of infective endocarditis are diverse: weight loss, malaise, fevers, and dyspnea are common. On the one hand, the clinical manifestations may reflect the role of cachectin/TNF, interleukin 1, and recurrent bacteremias; on the other, they may represent the hemodynamic consequences, often aggravated by the valvular damage. Systemic emboli, both infected and sterile, are often accompanied by splenomegaly, heart murmurs, and multiorgan dysfunction. Clubbing is present in up to 20 percent of cases, and cutaneous manifestations of embolic infection in up to 50 percent. Major emboli and congestive heart failure occur in up to a third of patients each.

The lungs are usually involved in infective endocarditis secondary to left ventricular failure that is caused by dysfunction of the mitral or aortic valves, myocarditis, or cardiac ischemia; in addition, tachycardia, fever, and hypotensive episodes contribute to the cardiac abnormalities. However, direct pulmonary involvement is common in right-sided (e.g., tricuspid valve) disease or in congenital cardiac anomalies with left-to-right shunting, e.g., tetralogy of Fallot. In this setting, pulmonary emboli, followed by acute pneumonia or lung abscess, are common. Pleural embolic seeding is also frequent with the subsequent development of pleural effusions and empyema (Fig. 89-5).

Intravenous drug abusers (Chapter 90) are most often affected by the pulmonary complications of IE: tricuspid valvular involvement occurs in over half of the patients, with or without infection of other heart valves. The clinical presentation is often that of a young person with dyspnea of sudden onset, pleurisy, fever, or occasionally hemoptysis. Cutaneous manifestations of sepsis and infected injection sites are common. The patient generally develops radiographic evidence of septic embolic involvement of the lung (pneumonia, pulmonary infarction, pleural effusion) during the early part of the hospitalization (Fig. 89-6). Tricuspid insufficiency can be demonstrated only in a minority of these individuals. Pulmonary

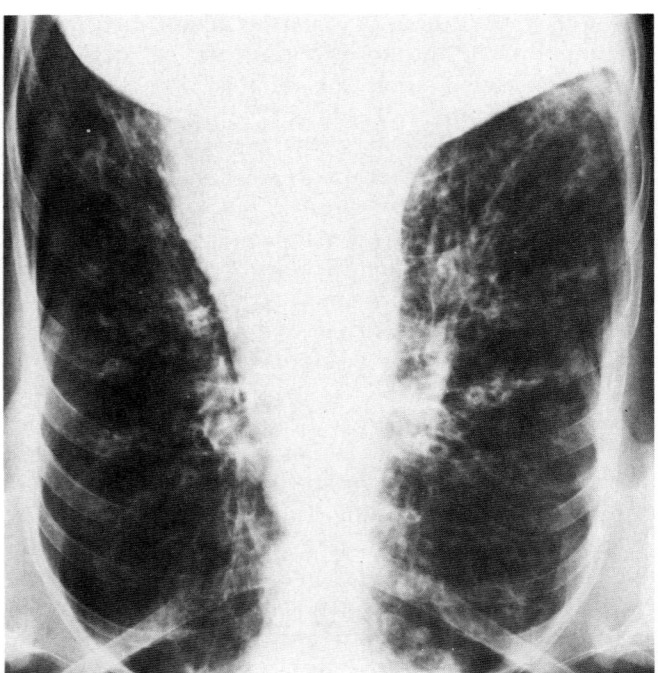

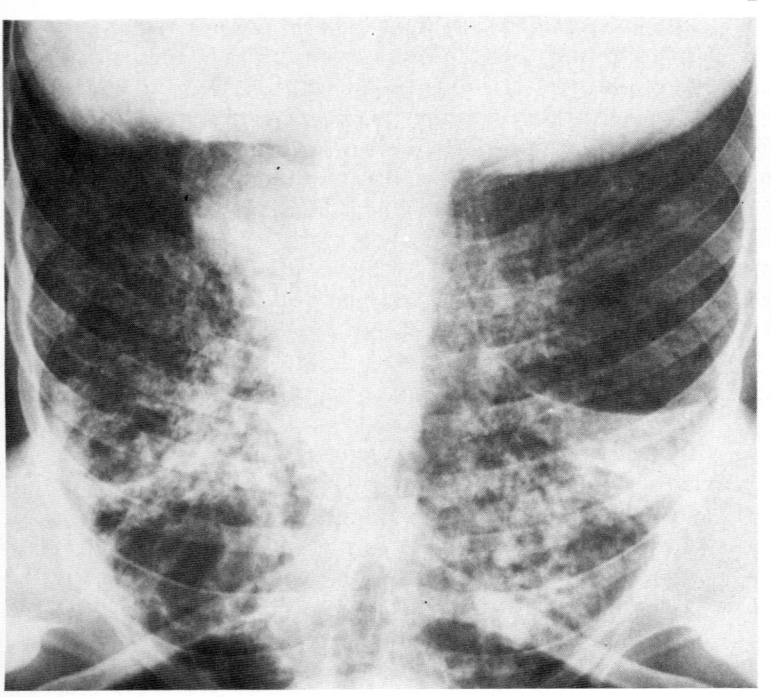

FIGURE 89-6   Right-sided *S. aureus* endocarditis in a heroin abuser with multiple pulmonary abscesses due to septic emboli (A). The distribution of lung involvement contrasts with the patchy pneumonic picture of miliary (i.e., bacteremic) tuberculosis (B).

involvement can be worsened by the presence of talc, cotton fibers, or other impurities in the intravenous drug mixture. "Skin poppers" who inject narcotics subcutaneously are also subject to right-sided IE. All injectable illicit drugs are potentially contaminated; local infection of the skin (abscesses) or veins (thrombophlebitis) are common and may require surgical intervention for cure. Therapy is guided by the results of multiple blood cultures drawn sterilely, during the first 24 h of hospitalization. However, in the gravely ill patient, the empiric administration of broad-spectrum intravenous antibiotics—directed at both gram-negative and gram-positive bacteria—is necessary in the acute setting. However, even in these patients, blood cultures should be drawn before starting antibiotics parenterally. Peripheral sites of infection (e.g., skin lesions, infected veins) often yield the organisms, and a Gram stain of the blood buffy coat is sometimes helpful in directing therapy. In the addict, the organisms responsible for IE include *S. aureus*, *P. aeruginosa*, *Candida albicans*, other gram-negative aerobes, anaerobes, and occasionally multiple organisms are isolated. The spectrum of organisms seen in infections in the intravenous drug user has been greatly expanded due to the susceptibility of this population to the development of opportunistic infection due to AIDS.

Fungal endocarditis is common not only in the drug addict population but also in patients who have recently undergone cardiac surgery, in immunocompromised patients, and in those who have had prolonged exposure to intravenous central catheters for monitoring, therapy, or hyperalimentation (Figs. 89-6 and 89-7). The development of fever and systemic signs may be quite insidious in these patients; until embolic phenomena occur, fungal blood isolates are often disregarded as contaminants of the cultures. After cardiac surgery, infections have been encountered with *Aspergillus* as well as *Candida* species, probably reflecting nosocomial sources for the fungi. In the immunocompromised patient, unusual agents, i.e., the *Mucor* agents or *Trichosporon beigelii*, are also being recognized. The development of fungal pneumonia in the addict is probably related to the presence of fungal contaminants in the marijuana and cocaine preparations used. In these individuals, direct inhalation and/or sinusitis may be the source of a bacteremic infection.

Intravascular infection of the venous circulation, followed by pulmonary embolization, occurs in association with thrombosis of the deep veins of the pelvis or legs, or in the presence of vein grafts and intravascular prosthetic devices (Fig. 89-4). Septic thrombophlebitis is a major cause of secondary lung abscess, usually presenting as a single area of pneumonitis in contrast to the multiple peripheral lesions seen in bacteremic disease. Possibly because of the tendency of emboli to lodge distally in the pulmonary circulation, approximately one-third are complicated by the development of empyema and, occasion-

ally, by bronchopleural fistula. Invasive organisms, i.e., *Staphylococcus*, *Streptococcus*, *Klebsiella*, and *E. coli*, tend to involve the pleural space in the course of bacteremic pneumonia. Embolic infection is also a complication of prolonged intravenous therapy. Contamination of catheters, e.g., Hickman, Broviac, and Swan-Ganz lodged in the right atrium or superior vena cava, occurs in up to 10 percent of patients; this contamination is accompanied by bacteremia or fungemia in about 3 patients per 1000 catheter-use days. The initial therapy for catheter-related infection is to remove the device. However, the difficulty in recognizing that systemic infection exits, coupled with the tendency to use these devices in patients in whom venous access is difficult, tends to delay removal. Infection due to the catheter cannot be treated successfully without its removal. The development of an infected thrombus on a subclavian catheter may require surgical intervention to remove the infected line and to relieve vascular obstruction. In the immunocompromised patient these infections are associated with a high mortality. Because of the relative absence of inflammatory signs in the neutropenic host, infection can progress insidiously before it is recognized. A typical example of this phenomenon was observed in a patient with acute myelogenous leukemia in whom a Hickman catheter was placed to allow venous access for chemotherapy and for hyperalimentation. The cannula became infected with *Trichosporon beigelii*, and disseminated infection with this fungus was unresponsive to therapy by the time it was recognized, even after the infected line was removed (Fig. 89-7). The first evidence of systemic infection was the development of pneumonia with pleural effusion. In the course of a single day, the full-blown picture of ARDS developed in association with a persistent neutropenia, i.e., fewer than 500 polymorphonuclear leukocytes per cubic millimeter. Prominent among the postmortem findings was a necrotizing, hemorrhagic pneumonitis and fungal seeding throughout the vascular tree. Although catheter-induced bacteremia is usually uncomplicated, it can result in endocarditis or in clinically significant systemic infections.

Another source of bacteremia, direct infection of the arterial wall (endarteritis), is uncommon unless atherosclerotic or aneurysmal injury has preceded it. High-grade bacteremia and systemic signs similar to those of infective endocarditis then ensue. More common is infection of prosthetic vascular grafts, secondary to surgical contamination, incomplete coverage of the device by vascular endothelium, fibrin deposition, and occasionally adherence of adjacent organs (bowel or ureter) accompanied by leakage of organisms across the graft-vessel wall. Graft anastomoses are the most susceptible to colonization with organisms, and those in the inguinal region are the most often affected. As a rule, the infecting organism is *S. aureus*, but *E. coli* is more common in the setting of intra-

abdominal infection. The clinical manifestations are those of either a chronic infection or a draining abscess, or the development of a false aneurysm at an anastomotic site. Infections of prosthetic cardiac valves also afford a nidus for infection within the bloodstream; the resultant bacteremia and systemic manifestations resemble those of infective endocarditis. Pulmonary involvement is common in infections of venous filters that are placed in the inferior vena cava to prevent pulmonary emboli from the deep veins of the pelvis and legs. Infections of these devices is complicated, on the one hand, by their tendency to cause septic emboli and obstruction of the vena cava and, on the other, by the extreme difficulty of removing them once they become embedded in the vascular intima. Treatment is generally based on the supposition that the infection is not of the device itself but rather of the attached clot and debris. In fact, antibiotics and anticoagulation are generally successful in treating these infections, and very few of them are actually removed.

Occult Infection: Burns, Sickle Cell Anemia, Alcoholism

The ability of organisms carried by the bloodstream to reach, and to infect, the pulmonary parenchyma has been considered above. Secondary infection of the lungs by bacteremias initiated by pneumonias are also common. More often, however, the physician is confronted by the development of pulmonary symptoms or by radiologic evidence of pulmonary disease in the absence of evident bacteremia. In these patients, the lungs are often seeded by pathogenic bacteria from unknown primary sites of infection.

Striking examples of occult infections that affect the lungs are seen in patients with burns, sickle cell disease, and alcoholism. As a rule, patients with full-thickness burns receive at least one prophylactic dose of penicillin at the time of admission to avoid acute streptococcal infection of the skin and bloodstream. Antibiotics are also administered prophylactically before manipulation of burned skin, debridement, or skin grafting procedures to deal with anticipated bacteremia. The antibiotics used tend to reflect the common infecting flora of the burns treated at a given medical center; they also determine which resistant organisms will become the colonizing agents of the injured skin. Before the advent of topical antibacterial therapy, local infection used to be responsible for the progression of a partial thickness burn to a fully necrotic dermis. Topical therapy is aimed at the reduction of the bacterial burden of the injured skin: silver sulfadiazine is more effective against gram-negative organisms, whereas mafenide acetate is better against the gram-positive bacteria. The best method for reducing infection is to cover the burned area with skin autografts or allografts as soon as possible after the patient has been stabilized hemodynamically.

In burn patients, colonization with antibiotic-resistant organisms and cross-contamination is common despite intensive isolation procedures. Superinfection is often with S. aureus, P. aeruginosa, and Candida species. The mortality of burns relates to the level of infection of the viable tissues that surround the burn site. Quantitative bacterial cultures of biopsies taken of burned tissues have demonstrated a correlation between the type and the number of organisms isolated from the skin and those that, ultimately, cause death. Because burn patients with over 40 percent body burns do not adequately mobilize neutrophils, either locally or systemically, these individuals are effectively immunosuppressed. Bacteremia and hematogenous infection, notably of the lungs, are common. Because of the poor neutrophil response, bronchopneumonia can occur without infiltrates on the chest radiographs. An example of the development of pneumonia in the absence of an appropriate local leukocyte response is shown in Fig. 89-3. In these patients, subtle changes in either the skin wounds (i.e., discoloration, weeping, and hemorrhage) or in the hematologic parameters (i.e., new coagulation defects, abnormal white blood cell counts in the peripheral blood, or abnormal liver function tests) or abnormalities in the chest radiograph are a basis for concern. Excision of infected tissues or of the sites responsible for the disseminated infection may be necessary.

Complications of the prolonged use of intravenous catheters is also common in the burn patient. Venous access is always difficult to achieve in burn patients, and transient bacteremias are common. Suppurative thrombophlebitis occurs frequently even without catheter infection and is difficult to detect under burned skin. Fungal endocarditis has been observed as a result of right atrial cannulae placed during a period of unsuspected fungemia (Fig. 89-5). Fungal growth in blood cultures is often slow; intermittently positive cultures for common clinical laboratory contaminants, e.g., Candida and Aspergillus, may be ignored. Because the signs of infection may be muted in these patients, it may progress unnoticed. Inhalational burn injury of the lungs, resulting in atelectasis, edema, decreased mucociliary function or ARDS, promotes the rapid development of pneumonia. Necrotic muscle caused by burns is often infected. If so, the infected muscle or fascia must be resected to save viable tissues and to prevent dissemination of infection.

Two groups of individuals with phagocytic and opsonic immune dysfunction are markedly susceptible to lung injury during infection: the individual with sickle cell anemia and the alcoholic. Because of splenic dysfunction, infarction, or spontaneous amputation, the individual with sickle cell anemia has a heightened susceptibility to infection with "encapsulated" organisms that require specific antibody and splenic function for their clearance, e.g., S. pneumoniae, Haemophilus influenzae, and Neisseria meningitidis. If untreated, these infections may

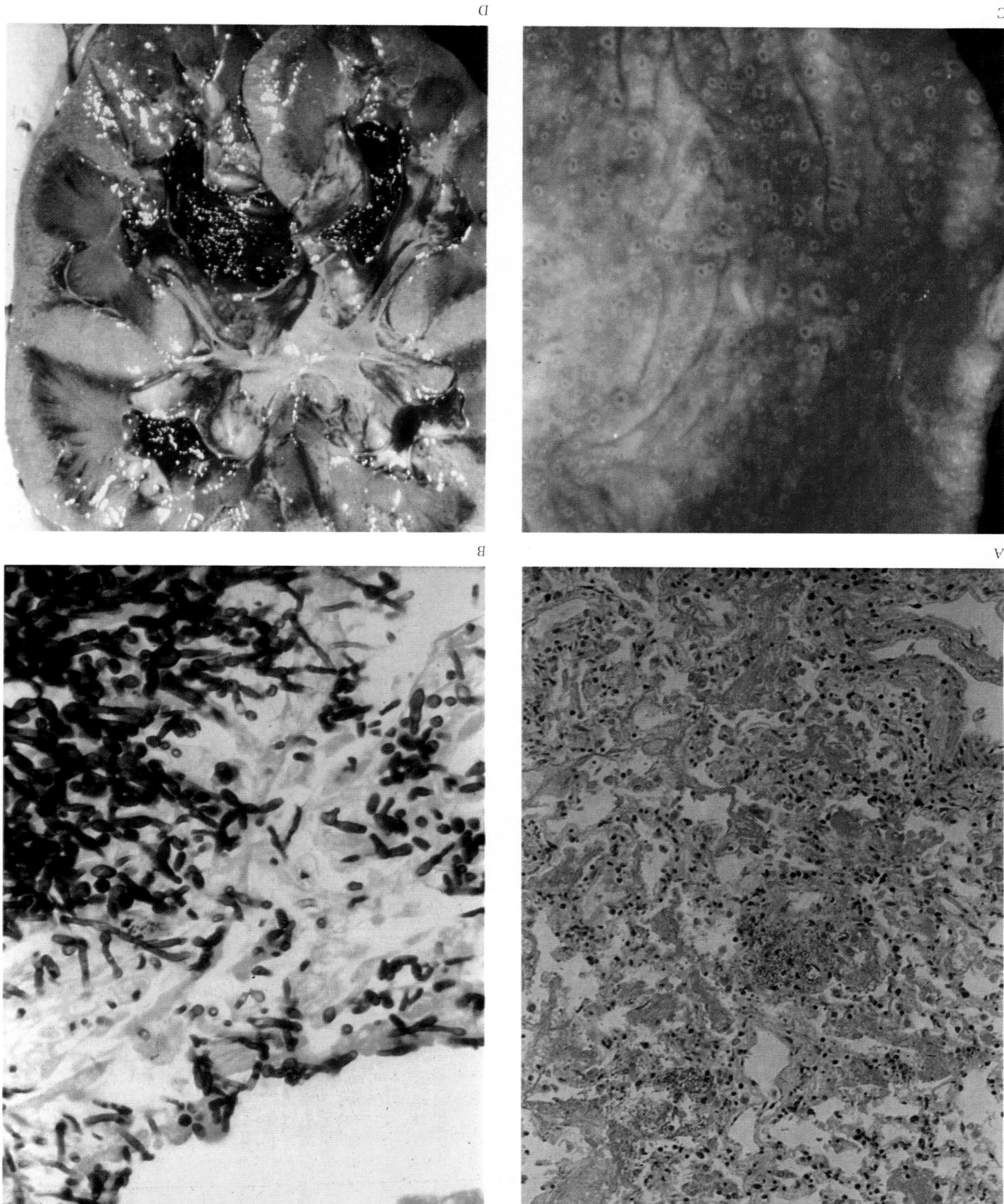

C

D

A

B

progress to pneumonia, meningitis, bacteremia, and death. Penicillin prophylaxis has been recommended for children with sickle cell anemia to prevent pneumococcal bacteremia. These patients also develop sickle "crises" during infection; vasoocclusive episodes may cause bone and joint pain and injure the kidneys, liver, and brain. Gallbladder disease, hepatic and bone marrow infarction, abscess formation in devitalized tissues, and recurrent skin ulceration increase vulnerability to systemic infection. The lungs sometimes undergo sterile infarction either from small vessel thrombosis or from emboli that originate in infarcted bone marrow. Recurrent infarction and infection may cause pulmonary scarring extensive enough to cause pulmonary hypertension. Systemic viral infections, pneumonias, trauma, or dehydration may all initiate a "sickle crisis." Pleurisy is a common complaint

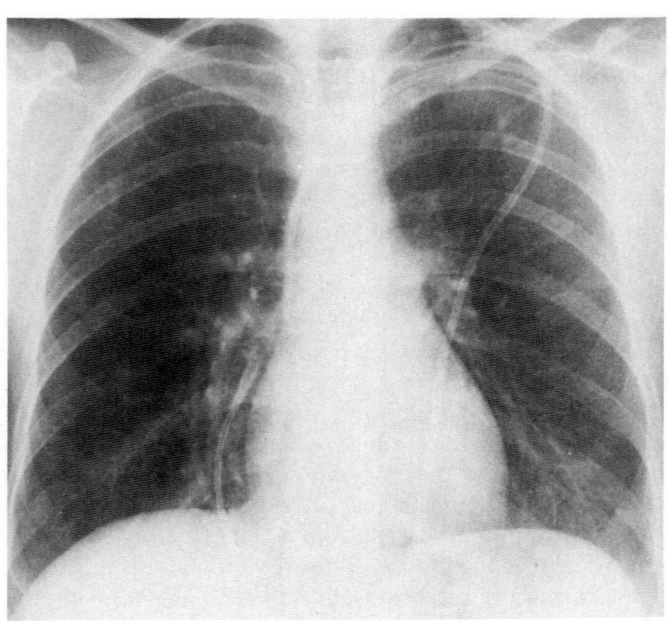

E

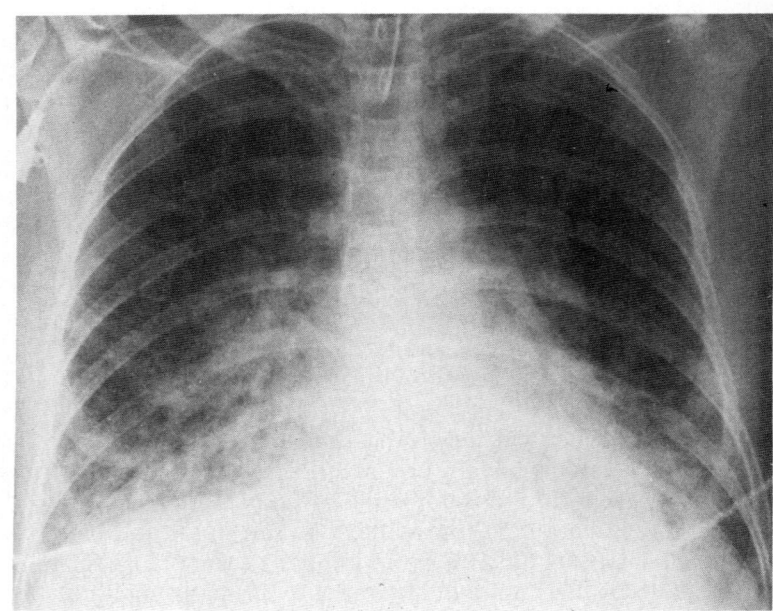

F

FIGURE 89-7 Catheter-related fungal pneumonia and hemorrhage. A 46-year-old woman with acute myelogenous leukemia developed fungemia with *T. beigelii* related to an infected Hickman catheter site. *Facing page (A–D).* Metastatic bronchopneumonia (A) was due to fungus (B). Ulceration of the gastric mucosa (C) and DIC with renal hemorrhage (D) also occurred. Over a period of 7 days, her chest radiograph progressed from essentially clear (E), to patchy bronchopneumonia (F), and finally to a picture of diffuse infiltrates and the adult respiratory distress syndrome (G).

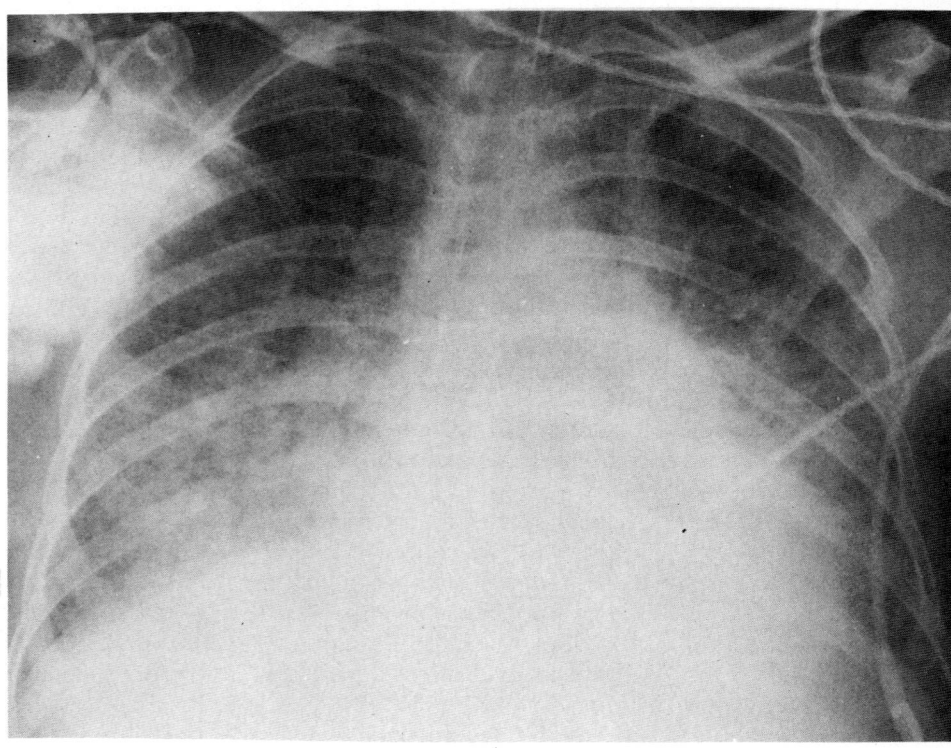

G

because of multiple, pleural-based infarcts. As soon as appropriate samples for culture have been taken, antibiotic therapy, using ampicillin and/or erythromycin, is begun in anticipation of the pathogens apt to be encountered, including *H. influenzae, S. pneumoniae, Mycoplasma pneumoniae,* and *Legionella* species. *S. aureus* may also complicate skin or bone infections.

The alcoholic, particularly if cirrhotic, suffers from a series of immune deficits. The presence of portal venous hypertension predisposes to intermittent bacteremias, presumably due to colonic flora leaking across the edematous bowel wall. Because of the portal bacteremias, the hepatic fibrosis and inflammation, and the splenic dysfunction, the alcoholic is prone to systemic bacteremias. These bacteremias are poorly cleared due to systemically diminished phagocytic function. Should endotoxemia occur, it is likely to persist as a consequence of the compromised metabolic functions of the liver. A serum inhibitor of neutrophil chemotaxis, the acute neutrophil dysfunction seen in the presence of alcohol, a mild chronic neutropenia, and a decreased ability to mobilize immune responses to new antigens combine to reduce the efficacy of the alcoholic's inflammatory response. The alcoholic tends to seek medical help later than do other patients, and, thus, tends to have more advanced infection at the time of presentation to the hospital. The organisms causing bacteremia are the same as those in the sickle cell patient; *Klebsiella* or *E. coli* are more often responsible for bacteremia in these patients than are other gram-positive organisms. The oropharynx of the alcoholic who experiences recurrent pneumonias and who has poor dentition becomes colonized with antibiotic-resistant, gram-negative organisms in addition to the resident anaerobic flora. In these patients, bacteremia may follow aspiration of oropharyngeal organisms, especially after a bout of deep intoxication. Trauma is common in these patients, and secondary infection of hematomas surrounding clavicular and rib fractures occurs quite often. Bacteremia due to an unusual aerobic gram-negative bacillus called DF-2 (dysgonic fermenter) has been recognized in alcoholic and splenectomized patients in association with animal bites. This organism may be recognized on a Gram stain of the peripheral blood buffy coat, and it grows poorly in traditional culture media. It is notable for its association with DIC and shock. Penicillin or ampicillin therapy will generally be successful and will also cover *Pasteurella multocida* infection.

Infection in the immunocompromised individual is discussed elsewhere (Chapter 109). The diminished inflammatory response in these patients often reduces the symptoms of infection. This group represents a spectrum of susceptible hosts from the diabetic to the neutropenic host. Nonetheless, in all these individuals, bacteremias and fungemias due to thrombophlebitis, catheter infection, rectal lesions, sinusitis, bed sores and skin cracks,

gallbladder disease, or urinary tract infection are life-threatening. In over half of the neutropenic patients with fever, infection is the source of fever, and over half of those who die of infection will succumb to pneumonia. These patients are often colonized with antibiotic-resistant organisms. Spontaneous bacteremias and mucosal ulcerations are common in those with marked neutropenia. Prevention of infection is the hallmark of successful care. Dual infection is often observed in these hosts. For example, gastrointestinal infection with *Strongyloides stercoralis* in these patients is often accompanied by gram-negative bacteremia and, occasionally, by pulmonary eosinophilia.

Some special hosts manifest a propensity for simultaneous pulmonary and systemic infections. While the causative relationship remains unclear, cytomegalovirus infection frequently coexists with *Pneumocystis carinii* or mycobacteria in pneumonias that occur in AIDS. In the AIDS patient, systemic infection with cytomegalovirus, mycobacterial species, or *Cryptococcus neoformans* may present with significant lung involvement. Nonspecific interstitial pneumonitis may reflect systemic infection with the *human immunodeficiency virus (HIV)* in AIDS or resolving infection due to *Pneumocystis* or other pathogens. Recent studies of the newborn infant (who has yet to develop mature immune responses) suggest that pulmonary changes are usually the first signs of neonatal sepsis. These infants develop tachypnea, cyanosis, nasal flaring, diffuse pulmonary infiltrates, and pleural effusions on the chest radiographs; sepsis may progress to cardiac failure and death within hours. The development of neutropenia in the early phase of the disease is a poor prognostic sign. Many of these infections are due to group B streptococci, thought to be derived from the colonized mother. The lungs develop hyaline membranes and alveolar exudates with proteinaceous fluid, bacteria, granulocytes, and hemorrhage. These changes are indistinguishable from those of endotoxic shock lung. The mediator of this injury is thought to be an extracellular bacterial toxin, including a polysaccharide surface antigen from the group B streptococcus. This exotoxin appears to act much like bacterial endotoxin. Ampicillin is used for prophylaxis in colonized pregnant women.

TREATMENT OF SYSTEMIC INFECTIONS INVOLVING THE LUNGS

The patient with systemic infection who also has pulmonary disease is often critically ill. Treatment of the illness is greatly simplified if, before starting antibiotic therapy, bacteriologic evidence of the source can be established and the antibiotic sensitivities of the organisms responsible for the infection can be determined. In the case of a localized abscess or of a collection of infected fluid under pressure, initial empiric therapy is usually directed at the

bacteremia with coverage of the likely pathogens based on the location of the infection. If the patient can be stabilized in 1 to 2 h by medical therapy alone, surgical intervention may be avoided. However, the reversibility of septic shock falls with time. In the immunocompromised host, surgical drainage of infected tissues is essential. In the inoperable patient, e.g., the patient with life-threatening cardiac disease, temporizing measures such as drainage via catheters or cholecystotomy may be the best option. In many patients, opposing hemodynamic forces are active: sepsis which causes peripheral vasodilatation, and dehydration and hypovolemia which tend to increase the peripheral vascular resistance. Rehydration is usually appropriate. Empiric antibiotic therapy, using antistaphylococcal and anti-gram-negative bacterial coverage, suffices unless a suspected source exists for anaerobic (e.g., abdominal), resistant gram-negative or fungal (e.g., nosocomial) organisms, or central nervous system infection exists. It cannot be overemphasized that therapy can be tailored to the patient's needs only if the proper cultures are obtained before antibiotic therapy is initiated. Occasionally, lung abscesses or empyemas develop despite appropriate therapy and require a drainage procedure to ensure resolution.

A few infections that involve the respiratory system should be considered to be life-threatening emergenices. These infections (Table 89-4) merit consideration in any patient with deterioration of respiratory function without a clear etiology (e.g., pneumothorax or cardiac disease). The recognition of these entities may be lifesaving in the tenuous patient, most notably those with head and neck infections, paralytic disease, or underlying immune compromise.

BIBLIOGRAPHY

Bachofen M, Weibel ER: Alterations of the gas exchange apparatus in adult respiratory insufficiency associated with septicemia. Am Rev Respir Dis 116:589–615, 1977.
  Morphometry and electron micrographs of tissues from shock lung patients give insights into the development of ARDS.

Bessa SM, Dalmasso AP, Goodale RL: Studies on the mechanism of endotoxin-induced increase in alveolocapillary permeability. Proc Soc Exp Biol Med 147:701–705, 1974.
  Investigation of the role of complement in the development of shock lung reveals differences between species and protection by pretreatment with corticosteroids. The effects of endotoxin on endothelial cells is independent of complement activation.

Beutler B, Cerami AC: Cachectin and tumor necrosis factor as two sides of the same biologic coin. Nature 320:584–588, 1986.
  An overview of the activities of cachectin/TNF.

Beutler B, Krochin N, Milsark IW, Wedke C, Cerami AC: Control of cachectin (tumor necrosis factor) synthesis: Mechanisms of endotoxin resistance. Science 232:977–980, 1986.
  The role of endotoxin in the transcription and translation of the cachectin gene is evaluated. A possible mechanism for the role of steroids in sepsis is proposed.

Brigham KL, Meyrick B: Interactions of granulocytes with the lungs. Circ Res 54:623–635, 1984.
  This review correlates the histopathologic features of experimental endotoxic lung with the observed physiological alterations.

Brigham KL, Woolverton WC, Blake LH, Staub NC: Increased sheep lung vascular permeability caused by *Pseudomonas* bacteremia. J Clin Invest 54:792–804, 1974.
  Minor increases in lung vessel permeability are inapparent during bacteremia due to the great capacity of pulmonary lymphatics.

Brogden KA, Cutlip RC, Lehmkuhl HD: Complexing of bacterial lipopolysaccharide with lung surfactant. Infect Immunol 52:644–649, 1986.
  Complexing of endotoxin with surfactant may augment the toxicity of the endotoxin as well as altering the surface activity of the surfactant.

Broome CU, Reingold AL: Current issues in toxic shock syndrome, in Remington J, Swartz MN (eds), *Current Clinical Topics in Infectious Disease (5)*. New York, McGraw-Hill, 1984, pp 65–85.
  The authors review the current information on the epidemiology and clinical features of toxic shock syndrome.

Carton RW: Pulmonary complications of sickle-cell disease. J Respir Dis 7:73–80, 1986.
  The prolonged survival of sickle cell anemia patients allows the development of progressive pulmonary dysfunction. A heightened susceptibility to infection increases the incidence of pulmonary infection and infarction in this population.

Dinarello CA: Interleukin-1. Rev Infect Dis 6:51–95, 1984.
Interleukin 1 is a key mediator of host responses to microbial invasion. This exhaustive review describes many of this hormone's effects.

Dinarello CA, Cannon JG, Wolfe SM, Bernheim HA, Beutler B, Cerami AC, Figari IS, Palladino MA Jr, O'Connor JV: Tumor necrosis factor (cachectin) is an endogenous pyrogen and induces production of interleukin 1. J Exp Med 163:1433–1450, 1986.
The interplay of the mediators of infectious injury is clarified. Multiple factors with overlapping effects contribute to the systemic manifestations of infection.

Dunn MM, Toews GB, Hart D, Pierce AK: The effects of systemic immunization on pulmonary clearance of Pseudomonas aeruginosa. Am Rev Respir Dis 131:426–431, 1985.
Humoral immunity may play a role in protecting the lung from bacteremic invasion and growth.

Gaston MH, Verter JI, Woods G, Pegelow C, Kelleher J, Presbury G, Zarkowsky H, Vichinsky E, Iyer R, Lobel JS, et al: Prophylaxis with oral penicillin in children with sickle cell anemia. N Engl J Med 314:1593–1599, 1986.
The morbidity of bacteremia due to S. pneumoniae in sickle cell anemia patients may be ameliorated by penicillin prophylaxis in children.

Glauser FL, Fairman RP: The uncertain role of the neutrophil in increased permeability pulmonary edema. Chest 88:601–607, 1985.
This review discusses the available data in relation to five models for the role of neutrophils in adult respiratory distress syndrome and shock lung.

Horan TC, White JW, Jarvis WR, Emori TG, Culver DH, Munn VP, Thornsberry C, Olson DR, Hughes JM: Nosocomial infection surveillance, 1984, Centers for Disease Control. CDC Surveillance Summaries, 1986, 35:17SS–29SS, 1986.
Nosocomial infection varies by size and type of medical facility. The incidences of the specific sites, organisms, and outcomes of these infections are summarized.

Johanson WG, Pierce AK, Sanford JP: Changing pharyngeal bacterial flora of hospitalized patients: Emergence of gram-negative bacilli. N Engl J Med 281:1137–1140, 1969.
The prevalence of gram-negative bacilli in oropharyngeal flora remained low in hospitalized normal individuals but increased markedly in patients with illnesses of varying severity, presumably reflecting impaired pharyngeal clearance in the patients.

Kaplan RL, Sahn SA, Petty TL: Incidence and outcome of the respiratory distress syndrome in gram-negative sepsis. Arch Intern Med 139:867–869, 1979.
The development of ARDS is associated with preexisting cardiac disease, hypotension, and evidence of disseminated intravascular coagulation.

McCabe WR, Treadwell TL, DeMaria A: Pathophysiology of bacteremia. Am J Med 75S:7–18, 1983.
An excellent review of the predisposing factors to bacteremia and its clinical outcome. This symposium includes reviews of host factors in infection and methods for the improved detection of bacteremia and fungemia.

Morrison DC: Bacterial endotoxins and pathogenesis. Rev Infect Dis 5:S733–747, 1983.
The endotoxin-unresponsive C3H/HeJ mouse model is used to study the effects of bacterial endotoxins and their role in bacterial shock.

Nawroth PP, Bank I, Handley D, Cassimeris J, Chess L, Stern D: Tumor necrosis factor/cachectin interacts with endothelial cell receptors to induce release of interleukin 1. J Exp Med 163:1363–1375, 1986.
Tumor necrosis factor can bind specifically to endothelium and initiate a cascade of inflammatory and coagulant events on the endothelial surface. These events may be central to the response of the host to sepsis and neoplasia.

Nishijima H, Weil MH, Shubin H, Cavanilles J: Hemodynamic and metabolic studies on shock associated with gram negative bacteremia. Medicine 52:287–294, 1973.
Clinical and physiological studies of 32 patients with bacteremia and circulatory shock.

Parillo JE, Burch C, Shelhamer JH, Parker MM, Natanson C, Schuetie W: A circulating myocardial depressant substance in humans with septic shock. J Clin Invest 76:1539–1553, 1985.
A serum factor isolated from bacteremic patients was able to reduce myocardial cell contractility and may play a role in the depression of the ejection fraction in septic shock.

Proctor RA, Will JA, Burhop KE, Raetz CRH: Protection of mice against lethal endotoxemia by a lipid A precursor. Infect Immunol 52:905–907, 1986.
A major biosynthetic precursor of lipid A called lipid X mimics many features of endotoxin, but does not cause a shock syndrome.

Pruitt BA Jr, Flemma RJ, DeVincenti FC, Foley FD, Mason AD Jr, Young WG Jr: Pulmonary complications in burn patients: A comparative study of 697 patients. J Thorac Cardiovasc Surg 59:7–20, 1970.
A review of the infectious and noninfectious lung injuries associated with thermal burns.

Root RK, Sande MA (eds): Septic Shock, in *Contemporary Issues in Infectious Diseases (4)*. New York, Churchill-Livingstone, 1985.
This group of papers gives an overview of the systemic effect of gram-negative bacterial infection.

Scheld WM, Sand MA: Endocarditis and intravascular infections, in Mandell GL, Douglas RG Jr, Bennett JE (eds), *Principles and Practice of Infectious Diseases*, 2d ed. New York, Wiley, 1985, pp 504–530.
This chapter gives an extensive treatment to the clinical and microbiologic characteristics of infective endocarditis.

Seeger W, Bauer M, Bhakdi S. Staphylococcal alpha-toxin elicits hypertension in isolated rabbit lungs. J Clin Invest 74:849–858, 1984.
The triggering of the arachidonic acid cascade by alpha-toxin is mediated by nonphysiological calcium channels in pulmonary endothelial cells.

Seeger W, Stohr G, Wolf HRD, Neuhof H: Alteration of surfactant function due to protein leakage: Special interaction with fibrin monomer. J Appl Physiol 58:326–338, 1985.
Protein leakage into the alveolar space alters the surface activity of surfactant and the pressure-volume characteristics of the lungs.

Seeger W, Walmrath D, Neuhof H, Lutz F: Pulmonary microvascular injury induced by *Pseudomonas aeruginosa* cytotoxin in isolated rabbit lungs. Infect Immunol 52:846–852, 1986.
In isolated perfused rabbit lungs, Pseudomonas cytotoxin induces an acute lung injury with a progressive rise in pulmonary vascular resistance which was only partially reversible.

Shennib H, Chiu RC-J, Mulder DS, Richards GK, Prentis J: Pulmonary bacterial clearance and alveolar macrophage function in septic shock lung. Am Rev Respir Dis 130:444–449, 1984.
Alveolar macrophage function is depressed during septic shock and contributes to a decrease in bacterial clearance from the lung. This depression will enhance the pathogenicity of embolized or aspirated bacteria.

Soave R, Murray HW, Litrenta MM: Bacterial invasion of pulmonary vessels. Pseudomonas bacteremia mimicking pulmonary thromboembolism with infarction. Am J Med 65:864–867, 1978.
An illustration of the propensity of P. aeruginosa for invading blood vessels and causing necrosis of the vessel wall.

Sorensen GK, Redding GJ: Cardiopulmonary effects of sepsis in the newborn. Sem Respir Med 6:141–147, 1984.
The pathologic and physiological changes associated with neonatal sepsis are most pronounced in the lungs.

Stamler J, Rodbard S, Katz LN: Blood pressure and renal clearances in hypertensive dogs following tissue injury. J Exp Med 160:21–30, 1950.
Early research into the mechanisms of the hypotensive effect or tissue necrosis suggested that ischemic, traumatic, and infectious tissue injuries share nonspecific mechanisms which cause hemodynamic changes.

Suffredini AF, Ognibene FP, Lack EE, Simmons JT, Brenner M, Gill VJ, Lane HC, Fauci AS, Parrillo JE, Masur H, Shelhamer JH: Nonspecific interstitial pneumonitis: A common cause of pulmonary disease in the acquired immunodeficiency syndrome. Ann Intern Med 107:7–13, 1987.
Nonspecific interstitial pneumonitis was seen in 38 percent of patients with AIDS over a 4-year period. The etiology of this inflammatory pattern remains unclear. In pediatric AIDS, interstitial pneumonitis without an etiology is second only to Pneumocystis carinii pneumonia in terms of the frequency of pathologic diagnosis.

Suttorp N, Seeger W, Uhl J, Lutz F, Roka L: Pseudomonas aeruginosa cytotoxin stimulates prostacyclin production in cultured pulmonary artery endothelial cells: Membrane attack and calcium influx. J Cell Physiol 123:64–72, 1985.
An investigation of the effects of highly purified cytotoxin from P. aeruginosa on cultured pulmonary arterial endothelium. Apparently the cytotoxin triggers the arachidonic acid pathway via calcium influx through toxin-created transmembrane lesions.

Winslow EJ, Loeb HS, Rahimtoola HH, Kamath S, Gunnar RM: Hemodynamic studies and results of therapy in 50 patients with bacteremic shock. Am J Med 54:421–432, 1973.

Differences between gram-positive and gram-negative infections and factors related to survival are discussed. Comments are made about the use of pressor agents and the role of corticosteroids in the therapy of bacteremia.

Young LS, Stevens P, Ingram J: Functional role of antibody against "core" glycolipid of Enterobacteriaceae. J Clin Invest 56:850–861, 1975.

These experiments helped to establish the central role of lipid A derivatives of endotoxin in the septic shock syndrome.

Chapter 90

Pulmonary Complications of Drug Abuse

M. Henry Williams, Jr.

Drug Overdose
    Alveolar Hypoventilation
    Pulmonary Edema

Pulmonary Infections

Septic Pulmonary Embolism

Pulmonary Hypertension

Bronchitis, Emphysema, and Asthma

Tuberculosis

Direct Injury to the Lungs

The respiratory system can be damaged directly and indirectly by the use and abuse of a variety of substances. On the one hand is alcohol abuse that affects 5 to 10 percent of the adult population, impairing defense mechanisms and predisposing to aspiration. On the other are central nervous system depressants and stimulants, analgesics, hallucinogens, and all sorts of drug combinations that can derange defense mechanisms, suppress protective reflexes, depress the ventilation to the point of respiratory arrest, and upset mentation so that damage is done to the respiratory system. Moreover, consequences of substance abuse often depend on the route of administration: when administered intravenously, the untoward consequences of street drugs are often compounded, and even upstaged, by the foreign material injected along with it.

Individuals addicted to narcotic drugs suffer a variety of pulmonary diseases, including pneumonia, empyema, lung abscess, and bronchiectasis. As a rule, these do not differ importantly from the corresponding disease in non-addicted subjects. In contrast, septic pulmonary embolism is a specific and serious complication of drug abuse. Older addicts with chronic bronchitis and emphysema are particularly prone to the development of ventilatory failure brought on by narcotics and other agents that depress the central nervous system. Patients in whom methadone has been substituted for heroin in the treatment of drug addiction are candidates for the same complications. Because of poor life-style, impaired defense mechanisms,

and bad habits, drug addicts are particularly vulnerable to the development of tuberculosis; once they have acquired tuberculosis, their behavior patterns often interfere with adherence to antituberculosis regimens.

The respiratory system can be assaulted by drugs in two ways: inhalation and intravenous injection. The major injury is inflicted by agents injected intravenously. A variety of foreign particles, including talc and cotton, may be injected with the drug and produce miliary pulmonary emboli that, in turn, stimulate the formation of granulomas. Particulate matter usually accompanies the intravenous injection of preparations designed to be used orally or inhaled. The ensuing clinical picture can mimic primary pulmonary hypertension. Agents such as heroin and methadone, which are concentrated in the lungs, probably also directly damage the pulmonary parenchyma. The use of heroin often is associated with abnormalities of pulmonary function, and even with bullous emphysema, changes that cannot be ascribed to particular embolization.

DRUG OVERDOSE

If the dose is sufficient, any of the central nervous system depressants or narcotics can derange respiratory control. Among the depressants encountered in drug abuse are phenobarbital ("nembies"), secobarbital ("reds"), amobarbital ("blues"), seco/amobarbital ("rainbows"), methaqualone ("love drug"), and chlordiazepoxide ("green and whites"). Among the narcotics, heroin ("junk"), methadone ("dollies"), and pentazocine ("Ts") are prominent. Injected materials include ground pills and contents of inhalers. But, as far as the respiratory system is concerned, overdose from either intravenous or intranasal administration of heroin, or from the oral administration of methadone, is the most serious form of drug abuse.

Alveolar Hypoventilation

In contrast to the coma without significant hypoventilation that generally results from barbiturate overdosage, alveolar hypoventilation is an extremely common and serious component of drug overdose with heroin and methadone. In both human beings and experimental animals, barbiturates produce surgical anesthesia without significant hypoventilation. In most patients with heroin or methadone overdose, the administration of a narcotic antagonist, such as nalorphine, is followed by return of consciousness and restoration of normal ventilation so that intubation and artificial ventilation are unnecessary. Indeed, in large centers, many patients are managed satisfactorily in the emergency room without hospitalization. Vomiting is extremely common in the course of developing, or recovering from, an overdose, and aspiration pneu-

monia is a frequent complication. A chest radiograph is mandatory to assess this possibility. Other pulmonary infections may appear some time after the episode of drug overdose but not often enough to warrant prophylactic use of antibiotics.

Pulmonary Edema

The most important and least understood feature of overdose with heroin or methadone is pulmonary edema (Fig. 90-1). Practically all patients who die of overdose with these drugs have pulmonary edema at autopsy; so do most patients treated in an emergency room for overdosage with these drugs. However, pulmonary edema is not an inevitable result of an overdose: many patients in whom hypercapnia and hypoxemia are severe respond promptly to a narcotic antagonist without developing pulmonary edema.

The clinical picture after overdosage with heroin is fairly stereotyped: generally, within 2 h after the intravenous injection of heroin, the patient is brought to the emergency room comatose and cyanotic. Respiratory depression is severe; the respiratory rate is often less than five breaths per minute. Bilateral, diffuse rales are heard over the lungs; frothy sputum, sometimes blood-tinged, is often evident at the mouth; and a chest radiograph reveals diffuse alveolar infiltrates, while the cardiac silhouette is normal in size and appearance.

The etiology of this type of pulmonary edema is not clear. That it is related to administration of excessive amounts of narcotic is suggested by the occurrence of small epidemics of pulmonary edema in which the common denominator appears to be the sharing of a batch of heroin which is stronger than expected, or by its appearance in an inexperienced individual who has self-administered a dose of drug to which he, or she, has not built up tolerance. An allergic reaction is highly unlikely since subsequent injections of heroin are not likely to cause recurrences of pulmonary edema, and pulmonary edema sometimes occurs after the first trial of the drug. Nor is particulate embolization a serious consideration since pulmonary edema has also occurred after intranasal and oral administration of the drug.

In many respects, the pulmonary edema resembles high altitude pulmonary edema. Consequently, the suggestion has been made that hypoxia, secondary to alveolar hypoventilation, is the common denominator in both. Unfortunately, this hypothesis does not seem to hold

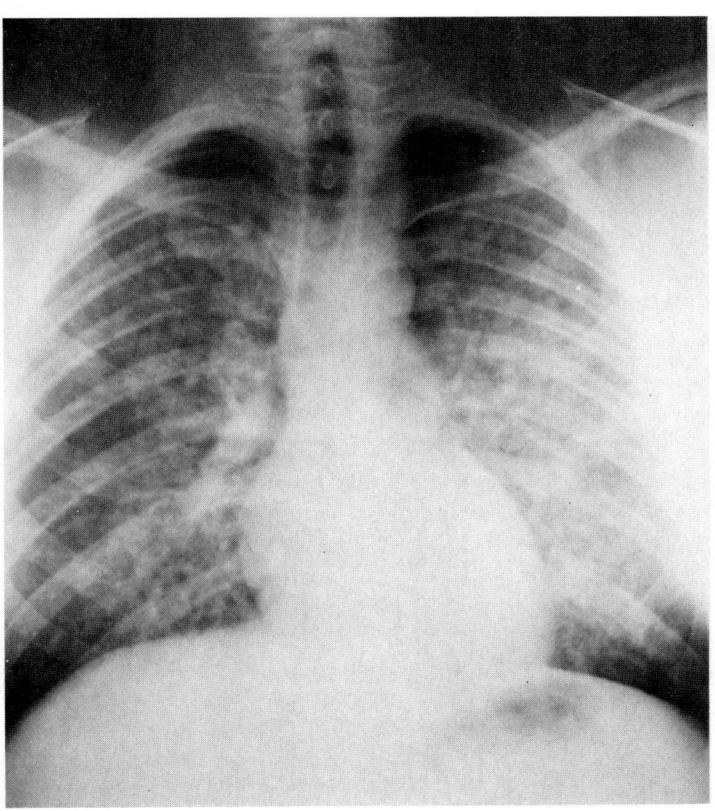
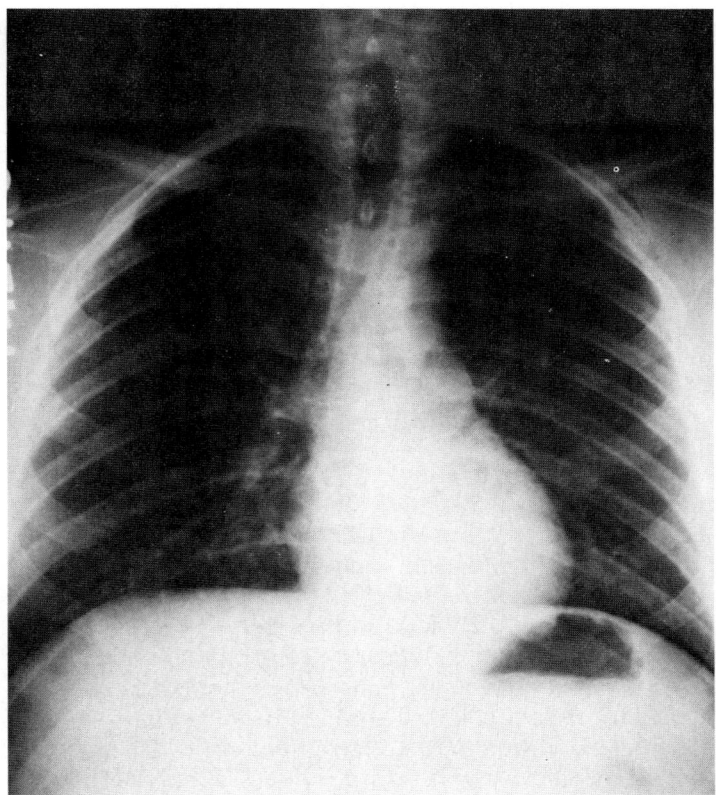

A   *B*

FIGURE 90-1   Heroin pulmonary edema. Radiographs of the chest in a 22-year-old patient on presentation in the emergency room after intravenous injection of heroin.   *A*. Extensive alveolar infiltrates with a normal cardiac silhouette. *B*. Forty-eight hours later showing complete resolution of the pulmonary edema.

water since hypoxia does not cause pulmonary capillary vessels to leak. Although overdose with many other drugs, including barbiturates, may be associated with pulmonary edema, it is most uncommon for patients with severe hypoxemia secondary to hypoventilation to develop pulmonary edema.

Another line of speculation concerning pathogenesis resembles in many ways a prevalent notion about pathogenesis of neurogenic pulmonary edema: according to this hypothesis, a trigger (hypoxia or a drug in the case of narcotic overdosage) acts on the central nervous system to cause systemic venoconstriction, massive shifts of intravascular volume from systemic veins to the pulmonary circulation, severe pulmonary capillary hypertension, and exudation of fluid into the interstitium and alveoli. In keeping with this hypothesis is the high concentration of proteins in the edema fluid and the rapid development of pulmonary edema after narcotic overdosage. However, no direct experimental evidence exists to support this hypothesis.

Finally, a direct action of heroin on pulmonary capillaries has not been excluded. Unfortunately, intensive efforts to reproduce this condition in experimental animals, ranging from mice to baboons, have been consistently unsuccessful, raising the possibility that some peculiar characteristics, either of the human pulmonary circulation or of the central vasomotor regulatory system, may make this reaction unique to human beings.

Treatment is directed at restoring consciousness and stimulating respiration; serial determinations of arterial blood gases provide a useful guide to therapy. In most patients, arterial blood-gas analysis reveals severe hypoxemia (P_{O_2} from 30 to 50 mmHg) and hypercapnia. A narcotic antagonist is the principal recourse in therapy; oxygen and artificial ventilation are administered if needed. In many subjects, administration of nalorphine promptly improves consciousness, restores normal ventilation and, in conjunction with an O_2-enriched mixture delivered by mask, leads to adequate arterial oxygenation.

About 20 percent of patients who have taken an overdose of heroin present with apnea. These require emergency intubation and artificial ventilation using O_2-enriched inspired gas mixtures. In most instances, the endotracheal tube can be removed in a few hours. The rare patient who fails to respond may require artificial ventilation, using positive end-expiratory pressure (PEEP) for several days. Serial determinations reveal that the arterial P_{CO_2} returns to normal, and the arterial P_{O_2} exceeds 70 mmHg, within 24 h; within 48 h, the radiographic abnormalities are often gone. The vital capacity improves much more slowly: it begins to increase within 1 to 2 days but returns to its maximal level only after several days; the low vital capacity probably represents persistent interstitial edema. In our experience with over 40 patients treated for heroin pulmonary edema, there has been no mortality.

It is clear that if treatment can be applied in time, the condition, no matter how extensive, is completely reversible.

A number of patients have developed pulmonary edema after ingesting methadone. The condition is similar to that which follows an overdose with heroin except that there is generally a longer period between ingestion of drug and development of symptoms; correspondingly, the clearing of the chest radiograph is slower, and arterial blood gases take longer to return to normal levels.

PULMONARY INFECTIONS

The most serious infections that strike drug users are associated with the acquired immunodeficiency syndrome (AIDS). In our hospitals in the Bronx, AIDS is more often related to intravenous drug abuse than to homosexuality. A drug user who presents with fever, constitutional symptoms, and even a suggestion of a pulmonary infiltrate requires immediate hospitalization. Since *Pneumocystis carinii* is the most common infection, and since it may progress with devastating rapidity, it is our practice to institute therapy with trimethoprim and sulfamethoxazole immediately and to perform bronchoscopy as soon as possible. In most instances, a touch preparation reveals the diagnosis immediately. Other agents that may cause infection singly, or in combination, include mycobacteria and fungi. *Avium* infections are so common that if an acid-fast organism is found, it should be treated with a regimen containing ansamicin and clofazimine pending cultural identification. Usually the initial infection or infections can be treated successfully. But, once this syndrome has become apparent the prognosis becomes very poor because of recurrent infections or, rarely, the development of Kaposi's sarcoma. Undoubtedly, a great many more drug users have immunologic deficiencies without manifesting the full-blown syndrome. However, at present, it is not possible to identify these individuals and it cannot be predicted how likely it is that they will develop AIDS.

Bacterial pneumonia is also a common cause of hospitalization for drug addicts. Since about one-half of the patients are also chronic alcoholics, it is likely that alcohol, with its known effects on inhibiting phagocytosis, mucociliary clearance, leukocytosis, and possibly other aspects of host defense, is a major contributing factor. Treatment is not different than for the nonaddict: the initial selection of antibiotics is based on the Gram stain of the sputum; subsequent judgment is based on blood and sputum cultures. We have encountered small numbers of patients with empyema and lung abscess who have also responded in the usual fashion to conventional therapy. In some instances, empyema may be extensive with large multiloculated collections of thick pus that are often asso-

ciated with bronchopleural fistula. These patients require extensive antimicrobial therapy using appropriate drugs, chest tubes and, often, open drainage and decortication. Not infrequently, these patients, who tend to neglect themselves and their health, only seek medical treatment after developing rather extensive illness over a long time. Among our patients with lung abscess, about two-thirds give a history of coma prior to admission: the others are alcoholic. It is quite likely that, as in other patients, the lung abscess is the result of necrotizing aspiration pneumonia; in most instances, it responds satisfactorily to the administration of penicillin.

Bronchiectasis may pose a particular problem because it is often difficult to implement an essential feature of therapy, i.e., adequate and sustained postural drainage.

SEPTIC PULMONARY EMBOLISM

Septic pulmonary emboli present with a characteristic history of fever, associated with chest pain, and hemoptysis. Often there is evidence of skin infection. The chest radiograph reveals multiple thin-walled cavities scattered throughout the lung fields. Some patients present with bronchopneumonia but fail to respond to antibiotics. The chest radiograph then discloses new infiltrates, and tomograms reveal multiple hazy densities and cavities that are often missed on the conventional radiograph (Fig. 90-2). Tomograms should be obtained when septic pulmonary emboli are suspected. Septic pulmonary emboli commonly result from and may be the only manifestation of right-sided staphylococcal endocarditis. Even though staphylococci are not isolated from the blood in about one-half of the patients, and even though many of them do not reveal definite evidence of bacterial endocarditis, e.g., systemic embolization or changing heart murmurs, all patients with septic emboli should be treated as if they had staphylococcal bacterial endocarditis, by administering a penicillinase-resistant penicillin for 4 to 6 weeks. In response to effective antimicrobial therapy, systemic symptoms disappear within a few days, and the chest radiographs clear progressively during the next few weeks.

PULMONARY HYPERTENSION

One important complication of drug abuse is pulmonary hypertension secondary to embolization of particulates, generally oral agents that have been ground up and injected intravenously. Some patients develop cor pulmonale and right ventricular failure; in others who discontinue intravenous use of drugs the level of pulmonary hypertension decreases. The drug that has been employed

most frequently is pentazocine, and the embolic material is usually talc (Fig. 90-3); but cotton, cellulose, and other agents have also been implicated. The anatomic lesions in the parenchyma and pulmonary microcirculation resemble those of primary pulmonary hypertension plus inflammatory reactions to the foreign material (Fig. 90-4). Patients present with signs and symptoms of pulmonary hypertension, e.g., at rest and on exertion, and chest pains (Chapter 64). Pulmonary function tests are often virtually normal (Fig. 90-5), except for the diffusing capacity which is almost invariably subnormal (Fig. 90-6). The reduction in diffusing capacity affects exclusively the "membrane component" and seems attributable to a combination of granulomatous interstitial disease and pulmonary vascular occlusion. No consensus exists about whether the decrease in diffusing capacity correlates with the increase in pulmonary arterial pressure.

BRONCHITIS, EMPHYSEMA, AND ASTHMA

For many years, an elderly addict was a rarity. But, there is now a sizable number of elderly patients who have used narcotics for years and have developed some of the pulmonary diseases encountered in the non-drug-abusing older population. Prominent among these is obstructive airways disease, since many of the older addicts are long-standing heavy smokers and they are disinclined either to stop smoking or to adhere to a continuing medical program of antibiotics and bronchodilators. Although the acute administration of either drug can cause alveolar hypoventilation, respiratory sensitivity is more apt to return to normal in the morphine addict than in the methadone addict; in the latter, respiratory depression often becomes persistent. As a result, many addicts who are treated with methadone continue to have hypercapnia and a diminished ventilatory response to CO_2 after months of maintenance therapy. This may represent a limitation to the use of methadone in patients with chronic bronchitis and emphysema. If the narcotic is used, continuing alertness is required to avoid serious alveolar hypoventilation and ventilatory failure.

Bullous emphysema also occurs in drug addicts. In a group of illicit drug users, the frequency was 1.6 percent. Characteristically, the bullae were large and confined to the upper lobes. In this population, bullous emphysema may result either from the direct effect of heroin on the lung or from unrecognized, subclinical necrotizing infections that are so common in addicts.

Asthma does not appear to be unduly prevalent among addicts. Even though the asthmatic feels better after taking heroin, probably because of relief of anxiety and tension, asthma in the addict poses no special problems in management.

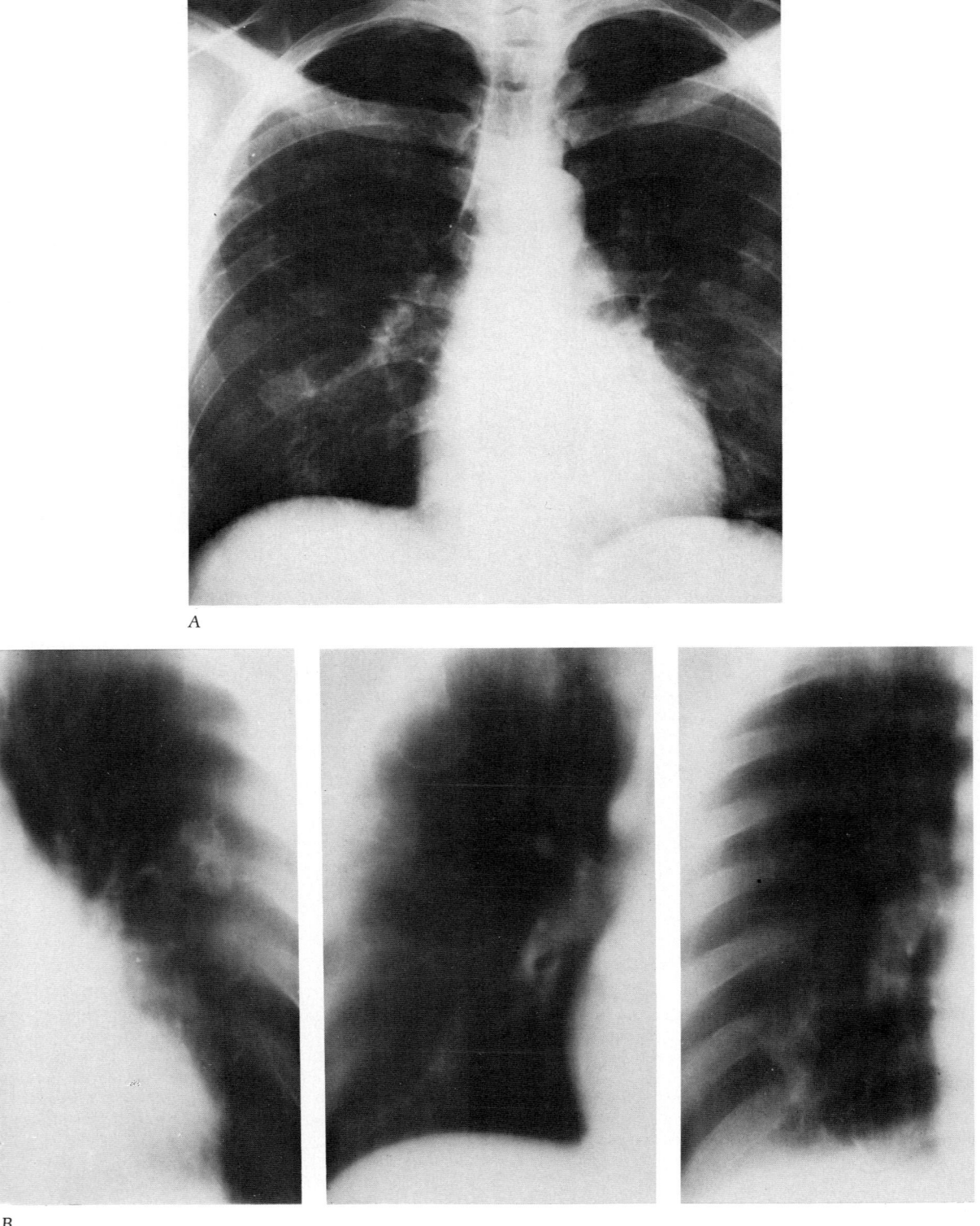

A

B

FIGURE 90-2 Septic pulmonary emboli. *A.* Multiple areas of infiltration and cavitation in a 38-year-old addict with herelia septicemia. *B.* The cavitary lesions are more evident on the tomographic cuts.

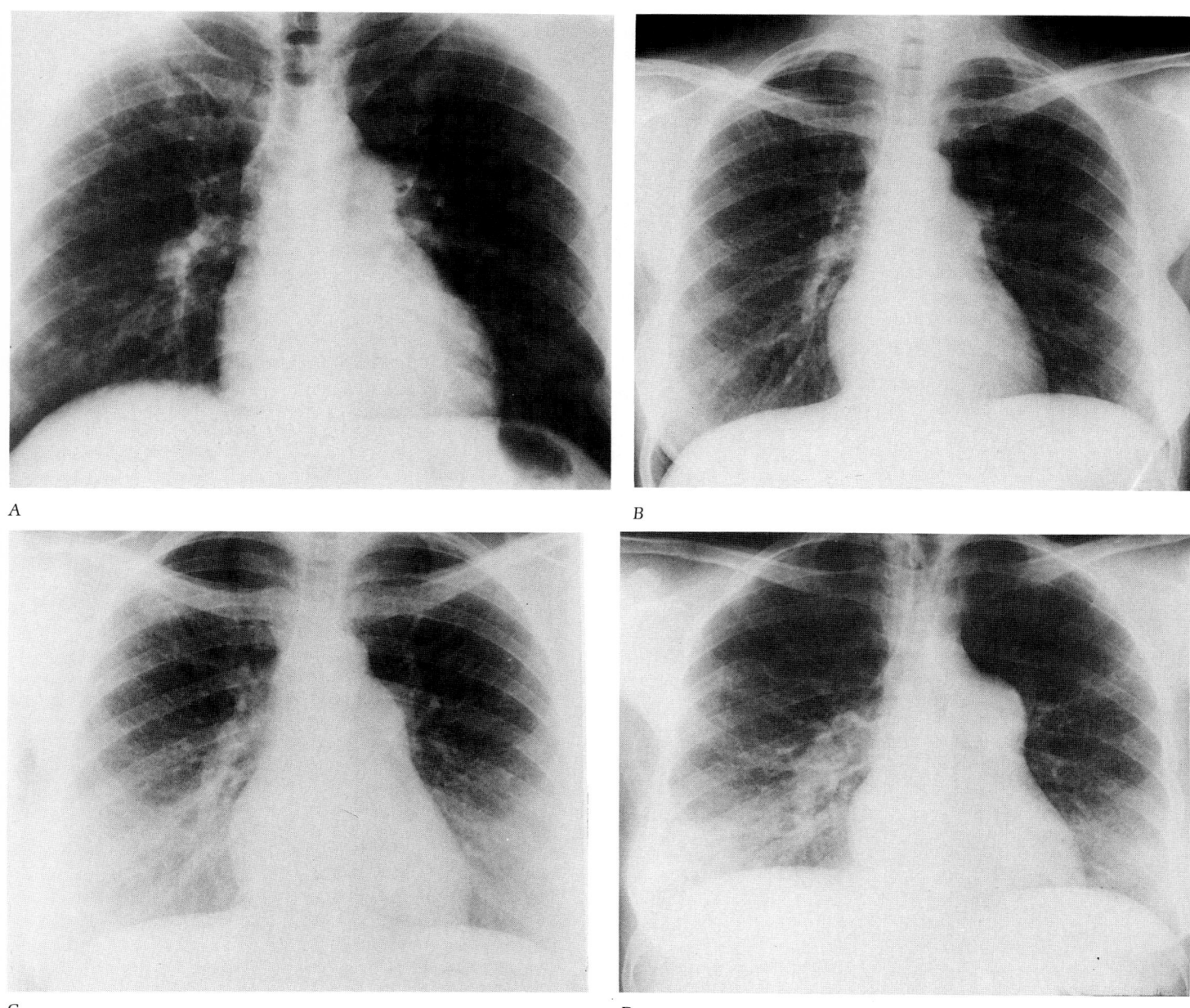

FIGURE 90-3 Pulmonary hypertension due to talc. *A.* 39-year-old heroin abuser who had self-administered heroin intravenously for years prior to present admission. Over 2½ years, pulmonary arterial pressure had increased from 57/34 to 85/40 mmHg. Pulmonary vasodilator trials were ineffective. Open lung biopsy showed intimal proliferation and medial hypertrophy; birefringent material, consistent with talc crystals, was found free and in many foreign-body giant cells. *(Courtesy of Dr. D. Murphy.)* *B.* On admission. 30-year-old female heroin abuser with 15-year history of intravenous and subcutaneous self-administration of methylphenidate (Ritalin) and pentazocine (Talwin). Progressive enlargement of central pulmonary arteries over a 3½ year period. *C.* Two and one-half years later. An infiltrate is present at the right lung base. *D.* Three and one-half years later. Progressive reticular nodular disease is evident.

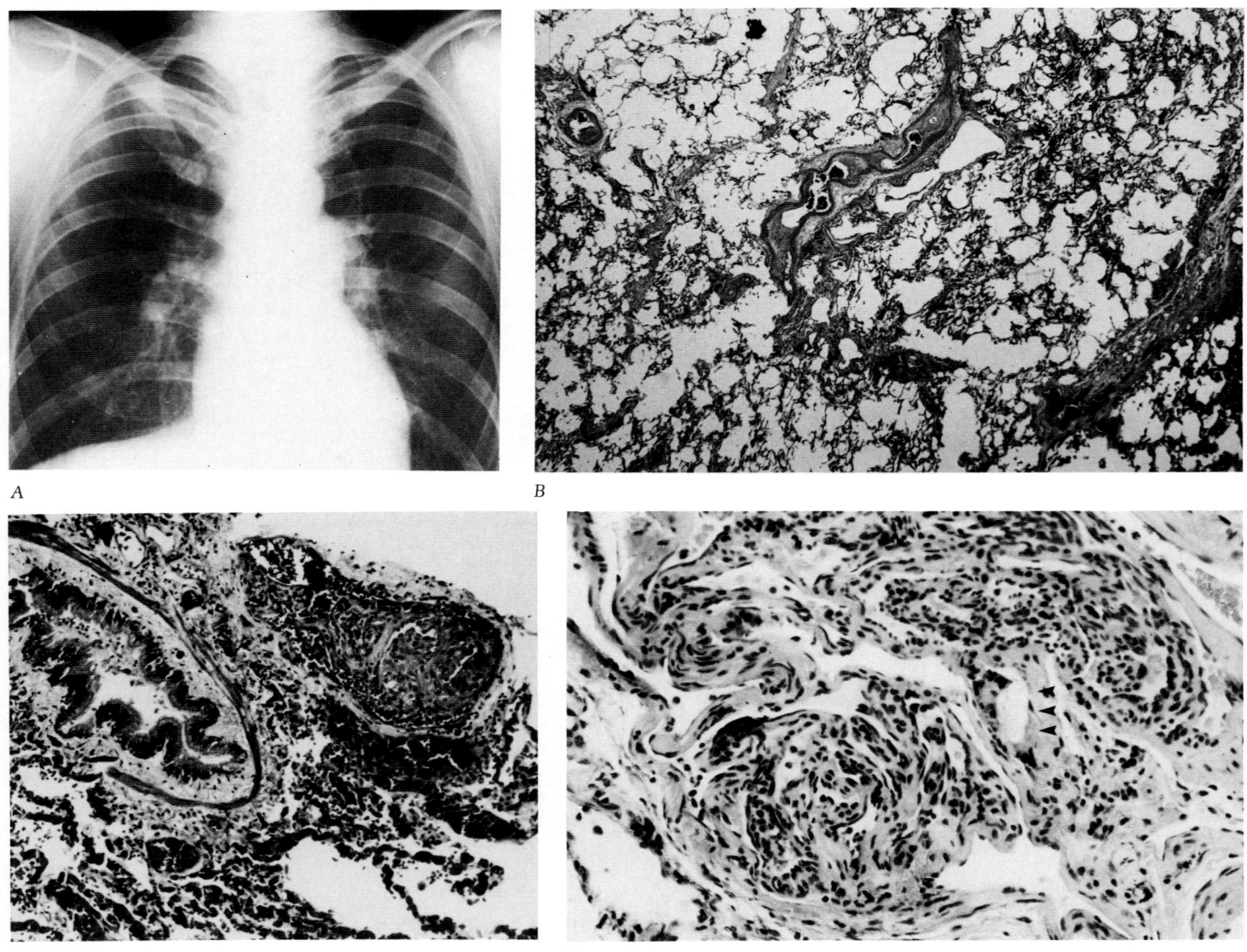

A

B

C

D

FIGURE 90-4 Pulmonary hypertension secondary to intravenous drug abuse that began with "cold shaking" 15 years before death in right ventricular failure. *A.* Chest radiograph. The central pulmonary arteries are enlarged, whereas the peripheral pulmonary vasculature is attenuated. Pulmonary arterial pressure of 90/40 mmHg associated with normal left-sided cardiac pressures. Diffusing capacity, 58 percent of predicted. *B.* Autopsy. Scanning view of the lung. Prominent vascular lesions coexist with minimal interstitial disease. The vascular lesions include intimal proliferation and fibrosis *(upper left and center)* and an angiomatoid lesion *(lower right).* H&E, ×26. *C.* Autopsy. Angiomatoid lesion with multiple channels adjacent to an artery that shows intimal proliferation and fibrosis. H&E, ×150. *D.* Autopsy. Early plexiform lesion illustrating multiple endothelial channels. Birefringent foreign material is also present (arrowheads). *(Courtesy of Dr. R. Goldring and E. Fazzini.)*

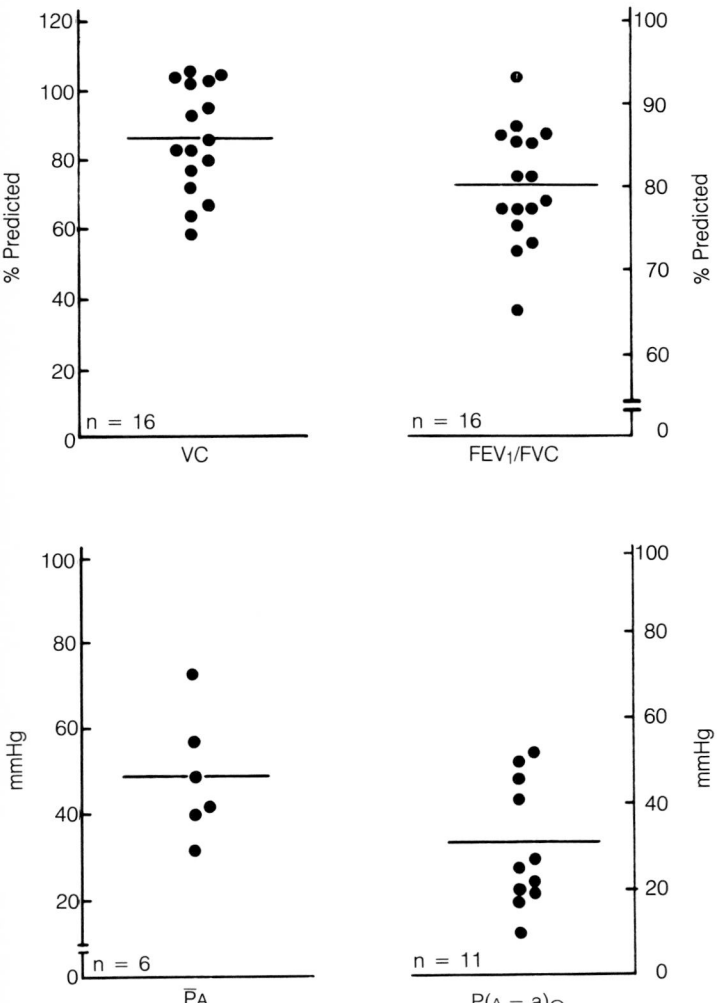

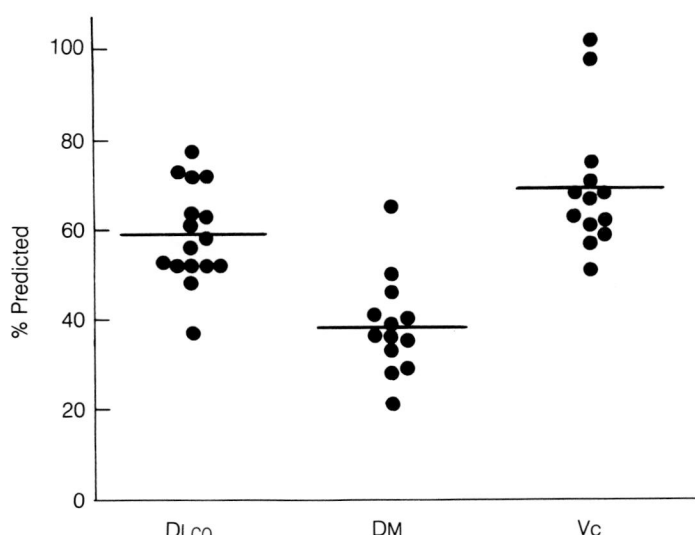

FIGURE 90-6   The diffusing capacity for carbon monoxide (D_{LCO}) in pulmonary hypertension secondary to intravenous drug abuse. The diffusing capacity is decreased in all patients, averaging 58 percent of predicted. The reduction in the membrane component (D_M) is large, whereas the capillary blood volume (V_c) is well preserved. *(From Frimer et al., 1985.)*

FIGURE 90-5   Pulmonary function tests in pulmonary hypertension secondary to intravenous drug abuse. In the six patients subjected to cardiac catheterization *(lower left)*, the mean pulmonary arterial pressure averaged about 50 mmHg. The vital capacity (VC) and flow rates (FEV$_1$/FVC) and the alveolar-arterial difference in P_{O_2} [$P(A-a)_{O_2}$] are near normal.

TUBERCULOSIS

Although tuberculosis may not be more prevalent among drug addicts than among other individuals from a similar socioeconomic class, the disease in drug addicts is often protracted and drug-resistant because of their failure to adhere to an effective program of prolonged antimicrobial therapy. At the Bronx Municipal Hospital Center, drug addiction used to be an important and common cause of premature discharge from the hospital, resulting in inadequate therapy for tuberculosis, progression and relapses of the disease and, in all likelihood, infection of other individuals in the community. This deplorable situation was dramatically improved by the introduction of a combined program of methadone maintenance and antituberculosis therapy.

DIRECT INJURY TO THE LUNGS

Chronic drug abusers are apt to have abnormal pulmonary function. The most common abnormality in pulmonary function in drug abusers is regional inhomogeneity in ventilation and perfusion. This inhomogeneity can be displayed by lung scanning using radioisotopic tracers. Perfusion abnormalities are more common than ventilation abnormalities, presumably as a consequence of injury to small vessels.

Focal abnormalities of the lungs occur in different forms. Notable among these is bullous disease which has complications of its own, including infection, hemoptysis, pneumothorax, or progressive enlargement to compress normal lung.

BIBLIOGRAPHY

Arnett EN, Battle WE, Russo JV, Roberts WC: Intravenous injection of talc-containing drugs intended for oral use. A cause of pulmonary granulomatosis and pulmonary hypertension. Am J Med 60:711–718, 1976.
  Review of the literature on this interesting condition, which may simulate primary pulmonary hypertension, is supplemented by two more well-documented cases.

Camargo G, Colp C: Pulmonary function studies in ex-heroin users. Chest 67:331–334, 1975.
  A study of former intravenous drug users revealed reduction of diffusing capacity.

Cucco RA, Yoo OH, Cregler L, Chang JC: Nonfatal pulmonary edema after "freebase" cocaine smoking. Am Rev Respir Dis 136:179–181, 1987.
  An unusual instance of a patient who developed acute pulmonary edema after smoking "freebase" cocaine.

Douglass RE, Levison MA: Pneumothorax in drug abusers. An urban epidemic? Am J Surg 52:377–380, 1986.
  At the Detroit Receiving Hospital, of 525 diagnoses of pneumothorax between January 1, 1982, and December 31, 1984, 113 (21.5 percent) occurred as a result of drug abuse in 84 patients.

Duberstein JL, Kaufman DM: A clinical study of an epidemic of heroin intoxication and heroin-induced pulmonary edema. Am J Med 51:704–714, 1971.
  A large series of drug overdoses from a municipal hospital in New York emphasizes the need for prompt diagnosis and treatment.

Frand UI, Shim CS, Williams MH Jr: Heroin-induced pulmonary edema. Ann Intern Med 77:29–35, 1972.
  Serial studies of pulmonary function revealed prompt improvement of arterial blood gases and slower increase of vital capacity and diffusing capacity.

Frand UI, Shim CS, Williams MH Jr: Methadone-induced pulmonary edema. Ann Intern Med 76:975–979, 1972.
  Since pulmonary edema can occur after an overdose with an oral agent, embolic occlusion of pulmonary arteries is not a likely cause.

Frimer RB, Rapoport DM, Epstein H, Goldring RM: Diffusing capacity and its partition in the evaluation of unexplained pulmonary hypertension. Am Rev Respir Dis 131:402a, 1985.
  Lung volumes, flow rates, and alveolar-capillary gas exchange related to the level of pulmonary hypertension. In contrast to other reports, the reduction in diffusing capacity did not correlate with the level of pulmonary hypertension.

Goldstein DS, Karpel JP, Appel D, Williams MH Jr: Bullous pulmonary damage in users of intravenous drugs. Chest 89:266–269, 1986.
  Among a large group of users of illicit intravenous drugs, the incidence of bullous pulmonary damage was noted to be 2 percent (6/387). The bullae were large and confined to the upper lobes.

Harley DP, White RA, Nelson RJ, Mehringer CM: Pulmonary embolism secondary to venous thrombosis of the arm. Am J Surg 147:221–224, 1984.
  Pulmonary embolism is an infrequent complication of axillary and subclavian vein thrombosis. Drug abuse is one cause of this type of thrombosis.

Itkonen J, Schnoll S, Daghestani A, Glassroth J: Accelerated development of pulmonary complications due to illicit intravenous use of pentazocine and tripelennamine. Am J Med 76:617–622, 1984.
  The natural history and prevalence of pulmonary gas-exchange abnormalities resulting from intravenous drug abuse were studied. In 45 individuals, 20 of whom used a mixture of the synthetic opiate pentazocine and the antihistamine tripelennamine ("Ts" and "Bs"), low values for diffusing capacity and abnormal responses to exercise testing were common.

Jaffe RB, Koschmann EB: Septic pulmonary emboli. Radiology 96:527–532, 1970.
  Seventeen cases of septic pulmonary emboli highlight the prompt development of cavitation in these lesions.

Marks CE, Goldring RM: Chronic hypercapnia during methadone maintenance. Am Rev Respir Dis 108:1088–1093, 1973.
  Methadone maintenance may be associated with chronic CO_2 retention due to suppression of respiratory drive. This may be a problem in patients with coexistent chronic obstructive lung disease.

May DC, Helderman JH, Eigenbrodt EH, Silva FG: Chronic sclerosing glomerulopathy (heroin-associated nephropathy) in intravenous T's and Blues abusers. Am J Kidney Dis 8:404–409, 1986.
> *The intravenous (IV) use of pentazocine (Talwin) and tripelennamine (pyribenzamine) has become a major form of drug abuse in the midwestern United States. Complications of this abuse include psychotic reactions, acute pulmonary insufficiency, convulsions, and various infections. In three patients, the IV use of these agents was associated with the nephrotic syndrome and renal histopathologic findings similar to those reported in heroin addicts with the so-called heroin-associated nephropathy.*

Robertson CH Jr, Reynolds RC, Wilson JE III: Pulmonary hypertension and foreign body granulomas in intravenous drug abusers. Am J Med 61:657–664, 1976.
> *Four patients with foreign-body granulomas due to intravenous injection of oral drugs revealed a direct relationship between the degree of pulmonary hypertension and reduction of the diffusing capacity.*

Soin JS, Wagner HN Jr, Thomashaw D, Brown TC: Increased sensitivity of regional measurements in early detection of narcotic lung disease. Chest 67:325–330, 1975.
> *Perfusion and ventilation defects are surprisingly common in intravenous drug users, even when pulmonary function and arterial blood gases are normal.*

Stover DE, White DA, Romano PA, Gellene RA, Robeson WA: Spectrum of pulmonary diseases associated with the acquired immune deficiency syndrome. Am J Med 78:429–437, 1985.
> *This 4-year experience with 130 patients with AIDS reveals the full panorama of pulmonary complications.*

Theodore J, Robin ED: Speculations on neurogenic pulmonary edema (NPE). Am Rev Respir Dis 113:405–411, 1976.
> *The sudden onset of pulmonary edema after head injury and, perhaps, after heroin overdose may be due to systemic venoconstriction with major shifts of intravascular volume into the lung.*

Williams MH Jr: Heroin pulmonary edema. Am J Clin Res 1:107–108, 1970.
> *A direct effect of heroin on pulmonary capillaries, thereby increasing permeability, may be the mechanism for heroin pulmonary edema.*

Nontuberculous Infections of the Lungs: Specific Disorders

Chapter 91

Pneumonias Caused by Gram-Positive Bacteria

David S. McKinsey / Alan L. Bisno

A variety of gram-positive organisms are associated with human pneumonia. Some, such as *Mycobacterium tuberculosis* and *Nocardia asteroides*, are considered elsewhere in this book. Among the gram-positive cocci, *Streptococcus pneumoniae*, *Staphylococcus aureus*, and *Streptococcus pyogenes* have been singled out for consideration in this chapter; the gram-positive anaerobic cocci commonly encountered in aspiration pneumonia are considered in Chapter 56. Among the bacilli, *Bacillus anthracis* is also considered in this chapter.

STREPTOCOCCUS PNEUMONIAE

S. pneumoniae (the "pneumococcus") is the most common cause of community-acquired bacterial pneumonia.

The organism may on occasion also be a cause of nosocomial pneumonia, especially in elderly, debilitated patients. Despite major advances in the diagnosis, treatment, and prophylaxis of pneumococcal pneumonia, this entity has been estimated to account for up to 30,000 deaths annually in the United States and is a major source of morbidity and mortality throughout the world.

Historical Perspective

S. pneumoniae was simultaneously identified by Pasteur and by Sternberg in 1881. Two years later, Friedlander noted the association of this organism with lobar pneumonia. In the early 1900s, Neufeld discovered the presence of distinct pneumococcal serotypes. This finding led to the development of type-specific antisera, the first specific form of therapy for the disease. Following the purification of pneumococcal capsular polysaccharide in the early 1940s, a polyvalent vaccine was developed, but its use was discontinued when penicillin became available for civilian use and was found to be extremely effective in the treatment of pneumococcal infections. The vaccine was reintroduced in the 1970s after clinical studies demonstrated that the morbidity and mortality rates of bacteremic pneumococcal infections remained high despite the availability of seemingly effective antibiotics. In the 1970s and 1980s, the appearance of multiply antibiotic resistant strains of *S. pneumoniae* has become a matter of concern.

Microbiology

S. pneumoniae (formerly *Diplococcus pneumoniae*) is the causative agent of pneumococcal pneumonia. This organism is an encapsulated gram-positive coccus which measures 0.5 to 1.25 μm in diameter and is characteristically lancet-shaped. The composition of the organism's polysaccharide capsule varies among the different serotypes. Pneumococci typically associate in pairs, but may occur singly or in short chains.

Pneumococci are facultative anaerobes. When cultivated on blood agar plates at 37°C, young colonies are circular and glistening and measure approximately 1 mm in diameter. If incubated under aerobic conditions, they are surrounded by a zone of α hemolysis. Pneumococci can be differentiated from other α-hemolytic streptococci by their susceptibility to Optochin (ethylhydrocupreine), their solubility in bile, and their high degree of virulence in mice. When type-specific antipneumococcal serum is added to specimens containing pneumococci of the homologous serotype, the optical density of the organisms' capsules is altered, causing them to appear swollen and distinct. This test, known as the *quellung reaction*, not only enables the differentiation of pneumococci from other streptococci, but also allows the separation of pneumococci into more than 80 distinct serotypes.

Epidemiology

Because pneumococcal pneumonia is not a reportable disease in the United States, exact incidence figures are unavailable. The annual incidence has been estimated by the U.S. Centers for Disease Control at between 0.68 and 2.6 cases per 1000 population. Pneumococcal pneumonia is more common in males than females, and its incidence increases with advancing age. A variety of medical illnesses predispose to pneumococcal pneumonia, as discussed below. There is seasonal variation in the incidence of the disease; most cases occur in the winter or early spring.

CARRIAGE

S. pneumoniae often constitutes part of the microbial flora of the upper respiratory tract. Asymptomatic carriage rates in the general population are highly variable and are dependent on such factors as age and environment. A study in Charlottesville, Virginia, demonstrated that carriage rates ranged from 6 percent in childless adults to 38 percent in preschool children. In contrast, rates as high as 70 percent have been reported in certain closed populations such as military recruits. In general, carriage rates diminish with advancing age and are highest during the winter months.

RISK FACTORS

Several conditions are associated with an increased risk of pneumococcal pneumonia. Viral upper respiratory infections are reported as an antecedent event in a high percentage of cases. Conditions which are conducive to the aspiration of nasopharyngeal contents into the lungs, e.g., alcoholism and chilling, are common concomitants of pneumococcal pneumonia. Because fluid-filled alveoli are more susceptible to infection, there is an increased risk of pneumonia in persons with congestive heart failure, viral pneumonia, or noxious gas exposure. Several chronic medical illnesses are associated with an increased risk of pneumococcal infection, including multiple myeloma, splenic dysfunction, sickle cell disease, and chronic pulmonary disease. In addition, individuals who have undergone splenectomy or renal transplantation are predisposed to pneumococcal infections.

PNEUMOCOCCAL SEROTYPES

More than 80 pneumococcal serotypes have been identified; however, only a limited number of serotypes account for the majority of infections. Approximately 80 percent of cases of pneumococcal pneumonia in adults are caused by serotypes 1, 3, 4, 6, 7, 8, 9, 12, 14, 18, 19, or 23. The mortality rates from infections caused by the different serotypes are highly variable. For example, in one major study, bacteremic type III infections were found to carry a mortality rate of 55 percent, compared to an overall rate of 17 percent for all bacteremic pneumococcal infections.

Pathophysiology

Patients who develop pneumococcal pneumonia are usually colonized with a virulent strain of the organism and generally have impaired local host defense mechanisms, either due to transient derangements or chronic medical illnesses. Under these circumstances, virulent pneumococci can be aspirated from the nasopharynx into the alveoli, after which pneumococcal pneumonia develops in a characteristic fashion. The presence of bacteria in the alveoli elicits an outpouring of serous fluid, which supports replication of the organisms and, in addition, transports them outward via the pores of Kohn to adjacent alveoli. The spread of edema fluid continues until it is halted by anatomic barriers such as the visceral pleura or the pericardium. Within a few hours, alveoli become consolidated with polymorphonuclear leukocytes and erythrocytes. In the later stages of infection, macrophages migrate into the alveoli and ingest the remaining debris. Because the alveolar walls are not destroyed, the pulmonary parenchyma is usually normal following resolution of the infection.

As with other forms of aspiration pneumonia, pneumococcal pneumonia typically involves the dependent portions of the lungs. The infection is confined to a single lobe in the majority of cases. Interlobar spread, however, can occur if infected edema fluid flows from the bronchus of an involved lobe into that of an uninvolved lobe. Multilobar involvement occurs in approximately 20 to 30 percent of cases. Pneumococci can gain access to the pleural or pericardial spaces via direct spread from the pulmonary parenchyma, resulting in empyema or purulent pericarditis.

Lymphatic drainage of organisms occurs early in the course of the illness. If regional lymph nodes are unable to contain the infection, organisms enter the bloodstream. Bacteremia occurs in about 25 to 30 percent of patients and is usually associated with the more virulent serotypes. Bacteremia sometimes results in metastatic foci of infection, such as meningitis, septic arthritis, endocarditis, and endophthalmitis, or, rarely, peritonitis.

In the early stages of infection, phagocytosis is dependent on activation of the alternative complement pathway by components of the pneumococcal cell wall. Type-specific anticapsular antibodies appear 5 to 10 days after the onset of infection. The appearance of such opsonic antibodies, which markedly enhance phagocytosis of pneumococci, correlates temporally with the clinical "crisis" observed in the pre-antibiotic era, during which the patient undergoes an abrupt and striking improvement.

Clinical Manifestations

Few diseases have a clinical course that is as dramatic and as highly characteristic as that of pneumococcal pneumonia in its classic form. The illness often occurs shortly after an upper respiratory infection. Its onset is abrupt and is frequently manifested by a severe shaking chill (the "herald chill") which lasts for up to an hour. Shortly thereafter, the patient develops fever of 103 to 106°F, marked tachycardia and tachypnea, a dry cough, and severe pleuritic chest pain. Nausea and vomiting occur in about a third of patients. By the second or third day of the disease, the patient is acutely ill, with prominent malaise, weakness, and prostration. Marked respiratory distress is occasionally present, in part because of severe chest pain which leads to splinting of the chest wall. The cough, which is initially dry, becomes productive of thick, tenacious sputum which is "rusty" in appearance due to intra-alveolar hemorrhage.

On examination, the patient appears toxic and is in moderate to severe respiratory distress. The temperature, pulse rate, and respiratory rate are elevated, often markedly so. There is prominent diaphoresis. Many patients have herpes labialis. Respirations are shallow, and expiratory grunting is present.

In established cases of pneumococcal pneumonia, examination of the chest often reveals evidence of voluntary splinting of the muscles of the chest wall and consolidation of the involved area of the lung. Movement of the involved hemithorax is restricted to varying degrees. On palpation, there is increased tactile fremitus and occasionally a palpable rub over the area of involvement. Dullness to percussion can be detected in cases in which extensive consolidation is present. Auscultation over the involved area of lung may reveal coarse inspiratory rales, increased vocal fremitus, bronchial breath sounds, egophony, and a localized pleural friction rub. These auscultatory findings may be obscured, however, in the presence of a sizable pleural effusion or empyema.

Although the "classic" presentation of pneumococcal pneumonia was common in the preantibiotic era, the signs and symptoms of patients presenting with the disease in the 1980s are often much more muted. A minority of hospitalized patients describe chills or pleuritic chest pain, and even such cardinal manifestations as fever and sputum production are not invariably present. In elderly or debilitated patients, localizing signs of infection are sometimes absent, and mental status abnormalities may be the most striking finding.

Clinical Course

In an untreated case of pneumococcal pneumonia, the patient is acutely ill for 5 to 10 days, after which in surviving patients the infection either resolves promptly by "crisis" or subsides more gradually by "lysis." Patients who receive penicillin therapy usually improve quickly. Defervescence often occurs within 24 to 36 h. However, even in appropriately treated, uncomplicated cases, fever may take several days to resolve. It is unnecessary to alter therapy in such cases. More worrisome is the recurrence of fever following an initial response to therapy. Among the causes of recurrent fever are extrapulmonary foci of infection (see "Complications," below), bronchial obstruction by tumor or foreign body, drug fever, thrombophlebitis at sites of intravenous infusion, misidentification of the original infecting organism, superinfection, or, rarely, antibiotic resistance.

Complications

Patients with pneumococcal pneumonia may develop a wide variety of local or distant complications. Pleural effusions are the most common local complications. Such effusions are exudative in nature and are usually small and self-limited. Although most effusions are sterile, empyema develops on occasion, usually in cases in which antimicrobial therapy is delayed or inadequate. Empyema should be suspected in patients with pleural effusions who have persistent fever and leukocytosis, and thoracentesis should be performed in all such patients. Pneumococcal pericarditis, once the most common form of bacterial pericarditis, is now a rare complication. Suggestive clinical features include persistent fever, tachycardia, chest pain, a pericardial friction rub, and radiographic evidence of an enlarging cardiac silhouette.

Pneumococcal meningitis results from bacteremic spread of organisms to the meninges. A high index of suspicion must be maintained for this life-threatening condition, particularly in elderly or debilitated patients in whom the clinical features may not be clear-cut, and confusion or agitation may be attributed to other causes. Less common metastatic complications of pneumonia include infective endocarditis, septic arthritis, and endophthalmitis.

A variety of nonsuppurative complications have been reported. Jaundice has been noted in up to 26 percent of patients with lobar pneumonia in some series, usually in association with right lower lobe consolidation. In such patients, right upper quadrant tenderness and hepatomegaly are prominent findings, occasionally to such a degree that the pneumonia is overlooked while diagnoses of acute cholecystitis, hepatitis, or cholangitis are entertained. The pathophysiology of jaundice associated with pneumococcal pneumonia is unclear. There is often evidence of both hepatocellular injury and intrahepatic cholestasis. In some cases, hemolysis due to glucose-6-phosphate dehydrogenase deficiency may be a contributing cause. Other complications which have been reported include adult respiratory distress syndrome, rhabdomyolysis, and the syndrome of inappropriate secretion of antidiuretic hormone.

Prognosis

In the preantibiotic era, pneumococcal pneumonia was a dreaded disease with a mortality rate approaching 30 percent. Following the introduction of penicillin, the overall mortality rate has fallen to approximately 5 percent in nonbacteremic cases and 17 percent in bacteremic cases. There is considerable variation in prognosis among different patient subgroups. Mortality rates are higher in infants, the elderly, alcoholics, women in late pregnancy, and individuals with chronic underlying medical illnesses. Cases associated with leukopenia, multilobar involvement, or extrapulmonary complications carry a considerably increased mortality rate.

Diagnosis

Although the diagnosis of pneumococcal pneumonia may be strongly suggested by the clinical picture, a variety of laboratory tests are helpful in confirming the diagnosis.

It is important to obtain an adequate sputum specimen and to culture the blood and, if present, pleural fluid early in the course of the illness, prior to the institution of antimicrobial therapy. Though the diagnosis can be confirmed only by the isolation of *S. pneumoniae* from blood, pleural fluid, or lung tissue, a positive sputum Gram stain can rapidly provide strong presumptive evidence of pneumococcal pneumonia. To be accepted as adequate, the expectorated sputum specimen must contain numerous polymorphonuclear leukocytes (unless the patient is neutropenic) and few epithelial cells, to assure that one is not simply examining oropharyngeal contents. The presence of lancet-shaped, gram-positive diplococci in close association with leukocytes (Fig. 91-1) is highly suggestive of pneumococcal infection and correlates with a favorable clinical response to antipneumococcal therapy. A nega-

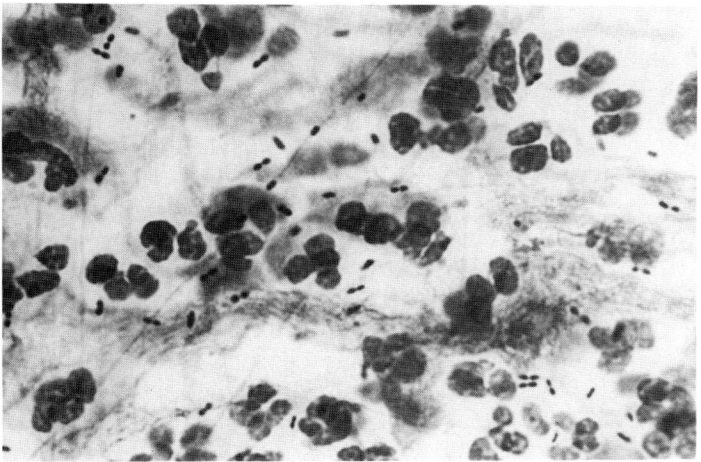

FIGURE 91-1 Sputum Gram stain from patient with pneumococcal pneumonia. Numerous lancet-shaped diplococci are seen in association with polymorphonuclear leukocytes. ×565.

tive Gram stain does not exclude the possibility of pneumococcal pneumonia. The sputum culture is of much less value than the Gram stain in the diagnosis of pneumonia. False-negativity rates of up to 50 percent have been reported. Moreover, in one series of patients with bacteremic pneumococcal pneumonia, over one quarter of sputum cultures grew potential pathogens other than *S. pneumoniae.*

Unfortunately, adequate sputum specimens are difficult to obtain in many patients, particularly those who are elderly, debilitated, and/or dehydrated. In selected patients in whom the differential diagnosis is particularly challenging, sputum specimens may be obtained via invasive techniques such as bronchoscopy (using a protected catheter tip to avoid oropharyngeal contamination) or rarely transtracheal aspiration. The decision to employ the latter technique, however, must be individualized and must take into account the experience of the operator in performing the procedure and the risk of potentially serious complications.

Counterimmunoelectrophoresis (CIE) is a rapid technique for the detection of pneumococcal polysaccharide in sputum, blood, urine, or cerebrospinal fluid. The major advantages of the test include its rapidity (1 h) and sensitivity (up to 80 percent for sputum specimens in some series). CIE results often remain positive for up to a week following the initiation of treatment, because of delayed clearance of pneumococcal polysaccharide. Although CIE is a promising technique, the required polyvalent pneumococcal antiserum is unavailable in many centers. The utility of the test is further hampered by the fact that positive results may be obtained in colonized patients without pneumonia.

A variety of nonspecific laboratory abnormalities are observed in patients with pneumococcal pneumonia. These include leukocytosis, often with a shift to the left; elevation of the erythrocyte sedimentation rate; and either hypernatremia or hyponatremia, reflecting varying degrees of dehydration and sodium depletion related to fever, vomiting, or ileus. Arterial blood gases reveal varying degrees of hypoxemia. Leukopenia is sometimes observed in patients with overwhelming infections. Liver function tests are occasionally abnormal, usually in a mixed hepatocellular and cholestatic pattern.

Chest radiographic findings are variable. In patients with full-blown lobar pneumonia, there is opacification of the involved area, and air bronchograms are present (Fig. 91-2). In recent years, lobar pneumonia has been seen less frequently; bronchopneumonia, manifested by multiple patchy infiltrates, has been a more common radiographic finding. Pleural effusions are detected in about 10 percent of cases. Necrotizing or cavitating lesions occur only rarely in pneumococcal pneumonia.

Pulmonary infiltrates are often masked in patients who are dehydrated and may not become apparent until

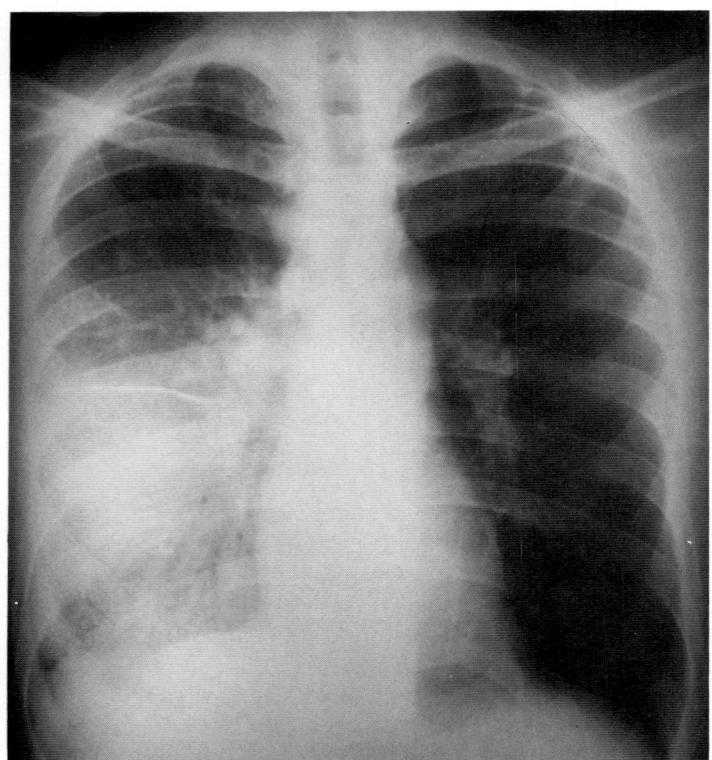

FIGURE 91-2 Chest radiograph from 38-year-old man with bacteremic pneumococcal pneumonia. There is extensive consolidation of right lower lobe with air bronchograms and partial obscuration of right hemidiaphragm. *(Courtesy of Cynthia Cofer, M.D.)*

the patient receives fluid replacement. Therefore, the absence of an infiltrate on initial chest radiograph does not unequivocally exclude the possibility of pneumonia.

Radiographic resolution of pneumococcal pneumonia is often delayed, even when there is prompt clinical improvement. Over one-half of patients have persistent radiographic abnormalities 4 weeks after the episode of pneumonia has resolved. However, if infiltrates persist for more than 8 weeks, the patient should be investigated for specific causes of treatment failure, such as malignancy, empyema, or bronchopleural fistula.

Differential Diagnosis

Pneumonia due to *S. pneumoniae* must be differentiated from that due to other agents which commonly cause community-acquired pulmonary infection, such as *Legionella pneumophila* and *Mycoplasma pneumoniae*. There are many overlapping features among these diseases. Pneumococcal infection characteristically presents with lobar or segmental consolidation. Legionnaires' disease more often presents with multiple organ system involvement, and there is a significantly higher incidence of hematuria, unexplained mental status alterations, and ele-

vation of hepatocellular enzymes. *Mycoplasma* pneumonia is a more indolent illness which rarely causes lobar consolidation, and it occurs year-round without any distinct seasonality.

Several other microorganisms can cause pulmonary infections which simulate pneumococcal pneumonia. *Klebsiella pneumoniae* causes necrotizing lobar pneumonia which often involves the upper lobes; patients may produce an extremely mucoid "currant jelly" type of sputum. *Hemophilus influenzae* and *Neisseria meningitidis* are relatively rare causes of pneumonia, but pulmonary infections caused by these organisms are clinically indistinguishable from pneumococcal pneumonia. Infections due to *Staphylococcus aureus*, *Streptococcus pyogenes* (see "Streptococcus Pyogenes," below), or *Mycobacterium tuberculosis* can at times also mimic pneumococcal pneumonia. This broad differential diagnosis underscores the importance of obtaining adequate bacteriologic studies in patients with pneumonia.

In addition several noninfectious diseases must be considered. Pulmonary infarction can cause fever, pleuritic chest pain, dyspnea, and hemoptysis, but the degree of systemic toxicity (chills, high fever, striking leukocytosis) is generally less than in classic pneumococcal lobar pneumonia. Occasionally, pulmonary angiography is necessary to differentiate between the two conditions. Pneumococcal pneumonia can also be mimicked by pulmonary manifestations of atelectasis, malignancy, systemic lupus erythematosus, congestive heart failure, uremia, or sickle cell disease, and by intra-abdominal infections involving the subdiaphragmatic spaces.

Treatment

Pneumococcal pneumonia is a potentially life-threatening illness, and its victims require excellent supportive care as well as appropriate antimicrobial therapy. The majority of patients should be hospitalized, although young, otherwise healthy individuals with mild infections can sometimes be managed as outpatients. Hospitalized patients should be confined to bed and monitored carefully. Fluid and electrolyte status require particular attention, since fever, diaphoresis, vomiting, and/or ileus can result in significant dehydration and electrolyte imbalances. Hypotensive patients generally require intravascular pressure monitoring. Arterial blood gases should be monitored, particularly if there is a history of underlying pulmonary disease, and supplemental oxygen should be administered as needed.

Pleuritic chest pain can be quite severe, and potent analgesic agents are often necessary to control it. Codeine may suffice in milder cases, but parenteral meperidine or morphine sulfate may be required. In such instances, care should be taken to avoid significant respiratory depression, especially in elderly individuals.

Because the indiscriminate use of antipyretics masks the fever curve and subjects the patient to frequent uncomfortable temperature swings, their use should generally be minimized. Certain patients with high and prolonged fever will clearly require judicious use of antipyretics. Otherwise, the primary indication for antipyretics is for the prevention of fever-induced tachycardia in patients who tolerate tachycardia poorly because of cardiac disease or advanced age.

Alcoholics with pneumococcal pneumonia require particular attention because of the risk of delirium tremens in such patients. Prophylactic benzodiazepines are generally advisable. Should mental status aberrations or other unexplained neurologic abnormalities occur, lumbar puncture may be necessary to rule out meningitis.

Patients in whom pneumonia is complicated by empyema require drainage procedures in addition to antimicrobial therapy. Most empyemas can be drained successfully by chest tube thoracostomy, although open drainage procedures are occasionally necessary.

Appropriate antimicrobial therapy of pneumococcal pneumonia decreases the duration and severity of the illness, reduces overall mortality, and greatly lessens the risk of local and metastatic complications. Since its introduction in the 1940s, penicillin has been the agent of choice for the treatment of infections caused by S. pneumoniae. A great majority of strains are exquisitely sensitive to penicillin, being inhibited by serum levels of 0.02 μg/ml or less. However, in recent years, a few penicillin-resistant strains have been isolated, as discussed below.

Most patients with pneumococcal pneumonia require parenteral penicillin therapy. Recommended regimens include procaine penicillin G, 600,000 units intramuscularly every 12 h, or aqueous penicillin G, 1 million units intravenously every 4 to 6 h. In contrast, patients who are hypotensive or who have complications such as meningitis or endocarditis should receive high-dose intravenous penicillin (18 to 20 million units per day in adults). Patients with mild, uncomplicated cases of pneumococcal pneumonia can be treated with oral penicillin V, 500 mg four times daily. There has been an increasing tendency among more junior physicians to use very high doses of penicillin for the treatment of pneumococcal pneumonia. Controlled trials, however, have shown no differences in outcome between nonhypotensive patients treated with twice-daily intramuscular procaine penicillin G and those treated with high-dose intravenous therapy. This is to be expected, given the exquisite sensitivity of most strains of S. pneumoniae to penicillin. Antibiotic therapy should be continued for 7 to 10 days. After the patient has been afebrile for three days, it is reasonable to discontinue parenteral antibiotics and begin oral antibiotics.

In the penicillin-allergic patient, erythromycin or vancomycin are appropriate alternatives. In adult patients, erythromycin may be administered intravenously in a dose of 500 mg every 6 h. Oral erythromycin can be given to patients who are less acutely ill. The dose is 400 to 500 mg every 6 h, depending on the preparation chosen. When vancomycin is used in the treatment of pneumonia, it must be given intravenously. The usual dosage is 500 mg every 6 h or 1 g every 12 h for normal-sized adults. The dose must be decreased proportionately in children and in patients with renal failure. In persons whose allergic history is that of a mild and delayed skin rash, a first-generation cephalosporin may be considered. Cephalosporins should not, however, be used in patients with a history of immediate-type hypersensitivty reactions to β-lactam antibiotics.

Penicillin-Resistant *S. Pneumoniae*

For more than 25 years following the introduction of penicillin, all S. pneumoniae strains were exquisitely susceptible to it. In 1967, however, the first "relatively penicillin-resistant" (RPR) strain was identified. By definition, such strains have a minimum inhibitory concentration (MIC) to penicillin between 0.1 to 1.0 μg/ml, in contrast to the usual MIC below 0.02 μg/ml. RPR isolates have been reported from South Africa, Australia, New Guinea, England, Canada, the United States, and France. Reported prevalence rates vary widely. RPR was identified in 3.7 percent of S. pneumoniae isolates in a nationwide screening program in the United States. Elsewhere, rates as high as 13.5 percent have been reported. The prevalence of RPR strains of S. pneumoniae appears to be steadily increasing.

Of even greater concern were reports in 1977 from Durban and Johannesburg, South Africa, of infections due to highly penicillin-resistant strains (MIC greater than 1.0 μg/ml). These organisms were also resistant to a variety of other antibiotics, including other β-lactam agents, erythromycin, clindamycin, tetracycline, and trimethoprim-sulfamethoxazole. Five different antimicrobial susceptibility patterns were identified. Although such multiply resistant isolates fortunately have remained rare, there have been a few additional reports of both community-acquired and nosocomial infections due to highly resistant strains in France, South Africa, and the United States.

Both relative and high-level penicillin resistance are thought to result from chromosomally mediated alterations in bacterial penicillin-binding proteins. Under experimental conditions, penicillin resistance has been shown to result from exposure of organisms to progressively greater concentrations of penicillin.

Because the MICs of RPR S. pneumoniae remain well below achievable serum penicillin levels, most infections caused by these organisms are theoretically curable with high-dose penicillin therapy. However, a few treatment failures have been reported, particularly in the setting of concomitant meningitis. In contrast, high-dose penicillin is consistently ineffective against highly resistant strains.

In general, documentation of penicillin resistance should prompt use of another agent to which the organism is susceptible in vitro. The only antibiotic to which such strains have been universally susceptible is vancomycin. In addition, some isolates have been susceptible to erythromycin, chloramphenicol, tetracycline, and/or rifampin. In treating infections caused by penicillin-resistant S. pneumoniae, the clinician must be guided by results of in vitro susceptibility tests and by the patient's response to therapy. The necessity for routine antimicrobial susceptibility testing of S. pneumoniae isolates depends upon the prevalence of antibiotic-resistant strains in a given geographic locale.

Pneumococcal Vaccine

Efforts to produce an effective vaccine against S. pneumoniae date to 1911, when whole bacterial cell preparations were tested in South African gold miners. Such vaccines proved to be of limited efficacy. In the 1940s, following the identification and purification of pneumococcal capsular polysaccharides, a polyvalent pneumococcal polysaccharide vaccine was developed. In independent studies among military recruits and hospitalized elderly patients, the vaccine was immunogenic and was protective against infection. In 1945, a six-valent vaccine was licensed, but interest in the vaccine waned after penicillin became widely available. After 2 years, the manufacturer ceased production of the vaccine.

Landmark studies conducted between 1952 and 1962 by Austrian and Gold led to reconsideration of the role of a pneumococcal vaccine. These studies demonstrated that despite the widespread use of penicillin, the prevalence and case fatality rate of bacteremic pneumococcal infections remained high, particularly among certain high-risk populations. Furthermore, the majority of cases were caused by a limited number of serotypes.

A new vaccine was developed in the 1970s, and several efficacy trials were undertaken. The vaccine was shown to be immunogenic among healthy adults, and efficacy rates of 76 to 92 percent were demonstrated among South African gold miners. Based on these findings, a 14-valent pneumococcal polysaccharide vaccine was licensed in 1977, which was replaced by a 23-valent vaccine in 1983. The current vaccine contains 25 μg each of 23 polysaccharide antigens (Danish types 1, 2, 3, 4, 5, 6B, 7F, 8, 9N, 9V, 10A, 11A, 12F, 14, 15B, 17F, 18C, 19A, 19F, 20, 22F, 23F, 33F). These 23 serotypes accounted for 87 percent of cases of bacteremic pneumococcal pneumonia reported to the Centers for Disease Control in 1983.

In recent years, however, new questions have been raised about the efficacy of the pneumococcal vaccine, particularly in the high-risk groups who would most benefit from an effective vaccine.

Although the vaccine has been demonstrated to be highly immunogenic and protective in healthy young men, it is less effective in young children, immunocompromised patients, and the elderly. Children under the age of 2 do not mount an adequate antibody response to polysaccharide antigens, so it is not surprising that the vaccine has been ineffective in this patient population. Studies of vaccine immunogenicity in immunocompromised adults have demonstrated impaired antibody response to pneumococcal polysaccharide in patients with chronic renal failure, multiple myeloma, nephrotic syndrome, renal allografts, and Hodgkin's disease. Moreover, a recent large cooperative study demonstrated that the majority of "high-risk" persons over the age of 55 (i.e., those with chronic pulmonary, cardiac, hepatic, or renal dysfunction, diabetes mellitus, or alcoholism) did not develop antipneumococcal antibodies after receiving the vaccine.

Vaccine efficacy in patients at increased risk of pneumococcal infections has been difficult to assess. In two large, randomized trials involving elderly patients, there were too few cases of bacteremic illness to allow meaningful statistical analysis of vaccine efficacy. However, there was no reduction in morbidity or mortality due to pneumococcal infections in vaccinated patients versus controls. In the cooperative study described above, there was no reduction in incidence of pneumococcal infections in vaccinated high-risk patients, compared to unvaccinated controls.

Because of the limited number of conclusive clinical trials, alternative methods have been used to assess vaccine efficacy. One study retrospectively analyzed the distribution of pneumococcal serotypes causing infections in vaccinated patients and compared them to serotypes in unvaccinated persons. Serotypes included in the vaccine were isolated much less often in vaccinated than in unvaccinated persons; overall vaccine efficacy was estimated at 64%. A well-designed case-control study demonstrated vaccine efficacy of 77 percent in patients with underlying medical illnesses such as diabetes mellitus, chronic pulmonary disease, congestive heart failure, alcoholism, and chronic renal failure; efficacy was 70 percent in persons over 55 years of age. Not surprisingly, no efficacy was demonstrated in highly immunocompromised patients.

Despite limited and conflicting data on the vaccine's efficacy in high-risk groups, most authorities, including the Immunization Practices Advisory Committee of the Centers for Disease Control, continue to recommend its use in patients at increased risk of pneumococcal infection. We heartily concur. The vaccine is safe, inexpensive, and potentially effective against approximately 90 percent of serotypes causing bacteremic pneumococcal infections. Current recommendations call for the immunization of persons over 2 years of age who have sickle cell disease, anatomic or functional asplenia, cerebrospinal fluid leaks, nephrotic syndrome, or other conditions associated with immunosuppression. Additional indications for immuni-

zation in adults include alcoholism, multiple myeloma, Hodgkin's disease, renal failure, or chronic cardiac or pulmonary disease. In addition, it is recommended that all adults over age 65 receive the vaccine.

The vaccine is given as a single intramuscular injection. Since its safety in pregnant women has not been established, its use should be avoided in this patient population. In about half of vaccine recipients, local tenderness occurs; fewer than 5 percent develop transient fever or myalgias. Because detectable antibody responses to pneumococcal polysaccharide persist for many years, and because occasional severe reactions have occurred following administration of a second vaccine dose, routine reimmunization is not recommended at this time. Recommendations for selective reimmunization of certain high-risk groups may be forthcoming, however, as additional experience with the vaccine is gained.

STAPHYLOCOCCUS AUREUS

Staphylococcal pneumonia is a relatively uncommon disease which nevertheless occurs in a wide variety of clinical settings and has protean clinical manifestations. In its most severe form, it is a fulminating, devastating illness which is associated with a high mortality rate.

Microbiology

S. aureus is a gram-positive coccus which measures 0.8 to 1.0 μm in diameter and often occurs in grapelike clusters. When grown on blood agar plates, colonies appear smooth and round, measure 1 to 4 mm in diameter, and are usually golden yellow. Staphylococci produce a variety of toxins and extracellular enzymes; the presence of the extracellular enzyme coagulase enables the rapid differentiation of S. aureus from other species of staphylococci.

Epidemiology

S. aureus is an ubiquitous microorganism which frequently colonizes human skin and mucous membranes. Approximately 15 percent of adults are persistent nasal carriers, and transient carriage is common among the remainder of the population. Most cases of staphylococcal pneumonia are presumed to occur in previously colonized individuals. In previously healthy children or adults, staphylococcal pneumonia occurs as a complication of influenza A infection. There have been rare reports of transmission of S. aureus via droplet spread of the organisms from colonized infants who developed concomitant viral upper respiratory infections.

Pathophysiology

Staphylococcal infection can be established in the lower respiratory tract via either of two mechanisms. *Bron-chogenous spread* of organisms results from aspiration of infected nasopharyngeal secretions into the lungs and is the basis of postinfluenza pneumonia. Individuals with anatomic abnormalities of the respiratory tract and those who are immunosuppressed due to underlying diseases or immunosuppressive medications are also predisposed to infection by the bronchogenous route.

Hematogenous spread results from the release of staphylococci into the bloodstream from an intravascular focus. Organisms are transported via the pulmonary circulation to one or more areas of the lung, where infection is established. Persons at high risk for hematogenous staphylococcal pneumonia include intravenous drug abusers, hemodialysis patients, persons with infected intravascular devices, and patients with suppurative thrombophlebitis.

Regardless of the route of entry, S. aureus elicits an intense inflammatory response in the lung manifested by polymorphonuclear leukocytic infiltration, local edema, and hemorrhage. In severe infections, there is extensive tissue necrosis with destruction of alveolar walls. Because inhaled air can enter these damaged alveoli but cannot escape, air-filled cavities are sometimes created. Thin-walled air-filled cavities called "pneumatoceles" are highly characteristic of staphylococcal pneumonia, particularly in children. In adults, thick-walled abscess cavities are a more common finding.

Clinical Manifestations

The clinical presentation of staphylococcal pneumonia is highly variable, depending on the age and previous health status of the patient. Because there are no unique manifestations of staphylococcal pneumonia to differentiate it from other bacterial pneumonias, correct diagnosis requires a high index of suspicion.

In children less than 1 year old, staphylococcal pneumonia is almost always related to an antecedent episode of influenza or measles and is manifested by an unexpected deterioration in the infant's condition shortly following an upper respiratory infection. Typical findings include high fever, tachypnea, grunting respirations, and cough. Examination usually reveals diminished breath sounds and localized rales over the area of involvement. Pleural effusions occur in the majority of cases, and empyema and pneumothorax are not uncommon.

Similarly, staphylococcal pneumonia in previously healthy adults almost always occurs as a complication of influenza A. In a classic monograph published in 1919, Chickering and Park were the first to provide a detailed description of the clinical features of postinfluenza staphylococcal pneumonia. Their observations, quoted below, remain pertinent today.*

---

*JAMA 72:617–629, March 1, 1919. Copyright 1919, American Medical Association.

The onset of S. aureus pneumonia is almost always insidious and rarely accompanied by the chill and localized pain of a typical lobar pneumonia, though the course of the disease is extremely rapid. The facies, the anxious expression, and deep cyanosis suggest a grave prognosis from the onset, at a period when physical signs of pulmonary involvement are but scanty. Herpetic eruptions on the lips are scarcely ever noted, nor is delirium present except rarely. Usually the mind is clear almost to the end. Occasionally pleuritic pain is complained of, but this is not usual. It is the picture of a general septicemia. The fever on the whole is high, ranging between 104 and 106, with frequent remissions to 101. These patients rarely have the painful and labored breathing seen in pneumococcus infections.

Clinical examination of the chest of the average case reveals a very atypical type of pneumonic involvement. Signs of congestion of both lower lobes are found frequently, though in the majority of cases a diffuse process in all the lobes may be present. At the onset, only slightly diminished resonance to percussion may be elicited, with diminished breath sounds and many coarse and fine moist rales. But rarely are there signs of pure consolidation of one or more lobes, and then only late in the disease. Frequently there is an abundance of coarse moist rales heard throughout the chest.

Staphylococcal pneumonia is not always associated with an antecedent viral infection. It may occur, apparently de novo, in chronically ill or immunocompromised patients. The clinical picture in such patients ranges from a subacute, smouldering infection to an acute, life-threatening illness as described above. In all forms of staphylococcal pneumonia, pleural effusion and empyema are common complications. Bacteremia has been reported in approximately 20 percent of cases.

Patients who acquire staphylococcal pneumonia by the hematogenous route typically have a subacute pulmonary illness manifested by fever, cough, and dyspnea. They occasionally develop hemoptysis or pleuritic chest pain. The illness tends to be milder than bronchogenous pneumonia.

Diagnosis

Initial presumptive diagnosis hinges upon the epidemiologic and clinical features of the case plus accurate interpretation of the sputum Gram stain. The latter characteristically reveals gram-positive cocci in clusters or tetrads in close association with polymorphonuclear leukocytes (Fig. 91-3). Because the organisms often remain viable for several hours following phagocytosis, intracellular bacteria are occasionally observed.

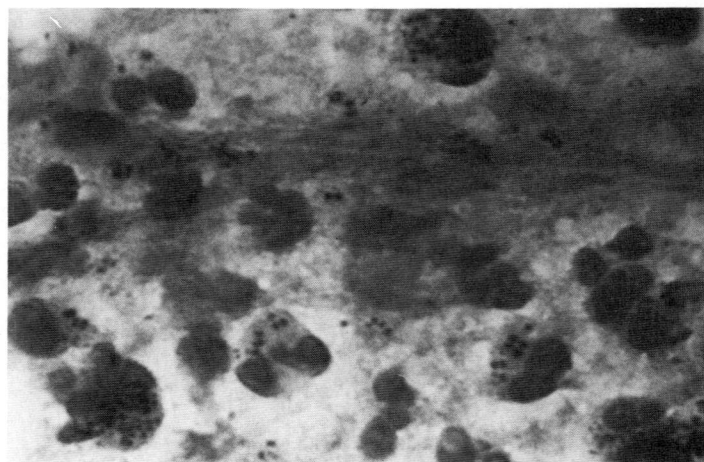

FIGURE 91-3 Sputum Gram stain from patient with staphylococcal pneumonia, demonstrating numerous intracellular cocci in tetrads and clusters. ×565.

Confirmation of the diagnosis of staphylococcal pneumonia requires isolation of the organism from blood, pleural fluid, or lung tissue. In the absence of such evidence, a variety of other laboratory tests are helpful in providing a presumptive diagnosis.

Antibodies to teichoic acid, a component of the staphylococcal cell wall, are present in a variety of deep-seated staphylococcal infections, including pneumonia. Serologic testing for teichoic acid antibodies is probably most helpful in cases in which bacteriologic studies are negative.

Radiographic abnormalities are variable. Most commonly, single or multiple patchy areas of bronchopneumonia appear; they rapidly enlarge, cavitate, and form air-filled cavities (either pneumatoceles or thick-walled abscess cavities) (Figs. 91-4 and 91-5). Localized areas of consolidation are relatively unusual. Pleural effusions are common, particularly in infants.

Treatment

Patients with staphylococcal pneumonia are usually critically ill. Even with appropriate therapy, the mortality rate can be as high as 50 percent. As with pneumococcal pneumonia, successful management requires both intensive supportive care and appropriate antimicrobial therapy.

Despite the availability of a variety of effective antimicrobial agents, treatment of staphylococcal pneumonia is often challenging, in part because of variable antibiotic resistance patterns. Although penicillin is the agent of choice against susceptible strains, almost all strains of S. aureus are now highly penicillin-resistant owing to plasmid-mediated penicillinase production. Therefore, initial therapy of staphylococcal pneumonia should always include either a penicillinase-resistant penicillin

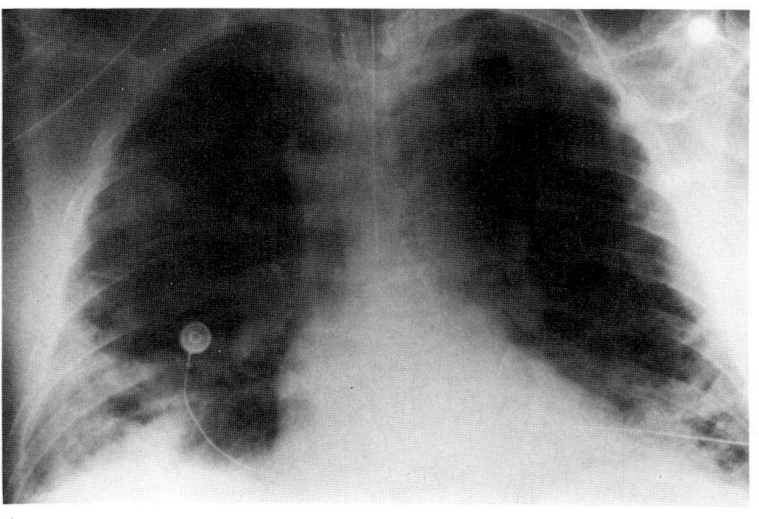
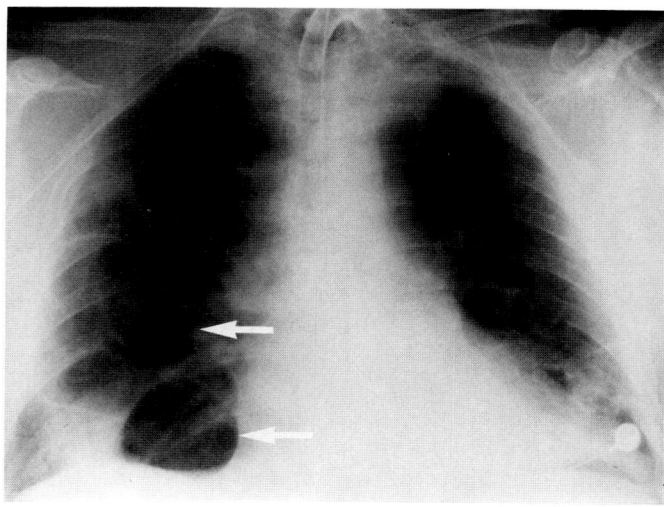

A   B

FIGURE 91-4 Serial chest radiographs from 58-year-old man with bronchogenous staphylococcal pneumonia superimposed on chemical pneumonitis secondary to inhalation of ammonia and chlorine gas. A. Infiltrates in both lower lobes and right mid-lung field with early cavitation in right lower lobe. B. Same patient 18 days later. Note two large pneumatoceles.

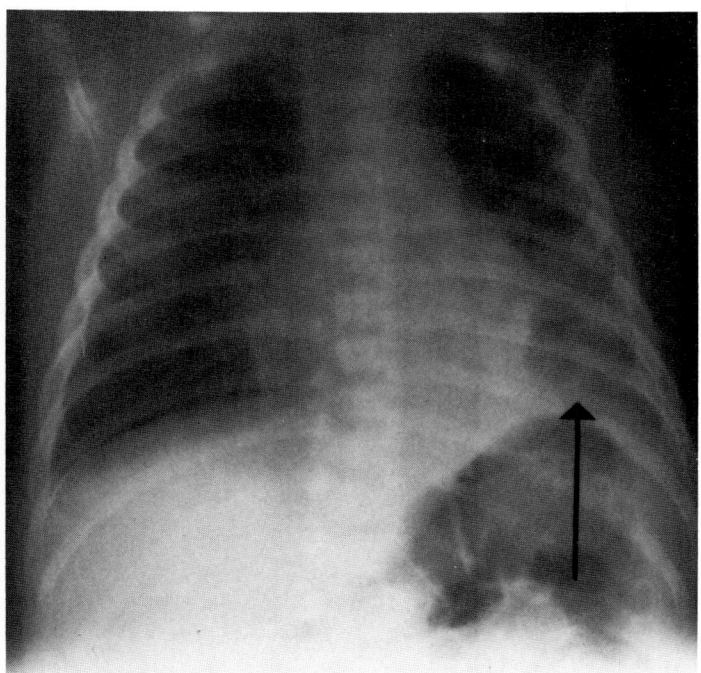

FIGURE 91-5 Chest radiograph from 1-month-old male with staphylococcal pneumonia involving the left lower lobe. A large pneumatocele is present (arrow) with two superimposed smaller pneumatoceles. *(Courtesy of Sarah Fitch, M.D.)*

(nafcillin, methicillin, or oxacillin) or vancomycin, all of which are highly active against S. aureus. Specific therapy can then be instituted once the results of antimicrobial susceptibility testing are available. The recommended dose of the penicillinase-resistant penicillins is 1.5 to 2 g intravenously every 4 h. Vancomycin may be

given to adults with normal renal function at a dose of 500 mg intravenously every 6 h or 1 g every 12 h. The optimum duration of antimicrobial therapy has not been established. Because staphylococcal pneumonia tends to be a serious, deep-seated infection which is slow to respond to therapy, a 4-week course of antibiotics may be required. If the patient improves promptly, treatment can be completed with dicloxacillin, an oral agent which is well absorbed and attains high blood levels.

The emergence of methicillin-resistant strains of S. aureus (MRSA) in recent years has posed a special therapeutic problem. Although such strains as yet represent a small proportion of isolates in the community, they are important nosocomial pathogens and have been reported with increasing frequency in Europe and the United States. MRSA are resistant to all penicillins and cephalosporins. The agent of choice for the treatment of MRSA infections is vancomycin, to which such organisms have been universally susceptible.

Tolerance, defined as a wide (10- to 32-fold or more) dissociation between a cell-wall-active antibiotic's bacteriostatic and bactericidal activity against a susceptible microorganism, is a recently described phenomenon of uncertain clinical significance. Up to 30 percent of S. aureus strains in some series have been found to exhibit tolerance, usually to penicillinase-resistant penicillins, but also to vancomycin on occasion. Because of the life-threatening nature of staphylococcal pneumonia, it seems reasonable to test isolates for minimum bactericidal as well as minimal inhibitory concentrations of antistaphylococcal β-lactam antibiotics and to treat infections caused by tolerant strains with combination therapy, including an aminoglycoside antibiotic (i.e., gentamicin or

tobramycin). Clinical data are lacking, however, to indicate that such a course of action is beneficial in staphylococcal pneumonia.

Rifampin, a highly effective antistaphylococcal antibiotic which penetrates well into leukocytes and tissues, has been used at times as ancillary therapy for staphylococcal infections. Its role, if any, in treatment of life-threatening cases of staphylococcal pneumonia remains undefined.

Penicillin-allergic patients can be treated cautiously with a first-generation cephalosporin, using the guidelines set forth above. If there is a history of an immediate hypersensitivity reaction, vancomycin is the agent of choice.

STREPTOCOCCUS PYOGENES

Pneumonia due to S. pyogenes was once a common epidemic infection among military recruits but has become a rare entity since the advent of penicillin. Streptococcal pneumonia is usually related to an antecedent episode of influenza, measles, or varicella. The illness is characterized by the abrupt onset of fever and chills, followed by dyspnea, cough, blood-streaked sputum production, and pleuritic chest pain. Chest radiographs generally reveal evidence of bronchopneumonia; lobar consolidation is uncommon. Bacteremia is present in approximately 10 to 15 percent of cases. Up to 40 percent of patients develop empyema, which is manifested by large pleural effusions containing thin, serosanguinous pleural fluid. Appropriate therapy of streptococcal pneumonia includes chest-tube drainage of empyema fluid and administration of procaine penicillin G, 4 to 6 million units per day divided into two to four intramuscular injections. Alternatively, the same dose of aqueous penicillin G can be administered intravenously. Therapeutic options in the peni-

cillin-allergic patient are identical to those described above for pneumococcal pneumonia.

BACILLUS ANTHRACIS

Inhalation anthrax (*woolsorter's disease*) is a rare entity which is primarily of historical interest. Less than 20 cases have been reported in the United States in the twentieth century. The disease occurs sporadically (or rarely in epidemics) as a result of inhalation of B. anthracis spores from imported goat hair. It primarily afflicts textile mill workers, tannery employees, or laboratory personnel.

Following inhalation of B. anthracis spores into the alveoli, the spores are ingested by alveolar macrophages and transported to the mediastinal lymph nodes. Organisms rapidly multiply and produce toxin, which causes extensive mediastinal edema, hemorrhage, and necrosis. Organisms then enter the bloodstream and are widely disseminated; meningeal involvement occurs in approximately 50 percent of cases.

Inhalation anthrax is a biphasic illness. The initial phase consists of nonspecific flulike symptoms including low-grade fever, malaise, myalgias, nonproductive cough, and occasionally a sensation of chest pressure. After a few days, the patient spontaneously improves, only to enter the second phase of the illness and deteriorate abruptly. At this stage of the disease, there is prominent dyspnea and occasionally stridor due to tracheal compression by enlarged mediastinal nodes. Vasomotor collapse often ensues rapidly. Chest radiographs almost always reveal prominent widening of the mediastinum.

Because of the rarity of this disease, there have been no controlled trials to guide treatment decisions. Recommended therapy consists of intravenous aqueous penicillin G, 2 million units every 2 h. Even with aggressive treatment, few patients survive.

BIBLIOGRAPHY

American College of Physicians, Health and Public Policy Committee: Pneumococcal vaccine. Ann Intern Med 104:118–120, 1986.
Recommendations for populations to be vaccinated.

Austrian R: Pneumococcal pneumonia. Diagnostic, epidemiologic, therapeutic and prophylactic considerations. Chest 90:738–743, 1986.
A perspective on the use of pneumococcal vaccine.

Austrian R: A reassessment of pneumococcal vaccine. N Engl J Med 310:651–653, 1984.
A review of available data on the efficacy of pneumococcal vaccine and a discussion of the role of the vaccine in the 1980s.

Austrian R., Gold J: Pneumococcal bacteremia with especial reference to bacteremic pneumococcal pneumonia. Ann Intern Med 60:759–776, 1964.
A landmark study which demonstrated the persistently high case fatality rates of bacteremic pneumococcal infections despite the availability of effective antimicrobial agents.

Barrett-Connor E: The nonvalue of sputum culture in the diagnosis of pneumococcal pneumonia. Am Rev Respir Dis 103:845–848, 1971.
  In this study, sputum cultures failed to yield S. pneumoniae in approximately 50 percent of cases of bacteremic pneumococcal pneumonia.

Basiliere JL, Bistrong HW, Spence WF: Streptococcal pneumonia: Recent outbreaks in military recruit populations. Am J Med 44:580–589, 1968.
  A review of the epidemiologic and clinical aspects of an epidemic of streptococcal pneumonia among military recruits.

Boerner DF, Zwadyk P: The value of the sputum Gram's stain in community-acquired pneumonia. JAMA 247:642–645, 1982.
  Sputum Gram stains revealed gram-positive diplococci in over one-half of patients with community-acquired pneumonia. This finding strongly correlated with a favorable response to specific antipneumococcal therapy.

Bolan G, Broome CV, Facklam RR, Plikaytis BD, Floser DW, Schlech WF: Pneumococcal vaccine efficacy in selected populations in the United States. Ann Intern Med 104:1–6, 1986.
  Based on an alternative retrospective method of assessing pneumococcal vaccine efficacy in certain patient populations (persons over 2 years old without serious underlying immunodeficiency), average overall vaccine efficacy was 64 percent.

Brachman PS: Inhalation anthrax. Ann NY Acad Sci 353:83–93, 1980.
  A review of the history, clinical aspects, and pathogenesis of inhalation anthrax.

Brewin A, Arango L, Hadley WK, Murray JF: High-dose penicillin therapy and pneumococcal pneumonia. JAMA 230:409–413, 1974.
  There were no differences in outcome between patients with pneumococcal pneumonia who received 1.2 million units of procaine penicillin G daily and those treated with 20 million units of aqueous penicillin G daily.

The British Thoracic Society and the Public Health Laboratory Service: Community-acquired pneumonia in adults in British hospitals in 1982–83: a survey of aetiology, mortality, prognostic factors and outcome. Q J Med 62:195–220, 1987.
  Four hundred and fifty-three adults in 25 British hospitals entered a prospective study of community-acquired pneumonia. In about two-thirds of the patients, the causative agent was proved, or strongly suspected, to be Streptococcus pneumoniae. The authors recommend that antibiotics be given as early as possible to cover S. pneumoniae; in addition, M. pneumoniae during outbreaks, and S. aureus during influenza epidemics.

Centers for Disease Control: Update: Pneumococcal polysaccharide vaccine usage—United States. Recommendations of the Immunization Practices Advisory Committee. Ann Intern Med 101:348–350, 1984.
  The most recently revised recommendations for pneumococcal vaccine usage.

Chickering HT, Park JH: Staphylococcus aureus pneumonia. JAMA 72:617–626, 1919.
  The original and classic description of postinfluenza staphylococcal pneumonia.

Glupczynski Y, Lagast H, Van der Auwera P, Thys JP, Crokaert F, Yourassowsky E, Meunier-Carpentier F, Klastersky J, Kains JP, Serruys-Schoutens E et al.: Clinical evaluation of teicoplanin for therapy of severe infections caused by gram-positive bacteria. Antimicrob Agents Chemother 29:52–57, 1986.
  Teicoplanin was evaluated in 47 patients with severe infections. Teicoplanin is a potentially effective and well-tolerated antimicrobial agent for therapy of nonbacteremic infections caused by gram-positive bacteria.

Harper TE, Christensen RD, Rothstein G, Hill HR: Effect of intravenous immunoglobulin G on neutrophil kinetics during experimental group B streptococcal infection in neonatal rats. Rev Infect Dis 8:S401–S408, 1986.
  A modified form of serum immunoglobulin G (pH 4.25) was tested for its effect on neutrophil kinetics and survival rates in neonatal rats with type III, group B streptococcal pneumonia and sepsis. Immunoglobulin facilitated the neutrophil inflammatory response: neutrophils were released more rapidly from the storage pool and accumulated more quickly at the site of bacterial inoculation. Immunoglobulin recipients did not develop neutropenia or depletion of the neutrophil storage pool.

Helms CM, Viner JP, Sturm RH, Renner ED, Johnson W: Comparative features of pneumococcal, mycoplasmal, and Legionnaires' disease pneumonias. Ann Intern Med 90:543–547, 1979.
  Patients with Legionnaires' disease are more likely to present with multiple organ system involvement, hematuria, or unexplained mental status alterations than are patients with pneumococcal or mycoplasma pneumonia.

Hendley JO, Sande MA, Stewart PM, Gwaltney JM: Spread of Streptococcus pneumoniae in families. I. Carriage rates and distribution of types. J Infect Dis 132:55–61, 1975.

Using the best available methods for documenting pneumococcal colonization, rates ranged from 6 percent in childless adults to 38 percent in preschool children.

Jacobs MR, Koornhof HJ, Robins-Browne RM, Stevenson CM, Vermaak ZA, Freiman I, Miller GB, Witcomb MA, Isaacson M, Ward JI, Austrian R: Emergence of multiply resistant pneumococci. N Engl J Med 299:735–740, 1978.

An extensive investigation of patients and hospital staff members in Johannesburg, South Africa, which documented the increasing prevalence of multiply antibiotic-resistant pneumococci.

Jay SJ, Johanson WG, Pierce AK: The radiographic resolution of Streptococcus pneumoniae pneumonia. N Engl J Med 293:798–801, 1975.

Over one-half of patients with pneumococcal pneumonia had persistent radiographic abnormalities 4 weeks after the episode of pneumonia resolved. An appropriate interval for follow-up chest radiographs is 6 weeks.

Krook A, Fredlund H, Holmberg H: Diagnosis of pneumococcal pneumonia by detection of antigen in saliva. Eur J Clin Microbiol 5:639–642, 1986.

A sandwich enzyme-linked immunosorbent assay was used for the detection of pneumococcal C polysaccharide in saliva samples from patients with radiologically verified pneumonia. The authors conclude that the detection of pneumococcal C polysaccharide in saliva offers a valuable complement to conventional diagnostic methods for pneumococcal pneumonia.

Macfarlane JT, Finch RG, Ward MJ, Macrae AD: Hospital study of adult community-acquired pneumonia. Lancet 2:255–258, 1982.

Pneumococcal pneumonia accounted for 76 percent of 127 consecutive cases of community-acquired pneumonia in adults.

Musher DM, McKenzie SO: Infections due to Staphylococcus aureus. Medicine 56:383–409, 1977.

An extensive review of the clinical aspects of infection due to S. aureus, which includes a discussion of 20 patients with staphylococcal pneumonia.

Ort S, Ryan JL, Barden G, D'Esopo N: Pneumococcal pneumonia in hospitalized patients: Clinical and radiological presentations. JAMA 249:214–218, 1983.

An informative study of 94 patients with pneumococcal pneumonia who were hospitalized in the late 1970s. Sixty-one percent of the patients had bronchopneumonia, and in many cases, "classic" findings of pneumococcal pneumonia were lacking.

Pauluzzi S, Del Favero A, Menichetti F, Baratta E, Moretti VM, Di Filippo P, Pastici MB, Guerciolini R, Patoia L, Frongillo RF: Treatment of infections by staphylococci and other gram-positive bacteria with teicoplanin: an open study. J Antimicrob Chemother 20:431–438, 1987.

Teicoplanin, 200–400 mg (3–6 mg/kg) daily IV or IM, was used to treat 71 episodes of infection. The average duration of treatment was 22 days. Teicoplanin is an effective and well-tolerated antibiotic for infections by gram-positive bacteria, and it is effective against methicillin-resistant staphylococci.

Polsky B, Gold JW, Whimbey E, Dryjanski J, Brown AE, Schiffman G, Armstrong D: Bacterial pneumonia in patients with the acquired immunodeficiency syndrome. Ann Intern Med 104:38–41, 1986.

Eighteen episodes of community-acquired bacterial pneumonia were diagnosed in 13 patients among 336 with the acquired immunodeficiency syndrome (AIDS). Bacterial pathogens isolated in 16 of 18 episodes were Haemophilus influenzae in 8, Streptococcus pneumoniae in 6, group B streptococcus in 1, and Branhamella catarrhalis in 1. Bacteria associated with B-cell defects should be anticipated with formulating empiric antibiotic therapy, pending a definitive diagnosis, for pulmonary infiltrates in patients with AIDS.

Schmid RE, Anhalt JP, Wold AD, Keys TF, Washington JA: Sputum counterimmunoelectrophoresis in the diagnosis of pneumococcal pneumonia. Am Rev Respir Dis 119:345–348, 1979.

Sputum counterimmunoelectrophoresis was positive in 86 percent of patients with definite or probable pneumococcal pneumonia. However, the false-positivity rate of CIE was 29 percent.

Shapiro ED, Clemens JD: A controlled evaluation of the protective efficacy of pneumococcal vaccine for patients at high risk of serious pneumococcal infections. Ann Intern Med 101:325–330, 1984.

A case-control study of pneumococcal polysaccharide vaccine efficacy which demonstrated protective efficacy of 77 percent in patients at moderately increased risk of infection, 70 percent in persons over 55 years of age, and 0 percent in severely immunocompromised patients.

Simberkoff MS, Cross AP, Al-Ibrahim M, Baltch AL, Geiseler J, et al: Efficacy of pneumococcal vaccine in high-risk patients. N Engl J Med 315:1318–1327, 1986.
A prospective, randomized, placebo-controlled trial of the efficacy of pneumococcal vaccine in high-risk patients. There was no reduction in incidence of pneumococcal infections in vaccine recipients.

Sisk JE, Riegelman RK: Cost effectiveness of vaccination against pneumococcal pneumonia: an update. Ann Intern Med 104:79–86, 1986.
An update of a 1978 cost-effectiveness analysis of vaccination against pneumococcal pneumonia. Current levels of vaccination appear to be too low considering the potential health benefits and cost-effectiveness.

Tugwell P, Williams AO: Jaundice associated with lobar pneumonia. Q J Med 46:97–118, 1977.
An extensive investigation of Nigerian patients with jaundice associated with pneumococcal pneumonia. Hemolysis due to glucose-6-phosphate dehydrogenase deficiency was a common finding.

Tuomanen E, Rich R, Zak O: Induction of pulmonary inflammation by components of the pneumococcal cell surface. Am Rev Respir Dis 135:869–874, 1987.
Using a rabbit model of experimental pneumonitis, the authors investigated the components on the surface of the pneumococcus that incite pulmonary inflammation. The authors propose that pulmonary inflammation during pneumococcal pneumonia arises in large part from the interaction of the bacterial cell wall with complement and noncomplement-mediated host defenses.

Williams JH Jr, Moser KM: Pneumococcal vaccine and patients with chronic lung disease. Ann Intern Med 104:106–109, 1986.
The authors conclude that routine vaccination of all patients with chronic lung disease is not warranted.

Woodhead MA, MacFarlane JT: Comparative clinical and laboratory features of legionella with pneumococcal and mycoplasma pneumonias. Br J Dis Chest 81:133–139, 1987.
The clinical and laboratory features of 83 cases of community-acquired pneumococcal pneumonia, 79 cases of legionella pneumonia, and 62 cases of mycoplasma pneumonia were compared. No unique features were found in any group.

Zeluff B, Catchpole M, Lowe P, Koornhof H, Gentry L: Cefadroxil compared with cefaclor in the treatment of streptococcal pneumonia in adults. Drugs 32:39–42, 1986.
103 young male Black African gold miners with pneumococcal pneumonia confirmed by culture or serology were randomly assigned to receive the long-acting oral cephalosporin cefadroxil 1 g every 12 h or cefaclor 500 mg every 8 h for 10 days. Both displayed effective antimicrobial activity and low toxicity in the treatment of pneumococcal pneumonia.

Chapter 92

Pneumonias Caused by Gram-Negative Aerobic Organisms

Alan K. Pierce

Community-Acquired Pneumonia
Hemophilus influenzae Pneumonia
Klebsiella Pneumonia
Chronic Klebsiella Pneumonia
Other Community-Acquired Pneumonias
Hospital-Acquired (Nosocomial) Pneumonia
Organisms with Specific Epidemiologic Features
Pertussis (Whooping Cough)
Tularemia
Melioidosis
Plague
Pleuropulmonary Involvement of Systemic Infectious Agents
Salmonella
Brucellosis
Glanders

Pneumonias due to gram-negative aerobic bacilli may be divided into groups: those that are community-acquired, those that are hospital-acquired, and those with specific epidemiologic features. The distinctions are based on the differing incidences and clinical characteristics of gram-negative bacillary pneumonias. Either community- or hospital-acquired pneumonias may result from the same bacterial species. On occasion, additional gram-negative species may cause pulmonary infection under the appropriate epidemiologic circumstances.

Although exact prevalence data are not available, it is probable that Hemophilus influenzae is the most frequent cause of community-acquired pneumonia due to gram-negative bacilli. These pleomorphic coccobacilli are non-motile and non-spore-forming, and they grow best on chocolate agar.

Three additional families of aerobic gram-negative bacilli (Enterobacteriaceae, Pseudomonadaceae, and Achromobacteraceae) may cause community- or hospital-acquired pneumonia. Genera included among the Enterobacteriaceae include Klebsiella, Enterobacter, Escherichia, Arizona, Citrobacter, Edwarsiella, Hafnia, Serratia, Proteus, and Providence. The term coliform refers to some genera of this family including Klebsiella, Escherichia, and Enterobacter, the most common of these gram-negative bacilli implicated in both community- and hospital-acquired pneumonias. Other genera of this family are more commonly associated with hospital-acquired disease. The other two families of bacteria are also more commonly associated with hospital-acquired pneumonia. Their genera include Pseudomonas aeruginosa, P. maltophilia, P. cepacia, P. stutzeri, Acinetobacter lwoffi, A. anitratus, Moraxella, Alcaligenes, Flavobacterium, and Aeromonas hydrophila. All these bacteria are gram-negative, non-spore-forming bacilli which may be readily cultured on ordinary laboratory media. Many of them are natural commensals in the intestinal tract of humans and animals and are found regularly in feces.

COMMUNITY-ACQUIRED PNEUMONIA

Although the organism Hemophilus influenzae was described in 1893, the first well-documented case of this gram-negative bacillus causing pneumonia in an adult did not appear until 1942. Only a few reports of this pathogen causing adult pneumonia were published before the 1970s, and H. influenzae was considered a rare cause of this illness. Subsequently, increasing numbers of cases have been reported, especially since 1977. Reasonable estimates suggest that H. influenzae now causes 10 to 15 percent of bacterial pneumonias among adults who are sufficiently ill to be admitted to a hospital. It is likely that a part of this increase in incidence is apparent owing to more frequent recognition of this pathogen because of improved cultural techniques. However, even in hospitals which have not changed bacteriologic methodology, there has been an increased number of reported cases. It has been suggested that the increased incidence is due to a declining immunity of adults to H. influenzae in recent years. Early antimicrobial therapy of childhood infections has been proposed as the cause of decreased production of protective antibodies.

Hemophilus influenzae Pneumonia

PATHOLOGY

The gross and microscopic changes in the lungs due to H. influenzae are similar to those caused by Streptococcus pneumoniae and which have been outlined in Chapter 91. Differentiation may be made only by observation of the organisms in tissue sections or by culture of the causative organism.

CLINICAL MANIFESTATIONS

Pneumonia due to *H. influenzae* is more common among older persons, especially men: two-thirds of patients are over 50 years of age. Most patients have a chronic illness. Chronic obstructive pulmonary disease is present in about one-half of persons who develop this type of pneumonia and chronic alcoholism in about one-third. It should be emphasized, however, that pneumonia due to *H. influenzae* may occur in young adults and in persons who have no chronic disability. The onset of symptoms is abrupt. On average, patients are sufficiently ill to seek medical aid within 2 days, although it has been reported that pneumonias due to nontypable strains have a mean duration of symptoms of five days. The most common symptoms are shaking chills (45 percent), fever, cough productive of purulent sputum, dyspnea, and pleuritic pain (35 percent). On physical examination these patients usually appear acutely ill with fever, tachypnea, and apparent dyspnea. Findings in the chest are usually limited to the lower lobes. Rales are the most frequent abnormality with signs of consolidation in about one-third. None of these historical or physical findings separates pneumonia due to *H. influenzae* from the more common pneumonia due to *Streptococcus pneumoniae*. However, about 25 percent of patients with *H. influenzae* pneumonia develop pleural effusions, some of which are present at time of admission. This incidence of pleural disease is somewhat higher than occurs with the pneumococcus. Almost all these fluids are sterile, parapneumonic effusions.

LABORATORY AND RADIOGRAPHIC FINDINGS

Most patients with *H. influenzae* pneumonia have a leukocytosis with a median white blood cell count of 13,500 per cubic millimeter. Leukopenia is a serious prognostic sign. Gram-stained sputum in an area with a predominance of polymorphonuclear leukocytes may demonstrate large numbers of small, gram-negative coccobacilli with no other bacterial forms seen. However, many reports indicate that the gram-stained sputum may be misinterpreted as showing gram-positive diplococci when the specimen has not been adequately decolorized. Other reports indicate frequent failure to identify *H. influenzae* even in adequately stained sputum. Thus the correct diagnosis may not be suspected until cultures become available. When appropriate media are used, blood cultures are positive in approximately 20 percent of patients and sputum cultures in about 70 percent.

Radiographic infiltrates are much more frequent in lower than upper lobes. Infiltrates in both lower lobes is not uncommon. In about 75 percent of cases the infiltrate is a patchy bronchopneumonia; in the remainder it is a more dense consolidation conforming to a segmental or lobar distribution. These findings do not differentiate *H. influenzae* from pneumococcal pneumonia. As indicated previously, up to 25 percent of patients have pleural effusions; most of these develop after hospitalization. Lung necrosis with cavitation has been reported only rarely.

TREATMENT AND PROGNOSIS

There are six encapsulated and, therefore, typable strains of *H. influenzae*. Until recently it was thought that most adult pneumonias are due to type b, the causative strain of most childhood infections. It has now become apparent that most adult disease is due to unencapsulated and, therefore, nontypable strains. This distribution of types may influence the choice of the antimicrobial used for therapy, since about 20 percent of type b strains are resistant to ampicillin, while most nontypable strains in the United States are sensitive.

Ampicillin is reasonable therapy for *H. influenzae* pneumonia in adults in hospitals in which a high incidence of resistance has not been demonstrated. The optimal dose has not been investigated, but 6 g per day administered parenterally in divided doses has been reported to be successful. For patients who are profoundly ill, or in hospitals with a high fraction of strains resistant to ampicillin, chloramphenicol 2 to 3 g per day is probably the treatment of choice. Trimethoprim-sulfamethoxazole and third-generation cephalosporins may also be effective, but their use has not been documented in substantial series. Most patients respond promptly to therapy and become afebrile within 72 h. The mortality rate in recent series has been reported to be 25 percent. Many of the patients, however, were treated with inappropriate antimicrobials at the outset. Additional mortalities occurred owing to the underlying condition that predisposed to the pneumonia. In one report of 30 patients treated with appropriate antimicrobials at the time of admission, the mortality was only 6.6 percent.

Klebsiella Pneumonia

Gram-negative bacilli were not a frequent cause of community-acquired pneumonia until relatively recently. The most common was pneumonia due to *Klebsiella pneumoniae* which accounted for 0.5 to 5.0 percent of all community-acquired pneumonias requiring hospitalization. There is now a growing awareness that a larger spectrum of gram-negative organisms, especially other coliform bacteria, may cause pneumonia in the community. The incidence of pneumonia due to these organisms probably varies among hospitals, depending on the population served. Elderly and chronically ill persons, especially those living in nursing homes, are at greatest risk, and hospitals serving large numbers of such patients have the greatest incidence. It is reasonable to estimate that, on average, these gram-negative bacilli cause 15 percent of community-acquired pneumonias among adults who are sufficiently ill to require hospitalization. Among these pathogens,

K. pneumoniae sometimes causes the most distinctive clinical presentation, and this is described first.

PATHOLOGY

Experimental infection due to *K. pneumoniae* (Friedländer's bacillus) begins in a lobular distribution and spreads rapidly in much the same manner as that described for pneumococcal pneumonia. The outer margin is characterized by a zone of edema fluid in which the organisms multiply freely. The fluid mechanically transports the organisms to contiguous areas of lung, and in extensive disease endobronchial dissemination may occur to more remote areas. Inside the outer edema zone there is a zone of early consolidation with many polymorphonuclear leukocytes in addition to the bacteria; little phagocytosis is apparent. In the inner zone there is more marked consolidation with large numbers of phagocytes, most of which are polymorphonuclear leukocytes, with some mononuclear cells. Phagocytosis is marked in some areas of consolidation, while in others organisms are apparently multiplying freely. In comparison with pneumococcal pneumonia, there are more organisms in the zone of consolidation. Additionally, there is evidence of destruction of alveolar walls and of fibroblastic activity.

Pneumonia due to *K. pneumoniae* has a predilection for upper lobes, especially the right upper lobe (Fig. 92-1). In fatal cases an entire lobe is most commonly involved with a reddish gray consolidation. The pleural surface is covered with a fibrinous exudate. Cavity formation is common and may be extensive with virtual destruction of the normal architecture of the lobe. Microscopically the consolidated areas demonstrate alveoli filled with an exudate containing both polymorphonuclear leukocytes and mononuclear cells. The walls of abscess cavities are formed by granulation tissue, partially epithelialized alveolar remnants, and fibrous tissue.

CLINICAL MANIFESTATIONS

Pneumonia due to *K. pneumoniae* most commonly occurs in middle-aged or elderly patients. It is much more common in men than women. Almost all patients have some underlying chronic disease, and in approximately two-thirds it is alcoholism. The other frequent predisposing conditions are chronic bronchopulmonary disease and diabetes mellitus.

The onset of *Klebsiella* pneumonia does not differentiate it from the more common pneumococcal pneumonia. The onset is usually abrupt (90 percent) with true rigors (60 percent), fever to 104°F, cough productive of sputum (90 percent), and pleuritic chest pain (80 percent). The patient is typically extremely ill. The sputum is frequently a thick, gelatinous, bloody mucus which the patient may have difficulty in expectorating. However, this typical, brick-red sputum is not present in a sufficient fraction of patients for it to be a reliable differential diagnostic sign. Frank hemoptysis may occur. Examination reveals an acutely ill, febrile patient with tachypnea and apparent dyspnea. The chest demonstrates signs of consolidation over the involved lobe or lobes. Findings of pleural effusion may be present when the patient first presents.

LABORATORY AND RADIOGRAPHIC FINDINGS

Most patients with *Klebsiella* pneumonia have a leukocytosis, but up to one-quarter have a normal leukocyte count. Neutropenia is a grave prognostic sign. Gram stain of expectorated sputum typically reveals short, thick, gram-negative bacilli with large capsules. However, in many patients the organism may be seen only rarely or not at all. In most cases the organism is subsequently reported as present in initial sputum cultures. Blood cultures are positive in up to 25 percent of patients.

Most commonly the chest radiograph demonstrates a dense lobar or segmental consolidation, most frequently of the right upper lobe (Fig. 92-1). In some cases the distribution is bronchopneumonic, and bilateral perihilar infiltrates have been reported. As in other bacterial pneumonias, a moderate amount of volume loss may occur in the involved lobe. Occasionally there is an expansion of the involved lobe with bulging of the adjacent fissures; this feature is highly suggestive of *Klebsiella* pneumonia. Lung necrosis with abscess formation occurs in up to 50 percent of surviving patients and may be radiographically demonstrable within 4 days of onset of the disease. The cavities frequently are quite large and may involve an entire lobe. Empyema occurs in up to one quarter of cases.

TREATMENT AND PROGNOSIS

Untreated *Klebsiella* pneumonia is fatal in from 50 to 97 percent of cases. Adequate antimicrobial therapy reduces the mortality to the range of 20 to 50 percent. Advanced age, severe underlying disease, leukopenia, and bacteremia are correlated with a fatal outcome. Supportive care including oxygenation and maintenance of clear airways is important; the mode of death frequently suggests inadequate removal of tenacious secretions. Antimicrobial therapy is directed by in vitro sensitivity testing when these become available. At the outset, however, the bacterial etiology of the pneumonia is not known, and empiric therapy is necessary. A combination of two antimicrobials, each of which has a broad spectrum of activity, is recommended. An aminoglycosidic antibiotic, amikacin, gentamicin, or tobramycin, which has been shown to have the fewest resistant organisms at the hospital to which the patient is admitted, is one of the antimicrobials usually chosen. If the patient is only moderately ill, a first- or second-generation cephalosporin is reasonable for the second antibiotic; but for critically ill patients, a third-generation cephalosporin may be desirable.

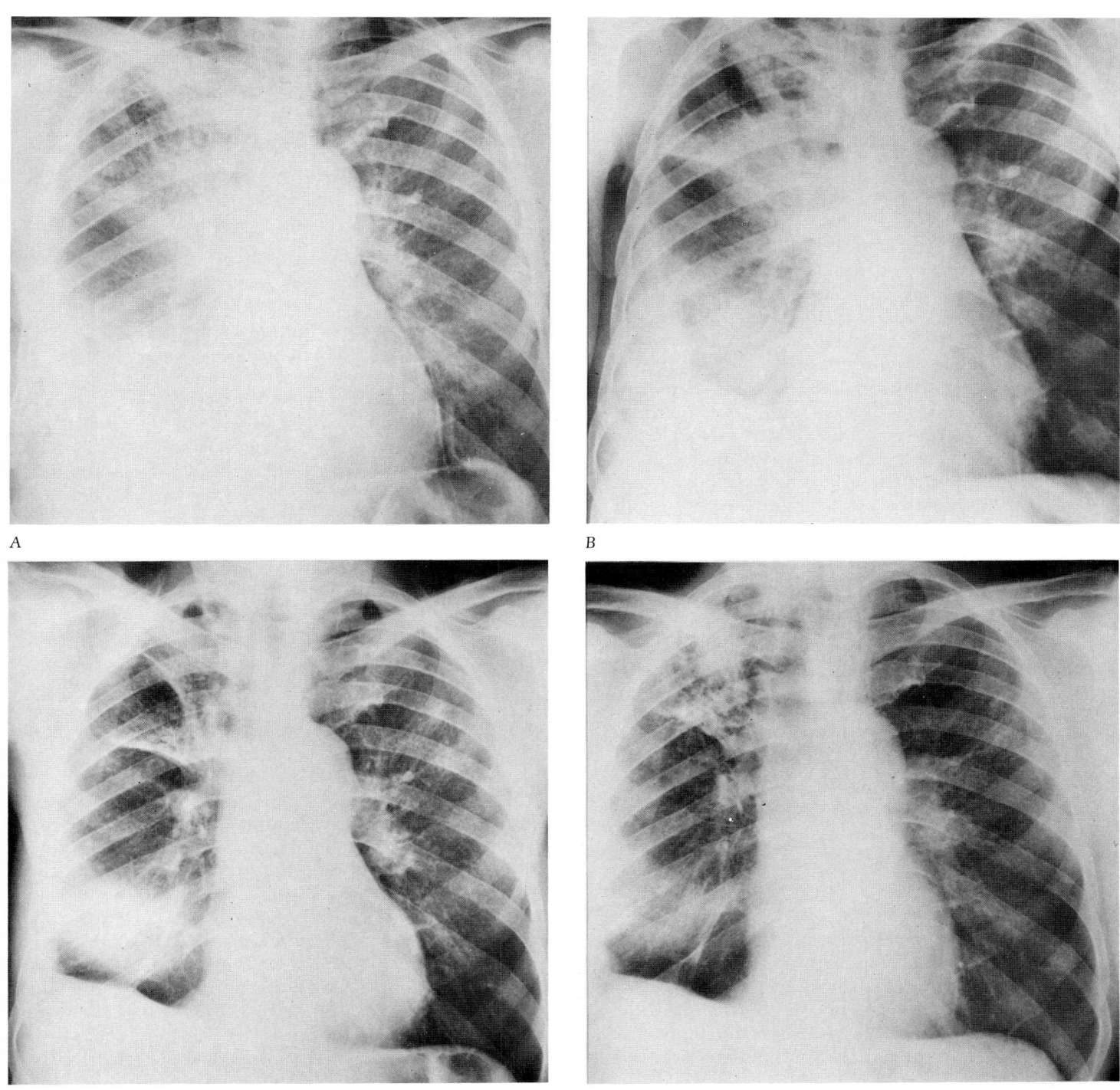

FIGURE 92-1 *Klebsiella* pneumonia in a 64-year-old man with acute onset of cough, productive of yellow-green, thick sputum, fever, and chest pain over the right anterior chest. Sputum, blood, and urine contained Freidländer's bacilli.   *A.* On admission (2 days after onset). Consolidation of right upper lobe with scattered miliary densities throughout both lung fields. Right empyema.   *B.* One week after admission. Resolution and cavitation in right upper lobe.   *C.* Four months later. Residual scarring and cavitary lesions in right upper lobe. Thickened pleura on the right.   *D.* Five years later. Chronic cavities and thickened pleura on right. Question of "fungous ball" in right upper lobe (opaque area beneath clavicle).

Chronic *Klebsiella* Pneumonia

Although *Klebsiella* pneumonia most commonly presents in a fulminant manner, occasionally it occurs as an indolent lung abscess. In the preantimicrobial era, chronic lung abscess sometimes followed acute *Klebsiella* pneumonia; this remains a potential development among inadequately treated patients. However, indolent pneumonia with abscess formation may occur without an antecedent acute phase. The disease, as are the more common abscesses due to anaerobic organisms, is most frequent in alcoholic patients. Mild symptoms of low-grade fever, cough, and weight loss may be present for days to weeks before the patient seeks medical advice.

The chest radiograph reveals a pulmonary infiltrate with abscess formation. There are no features which distinguish it from pneumonia with abscess due to anaerobic organisms. Expectorated sputum may reveal the organisms, but such is frequently disregarded until the abscess fails to respond to penicillin. Direct culture of the abscess fluid by means of transthoracic aspiration or fiberoptic bronchoscopy to reveal *Klebsiella* in pure growth may be necessary for a convincing diagnosis.

Therapy with antimicrobial drugs to which the organisms are sensitive in vitro is usually successful without the need for mechanical drainage of the abscess. However, prolonged antibiotic administration may be necessary.

Other Community-Acquired Pneumonias

Most bacterial pneumonias are caused by organisms which colonize the upper airways and are inoculated into the lung by aspiration during sleep. Since gram-negative aerobic bacilli, except *H. influenzae*, do not frequently colonize the upper airways of healthy persons, normal adults are at very low risk of developing pneumonia from these organisms. The increased prevalence of community-acquired gram-negative bacillary pneumonias has occurred in patients with chronic debilitating diseases such as chronic obstructive pulmonary disease, heart diseases, malignancies, neurologic diseases, alcoholism, and renal failure. The oropharyngeal flora of such patients regularly includes gram-negative bacilli.

The most common pathogens causing pneumonia among these patients are *K. pneumoniae, E. coli,* and *Enterobacter aerogenes.* For patients who have been residing in nursing homes, additional pathogens including *Pseudomonas aeruginosa* are also frequently implicated. The clinical syndromes caused by these organisms, including *K. pneumoniae,* may be indistinguishable, and a correct diagnosis may depend on results of cultures of sputum, transtracheal aspirates, blood, or empyema fluid. Indeed, it is common to recover more than one pathogen from sputum cultures, and the role of each organism cannot be determined.

PATHOLOGY

E. coli pneumonia is most commonly a diffuse lower lobe bronchopneumonia. Alveolar septa are thickened by edema, capillary engorgement, and a mononuclear infiltrate, and there is some cuboidal metaplasia of alveolar walls. Alveoli are filled with edema fluid and a moderate number of mononuclear cells. Abscess cavities of moderate size may be present, consisting of alveolar wall necrosis, edema fluid, and large numbers of polymorphonuclear leukocytes. The pleura is fibrotic and thickened by a moderate number of mononuclear cells and small lymphocytes, and a purulent effusion may be present.

Pneumonia due to Pseudomonadaceae is most commonly a diffuse bronchopneumonia involving several lobes. Alveolar septa are thickened by cellular infiltrates of mononuclear cells and polymorphonuclear leukocytes and by fibrous tissue. Multiple small microabscesses are scattered throughout the involved lung with necrosis of alveolar walls and cellular infiltrate. Pleural adhesions and small pleural effusions are common.

Pneumonia due to *Proteus* may cause a dense, lobar consolidation, most commonly of the right upper lobe. Alveolar septa are thickened by capillary congestion and fibrosis with scattered macrophages filled with hemosiderin. Alveolar spaces are filled with edema fluid and a mixed exudate of mononuclear cells and polymorphonuclear leukocytes. Cavities tend to be multiple and large and demonstrate mononuclear cells and polymorphonuclear leukocytes in various stages of degeneration. Only occasional pleural adhesions are found, and pleural effusions are not common.

CLINICAL MANIFESTATIONS

As has been emphasized, the great majority of all patients with community-acquired, gram-negative bacillary pneumonia are chronically ill, and most are old. The onset of illness may be similar to that of any aerobic bacterial pneumonia with shaking chills, fever, cough productive of purulent sputum, and pleuritic chest pain. However, atypical presentations in this population are not unusual, and the clinical signs and symptoms may be subtle. Chills occur in only about 30 percent of patients. Fever may be low-grade or even absent in some patients. Relative bradycardia and an alteration in diurnal temperature patterns with the peak temperature in early morning are thought to suggest *Pseudomonas* pneumonia. Cough may be mild or absent, and many debilitated patients are unable to produce sputum. Pleural chest pain occurs in the minority. Indeed, nonpulmonary symptoms such as anorexia, weakness, lethargy, or confusion may dominate the clinical presentation. Physical findings are difficult to elicit, particularly if the patient cannot cooperate or has chronic obstructive lung disease. Tachypnea may be the major

finding suggesting pneumonia. Rales are heard in over half of the patients, but signs of consolidation occur in only about 30 percent. Findings of a pleural effusion occur in approximately 40 percent of patients with *E. coli* pneumonia, but it is rarely present at time of admission. Pleural effusions are more common in *Pseudomonas* pneumonia but are less common in that due to *Proteus*.

LABORATORY AND RADIOGRAPHIC FINDINGS

Most patients with gram-negative bacillary pneumonia demonstrate leukocytosis, most commonly in the range of 15,000 to 20,000 cells per cubic millimeter. Expectorated sputum frequently reveals gram-negative bacilli on direct stain, and the organisms are usually cultured from the original specimen. Blood cultures are positive in approximately 25 percent of patients with pneumonia due to *Klebsiella*, 20 percent due to *E. coli* or *Enterobacter*, and 50 percent due to *Pseudomonas*.

Chest radiographs are not usually specific for the causative organism. Bronchopneumonia without lobar or segmental consolidation is the usual finding. The infiltrates may be unilateral or bilateral and most commonly involve the lower lobes. In some instances, however, a more specific pattern may be recognized. Chest radiographs of patients with *E. coli* pneumonia may reveal lower lobe bronchopneumonia which may be unilateral or bilateral. Moderate-sized abscess cavities are common. Empyema is common and may be quite large; it is usually unilateral on the side with the greater parenchymal infiltrate. *Pseudomonas* pneumonia may appear radiographically as diffuse, bilateral bronchopneumonia involving several lobes. The infiltrates frequently appear as nodules 0.5 to 2 cm in diameter which tend to coalesce into larger infiltrates with time. Small abscess cavities are common. Pleural effusions are usually small and may be present on admission. *Proteus* pneumonia may present with a radiographic appearance similar to that of classic *Klebsiella* pneumonia, with volume loss of the involved lobe a common feature. Pleural effusions are rare.

TREATMENT AND PROGNOSIS

Mortality rates are high for patients with community-acquired, gram-negative bacillary pneumonia, especially when bacteremia is present. Since these patients are usually seriously ill before the onset of pneumonia, the relative contribution of the infection is not always clear. However, the mortality is markedly higher in patients in whom appropriate antimicrobial therapy is delayed or never administered, indicating a significant role of the infection in many deaths. Mortality rates of 30 to 40 percent for the Enterobacteriaceae, 70 to 80 percent for Pseudomonadaceae, and 25 percent for other aerobic gram-negative organisms may be expected. Survival beyond hospitalization is even lower owing to the associated diseases.

As indicated in the section on *Klebsiella* pneumonia, initial therapy is empiric. The recommendations in that section are reasonable for patients who have not been institutionalized before admission. Among patients from nursing homes the incidence of pneumonia due to organisms other than the coliform bacteria, such as *Pseudomonas aeruginosa*, is higher. An antimicrobial regimen incorporating an agent against this organism is reasonable. This includes an aminoglycosidic antibiotic and a third-generation cephalosporin such as cefoperazone or ceftazidime, or an aminoglycosidic agent and an antipseudomonal penicillin such as mezlocillin, azlocillin, or piperacillin. Clinical trials have utilized third-generation cefalosporins, such as those above, or the newer class of antimicrobials, the carbapenems, as the single antimicrobial administered, but there are insufficient data to recommend this therapy at present. In geographic areas where *Legionella pneumophilia* occurs frequently, the addition of 4 g per day of erythromycin should be considered.

HOSPITAL-ACQUIRED (NOSOCOMIAL) PNEUMONIA

Hospital-acquired pneumonias are those that develop in hospitalized patients in whom the infection was not present at the time of admission, and hence they are not manifest in the first 72 h of hospitalization. Nosocomial pneumonias occur in approximately 1 percent of all patients. Among the more severely ill hospitalized patients, those admitted to an intensive-care unit (ICU), the incidence is about 12 percent. Approximately 55 percent are caused by gram-negative bacilli, and among ICU patients these organisms are even more prevalent. Any of the genera and species of the previously indicated families of organisms may be implicated. The most common are *Klebsiella* species, *Pseudomonas aeruginosa*, *Enterobacter* species, *E. coli*, *Proteus* species, and *Serratia* species. Frequently more than one species is recovered from respiratory secretions, and the role of each cannot be determined with certainty. Indeed, the organisms identified in tracheobronchial secretions may not correlate with those grown from the more reliable culture sites of blood, pleural fluid, percutaneously aspirated lung material, or endobronchial brushings.

EPIDEMIOLOGY

It has been indicated in a previous section that most pneumonia probably is caused by organisms from the oropharynx. Gram-negative bacilli are found only rarely in this location in normal persons. Chronically or severely ill persons lose effective pharyngeal clearance mechanisms allowing colonization with gram-negative bacilli, and hence these patients are at risk for developing pneumonia due to these organisms. The patients most likely to be colonized are those with features suggesting a severe primary

illness such as hypotension, coma, azotemia, acidosis, or endotracheal intubation; the incidence of colonization in such patients approaches 75 percent. Since clusters of patients within an intensive-care unit may be colonized simultaneously with the same species of gram-negative bacilli, the bacteria may, in part, be transmitted from patient to patient within the hospital setting. However, approximately 20 percent of the patients are colonized at the time of admission, and others are colonized with organisms not recovered from other patients, suggesting that many people are colonized by organisms indigenous to themselves. The gastrointestinal tract may be the primary source in these latter patients. Hospital-acquired pneumonia also may be associated with contaminated respiratory therapy equipment. The unique feature of such equipment is its capability of suspending bacteria in sufficiently small droplets to be deposited in terminal lung units where the potential for causing pneumonia is greatest. Equipment incorporating nebulizers, i.e., aerosol generators, has been especially incriminated in this regard. Contamination of nebulizers is virtually always by aerobic gram-negative bacilli. However, pneumonia due to such equipment is unnecessary, since practical methods of decontamination exist. To be effective, decontamination must be carried out at least once every 24 h, and the equipment must be monitored on a periodic basis to ensure sterility.

CLINICAL FEATURES

Patients without antecedent pulmonary or infectious disease may have signs and symptoms similar to those indicated for community-acquired pneumonia. However, in many critically ill patients the primary disease may mask or simulate the occurrence of bacterial pneumonia, making a definitive diagnosis difficult. These patients frequently are unable to report symptoms accurately. Fever, leukocytosis, antecedent radiographic abnormalities, and purulent sputum may be part of the primary disease process. Gram-negative bacilli in sputum are found in a high fraction of these patients in the absence of clinical pneumonia. In these circumstances an infection is suggested by (1) the radiographic appearance of a new or progressive pulmonary infiltrate, (2) fever, (3) leukocytosis, and (4) purulent tracheobronchial secretions. Utilizing these criteria, however, there is a 30 percent false-positive and false-negative rate of diagnosis.

Patients suspected of developing a hospital-acquired pneumonia should be treated from the outset with broad antimicrobial coverage appropriate for gram-negative and gram-positive (staphylococcal, pneumococcal) organisms. The recommendations for antimicrobials to be used for empiric therapy for community-acquired pneumonia patients from nursing homes is reasonable. If specific coverage for S. aureus is deemed necessary in a hospital with a significant incidence of methicillin-resistant *Staphylococcus aureus* strains, vancomycin, 1.0 g IV every 12 h, should be added.

ORGANISMS WITH SPECIFIC EPIDEMIOLOGIC FEATURES

Pertussis (Whooping Cough)

Pertussis (whooping cough) is a highly contagious, acute respiratory illness primarily affecting infants and young children. The causative organism is *Bordetella pertussis*, although *B. parapertussis* and *B. bronchiseptica* may cause similar clinical syndromes. These organisms are small, nonmotile, gram-negative bacilli 0.5 to 1.0 μm in length. Special medium (Bordet-Gengou) is required for cultural isolation.

PATHOLOGY

Pathologic changes in fatal cases are predominantly in the bronchi and bronchioles. The gram-negative organisms are found in large numbers among the cilia of intact epithelial cells. Bronchial and bronchiolar walls are infiltrated with lymphocytes and plasma cells, and the epithelium shows patchy destruction and detachment. Peribronchiolar infiltration of lymphocytes gives the appearance of an interstitial pneumonia. Small airways are obstructed with mucopurulent exudate, and secondary changes of patchy atelectasis or overdistended alveoli occur.

CLINICAL MANIFESTATIONS

Whooping cough is transmitted by droplet infection. The attack rate is very high for a bacterial disease, up to 90 percent among susceptible family members. After an incubation period of 1 to 2 weeks the clinical disease typically occurs in three stages, each of approximately 2-week duration. The catarrhal stage cannot be distinguished from a viral respiratory infection. The patient may have a low-grade fever with sneezing, injected conjunctivas, and a cough which is worse at night. In the paroxysmal stage the cough becomes more severe. The paroxysm is a series of short coughs of increasing severity followed by a large inspiration which produces the characteristic "whoop." Expectoration of tenacious mucus frequently occurs, and vomiting at the end of paroxysm is not unusual. Between paroxysms, which may occur every half-hour, the patient may feel relatively well. During this phase the patient is afebrile unless a secondary bacterial pneumonia or otitis media occurs. Physical examination of the chest usually reveals only scattered rhonchi, but there may be signs, such as periorbital edema and conjunctival petechiae, of the increased venous pressure which occurs during a par-

oxysm. During the convalescent stage the paroxysms gradually become less frequent and less severe and slow recovery ensues.

LABORATORY AND RADIOGRAPHIC FINDINGS

The leukocyte count is typically 15,000 to 30,000 per cubic millimeter, but counts may reach 100,000 cells per cubic millimeter. As many as 80 percent of the cells are mature lymphocytes. A high fraction of polymorphonuclear leukocytes suggests a secondary bacterial infection. Mucus for bacteriologic identification of *B. pertussis* is obtained from the nasopharynx by a swab passed through the nares. The material is plated directly on Bordet-Gengou medium, which must be incubated for at least 72 h. Nasopharyngeal mucus may also be smeared on glass slides, fixed, and stained with *B. pertussis*-specific, fluorescein-conjugated antiserum and examined under fluorescent microscopy for the presence of organisms.

The chest radiograph is usually normal. Occasionally there are moderate interstitial infiltrates or hilar adenopathy.

TREATMENT AND PROGNOSIS

Antimicrobial drugs are ineffective in altering the course of pertussis after the paroxysmal stage of illness has developed but may be effective in prophylaxis of exposed susceptible individuals or in aborting the disease if given in the catarrhal stage. Further, even in the paroxysmal stage, antimicrobial drugs decrease the time that the organisms may be recovered from the nasopharynx and thus probably decrease the infectiousness of the patient for other persons. Erythromycin is the drug of choice; oxytetracycline and chloramphenicol are also effective. The dose of each is 50 mg/kg of patient weight per day in four divided doses. Duration of treatment is 7 to 10 days.

Hyperimmune human γ-globulin has also been recommended in the dose of 1.25 to 2.5 ml intramuscularly for three successive days. However, such therapy has not been demonstrated to alter the course of disease when given in the paroxysmal stage and does not decrease the time of recovery of the organisms from the nasopharynx.

The mortality rate from pertussis is low. Deaths usually occur in patients under 1 year of age and are usually related to secondary bacterial infections.

Tularemia

Tularemia is a systemic infectious disease which may cause pneumonia or pleural effusion as one of its manifestations. It is transmitted to humans by handling or eating infected rabbits or other rodents; by bites of infected arthropods such as ticks or deer flies; or by inhalation of organisms, especially in bacteriology laboratories. *Francisella tularensis*, the causative organism, is a gram-nega-

tive, nonmotile, pleomorphic coccobacillus that grows readily on specialized culture media such as blood-glucose-cysteine agar.

PATHOLOGY

In fatal cases with pneumonia the lung is covered by a fibrinopurulent exudate, and there may be a pleural effusion. The cut lung has gray-white nodules which may coalesce into lobar consolidation. The areas of consolidation may break down into abscesses filled with caseous material. Regional lymph nodes are usually enlarged and may have similar abscesses.

Microscopically there are areas of necrosis with pale outlines of the alveolar structure remaining. Surrounding the necrotic areas the major cellular response is of mononuclear cells and lymphocytes. The outer zone of involvement contains alveoli filled with fibrinous exudate with fewer mononuclear cells and some polymorphonuclear leukocytes. Many arteries demonstrate endarteritis, and thrombosis may occur in the areas of necrosis.

CLINICAL MANIFESTATIONS

The incubation period is 2 to 10 days. Early symptoms in all forms of tularemia include headache and fever. The onset may be fulminant, or it may be less striking, and the patient may have been ill for several days or even weeks before seeking medical attention.

Patients with tularemia may present with one of several distinctive syndromes. In ulceroglandular tularemia a reddish papule that may ultimately ulcerate occurs on the skin at the portal of entry of the organisms. Regional lymph nodes are enlarged and tender, and after several days these nodes may become fluctuant and may drain. Generalized lymphadenopathy also occurs. Systemic symptoms may be mild or severe. Glandular tularemia is a similar syndrome without a specific skin lesion to indicate the portal of entry. In oculoglandular tularemia the patient experiences ocular pain, photophobia, itching, lacrimation, and mucopurulent discharge. Small granulomatous lesions which may eventually ulcerate occur on the conjunctivas or cornea. Regional lymph nodes become enlarged and may ultimately become fluctuant and drain. In typhoidal tularemia no portal of entry of the organisms may be apparent, or there may be buccal or pharyngeal ulceration. These patients are characteristically extremely ill with high fever, gastrointestinal symptoms, delirium, stupor, or coma. Pneumonia may occur with any of these syndromes or may occur independently of any other symptom complex.

The type of pulmonary disease caused by tularemia is extremely varied and is not sufficiently specific to suggest the diagnosis in the absence of cutaneous or lymphatic findings. Most patients have chills, fever, and systemic signs of toxicity. Cough is frequently severe and nonpro-

ductive early with subsequent production of mucoid or mucopurulent sputum. Mild hemoptysis is common. Pleuritic chest pain may occur. In patients who have been ill for days to weeks before presenting to a physician weight loss is common, and the history is suggestive of pulmonary tuberculosis. Chest findings on physical examination are similarly varied, but findings frequently are minimal relative to radiographic abnormalities.

LABORATORY AND RADIOGRAPHIC FINDINGS

The blood leukocyte count is usually normal or low. Early in the illness *F. tularensis* may be recovered from the local ulcer or from regional lymph nodes in ulceroglandular tularemia. Organisms may also be recovered from the nasopharynx, sputum, or pleural fluid. Recovery from blood cultures is rare. Since tularemia may be acquired by inhalation of the organisms, culture material must be handled with care.

The diagnosis in most recently reported cases has been made by serum agglutination testing. Specific agglutinins appear approximately 8 to 10 days after the onset of illness. Maximal titer levels usually occur in about 4 weeks and remain elevated for a protracted interval. As in most serologic testing, a rising titer is most helpful, but absolute levels of 1:160 or greater are considered diagnostic. Patients with brucellosis may have cross-agglutination.

The radiographic manifestations of tularemia are extremely varied. The most common appearance is a localized bronchopneumonia, but lobar consolidation is also frequent. Hilar adenopathy in association with a parenchymal infiltrate is very common, and hilar or mediastinal adenopathy may occur independently. Apical infiltrates resembling tuberculosis are not uncommon. Abscess cavities may occur with any type of infiltrate but are not common. Some patients have radiographic infiltrates which are oval in shape; these may be single or multiple. Even miliary infiltrates have been reported. Pleural effusions may occur during the course of any of the types of parenchymal infiltrates.

TREATMENT AND PROGNOSIS

Streptomycin is the antimicrobial drug of choice for tularemia. A satisfactory regimen is 0.5 g intramuscularly every 12 h for adults for 10 days. A rapid response to therapy is usual with most patients afebrile in 48 to 72 h. Gentamicin (3.0 mg/kg per day IM) or kanamycin (15 mg/kg per day IM) produce similar results. Tetracycline and chloramphenicol also may cause prompt improvement, but relapses may occur after discontinuation of therapy unless treatment consists of 2.0 g daily for 15 days.

Deaths among patients treated with streptomycin are rare. A trial of such therapy is reasonable for persons with pneumonia who have the appropriate epidemiologic history and have not responded to penicillin, especially in the southern or western United States.

Melioidosis

Melioidosis is an infectious disease of tropical countries which is observed in the United States only in persons with a history of travel to endemic areas. Presently recognized endemic areas include southeast Asia and Madagascar, with sporadic cases reported from Central and South America, the West Indies, Australia, Guam, Korea, the Philippines, and Turkey. The disease is caused by *Pseudomonas pseudomallei,* a gram-negative, motile, bipolar-staining bacillus that grows well on ordinary laboratory media. Because the organism may not be identified correctly unless culture media are specifically processed, the clinician should inform the bacteriologist when this diagnosis is being considered.

PATHOLOGY

Melioidosis may occur as an acute fulminant or as a chronic indolent disease. Occasionally the chronic form may exacerbate into the acute form. In the acute form the lungs typically demonstrate multiple, widespread, slightly raised, yellowish white areas measuring from 1 mm to several centimeters in diameter. Some foci have cavities containing yellow-green material. The pleural spaces may contain serosanguineous fluid and foci of fibrinous pleuritis. Microscopically, the foci in the lungs demonstrate extensive cellular destruction with microabscess formation. Cellular reaction includes polymorphonuclear leukocytes, lymphocytes, and macrophages, and extensive hemorrhage is common. The most striking histologic feature of the lesions is marked karyorrhexis. Similar lesions are observed throughout other viscera, especially the liver, spleen, bone marrow, lymph nodes, adrenals, and kidneys.

In the chronic form of melioidosis, pulmonary findings are usually upper lobe fibrocavitary lesions. The cavities frequently are thin-walled. Histologically there is extensive fibrosis and infiltrates of chronic inflammatory cells. Granuloma formation is not a feature of the disease.

CLINICAL MANIFESTATIONS

It has been reported that 1 to 2 percent of uninjured American troops formerly stationed in Vietnam and up to 7 percent of troops injured in Vietnam have significant agglutinin titers to *P. pseudomallei.* Since clinical disease may occur from months to years after residence in an endemic area, these persons are considered to be at risk for developing melioidosis. Acute or chronic illness may occur after such a latent interval.

The acute, septicemic form of the disease may begin with no recognized precipitating event, but in many pa-

tients there is antecedent surgery, trauma, or intercurrent illness. Symptoms begin abruptly with shaking chills, high fever, and marked prostration. Although some patients have no localizing findings, pulmonary symptoms predominate in most. These include cough, dyspnea, pleuritic chest pain, and hemoptysis. Bacteremia disseminates the organisms widely, and extrapulmonary abscesses may develop, especially in the liver, spleen, bone marrow, lymph nodes, skin, and subcutaneous tissues. If the patient survives the first few days of illness, symptoms relating to the extrapulmonary abscesses become apparent.

The chronic form of illness may occur in survivors of the acute form or may occur without recognized antecedent illness. This phase of the illness may be manifested by chronic visceral or cutaneous abscesses with sinus tracts draining purulent material. However, in this country the most frequently reported form is chronic pulmonary disease. In this type of disease the patient presents with a history of days to weeks of fever, productive cough, and weight loss simulating the history of pulmonary tuberculosis. Pleuritic chest pain occurs in about one-half of the patients and mild hemoptysis in about one-third. Dyspnea is rarely a feature of this form of the disease.

LABORATORY AND RADIOGRAPHIC FINDINGS

The blood leukocyte count is normal or moderately elevated. Neutrophilia tends to occur in the acute but not the chronic cases. Sputum cultures most commonly reveal *P. pseudomallei* when it is specifically sought. Blood cultures are frequently positive in the acute but not in the chronic disease. Serum agglutinins against the organism are not demonstrable in the acute disease but are present at greater than 1:40 titers in most patients with chronic pulmonary melioidosis. Agglutination titers remain elevated for protracted intervals despite successful therapy.

Patients with acute melioidosis may have a normal chest radiograph. In those patients with pulmonary involvement, the radiographic pattern tends to consist of widespread, irregular, nodular densities a few millimeters in diameter which become larger and coalesce with time. Cavitation is common, and pleural effusion is not rare. In chronic disease the radiographic infiltrate is usually nodular, and cavitation occurs in approximately 70 percent. The cavities, which may be multiple, are 2 to 7 cm in diameter; they tend to be thin-walled and have no air-fluid levels. Since these findings are almost always in upper lobes, the radiographic appearance suggests tuberculosis. Pleural effusions are unusual in the chronic form of the disease.

TREATMENT AND PROGNOSIS

Almost all untreated patients with acute melioidosis die, although a few survive with a chronic illness, usually with multiple visceral abscesses. Mortality among antibiotic-treated patients has been reported to be 30 percent. Survival rates among U.S. Army personnel in Vietnam were evidently higher, but acute and chronic cases were not clearly separated. Mortality from chronic pulmonary melioidosis is rare.

P. pseudomallei is usually sensitive in vitro to tetracycline, chloramphenicol, sulfonamides, and the combination of trimethoprim and sulfamethoxazole. The organism is partially resistant to ampicillin, penicillin G, rifampin, nalidixic acid, gentamicin, and tobramycin. It is resistant to cephalothin, lincomycin, vancomycin, streptomycin, colistin, and polymyxin B. Treatment of acute cases with the combination of tetracycline, chloramphenicol, and sulfonamide early and protracted administration of tetracycline and sulfonamide usually is recommended. Treatment of chronic pulmonary melioidosis with tetracycline alone, with tetracycline and chloramphenicol or sulfonamide, and with trimethoprim and sulfamethoxazole has been demonstrated to be satisfactory. Antimicrobial therapy must be continued for weeks to months. If chloramphenicol is used for such protracted intervals, the physician must be alert to the possibility of hematologic or neural toxicity. In patients with residual cavitary lesions at 6 months, resection of the involved lobe may be necessary.

Plague

Plague is an acute infectious disease which may occur as a systemic illness only incidentally causing pneumonia, *bubonic plague,* or as a primary pneumonia resulting from the inhalation of infectious aerosols from patients with pulmonary involvement, *pneumonic plague.* Its natural reservoir is in rats and other rodents from which it occasionally spreads to humans through the bite of rat fleas. The disease is endemic in rodents in several geographic areas including the western United States. The causative organism, *Yersinia pestis,* is a coccoid-to-large ovoid gram-negative bacillus which grows slowly on ordinary laboratory media and which demonstrates bipolar staining causing a "safety pin" appearance.

PATHOLOGY

Regional lymph nodes in the bubonic form demonstrate a hemorrhagic reaction with infiltration of polymorphonuclear leukocytes. The lesion progresses to necrosis and suppuration. A gelatinous edema of surrounding connective tissue occurs. Other organs demonstrate vascular congestion and hemorrhages.

Plague pneumonia secondary to systemic disease begins as perivascular reaction with inflammation and colonies of *Y. pestis.* Later in the course both primary and secondary pneumonia cause lobular or lobar pneumonia with gross hemorrhage and inflammatory cell infiltrates.

Large amounts of bloody, watery mucus are present in which the organisms may be profusely demonstrated.

CLINICAL MANIFESTATIONS

The incubation period of bubonic plague is 1 to 5 days. The onset of illness is abrupt with high fever, malaise, and prostration. In untreated persons fulminant bacteremia ensues in 2 to 6 days resulting in apathy, confusion, and oliguria. An extremely rapidly progressive bilateral pneumonia may occur during this stage, which is typically fatal within 2 days. The diagnosis is suggested by the epidemiologic history and typical bubo. A single lymph chain is usually involved. In most instances it is the inguinal or femoral nodes, but axillary or cervical nodes may be the primary site, especially in women and children. The bubo may be a single enlarged lymph node, or several contiguous nodes may be involved. It is exquisitely tender and the overlying skin is tense and purple. The surrounding skin has a pink cyanotic color.

Pneumonic plague occurs by inhalation of infected respiratory droplets among contacts of patients with pneumonia secondary to bubonic plague. These persons then propagate the disease to their contacts. The attack rate among contacts is very high, especially if environmental humidity is high. The onset of plague pneumonia is even more dramatic than bubonic plague with high fever, tachycardia, tachypnea, and anxiety. During the first few hours pulmonary symptoms may be absent, or the patient may complain of pleuritic or substernal chest pain. An early nonproductive cough is followed by production of larger and larger amounts of bloody, thin sputum. The entire course of pneumonic plague from onset to death is usually less than 48 h.

LABORATORY AND RADIOGRAPHIC FINDINGS

Blood leukocytes are usually increased to 12,000 to 15,000 cells per cubic millimeter with a predominance of polymorphonuclear leukocytes. *Y. pestis* may usually be cultured from aspirates of the bubo, sputum, and blood; however, the incubation period on media of 48 to 96 h is too long to withhold treatment in suspected cases.

The radiographic appearance of the chest is characterized only by rapidly advancing infiltrates. There is a nonsegmental alveolar density which may progress to the appearance of diffuse, bilateral pulmonary edema.

TREATMENT AND PROGNOSIS

Antimicrobial therapy must be begun in suspected cases based on epidemiologic and clinical grounds. A delay of only a few hours may result in a fatal outcome. When antimicrobial therapy is not begun in the first 12 to 18 h after the onset of fever in patients with plague pneumonia, the mortality approaches 100 percent. Conversely, treatment during the bubo stage results in a mortality of less than 5 percent.

Streptomycin in combination with tetracycline or chloramphenicol is recommended. Streptomycin 2 to 4 g in divided doses is administered for the first 3 days followed by 1 to 2 g daily for an additional 7 days. Tetracycline or chloramphenicol in doses of 6 g daily for the first 2 days followed by 50 mg/kg per day in divided doses for an additional week has been recommended. At the outset the drug is administered intravenously and subsequently by mouth.

Patients with plague pneumonia should have strict respiratory isolation. Contacts, including all medical personnel, should be treated with 0.5 g tetracycline every 6 h for at least 5 days.

PLEUROPULMONARY INVOLVEMENT OF SYSTEMIC INFECTIOUS AGENTS

Salmonella

Occasional cases of pneumonia or empyema due to *Salmonella* are reported. The clinical signs and symptoms are quite varied. On the average, a subacute disease of several days' duration is reported. The most common symptoms are chills, fever, anorexia, weight loss, and abdominal pain. Diarrhea is inconstant. Abnormal physical findings usually are limited to the thorax. Segmental or lobar pneumonia with abscess formation is the most common manifestation with no apparent predilection for a particular segment. Empyema is not uncommon.

The diagnosis is made by culture of *Salmonella* from sputum or pleural fluid, or it may be suggested by recovery of the organism from feces or urine. Blood cultures are not likely to yield the organism. Blood agglutinins may be helpful if an absolute titer of 1:160 or a fourfold rise in titer is observed, but only a few *Salmonella* species are included in most laboratories' antisera. The treatment of choice is chloramphenicol 50 mg/kg per day in four divided doses. Several weeks of therapy may be necessary.

Brucellosis

Undulant fever, a disease due to *Brucella abortus, B. melitensis,* or *B. suis* and transmitted to humans through contact with infected livestock or ingestion of their products, may be associated with respiratory symptoms. Most commonly the disease has an insidious onset with low-grade fever, headache, weakness, arthralgias, low back pain, and sweats. Occasionally the onset is abrupt with fever, chills, and prostration. With either onset, up to 15 percent of the patients develop a protracted cough and physical findings of wheezes and rhonchi. Occasional patients may demonstrate hilar adenopathy and perihilar infiltrates radiographically. These changes may persist for protracted in-

tervals. Even more unusual is the occurrence of pleural effusions.

The diagnosis is suggested by the epidemiologic history; approximately one-half of the patients have lymphadenopathy, and one-third have hepatomegaly or splenomegaly. In the acute type of disease, blood cultures may be positive, and the organisms occasionally are recovered from sputum or pleural fluid. Agglutinating antibodies in titers of 1:80 or greater are present in most patients with chronic disease.

Tetracycline, 2 g daily in four divided doses for 3 weeks is usually successful therapy. In acutely ill patients, streptomycin, 1 g daily intramuscularly, may be given in addition for the first few days of therapy. Some patients suffer a subsequent relapse requiring retreatment.

Glanders

Glanders is an infectious disease of horses, mules, and donkeys caused by *Actinobacillus mallei*. It has been eliminated in the United States by destruction of infected animals. It may occur as a fulminant febrile disease or as a chronic, relapsing disease. Its features include nasal cellulitis with destructive ulcers and cutaneous cellulitis with ulceration and lymphadenopathy. Pulmonary involvement with necrotizing pneumonia and empyema is common.

The diagnosis is made by cultural isolation of *A. mallei* from involved tissues. Little definitive evidence is available about the response to therapy. The combination of streptomycin and tetracycline is recommended.

BIBLIOGRAPHY

Bartlett JG, O'Keefe P, Tally FP, Louie TJ, Gorbach SL: Bacteriology of hospital-acquired pneumonia. Arch Intern Med 146:868–871, 1986.
  Nosocomial pneumonia was judged directly responsible for lethal outcome of 19% of patients and a contributing factor to death in another 13%.

Bass JW, Klenk EL, Kotheimer JB, Linnemann CC, Smith MHD: Antimicrobial treatment of pertussis. J Pediatr 75:768–781, 1969.
  This study establishes that erythromycin is the most effective antimicrobial treatment of pertussis.

Berger R, Arango L: Etiologic diagnosis of bacterial nosocomial pneumonia in seriously ill patients. Crit Care Med 13:833–836, 1985.
  This study emphasizes the difficulty in making a precise diagnosis of the microbiologic cause of nosocomial pneumonia.

Campbell GD, Woods DE: The diagnosis of gram-negative bacillary pneumonia in an animal model using a competitive ELISA technique to detect the presence of lipid A. Am Rev Respir Dis 133:861–865, 1986.
  Using an ELISA procedure for quantitation of lipid A in pulmonary lavage fluid the presence or absence of pneumonia caused by gram-negative bacilli organisms could be demonstrated in laboratory animals.

Conrad FG, LeCocq FR, Krain R: A recent epidemic of plague in Vietnam. Arch Intern Med 122:193–198, 1968.
  This excellent review of the epidemiologic and clinical manifestations of plague includes both the primary and secondary pneumonia forms.

Driks MR, Craven DE, Celli BR, Manning M, Burke RA, Garvin GM, Kunches LM, Farber HW, Wedel SA, McCabe WR: Nosocomial pneumonia in intubated patients given sucralfate as compared with antacids or histamine type 2 blockers. The role of gastric colonization. N Engl J Med 317:1376–1382, 1987.
  The authors studied the rate of nosocomial pneumonia among 130 patients given mechanical ventilation in an intensive care unit who were receiving as prophylaxis for stress ulcer either sucralfate (n = 61), which does not raise gastric pH, or conventional treatment with antacids, histamine type 2 (H2) blockers, or both (n = 69). They conclude that in patients receiving mechanical ventilation, the use of a prophylactic agent against stress-ulcer bleeding that preserves the natural gastric acid barrier against bacterial overgrowth may be preferable to antacids and H2 blockers.

Everett ED, Nelson RA: Pulmonary melioidosis. Am Rev Respir Dis 112:331–340, 1975.
  This series of 39 cases of pulmonary melioidosis describes the clinical course of the most common form of this infection seen in the United States.

Gardner WG: Multicentered clinical evaluation of cefoperazone for the treatment of lower respiratory tract infections. Rev Infect Dis 5 (Suppl):S137, 1983.
  This study summarizes the use of a single third-generation cephalosporin, cefoperazone, in the treatment of lower respiratory tract infection.

Garibaldi RA: Epidemiology of community-acquired respiratory tract infections in adults. Am J Med 78 (Suppl 6B):32–37, 1985.
  This review emphasizes the spectrum of bacterial agents causing community-acquired pneumonia.

Karnad A, Alvarez S, Berk SL: Pneumonia caused by gram-negative bacilli. Am J Med 79 (Suppl 1A):61–67, 1985.
  These authors emphasize that the clinical signs of gram-negative bacillary pneumonia are frequently subtle in elderly, debilitated patients.

Lerner AM: The gram-negative bacillary pneumonias. Dis Month 27:1–56, 1981.
  This extensive review of gram-negative bacillary pneumonia reports the experience of one of the major contributors to an understanding of these infections.

Levin DC, Schwarz MI, Matthay RA, LaForce FM: Bacteremic Hemophilus influenzae pneumonia in adults. A report of 24 cases and a review of the literature. Am J Med 62:219–224, 1977.
  This report of 24 cases of pneumonia in adults due to H. influenzae was the first of several recent series indicating an increasing prevalence of this infection. Since the culture techniques in the hospitals in which these patients were treated had not changed in over 10 years, the authors' data indicate a true increase in the incidence of this infection.

Miller RP, Bates JH: Pleuropulmonary tularemia. A review of 29 patients. Am Rev Respir Dis 99:31–41, 1969.
  Based on their personal experience with 29 patients with tularemia pneumonia, these authors emphasize the variable clinical presentation of patients with this infection.

Musher DM, Kubitschek KR, Crennan J, Baughn RE: Pneumonia and acute febrile tracheobronchitis due to Haemophilus influenzae. Ann Intern Med 99:444–450, 1983.
  These investigators report an increasing prevalence of pneumonia due to nontypable H. influenzae relative to typable strains.

Pennington JE: Gram-negative bacterial pneumonia in the immuno-compromised host. Semin Respir Infect 1:145–150, 1986.
  A review of mechanisms involved and their implications for prevention and treatment.

Pfischner WCE Jr, Ishak KG, Neptune EM Jr, Fox SM III, Farid Z, Norel Din G: Brucellosis in Egypt. A review of experience with 228 patients. Am J Med 22:915–919, 1957.
  Reports the signs, symptoms, and clinical course of 228 patients with brucellosis and clearly defines the predominance of musculoskeletal symptoms relative to pulmonary symptoms.

Pierce AK, Sanford JP: Aerobic gram-negative bacillary pneumonias. Am Rev Respir Dis 110:647–658, 1974.
  Reviews not only the clinical manifestations of pneumonia due to gram-negative bacilli but also data relative to colonization of the oropharynx which predisposes patients to these pathogens.

Reed WP: Indolent pulmonary abscess associated with Klebsiella and Enterobacter. Am Rev Respir Dis 107:1055–1059, 1973.
  A report of three well documented cases of indolent pulmonary abscesses associated with Klebsiella or Enterobacter emphasizing the suggestive clinical features of this infection.

Salata RA, Gebhart RL, Palmer DL, Wade BH, Scheld WM, Groschel DHM, Wenzel RP, Mandell GL, Duma RJ: Pneumonia treated with imipenem/cilastatin. Am J Med 78 (Suppl 6A):104–109, 1085.
  This study reports the use of single agent therapy with imipenem in patients with nosocomial and community-acquired infections. This monotherapy was successful except in the case of disease associated with Pseudomonas aeruginosa.

Salata RA, Lederman MM, Shlaes DM, Jacobs MR, Eckstein E, Tweardy D, Toossi Z, Chmielewski R, Marino J, King CH et al: Diagnosis of nosocomial pneumonia in intubated intensive care unit patients. Am Rev Respir Dis 135:426–432, 1987.
  The authors studied 51 intubated, intensive care unit patients prospectively by serial examinations of tracheal aspirates for elastin fibers, graded Gram stains, and quantitative bacterial cultures in conjunction with clinical and radiologic observations. Patients with infection, as distinct from colonization, had new or progressive pulmonary infiltrates plus 1 of the following: positive blood culture results, radiographic evidence of cavitation, or histologic evidence of pneumonia, or 2 or more of the following: new fever, new leukocytosis, or grossly purulent tracheal aspirates. Infected patients had a longer duration of intubation, higher Gram stain grading for neutrophils or bacteria, higher bacterial colony counts, and more frequent detection of elastin fibers in tracheal aspirates.

Sanford JP: Tularemia. JAMA 250:3225–3226, 1983.
   This succinct paper outlines the clinical presentations of tularemia and the presently accepted antimicrobial regimens used in its treatment.

Stoutenbeek CP, van Saene HK, Miranda DR, Zandstra DF, Langrehr D: Nosocomial gram-negative pneumonia in critically ill patients. A 3-year experience with a novel therapeutic regimen. Intensive Care Med 12:419–423, 1986.
   The authors investigated the efficacy of selective decontamination of the oral cavity and GI-tract in the treatment of established gram-negative pneumonia in critically ill, mechanically ventilated patients with pneumonia caused by Enterobacteriaceae or Pseudomonadaceae. Eradication of pathogens from the respiratory tract was achieved in 24 of the 25 patients within 9 days (median 5 days); the cure rate was 96%.

Trenholme GM, Pollage JC, Karakusis PH: Use of ceftazadime in the treatment of nosocomial lower respiratory tract infections. Am J Med 79 (Suppl 2A):32, 1985.
   This study reports the use of a third-generation cephalosporin, ceftazadime, as monotherapy for nosocomial pneumonia.

Weiss W, Eisenberg GM, Flippin HF: *Salmonella* pleuropulmonary disease. Am J Med Sci 233:487–496, 1957.
   These authors report the signs and symptoms of Salmonella pleuropulmonary disease.

Yangco BG, Palumbo JA, Nolen T, Lifland PW, Schleupner CJ: Comparative multicentre evaluation of the safety and efficacy of ceftazidime versus cefamandole for pneumonia. J Antimicrob Chemother 18:521–529, 1986.
   Ceftazidime and cefamandole were compared in a randomized multicenter trial in hospitalized patients with pneumonia.

Chapter 93

Anaerobic Infections of Lungs and Pleura

Sydney M. Finegold

Predisposing Conditions

Pathogenesis and Pathology

Clinical Expressions

Bacteriology

Diagnosis

Therapy

Prevention

Although anaerobic infections of the lung and pleural space are relatively common, they are frequently overlooked. In lung abscess and in infection following aspiration pneumonia, anaerobes are recoverable from more than 90 percent of patients. Moreover, in these disorders, one-half to two-thirds of the cultures yield only anaerobic bacteria. Empyema that is not related to previous surgery involves anaerobes 75 percent of the time; in about one-half of these patients, only anaerobes are isolated. Because of difficulties inherent in obtaining proper specimens for diagnosis of anaerobic pulmonary infection, the presence of this type of infection is often not proved even though it is suspected.

In the years before antimicrobial agents were introduced, autopsies and surgical specimens provided important information about the natural history of untreated anaerobic infections of the lungs and pleural space. Soon after the introduction of antimicrobial agents, the literature about proved anaerobic pleuropulmonary infections became relatively sparse. Indeed, the literature of that period conveyed the impression that aspiration pneumonia, necrotizing pneumonia, lung abscess, and empyema were being caused by various aerobic and facultative bacteria rather than by anaerobes. However, this misconception was dispelled by the introduction of percutaneous transtracheal aspiration to bypass normal oropharyngeal flora and by the use of improved techniques to transport specimens to the laboratory under anaerobic conditions.

One other factor accounting for difficulty in diagnosis of anaerobic pleuropulmonary infection in the antimicrobial era should be noted. Before antimicrobial drugs were available, infections of the pharynx and tonsils caused by *Fusobacterium necrophorum* were relatively common and were often complicated by septic thrombophlebitis, bacteremia, and metastatic infection, the last frequently involving the lung and pleural space. This type of infection is seldom encountered today, probably because of widespread use of antibiotics in the treatment of upper respiratory tract infection. Moreover, bacteremia in the course of anaerobic pleuropulmonary infection is now quite uncommon.

PREDISPOSING CONDITIONS

By far the most important underlying mechanism for anaerobic infection of the lung or pleural space is aspiration, usually related to altered consciousness. Common etiologies of altered consciousness in patients who develop anaerobic pleuropulmonary infection are alcoholism, cerebrovascular accident, general anesthesia, drug overdose or addiction, and seizure disorder. Other factors leading to aspiration include dysphagia, due either to esophageal or neurologic disease, intestinal obstruction, and tonsillectomy or tooth extraction.

The second most important factor predisposing to anaerobic pulmonary infection is periodontal disease or gingivitis. Other underlying processes include bronchogenic carcinoma, bronchiectasis, pulmonary embolism with infarction, subphrenic abscess or other intra-abdominal infection, and metastatic infection in the course of bacteremia. Alcoholism, in addition to being responsible for aspiration, may contribute to anaerobic pleuropulmonary infection by interfering with host defense mechanisms in the lung. The compromised host is susceptible to anaerobic infection as well as to many other types of infection. For example, several cases of anaerobic pulmonary infection have been reported in patients who have undergone cardiac transplantation.

PATHOGENESIS AND PATHOLOGY

The most common site of anaerobic pulmonary infection is the posterior segment of the right upper lobe (Fig. 93-1); the same segment on the left is less commonly affected. Next in frequency of involvement are the apical segments of the lower lobes. These segments are dependent, and the distribution relates to the important role of aspiration or inhalation in the pathogenesis of this disorder. Normally, inhaled material is dealt with by ciliary action, cough, and alveolar macrophages. If the protective mechanisms are ineffective, infection may result. Thick or particulate matter and foreign bodies are not easily removed and may lead to bronchial obstruction and atelectasis. In aspiration pneumonia, gastric acid and enzymes may be primary injurious agents.

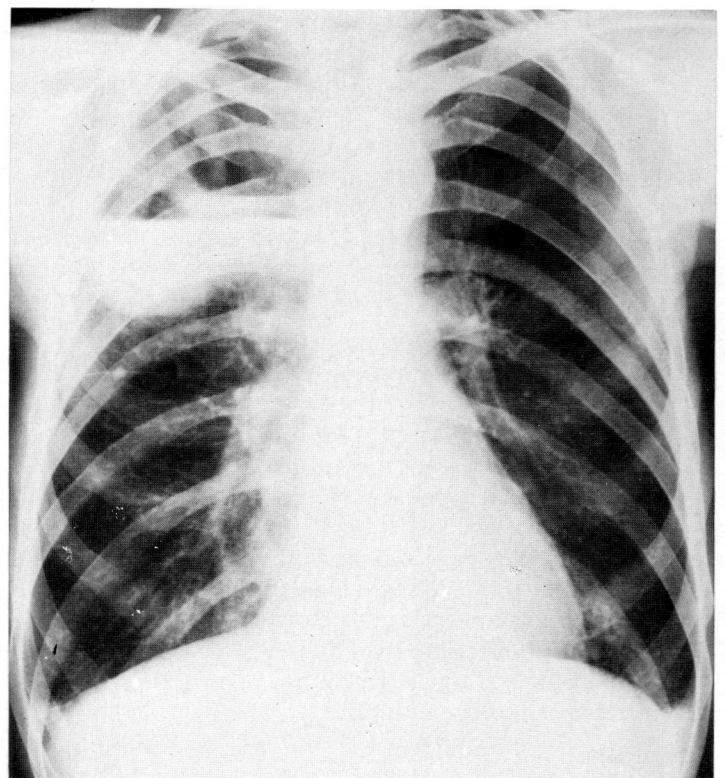
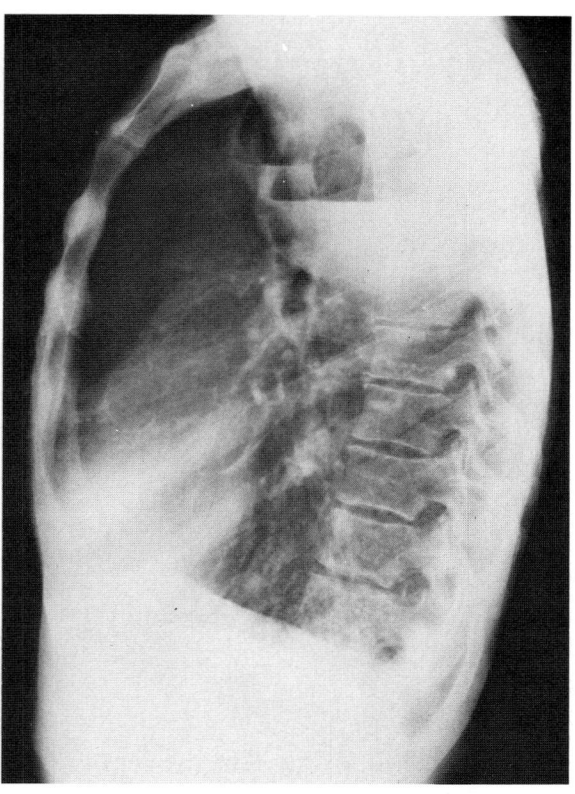

A   B

FIGURE 93-1   Anaerobic pneumonia with abscess formation in a 48-year-old alcoholic man. The abscesses are located in the posterior segment of right upper lobe, a dependent segment.

Subdiaphragmatic infection may extend to the lung or pleural space by way of lymphatics, directly through the diaphragm or defects in it, or by way of the bloodstream. Infection may arise in or behind an obstructing neoplasm. Although the virulence of the infecting organism(s) may contribute to the nature and extent of the infective process, this factor is usually unimportant in anaerobic infections, with the possible exception of *F. necrophorum*. However, the number of the organisms that are aspirated may be an important factor.

In the early stages of infection, the pathology is essentially that of an ordinary pneumonia. Later, necrosis supervenes upon the inflammation, and cavitation or abscess formation takes place. Subsequently, the abscess cavity may become partially lined with regenerated epithelium, and local bronchiectasis and emphysema may develop.

CLINICAL EXPRESSIONS

The classic patient with *bronchiectasis*, which is now uncommon, produced copious amounts of foul-smelling sputum, which layered; mixed anaerobic infection was characteristic even though the anaerobes were often only secondary invaders.

Septic pulmonary emboli (Fig. 93-2), secondary to septic thrombophlebitis associated with anaerobic infection elsewhere in the body, was not uncommon prior to the advent of antimicrobial therapy. Most often, the primary lesions were tonsillar or pharyngeal infections and pelvic infections. This type of process is now uncommon. Septic emboli, as well as secondary infection of bland pulmonary infarcts, can lead to *lung abscess*, often multiple. This type of secondary lung abscess is discussed in Chapter 110.

Most often, the parenchymal involvement in anaerobic pulmonary infection begins as a pneumonia without excavation, as a lung abscess (Fig. 93-1) (arbitrarily defined as a cavity 2 cm or greater in diameter), or as a *necrotizing pneumonia* (multiple excavations less than 2 cm in diameter) (Fig. 93-3). Essentially, these lesions are different stages, or expressions, of the same fundamental process that follows aspiration. Therefore, early in the course of illness, pneumonia is apt to be present without excavation or abscess formation; pneumonia may progress to either of the other entities, particularly if appropriate therapy is delayed. These may eventuate in extensive destruction of lung—*pulmonary gangrene* (Fig. 93-4). Any of these three basic presentations may be complicated by pleural *empyema* (Fig. 93-5).

The designation *aspiration pneumonia* refers to three

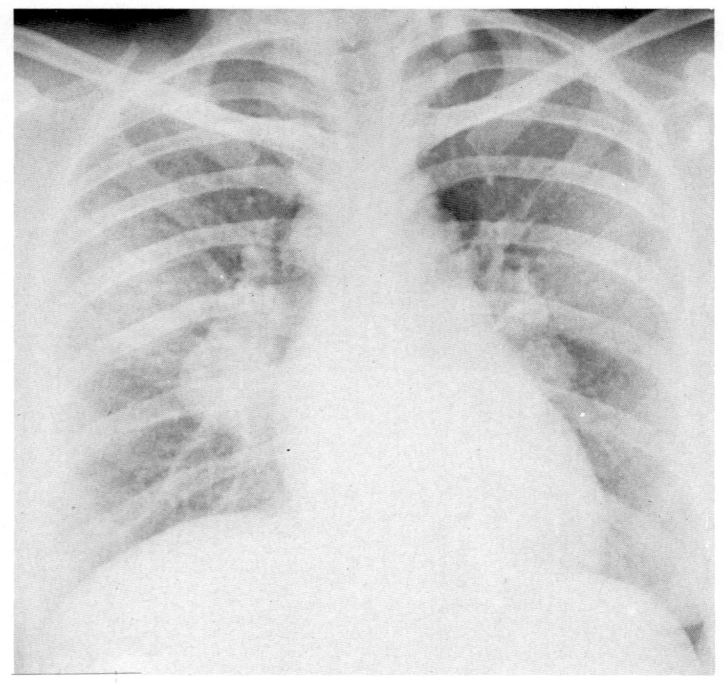

A

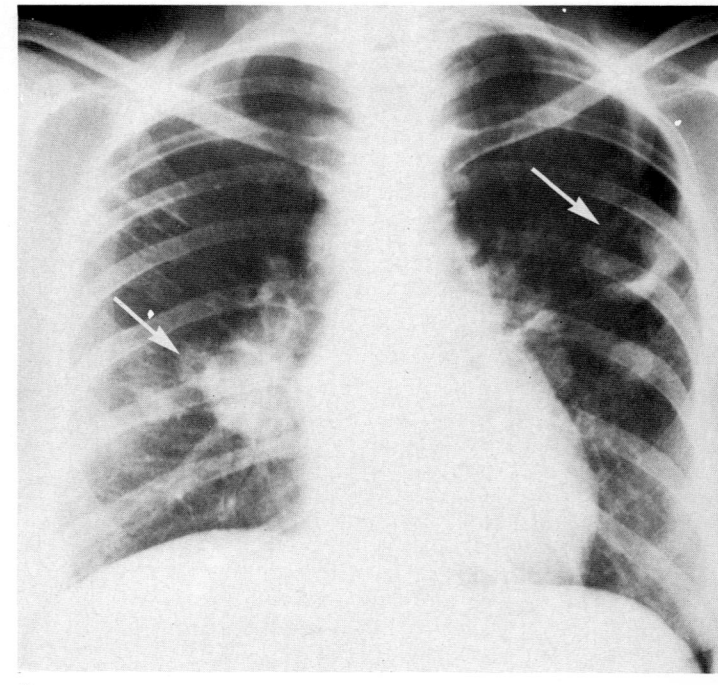

B

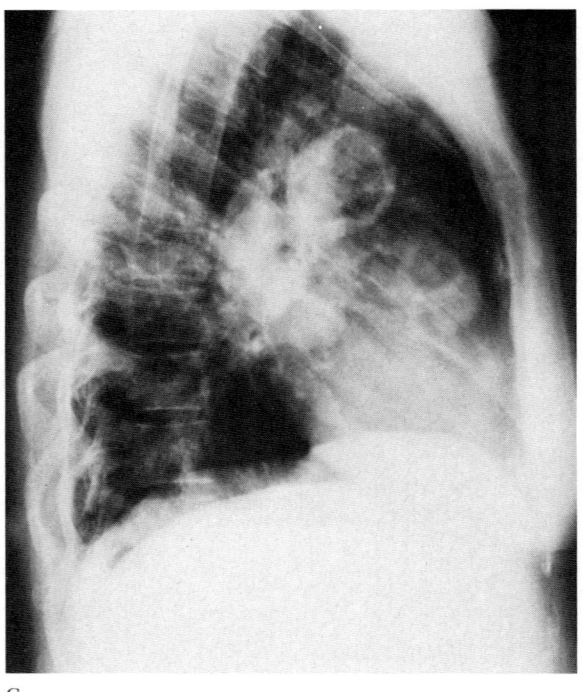

C

FIGURE 93-2 Septic emboli in a patient with asymptomatic sarcoidosis and history of pyelonephritis. Thirty-three-year-old woman admitted for headache, fever, and backache after spontaneous abortion. *Pseudomonas* grown from sputum culture. *A.* Chest radiograph before onset of present illness. Bilateral hilar adenopathy of Boeck's sarcoid. *B.* Posteroanterior view of chest shows bilateral cavitary lesions (arrows). *C.* Lateral view. The lesions are more dramatically seen.

different types of processes. The first is the aspiration of particulate matter of sufficient size and volume to plug bronchi and/or to cause asphyxiation; the second type, *Mendelson's syndrome*, is a chemical pneumonia related to gastric acidity and perhaps enzymes. Infection may complicate either of the above events but often does not. For example, bacterial pneumonia developed in only 8 of Mendelson's original 66 patients. The third type does not

involve either mechanical obstruction or chemical pneumonia and also may or may not be followed by infection subsequent to the aspiration.

Anaerobic pneumonia without necrosis or abscess formation is by far the most easily overlooked of all anaerobic pleuropulmonary infections because three very important clues to anaerobic infection are generally absent, i.e., foul-smelling discharge, tissue necrosis, and subacute

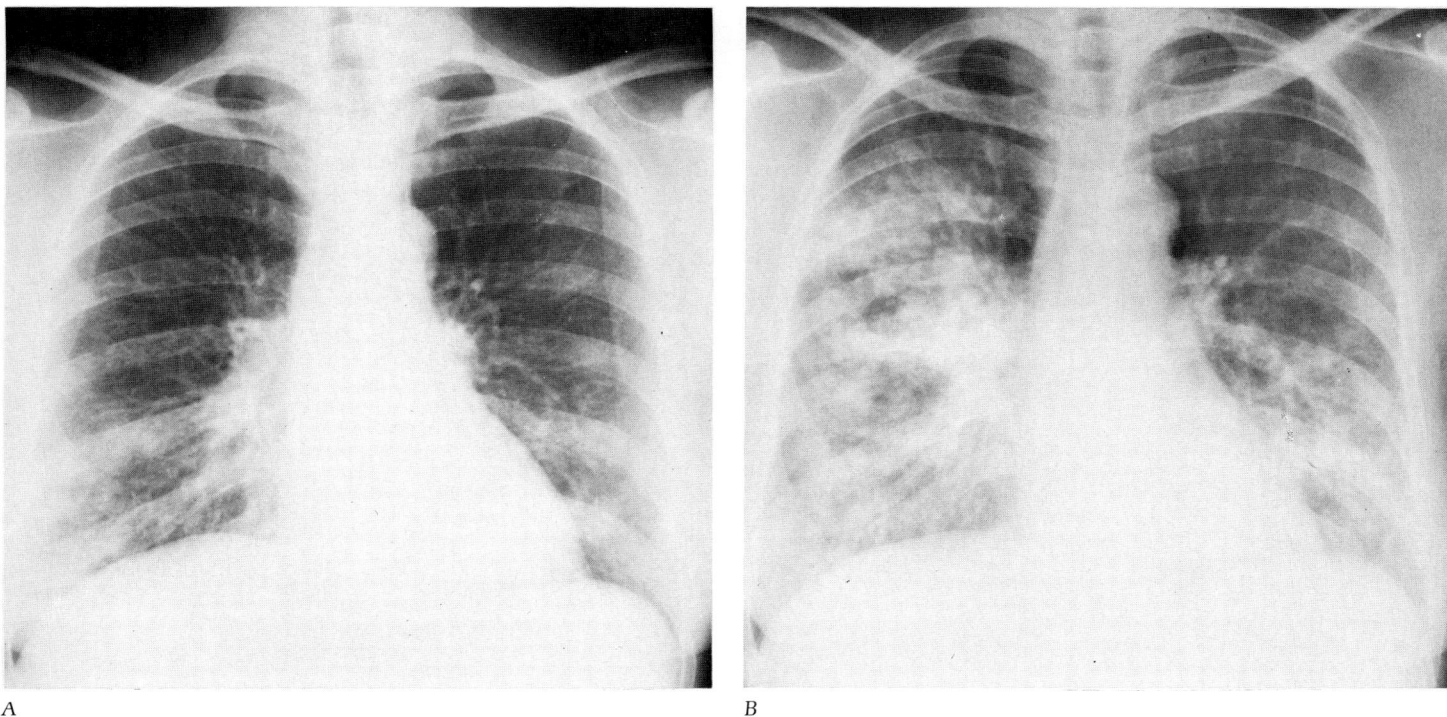

FIGURE 93-3 Fulminating anaerobic pneumonia in a 44-year-old woman with onset of pneumonia 6 days prior to admission. *A.* Day of admission. Patchy consolidation in right lower lung field and behind the cardiac silhouette. *B.* Next day (2 days before death). Extensive patchy alveolar infiltrates bilaterally with areas of rarefaction on right suggestive of cavitation.

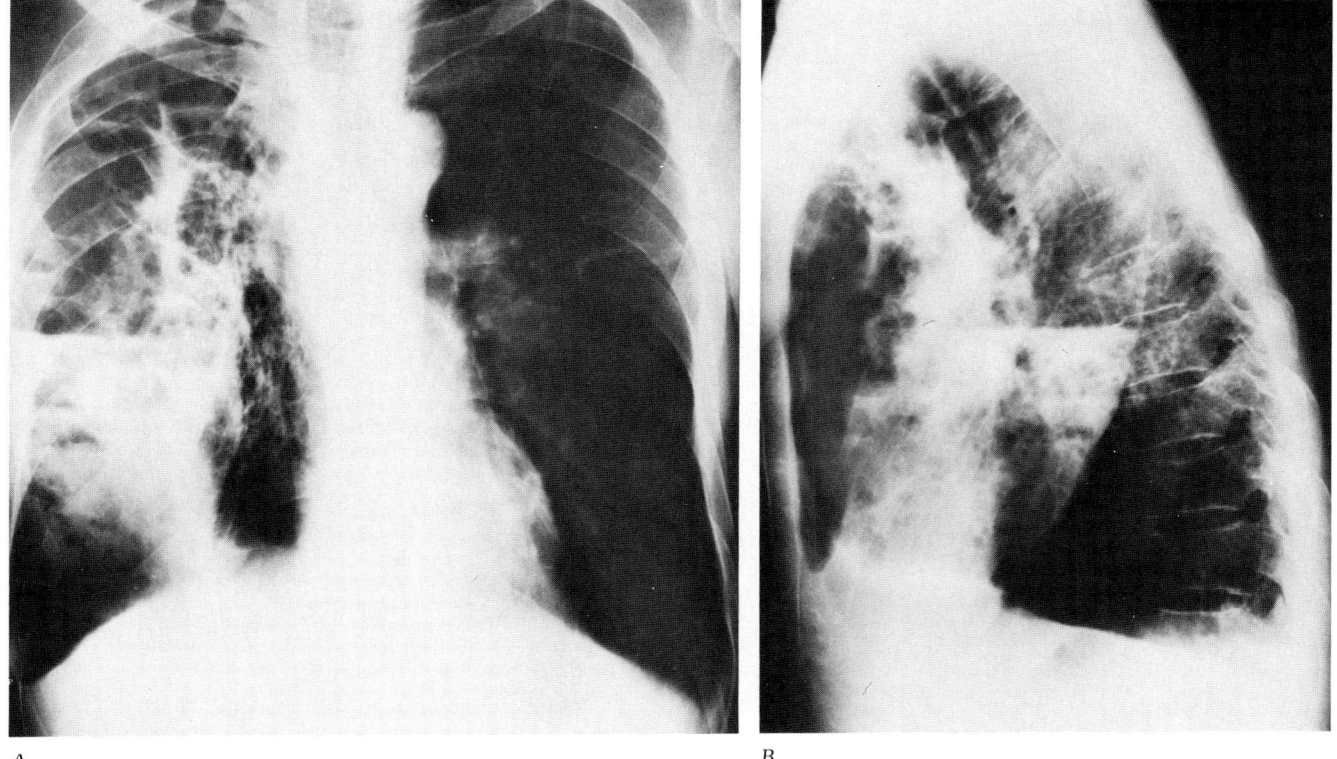

FIGURE 93-4 Gangrene of the lung after aspiration, anteroposterior *(A)* and lateral *(B)* views. The extensive cavitation is the result of a rapidly spreading necrotizing pneumonia in a 65-year-old man. Vascular thrombosis in an area of consolidated lung presumably caused necrosis and sloughing of devitalized parenchyma, leading to an extreme form of anaerobic lung abscess.

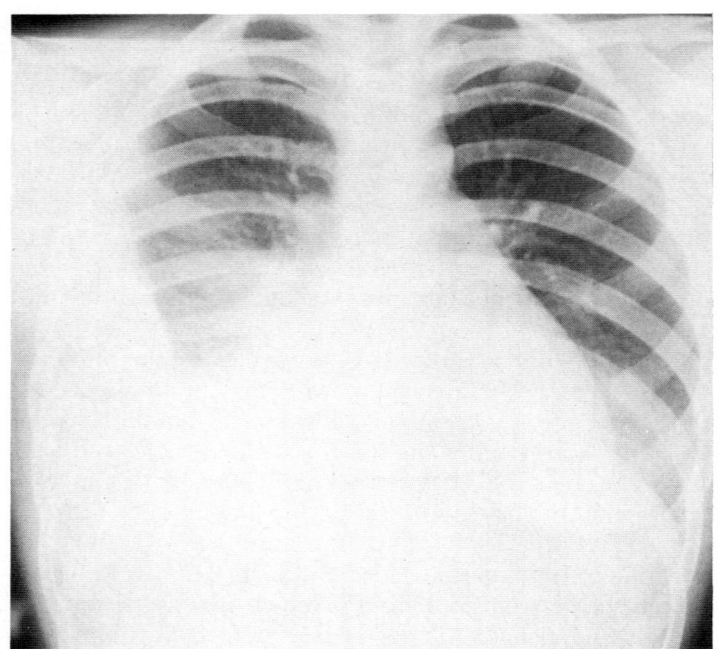

FIGURE 93-5 Large putrid empyema accompanying a right middle lobe pneumonia.

Virtually all cases of anaerobic empyema have associated parenchymal disease. Aspiration, again, is the predominant predisposing mechanism, but in some patients anaerobic empyema results from the spread of subphrenic or other infradiaphragmatic infection. Patients with empyema have usually been sick for at least a week and often for several weeks before they come to the physician. More than one-half of them have experienced loss of weight and have a relatively high fever and leukocytosis. In virtually all patients, the empyema fluid is purulent or becomes purulent; it is often loculated. The prognosis varies with the extent and severity of the underlying parenchymal process, but it is generally good when appropriate management is instituted without undue delay.

Anaerobic bacteria may also be involved in secondary infection of lung cysts, cavities, or tumors. In the last case, the infection may be within the tumor tissue itself or distal to an obstructing carcinoma. Although anaerobic infection sometimes follows thoracotomy or a penetrating wound of the chest, this sequence is quite uncommon.

Anaerobic pulmonary and pleural processes rarely extend to the chest wall unless associated with actinomycosis, tuberculosis, or tumor.

BACTERIOLOGY

The role of *Actinomyces, Arachnia,* and spirochetes in pleuropulmonary infection is discussed in Chapter 99 in this book.

The bacteriology of *aspiration pneumonia* is noted in Tables 93-1 and 93-2. The bacteriology depends on where the patient happens to be at the time of aspiration. Those who aspirate while in the community are likely to have only anaerobes recovered on culture, whereas those who aspirate while in the hospital often have mixtures of anaerobes and aerobes or facultatives, or of the latter groups alone. The aerobes or facultatives recovered in the hospitalized patient include many potential pathogens from the hospital environment, such as *Staphylococcus aureus, Klebsiella, Enterobacter* and other Enterobacteriaceae, and *Pseudomonas.* This reflects colonization of the upper

or indolent course. The major clue to the presence of anaerobic infection is a history of antecedent aspiration or suspected aspiration. Unless a complicating empyema is present, percutaneous transtracheal aspiration is generally required if suitable material is to be obtained for culture. Accordingly, many instances of aspiration pneumonia are overlooked, particularly when aspiration is unsuspected.

Anaerobic pneumonia is usually characterized by an acute course and a rapid response to proper therapy. In this respect, it differs from other types of anaerobic pulmonary infection in which chronic manifestations are the rule. Occasionally, anaerobic pneumonia persists for months without evidence of tissue necrosis. The prognosis in anaerobic pneumonia is good unless the aspiration pneumonia is a complication of a severe underlying condition.

TABLE 93-1
Bacteriology of Aspiration Pneumonia in 70 Patients—Overall Data

Bacteriologic Results	Hospital-Acquired	Community-Acquired	Percent of Total Cases
Only anaerobes recovered	7	25	46
Anaerobes and aerobes or facultatives recovered concurrently	19	10	41
Only aerobes or facultatives recovered	6	3	13
Total cases	32	38	

SOURCE: Based on data in Bartlett, Gorbach, Finegold, 1974.

TABLE 93-2
Bacteriology of Aspiration Pneumonia in 70 Patients—Specific Data

Bacteriologic Results	No. of Patients
Anaerobic isolates	
Bacteroides melaninogenicus group	27(1)*
B. fragilis group	10
Other *Bacteroides* (*B. oralis*, *B. corrodens* or *B. gracilis*, *B. pneumosintes*)	12
Fusobacterium nucleatum	19
F. necrophorum	1
Unidentified anaerobic gram-negative rods	4(1)
Peptostreptococcus	34(6)
Microaerophilic streptococcus	9(1)
Veillonella	4
Gram-positive non-spore-forming rods (*Eubacterium*, *Propionibacterium*, *Bifidobacterium*)	14
Clostridium	2
Aerobic and facultative isolates	
Staphylococcus aureus	11(2)
Streptococcus pneumoniae	11(2)
Other streptococci	5
Enterobacteriaceae	19(2)
Pseudomonas (*P. aeruginosa* and *P. maltophilia*)	8

*Parentheses indicate number of organisms recovered in pure culture.

SOURCE: Based on data in Bartlett, Gorbach, Finegold, 1974.

respiratory tract with these potential pathogens from the hospital setting and must be taken into account in devising therapeutic regimens. The bacteriology of aspiration pneumonia (Table 93-2) is typical of the bacteriology of anaerobic pleuropulmonary infections in general. The most frequent isolates are the *Bacteroides melaninogenicus* group, *Fusobacterium nucleatum*, *Peptostreptococcus*, and microaerophilic streptococci (Figs. 93-6 and 93-7). In early studies, the *B. fragilis* group was isolated from 15 to 20 percent of patients with anaerobic pleuropulmonary infections. However, later studies employing newer techniques and utilizing newer taxonomic criteria found *B. fragilis* group isolates in only 5.2 percent of 135 patients with anaerobic pleuropulmonary infection (based on percutaneous transtracheal aspirates and pleural empyema specimens). In this same study, 31 percent of appropriate specimens from patients with anaerobic pleuropulmonary infection yielded less commonly encountered gram-negative bacilli such as *B. oris*, *B. buccae*, *B. ureolyticus* (most of which were subsequently reidentified as *B. gracilis*), *B. bivius*, *B. disiens*, *F. gonidiaformans*, and *F. naviforme*. The *B. fragilis* group is important because of its resistance to penicillin G and sometimes other antimicrobial agents. Less well known is the fact that a number of the other organisms noted above show

significant resistance to penicillin G and also to other agents on occasion.

The bacteriology of *lung abscess* differs in terms of the numerous organisms other than anaerobes that may be involved in its etiology on occasion. It is clear that lung abscess is primarily an anaerobic infection. In one prospective study of 26 patients studied by transtracheal aspiration, 24 yielded anaerobic bacteria (including microaerophilic streptococci). However, certain nonanaerobic organisms can cause lung abscess (or necrotizing pneumonia), with or without empyema. Included are *Staphylococcus aureus*, *Streptococcus pyogenes*, *K. pneumoniae*, and *P. aeruginosa*. It is said that pneumococci of type 3 can, rarely, cause lung abscess. Infrequently, other gram-negative bacilli such as *Escherichia coli* and perhaps *Proteus* may cause pulmonary necrosis. Uncommon but important causes of cavitating pneumonia are *Nocardia asteroides*, *Legionella*, and the agents of melioidosis and glanders. Tuberculosis may cause necrotizing pneumonia, and certain fungal infections may result in this also. *Entamoeba histolytica* is an important, but uncommon, cause of lung abscess, almost always in the basilar portion of the right lower lobe.

Empyema involves anaerobic bacteria commonly, as noted earlier, but it is not primarily an anaerobic process. Overall, the most common cause of thoracic empyema is *Staphylococcus aureus*. Various gram-negative aerobic or facultatively anaerobic bacilli, particularly *P. aeruginosa*, and also *Escherichia coli*, *Klebsiella* species, and *Proteus* species may cause thoracic empyema as can various streptococci (viridans and enterococcal groups and *Streptococcus pyogenes*), *Mycobacterium tuberculosis*, *Nocardia asteroides*, and various fungi.

Table 93-3 correlates the infecting organisms with the various conditions underlying anaerobic pleuropulmonary infection. The major source of the *B. fragilis* group is peritoneal infection or a source in the bowel. However, a significant number of instances of infection involving this organism followed aspiration or middle ear infection. As noted previously, *F. necrophorum* is seen particularly in association with tonsillitis. Most infections involving *Clostridium* are related to chest trauma or surgery. Anaerobic pleuropulmonary infection secondary to pelvic infection is apt to involve anaerobic gram-positive cocci or *F. necrophorum*.

DIAGNOSIS

Because aspiration pneumonia, lung abscess, and empyema that are not related to prior surgery are usually anaerobic infections, the presence of one of these conditions should suggest the likelihood that the process is an anaerobic infection. Foul- or putrid-smelling sputum or empyema fluid is pathognomonic of anaerobic pleu-

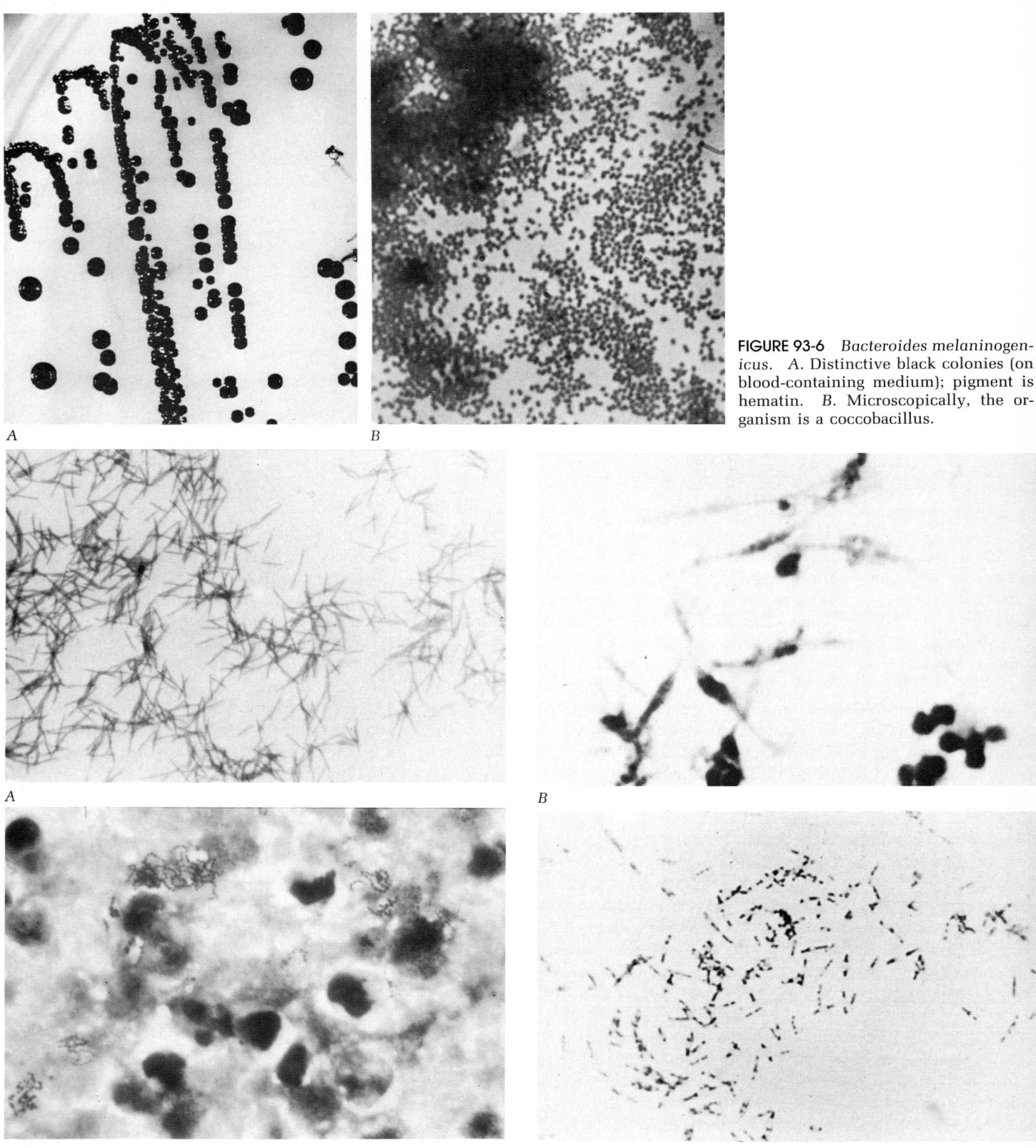

FIGURE 93-6 *Bacteroides melaninogenicus.* *A.* Distinctive black colonies (on blood-containing medium); pigment is hematin. *B.* Microscopically, the organism is a coccobacillus.

FIGURE 93-7 Bacteriology of aspiration pneumonia. *A. Fusobacterium nucleatum,* microscopic morphology. Organism is thin and delicate. Gram-negative bacillus with tapered ends (sometimes filamentous). *B.* Pleomorphic gram-negative bacillus with filaments containing swollen portions and with large round bodies. This appearance is seen with *F. necrophorum, F. mortiferum,* and *F. varium.* *C.* Pus showing microaerophilic streptococcus. *D.* Microscopic morphology of *Bacteroides fragilis.* Organism is an irregularly stained, gram-negative rod. Bipolar staining, when present, is suggestive of this organism.

TABLE 93-3

Correlation of Infecting Organism and Conditions Underlying Anaerobic Pleuropulmonary Infection

Bacteria	Aspi-ration	Tonsil-litis, Tonsil-lectomy	Gingivitis, Dental Extraction, Pyorrhea	Otitis Media, Mastoid-itis	Bronchi-ectasis	Broncho-genic Carcinoma	Chest Trauma, Thora-cotomy	Peritoneal Infection or Source in Bowel	Pelvic Infection
Bacteroides fragilis group	11	1	0	7	3	1	3	16	1
B. melaninogenicus group	13	0	7	0	2	0	0	2	0
Fusobacterium nucleatum	24	2	7	2	4	4	4	6	1
F. necrophorum	2	45	2	0	1	2	0	5	4
Peptostreptococcus	27	5	9	4	4	2	10	6	8
Microaerophilic streptococcus	17	0	5	0	0	4	0	5	1
Anaerobic non-spore-forming catalase-negative gram-positive rods	6	1	0	3	1	2	1	3	0
Clostridium	6	3	1	0	0	0	15	7	1

SOURCE: Based on data in Finegold, 1977.

ropulmonary infection if one can rule out an anaerobic dental or oral infection. However, the absence of a foul odor does not exclude the possibility of anaerobic infection since certain anaerobes (particularly some of the cocci) do not produce the end products of metabolism responsible for this type of odor. Moreover, in some instances, communication is lacking between the site of the lesion and the tracheobronchial tree. In general, discharges from approximately one-half of patients with anaerobic pleuropulmonary infection will exhibit the foul odor. The presence of certain conditions which typically underlie anaerobic pleuropulmonary infection (e.g., aspiration or suspected aspiration, or periodontal disease) constitutes an important clue to the likely role of anaerobes in pleuropulmonary infection.

Abscess formation, or other evidence of tissue necrosis, is not specific but is so common in anaerobic infection that it raises the possibility of anaerobes. Rapid cavitation within a dense segmental consolidation suggests anaerobic infection; rapidly enlarging multiple nodular lesions, with or without cavitation, also raise this possibility. Although anaerobic pulmonary infections sometimes are acute and fulminating, almost two-thirds of them have a subacute or chronic presentation. Aside from mycobacterial infections, this type of course is relatively unique among bacterial infections of the lung. Pyopneumothorax, in the absence of bronchopleural fistula or prior thoracentesis, suggests the possibility of gas formation by bacteria involved in the infection; although it is not specific for anaerobic infection, it is suggestive of it. Certain anaerobes, particularly *F. nucleatum* and the *B. melaninogenicus* group, exhibit morphology which is unique enough to suggest their identity (Figs. 93-4 and 93-5). Finally, failure

to recover a likely pathogen on aerobic culture of appropriate material raises the possibility of anaerobic involvement.

The importance of proper specimen collection and transport in diagnosing anaerobic pleuropulmonary infection cannot be overemphasized. When empyema or bacteremia complicates anaerobic pulmonary infection (bacteremia is no longer common in this setting), obtaining a reliable specimen for culture free of normal flora is no problem. Coughed sputum is not suitable for diagnosis of anaerobic pulmonary infection because of the prevalence of large numbers of anaerobes as normal flora in the mouth and upper respiratory tract (Fig. 93-8). Accordingly, this indigenous flora must be bypassed. Unless con-

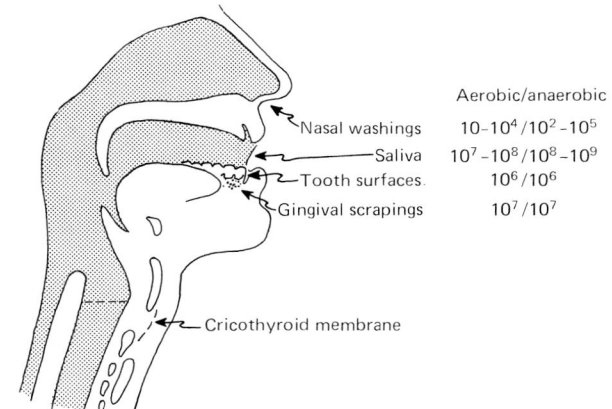

FIGURE 93-8 Sagittal section illustrating presence of large numbers of organisms, including anaerobes, as indigenous flora in upper respiratory tract. (Values given as number of aerobic/anaerobic organisms per milliliter.) *(Courtesy of P. D. Hoeprich.)*

traindications exist to percutaneous transtracheal aspiration, this procedure is the easiest, safest, and most dependable way of obtaining a proper specimen (Fig. 93-9). Percutaneous transthoracic aspiration (direct lung puncture) may also be used. Specimens obtained by way of a rigid bronchoscope are not suitable, but specimens collected through a fiberoptic bronchoscope, using a plugged double lumen sampling catheter and special precautions, may be useful when quantitative anaerobic culture is employed. It is essential that material obtained for

culture be placed under anaerobic conditions promptly prior to transport to the laboratory. A syringe technique illustrated in Fig. 93-10A may be used, providing the specimen can be delivered to the laboratory and set up in culture within 20 to 30 min. It is imperative that all bubbles of air be eliminated from the syringe and needle. It is generally preferable to transfer the material to be cultured from the syringe to a tube that has been gassed out with O_2-free gas for transport of the specimen to the laboratory (Fig. 93-10B).

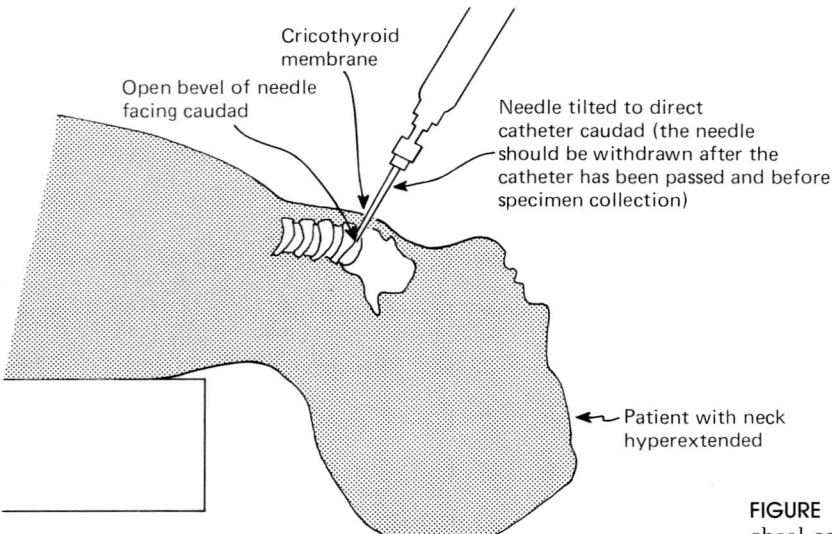

FIGURE 93-9 Diagrammatic illustration of procedure of transtracheal aspiration. *(Courtesy of J. G. Bartlett.)*

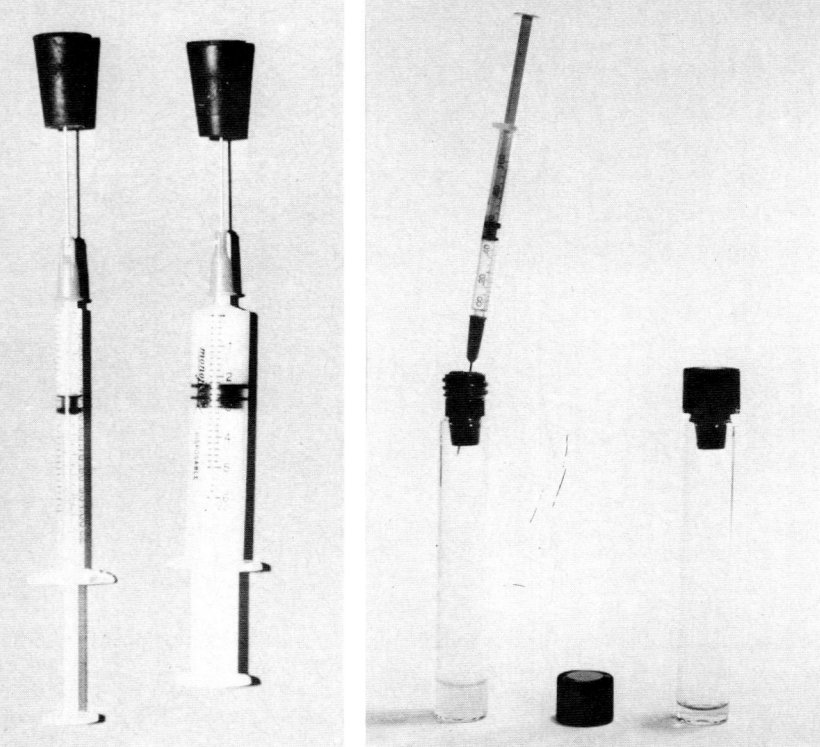

A   *B*

FIGURE 93-10 Transport of anaerobic specimens. *A*. Syringe technique. *B*. Tube with O_2-free atmosphere. A small amount of nonnutritive fluid in the tube contains resazurin, an oxidation-reduction indicator.

THERAPY

Penicillin has ordinarily been the drug of choice for anaerobic infections of the lung and pleural space. With the exception of the *B. fragilis* group, the majority of anaerobes recovered in this setting are susceptible to penicillin G. However, this situation is in the process of change. An increasing number of anaerobes are producing β lacta-

mases and, accordingly, showing increasing levels of resistance to penicillin G. At this time, penicillin G is still the drug of choice for anaerobic pleuropulmonary infection, but it should be used in high dosage (12 to 18 million units per day IV in average size adults with normal renal function), and other drugs should be used together with penicillin, at least initially, in patients who are seriously ill. In the latter patients, metronidazole (2 g per day in

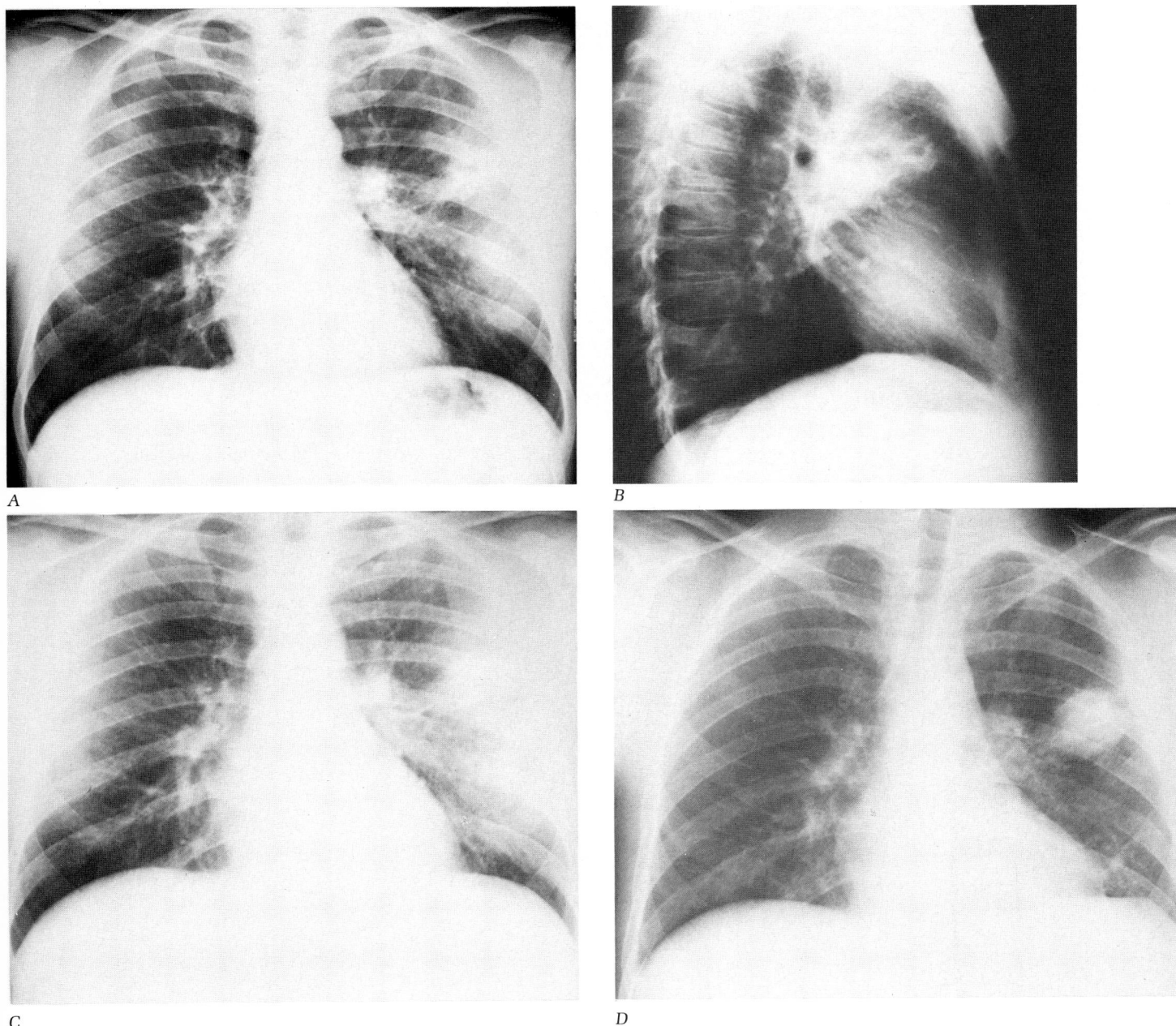

FIGURE 93-11 Lung abscess, inadequately treated. Twenty-nine-year-old alcoholic with anaerobic lung abscess. *A.* On admission. Radiolucent area in midst of consolidation in the left upper lung field. *B.* Lateral view demonstrates multiple cavities. Patient treated for 5 days with penicillin, 6 million units per day administered intravenously. Same dosage by mouth for next 10 days. *C.* Two weeks after admission. Infiltrate persists. No cavity is visible. *D.* Six weeks after treatment with penicillin stopped. Recurrence of abscess in same area. Marked pleural reaction in vicinity.

four divided doses) should be used in addition to penicillin G in order to cover β-lactamase-producing organisms. In certain locales, there is significant resistance of the *B. fragilis* group to clindamycin and cefoxitin. Other alternatives include ticarcillin plus potassium clavulanate, imipenem, and chloramphenicol. In patients who are acutely ill, therapy should be extensive and, ordinarily, prolonged. This type of infection tends to relapse if treatment is stopped too soon (Fig. 93-11). In individuals who have aspirated in the hospital setting, therapy should also include drugs appropriate for the aerobic and facultative bacteria (chiefly *Staphylococcus aureus* and various gram-negative bacilli, including Enterobacteriaceae and *Pseudomonas*) that may commonly be encountered along with the anaerobes. Table 93-4 shows the susceptibility of the major anaerobic bacteria to a variety of agents which may be useful in infections with these organisms.

As in other types of infection, relief of obstruction and provision of drainage may be very important elements in determining a satisfactory response. Thus intrabronchial foreign bodies must be removed, and empyema must be drained. Surgical drainage may be required for empyema; open thoracotomy with rib resection is usually the specific procedure of choice when the fluid is frankly purulent. All loculated areas must be opened to effect good drainage. On the other hand, surgery is rarely indicated for lung abscess (except if there is an associated tumor) and, indeed, is usually *contraindicated* because spillage of abscess contents into other segments during surgery may lead to spread of disease or asphyxiation. On occasion, bronchoscopy may be a useful adjunct to postural drainage in order to effect good drainage of lung abscesses.

PREVENTION

Since aspiration and periodontal disease or gingivitis are important underlying causes of anaerobic pulmonary infection, attention is directed to these abnormalities in considering prevention of anaerobic infections. Avoiding aspiration in predisposed individuals is difficult. Proper positioning of a patient during anesthesia helps. Proper management of periodontal disease and of gingivitis minimizes anaerobic pulmonary infection secondary to this type of process. Adrenocorticosteroids are commonly recommended in patients who have aspirated gastric contents; the value of this intervention is uncertain. Also doubtful is the value of administering prophylactic antimicrobial agents following aspiration of gastric contents. The early institution of therapy with appropriate antimicrobials, if there is evidence of a superimposed bacterial infection in patients who have previously aspirated, seems to be the most rational approach.

TABLE 93-4

Susceptibility of Anaerobes to Antimicrobial Agents

Bacterium	Chloram-phenicol	Clinda-mycin	Erythro-mycin	Metroni-dazole	Cefoxitin	Penicillin G	Piperazine, Ureido, and Carboxy Penicillins	Tetra-cycline	Vanco-mycin
Microaerophilic and anaerobic cocci	+++	++ to +++	++ to +++	++	+++	+++ to ++++	+++	+ to ++	+++
Bacteroides fragilis group	+++	++ to +++	+ to ++	+++	++ to +++	+	++ to +++	+ to ++	+
B. melaninogenicus group	+++	+++*	++ to +++	+++	+++*	++ to +++	+++*	++	+
Fusobacterium varium	+++	+ to ++	+	+++	+++*	+++*	+++*	++	+
Other *Fusobacterium* spp.	+++	+ to ++	+	+++	+++†	++++	+++†	+++	+
Clostridium perfringens	+++	+++†	+++	+++	+++	++++*	+++	++	+++
Other *Clostridium* spp.	+++	++	++ to +++	+++	+ to ++	+++	+++	++	++ to +++
Actinomyces	+++	+++	+++	+	+++	++++	+++	++ to +++	++

*A few strains are resistant.

†Rare strains are resistant.

NOTE: Aminoglycosides, such as gentamicin and kanamycin, are generally quite inactive against the majority of anaerobes. The activity of erythromycin varies significantly according to the testing procedure. Erythromycin and vancomycin are not approved by the Food and Drug Administration for anaerobic infections. ++++ = drug of choice; +++ = good activity; ++ = moderate activity; + = poor or inconsistent activity. There is no difference in activity between drugs rated +++ and those rated ++++; the symbol ++++ indicates a drug with good activity, good pharmacologic characteristics, and low toxicity.

BIBLIOGRAPHY

Bartlett JG: Anaerobic bacterial infections of the lung. Chest 91:901–909, 1987.
   An update on approaches to diagnosis and treatment.

Bartlett JG, Gorbach SL, Finegold SM: The bacteriology of aspiration pneumonia. Am J Med 56:202–207, 1974.
   A prospective bacteriologic study of 54 patients with aspiration pneumonia.

Bartlett JG, Gorbach SL, Thadepalli H, Finegold SM: The bacteriology of empyema. Lancet 1:338–340, 1974.
   A bacteriologic study of 83 patients with empyema in three hospitals with anaerobic bacteriology research laboratories.

Bartlett JG, Rosenblatt JE, Finegold SM: Percutaneous transtracheal aspiration in the diagnosis of anaerobic pulmonary infection. Ann Intern Med 79:535–540, 1973.
   Transtracheal aspiration was carried out in 91 patients with various pulmonary conditions; 33 yielded anaerobes on culture.

Brock RC: *Lung Abscess.* Springfield, Ill, Charles C Thomas, 1952.
   A classic text on lung abscess.

Brook I: Direct and indirect pathogenicity of anaerobic bacteria in respiratory tract infections in children. Adv Pediatr 34:357–377, 1987.
   A recent increase in numbers of beta-lactamase producing strains of anaerobic gram-negative bacteria in respiratory tract infections has been associated with increased failure rates of penicillins in eradication of these infections. Not only do these organisms survive penicillin therapy but they also protect penicillin susceptible pathogens from that drug. Appropriate antimicrobial therapy should be directed against all pathogens in mixed infections.

Brook I, Finegold SM: Bacteriology of aspiration pneumonia in children. Pediatrics 65:1115–1120, 1980.
   Aspiration pneumonia in children, as in adults, commonly involves anaerobic bacteria. When aspiration occurs in a medical institution, nosocomial pathogens which are aerobic or facultative will also often be involved, in both children and adults.

Bynum LJ, Pierce AK: Pulmonary aspiration of gastric contents. Am Rev Respir Dis 114:1129–1136, 1976.
   A retrospective analysis of 50 patients who had been observed to aspirate gastric contents.

Finegold SM: *Anaerobic Bacteria in Human Disease.* New York, Academic, 1977.
   A very extensive review of the literature on the role of anaerobic bacteria in infection of all types, together with observations from the author's experience.

Finegold SM: Increasing resistance in anaerobes. Infect Surg 33:332–335, 338, 1984.
   Review of recent experience with increasing resistance of anaerobic bacteria to antimicrobial agents.

Finland M, Barnes MW: Changing ecology of acute bacterial empyema: Occurrence and mortality at Boston City Hospital during 12 selected years from 1935 to 1972. J Infect Dis 137:274–291, 1978.
   A classic paper on the changing etiology and ecology of empyema over the years.

George WL, Kirby BD, Sutter VL, Citron DM, Finegold SM: Gram-negative anaerobic bacilli: Their role in infection and patterns of susceptibility to antimicrobial agents. II. Little-known Fusobacterium species and miscellaneous genera. Rev Infect Dis 3:599–626, 1981.
   Review of the authors' experience over 6 years and an extensive literature review covering 20 infrequently reported species of Fusobacterium and other gram-negative anaerobic rods.

Johnson CC, Reinhardt JF, Edelstein MAC, Mulligan ME, George WL, Finegold SM: *Bacteroides gracilis,* an important anaerobic bacterial pathogen. J Clin Microbiol 22:799–802, 1985.
   B. gracilis, previously classified with B. ureolyticus, proves to be much more virulent and resistant to antimicrobial agents.

Kirby BD, George WL, Sutter VL, Citron DM, Finegold SM: Gram-negative anaerobic bacilli: Their role in infection and patterns of susceptibility to antimicrobial agents. I. Little-known Bacteroides species. Rev Infect Dis 2:914–951, 1980.
   The role in infection and antimicrobial susceptibility of 17 species of Bacteroides was studied; they proved to be more common than had been appreciated.

Wimberley N, Faling LJ, Bartlett JG: A fiberoptic bronchoscopy technique to obtain uncontaminated lower airway secretions for bacterial culture. Am Rev Respir Dis 119:337–342, 1979.
   In vitro studies and a preliminary clinical trial of a double lumen catheter for sampling lower respiratory tract secretions with minimal upper airway bacterial contamination.

Chapter 94

Unusual Bacterial Pneumonias

Arnold N. Weinberg

Pneumonias Caused by Obligate Human Parasites
   Neisseria Meningitidis
   Branhamella (Neisseria) Catarrhalis

Environmental and Animal Product Pneumonias
   Anthrax Respiratory Disease
   Pneumonia Due to *Brucella* Species
   Pneumonia Due to *Pseudomonas Pseudomallei*
   Pulmonary Infections Due to *Yersinia Enterocolitica*

Zoonotic Bacterial Pneumonias
   Pasteurella Multocida Respiratory Infections
   Pneumonia Due to *Yersinia Pestis*
   Pneumonia Due to *Francisella Tularensis*

A decade has passed since the epidemic of acute respiratory disease erupted among delegates to the American Legion convention in Philadelphia. A ripple effect of that experience has been the intensified efforts physicians have made to sharpen their diagnostic skills when confronted by patients with obscure pneumonias. Many different microorganisms can infect the lungs, but routes of spread are few, clinical presentations overlap, radiologic changes are often nonspecific, and pathophysiological mechanisms are limited. Making a clinical diagnosis of pneumonia is relatively easy, but defining the etiologic agent can be difficult. The search for the *specific etiologic agent* is driven by a number of compelling issues, including: the desire to use specific therapy for a specific pathogen; the potential for progressive respiratory impairment when the wrong antibiotic is used; and epidemiologic concerns in the family, in the hospital community, and in the public at large for isolation and containment.

This discussion of "unusual bacterial pneumonias" focuses on a limited number of microorganisms and not on an exhaustive list of possible causative agents. The unique properties of these bacteria exemplify how bacteriology, ecology, epidemiology, and pathogenesis relate to the clinical pneumonia described and how these properties serve as helpful clues to earlier diagnosis and, therefore, specific therapy.

The diseases to be described in this chapter include examples of those caused by human commensals, by environmental microorganisms, and by bacteria intimately associated with domestic or wild animals. Some of the distinguishing epidemiologic characteristics of these agents are listed in Table 94-1.

PNEUMONIAS CAUSED BY OBLIGATE HUMAN PARASITES

As discussed in Chapter 95, the majority of bacterial pneumonias are caused by obligate human commensals that are easy to isolate, like *Streptococcus pneumoniae*. Among the less common causes of pneumonia due to human commensals, *Neisseria meningitidis* (the meningococcus) and *Branhamella* (formerly *Neisseria*) *catarrhalis* stand out as pathogens or opportunists that may escape bacteriologic identification and therefore present problems in diagnosis and therapy.

Neisseria Meningitidis

During the influenza viral pandemic of 1918–1919, *N. meningitidis* was an important respiratory pathogen. Afterward, few references to the meningococcus appeared in the medical literature of bacterial pneumonias, as reports of meningococcal disease focused on its role in causing meningitis. With the advent of improved bacteriologic techniques, over 100 cases of *N. meningitidis* pneumonia have been reported during the last decade. It remains to be established whether this is a true increase in incidence or reflects greater awareness on the part of physicians.

BACTERIOLOGY AND IMMUNOLOGY
Bacteriology
Neisseria are oxygen-requiring, gram-negative staining cocci recognized by their characteristic pairing as kidney-shaped diplococci. They are fastidious, succumbing rapidly to the external environment and to dry or cold conditions. Although *Neisseria* can grow on blood agar, optimal conditions include enriched media, like chocolate agar, and incubation in an atmosphere of 6% CO_2 at 35 to 37°C with 50 percent humidity. *N. meningitidis* is distinguishable from other *Neisseria* species that are residents of the oral-respiratory region by sugar-fermentation reactions and by serologic identification, which depends on specific capsular polysaccharides. Isolation and identification of *N. meningitidis* in sputum is facilitated by the use of a selective medium, like modified Thayer-Martin agar (MTM), which contains antibiotics that will suppress more rapidly growing microorganisms. The presence of *Neisseria*-like diplococci in a Gram-stained smear of sputum should provide the impetus to culture the specimen on MTM agar as well as on less selective media like blood and chocolate agar (Fig. 94-1).

TABLE 94-1
An Overview of Unusual Pneumonias

Environmental Niche	Microorganism	Disease	Epidemiologic Associations	Distribution
Obligate human parasite	*Neisseria meningitidis*	Meningococcal pneumonia	*Airborne*, human to human; postviral, nosocomial	Humans worldwide
	Branhamella catarrhalis	Branhamella pneumonia	*Aspiration*, especially individuals with underlying lung disease	Humans worldwide
Soil, stagnant water and inert animal products	*Bacillus anthracis*	Inhalation anthrax or woolsorter's disease	*Industrial*; use of animal products in hobbies	Worldwide in warmer regions
	Brucella species	Brucellosis	*Ingestion* or *contact* with infected animal products	Worldwide
	Pseudomonas pseudomallei	Melioidosis	Direct penetrating *contact* with soil, water	Latitude 20°N to 20°S, especially rural Asia
	Yersinia enterocolitica	Yersiniosis	*Ingestion* contaminated foods, water; Cirrhosis	Worldwide
Live animal contact or via arthropod	*Francisella tularensis*	Tularemia	*Contact* with animals, birds, or arthropods	North America, Europe, Asia
	Pasteurella multocida	Pasteurellosis	Feline and dog *contact*; chronic lung disease	Worldwide
	Yersinia pestis	Plague	*Contact* with rodents, fleas; *Contact* with plague pneumonia case	Worldwide, including Asia, southwest U.S.

N. *meningitidis* is a typical gram-negative organism containing a potent lipopolysaccharide "endotoxin" in the outer membrane layer of the cell envelope. Exterior to this layer is a polysaccharide capsule, by which N. *meningitidis* can be separated into at least 13 chemically defined serogroups. Groups A, B, C, X, Y, Z, and W-135 are currently the most important clinically.

Immunology

Immunity to meningococci is complex. Bactericidal antibody, present in the newborn, disappears by approximately 6 months of age. During childhood and adolescence, overt disease and subclinical encounters with various capsular strains of N. *meningitidis*, as well as with nonpathogenic *Neisseria* species, leads to stimulation of bactericidal antibody. Facilitated by terminal complement components C5 to C8, this can result in immune lysis of organisms. Antibodies to certain outer membrane proteins and to a variety of envelope antigens of *Escherichia coli* and other commensals cross react with antigens from N. *meningitidis*. Individuals lacking bactericidal or capsular antibody to a specific serogroup are susceptible to colonization and to disease caused by that serogroup. With increasing age, acquisition of protective antibodies is associated with less likelihood of developing clinical disease.

EPIDEMIOLOGY

Nasopharyngeal carriage of various serogroups of meningococci occurs in approximately 5 to 15 percent of individuals. Convening and crowding large numbers of young individuals from widely separated geographic areas, as occurs in the military or in boarding schools, can result in significant and rapid spread of an individual serogroup from a few asymptomatic carriers to many susceptibles. A case of meningococcal disease in a family setting is often associated with an increased prevalence of meningococcal isolation from relatives with symptoms of upper respiratory infection. In the military experience carrier rates can rapidly approach 100 percent followed by many cases of meningitis.

Respiratory disease due to meningococci was recognized early in the twentieth century, especially during the influenza pandemic of 1918–1919. Then in the mid-1970s outbreaks of serogroup Y meningococcal pneumonia occurred in military installations. Over the past decade isolated respiratory disease, primarily due to serogroups Y and W-135, has been detected in civilian populations and nosocomially in individuals in contact with an index case. Spread is probably by aerosol droplets during close contact, since drying rapidly kills meningococci. Individuals ill with influenza or adenoviral respiratory infections

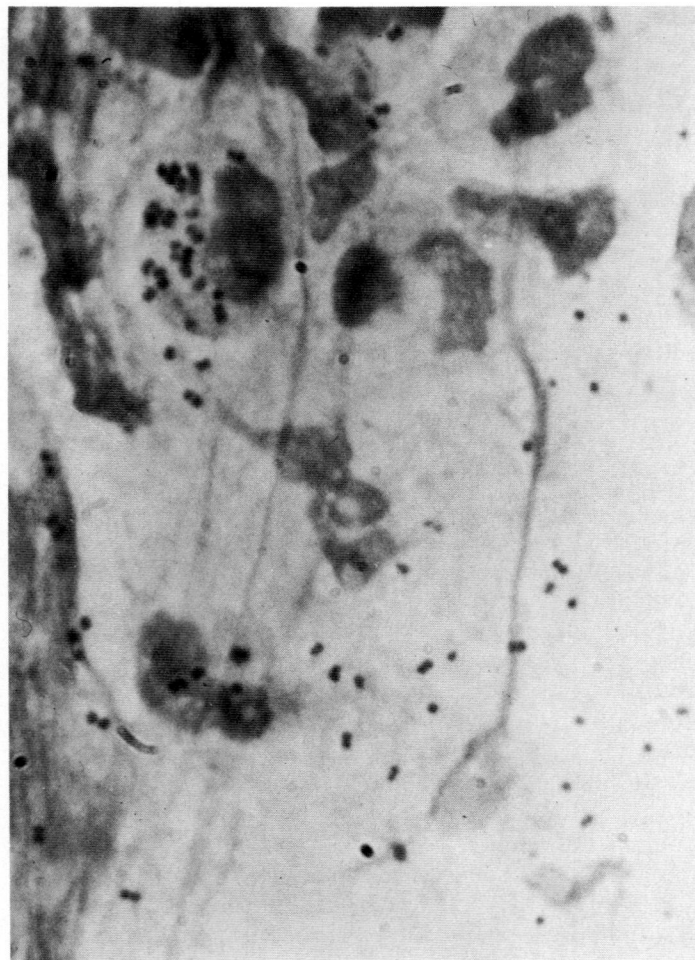

FIGURE 94-1 Gram stain of expectorated sputum from a patient with proven *Branhamella* pneumonia. In this black and white photomicrograph, the distinguishing features include the presence of morphologic kidney-shaped diplococci (gram-negative) associated with polymorphonuclear leukocytes. This appearance suggests *Neisseria* or *Branhamella* infection.

appear to be more susceptible, just as occurs with other respiratory pathogens like *S. pneumoniae* and *Staphylococcus aureus.*

PATHOGENESIS AND PATHOPHYSIOLOGY

Initiation of infection begins when an encapsulated strain colonizes the nasopharynx of an individual lacking immunity to that serogroup. Attachment to mucosal cells is facilitated by filamentous pili and perhaps by the action of bacterial IgA1 protease. The lower respiratory tract is invaded by aspiration or inhalation of droplet particles. A preceding viral infection can stimulate excessive airway secretions, damage surface epithelial structures, and interfere with clearance of microorganisms. Septicemia, petechial eruptions, meningitis, diffuse intravascular coagulation (DIC), and adult respiratory distress syndrome (ARDS) rarely accompany pneumonia, supporting the

presumed aspiration mechanism. Bronchopneumonia, lobar extension, and necrosis and abscess formation are seen. Modern pathologic correlations are lacking since there are no animal models of meningococcal pneumonia and histopathologic material is essentially nonexistent.

CLINICAL AND RADIOLOGIC FEATURES

Clinical Features
The clinical presentation of meningococcal pneumonia resembles that of pneumococcal infection. Productive cough, pleuritic pain, chills, and fever are associated with physical changes of rales with consolidation. In contrast to pneumococcal disease, pleural rubs and hemoptysis are unusual. Suspicion of meningococcal disease is enhanced if many cases of bacterial pneumonia erupt in closed populations like military or school groups or among individuals in a hospital setting. Pharyngitis is often an early complaint.

Radiology
Radiologic findings are nonspecific and include patchy bronchopneumonia and lobar airspace infiltrates, usually located in a lower or right middle lobe, accompanied by an effusion in about 20 percent of cases. Occasionally the radiologic appearance resembles diffuse pulmonary edema or the antecedent viral infection.

DIAGNOSTIC FEATURES

Diagnosis depends on isolation of predominantly *N. meningitidis* from a carefully collected sputum specimen that has characteristic gram-negative diplococci among polymorphonuclear leukocytes on the stained smear (Fig. 94-1). Attention to these criteria is essential, since pathogenic and nonpathogenic *Neisseria* are part of the normal respiratory flora. Invasive procedures, like transtracheal aspiration, are not necessary if a valid sputum is available, and the Gram-stain appearance prompts culturing the specimen on Thayer-Martin medium. Alternative methods of identification include the capsular swelling technique (quellung), latex bead coagglutination, and fluorescent antibody staining. Recent purification of all of the major group-specific capsular polysaccharides should lead to expansion of these rapid diagnostic methods. Blood and CSF cultures are rarely positive in meningococcal respiratory disease (Table 94-2).

TABLE 94-2
Diagnosing Meningococcal Pneumonia

Antecedent viral respiratory infection
Multiple community or hospital respiratory cases
Purulent or frothy sputum
Kidney-shaped, gram-negative diplococci on smear (Fig. 94-1)
Culture sputum on Thayer-Martin medium
Incubation with CO_2 enrichment

DIFFERENTIAL DIAGNOSIS

Respiratory infections due to other causes, especially involving multiple cases, must be considered in the differential diagnosis.

Viral Pneumonia

Acute respiratory infections affecting a number of individuals, especially under institutional or crowded circumstances, can be caused by viral agents like influenza A or B or adenoviruses. Diagnosis is usually confirmed by the epidemiologic and clinical circumstances, a nonspecific sputum examination, absent or interstitial infiltrates radiologically, and paired serologic titers.

Mycoplasma pneumonia

The illness is often biphasic with upper respiratory inflammation and headache prominent early symptoms and, occasionally, bullous tympanitis producing severe ear pain. The sputum is often purulent, with a mixture of polymorphonuclear neutrophil leukocytes (PMNs) and mononuclear cells, but no dominant microorganism is observed. Diagnosis is usually confirmed by a cold agglutinin titer of 1:32 or greater or a rising titer of complement-fixing antibody. When multiple cases occur in a closed community, they usually erupt over many weeks rather than days to a few weeks.

Pyogenic Pneumonia

Acute bacterial pneumonias often follow in the wake of viral respiratory infections. S. pneumonia and S. aureus infections are differentiated by microscopic examination, culture of sputum, and the results of blood cultures. In hospitals, especially among immunocompromised patients or individuals attached to respirators, a variety of gram-negative microorganisms can produce pneumonia. *Hemophilus influenzae* infections can usually be suspected, but B. catarrhalis looks like *Neisseria* morphologically and may not respond to penicillin treatment (see below).

Rocky Mountain Spotted Fever

Acute respiratory failure secondary to small vessel endothelial cell damage or to ARDS can complicate this rickettsial disease. A petechial or morbilliform eruption is usually seen on the extremities. With meningococcal respiratory disease, a rash is rarely seen.

TREATMENT AND PREVENTION

Treatment

Low-dose penicillin is effective for most cases, although those complicated by cavitation or empyema should be treated with a minimum of 6 million units daily. Individuals allergic to penicillin can be given chloramphenicol, 2 to 3 g in four to six divided doses. The third-generation cephalosporins also are effective, although their use in respiratory disease is limited. In contrast to meningitis or meningococcemia, respiratory infections appear to respond uniformly well to treatment.

Prevention

Meningococci spread via aerosols, so isolation of suspected cases is essential, usually for the first 24 h of treatment. Chemoprophylaxis and immunoprophylaxis have been found effective in epidemics of meningitis, but no data are available for respiratory disease protection. Penicillin, the drug of choice for treating active disease, does not reliably eradicate the carrier state or protect intimately exposed contacts. Rifampin, probably due to transport into oral and respiratory tract secretions in high concentrations, is an effective prophylactic agent. The usual protective dose is 600 mg orally, twice daily for 2 days. Minocycline is also found in upper respiratory secretions in high concentrations and is a useful alternative to rifampin. Labyrinthitis, a frequent toxic side effect, obviates wider use of this agent, however.

Immunoprophylaxis has been safe and effective when given systematically to large at-risk groups in military installations, schools, day-care centers or in defined communities. A quadrivalent vaccine, containing serogroups A, C, Y, and W-135, is commercially available, and an octavalent preparation is in development. Although groups Y and W-135 isolates have commonly been causal, there is no data for efficacy of the vaccine for respiratory infections. Children below the age of 2 years respond poorly to the group C vaccine and unpredictably to the other polysaccharide products. This younger age group remains vulnerable at present, and protection must be provided, when necessary, with chemoprophylaxis. Immunizing individuals with influenza viral vaccines should eliminate some cases of secondary bacterial infections, including those caused by N. meningitidis.

Branhamella (Neisseria) Catarrhalis

Formerly considered a nonpathogenic respiratory commensal, B. catarrhalis has aroused renewed interest as an opportunist and primary pathogen. Resemblance to *Neisseria* on Gram stain, and penicillin resistance of many clinically significant isolates are features that encourage inclusion in this section.

BACTERIOLOGY

Branhamella are gram-negative cocci that pair as kidney-shaped diplococci; hence they can't be distinguished morphologically from *Neisseria*. Biochemical studies lead to a reclassification of these microorganisms to the genus *Branhamella*. With further refinements, their shaky taxonomic status has been stabilized, and they are classified as *Moraxella (Branhamella) catarrhalis* in the newest edition of *Bergey's Manual of Systemic Microbiology*. Clinical microbiologists and clinicians accept changes slowly, so reference to the designation most familiar in contemporary medical literature and practice is used here.

The organisms grow well on nonselective media such as sheep blood agar and enriched chocolate agar, espe-

cially in an atmosphere with added CO_2. Growth of *Branhamella* is variable on selective media like MTM, in contrast to pathogenic *Neisseria*, which thrives on that medium. *Branhamella* fail to utilize a variety of sugars. These and other biochemical tests help to distinguish them from *Neisseria* and other *Moraxella* microorganisms. Many clinical isolates produce β-lactamase and, therefore, are resistant to penicillins.

EPIDEMIOLOGY

A member of the resident microflora of the nasopharynx and pharynx, *B. catarrhalis* can also colonize the mucosa of the genital tract. In individuals with chronic lung disease it can be found along with other bacteria in respiratory secretions. The extent of colonization of mucous surfaces in healthy or diseased individuals is not known. There is no evidence for human-to-human transmission although infections in the hospital setting are common, probably related to antimicrobial drug selective pressures. In normal children and adults, otitis media, sinusitis, and laryngotracheobronchitis probably result from direct spread from colonized mucosal surfaces. This view is supported by finding mixed infections with other commensals, like *H. influenzae* and mouth anaerobes.

PATHOGENESIS AND PATHOPHYSIOLOGY

In contrast to pathogenic *Neisseria*, *Branhamella* lack antiphagocytic capsules and IgA proteases. They have outer-envelope lipopolysaccharide endotoxin, characteristic of all gram-negative microbes, but no specific pathogenic factors have been described.

The mechanism of initiation of respiratory disease appears to be primarily related to underlying obstruction and chronic inflammation. Aspiration of nasopharyngeal secretions, stimulated by an acute viral upper respiratory infection, is the most common proposed pathophysiological factor. Contributing conditions that are immunocompromising, like steroid therapy, malignancy, hypogammaglobulinemia, and neutropenia, are present in a large number of patients. Paranasal sinus and ear infections occur predominantly in children, probably related to compromised drainage ducts in anatomically crowded areas. Rarely, *Branhamella* produce primary invasive diseases outside the respiratory tract, including meningitis, endocarditis, septic arthritis, and in immunocompromised patients, septicemia.

CLINICAL AND RADIOLOGIC FEATURES

Clinical Features

The majority of individuals who develop respiratory infections are adults with chronic lung disease associated with smoking, industrial exposures, or bronchitis and bronchiectasis. Purulent bronchitis or bronchopneumonia can follow an intercurrent viral infection. Respiratory distress may be present, related to the acute process, with bronchospasm and fever superimposed on the chronic underlying disease. Signs of consolidation or pleural fluid may be present along with persistent obstructive changes. Evidence has been accumulating recently that normal adults may develop primary laryngitis and children a nonproductive cough as other manifestations of clinical respiratory tract disease.

Radiology

The radiologic appearance is influenced by the underlying chronic lung disease. No acute changes may be observed, but usually increased markings are seen superimposed upon the findings of obstructive lung disease and fibrosis. Patchy consolidation is often noted. Lobar infiltrates, cavitation, and pleural effusions are distinctly unusual findings and suggest mixed infection or other complications of the underlying disease.

DIAGNOSTIC FEATURES

The unique feature in cases of *B. catarrhalis* respiratory infections is the finding of gram-negative kidney-shaped diplococci associated with polymorphonuclear exudate cells (Fig. 94-1). Diagnosis depends on careful examination of an adequate expectorated sputum sample and culturing the specimen on nonselective blood and enriched chocolate agar as well as on selective MTM. The use of multiple media assures that these fastidious organisms will be identified in a crowd of other commensals, and their presence must be considered significant in designing treatment programs. Blood cultures should be obtained in cases associated with immunosuppression or malignancy, and pleural effusions aspirated and examined bacteriologically. Transtracheal aspiration rarely adds to the examination of an adequate expectorated sputum. Serologic methods are not available to help verify a pathogenic role for *Branhamella* in mixed infections (Table 94-3).

DIFFERENTIAL DIAGNOSIS

The major diagnostic confusion results from the presence in sputum of *Neisseria* species and other potential pathogens like *S. pneumoniae* or *H. influenzae*. In patients with chronic lung disease, mixed infections make it impossible to ascribe pathogenicity to a single unique pathogen. Coccobacillary microorganisms, or gram-negative bacilli that demonstrate bipolar staining (e.g., *Brucella*, *Pasteurella*), can be confused with *B. catarrhalis*.

TABLE 94-3
Diagnosing Branhamella Pneumonia

Underlying chronic lung disease

History of aspiration

Kidney-shaped, gram-negative diplococci on smear (Fig. 94-1)

Culture sputum on sheep blood and enriched chocolate media

Culture sputum on selective modified Thayer-Martin medium

TREATMENT

As the pathogenic role for *B. catarrhalis* was recognized, it became apparent that many isolates produced β-lactamase and were resistant to penicillin and ampicillin. Numerous treatment failures with penicillins have been described, often with dramatic improvement once an alternative antibiotic was administered. β-Lactamase production is present in approximately 75 percent of isolates from middle ear, sinus, and nasopharyngeal locations in children. In adults with bronchopulmonary disease the range is broader. From 10 to 100 percent of isolates are penicillin-resistant. Of 994 strains randomly collected in Sweden, without regard to clinical significance, 35 percent produced β-lactamase. Therapy should, therefore, be initiated with either a second-generation cephalosporin like cefuroxime, erythromycin, the combination of amoxicillin-clavulanic acid (Augmentin), or trimethoprim-sulfamethoxazole until β-lactamase activity is determined. Supportive therapy with adequate hydration, bronchodilators, and other measures directed at the underlying respiratory disease are essential for a successful outcome.

ENVIRONMENTAL AND ANIMAL PRODUCT PNEUMONIAS

The discussion in this section focuses on four diseases that are spread to humans predominantly from contact with contaminated soil, water, foods, or animal structural elements. Epidemiologic and ecologic aspects are essential to understanding how humans become infected. The diagnosis usually depends upon a careful history. Once alerted, the clinician can request those studies that can reveal the cause of an obscure disease.

Anthrax Respiratory Disease

Inhalation anthrax was a common enough disease in the nineteenth and early twentieth centuries to be referred to variously as *Bradford disease*, after the English town, and *woolsorter's disease* for the epidemiologic association with the sheep industry. Fortunately, inhalation anthrax has become a rare disease, and reports available in the western literature number only seven (2 in the United States) during the past 15 years and fewer than 50 cases since the early part of the century. The potential exposure of susceptible individuals to *Bacillus anthracis* spores argues for including this devastating, usually lethal, disease here.

BACTERIOLOGY

B. anthracis is a large (red cell diameter) square-ended bacillus that stains gram-positive and has a tendency to form chains. Growth on sheep blood agar results in dull, sticky, irregularly shaped colonies within 24 h. The organism possesses a polyglutamic acid capsule, produces a complex potent exotoxin and, under adverse conditions, forms highly refractile spores that are very resistant to temperature and moisture extremes. Over a century ago, Louis Pasteur used serial passage at 43°C to develop an effective, safe vaccine for animals, and it is now known that toxin production is mediated by a temperature-sensitive plasmid.

ECOLOGY AND EPIDEMIOLOGY

Ecology

Anthrax is primarily a disease of herbivores. The resistant spores are present after animals dying of the disease contaminate the soil, especially in regions termed *incubator areas*. These "hot spots" are found in milder regions of the United States, like Oklahoma, Texas, and California. The optimal conditions for germination of spores and multiplication of bacilli include alkaline soils containing adequate calcium, low areas that are wet for prolonged periods, thick vegetation that produces heat with decay, and periods of extreme drought after a rainy season. Animals grazing in these "bad" fields can inhale or ingest spores or pick them up on their fur. The cycle is completed when an animal develops the disease and dies, returning organisms to the soil where they eventually sporulate.

Epidemiology

Inhalation anthrax rarely occurs from contact with live infected animals, and there is no human-to-human transmission. Working in the animal hide industry, being exposed to bone meal fertilizer, and using imported raw wool in home crafts can lead to inhalation of spores and clinical disease in susceptible individuals. The unvaccinated repair person who occasionally enters a goat wool processing plant is at greatest risk for an inhalation exposure.

PATHOGENESIS AND PATHOPHYSIOLOGY

Inhalation results in activation of bronchial clearing mechanisms and entrapment of spores in hilar and mediastinal nodes, where reversion to vegetative bacilli can occur. The polyglutamic acid capsule is antiphagocytic, and the extracellular microorganisms produce a tripartite protein exotoxin that leads to profound local edema acutely, accompanied by hemorrhage in the mediastinum and hilar area. Compromise of airflow results. Recent studies have elucidated the mechanism of edema formation. The *protective antigen* fragment of the toxin is the binding domain, essential for cell penetration by the *edema factor* portion of the molecule. Edema factor is a potent adenylate cyclase. Activation within mammalian

cells results in production of cyclic AMP, and the resultant flux of sodium, potassium, and water leads to profound local edema. When this process takes place in hilar and mediastinal nodes and surrounding tissues, profound airway obstruction ensues, with pooling of secretions and, if the patient survives, secondary bacterial pneumonia. The pathogen rarely invades lung tissue, as death from asphyxia occurs rapidly, usually associated with pleural effusions (secondary to lymphatic obstruction) and hemorrhagic septicemic lesions in many organs, including the central nervous system.

CLINICAL AND RADIOLOGIC FEATURES

Clinical Features

The onset of inhalation anthrax is insidious, usually resembling a nonspecific febrile influenzalike illness. Malaise and muscle aches, mild headache, coryza, pharyngitis, and chest pains have been described as early features. Cough, if present, is usually mild and nonproductive, and fever is low-grade. At this stage it is hardly possible for the physician to entertain a presumptive or possible diagnosis of anthrax *unless* a history of industrial or craft-related exposure to imported animal hair or hides or to animal products like bone meal is obtained. A number of the nonspecific features described above may be relevant. Watery nasal discharge can be indicative of nasal or paranasal sinus edema. Cough may represent hilar and mediastinal node swelling, and careful auscultation may reveal prolonged expiration or wheezes. Chest pain may be the first clue that hilar-mediastinal inflammation is present.

Within hours to a few days, the mild complaints *abruptly* worsen and acute airway obstructive features dominate the clinical picture. Any activity precipitates severe dyspnea, stridor, and wheezing. Involvement of the nervous system (hemorrhagic meningitis) and hypoxemia result in decreasing levels of consciousness. Edema of the pharynx, neck, and anterior chest may develop. Chest pain, fever, and cyanosis are progressive changes. Worsening airway obstruction can lead to intercostal space retraction, and pleural effusions are noted on examination. Death usually occurs within hours to a day once acute respiratory symptoms are present.

Radiology

Inhalation anthrax is primarily a mediastinitis, and the radiologic features mostly reflect the pathologic findings. Widening of the mediastinum or prominence of hilar nodes is the earliest radiographic finding, sometimes accompanied by pleural effusions. In advanced cases the mediastinal shadow is greater than 9 cm in width and sharply demarcated from surrounding lung tissue due to absence of airspace consolidation. There may be perihilar and peribronchial streaking associated with edema and hemorrhage.

DIAGNOSTIC FEATURES

A physician alerted to the possibility of inhalation anthrax has few laboratory studies to rely on. Nasal secretions and sputum rarely reveal the characteristic bulky gram-positive bacilli. Half of the reported cases of inhalation disease are complicated by meningitis, and hemorrhagic cerebrospinal fluid with observable organisms will confirm the diagnosis. There are no available data on examining buffy-coat smears, and therapy must be instituted before blood culture results become available. Unfortunately, the most commonly recognized form of anthrax, the cutaneous chancreform necrotic lesion, is not usually seen in inhalation cases.

The differential diagnosis includes other causes of acute mediastinitis, like esophageal perforation. Tuberculosis and histoplasmosis rarely produce *acute* respiratory failure as part of hilar and mediastinal node involvement. Lymphoproliferative diseases, like nodular sclerosing Hodgkin's, evolve at a slower pace. Chest wall and neck edema, associated with acute breathing difficulties, can accompany diphtheria or *Streptococcus pyogenes* pneumonia, and bilateral pleural effusions may be an early manifestation of streptococcal pneumonia. Acute epiglottitis is usually a disease of preteen children, and a large epiglottis can be seen by direct examination or a lateral radiograph of the neck.

TREATMENT AND PREVENTION

Treatment

Intravenously administered penicillin is the treatment of choice. Chloramphenicol or tetracycline are effective substitutes in penicillin-allergic individuals. (See Table 94-4 for specific dosage recommendations.) Unfortunately, the lower airway obstructive manifestations are not reversible once acute respiratory manifestations have developed. Assisted ventilation, drainage of pleural effusions, and use of diuretics are all reasonable support efforts, but they are generally not successful.

Prevention

Mortality in inhalation anthrax approaches 100 percent of cases, compared to a rare death from cutaneous disease. In the animal hide hair industry, prevention is the cornerstone of dealing with anthrax. Plant workers and others in contact with potentially infected animal products should be immunized with the currently available vaccine. Animal products imported from endemic regions of the world, like the Near East and the Indian subcontinent, are steam sterilized, and modern ventilation is in the workplace. At risk individuals, then, are people who service these plants, such as ventilation repairers and other transients. Bone meal is another vehicle for carrying inert spores; it should be treated by heat sterilization prior to packaging for use by commercial and home gardeners.

TABLE 94-4
Diagnostic Studies and Treatment Recommendations in Zoonotic Pneumonias

Disease	Gram-Stain Morphology	Culture Methods	Identifying Tests	Therapy Total Dose/Number of Doses*
Anthrax	*Large* gram + bacillus (rarely seen)	BAP†, blood cultures	FA	PCN (12–18 mu/6) **or** CL (4–6 g/6)
Brucellosis	*Small* gram − coccobacillus (rarely seen)	Media enriched with serum, $CO_2 + O_2$	Rise in AA	SM (1 g/2) **and** T (2 g/4) **or** TMP-SMX (480 mg + 2.4 g/3)
Melioidosis	Bipolar staining gram − bacillus	BAP, MAC	Morphology, FA, AA	TMP-SMX (640 mg + 3.2 g/4) **and** Ceftazidime (6–9 g/3) **or** CL (4–6 g/4) **or** T (3 g/4)
Pasteurellosis	*Small* bipolar staining gram − bacillus	BAP, CO_2	Inhibited by MAC, biochem. tests	PCN **or** A (6 mu **or** 8 g/4) **or** Cefotaxime (6–8 g/4) **or** CL (3 g/4)
Plague	*Enteric* bipolar staining gram − bacillus	BAP, MAC, enteric media, blood cultures	Biochem. tests, FA, AA	SM (2 g/2) **and** T (2–3 g/4) **or** CL (4–6 g/4)
Tularemia	*Small* gram − coccobacillus	Enriched media cysteine, serum	FA, AA, rarely cultured	SM **or** gentamicin (2 g/2 **or** 4.5 mg/kg/3) **or** CL (3–4 g/4) **or** T (2 g/4)
Yersiniosis	*Enteric* gram − bacillus	BAP, MAC, enteric media, blood cultures	Biochem. tests, motility 25°C	A (8 g/4) **or** 2d or 3d gen. cephalosp. (6–8 g/4)

*Expressed as million units (mu), grams (g), or milligrams (mg) divided by *number* of doses in 24 h.

†BAP = blood agar; MAC = MacConkey agar; FA = fluorescent antibody; AA = agglutinin antibody; PCN = penicillin; CL = chloramphenicol; SM = streptomycin; T = tetracycline; TMP-SMX = trimethoprim-sulfamethoxazole; A = ampicillin.

Those who import raw craft yarn from endemic areas are at special risk unless the rules for commercial hide sterilization are also imposed on casual imports as well.

Pneumonia Due to *Brucella* Species

Of the approximately 200 cases of brucellosis that are reported yearly in the United States, acute respiratory manifestations are usually insignificant. Brucellosis is often, however, a prolonged and perplexing illness, and in chronic cases pleurisy, hilar adenopathy, and nodular lung lesions are encountered. Exposure to animals or to animal foods or residence in an endemic region is usually present when sought for in the history.

BACTERIOLOGY

Brucellae are small coccobacillary, gram-negative, nonmotile, aerobic, nonencapsulated organisms of uncertain genus. Carbon dioxide is essential for growth of *Brucella abortus*, and all four pathogenic species require growth medium enriched with vitamins and serum. Using a battery of biochemical, metabolic, and immunologic criteria, brucellae pathogenic for humans can be speciated as *B. abortus*, *B. suis*, *B. melitensis*, and *B. canis*. In general the species designation corresponds to the animal usually colonized or diseased.

ECOLOGY AND EPIDEMIOLOGY

Ecology
Brucella species are distributed worldwide, wherever their natural hosts reside. Infection and disease occur primarily in domestic animals in geographic regions like the Mediterranean littoral (*B. melitensis*), worldwide except areas of Europe and Japan (*B. abortus*), midwestern United States (*B. suis*), and North and Latin America (*B. canis*). Spread from one region to another occurs with live animal transfers and when infected animal products are commercially or privately shipped. Rigorous control measures such as herd inspections and vaccination procedures have dramatically reduced enzootic and epizootic disease in many geographic regions.

Epidemiology
The epidemiology of brucellosis is intimately related to the association of susceptible individuals with infected animals and animal products. Abattoir workers (especially slaughterers) and others in the meat processing industry, farmers, dairy workers, veterinarians, and bacteriology laboratory technicians account for the majority of cases in the United States and the preponderance of male victims. Also at risk are travelers to endemic regions who eat local foods and individuals who consume imported goat cheese, sausage, and other unpasteurized edibles.

The organisms are usually acquired by ingestion, through skin abrasions and lacerations, or via conjunctival inoculation. Recent evidence indicates that aerosol spread can be a route in abattoir workers. No human-to-human transmission has been reported.

PATHOGENESIS AND PATHOPHYSIOLOGY

Organisms invade the local reticuloendothelial system (RES) and lymph nodes, followed by bacteremic spread to many organs during the following weeks. There is increasing evidence that the aerosol route may be especially efficient as a portal of entry. The distribution of nodular lesions in lung tissue is primarily in basal segments, however, which argues for bacteremia rather than primarily an inhalation mechanism for most cases of pulmonary disease.

A race between bacterial growth and the development of cell-mediated immunity ensues, primarily in lymph nodes and the RES. Like tuberculosis, the end result is often containment within granulomas that eventually become fibrotic or calcify. Species and strain differences account for the wide variety of tissue reactions encountered including granulomas, necrosis, and abscess formation. Smooth variants appear to be more virulent than rough forms and may contain polysaccharide polymers in their superficial envelope that, like true capsules, inhibit phagocytosis and intracellular destruction. Lipopolysaccharide endotoxin is present in the cell envelope and may be responsible for profound metabolic and cardiovascular effects initially and as organisms are killed during therapy. *Brucella* species are able to survive within unsensitized macrophages and can destroy these cells while escaping host antibodies and antibiotic therapy. As macrophages become activated, they develop the capacity to rapidly kill ingested *Brucella* organisms. The development of host immunity appears to be primarily cell-mediated just as in *Mycobacterium tuberculosis* disease. Impairment of cell-mediated immunity can lead to activation of latent *Brucella* or to greater susceptibility and severity of a primary infection.

CLINICAL AND RADIOLOGIC FEATURES

Clinical Features
The clinical expression of brucellosis is dominated by nonspecific flulike constitutional manifestations, including fever and headache. Nonproductive cough has been described in from 10 to 33 percent of cases, but other indicators of respiratory involvement are rarely or poorly described. In one review of 59 cases, dyspnea and pleuritic chest pain were present in 10 percent of the patients. Hoarseness, bronchitis, and rarely mucopurulent, purulent, or hemorrhagic sputum have been noted. Only one patient with verified pulmonary involvement was described in a review of 160 acute and subacute cases of

brucellosis reported in 1974. Most modern reports lack clinical details and physical findings of respiratory disease.

Radiology
The most frequent radiologic findings have been perihilar and peribronchial infiltrates or solitary granulomas. Unilateral hilar adenopathy, nodular basilar infiltrates, and pleural effusions occur occasionally.

DIAGNOSTIC FEATURES

During the acute illness or in relapse, blood cultures may be positive, especially if kept for a minimum of 14 days. In the presence of an infiltrate or pleural effusion, material for Gram stain and culture should be obtained, even though the yield from these studies is small. A positive culture may be obtained from a lymph node or pulmonary granuloma biopsy. In most cases the diagnosis is made by a fourfold rise or a single value of $\geq 1:160$ in the agglutination titer. Occasionally "inhibitory" or blocking antibodies are present in the serum and a positive titer will be discovered only if the serum is further diluted (so-called prozone phenomenon). The standard tube agglutination test utilizes *B. abortus* as the antigen and will detect antibodies to *B. suis* and *B. melitensis*, but not to *B. canis*. Diagnostic confusion and multiple alternative diagnoses are the rule in cases of brucellosis. Acute disease can be confused with miliary tuberculosis, endocarditis, tularemia, disseminated histoplasmosis, and lymphoproliferative diseases. Subacute and chronic cases must be differentiated from subacute bacterial endocarditis (SBE), tuberculosis, histoplasmosis, and other systemic fungal infections and sarcoidosis.

TREATMENT AND PREVENTION

Treatment
The combination of streptomycin and tetracycline daily for 1 month has been the most effective therapy with the fewest relapses. Gentamicin has been successfully substituted for streptomycin. Experience with trimethoprimsulfamethoxazole is encouraging, with an extremely low relapse rate. (See Table 94-4 for dosage details.)

Prevention
Preventive measures for cattle have been successful utilizing vaccination programs and destruction of diseased animals. Quarantine and inspection activities have diminished the risk of importing infected animals into the United States, and this reduction in disease in cattle has resulted in a decline in human cases. The program for *B. suis* eradication has been ineffective, and human cases of *B. suis* now outnumber those due to *B. abortus*. The efficacy of human vaccines is marginal. Education programs for workers in abattoirs have been aimed at protecting and preventing skin lacerations and eye contamina-

tion. Deployment of more experienced workers in killing rooms assures that immune (from subclinical exposures) skilled individuals will be involved in the most contaminated areas.

Pneumonia Due to *Pseudomonas Pseudomallei*

Melioidosis is primarily an acute necrotizing pneumonia or a chronic fibronodular cavitating process indistinguishable from tuberculosis. A disease of tropical latitudes, most cases have been described from southeast Asia, associated with rural settings. *P. pseudomallei* infection has been seen almost exclusively in this country after a latent period of months to years in military personnel returning from regions like Vietnam and in refugees from endemic areas.

BACTERIOLOGY

The organism is an aerobic, bipolar-staining, gram-negative bacillus that is motile and lacks a well-defined outer capsule. Like other pseudomonas, it grows well on minimal as well as enriched media, including blood and Mac-Conkey agar used in most routine laboratories. Typical colonies are distinctive in appearance, rough or wrinkled, and cream to orange in color; they may resemble a flower with folds radiating from a central core. Colonies have the typical musty, fruity odor of the family but lack pyocyanin and other pigments that characteristically stain the surrounding medium. Identification rests on a battery of biochemical reactions, and confirmation is based on agglutination or fluorescent antibody studies.

ECOLOGY AND EPIDEMIOLOGY

Ecology
P. pseudomallei occupies an environmental niche that includes moist soils, rice paddies, and other stagnant water in tropical and subtropical regions, approximately subtended by latitude 20° north to 20° south. Evidence of subclinical and clinical disease occurs in wild and domestic animal populations, as well as in humans living permanently or transiently in rural endemic areas, especially in southeast Asia and northeast Australia. As many as 10 to 30 percent of native populations have evidence of prior infection from serologic data. Approximately 1 to 2 percent of healthy American military personnel present in southeast Asia has antibodies, and almost 9 percent of wounded soldiers who served in Vietnam have titers for *P. pseudomallei*. A significant number of the approximately 3 million American soldiers who fought in the region constitute a reservoir of latent disease that, like tuberculosis, can become active even decades later, far removed from an endemic area. Refugees from southeast Asia represent another important group of carriers.

Epidemiology
Transmission is mainly by direct contact with contaminated soil or water through minor abrasions or major wounds. Ingestion and inhalation are probably less frequent modes of spread, but common source outbreaks occur in animals and humans. Animal-to-human disease has not been described, and the only reported human-to-human spread has been associated with Foley catheter contamination and venereal transmission. In endemic regions lack of previous exposure and debilitating circumstances, including malnutrition and uncontrolled diabetes, may increase susceptibility to infection and disease.

PATHOGENESIS AND PATHOPHYSIOLOGY

There is no information available on the mechanisms of pathogenicity of *P. pseudomallei*, although crude thermolabile cell-free extracts have produced necrotic lesions in experimental animals. The absence of an antiphagocytic capsule and a potent endotoxin have been noted. Acute infections are associated with necrotic, polymorphonuclear leukocyte (PMN) containing lesions in lung and in other tissues. Chronic infections, especially involving the respiratory tract, resemble tuberculosis with granuloma formation, Langhans' or foreign-body giant cells, central caseation necrosis, and occasionally a PMN response in the necrotic area. Activation of latent infection after a period of months to even decades occurs. This awakening can be in the wake of influenza and other acute infections, acute stress (trauma, thermal burn, surgery, etc.), and immunosuppressing illnesses or therapies, but spontaneous activation also occurs. The location of dormant microorganisms and the specific molecular events that stimulate recurrent diseases is unknown.

An antecedent local infection in an area of broken skin can be followed by acute septicemia in nonimmune individuals. Initial pulmonary lesions occur predominantly in the better vascularized basal segments, but eventually other areas of the lungs and other tissues are involved. Subacute and chronic disease may result from a subclinical primary focus and is often localized in apical segments, resembling tuberculosis in location and propensity for granuloma formation and cavitation. Subpleural involvement can result in empyema or sympathetic sterile effusions.

CLINICAL AND RADIOLOGIC FEATURES

Clinical Features
Primary melioidosis occurs within a few days to 2 weeks of exposure, usually in individuals present in or recently from an endemic area. Military personnel with outdoor injuries constitute a potential group for delayed active disease. In the United States the acute phase of melioidosis is rarely seen. The portal of entry may be pres-

ent as a small necrotic skin lesion in an area of known trauma, with accompanying cellulitis or lymphangitis. In addition to marked toxicity and high fevers, the respiratory complaints include cough, dyspnea, pleuritic pain, and purulent sputum. Bibasilar rales may be heard, but objective findings are often minimal in the face of severe toxicity. Mortality approaches 75 percent, even when the diagnosis is suspected and appropriate therapy immediately instituted.

Milder types of subacute and chronic pneumonia are usually seen in patients developing clinical illness after leaving an endemic area. In addition to fever, productive cough, and pleuritic pain, many patients experience marked weight loss and a clinical picture resembling tuberculosis or fungal disease. Secondary skin manifestations are rarely seen, unless bacteremia ensues. Physical changes are often subtle but can include localized rales, a pleural friction rub, signs of an effusion, and manifestations of disease localized to soft tissues, lymph nodes, bones, or joints.

Radiology

Radiologic findings reflect the stage of disease present. In acute fulminant infections, airspace disease can be absent or miliary to larger nodular densities seen in basal segments. In subacute and chronic cases, fibronodular, or cavitary apical lesions are found.

DIAGNOSTIC FEATURES

Melioidosis should be seriously entertained in any febrile patient with a history of residence in a major endemic region like southeast Asia or northeast Australia. If sputum is available, the gram-negative bipolar staining bacilli may be seen, and the organisms can be readily cultured and identified by the routine laboratory. Blood and urine cultures are frequently positive in acute cases. In more indolent infections, biopsy may be necessary. Serologic studies can be helpful in active and recrudescent disease. A specific IgM immunofluorescence test is often positive in recent infections and recrudescent disease. Complement fixation and indirect hemagglutination tests are available and require testing of paired sera over several weeks to confirm active disease.

DIFFERENTIAL DIAGNOSIS

Acute fulminating infections with pneumonia, in patients from southeast Asia, may be due to traditional bacteria and viruses, but may also be caused by infection with *Yersinia pestis* (plague) and *Francisella tularensis* (tularemia) (see below).

Chronic forms of melioidosis resemble tuberculosis and fungal infections such as histoplasmosis and blastomycosis. Occupation, travel, and history of prior respira-

tory illness should help to clarify the etiology. Confirmation usually requires biopsy with special stains and culture, or serologic data.

TREATMENT AND PREVENTION

Treatment

Recommendations for therapy of acute septicemic melioidosis must be couched in cautious statements. During the Vietnam War mortality rates of greater than 50 percent occurred, even using massive doses of three drug regimens. In subacute and chronic pneumonias, and recrudescent disease, cure rates approach 100 percent. Treatment must be prolonged, and surgical intervention for drainage or removal of cavitary lesions is sometimes necessary.

During the past decade a number of encouraging reports have confirmed the efficacy of trimethoprim-sulfamethoxazole for acute and other forms of respiratory disease. Limited experience with the third-generation cephalosporins indicates that ceftazidime may be the most effective newer antimicrobial for treating severe disease. In selected patients results have supported the continued usefulness of the tetracyclines and chloramphenicol. In vitro data for the fourth-generation penicillin, piperacillin, are encouraging, but no clinical experience with this agent is available. In most instances *P. pseudomallei* is resistant to the other penicillins, first- and second-generation cephalosporins, erythromycin and, excepting kanamycin, the aminoglycosides.

Although contemporary experience is limited, and in vitro data must serve as a guide, suggested recommendations for acute and chronic infections are outlined in Table 94-4. It should be emphasized that this is a controversial area, that dosages are enormous and drug toxicity can limit the usefulness of many recommended agents. Modifications in these programs must be guided by clinical circumstances and await more definitive studies.

Prevention

There are no prophylactic antimicrobial studies available, nor has a vaccine been developed. Individuals traveling, working, or living in endemic regions should be advised of this soil- and water-dwelling organism. Care and caution should be used to avoid traumatic injuries, and any wounds contaminated with soil or stagnant water should be assiduously cleansed.

Pulmonary Infections Due to *Yersinia Enterocolitica*

The majority of infections caused by *Y. enterocolitica* involve the gastrointestinal tract, causing a self-limited gastroenteritis or appendicitis-mimicking mesenteric and terminal ileum adenitis. Septicemias and involvement of the lungs and other viscera are extremely rare, usually occur-

ring in individuals suffering from cirrhosis or who are immunocompromised.

Yersiniae belong to the family Enterobacteriaceae. *Y. enterocolitica* is a gram-negative, facultative bacillus that resembles many other enteric microbes. Identification procedures include the ability to grow and exhibit motility at room temperature plus a battery of biochemical and serologic tests. Although occasionally overlooked in stool because it is confused with many other members of the fecal flora, the organism is readily identified in blood and respiratory specimens. Most strains are nonlactose or slow lactose fermenters, causing confusion with *Y. pestis,* *Salmonella, Shigella,* and several other members of the Enterobacteriaceae family. Cold enrichment techniques and highly selective media, extensively used to identify this organism in fecal specimens, are not necessary in nonfecal material. Multiple serotypes and biotypes, with distribution in geographically distinct regions, have been described.

Y. enterocolitica has been isolated from a variety of rodents and other wild animals, and from cats and dogs. There is little evidence for direct transmission or for spread among people other than by the fecal-oral route. Most cases occur singly, but epidemics involving families and hundreds of people have been described. Disease is initiated by ingestion of contaminated milk or other food. Most cases of respiratory disease have been reported in immunocompromised hosts, alcoholics, and cirrhotics.

Direct aspiration may be the mechanism for initiation of pulmonary disease, following an initial pharyngeal focus. Bacteremia can complicate pharyngeal disease, although the most likely mechanism involves ulceration of Peyer's patches in the terminal ileum, mesenteric adenitis, and portal bacteremia. Systemic shunting to the lungs can follow, especially in cirrhotics, the group that most frequently develops septicemia. Mechanisms of pathogenesis are not clarified, but strains virulent for animals and causing human disease have plasmid-mediated V and W envelope antigens, temperature-sensitive calcium dependency (like *Y. pestis*), a factor that enhances cell penetration, and endotoxin. An enterotoxin, similar to stable toxin of *E. coli,* is also produced, but an extragastrointestinal role has not been established for this material. The development of immune-complex manifestations like erythema nodosum and nonsuppurative polyarthritis may contribute to pathogenicity.

During the past decade, concomitant with greater recognition of this pathogen as a cause of gastroenteritis, cases of pneumonia and lung abscess have been reported. Respiratory infections occur in association with an acute febrile septicemic illness or as a primary respiratory process, with cough, dyspnea and signs of consolidation. The history is usually vague for gastrointestinal symptoms, animal exposures, or unusual food intake. There may be signs of increasing hepatic failure with ascites or peritoni-

tis in patients with underlying cirrhosis. Radiologic findings include nodular basilar densities consistent with septicemic spread, dependent segment infiltrates suggesting an aspiration mechanism, occasionally with cavitation, and fluffy widespread densities consistent with septic emboli.

The diagnosis often depends on information obtained from blood or sputum cultures. Entericlike, gram-negative bacilli can be seen in sputum. Pharyngeal cultures should be done if signs of local inflammation are present. Suppurating nodes and peritoneal or joint fluids are other sources of material that may contribute to the diagnosis when sputum is not available.

Cases of respiratory infection have responded well to a variety of antibiotics, including ampicillin or second-generation cephalosporins. Third-generation cephalosporins, chloramphenicol, and aminoglycosides are also effective. Underlying diseases influence the outcome, but when pneumonia is the major problem, prognosis is excellent. Treatment is usually continued for a total of 3 to 6 weeks. (See Table 94-4 for dosage details.)

Preventive measures include avoiding rodent or domestic animal contamination of food and water supplies. Opportunities for susceptible individuals to come in contact with this zoonotic microorganism may be increasing as well, and immunocompromised people look to natural foods and mineral waters for improved health.

ZOONOTIC BACTERIAL PNEUMONIAS

A wide variety of domestic and wild vertebrates are colonized by bacteria capable of producing pneumonia in humans. In this section three diseases that illustrate the mechanisms for dissemination and the characteristic features of respiratory involvement are described. There are few unique distinguishing clinical features that reveal the etiology of these infections. Clues derived from a careful history of travel, occupation, hobbies, and animal and arthropod contact, however, are invaluable aides to the correct diagnosis and therapy and can be lifesaving.

Pasteurella Multocida Respiratory Infections

Pasteurella multocida is a common commensal of the oral cavity of most felines and many dogs and a frequent respiratory pathogen in animals and birds. In the United States the domestic associations are responsible for many cases of cellulitis following cat or dog bites. Respiratory infections are rarely reported, with fewer than 50 cases on record. Sputum isolates, however, are not infrequent in individuals with chronic pulmonary disease.

BACTERIOLOGY

P. multocida is a small gram-negative bipolar staining coccobacillary organism that resembles *Hemophilus* species.

Rapid growth on blood agar and inhibition by MacConkey medium help to separate this microorganism from other common components of the respiratory flora.

ECOLOGY AND EPIDEMIOLOGY

In cats and other felines the organism resides periodontally in the anterior regions of the mouth. Isolates from dogs are characteristically from the posterior pharynx. Many birds and domestic and wild animals worldwide harbor this organism as a commensal in the oral or gastrointestinal areas. *P. multocida* is occasionally found in the secretions of individuals with chronic lung disease, especially with bronchiectasis, often without a history of animal contacts. No human-to-human transmission has been documented. The organism can survive in soil and water for upward of 3 weeks, and in animal carcasses for approximately 2 months.

PATHOGENESIS AND PATHOPHYSIOLOGY

Pathogenic strains have a polysaccharide capsule that inhibits phagocytosis, and they contain endotoxin in the cell envelope. Exotoxins and other pathogenicity-promoting factors have not been identified. Almost all patients who develop respiratory infections have underlying chronic pulmonary disease. Aspiration probably initiates active infection. Necrosis and lung abscess, empyema, septicemia, and transbronchial spread to other lung segments have been described.

CLINICAL AND RADIOLOGIC FEATURES

The clinical features of *P. multocida* respiratory disease include worsening of the patient's baseline respiratory function, especially when high fever, tenacious secretions, and pleural effusions develop. Radiologic changes include lobar, multilobar, or diffuse patchy infiltrates, usually sparing the upper lobes, superimposed on underlying chronic lung disease (Fig. 94-2). Effusions have been noted in approximately 20 percent of cases.

DIAGNOSTIC FEATURES

The diagnosis depends upon isolating the organism from sputum, pleural fluid, or blood. The pathogen can usually be identified by the routine methodology of the diagnostic laboratory. The bipolar, gram-negative staining bacilli resemble *Brucella* species, *Yersinia pestis*, *Francisella tularensis*, *P. pseudomallei*, and *Hemophilus* species.

TREATMENT

The majority of strains are exquisitely susceptible to penicillin or ampicillin. The third-generation cephalosporin, cefotaxime, is as active as penicillin and more potent than earlier generation relatives. Tetracycline and chloram-

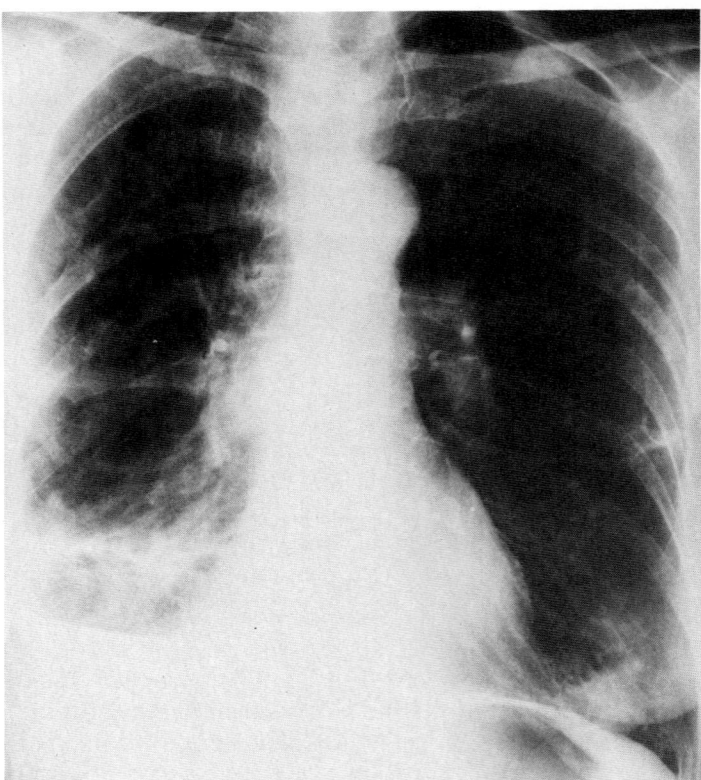

FIGURE 94-2   Bilateral pneumonia due to *Pasteurella multocida* in a 69-year-old woman suffering from chronic obstructive pulmonary disease and a prior right lower lobectomy for carcinoma. Infiltrates disappeared with penicillin therapy.

phenicol are useful when a history of immediate allergic reactions precludes use of a β-lactam agent. Oral preparations of cephalosporins and penicillins are not recommended for treating pneumonias due to *P. multocida*. (See Table 94-4 for specific dosages of useful agents.)

Pneumonia Due to *Yersinia Pestis*

This organism left an indelible mark on humanity long before its late nineteenth century isolation and characterization. The cause of three major pandemics from the sixth through the nineteenth centuries A.D., pulmonary disease in a few victims lead to aerosol spread to countless others, resulting in acute primary pneumonia and the "black death" of epidemic plague. In the United States approximately 20 cases of plague are reported yearly, of which 20 percent have lung involvement. Early recognition and specific therapy, combined with isolation procedures and appropriately directed prophylaxis of contacts, should help maintain a record of no human-to-human transmission since the 1920s.

BACTERIOLOGY

Y. pestis is a bipolar staining, gram-negative bacillus closely related to *E. coli* and other Enterobacteriaceae. It grows well on blood or MacConkey agar and is identified definitively using differential biochemical tests, agglutination reactions, and direct fluorescent antibody staining.

ECOLOGY AND EPIDEMIOLOGY

Ecology
In the United States *Y. pestis* is endemic in rock squirrels, prairie dogs, and other ground animals. Spread among animals occurs via several species of rodent fleas. Domestic animals that wander outdoors, like cats, can become infected by direct contact with sick rodents or via rodent flea bites. In addition, cats and dogs can inadvertently bring fleas home. Occasionally rodent die-offs, called epizootics, occur, and many dead animals can be found with viable organisms in carcasses and in the soil surrounding ground dwellings.

Epidemiology
In the United States spread to humans occurs in the endemic areas west of the Rockies, especially in California, northern Arizona and New Mexico, when a thirsty flea feeds upon a susceptible person. Living or working in proximity to local enzootic "hot spots" places certain groups like American Indians, geologists, hikers, veterinarians, and pet owners at risk. Bubonic and cutaneous plague is usually acquired by contact with infected fleas, but aerosols from ill animals or from carcasses can lead to primary pneumonia, pharyngitis, or conjunctivitis. Several cases of cat-to-human aerosol spread have been described in the past decade. The great fear of physicians caring for patients with respiratory involvement is the potential for rapid airborne dissemination, especially during coughing and face-to-face contacts.

PATHOGENESIS AND PATHOPHYSIOLOGY

Once the organism gains access to human tissues at 37°C, rapid multiplication occurs with formation of a polysaccharide capsule. The capsule imparts virulence properties that include resisting phagocytosis and persistence of bacteria within nonsensitized monocytes. Virulence factors impacting on the host also include a potent endotoxin and V and W antigens of the cell envelope, which also influence intracellular survival. Bacteremic spread usually follows initial multiplication in regional nodes or at the local flea bite site. *Secondary pneumonia* involving the well-perfused basal segments can follow. Theoretically, when an individual with plague pneumonia coughs, there may be aerosol spread to individuals in proximity, resulting in *primary pneumonia*. Occasionally, ingested organisms can infect the nasopharynx with resulting adult respiratory distress syndrome.

CLINICAL AND RADIOLOGIC FEATURES

Clinical Features
The clinical presentation of pneumonia depends on the mechanism of spread. In contemporary experience in the United States, cases have all been secondary to bubonic plague or to primary septicemia without an overt skin lesion. The onset of respiratory disease follows after days to a week of a febrile illness, and is ushered in by the gradual onset of cough, dyspnea, and increasing toxicity. A hemorrhagic productive cough, pleurisy, and increasing respiratory distress are additional symptoms. The unique feature in most cases of pneumonia is the epidemiologic association with classic bubonic plague in a person recently in an endemic area. From cases of primary inhalation pneumonia described previously, exposure to an index case may be followed by the rapid development of a fulminating respiratory illness with dyspnea, cyanosis, and thin, watery sputum that rapidly becomes hemorrhagic. The clinical picture is not unlike overwhelming pneumococcal pneumonia with marked toxicity and mental torpor associated with progressive cyanosis.

Radiology
The radiologic features of secondary pneumonia include basal segment nodular to hazy airspace infiltrates, hilar and mediastinal node hypertrophy, and occasionally pleural effusions. In primary pneumonia, infiltrates may be minimal during the first 24 h followed by progressive airspace disease resembling ARDS or pulmonary edema.

DIAGNOSIS AND DIFFERENTIAL DIAGNOSIS

The presence of characteristic bipolar staining, gram-negative bacilli in sputum supports the diagnosis. Cultures of blood, sputum, and lymph node aspirates often yield positive results. Direct fluorescent antibody staining, if available, can provide immediate etiologic confirmation. Other acute respiratory infections caused by microorganisms that appear as gram-negative bacilli with bipolar staining must be considered, including *F. tularensis*, and *P. multocida*.

TREATMENT AND PREVENTION

Treatment
The combination of streptomycin and tetracycline has been the treatment of choice for serious plague infections. Gentamicin can be substituted for streptomycin if intravenous therapy is necessary. In patients with impaired renal function chloramphenicol should be used in place of tetracycline. (See Table 94-4 for dosage schedules.)

Prevention
Individuals suspected of having plague pneumonia should be rapidly isolated, and strict contact and respiratory and conjunctival precautions should be instituted.

Anyone exposed face-to-face with a coughing patient, including health care workers, should be given preventive tetracycline, 2 g daily, divided into four doses for 5 to 10 days. Isolation procedures are continued until productive cough is no longer present or sputum cultures are negative for *Y. pestis.*

A vaccine is available for laboratory workers and others with frequent exposure to the microorganism or to hyperendemic areas. Careful surveillance of ground rodent populations, posting warnings in endemic regions, watching for die-offs that indicate epizootic spread, and spraying for local flea control may also be effective preventive measures.

Pneumonia Due to *Francisella Tularensis*

Tularemia is a common zoonotic disease in the United States. The etiologic agent, *F. tularensis*, is ubiquitous, distributed among many species of wild and domestic animals and birds. Bloodsucking arthropods serve an important role in transmission. Like plague, the major clinical manifestations involve skin lesions and draining regional lymph nodes. Pulmonary involvement occurs secondary to bacteremia or as a primary inhalation or aspiration pneumonia. Approximately 150 cases occur in the United States yearly. Pulmonary involvement is seen in 10 to 15 percent of ulceroglandular cases and in greater than 50 percent of patients with the typhoidal syndrome.

BACTERIOLOGY

F. tularensis is a fragile-appearing, gram-negative coccobacillary organism that grows poorly on artificial media unless fortified with serum and cysteine (or sulfhydryl compounds). The potential for laboratory-acquired inhalation or ingestion-associated disease is great. Most routine laboratories will not attempt to culture the organism, leaving this to special reference centers. Identification is on the basis of morphologic and biochemical determinants, but direct fluorescent staining or agglutination reactions with specific antisera are also useful.

ECOLOGY AND EPIDEMIOLOGY

Ecology

The organism is found in nature associated with over 100 species of wild and domestic animals and birds, but most clinical cases involve contact with rabbits, squirrels, or arthropods. Aquatic mammals and their immediate water and mud living environments can also be contaminated with *F. tularensis.* Bloodsucking arthropods, especially ticks and deerflies, act as reservoirs capable of harboring the pathogen for long periods and are responsible for dissemination among wildlife species.

Epidemiology

Most human cases are acquired from contact with infected animals during hunting, trapping, and other outdoor pursuits, especially during colder months. In more southern areas, or in the summer season in northern latitudes, bloodsucking arthropods constitute a significant mode of spread. Ingestion of contaminated food, animal bites, conjunctival contact, and aerosol dissemination are also important mechanisms for acquiring the pathogen. Human-to-human transmission is not recognized in contrast to the significant theoretical potential for spread of pneumonic plague.

PATHOGENESIS AND PATHOPHYSIOLOGY

F. tularensis contains a number of protein and polysaccharide antigens in the cell envelope and an endotoxin component that is similar to endotoxins of other gram-negative microorganisms. There is very little known about other mechanisms of pathogenesis. The organism is capable of remaining viable in RES cells of nonimmune individuals and in macrophages that have not been stimulated by recent prior exposure to intracellular pathogens. As few as 10 to 50 organisms can initiate disease following cutaneous penetration or by inhalation, but a significant number are required when the challenge is through ingestion. Local growth usually is followed by regional node suppuration and occasionally bacteremic dissemination to many organs, including the lungs. Rhabdomyolysis of uncertain cause may accompany bacteremia and pneumonia. Ingestion may result in pharyngeal infection, involvement of the gastrointestinal tract, or subclinical disease followed by the typhoidal syndrome. Primary pneumonia follows inhalation of organisms, resulting in multiple areas of inflammation, necrosis, and a tendency to granuloma formation.

CLINICAL AND RADIOLOGIC FEATURES

Clinical Features

Respiratory disease is heralded by the onset of a nonproductive cough, usually in a febrile patient ill with the ulceroglandular form of tularemia. In the absence of a local chancreform lesion or tender swollen lymph node (bubo), the disease may be dominated by constitutional symptoms with high fever and shaking chills (typhoidal tularemia). Pneumonia following an inhalation exposure results in cough, dyspnea, and occasionally pleurisy. Respiratory disease can be subtle, and the diagnosis apparent only if a chest radiograph is done.

Radiology

Radiologic changes include evidence of parenchymal and pleural disease, which is often out of proportion to the physical findings. Diffuse areas of bronchopneumonia occur, with hilar node enlargement. Unilateral or bilateral pleural effusions are often noted (Fig. 94-3). Central oval infiltrates, described as characteristic in early reports, are seldom observed today. Lobar airspace disease and lung

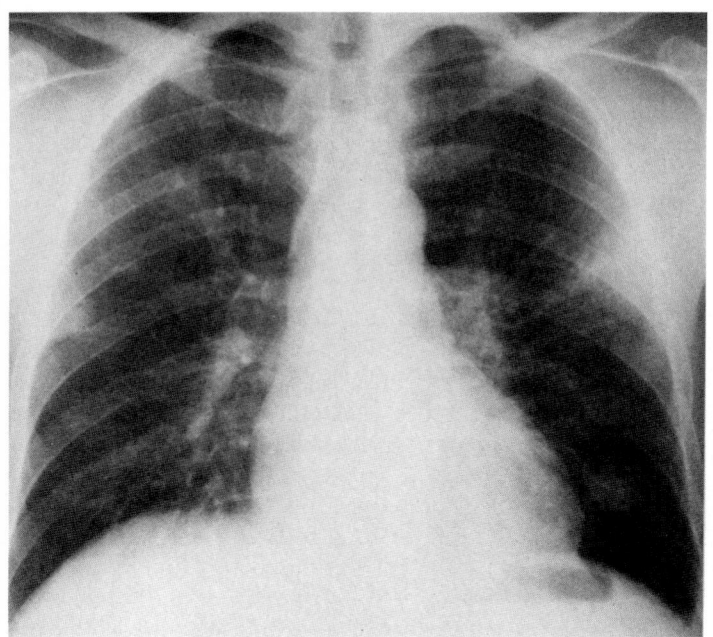

FIGURE 94-3 Patchy nodular and bronchopneumonia, hilar adenopathy, and left pleural effusion due to *Francisella tularensis* in a 38-year-old veterinarian exposed to a cat dying with a respiratory infection. All the findings resolved with tetracycline therapy.

abscess are unusual additional patterns that have been described.

DIAGNOSIS AND DIFFERENTIAL DIAGNOSIS

Diagnostic Features
Any febrile patient with animal or arthropod exposure in an endemic region, especially presenting with a skin lesion or tender lymph node, should be evaluated for tularemia. Respiratory involvement is confirmed by radiographic study. Cough, when present, is usually nonproductive, and blood cultures are seldom positive. Characteristic organisms are rarely seen in pleural fluid or aspirates of suppurating nodes. Direct fluorescent antibody staining of exudates can confirm the diagnosis, but this method is not widely available. Serologic agglutination testing of paired sera is usually necessary for diagnostic confirmation, but a single convalescent titer of 1:160 or greater is considered highly suspicious for active disease. An elevated blood level of creatine phosphokinase (CPK) is a clue that tularemia-induced rhabdomyolysis is the cause of the acute infection, especially in highly endemic areas. Skin testing can be helpful in diagnosis, but the antigen is not commercially available.

Differential Diagnosis
Among the respiratory infections that are confused with tularemia, nonbacterial diseases, which are also associated with outdoor and animal exposures like psittacosis and Q fever, are especially important. Legionnaires' disease and mycoplasma pneumonias can present with similar clinical courses, without diagnostic sputum. Plague, tuberculosis, and systemic fungal infections produce a spectrum of acute to chronic respiratory manifestations that can be confused with pulmonary tularemia.

TREATMENT AND PREVENTION

Treatment
Streptomycin was the first effective antibiotic for treating all forms of tularemia and still remains the agent of choice. Gentamicin appears to be equally potent and has the advantage of a broader spectrum of activity if initiating treatment when the etiologic diagnosis is less secure. Additionally, it can be given intravenously, and blood levels can be monitored. Recent experience confirms that results of therapy are optimal when an aminoglycoside is chosen early in the clinical illness. Tetracycline and chloramphenicol are useful alternatives when an aminoglycoside is contraindicated, but relapse rates are higher, especially when tetracycline is given for less than 2 weeks. The prognosis is excellent with appropriate antimicrobial therapy. (See Table 94-4 for specific dosages.)

Prevention
Cautious practices are required when dealing with animals and their carcasses. Using gloves, cooking wild animal meat thoroughly, and wearing protective clothing and repellants to avoid sucking arthropods are helpful measures. Immunoprophylaxis with an attenuated strain is in the developmental stage and, when available, may be effective in protecting high-risk individuals like hunters, trappers, and selected laboratory personnel.

BIBLIOGRAPHY

Alsofrom DJ, Mettler FA, Mann JM: Radiographic manifestations of plague in New Mexico, 1975–1980. Radiology 139:561–565, 1981.
  A radiologically oriented review of 42 well-documented cases from the past decade, with excellent clinical correlations.

Barnes PF, Appleman MD, Cosgrove MM: A case of melioidosis originating in North America. Am Rev Respir Dis 134:170–171, 1986.
  A case of melioidosis is described in a patient from Mexico.

Buchanan TM, Faber LC, Feldman RA: Brucellosis in the United States, 1960–1972. Medicine 53:403–413, 1974.
A study of an epidemic of 160 cases of brucellosis at one abattoir illustrates the paucity of respiratory signs and symptoms except for cough (present in 23 percent) and documented pneumonia (one case).

Cropp AJ, Gaylord SF, Watanakunakorn C: Case Report: Cavitary pneumonia due to *Yersinia enterocolitica* in a healthy man. Am J Med Sci 288:130–132, 1984.
A survey of respiratory disease associated with Yersinia enterocolitica including underlying disease, laboratory data, and brief remarks on therapy.

Doern GV: *Branhamella catarrhalis*—An emerging human pathogen. Diag Microb Infect Dis 4:191–201, 1986.
An up-to-date review of all facets of the bacteriology and clinical impact of B. catarrhalis, including respiratory disease, with a complete bibliography.

Evans ME, Gregory DW, Schaffner W, McGee ZA: Tularemia: A 30-year experience with 88 cases. Medicine 64:251–269, 1985.
From the area of the United States where tularemia is most prevalent, this extensive article considers all facets of epidemiology and clinical disease, including pulmonary aspects as well as diagnostic tests and therapy.

Everett ED, Nelson RA: Pulmonary melioidosis. Am Rev Respir Dis 112:331–340, 1975.
A clinical report of 39 cases from the military experience in Vietnam, with an excellent discussion of the subacute and chronic presentation of a tuberculosislike syndrome.

Greer AE: Pulmonary brucellosis. Dis Chest 29:508–519, 1956.
The most recent analysis of a large number of cases of the respiratory manifestations of brucellosis; for reference when evaluating isolated occasional reports of the past decade.

Hager H, Verghese A, Alvarez S, Berk S: *Branhamella catarrhalis* respiratory infections. Rev Infect Dis 9:1140–1149, 1987.
In addition to six personally studied cases, the authors report on a review of 429 patients with Branhamella lower respiratory infections. The findings confirm the importance of underlying pulmonary disease in the background of most patients and the contribution of immunosuppressive medications and illnesses to susceptibility. Bacteriologic findings analyze mixed infections, too, and antibiotic sensitivities are detailed.

Meyer KF: Pneumonic plague. Bact Rev 25:249–261, 1961.
An extensive and thoughtful review of the respiratory manifestations of plague, including studies of experimental pneumonia and clinical details of primary and secondary respiratory infections.

Miller RP, Bates JH: Pleuropulmonary tularemia. Am Rev Respir Dis 99:31–41, 1969.
An excellent, detailed review of the pulmonary manifestations of tularemia; well-illustrated with radiographs and including a discussion of arthropod-borne cases.

Nelson SC, Hammer GS: *Pasteurella multocida* empyema: Case report and review of the literature. Am J Med Sci 281:43–49, 1981.
A full discussion of the pleural manifestations of P. multocida, with a review of patient backgrounds and reported cases from the literature.

Penn RL, Kinasewitz GT: Factors associated with a poor outcome in tularemia. Arch Intern Med 147:265–268, 1987.
A review of 28 cases, focusing on the factors that are associated with severe disease and poor outcome, stressing the importance of early suspicion of tularemia and prompt use of an aminoglycoside like streptomycin or gentamicin.

Plotkin SA, Brachman PS, Utell M, Bumford FH, Atchison MM: An epidemic of inhalation anthrax, the first in the twentieth century. Am J Med 29:992–1000, 1960.
An important clinical report of a very rare manifestation of anthrax, with radiographs and clinical observations of five cases graphically depicting this catastrophic disease.

Polsky B, Gold JW, Whimbey E, Dryjanski J, Brown AE, Schiffman G, Armstrong D: Bacterial pneumonia in patients with the acquired immunodeficiency syndrome. Ann Intern Med 104:38–41, 1986.
Eighteen episodes of community-acquired bacterial pneumonia were diagnosed in 13 patients among 336 with the acquired immunodeficiency syndrome (AIDS). Bacterial pathogens isolated in 16 to 18 episodes were Haemophilus influenzae in 8, Streptococcus pneumoniae in 6, group B streptococcus in 1, and Branhamella catarrhalis in 1.

Robinson A, Johnson PC, Griffith SB: Clinical interpretation of beta-lactamase-producing strains of Branhamella catarrhalis in sputum Gram's stain and culture. Am J Clin Pathol 87:498–503, 1987.
> *Sputum Gram stain and culture results suggesting significant infection with β-lactamase-producing strains of B. catarrhalis should be interpreted with caution.*

Rubin SA: Radiographic spectrum of pleuropulmonary tularemia. Am J Roentgenol 131:277–281, 1978.
> *A valuable report focusing on radiographic findings and including patients without respiratory symptoms.*

Slevin NJ, Aitken J, Thornley PE: Clinical and microbiological features of Branhamella catarrhalis bronchopulmonary infections. Lancet 1:782–783, 1984.
> *A recent experience of 101 adult cases of B. catarrhalis bronchopulmonary disease from a general hospital, with details of underlying disease, bacteriology, and antimicrobial susceptibility and stressing the emergence of β-lactamase-producing strains with resulting treatment failures using penicillin-ampicillin.*

Spotnitz M, Rudnitzky J, Rambaud JJ: Melioidosis pneumonitis. JAMA 202:126–130, 1967.
> *A very sound clinical report from the military experience in Vietnam focusing on the subacute form of the disease in nine patients.*

Syrjala H, Sutinen S, Jokinen K, Nieminen P, Tuuponen T, Salminen A: Bronchial changes in airborne tularemia. J Laryngol Otol 100:1169–1176, 1986.
> *In seven patients with "typhoidal tularemia", four of whom has had exposure to Francisella tularensis by inhalation, pathologic changes were found in the airways during diagnostic bronchoscopy.*

Teutsch SM, Martone WJ, Brink EW, Potter ME, Eliot G, Hoxsie R, Craven RB, Kaufman AF: Pneumonic tularemia on Martha's Vineyard. N Engl J Med 301:826–828, 1979.
> *A detailed report describing inhalation tularemia in seven patients with information on the circumstances of dissemination by the aerosol route.*

Vessal K, Yeganehdoust J, Dutz W, Kohout E: Radiological changes in inhalation anthrax: A report of radiological and pathological correlation in two cases. Clin Radiol 26:471–474, 1975.
> *A brief but detailed description of the radiologic clues in inhalation anthrax, focusing on the early sign of widening of the mediastinum with smooth sharp demarcation from adjacent lung tissue.*

Weber DJ, Douglass LE, Brundage WG, Stallkamp TC: Acute varieties of melioidosis occurring in U.S. soldiers in Vietnam. Am J Med 46:234–244, 1969.
> *A discussion of the devastating acute septicemic form of melioidosis contrasted with subacute cases; emphasis is on the urgency of antimicrobial therapy using massive doses of drugs.*

Weber DJ, Wolfson JS, Swartz MN, Hooper DC: Pasteurella multocida infections. Medicine 63:133–154, 1984.
> *An exhaustive recent review of cases from the Massachusetts General Hospital, including a thoughtful discussion of the respiratory disease, bacteriology, ecology of the pathogen, and therapy.*

Weinberg AN: Pneumonia due to Neisseria meningitidis, in Weinstein L, Fields BN (eds), Seminars in Infectious Disease, vol 8. New York, Thieme-Stratton, 1983, pp 147–158.
> *A recent review of the literature of meningococcal respiratory infections including an update on bacteriology, serogroups, epidemiology, pathogenesis, and a summary of contemporary cases.*

Chapter 95

Community-Acquired Pneumonia

Cyrus C. Hopkins

Pneumonia is a parenchymal infection of the lung that is distinguished from infections of the larger airways alone, e.g., tracheobronchitis, even though many of the same organisms cause both conditions. Pneumonia that develops outside the hospital, without iatrogenic or invasive procedures, is considered to be community-acquired. Most community-acquired pneumonias are caused by a few agents which often produce a predictable clinical pattern.

ACQUISITION AND PATHOGENESIS

Several routes can be involved in establishing a site of parenchymal lung infection. Among these are aspiration, droplets, airborne transmission, and hematogenous spread. The most common of these for bacterial pneumonias is *aspiration* of small numbers of organisms from the pharynx. Both the upper and lower respiratory tracts have a variety of defenses against this source of contamination of pulmonary parenchyma. Usually they are very effective. Although small amounts of pharyngeal fluid find their way into the lower respiratory tract quite regularly, especially during sleep (microaspiration), tracheobronchitis and pneumonia are relatively uncommon. However, alterations in host defenses can lead to pneumonia. Indeed, these alterations are perhaps more important than the intrinsic virulence of pharyngeal organisms themselves, at least for the common bacterial pneumonias acquired by this route.

Droplets can be responsible for the spread of some organisms from one patient to another, especially for viral and mycoplasmal infections. This type of transmission requires close contact between individuals and exchange of respiratory secretions, with or without interposition of infected fomites. In such situations, the infection may first be deposited on nasal or pharyngeal mucosa, whence it is subsequently aspirated into the lung.

Airborne transmission is not involved in the most common causes of pneumonia, though a few important diseases are spread by an airborne route.

Finally, *hematogenous spread* of organisms can occur, involving the lungs from infections elsewhere. The most common source for this type of spread is either the abdominal or pelvic veins or right-sided endocarditis. Combinations of these routes can also occur, as when a pulmonary infarction becomes secondarily infected.

ETIOLOGY AND FREQUENCY

Streptococcus pneumoniae ("pneumococcus") is the most common single etiologic agent, compromising more than half of all community-acquired pneumonias. Other agents, notably *Mycoplasma pneumoniae* and *Legionella pneumophila*, or viral infections are less common. Other uncommon but important causes of bacterial pneumonias are *Hemophilus influenzae*, *Staphylococcus aureus*, and a number of gram-negative bacilli, especially *Klebsiella pneumoniae*.

Although viral infections of the upper respiratory tract are frequent, they do not often cause pneumonia, especially in the adult.

Other etiologic agents, such as *Legionella pneumophila*, have caused either outbreaks or sporadic cases, but these are exceptions. Even in situations of unusual exposure or of immunocompromise, the commonest etiologies still occur most often. For example, even though the immunocompromised patient is a better candidate for an "opportunistic" pneumonia than is the normal individual, the commonest community-acquired pneumonias in immunocompromised patients are those commonly seen in the normal population.

CLINICAL PRESENTATION

Certain clinical features are common to all pneumonias, although they may differ considerably in degree: (1) respiratory distress, which is manifested either as dyspnea, or as tachypnea or alterations in blood gases; (2) increased airway or respiratory secretions, often manifested by increased cough and sputum production; and (3) the systemic response, which may include fever, chills, malaise, fatigue, and leukocytosis. Specific systemic signs or signs of infection in other organ systems are helpful in differential diagnosis and in the choice of therapy.

The features most useful in diagnosis are the anatomic pattern as observed on chest radiograph, the acuity of illness, and the sputum examination. Taken together, these usually constitute a consistent pattern of presentation for the most important etiologic agents (Table 95-1), even though there are many exceptions and any single feature taken out of context may be misleading.

Radiology

A chest radiograph showing some kind of parenchymal involvement is virtually required to establish the existence, as well as the nature, of pneumonia. The different etiologic agents can cause anatomic differences in the pattern of disease on the chest radiograph. Although these radiologic patterns are far from specific, they may exclude certain etiologic possibilities. For example, the finding of a consolidated lobe mitigates strongly against uncomplicated viral pneumonia, especially if cavitation is also present. In addition, the nature of the infiltrate is generally reflected in the findings on physical examination.

LOBAR CONSOLIDATION

Lobar consolidation features prominently early in the course of certain bacterial infections, especially pneumococcal (or rarely, streptococcal) infections; in these types of pneumonia, rapid spread of early watery infiltrate can occur throughout the lobe without respect to segmental boundaries. Certain gram-negative pneumonias, e.g., *Klebsiella* pneumonia, can also present with a homogeneous lobar infiltrate. In either instance, the abundant exudate filling the lobe may result in an apparent enlargement or swelling of the lobe, producing a "bulging fissure" at its margin. This radiographic appearance is uncommon with other bacterial infections, and essentially does not occur with viral infection.

TABLE 95-1
*Paradigmatic Patterns of Pneumonia**

Type	Clinical Presentation	Chest Radiograph	Sputum Gram Stain — Cells	Sputum Gram Stain — Organisms
Lobar pneumonia (Pneumococcal; streptococcal; *Hemophilus,* especially in children)	Acute	Lobar, homogeneous without destruction	Polymorphonuclear leukocytes	Helpful, if abundant, diagnostic or atypical
Bronchopneumonia [Pneumococcal; *H. influenzae* (especially in adults with bronchitis); *S. aureus*]	Acute	Patchy With or without destruction, depending on organism	Polymorphonuclear leukocytes	Helpful, if abundant, diagnostic or atypical
Legionella	Short prodrome, then acute	Patchy, nodular, progressing consolidation to multiple lobes	Few to no polymorphonuclear leukocytes	Mixed normal flora
Mycoplasma	Acute to subacute	Often segmental, patchy or diffuse; without destruction	Few polymorphonuclear leukocytes	Mixed normal flora
Viral	Acute or biphasic	Diffuse, interstitial, or small; patchy and focal without destruction	Few to no polymorphonuclear leukocytes	Mixed normal flora

*The patterns outlined are stereotypical for the more common types of pneumonia. In practice, considerable overlapping occurs. Therefore, these patterns are most useful as points of departure in differential diagnosis.

BRONCHOPNEUMONIA

Bronchopneumonia, or patchy, inhomogeneous infiltrates, especially in dependent lobes, is another common pattern seen in pneumococcal infection. It is usually associated with abnormal airways, e.g., as a complication of chronic bronchitis or bronchiectasis, or due to organisms such as *Staphylococcus aureus* or *Hemophilus influenzae*. Part of the reason for the association between these organisms and the bronchopneumonic pattern is that the pneumonia often follows infection with the influenza virus. *Hemophilus* infections are also associated with bronchopneumonia because the abnormal tracheobronchial tree of patients with chronic bronchitis and bronchiectasis is often colonized with *H. influenzae*. In these infections, the signs of consolidation are often incomplete. More prominent are signs of airway involvement, e.g., rhonchi, with or without bronchospasm. Multiple smaller patchy infiltrates are found, less often, in viral infections.

INTERSTITIAL INFILTRATES

With few exceptions, e.g., *Hemophilus*, bacterial infections rarely cause interstitial infiltrates. Interstitial responses are much more commonly associated with viral or mycoplasmal infection.

GRANULOMATOUS DISEASE

Granulomatous disease is an entirely different category. Although usually defined in pathologic terms, certain clinical characteristics, e.g., tuberculosis of the upper lobes, are more often associated with it. This type of pneumonia is commonly slow and indolent; it infrequently presents as acute pneumonia.

NECROSIS

Cavitation, or abscess formation secondary to necrosis, is a more frequent complication of some etiologies than of others. Staphylococcal infections tend to cause necrosis, with rapidly progressive destruction and formation of lung abscess; in children, the residua of staphylococcal infection take the form of multiple, small thin-walled abscesses, i.e., pneumatoceles. Abscess formation may also follow gram-negative bacillary infections, particularly *Klebsiella* pneumonia; pneumococcal infections almost never form abscesses. As a rule, viral, *Mycoplasma* and *Legionella* infections also do not cause necrosis and abscesses.

Destructive infections followed by abscess formation sometimes follow aspiration of mixed flora, containing oral anaerobes, often in association with an aspirated foreign body, or inadequately drained secretions. These generally present more indolently than do the acute pneumonias.

LOBAR DISTRIBUTION

Since many bacterial infections are the result of aspiration, i.e., of microaspiration, most sites of bacterial infection are in dependent portions of the lung: for patients who aspirated while supine, the localization tends to be in lower lobes, or in the posterior portions of the upper lobes; in contrast, upper lobe infections more often reflect granulomatous disease, probably a consequence of a favored locus for growth after seeding by a bacteremic episode, or a structurally abnormal bronchial tree. Infiltrates that are diffuse and centrally located are less likely to be bacterial in origin.

UNUSUAL PATTERNS

Specific alterations in the patterns described above may be important. For example, in patients with chronic obstructive airways disease, the characteristic lobar pattern of pneumococcal pneumonia may be totally obscured. Recurrent pneumonias in a single lobe or segment may signal a local bronchial defect; recurrent pneumonias in different parts of the lung suggest defects either in upper airway defenses, e.g., recurrent aspiration, or in systemic host defenses.

Speed of Development

Many bacterial pneumonias, especially pneumococcal, are *acute* processes, with development of high fever and systemic signs very early in the illness; in contrast, *Mycoplasma* pneumonias are often more subacute in onset, with cough and respiratory symptoms appearing gradually and progressively over several days. These must also be distinguished from a number of other infections of a much more chronic nature, which may represent either a more indolent organism, e.g., tuberculosis or fungal infection, or a more walled-off process, e.g., lung abscess. A biphasic illness may suggest either a viral illness or, more often, bacterial superinfection of either viral or other bacterial infection.

Sputum

The nature and extent of sputum production is an essential part of the clinical assessment.

ACUTE PNEUMONIA

Acute pneumonia with purulent sputum is nearly always a manifestation of acute bacterial infection. Although distinction between likely agents may not be possible, correlation should be attempted between the Gram stain and culture results on the one hand, and the radiologic picture on the other.

SUBACUTE PNEUMONIAS

Subacute pneumonias, accompanied by purulent sputum, may also represent bacterial pneumonia; other clues, such

as leukocytosis and the Gram stain of the sputum, may be helpful in making the diagnosis of a bacterial pneumonia. But, when sputum is not purulent or absent, the question arises of nonbacterial etiologies, including viral, *Mycoplasma*, or sometimes *Legionella* infection.

CHRONIC PNEUMONIAS

Chronic pneumonias, or infiltrates that accompany chronic illnesses, occur in a variety of infections. The differential diagnosis of these infections is long, ranging from tuberculosis and fungal infections on the one hand, to lung abscesses on the other. As a rule, these agents do not weigh heavily in the acute differential diagnosis of the acute illnesses described above.

Special Settings

The history or physical examination may redirect diagnostic thinking, primarily by raising the index of suspicion that atypical or unusual organisms may be involved (Table 95-2). Striking examples of unusual etiologies occur at the extremes of age: infections in childhood (less often in the elderly) often involve *H. influenzae*; also, elderly individuals, even outside hospitals, often have gram-negative bacillary pneumonias or staphylococcal infection.

Infection elsewhere in the respiratory tract predisposes the lower respiratory tract to infection with the same organism; chronic or recurrent sinusitis may be a clue either to a responsible organism or to an unusual predisposing anatomic defect. Finally, immunocompromised patients are also encountered in community populations, particularly in recent years as the number of patients with AIDS has increased. Also, depending on the setting and the differential white blood cell counts, unexplained granulocytopenia may represent either a predisposing factor or a complication associated with a poor prognosis.

Alcoholism represents a particular risk. Alcoholic intoxication acutely increases the risk of aspiration. Furthermore, alcoholics seem to be at higher risk of developing pneumonia with gram-negative bacilli, probably because of an increased incidence of pharyngeal colonization with these organisms.

Special exposures must be taken into account in the differential diagnosis. Among these are exposure to large amounts of dust from sources as varied as the destruction of buildings on the one hand, to foundries on the other; or from droplets that originate in such divergent sources as cooling towers and hot tubs. Exposure to animals, including pets, well or ill, or contact with other persons who have respiratory infections may provide important clues.

Institutions in which conditions are crowded, or into which an influx of persons has occurred, may be the seat of different kinds of infections. Schools and mili-

TABLE 95-2

Atypical Historical Features

Atypical Features	Etiologic Organisms
Underlying conditions	
Extremes of age	
Neonates	Gram-negative bacilli, streptococci
Children	(Viral and *Mycoplasma* infections more common)
	H. influenzae
Elderly	Gram-negative bacilli (especially *Klebsiella*), *S. aureus*, perhaps *H. influenzae*
Alcoholism	*Klebsiella pneumoniae*
	Gram-negative bacilli
Bronchitis	*H. influenzae*, Pneumococcus
Recent influenza	*S. aureus*, *H. influenzae* (but pneumococci most common)
Cystic fibrosis	*P. aeruginosa*
Immunocompromised host	*P. carinii* and a huge range of fungal, viral, mycobacterial, and other bacterial infections (further invasive diagnostic techniques usually required)
Unusual exposure	
Aerosols of fluid	Gram-negative bacilli, e.g., *Pseudomonas*, and *Legionella*, depending on source of fluid
Sources of dust (including building destruction)	Fungal infection or reaction depending on geography (*Histoplasma*, coccidioidomycosis) or immunocompromise (*Aspergillus*, cryptococcosis) or rarely (foundry exposure), *Acinetobacter*
Wild animal sources	Zoonoses of a wide variety including leptospirosis, Q fever, tularemia, plague
Birds	Psittacosis

tary institutions spawn outbreaks of mycoplasmal or viral infection.

Involvement of sites other than the lungs occasionally provides an important clue that a particular patient does not fit into one of the more usual categories. For example, even though jaundice does occur in the course of severe pneumococcal pneumonia, it is uncommon. In contrast, manifestations of antecedent hepatic disease—as well as of antecedent renal or gastrointestinal disease—raise the prospect of Legionnaires' disease. Also, extrapulmonic manifestations are common in *Mycoplasma* pneumonia and can be exceedingly pleomorphic. A primary source found outside the lungs raises the possibility of hematogenous infection, whereas evidence of metastatic seeding of other sites (especially of the meninges) may also redirect diagnostic thinking.

DIAGNOSIS

It is not possible to establish an etiologic diagnosis on clinical and radiologic grounds alone. Although a purely empirical approach will succeed in some cases, documentation of etiology by laboratory support should be attempted to avoid subsequent problems and complications.

Blood Culture

A reliable identification of a specific etiology for a bacterial infection is either a positive blood culture, or a positive culture or Gram stain of another body fluid, e.g., pleural fluid. However, though bacteremia may occur often in pneumococcal pneumonia, in most patients blood culture is negative. Nevertheless, in the severely ill patient, blood cultures should be obtained, since if positive they are specific and helpful in prognosis and management.

Sputum Culture

It is important to obtain sputum or tracheal secretions for bacteriologic examination; the examination should always include Gram stain as well as culture. Gram stain is helpful both for identifying polymorphonuclear leukocytes and for recognizing organisms. The polymorphonuclear leukocytes serve to identify the sputum as of good quality, i.e., that it is likely to have come from an inflammatory focus, and also increase the likelihood that the inflammation is bacterial, or pyogenic, in origin.

Questions have been raised about the validity of the Gram stain of sputum in identifying pneumococcal pneumonia. Nonetheless, the bacterial flora seen may help define the etiologic agent. Even though the specificity and sensitivity of culture are both low, the Gram stain adds an important piece of information to the other clinical findings. For pneumococcal infection, the Gram stain is more sensitive than culture, and it allows early suspicion of other, nonpneumococcal, etiologies. The finding of gram-positive cocci in clusters lends support to the diagnosis of staphylococcal infection. Identifying the small gram-negative coccobacillary forms of *Hemophilus* infection or the plump gram-negative rods of *Klebsiella* infection also helps to establish diagnosis and direct treatment. Finally, in seeking special organisms, e.g., *Legionella* or acid-fast mycobacteria, special stains of sputum or tracheal secretions may be important.

The challenge recently posed to the accuracy or reliability of sputum Gram stain has raised the question of what to do if sputum is not readily available. Often, in the absence of sputum, transtracheal aspiration is recommended. However, in many instances, this step can be bypassed by instituting empiric treatment (after cultures of likely sources of organism have been obtained) based on clinical and statistical considerations. Transtracheal aspiration, especially in inexperienced hands, is a potentially hazardous technique. Invasive techniques should be reserved for situations in which differential diagnosis is difficult, e.g., as in immunocompromised patients, or if there is a clear need to document the nature of anaerobic organisms without risk of pharyngeal contamination, or if the disease progresses despite empiric treatment. However, in the immunocompromised patient, open lung biopsy is probably a more productive technique.

Peripheral Techniques

Some infections, including *S. pneumoniae*, *H. influenzae*, and cryptococcal infections, may release from the organisms antigens which may be identified in sputum, blood, or urine. Although these tests occasionally help resolve a diagnostic dilemma, they are infrequently used clinically. Search for antigen in sputum, as in techniques available for *Legionella* or mycobacterial infection, are neither easy nor reliable when obtained from heavily contaminated sources such as sputum.

Serology

Serologic techniques are generally not helpful, since specific results are not available for weeks; moreover, they are available primarily for the less common *Mycoplasma* or viral infections. Even the less specific "cold agglutinins" will appear in only 50 percent of patients with *M. pneumoniae* infection, and only after 7 to 10 days.

COMPLICATIONS

The possibility of complications should be considered from the onset of the pneumonia, particularly since some will either change the diagnostic considerations or require different modes of therapy. A logical sequence of this consideration might include the following:

1. *Local destruction*, with abscess formation, which to some extent will modify the differential diagnosis by limiting the etiologic possibilities. Abscesses often require consideration of the adequacy of drainage.
2. *Local extension* to pleural, or less often, the pericardial space, particularly if processes are lobar or necrotizing. Pleural effusions of small size occur in many pneumonias, including viral and *Mycoplasma* pneumonias, but larger effusions, of a size which can be easily tapped with a high degree of safety, are much more commonly associated with bacterial infection. A large effusion should be tapped for two reasons: the fluid often documents the presence and nature of infection, and provides an important source of material for culture or for special tests, e.g., fluorescent antibody search for *Legionella pneumophila*; in addition, it pro-

vides data that help in distinguishing effusion from empyema and in deciding about drainage.

3. *Hematogenous extension* to other sites, of which the most dangerous is the meninges. In critically ill patients, especially children, meningeal signs should be carefully sought and mental status carefully evaluated. If there is any doubt, in children or in adults, lumbar puncture should be performed, since meningitis significantly alters the drug or dose of the antibiotic selected. While the seeding of other sites is a possibility, particularly in the case of staphylococcal bacteremia, these are rarely identified in the initial evaluation.

4. *Progression of radiologic picture* may or may not represent a complication. Several different patterns of progression may be observed. In some patients, particularly if dehydrated when first seen, the infiltrates often become more prominent in the first few days of therapy as fluid replacement is undertaken. On the other hand, true progression, especially if other parameters of infection remain abnormal (or become worse), is an important indication that treatment has failed, and requires reevaluation of the diagnosis.

TREATMENT

Several elements enter into plans for treatment. Systemic support and correction of chemical and cardiovascular abnormalities are fundamental as is close attention to ventilatory status. A decision about hospitalization rests on the clinical state and whether oral antibiotics can be used.

Antibiotics are the mainstay of therapy. Certain generalizations about their use can be made as follows.

Acute Illness (Purulent Sputum, Diagnostic Chest Radiograph)

In the presence of lobar consolidation, penicillin or erythromycin may be used. Penicillin is particularly indicated if the acuity of illness, purulence (or bloodiness) of sputum, and radiographic pattern make pneumococcal pneumonia the likely etiology.

If Gram stain clearly suggests other etiologies, especially *Staphylococcus, Hemophilus,* or gram-negative bacillary involvement, or if the history or background makes these more likely, coverage should be expanded. Coverage which requires two agents, without Gram stain or cultural support, is rarely indicated, and a penicillinase-resistant penicillin (nafcillin, oxacillin) or a first-generation cephalosporin, usually suffices. Cephalosporins should not be used if pneumococcal disease is likely, even without documented meningitis at the time of diagnosis, since they will neither prevent nor treat meningeal seeding.

Subacute Illness (Less Purulent Sputum)

Unless the chest radiograph is suggestive of other processes (e.g., abscess, or tuberculosis), particularly in the presence of bilateral and interstitial infiltrates, the question of *Mycoplasma* pneumonia should be seriously considered, and erythromycin should be started. In many instances, the clinical picture of viral pneumonia is indistinguishable from that of *Mycoplasma* pneumonia; unfortunately, therapy for viral lower respiratory infections is not available. However, since there is no specific test to exclude or confirm *Mycoplasma* infection, treatment should be continued. Erythromycin, of course, is also appropriate therapy for pneumococcal pneumonia.

Biphasic or Progressive Illness

Progression of disease or failure to respond within 2 to 3 days suggests inappropriate therapy (or diagnosis), and the clinical and laboratory evidence should be reviewed, bearing in mind that some diseases (e.g., mycoplasmal, viral, or *Legionella*) may be impossible to document using routine tests. Since recommended doses for severe *Legionella* infection are higher than those commonly used for viral or *Mycoplasma* pneumonia, if a change in therapy is undertaken empirically, higher doses of erythromycin should be used. Biphasic illness, however, may also suggest superinfection. In community-acquired pneumonias, perhaps the most common situation for this is bacterial superinfection of antecedent viral, especially influenza, infection. The diagnostic principles are the same as those above. What is important is the willingness to reobtain and reevaluate the diagnostic data when a previously stable, or improving, patient suddenly becomes worse.

Further therapeutic issues include two techniques which are often used because they seem logical, but are of undocumented value: (1) humidification of the airways, primarily to loosen respiratory secretions, is often undertaken even though this practice has not been subjected to critical evaluation, and (2) chest physical therapy, with percussive techniques and postural drainage. Assessment of this practice indicates that in uncomplicated pneumonia, the procedure is not helpful. The possibility remains that subsets of patients do exist for whom chest physical therapy would be helpful. For example, it seems reasonable in those in whom the procedure yields large volumes of purulent sputum.

PREVENTION

Even in the initial evaluation of patients with community-acquired pneumonia, thoughts of prevention should come to mind. The possibility that many instances of pneumococcal pneumonia, or bacterial pneumonias which follow

influenza, may be preventable, may remind us to use pneumococcal vaccine, or influenza vaccine in the future.

Finally, it should be recalled at the time of hospitalization that a few of these pneumonias are communicable. Most are not likely to cause nosocomial disease in patients or staff if appropriate precautions are promptly begun. Precautions may need to be quite stringent, as for staphylococcal pneumonia, or directed particularly at airborne disease, as in tuberculosis. Finally, handwashing and awareness of the details of droplet transmission and contamination of fomites may serve to interrupt an important part of the transmission of these infections.

BIBLIOGRAPHY

Austrian R, Gold J: Pneumococcal bacteremia with special reference to bacteremic pneumococcal pneumonia. Ann Intern Med 60:759–776, 1964.
   Older experience describing 529 bacteremic cases, but the classic description from which much of our thinking about incidence and risk of type and of complication is drawn.

Barrett-Connor E: The non-value of sputum culture in the diagnosis of pneumococcal pneumonia. Am Rev Respir Dis 103:845–848, 1971.
   One of the first, and frequently cited, entries into the recent debate about accuracy of established diagnostic procedures. While discouraging the use of the random sputum culture for confirming pneumococcal pneumonia, it provides support for the use of Gram stain.

Brown RB, Sands M, Ryczak M: Community-acquired pneumonia caused by mixed aerobic bacteria. Chest 90:810–814, 1986.
   Mixed bacterial pneumonia caused by organisms other than anaerobes has been infrequently reported. This paper describes six cases and reviews the literature.

Ebright JR, Rytel MW: Bacterial pneumonia in the elderly. J Am Geriatr Soc 28:220–223, 1980.
   Even excluding patients from nursing homes, the proportion of patients over age 65 with gram-negative bacillary pneumonia is markedly increased (21 percent) with high associated morbidity.

Fekety FR, Caldwell J, Gump D, Johnson JE, Maxson W, Mulholland J, Thoburn R: Bacteria, viruses, and mycoplasmas in acute pneumonia in adults. Am Rev Respir Dis 104:499–507, 1971.
   One hundred cases of adult pneumonia were carefully studied. Sixty-two were felt to be pneumococcal, 34 were unknown, though at least preceding infection with a viral agent was identified serologically in 17. The serologic diagnosis of Mycoplasma was made in eight.

Fick RB Jr, Reynolds HY: Changing spectrum of pneumonia—News media creation or clinical reality? Am J Med 74:1–8, 1983.
   Though the factual base is weakened by its use of discharge diagnoses, this extended editorial emphasizes the increased complexity, and possible recent changes, of the etiologic agents.

Garb JL, Brown RB, Garb JR, Tuthill RW: Differences in etiology of pneumonias in nursing home and community patients. JAMA 240:2169–2172, 1978.
   Compares 35 elderly patients from the community with patients from nursing homes. The latter had more likely received prior antibiotics (47 percent versus 6 percent), and more commonly had Klebsiella (40 percent versus 9 percent) or staphylococcal pneumonia (26 percent versus 14 percent).

Graham WGB, Bradley DA: Efficacy of chest physiotherapy and intermittent positive-pressure breathing in the resolution of pneumonia. N Engl J Med 299:624–627, 1978.
   A randomized trial of 54 patients with uncomplicated pneumonia, showing no benefit of chest physiotherapy.

Huxley EJ, Viroslav J, Gray WR, Pierce AK: Pharyngeal aspiration in normal adults and patients with depressed consciousness. Am J Med 64:564–568, 1978.
   Forty-five percent of normal subjects aspirate indium-labeled pharyngeal secretions during sleep; 70 percent of patients with depressed consciousness did so.

Kroboth FJ, Yu VL, Reddy SC, Yu AC: Clinicoradiographic correlation with the extent of Legionnaires' disease. AJR 141:263–268, 1983.
   Thirty-four cases carefully described from the Pittsburgh experience, emphasizing the patchy early infiltrate progressing often to consolidation and bilateral disease.

Levin D, Schwarz M, Matthay R, LaForce FM: Bacteremic *Hemophilus influenzae* pneumonia in adults. A report of 24 cases and a review of the literature. Am J Med 62:219–224, 1977.
  Twenty-four cases are described, emphasizing the variable chest radiographs (consolidation in 38 percent) and complications. Seventy-five percent had the organism suggested on Gram stain, though sputum cultures were often negative.

Mufson MA: Pneumococcal infections. JAMA 246:1942–1948, 1981.
  A good, brief general review of the most common cause of community-acquired pneumonia.

Murphy TF, Henderson FW, Clyde WA Jr, Collier AM, Denney FW: Pneumonia: An eleven-year study in a pediatric practice. Am J Epidemiol 113:12–21, 1981.
  An 11-year study in a pediatric group practice, serving to illustrate the frequency of pneumonia in children less than 7 years old, and the predominance of viral and mycoplasmal etiologies.

Murray HW, Masur H, Senterfit L, Roberts RB: The protean manifestations of *Mycoplasma pneumoniae* infection in adults. Am J Med 58:229–242, 1975.
  Review of the described clinical features, emphasizing the variety of extrapulmonic symptoms and signs and the variability of chest radiologic findings.

Ort S, Ryan JL, Barden G, Desopo N: Pneumococcal pneumonia in hospital patients: Clinical and radiologic presentations. JAMA 249:214–218, 1983.
  Reviewing the clinical and radiologic features of 94 patients, pointing out that the majority presented with bronchopneumonia (61 percent).

Perlino CH: Laboratory diagnosis of pneumonia due to *Streptococcus pneumoniae*. J Infect Dis 150:139–144, 1984.
  Use of Quellung reaction and Gram-stain-directed sputum culture were both positive in cases of pneumonia confirmed to be pneumococcal. The latest in a long series of articles debating the use of Gram stain and culture.

Rose HD, Franson TR, Sheth WK, Chusid MJ, Macher AM, Zeirdt CH: Pseudomonas pneumonia associated with use of a home whirlpool spa. JAMA 250:2027–2029, 1983.
  A case report of a single patient, but a well-documented example of the relationship of ecology to unusual causes of pneumonia.

Tew J, Calenoff L, Berlin BS: Bacterial or nonbacterial pneumonia: Accuracy of radiographic diagnosis. Radiology 124:607–612, 1977.
  Thirty-one cases were reviewed radiologically. Accuracy of diagnosis with respect to viral-versus-bacterial etiology was accurate only 65 percent of the time, emphasizing the need to combine radiologic with other clinical data.

Woodhead MA, Macfarlane JT: Legionnaires' disease: a review of 79 community acquired cases in Nottingham. Thorax 41:635–640, 1986.
  Seventy-nine cases of sporadic, community-acquired Legionnaires' disease are reviewed. Of the features noted on admission, only a high plasma urea concentration was significantly associated with death.

Yu VL, Kroboth FJ, Shonnard J, Brown A, McDearman S, Magnussen M: Legionnaires' disease: New clinical perspective from a prospective pneumonia study. Am J Med 73:357–361, 1982.
  L. pneumophila proves to be the most common single-agent cause of pneumonia in Pittsburgh, though two-thirds of their cases were nosocomial in origin. It is not necessarily associated with abdominal signs and symptoms.

Ziskind MM, Schwarz ML, George RB, Weill H, Shames JM, Herbert ST, Ichinose H: Incomplete consolidation in pneumococcal lobar pneumonia complicating pulmonary emphysema. Ann Intern Med 72:835–839, 1970.
  An attempt to sort different radiologic patterns seen in pneumococcal pneumonia. Emphasizes caution in radiologic diagnosis: under age 40, lobar patterns were almost always seen; over 40, with emphysema, a much more heterogenous pattern.

Chapter 96

Chronic Bronchitis

Ira B. Tager

DEFINITION

Chronic bronchitis was defined in the 1950s by the presence of cough and phlegm for 3 months per year for more than two consecutive years. This restrictive definition, an outgrowth of epidemiologic studies, focused on symptoms that are secondary to hypersecretion of mucus by cells lining the airways. However, despite this attempt to narrow the definition of chronic bronchitis, in popular usage, "chronic bronchitis" has continued to be synonymous with a spectrum of airways disease that ranges on the one hand from simple mucous hypersecretion and on the other to airflow obstruction (generally defined by a low FEV_1, i.e., usually less than 65 percent of predicted values corrected for age, sex, and height, or by a low FEV_1/ FVC ratio).

This dichotomy has promoted ambiguity in the definition of chronic bronchitis and clouded interpretation of research that presupposes that mucous hypersecretion is relevant to the problem of airflow obstruction, which is clinically more important. Indeed, it now seems clear that neither the presence nor the course of mucous hypersecretion is related either to the rate of deterioration in lung function (as defined by a long-term decline in FEV_1) or to mortality from airflow obstruction. Usage of the more restrictive definition of chronic bronchitis is further complicated by the fact that, in epidemiologic studies, cough and phlegm are important symptoms in some patients with asthma and that complaints of wheezing are often elicited in individuals who do not have asthma. These prospects

for imprecision in diagnosis impact on the interpretation of data that relate to the treatment of chronic bronchitis.

To circumvent ambiguities inherent in the term *chronic bronchitis*, this chapter distinguishes, whenever possible, between mucous hypersecretion and airways obstruction. When the term chronic bronchitis is used, it refers to the spectrum of diseases in which mucous hypersecretion is the predominant feature. In this usage, it does not take into account evidence of airways obstruction; it also excludes bronchospasm as the dominant feature of the disease.

EPIDEMIOLOGY

Chronic bronchitis is a common disease. In 1981, there were at least 8 million persons in the United States with chronic bronchitis. Prevalence rates for chronic bronchitis range from 3.6 percent at ages 45 to 64 to 4.5 percent at ages over 65 years. As a cause of mortality, chronic bronchitis (with or without emphysema) ranks fifth (3.3 percent of total deaths), and its frequency has been increasing steadily over the past two and one-half decades. Between 1979 and 1983, mortality from chronic bronchitis increased by 19.2 percent; most of this increase occurred in persons 55 years of age and older. In the age group 45 to 54 years, mortality for females approached that of males, suggesting that the excess male mortality from chronic bronchitis reported in the past may have been due to marked differences between the smoking habits of older men and women, a suggestion in keeping with the increase in smoking by women during the past two decades.

Cigarette smoking is the most important factor associated with the occurrence of mucous hypersecretion and airflow obstructive diseases. In the United States, 80 to 90 percent of these entities can be attributed to cigarette smoking. In both men and women, the occurrence of chronic cough and phlegm increases with increasing cigarette use. Heavy smokers (20 to 25 cigarettes per day) in all age groups and in both sexes are four to five times more likely to report chronic cough and/or phlegm than are individuals who have never smoked cigarettes; cessation of smoking is accompanied by a return toward the lower frequencies of these symptoms in those who have never smoked. Abnormalities in pulmonary function, as reflected in the FEV_1, and in other tests of small airway function, have shown dose-response relationships with lifetime cigarette smoking. Teenagers and young adults who smoke have lower levels of pulmonary function than do those who have never smoked. In longitudinal studies, active smokers have been found to undergo decrements in FEV_1 that are two to three times as great as those of persons who have never smoked. Finally, eight major prospective studies, which have involved 17 million person-years of follow-up and 330,000 deaths, have shown that

TABLE 96-1

Risk Factors for Mucous Hypersecretion and/or Chronic Airflow Obstruction in Adults

Established factors
    Cigarette smoking (active)
    α_1-Antitrypsin deficiency
Factors for which some data suggest increased risk
    Age
    Air pollution
    Alcohol
    Atopy, allergy, or hypersensitivity (bronchial hyperreactivity)
    Childhood respiratory illness
    Environmental pollution (macroenvironmental)
    Familial and/or household (microenvironmental)
    Genetic (e.g., ABH secretor status, other not defined)
    Occupation
    Respiratory illness history in adulthood
    Sex (male > female)
    Social class

SOURCE: Adapted from U.S. Department of Health, Education and Welfare, 1984, and Speizer and Tager, 1979.

male cigarette smokers are 3.5 to 25 times more likely (depending on the amounts smoked) to die of chronic bronchitis and/or emphysema than are nonsmokers; the data are similar for women, although the number of women included in these studies is fewer than the number of men. Smoking cessation is associated with a reduction in mortality risk from chronic bronchitis and/or emphysema that is directly related to the number of years since cessation of smoking.

Many factors other than cigarette smoking have been extensively investigated for their roles in causing mucous hypersecretion and chronic airflow obstruction—either directly or by modification of the risk due to cigarette smoking. Of these, only the Pi ZZ genotype of α-antitrypsin deficiency has been shown clearly to be associated with the occurrence of chronic airflow obstruction, independently and interactively with cigarette smoking (Table 96-1); no such association could be shown between Pi ZZ genotype and mucous hypersecretion. One other exception may be sex; even after adjustment for smoking habits, males still manifest higher rates of mucous hypersecretion than do women.

PATHOGENESIS, PATHOPHYSIOLOGY, AND NATURAL HISTORY

Early epidemiologic studies by British epidemiologists suggested that mucous hypersecretion resulted from exposure to a variety of inhaled irritants, e.g., cigarette smoke and air pollutants. A sequence was then pictured in which increased mucous production was associated with blockage of airways and reduced clearance of mucus, thereby setting the stage for recurrent infections; in turn, the repeated infections were presumed to damage the pulmonary airways and cause destruction of airspaces, thereby culminating in irreversible airflow obstruction. The implications of this hypothesis were that if one removed the irritants and treated the infections, the development of airflow obstruction could be prevented or arrested. A great deal of the subsequent body of data concerning the role of infectious agents in the pathogenesis of chronic bronchitis, and of treatment designed to control the infection, is based on this hypothesis. However, mucous hypersecretion and episodes of chest illness have not proved to be causally related to the origins and perpetuation of the obstructive abnormality.

Nor have epidemiologic studies succeeded in establishing other pathogenetic mechanisms. For example, the idea that smoking sometimes initiates two parallel processes, i.e., mucous hypersecretion and airflow obstruction, has not stood up to testing. Also unproven is a third hypothesis that invokes allergic hypersensitivity of the airways to a variety of insults. According to this proposal, mucous hypersecretion is one manifestation of this hypersensitivity, and increased responsiveness of the airways to histamine is another; recurrent infections are believed to be secondary to bronchoconstriction which, in turn, decreases the capability of the airways to clear microbial agents. This proposed sequence clearly resembles that used to explain extrinsic asthma. However, tests of this hypothesis, using epidemiologic and clinical approaches, have not settled the issue.

The epidemiologically based hypotheses discussed above consider chronic airflow obstruction without regard to the underlying pulmonary pathology. Another important hypothesis that derives from the lesions of emphysema (see below) that occurs in some patients with chronic bronchitis is the protease-antiprotease hypothesis of emphysema. This topic is discussed fully elsewhere (see Chapter 74). According to this hypothesis, cigarette smoke disrupts the normal homeostatic mechanisms that protect the lung from damage by a variety of proteolytic insults. Although this hypothesis has considerable appeal and much data to support it, it is still speculative. Furthermore, even if this hypothesis does provide a major explanation for the mechanism by which cigarette smoke exerts its deleterious effects, it offers incomplete insight into the considerable variability in risk among smokers of developing clinically significant chronic airflow obstruction. The extent to which subtle variations in inhalation patterns, e.g., volume and duration, the tar content of cigarettes, exposure to other noxious environmental stimuli, and "constitutional" factors contribute to this variability is unknown.

As a rule, in patients with chronic mucous hypersecretion the size of the tracheobronchial seromucous glands is increased as is the proportionate volume of the mucus-secreting, as compared with the serous-secreting, portions of these glands. As expected, the frequency of clinical manifestations of mucous hypersecretion parallels that of cigarette smoking. Metaplasia of goblet cells in central airways occurs occasionally, but this abnormality appears to be related more closely to clinical manifestations of airflow obstruction than to clinical manifestations of mucous hypersecretion.

Clinical-physiological-pathologic correlations have led to the prevalent current idea that the primary pathophysiological event in the development of chronic airflow obstruction takes place in the small airways of the lung (nonalveolated airways smaller than 2 mm in internal diameter) (Table 96-2). The initial lesion is presumed to be a respiratory bronchiolitis (aggregations of pigmented macrophages in and around first- and second-order respiratory bronchioles with inflammation of adjacent bronchiolar and alveolar walls) that is seen principally, but not exclusively, in the small airways of smokers. In turn, the initial respiratory bronchiolitis is postulated to result in squamous metaplasia, denuded epithelium, mural fibrosis, goblet cell metaplasia, and intraluminal mucus and hypertrophied airway muscle—which also contribute to the physiological evidence for small airways disease. In older smokers, airways <400 μm are also narrowed or reduced in number. These abnormalities may also be responsible for the obstructive defect but, as a rule, inflammation per se is sufficient.

Respiratory bronchiolitis may also be the initial lesion of centrilobular emphysema, which is common in smokers, since (1) distribution of the bronchiolitis in the lung parallels that of centrilobular emphysema, (2) respiratory bronchiolitis temporally precedes the occurrence of centrilobular emphysema, and (3) centrilobular emphysema begins at the site that corresponds to the respiratory bronchiolitis. Progression of these various processes eventually culminates in clinically and physiologically significant airflow obstruction in smokers destined to develop this problem.

The extent to which factors other than smoking contribute to the above processes has not been studied. Moreover, although stopping smoking is associated with improved lung function, the few available data on pathology have failed to show concomitant improvement in the inflammatory lesion.

A plausible synthesis of the hypothesis and pathophysiological data considered above into a coherent theory of the natural history of chronic bronchitis is shown in Fig. 96-1. FEV$_1$ is used in this figure since it is the test most commonly used in epidemiologic and clinical studies of airways obstruction. The influence of cigarette smoking, and of stopping smoking, features prominently in the various pathways shown in this figure.

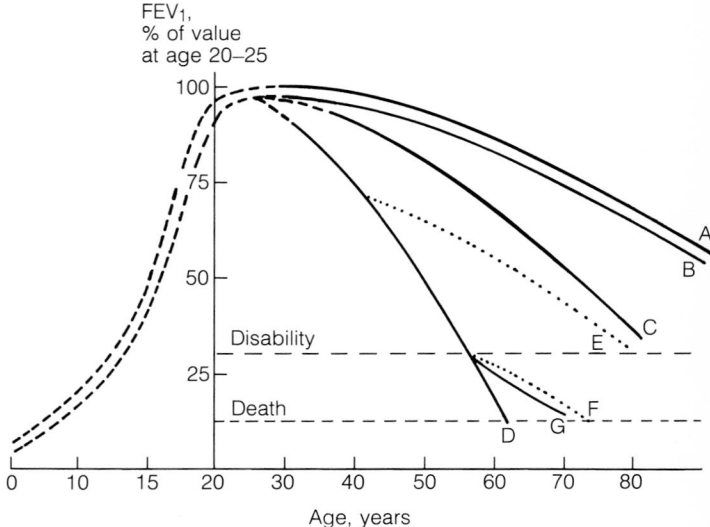

FIGURE 96-1 Potential pathways in the evolution of chronic bronchitis. Curve A: *Adult non-smokers.* There is a slow rate of decrease in FEV$_1$ (20 to 30 ml/year), but it never reaches levels associated with disability or death. Curves B and C: *Most cigarette smokers (70 to 80 percent).* The rate of decrease is either normal (curve B) or somewhat increased (curve C), but disabling obstructive airways disease does not develop. Curve D: *Remaining cigarette smokers (20 to 30 percent).* For unknown reasons, FEV$_1$ decreases at a sufficiently rapid rate (60 to 80 ml/year) for clinically evident obstructive airways disease to appear. Curve E: *Early cessation of smoking.* By stopping smoking early in life, disability may be prevented and lost pulmonary function may be recovered. Curve F: *Cessation of smoking in disabled persons.* Sometimes the rate of decrease in pulmonary function is slowed (curve F) but more often the rate of decrease continues (curve D) resulting in death from chronic obstructive airways disease. Curve G: *Survivors after 10 years of disability.* For those who survive for as long as 10 years after disability starts, the rate of decrease in FEV$_1$ slows regardless of smoking status. (*From Speizer and Tager, 1979, with permission.*)

TABLE 96-2

Pathophysiological Correlates of Chronic Mucous Hypersecretion and Chronic Airflow Obstruction

Chronic mucous hypersecretion
  Tracheobronchial seromucous gland enlargement
  Increased volume density of tracheobronchial mucous glands
Chronic airflow obstruction
  Inflammation of small airways (respiratory bronchiolitis)
  Bronchiolar narrowing
  Goblet cell metaplasia
  Intraluminal obstruction of small airways (mucus, increased muscle, obliteration or collapse of bronchioles, emphysema)

SOURCE: Adapted from Thurlbeck, 1980.

CLINICAL MANIFESTATIONS AND DIAGNOSIS

The clinical presentation and diagnosis of chronic bronchitis usually offer little problem for the physician. The patient is most likely to present with complaints of shortness of breath, with or without complaints of wheeze, cough, and phlegm. Typically, symptoms are episodic, especially those related to mucous hypersecretion. Careful questioning often reveals a baseline level of persistent symptoms that is punctuated by periods of increasing mucous hypersecretion, followed by the appearance of, or worsening of, shortness of breath. During an acute exacerbation, patients not infrequently report an increase in the purulence of the sputum, often unaccompanied by signs or symptoms of respiratory infection.

The criteria for the diagnosis of the hypersecretion and obstructive components of the chronic bronchitis complex appear in Table 96-3. For the diagnosis of the chronic mucous hypersecretion component, cough and phlegm remain the sine qua non. However, complaints of wheeze may be as frequent as cough and phlegm and may also occur without them. Similarly, chronic cough occurs in some patients who do not produce phlegm; in these patients, an atypical presentation of adult-onset asthma may need to be considered. A standardized epidemiologic questionnaire may be helpful in distinguishing between those who have the usual presentations of chronic bronchitis that are considered in this chapter and others in which bronchospasm features so prominently as to suggest the clinical diagnosis of asthma. Past emphasis on the presence or absence of purulent sputum no longer seems to be as important for the diagnosis of chronic bronchitis as does the carefully detailed record of presenting symptoms.

In contrast to the clinical criteria for the diagnosis of mucous hypersecretion, the diagnosis of chronic airflow obstruction is, in part, arbitrary, relying heavily on the determination of FEV_1. The usual cutoff for FEV_1 of 65 percent of predicted (corrected for age, height, and sex) is derived both from the Gaussian distribution of values of FEV_1 (expressed as percent of predicted) and from the epidemiologic data that relate the rates of decline in FEV_1 to time (see above). Sixty-five percent represents approximately two standard deviations from the mean value of 100 percent predicted. Therefore, even though most patients who have FEV_1 values below this level will have clinically significant obstruction to airflow, interpretation of the percent predicted value must take into account the statistical origins of this cutoff and, therefore, the possibility that a few patients—especially those without symptoms—may not have disease.

Tests of small airways disease [e.g., airflows at the mid- and low-lung volume range of maximum expiratory flow-volume (MEFV) curves, slope of phase III of the single-breath nitrogen washout curve, closing volumes/capacity] have been investigated in an effort to improve diagnostic sensitivity. Although these tests are more sensitive to FEV_1 for the detection of abnormalities in small airways, most studies have failed to demonstrate that these tests are any better than FEV_1 for the identification of patients who are likely to develop clinically significant disability or mortality from impairment of lung function. Thus, they are not used for routine diagnosis and follow-up.

Whether FEV_1 should be determined routinely in all middle-aged and older patients who visit a physician has not been settled. However, it does seem reasonable that all patients who are currently smoking cigarettes should be screened. Patients in their fifth and sixth decades in whom the FEV_1 percent predicted is less than 80 to 85 percent (approximately one standard deviation below the mean) should be singled out for intensive efforts at smoking cessation.

TABLE 96-3
Criteria for Diagnosis of Chronic Bronchitis

Mucous hypersecretion
  Cough and phlegm for 3 months out of the year for 2 consecutive years
    Time of day not critical (morning "smokers cough" not required)
    Season not critical
    Wheeze not part of formal definition
    Quality of sputum (clear, mucopurulent, purulent) not critical
Chronic airflow obstruction
  Age, height, and sex adjusted level of FEV_1 of less than 65 percent of predicted
  FEV_1/FVC ratio of less than 70 percent of predicted (used less frequently than FEV_1)

MANAGEMENT

This chapter focuses on three areas of management that relate directly to the epidemiologic hypotheses about the natural history of chronic bronchitis and the role of acute exacerbations of chronic bronchitis: (1) respiratory tract infections, (2) glucocorticosteroids, and (3) bronchodilators. However, since the natural history of chronic bronchitis is dominated by the effects of cigarette smoking, physician attempts to promote cessation of smoking are indispensable for the rational management of patients with chronic bronchitis. Cessation of smoking has been associated with a number of improvements in the manifestations of chronic bronchitis: (1) diminution and/or resolution of the signs of mucous hypersecretion and of the acute exacerbations associated with these symptoms, (2)

reversal of abnormalities in the function of small airways that are thought to be the antecedent pathophysiological abnormalities in clinical chronic airflow obstruction, and (3) reduction in the average rates of annual decline in FEV_1 across a side range of functional impairment. (Some recent data suggest a small recovery of level of function in persons who have recently ceased to smoke.)

Efforts at smoking cessation have met with limited success. But patients with pulmonary disease do appear to be more likely to achieve at least short-term cessation than persons without such disease. Motivation of the patient by the physician and continued patient counseling do have small but measurable effects. Apparently, physicians can be most effective in terms of smoking cessation when they are part of an effort that includes programs specifically tailored to smoking cessation. In addition, the judicious use of nicotine chewing gum, in conjunction with a counseling program, may increase the likelihood of long-term smoking cessation.

RESPIRATORY TRACT INFECTIONS

Several issues relate to the management of respiratory infections as causes of acute exacerbations of chronic bronchitis: (1) the extent to which infections are the cause of acute exacerbations, (2) the susceptibility of patients with chronic bronchitis to respiratory infection and the types of infections involved, (3) the efficacy of antimicrobial therapy in the control of the signs and symptoms of acute infection, and (4) the relationship between acute exacerbations triggered by infections and their treatment to the long-term natural history of chronic airflow obstructions.

Many investigators have identified an increased frequency of *Hemophilus influenzae* and *Streptococcus pneumoniae* in secretions from the lower respiratory tract of patients with chronic bronchitis, usually in those with the more severe manifestations of disease in terms of airflow obstruction and of purulent mucous hypersecretion. Early on, serologic tests also provided some support for the idea that *H. influenzae* and *S. pneumoniae* were responsible for the increased purulence of the sputum during an exacerbation of chronic bronchitis. However, subsequent prospective studies have either failed to confirm the serologic findings of the earlier studies or have suggested a complex interaction between the occurrence of a viral infection and serologic evidence of infection with these bacteria. No consistent associations with other bacteria have been reported.

Viruses and *Mycoplasma pneumoniae* have also been implicated as causes of acute exacerbations. Serologic studies suggest that patients with chronic bronchitis are more susceptible to infection with common respiratory viruses and possibly with *M. pneumoniae*. Viral infections are far more common than *M. pneumoniae* infec-

tions; together they account for less than half of all exacerbations. Acute exacerbations sometimes also occur in patients who have no evidence of infection. Although the reason for this discrepancy is unknown, undoubtedly some of these exacerbations are due to infections that were not detected by the diagnostic procedures.

The most stringent test of the role of infectious agents as causes of acute exacerbations of chronic bronchitis relates to attempts at therapy. Since antiviral agents either are not available or have not been studied extensively, most data relate to antibacterial agents. Such agents have been used in an attempt to control acute symptoms, to prevent recurrent exacerbations, and to reduce long-term declines in lung function.

Interpretation of the data about the efficacy of antibiotics to control acute exacerbations is controversial: most studies have either been uncontrolled or have not included a placebo group. Among the few that were blinded and placebo-controlled, and conducted in patients with a moderate to severe exacerbation but with no evidence of pneumonia (usually hospitalized patients), the results were equivocal; at best they suggested a very limited benefit. This is not surprising since most infectious exacerbations are of viral etiology.

Well-controlled studies are available concerning the use of antibiotics to prevent recurrent episodes of exacerbations of chronic bronchitis. They have almost consistently failed to show any benefit, either in terms of significant reduction in the number of episodes of exacerbation or in slowing the rate of decline of the FEV_1. These observations and others that have evaluated the effect of specific infections, e.g., influenza virus infection or the occurrence of *S. pneumoniae* in sputum, suggest that episodes of infection are not important determinants of functional deterioration.

Table 96-4 suggests an approach to the use of antibiotics in managing acute exacerbations of chronic bronchitis

TABLE 96-4

Suggested Approach for Use of Antibiotics for Management of Acute Exacerbations of Chronic Bronchitis

Routine Gram stain and culture *not* necessary

Advice on smoking cessation (at least reduction)

Observation of patient for 3–5 days (arbitrary) to determine if improvement occurs without antibiotics

If no improvement or worsening, e.g., ↑ shortness of breath, ↑ sputum ± purulence, deterioration of oxygenation ($\downarrow Pa_{O_2}$ or O_2 saturation), deterioration of ventilation ($\uparrow Pa_{CO_2}$), onset or worsening of systemic symptoms (e.g., fever, anorexia, etc.)

Tetracycline 250 mg PO qid (doxycycline reserved for patients with renal impairment)

Erythromycin 250 mg PO qid

Discontinue after 7 days and reevaluate if no improvement or continued worsening

(assuming that pneumonia has been ruled out by a chest radiograph). Since only erythromycin and tetracycline have proven to be efficacious against M. pneumoniae as well as to have some effect against S. pneumoniae (both agents) and H. influenzae (tetracycline), no other alternatives are offered in Table 96-4. For patients who cannot tolerate these agents, any antibiotic with activity against S. pneumoniae and H. influenzae may be substituted. It should be noted that β-lactamase-producing strains are infrequent among the nonencapsulated isolates of H. influenzae obtained from some patients with chronic bronchitis. Therefore, ampicillin is preferable to the more expensive or toxic alternatives.

GLUCOCORTICOSTEROIDS

The use of glucocorticosteroids in the treatment of chronic bronchitis can be traced to the suspicion that the anti-inflammatory properties of the agents might be beneficial and to the documented improvement that followed the use of these agents in patients with asthma. In a single, well-controlled study that used methylprednisolone (0.5 mg/kg every 6 h IV for 3 days) to treat an acute exacerbation, the steroid-treated patients manifested an increase in FEV_1. Mortality could not be assessed, and no data were provided about the length of hospitalization. Neither the alveolar-arterial P_{O_2} difference nor the arterial P_{CO_2} showed greater improvement in the steroid-treated group. Therefore, the role of glucocorticosteroids in the management of acute exacerbation of chronic bronchitis has only been inadequately studied; glucocorticosteroids cannot be considered as part of standard therapy.

In individuals with stable chronic bronchitis, many more data are available. Most controlled studies have concluded that only a minority of patients with chronic bronchitis are apt to respond to glucocorticosteroids. Unfortunately, no consensus exists about the indices by which responsive patients can be preselected. Among the potential predictors tested were the following: response to bronchodilators, sputum or blood eosinophilia, wheeze (by history or examination), personal or family history of asthma, and pre-therapy pulmonary function testing. Moreover, only the short-term response of pulmonary function and of symptoms to glucocorticosteroids has been tested. Therefore, whether this type of therapy affects the long-term rate of decline in pulmonary function is unknown.

Because of the subjective nature of respiratory symptoms, and the difficulty in quantifying them, the response of symptoms to glucocorticosteroids has not been extensively studied. In the few studies that have been done, symptoms (usually wheeze or shortness of breath) have not correlated well with the results of standard tests of pulmonary function, e.g., FEV_1. Virtually no data are

TABLE 96-5

Suggested Guidelines for Use of Glucocorticosteroids in Patients with Stable, Severe Chronic Bronchitis with Airflow Obstruction

Make multiple measurements of FEV_1 over 2–3 month period prior to starting treatment to identify "best" level of function

Two-week trial of prednisone (or equivalent) at 30 mg/day

Continue: if FEV_1 improves 25–30% over "best" pretreatment FEV_1

    Taper to lowest effective daily or qod dose

    Continue with oral in preference to inhaled steroid*

Discontinue (at 2 weeks) if (1) FEV_1 improves less than 25% of "best" pretreatment FEV_1; (2) unacceptable side effects

Discontinue at intervals to determine if patient still requires steroids to maintain optimal level of function

---

* The few studies that have evaluated inhaled steroids have shown even fewer consistent effects than will oral agents.

available with regard to effects on mucous hypersecretion (cough and phlegm).

In essence, recommendations about the use of glucocorticosteroids can be only tentative, since there is no unanimity about their effectiveness and no set of indices predict reliably which patients will respond. However, any patient with severe obstruction to airflow should be considered to be a candidate for treatment, and an attempt should be made to determine if a response will occur. This recommendation is restricted to patients with severe disease (FEV_1 usually <1 to 1.5 L) because studies have not been done in patients with moderate functional impairment, nor have data been generated to evaluate whether the natural history of chronic bronchitis is influenced by steroid therapy. It can also be argued that only patients who have ceased to smoke should be considered for such therapy in view of the overwhelming effects of cigarettes on symptoms and the rate of decline of lung function. The suggested management strategy in Table 96-5 is distilled only from recommendations made on the basis of properly blinded, controlled trials.

BRONCHODILATORS

Recommendations for the rational use of bronchodilator therapy in patients with chronic bronchitis cannot be made on any firm grounds. Because of the limitations of current data, the decision to use these agents is purely empirical. (See Chapter 80 for types of agents, dosage, and route of administration.) Before embarking on their use, a 3- to 6-month period of close observation (monthly evaluation of function and symptoms) should be undertaken to assess the variability of the patient's symptoms and level of function and to stop the patient from smoking. Some

objective measure of the patient's exercise capacity should be undertaken, e.g., a 12-min, measured walk or progressive cycle ergometry. If a decision is made to use a bronchodilator (see Chapter 80 for preferred methods and techniques of administration), all these parameters should be reassessed frequently over several months to determine to what extent any observed improvement in function is paralleled by improvement in the patient's symptoms and objective measures of performance. If little correlation is found, or there has been no improvement in function, the therapy should be discontinued.

BIBLIOGRAPHY

Albert RK, Martin TR, Lewis SW: Controlled clinical trial of methylprednisolone in patients with chronic bronchitis and acute respiratory insufficiency. Ann Intern Med 92:753–758, 1980.
  Randomized, double-blind, controlled trial of IV methylprednisolone in severe obstructive chronic bronchitis in exacerbation. Data show marginal benefit for treated group in terms of more rapid and larger increases in FEV$_1$ over first 72 h of hospitalization.

Anthonisen NR, Manfreda J, Warren CP, Hershfield ES, Harding GK, Nelson NA: Antibiotic therapy in exacerbations of chronic obstructive pulmonary disease. Ann Intern Med 106:196–204, 1987.
  A randomized, placebo-controlled study of a 10-day course of antibiotics (trimethoprim, sulfamethoxazole, amoxicillin, or doxycycline) in patients experiencing exacerbations of chronic obstructive pulmonary disease. Those with increased dyspnea, sputum volume, and sputum production showed greater resolution of symptoms. Other types of exacerbations including those with wheeze were not benefited.

Burrows B, Lebowitz M: Characteristics of chronic bronchitis in a warm, dry region. Am Rev Respir Dis 112:365–370, 1975.
  Population-based study of 3167 people in Tucson, Arizona, to identify distribution of and interrelationships between chronic respiratory symptoms.

Dodge R, Cline MG, Burrows B: Comparisons of asthma, emphysema, and chronic bronchitis diagnoses in a general population sample. Am Rev Respir Dis 133:981–986, 1986.
  This report is an analysis of cases of obstructive airways disease diagnosed during the first 8 years of a community study. A majority of subjects who developed emphysema were males, whereas 72.8% of the asthma and chronic bronchitis subjects were female. Physician bias may result in labeling male patients as emphysematous and female patients as asthmatic or bronchitic.

Eaton ML, McDonald FM, Church TR, Niewoehner DE: Effect of theophylline on breathlessness and exercise tolerance in patients with chronic airflow obstruction. Chest 82:538–542, 1982.
  Placebo-controlled, randomized trial of oral theophylline in patients with severe airflow obstruction. Representative of other such studies that show with theophylline small improvements in forced expiratory volumes that are not correlated with symptomatic improvement in patients.

Ferris BG: Epidemiology Standardization Project. Am Rev Respir Dis 118:1–111, 1978.
  A comprehensive statement of the criteria for pulmonary function testing and questionnaire structure that is geared toward epidemiology studies. However, the monograph has important guidelines for the collection of data for individual patients.

Fletcher CM: Terminology in chronic obstructive lung diseases. J Epidemiol Commun Health 32:282–288, 1978.
  Historical review of the origins of the various diagnostic labels used to refer to chronic obstructive lung disease. Provides excellent perspective on problems of nosology for chronic bronchitis, emphysema, and asthma.

Fletcher C, Peto R, Tinker C, Speizer FE: The Natural History of Chronic Bronchitis and Emphysema. New York, Oxford University Press, 1976.
  A comprehensive presentation of a test of the "British" hypothesis of the pathogenesis of chronic bronchitis based on the long-term follow-up of a group of British workingmen. Concludes that cigarette smoking is the major cause of mucous hypersecretion and airflow obstruction, but the latter two are not part of a single disease process.

Gump DW, Philips CA, Forsyth BR, McIntosh K, Lamborn DR, Stouch WH: Role of infection in chronic bronchitis. Am Rev Respir Dis 113:465–474, 1976.
  Intensive, 4-year follow-up study of 25 patients with chronic bronchitis that demonstrates predominance of viruses as etiologic agents in acute exacerbations. Data also demonstrate that even with intensive follow-up and extensive microbial surveillance, only a minority of acute exacerbations can be attributed clearly to a respiratory pathogen.

Higgins MW, Keller JB, Landis JR, Beaty TH, Burrows B, Demets D, Diem JE, Higgins ITT, Lakatos E, Lebowitz MD, Menkes H, Speizer FE, Tager IB, Weil H: Risk of chronic obstructive pulmonary disease. Am Rev Respir Dis 130:380–385, 1984.
> *A prospective, population-based test of a model to predict the occurrence of FEV_1 less than 65 percent predicted during a 10-year follow-up. Cigarette consumption, level of FEV_1 10 years previously, and age were the only significant predictors of abnormal function.*

Janoff A: Elastases and emphysema: Current assessment of the protease-antiprotease hypothesis. Am Rev Respir Dis 132:417–433, 1985.
> *A comprehensive review of the role of elastase in the pathogenesis of pulmonary emphysema and the pathways through which cigarette smoke may exert its deleterious effects.*

Jeffery PK: Anti-inflammatory drugs and experimental bronchitis. Eur J Respir Dis 146:245–257, 1986.
> *Using an experimental model of chronic bronchitis in rats, the author finds that cigarette-smoke-induced bronchitis can be inhibited by the concomitant administration of certain agents (indomethacin, fluriprofen, or N-acetylcysteine).*

Johnston RN, McNeill RS, Smith DH, Legge JS, Fletcher F: Chronic bronchitis: Measurements and observations over ten years. Thorax 31:25–29, 1976.
> *Follow-up at 10 years to an earlier report at 5 years of follow-up that had suggested benefit of antibiotic treatment in terms of reduced decline in FEV_1. Ten-year follow-up failed to show sustained benefit. Points out importance of need for long period of follow-up data before conclusion about effects of antibiotics on function can be evaluated.*

Kauffmann F, Drouet D, Lellouch J, Brille D: Twelve years of spirometric changes among Paris area workers. Int J Epidemiol 8:201–212, 1979.
> *Population-based, longitudinal study of 575 workingmen with extensive analysis of factors associated with accelerated decline of FEV_1.*

Lakshminarayan S: Ipratropium bromide in chronic bronchitis/emphysema. A review of the literature. Am J Med 81:76–80, 1986.
> *A review of the literature on the efficacy of ipratropium bromide in chronic obstructive pulmonary disease. Several studies comparing ipratropium with sympathomimetic agents or methylxanthines in patients with chronic bronchitis or emphysema have shown at least an equal and in most instances a superior bronchodilator action with ipratropium. Other papers in this volume evaluate ipratropium in other airway disorders.*

MacNee W, Connaughton JJ, Rhind GB, Hayhurst MD, Douglas NJ, Muir AL, Flenley DC: A comparison of the effects of almitrine or oxygen breathing on pulmonary arterial pressure and right ventricular ejection fraction in hypoxic chronic bronchitis and emphysema. Am Rev Respir Dis 134:559–565, 1986.
> *Chronic administration of almitrine bismesylate, a new, orally administered respiratory stimulant, improves arterial blood gas tensions in patients with chronic bronchitis and emphysema but increases mean pulmonary arterial pressure.*

Mendella LA, Manfreda J, Warren CP, Anthonisen NR: Steroid response in stable chronic obstructive pulmonary disease. Ann Intern Med 96:17–21, 1982.
> *Double-blind, crossover study of methylprednisolone in patients with stable chronic bronchitis. Illustrates need from multiple pretreatment measures of function and the fact that only a minority subset of patients will respond.*

Mitchell DM, Rehahn M, Gildeh P, Dimond AH, Collins JV: Effects of prednisolone in chronic airflow limitation. Lancet 2:193–196, 1984.
> *Double-blind, crossover study of prednisolone in patients with stable chronic bronchitis that makes important points about the evaluation of glucocorticosteroids. Unlike most, contains some evaluation of symptoms as well as function.*

Monto AS, Higgin MW, Ross HW: The Tecumseh Study of respiratory illness. VIII. Acute infection in chronic respiratory disease and comparison groups. Am Rev Respir Dis 111:27–36, 1975.
> *A population-based, controlled study of the microbial causes of acute exacerbations in individuals with chronic lung disease. Demonstrates that only a minority of acute exacerbations of chronic bronchitis are associated with an identifiable microbial agent and that viruses with M. pneumoniae, and not H. influenzae, and S. pneumoniae, are the likely etiologic agents. Typical of most prospective studies conducted over the past 15 years.*

Nicotra MB, Rivera M, Awe RJ: Antibiotic therapy of acute exacerbations of chronic bronchitis. Ann Intern Med 97:18–21, 1982.
> *Double-blind, placebo-controlled trial of tetracycline in 40 patients hospitalized for an acute exacerbation of chronic bronchitis. Only marginal benefit in treatment group expressed as slightly greater increase in Pa_{O_2} after 7 days of treatment.*

Petersdorf RG, Featherstone HJ: New antimicrobial drugs and their value in the treatment of respiratory infections. Am Rev Respir Dis 117:1139–1140, 1978 (letter).
> *This and an accompanying letter highlight the controversy that still persists in regard to the use of antibiotics in the management of acute infections. These authors conclude that despite the inadequacies of the data, antibiotics should be considered in treatment. (See additional accompanying letter on page 1139.)*

Peto R, Speizer FE, Cochrane AL, Moore F, Fletcher CM, Tinker CM, Higgins ITT, Gray RG, Richards SM, Gilliland J, Norman Smith B: The relevance in adults of airflow obstruction, but not of mucus hypersecretion, to mortality from chronic lung disease. Am Rev Respir Dis 128:491–500, 1983.
> *Extensive analysis of relationship of mucous hypersecretion to mortality from airflow obstruction based on 20 to 25 years of follow-up of 2718 males in Britain.*

Ramsdale EH, Morris MM, Roberts RS, Hargreave FE: Bronchial responsiveness to methacholine in chronic bronchitis: Relationship to airflow obstruction and cold air responsiveness. Thorax 39:912–918, 1984.
> *Study of 27 patients with chronic bronchitis and a broad range of functional impairments which illustrates differential response to methacholine and cold air. Good discussion of data on bronchial hyperreactivity in chronic bronchitis with good bibliography.*

Reid LM: The pathology of obstructive and inflammatory airway disease. Eur J Respir Dis 147:26–37, 1986.
> *Chronic bronchitis, bronchiolitis, bronchiectasis, and asthma are reviewed with respect to morphology and the role of inflammation.*

Speizer FE, Tager IB: Epidemiology of chronic mucous hypersecretion and obstructive airways disease. Epidemiol Rev 1:124–142, 1979.
> *A critical review of the data that link various epidemiologic factors to the occurrence of mucous hypersecretion and chronic airflow obstruction.*

Tager IB, Speizer FE: Role of infection in chronic bronchitis. N Engl J Med 292:563–571, 1975.
> *An extensive review of data on the role of infection in the pathogenesis and management of chronic bronchitis. Although 10 years old, the conclusions are still valid, and little data of striking importance have appeared since its publication.*

Taylor RG, Joyce H, Gross E, Holland F, Pride NB: Bronchial reactivity to inhaled histamine and annual rate of decline in FEV_1 in male smokers and ex-smokers. Thorax 40:9–16, 1985.
> *Prospective study of 227 males over 7.5 years. Data show accelerated decline in FEV_1 in smokers with PC20 histamine less than 16 mg/ml. Methodologic limitations permit causal as well as noncausal inferences.*

Thurlbeck WM: Smoking, airflow limitation, and the pulmonary circulation. Am Rev Respir Dis 122:183–186, 1980.
> *An editorial summary of important work on pathophysiology of chronic airflow limitation. Focus is on significance of inflammation of small airways as the principal lesion in the pathophysiology of chronic airflow obstruction.*

Traver GA, Cline MG, Burrows B: Predictors of mortality in chronic pulmonary disease: A 15-year follow-up study. Am Rev Respir Dis 119:895–902, 1979.
> *A 15-year follow-up of 200 patients with initial $FEV_1/FVC < 60$ percent of predicted. Explores the value of a larger number of clinical findings in the prediction of survival in patients with severe chronic airflow obstruction.*

U.S. Department of Health, Education and Welfare. The Health Consequences of Smoking-Chronic Obstructive Lung Disease, 1984. US GPI, Washington, D.C., 1984.
> *A comprehensive report on the relationship of cigarette smoking to mucous hypersecretion and airflow obstructive disease. Extensive epidemiologic, physiological, and pathologic data are succinctly summarized and supplemented with an exhaustive list of references.*

Chapter 97

Bronchiectasis

Morton N. Swartz

Bronchiectasis is a chronic abnormal dilatation and distortion of bronchi caused by destruction of the elastic and muscular components of the bronchial walls. This is basically an anatomic definition. Usual clinical features include those of chronic or recurrent pulmonary infections: cough, copious mucopurulent sputum, fetid breath. Dilatation of bronchi can also occur in chronic bronchitis. Distinction between the two processes then becomes a matter of the degree and extent of the abnormality (milder and more generalized in chronic bronchitis). True bronchiectasis is permanent and should be distinguished from the reversible changes of pneumonia, tracheobronchitis, and atelectasis; these conditions may cause abnormalities on bronchography simulating bronchiectasis if this procedure is performed during or shortly after the acute pulmonary process.

PREVALENCE

Bronchiectasis, a common disabling and often fatal illness in the preantibiotic era, has become a comparatively rare disease over the past three decades in developed countries. This change stems, in a large measure, from the greater availability of antibiotics for the treatment of respiratory tract infections and from the widespread use of immunization in childhood, particularly against pertussis and measles. For a group of children's hospitals in the United Kingdom, Field found that the admission rate for patients with bronchiectasis had decreased from about 48 per 10,000 admissions to about 10 per 10,000 admissions between 1952 and 1960. At the Boston Children's Hospital, the number of new cases of bronchiectasis associated with infection (pneumonia, pertussis, measles, etc.) seen in a 5-year period (1946 to 1950) had declined from 47 to

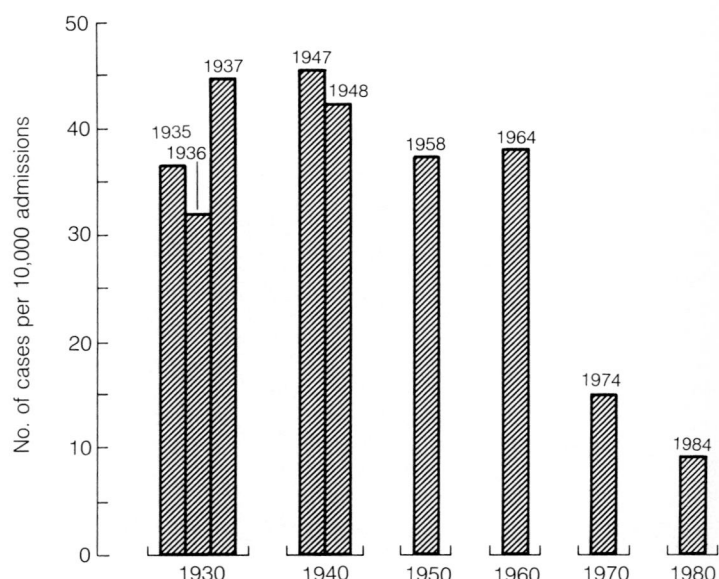

FIGURE 97-1 Annual incidence of bronchiectasis among patients admitted to Massachusetts General Hospital (MGH) during the decades from the 1930s to 1980s. The specific years for which data are illustrated are noted at the top of each of the bars.

only 2 cases a decade later (1956 to 1960). At the Massachusetts General Hospital, the number of patients with bronchiectasis per 10,000 admissions had declined from 45 in 1947 to about 9 in 1984 (Fig. 97-1). Currently, at this hospital only one to five bronchograms are done annually to establish a diagnosis of bronchiectasis.

PATHOLOGY

The abnormal bronchial dilatation in bronchiectasis involves principally the medium-sized bronchi but extends to the more distal bronchi and bronchioles as well. The airways are markedly dilated, sometimes as much as four times their normal diameter. On gross examination, the bronchi and bronchioles are usually so prominent as to be visible all the way to the pleural surface. This is in contrast to the normal lung in which the bronchioles can be followed by gross dissection only to a point 2 to 3 cm from the pleura. Bronchiectatic segments commonly are filled with purulent secretions, and the mucosal surface is swollen, inflamed, and often ulcerated. The bronchial epithelial lining may have a "polypoid" appearance as a result of prominent subjacent granulation tissue formation. Further distortion of the bronchial lumen is produced by exaggerated, transverse ridging of the encircling bronchial smooth muscle (Fig. 97-2) and by the pitted appearance caused by dilated bronchial mucous glands and ducts. With severe and extensive involvement, an almost cystic pattern is evident on the cut surface of the lung (Figs. 97-3 and 97-4) and may be evident on chest radiograph. As infection continues and spreads in the bronchial wall, the epithelial lining is denuded and elastic tissue, smooth muscle, and even surrounding cartilage are distorted and destroyed (Fig. 97-5). Focal lung abscesses may develop as a result of the necrotic process beginning in the bronchial walls. In more chronic bronchiectasis, marked fibrosis

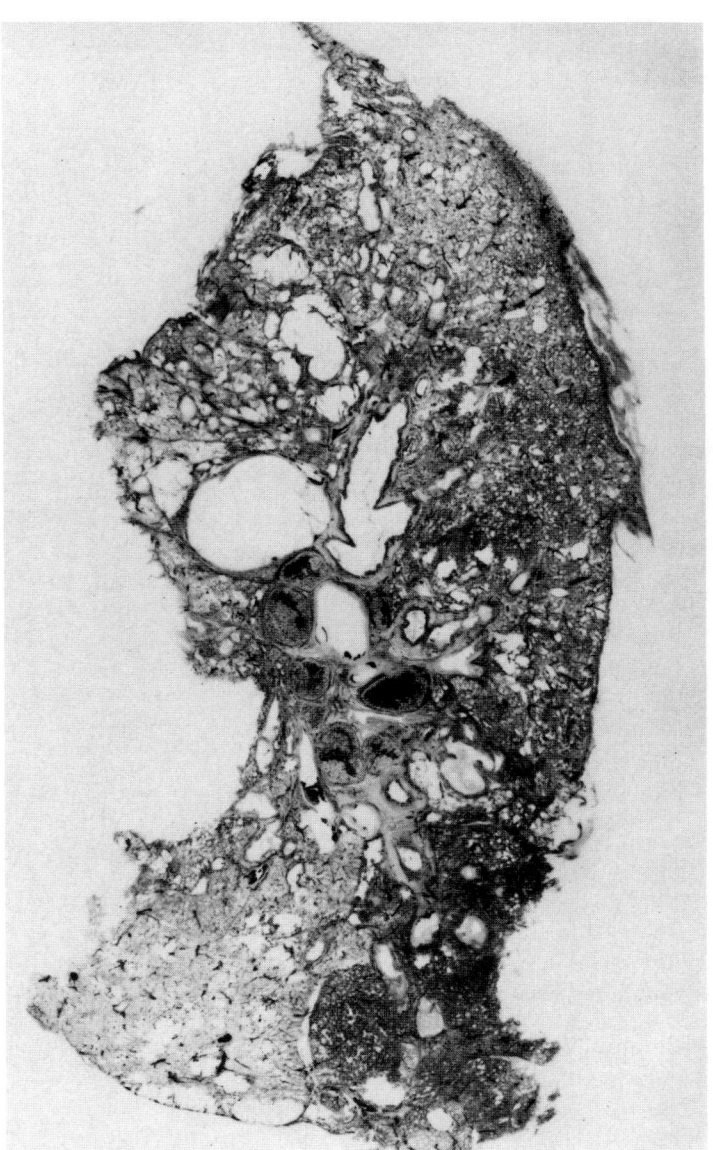

FIGURE 97-3 Gough section of lung of 59-year-old patient with a long history of recurrent pneumonias and chronic bronchiectasis who died with cor pulmonale. Enlarged hilar nodes and severe bronchiectasis, particularly in the mid-lung fields, are evident. Large sacs, up to 4 cm in diameter, appear grossly to be continuous with the bronchi.

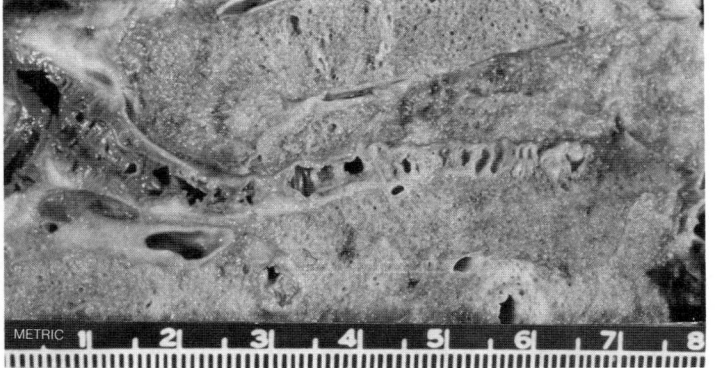

FIGURE 97-2 Gross section of lung showing cylindrical bronchiectasis. The dilated bronchus with thick intraluminal secretions and thickened walls shows transverse ridging due to muscle and cartilage changes.

occurs in and surrounding bronchial walls, replacing muscle, mucous glands, and cartilage.

Circulatory changes may develop in the lung as a consequence of bronchiectasis. Morphologically, bronchial arteries may be considerably enlarged (up to three times their normal caliber of 1.5 mm) and tortuous in patients with extensive bronchiectasis. This is believed due to the development of extensive anastomoses between the bronchial and pulmonary arterial circulations at the precapillary levels in the extensive granulation tissue in the walls

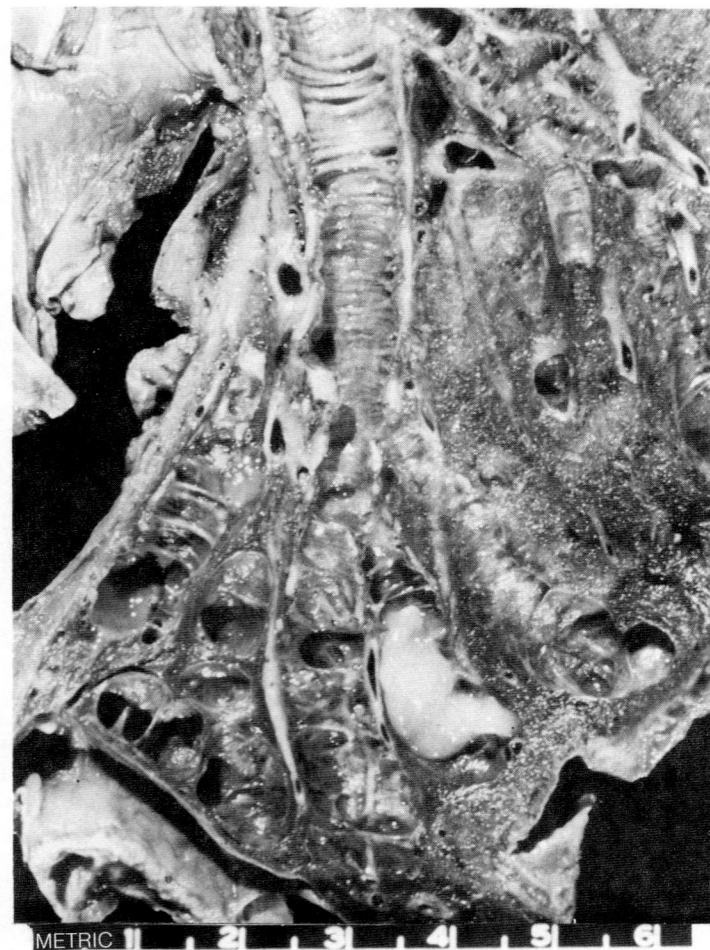

FIGURE 97-4 Severe saccular bronchiectasis with atelectasis and consolidation and cystic bronchi extending close to pleural surface.

of bronchiectatic airways. Evidence for such collateral circulation has been found on pathologic examination of bronchiectatic lung and by angiographic demonstration of bronchopulmonary anastomoses. Once such anastomotic channels are enlarged sufficiently, shunting of oxygenated blood from the higher-pressure systemic bronchial (or intercostal) arteries into the lower-pressure pulmonary circulation occurs. Measurement of such aortopulmonary collateral flow by dye dilution methods indicates that it may amount to 3 to 12 percent of pulmonary flow. The extent of collateral flow roughly correlates with the extent of bronchiectasis.

Bronchiectasis is bilateral in about 30 percent of patients. The lower lobes are those most frequently involved. The left lower lobe is involved over three times as frequently as the right. This may be because (1) the right bronchus is more readily drained by virtue of being a continuation of the trachea, (2) there is slight compression of the left bronchus where it is crossed by the left pulmonary artery, and (3) the left bronchus is narrower than the right.

In 50 to 80 percent of patients with bronchiectasis of the left lower lobe severe enough to have warranted resection, the lingula was involved as well. In left lower lobe bronchiectasis, the segmental involvement is unequal, e.g., the posterior basal segment is almost always diseased and the apical segment is spared in 75 percent of cases.

Classification

Bronchiectasis may be classified in a variety of ways: by pathogenetic mechanisms or predisposing factors, by bronchographic findings, or by gross and microscopic appearance on pathologic examination. All provide valuable information for the clinician and insights into pathogenesis and pathophysiological consequences. Since the investigations of Reid in 1950 have provided a correlation between bronchographic findings and pathologic (gross and microscopic) changes in resected bronchiectatic lobes, it is described here. It is the most widely used classification employed by pulmonologists, radiologists, and pathologists. Classification of bronchiectasis by predisposing factors is considered in a later section.

CYLINDRICAL BRONCHIECTASIS

On bronchogram, the bronchi are regularly outlined (tubular) and not greatly increased in diameter; their walls are straight. The involved bronchi come to an abrupt, squared end rather than taper gradually (Fig. 97-6). The anatomic changes occurring in the bronchial tree can also be evaluated by examining the number of subdivisions of the bronchial tree in the bronchiectatic segment (e.g., posterior basal segment of the left lower lobe) extending down to the respiratory bronchioles leading to the costal surface. In normal adult lung, the posterior basal bronchus has approximately 20 subdivisions, and this number is roughly the same in cylindrical bronchiectasis of the same pulmonary segment. Although the number of subdivisions in cylindrical bronchiectasis appears normal as viewed by dissection and microscopic examination of excised lobes, on bronchography prior to surgical resection the number of subdivisions is markedly reduced. This discrepancy stems from obstruction to filling by radiocontrast material caused by thick secretions, bronchial casts, and inflammatory edema of the bronchial walls of the peripheral bronchial tree.

VARICOSE BRONCHIECTASIS

On bronchogram, the bronchi are generally dilated and irregular in form and size. Unlike normal bronchi, they do not taper in diameter as they extend peripherally. Their terminations are distorted and characteristically bulbous (Fig. 97-7). Their irregular bulging contour is highly reminiscent of the appearance of saphenous varicosities. The average number of bronchial divisions is reduced on mi-

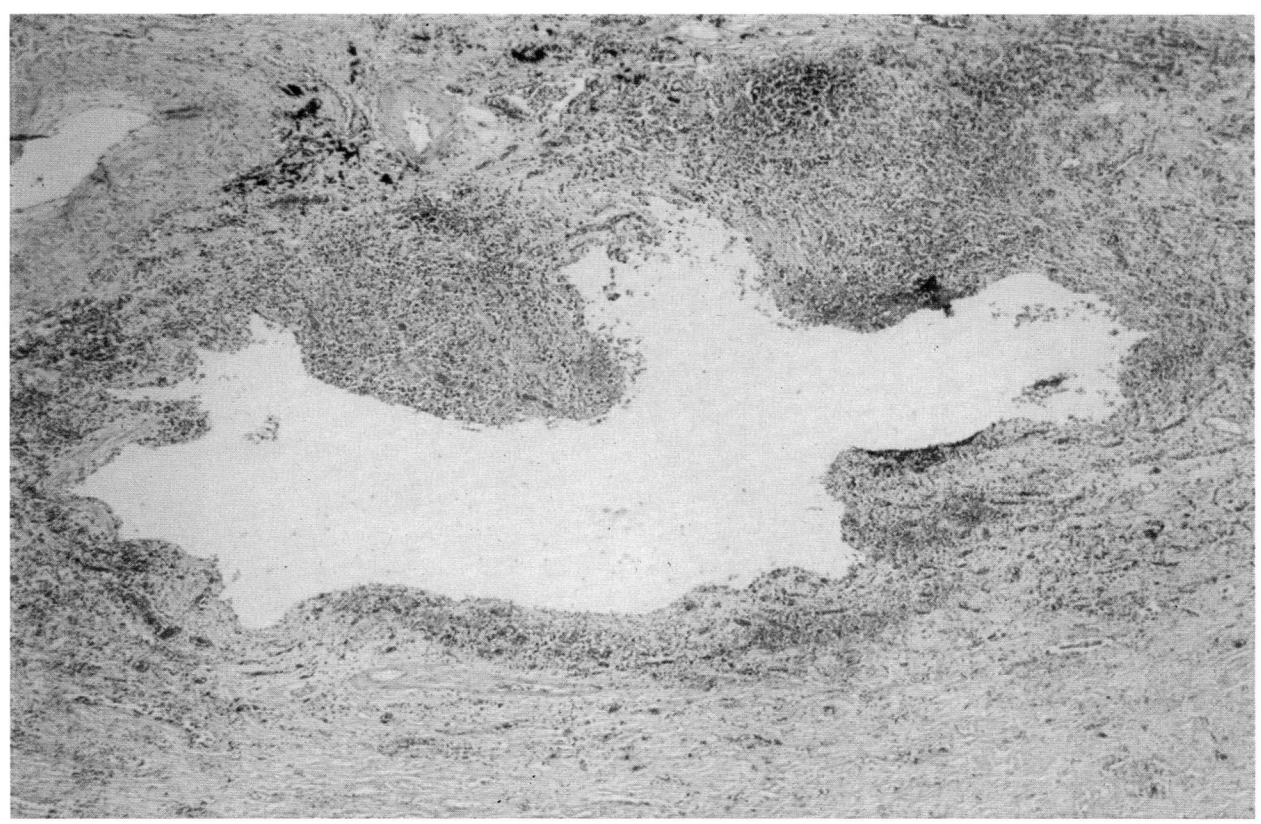

FIGURE 97-5 Microscopic section of lung of patient with bronchiectasis. Lining of small bronchus is totally denuded of surface epithelium. There is extensive surrounding inflammation with numerous capillaries and polypoid excrescences extending into the lumen. (H&E, ×100).

croscopic examination to about half the number present in normal lung. In many areas the bronchial lumen is totally obliterated by fibrous tissue containing bundles of muscle fibers, elastic tissue, and even remnants of the cartilaginous plates of the former bronchial wall. This fibrotic replacement of bronchial lumen may extend for a short distance, and further on the peripheral remnants of the bronchial tree may be distinguishable. Some of the distal bronchial remnants become epithelium-lined, fluid-filled cysts. In other areas, medium-sized bronchi terminate in dense fibrous tissue which extends cordlike along the route of the former bronchus.

SACCULAR (CYSTIC) BRONCHIECTASIS

On bronchogram, the bronchi are dilated, and this ballooning in outline (Fig. 97-8) increases as they progress to the lung periphery almost to the pleural surface. The number of bronchial subdivisions present on microscopic examination is sharply reduced (one-fourth to one-fifth the number found normally). Saccular bronchiectasis was formerly thought to involve smaller bronchioles because of the location of the bronchiectatic pus-filled cavities

(saccules) adjacent to the pleura. However, this view is not supported by the findings on pathologic examination of resected lobes where the fifth subdivision (20 subdivisions in normal lung) of the dilated bronchial tree is the terminal one, ending blindly immediately subjacent to the pleura. The "saccules" are the terminations of the diseased segments of the bronchial tree, with all the more peripheral branches destroyed beyond recognition or totally fibrosed. The larger presaccular bronchi are not dilated despite marked inflammation in the bronchial walls. The most prominent change in these bronchi is polyposis of bronchial epithelium, with numerous large fronds often causing bronchial obstruction. The saccular shape of the bronchiectatic airways probably results from (1) extension of the inflammation of the bronchial walls to supporting structures and surrounding pulmonary parenchyma, which are destroyed or undergo fibrosis, and (2) partial obstruction of presaccular bronchi by polyposis of its mucosa, preventing drainage of the saccular bronchi, which become distended with pus. Squamous metaplasis is common in saccular bronchiectasis but uncommon in other forms of bronchiectasis.

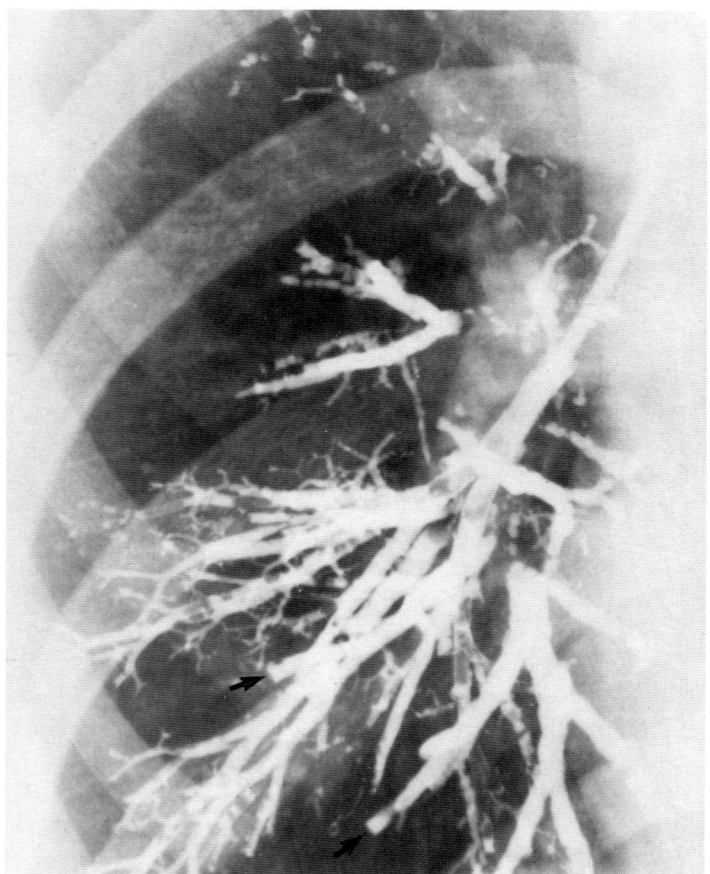

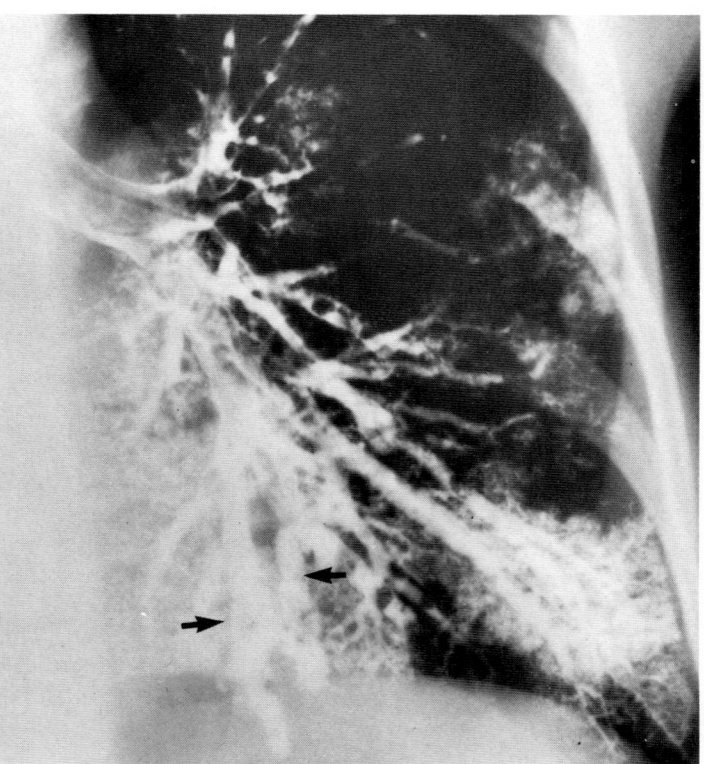

FIGURE 97-7 Bronchogram showing varicose bronchiectasis of basal segments of left lower lobe (arrows). *(Courtesy of Dr. T. McLoud.)*

FIGURE 97-6 Bronchogram demonstrating cylindrical bronchiectasis in some of lower lobe bronchi. Note the mild increase in diameter and blunt squared ends of bronchi (arrows). *(Courtesy of Dr. T. McLoud.)*

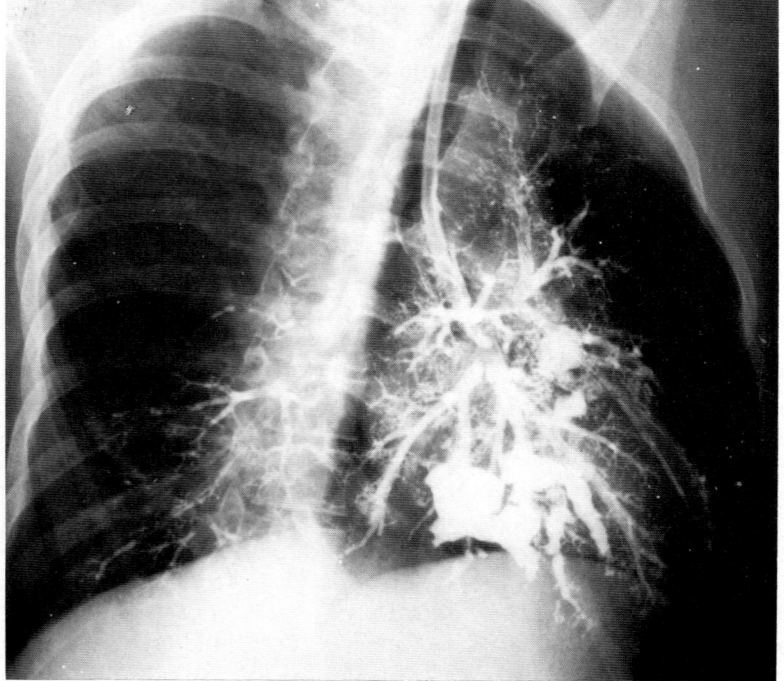

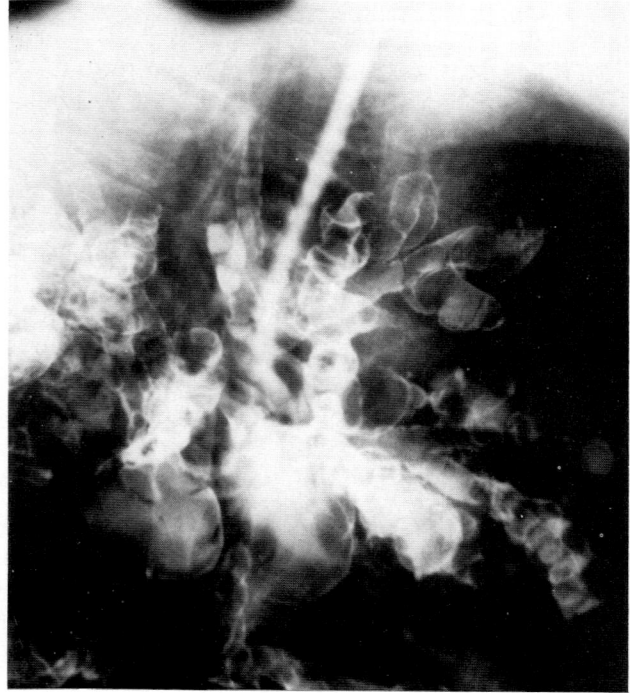

A   *B*

FIGURE 97-8 Bronchograms showing saccular (cystic) bronchiectasis. A. Saccular bronchiectasis of left lower lobe in a young man. *(Courtesy of Dr. C. Hales.)* B. Severe saccular bronchiectatic changes shown on this close-up view were widespread in both lungs. *(Courtesy of Dr. T. McLoud.)*

Other Pathologically Defined Forms of Bronchiectasis or Pathologically Similar Conditions

FOLLICULAR BRONCHIECTASIS

Follicular bronchiectasis is defined not by clinical or radiologic grounds but by strictly histologic criteria. The most prominent feature is the formation of lymphoid follicles and nodes in the walls of bronchi and bronchioles and in adjacent pulmonary parenchyma. Hilar lymph node enlargement is usually present. Involvement may be localized to a single bronchopulmonary segment or may include an entire lobe or several lobes. Associated with lymph follicle formation, elastic tissue is lost; with more extensive involvement, widespread destruction of smooth muscle and cartilage follows. Subepithelial lymph follicles produce partial obstruction of bronchial lumina and compress the openings of peripheral branches of diseased bronchi. The principal lesions develop in smaller bronchi, bronchioles, and adjacent alveoli. With more extensive inflammation, the distal bronchial tree is obliterated and the more proximal bronchi become involved with destruction of surrounding supporting tissues. Mucous gland ducts enlarge as a result of this circumbronchial necrosis and form part of the weakened bronchial or bronchiolar wall. Interstitial pneumonia is very frequently also present. The bronchographic picture can be that of any of the three types of bronchiectasis described above, depending on the severity of the process. Follicular bronchiectasis has been described primarily as a consequence of either a childhood viral infection (measles, adenovirus, or herpes simplex) or a bacterial infection (pertussis or a primary bronchopneumonia).

Follicular bronchiectasis may be accompanied by prominent lymphoid bronchiolectasis. The latter should be distinguished from another process, follicular bronchitis-bronchiolitis, which is characterized by abundant peribronchiolar lymph follicles compressing the bronchiolar lumen to a slitlike opening, acute purulent exudate in the bronchiolar lumen, and disruption of the reticular layer of the bronchiolar wall in the absence of chronic obstructive pulmonary disease or bronchiectasis. Follicular bronchitis-bronchiolitis occurs in the setting of collagen vascular disease (particularly rheumatoid arthritis and Sjögren's syndrome), immunodeficiency syndromes, and hypersensitivity states with eosinophilia.

CONGENITAL BRONCHIAL CYSTS OR CONGENITAL (BRONCHIAL) CYSTIC DISEASE

These congenital cysts in the pulmonary parenchyma represent developmentally abnormal bronchial wall structures, partially or completely filled with mucus and lined by respiratory tract epithelium. Histologically, they may mimic bronchiectasis. They occur in two forms: (1) *Central congenital cysts.* These are usually solitary, lack connection with their parent bronchus, and do not communicate with the distal alveolar parenchyma. The lumen is lined with respiratory epithelium, and the walls contain mucous glands, elastic tissue, muscle, and cartilage. If they become infected, communication with the proximal tracheobronchial tree may become established. Under these circumstances, the intraluminal mucus is replaced by pus, and the cysts may become distended with air as a result of a check-valve mechanism. (2) *Peripheral congenital cysts.* These are frequently multiple and represent a defect in bronchial maturation at a later stage in fetal development. They usually lack mucous glands, are lined by nonciliated columnar epithelium, and contain serous fluid; their walls contain much elastic tissue and a few abnormal cartilaginous plates. If infection occurs in these cysts, their congenital nature may be completely obscured, and the process resembles bronchiectasis by virtue of the inflammation, loss of respiratory epithelium, and apparent loss of much of the supporting cartilage.

INTRALOBAR BRONCHOPULMONARY SEQUESTRATION

This congenital malformation consists of a detached segment of pulmonary tissue, adjoining normal lung and covered by the same visceral pleura, which receives its blood supply from an anomalous artery taking origin from the aorta or one of its branches. Pneumonia in the sequestered segment is common in adults. The involved area contains cystic spaces which are lined by ciliated columnar or flattened epithelium and are filled with mucus, or pus when infected. Ordinarily, since there is no normal bronchial connection with the sequestered lung, the latter is not air-containing. With infection, communication often develops between the cystic, sequestered area of lung and the bronchial tree. Inflammatory cells are present in the cyst walls, which lack cartilage (a bronchial wall component often totally obliterated in bronchiectasis) and mucous glands.

PATHOGENESIS AND PREDISPOSING FACTORS

The proximate cause of bronchiectasis is almost universally a necrotizing infection (or a sequence of multiple infections) involving the tracheobronchial walls and surrounding pulmonary parenchyma. In years past, since its manifestations first appeared in childhood, bronchiectasis was considered to be predominantly a congenital disease due to some anatomic or functional abnormality of bronchi and bronchioles that predisposed to chronic infection. It now appears that "congenital" bronchiectasis is quite rare and due to definable abnormalities in tracheobronchial cartilage structure, defects in ciliary structure and function, alterations in the character of upper respiratory tract mucus, etc. (Table 97-1). The sharp decline in the prevalence of bronchiectasis following the introduction of modern antimicrobial therapy and widespread use

TABLE 97-1
Predisposing Factors for Bronchiectasis

Categories	Specific Entities	Categories	Specific Entities
Bronchopulmonary infections		Congenital anatomic defects (cont.)	
Childhood diseases	Pertussis; measles	Vascular	Pulmonary (intralobar) sequestration; pulmonary artery aneurysm
Other bacterial infections	Infections due to S. aureus, Klebsiella, M. tuberculosis, H. influenzae	Lymphatic	Yellow-nail syndrome
Other viral infections	Infections due to adenovirus (particularly types 7 and 21), influenza, herpes simplex; viral bronchiolitis	Immunodeficiency states IgG deficiency	Congenital (Bruton's type) agammaglobulinemia; selective deficiencies of subclasses (IgG2, IgG4); acquired immune globulin deficiency
Miscellaneous infections	Mycotic infections (histoplasmosis); ? mycoplasmal infections	IgA deficiency	Selective IgA deficiency ± ataxia-telangiectasia syndrome
Bronchial obstruction		Leukocyte dysfunction	Chronic granulomatous disease
Foreign body aspiration	Peanut; chicken bone; grass inflorescence, etc.	Hereditary abnormalities	
Neoplasms	Laryngeal papillomatosis; adenomas; bronchogenic carcinoma	Ciliary defects of respiratory mucosa	Kartagener's syndrome; immotile cilia syndrome; ciliary dyskinesis
Hilar adenopathy	Tuberculosis; histoplasmosis; sarcoid	α_1-Antitrypsin deficiency	Production of abnormal antitrypsin molecules; failure of gene transcription
Mucoid impaction	Allergic bronchopulmonary aspergillosis; bronchocentric granulomatosis; postoperative mucoid impaction	Cystic fibrosis (mucoviscidosis)	Typical early childhood syndrome; adolescent presentation with solely pulmonary symptoms
Chronic obstructive pulmonary disease	Chronic bronchitis; bronchial asthma	Miscellaneous disorders	
Acquired tracheobronchial disease	Relapsing polychondritis; tracheobronchial amyloidosis	Young's syndrome	Obstructive azoospermia with sinopulmonary infections
Congenital anatomic defects		Recurrent aspiration pneumonias	Alcoholism; neurologic disorders; lipoid pneumonia
Tracheobronchial	Bronchomalacia; bronchial cysts; cartilage deficiency (Williams-Campbell syndrome); tracheobronchomegaly (Mounier-Kuhn syndrome); ectopic bronchus; endobronchial teratoma; tracheo-esophageal fistula	Inhalation of irritants	Ammonia, nitrogen dioxide, or other irritant gases; smoke; talc; silicates; detergents
		Following combined heart-lung transplantation	Associated with obliterative bronchiolitis

of immunization for childhood diseases strongly suggests that infection, per se, is responsible for the majority of cases of this disease. Such a steep decline in frequency over the span of a few decades would be difficult to reconcile with a putative congenital defect. The question might then be asked as to whether there exists such an entity as congenital bronchiectasis. The term would most reasonably be applied to the small number of cases of congenital or hereditary disorders in which there is a high incidence of secondary bronchiectasis (Table 97-1). Even with such predisposing factors as congenital anatomic defects, congenital immunoglobulin deficiencies and respiratory tract dysfunction due to hereditary ciliary defects, cystic fibro-

sis, or α_1-antitrypsin deficiency, the associated bronchiectasis is thought to develop early in childhood rather than be present at birth.

The basic element in the development of ordinary acquired bronchiectasis appears to be inflammatory destruction of the components (elastic tissue, smooth muscle, cartilage) of the bronchial wall (see "Pathology," above). As a consequence of this inflammatory reaction, alterations develop in the configuration of the involved bronchi secondary to pressure changes occurring on respiration and coughing as well as secondary to peribronchial fibrosis. The result is the distortion and ballooning of the diseased bronchi. A requirement for such a definition of

acquired bronchiectasis is microscopic evidence of inflammatory destruction of the walls of ectatic bronchi. The term *congenital bronchiectasis* might reasonably apply then in infants and young children to regional clusters of ectatic bronchi, the walls of which show no significant evidence of inflammation. Culiner considered three congenital processes characterized by areas of dilated or cystic bronchi (*bronchial cysts, intralobar pulmonary sequestration,* and *congenital cystic bronchiectasis*) to be variants of a single group of anomalies. In congenital cystic bronchiectasis, in contrast to the other two entities, the bronchial cysts are not usually isolated from the remainder of the bronchial tree but rather represent ectatic bronchial canalization in continuity with normal segmental bronchi. Lower lobes from children with such anomalies and lacking evidence of inflammation have occasionally been observed and might qualify for the designation *congenital bronchiectasis.* With time, infection develops in these areas, eliminating mural inflammation as a discriminant between acquired and congenital bronchiectasis.

A genetic predisposition to bronchiectasis has been suggested by its apparently increased incidence in certain racial groups. In the United States, the prevalence of bronchiectasis is about 60 per 100,000 population. Among Polynesians in Western Samoa the incidence, based on detection of gross disease by radiologic screening, is an order of magnitude higher. Similarly, the annual incidence rate of bronchiectasis among native Alaska Indians and Inuits is high, 6.8 cases per 10,000 children aged 0 to 10 years compared to 1.06 per 10,000 children in Scotland. However, factors other than ethnic ones may play the primary role in these geographic areas: inadequate diet, crowded living conditions (contributing to increased numbers of respiratory infections), and lack of medical attention and antimicrobial therapy (allowing progression of acute bronchopulmonary infections to a chronic destructive state). At present, such issues preclude assigning any specific role of genetic factors to these cases of bronchiectasis. It is of interest to note, however, that abnormal cilia have been observed on electron microscopic examination of respiratory tract epithelium of a high percentage of Polynesians with bronchiectasis. Dextrocardia, however, is not associated with bronchiectasis in these patients.

Infections

In the first half of the century, prior to extensive immunization against pertussis and measles, a variety of pulmonary infections during childhood were associated with subsequent bronchiectasis (Table 97-1). Severe preceding lower respiratory infections have been reported in as many as 69 percent of cases of childhood bronchiectasis, whereas antecedent aspirational events occurred in 16 percent, and the predisposing factor in the remaining 15 percent was a congenital disorder. Studies by Ogilvie earlier in this century suggested that the initiating infection is not necessarily a severe one: in 66 percent of cases, the symptoms of bronchiectasis dated from the first 5 years of life, and in 43 percent of the cases the onset had been insidious and could not be related to any specific event.

MEASLES

The association of measles with bronchiectasis is much less prominent now in the United States than formerly. In the 1960s and 1970s, 14 percent of cases of childhood bronchiectasis appeared to have been associated with antecedent measles. In underdeveloped countries, this association is currently much more prominent. Follicular bronchiectasis is generally considered to be a complication of measles, pertussis, or influenza viral pneumonia. The presence of extensive peribronchial inflammation as well as striking proliferation of bronchial and bronchiolar epithelium in fatal cases of measles pneumonia is consistent with the concept of acute bronchial damage which might progress to follicular bronchiectasis. In children dying within a month of onset of measles, other etiologies for complicating necrotizing bronchopneumonia have been observed. These include infections due to adenovirus, *Herpesvirus,* and bacteria (*Staphylococcus aureus, Klebsiella, Pseudomonas*). In other children recovering from such infections, the bronchial damage is presumed to lead to varying degrees of follicular bronchiectasis, accentuated by subsequent lower respiratory tract infections. In some instances, persisting viral infection may be a factor in the extensive lymphoid aggregates characterizing follicular bronchiectasis.

PERTUSSIS

Secondary necrotizing bacterial pneumonia is an important factor in the development of bronchiectasis following whooping cough. However, pertussis itself can produce a necrotizing bronchitis. In the course of pertussis, inspissated mucus and debris may produce resorptive atelectasis in infants and young children and serve as an additional contributing factor in postpertussis bronchiectasis.

OTHER BACTERIAL PULMONARY INFECTIONS

The bacterial pneumonias that appear to predispose to the development of subsequent bronchiectasis are usually necrotizing processes due to species such as *S. aureus, Klebsiella pneumoniae,* and *Pseudomonas aeruginosa.* Lobar pneumonia due to *Streptococcus pneumoniae,* which is not ordinarily destructive of tissue and heals without significant scarring, is not likely to render the bronchial tree susceptible to subsequent bronchiectasis. *S. pneumoniae,* however, may colonize the bronchial tree in some patients with bronchiectasis. *Hemophilus influenzae* type B can cause invasive pneumonias in infants and children but appears to play no important role in

bronchiectasis. On the other hand, unencapsulated *H. influenzae* are very commonly present in the sputa of patients with bronchiectasis, as colonizers, and also as contributors to chronic progressive infection of the bronchial tree.

Necrotizing Pneumonia Due to Anaerobic Bacteria

Anaerobic necrotizing pneumonia is usually of aspirational origin or a consequence of bronchial obstruction. The necrotizing nature of the process is reflected by the frequent progression to parenchymal destruction (pulmonary gangrene), to lung abscess, to putrid empyema, and to chronic bronchiectasis in some instances. The bacteria involved consist of a mixture of facultative and obligately anaerobic species indigenous to the oral cavity.

Tuberculosis

The pathogenesis of so-called tuberculous bronchiectasis may take several forms. (1) A marked degree of caseation necrosis of bronchial walls can occur, particularly when upper lobes are involved. Tuberculous granulomatous inflammation can be observed at the distal end of some saccular lesions, suggesting that at least in some cases bronchiectasis represents extension of an initial tuberculous bronchitis. (2) Scarring of an initial tuberculous involvement of larger bronchi can produce bronchial stenosis. Mixed bacterial infection and retained purulent secretions can then produce bronchiectasis as might occur following any other type of bronchial obstruction. (3) Extraluminal obstruction of larger bronchi by tuberculous hilar lymphadenopathy can produce the same consequences as intraluminal obstruction and eventuate in bronchiectasis. As with bronchostenotic tuberculosis, the inflammatory destruction of bronchial walls is to a large measure related to bacterial infection (indigenous upper respiratory tract flora or superimposed pyogens such as *S. aureus*) rather than to *Mycobacterium tuberculosis*. (4) Some or all of the bronchiectatic sacs in the upper lobes may represent healing or healed tuberculous cavities that have become partially relined with ciliated epithelium. Such cavities may or may not have established continuity with the bronchial tree.

Mycotic Infections

Pulmonary histoplasmosis is probably the best example of a primary pulmonary mycotic infection that can predispose to bronchiectasis. The sequence here is that of hilar lymphadenopathy, bronchial obstruction, and secondary bacterial inflammation with resultant ectasia of bronchial walls.

Bronchial Obstruction

A variety of mechanisms have been proposed for the development of "atelectatic bronchiectasis," the form of bronchiectasis associated with bronchial obstruction. It has been suggested that collapse follows bronchial obstruction and the bronchi proximal to the obstruction would then be subject to strong dilating forces caused by the pressure difference between atmospheric pressure in the bronchi and negative pressure in the pleural space. It was also thought that traction on more distal airways due to the collapse of surrounding, normally cushioning alveoli would contribute to bronchial dilatation following obstruction of peripheral bronchi. Whitwell offered evidence against the latter pathogenetic mechanism from studies of follicular and saccular bronchiectasis where obstruction of peripheral bronchi was almost uniformly present. In the lung units involved, atelectasis was absent. Collateral airdrift or ventilation, the passage of air to alveoli other than by direct airway connections, appeared to account for this. Adequate collateral air circulation is provided under these circumstances by several possible routes: (1) pores of Kohn (circular openings in the walls between adjoining alveoli) and (2) canals of Lambert (epithelium-lined tubules between preterminal bronchioles and surrounding alveoli; not only those in normal sequence to the particular preterminal bronchiole but also those normally aerated via other preterminal bronchioles).

Evidence indicates that bronchial obstruction, per se, does not cause bronchiectasis but rather facilitates its development by interfering with bronchial clearance and encouraging bacterial infection. Ligation of bronchi of rabbits, causing bronchi to fill with secretions, does not produce bronchiectasis unless infection occurs spontaneously or is intentionally introduced. Ligation of bronchi of rats, which have an indigenous bronchial flora, commonly leads to bronchial infection and bronchiectasis, unless infection is initially controlled by appropriate antibiotic administration.

In contrast to the frequency of bronchiectasis following atelectasis and infection secondary to bronchial obstruction, bronchiectasis has been a rarity after collapse of the lung due to hydrothorax or therapeutic pneumothorax. The explanation probably lies in the absence of bronchial infection in the latter.

FOREIGN BODY BRONCHIECTASIS

Bronchiectasis may develop many years following unrecognized aspiration of a foreign body such as a chicken bone, pipe stem, or peanut. Such postobstructive bronchiectasis is a localized rather than a diffuse process. Bronchiectasis can be produced in animals 2 to 8 weeks following introduction of sterile foreign bodies into the bronchial tree. Obstructive emphysema, atelectasis, and infection precede the development of chronic inflammation and ensuing bronchiectasis.

A particularly difficult to diagnose type of foreign body aspiration in children is that of a grass inflorescence (flowering head). It is less likely to cause immediate respi-

ratory symptoms than does aspiration of an inorganic foreign body or a peanut by virtue of being relatively inert; also, the configuration of a grass inflorescence is less likely to completely occlude a bronchus or produce a ball valve obstruction. Such grass heads commonly migrate into segmental bronchi, where they are extremely difficult to visualize on bronchoscopy. Months later chronic cough, recurrent pneumonias, and hemoptysis herald the development of localized progressive bronchiectasis.

NEOPLASMS

Various endobronchial tumors such as adenomas and carcinomas can be associated with localized bronchiectasis. Laryngeal papillomas with papillomatosis of the lower respiratory tract may produce bronchial obstruction and resultant bronchiectasis.

MUCOID IMPACTION

Allergic Bronchopulmonary Aspergillosis (ABPA)
The principal features of ABPA are episodic wheezing and bronchial obstruction, recurrent febrile episodes, peripheral blood eosinophilia, intermittent pulmonary infiltrates, and expectoration of mucous plugs containing eosinophils and *Aspergillus* species (usually *A. fumigatus*). Laboratory findings include elevated levels of IgG and serum precipitins against *Aspergillus* antigens, and immediate wheal and flare and type III skin test reactivity. Invasive bronchopulmonary aspergillosis does not develop; the fungus remains within the bronchial lumen. The underlying pathogenesis of ABPA appears to be an allergic response to the presence of *Aspergillus* species in the bronchial tree. A type I hypersensitivity reaction, mediated by IgE, is responsible for bronchospasm; a type III (Arthus') reaction, mediated by immune complexes, is thought to be responsible for bronchial and peribronchial inflammation. The latter is manifest radiologically as acute patchy infiltrates, particularly in the upper lobes, and as the so-called tram-line shadows, which are transitory thin parallel line densities, probably representing edema of bronchial walls. Cylindrical bronchiectasis may complicate ABPA, developing in bronchial segments that have previously been sites of transient infiltrations and sites of *Aspergillus* antigen in mucous plugs (mucoid impaction). The bronchiectasis of ABPA is characteristically a proximal bronchiectasis; lesser bronchi and bronchioles are distally more normal in contrast to the pattern generally seen with usual infectious bronchiectasis.

Chronic Obstructive Airways Disease
Bronchiectasis can complicate diffuse obstructive airways diseases such as asthma and chronic bronchitis. Hypertrophy of mucous glands and hypersecretion of mucus is characteristic of chronic bronchitis. In the early stages of this condition, the bronchographic findings are those of incomplete peripheral filling, most likely representing partial or complete obstruction by mucus of the smallest peripheral bronchi. With continued infection and intermittent mucoid impaction, bronchial inflammation can gradually progress to bronchiectasis.

Congenital Anatomic Defects

Although a congenital basis for most cases of bronchiectasis was suggested and supported by many in the first half of this century, current evidence does not sustain this concept. The congenital anatomic defect may be categorized as tracheobronchial, vascular, and lymphatic.

TRACHEOBRONCHIAL

Congenital Bronchial Cartilage Deficiency (Williams-Campbell Syndrome)
A small number of patients with bronchiectasis develop respiratory symptoms in the first year of life (or even first weeks) as a result of specific anatomic defects. Children with the rare Williams-Campbell syndrome have the clinical features of bronchiectasis (persistent cough, sputum production, recurrent pulmonary infections, and clubbing); the bronchographic findings are those of airway dilations on inspiration and almost complete airway collapse on expiration of the second- to eighth-order bronchi.

Anatomic features of the Williams-Campbell syndrome include: (1) deficiency of bronchial cartilage extending proximally to the first and second segmental divisions, but presence of intact cartilaginous plates at bronchial bifurcations out to seventh-order divisions; (2) absence of destruction of other (noncartilaginous) bronchial wall structures by inflammation; and (3) uniform, bilateral distribution of the process. In addition to these anatomic features which distinguish this process from the more common forms of bronchiectasis, bronchographic findings early in the course of the disease have been much more marked and extensive than would have been anticipated on the basis of the duration and severity of infection. Proximal extension of the bronchiectatic lesions to the second-order bronchi would be most unusual in acquired bronchiectasis and serves to distinguish this disease. Whether true bronchiectasis is present at birth or whether it develops rapidly very early in life as a consequence of congenital bronchomalacia is not known.

Tracheobronchomegaly (Mounier-Kuhn Syndrome)
This very rare disorder of the lower respiratory tract consists of marked dilatation of the trachea and central bronchi, associated with repeated episodes of pulmonary infections. Beyond the involved major bronchi the transition is abrupt to normal caliber airways. Symmetric saccular bronchiectasis is frequently present. Widening of the tracheal air column is evident on posteroanterior radi-

ographs of the chest. On bronchography, saccular out-pouchings of the lumen between the cartilage rings of the dilated trachea and major bronchi are visible. They represent protrusions of redundant mucosa between the transverse bundles of trachealis muscle fibers, which connect the posterior ends of the U-shaped tracheal cartilages.

Limited pathologic study suggests the underlying process is a primary atrophy of the elastic tissue and smooth muscle of the trachea and major bronchi.

Clinically, most patients with this syndrome present in adult life, but occasional cases have been diagnosed in infants. The distinctive features are those of tracheobronchomegaly associated with symmetric involvement of the bronchial tree in varicose and saccular bronchiectasis. In addition, the marked pliability of the airways and redundancy of mucosa may produce obstructive airways disease as a consequence of airway collapse during expiration.

VASCULAR

Bronchopulmonary (Intralobar) Sequestration
This topic has been considered above (see "Intralobar Bronchopulmonary Sequestration").

LYMPHATIC

"Yellow-Nail" Syndrome
This very rare syndrome involves the combination of lymphedema of the lower extremities, recurrent pneumonia and bronchiectasis, and yellow discoloration of the nails. No clear common thread has been uncovered to account for this bizarre combination of abnormalities, although some form of lymphatic obstruction has been suggested. Pathologic examination of excised lobes has shown only advanced stages of conventional bronchiectasis.

Immunodeficiency States

Bronchiectasis is more often associated with defects in humoral than cellular immunity.

IgG DEFICIENCY

Repeated infections with invasive pyogenic bacteria such as pneumococci, streptococci, and *H. influenzae* characterize X-linked agammaglobulinemia. Bruton's original patient had had 19 episodes of pneumococcal sepsis by 8 years of age. The most common types of infection in patients with this form of immunodeficiency are sinusitis, pneumonia, otitis, bacteremia, meningitis, and furunculosis. If untreated, recurrent episodes of pulmonary infection in boys with this condition often progress to chronic bronchiectasis. Replacement of gamma globulin prevents recurrent infection and the ultimate development of chronic pulmonary disease. Occasionally, children with

normal levels of total IgG have selective deficiencies of IgG subclasses (IgG2, IgG4, IgG3) and are subject to recurrent sinopulmonary infection, sometimes progressing to chronic bronchiectasis. Such IgG subclass deficiency should be considered in any child or young adult with otherwise unexplained recurrent sinopulmonary infections and bronchiectasis. Similar problems or pulmonary infections and bronchiectasis occur in patients (males or females) at any age who develop common variable immunodeficiency.

OTHER IMMUNODEFICIENCIES

Recurrent sinopulmonary infections are frequent in patients with selective IgA deficiency. Occasional patients go on to develop bronchiectasis, particularly if levels of an IgG subclass (IgG2 or IgG3) are also reduced. The rarer isolated IgE and isolated IgM deficiencies have occasionally been complicated by chronic pulmonary infections and bronchiectasis. The so-called bare lymphocyte syndrome, a failure of lymphocytes to express cell surface histocompatibility antigens (HLA-A, HLA-B, etc.), may, in some patients, be associated with immunodeficiency and be manifest as recurrent sinopulmonary infections and progressive diffuse bronchiectasis.

Recurrent infections occurring in patients with chronic granulomatous disease, a group of disorders characterized by defects in oxygen-dependent neutrophil microbicidal activity, include pneumonia and lung abscess. Pulmonary fibrosis and bronchiectasis may follow a prolonged course of repeated infections. However, bronchiectasis appears to be a less common complication of this condition than might be expected.

Hereditary Abnormalities

An impressive array of genetic defects are associated with clinical syndromes in which bronchiectasis is sometimes a striking feature.

CILIARY DEFECTS OF RESPIRATORY MUCOSA

Immotile Cilia Syndrome (Dyskinetic Cilia Syndrome)
In humans, ciliated epithelium lines the nasal cavity, paranasal sinuses, middle ear, respiratory tract down to the level of the respiratory bronchioles (see Chapter 2), cerebral ventricles, and oviducts; in addition, corneal cells lining the anterior chambers each bear a solitary cilium. In the respiratory tract, coordinated beating of the cilia mechanically assists clearance of the airways of aggregates of bacteria and phagocytic cells. On electron microscopy, cross-sectional structure of the central core (axoneme) of a respiratory tract cilium is highly ordered; nine peripheral pairs of microtubules surround a central microtubular doublet ("9 + 2 pattern") (Fig. 97-9). Each peripheral pair of microtubules is connected to adjacent doublets by

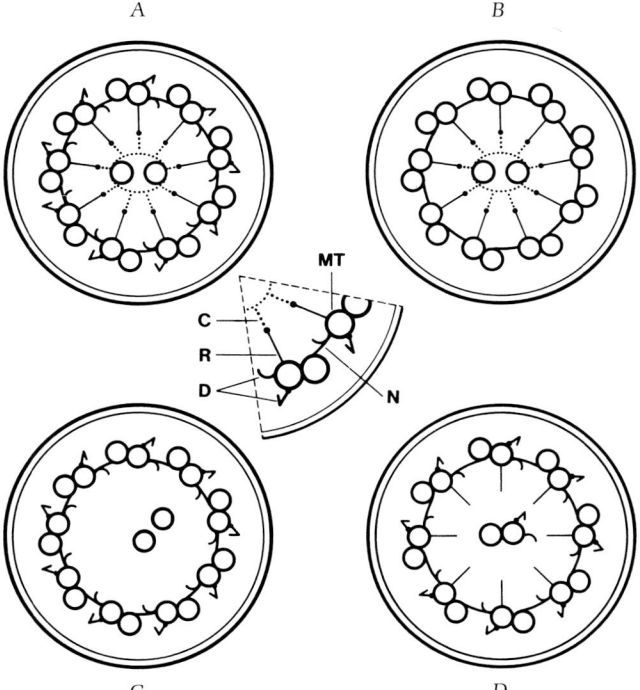

FIGURE 97-9 Schematic cross section views of cilia. *A.* Normal cilium with nine outer pairs of microtubules (MT) distributed symmetrically about a central pair, which is ringed by a central sheath (C). The outer pairs of microtubules are connected to each other by nexin links (N). Radial spokes (R) connect each of the outer pairs to the central sheath. As a consequence of this binding of the pairs of microtubules, their shortening is translated into bending motion. The driving energy for the shortening of the MT is provided by ATP hydrolysis catalyzed by the ATPase located in the dynein arms (outer and inner; designated D in inset). *B to D* represent various forms of congenital ciliary defects. *B.* Immotile cilia lacking dynein arms. *C.* Immotile cilia with missing radial spokes; central pair is eccentrically placed. *D.* Another type of cilia (immotile) defect in which the abnormality is a transposition of an outer microtubular pair to the central position. As a result, only eight pairs of microtubules are present in the peripherally placed array. At the more proximal portion of the cilium (near the cell surface), the appearance may be that of nine normal peripheral microtubular pairs without a central pair. Inset indicates various components (MT, C, R, D, N) of the cilial structure. *(Modified from Davis et al., 1983.)*

nexin links. Appended symmetrically to the comparable microtubule of each peripheral doublet are two hooklike structures (inner and outer dynein arms). The dynein arms are made up of the protein dynein, which has ATPase activity, and are oriented in a clockwise direction. Surrounding the central pair of tubules is a sheath, and a series of radial spokes connects the central tubules to each of the outer doublets. The same anatomic features are evident in the tails of spermatozoa.

The rhythmic motion of cilia effecting mucociliary transport in the respiratory tract is produced by the linking via dynein arms of one pair of outer tubules to the adjacent doublet and the sliding of actin filaments of the

microtubular pairs past each other, much as occurs with actin and myosin in muscle. The hydrolysis of adenosine triphosphate by the dynein ATPase powers this reaction. Since the outer filaments are tied together by nexin links and tied to the central sheath by radial spokes, the sliding of the microtubule pairs is converted to a bending motion of the ciliary shaft. The direction of bending is dictated by the relationship of the peripheral tubules vis-a-vis the central tubules. Coordinated bending of sheets of cilia on respiratory epithelial cells is necessary to move the overlying mucous blanket. This is made possible by orientation of central doublet pairs within 25° of each other.

The immobile cilia syndrome is a genetic disorder (frequently seen among siblings in areas where consanguinity is high) whose molecular lesion produces immotile or otherwise defective cilia. As a result of the wide distribution of cilia, symptoms produced include sinusi-

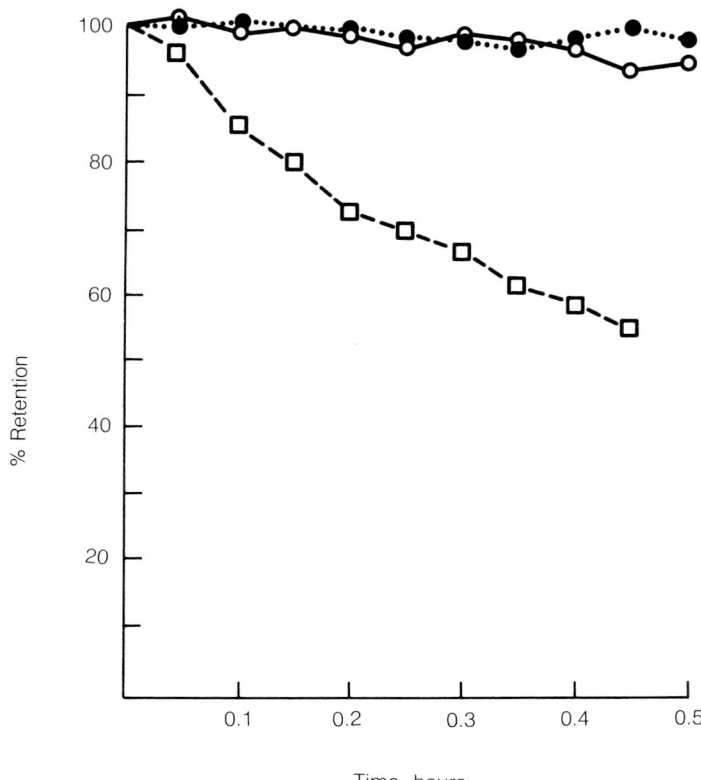

FIGURE 97-10 Nasal mucociliary transport as measured by removal of a 0.02-ml droplet of ^{99m}Tc-labeled albumin from the nasal cavity over 30 min. Clearance of radioactivity is calculated from the radioactivity (disintegrations per minute) retained in the nasal cavity as a percentage of the initial dpm measured (percent retention). ● = Mean clearance curve for four patients with bronchiectasis and chronic sinusitis and immotile cilia (but without situs inversus). ○ = Mean clearance curve for six patients with Kartagener's syndrome. □ = Mean clearance curve for 13 normal subjects. Pulmonary mucociliary transport was similarly deficient in patients with the immotile cilia syndrome, both those with and without Kartagener's syndrome. *(Modified from Rossman et al., 1980.)*

tis, otitis, chronic rhinitis, chronic or recurrent bronchitis, bronchiectasis, male sterility, corneal abnormalities (malformations), and impaired olfactory function. The concept of an immotile cilia syndrome stemmed from initial observations by Petersen and Afzelius in several infertile men of the production of spermatozoa that were living but whose tails were stiff, straight, and immotile. The structure of the spermatozoa was relatively normal except for the absence of dynein arms. These patients had had frequent colds, otitis media, and pneumonias, as well as chronic sinusitis and bronchitis since childhood. Bronchial cilia from such patients had a similar abnormal ultrastructure and absence of dynein arms, and they were immotile.

The criteria for diagnosis of the immotile cilia syndrome include: (1) clinical manifestations of recurrent and chronic upper and lower respiratory tract infections such as rhinitis, sinusitis, otitis, bronchitis, and bronchiectasis; (2) absence or near absence of tracheobronchial or nasal mucociliary transport (Fig. 97-10); (3) total or near total absence of dynein arms of the cilia in nasal or bronchial mucosa; rarely, ultrastructural axonemal defects other than absent dynein arms such as absent or defective radial spokes or transposition of a peripheral microtubular doublet to the center of an axoneme are associated with the syndrome; and (4) sterility in males associated

with living but immotile spermatozoa with similar axonemal ultrastructural abnormalities. In women, reduced fertility is a feature as well. The term *immotile cilia syndrome* is generally used to describe this tetrad of clinical and laboratory findings associated with dynein-deficient cilia. However, the terms *ciliary dyskinesia syndrome* or *dyskinetic cilia syndrome* have been suggested as a result of the finding that the cilia in some patients with this syndrome, although anatomically abnormal, are in fact motile, albeit with abnormal motions.

The frequency of bronchiectasis in the immotile cilia syndrome is high, about 30 percent, but the long-term prognosis for patients is relatively good, some patients living to an advanced age. Some patients over 35 years of age with this syndrome show on pulmonary function testing only mild to moderate airways obstruction. Exacerbations of infections tend to be more severe in late childhood and adolescence; in adult years, there may be an amelioration of symptoms.

Kartagener's Syndrome

The triad of bronchiectasis, sinusitis, and situs inversus (Kartagener's syndrome) (Fig. 97-11) is a subset of the immotile cilia syndrome and occurs in about 50 percent of patients with this cilial dysfunction syndrome. How the

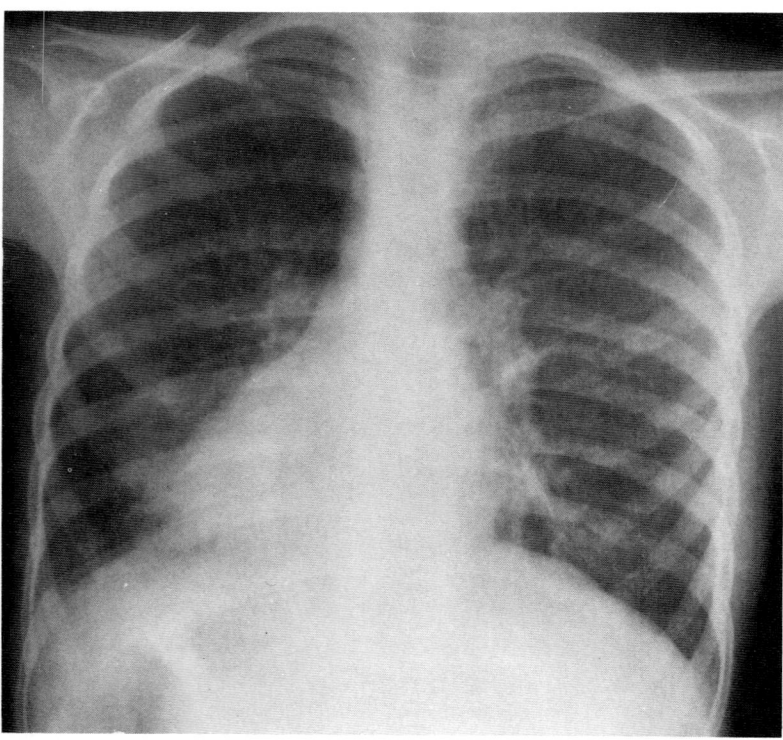

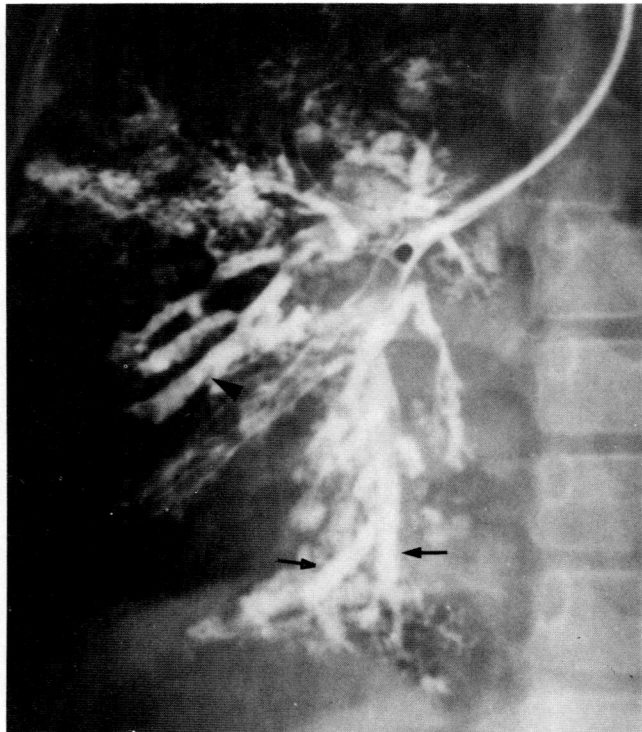

A   B

FIGURE 97-11   Young girl with Kartagener's syndrome.   *A.* Chest radiograph at age 5 years showing dextrocardia, as part of situs inversus, and right lower lung infiltrate.   *B.* Bronchogram performed at age 8 years showing varicose bronchiectasis of bronchi to lower lobe (arrows) and of bronchi that represent lingular equivalents (arrowhead). *(Courtesy of Dr. D. Kushner.)*

situs inversus of Kartagener's syndrome fits into the cilial dysfunction syndrome is unclear. Afzelius has postulated that in normal embryos the cilia on epithelia have fixed positions and direction of beating. As a result, in the normal course of development the cilia are presumed to cause the embryonic viscera to bend into a right-handed helical configuration, shifting the heart to the left. In the absence of ciliary function, whether the embryonic viscera would make a right-handed twist (to normal situs) or a left-handed twist or malrotation (to situs inversus) would be determined solely by chance. In keeping with this postulate is the fact that among siblings with the immotile cilia syndrome about half have complete and half have partial (no situs inversus) Kartagener's syndrome.

Kartagener's syndrome affects about one individual in 68,000 and appears to be inherited as an autosomal recessive trait. Of patients with bronchiectasis who have been studied, about 1.5 percent have Kartagener's triad. Of individuals with situs inversus, about 15 percent have the complete Kartagener's syndrome. Essentially all patients with Kartagener's syndrome have immotile cilia with obvious ultrastructural defects (usually absent or defective dynein arms) in the ciliary axoneme. However, a patient with Kartagener's syndrome has been described with no obvious ciliary abnormality on electron microscopy. It is very likely that the defect here is a functional abnormality in the cilia, perhaps in the dynein ATPase or other enzymatic constituent.

Among Polynesians, New Zealand Maoris, and Samoan Islanders, bronchiectasis is a common problem. It is often associated with sinusitis, impaired mucociliary clearance, and immotile spermatozoa. On electron mi-croscopy of bronchial or nasal ciliated epithelium, dynein arms are either absent or incomplete. Unlike the case in Europeans or Americans, however, these abnormalities are not associated with dextrocardia, and this fact is an argument against Afzelius's postulate. The ciliary microstructural abnormalities observed among Polynesians are more varied than those seen in Kartagener's syndrome. In addition to lack of dynein arms, these include cilia with missing, misplaced, or supernumerary tubules and compound cilia (containing several axonemes) (Fig. 97-12). Perhaps the mutation in the Polynesians is distinct from that in Europeans with Kartagener's syndrome.

In addition to anomalies of the bronchial ciliary apparatus that are congenital, acquired ones also occur. The latter, by compromising mucociliary clearance, may predispose to recurrent or prolonged pulmonary infections and, in this way, ultimately lead to bronchiectasis (an as yet unproven hypothesis). Dysmorphic changes in ciliary ultrastructure of respiratory epithelia, particularly microtubular additions or deletions in the 9 + 2 pattern, have been observed focally during viral illnesses (Fig. 97-12). These include infections due to influenza, parainfluenza, adenovirus, and respiratory syncytial virus. Similarly, in several young children with recurrent undefined lower respiratory infections or, in one instance *Mycoplasma pneumoniae* infection, ciliary abnormalities such as megacilia, fused cilia, disorganized axonemes, and partial lack of dynein arms have been observed in bronchial epithelium. Such infection-related changes appear to operate at the level of microtubule assembly during the course of cilioneogenesis. Normal organization of epithelium and ultrastructure of cilia is restored by 10 weeks following infection.

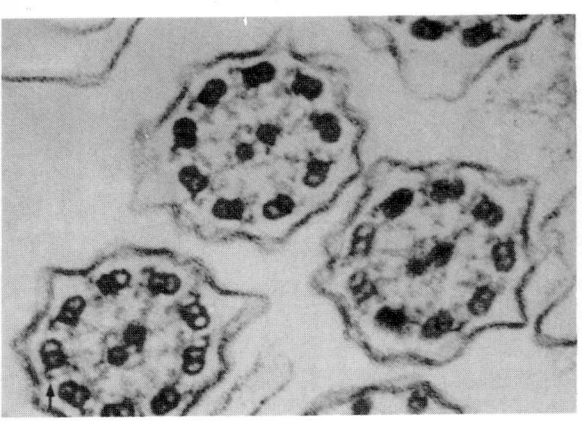 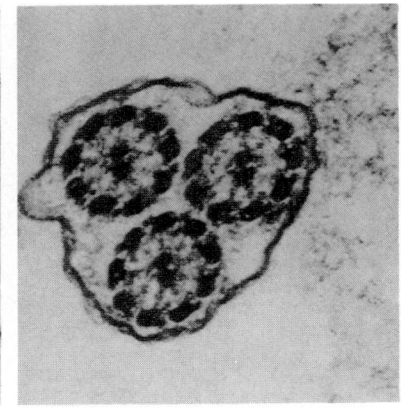 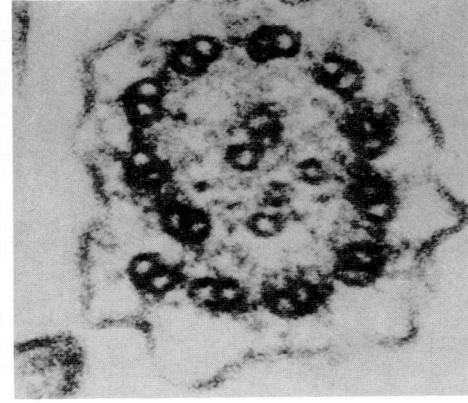

A   *B*   *C*

FIGURE 97-12 Electron micrographic cross sections of cilia from human conducting airways. *A.* Cross section of cilia from a healthy individual showing the normal 9 + 2 microtubular pattern as well as the appropriate parallel alignment of the central pairs of microtubules of adjacent cilia. The small arrow points to the outer dynein arm of one of the peripheral microtubular pairs. *B.* A compound cilium, one of the many abnormalities observed in respiratory tract cilia of Polynesians with bronchiectasis or in normal individuals in association with acute viral respiratory tract infections. *C.* A cilium with marked configurational alterations, again consistent with the varied aberrations observed in Polynesians with bronchiectasis and normal individuals following acute viral respiratory tract infections. (*A* and *B*, approximately ×100,000; *C*, ×216,000). (*Courtesy of Dr. G. R. Dickersin.*)

α_1-ANTITRYPSIN DEFICIENCY

Patients with severe deficiency of the major serum protease inhibitor, α_1-antitrypsin, are particularly susceptible to the development of panlobular emphysema (see Chapter 74). Approximately 2 percent of patients with emphysema have a hereditary deficiency of α_1-antitrypsin. Some patients with the deficiency develop the pulmonary complication of chronic bronchitis or, occasionally, bronchiectasis.

CYSTIC FIBROSIS (MUCOVISCIDOSIS)

Cystic fibrosis currently is the principal predisposing factor in at least half the cases of bronchiectasis identified in the first two decades of life. It is a heritable (autosomal recessive) disease of eccrine and exocrine glands characterized by unusually viscid mucous secretions that cause chronic pulmonary disease and pancreatic insufficiency as major organ dysfunctions, but other manifestations as well. Almost 95 percent of the mortality is a consequence of infection and chronic *destructive* pulmonary disease (see Chapter 78).

Viscid secretions characterizing this disease produce extensive peripheral small airways obstruction and air trapping. Recurrent episodes of viral bronchiolitis and bacterial bronchitis increase the obstructive changes. Chronic infection takes over, with secretions and inflammatory exudate blocking larger bronchial subdivisions, and eventuates in bronchiectasis. Thereafter, progressive disease is characterized by recurrent flareups of bronchitis and bronchopneumonia.

The changes of cystic bronchiectasis were noted radiographically in 64 percent of 200 adults with cystic fibrosis reviewed by di Sant'Agnese and Davis; another report of 50 patients indicated that 90 percent of the adults with cystic fibrosis had the specific radiologic features of bronchiectasis. Bronchiectasis is found on pathologic examination of essentially all autopsied patients who are over 6 months of age. Peribronchial or focal pneumonia, sometimes with areas of abscess formation, is often present at autopsy. Bronchial lymph node enlargement is usually present.

Pulmonary function tests in advanced cystic fibrosis show the findings predominantly of obstructive airways disease, or sometimes of a mixed obstructive-restrictive process reflecting the onset of fibrosis. An increased alveolar-to-arterial difference in P_{O_2} reflects uneven alveolar ventilation in the face of normal perfusion. With progression of pulmonary involvement and partial obstruction of large bronchi, expiratory flow rates decrease and both residual and total lung volumes increase. Arterial hypoxemia, pulmonary hypertension, and hypercapnia ensue. In more than 70 percent of patients, cor pulmonale develops eventually.

As patients with cystic fibrosis grow older, hemoptysis occurs with increasing frequency. Active bronchiectasis is the cause of the hemoptysis. The pathogenetic factors of the hemoptysis include: (1) destruction of lung tissue and erosion of blood vessels by active infection, (2) increased tortuosity and size of bronchial arteries, (3) increase in bronchial arterial circulation in the peribronchial granulation tissue, and (4) pulmonary arterial hypertension. Most major bleeding takes origin from the bronchial circulation.

Radiographic Findings

The early radiographic changes of cystic fibrosis in childhood are usually secondary to mucous plugging of small airways and consist of hyperinflation and bronchial wall thickening. With recurrent infections, patchy pulmonary infiltrates, atelectasis, and further hyperinflation are observed. Lobar atelectasis occurs often during the initial episode of clinical pulmonary disease and is most common in the upper right lobe. Initially, some of the radiologic changes clear with antibiotic treatment of intercurrent infections. As the pulmonary disease advances, the typical radiologic changes seen with chronic bronchiectasis become more evident: mucous plugs, mucoid impaction, pus-filled bronchi, thickened bronchial walls, and dilated bronchial (ring) shadows (Fig. 97-13). Additional

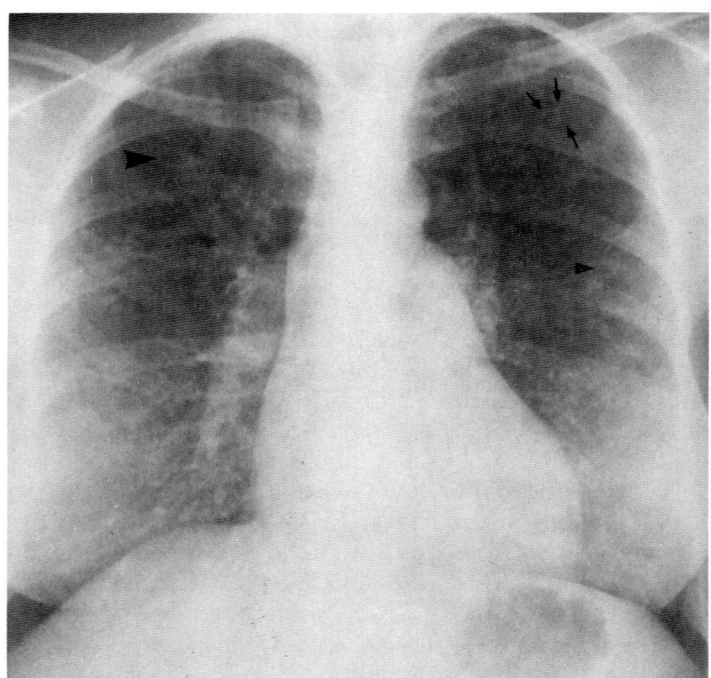

FIGURE 97-13 Chest radiograph of 17-year-old young woman with cystic fibrosis. The large arrowhead in right upper lobe indicates a ring shadow. In the left upper lobe, the two arrows pointing down indicate the upper aspect of a tram line (thickened bronchial walls displayed longitudinally); the arrow pointing up indicates the inferior wall of the same bronchus. The small arrowhead in the left midlung field indicates a nodular density, probably an area of mucoid impaction.

linear, nodular, or irregular densities, not readily identified as bronchi or bronchial walls, can be seen in otherwise clear parts of the lung. Large (2 cm or more in diameter) thin-walled air-filled cysts (bullae) may appear in the upper lobes over the course of several years. Pneumothorax and pneumomediastinum may occur as complications.

Bacteriology of Pulmonary Infections in Cystic Fibrosis

The pulmonary pathogens of clinical importance in cystic fibrosis have changed over time. Prior to 1950, S. aureus was the predominant organism, isolated from the sputum or pharynx of 80 percent of children under 12 months of age with cystic fibrosis. Two decades later, this figure had declined to 30 percent; and currently, S. aureus is isolated from the sputum of fewer than 20 percent of children and young adults with cystic fibrosis. Although *H. influenzae* type B is an important respiratory tract pathogen in children and unencapsulated *H. influenzae* is a common colonizer and potential pathogen in the lower respiratory tract of adults with chronic bronchitis, its prevalence in sputum cultures of children with cystic fibrosis is less than 15 percent.

At present, the leading pulmonary pathogen in patients with cystic fibrosis who have chronic pulmonary disease (bronchitis, bronchiolitis, and bronchiectasis) is *P. aeruginosa*. Prevalence studies indicate colonization rates as high as 60 to 90 percent. Undoubtedly contributing to this frequency of colonization by *P. aeruginosa* are many factors. Among the most important are the ubiquity of this species in the environment and the selective pressure exerted by chronic antibiotic therapy with oral drugs with efficacy against the usual respiratory tract pathogens operative in the community, but not against *P. aeruginosa*.

Initially, colonization of the lower respiratory tract of patients with cystic fibrosis by *P. aeruginosa* involves run-of-the-mill strains that exhibit nonmucoid colonial morphology. Ultimately, mucoid strains exhibiting a shiny appearance due to profuse production of an exopolysaccharide, alginate, appear and predominate. Adherence of nonmucoid *P. aeruginosa* to respiratory epithelium is mediated by *Pseudomonas* pili, and for this to occur the cell surface layer of fibronectin must be depleted. The proteases in sputum of cystic fibrosis patients may facilitate initial adherence of *P. aeruginosa* by degrading fibronectin. On the other hand, adherence of mucoid *Pseudomonas* to respiratory tract epithelium appears to be mediated by the exopolysaccharide of the organism. The abundant alginate produced by the bacteria undoubtedly complicates mechanical clearance of secretions in the bronchial tree. In addition, it appears to impair polymorphonuclear leukocyte function and to act as a barrier to bactericidal antibodies. *P. aeruginosa*, both mucoid and nonmucoid, produces a variety of toxins that undoubtedly contribute in varying degrees to the production of bronchiectasis and continuing damage to bronchopulmonary tissues. These toxins include: (1) exotoxin A, an inhibitor of protein synthesis with cytotoxic and necrotizing effects; (2) exotoxin S, also an inhibitor of protein synthesis; and (3) proteases, particularly an alkaline protease and elastase, which can cleave complement components (and thus inhibit opsonization and chemotaxis) and IgG and IgA, destroy connective tissue components, and stimulate profuse mucin production.

Production of alginate by isolates of *P. aeruginosa* from patients with cystic fibrosis of long standing is common (more than 80 percent of isolates) in contrast to isolates of *P. aeruginosa* from other infections (2.5 percent). Isolation of mucoid strains of *P. aeruginosa* repeatedly from bronchial secretions of patients with a chronic pulmonary process indicates cystic fibrosis or bronchiectasis of some other causation.

In recent years, *Pseudomonas cepacia* has emerged as a pathogen with an increasing prevalence (up to 15 to 20 percent in some centers) in patients with cystic fibrosis. Some features of this organism in the setting of cystic fibrosis warrant concern: (1) its capacity to spread from patient to patient both in and out of hospital, (2) its association with more severe lung disease and with accelerated clinical deterioration in some patients (accompanied by necrotizing pneumonia and even bacteremia, features not ordinarily observed with *P. aeruginosa* infections in cystic fibrosis), and (3) its resistance to aminoglycosides and to most β-lactam antipseudomonal antibiotics. (The only antibiotics to which *P. cepacia* has been susceptible in the past have been trimethoprim-sulfamethoxazole and, occasionally, chloramphenicol; recently developed antibiotics such as ceftazidime, imipenem, aztreonam, and ciprofloxacin have shown some in vitro activity.)

Up to 50 percent of patients with cystic fibrosis carry Enterobacteriaceae (*Escherichia coli*, *Klebsiella*, etc.) in their sputum from time to time. In occasional patients, mucoid variants of *E. coli*, producing exopolysaccharide composed of colanic acid rather than the alginic acid characteristic of mucoid strains of *P. aeruginosa*, are isolated.

Miscellaneous Disorders

YOUNG'S SYNDROME

Young's syndrome consists of a combination of obstructive azoospermia (with normal spermatogenesis) and chronic sinopulmonary infections. This syndrome is distinguished from the immotile cilia syndrome by its lack of ultrastructural ciliary abnormalities and from cystic fibrosis by its lack of family history and the presence of normal sweat electrolytes and pancreatic enzyme secretion. Young's syndrome appears to be more common than the immotile cilia syndrome. Thirty to seventy percent of patients with this syndrome have bronchiectasis. The other

patients have clinical evidence of chronic bronchitis. The sinopulmonary infections appear in childhood, become milder in adult life, and do not attain the severity usually observed in cystic fibrosis or the immotile cilia syndrome. Respiratory function shows only mild impairment (increase in residual volume and decrease in FEV_1). Although a productive cough is usual, the raising of copious amounts of purulent sputum is uncommon. Rales are audible in a minority of patients, and manifestations of advanced chronic pulmonary disease, such as clubbing, cyanosis, and cor pulmonale, are usually lacking. Decreased tracheobronchial mucociliary clearance of inhaled particles has been reported in the few patients who have been studied.

Since the pulmonary manifestations of Young's syndrome are mild and nonspecific, the diagnosis is most often made when the patient seeks medical attention for infertility. Testicular function is normal. Anatomically normal spermatozoa are present in distended epididymal heads, and the middle region of the epididymis is obstructed by amorphous material.

Role of Elastase and Proteases in Airway Damage

Proteolytic enzymes have been implicated in the pathogenesis of the destructive changes in several chronic lung diseases. Among these are diseases, such as bronchiectasis, in which pathologic changes occur in the bronchial epithelium exposed to purulent secretions potentially rich in such proteases, including elastase, collagenase, and cathepsin G. Polymorphonuclear leukocytes contain and release such neutral proteases which are able to act on and destroy elastin, collagen and proteoglycans, all important structural components of the lung and bronchial tree. Purified granulocyte elastase can directly damage bronchial epithelium and inhibit normal ciliary action. In addition to their action on structural proteins of the lung, granulocyte proteases can inactivate complement component C3 and IgG and IgM immunoglobulins. In patients with bronchiectasis, elastolytic activity is an almost constant feature of purulent secretions. Purulent bronchial secretions from patients with cystic fibrosis and *P. aeruginosa* infection of the airways have markedly higher levels of granulocyte elastase activity than do bronchial secretions of other patients with bronchiectasis and exacerbations of chronic bronchitis. The latter two groups have more elastase activity in bronchial secretions than do patients without bronchial infection. Whether this strikingly higher level of granulocyte elastase activity in patients with cystic fibrosis is intrinsic to that disease or merely represents a measure of the severity of bronchiectasis and purulence of bronchopulmonary secretions in that disease is unclear. The presence of high levels of granulocyte elastase in the bronchial secretions of patients with cystic fibrosis indicates an imbalance between

this protease and the antiproteases in the lung such as α_1-antitrypsin. The α_1-antitrypsin in purulent bronchial secretions is present in an inactive form. Whether this is due to the action of oxidants released by granulocytes during phagocytosis or due to cleavage by *P. aeruginosa* elastase is not known.

CLINICAL FEATURES

In the preantibiotic era, when bronchiectasis was much more common, symptoms began in the first decade of life; indeed, in 60 to 90 percent of patients, symptoms were evident by 5 years of age. The common initiating events were infections such as measles, pertussis, necrotizing pneumonia, or tuberculosis. Since the incidence of several of these infections has been sharply reduced by immunization and since progressive destruction of lung parenchyma in others has been almost eliminated by the use of antimicrobial agents, the clinical setting of the disease has changed. Currently, many children or young adults with bronchiectasis have some inherited anatomic or functional abnormality; about half the cases have cystic fibrosis. Although most cases of cystic fibrosis present in early childhood, the diagnosis is not made in about 20 percent of the cases until after the age of 15 years, when significant chronic symptoms develop.

Cough, sometimes in paroxysms, is almost invariably present and may be the only symptom for years in childhood. Purulent sputum production, frequently worse in the morning having accumulated during recumbency in sleep, is present in over 90 percent of patients. Occasionally, expectoration is not a feature or is not persistent, and "dry phases," periods when sputum is mucoid rather than purulent, occur. Sometimes, but by no means exclusively, these changes occur following antimicrobial therapy. The volume of sputum produced in older children and adults with advanced untreated disease, rarely seen nowadays, can be prodigious: up to 600 ml per day. In the preantibiotic era, fetid sputum and foul odor of the breath was observed in about 25 percent of patients, but this is unusual today. The classic characterization of bronchiectatic sputum involves description of the separation of a 24-h collection of sputum into three layers: (1) an upper, colorless or slightly greenish brown one containing air bubbles, pus, and mucus; (2) a middle, thin mucoid layer similar to the first but containing less air; and (3) a lower layer comprising a thick greenish sediment made up of pus cells, debris, fibrin, bronchial plugs, and sometimes fatty acid crystals and elastic fibers. These findings are less commonly observed in the antibiotic era as early antibiotic therapy and postural drainage reduce sputum volume, purulence, and secondary overgrowth of anaerobic bacteria.

Exacerbations of bronchiectasis, induced by intercurrent viral bronchiolitis, bacterial bronchitis, or bronchial plugging, may be accompanied by fever (about one-third of cases), increased cough, sputum production, and shortness of breath. Multiple recurrent episodes are associated with anorexia and weight loss as well. Hemoptysis occurred in 40 to 70 percent of cases during the preantibiotic era; it occurs less commonly now that exacerbations of the disease can be treated by antimicrobials. So-called dry bronchiectasis is uncommon and may exhibit no symptoms other than occasional hemoptysis. Investigation may then reveal bronchiectatic changes on bronchography or CT scanning. Upper lobe involvement is more common in this syndrome. Bronchostenosis, sometimes due to endobronchial tuberculosis, may underlie the bronchiectatic process. Wheezing and dyspnea are associated with exacerbations at first but become more persistent as the bronchiectasis progresses.

Sinusitis may be associated with bronchiectasis, particularly in congenital predisposing syndromes such as cystic fibrosis, Young's syndrome, Kartagener's syndrome, and various immunoglobulin deficiencies.

Involvement of many lobes is a feature of bronchiectasis complicating cystic fibrosis. Early and predominant involvement of upper lobes, particularly on the right, is more characteristic of this condition than of classic preantibiotic era bronchiectasis where involvement was more frequent in the lower lobes (and middle lobe) and in the left lung particularly. In an occasional patient, "pleurisy" may be the presenting or most prominent symptom.

Most patients with bronchiectasis have abnormalities on physical examination. The most important finding is the presence of persistent "moist" crackles over the involved lobes. The crackles are medium-to-coarse, start early in inspiration, continue to mid-inspiration, and fade out by the end of inspiration. In contrast, the crackles of fibrosing alveolitis may begin in either the early or midphase of respiration, are fine and "close to the ear," and continue to the end of inspiration. Diffuse rhonchi and a prolonged expiratory phase of respiration may be present. Dullness and decreased breath sounds are sometimes present over extensively involved lobes. With complicating pneumonia, or sometimes even in its absence, bronchovesicular or bronchial breath sounds may be a feature. Decreased respiratory expansion of the lungs is evident in patients with more advanced disease and with complicating emphysema. Hyperexpansion may be evident, particularly in children who may develop a barrel chest.

Clubbing of the fingers and cyanosis was common (40 percent of cases) in the preantibiotic era. By the 1960s, clubbing was observed in only 7 percent of cases. In advanced and ultimately fatal cases of bronchiectasis in the past, cor pulmonale occurred in 10 to 22 percent of cases. It is now less common a complication than in the past, except perhaps in patients with cystic fibrosis and extensive bronchopulmonary damage. Secondary amyloid disease is now very rare even with long-standing bronchiectasis.

Occasionally, other diseases occur at a possibly increased frequency in patients with severe bronchiectasis. Some are categorized as immunologic disorders. These include idiopathic ulcerative colitis, cutaneous vasculitis, and autoimmune thyroiditis.

RADIOGRAPHIC FINDINGS

Chest Radiography

The routine chest radiograph commonly does not show distinctive changes; it may be totally unremarkable, particularly in early bronchiectasis. The earliest change observed may be a nonspecific increase in peribronchial markings in specific segments of the lung. Of more diagnostic significance is the appearance of "tubular shadows": paired parallel or slightly tapered line shadows, extending distally, sometimes branching, and following a bronchovascular distribution. These line shadows (tram lines) outlining the involved bronchi are produced by thickened bronchial walls, peribronchial fibrosis, and adjacent alveolar collapse. These same structures, when viewed in cross section, may appear as peripheral rounded or irregularly nodular densities or as ring shadows. As bronchiectasis becomes more chronic, associated atelectasis becomes more marked, resulting in crowding together of numerous tubular shadows, usually in the lower lobes. Loss in lung volume may be extensive enough to cause shift in position of a fissure or hemidiaphragm, or deviation of the trachea. When thickened bronchiectatic segments become filled with retained secretions or pus, they form homogeneous radiodense bands which have been referred to as *mucoid impaction* or, when branched, as *gloved finger* shadows.

With advanced saccular bronchiectasis, large cystic air-containing areas (with or without fluid levels) representing dilated terminations of abnormal bronchi can be seen (Fig. 97-14). Since they communicate with the proximal airways, these cysts, unlike those in patients with emphysematous bullae, can enlarge on inspiration and diminish on expiration. In very severe disease, a coarse honeycomb pattern is observed. The rarefied areas here, in contrast to the cystic spaces representing dilated bronchial termini, do not fill with contrast on bronchography. These areas represent emphysematous regions surrounded by fibrosis rather than dilated bronchi.

Compensatory hyperinflation of the remainder of the lung is common. This may be particularly prominent in patients with cystic fibrosis where it may be evident relatively early. Patchy areas of bronchopneumonia may punctuate the course of bronchiectasis, particularly in patients with cystic fibrosis. Hilar lymphadenopathy may

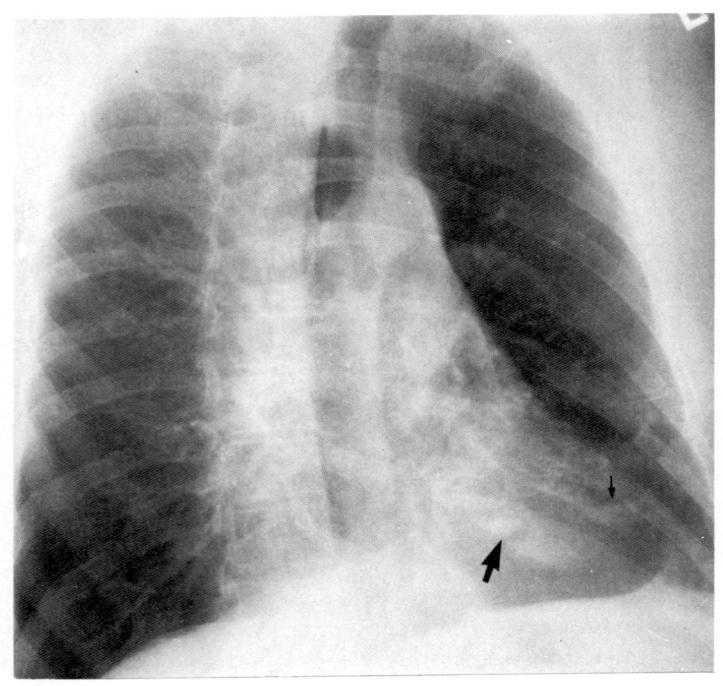
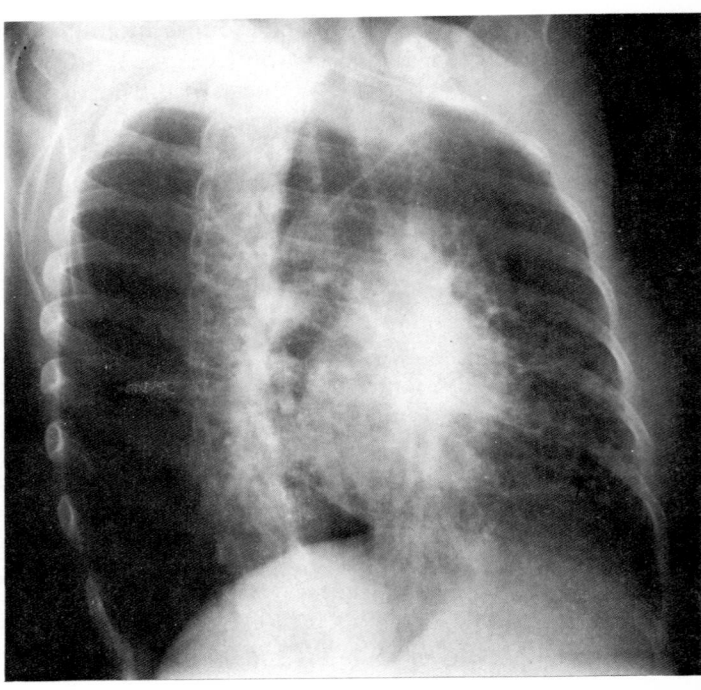

A

B

FIGURE 97-14 Plain chest radiographs of two patients with saccular bronchiectasis. *A.* Large fluid-filled cystic bronchial termini. Large arrow points to inferior edge of fluid-filled dilated bronchus. Smaller arrow points to air-fluid level in cystic bronchial terminus. *B.* Oblique view of chest radiograph demonstrating multiple cystic areas in the lower half of the lung beyond the heart border. The small arrow points to a cystic area with thickened walls, indicating active inflammation in the involved region.

be visible, both in a causative role (producing bronchial obstruction and resulting bronchiectasis) and as a consequence of the chronic infection that characterizes established bronchiectasis.

Bronchography

The finding on plain film of structures representing the parallel walls of dilated bronchi provides presumptive evidence of bronchiectasis. However, in 7 to 20 percent of patients with established bronchiectasis, conventional radiographs show no such abnormalities. For diagnosis in such patients with a clinical history suggesting bronchiectasis but a normal chest radiograph, and for the accurate definition of the extent and type of bronchiectasis (particularly if surgery is being considered), bronchography has been required. Computed chest tomography may replace bronchography in some instances (vide infra).

Several technical considerations are important in evaluating bronchial shadows on bronchograms. Tubular shadows outlining bronchial walls contain air in the lumen. If such shadows end abruptly, they usually suggest that air is passing freely to the periphery but that there is insufficient contrast to coat the more peripheral extent of the bronchus; this does not indicate bronchial obstruction. Solid shadows in the bronchi may be produced because of the presence of too much contrast me-

dium and no air in the lumen, even though peripheral filling is complete. True nonfilling of peripheral bronchi may be due to bronchial obstruction or to focal areas of retained secretions. To minimize the latter, bronchography should be performed only after adequate postural drainage and antibiotic therapy. Fiberoptic bronchoscopy has made it possible to perform more selective segmental bronchography with less adverse effects and discomfort. This procedure may be of particular help in evaluating a patient with recurrent hemoptysis where bronchoscopy shows the bronchopulmonary segment that is the site of bleeding but no endobronchial lesion is observed ("dry bronchiectasis").

The bronchographic features of *cylindrical bronchiectasis* (Fig. 97-6) include regularly outlined dilated bronchi with not greatly increased diameters peripherally, abrupt ending of bronchiectatic segments with little or no peripheral filling, and crowding of bronchiectatic segments. Obstructed bronchi in cylindrical (and other types of) bronchiectasis may show air bubbles in the intraluminal contrast medium since the air cannot enter the smaller bronchi. *Varicose bronchiectasis* is characterized by bronchial dilatation that is somewhat greater than that of cylindrical bronchiectasis. In addition, local constrictions cause irregularities in the outline of bronchi, giving an appearance akin to that of varicose veins (Fig. 97-7). Involved bronchial segments show bulbous terminations

with failure of peripheral filling. In *saccular bronchiectasis*, bronchi exhibit a ballooned outline. Cystic spaces containing contrast material (Fig. 97-8) or exhibiting air-fluid levels may be present.

"PSEUDOBRONCHIECTASIS" (REVERSIBLE BRONCHIECTASIS)

Pneumonia may produce changes in the bronchial tree acutely with subsequent resolution. Bachman et al. performed bronchograms on 60 young soldiers with radiographically proven pneumonia and no prior history of pulmonary disease. Bronchography was performed after the acute illness (1 to 8 weeks after onset) but usually before resolution of the pulmonary infiltrate. Twenty-five of the patients showed bronchial abnormalities. Of 16 patients with initial bronchial abnormalities who were followed with repeated bronchograms (seven with considerable widening of bronchi considered to be radiographically consistent with bronchiectasis and nine with milder bronchial abnormalities), 10 showed return of the bronchogram to normal within 4 months. Thus, in a patient with a chronic productive cough and pneumonia, who is suspected of having bronchiectasis, bronchography should be postponed for at least 4 months after the acute pneumonia. Otherwise, reversible dilatation of segmental bronchi without destruction, changes that often occur in acute pneumonia, may be erroneously attributed to irreversible cylindrical bronchiectasis.

Reversible bronchiectasis also can occur in the setting of acute bronchial obstruction. Acute extensive cystic bronchiectasis has followed traumatic stenosis of a bronchus 4 weeks after closed chest trauma. Resection of the stenotic segment produced nearly complete reversal of the bronchographic abnormalities in 8 days and total recovery in a month. Presumably, the initial changes were due to bronchial dilatation secondary to retained secretions and to atelectasis caused by the bronchostenosis. Since secondary infection was not introduced, the changes were reversible on relieving the obstruction.

BRONCHOGRAPHIC CHANGES IN CHRONIC BRONCHITIS

A variety of bronchographic changes can be observed in patients with chronic bronchitis and should be distinguished from the changes of bronchiectasis. These include: (1) lack of parallelism of the walls of medium-sized bronchi; (2) lack of full delineation of distal parts of bronchial tree, likely due to mucus obstructing small peripheral airways; and (3) mucosal pouches arising from sides of larger bronchi, representing either enlarged mouths of hypersecreting mucous glands or mucosal ridging. With advanced disease, "peripheral pools" (emphysematous spaces filled with contrast) and a "concertina" appearance (due to structural changes in the bronchial wall) can be observed.

Computed Tomography

Computed tomography (CT) can be useful in the diagnosis of bronchiectasis. It appears to be of value in the diagnosis of cystic bronchiectasis and in defining the anatomic extent of the process. It appears to be less reliable in the diagnosis of cylindrical and varicose forms of the disease. The CT changes in cystic bronchiectasis include: (1) markedly dilated bronchi, (2) air-fluid levels in bronchi, (3) "strings of cysts" (linear arrays of consecutive cystic dilatations of a bronchus visualized in a horizontal course), and (4) "cluster of cysts" (dilated bronchi in groups mimicking a cluster of grapes) (Fig. 97-15). Cylindrical bronchiectasis is characterized by smooth dilatation of bronchi (tram lines) extending to the periphery, thickened bronchial walls, or the presence of dilated bronchi in the periphery. In varicose bronchiectasis, the bronchi are more dilated than in cylindrical bronchiectasis and exhibit a beaded appearance. Visualization of dilated bronchi with thickened walls in the lung periphery must be interpreted with caution as a feature of bronchiectasis on CT, since pneumonia or other causes of parenchymal consolidation can produce a similar picture in the absence of bronchiectasis.

PATHOPHYSIOLOGICAL CHANGES

Pulmonary Function

Although there is no specific pattern of pulmonary function associated with bronchiectasis, a variety of abnormal-

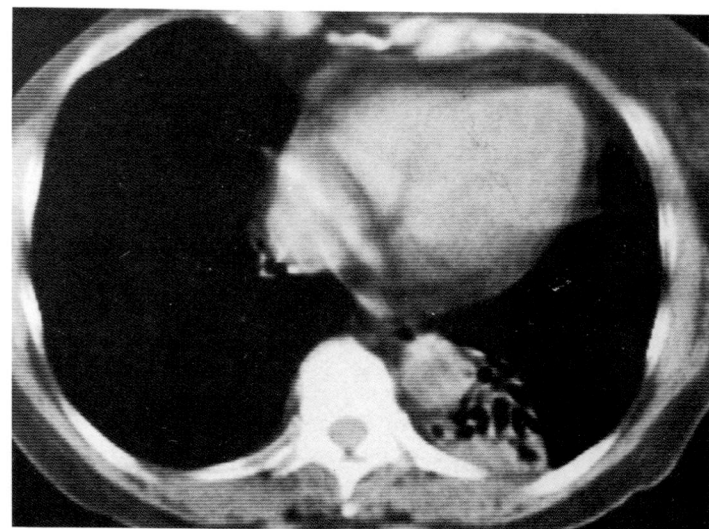

FIGURE 97-15 CT scan of chest showing a grapelike cluster of dilated bronchi characteristic of cystic bronchiectasis in an atelectatic left lower lobe. *(Courtesy of Dr. T. McLoud.)*

ities are commonly seen. The degree of impairment depends not only on the nature and extent of the morphologic abnormalities in the involved areas but also on the presence or absence of associated disease (chronic bronchitis, emphysema) elsewhere in the smaller airways and lung parenchyma. Patients with very localized bronchiectasis without chronic bronchitis have little dysfunction. However, there is not always a direct correlation between the number of involved bronchial segments or the type of anatomic change (cylindrical, etc.) and the dysfunction measured.

Patients with severe bronchiectasis show impaired airway dynamics similar to patients with chronic bronchitis and emphysema. In normal individuals, forced expiration or cough produces a proportionate narrowing throughout the bronchial tree. In patients with saccular and varicose bronchiectasis, cough produces a disproportionate, premature collapse of the large (usually lower lobe) bronchi causing obstruction to airflow and possibly contributing to air trapping. Inflammatory changes of chronic bronchitis are presumed responsible for the weakening of the proximal bronchi producing this phenomenon. As a consequence of airflow obstruction and reduced effectiveness of cough, bronchopulmonary toilet is impaired. Retained secretions predispose to further infection, and peribronchial inflammation extends.

In most patients with diffuse involvement, pulmonary function tests show a pattern of airways obstruction: reduced FVC, FEV_1, FEV_1/FVC, $FEF_{25-75\%}$ and increased residual volume. Abnormal maximum expiratory flow volume tracings at low lung volumes and other studies (closing volume, frequency dependence of dynamic compliance) can be helpful in detecting diffuse involvement of small airways. In some patients, particularly those with considerable associated atelectasis and fibrosis, abnormalities (e.g., decreased VC and FRC, reduced specific compliance) are of a mixed obstructive-restrictive pattern or a largely restrictive one.

Reduced regional ventilation (^{133}Xe), a lesser degree of reduction in perfusion, and decreased ventilation-perfusion ratios are observed in areas of bronchiectatic involvement. Additional evidence of ventilatory dysfunction includes increased dead-space ventilation and abnormal N_2 washout studies. Generally, the disturbances in overall lung function are more dependent on the extent of involvement (and associated bronchitis) than on the anatomic type of bronchiectasis. With progressive or extensive bronchiectasis, arterial hypoxemia may develop secondary to abnormalities in gas exchange in adjacent areas. Carbon dioxide retention occurs only in patients in whom bronchiectasis is associated with severe obstructive airways disease, generally severe chronic bronchitis and advanced emphysema.

Tracheobronchial Clearance

In patients with bronchiectasis, as in patients with chronic bronchitis, inhaled aerosol particles are deposited in more central bronchi than in the case of normal individuals. This has been ascribed to more turbulent airflow in obstructed large bronchial segments. In addition, particle clearance is impaired. A number of abnormalities can contribute to such impairment: (1) loss of normal ciliated epithelium from the lining of involved bronchi, (2) hereditary ciliary defects (immotile cilia syndrome, Kartagener's syndrome), and (3) altered mucous blanket of the bronchial tree.

Mucociliary transport (MCT) can be accurately measured by monitoring over several hours the disappearance of ^{99m}Tc-human serum albumin aerosol deposited as a bolus in the large airways. Rapid loss of radioactivity from the lung occurs in normal individuals, but marked retention of the radioactive particles is characteristic of patients with Kartagener's syndrome and bronchiectasis.

Several features of bronchiectasis alter the character and viscosity of the sputum produced. The purulent sputum is more viscid, particularly as a result of its deoxyribonucleic acid content and disulfide linkages of proteins, resulting in slower MCT. This property is not specific for the purulent sputum of bronchiectasis. Patients with bronchiectasis also produce mucoid sputum. The submucosal glands of the bronchi are hyperactive and, unlike other hypersecretory states, the ratio of serous to mucous cells is not decreased. Purulent bronchial secretions from patients with cystic fibrosis (and accompanying bronchiectasis) contain granulocyte neutral proteases which are able to cleave major structural proteins (collagen, elastin, proteoglycans) of the lung as well as inactivate opsonins such as C_3, IgG, and IgM. Enhancing the proteolytic capability of the purulent bronchial secretions in cystic fibrosis is the *P. aeruginosa* elastase. This enzyme is capable of destroying the two principal inhibitors of granulocyte proteases in the lung (α_1-antitrypsin and bronchial mucosal protein inhibitor). Thus, the synergistic effect of this infecting organism and the proteolytic activity of polymorphonuclear leukocytes of the inflammatory response contributes in a major way to the progressive destruction of structural bronchial and parenchymal proteins and to the advance of the inflammatory process in bronchiectasis.

Hemodynamic Changes

Hemodynamic changes in bronchiectasis are of several types. Extensive systemic-to-pulmonary anastomoses occur at the precapillary level in the granulation tissue about bronchiectatic segments. Such anastomoses can lead to bronchial artery enlargement and left-to-right shunts. This is not an important contributor to the pulmo-

nary hypertension and ultimate cor pulmonale that develops in relatively few patients with severe bronchiectasis. If pulmonary hypertension should develop, hypoxia, generally attributable to a severe underlying chronic bronchitis and emphysema, has a major etiologic role.

DIAGNOSIS

Diagnosis comprises two elements: the identification of bronchiectasis as the cause of suppurative bronchopulmonary disease and the ascertainment of any predisposing process. The history of chronic cough, purulent sputum, recurrent exacerbations of bronchitis, recurrent pneumonias, or recurrent hemoptyses in a patient with a chest radiograph showing increased and crowded pulmonary markings (including tram lines, ring densities, or cystic areas with fluid levels) effectively makes the clinical diagnosis of bronchiectasis. In less clear-cut cases or where definition of the extent of involvement is important, CT of the chest can be a helpful noninvasive means of diagnosis. The gold standard for diagnosis in patients in whom there is uncertainty about the presence of bronchiectasis, or where surgery is being considered, remains bronchography.

Bronchography

The role of bronchography in diagnosis has declined strikingly as a result of the better appreciation of the radiologic findings of this disease on plain chest films and the use of chest CT for diagnosis. Nonetheless, bronchography remains the procedure of choice to assess the extent of the process, to confirm the diagnosis in a doubtful case (e.g., dry bronchiectasis with recurrent hemoptysis), or to evaluate the bronchial tree where a congenital defect may be a predisposing factor.

Adverse effects may accompany bronchography. These include possible allergic reactions to the topical anesthetic or iodine-containing contrast material, impairment of ventilation due to the filling of bronchi with contrast, or segmental pulmonary collapse, particularly in children who have undergone general anesthesia with a readily diffusible gaseous agent. In patients with considerably impaired pulmonary function, bronchography should be avoided.

Bronchoscopy

Bronchoscopy is not of value in directly diagnosing bronchiectasis, but it may be of value in defining the presence of an obstructing lesion responsible for localized segmental bronchiectasis or in defining the bronchopulmonary segment that is the source of recurrent hemoptysis in a patient without a discernible endobronchial lesion but with bronchiectasis. Bronchography via fiberoptic bron-

choscopy can be helpful in confirming the presence of localized bronchiectasis and has the advantage in this circumstance of selective instillation of contrast and less likelihood of inducing hypoxia in a patient with diminished respiratory reserve.

Computed Tomography

Chest CT may provide a useful noninvasive means of establishing the diagnosis of saccular bronchiectasis and defining its anatomic extent. It appears to be less reliable in detecting cylindrical, or possibly varicose, changes. The ability to identify a bronchus on CT depends on its size and orientation. Horizontally oriented bronchi are more readily visualized and evaluable than bronchi with vertical courses. Since the basilar segmental bronchi, apical bronchi, bronchus intermedius, and lower lobe bronchi are seen only on cross section, cylindrical or mild varicose changes there may be more readily overlooked than similar changes in the lingular or right middle lobe bronchi.

Bacteriologic Findings

Definitive delineation of the bacteriology of bronchiectasis has not been accomplished. Many of the studies of bronchiectasis in the first half of this century when the disease was more common suffered from the fact that they were retrospective, that they antedated modern techniques for anaerobic bacteriology, and that their data were derived from culture of sputum (readily contaminated with oropharyngeal flora on passage through the oral cavity). Accurate information from transtracheal aspiration and culture of resected lung are not at hand. Available data indicate the frequent presence of *H. influenzae* (usually unencapsulated), and *Streptococcus pneumoniae* in the sputum of patients with bronchiectasis in addition to normal components of the oropharyngeal flora. Suppurative pneumonias following measles and predisposing to bronchiectasis have been due to *S. aureus, K. pneumoniae*, and *P. aeruginosa*. In bronchographically confirmed "pseudobronchiectasis" following pneumonia, the etiologies have been either *Streptococcus pyogenes* or "atypical pneumonia." In the antibiotic era, the organisms isolated from patients with bronchiectasis can show shifts in the resident bronchial species as a result of antibiotic selective pressure. Mucoid strains of *P. aeruginosa* have been isolated from patients with bronchiectasis who do not have cystic fibrosis. As noted earlier in this chapter, in cystic fibrosis patients initial sputum isolates are often *H. influenzae* or *S. aureus*. Later in the course of the disease, Enterobacteriaceae, mucoid strains of *P. aeruginosa*, or *P. cepacia* tend to predominate, to a large measure influenced by antimicrobial selective pressure.

Anaerobic bacteria undoubtedly play an important primary or contributory role in some cases of bronchiecta-

sis. Evidence for this includes: (1) the foul, putrid odor of the sputum of some patients; (2) the fact that bronchiectasis has sometimes followed necrotizing aspiration pneumonias associated with oral anaerobes (*Bacteroides melaninogenicus, Fusobacterium necrophorum*, peptococci, peptostreptococci, etc.); (3) the finding at autopsy in the preantimicrobial era of fusiform bacteria and spirochetes in stained sections of bronchiectatic segments; (4) the isolation from bronchiectatic lobes removed at surgery during the preantibiotic era of fusobacteria, always in association with facultative cocci; and (5) the occasional complication of bronchiectasis by brain abscess due to mixed anaerobes.

Other Laboratory Studies

Gram-stained smear of sputum shows numerous polymorphonuclear leukocytes and mixed bacterial flora, often including fusiform bacteria as well as a variety of gram-negative rods and gram-positive cocci. In some, there may be no single predominating organism; in others, the predominating organism may vary. Leukocytosis is variable and may be associated with an exacerbation. Anemia of chronic infection is present with long-standing disease. Since cystic fibrosis may be manifest primarily as bronchiectasis appearing in late adolescence or early adult life, a sweat chloride test should be performed in patients of such an age in whom there is no evidence of antecedent pneumonia, obstructing lesion, or other evident predisposing cause of bronchiectasis. Serum immunoglobulins should be determined in a young patient, particularly a young male, with recurrent pneumonias and bronchiectasis. The electrocardiogram may show evidence of cor pulmonale in the presence of advanced disease.

DIFFERENTIAL DIAGNOSIS

There are two aspects to the differential diagnosis of bronchiectasis. The first relates to distinguishing this disease from other processes that may produce a similar constellation of symptoms, physical findings, and radiographic changes. The second relates to defining whether any of the numerous predisposing conditions producing secondary bronchiectasis are present.

Chronic bronchitis is the most common disease which closely resembles bronchiectasis in symptomatology, physical findings, and abnormal pulmonary function tests. Bronchiectasis may be accompanied by small airways disease, and reciprocally, localized bronchiectatic areas can develop in the setting of chronic bronchitis and emphysema. The presence of tram-line and ring shadows on chest radiographs is more suggestive of bronchiectasis, but bronchographic visualization may be the only means to distinguish between these two processes. Allergic bronchopulmonary aspergillosis, a form of hypersensitivity lung disease, is characterized by episodic wheezing, expectoration of mucous plugs, intermittent pulmonary infiltrates, and irregularly dilated proximal bronchi that connect with normal bronchi and bronchioles peripherally. In contrast, in bronchiectasis the sputum is usually more abundant and purulent, and the involvement is in the more distal bronchial tree. The distinction between these two conditions may be blurred by the fact that cylindrical bronchiectasis may complicate long-standing ABPA. Other entities that should be distinguished from bronchiectasis include bronchiolitis obliterans, recurrent episodes of pneumonia, and organized or unresolved pneumonia.

Productive cough, dyspnea, and occasional hemoptyses, clinical manifestations of bronchiectasis, occur also in a relatively rare pulmonary disease known as the unilateral hyperlucent lung (Swyer-James or Macleod's syndrome). The diagnosis is usually made on the basis of radiographic findings of hyperlucency of a lung or lobe resulting from air trapping (particularly during expiration) and decreased pulmonary vascular markings in the involved area. This condition appears to be a consequence of bronchiolitis obliterans resulting from viral or bacterial infection in childhood, eventuating in subsequent underdevelopment of the involved portion of lung. Decreased pulmonary artery size reflects decreased flow and is an effect rather than a cause of the findings in this disease. Decreased ventilation and perfusion is present in the affected area on radionuclide lung scans. Bronchograms show dilated and beaded-appearing smaller bronchi consistent with bronchiectasis.

Pulmonary sequestration is suspected in a patient with recurrent infiltrates about a single chronically involved area containing cystic spaces in a basilar segment of a lower lobe. A clue as to diagnosis may be provided by the presence of a continuous bruit over the chest or axilla on the involved side due to shunting of blood from systemic artery to pulmonary vein in the intralobar sequestration.

Numerous congenital abnormalities of the tracheobronchial tree, acquired obstructive bronchial lesions and destructive parenchymal processes, and various inherited disorders predisposing to bronchiectasis should be considered in the evaluation of a patient with this disease (see "Pathogenesis and Predisposing Factors," above) (Table 97-1).

COMPLICATIONS AND PROGNOSIS

The principal complications of bronchiectasis are progressive suppuration, hemoptysis and major pulmonary hemorrhage, obliteration of peripheral airways with associated extensive bronchitis and emphysema, and chronic respiratory insufficiency and cor pulmonale. Continued

active suppuration has been more readily controlled in the antibiotic era, but recurrent episodes of bronchopneumonia and exacerbations of chronic bronchial infections (often due to antibiotic-resistant organisms such as *P. aeruginosa* in patients with cystic fibrosis) are still frequent in occasional patients. Metastatic brain abscess is now a rare complication because of better control of active pulmonary infection with antimicrobials. In rare instances, pulmonary hemorrhage can be major, requiring surgery, or can be massive with death due to exsanguination or asphyxiation. The greatest disability stems from the combination of bronchiectasis and emphysema producing chronic respiratory failure. Now with better control of its suppurative aspects, bronchiectasis is rarely complicated by amyloidosis.

Over time, despite repeated antibiotic administration, the process could advance in bronchial segments already involved. In the preantibiotic era, spread of the process from involved segments or lobes to other pulmonary segments appeared to follow bronchopulmonary aspirational events which produced new foci of pneumonia. In the antibiotic era, such spread to previously normal segments is unusual, unless bronchiectasis has developed in the setting of a diffuse predisposing process such as cystic fibrosis or the immotile cilia syndrome. Even with such underlying disease where bronchiectasis may be extensive, appropriate use of antibiotics may control symptoms, slow progression, and render surgery unnecessary. Indeed, now about 50 percent of patients with cystic fibrosis survive to 20 years of age or older.

Patients with childhood bronchiectasis often tend to improve during their teens and twenties and may remain relatively stable thereafter. Even in the preantibiotic era, cases of bronchiectasis could be compatible with longevity. Laennec's famous patient, a piano teacher with chronic productive cough since age 16, continued her occupation and died at age 82. At autopsy she had gross bronchiectasis involving four lobes.

TREATMENT

The aim of treatment is control of symptoms and prevention of progression. In addition to measures directed at specific predisposing conditions (removal of obstructing endobronchial lesions, gamma globulin replacement for immunoglobulin deficiency), treatment consists of control of infection and basic supportive measures to provide good pulmonary toilet and relief of bronchospasm and small airways disease.

There are several elements in control of infection. Appropriate immunizations against potential pulmonary pathogens (influenza vaccine, pneumococcal vaccine) should be performed. In children, the basic immunizations against childhood diseases (measles, pertussis) that

can predispose to bronchiectasis should have been carried out. Prompt antimicrobial treatment of superimposed acute pneumonitis or acute febrile exacerbations of bronchitis is indicated. Guidance in antibiotic selection is provided by evaluation of Gram-stained smears of sputum and results of sputum culture. Based on the frequent isolation of *H. influenzae*, pneumococci, or mixed oral flora, initial treatment with ampicillin, amoxicillin, or trimethoprim-sulfamethoxazole may be sufficient. The presence of *S. aureus* warrants the use of a penicillinase-resistant penicillin such as oxacillin or nafcillin. In patients with cystic fibrosis where *P. aeruginosa* may be the dominant bacterial flora during an acute episode of clinical infection, treatment usually requires the use of ticarcillin (or one of the ureidopenicillins) in combination with an aminoglycoside. Third-generation cephalosporins with anti-

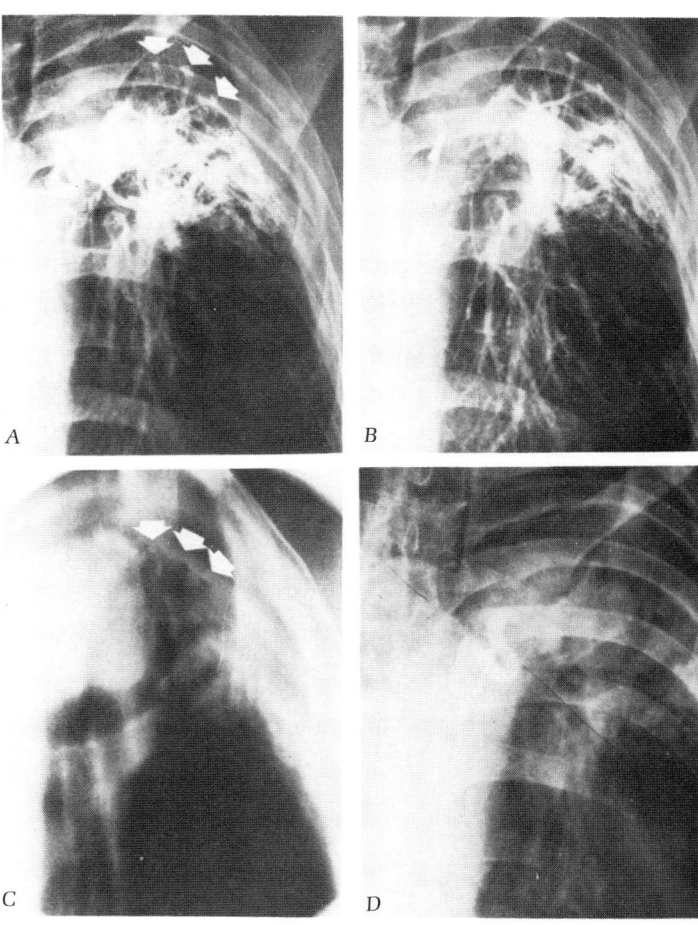

FIGURE 97-16 Hypervascularity about bronchiectatic lesions demonstrated on bronchial arteriography. *A.* Arterial tufts (arrows) in periphery of left upper lobe bronchiectasis. *B.* Extensive bronchial to pulmonary arterial shunting with prominent opacifications of left pulmonary artery. *C.* Tomographic view of the cystic dilated left upper lobe bronchi (arrows). *D.* Angiographic view showing occlusion of the left bronchial artery after embolization. *(Reproduced from Uflacker et al., 1983.)*

pseudomonal activity (e.g., ceftazidime) may be of value in treating infections due to resistant *P. aeruginosa*. Although ceftazidime has been used successfully as monotherapy, combination with an aminoglycoside is probably preferable to avoid selection of resistant strains during acute pulmonary infections severe enough to require hospitalization.

In patients with bronchiectasis whose cough and sputum volume and purulence increase but whose illness does not require hospitalization, oral therapy with ampicillin, tetracycline, or trimethoprim-sulfamethoxazole is reasonable during the symptomatic exacerbation. Therapy may be initiated similarly at the onset of a viral upper respiratory infection or with symptomatic sinusitis. In some patients with bronchiectasis, as in some patients with chronic bronchitis, such exacerbations are frequent and debilitating. Suppressive prophylactic antimicrobial therapy with one of the aforementioned drugs during the winter season may be warranted in selected patients.

Pulmonary toilet by postural drainage and chest percussion is of major importance in management, particularly in patients with sputum volumes greater than 30 to 50 ml per day. Bronchoscopy is not indicated to assist in removal of secretions, only for removal of a foreign body or bronchial plug. Hydration should be well maintained to avoid inspissation of secretions. Inhalation of a nebulized mist may sometimes be useful in loosening secretions.

Bronchodilators may be helpful because of the associated diffuse small airways disease; improved mucociliary clearance and removal of pooled secretions may follow. However, in occasional patients, reduction in bronchomotor tone may inhibit the cough reflex and promote further pooling of secretions with resultant deterioration of pulmonary function. Smoking should be proscribed.

Medical management is satisfactory in most patients with bronchiectasis. Surgical resection is reserved primarily for young patients with troublesome symptoms (severe cough, recurrent pneumonias, profuse purulent sputum) that persist despite conservative management and interfere with normal life. Such patients with localized disease can be cured by segmental resection or lobectomy; patients with extensive disease are less likely to benefit, although bilateral resections have been successful when the remaining lung is essentially uninvolved. Another indication for surgical resection is major hemorrhage from an eroded vessel in a bronchiectatic segment. The principal source of bleeding in patients with major hemoptyses, with the rare exception of the patient with a Rasmussen aneurysm of the pulmonary artery in a tuberculous cavity, is from a branch of a bronchial artery. Bronchial arteriography and embolization (Fig. 97-16) has been used to control massive or repeated hemoptysis in about 35 reported patients with bronchiectasis. This procedure may be indicated for patients who are not surgical candidates by virtue of diffuse involvement of both lungs (e.g., patients with advanced cystic fibrosis) or as a temporizing measure for patients who require immediate stabilization in preparation for later elective surgery. Cessation of major bleeding has been achieved in 12 of 13 patients with cystic fibrosis by this procedure, although minor hemoptyses later recurred in five. The presence of a spinal radicular artery arising from a bronchial artery is considered a contraindication to embolization because of risk of spinal cord injury.

BIBLIOGRAPHY

Afzelius BA: "Immotile-cilia" syndrome and ciliary abnormalities induced by infection and injury. Am Rev Respir Dis 124:107–109, 1981.
Distinctions are made between ciliary abnormalities due to inborn errors (ciliary mutants) and those due to acquired lesions in the respiratory tract.

Bachman AL, Hewitt WR, Beekley HC: Bronchiectasis. A bronchographic study of sixty cases of pneumonia. Arch Intern Med 91:78–96, 1953.
Bronchograms were performed on young adult patients from 1 to 8 weeks after onset of pneumonia. Changes of reversible bronchiectasis were found in 25 of 60 patients studied.

Barton AD, Lourenço RV: Bronchial secretions and mucociliary clearance. Biochemical characteristics. Arch Intern Med 131:140–144, 1973.
The composition of the normal respiratory tract mucous blanket is compared with changes observed in purulent secretions. Possible effects on mucociliary transport are considered.

Bass H, Henderson JAM, Hecksher T, Oriol A, Anthonisen NR: Regional structure and function in bronchiectasis. Am Rev Respir Dis 97:598–609, 1968.
Regional lung functions were compared with bronchographic findings in eight patients with bronchiectasis. Regions demonstrating bronchiectasis showed reduced ventilation, lowered ventilation-perfusion ratios, and mildly reduced perfusion.

Carson JL, Collier AM, Hu SS: Acquired ciliary defects in nasal epithelium of children with acute viral upper respiratory infections. N Engl J Med 312:463–468, 1985.

This careful study documents the occurrence of a variety of nasal ciliary ultrastructural abnormalities with viral respiratory infections. Reestablishment of normal epithelial organization and ciliary ultrastructure occurred 2 to 10 weeks following infection.

Cherniack NS, Carton RW: Factors associated with respiratory insufficiency in bronchiectasis. Am J Med 41:562–571, 1966.

Lung function was measured in 42 patients with proven cystic and cylindrical bronchiectasis. Abnormalities observed included reduced maximum breathing capacity, elevated pulmonary resistance, and an increased ratio of residual volume to total lung capacity.

Chipps BE, Talamo RC, Winkelstein JA: IgA deficiency, recurrent pneumonias, and bronchiectasis. Chest 73:519–526, 1978.

The report of a case of bronchiectasis associated with IgA deficiency. This association and the other conditions predisposing to bronchiectasis are reviewed.

Culiner MM: Intralobar bronchial cystic disease, the "sequestration complex" and cystic bronchiectasis. Dis Chest 53:462–469, 1968.

The relative similarities (and differences) pathogenetically and pathologically between cystic bronchiectasis, intralobar sequestration, and simple bronchial cystic disease are considered here.

Davis PB, Hubbard VS, McCoy K, Taussig LM: Familial bronchiectasis. J Pediatr 102:177–184, 1983.

A very clearly written review of the various congenital disorders predisposing to bronchiectasis.

di Sant'Agnese PA, Davis PB: Cystic fibrosis in adults. Am J Med 66:121–132, 1979.

An authoritative review of the clinical and laboratory findings in more than 200 adult patients with cystic fibrosis. Pulmonary findings are well detailed. Bronchiectasis (cystic) was present in 64 percent of the cases that had been evaluated.

Drapanas T, Siewers R, Feist JH: Reversible poststenotic bronchiectasis. N Engl J Med 275:917–921, 1966.

A case report demonstrating dramatic reversal of marked saccular and cylindrical bronchiectasis following resection of an acute posttraumatic bronchial stenosis.

Eliasson R, Mossberg B, Camner P, Afzelius BA: The immotile-cilia syndrome: A congenital ciliary abnormality as an etiologic factor in chronic airway infections and male sterility. N Engl J Med 297:1–6, 1977.

A well-illustrated report of six patients with recurrent pulmonary infections (proven bronchiectasis in three) who were shown to lack dynein arms in cilia (and sperm tails) and to exhibit delayed mucociliary transport. Four of the patients had Kartagener's syndrome.

Ellis DA, Thornley PE, Wightman AJ, Walker M, Chalmers J, Crofton JW: Present outlook in bronchiectasis: Clinical and social study and review of factors influencing prognosis. Thorax 36:659–664, 1981.

A follow-up (mean duration 14 years) study of 116 patients with proven bronchiectasis. Cor pulmonale was present in 37 percent of the 22 patients who had died.

Fellows KE, Khaw KT, Schuster S, Shwachman H: Bronchial artery embolization in cystic fibrosis; technique and long-term results. J Pediatr 95:959–963, 1979.

This study reports the successful interruption by bronchial artery embolization of major bronchial hemorrhage in 12 of 13 patients with cystic fibrosis. Five of the thirteen patients did have recurrence of minor hemoptysis over the follow-up period which ranged from 1 to 30 months.

Field CE: Bronchiectasis. Third report on a follow-up study of medical and surgical cases from childhood. Arch Dis Child 45:551–561, 1969.

This longitudinal study of children shows a striking decline in the hospital admission rate for bronchiectasis between 1952 and 1960 in five major children's hospitals in England and Scotland. This coincided with the period when broad spectrum antibiotics (particularly tetracyclines) became available for widespread use.

Fraser RG, Macklem PT, Brown WG: Airway dynamics in bronchiectasis. A combined cinefluorographic-manometric study. Am J Roentgenol 93:821–835, 1965.

Bronchograms of 17 patients with bronchiectasis were studied cinefluorographically. Some showed a normal pattern: cough produced a proportionate reduction in caliber through the length of the bronchial tree. Others showed disproportionate changes: cough produced collapse of lobar bronchi with little or no change in diameter of bronchiectatic segments.

Fraser RG, Pare JAP: Roentgenologic signs in the diagnosis of chest disease, in *Diagnosis of Diseases of the Chest*, 2d ed. Philadelphia, Saunders, 1977, pp 518–525.
> *An authoritative review of the changes on plain chest radiograph observed in bronchiectasis and chronic bronchitis.*

Fraser RG, Pare JAP: Diseases of the airways, in *Diagnosis of Diseases of the Chest*, 2d ed. Philadelphia, Saunders, 1977, pp 1443–1456.
> *An excellent description of the bronchographic changes of cylindrical, varicose, and saccular (cystic) bronchiectasis.*

Friedman PJ, Harwood IR, Ellenbogen PH: Pulmonary cystic fibrosis in the adult: Early and late radiologic findings with pathologic correlation. AJR 136:1131–1144, 1981.
> *A very detailed analysis of the radiographic changes observed in adult patients with cystic fibrosis. In 90 percent of cases, characteristic radiographic findings of bronchiectasis were observed.*

Gay S, Dee P: Tracheobronchomegaly—the Mounier-Kuhn syndrome. Brit J Radiol 57:640–644, 1984.
> *A striking bronchographic demonstration of the marked dilatation of the trachea and central bronchi, the mucosal protrusion through tracheal rings, the abrupt transition to normal caliber of terminal airways, and the association with bronchiectasis that are features of this unusual syndrome.*

Glimp RA, Bayer AS: Fungal pneumonias. Part 3. Allergic bronchopulmonary aspergillosis. Chest 80:85–94, 1981.
> *A comprehensive review of the clinical, mycologic, and immunologic features of allergic bronchopulmonary aspergillosis.*

Gregg I, Trapnell DH: The bronchographic appearance of early chronic bronchitis. Br J Radiol 42:132–139, 1969.
> *A bronchographic study of 39 patients with early chronic bronchitis who did not have associated bronchiectasis. Incomplete peripheral filling was the most common abnormality. Dilatation of the mouths of mucous glands of the larger bronchi was also observed.*

Handelsman DJ, Conway AJ, Boylan LM, Turtle JR: Young's syndrome. Obstructive azoospermia and chronic sinopulmonary infections. N Engl J Med 310:3–9, 1984.
> *A disease entity whose clinical features resemble cystic fibrosis and immotile-cilia syndrome is described. The basis of bronchiectasis is unclear. The azoospermia is due to obstruction of the epididymis by inspissated secretions.*

Holmes LB, Blennerhassett JB, Austen KF: A reappraisal of Kartagener's syndrome. Am J Med Sci 255:13–28, 1968.
> *The clinical features of Kartagener's syndrome are described in 13 patients. Phenotypic variations of the syndrome are noted.*

Jederlinic PJ, Sicilian LS, Baigelman W, Gaensler EA: Congenital bronchial atresia. A report of 4 cases and a review of the literature. Medicine (Baltimore) 66:73–83, 1987.
> *The clinical, radiographic, and pathologic findings in 82 patients with congenital bronchial atresia (CBA) are reviewed, and four cases are added. Computed tomography is diagnostic. The differential diagnosis often includes allergic bronchopulmonary aspergillosis, cystic bronchiectasis, bronchogenic cysts, and intrapulmonary sequestration.*

Kaschula ROC, Druker J, Kipps A: Late morphologic consequences of measles: A lethal and debilitating lung disease among the poor. Rev Infect Dis 5:395–404, 1983.
> *A suggestive causal relationship to measles was suggested in 20 of 57 new cases of bronchiectasis in children in South Africa. Further, the authors suggest that intercurrent adenovirus and herpesvirus infections following measles are important initiators of follicular bronchiectasis in childhood.*

Konietzko NFJ, Carton RW, Leroy EP: Causes of death in patients with bronchiectasis. Am Rev Respir Dis 100:852–858, 1969.
> *A study of 62 patients with bronchiectasis from 1956 to 1968. It appears that bronchopulmonary infections have declined strikingly as a cause of death, and cor pulmonale (and other cardiovascular diseases) have increased in importance.*

Lewiston NJ: Bronchiectasis in childhood. Pediatr Clin North Am 31:865–878, 1984.
> *An excellent broad overview of childhood bronchiectasis with emphasis on pathogenesis, clinical features, diagnosis, and treatment. Bibliography is extensive.*

Liebow AA, Hales MR, Lindskog GE: Enlargement of bronchial arteries, and their anastomoses with pulmonary arteries in bronchiectasis. Am J Pathol 25:211–233, 1949.
This is the classic paper demonstrating anatomically the prominent bronchial artery collaterals in cases of bronchiectasis.

Lopez-Vidriero MT, Reid L: Chemical markers of mucous and serum glycoproteins and their relation to viscosity in mucoid and purulent sputum from various hypersecretory diseases. Am Rev Respir Dis 117:465–477, 1978.
Alterations in concentrations of chemical constituents (fucose, mannose, α-acetyl neuraminic acid) in the purulent sputum of patients with bronchiectasis are described.

Muller NL, Bergin CJ, Ostrow DN, Nichols DM: Role of computed tomography in the recognition of bronchiectasis. AJR 143: 971–976, 1984.
The value and limitations of CT in the diagnosis of bronchiectasis is discussed based on studies of 11 patients with this disease. The authors suggest that CT may be useful in the diagnosis of cystic bronchiectasis but is of less value in detecting cylindrical and varicose bronchiectasis.

Ogilvie AG: The natural history of bronchiectasis—A clinical, roentgenologic and pathologic study. Arch Intern Med 68:395–465, 1941.
A classic study of bronchiectasis, written when this disease was a common clinical problem. The discussion of pathology is particularly informative.

Perry KMA, King DS: Bronchiectasis. A study of prognosis based on a follow-up of 400 patients. Am Rev Tuberc 41:531–548, 1940.
A clinical study of a large number of patients with bronchiectasis studied in the preantibiotic era. There is detailed analysis of the lobes involved, clinical course and complications, and the use of surgery in treatment.

Reid LM: Reduction in bronchial subdivision in bronchiectasis. Thorax 5:233–247, 1950.
An excellent study of the pathologic changes in bronchiectasis providing correlation with the bronchographic description of cylindrical, varicose, and saccular forms of the disease. A reduction in the number of bronchial subdivisions in saccular and varicose, but not cylindrical, bronchiectasis is described.

Reid LM: The pathology of obstructive and inflammatory airway diseases. Eur J Respir Dis 147:26–37, 1986.
The diseases included are chronic bronchitis, bronchiolitis, bronchiectasis, and asthma. The term bronchiectasis is used to describe bronchial or bronchiolar distortion and scarring.

Rivera M, Nicotra MB: Pseudomonas aeruginosa mucoid strain. Its significance in adult chest disease. Am Rev Respir Dis 126:833–836, 1982.
The authors reviewed 31 patients from whose sputum mucoid strains of Pseudomonas aeruginosa were isolated. Only two of the patients were considered to have cystic fibrosis. The remainder of the patients had chronic pulmonary disease, and the common feature was bronchiectasis.

Rosenzweig DY, Stead WW: The role of tuberculosis and other forms of bronchopulmonary necrosis in the pathogenesis of bronchiectasis. Am Rev Respir Dis 93:769–785, 1966.
The thesis is advanced that necrotizing pulmonary tuberculosis can produce bronchial dilatation which subsequently may or may not become secondarily infected.

Rossman CM, Forrest JB, Ruffin RE, Newhouse MT: Immotile cilia syndrome in persons with and without Kartagener's syndrome. Am Rev Respir Dis 121:1011–1016, 1980.
A group of patients is described in whom bronchiectasis, impaired mucociliary transport, and lack of ciliary dynein arms are features but in whom situs inversus is absent.

Sanderson JM, Kennedy MCS, Johnson MF, Manley DCE: Bronchiectasis: Results of surgical and conservative management. A review of 393 cases. Thorax 29:407–416, 1974.
The authors consider the various indications for surgical treatment of bronchiectasis.

Schreiber JR, Goldman DA: Infections complicating cystic fibrosis, in Remington JS, Swartz MN (eds), Current Clinical Topics in Infectious Disease-7. New York, McGraw-Hill, 1986, pp 51–81.
A thorough review of the pulmonary infections complicating cystic fibrosis with particular emphasis on the bacteriologic findings and antimicrobial therapy.

Silverman PM, Godwin JD: CT/bronchographic correlations in bronchiectasis. J Comput Assist Tomogr 11:52–56, 1987.
Computed tomography was compared with bronchography to assess the utility of CT in diagnosing and determining the extent of bronchiectasis.

Simila S, Linna O, Lanning P, Heikkinen E, Ala-Houhala M: Chronic lung damage caused by adenovirus type 7: A ten-year follow-up study. Chest 80:127–131, 1981.
Adenovirus pneumonia is described as a predisposing factor leading to subsequent bronchiectasis. Early bronchiolar obstruction (obliterating bronchiolitis) is considered as contributing to this sequence.

Sobonya RE, Taussig LM: Quantitative aspects of lung pathology in cystic fibrosis. Am Rev Respir Dis 134:290–295, 1986.
The lungs of nine patients with cystic fibrosis were studied by morphometric techniques to determine the amount of bronchiectasis, emphysema, pneumonia, bronchial gland enlargement, and small airways narrowing and density. Bronchiectasis was present in all children, but the amount of bronchiectasis did not appear to increase with age.

Stockley RA: Bronchiectasis—new therapeutic approaches based on pathogenesis. Clin Chest Med 8:481–494, 1987.
This article highlights several new concepts in the pathogenesis of bronchiectasis and proposes a hypothesis that could explain the deterioration seen in some of the patients.

Suter S, Schaad UB, Roux L, Nydegger UE, Waldvogel FA: Granulocyte neutral proteases and Pseudomonas elastase as possible causes of airway damage in patients with cystic fibrosis. J Infect Dis 149:523–531, 1984.
The results of this study indicate that large amounts of free granulocyte elastase are present in the bronchial secretions of patients with cystic fibrosis infected with P. aeruginosa. At the same time, concentrations of antiproteinases in the bronchial secretions are reduced. Antimicrobial therapy results in lowered granulocyte elastase activity and increased concentrations of several antiproteinases in bronchial secretions.

Trapnell DH, Gregg I: Some principles of interpretation of bronchograms. Br J Radiol 42:125–131, 1969.
A very helpful introduction to what to look for and why in interpreting bronchograms. Technical aspects that may cause misinterpretation are indicated.

Uflacker R, Kaemmerer A, Neves C, Picon PD: Management of massive hemoptysis by bronchial artery embolization. Radiology 146:627–634, 1983.
A very well-illustrated (bronchial arteriograms) article reviewing the results of treating 33 patients with major hemoptyses by embolization directed by selective bronchial arteriography. Control of hemoptysis was achieved in 82 percent of patients.

Wayne KS, Taussig LM: Probable familial congenital bronchiectasis due to cartilage deficiency (Williams-Campbell syndrome). Am Rev Respir Dis 114:15–22, 1976.
This is a detailed clinical report of two cases (in siblings) of this rare syndrome of congenital deficiency of bronchial cartilage associated with bronchiectasis. The authors favor a congenital basis for this variety of bronchiectasis because of the familial pattern and the onset of symptoms in early childhood.

Wentworth P, Gough J, Wentworth JE: Pulmonary changes and cor pulmonale in mucoviscidosis. Thorax 23:582–589, 1968.
Large Gough sections of lungs of eight patients with cystic fibrosis were examined. Prominent changes included those of diffuse and marked bronchiectasis, pronounced peribronchial granulation tissue, and dilatation of the pulmonary arterial system.

Whitwell F: A study of the pathology and pathogenesis of bronchiectasis. Thorax 7:213–239, 1952.
An excellent review of the pathology of bronchiectasis based on examination of 200 operative specimens. This study also considers the pathogenesis of the disease. The description of the pathologic entity "follicular bronchiectasis" is particularly illuminating.

Wilson JF, Decker AM: The surgical management of childhood bronchiectasis. A review of 96 consecutive pulmonary resections in children with nontuberculous bronchiectasis. Ann Surg 195:354–363, 1982.
A review of the results of 96 pulmonary resections in 195 Alaskan native children with nontuberculous bronchiectasis performed over a 24-year period. Surgical indications are defined in detail.

Chapter 98

Respiratory Viral Infections

R. Gordon Douglas, Jr. / Paul J. Edelson

About 300 million cases of acute respiratory disease occur in the United States each year, accounting for about 150 million visits to physicians. The cost of these illnesses exceeds $1 billion, exclusive of time lost from work.

EPIDEMIOLOGY

The incidence of respiratory disease varies with both age and sex. Children under the age of 6 have about a three-fold greater incidence of acute respiratory disease than adults. In infancy the incidence of lower respiratory disease is higher among boys than girls, but above the age of 6 years both the incidence and duration of acute respiratory infections is higher in females.

At least seven distinct clinical syndromes that result from viral infection of the respiratory tract can be identified: rhinitis (common cold), pharyngitis, laryngitis, laryngotracheobronchitis (croup), tracheobronchitis, bronchiolitis, and pneumonia. Each of these clinical syndromes may occur alone; some may also occur in combination. Each clinical entity can be caused by more than one virus, and each virus can cause more than one clinical disease. Therefore, clinical signs and symptoms are not sufficient criteria for making an etiologic diagnosis in viral respiratory disease.

There are, however, some practical approaches to the clinical diagnosis of viral respiratory disease. First, certain syndromes are so characteristically associated with only one or two viruses as to make the clinical picture almost pathognomonic, as in the case of croup or of bronchiolitis. Second, many of these agents have such distinctive epidemiologic patterns that by taking into account such factors as age, season, community data on viral activity, and special features (such as a hospital nursing home setting, or disease in military recruits) it is possible to make a well-informed etiologic guess. For example, the "winter infantile wheezing" syndrome is very likely to represent infection with respiratory syncytial or parainfluenza 3 virus. Or, although several different agents can cause the common cold syndrome, rhinovirus activity generally peaks in early fall and again in late winter or early spring; parainfluenza viruses are the cause of a second peak later in the fall; up to a quarter of colds in January and February in the northern temperate zone are due to coronaviruses; or, again, adenoviruses are an important cause of lower respiratory tract disease, including pneumonia, in military recruits, but among civilian populations they are primarily pediatric respiratory pathogens. Last, for certain common agents it is now possible to establish a laboratory identification within several hours, making a confirmed etiologic diagnosis available at the time of treatment.

Viruses

Viruses of six major families, including over 200 serologically distinct agents, cause acute disease of the respiratory tract (see Table 98-1). In addition, other viruses may be implicated in some cases of otitis or sinusitis, and the papilloma virus is responsible for laryngeal papillomatosis.

These viruses include both RNA and DNA viruses, both enveloped and nonenveloped viruses, viruses with segmented genomes, and those with a continuous genome. However, for all their molecular differences, their modes of infection and the pathophysiology of the diseases they cause fall into a relatively restricted set of patterns.

Transmission

Respiratory viruses can be transmitted in one of three ways: by large droplets, by small droplets, and by direct contact. Large-particle aerosols (greater than 10 μm in diameter) travel only a few feet before settling, limiting transmission to those in close contact with an infected individual. Although this pattern may occasionally be a mechanism for transmission of viral disease, it does not appear to be an important route for transmission of the common respiratory pathogens.

Small-droplet aerosols, on the other hand, play an important role in transmission of adenovirus, influenza A and B, and some Coxsackie viruses. Small particles can travel considerable distances from person to person and therefore can inoculate a large number of individuals simultaneously. Unlike the large-particle aerosols which are often deposited in the naso- and oropharynx, small droplets will often reach and directly inoculate the lower respiratory tract epithelium.

Direct hand-to-hand or hand-to-fomite-to-hand transmission with subsequent self-inoculation of conjunctival or nasal membranes is a major mechanism for transmission of the rhinoviruses and respiratory syncytial virus. Thus, in the hospital, hand washing and decontamination of environmental surfaces are more effective ways of limiting the spread of these agents than are such typical respiratory precautions as the use of masks and gowns, and isolation of patients behind closed doors.

Pathophysiology

Clinical infection may be initiated by one or a small number of viral particles. The route of spread and site of inoculation may account for the occurrence of prodromal symptoms before the development of the classic illness. For example, primary inoculation of respiratory syncytial virus onto conjunctival or nasal membranes probably accounts for the upper respiratory prodrome which often precedes the development of bronchiolitis and pneumonia with that agent. On the other hand, because influenza virus often initially infects the lower respiratory tract, the first signs of influenza infection are pulmonary and systemic.

In general, infection with these agents is limited to the respiratory tract. Although it is not unusual for some agents to extensively involve both the upper and lower tracts, it is rare to find extrarespiratory spread of virus. The systemic and constitutional signs characteristic of infection with some of these agents should not be misinterpreted as representing either a viremia or extrarespiratory spread; they are more likely to result from the liberation of such soluble mediators of the inflammatory process as interferon. The major exception to this rule is adenovirus, where extrapulmonary infection, for example cystitis, is not uncommon.

The signs and symptoms of viral respiratory infection derive from two major local processes, viral cytopathic effects and the inflammation they trigger. Most clinical signs and symptoms are accounted for by the direct viral cytopathic effects, as illustrated by the direct correlation between the titers of rhinovirus or influenza virus in nasal washes and the severity of disease. However, host responses clearly contribute to the clinical picture in bronchiolitis, for example, where specific antiviral IgE may mediate the release of bronchoconstrictive agents such as prostaglandin E_2 and $F_{2\alpha}$ and SRS-A. In addition, viral damage to the mucociliary escalator and to pulmonary macrophages and neutrophils probably accounts for the phenomenon of secondary bacterial infection that follows infection with such agents as influenza virus.

TABLE 98-1
Human Respiratory Viruses

Family	Genus	Types and Groups
Orthomyxoviridae	Influenzavirus	Influenza virus types A, B, and C
4-Paramyxoviridae	Paramyxovirus	Parainfluenza virus types 1–5
	Pneumovirus	Respiratory syncytial virus
Picornaviridae	Rhinovirus	105 serotypes
	Enterovirus	Group A Coxsackie, 23 types
		Group B Coxsackie, 6 types
		Echovirus, 31 types
		Enterovirus, 3 types
Coronaviridae	Coronavirus	3 types
Adenoviridae	Mastadenovirus	31 serotypes
Herpetoviridae	Herpesvirus	Herpes simplex virus types 1, 2
		Epstein-Barr virus

SOURCE: Douglas RG Jr, in Galasso GJ et al. (eds), *Antiviral Agents and Viral Diseases of Man.* New York, Raven, 1984.

Laboratory Diagnosis of Viral Respiratory Disease

The cornerstone of laboratory diagnosis of viral disease is isolation and identification of the virus in cell culture. Although in the past embryonated eggs were frequently used for viral isolation, this method has been replaced largely by modern cell culture techniques. There are three requirements for the successful isolation of a viral agent in culture: a satisfactory clinical specimen containing infectious virions, a permissive cell system allowing the virus to multiply, and a method for detecting viral growth in culture.

While some viruses are very hardy, many of the respiratory viruses will not tolerate freezing or drying. In addition, clinical specimens may contain such natural antiviral substances as proteases and antibody, or they may be contaminated by bacterial flora which can overgrow stored specimens and destroy inoculated cells in culture. Therefore, gentle handling of specimens, use of appropriate viral carrying media, and prompt inoculation into a suitable cell type are essential for the reliable isolation of viruses from clinical samples. In the absence of specific recommendations to the contrary, the most reliable way of handling specimens for viral culture when prompt inoculation is not possible is to hold them in viral carrying medium on wet ice or in a refrigerator. However, some viruses, including respiratory syncytial virus, will not tolerate even these conditions for more than 4 to 6 h.

Some viruses, such as the herpesviruses, will give a positive culture result within 72 h. Many viruses, however, require considerably longer times for isolation and identification. For a few viruses, rapid techniques that can provide a viral diagnosis within a few hours have been developed. Originally these systems used fluorescence microscopy to detect viral antigens, but this technique has largely been replaced by enzyme-linked immunosorbent assay (ELISA) systems. Commercial kits are now available for the rapid detection of respiratory syncytial virus, and tests for the influenza and parainfluenza viruses are under development.

Detection of serum antibody responses by serologic tests has a small role to play in the routine diagnosis of viral respiratory disease.

INFLUENZA

Epidemiology

Influenza is the most common cause of lower respiratory tract infection in the United States. About 48 million cases of influenza occur in the United States each winter, accounting for about 3.9 million hospitalizations and 20,000 deaths. The burden of the disease falls most heavily on people at the two extremes of age, those under 5 or over 65 years, and on those with preexisting cardiac or pulmonary disease.

Type A influenza virus infection occurs most frequently and is responsible for the greatest amount of morbidity and the largest number of deaths. Type A disease occurs every year, with epidemic numbers of cases every 3 or 4 years and pandemic outbreaks every 10 to 30 years. Excess influenza and pneumonia mortality is most closely associated with these pandemic outbreaks. Type B disease occurs every 2 to 4 years, but it does not cause pandemics. Type C rarely causes detectable disease.

Influenza virus is a negative-strand enveloped RNA virus, with a segmented genome composed of eight separate genes (seven in the case of type C). Types A and B virus display on their surface a *hemagglutinin* and a *neuraminidase*. These proteins show a remarkable capacity for antigenic variation, which accounts for the unique epidemiology of influenza.

Two sorts of antigenic changes among influenza virus are recognized: *antigenic drift* and *antigenic shift*. *Antigenic drift* occurs with both type A and type B viruses and refers to the emergence of minor antigenic differences among the viral hemagglutinins and neuraminidases, developing every winter as the result of immunologic selection pressures. These differences represent spontaneous point mutations in the viral genome. It is thought that the epidemic waves of disease which occur every few years represent the ascendance of new subtypes emerging through this process of antigenic drift.

Antigenic shift, a process which is associated with only type A virus, represents the emergence of a new viral subtype with an antigenically distinct hemagglutinin or neuraminidase or both. Such new subtypes are believed to result from reassortment occurring when two different viral subtypes simultaneously infect the same cell, leading to the production of hybrid progeny carrying genetic material from each parental subtype. These changes can occur because the genome is segmented, so that independent assortment of viral genes is possible. Few persons will have protective immunity against a newly produced subtype, making it possible for its emergence to be associated with pandemic outbreaks of the kind seen once a decade or so ago. To date, three hemagglutinins (H1, H2, H3) and two neuraminidases (N1, N2) have been observed among human influenza A viruses. Subtypes are named by their hemagglutinin and neuraminidase, e.g., H1N1, H3N2, etc., and strains within a subtype by year and site of isolation, e.g., A/Bangkok/79 H3N2.

Pathophysiology

Influenza is transmitted in small-particle aerosols produced when respiratory secretions are vigorously coughed. The ability of these aerosols to remain suspended in the air for hours accounts for the point-source pattern and explosive spread of influenza infection. Because of the small size of these infectious droplets, when

the aerosols are inhaled, the upper respiratory tract may be completely bypassed and primary inoculation of the virus occurs instead in the ciliated epithelium of the lower respiratory tract. Only one infectious unit, presumably one virus, is required to infect a susceptible person.

Disease in both airways and airspace is present in most patients with influenza. The infection is usually cytotoxic to infected cells, causing cellular debris to accumulate in airspaces and to obstruct small airways. The inflammatory process brings cells and fluid to the area, swelling the respiratory tissues and further compromising the airways. Additionally, certain inflammatory mediators liberated during this process have direct effects on airway smooth muscle, leading to bronchoconstriction and further compromise of airway flows.

Clinical Picture

Although there may be a 2- to 3-day prodromal period, the onset of clinical disease is often quite abrupt. Influenza is more commonly associated with extrarespiratory and systemic symptoms than are the other respiratory viruses. The "flu" syndrome includes fever above 101.4°F, headache, myalgias, muscle tenderness, and arthralgias. In severe cases, these symptoms are associated with elevated serum levels of creatine phosphokinase (CPK) and myoglobinuria. Photophobia, conjunctivitis, and "gritty" eyes are not unusual, and many patients will also complain of anorexia or nausea. Diarrhea is primarily associated with type B infection, and is especially common in children.

Respiratory symptoms, including a dry cough, often associated with substernal burning, a scratchy throat, and a watery nasal discharge, usually last 3 to 5 days, followed by the resolution of fever over a 1- to 2-day period. Convalescence, however, may take several weeks. Hyperreactive airway disease may be a part of the clinical picture at any stage, but it is of particular importance during the convalescent phase, where it may be manifested by a chronic cough rather than wheezing, in a picture of what has been called *cough-equivalent* bronchospasm. In these cases, the cough will often respond to bronchodilator therapy.

Diagnosis

Laboratory studies are of great importance in defining the severity of disease and detecting secondary bacterial infection, but the diagnosis of influenza may be made often on clinical grounds during epidemics. Confirmation by viral culture or serologic methods is of epidemiologic importance, of value in cases of atypical or severe disease, and of use in detection of sporadic cases. Rapid diagnostic techniques for influenza are in development, but they are not yet commercially available.

Complications

There are three major respiratory complications of influenza: tracheobronchitis, primary influenza pneumonia, and secondary bacterial pneumonia.

Tracheobronchitis is usually associated with clinical signs of lower respiratory tract involvement in the face of a normal chest radiograph. Individuals who may be otherwise healthy will note an exacerbation of their previously dry cough, with the production of frothy or blood-tinged sputum. Although symptoms may persist for up to 3 weeks, tracheobronchitis generally has a good prognosis and should not be confused with the far more serious complications of primary influenza pneumonia or secondary bacterial pneumonia, described below.

Primary influenza pneumonia refers to a clinical syndrome of rapidly progressive pulmonary involvement, usually occurring in a high-risk individual and often proceeding relentlessly to a fatal outcome. Individuals with preexisting pulmonary disease or cardiac valvular disease are at the greatest risk. Pregnant women have also been at increased risk during some outbreaks, but the risk seems unrelated to the stage of pregnancy and cannot be directly related to the altered mechanics of breathing characteristic of late pregnancy.

The patient develops increasing respiratory distress, associated with the production of frothy, blood-tinged sputum, 24 to 48 h after the onset of typical influenza. Unlike patients with tracheobronchitis, persons with primary influenza pneumonia appear seriously ill, extremely dyspneic, and often deeply cyanotic. Auscultation reveals diffuse fine rales and wheezes, but no evidence of consolidation, and the chest radiograph is consistent with pulmonary edema or interstitial pneumonia. The white blood cell count may be elevated, and an increase in immature neutrophils is not unusual and should not be misinterpreted as indicating a bacterial etiology. Occasionally leukopenia is seen, particularly in individuals with combined viral and bacterial infection, and is a poor prognostic sign. Perhaps the single most valuable laboratory test is the examination of a Gram-stained smear of sputum. The specimen should have few if any neutrophils, and there will be no predominant bacterial species.

The characteristic clinical course of influenza pneumonia is one of progressive hypoxemia, despite high ambient oxygen pressures and mechanical ventilation. Mortality is high, with most patients dying with a picture of adult respiratory distress syndrome. Although there is no response to antibiotics, it may at times be difficult to exclude concomitant bacterial infection for which antibiotics are necessary. Newer antiviral agents (see below) may have an important role to play in treating this disease.

Secondary bacterial pneumonia occurs far more often than primary influenza pneumonia. Although it also

has a predilection for older individuals with chronic pulmonary disease, it is not unusual for it to occur in an otherwise healthy young adult. It was a leading cause of death in the 1918 influenza pandemic and the leading complication in the pandemic of 1957–1958.

Persons with secondary bacterial pneumonia report a "relapse" of symptoms 1 to 4 days into their convalescence from what had until then appeared to be a typical case of influenza. They develop a heavy, productive cough and usually have evidence of a new consolidation on physical examination or by radiograph.

Although *Staphylococcus aureus* is most characteristically associated with postinfluenza bacterial pneumonia, far more cases are caused by the pneumococcus. β-Hemolytic streptococci and *Haemophilus influenzae* should also be considered. Gram-negative enteric organisms, such as *Klebsiella* and *Enterobacter*, may be important in individuals in intensive-care units and in residents of nursing homes. The sputum Gram stain is often very helpful in distinguishing this complication from influenza pneumonia and in suggesting the likely organism. Prompt therapy with appropriate antibiotics may be lifesaving.

Extrapulmonary complications of influenza characteristically involve the heart, the nervous system, and the liver. Myocarditis has been reported with both influenza A and B infections, and it may be associated with some cases of sudden death in otherwise healthy young adults during influenza season. This uncommon, but obviously frightening, possibility has inspired the advice to individuals who maintain a regular aerobic exercise schedule that strenuous exercise should be suspended when one has a viral respiratory illness or, more memorably, "When your nose runs, you shouldn't." Neurologic complications of influenza may affect almost any level of the nervous system, from encephalitis through transverse myelitis, to radiculitis and Guillain-Barré syndrome. Reye's syndrome is particularly a complication of influenza B infection. Although many cases have been reported in which there was no exposure to aspirin, aspirin use increases the risk of clinical disease and it is prudent to recommend the use of antipyretics and analgesics that do not contain aspirin to treat children during influenza season.

Therapy

For most individuals, bed rest and symptomatic relief are all that is necessary. However, high-risk individuals, the very young, the elderly, and those whose illness has been aggravated by either pulmonary or extrarespiratory complications may require hospitalization.

The keystone of in-hospital management of influenza is oxygen. Every patient hospitalized with influenza should be assumed to be hypoxemic, and supplemental oxygen should be considered part of the immediate management, provided that one observes the appropriate cautions concerning the use of oxygen in individuals with chronic carbon dioxide retention whose respiratory drive may be maintained only by hypoxemia. In general, however, these individuals quickly require mechanically assisted ventilation, making the issue of respiratory drive moot.

The antiviral drug amantadine (1-adamantanamine hydrochloride, Symmetrel), which is highly active in vitro against influenza A virus, has been available in the United States for several years for the prevention of influenza A infection. More recently, it has also been recommended for use in the treatment of established infection, provided it is begun within the first 72 h of illness. Amantadine reduced both the extent and duration of fever and has a moderate ability to relieve systemic symptoms of influenza infection. Some data suggest that amantadine also promotes a more rapid resolution of respiratory symptoms and a reduction in viral shedding. The dosage is 200 mg PO initially, and then 100 mg once daily (just as effective as the 100 mg bid dosing currently recommended by the manufacturer) for the duration of fever, which is usually 3 to 5 days. Dosing must be adjusted in patients with renal insufficiency.

The major drawback to the use of amantadine is the occurrence of unpleasant neurologic side effects, including dizziness, insomnia, attention difficulties, and extrapyramidal symptoms. Although these effects are reversible when the drug is discontinued, they are particularly troublesome in the elderly, who are the major group of recipients of amantadine. Rimantadine, a congener of amantadine which is not yet approved for use in this country, appears to be just as effective but is much less able than amantadine to penetrate the central nervous system and thus does not produce neurologic side effects.

Another antiviral, ribavirin (1-β-D-ribofuranosyl-1,2,4-triazole-3-carboxamide, Virazole), although not yet approved for use in influenza in this country, appears promising for the therapy of both influenzas A and B. When administered in a small-particle aerosol it has been shown to be effective virologically and clinically in both experimental and natural influenza infection. Although the principal toxicity of the systemically administered drug is a reversible anemia, this effect is not seen with aerosol administration.

Prevention

Administration of inactivated influenza vaccine is an important way to modify both the incidence and severity of disease. Efficacy rates for vaccine of 67 to 92 percent have been reported in various studies. Vaccination programs are particularly likely to benefit individuals in

nursing homes, where influenza attack rates may be as high as 60 percent and case-fatality ratios as high as 30 percent. Because of the constantly changing antigenic characteristics of human influenza viruses, vaccine composition must be modified annually, and individuals require annual reimmunization with newly dominant strains. The Centers for Disease Control have recommended that attention be focused on certain high-risk target groups (see Table 98-2).

It is currently recommended that anyone over the age of 12 years receive a single 0.5-ml dose of *either* the whole virion or the split virion preparation. Children from 3 to 12 years should receive two doses of 0.5 ml of the split virus preparation only, separated by 4 weeks or more. Infants 6 to 35 months old should receive two doses of 0.25 ml of the split virus preparation, separated by 4 weeks or more. However, these recommendations may be modified in future years for different vaccine formulations.

Amantadine may also be used for prophylaxis, either alone or in conjunction with an immunization program. It may be useful in certain high-risk individuals who cannot receive influenza vaccine, and as an adjunct to vaccination programs to control institutional outbreaks, or in case of severe epidemic outbreaks, during the 2 weeks necessary for immunization to take effect. The dose is 100 mg PO per day.

Once the needs of these three groups are addressed, high priority should also be given to

1. Otherwise healthy individuals over the age of 65
2. Adults and children with chronic metabolic diseases (including diabetes mellitus), renal disease, anemia, immunosuppression, or asthma who have required regular medical follow-up or hospitalization in the preceding year

GENERAL POPULATION

Physicians should immunize any persons in their practice who want to reduce their risk of acquiring influenza. Persons providing essential community services (e.g., firefighters, police officers, health care personnel) should be considered for targeted vaccination to minimize possible disruption of essential services during severe epidemics.

PREGNANT WOMEN

Pregnancy is not itself considered an indication for high priority vaccination. The vaccine is generally considered safe for use in pregnancy, but waiting until the second or third trimester to administer it may be prudent.

PERSONS WHO SHOULD NOT BE VACCINATED

The vaccine should not be administered to anyone with a history of anaphylactic hypersensitivity to eggs. This in-

TABLE 98-2
Current Centers for Disease Control Recommendations on the Use of Influenza Virus Vaccine in Selected Populations

Highest priority
1. Adults and children with chronic disorders of the cardiovascular or pulmonary systems that are severe enough to have required regular medical follow-ups or hospitalization during the preceding year.
2. Residents of nursing homes and other chronic-care facilities (i.e., institutions housing patients of any age with chronic medical conditions). Infection control programs in these institutions should make their goal immunization of no fewer than 80% of residents.

High priority
1. Physicians, nurses, and other personnel who have extensive contact with high-risk patients (including both primary care personnel and certain specialty staff, and staff of intensive-care units, including neonatal intensive-care units).

SOURCE: Adapted from Morbidity and Mortality Weekly Reports 33:253–260, 265–266, 1984.

cludes individuals who, on eating an egg, develop swelling of the lips or tongue or experience acute respiratory distress or collapse. Persons with intercurrent acute febrile illnesses should not be immunized until their symptoms have abated.

BRONCHIOLITIS AND VIRAL PNEUMONIA

Etiology

Respiratory syncytial virus (RSV), parainfluenza types 1 and 3, and *Mycoplasma pneumoniae* together account for 75 percent of winter lower respiratory tract infections in children. However, each of these causes of atypical pneumonia is most important in a different age group. RSV is the major cause of viral pneumonia in children under age 2. Parainfluenza types 1 and 3 are most important between ages 2 and 5. *M. pneumoniae* is the leading cause beyond the age of 5, followed by influenza A and B. The parainfluenza viruses also contribute cases to the youngest age group, whereas the adenoviruses cause a severe but uncommon type of pneumonia in all age groups.

Epidemiology

RSV is the most important winter respiratory pathogen of infancy and early childhood, estimated to be responsible for 134 cases per 1000 children per year in private practices in the United States. For children under 1 year of age, the attack rate may be as high as 50 percent, and nearly all children are seropositive by age 3. Since RSV infection does not produce absolute immunity, individuals continue to have mildly symptomatic or asymptomatic infections through adulthood. However, lower respiratory

tract involvement is confined to children under the age of 2, and, occasionally, to the elderly. Although distinct viral types are not recognized for RSV, recent studies using monoclonal antibodies suggest that there may be antigenically distinct subtypes of RSV and that repeated infection may be at least partly due to exposure to different antigenic variants.

RSV is the only respiratory virus which causes major epidemics every year. It generally occurs in midwinter in the temperate and subtropical zones; smaller outbreaks may also occur in late spring. The phenomenon of *viral interference* is seen epidemiologically with each of the viral respiratory pathogens, except parainfluenza 3. Thus, during the winter, it is not unusual to see RSV disease abate or disappear in the community while influenza A or B is active, only to have RSV activity resume its epidemic levels once influenza has gone.

Poverty, poor housing, and large families all appear to be important risk factors for both incidence and severity of disease. Toddlers attending day-care programs have an exceptionally high attack rate, with 98 percent of children experiencing at least one attack, and 65 percent having three or more episodes. RSV is also coming to be recognized as a significant respiratory pathogen in the elderly and in patients with chronic obstructive lung disease or cystic fibrosis. There is some evidence that asymptomatic carriage occurs in adults, but recovery of virus from an asymptomatic child is rare.

Pathophysiology of Infection

RSV is a medium-size enveloped RNA virus generally grouped with the paramyxoviruses, but assigned its own specific genus: Pneumovirus. The virion has three major viral proteins, a *nucleocapsid* and two *membrane* proteins, one of which is glycosylated.

The incubation period for experimental infection in adult volunteers is 5 days; in natural infection it is estimated as 2 to 8 days. Infection results from inoculation of the conjunctivae or nasal mucosa; oral mucous membranes are not susceptible to infection.

As infection spreads along the respiratory mucosa, it provokes peribronchial mononuclear cell infiltrates and necrosis of the epithelium of small airways, which leads to plugging of their lumens, air trapping, and eventually wash-out atelectasis. There is also a lymphocytic peribronchiolar infiltrate with edema of the walls, including the submucosa and adventitia. As the infection progresses, there is necrosis and sloughing of the bronchiolar epithelium and increased mucus production, both of which contribute to further airway obstruction, leading to atelectasis and ventilation-perfusion mismatch.

While histologic recovery may begin within a few days, ciliated epithelium may not begin to replace necrotic areas for 2 weeks, and complete healing can take more

than a month. Enlarged submucosal glands, augmented goblet cells, and muscular hypertrophy may persist for some time.

Clinical Presentations

Although bronchiolitis is the most characteristic presentation of RSV infection, more children with RSV have pneumonia without clinically evident bronchospasm. About one-third of children present with bronchiolitis, whereas nearly half have simply pneumonia.

Bronchiolitis is clinically detectable airway hyperreactivity occurring in infants and resulting from a respiratory infection. The characteristic symptoms are tachypnea, wheezing, and evidence of respiratory distress, including nasal flaring and intercostal and substernal retractions. The chest radiograph shows hyperinflation with air trapping. Peribronchial cuffing is characteristic, and scattered infiltrates are common. With severe distress air may appear in the mediastinum.

In the case dominated by pneumonia, tachypnea and distress are characteristic, but wheezing may be absent, and the expiratory phase is not prolonged. Chest radiograph is less likely to show air trapping and more likely to show diffuse pulmonary infiltrates.

Many children will have elements of each of these clinical pictures. The most important difference between these two presentations is that bronchiolitis is typically seen in the infant, while pneumonia alone is more common in the toddler. Most of the differences in course, complications, and outcome between these two clinical forms are really a reflection of these age-related differences.

Nearly every child with RSV infection ill enough to require hospitalization has cough, tachypnea, and copious respiratory secretions. A rash, ranging from mild erythema to a confluent maculopapular reaction, and occurring several days into the illness, is not uncommon, but fever beyond the first day, conjunctivitis, and otitis are, occurring in fewer than 10 to 15 percent of children.

Although upper respiratory symptoms, particularly coryza, are most characteristic of infection in the adult, it is not unusual for RSV infection in the infant to begin as an upper respiratory infection (URI). One should be alert to the possibility of pneumonia in any infant under 6 months of age whose winter cold progresses to tachypnea and distress. This progression is often heralded by the development of a cough.

Croup is an uncommon clinical manifestation of RSV infection, with only about 5 percent of infections presenting this way. Central nervous system manifestations, including myelitis, ataxia, hemiplegia, and facial palsy, have been reported in occasional cases. Isolated cases of myocarditis, including some with complete heart block, have also been ascribed to RSV infection.

Laboratory Studies

The most important use of radiograph and laboratory studies is to exclude bacterial causes of pneumonia. As described above, nearly every child ill enough to be hospitalized will have an abnormal chest radiograph. Lobar consolidations are seen in about 20 percent of patients, but areas of collapse or hyperlucency, abscess cavities, fluid in the chest, or "white-out" are not seen with uncomplicated RSV pneumonia.

White blood cell counts, though normally somewhat higher in the infant than the adult, nonetheless are rarely above 12,500 cells per cubic milliliter or show more than a modest left shift in the absence of secondary bacterial disease. Most children are mildly or moderately hypoxemic, but arterial P_{O_2} tensions below 70 mmHg are quite uncommon, as are hypercapnia and respiratory acidosis. Abnormalities of gas exchange are persistent, however, and most infants are hypoxemic at discharge and may continue to be so for several weeks.

Special Presentations in Early Infancy

In addition to the pneumonic and bronchiolitic presentations, there are two other presentations reported in infants under 3 months of age: one is the development of apnea; the other is a clinical picture of sepsis.

Apnea develops in association with RSV infection in infants who were considerably premature and who often have a history of neonatal apnea. Initially there may be no other evidence of respiratory disease, and these children may be admitted as having suspected "near-sudden infant death syndrome." One of the reasons it is important to recognize those children in whom RSV is the etiologic agent is that their prognosis both in hospital and at home is excellent. The apneic episodes will usually stop within the first 24 h, and they do not recur during the illness. These children do not need to be monitored at home and do not appear to be at increased risk for further apneic episodes with subsequent respiratory infections.

The *viral sepsis* presentation, however, while much less common than the presentation with apnea, is far more ominous. The leading symptoms are lethargy, poor feeding, and irritability—the characteristic clinical triad of neonatal sepsis. Some will also have a rash and fever. Respiratory signs and symptoms are generally absent, though occasionally apnea may be present. The picture appears much more frequently in premature infants, and unexpected deaths have occurred in several of these children. During the winter months, it is not unusual for nosocomial outbreaks of RSV infection to occur in neonatal intensive-care units, and one should particularly consider this diagnosis in a hospitalized premature infant who has undergone a precipitous clinical deterioration during RSV season.

Viral Diagnostic Studies

For years, cell isolation of RSV in cell culture systems was the only way to establish a diagnosis. RSV will grow in a wide variety of human and animal cells, but cytopathic effects are best seen in the human continuous cell lines, particularly in HEp-2 cells. Cultures are often positive in 2 to 5 days, provided the samples have been carefully handled and promptly inoculated. RSV is quite sensitive to both freezing and drying, and for reliable results cultures should be inoculated immediately.

Rapid viral diagnostic studies, either by fluorescence microscopy, or more recently by ELISA, have made a tremendous impact on the diagnosis and management of the hospitalized child with RSV. These tests can be carried out on respiratory secretions in 3 to 4 h, using commercial reagents which have excellent specificity (>95 percent) and good sensitivity (>90 percent). They are extremely convenient for clinical decision making, and some have now supplanted virus culture as the diagnostic "gold standard." Their availability has become particularly important now that specific antiviral chemotherapy for RSV is available.

Management

The overwhelming majority of children with RSV infection can be cared for at home with humidification and symptomatic therapy. About 1 percent of cases require hospitalization. These are primarily infants under 6 months of age—the median age for admissions at our institution is 3 months—or children who fall into a high-risk category.

High-risk children are those with underlying cardiac or pulmonary disease, children with immunodeficiencies, and those with neuromuscular disorders that limit their respiratory effort. The major diagnoses that contribute to this group are bronchopulmonary dysplasia, a sequela of severe neonatal respiratory distress syndrome, and congenital cardiac diseases, particularly those varieties associated with intrapulmonary shunting or pulmonary hypertension.

While the case fatality rate for hospitalized infants with uncomplicated RSV infection has been estimated at 1 to 5 percent, in children with congenital cardiac disease it is more than 30 percent. It is not uncommon for the increasing respiratory deterioration characteristic of RSV infection in these children to be misinterpreted as worsening of their underlying cardiac disorder. During the winter months, it is important to consider RSV infection in any child with cardiac or pulmonary disease who deteriorates clinically or whose chest radiograph shows new pulmonary infiltrates.

The keystone of management of the child with RSV infection who is sick enough to be hospitalized is supple-

mental oxygen. The child's tachypnea is a sensitive indicator of hypoxemia and should be followed in addition to blood-gas determinations as a guide to the amount of oxygen required. The role of bronchodilators in RSV pneumonia is less clear. It has been argued that, because small airway resistance so dominates the clinical picture of RSV pneumonia and because these branches lack significant amounts of smooth muscle, it is inappropriate to use bronchodilators, particularly theophylline or other β-adrenergic agents, in treating children with RSV infection. In fact, at one time the responsiveness to bronchodilators was considered a key diagnostic point in distinguishing an asthmatic episode from bronchiolitis. However, there is some clinical experience that certain children with RSV infection can benefit from bronchodilator therapy, provided that dosing and drug levels can be carefully monitored to avoid potentially serious side effects. There is also renewed interest in using other medications effective in asthma in some of these children.

Undoubtedly the single most important advance in the management of RSV infection is the recent introduction of the wide-spectrum antiviral agent ribavirin. This agent, which interferes with the capping process required for the production of viral message, is active in vitro against a wide range of RNA and DNA viruses, including most of the common respiratory viruses. It is effective therapy for RSV pneumonia and bronchiolitis in both high- and low-risk hospitalized patients, reducing viral shedding, limiting the severity of symptoms, and reducing the total duration of illness. In high-risk patients it has been especially important in limiting the progression of illness and reducing the need for mechanical ventilation.

Secondary bacterial infections rarely complicate RSV pneumonia, and in double-blind clinical studies antibiotics have provided no benefit.

Control and Prevention

There is currently no vaccine available for widespread prophylaxis. Earlier efforts with a killed-virus vaccine stimulated high antibody levels in vaccinees but led to more severe illness with subsequent natural infection.

Because RSV is so widespread each winter, there is no practical way, and in many cases little need, to prevent infant exposures. However, it is possible to reduce the risk of infection in the high-risk groups. We recommend avoiding all elective admissions during RSV season for infants with congenital cardiac or chronic pulmonary disease. When such children must be admitted, they should not share a room with children with bronchiolitis or pneumonia. As transmission of RSV is accomplished almost entirely by contact, it is important to reemphasize the need for hand washing for all staff, particularly for those caring for children with respiratory infection.

Outcome

There are two issues regarding the consequences of RSV infection. First is the question of whether children with RSV bronchiolitis are more likely to experience subsequent episodes of bronchospasm. Second is the question of whether RSV infection, in certain children, can lead to long-term pulmonary abnormalities.

As yet, neither of these issues has been definitively addressed. Recent follow-up studies, extending over periods of up to 10 years, show that among children previously hospitalized with bronchiolitis there is an association between an increased sensitivity to methacholine challenge and a history of recurrent bronchiolitis. It is not clear whether this means that repeated respiratory infection leads to long-term bronchial hyperreactivity or whether children with preexisting bronchial hyperreactivity are more likely to respond to respiratory viral infection with bronchoconstriction.

LARYNGOTRACHEOBRONCHITIS AND CROUP

Etiology

The parainfluenza viruses are the most commonly identified causes of laryngotracheobronchitis (LTB) and croup. Although there is no strict relationship between specific viral types and particular clinical pictures, parainfluenza type 1 is the leading cause of croup, whereas type 3 is more commonly associated with LTB. In the United States it is the type 1 virus which is responsible for the characteristic biannual winter outbreaks of croup and LTB in children. Type 2 virus, less commonly isolated than types 1 or 3, is most often associated with mild upper respiratory infection, although it has occasionally been associated with small outbreaks of lower respiratory tract disease. Type 4 virus has been associated with only mild, sporadic upper respiratory disease.

Both influenza A virus (H2N2, H3N2, and H1N1) and influenza B virus have been associated with severe LTB or croup. Respiratory syncytial virus and lower numbered serotypes of adenovirus are also frequently isolated from patients with LTB. Isolations of rhinoviruses, enteroviruses, herpes simplex virus, and reoviruses have been reported occasionally, but the etiologic significance of these isolates is uncertain.

Bacterial infections, inflammatory processes, and trauma may also cause the croup syndrome. Diphtheritic croup was not unusual in prevaccine days. Foreign-body aspiration, smoke inhalation, ventilatory intubation, hereditary angioneurotic edema, or anaphylaxis may also be responsible for rapidly developing respiratory obstruction manifested as cough, hoarseness, dyspnea, and inspiratory stridor. However, these conditions do not cause the

fever or catarrhal symptoms usually associated with viral respiratory disease.

Pathophysiology

Parainfluenza virus infection begins in the nasal or pharyngeal mucosa. Virus spreads cell-to-cell within the ciliated epithelium as the infection extends caudally toward the bronchi. Along its path edema and hyperemia develop, and the airway itself becomes narrowed by the swollen epithelium. Swelling of the vocal cords, or of the aryepiglottic folds, may cause hoarseness or loss of voice. In organ culture, infection can also lead to inhibition of ciliary action, cell death, and even invasion into the lamina propria. Necrotic debris desquamating into the airways further obstructs airflow and probably accounts for much of the patchy atelectasis which develops in more severe cases. Inflammatory and immunologic responses, particularly the local production of antiviral IgE, may further contribute to airway narrowing and hyperreactivity by triggering the production of prostanoids and liberating histamine and other bronchostrictive agents. With severe infection, both airway obstruction and ventilation-perfusion imbalance caused by intrapulmonary shunting can lead to hypoxemia and air hunger. Severe airway obstruction also leads to retention of carbon dioxide and ventilatory failure.

Although symptomatic reinfection with the same viral type does occur, even in individuals with circulating type-specific antibody, the amelioration of symptoms in adults as compared with children suggests that partial immunity does develop, and there are data suggesting that local secretory antibodies confer resistance to homotypic rechallenge.

Clinical Presentation

Although much has been made of the differences between LTB on the one hand, and croup on the other, these are two ends of a single clinical spectrum, and elements of both processes are often present at the same time. For most patients, the illness begins with cough, hoarseness, and fever which may go on for 2 or 3 days. In some patients, symptoms and signs of lower respiratory tract disease, including wheezing, air trapping, and hypoxemia, will dominate the clinical picture. Others, however, will go on to develop the brassy, barklike cough and inspiratory stridor characteristic of croup.

Croup generally affects children 3 months to 3 years old. Typically, it shows a nocturnal pattern of exacerbation; the child's symptoms wane each morning, only to return again at night. This cyclic pattern usually continues for three or four nights, with children reaching the peak of symptoms on the second or third evening.

LTB, on the other hand, shows a more clearly mono-tonic period of worsening over 3 to 4 days, followed by several days of improvement, although some individuals may be symptomatic for as long as 2 weeks.

Differential Diagnosis

There is very little difficulty in recognizing these diseases during epidemic periods. Respiratory symptoms dominate the clinical picture. Patients will often be only minimally toxic, and high fevers are not typical of uncomplicated viral LTB or croup.

Croup should be easy to distinguish from noninfectious causes of upper airway obstruction, as these are not associated with such prodromal symptoms as coryza or fever. The most important condition to distinguish is acute infectious *epiglottitis*, a rapidly progressing bacterial infection of the epiglottis which may lead to complete airway obstruction within a period of several hours. Epiglottitis is a medical emergency; immediate recognition and prompt establishment of a secure airway can be lifesaving. Patients with epiglottitis are typically older (3 to 6 years) than those with croup, and it may even occur in adults. Persons with epiglottitis usually present to a physician within 12 h of the onset of symptoms with an initial complaint of severe throat pain. Swallowing is often so painful that they are forced to drool. Many are, or quickly become, air-hungry. They often refuse to lie down, preferring to sit upright with chin jutting forward in an effort to keep the epiglottis from obstructing the trachea.

Diagnostic Studies

The diagnosis of LTB or croup is usually made quite easily on clinical grounds, and laboratory studies are of most use in excluding secondary bacterial complications. Most patients show a normal or only modestly elevated white blood count, with no increase in immature forms. A substantial leukocytosis should raise the question of bacterial infection, either bacterial superinfection complicating a viral process or bacterial epiglottitis.

Radiologic studies are also of limited value in uncomplicated croup and LTB. Epiglottitis produces a very characteristic bulge into the tracheal air column which is readily recognized on a lateral neck film. However, radiologic studies to confirm a suspected case of epiglottitis often require the patient to be away from medical observation and resuscitative equipment for an extended period of time and may seriously delay the urgent placement of an airway. The diagnosis of epiglottitis should be made in the operating room where controlled laryngoscopy and placement of a nasal airway can be accomplished quickly and safely. Attempts to see the epiglottis in the office or emergency room are very dangerous, as depressing the tongue may precipitate pharyngeal spasm and total airway obstruction.

Viral Diagnostic Studies

The standard for establishing a viral diagnosis is isolation of the agent in cell cultures, usually primary monkey kidney cells. Both nasopharyngeal and oropharyngeal secretions should be collected in as great a quantity as possible and inoculated promptly into cell cultures. Because viral shedding may persist for weeks, it is worthwhile collecting respiratory secretions even several days into the illness. Cytopathic effect is not generally observed in culture, but infectivity is detected by hemadsorption using guinea pig red blood cells. In some cases it may take as long as 3 weeks for a culture to become positive.

Rapid viral diagnostic techniques, using either immunofluorescent microscopy or ELISA, are currently in development and are likely to soon become part of the routine diagnostic approach.

Treatment

Until recently, the mainstays of therapy for both LTB and croup have been symptomatic measures. LTB generally requires little more than an antipyretic and occasionally a cough suppressant. Croup responds well to humidified air, and a favorite therapy is to have the patient spend 15 to 20 min in a bathroom which has been steamed up by running hot water in the shower. A patient who becomes or remains agitated despite this measure should be seen promptly and evaluated for epiglottitis, regardless of a lack of any other characteristic symptoms.

While parainfluenza infections are not usually serious in otherwise healthy individuals, in persons with preexisting cardiac or pulmonary disease they can be life-threatening. Nearly all patients with croup are hypoxemic, and oxygen is a mainstay of therapy. As judged in double-blind placebo-controlled studies, racemic epinephrine, administered by aerosol with or without IPPB, is effective in providing prompt symptomatic relief for the more severely ill patient, although this therapy has no effect on arterial oxygen tension or on the speed with which the disease resolves. The use of steroids in this illness is still hotly debated; we do not recommend their use in the routine management of infectious croup.

Although specific therapy for the parainfluenza viruses is still in the experimental stage, antiviral agents are clearly on the horizon for use in these infections. Ribavirin, a drug approved for use in RSV infections, has in vitro activity against parainfluenza, types 1, 2, and 3, and appears to halt viral shedding in natural infection with these agents. No systematic studies of its clinical efficacy against these agents have yet been reported.

Outcome of Infection

In otherwise healthy individuals, parainfluenza infection is a self-limited illness with no evident sequelae, although few long-term studies of large numbers of infants and children with parainfluenza infection have been done. Chronic respiratory infection with parainfluenza virus has been described in some children with antibody-deficiency syndromes, but even in these patients it is uncertain whether the infection leads to long-term damage.

Although there is no evidence that parainfluenza infection leads to permanent pulmonary damage, many children will have temporary hyperreactive airway disease for months after their infection has resolved. Some of these patients may need bronchodilator therapy when they develop subsequent respiratory infections.

Prevention

The parainfluenza viruses are widespread agents, making prophylaxis nearly impossible. Nosocomial spread can, however, be limited to some extent by maintaining contact precautions, encouraging hand washing, cohorting children hospitalized with viral LTB or croup, and in particular limiting their contact with children who have preexisting cardiac or pulmonary disease.

THE COMMON COLD

Although the term *common cold* is often used interchangeably with URI, the former is a distinct clinical syndrome and should not be used to refer to any infection of the upper respiratory tract. The common cold is a self-limited syndrome of nasal stuffiness, watery nasal discharge, sneezing, and scratchy throat. A nonproductive cough is common. Systemic symptoms are mild, and low-grade fever is present in about 10 percent of cases.

In children, rhinovirus and coronavirus infections account for the majority of cases in which an etiologic agent can be identified. Although these, too, are the leading agents in adults, the latter also develop colds when infected with such agents as respiratory syncytial virus or the parainfluenza viruses, which cause lower respiratory tract disease in children.

Rhinoviruses

The rhinoviruses are small RNA viruses of the picornavirus family. Over 100 serotypes are responsible for one-third to one-half of all colds in adults, but at any one time only a small number of serotypes will be active in a given locale. Although infections occur year-round, they are most common in fall and spring. Frost shrewdly recognized some years ago that the epidemic curve of the common cold was actually composed of many miniepidemic peaks, leading him to conclude that cold outbreaks represent concomitant activity by several different agents, rather than wide-scale activity by one or a few viruses as occurs in influenza or RSV epidemics.

The rhinoviruses spread in small groups, in schools, and especially in families, where secondary attack rates can be as high as 30 to 50 percent. Children are the major "introducers" of infection into the family, and large families have twice as many colds as small families. In about one-fourth of cases infection is inapparent. The rhinoviruses are spread by contact rather than via aerosols. The virus in nasal secretions contaminates the hands of contacts who then inoculate themselves by touching their nasal mucosa or conjunctivae.

Symptoms develop after a 2- to 4-day incubation period, are most severe on days 2 and 3, and generally subside by 1 week. However, it is not unusual for symptoms to last as long as 1 month. Rhinovirus usually does not infect the lower respiratory tract, and, in the absence of other signs of pulmonary involvement, the prominent cough it often causes should not be misinterpreted to indicate lower tract involvement. Rhinovirus infection is not more severe in children, although it may precipitate bronchospasm in asthmatics. Rhinovirus infection has been associated with acute exacerbations in persons with chronic lung disease, and in these patients pulmonary flow rates may remain abnormal for months.

The differential diagnosis includes infection with coronavirus, respiratory syncytial virus, parainfluenza viruses, and, in fact, any respiratory virus. In susceptible patients, measles should be kept in mind, as the measles prodrome of cough, coryza, and conjunctivitis may sometimes be confusing until the characteristic rash appears. There is little need for laboratory studies in persons with the common cold. There is a moderate neutrophilia early in the illness and a mild elevation in the sedimentation rate in about one-third of patients.

Viral cultures are not routinely done. No single cell or organ culture system is optimal for recovering all serotypes, and it may be necessary to inoculate a panel of human and monkey cells and fetal tracheal organ cultures. The virus grows best at reduced temperatures, and cultures are kept at 33 to 34°C. The best source of virus is nasal washings.

Although more than $500 million is spent each year on cold remedies, there is no specific therapy for the common cold. Although several potential antivirals have in vitro activity against rhinovirus, none has yet been shown effective in patients. As antibody responses develop after clinical symptoms have resolved, nonantibody mechanisms such as interferon must play the major role in controlling infection. Large doses of interferon intranasally can reduce the quantity and duration of viral shedding, but they have only modest clinical benefit and can cause nasal stuffiness and bleeding, which may be as unpleasant as a cold itself. Interferon inducers are not effective. Treatment is directed toward symptomatic relief.

Prevention of colds remains elusive. Some practical measures include disinfection of fomites, containment of secretions, and hand washing. Avoiding chills does not reduce the likelihood of developing a cold. There are no vaccines. Recently, studies have shown that short-term use of topical α-interferon is effective prophylaxis for family contacts.

Coronaviruses

Coronaviruses are medium-size RNA viruses with some resemblances to the myxoviruses. Human pathogens are classified in four groups, but serologic reagents are available only for two, group I whose prototype strain is 229E, and group II whose prototypes are OC38 and OC43.

Coronavirus is responsible for 5 to 15 percent of colds, with peaks of activity occurring in late winter or early spring every 2 to 3 years. Half the infections are asymptomatic, and even symptomatic infections may not be associated with an antibody titer rise. Children begin to develop antibodies to coronavirus in the first year of life, and 70 percent of adults are seropositive. Symptomatic reinfections are common.

The speed and intensity of urban outbreaks suggests that coronaviruses are transmitted by small-particle aerosols. The virus replicates in respiratory epithelium, with a 2- to 4-day incubation period. In experimental infection, it causes an afebrile illness with profuse nasal discharge lasting about a week. Although in animals coronaviruses can cause disseminated infection, there is no evidence that it can cause lower respiratory tract or systemic disease in humans. Treatment is symptomatic.

Enteroviruses

Although the most important target of the enteroviruses, including echoviruses and Coxsackie viruses, is the central nervous system, most of the enteroviruses can cause an afebrile or febrile respiratory infection, including hand-foot-mouth disease, herpangina, and epidemic pleurodynia (Bornholm disease). They cause fewer than 5 percent of all common colds and may be responsible for a rare case of pneumonia. They are most active during the summer.

BIBLIOGRAPHY

Breinig MK, Zitelli B, Starzl TE, Ho M: Epstein-Barr virus, cytomegalovirus, and other viral infections in children after liver transplantation. J Infect Dis 156:273–279, 1987.
  In 51 consecutive pediatric patients, the frequency and morbidity of viral infections after liver transplantation was comparable to that seen in adult transplant recipients except that fewer pediatric than adult transplant patients experienced primary CMV infection.

Couch RB, Kasel JA: Immunity to influenza in man. Annu Rev Microbiol 37:529–549, 1983.
An excellent review of host defenses in influenza.

Denny FW, Murphy TF, Clyde WA Jr, Collier AM, Henderson FW: Croup: An 11-year study in a pediatric practice. Pediatrics 71:871–876, 1983.
Epidemiology and etiologies of pediatric laryngotracheobronchitis.

Douglas RG Jr: Respiratory diseases, in Galasso GJ, Merigan C, Buchanan R, (eds), *Antiviral Agents and Viral Disease of Man*, 2d ed. New York, Raven, 1984, pp 313–367.
A useful overview.

Douglas RG Jr: Pathogenetic mechanisms in viral respiratory tract infections, in Sande M, et al., *Respiratory Infections*. London, Churchill-Livingstone, 1986, pp 25–46.
Up-to-date summary of the pathophysiology of viral respiratory infection.

Finland M, Parker F, Barnes M, Joliffe LS: Acute myocarditis in influenza A infections. Am J Med Sci 209:455–468, 1945.
Two cases in which the virus was recovered from the myocardium.

Glezen WP: Serious morbidity and mortality associated with influenza epidemics. Epidemiol Rev 4:25–44, 1982.
Surveys the burden of disease associated with influenza.

Glezen WP, Denny FW: Epidemiology of lower respiratory disease in children. N Engl J Med 288:498–505, 1973.
An expert review of the subject.

Gundelfinger BF, Stille WT, Bell JA: Effectiveness of influenza vaccines during an epidemic of Asian influenza. N Engl J Med 259:1005–1009, 1958.
Efficacy of 90 percent was documented in this study.

Hall CB, Douglas RG, Simons RL, Geiman JM: Interferon production in infants and children with respiratory syncytial virus, influenza, and parainfluenza virus infections. J Pediatr 93:28–32, 1978.
Interferon may have a larger role to play in influenza and parainfluenza infection than in infection with RSV.

Hall CB, McBride JT, Walsh EE, Bell DM, Gala CL, Hidreth S, Ten Eyck LG, Hall WJ: Aerosolized ribavirin treatment of infants with Respiratory Syncytial Viral infection. N Engl J Med 308:1443–1447, 1983.
Effective antiviral therapy, judged in a double-blind placebo-controlled study.

Hall CB, Powell KR, MacDonald NE, Gala CL, Menegus ME, Suffin SC, Cohen HJ: Respiratory syncytial viral infection in children with compromised immune function. N Engl J Med 315:77–81, 1986.
For 10 winters, 608 children five years old or younger who were hospitalized with respiratory syncytial virus (RSV) infection were prospectively studied to evaluate the relation between their immune status and the severity of their infection. The findings indicate that children receiving chemotherapy for cancer and those with immunodeficiency disease are at risk for complicated or fatal infections from RSV.

Hayden FG, Albrecht JK, Kaiser DL, Gwaltney JM Jr: Prevention of natural colds by contact prophylaxis with intranasal alpha-2-interferon. N Engl J Med 314:71–75, 1986.
Topical interferon was highly effective when used in postexposure prophylaxis.

Institute of Medicine: New Vaccine Development: Establishing Priorities, vol 1, Diseases of Importance in the United States. Washington, DC, National Academy of Sciences, 1985, pp 342–364.
A summary of the economic costs of viral respiratory infection and the possible role of vaccines in public health control strategies.

Kilbourne ED (ed): *The Influenza Viruses and Influenza*. New York, Academic, 1975.
Excellent and authoritative.

Knight V, Fedson D, Baldini J, Douglas RG Jr: Amantadine therapy of epidemic influenza A2 (Hong Kong). Infect Immunol 1:200–204, 1970.
Therapeutic use of amantadine in influenza.

Knight V, McClung HW, Wilson SZ, Waters BK, Quarles JM, Cameron RW, Greggs SE, Zerwas JM, Couch RB: Ribavirin small-particle aerosol treatment of influenza. Lancet 2:945–949, 1981.
Effective in a randomized, placebo-controlled study, including one patient with primary influenza pneumonia.

Lennette EH, Schmidt NJ (eds): *Diagnostic Procedures for Viral, Rickettsial and Chlamydial Infections,* 5th ed. Washington, DC, American Public Health Association, 1979.
  Authoritative manual of diagnostic clinical virology.

Little JW, Hall JW, Douglas RG Jr, Mudholkar GS, Speers DM, Patel K: Airway hyperreactivity and peripheral airway dysfunction in influenza A infection. Am Rev Respir Dis 118:295–303, 1978.
  Bronchospasm may be an important clinical problem in viral lower respiratory tract disease.

Loughlin GM, Taussig LM: Pulmonary function in children with a history of laryngotracheobronchitis. J Pediatr 94:365–369, 1979.
  Possible relation between airway hyperreactivity and repeated episodes of viral lower respiratory tract infections.

Louria DB, Blumenfeld HL, Ellis JT, Kilbourne ED, Rogers DE: Studies on influenza in the pandemic of 1957–58. II. Pulmonary complications of influenza. J Clin Invest 38:213–265, 1959.
  An excellent study of a modern (1957–1958) pandemic (Hong Kong flu).

Mills EL: Viral infections predisposing to bacterial infections. Annu Rev Med 35:469–479, 1984.
  Reviews the pathophysiology of secondary bacterial infection.

National Institutes of Health Consensus Development Conference: Amantadine: Does it have a role in the prevention and treatment of influenza? Ann Intern Med 92:256–258, 1980.
  The consensus recommends use of amantadine in both prophylactic and therapeutic situations.

National Institutes of Health Consensus Development Conference: Diagnosis and treatment of Reye's syndrome. JAMA 246:2441–2444, 1981.
  The relation to influenza and aspirin use.

Rapkin RH: The diagnosis of epiglottitis: Simplicity and reliability of radiographs of the neck in the differential diagnosis of the croup syndrome. J Pediatr 80:96–98, 1972.
  Describes the "thumb sign" indicating a swollen epiglottis imposing on the tracheal air column.

Stuart-Harris C: The present status of live influenza virus vaccine. J Infect Dis 142:784–793, 1980.
  A good summary of the problems and prospects.

Taussig LM, Castro O, Beaudry PH, Fox WW, Bureau M: Treatment of laryngotracheobronchitis (croup). Use of intermittent positive-pressure breathing and racemic epinephrine. Am J Dis Child 129:790–793, 1975.
  Epinephrine is effective for symptomatic management of infectious croup.

Tyerar FJ: Report of a workshop on respiratory syncytial virus and parainfluenza viruses. J Infect Dis 148:588–597, 1983.
  Excellent recent summary of the state of knowledge of these agents.

Wingfield WL, Pollack D, Grunert RR: Therapeutic efficacy of amantadine HCl and rimantadine HCl in naturally occurring influenza A2 respiratory illness in man. N Engl J Med 281:579–584, 1969.
  Amantadine is effective for treating influenza A infection.

Winterbauer RH, Ludwig WR, Hammar SP: Clinical course, management, and long-term sequelae of respiratory failure due to influenza virus pneumonia. Johns Hopkins Med J 141:148–155, 1977.
  A very useful clinical summary, though too old to include specific antiviral chemotherapy.

Chapter 99

Actinomyces, Arachnia, and Nocardia

Gregory A. Filice / Donald Armstrong

ACTINOMYCES AND ARACHNIA

Actinomycosis is an indolent disease characterized by necrosis of tissue and a pyogenic response followed by intense fibrosis. Occasionally, the pus contains minute yellow granules made up of clumps of *Actinomyces* filaments. Actinomycosis is usually caused by *Actinomyces israelii*, but other species of *Actinomyces* and *Arachnia propionica* are occasionally implicated. Since the different species are associated with clinically similar disease, they will be considered together. Actinomycosis usually takes one of three forms, cervicofacial, pulmonary, or abdominal. Only pulmonary actinomycosis is considered in detail in this chapter.

Epidemiology and Pathogenesis

Pathogenic species of *Actinomyces* and *Arachnia* are strict or facultative anaerobic bacteria that normally inhabit anaerobic niches in the human oral cavity. Thoracic actinomycosis often occurs in people with carious teeth and periodontal disease where numbers of these bacteria are increased. Aspiration of infective material is the probable inciting event. Spread to the mediastinum is usually from pulmonary or, less commonly, cervicofacial disease. Actinomycosis occurs throughout the world. Males are affected more often than females, and the disease affects people of all ages.

The typical lesion consists of one or more abscesses, filled with neutrophils and surrounded by dense fibrous tissue. Macrophages, plasma cells, and lymphocytes are numerous in the periphery of lesions. Giant cells are uncommon, and epithelioid granulomas are exceedingly rare. In the lung, consolidation can occur without macroscopic abscess formation. Sputum is usually white or yellow and has no distinctive odor. Malodorous sputum should suggest the presence of another anaerobic organism, possibly in combination with *Actinomyces* or *Arachnia*.

In tissue, *Actinomyces* organisms tend to grow in dense microcolonies or granules that may reach 4 mm in size. These are often called sulfur granules because they are usually yellow, although they do not contain much sulfur. Neutrophils surround the granules, but the granules themselves contain only bacteria and amorphous material.

Actinomycosis often spreads without regard for anatomic tissue planes. Disease often extends to involve nearby structures, and fistulae or abscesses may appear at unexpected sites far from primary lesions. Skin, subcutaneous tissue, and bone are frequently involved.

Lesions of actinomycosis often contain other bacteria, sometimes referred to as *concomitant bacteria*, which may contribute to the pathogenesis. Generally, the concomitant bacteria are from the same oral mucosal niches as the *Actinomyces* organisms. The relationship between one such bacterium, *Actinobacillus actinomycetemcomitans*, and actinomycosis is so close that isolation of *A. actinomycetemcomitans* should always lead to a careful search for *Actinomyces*.

Clinical Manifestations

Pulmonary disease begins insidiously with cough, sputum production, fever, and weight loss. Hemoptysis and pleuritic pain each occur in a minority of cases. Leukocytosis, neutrophilia, and moderate anemia are common. Symptoms are often surprisingly mild for the extent of disease. In advanced cases, clubbing, pulmonary osteoarthropathy, or amyloidosis may occur.

Mediastinal involvement is common, and pericarditis and the superior vena cava syndrome have each been reported. Empyema is common. Pulmonary lesions may burrow through the chest wall to drain, or to involve other chest wall structures which should strongly suggest the diagnosis. Rib involvement typically produces a peculiar "wavy periostitis." Other adjacent structures that may be involved include the shoulder girdle, sternum, and thoracic vertebrae. Involved vertebrae characteristically appear mottled because of parallel processes of resorption and new bone formation. Spread to adjacent vertebrae and intervertebral disk space narrowing are distinctly unusual, whereas they are common with pyogenic and tuberculous osteomyelitis.

On radiographs, infiltrates are often dense and well circumscribed (Fig. 99-1). Since symptoms are often mild,

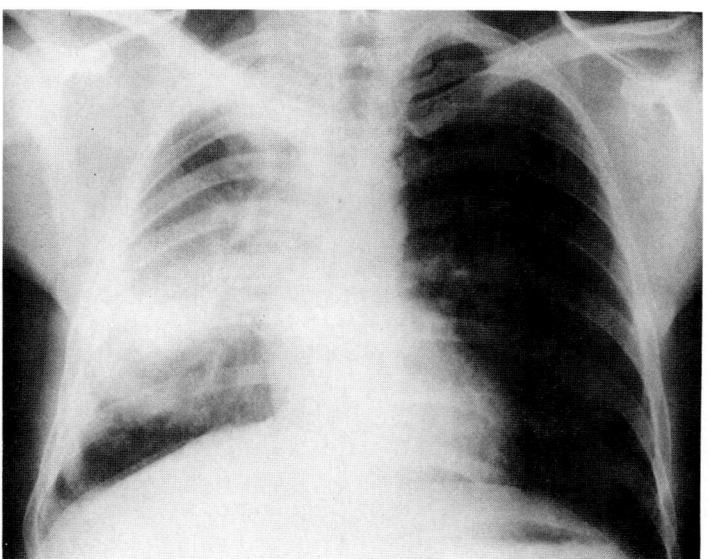

FIGURE 99-1 Extensive infiltrates in the right lung illustrate the marked density characteristic of pulmonary actinomycosis. *(By permission, Grune & Stratton.)*

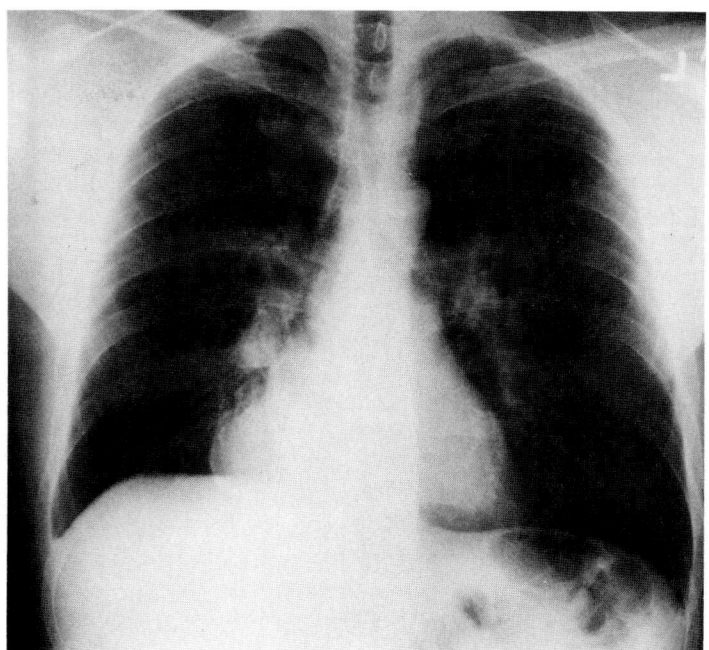

A

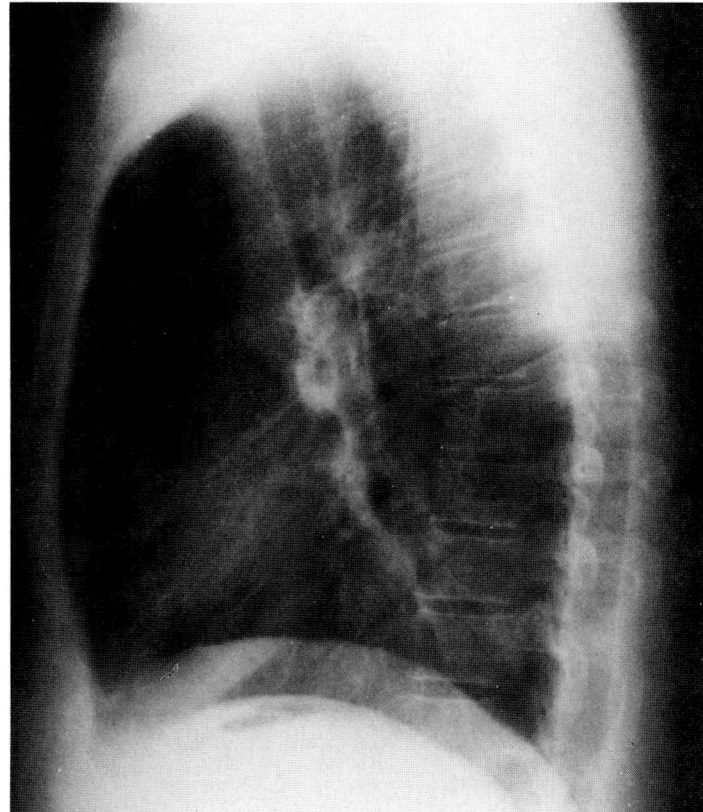

B

FIGURE 99-2 *A, B.* The dense, round infiltrate in the right lower lobe suggested carcinoma, but it proved to be due to actinomycosis.

the radiographic appearance often suggests a diagnosis of lung cancer (Fig. 99-2). Cavities are observed in about half of the cases and tend to be small. Because of the lack of regard for anatomic barriers, actinomycosis may involve multiple lobes by spread through interlobar fissures. Other patterns that may occur include fibronodular (Fig. 99-3) or alveolar infiltrates. Occasionally, erosion of a blood vessel results in miliary disease.

Diagnosis

Diagnosis is difficult because the organisms are part of the normal upper respiratory flora. A positive sputum culture has no clinical significance. The presence of granules in sputum is highly suggestive of the diagnosis, but they are infrequent. A search should be made in suspect cases. If the diagnosis cannot be made by simpler means, transthoracic needle aspiration, transbronchial biopsy, or open lung biopsy should be performed. Which of these procedures is performed should depend on the nature and location of the lesion, the condition of the patient, and the expertise available within the institution. Transbronchial biopsy has the disadvantage that specimens may be contaminated by upper respiratory secretions and reliance must be placed on histologic examination of tissue.

If there is a fistula, the presence of granules in secretions is a strong clue to the diagnosis. If granules are not immediately apparent in discharge from a wound, they can often be trapped in a gauze dressing. Suspect granules should be placed in water or KOH or Gram-stained and then should be examined for the presence of typical

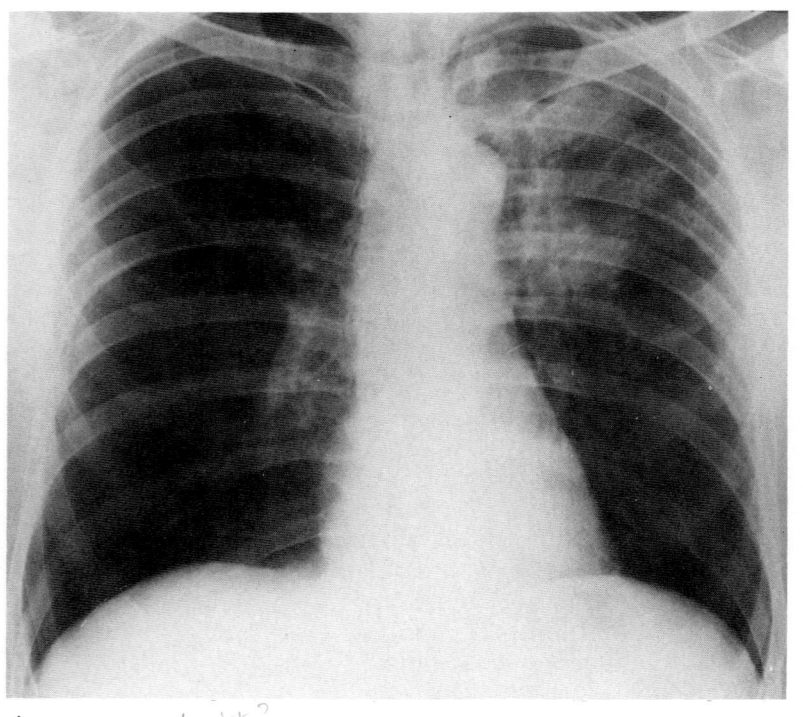
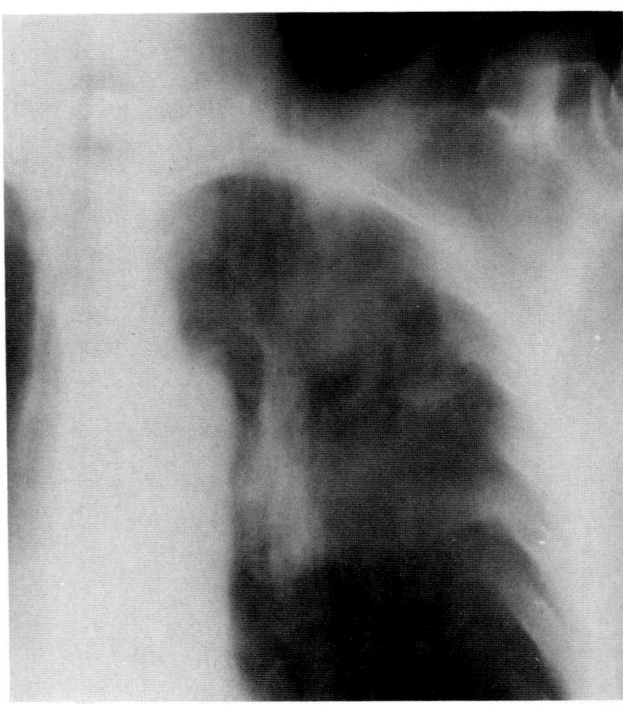

A   B

FIGURE 99-3 *A.* Right upper lobe fibronodular infiltrate due to pulmonary actinomycosis. *B.* Tomography revealed the nodular nature of the infiltrate. *(By permission, Grune & Stratton.)*

branching filaments. The bacteria can be cultured from a granule if they have not succumbed to oxygen exposure.

In tissues, secretions, or granules, *Actinomyces* and *Arachnia* are long, branching, beaded gram-positive filaments 0.2 to 0.5 μm in width and up to 50 μm in length. With age or under adverse conditions, the organisms may break up into coccobacillary forms, and they may appear to be gram-negative. The beaded appearance and the occurrence of gram-positive segments interspersed with gram-negative ones may give the impression of many bacilli and cocci lined up end to end. *Actinomyces* filaments can also be seen in KOH preparations. They are rarely acid-fast; the presence of acid-fast organisms should suggest *Mycobacterium* or *Nocardia*. *Actinomyces* stain with methenamine silver and periodic acid-Schiff stains.

Cultures should be made from involved tissue or normally sterile body secretions. Material for culture should be kept strictly anaerobic and inoculated promptly. The yield is greatest from pieces of tissue, next best from tubes of pus, and poorest from swabs. If a specimen cannot be delivered to a laboratory immediately, a microbiologist should be consulted concerning use of a transport medium or inoculation at the bedside. Media known to support the growth of *Actinomyces* must be used. Prior antimicrobial therapy often makes cultures negative, and specimens should be obtained before such therapy is given.

Therapy

Penicillin is the drug of choice. In severe cases, it should initially be given intravenously in high doses, 10 to 20 million units per day. Then, therapy should be continued with oral penicillin in maximal tolerated doses. Tetracycline and clindamycin have also been used with good results.

In vitro tests of susceptibility of *Actinomyces* to antimicrobials are still in the developmental stage. Penicillin, erythromycin, cephaloridine, minocycline, rifampin, and clindamycin are very active. Organisms are inhibited by achievable concentrations of cephalothin, ampicillin, tetracycline, doxycycline, and chloramphenicol. A few strains are susceptible to sulfamethoxazole. Notably, metronidazole is ineffective.

Other bacteria frequently accompany *Actinomyces* in tissue and may contribute to the pathogenesis of the disease. The antimicrobial susceptibilities of these organisms often differ from those of *Actinomyces*. It is usually not necessary to add additional antimicrobial drugs to treat these associated organisms. They may contribute to the pathogenesis, but *Actinomyces* are essential, and successful treatment of *Actinomyces* along with appropriate surgical drainage usually cures the disease.

Surgery should be used as it is for bacterial diseases of the chest in general. Empyemas should be drained. Surgery is sometimes required to relieve obstruction of mediastinal structures.

Actinomycosis has a marked tendency to relapse, and therapy should be continued for from 6 to 12 months. The exact duration should depend on the extent of the disease within and outside the chest and the response to treatment. With prompt diagnosis and appropriate treatment, approximately 90 percent of patients are cured.

NOCARDIA

Pulmonary nocardiosis is a subacute or chronic pneumonia caused by the aerobic actinomycete, *Nocardia asteroides*, or less commonly, N. *brasiliensis* or N. *caviae*. N. *asteroides* frequently disseminates to other sites or is associated with mycetoma, skin and connective tissue infection after transcutaneous inoculation, or keratitis, but these diseases are beyond the scope of this chapter.

Epidemiology and Pathogenesis

Nocardia are common, worldwide inhabitants of soil, where they contribute to decay of organic matter. In the soil, *Nocardia* form aerial mycelia, and it is thought that pneumonia follows inhalation of fragmented mycelia. The disease occurs worldwide. It was estimated in 1974 that between 500 and 1000 cases of *Nocardia* infection are diagnosed each year in the United States, 85 percent of them pulmonary and/or systemic. The disease usually occurs in adults, and males are affected twice as often as females. There is no well-documented seasonality.

About half of reported cases are in otherwise healthy people, but the incidence is greater in people with deficient host defenses. The most common deficiency is of cell-mediated immunity, but nocardiosis has also been associated with pulmonary alveolar proteinosis, chronic granulomatous disease, and pulmonary tuberculosis.

The typical lesions of nocardiosis are abscesses which are extensively infiltrated with neutrophils. There is usually extensive necrosis. Granulation tissue often surrounds the lesions, but extensive fibrosis or encapsulation is rare. Microcolonies (granules) are occasionally observed in histologic preparations but are almost never discharged from lesions. Rarely, epithelioid granulomas are observed in the central nervous system. Pulmonary infection disseminates in one-half of cases, most commonly to brain, skin and subcutaneous tissues, and kidneys.

Clinical Manifestations

Pulmonary nocardiosis is usually subacute or chronic; patients typically present after symptoms have been present for several days or weeks. Cough is a prominent symptom and is often productive of small amounts of sputum which is not malodorous. Fever, anorexia, weight loss, and malaise are common, but dyspnea, pleuritic pain, and hemoptysis are not. Remissions and exacerbations lasting

for days or weeks are frequent. Tracheitis, bronchitis, mediastinitis, pericarditis, endocarditis, and direct spread through the chest wall are uncommon manifestations of nocardiosis.

Radiographic patterns are variable. Infiltrates and nodules are common (Fig. 99-4). Infiltrates may be of any size and are usually of at least moderate density. Empyema is present in one-third of cases. Cavitation is common (Fig. 99-4), and the radiographic appearance may suggest anaerobic lung abscess or a tumor. The radiographic appearance and clinical picture may suggest pulmonary tuberculosis or fungal pneumonia, but volume loss and fibrosis are usually less prominent with nocardiosis.

Nocardia species sometimes colonize patients without producing disease. Most of the time, such patients have abnormal airways or pulmonary parenchyma. Factors that should influence the interpretation of a positive sputum culture in the absence of obvious nocardial disease are the clinical presentation, the presence or absence of *Nocardia* on Gram stain, and the ability to isolate *Nocardia* in multiple cultures. A positive sputum culture in the presence of symptoms and signs of pulmonary infection must be taken seriously. A positive sputum culture in an immunosuppressed patient usually reflects disease and not colonization.

In one-half of all cases of pulmonary nocardiosis there is disease outside the lungs. Central nervous system disease is the most common manifestation of disseminated disease and occurs in one-fourth of all cases of pul-

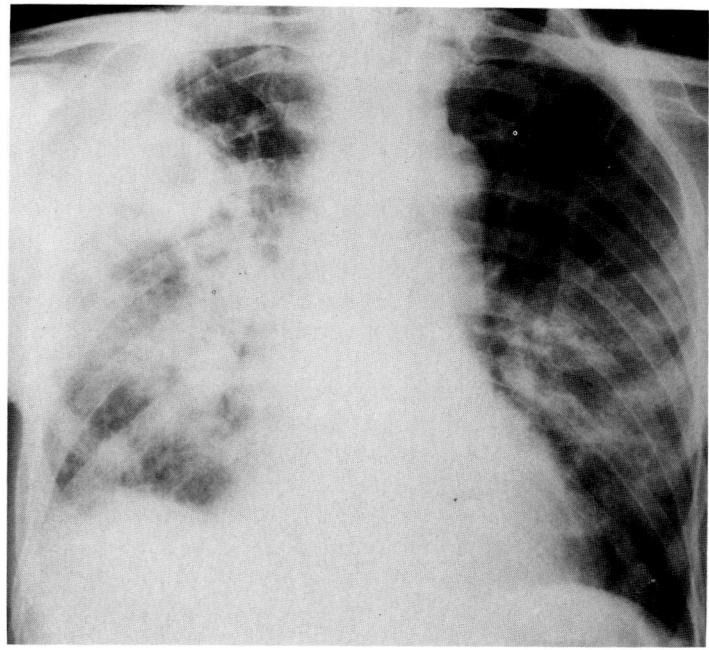

FIGURE 99-4 Pulmonary nocardiosis. Irregular infiltrates were present bilaterally. A large cavity was apparent in the right upper lobe. *(By permission, Grune & Stratton.)*

monary nocardiosis. Other common sites of dissemination include the skin and subcutaneous tissues, kidneys, bone, and muscle. Local infection from transcutaneous inoculation is common, but the physician should be aware that a lesion in skin or soft tissue may simply be the most obvious manifestation of pulmonary nocardiosis.

Diagnosis

Examination of sputum is the first step when pulmonary nocardiosis is suspected. However, sputum smears are often negative. Sputum cultures are positive more often, but colonies may not be apparent for days or weeks (see below). If multiple sputum examinations do not yield the diagnosis in a suspected case, and the diagnosis cannot be made easily from lesions elsewhere in the body, more invasive diagnostic procedures should be performed. Transtracheal aspiration, bronchoscopy, needle aspiration, and open lung biopsy are all useful. Which alternative is best depends on the location and nature of the lesions, the severity and tempo of the illness, and the expertise that is available for the more invasive procedures. *Nocardia* are commonly associated with cellulitis in the tissues overlying the cricothyroid membrane after transtracheal aspira-

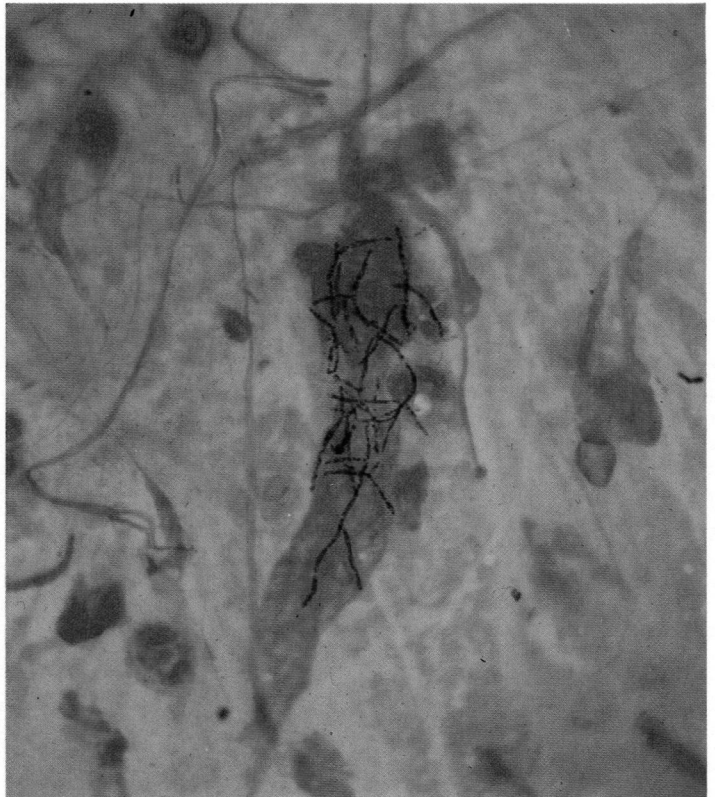

FIGURE 99-5 *Nocardia asteroides* in a gram-stained smear of sputum. The neutrophils give an indication of the scale.

tion, and this should lead to the choice of another procedure if nocardiosis is strongly suspected.

Nocardia are thin, crooked, branching filaments that are weakly to strongly gram-positive and appear beaded (Fig. 99-5). Most *Nocardia* in clinical specimens are acid-fast if a weak acid is used for decolorization as with the modified Kinyoun, Ziehl-Neelsen, or Fite-Faraco methods. They usually lose their acid fastness in laboratory culture. With these methods, *Actinomyces* and *Streptomyces* are not acid-fast. *Nocardia* may stain with silver stains, but other common clinical stains are not helpful.

Nocardia grow readily on most nonselective laboratory media, but they grow more slowly than most bacterial pathogens. The laboratory should always be alerted when nocardiae are suspected so that cultures will be kept longer than usual and so that the likelihood of isolating nocardiae will be maximized. *Nocardia* grow on nonselective mycobacterial and fungal media, but they may not survive harsh sputum digestion procedures. Routine blood cultures are usually negative, but if biphasic culture bottles are inoculated and incubated aerobically for up to 30 days, *Nocardia* can sometimes be isolated from blood.

Therapy

Sulfonamides are the antimicrobials of choice, and 6 to 12 g of sulfisoxazole or sulfadiazine should be given daily in four to six divided doses. In difficult cases, sulfonamide levels should be measured and dosages should be adjusted to keep serum levels between 100 and 150 μg/ml. Many patients have been treated with the combination of sulfamethoxazole and trimethoprim, but it is unclear whether the combination is superior to the use of sulfonamides alone. If the combination is selected, 5 to 20 mg of trimethoprim and 25 to 100 mg of sulfamethoxazole per kilogram per day should be given in two or three divided doses.

There is much less experience with other antimicrobials. Nonetheless, it appears that minocycline is the most effective orally administerable alternative to sulfonamides. Minocycline should be given in doses of 100 to 200 mg twice a day. Other tetracyclines are less effective or inadequately tested. Success with amikacin has been reported for a few cases, but amikacin must be administered parenterally; 5 to 7.5 mg of amikacin per kilogram should be given every 12 h. Serum levels should be monitored with prolonged therapy, in the face of diminished renal function, or in the elderly.

In vitro tests of susceptibility of *Nocardia* species to antimicrobials are still under development, and the clinical relevance of these tests is unclear. They suggest that several newer β-lactam antibiotics are quite active and that clavulanic acid enhances the activity of ampicillin, but there is almost no published clinical experience with these drugs.

Surgery is used as it is for other infectious diseases of the chest. Empyemas should be drained. Lung abscesses usually respond to antimicrobial therapy alone.

Immunosuppressive therapy increases the risk of nocardiosis, but it is not clear that continued immunosuppressive therapy interferes with successful treatment. Many patients must continue immunosuppressive therapy for maintenance of a transplanted organ or treatment of an underlying disease. In other cases, it seems prudent to reduce or eliminate immunosuppressive therapy if possible.

Long courses of antimicrobial therapy are necessary to prevent relapse. For nonimmunosuppressed patients, treatment of pulmonary nocardiosis should be continued for 6 to 12 months. Central nervous system disease requires treatment for 1 year unless all apparent disease has been excised, in which case 6 months should be sufficient. Immunosuppressed patients with pulmonary nocardiosis should be treated for 1 year. In occasional patients, much longer durations are necessary. Patients should be carefully followed during therapy and for at least 6 months for signs of relapse after therapy is stopped. With prompt diagnosis and appropriate treatment, survival of pulmonary nocardiosis is to be expected in more than 95 percent of patients.

Nocardiosis is rare in an otherwise healthy child, and its occurrence in this setting may be a clue to the presence of chronic granulomatous disease. The phagocytes of such a child should be tested for the adequacy of their respiratory burst.

BIBLIOGRAPHY

Actinomyces and *Arachnia*

Allen HA III, Scatarige JC, Kim MH: Actinomycosis: CT findings in six patients. AJR 149:1255–1258, 1987.
A retrospective review of CT scans in six proved cases revealed a spectrum of findings, including soft-tissue mass with various degrees of infiltration and abscess formation.

Bates M, Cruickshank G: Thoracic actinomycosis. Thorax 12:99–124, 1957.
A review of 85 cases and of the literature.

Brock DW, Georg LK, Brown JM, Hicklin MD: Actinomycosis caused by *Arachnia propionica*. Report of 11 cases. Am J Clin Pathol 59:66–77, 1973.
A clinical and microbiologic analysis of cases caused by A. propionica.

Brown JR: Human actinomycosis. A study of 181 subjects. Hum Pathol 4:319–330, 1973.
A review with emphasis on pathologic features.

Cope Z: *Actinomycosis.* London, Oxford University Press, 1938.
A classic monograph with detailed descriptions of cases that occurred before the antimicrobial era.

Flynn MW, Felson F: The roentgen manifestations of thoracic actinomycosis. Am J Roentgenol 110:707–716, 1970.
A review of 15 cases with emphasis on radiographic features.

McQuarrie DG, Hall WH: Actinomycosis of the lung and chest wall. Surgery 64:905–911, 1968.
A review of 28 cases with emphasis on clinical features and diagnosis.

Oddo D, Gonzalez S: Actinomycosis and nocardiosis. A morphologic study of 17 cases. Pathol Res Pract 181:320–326, 1986.
The clinicopathologic features of 17 cases are reported. Actinomycosis was frequently observed as a secondary and localized infection, often with lung involvement, especially in residual cavities or bronchiectasis, whereas nocardiosis was observed as an opportunistic infection in the three cases studied.

Smego RA Jr: Actinomycosis of the central nervous system. Rev Infect Dis 9:855–865, 1987.
A review of 70 cases of CNS actinomycosis was conducted in an effort to characterize clinicopathologic features and identify patients with a high risk of death from infection. Most infections developed from distant sites (lung, 19 cases; abdomen, four; pelvis, three) or contiguous foci (ear, sinus, and cervicofacial region, 21 cases).

Nocardia

Angeles AM, Sugar AM: Rapid diagnosis of nocardiosis with an enzyme immunoassay. J Infect Dis 155:292–296, 1987.
Using a previously identified Nocardia asteroides-specific protein, the authors developed an enzyme immunoassay for the rapid diagnosis of nocardiosis. This assay represents a highly sensitive and specific serodiagnostic tool for evaluating patients with possible nocardiosis.

Arroyo JC, Nichols S, Carroll GF: Disseminated *Nocardia caviae* infection. Am J Med 62:409–412, 1977.
A case report and review of the literature on infection with N. caviae.

Chazen G: *Nocardia.* Infect Control 8:260–263, 1987.
A review of the laboratory and clinical approaches to diagnosis and treatment using trimethoprim and sulfamethoxazole.

Feigin DS: Nocardiosis of the lung: Chest radiographic findings in 21 cases. Radiology 159:9–14, 1986.
A review of the pulmonary radiologic manifestations of nocardial infection based on a large experience. The series included otherwise healthy individuals as well as immunocompromised patients.

Filice GA, Simpson GL: Management of *Nocardia* infections, in Remington JS, Swartz MN (eds), *Current Clinical Topics in Infectious Diseases.* New York, McGraw-Hill, 1984, pp 49–64.
A detailed discussion of therapy.

Frazier AR, Rosenow EC III, Roberts GD: Nocardiosis. A review of 25 cases occurring during 24 months. Mayo Clin Proc 50:657–663, 1975.
A review with emphasis on patients with colonization of the respiratory tract and no apparent nocardial disease.

Goldstein FW, Hautefort B, Acar JF: Amikacin-containing regimens for treatment of nocardiosis in immunocompromised patients. Eur J Clin Microbiol 6:198–200, 1987.
Eight patients with disseminated infections due to multiresistant Nocardia asteroides were administered amikacin in combination with other effective antibiotics for a duration of 2 to 12 months. Seven patients were considered cured at follow-up after 2 years.

Grossman CB, Bragg DG, Armstrong D: Roentgen manifestations of pulmonary nocardiosis. Radiology 96:325–330, 1970.
A review of radiographic features.

Palmer DL, Harvey RL, Wheeler JK: Diagnostic and therapeutic considerations in *Nocardia asteroides* infection. Medicine 53:391–401, 1974.
A review of 13 cases and of the literature.

Rodriguez JL, Barrio JL, Pitchenik AE: Pulmonary nocardiosis in the acquired immunodeficiency syndrome. Diagnosis with bronchoalveolar lavage and treatment with non-sulphur containing drugs. Chest 90:912–914, 1986.
A patient with the acquired immunodeficiency syndrome (AIDS) who developed Pneumocystis carinii pneumonia and pulmonary nocardiosis.

Simpson GL, Stinson EB, Egger MJ, Remington JS: Nocardial infections in the immunocompromised host: A detailed study in a defined population. Rev Infect Dis 3:492–507, 1981.
A description of 21 cases in heart transplant recipients who were treated with sulfisoxazole.

Smeal WE, Schenfeld LA: Nocardiosis in the community hospital. Report of three cases. Postgrad Med 79:77–82, 1986.
In North America, the most common presentation is that of primary subacute pneumonia. In Central and South America, primary cutaneous infections are more common.

Smego RA, Gallis HA: The clinical spectrum of *Nocardia brasiliensis* infection in the United States. Rev Infect Dis 6:164–180, 1984.
A review of seven cases and the literature on infection with N. brasiliensis.

Smego RA, Moeller MB, Gallis HA: Trimethoprim-sulfamethoxazole therapy for *Nocardia* infections. Arch Intern Med 143:711–718, 1983.
A description of 19 patients treated with trimethoprim and sulfamethoxazole.

Young LS, Armstrong D, Blevins A, Leiberman P: *Nocardia asteroides* infection complicating neoplastic disease. Am J Med 50:356–366, 1970.
A review with emphasis on disease in patients with neoplastic disease and on patients with colonization of the respiratory tract and no apparent nocardial disease.

Chapter 100
Rickettsial Pneumonias

Theodore E. Woodward

Definition

Routes of Infection and Pathogenesis

Pathologic Physiology

Pathology
    Epidemic Typhus
    Rocky Mountain Spotted Fever
    Scrub Typhus Fever
    Q Fever

Clinical Manifestations
    Q Fever
    Epidemic, Murine, Scrub Typhus, and Rocky Mountain
      Spotted Fevers

Treatment

Human rickettsial diseases consist of several clinical entities caused by rickettsiae, which are obligate intracellular parasites appearing microscopically as pleomorphic coccobacilli. Each rickettsia pathogenic for humans reproduces in one or more species of arthropods as well as in animals and humans. Most rickettsiae are present in nature involving a cycle of an insect vector and an animal; human infection is unnecessary for maintenance of the cycle. Epidemic typhus fever differs from most rickettsioses because the natural cycle of infection involves only humans and the louse; an animal reservoir has not been fully established.

The rickettsioses fall into four principal groups based on their clinical manifestations, epidemiologic considerations, and underlying immunologic features. A compendium of general information on the rickettsial diseases to be discussed is given in Table 100-1. Specific therapeutic measures are not given since each rickettsial infection responds to tetracyclines or chloramphenicol. Procedures for isolation of rickettsiae are also omitted because the techniques utilized are specialized and potentially hazardous. Serologic methods and immunofluorescence techniques are useful and practical diagnostic methods.

DEFINITION

Rickettsial diseases are acute, specific infections usually characterized by a sudden onset of fever, malaise, severe headache, weakness, myalgia, anorexia, prostration, and a generalized macular or maculopapular cutaneous rash, which appears on the third to sixth days of illness (average four) and is terminated by rapid lysis in about 2 weeks (Fig. 100-1). These features typify Rocky Mountain spotted fever and epidemic, murine, and scrub typhus fevers; fatality rates may reach 20 percent or more. Q fever is of shorter duration and usually is not associated with an exanthem. Often it is associated with an acute interstitial pneumonitis. Vegetative endocarditis and granulomatous hepatitis are chronic forms of Q fever.

ROUTES OF INFECTION AND PATHOGENESIS

Human rickettsioses develop following infection through the skin or the respiratory tract. Agents of epidemic typhus and Rocky Mountain spotted fever are introduced through the bite of the infected arthropod vector. Tick and mite vectors which transmit the agents of spotted fever and scrub typhus, inoculate the rickettsiae directly into the dermis during feeding. The louse or flea which transmits the agents of epidemic or murine typhus, respectively, deposits infected feces on the skin; infection occurs when organisms are rubbed into the puncture wound made by the arthropod. Fatal human rickettsial infections have occurred after inhalation of infected aerosols, particularly among laboratory investigators, although this is an uncommon mode of natural transmission. Inhalation of dried rickettsial-laden feces can cause human infections.

The rickettsiae of Q fever gain entry via the respiratory tract by inhalation of infected dust, by handling infected materials, and possibly by drinking milk contaminated with *Coxiella burnetii*. Several species of ticks are naturally infected; sheep, goats, and cows are naturally infected in North America and Europe. The airborne route of dried contaminated material seems the most likely. Person-to-person transmission does not occur.

Rickettsiae probably multiply at the original site of entry in most instances. Local lesions occur with some regularity in scrub typhus (Fig. 100-2), less commonly in Rocky Mountain spotted fever, and not in epidemic murine typhus or Q fever.

Volunteers infected with rickettsiae of either scrub typhus or Q fever develop rickettsemia late in the incubation period often several days before the onset of fever. Similar events probably occur in Rocky Mountain spotted fever and epidemic and murine typhus. Circulating rickettsiae can be detected during the early febrile period in practically all patients. Little is known about the pathogenesis of infection during the mid-incubation period, but

TABLE 100-1
Rickettsial Diseases

Type	Agent	Geographic Distribution	Arthropod	Mammal	Principal Means of Transmission to Humans	Weil-Felix Reaction	CF, MA, IFA, Reactions*	IF†
Rocky Mountain spotted fever	R. rickettsii	Western Hemisphere	Ticks	Wild rodents; dogs	Tick bite	Positive OX-19 OX-2	Positive group and type specific	Positive skin, tissues
Typhus fevers								
Epidemic	R. prowazekii	Worldwide	Body louse	Humans, flying squirrels	Infected louse feces into broken skin	Positive OX-19	Positive group and type specific	Positive skin, tissues
Murine	R. typhi (mooseri)	Worldwide	Flea	Small rodents	Infected flea feces into broken skin	Proteus OX-19	Positive group and type specific	Positive* skin, tissues
Scrub typhus (tsutsugamushi disease)	R. tsutsu-gamushi	Asia, Australia, Pacific Islands	Trombiculid mites	Wild rodents	Mite bite	Positive OX-K	Positive in adults, 50% of patients	Probably positive skin, tissues
Q fever	C. burnetii	Worldwide	Ticks	Small mammals, cattle, sheep, goats	Inhalation of dried infected material	Negative	Positive	Positive tissues

*CF = complement fixation; MA = rickettsial microagglutination; IFA = indirect fluorescent antibody.

†Rickettsiae have been visualized by indirect fluorescence techniques in skin biopsy specimens of patients with Rocky Mountain spotted fever; they are readily visualized in animal tissues.

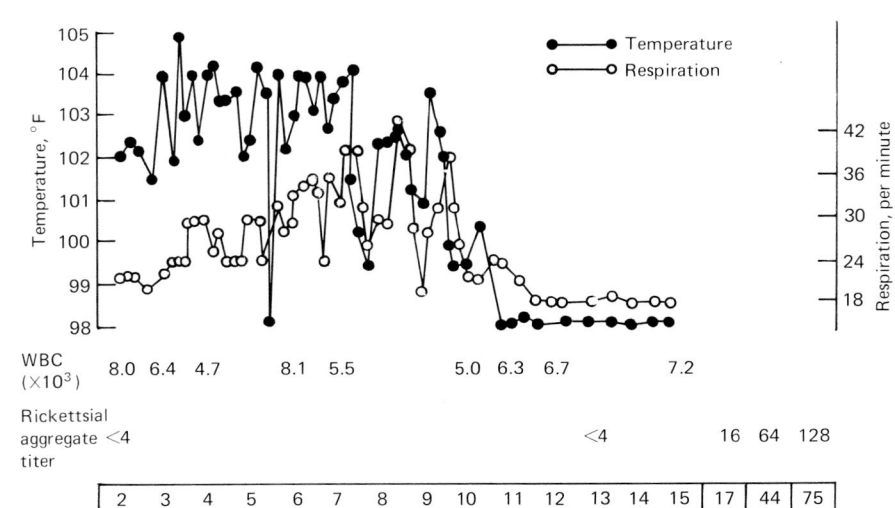

FIGURE 100-1 Q fever. Clinical chart of a 25-year-old man with sudden onset of illness. Mild cough and audible rales were noted on the fourth febrile day. Full recovery without specific treatment.

it is reasonable to assume that, during this time in patients with spotted and typhus fevers, a transient low-grade rickettsemia results from release of organisms multiplying at the initial site of infection. Infection may then spread to endothelial cells of the vascular tree, including the lungs. Vascular lesions developing at such sites account for pathologic changes, including the rash.

Proliferation of rickettsiae in endothelial cells of small blood vessels leads to their destruction and eventual disruption. Rickettsiae may exert a toxic effect on endothelial cells, and in mice the rickettsial toxin causes remarkable increase in capillary permeability, independent of proliferation. Later manifestations in rickettsial diseases may result from immunopathologic mechanisms

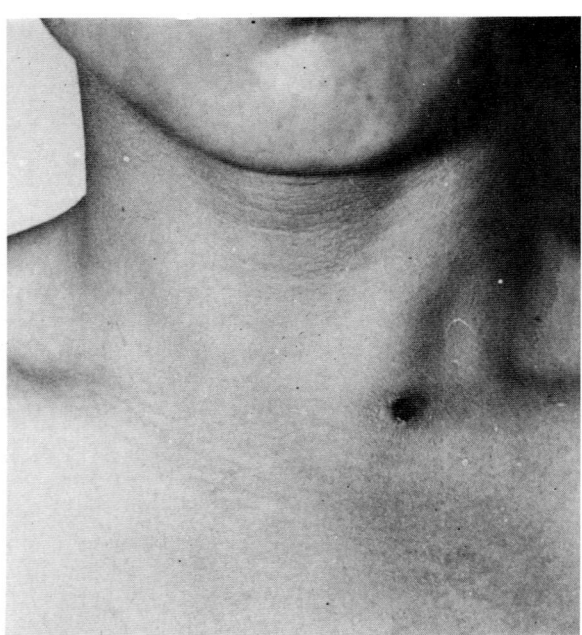

FIGURE 100-2 Scrub typhus. Classic eschar of scrub typhus (tsutsugamushi disease) which appeared at site of mite attachment. Note faint macular lesions on trunk and face.

since humoral antibodies are present during the second febrile week when increase in capillary permeability and vascular thrombosis and ecchymoses are greatest. Also, a delayed type of hypersensitivity occurs during infection.

The underlying cause of the toxic-febrile state that characterizes the rickettsial diseases is unknown. Several rickettsial species contain type-specific toxins that are lethal for mice; they may play a role in humans. Rickettsia-like bodies are seen within the cytoplasm of polymorphonuclear leukocytes in alveolar and bronchial exudate of fatal cases of epidemic typhus. They are also observed in large mononuclear cells and in thickened infiltrated septa but not in bronchial epithelium utilizing Giemsa and Gram stains.

Further support that *Rickettsia prowazekii* unaided by secondary bacterial infection may cause bronchopneumonia is found in animal experiments. Intranasal or intratracheal instillation of rickettsial suspensions in mice, rats, or rabbits results in extensive consolidation and multiplication of these microorganisms in inflammatory cells. Castaneda produced extensive hemorrhagic consolidation in lungs by intranasal inoculations. Polymorphonuclear leukocytes appeared in large numbers with rickettsiae visualized in bronchial epithelium and mononuclear and polymorphonuclear cells. Hence, secondary bacterial superimposed infections play no role in the specific lesions of rickettsial bronchopneumonia caused by *R. prowazekii.*

In murine typhus, a hacking, nonproductive cough is common and rapid respiration with overbreathing is fre-

quently observed; the most frequent findings are basilar crackling rales during the second febrile week. These are indicators of bronchiolitis with interstitial pneumonitis caused by the rickettsial agent.

After intranasal infections of white mice, the rickettsia of Q fever, *C. burnetii*, lodge in fixed and wandering cells of the reticuloendothelial system without cell damage. Ultrastructural and cytochemical studies show increased amounts of RNA in nucleoli, and *C. burnetii* are visible in lung alveolar macrophages. Tissue sections show *C. burnetii* localized within vacuoles and in cytoplasm of infected reticular cells; they visualize well with immunochemical techniques (fluorescent antibody). Inflammation develops slowly in mouse lungs with scant exudate consisting of macrophages in semicollapsed alveoli; *C. burnetii* appear free and in alveolar macrophages staining bright by the immunofluorescence technique.

PATHOLOGIC PHYSIOLOGY

Peripheral vascular collapse results in death in fulminating cases during the first week with capillary dilatation, pooling of blood without increased capillary permeability, or loss of fluid into extravascular spaces. As proliferative and thrombotic lesions develop in small vessels, anoxia occurs in the areas supplied, resulting in necrosis and increased capillary permeability with loss of water, electrolytes, proteins, and erythrocytes. This and other contributing factors result in a decrease in blood volume, serum proteins, and chloride together with an increase in extravascular space and clinical edema. Edema and anoxia of the myocardium are indicated by electrocardiographic changes. Liver function is diminished. The azotemia which develops in seriously ill patients appears to be prerenal. Clinical manifestations resulting from the peripheral vascular collapse are oliguria, anuria, azotemia, anemia, hypoproteinemia, hypochloremia, anoxia and edema of underlying tissues, and coma. In spotted fever and epidemic typhus patients with hemorrhagic skin lesions, a consumption type of coagulopathy is suggested by the presence of thrombocytopenia, hypofibrinogenemia, and other coagulation abnormalities. The above alterations are absent or minimal in mild cases or in those given specific treatment early.

PATHOLOGY

The basic changes in the spotted and typhus fever groups are vascular, with resultant widespread lesions in adjacent parenchymatous tissues throughout the body. They are most common in the skin, muscles, heart, lungs, and brain. The most conspicuous and diverse changes are

found in Rocky Mountain spotted fever. Here swelling, proliferation, and degeneration of endothelial cells occur, frequently with thrombus formation which partially or completely occludes the lumen (Fig. 100-3). Muscle cells of the arterioles undergo swelling with fibrinoid changes, and adventitial tissues are infiltrated with mononuclear leukocytes, lymphocytes, and plasma cells. The vascular damage is scattered along the arterioles, veins, and capillaries, with normal architecture prevailing throughout most of the vascular bed. Changes in epidemic and scrub typhus fevers resemble those in Rocky Mountain spotted fever, but thrombosis is uncommon and involvement of the musculature is rare.

Interstitial myocarditis occurs in each of these diseases but is usually most extensive in Rocky Mountain spotted fever and in scrub typhus. In the brain, glial nodules are found in all members of the group, but microinfarcts in brain tissue or in the myocardium are most often observed in spotted fever.

A rickettsial pneumonitis occurs, at least to some extent, in many patients with spotted or typhus fevers and is the characteristic pathologic change in patients with Q fever. The process is patchy and consists microscopically of areas of congestion and edema. Within the consolidated areas, alveoli are filled with compact fibrinocellular exudate containing lymphocytes, plasma cells, large mononuclear cells, and erythrocytes but few, if any, polymorphonuclear leukocytes.

Walker has described multifocal interstitial pneumonitis with mononuclear and lymphocytic infiltration in fatal cases of Rocky Mountain spotted fever. Rickettsiae are visualized in the pulmonary capillary endothelium by immunofluorescence. Nonproductive cough is an early clinical sign; pulmonary rales indicative of pneumonitis associated with interstitial edema occur later. After a

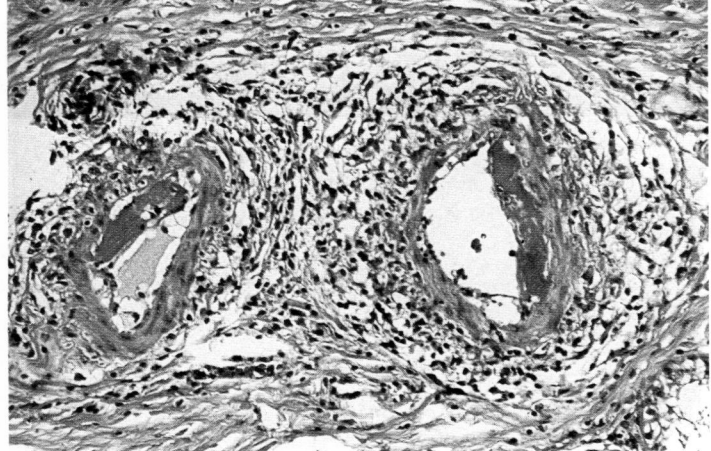

FIGURE 100-3 Rocky Mountain spotted fever. Specimen of skin on about the tenth day of illness showing two arterioles with a mural thrombus and perivascular reaction. ×215

week to 10 days of illness, the radiograph may show patchy infiltrates.

Rickettsiae can occasionally be observed microscopically in sections of tissue. However, failure to demonstrate them is of no diagnostic significance.

Epidemic Typhus

In his classic treatise, Wolbach stated that tracheobronchitis was so prevalent in the fatal cases studied to suggest that it was as "characteristic of the disease as with measles." Bronchopneumonia is a common occurrence in fatal cases, and there is good evidence of a specific rickettsial pneumonia as well as a terminal type of bronchopneumonia which typifies various diseases.

Rocky Mountain Spotted Fever

Pneumonia is a serious complication which may cause death in Rocky Mountain spotted fever. True rickettsial invasion of the lungs may occur accompanied by the production of scant, nonpurulent sputum. More common is pulmonary congestion as a sequel to interstitial edema; the protein-containing edema fluid is an excellent culture medium for conventional bacteria, and it may lead to the development of secondary pneumonitis. Pulmonary congestion may develop consequent to cardiac failure. Bronchopneumonia is a frequent finding in fatal cases of Rocky Mountain spotted fever.

Scrub Typhus Fever

Often the lungs of patients with fatal cases of scrub typhus fever show evidence of hemorrhagic pneumonia with the characteristic microscopic lesions of focal vasculitis and perivasculitis of smaller vessels consisting of accumulations of monocytes, plasma cells, and lymphocytes. The vascular lesions are less severe than in epidemic typhus. Interstitial pneumonitis occurs in most fatal cases. Often there is a superimposed secondary bronchopneumonia.

Q Fever

The acute form of Q fever is seldom fatal, and postmortem findings are based on only a few human postmortem examinations as well as studies of experimentally infected animals. In most human patients, death results from diffuse lobar pneumonia, which grossly resembles the consolidation of pneumococcal pneumonia. The mononuclear exudate resembles viral or psittacine pneumonia which differs from the polymorphonuclear reaction of *Diplococcus pneumoniae*. During the early stage of red hepatization, consolidation is uneven and the distribution of eosinophilic exudates within alveoli is sporadic. Large mononuclear macrophages show cytoplasmic vacuolation, other degenerative changes, and intense congestion of blood vessels throughout the consolidated area. In areas

of gray consolidation, thickened alveolar walls are infiltrated with macrophages, a smaller number of lymphocytes, plasma cells, and neutrophils. Necrotic areas and disruption of septa occur. Alveolar exudate consists mostly of vacuolated and degenerate macrophages; bronchioles contain similar exudates with mucosal degeneration. Edema and round cell infiltration are occasionally present in subpleural areas and in interlobular connective tissue. *C. burnetii* lie free and within macrophages in lung lesions.

Solitary lung masses called an *inflammatory pseudotumor*, which simulates a lung neoplasm, may develop during the course of Q fever pneumonitis. They resemble coin or mass lesions. The histologic findings are edematous bronchioles, partially or totally occluded by fibroblasts, and sparse collagen infiltrated with lymphocytes, plasma cells, and macrophages. In the alveoli, there are "foam cells" made up of obstructive organizing exudates.

Chronic endocarditis caused by *C. burnetii* is the principal cause of death in Q fever; chronic granulomatous hepatitis causes a lingering illness.

CLINICAL MANIFESTATIONS

Q Fever

The incubation period varies from 14 to 26 days, and the illness usually begins with headache, chilly sensations, fever, malaise, myalgia, and anorexia. The temperature ranges from 101 to 104°F; wide swings in fever are common. The entire course rarely exceeds 2 weeks and usually ranges from 3 to 6 days. During the early stages respiratory symptoms are not conspicuous. A dry cough and chest pain occur after about 5 days; at that time, rales are usually audible. The cough usually produces a small amount of mucoid sputum which is occasionally streaked with blood; *C. burnetii* have been recovered from the sputum but not visualized directly. In various outbreaks, more than 60 percent of patients showed pulmonary disease visible by radiograph indicating that pneumonitis is a common occurrence. Nonetheless, Q fever is a systemic illness of rickettsial etiology, and serious illnesses have occurred without pneumonitis present at any time.

Respiratory symptoms and physical findings produced by the lung lesion of Q fever are often minimal; during the peak of illness fine crepitant rales may be heard after deep inspiration. Dullness to percussion is occasionally elicited and may indicate consolidation or the presence of pleural effusion. *C. burnetii* has been isolated from pleural fluid. Other clinical signs are a relative bradycardia, hepatomegaly, and splenomegaly, none of which often occur simultaneously.

The radiographic findings are often indistinguishable from those of viral, primary, atypical pneumonia and may closely resemble pneumococcal pneumonia. Infiltrations are usually present by the third to fourth days of disease, first as patchy areas of consolidation involving a portion of one lobe giving a homogeneous ground glass appearance. The lesions tend to occur in the peribronchial and alveolar tissues rather than the hilar regions and often in the lower lobes. These manifestations persist beyond the febrile period and may appear in patients who are unaware of pulmonary involvement. Segmental or lobar infiltrations occur more commonly in Q fever than in many atypical pneumonias. The sputum of patients with pneumococcal lobar pneumonia differs significantly from that of patients with Q fever: in Q fever, small amounts of mucoid sputum are produced and the sputum is occasionally streaked with blood and contains a few mononuclear cells; in contrast, the sputum in pneumococcal pneumonia, although also mucoid, is often rusty and contains leukocytes, erythrocytes, and identifiable *D. pneumoniae*.

In one series of 115 patients, 97 showed radiographic evidence of pneumonitis of the atypical type; of these 97 patients, abnormal lung findings were noted in 89 as well as in 10 whose chest films were normal. Three deaths occurred in patients with Hodgkin's disease, healed myocardial infarction, and chronic recurring illness, respectively.

Occasionally a homogeneous localized infiltration may resemble a tumor mass. Diagnosis is confirmed by use of serologic reactions which show antibodies to phase II antigens; *C. burnetii* may be visualized in infected tissues by immunofluorescence techniques.

Epidemic, Murine, Scrub Typhus, and Rocky Mountain Spotted Fevers

The clinical manifestations of epidemic, murine, scrub typhus, and Rocky Mountain spotted fevers are similar (Fig. 100-4). Cough occurs after several days of illness and

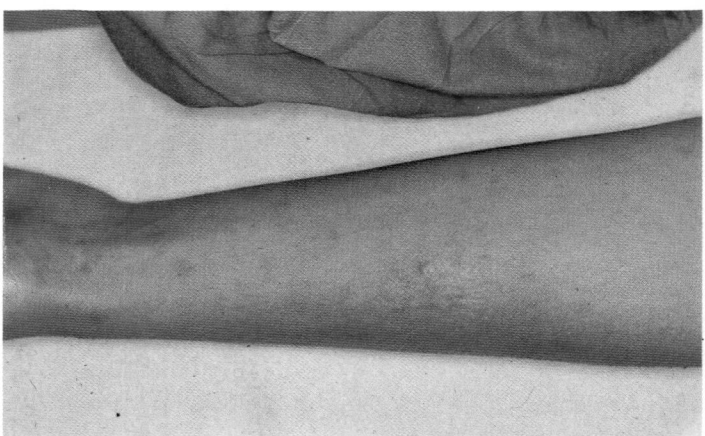

FIGURE 100-4 Rocky Mountain spotted fever. Characteristic early pink macular rash on the forearm on about the fourth day of illness.

is attributable to bronchiolitis, which typifies these major rickettsioses. The cough is usually nonproductive but may become persistent, accompanied by rapid, shallow respirations. As the illness progresses, there may be signs of pulmonary infiltration with moist or crepitant rales. Tachypnea may increase, and in seriously ill patients the lips and nails may become deeply cyanotic, signs which are attributable to vascular abnormalities as much as to the pulmonary changes. During the stages of vascular decompensation and leakage, there may be signs of pulmonary congestion, which usually is the result of a specific rickettsial pneumonitis. Added to these types of lung involvement is pulmonary edema attributable to cardiac decompensation or increased capillary permeability, which requires conventional types of treatment. Pulmonary edema is particularly prone to develop after the injudicious use of intravenous fluids.

Chest radiographs occasionally reveal mottling in various areas of the lungs and signs of localized pneumonitis or bronchopneumonia. Occasionally there is lobar consolidation.

The sputum, when productive, is mucoid and consists of a few mononuclear cells and neutrophils. Rickettsiae are not visualized by conventional staining techniques.

When secondary bacterial pneumonia develops in fatal cases, it is caused by conventional bacteria; *D. pneumoniae* is the most common type. Specific antibacterial treatment is then given in keeping with the results of laboratory findings.

LABORATORY DIAGNOSIS

There are no specific hematologic findings in patients with rickettsial diseases. Normochromic anemia occurs in most severely ill patients, the leukocyte count is usually within the normal range, 6000 to 10,000 cells per cubic millimeter. Leukopenia is occasionally observed; in the presence of superimposed infections, such as pneumonia and extensive vascular lesions, moderate leukocytosis occurs. The differential blood count is usually normal.

In severely ill patients with extensive vascular lesions, thrombocytopenia is common. Other abnormalities in clotting mechanisms also occur. Among these are hypofibrinogenemia and prolonged prothrombin and partial thromboplastin times.

SPECIFIC DIAGNOSIS

Available confirmatory laboratory tests for rickettsial diseases include the Weil-Felix, complement fixation, rickettsial microagglutination, and indirect fluorescent antibody reaction, and more tedious isolation of causative rickettsiae in animals or tissue culture. With each of these procedures confirmatory results are available late in the illness when serious or irreversible vascular changes or death may have occurred.

R. RICKETTSII

R. rickettsii, the causative agent of Rocky Mountain spotted fever, has been identified in skin specimens obtained by biopsy of a macular lesion from patients as early as day 4 or as late as day 8 of illness. This technique will undoubtedly be adaptable to early confirmation of patients with epidemic and scrub typhus by biopsy of a skin lesion.

TREATMENT

The general principles of therapy are the same for the rickettsial diseases. These include: (1) antimicrobial therapy, (2) supportive measures, (3) skilled nursing to avoid complications, and (4) prompt recognition and treatment of complications. In mild cases, antimicrobial therapy supplemented by usual medical care generally suffices.

Specific treatment of the rickettsial diseases with antimicrobials was achieved with the development of chlortetracycline, oxytetracycline, and chloramphenicol in the late 1940s. Prompt usage of the proper antimicrobial agents is the cornerstone of treatment: it has shortened morbidity and has virtually eradicated mortality in this group of potentially severe diseases. As a rule, drugs of the tetracycline series are the antibiotics of choice. Chloramphenicol, although equally effective, is less favored because of the threat of aplastic anemia. Since neither of these categories of antimicrobials is rickettsicidal, arrest of the infection depends on the immune response of the patient.

In treating the usual rickettsial diseases, tetracycline HCl is usually given by mouth. As a rule, in adults, 2 g per day is administered in divided doses at 4- to 6-h intervals. Chloramphenicol is administered at the same time intervals for a total of about 4 g per day. Parenteral therapy is indicated if the patient cannot swallow. Special precautions about dosage are required in treating the newborn. The new lipotropic tetracyclines have abbreviated the management of certain rickettsial diseases (louse-borne typhus) but are less effective in others (scrub typhus). Standard texts should be consulted for details of specific treatment.

In the usual uncomplicated case, fever generally drops within 24 h and the patient becomes afebrile in 2 to 3 days (Fig. 100-1). In the severe rickettsioses complicated by pneumonitis, the antimicrobial agents should be tailored to the bacteriologic findings in the sputum. Infiltrates generally resolve within 2 to 3 weeks after institution of antibiotic therapy. Adjuvant therapy, in the form of high dose, short-term corticosteroid therapy, has been reported to exert dramatic effects in the severely ill patient with neurologic involvement. Among the dreaded complications are circulatory collapse, gangrene, and thrombophlebitis. Other disturbances, notably neurologic manifestations, usually resolve spontaneously during

convalescence. Fluid and electrolyte imbalances require careful correction to avoid volume overload and pulmonary edema. Severe agitation on the one hand and coma on the other require skilled nursing care to avoid a wide span of complications ranging from self-inflicted injury to decubitus ulcers, thrombophlebitis, hypostatic pneumonia, and endocarditis.

Oxygen therapy is necessary for support of the circulatory and lung abnormalities as indicated by clinical signs and alterations of blood gases. Always, the clinician should administer intravenous fluids judiciously in order to avoid the inadvertent development of pulmonary edema.

BIBLIOGRAPHY

Ariel BM, Khavkin TN, Amosenkova NI: Interaction between *Coxiella burnetii* and the cells in experimental Q-rickettsioses. Pathol Microbiol 39:412–423, 1973.
   A good description of the localization of C. burnetii in reticuloendothelial cells of white mice after intranasal inoculation. Ultrastructural cytochemical studies show RNA content in nucleoli and C. burnetii are visualized in living alveolar macrophages and reticular cells.

Beck MD, Bell SA, Shaw EW, Huebner RJ: Q fever studies in Southern California. Pub Health Rep 64:41, 1949.
   Report of Q fever in 115 patients with 97 showing radiographic evidence of pneumonitis. The abnormal lung findings are reported.

Castaneda MR: Experimental pneumonia produced by typhus rickettsiae. Am J Pathol 15:467, 1939.
   Description of the method of producing pneumonitis in animals as a means of vaccine production.

Commission on Acute Respiratory Diseases, Fort Bragg, North Carolina: A laboratory outbreak of Q fever caused by the Balkan Grippe strain of *Rickettsia burnetii*. Am J Hyg 44:123–157, 1946.
   Excellent description of the epidemiology, extent, and duration of various clinical signs, radiographic findings, and diagnosis. Authors report isolation of C. burnetii from pleural fluid.

Donohue JF: Lower respiratory tract involvement in Rocky Mountain spotted fever. Arch Intern Med 140:223–227, 1980.
   A good description of the lower respiratory tract involvement in Rocky Mountain spotted fever, including a discussion of the noncardiac pulmonary edema.

Hand WL, Miller JB, Reinarz, JA, Sanford JP: Rocky Mountain spotted fever. Arch Intern Med 125:879–882, 1970.
   A discussion of Rocky Mountain spotted fever as a vascular disorder with emphasis upon the need to avoid an intravenous overload.

Harrell GT: Rocky Mountain spotted fever. Medicine 28:333, 1949.
   A classic description of the fundamental clinical manifestations of Rocky Mountain spotted fever and the underlying pathophysiologic mechanisms.

Huebner RJ, Jellison WL, Beck MD: Q fever: A review of current knowledge. Ann Intern Med 30:495–509, 1949.
   A good discussion of the clinical features of Q fever and the pulmonary manifestations, including pleural effusion.

Janigan DT, Marrie TJ: An inflammatory pseudotumor of the lung in Q fever pneumonia. N Engl J Med 308:86–88, 1983.
   A case report of a solitary lung mass during the course of Q fever which resembled a localized neoplasm.

Marrie TJ, Haldane EV, Noble MA, Faulkner RS, Martin RS, Lee SH: Causes of atypical pneumonia: Results of a 1-year prospective study. Can Med Assoc J 125:1118–1123, 1981.
   In a protocol study of cases of atyical pneumonia over a 1-year period, an etiologic agent was established in 16 cases: Legionella pneumophila in 8, Coxiella burnetti in 3, Chlamydia trachomatis in 2, Mycoplasma pneumoniae in 1, and para-influenza 3 virus in 1.

Marrie TJ, Schlech WF III, Williams JC, Yates L: Q fever pneumonia associated with exposure to wild rabbits. Lancet 1:427–429, 1986
   Four patients with atypical pneumonia and a history of exposure to wild rabbits were found to have antibodies to Coxiella burnetii but not to the other organisms also commonly associated with atypical pneumonia.

Pathology of epidemic typhus: Report of fatal cases studied by United States of America Typhus Commission in Cairo, Egypt, during 1943–45. AMA Arch Pathol 56:397–435, 512–553, 1953.
> *A thorough description of the pathologic changes in epidemic typhus fever based on 25 fatal cases studied by the USA Typhus Commission during World War II. Leading pathologists contributed to the study.*

Sawyer LA, Fishbein DB, McDade JE: Q fever: Current concepts. Rev Infect Dis 9:935–946, 1987.
> *A review of etiology, clinical manifestations, diagnosis, treatment, and prevention.*

Spicknall CG, Huebner RJ, Finger JA, Blocker WP: Report of an outbreak of Q fever at the National Institutes of Health. I. Clinical features. Ann Intern Med 27:28–40, 1947.
> *Description of a laboratory outbreak of Q fever with emphasis on clinical features. Isolation of C. burnetii from sputum.*

Walker DH, Bradford WD: Rocky Mountain spotted fever in childhood. Perspect Pediatr Pathol 6:35–61, 1981.
> *A comprehensive description of the pathologic changes, and the pathophysiologic mechanisms of Rocky Mountain spotted fever. This includes a good description of the lung findings.*

Walker DH, Crawford CG, Cain BG: Rickettsial infection of the pulmonary microcirculation: The basis for interstitial pneumonitis in Rocky Mountain spotted fever. Hum Pathol 11:263–272, 1980.
> *An important paper for the understanding of pulmonary involvement in rickettsial disorders.*

Wisseman CL Jr: Rickettsial disease, in Wyngaarden J, Smith LH Jr (eds), *Cecil's Textbook of Medicine*, 17th ed. New York, Saunders, 1985, pp 1672–1686.
> *A concise but comprehensive overview of rickettsial disorders with primary focus on nonrespiratory aspects.*

Wolbach SB, Todd JL, Palfrey FW: The etiology and pathology of typhus. League of Red Cross Societies, Harvard University Press, Cambridge, Mass, 1922.
> *The classic treatise on the cause and pathologic changes in epidemic typhus with correlation of clinical manifestations and histologic findings. Rickettsiae are shown in tissues stained by conventional methods.*

Woodward TE: The rickettsioses, in Braunwald E, Isselbacher KJ, Petersdorf RG, Wilson JD, Martin JB, Fauci AS (eds), *Harrison's Principles of Internal Medicine*, 11th ed. New York, McGraw-Hill, 1987, pp 747–757.
> *A general description of the rickettsial diseases including historical contributions, etiology, pathogenesis, pathologic changes, clinical manifestations, epidemiology, and management.*

Woodward TE, Pedersen CE Jr, Oster CN, Bagley LR, Romberger J, Snyder MJ: Prompt confirmation of Rocky Mountain spotted fever: Identification of rickettsiae in skin tissues. J Infect Dis 134:297–301, 1976.
> *Initial paper to report the visualization of R. rickettsii (cause of Rocky Mountain spotted fever) in skin specimens obtained by biopsy and stained by immunofluorescence techniques.*

Chapter 101

The Atypical Pneumonias

Thomas W. Nash / Henry W. Murray

The term *atypical pneumonia* entered our lexicon in the mid-1930s to help draw the distinction between those pneumonias which presented in the traditional clinical fashion and those which did not. Typical (classic) bacterial pneumonias present with rigors, fever, a productive cough, pleuritic chest pain, and lobar infiltrates. Atypical pneumonias commonly present in a less acute or dramatic fashion (similar to viral pneumonias) with a nonproductive cough, milder symptoms, and nonlobar infiltrates.

This clinical distinction is epidemiologically misleading, however, since the atypical pneumonia syndrome (including Legionnaires' disease) is actually more common than the typical pneumonias. The origin of this paradox derives largely from the evolution of the diagnostic microbiology laboratory. The bacterial agents of typical pneumonia (e.g., *Streptococcus pneumoniae, Hemophilus influenzae, Staphylococcus aureus*) were discovered first, whereas the isolation and characterization of the agents responsible for the atypical pneumonias *(Mycoplasma pneumoniae, Chlamydia, Coxiella burnetti)* required considerably more sophisticated science. Indeed, one of the principal pathogens in the atypical pneumonia syndrome, *Legionella pneumophilia*, was not identified until the late 1970s. Despite thorough evaluation, moreover, no etiologic agent can be identified in more than 50 percent of cases of atypical pneumonia. Pneumonias caused by *M. pneumoniae, Chlamydia* species, and *C. burnetti* have, however, been well characterized.

MYCOPLASMA PNEUMONIAE

M. pneumoniae has traditionally been regarded as a seasonal respiratory tract pathogen of children and young adults. More recent experience, however, indicates that this organism is also an important year-round cause of pneumonia and upper respiratory tract infections in adults of all age groups. In addition, it now appears clear that *M. pneumoniae* infection can also be associated with a wide spectrum of both pulmonary and extrapulmonary syndromes that may be benign and self-limited, moderately troublesome, or sometimes life-threatening. On occasion, extrapulmonary manifestations may actually overshadow or occur in the absence of symptomatic respiratory tract involvement.

The Organism

M. pneumoniae is a procaryote that is bound by a single triple-layered membrane, stains gram-negative, exhibits hemadsorption, and produces a peroxide hemolysin. The organism is 10×200 nm in size, appears filamentous, and readily grows on artificial media supplemented with yeast and other factors. On its end, there is a neuraminic acid receptor site for attachment to membranes of host cells such as erythrocytes and respiratory tract epithelium. Unlike true bacteria, *M. pneumoniae* cannot synthesize a cell wall; therefore, it is resistant to penicillin and other cell-wall-active antibiotics.

A *Mycoplasma* was the first organism identified as an etiologic agent of the atypical pneumonia syndrome. Historically, this microbe was first termed the *pleuropneumonia-like* organism (PPLO) and later the *Eaton agent*—named for the investigator who in 1944 inocu-

lated hamsters with filtered secretions from patients with atypical pneumonia and reproduced the illness in the animals. *M. pneumoniae* is the species responsible for human respiratory illness. Other species of *Mycoplasma* (e.g., *M. hominis*) and a species of the related genus *Ureaplasma* (*U. urealyticum*) are important agents of human genitourinary disease.

Epidemiology

Although the incidence of *M. pneumoniae* infection has been reported to increase during the late summer and fall, there is little hard evidence to indicate any seasonality. From a longitudinal study in Seattle from 1963 to 1979, it appears that *M. pneumoniae* was responsible for approximately 15 percent of community-acquired nonepidemic pneumonias. Most cases occur in children and young adults (ages 5 to 20). Aging, though, offers no barrier to infection since *M. pneumonia* has been implicated in 4 to 40 percent of pneumonias in adults. Horizontal spread is common and requires close contact. Enclosed populations (e.g., college students, military recruits, or families) appear to be particularly prone to *M. pneumoniae* infection. Outbreaks in these settings account for much of the higher incidence figures.

Pathogenesis

Infection appears to be acquired via inhalation of infected material after exposure to an acutely ill, coughing individual. Intense exposure is probably necessary for acquisition of infection. Nasopharyngeal carriers of *M. pneumoniae* whose clinical illness has resolved do not appear to transmit the organism readily.

Since fatal cases of *M. pneumoniae* pneumonia are rare, there is little pathologic data from which to draw pathogenetic inferences. In fatal cases, interstitial and alveolar pneumonitis, bronchitis, and bronchiolitis can be found. Histologic findings have included tracheal and bronchial mucosal hyperemia, alveolar exudates comprising principally mononuclear inflammatory cells, plasma cell interstitial space infiltration, and accumulation of monocytes and macrophages in the bronchial epithelial submucosa. Studies using an experimental animal model have demonstrated that *M. pneumoniae* binds via neuraminic acid receptors to respiratory tract epithelial cells and initiates injury to local mucosal cells with resultant stasis of cilia. *M. pneumoniae* may also penetrate the bronchial mucosa. Polymorphonuclear leukocytes are attracted to deciliated cells, and leukocyte products probably contribute to or perpetuate the superficial inflammatory process.

Cell injury may also be mediated by hydrogen peroxide or superoxide anion which can be elaborated by the organism. However, the amounts of these oxidants that are produced are probably too small to account for the extent of cellular damage. Recent evidence also suggests that *M. pneumoniae* has the ability to decrease the activity of a target cell's catalase (the endogenous enzyme that detoxifies hydrogen peroxide), thereby rendering the host cell more susceptible to the toxicity of hydrogen peroxide.

There is a body of evidence that suggests that immune mechanisms, rather than actual direct infection, play a role in the development of clinically apparent *M. pneumoniae* pneumonia as well as in some of the extrapulmonary complications. For example, *M. pneumoniae* is rarely isolated from nonrespiratory sites despite its ability to cause disease in practically any organ, body fluid, or mucosal or serosal surface. In addition, severe illness due to *M. pneumoniae* is observed almost exclusively in immunocompetent patients. Conversely, in our experience and in that of others, *M. pneumoniae* is an exceedingly infrequent cause of serious disease in patients with an impaired immune system. Further, in one study, clinical pneumonia did not develop in children with immunodeficiency syndromes who had acquired *M. pneumoniae* respiratory tract infections.

M. pneumoniae can stimulate T lymphocytes and activate B cells. These findings may in part explain the occurrence of circulating immune complexes in up to 40 percent of infected patients. These immune complexes as well as the well-documented development of autoantibodies to various tissues (including lung, heart, brain, liver, kidney, and smooth muscle) during *M. pneumoniae* infection may contribute to target organ injury or inflammation. In one study, the titer of circulating immune complexes could be directly correlated with the severity of respiratory tract disease. In experimental *M. pneumoniae* infection, antithymocyte globulin has been shown to abrogate or diminish the severity of disease, and corticosteroids have been used with success to modify some of the severe effects of infection with this organism. These observations support the hypothesis that the vigor of the host immune response may explain in part why some patients with *M. pneumoniae* infection develop pneumonitis rather than bronchitis alone and why some experience extrapulmonary complications. Repeated subclinical *M. pneumoniae* infections with subsequent sensitization of immune effector cells may thus be a factor in the development of serious illness. This theory, though, is in conflict with other observations that antibody to *M. pneumoniae* confers protection against infection and may alter the severity of the illness (see "Immunity").

Immunity

Resistance to and recovery from infection appears to be related to the production of specific IgG and IgA antibody. IgG can mediate lysis of the organism with complement or can facilitate attachment to or destruction of *M. pneumoniae* by mononuclear phagocytes, alveolar macrophages, and polymorphonuclear cells. IgA antibody can inhibit

the binding of *M. pneumoniae* to respiratory tract epithelium. Circulating antibody to *Mycoplasma* appears to increase host resistance against infection. However, this protection is not absolute, and reinfection can occur. In documented cases of reinfection, the clinical illness is typically mild. Mycoplasma organisms appear to persist longer in patients with immune deficiency syndrome so cell-mediated immune mechanisms may also play a role in host defense.

The rate of decay of serum antibody has been observed to depend on the age of the patient and the severity of the illness. Antibody titers decrease most rapidly in young children and in patients with mild disease and persist longer in those with pneumonia. The duration of antibody persistence has not been fully defined, but in adults, antibodies detected by complement fixation typically last at least 10 years and probably longer.

Pulmonary Manifestations

UNCOMPLICATED PNEUMONIA (SEE TABLE 101-1)

After exposure, the incubation period for most mycoplasmal infections is 14 to 21 days. In contrast to most cases of psittacosis and Q fever which begin with an abrupt onset

TABLE 101-1
Symptoms and Signs in Five Series of Patients with M. Pneumoniae Pneumonia

Series	A	B	C	D	E
No. of patients	109	90	200	175	40
Symptoms	% of Patients				
Fever (>38.9°C)	100	50	74	72	
Chills	73	65	58	78	
Headache	72	40	64	85	25
Cough	100	95	100	93	75
Purulent sputum		20	49		18
Hemoptysis		5			2
Chest pain		30	2	42	
Sore throat	41	25	53	53	25
Rhinorrhea	17	25	25	49	40
Earache		2	35		15
Malaise		40	89	74	60
Anorexia				36	25
Nausea/vomiting	44		29		15
Diarrhea			16		12
Myalgias/arthralgias		20		45	15
Signs					
Rales	82	60		84	
Pharyngitis	57			12	
Lymphadenopathy	28	40		18	19
Myringitis					12
Rash			16		28

and impressive symptoms, illness due to *M. pneumoniae* commonly begins insidiously with a 2- to 5-day prodrome of fever, malaise, and headache.

Most infected patients develop pharyngitis or tracheobronchitis. Clinically apparent pneumonia occurs in only 10 percent of cases and is usually mild. In patients with pneumonia, cough is the prominent symptom and is typically nonproductive. If obtained, sputum can appear purulent in up to one-third of cases. Although hemoptysis and pleuritic chest pain are rare, *M. pneumoniae* pneumonia may occasionally mimic pulmonary embolism with infarction. Rales and rhonchi are common physical findings. Occasional cases can simulate bacterial lobar infection, but signs of airspace consolidation are infrequent. In 25 to 50 percent of patients with pneumonia, there are upper respiratory tract signs and symptoms, including sore throat, rhinorrhea, and earache. Although up to one-third of patients have the last complaint, objective myringitis with tympanic membrane bullae (sometimes with hemorrhage) is seen in only 15 to 20 percent of patients. Musculoskeletal and gastrointestinal symptoms are common but minor. Additional, but less often encountered findings in patients with *M. pneumoniae* pneumonia include cervical lymphadenopathy, sinusitis, conjunctivitis, rashes, and pulse-temperature dissociation. Generalized lymphadenopathy and splenomegaly are rare. *M. pneumoniae* infection may also precipitate respiratory deterioration and/or bronchospasm in patients with chronic obstructive lung disease.

Within 3 to 10 days in untreated cases, fever, headache, and malaise resolve. Cough and rales dissipate more slowly and parallel the clearing of the chest radiograph. Despite appropriate therapy, clinical relapses with reappearance of symptoms and infiltrates may occur 7 to 10 days after an initial response. Moreover, progression of pulmonary infiltrates to involve new parenchymal areas may also occur during therapy.

PLEURAL EFFUSIONS

Although once considered rare in *M. pneumoniae* infection, pleural effusions actually occur in up to 25 percent of patients (Fig. 101-1). Effusions typically are small, unilateral, and transient. Lateral or decubitus radiographic views are usually required to demonstrate the fluid. Bilateral or massive effusions are very unusual but may occur and take 3 to 4 weeks to resolve.

Pleural fluid accompanying *M. pneumoniae* pneumonia usually has the characteristics of an exudate with a normal glucose level, elevated protein, and variable numbers (up to 40,000 per cubic millimeter) of both polymorphonuclear leukocytes and mononuclear cells. When done, pleural biopsies have shown no remarkable abnormalities. Isolation of *M. pneumoniae* from pleural fluid is difficult, and positive cultures are exceedingly rare.

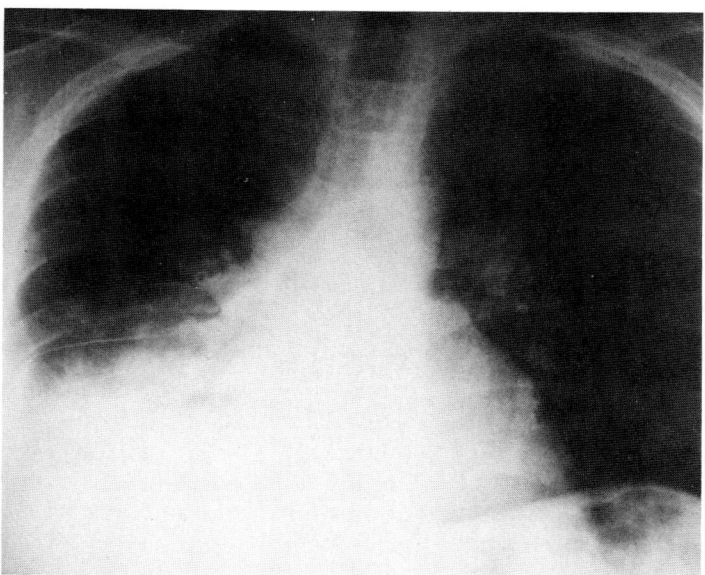

FIGURE 101-1 Chest radiograph of a 23-year-old man with serologically confirmed *M. pneumoniae* showing a right middle lobe infiltrate and large right pleural effusion. Right lateral decubitus view showed freely layering fluid. *M. pneumoniae* was isolated from this patient's sputum but not from the pleural fluid. *(Reprinted with permission from Murray HW, Masur H, Senterfit LB, Roberts RB: The protean manifestations of Mycoplasma pneumoniae infection in adults. Am J Med 58:229, 1975.)*

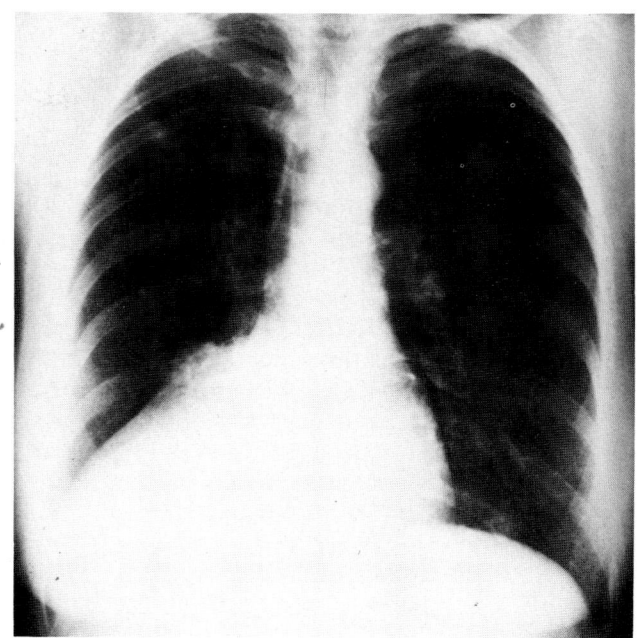

FIGURE 101-2 Chest radiograph of a 35-year-old woman with serologically confirmed *M. pneumoniae* pneumonia showing collapse of the right lower lobe. Resolution required 6 weeks. *(Reprinted with permission from Murray HW, Tuazon CU: Atypical pneumonias. Med Clin North Am 64:507, 1980.)*

COMPLICATED PULMONARY INFECTIONS

Although usually benign and self-limited, *M. pneumoniae* pulmonary illness can be severe and even catastrophic. Patients with sickle cell anemia may develop protracted high fever, marked leukocytosis (greater than 50,000 per cubic millimeter), multilobe involvement, large pleural effusions, and pleuritic pain. Fulminant respiratory failure leading to the adult respiratory distress syndrome (occasionally fatal) has also been reported.

Mixed infection with respiratory viruses (e.g., influenza and adenovirus) has been observed, as has coinfection or superinfection with bacterial pathogens including *Legionella pneumophila*.

A few cases of lung abcess in patients with laboratory-confirmed *M. pneumoniae* infection have been reported, and these responded slowly to treatment. Other pulmonary complications or findings have included residual pleural scarring, the hyperlucent lung syndrome, pneumatoceles, hilar adenopathy, lobar collapse (Fig. 101-2), and presentation as a mediastinal mass.

Extrapulmonary Manifestations

There are a host of potentially serious nonrespiratory complications that patients with *M. pneumoniae* infection can develop, and, as illustrated in Table 101-2, virtually any organ system may be involved.

TABLE 101-2

Extrapulmonary Manifestations of M. Pneumoniae Infections

Hematologic	Autoimmune hemolytic anemia, thrombocytopenia, disseminated intravascular coagulation
Gastrointestinal	Gastroenteritis, anicteric hepatitis, pancreatitis
Musculoskeletal	Arthralgias, myalgias, polyarthritis
Dermatologic	Various rashes, erthyema nodosum and multiforme, Stevens-Johnson syndrome
Cardiac	Pericarditis, myocarditis, pericardial effusion, conduction defects
Neurologic	Meningitis, meningoencephalitis, transverse myelitis, peripheral and cranial neuropathy, cerebellar ataxia
Miscellaneous	General lymphadenopathy, splenomegaly, interstitial nephritis, glomerulonephritis, arthritis, fevers of unknown origin

HEMATOLOGIC

Autoimmune hemolytic anemia is probably the best recognized among the extrapulmonary manifestations of *M. pneumoniae* infection. In 40 to 75 percent of patients, the infection results in the production of a monoclonal IgM antibody that can agglutinate erythrocytes at 4°C. In vivo, these antibodies bind to the I antigen of the erythrocyte

surface as the red blood cells traverse the cooler areas of the body (extremities, nose, ear). Antibody-mediated fixation of complement to the erythrocyte surface occurs and is responsible for the positive Coombs' test (seen in over 80 percent of patients with *M. pneumoniae* infection) as well as hemolysis. Mild subclinical hemolysis is common, and reticulocytosis can be detected in up to 64 percent of cases. Hemolysis severe enough to produce clinical anemia is, however, rare. When it occurs, treatment should be instituted with warmed packed red blood cell transfusions and systemic corticosteroids. Severe hemolysis usually occurs 2 to 3 weeks after the onset of clinical illness, and it usually coincides with recovery from pneumonia and the presence of high cold agglutinin titers—typically ≥1:1000, although cases with lower antibody titers have been reported. The agglutination potential of these cold-induced antibodies can, on rare occasions, be responsible for Raynaud's phenomenon, acrocyanosis, and disseminated intravascular coagulation with thrombocytopenia and renal failure.

GASTROINTESTINAL

Anorexia may persist for several weeks, but most other gastrointestinal symptoms, such as nausea, vomiting, and diarrhea (Table 101-1), resolve promptly. Anicteric hepatitis and acute pancreatitis have been reported to develop during the course of *M. pneumonia* infection.

MUSCULOSKELETAL

Nonspecific myalgias and arthralgias occur in up to 40 percent of patients with *M. pneumoniae* pneumonia. A prominent rheumatic syndrome with acute arthritis or severe arthralgias may also develop during the first 2 weeks of respiratory illness. Involvement can be migratory and polyarticular, and the large joints are most often affected. Synovial effusions and morning stiffness may both be troublesome, and resolution of joint complaints may be slow.

DERMATOLOGIC

A variety of mucocutaneous lesions can complicate *M. pneumoniae* infection. In up to 25 percent of patients, skin lesions occur during the first or second week of respiratory symptoms. The various rashes include macular, petechial, or morbilliform eruptions as well as erythema nodosum, urticaria, and erythema multiforme; they are usually transient and typically not of much clinical significance. On occasion, however, extensive vesicular skin eruptions with mucous membrane involvement, ulcerative stomatitis, conjunctivitis, and urethritis (the Stevens-Johnson syndrome or erythema multiforme major) may develop. *M. pneumoniae* has been isolated from fluid

from both bullous and vesicular skin lesions. This severe dermatologic complication typically develops within the first two weeks of infection and takes weeks (up to 9 weeks) to resolve. Therapy with tetracycline, effective in the pulmonary lesions, has little clear benefit for the skin lesions which may require systemic corticosteroids.

CARDIAC

Once thought rare, cardiac involvement in *M. pneumoniae* infections may not be unusual. In one prospective study, up to 7.5 percent of patients with illness due to *M. pneumoniae* developed pericarditis or myopericarditis. Cardiac involvement, which can occur in the absence of pulmonary infiltrates, is commonly mild and clinically silent. Pericardial abnormalities range from asymptomatic EKG abnormalities to large effusions. Myocardial dysfunction, congestive heart failure, and rhythm and conduction disturbances, including complete heart block, may occur. Rare patients are left with a chronic cardiomyopathy. In one patient, *M. pneumoniae* was isolated at autopsy from blood and pericardial fluid.

NEUROLOGIC

Central and peripheral nervous system disease is the most severe and potentially devastating nonpulmonary complication of *M. pneumoniae* infection. Aseptic meningitis is typically benign and transient. Meningoencephalitis occurs and can be associated with hemiplegia, coma, and residual neurologic impairment. Transverse myelitis, granulomatous cerebral angiitis, cerebellar ataxia (children), and acute psychosis have been documented. Peripheral and cranial neuropathies can be severe and lead to a disabling Guillain-Barré syndrome or prolonged nerve dysfunction.

Neurologic manifestations occur up to 4 weeks after the initial infection. In 20 percent of cases, there may be no evident pulmonary involvement. Cerebrospinal fluid usually reveals a mild pleocytosis (10 to 90 percent polymorphonuclear leukocytes) with a normal (rarely low) glucose and a normal or high protein level. Complement-fixing antibody may be found in the spinal fluid. No correlation has been found between the severity or the type of *M. pneumoniae* infection or the height of the cold agglutinin titer and the subsequent development or extent of neurologic manifestations. *M. pneumoniae* has been isolated from the spinal fluid from one patient, and, in another patient, organisms were identified in spinal fluid by indirect immunofluorescence. In no instance, however, has *M. pneumoniae* been isolated from the brain or other neural tissue, and brain biopsies and autopsy studies have not yielded firm pathogenetic clues. Thus, the pathogenesis of the neurologic complications of *M. pneumoniae* infection remains obscure. Speculative mechanisms include

intracerebral intravascular coagulation, direct invasion, neurotoxin elaboration, and immune complex deposition.

Miscellaneous Findings

Additional nonpulmonary manifestations of M. pneumoniae infection include pharyngitis, sinusitis, rhinitis, isolated (occasionally bullous) myringitis, inappropriate antidiuretic hormone secretion, tuboovarian abscess, and immune-complex-mediated interstitial nephritis and glomerulonephritis.

Although it is clear that multisystem involvement occurs with M. pneumoniae infection in a protean fashion, serious illness or mortality remains unusual. Since M. pneumoniae is seldom isolated from sites distant from the respiratory tract, the pathogenesis of most of these extrapulmonary manifestations remains to be clarified. It is important to note that appropriate antimicrobial therapy does not appear to influence either the development or the course of the systemic complications.

Laboratory Findings and Diagnostic Methods

The white blood cell count is greater than 10,000 per cubic millimeter in approximately 25 percent of patients with M. pneumoniae pneumonia. Counts as high as 25,000 to 56,000 per cubic millimeter have been recorded in unusually severe cases. Neutrophilia, lymphocytosis, and monocytosis may all occur, but leukopenia is rare. With the exception of occasional elevation in hepatic transaminases, routine blood studies are typically normal. Transient tuberculin anergy may develop. Electrocardiographic changes suggestive of pericarditis or myocarditis may also be noted.

Radiograph abnormalities in M. pneumoniae pneumonia are highly variable. Infiltrates characteristically are unilateral patchy areas of bronchopneumonia and involve the lower lobes in 75 to 90 percent of cases. Punctate mottling and centrally dense infiltrates may be helpful diagnostic signs. Lobar consolidations with upper lobe involvement and multilobe infiltrates are unusual. Radiographic abnormalities typically resolve within 10 to 20 days, but complete resolution may require 4 to 6 weeks. Residual chest radiographic abnormalities are rare.

The laboratory diagnosis of M. pneumoniae infection can be made either by isolation of the organism from an acutely ill individual or by demonstration of an appropriate rise in specific antibody titer. Since both techniques require several weeks for positive results, the diagnosis must initially be based on the characteristic history and appropriate clinical findings. Sputum Gram stains show a moderate number of leukocytes (either mononuclear or polymorphonuclear cells), but no predominant bacterial pathogen. Routine sputum cultures grow only normal throat flora. Finding sheets of polymorphonuclear cells on

Gram stain may indicate bronchial or alveolar septal necrosis due to M. pneumoniae, but it most often reflects a secondary bacterial infection.

Although not all clinical laboratories have facilities to culture these organisms, M. pneumoniae may be readily isolated from throat washings, sputum, or throat swabs. Seven to ten days after inoculation into broth media, typical colonies may be observed by means of a binocular microscope. A presumptive identification of M. pneumoniae is made if colonies show hemadsorption of red blood cells. Although results are seldom positive, attempts to isolate the organism from bodily fluids, skin lesions, clinically involved tissues, and abscess material should nonetheless be pursued. M. pneumoniae has occasionally been recovered from middle ear and skin vesicle fluid, and on rare occasion from blood, pericardial, pleural, spinal fluid, and a tuboovarian abscess.

Serology is the best method for diagnosing M. pneumoniae infection. Optimally, serum samples should be obtained during both the acute and convalescent periods. A fourfold rise in complement fixation antibodies in paired sera is diagnostic of recent infection. Complement fixation antibody titers begin to rise 1 week after infection and peak at 3 to 4 weeks. If only a convalescent sample is available, a titer of ≥1:64 is highly suggestive of recent M. pneumoniae infection. IgM cold agglutinin antibody also appears 7 to 9 days after infection, and titers peak 4 to 6 weeks later. One-third to three-fourths of patients will develop titers of ≥1:64 or a fourfold rise in cold agglutinins. Elevated cold agglutinin titers are not specific to M. pneumoniae infections and can be seen in a variety of other infections and neoplastic disorders. However, a fourfold rise in titer or a single titer of ≥1:64 in concert with an anti-M. pneumoniae complement-fixation antibody titer of ≥1:64 is diagnostic of M. pneumoniae infection. M. pneumoniae can also result in the development of autoantibodies including antinuclear antibody, a false-positive test for syphilis (VDRL), and, in 30 percent of patients, antibody to a streptococcal organism, Streptococcus MG.

Treatment

The resolution of fever, cough, and clinical signs of pneumonia, as well as the clearing of radiographic abnormalities can be hastened by oral tetracycline or erythromycin treatment (2 g per day). Therapy is usually given for 10 to 14 days. Like tetracycline and erythromycin, other agents including chloramphenicol, clindamycin, and the aminoglycosides are mycoplasmastatic in vitro. However, clinical experience with these agents either has been very limited or has shown them to be ineffective (e.g., clindamycin). The penicillins and cephalosporins are clearly ineffective. Clinical resistance to tetracycline has been observed in patients with M. pneumoniae pneumonia despite in vitro sensitivity of the isolates. These patients

respond to erythromycin. Erythromycin-resistant, tetracycline-sensitive organisms have also been described.

M. pneumoniae often persists in respiratory tract secretions despite both appropriate drug therapy and a prompt clinical response. In one study, approximately 50 percent of those originally culture-positive remained so 6 to 13 weeks after treatment. Perhaps for this reason, antibiotic therapy is generally considered to be ineffective in halting transmission of M. pneumoniae. In one study, prophylactic tetracycline therapy was unable to limit household spread of M. pneumoniae, but it may have attenuated the severity of the transmitted illness. Since there have been no additional studies with a similar outcome, there are no formal recommendations for prophylactic treatment of household or school contacts of those infected with M. pneumoniae.

CHLAMYDIA PNEUMONIA

Chlamydia are worldwide and important causes of human infection, but most chlamydial infections are nonpulmonary. For example, C. trachomatis is primarily a pathogen of the eye and genitourinary tract and is responsible for trachoma, lymphogranuloma venereum, and many, if not most, cases of nongonococcal urethritis and pelvic inflammatory disease. On rare occasions, C. trachomatis has been associated with pneumonia in neonates and immunocompromised adults. In contrast, C. psittaci is a primary pulmonary pathogen and is responsible for psittacosis—a human and avian infection.

The Organism

Chlamydiae are obligate intracellular parasites and are therefore unable to replicate in the extracellular environment. Despite viruslike characteristics, these organisms are classified as bacteria because they have a discrete cell wall, are sensitive to some antibacterial antibiotics, and contain DNA, RNA, and ribosomes (unlike viruses) and can therefore synthesize protein. These organisms are dependent on host cell machinery for generation of ATP.

The genus Chlamydia is divided into two species, C. psittaci and C. trachomatis, which share a common lipopolysaccharide antigen but can be differentiated by two characteristics: C. psittaci is resistant to sulfonamides and forms intracellular inclusions that do not stain with iodine; C. trachomatis is sensitive to sulfonamides and forms inclusions that contain glycogen and therefore stain with iodine.

C. psittaci infects both mammal and avian species. Humans are accidental hosts acquiring the organism through contact with infected birds. The major and primary hosts for C. trachomatis are humans, but one organism in this species has been recognized as a cause of mouse pneumonitis.

Chlamydia Psittaci

Psittacosis (parrot fever) is an avian infection caused by C. psittaci. Humans become infected through exposure to discharges of infected avian species. The human infection may be either a respiratory or a systemic disease. Psittacosis is an uncommon illness, but it is an important occupational hazard to people in the poultry business, as well as pet shop owners and workers, zoo workers, pigeon fanciers, bird owners, and veterinarians.

Epidemiology

Imported parrots were the first birds implicated in human infection, thus, the illness was named for the Greek word for parrot—psittakos. Since both psittacine and nonpsittacine birds may act as hosts, however, it has been suggested by some that ornithosis is a more appropriate term. Psittacosis occurs worldwide and has been identified in over 130 species of birds, including parrots, finches, canaries, sparrows, cockatiels, parakeets, lovebirds, cockatoos, doves, egrets, and gulls. The turkey serves as a major reservoir for occupational outbreaks in the United States; in Eastern Europe, the duck has been identified as a major vector.

Up to 30 percent of city pigeons have evidence of chlamydial infection. C. psittaci is present in the blood, tissues, feathers, and discharges of infected birds (often nestlings). It is a hardy organism and can remain infectious in dried fecal matter for months. Diseased birds frequently show only minimal evidence of illness, such as ruffled feathers, lethargy, and failure to eat. Although many of these young birds die promptly, survivors often become healthy carriers, discharging chlamydiae in their feces. Overcrowding, poor sanitation, improper feeding, and insufficient cage or pen conditions contribute to the development of the disease in pet birds in pet shops or during transport.

Two hundred thirty-six cases of psittacosis were reported to the Centers for Disease Control between 1975 and 1977. Forty-six percent of these cases occurred in bird owners, 13 percent in those involved in the poultry business, and 8 percent in pet shop workers. In 8 percent of cases, there was no known bird exposure. Over half of all cases were associated with exposure to psittacine birds. In Great Britain, the incidence of psittacosis appears to be increasing, and over 300 cases are reported yearly.

Although human infection usually follows inhalation of dried bird excreta, it may also be contracted by handling contaminated plumage or tissues or, rarely, from bites. Person-to-person transmission has been well documented, but it is considered rare and therefore respiratory precautions have not been routinely recommended. However, there has been a suggestion in some reports that nonavian transmission may occur. For example, in a recent outbreak of psittacosis in 24 boarding school inhabitants,

no avium point source could be identified. Over the past 15 years, in Great Britain, only 10 to 30 percent of cases of psittacosis could be linked to contact with birds. Human-to-human or animal-(sheep, cattle)-to-human transmission are potential nonavian routes for infection, but their importance and frequency will require further clarification.

Pathogenesis

After inhalation, the organism disseminates widely and eventually reaches the reticuloendothelial cells of the liver and spleen. After replication in local mononuclear phagocytes, *C. psittaci* spreads hematogenously to the lungs and other organs. Clinical illness begins only after this bacteremia, and therefore the incubation period is long—usually 1 to 2 weeks.

The initial pulmonary events are characterized by an outpouring of proteinaceous fluid and fibrin from capillary vessels filling alveoli and distending interstitial spaces. Polymorphonuclear leukocytes predominate in the early stages, but they soon disappear and are replaced by mononuclear cells and alveolar macrophages which become infected and contain cytoplasmic inclusions filled with replicating chlamydiae (Fig. 101-3). The affected areas, usually the dependent lobes, become consolidated with a rubbery gelatinous consistency. Septal necrosis and minor hemorrhage may occur, accounting for the occasional occurrence of hemoptysis seen clinically. Bronchi and bronchioles are largely unaffected, although the latter may be involved by a lymphocytic infiltrate. The

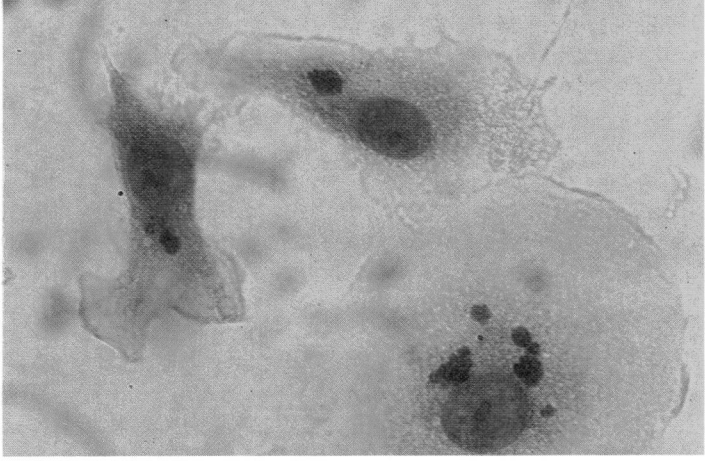

FIGURE 101-3   Bright-field photomicrograph showing *C. psittaci* replicating within normal human alveolar macrophages 20 h after in vitro challenge. Arrows indicate typical intracellular inclusions which contain numerous replicating chlamydiae. *(Reprinted with permission from Murray HW, Gellene RA, Libby DA, Rothermel ED, Rubin BY: Activation of tissue macrophages from AIDS patients: In vitro response of AIDS alveolar macrophages to lymphokines and interferon-γ. J Immunol 135:2374, 1985.)*

pleura are usually spared, but occasionally a fibrinous pleuritis has been noted.

Other pathologic changes include splenic enlargement, nonspecific splenic inflammation, reactive hepatitis, fatty degeneration and lymphocytic infiltration of the myocardium, and subendocardial hemorrhage, especially in the region of the mitral and aortic valves. In the kidney, tubular swelling or damage may occur. The central nervous system is usually unremarkable but edema, lymphocytic meningitis, and fibrinous or gelatinous arachnoiditis at the cerebral sylvian fissures have been described.

Clinical Features

GENERAL FEATURES AND PULMONARY MANIFESTATIONS

The clinical features of psittacosis are highly variable, but pulmonary symptoms usually predominate. The illness may vary from a mild and transient flulike syndrome to an acute disorder with high fever, severe headache, and a pneumonia that may progress to delirium, hypoxemia, and death.

The onset of the illness may be insidious but typically begins abruptly with chills, occasionally true rigors, fever up to 39 to 40°C, and diaphoresis. Pharyngitis, malaise, and arthralgia and severe myalgia, often in the back and neck, are common. Headache is frequent and is usually quite severe. The combination of headache and neck myalgia may mimic bacterial meningitis.

Cough usually develops after the initial symptoms have surfaced and is typically nonproductive and hacking. Occasionally, scanty mucoid or blood-streaked sputum may be produced. Auscultation characteristically reveals fine rales and, on occasion, signs of true consolidation. Pleuritic pain, pleural effusions, and friction rubs are unusual. The physical examination usually underestimates the extent of pulmonary involvement. As with other infections caused by intracellular organisms (Legionnaires' disease, typhoid fever, brucellosis), relative brachycardia (pulse-temperature dissociation) may be present.

EXTRAPULMONARY MANIFESTATIONS (SEE TABLE 101-3)

Psittacosis may also involve organs other than the lungs. In nonfatal cases, there have been reports of clinical and electrocardiographic evidence suggesting myocarditis. Endocarditis and pericarditis may occasionally occur.

Severe headache is a common but not universal symptom of psittacosis. Delirium, lethargy, and transient meningeal or focal neurologic signs may develop and can progress to coma. Rarely, a patient may present with seizures or even status epilepticus accompanied by electroencephalographic changes consistent with diffuse cerebral dysfunction.

Various hematologic abnormalities have been reported in patients with psittacosis. Anemia may develop,

TABLE 101-3
Extrapulmonary Manifestations of Psittacosis

Cardiac	Myocarditis, pericarditis, endocarditis
Neurologic	Headache, delirium—rarely, meningoencephalitis, seizures, focal neurologic signs, lymphocytic meningitis
Hematologic	Severe anemia, hemolytic anemia, positive Coombs' test, disseminated intravascular coagulation
Gastrointestinal	Hepatitis, pancreatitis, diarrhea, nausea
Renal	Proteinuria, oliguria, acute renal failure, nephritis
Miscellaneous	Splenomegaly, exudative tonsillitis, thyroiditis, fever of unknown origin, rash, arthritis

sometimes requiring transfusion. Hemolysis may occur, usually without the occurrence of cold agglutinins. Rarely, the Coombs' test is positive and persists for several months. Disseminated intravascular coagulation has been reported in fulminant cases.

Hepatitis and pancreatitis may complicate severe psittacosis. Pathologic studies have shown granulomatous hepatitis and, in patients dying of psittacosis, areas of focal hepatic necrosis. Acute pancreatitis has been reported in two severe cases.

Renal involvement has been manifested with proteinuria and oliguria. In an outbreak in 1930, pathologic studies reported cloudy swelling of renal parenchyma, glomerular congestion, and epithelial degeneration. Renal damage has been attributed to a possible direct toxic effect of the virulent chlamydial infection, although organisms have not been documented in kidney tissue.

Patients with psittacosis often have splenomegaly, considered by some as a most helpful diagnostic sign. A pale erythematous, macular, usually truncal rash similar to the evanescent rose spots of typhoid fever has been seen. Other dermatologic manifestations include measleslike eruptions, erythema nodosum, and vasculitis.

Laboratory and Radiographic Manifestations

There are no laboratory or radiologic abnormalities specifically associated with psittacosis. The leukocyte count is usually normal, although leukopenia and leukocytosis can occur. Sputum examination shows predominantly mononuclear cells. Other abnormalities include elevated transaminases and muscle enzymes, an occasional increase in serum bilirubin levels, and proteinuria. The cerebrospinal fluid is typically normal, although a mild lymphocytic pleocytosis may be detected.

Radiographic examinations of the chest show striking variability in the extent and character of infiltrates, which are generally bronchopneumonic in type. Chest films usually show patchy reticular infiltrates radiating from the hilar areas or involving the basilar lung segments (Fig. 101-4). Infiltrates are often unilateral but may be bilateral. Rarely, true lobar consolidation or pleural effusions have been seen. Because the physical examination of the chest is often unimpressive in patients with psittacosis, the clinician may be surprised by the extent of radiographic involvement.

Diagnosis

The protean manifestations of psittacosis render the diagnosis difficult to make on clinical grounds alone. A history of direct exposure to birds is an important clue to elicit especially if this occurred within the 1- to 2-week incubation period. The diagnosis is confirmed by the isolation of *C. psittaci* from sputum, tissue, or exudates.

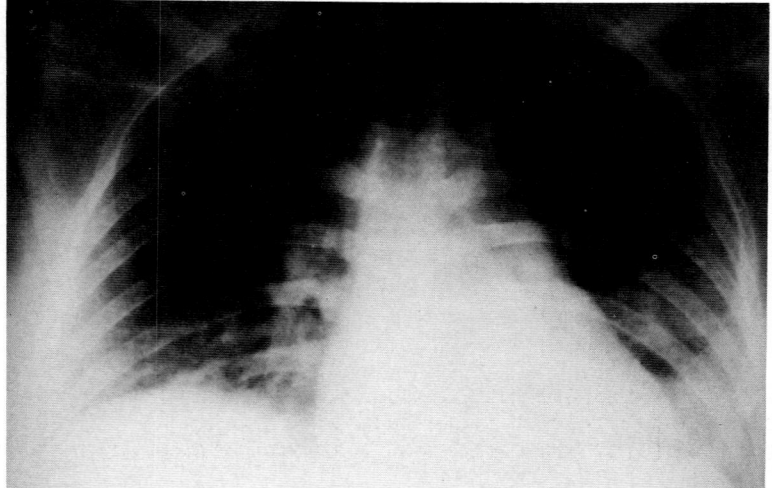 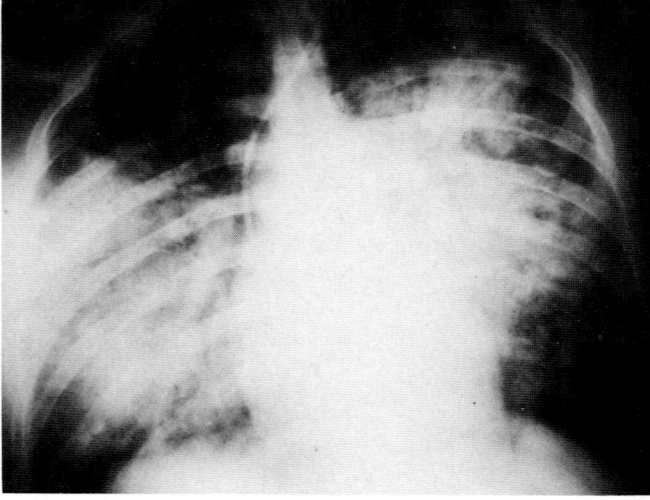

FIGURE 101-4 Chest radiographs of a 31-year-old pregnant woman with fulminant psittacosis. Admission chest film *(left)*. Chest film obtained 24 h later *(right)*. Infection due to *C. psittaci* was confirmed serologically.

Chlamydiae will not grow on routine media and instead require living cells for replication. Infected material can be inoculated onto cells in tissue culture or injected into mice (usually intraperitoneal injection). Bacteremia with *C. psittaci* has been documented on a few occasions. Because the isolation studies require laboratory expertise and are quite hazardous, serologic testing is the diagnostic method of choice. Antibodies to *C. psittaci* may be detected as early as the end of the first week of illness, but usually 2 weeks are needed for the antibody to appear. The serologic method most often used is the direct complement fixation test which detects antibodies against a heat-stable group antigen prepared from *C. psittaci*. Paired serum samples exhibiting a fourfold or greater rise in antibody titer is considered diagnostic. A titer of 1:16 during an acute pneumonic illness is presumptive evidence of disease. In untreated cases, antibody titers usually peak approximately 21 days after the onset of illness. Early treatment with tetracycline may delay the appearance of antibody for weeks. Cross-reactivity of *C. psittaci* with *Brucella*, *Coxiella burnetii*, and *Legionella pneumophila* may occur, and thus give false-positive complement fixation tests.

Pulmonary infections caused by *M. pneumoniae*, *C. burnetti*, *Francisella tularensis*, *L. pneumophila*, and by some viruses and fungi may mimic psittacosis. If pulmonary symptoms are less prominent or overshadowed, systemic febrile illnesses such as typhoid fever, tuberculosis, brucellosis, mononucleosis syndromes, infectious hepatitis, endocarditis, rheumatic fever, and sarcoidosis should be considered.

Thus, the diagnosis of psittacosis is usually based on an epidemiologic history of contact with avian species (patients should be carefully and repeatedly questioned); a clinical syndrome of high fever, severe headache, and relative bradycardia with nonbacterial pneumonia symptoms; and a fourfold rise in specific complement-fixation titer.

Treatment and Prevention

Although *C. psittaci* is sensitive to tetracycline and, to a lesser degree, to chloramphenicol and erythromycin, it has been difficult to measure the true efficacy of antibiotic therapy. Laboratory evidence and clinical experience, however, suggest that tetracycline is effective in the treatment of psittacosis. In most cases, response to tetracycline treatment may be slow and benefit may not be evident for several days. Thus, therapeutic trials with tetracycline cannot be relied on as a diagnostic maneuver. Tetracycline (2 to 3 g per day) should be continued for 10 to 14 days after defervescence. Before effective therapy was available, the mortality rate was 20 to 40 percent, but it has declined recently to as low as 1 percent. Relapse and reinfection can occur. Chronic carriage of the organism is rare but has been well documented in one patient over 10 years.

Problems in the prevention of psittacosis still exist. Historically, efforts to control psittacosis in humans have emphasized administrative procedures such as embargoes or bans on shipment of avian species. As a result of pressures from bird fanciers and the pet industry, importation of exotic birds has been reopened with the proviso that the birds be treated. Chlortetracycline-impregnated millet seeds are commercially available for the treatment of chlamydial infection in parakeets. Liquid vehicles have been developed for nectar-feeding birds, and medicated mash has been formulated for the treatment of larger psittacines such as parrots. These medicated feeds may be used therapeutically or prophylactically to eradicate latent chlamydial infection. In addition, the U.S. Public Health Service regulations require that imported psittacine species receive a 45-day course of chlortetracycline in a quarantine center licensed by the U.S. Department of Agriculture before being released for sale. Tetracycline feed does not affect organisms that have already contaminated the plumage. Smuggled birds are not affected by these measures.

Despite the above precautions, there has recently been a small increase in the number of human cases of psittacosis. Most of these are associated with contact in the commercial flow of the pet bird industry. The potential for point-source outbreaks in pet stores and department stores has been clearly documented. The absence of adequate monitoring may be a flaw in the current regulations concerning treatment of imported psittacines.

TWAR Infections

Recent reports from Europe, Japan, Taiwan, and the United States have implicated a new strain of *C. psittaci* (termed TWAR) that causes community-acquired lower respiratory tract infections in patients who do not have a history of exposure to birds. This organism's primary mode of transmission seems to be human to human. The prevalence of antibody to the TWAR strain in adult populations is in the 25 to 45 percent range, exceeding the antibody prevalence to all other *Chlamydia* strains in these populations. In seroepidemiologic studies of community-acquired pneumonias in adults, 10 to 21 percent of patients had serologic evidence of recent TWAR infection, suggesting that this organism is an important pulmonary pathogen.

Pulmonary infection caused by TWAR strains ranges from mild (pharyngitis, bronchitis) to severe illness (pneumonia). Severe and fatal pneumonia ascribed to TWAR has been reported in elderly patients. Most symptomatic patients complain of sore throat, fever, laryngitis, and a cough (often hacking, occasionally productive of purulent phlegm). Rales in the affected lobe and, on occasion, wheezing can be heard on examination. The respira-

tory illness produced by TWAR mimics the illness caused by *Mycoplasma* in many respects (prodromal pharyngitis, hacking cough, mild pneumonia). However, in contrast to *Mycoplasma*: (1) TWAR infections have not been associated with extrapulmonary signs or symptoms, and (2) TWAR infections seem to cause a more prolonged illness and are more likely to relapse. Relapse of pulmonary symptoms has been described in patients infected with TWAR who are treated with an anti-*Mycoplasma* regimen (erythromycin). Some of these patients have responded, subsequently, to tetracycline (2 g per day). Tetracycline (14-day course) may be a more appropriate regimen for TWAR infections. Clinical relapse and the need for prolonged therapy are likely related to the fact that TWAR, a *Chlamydia*, is an intracellular pathogen.

Diagnosis of TWAR infection can be made by isolation of the organism (cell culture technique) or serology. Neither methodology is routinely available at present.

Chlamydia Trachomatis Pneumonia

In contrast to *C. psittaci*, *C. trachomatis* is primarily a pathogen of humans. *C. trachomatis* usually causes ocular or genital infections, and pulmonary disease is an uncommon manifestation.

Pneumonitis caused by *C. trachomatis* typically affects infants 2 to 12 weeks old. The onset is gradual, and the course is characteristically protracted, lasting a month or longer. Most affected infants are afebrile. Initial symptoms are rhinitis with a mucoid nasal discharge or nasal obstruction. Later developments include a staccato cough that differs from pertussis in that there is no postcough whoop, tachypnea that can be profound, and rales. The chest radiograph usually reveals interstitial infiltrates and hyperinflated lungs but may show atelectasis, bronchopneumonia, or a reticulonodular pattern. Pleural reaction or lobar consolidation is extremely rare. Elevated IgG and IgM levels are noted as is mild eosinophilia. Approximately one-half of affected infants have clinical conjunctivitis. Myocarditis, pleural effusion, and apneic spells have been reported in association with *C. trachomatis* pneumonia. *C. trachomatis* has also been implicated in nonpneumonic illness such as nasopharyngitis, otitis media, and bronchitis.

Diagnosis of *C. trachomatis* infection can be made presumptively by identifying the characteristic inclusions in conjunctival or respiratory secretions or lung tissue or, more definitively, by culturing the organism from these materials. Elevated IgM antibody to the organism can also be detected.

In one series, *C. trachomatis* was cultured from either nasopharyngeal or tracheal aspirates in 18 of 20 infants with this syndrome. In the same series, *C. trachomatis* was recovered from 2 of 15 infants with nonocular nonpneumonic illnesses and from 10 of 12 infants with inclusion conjunctivitis but without lower respiratory tract illness. Infants with pneumonia differed from those with inclusion conjunctivitis alone in having significantly higher antibody levels against *Chlamydia*.

C. trachomatis is probably the most common etiologic agent in the diffuse pneumonitis syndrome of infants. In a recent prospective study of 104 infants with this syndrome, *C. trachomatis* was responsible for 25 percent of cases; the remainder were due to *Ureaplasma urealyticum*, cytomegalovirus, and *Pneumocystis carinii*. The clinical features and radiographic presentation of these pneumonias are indistinguishable. Diffuse pneumonitis in infants can be due to more than one pathogen; these multipathogen infections are not uncommon and are usually severe.

Therapy for the *C. trachomatis* syndrome in infants with either sulfisoxazole (100 mg/kg per day) or erythromycin ethyl succinate (40 mg/kg per day) for 2 to 3 weeks is effective.

In adults, *C. trachomatis* can cause a variety of respiratory tract infections ranging from pharyngitis to severe diffuse pneumonitis. The incidence of *C. trachomatis*-associated respiratory diseases in adults is unknown. Serologic evidence for *C. trachomatis* infection has been found in sporadically occurring cases of otherwise unexplained community-acquired pneumonia in normal adults. These patients present with a nonproductive or minimally productive cough, fever, myalgia, and, less commonly, rigors, hemoptysis, or pleuritic chest pain. Chest radiograph reveals patchy, streaky infiltrates with areas of platelike atelectasis. Involvement can be multi- or unilobar. Air bronchograms or pleural effusions are unusual.

C. trachomatis has been isolated from respiratory secretions and open lung biopsy specimens from immunocompromised adults. Presentations in this patient group have ranged from bronchitis and lobar pneumonia to severe diffuse interstitial pneumonitis. It appears that the severity of pulmonary infection is proportional to the degree of immunosuppression.

The histologic picture on lung biopsy specimens is one of interstitial inflammation which can be nodular in distribution and appearance. Lymphocytes and macrophages are prominent in this inflammatory reaction. Intracytoplasmic inclusions with *C. trachomatis* may not always be detected even if the organism has been cultured from these specimens. Concomitant infection with cytomegalovirus is common.

Therapy with erythromycin or a tetracycline appears to be effective. Whether this pneumonitis represents a newly acquired opportunistic infection or reactivation of a latent infection is still uncertain.

C. trachomatis also represents an occupational hazard to laboratory workers. Respiratory illness from laboratory exposure to the serotype of *C. trachomatis* that causes lymphogranuloma venereum has been documented. This infection resulted in interstitial pneumonia, pleural ef-

fusions, and mediastinal as well as supraclavicular lymphadenopathy. Pulmonary infection due to lymphogranuloma venereum stains of *C. trachomatis* is an extremely rare occurrence and, except for one or two occasions, does not occur outside a laboratory setting.

Q FEVER PNEUMONIA

Q fever was first described in 1935 in Australian abattoir workers in whom an unidentified organism was recovered from urine and blood. "Q" stood for query, since the etiology of the illness was unknown. The causative agent was subsequently isolated by Davis and Cox from ticks in Montana and was identified as *Rickettsia*-like by Burnet and Freeman. It was first named *Rickettsia burnetii* but now is most often referred to as *Coxiella burnetii*.

The Organism

C. burnetii is an obligate intracellular organism that differs in several major aspects from the other members of genus *Rickettsia*. It fails to evoke cross-reacting serum agglutinins to *Proteus* X strains (Weil-Felix reaction), is only rarely associated with a rash, and does not require an arthropod vector to maintain itself in nature. The organism has a spore stage and this may, in part, explain its hardiness. *C. burnetii* is highly resistant to physical and chemical agents such as toxic levels of heat, formaldehyde, and phenol. Viable *C. burnetii* have been recovered from fresh meat in storage after more than 1 month, animal blood, clay, or sand after 4 to 6 months, wool after 7 to 9 months, dry tick feces after 18 months, and tap water and milk after 30 to 42 months.

C. burnetii exhibit different antigens in different culture conditions (phase variation). Organisms in nature and isolated from laboratory animals have phase I antigens. Passage of phase I organisms in embryonated chicken eggs yields organisms with phase II antigens.

Epidemiology

The organism infects a wide variety of insects, rodents, and large domestic as well as wild animals. The disease is usually maintained in nature by animal-to-animal spread via ticks. In transmission to humans, the milk, feces, urine, placentas, and uterine discharges of infected sheep, goats, and cattle are most often implicated. In the United States, domestic livestock infection is common and subclinical. The resistance of *C. burnetii* to drying allows the dust in sheep pens and cattle sheds to become heavily contaminated, and human infection usually follows inhalation. The association with livestock need not be intimate. In one urban outbreak, the affected patients were exposed to *C. burnetii* only during their commute through a region with a livestock farm. Outbreaks have occurred in

wool and felt processing plants and tanneries and have been related to contaminated laundry and dusty straw used for packing. Airborne spread in one university medical research facility occurred in an environment where research with sheep was being conducted. Infection may also occur in laboratory workers; the handling of infected egg cultures or animals inoculated with the organism must always be considered hazardous.

Transmission by tick bite probably occurs as well. There is also evidence to suggest that Q fever may develop following the organism's penetration of skin abrasions or the conjunctivae. Person-to-person transmission of *C. burnetii* is unusual but has occurred, presumably via droplet spray and, on one occasion, via blood transfusion.

Human infection is rare in the United States. Approximately 20 to 60 cases of clinical illnesses are reported each year. Subclinical infections undoubtedly occur more frequently. Q fever is an important occupational hazard to abattoir workers and veterinarians. Cats may harbor *C. burnetii* and are a newly recognized and important animal vector. In one survey of Q fever in Nova Scotia, approximately 20 percent of patients had exposure to feline litters.

Pathogenesis

After inhalation, organisms multiply in the lung (or other sites of entry) followed by hematogenous spread to other organs. Later they may be excreted in the urine. Since Q fever is most often a benign illness, few patients have come to autopsy. Histologically, a mononuclear exudate helps to distinguish the process from a bacterial infection. Alveolar walls become thickened by infiltration with macrophages, lymphocytes, and plasma cells. The alveolar exudates are mostly composed of macrophages; polymorphonuclear leukocytes are conspicuously absent. The bronchiolar mucosa may be necrotic. Widespread lesions have been noted in the pericardium, spleen, liver, brain, kidney, and testis, and *C. burnetii* has been observed lying free within macrophages in various organs. In Q fever endocarditis, organisms may be isolated from or observed in valvular tissue and vegetations.

Clinical Features

The incubation period is usually 20 days, with a range of 2 to 5 weeks. The most common syndrome associated with *C. burnetii* infection is a self-limited, acute illness that is characterized by high fevers, severe headache, and myalgias. Less commonly, patients present with a sore throat, nausea, vomiting, rigors, diarrhea, confusion, and abdominal pain. Pulse-temperature dissociation may be detected.

In the vast majority of cases, Q fever is a benign, self-limited illness which resolves within 1 or 2 weeks with or without treatment. Although fever may persist for up to 3

months in atypical cases, patients are usually afebrile by the second week of illness. Sometimes, despite treatment, the course of Q fever may be complicated by extrapulmonary lesions, persistence of symptoms, or relapse. On occasion, the syndrome of chronic Q fever develops, with endocarditis being a prominent feature. *C. burnetii* infections may also be asymptomatic, being detected only by fortuitous serum antibody testing.

Pneumonia

The occurrence of pulmonary involvement in Q fever is highly variable and has been reported in 0 to 90 percent of cases. Geographic considerations appear to be important. Pneumonia is uncommon in Q fever in Australia (5 to 9 percent of cases) but more typical in Nova Scotia and California outbreaks (30 to 85 percent of cases). In a recent cluster of cases in a medical research facility, significant respiratory symptoms were notably rare. The cause(s) for this variable incidence of respiratory involvement is not apparent. Strain virulence differences have been reported and may be important. The inhaled inoculum may also be a factor. In one study, monkeys challenged with a large dose of *C. burnetii* organisms developed pneumonia, whereas monkeys that inhaled a small dose did not.

More than one-half of Q fever patients with pneumonia develop a nonproductive cough. Chest pain, frequently pleuritic, occurs in 15 to 45 percent of cases. The physical examination usually reveals fine rales and, at times, signs of consolidation. The exam typically underestimates the extensive infiltrates seen on the radiograph. Clinically, the pneumonia is usually mild and responds to therapy, but rapidly progressive, severe pneumonia can occur.

EXTRAPULMONARY MANIFESTATIONS (SEE TABLE 101-4)

Although pneumonia is the most common clinical presentation, Q fever is a true systemic infection that may produce disease in other organs. Hepatitis may be mild or can progress to jaundice, marked transaminase elevation and, rarely, death. Pathologic studies of the liver in these cases have revealed minimal to widespread parenchymal inflammation, necrosis, and granulomata. Organisms have

TABLE 101-4
Nonrespiratory Manifestations of Q Fever

Gastrointestinal	Hepatitis
Vascular	Thrombophlebitis, arteritis
Cardiac	Pericarditis, pericardial effusion, myocarditis, endocarditis
Ocular	Uveitis, iritis, optic neuritis
Neurologic	Meningitis, neuropathy
Miscellaneous	Otitis, arthritis, epididymitis, abortion, congenital malformations, fever of unknown origin

been demonstrated in the liver. Headache may be a prominent feature on presentation. Encephalitis, focal neurologic signs, and neuropathy have been reported but are rare. Vascular complications include thrombophlebitis with pulmonary embolism, arteritis, and thromboangiitis obliterans. Cardiovascular involvement has also been documented with pleuropericarditis, pericardial effusion, myocarditis, and endocarditis. The last is usually a manifestation of chronic Q fever and represents one of the causes of culture-negative endocarditis.

A number of hematologic abnormalities have been reported: bone marrow granulomata, histiocytic erythophagocytosis, hemolytic anemia, and a leukoerythroblastic peripheral blood picture. Additional nonrespiratory manifestations of Q fever include ocular disease (uveitis, iritis, optic neuritis), arthritis, otitis, epididymitis, abortion, and congenital malformations. Transient truncal erythematous macules have been observed on rare occasions. A few patients with Q fever fail to recover fully their general health and have experienced prolonged weakness, fatigue, weight loss, and vague aches.

C. burnetii may also persist in the liver (granulomatous hepatitis), osteomyelitis lesions, and vascular grafts and cause the chronic Q fever syndrome.

Laboratory and Radiographic Manifestations

Routine studies yield little helpful information. The white blood cell count is typically normal, or mildly elevated, with a slight shift to the left. The serum transaminase and alkaline phosphatase may be elevated. Gram stain of the sputum shows predominantly mononuclear leukocytes. Although headache and nuchal rigidity are often present, cerebrospinal fluid is usually unremarkable.

The chest radiographic abnormalities often resemble viral and *Mycoplasma* pneumonias with patchy infiltrates. However, in Q fever, the predominant pattern is alveolar rather than interstitial. Commonly, one can observe multiple, round 5- to 10-mm opacities of ground glass density, usually in the lower lobes. These lesions can be quite radio-dense and simulate coin or mass lesions (pseudotumors). Platelike linear atelectasis (again usually lower lobe) or partial or complete lobar consolidation can be seen. Pleural effusions occur in less than 10 percent of cases, and hilar adenopathy is rare. Infiltrates may take up to 10 weeks to resolve, but resolution in most cases is complete by 3 to 4 weeks.

Diagnosis

A history of direct or indirect exposure to livestock, ticks, or an ill patient with atypical pneumonia should arouse suspicion of Q fever. Moreover, one must be aware that Q fever may be a hazard of tourism since patients may have visited an endemic area and become infected before returning home. Medical centers engaged in research with

pregnant cats or livestock should be alert to the risk of Q fever.

The diagnosis is established either by isolation of *C. burnetii* or demonstration of a significant rise in specific antibody titer. *C. burnetii* has been recovered from blood, sputum, urine, spinal and pleural fluids, and tissue obtained by biopsy or at postmortem. If detected, rickettsemia can be found in the acute phase of the illness. Clinical materials may be inoculated into guinea pigs, hamsters, mice, or embryonated eggs. Animals are examined 4 to 6 weeks later for the presence of specific antibody. All isolation procedures are extremely hazardous and are not recommended routinely. Adequate safeguards must be in place.

Direct identification of *C. burnetii* in tissue may be accomplished by fluorescent antibody technique or by detecting intracytoplasmic organisms in macrophages by electron microscopy. Q fever pneumonia has also been diagnosed by transbronchial lung biopsy. Serologic diagnostic methods are simpler and safer and most often used to establish the diagnosis. Specific antibodies, identified by ELISA, complement fixation, microagglutination, and microimmunofluorescence, appear in humans 2 to 4 weeks after the onset of illness.

Antibody to phase II antigen usually exceeds antibody to phase I antigen in acute Q fever. A fourfold rise in IgG antibodies detected by complement function, microagglutination or immunofluorescence in paired acute and convalescent serum samples is diagnostic. IgM antibodies to *C. burnetii* can be found by a variety of techniques, including enzyme-linked immunosorbent assay (ELISA), and may persist in serum for up to 17 weeks after the onset of clinical illness. Detection of IgM antibody to *C. burnetii* is a particularly useful technique if only one serum sample is available. Weil-Felix agglutination tests are negative. A diagnosis of chronic Q fever is strongly supported by detecting antibody to phase I antigen in a titer of ≥1:200.

In considering the patient with suspected Q fever, the additional diagnostic considerations are numerous and depend on the mode of presentation. Pneumonia due to *C. burnetii* can be similar to tularemia (rural prevalence, animal exposure), Legionnaires' disease, psittacosis, influenza, and *Mycoplasma* pneumonia. If hepatitis or the extrapulmonary manifestations of chronic Q fever predominate, tuberculosis, brucellosis, neoplasm, endocarditis, typhoid fever, infectious mononucleosis, toxoplasmosis, leptospirosis, or histoplasmosis should be considered.

Treatment and Prevention

C. burnetii are sensitive in vitro to tetracycline and chloramphenicol. These antibiotics inhibit the growth of but do not kill these organisms. It is not clear whether therapy with these antibiotics alters the routine clinical course of the illness. In clinical practice, patients who are acutely ill or those with persistent symptoms or relapses are treated with antibiotics. Many patients with mild or subclinical illness improve without therapy or sequelae.

Tetracycline (2 g per day in divided doses) or doxycycline are the antibiotics of choice because of drug safety. Chloramphenicol is an effective alternative. Erythromycin also appears to have been used successfully in some patients (initially thought to have Legionnaires' disease) but the addition of rifampin was required in a few fulminant cases of progressive pneumonia. Tetracycline, doxycycline, trimethoprim-sulfamethoxazole and rifampin (in combination with one of the other antibiotics) are effective in Q fever endocarditis and chronic Q fever.

Measures to reduce the likelihood of infection in areas where Q fever is enzootic in domestic livestock are desirable. Milk should be boiled or pasteurized at high temperatures. Vaccines are currently undergoing investigation in field trials. Although the possibility of person-to-person transmission is not sufficient to warrant quarantine procedures, sputum, blood, urine, and other infected specimens, clothing, and autopsy material should be handled carefully.

BIBLIOGRAPHY

General

Massie TJ, Haldane EV, Noble MA, Faulkner RS, Martin RS, Lee SH: Causes of atypical pneumonia: Results of a one year prospective study. Can Med Assoc J 125(10):1118–1123, 1981.
   Twenty-seven consecutive "atypical" pneumonias were investigated over a 1-year period. Of note, three were due to C. burnetii and, in eleven, no cause could be identified.

Reiman HA: An acute infection of the respiratory tract with atypical pneumonia: A disease entity probably caused by a filterable virus. JAMA 251(7):936–944, 1984.
   Reprint of the landmark article, originally published in 1938, which was one of the earliest to characterize pneumonias as atypical.

Yung AP, Newton-John HF, Stanley PA: Atypical pneumonia: Recognition and treatment. Med J Aust 147:132–136, 1987.
> *Atypical pneumonia is a common clinical syndrome, the most common infectious causes of which are Mycoplasma pneumoniae, Chlamydia psittaci, Coxiella burnetii, and Legionella species.*

Mycoplasma Pneumoniae

Bayer AS, Galpin JE, Theofilopoules AN, Guze LB: Neurologic diseases associated with *Mycoplasma pneumoniae* pneumonias: Demonstration of viable *Mycoplasma pneumoniae* in cerebrospinal fluid and blood by radioisotopic and immunofluorescent tissue culture techniques. Ann Intern Med 94:15–80, 1981.
> *Viable mycoplasma were found in CSF during the acute neurologic syndrome which developed 25 days after the pneumonitis began.*

Case records of the Massachusetts General Hospital: Case 39-1983. N Engl J Med 309:782–789, 1983.
> *Discusses the hemolytic anemia associated with M. pneumoniae infection.*

Cassell GH, Cole BC: Myoplasmas as agents of human disease. N Engl J Med 304:80–89, 1981.
> *Review of pulmonary and nonpulmonary infections with 112 references.*

Fine NL, Smith LR, Sheedy IF: Frequency of pleural effusions in mycoplasma and viral pneumonias. N Engl J Med 283:790–793, 1970.
> *Six of twenty-nine patients with M. pneumoniae pneumonia had a pleural effusion.*

Foy HM, Kenny GE, Cooney MK, Allan ID: Long term epidemiology of infections with Mycoplasma pneumoniae. J Infect Dis 139:681–687, 1979.
> *Epidemiology of endemic and epidemic M. pneumoniae in Seattle, Washington, between 1963 and 1975.*

Foy HM, Ochs H, Davis SD, Kenny GE, Luce RR: *Mycoplasma pneumoniae* infections in patients with immunodeficiency syndromes. J Infect Dis 127:388–393, 1973.
> *These four patients had a modestly severe illness with cough but did not develop pneumonia.*

Koletsky RJ, Weinstein AJ: Fulminant *Mycoplasma pneumoniae* infection. Am Rev Respir Dis 122:491–496, 1980.
> *Mycoplasma pneumoniae can cause catastrophic illness. Discusses 11 cases.*

Murray HW, Masur H, Senterfit LB, Roberts RB: The protean manifestations of *Mycoplasma pneumoniae* infections in adults. Am J Med 58:229–241, 1975.
> *Extensive review of the pulmonary and nonpulmonary spectrum of signs and symptoms in M. pneumoniae infection.*

Smith CB, Golden CA, Tanner RE, Renzetti AD: Association of viral and *Mycoplasma pneumoniae* infections with acute respiratory illness in patients with chronic obstructive pulmonary diseases. Am Rev Respir Dis 121:225–232, 1980.
> *Viral infections predominated, but M. pneumoniae is an important pathogen.*

Psittacosis

Byrom NP, Wells J, Mair HJ: Fulminant psittacosis. Lancet 1:353–356, 1979.
> *Generally a mild illness, psittacosis can be overwhelming and produce multisystem failure.*

Hirshman JV: Psittacosis. Med Grand Rounds 1(1):57–66, 1982.
> *Thorough review with 49 references.*

Saikko P, Wang SP, Kleemola M, Brander E, Rusanen E, Grayston JT: An epidemic of mild pneumonia due to an unusual strain of *Chlamydia psittaci*. J Infect Dis 151:832–839, 1985.
> *Description of a community-acquired pneumonia, not associated with avian exposure, caused by a newly recognized strain of C. psittaci.*

Schaffner W, Drutz DJ, Duncan GW, Koenig MG: The clinical spectrum of endemic psittacosis. Arch Intern Med 119:433–443, 1967.
> *Nine illustrative case histories. Presentations often simulated bacterial pneumonias.*

C. trachomatis

Beem MO, Saxon EM: Respiratory tract colonization and a distinctive pneumonia syndrome in infants infected with *Chlamydia trachomatis*. N Engl J Med 296:306–310, 1977.
Clinical and serologic aspects of this syndrome in 20 infants.

Edelman RR, Hann LE, Simon M: *Chlamydia trachomatis* pneumonia in adults: radiographic appearance. Radiology 152:279–282, 1984.
Streaky, multilobar infiltrates were the common radiographic findings in six adults with this pneumonia.

Grayston JT, Kuo C, Wang S, Altman J.: A new *Chlamydia psittaci* strain (TWAR) isolated in acute respiratory tract infections. N Engl J Med 315:162–168, 1986.
TWAR is a common cause of upper respiratory tract infections in young adults.

Ito JI, Comess KA, Alexander ER, Harrison HR, Ray CG, Kiviat J, Subonya RE: Pneumonia due to *Chlamydia trachomatis* in an immunocompromised adult. N Engl J Med 307:95–98, 1982.
A case report of a patient with myeloblastic leukemia in whom immunosuppression was associated with pneumonia due to Chlamydia trachomatis.

Komaroff AL, Aronson MD, Schachter J: *Chlamydia trachomatis* infection in adults with community acquired pneumonia. JAMA 245:1319–1322, 1981.
A study of 52 adult patients admitted to the hospital over a 11-month period with symptoms suggesting pulmonary infection. Definite serologic evidence of recent chlamydial infection was found in 21 percent (4/19) of patients with pneumonia of unclear etiology, and in 0 percent (0/33) of patients with other pulmonary conditions. An additional three patients with pneumonia had suggestive serologic evidence of recent chlamydial infection.

Paran H, Heimer D, Sarov I: Serological, clinical and radiological findings in adults with bronchopulmonary infections caused by Chlamydia trachomatis. Isr J Med Sci 22:823–827, 1986.
A report of four cases of lower respiratory tract infection caused by Chlamydia trachomatis, three of whom had clinical and radiologic findings of atypical pneumonia.

Tack KJ, Rasp FL, Henlo D, Peterson TK, O'Leary M, Simmons RL, Sabeth LD: Isolation of *Chlamydia trachomatis* from the lower respiratory tract of adults. Lancet 1:116–120, 1980.
Three articles that describe C. trachomatis lower respiratory tract infections in adults. Severity of illness is related to the degree of immune compromise.

Q Fever

Marrie TJ: Q fever pneumonia. Med Grand Rounds 3:354–365, 1985.
Excellent and comprehensive review with chest radiograph, with 103 references.

Marrie TJ, Schlech WF III, Williams JC, Yates L: Q fever pneumonia associated with exposure to wild rabbits. Lancet 1:427–429, 1986.
Four patients with atypical pneumonia and a history of exposure to wild rabbits were found to have antibodies to Coxiella burnetii but not to the other organisms also commonly associated with atypical pneumonia.

Millar JK: The chest film findings in Q fever: A series of 35 cases. Clin Radiol 29:371–375, 1978.
Round opacities are characteristic.

Salmon MM, Howells B, Glencross EJ, Evans AD, Palmer SR: Q fever in an urban area. Lancet 1:1002–1004, 1982.
Only identifiable exposure for these patients was their daily commute past farms.

Spelman DW: Q fever: A study of 111 consecutive cases. Med J Aust 1:547–553, 1982.
Pneumonia is uncommon in Q fever and developed in only 8 of 111 cases.

Chapter 102

Legionnaires' Disease

Richard D. Meyer / Paul H. Edelstein

The term *Legionnaires' disease* refers to a distinct clinical entity characterized by a pneumonic illness with systemic manifestations caused by the gram-negative bacillus *Legionella pneumophila*. *L. pneumophila* also uncommonly causes extrapulmonary infection. Since at least 12 of the other 21 reported species of *Legionella* have also been shown to cause disease, it may be preferable to state the *Legionella* species causing disease regardless of clinical manifestations, for example, *L. micdadei* pneumonia. A mild nonpneumonic form of epidemic illness likely caused by certain *Legionella* species is known as *Pontiac fever*.

The 1976 epidemic of pneumonia in Philadelphia at an American Legion convention led to recognition and naming of the clinical entity of Legionnaires' disease and to later isolation and identification of the etiologic agent by workers at the Centers for Disease Control (CDC). These findings and the demonstration that *Legionella* had caused and currently causes both community-acquired and nosocomial disease indicate that it is neither a new nor an unusual infection.

ETIOLOGIC AGENTS

The agents of Legionnaires' disease are all members of the gram-negative bacterial family, Legionellaceae, which contains a single genus, *Legionella* (Table 102-1). *L. pneumophila* is the most common cause of pneumonia and other infections, followed by *L. micdadei*, *L. longbeachae*, and *L. dumoffii*. The remainder of the more than 25 species that have been frequently isolated are environmental isolates. It is incorrect to assume that species not yet isolated from human specimens are nonpathogenic, but it is probably reasonable to say that they will cause disease less frequently than *L. pneumophila*. Several of the species are in turn divided into serogroups. No evidence exists that infections caused by different serogroups or species require different treatment; therefore species and serogroup identification is of no clinical utility, although either may be very important for taxonomic and epidemiologic purposes.

The legionellae are gram-negative aerobic bacilli that utilize amino acids rather than carbohydrates for energy sources. L-cysteine is required for primary growth. None of the legionellae will grow on routine media used for culture of respiratory tract specimens such as blood agar media or MacConkey medium; rarely legionellae are recovered from nonselective chocolate agar medium supplemented with L-cysteine. The best growth medium is buffered charcoal yeast extract medium supplemented with α-ketoglutaric acid, which can be made semiselective for legionellae by addition of various antimicrobial drugs.

Species are differentiated from one another primarily by analysis of DNA hybridization, although many species can also be differentiated from one another by phenotypic characteristics. The most useful differential phenotypic characteristics include serotype, cellular fatty acid composition determined by gas-liquid chromatography, and cellular isoprenoid quinone (ubiquinone) composition determined by high-pressure liquid chromatography.

Considerable phenotypic overlap occurs between species, so it is often difficult to identify legionellae precisely to the species level.

MICROBIAL ECOLOGY

Treated and natural waters are the reservoirs for legionellae. These organisms are commonly found in

TABLE 102-1
Legionella Species and Serogroups

Species	No. of Serogroups	Comments
L. pneumophila	11	Most common clinical and environmental isolate
L. micdadei	1	Second most common clinical isolate; appears to affect a greater population of immunosuppressed patients than does L. pneumophila; also known as Pittsburgh pneumonia agent
L. longbeachae	2	Rare clinical isolate
L. dumoffii	1	Rare clinical isolate
L. gormanii	1	Rare clinical isolate
L. hackeliae	2	Rare clinical isolate
L. maceachernii	1	Rare clinical isolate
L. bozemanii	2	Uncommon clinical isolate
L. wadsworthii	1	Rare clinical isolate
L. rubrilucens	1	Red or yellow pigmentation; rare environmental isolate
L. erythra	1	Red or yellow pigmentation; rare environmental isolate
L. anisa	1	Rare environmental isolate
L. sainthelensi	1	Rare environmental isolate
L. spiritensis	1	Rare environmental isolate
L. parisiensis	1	Rare environmental isolate
L. cherrii	1	Rare environmental isolate
L. steigerwaltii	1	Rare environmental isolate
L. oakridgensis	1	Rare environemntal isolate
L. jordanis	1	Rare environmental isolate
L. jamestowniensis	1	Rare environmental isolate

freshwater lakes, ponds, stagnant rainwater, hot water heaters, air-conditioning cooling towers, and tap water. Pipes, other plumbing fixtures such as shower heads, and plumbing materials, particularly rubber washers, can all be colonized by legionellae. Water and fixtures colonized by legionellae also contain other microbial flora which provide nutrition. Hot water heaters and associated plumbing fixtures, and air conditioning cooling towers are probably the main organism amplifiers. Legionellae can be aerosolized from air-conditioning cooling towers, evaporative condensers, shower heads, faucets, humidifiers, and nebulizers; this probably represents the major mode of spread. A carrier state seems unlikely based on epidemiologic evidence, and asymptomatic colonization, if it occurs, is likely rare.

PATHOGENESIS AND IMMUNITY

Relatively little is known about the role of organism virulence factors in disease pathogenesis. A number of toxins are produced by L. pneumophila, which can cause hemolysis, cytolysis, malfunction of white blood cells, proteolysis, coagulation, and other in vitro phenomena. L. pneumophila and the majority of the other Legionella species studied produce species-specific β-lactamases.

L. pneumophila is a facultative intracellular parasite. Resistance to intracellular killing by inhibition of phagolysosomal fusion and intraphagosomal acidification are probably major virulence determinants. Immune or activated monocytes do, however, limit parasitism. The initial phagocytosis of L. pneumophila by monocytes occurs by an unusual mechanism of engulfment within a pseudopod coil. Legionellae adhere to a variety of cells cultured in vitro, including MRC-5 cells, a semicontinuous line of human embryonic lung fibroblasts, but the pathophysiological importance of this is unclear.

Several animal models of Legionnaires' disease exist, the best studied of which are in guinea pigs, rats, and non-human primates. Pneumonia is caused by aerosol or intratracheal delivery of bacteria in these models.

It is unclear whether the systemic manifestations of the disease are due to extrapulmonary infection or toxin elaboration. Bacteremia does occur and is a possible mode of spread. Extrapulmonary infection with inflammation has been documented in unusual instances involving the brain with leukoencephalopathy, lymph nodes, peritoneum, kidneys, liver, spleen, bone marrow, myocardium, paranasal sinus, skin and soft tissue, and arteriovenous fistula site.

PATHOLOGY

Legionella pneumonia begins as a subsegmental pneumonia that progresses to a segmental pneumonia and, in some cases, to lobar pneumonia. The hallmarks of pathologic examination in fatal cases are lobar, or less commonly segmental, consolidation. Pleuritis with pleural effusion, and hilar lymphadenopathy may also occur. Dense nodular outlines can be demonstrated with paper-mounted sections in some cases. Small macroscopic abscesses are seen uncommonly. Abnormalities due to Legionella outside the thorax are only uncommonly noted on gross examination. On microscopic examination there

is an acute purulent pneumonia with dense infiltration of intra-alveolar neutrophils and macrophages in varying states of lysis usually accompanied by a prominent fibrinous reaction; microabscesses are not uncommon. The larger airways and alveolar septa are spared.

Organisms are readily demonstrated in parenchymal tissue, less commonly in pleural tissue, and rarely in hilar lymph nodes. Extrapulmonary *L. pneumophila* has been detected by stains in the aforementioned sites, frequently associated with inflammation.

Routine tissue stains, including hematoxylin and eosin, Brown-Brenn and methanamine silver stains, do not usually show *Legionella*. Tissue imprints stained by the Brown-Brenn method may, however, show a few faintly staining gram-negative bacilli. The Kinyoun acid fast stain reacts with a minority of *L. micdadei* present and uncommonly even with a few *L. pneumophila* organisms. The Giménez stain of a tissue imprint of either fresh or fixed lung tissue is the best nonimmunologic method to demonstrate bacilli. The Dieterle silver impregnation stain or a modified Giménez stain, both of which are nonspecific, can be used for paraffinized tissue. Direct immunofluorescence examination is the most specific and sensitive means to visualize *Legionella* in tissues and blood fluids and is also suitable for either formalinized or deparaffinized specimens. Ultrastructural examination shows intracellular bacilli in phagosomes and/or cytoplasmic vacuoles.

EPIDEMIOLOGY

General

Sporadic cases surely outnumber defined outbreak cases even though sporadic cases are underreported. Over 20 nosocomial outbreaks of varying numbers of cases and duration have been reported from the United States and an additional 12 from Europe and Asia. Outbreaks in the United States and Europe have also been described as linked with other large buildings, particularly hotels and, less commonly, office buildings.

The initial CDC studies of the 1976 outbreak at the Philadelphia hotel and its environs with over 200 cases led to suspicion of airborne spread, which is compatible with later knowledge of contaminated water elsewhere. The usual incubation period for pneumonic disease was 2 to 10 days, with no person-to-person transmission. Milder illnesses without pneumonia also occurred. No standard methods then recovered *Legionella* from environmental sources, and no specimens were available later for retrospective culture when the etiology was known.

Subsequent nosocomial outbreaks that are noteworthy by the large numbers of patients involved are two outbreaks in Burlington, Vermont, at the same hospital in the 1970s, one with 225 confirmed cases over a 3-year

period at Wadsworth Veterans Administration Medical Center in Los Angeles, and the 1984 outbreak in Stafford, England, with over 100 cases during a short time period. Other outbreaks with varying numbers of patients have been described from widely scattered areas; usually, as in some of the aforementioned outbreaks, immunosuppressed patients are the first noted to have disease.

A remarkable building-associated outbreak occurred over a period of years in a hotel in Benidorm, Spain; eventually British and Spanish workers showed a link with contaminated potable water, and, for a couple sharing the same room, a greater risk of acquisition of pneumonia for the person who showered first in the morning.

Prevalence

NOSOCOMIAL DISEASE

In the previously cited outbreaks, *Legionella* have accounted generally for at least 10 percent of nosocomial pneumonia cases. The frequency of *Legionella* infections in the absence of outbreaks varies considerably and in some hospitals is very unusual despite conscientious efforts to diagnose cases. Early studies by the CDC estimated that overall *Legionella* accounts for about 10 percent of nosocomial pneumonia; recent estimates by others are lower. Risk factors for acquisition in diverse areas are immunosuppression (particularly corticosteroids), advanced age, male sex, underlying cardiopulmonary disease, smoking, renal failure, and duration of hospitalization. Attack rates in renal transplantation or bone marrow transplantation patients have been as high as 50 percent during an outbreak. Patients with hairy cell leukemia are very susceptible and acquired immunodeficiency syndrome (AIDS) patients have also contracted *Legionella* infection.

SPORADIC CASES

Serologic studies in adults have shown that *Legionella* caused 1 percent of community-acquired pneumonias that did not require hospitalization, 5 to 15 percent of patients admitted to hospital with pneumonia in different areas, and usually about 10 to 15 percent of so-called atypical pneumonia. *Legionella* infections in immunocompetent children do occur but are rare.

Most of the first 1005 sporadic cases of Legionnaires' disease reported to the CDC were found in the Northeast and Midwest and occurred between June and October. The age range in affected individuals was 16 months to 89 years. Patient risk factors were age >50 years, male sex, chronic renal disease necessitating dialysis or transplantation, diabetes mellitus, presence of cancer, use of immunosuppressive drugs, chronic bronchitis or emphysema, and smoking. Occupational risk has also been shown for employees in hospitals where nosocomial outbreaks have

occurred; cases in cooling tower workers have also been reported, although serosurveys have not shown increased antibody levels in other employees exposed to contaminated water.

Pontiac Fever

In July 1968 an illness that differed from pneumonic Legionnaires' disease by a shorter incubation period (mean of 36 h), occurrence exclusively in previously normal people, higher attack rate (up to 95 percent), more upper respiratory tract and neurologic symptoms, and no mortality occurred in a new county health department building in Pontiac, Michigan (Pontiac fever). Defective evaporative condenser discharge units of the air conditioner were found, and *L. pneumophila* serogroup I was later recovered. Subsequent outbreaks include two others that occurred in Vermont and Minnesota linked to whirlpool bath use. An outbreak that occurred in an automobile assembly plant in Windsor, Ontario, in 1981 was caused by *L. feeleii* found in lathe cooling oil; it involved over 300 ill people. Sporadic cases have been documented uncommonly. The pathogenesis of this form of illness is unknown; it may involve exposure to an inoculum lower than that required for development of pneumonia or, in other cases, may be similar to humidifier fever, which is probably caused by inhalation of bacterial toxins.

CLINICAL FEATURES

General

The usual incubation period for symptomatic disease is 2 to 10 days or so, and it may be shorter, especially in immunosuppressed patients and in patients with heavy exposure. Most symptomatic patients develop pneumonia, which is often severe. The range of infection varies, however, from asymptomatic seroconversion through mild disease to rapidly fatal pneumonia. Sero-prevalence studies that show high antibody levels in the general population with low prevalence of disease may indicate falsely high results because of cross-reactivity in the test.

Pneumonia

SYMPTOMS

The disease usually has gradual onset with predominant constitutional symptoms, but the onset may be more abrupt, especially in immunosuppressed patients. These initial symptoms often are malaise and lethargy, headache, weakness, myalgia, and anorexia. Upper respiratory symptoms are almost always absent. Fever is an early sign, and in some patients with nosocomial acquisition it may be noted before symptoms develop. It tends to rise in a stepwise fashion and become sustained. Most patients

then develop a dry nonproductive cough after a day or two of illness; this is not the usual chief complaint early. The sputum may be minimally purulent or bloody in over half of patients; this usually occurs several days into the illness. About a quarter to a third of patients complain of pleuritic pain. Shaking chills or true rigors usually occur in the first few days of illness and are recurrent in the absence of appropriate antimicrobial therapy. Other common complaints include diarrhea, nausea, vomiting, and headache. Diarrhea, which occurs in about half of cases, may be a prodromal symptom and, as the predominant complaint in unusual instances, distracts from consideration of pulmonary involvement. More commonly it occurs in the first 4 or 5 days of illness; it is usually watery, with three or four bowel movements per day. Anorexia occurs in most patients, but nausea and vomiting are seen in only about 25 percent of patients. Headache, often in association with confusion, is a common complaint, in some patients is very severe, and in very unusual instances is the chief complaint. Myalgia and arthralgia may occur in about a fifth of patients.

SIGNS

Fever is an early sign manifested by almost all patients and, in over 60 percent it is >40°C despite the use of antipyretic agents or corticosteroids. The fever frequently rises in a stepwise fashion, becomes sustained, and is associated in about 60 percent of cases with relative bradycardia.

Most patients appear rather toxic and diaphoretic when seen after a few days of illness. A small minority of patients (≈10 percent) may have a normal physical examination early. On physical examination the chest usually shows the most impressive findings. Early in the course of the disease, only scattered rales, rhonchi, or evidence of a small pleural effusion are frequently noted. Findings of consolidation are uncommon early, and a pleural rub is even less common. After progression of illness, striking findings of frank consolidation are almost always noted. Findings in the chest are usually proportional to those noted on chest radiograph; it is notable that some patients do not have a productive cough despite impressive clinical and radiographic evidence of consolidation. Massive pleural effusion and empyema have been noted, but are uncommon.

Nonspecific abdominal tenderness is found in a few patients, but not peritoneal signs. Splenomegaly is a rare finding. Abnormalities of mental status are common throughout the course and are found in about one-fourth of patients with pneumonia. Findings noted include confusion, disorientation, agitation, stupor, obtundation, coma, hallucinations, grand mal seizure, ataxia, dysarthria, and focal neurologic findings. Meningismus is a rare finding. Some patients develop retrograde amnesia for the illness.

Abnormalities of other systems, including hepatic, renal, hematologic, cardiac, and musculoskeletal, occur but are frequently noted only on laboratory examination. Some unusual features of *Legionella* infection that have been described are myositis, rhabdomyolysis, leukoencephalitis, pericarditis, prosthetic valve endocarditis, myocarditis, pericarditis, pancreatitis, visceral macroabscesses and microabscesses, wound infection, and pneumothorax. Extrapulmonary disease associated with pneumonia sometimes is apparent only weeks to months after resolution of pneumonia.

COURSES OF UNTREATED DISEASE

About 80 to 90 percent of patients without serious underlying diseases or immunosuppression recover without therapy or sequelae, although the illness may be quite severe or persist for over a week. Spontaneous recovery sometimes occurs by crisis on about days 6 to 8 of illness. Patients with serious underlying diseases, and/or who are being treated with glucocorticosteroids, have a significantly more severe clinical course. Forty to eighty percent of these patients may die of the infection, usually as a result of progressive pulmonary failure. All the complications associated with severe acute pulmonary failure may be seen, such as renal failure, severe hematologic abnormalities, cardiac failure, and obtundation.

Extrapulmonary Infections

Extrapulmonary disease caused by *Legionella* in the absence of pneumonia has been reported very uncommonly. Some cases seen in outbreaks in endemic areas have been diagnosed with clinical illness, laboratory confirmation, and negative findings on chest radiographs. Most of the additional nonpneumonia cases that have been reported have been documented only serologically and involve the central nervous system; these include focal neurologic findings, tremors, ataxia, peripheral neuropathies, and global dysfunction. Other sites have been paranasal sinuses, prosthetic valves, and wounds.

Other *Legionella* Infections

Pneumonia caused by other *Legionella* species seems to be usually clinically indistinguishable from that caused by *L. pneumophila*. Almost all cases caused by *L. micdadei*, however, have been nosocomial cases, and many have been in immunosuppressed patients. Some of these patients have had an indolent course and were afebrile despite the finding of nodular infiltrates; most, however, have had an abrupt onset of high fever and few other signs and symptoms, except for pleuritic pain in some. Many patients with *L. micdadei* pneumonia have had nodular pulmonary infiltrates of the type commonly seen with septic pulmonary embolism. *L. bozemanii* pneumonia

may differ by freshwater near-drowning having been a predisposing factor in two cases and by a high frequency of immunosuppressed patients among reported cases. Simultaneous infection with *L. pneumophila* and other *Legionella* species has been reported.

Pontiac Fever

Pontiac fever is characterized by the absence of fatality and lack of infiltrates on chest radiographs, although cough and many of the systemic symptoms common to Legionnaires' disease are seen; rales are sometimes noted. Neurologic complaints were very common in the Pontiac outbreak, but not in the Windsor outbreak or in a few sporadic cases.

DIAGNOSIS

Laboratory and Radiographic Findings

NONSPECIFIC LABORATORY FINDINGS

A number of nonspecific but frequently characteristic laboratory abnormalities occur in *Legionella* infections. The white blood cell count is very frequently elevated (WBC > 10,000 per cubic millimeter), with a left shift in about half to three-fourths of patients. Leukopenia and thrombocytopenia are observed in severe disease. Bone marrow examination has rarely shown the inhibition of myelopoiesis. Elevation of erythrocyte sedimentation rate occurs in most cases. Positive cold agglutinins and even cold agglutinin disease have also been observed in several cases. Disseminated intravascular coagulation occurs uncommonly. Elevations of lactic dehydrogenase and aspartate aminotransferase occur in over half of patients and that of alanine aminotransferase or alkaline phosphatase in slightly fewer. Bilirubin elevation is less common. Hypoxemia is usually in proportion to the degree of pulmonary involvement seen on chest radiograph. Hyponatremia, which is a nonspecific finding and may be due to the syndrome of inappropriate antidiuretic hormone secretion (SIADH) and/or to contributing diarrhea, occurs in about half of patients. Hypophosphatemia, presumably due to an accompanying *Legionella* bacteremia, occurs in a variable number of patients with no other explanation for it.

Abnormal renal findings include abnormal urinalysis with proteinuria, hyaline or granular casts, and less commonly hematuria. Renal failure in the absence of shock occurs quite uncommonly and is usually due to acute tubular interstitial nephritis and less commonly to acute tubular necrosis; it is least commonly associated with myoglobinuria and rhabdomyolysis.

Examination of pleural fluid, if present, usually shows a low-grade exudate; rarely, purulent findings are encountered. Examination of cerebrospinal fluid in patients with clinical neurologic abnormalities usually is

normal. Rarely, a small number (<100 cells per cubic millimeter) of cells are seen.

RADIOGRAPHIC FINDINGS

No radiographic findings are pathognomonic for *Legionella* infection. A usual early finding is an alveolar filling pattern with patchy or subsegmental distribution of consolidation. Progression within the same lobe is common. Spread to ipsilateral or, less commonly, contralateral areas may occur, and in a majority of cases seen, late, multilobe involvement is evident. Lower-lobe involvement is common. Pleural effusion may precede other radiographic findings or appear after the onset of parenchymal infiltrates; rarely, it occurs without a parenchymal infiltrate. Interstitial infiltrates may appear early, especially in immunosuppressed patients, but usually develop into consolidative infiltrates within days. Cavitation occurs uncommonly; a large majority of such cases have been in immunosuppressed patients (Fig. 102-1). Empyema thoracis is a rare complication that occurs in some untreated patients.

SPECIFIC LABORATORY DIAGNOSIS

Culture of respiratory tract specimens, including sputum, is overall the single best test for Legionnaires' disease (Table 102-2). This requires use of selective media and techniques when plating specimens from normally non-sterile sites.

Usually culture is combined with immunologic tests to detect whole bacterial cells in the same materials, using direct or indirect immunofluorescent microscopy. This has the advantage of being more rapid than culture techniques, but has the major disadvantage of being serogroup-dependent and of relatively low sensitivity. Determination of serum antibody titer is probably the least helpful test for individual cases, although it is an excellent epidemiologic tool in investigation of outbreaks. Serologic diagnosis, without confirmatory culture or immunofluorescent microscopic detection of bacteria, is more frequently false-positive than true-positive for most populations. Therefore, clinicians must question the diagnosis in such instances and regard "serologically proven" case reports of unusual manifestations of sporadic disease as being unproven. It must be emphasized that negative results of one or more of the laboratory tests do not exclude disease.

DIFFERENTIAL DIAGNOSIS

Many investigators believe that legionellae cause a rather typical illness, particularly in outbreaks. Others, however, have found no discriminating features compared to other pneumonias and dispute this. Certainly clinical diagnosis of *Legionella* infections is easier in an outbreak than in a nonepidemic setting. Likewise, it is easier to suspect in a pneumonia patient with multisystem abnormalities who

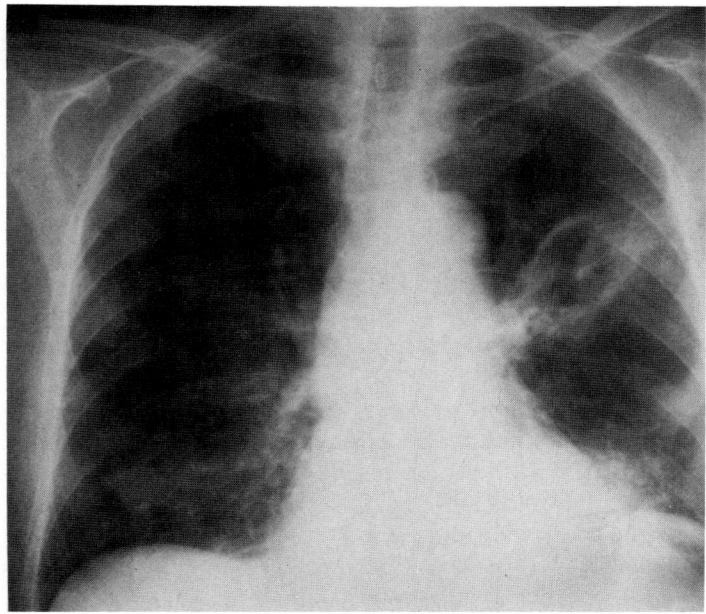

A   *B*

FIGURE 102-1   64-year-old man with steroid-dependent asthma developed fever, chills, and increased dyspnea 2 days before admission. Patient recovered after erythromycin and rifampin therapy. Rifampin was given for first $1\frac{1}{2}$ weeks and erythromycin for 2 months. Steroids were tapered to low dose. Culture of transtracheal aspirate yielded *L. pneumophila.*   *A.* On admission. Left upper lobe and smaller left lower lobe posterior segment infiltrate.   *B.* Progression to cavitation.

TABLE 102-2
Laboratory Diagnostic Tests for Legionnaires' Disease

Method	Suitable Specimens	Advantages	Disadvantages	Turnaround Time	Sensitivity	Specificity	Chances of False-Positive/False-Negative Results*
Culture	All lower respiratory tract secretions/tissues including sputum; blood, pleural fluid, abscesses; must be fresh; avoid collection in saline solutions	Independent of species or serogroup	Requires use of selective media and freshly collected, non-fixed specimens	2–7 days mean 3 days	? 80%–90% for sputum, TTA† >95% for lung tissue	100%	0% 10–20%
Immunofluorescent detection of bacteria	Same as for culture except for blood; can be fixed, although nonfixed specimens are best	Rapid	Technically demanding, serogroup specific; polyvalent antisera required	1–3 h	25% to 75% for sputum (mean 60%), >95% for lung tissue	95–99.9%‡	4–60%/17–35%
Antibody determination	Serum	Samples easy to obtain	Time consuming, requires use of multiple antigens and paired sera	Weeks§	60–70%	95–99%‡	25–60%/25–30%
Urinary antigen detection	Urine	Samples easy to obtain	Serogroup-specific, requires use of multiple antisera; unable to distinguish between acute and chronic (relapsing) disease; not available commercially	1 to 6 h	60–80%	98–99.9%	4–40%/17–30%

*With disease prevalence equal to 5%. Lowest estimate of false-positive rate is for highest estimated specificity, and lowest estimate of false-negative rate is for highest estimated sensitivity.

†Transtracheal aspirate.

‡Higher specificity estimate is for *L. pneumophila*, and lower one is for other *Legionella* species.

§Long turnaround time because of the need to test paired sera collected 2 to 6 weeks apart. The test itself takes less than 4 to 6 h to perform.

---

has no response after several days therapy with β-lactam agents and/or aminoglycosides than in a patient seen earlier. The diagnosis is favored if a patient has a progressively rising fever that becomes nonremitting, recurrent rigors, nonproductive or minimally productive cough in the face of consolidation, few or no bacteria or inflammatory cells seen in respiratory secretions, relative bradycardia, and severe prostration. Pneumococcal pneumonia differs from *Legionella* infection in that patients with lobar pneumococcal pneumonia usually have a single rigor, produce purulent sputum, and respond favorably to penicillin. Persistently dry hacking cough and, to a lesser degree, presence of upper respiratory tract signs and symptoms favor *Mycoplasma pneumoniae* pneumonia. Multiple system abnormalities may, however, occur in bacteremic patients with other causes of pneumonia or in patients with mycoplasmal infection, e.g., in the setting of a hemoglobinopathy.

Less common causes of atypical pneumonia should also be considered. Psittacosis is a consideration because about 20 percent of psittacosis patients have no history of bird exposure, the onset includes constitutional symptoms, relative bradycardia is commonly found, and the highly variable clinical features may include multisystem disease. Q fever may also have variable clinical manifestations with multisystem involvement. These two diseases are important considerations because empiric therapy would be tetracycline, rather than erythromycin. Early coccidioidomycosis, histoplasmosis, typhoid fever, leptospirosis, tularemia, and unusual pyogenic pathogens are additional possibilities. Dual infections occur, e.g., with pyogenic bacteria, especially in hospitalized patients.

THERAPY

General

Prudence dictates that respiratory isolation be used for patients with positive cultures or immunofluorescent examination until negative. Supportive therapy for hypoten-

sion, respiratory failure and, less commonly, renal failure is sometimes required. Immunosuppressive agents should be stopped or the dosage reduced to the lowest required for control of an underlying process, if at all possible. Corticosteroids should not be used except to treat adrenal insufficiency or for therapy of an underlying disorder.

Antimicrobial

Erythromycin alone or in combination with rifampin is the current drug of choice in treatment of *Legionella* infections. (Approval of the use of rifampin for this purpose by the Food and Drug Administration is pending.) This is supported by retrospective reviews, prospective clinical experience, and results of animal experiments. In the Philadelphia epidemic, the case fatality rate was lower with erythromycin than with tetracycline, and erythromycin was effective in the prospective experiences in the Los Angeles and Burlington outbreaks. Use of erythromycin has lowered the case fatality rate approximately fourfold in nosocomial cases.

Therapy with tetracycline and its congeners has led to variable results with both possible responses and definite failures. β-Lactam agents (penicillin; cephalosporins; the cefamycin, cefoxitin; the carbapenem, imipenem), as well as clindamycin and the aminoglycosides, should not be used to treat *Legionella* infections. Trimethoprim-sulfamethoxazole in a dose of 20 mg/kg per day trimethoprim component has been effective in animal models and in a few cases, but its exact role is not yet clear.

Clinical effectiveness appears to correlate with the ability of an antimicrobial to enter the alveolar macrophage, particularly in concentrations that are inhibitory. Thus, erythromycin and to a lesser degree tetracycline, which enter the alveolar macrophage at levels well above serum concentrations, are clinically effective. Rifampin and the experimental DNA-gyrase inhibitors, the quinolones (e.g., ofloxacin), also penetrate cells well, whereas β-lactam agents do not. Erythromycin, rifampin, doxycycline, trimethoprim-sulfamethoxazole and ofloxacin have all been effective to differing degrees in treatment of experimental *Legionella* pneumonia in animal models.

Erythromycin should be given in a dose of 2 to 4 g per day for at least 3 weeks to prevent relapse, usually explained on the basis of intracellular parasitism. Adults with mild illness may be treated with oral therapy up to 2 g per day and observed carefully. Moderately to severely ill adult patients should receive erythromycin intravenously for the first several days of therapy, or until the patient has a clinical response; then oral therapy may be substituted. Relapse after changing from intravenous to oral erythromycin therapy is occasionally seen. Rifampin in a dose of 300 to 600 mg twice per day should be considered as an adjunctive to erythromycin therapy if the patient is critically ill, is immunosuppressed, or has radio-graphic evidence of pulmonary cavities. Rifampin should not be given alone because of the possibility of emergence of resistance. Cavitary disease or empyema generally requires more prolonged therapy.

Doxycycline, which is lipid-soluble, is the preferred tetracycline drug if erythromycin cannot be given; it is given in a dose of 200 mg initially, then 100 mg in 12 h and then 100 to 200 mg daily thereafter. (Approval for the use of doxycycline for this purpose by the Food and Drug Administration is pending.) Consideration of rifampin use with doxycycline should be given for at least the first week of therapy in moderately severe to severely ill patients.

The clinical response to erythromycin therapy is usually prompt. Within the first 2 days after initiation of therapy, many patients begin to feel better and usually have a decrease in temperature. As with other bacterial pneumonias, pulmonary infiltrates and signs of pulmonary consolidation may continue to progress, while the patient manifests a clinical response. It is very unusual for a patient to have persistent fever, leukopenia, and confusion after more than 3 to 4 days of erythromycin therapy in appropriate dose. If this occurs, the diagnosis should be questioned, and superinfection or dual infection considered; if *Legionella* infection has been well documented, consideration should be given to adding rifampin therapy. Some immunosuppressed patients, particularly those with hairy cell leukemia, may have a prolonged febrile course despite optimal antimicrobial therapy.

PROGNOSIS, MORTALITY, AND SEQUELAE

Prognosis and case fatality rates are affected by presence and severity of underlying disease, if any, and by specific therapy given. Higher fatality rates were seen in the earlier epidemics, particularly nosocomial ones with patients with serious underlying disease. Overall mortality rates in sporadic cases are about 19 percent. Mortality rates in immunocompetent patients treated with erythromycin are about 5 percent. The case fatality rate in otherwise well patients who do not receive erythromycin therapy and in erythromycin-treated immunosuppressed patients is about 25 percent. Immunosuppressed patients who are not treated with erythromycin have a case fatality rate of about 80 percent.

Patients may complain of persistent fatigue and weakness for several months after completion of therapy or longer if not treated. Retrograde amnesia or persistent cerebellar ataxia may also be noted. Pulmonary fibrosis may follow recovery from respiratory failure. Radiographic resolution of pulmonary infiltrates is slow and may take from 3 weeks to 3 months or more after initiation of therapy.

BIBLIOGRAPHY

Brenner DJ, Steigerwalt AG, Gorman GW, Hazel WW, Bibb WF, Hackel M, Tyndall RL, Campbell J, Feeley JC, Thacker WL, Skaliy P, Martin WT, Brake BJ, Fields BF, McEachern HV, Corcoran LK: Ten new species of Legionella. Int J Syst Bact 35:50–59, 1985.
  Good review of taxonomy, with phenotypic characteristics of 22 species.

Edelstein PH: Control of Legionella in hospitals. J Hosp Infect 8:109–115, 1986.
  Prospective surveillance of immunocompromised patients with pneumonia is probably the most effective means to determine if a hospital is a source of Legionnaires' disease.

Edelstein PH, Calarco K, Yasui VK: Antimicrobial therapy of experimentally induced Legionnaires' disease in guinea pigs. Am Rev Respir Dis 130:849–856, 1984.
  Therapy of experimental pneumonia produced by intratracheal inoculation.

Fraser DW, Tsai TR, Orenstein W, Parkin WE, Beecham HJ, Sharrar RG, Harris J, Mallison GF, Martin SM, McDade JE, Shepard CC, Brachman PS: Legionnaires' disease: Description of an epidemic of pneumonia. N Engl J Med 297:1189–1197, 1977.
  Classic description of the first defined cases of Legionnaires' disease.

Garbe PL, Davis BJ, Weisfeld JS, Markowitz L, Miner P, Garrity F, Barbaree JM, Reingold AL: Nosocomial Legionnaires' disease: Epidemiologic demonstration of cooling towers as a source. JAMA 254:521–524, 1985.
  Example of excellent epidemiologic study, based on classic and molecular biology techniques. Stresses need to define exact source of epidemic.

Herwaldt LA, Gorman GW, McGrath T, Toma S, Brake B, Hightower AW, Jones J, Reingold AL, Boxer PA, Tang PW, et al: A new Legionella species, Legionella feeleii species nova, causes Pontiac fever in an automobile plant. Ann Intern Med 100:333–338, 1984.
  Most recent description of an outbreak of Pontiac fever, with good review of previous literature.

Horwitz MA: Phagocytosis of the Legionnaires' disease bacterium (Legionella pneumophila) occurs by a novel mechanism: Engulfment within a pseudopod coil. Cell 36:27–33, 1984.
  One of a series of elegant studies of bacteria and phagocyte interactions.

Kirby BD, Snyder KM, Meyer RD, Finegold SM: Legionnaires' disease: Report of sixty-five nosocomially acquired cases and review of the literature. Medicine (Balt.) 59:188–205, 1980.
  Review of clinical experience at Wadsworth VA Medical Center and the literature.

Kohler RB: Antigen detection for the rapid diagnosis of mycoplasma and Legionella pneumonia. Diagn Microbiol Infect Dis 4:47S–59S, 1986.
  Antigens can be detected in the urine of about 80% of patients with serogroup 1 Legionella pneumophila pneumonia and of some patients with serogroup 4 Legionella pneumophila and Legionella dumoffii pneumonia. The specificity of these assays is greater than 99%. Combining urinary antigen detection and direct fluorescent antibody examination of secretions increases the rapid diagnostic yield by 10–20%.

Korvick JA, Yu VL: Legionnaires' disease: An emerging surgical problem. Ann Thorac Surg 43:341–347, 1987.
  Legionnaires' disease is an important, although often overlooked, complication in the patient postoperatively. Patients undergoing a transplant procedure are at highest risk, but occurrence is common in the surgical patient undergoing general anesthesia, endotracheal intubation, or both.

Meyer RD: Legionella infections: A review of five years of research. Rev Infect Dis 5:258–278, 1983.
  General review and reference source.

Muder RR, Yu VL, Zuravleff JJ: Pneumonia due to the Pittsburgh pneumonia agent: New clinical perspective with a review of the literature. Medicine 62:120–128, 1983.
  Clinical description of large number of pneumonias caused by L. micdadei.

Neill MA, Gorman GW, Gibert C, Roussel A, Hightower AW, McKinney RM, Broome CV: Nosocomial legionellosis, Paris, France: Evidence for transmission by potable water. Am J Med 78:581–588, 1985.
  Epidemiologic analysis of outbreak site with multiple potential sources.

Parry MF, Stampleman L, Hutchinson JH, Folta D, Steinberg MG, Krasnogor LJ: Waterborne Legionella bozemanii and nosocomial pneumonia in immunosuppressed patients. Ann Intern Med 103:205–210, 1985.
  Description of largest number of L. bozemanii-caused pneumonias.

Saito A, Sawatari K, Fukuda Y, Nagasawa M, Koga H, Tomonaga A, Nakazato H, Fujita K, Shigeno Y, Suzuyama Y, et al: Susceptibility of *Legionella pneumophila* to ofloxacin in vitro and in experimental *Legionella* pneumonia in guinea pigs. Antimicrob Agents Chemother 28:15–20, 1985.
  Description of therapeutic potential for fluoroquinolones.

Shands KN, Ho JL, Meyer RD, Gorman GW, Edelstein PH, Mallison GF, Finegold SM, Fraser DW: Potable water as a source of Legionnaires' disease. JAMA 253:1412–1416, 1985.
  Description of use of hyperchlorination to control a nosocomial outbreak of Legionella infections.

Stout JE, Yu VL, Muraca P: Legionnaires' disease acquired within the homes of two patients. Link to the home water supply. JAMA 257:1215–1217, 1987.
  The first report that links acquisition of community-acquired Legionnaires' disease to contaminated water supplies within the homes of susceptible patients.

Thornsberry C, Balows A, Feeley JC, Jakubowski W: *Legionella*. Proceedings of the 2nd International Symposium, Washington, DC: American Society for Microbiology, 1984.
  Contains good review articles and results of environmental sources and modes of pathogenesis, and aspects of pathology.

Winn WC Jr: *Legionella* and Legionnaires' disease: A review with emphasis on environmental studies and laboratory diagnosis. CRC Crit Rev Clin Lab Sci 21:323–381, 1985.
  Detailed and complete review of environmental sources and modes of pathogenesis, and aspects of pathology.

Woo AH, Yu VL, Goetz A: Potential in-hosptial modes of transmission of *Legionella pneumophila*. Demonstration experiments for dissemination by showers, humidifiers, and rinsing of ventilation bag apparatus. Am J Med 80:567–573, 1986.
  Aerosolization of Legionella pneumophila by showers, humidifiers, and respiratory equipment rinsed in tap water was evaluated. Portable humidifiers rinsed in tap water readily generated aerosols of L. pneumophila, which disseminated through a two-bed patient room. Sterile water is recommended for rinsing ventilation bag apparatus and tubing.

Woodhead MA, Macfarlane JT: Legionnaires' disease: A review of 79 community acquired cases in Nottingham. Thorax 41:635–640, 1986.
  Seventy-nine cases of sporadic, community-acquired Legionnaires' disease are reviewed. Thirteen patients died. Of the features noted on admission, only a high plasma urea concentration was significantly associated with death.

Chapter 103

Pulmonary Aspergillosis

Steven M. Albelda / George H. Talbot

Mycology

Hypersensitivity Reactions to *Aspergillus*
   Allergic Bronchopulmonary Aspergillosis
   Bronchocentric Granulomatosis and Mucoid Impaction
     of the Bronchus
   Extrinsic Allergic Alveolitis
   Extrinsic Asthma

Saprophytic Colonization
   Aspergilloma

Invasive Aspergillosis
   Invasive Pulmonary Aspergillosis
   Chronic Necrotizing Pulmonary Aspergillosis

Pleural Aspergillosis

The term *pulmonary aspergillosis* refers to a spectrum of diverse lung disorders rather than to a single disease (Table 103-1). The clinical manifestations of disease are dependent not only on the pathogenic properties of the fungus but also on the immune status and on the underlying architecture of the lungs in the host. It is, therefore, possible for the same organism to produce hypersensitivity reactions, saprophytic colonization, or tissue invasion.

In reality, distinctions between these disorders are often blurred; some patients simultaneously demonstrate characteristics of more than one "disease," thereby defying simple categorization, whereas in others the pulmonary disease evolves from one apparent category to another. Nonetheless, despite these limitations, a classification system, such as the one described in Table 103-1, does prove a useful framework for an approach to a particular patient.

MYCOLOGY

Approximately 200 species of the genus *Aspergillus* have been identified. The most common pathogenic species are *A. fumigatus, A. flavus, A. niger,* and *A. terreus. Aspergillus* spores can be found in profusion where decaying vegetable matter provides a source of nutrition. Seasonal variation in the density of outdoor airborne spore levels may play a role in extrinsic hypersensitivity disease, but there is no convincing evidence of a seasonal variation in the incidence of invasive pulmonary aspergillosis, perhaps because filtration of hospital air by high efficiency particulate filters substantially reduces indoor spore counts. Spore counts on hospital wards vary for no apparent reason or in response to sporadic bursts of activity in the environment, such as vacuuming or cleaning. Persistently high levels of airborne spores can result from contaminated fireproofing, a contaminated ventilation system, or demolition and construction.

Aspergilli cultured on Sabouraud's dextrose agar or other fungal media grow as pigmented colonies with the uneven velvety surface characteristic of molds. Colony color is a helpful identifying feature, but precise speciation requires microscopic examination of the spore-bearing structure of the organism. Specimens from the patient, such as sputum, can be examined using a KOH prepara-

TABLE 103-1
Spectrum of Pulmonary Aspergillosis

Clinical Manifestation	Immune Status	Underlying Lung Architecture	Degree of Tissue Invasion
Hypersensitivity reactions			
Asthma	↑	Normal	None
Extrinsic alveolitis	↑	Normal	None
Allergic bronchopulmonary aspergillosis	↑	Excess airway mucus	None
Saprophytic colonization			
Aspergilloma	Normal	Preexisting cavity	None
Invasive disease			
Chronic necrotizing aspergillosis	↓	Normal	+
Invasive pulmonary aspergillosis	↓↓↓	Normal	+++

tion, with or without the addition of an ink stain. Fixed tissue specimens are best examined using a silver stain, although the periodic acid-Schiff stain is also useful. The hematoxylin and eosin stain and the tissue Gram stain are less sensitive. The organisms are visualized as 2.5 to 8.0 μm wide, septate hyphae that branch at acute angles. Spore-bearing structures are rarely seen in fixed tissue specimens.

HYPERSENSITIVITY REACTIONS TO *ASPERGILLUS*

Hypersensitivity reactions to *Aspergillus* species produce a number of clinical syndromes: allergic bronchopulmonary aspergillosis, bronchocentric granulomatosis, mucoid impaction of the bronchus, extrinsic allergic alveolitis, and extrinsic asthma. Table 103-2 summarizes the cardinal features of the three major manifestations of hyperimmune responses to *Aspergillus*. The manifestations of hypersensitivity that develop in a particular patient vary with the intensity of exposure to *Aspergillus* spores, the type of *Aspergillus* species encountered, and the immune state of the host.

Allergic Bronchopulmonary Aspergillosis

Allergic bronchopulmonary aspergillosis (ABPA), a complex hypersensitivity reaction to the presence of *Aspergillus* colonizing the bronchial tree, occurs almost exclusively in asthmatics. Although ABPA is still relatively unusual in the United States, the clinician must be aware of this entity because pulmonary fibrosis can result from unrecognized or inadequately treated disease.

PATHOPHYSIOLOGY

Allergic bronchopulmonary aspergillosis results from the immune responses to *Aspergillus* organisms that colonize the bronchial tree; most often, *A. fumigatus* is the cause. Usually, there is no evidence of tissue invasion. It is unclear whether fungal spores remain trapped within the bronchial lumen because of abnormally thick mucus present in certain asthmatic patients or whether the initial immunologic events assist in trapping the organism. In either case, fungal antigen stimulates the production of IgE and IgG antibodies: the IgE antibodies elicit a type I (immediate hypersensitivity) reaction, whereas the IgG antibodies result in the formation of immune complexes and Arthus' type III reaction. Inflammatory mediators from sensitized mast cells evoke bronchospasm, bronchial edema, and the accumulation of eosinophils, whereas the formation of immune complexes (probably in situ) leads to fixation of complement and the liberation of additional inflammatory mediators. An intense inflammatory reaction ensues that presumably causes bronchial damage, bronchiectasis and, in time, pulmonary fibrosis. Type IV reactions, involving cell-mediated immune responses, may add to the tissue damage.

Early in the disease, the bronchi are dilated and filled with mucus and exudate containing noninvasive fungal organisms. The bronchial mucosa manifests squamous metaplasia and is infiltrated by eosinophils, lymphocytes, and plasma cells. As the disease continues, bronchiectasis and pulmonary fibrosis develop.

CLINICAL COURSE

Because relatively few patients have been systematically followed for months to years, the natural history of pa-

TABLE 103-2
Hypersensitivity Reactions to Aspergillus

	Allergic Bronchopulmonary Aspergillosis	Extrinsic Allergic Alveolitis	Asthma
Pathology	Colonization of airways, viscid mucoid impaction, tissue eosinophilia	Lymphocytic infiltration of interstitium, non-caseating granuloma	Hypertrophied mucus glands
Radiographic features			
Early	Migratory peripheral infiltrates, atelectasis, bronchiectasis	Diffuse alveolar-interstitial infiltrates	Normal, hyperinflation
Late	Fibrosis	Reticulonodular interstitial opacities	Normal, hyperinflation
Skin test reactions to *Aspergillus* antigens			
Immediate	+ (90–100%)	Rarely +	+ (Up to 30%)
Delayed	+ (30–80%)	Rarely +	Rarely +
Peripheral eosinophilia	+ (90–100%)	Rare	Not unusual
IgG precipitins	+ (90%)	+ 100%	+ (Up to 25%)
Serum IgE levels	Markedly elevated (>2500 ng/ml)	Normal (up to 250 ng/ml)	Normal or modestly elevated (<1500 ng/ml)

tients with ABPA is not completely understood. However, a useful clinical staging system of ABPA was recently proposed by Patterson and colleagues (Table 103-3). This system recognizes five stages in the course of the disease. The *acute stage* is characterized by the paradigmatic symptoms, signs, and laboratory findings of ABPA: bronchospasm, eosinophilia, migratory infiltrates on the chest radiograph, positive skin test reactivity against *Aspergillus* antigens, and an increase in the concentration of IgE in serum.

After appropriate corticosteroid therapy, most patients enter a *remission stage* characterized by resolution of symptoms, clearing of pulmonary infiltrates, and a decrease in the IgE level in serum. Corticosteroid therapy can be slowly discontinued at this time. Some patients remain in a permanent or prolonged remission and require no further therapy, other than to control their asthma. In the *exacerbation stage*, some or all of the clinical and laboratory abnormalities of the acute stage recur. Treatment with steroids usually again causes an improvement. At this juncture, most patients with ABPA require long-term maintenance corticosteroids to control their asthma or to prevent exacerbation of ABPA or both *(corticosteroid-dependent asthmatic stage)*.

The *fibrotic lung disease stage* of ABPA, believed to occur after long-standing and/or inadequately treated disease, is characterized by both fibrotic lung changes and airway obstruction. The airway obstruction often has both reversible (corticosteroid responsive) and irreversible

components. In some patients, the disease progresses to cor pulmonale, respiratory failure, and death.

DIAGNOSIS

A number of clinical entities can be confused with ABPA. Among these are tuberculosis, cystic fibrosis, extrinsic allergic alveolitis, and other causes of eosinophilic lung disease. Perhaps the most difficult condition to distinguish from ABPA is atopic asthma accompanied by recurrent pneumonias.

Because no single clinical, radiographic, or laboratory finding is pathognomonic of ABPA, the diagnosis rests on the clinical picture and is generally ventured as a probability: the greater the number of features favoring the diagnosis, the more likely the diagnosis. Table 103-4 provides a summary of the diagnostic features of ABPA and estimates the prevalence of each manifestation in proved instances of ABPA.

Clinical Features

The symptoms of ABPA are nonspecific and depend on the stage and severity of the disease. Wheezing is present in most patients, but it cannot readily be differentiated from the underlying asthmatic condition. In addition, there may be fever, productive cough (often with blood-streaked sputum), weight loss, pleuritic chest pain, and general malaise. Expectorated sputum plugs are present in 20 to 60 percent of patients and suggest the diagnosis. Physical examination may be normal, but it usually re-

TABLE 103-3

Staging System for Allergic Bronchopulmonary Aspergillosis

Stage	Symptoms	Radiographic Features	Laboratory Features	Management
I. Acute	Fever, productive cough, wheezing	Pulmonary infiltrates, mucoid impaction	Blood eosinophilia, elevated serum IgE, positive skin test	Corticosteroids to achieve remission
II. Remission	Asymptomatic	Normal	Decrease in IgE and blood eosinophilia	Careful follow-up
III. Exacerbation	All or some of acute stage symptoms	All or some of acute stage findings	At least a doubling of IgE in asymptomatic patients and an increase in IgE in symptomatic patients	Re-treat with steroids to induce remission
IV. Corticosteroid dependent	Symptomatic steroid requiring asthma	Variable	Usually continued elevation of IgE	Long-term steroids to control asthmatic symptoms and keep IgE levels at baseline
V. Fibrotic	Severe dyspnea from fibrotic lung disease as well as bronchospasm	Pulmonary fibrosis	Restrictive plus reversible and irreversible obstructive changes on pulmonary function tests; may have continued increased IgE	Long-term corticosteroids

SOURCE: Modified from Patterson et al., 1982, and Mendelson et al., Chest 87:334, 1985.

TABLE 103-4
Diagnostic Criteria for Allergic Bronchopulmonary Aspergillosis

	Major	Minor	Approximate Prevalence, %
Clinical	Intermittent wheezing		100
		Sputum production	50–70
		Sputum plugs	30–70
		Hemoptysis	30–80
		Pleuritic chest pain	50
		Fever	30–70
Radiographic	Proximal bronchiectasis		40–80
	Migrating alveolar infiltrates		60–90
		Mucoid impaction	30
		Atelectasis	20–40
		Pseudohilar adenopathy	30
Laboratory	Peripheral eosinophilia		90–100
	IgG precipitins to *Aspergillus* antigens		70–90
	Elevated serum IgE (>1000 ng/ml)		80–100
	Immediate skin test reactivity to *Aspergillus* antigens		90–100
		Sputum eosinophilia	90–100
		A. fumigatus in sputum	50–80
		Dual skin test reactivity to *Aspergillus* antigens	30–80

SOURCE: Modified from Rosenberg M, et al: Ann Intern Med 86:405–414, 1977, and Chryssanthopoulos C, Fink J: J Asthma 21:41–51, 1984.

veals evidence of airway obstruction. Localized rales can be heard over areas of consolidation. Clubbing of the fingers may also be present in long-standing disease.

Radiographic Features
The radiographic findings in patients with ABPA arise from a number of pathologic processes. Inflammation and mucoid impaction in the airways can cause complete obstruction of a bronchus and lead to atelectasis. Because collateral air drift often prevents total lobar collapse, the impacted bronchus may appear on the chest radiograph as a distinctive lesion, i.e., a "full wine glass," "gloved finger," "V," "inverted V," "Y," or "toothpaste" shadow (Fig. 103-1). Mucoid impaction is often transient; sometimes it lasts for many months, producing a radiographic picture that mimics carcinoma.

The intense inflammatory reactions within the airways cause bronchial dilatation and thickening of the bronchial walls that are responsible for radiographic "tramline shadows," "parallel line shadows," or "ring shadows" (Fig. 103-1C). The development of proximal saccular bronchiectasis as the disease progresses causes characteristic changes in the conventional chest radiograph, on the computerized axial tomogram (Fig. 103-2A), and on the bronchogram (Fig. 103-2B and C). Proximal saccular bronchiectasis is sufficiently specific for ABPA to suggest the diagnosis strongly.

In addition to inflammatory responses in the airways, immune complex, and perhaps cell-mediated, immune reactions presumably occur in the pulmonary parenchyma. These processes lead to the ill-defined, patchy, alveolar infiltrates that are the most frequent radiographic manifestation of ABPA (Fig. 103-1A). The infiltrates are usually transient, but they may persist for six or more weeks; occasionally they cavitate. The infiltrates favor the upper lobes, and more than one infiltrate may be present at a given time. Although these infiltrates may be extensive, symptoms are generally mild or absent.

Less frequent abnormalities include local emphysema, perihilar pseudoadenopathy, and pneumothorax. In end-stage fibrotic disease, interstitial fibrosis is common, often associated with honeycombing of the lungs.

Laboratory Features
Although patients with ABPA do develop immunologic reactions to *Aspergillus* antigens, no test is specific for ABPA. Eosinophilia in sputum occurs in most patients, and *Aspergillus* can be cultured from respiratory secretions in up to one-half of them. Peripheral blood eosinophilia is almost invariable in untreated patients. Precipitating IgG antibodies against *Aspergillus* antigens are present in approximately 90 percent of patients; however, it must be kept in mind that similar precipitins can be found in up to 25 percent of asthmatics even though they have no other evidence of ABPA.

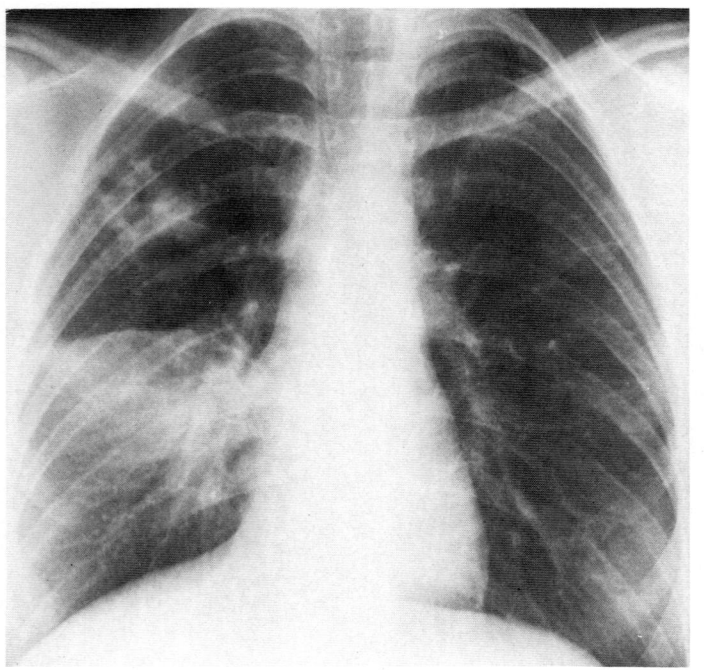

A

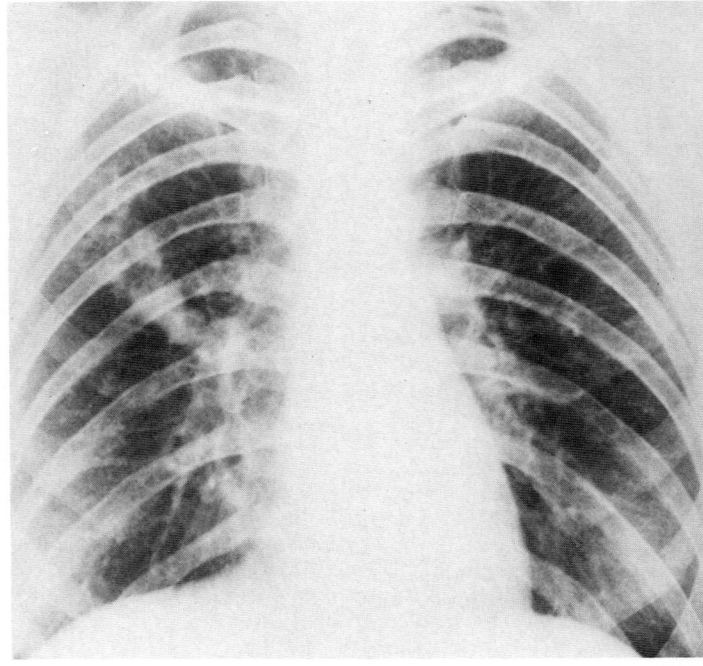

B

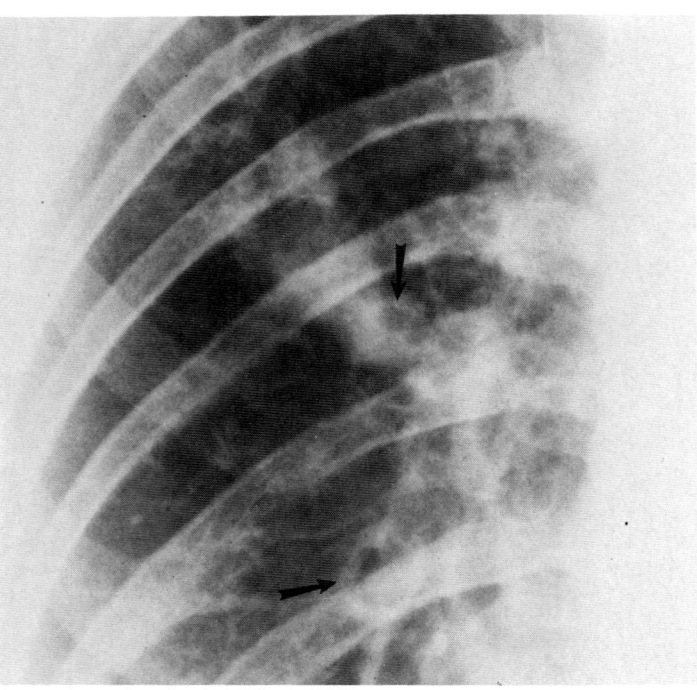

C

FIGURE 103-1   A 23-year-old female with documented allergic bronchopulmonary aspergillosis.   *A.* Chest radiograph shows mucoid impaction in right upper lobe and alveolar consolidation in right middle lobe.   *B.* Eight months later, alveolar consolidation has resolved and appearance of mucoid impaction in right upper lobe has changed.   *C.* Close-up of right lung from *B* shows "gloved finger" appearance of mucoid impaction as well as ring shadows (arrows) characteristic of bronchiectasis.

One of the most useful laboratory tests for both diagnosis and management of ABPA is measurement of total concentration of IgE in serum. In 75 to 90 percent of patients with ABPA, the serum levels are greatly increased, i.e., greater than 2500 ng/ml (normal: less than 250 ng/ml). Although the level of IgE in serum is also abnormally high in some asthmatic patients, the overlap between this group and patients with ABPA is small. Further distinc-

tion between ABPA and asthma is possible by determining the proportion of serum IgE specifically directed against *Aspergillus* antigens.

Two types of skin test reactions to *Aspergillus* antigens have been described in patients with ABPA: almost all manifest an immediate (type I) reaction, consisting of a cutaneous "wheal and flare" within 15 to 30 min of challenge; about 20 to 80 percent of these also manifest a de-

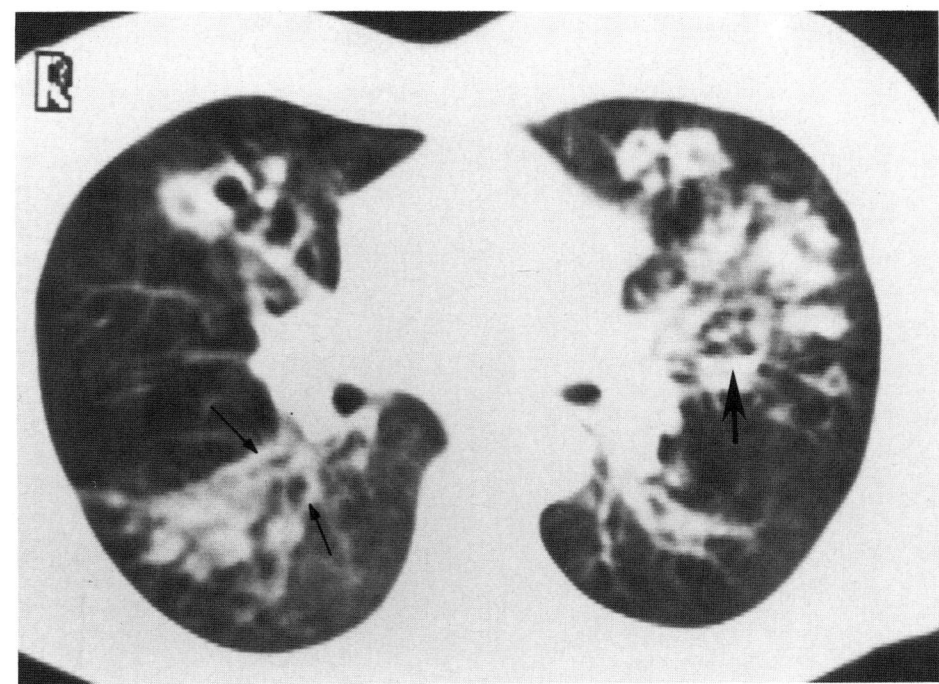

FIGURE 103-2 Proximal saccular bronchiectasis characteristic of allergic bronchopulmonary aspergillosis. *A.* Computed tomography reveals multiple rounded, dilated bronchi (small arrows); note air-fluid level (large arrow). *B* and *C.* Bronchography, viewed from the lateral position, from two different patients shows both normally tapering bronchi and bronchi with saccular widening (arrows).

A

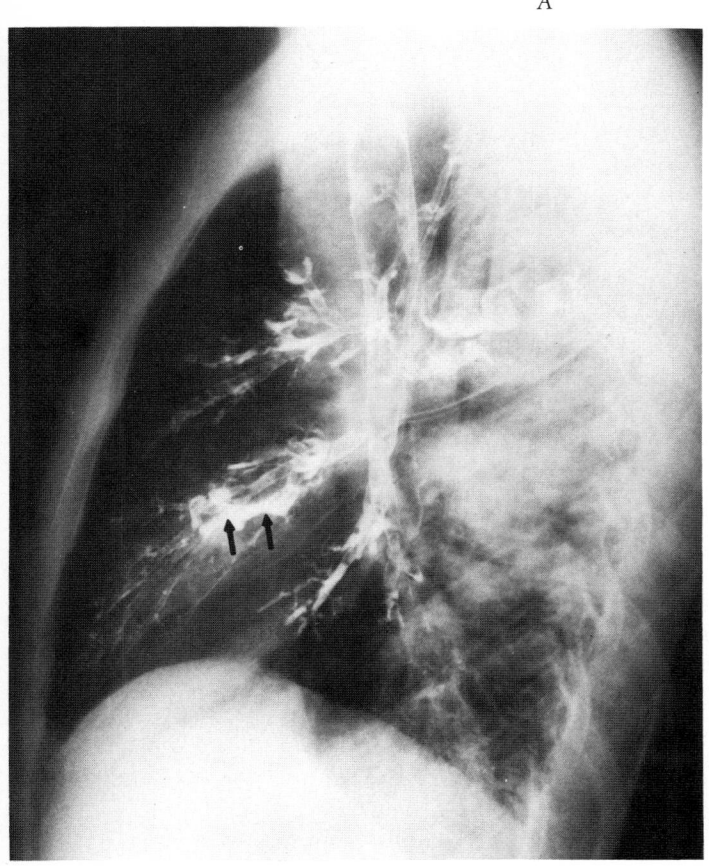

B

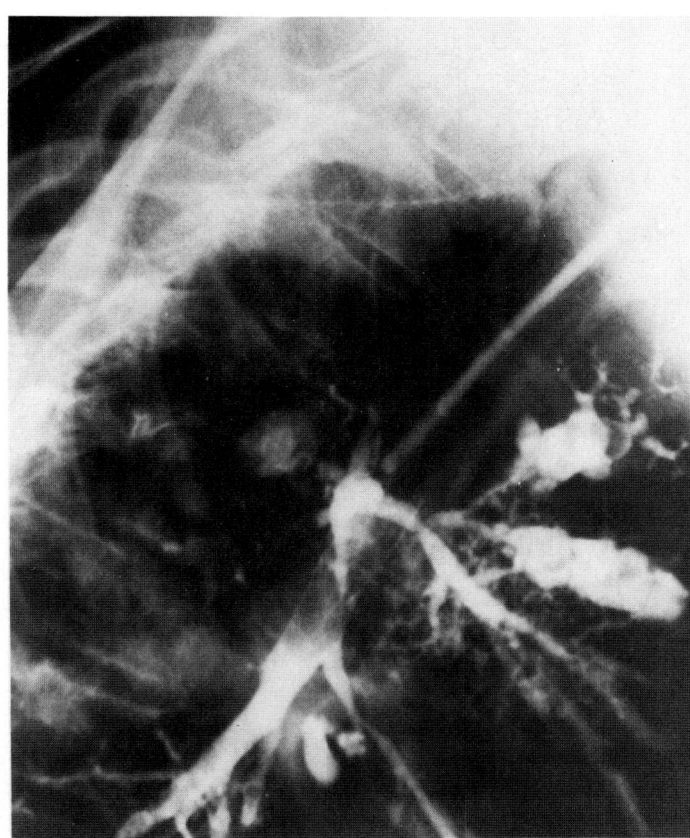

C

layed reaction (Arthus', type III), consisting of a hemorrhagic cutaneous lesion that occurs 4 to 10 h after challenge. Although immediate skin test positivity is of some use as a screening test—since its absence makes the diagnosis of ABPA unlikely—its practical value is limited by the high rate of positivity in asthmatics (up to 35 percent) and in other patients with chronic pulmonary disease (up to 20 percent).

Pulmonary function testing reflects both the stage of the disease and the activity of the underlying asthmatic state. Although the initial airway obstruction is reversible, it is often followed by increasing amounts of nonreversible obstruction and hyperinflation. As the disease progresses to the fibrotic stage, a restrictive pattern becomes superimposed on the obstructive changes.

TREATMENT

The treatment of ABPA is based on the assumption that the continued inflammation created by the immunologic reaction to intrabronchial *Aspergillus* organisms will lead both to further trapping of airway fungus and to permanent airway and parenchymal scarring. To date, corticosteroids are the only therapeutic agents shown to produce consistent clinical and radiographic improvements.

The use of corticosteroids is based on the understanding of the natural history of the disorder (Table 103-3). Inhaled steroid preparations are ineffective. Therefore, patients with acute disease are treated with 40 to 60 mg of oral prednisone per day. As the clinical symptoms and chest radiographs improve, the dose is decreased to 0.5 mg/kg body weight on alternate days. Alternate day therapy is usually continued for 3 months; the dose is then gradually tapered during the next 3 months. Levels of IgE in serum provide an excellent guide to the activity of the disease and should be determined frequently. If the patient remains in remission, no treatment is necessary other than that needed to treat the underlying asthmatic condition. Close follow-up is important because radiographic infiltrates and increased levels of IgE in serum occur in asymptomatic patients; asymptomatic or symptomatic exacerbations should be treated in the same way as the acute stage. However, most patients require maintenance corticosteroid therapy to control asthmatic symptoms, to prevent radiographic infiltrates, and to avoid marked increases in the level of total IgE in the serum. The minimum effective dose of steroids should be used, preferably an every other day regimen.

Other forms of therapy such as disodium cromoglycate and immunotherapy have not proved to be effective.

Bronchocentric Granulomatosis and Mucoid Impaction of the Bronchus

Bronchocentric granulomatosis is an unusual pathologic entity that is characterized by granulomatous destruction of pulmonary parenchyma around airways. Large and small airways are involved; the inflammation is intense and consists of a dense infiltrate of eosinophils, lymphocytes, and plasma cells surrounded by palisading epithelioid cells. The lumens of the airways are filled with necrotic material; blood vessels are not primarily affected. Radiographically, the disease most often appears in an upper lobe, either as a solitary nodule or an area of discrete consolidation. The diagnosis is usually made retrospectively, after the lesion has been resected.

Aspergillus hyphae have been identified within the lesion in 40 to 50 percent of patients with bronchocentric granulomatosis. Patients with bronchocentric aspergillosis are usually young, have a strong history of asthma, and manifest peripheral eosinophilia and positive skin tests to *Aspergillus*. They probably represent a subset of ABPA. However, it is unclear why they develop this peculiar localized pathologic reaction instead of the more generalized abnormalities seen in "classic" ABPA; the duration and intensity of exposure or their underlying lung architecture may be important factors. In the other patients with bronchocentric granulomatosis, the clinical syndrome is similar except for the absence of asthma or other evidence of immunologic reaction to *Aspergillus*; no antigen has been implicated in the pathogenesis of this disorder.

In patients who lack evidence of multiple lesions or systemic disease, resection of the diseased area effects a cure. But, corticosteroids are administered as for ABPA if multiple lesions are present, if there is evidence of a systemic immune response to *Aspergillus* (e.g., increase in the level of the total IgE in the serum) or a recurrence.

Extrinsic Allergic Alveolitis

Aspergilli, especially A. *clavatus*, sometimes serve as an inhaled antigen in producing extrinsic allergic alveolitis. This clinical syndrome is identical to that seen in reactions to many other organic dusts. In contrast to ABPA, there is no colonization of the bronchial tree by *Aspergillus* organisms. "Malt worker's lung" and some instances of "farmer's lung" are thought to be due to repeated challenge with *Aspergillus* antigens.

The immunopathogenesis of the syndrome is not completely understood. However, both cell-mediated immunity (type IV response) and immune-complex deposition (type III response) have been implicated. Pathologically, acute extrinsic alveolitis is characterized by infiltrates of lymphocytes primarily within the interstitial and peripheral airspaces. Small, noncaseating granulomas are common, vasculitis is absent, and airway involvement is minimal. Prolonged exposure leads to interstitial fibrosis.

An acute, heavy exposure elicits an influenzalike illness consisting of fevers, myalgias, cough, and shortness

of breath. Eosinophilia and bronchospasm are absent. In chronic exposures, constitutional symptoms are less common, but shortness of breath is more prominent. Radiographically, acute extrinsic alveolitis is characterized by diffuse alveolar-interstitial infiltrates; in the chronic illness, a fine reticulonodular interstitial infiltrate develops. IgG serum precipitins against the appropriate *Aspergillus* antigen are invariably present. Immediate and delayed skin test reactions occur occasionally. The concentration of IgE in serum is normal.

The acute disease undergoes spontaneous resolution when the patient is removed from exposure to sources of antigen. Corticosteroids seem to hasten resolution. Prevention of the chronic form of the disease requires avoidance of exposure.

Extrinsic Asthma

Few patients develop an allergic type of asthma after inhalation of *Aspergillus* spores even though 20 to 30 percent of asthmatics do have positive immediate skin test reactions to *Aspergillus* antigens. In contrast to other forms of *Aspergillus*-induced hypersensitivity reactions, the response appears to be mediated only by IgE (type I). The reaction does not cause long-term damage to the lungs.

SAPROPHYTIC COLONIZATION

Aspergilloma

A pulmonary mycetoma (or "fungus ball") is a mass of intertwined fungal elements lying free inside a pulmonary cavity that opens to the tracheobronchial tree. Although a number of fungi (such as the *Mucorales, Pseudoallescheria boydii,* or *Candida*) are occasionally responsible for the formation of a mycetoma, the most common cause is *Aspergillus.* It is worth emphasizing that an aspergilloma is due to saprophytic growth of fungus within a *previously formed* pulmonary cavity. It differs from the cavitary lesions seen in chronic necrotizing aspergillosis and invasive pulmonary aspergillosis in which the organism is involved in initiating the inflammatory process and in which cavitation is a consequence of local tissue necrosis.

PATHOPHYSIOLOGY

Presumably, any disease that causes pulmonary cavitation can predispose to the development of an aspergilloma. Traditionally, tuberculosis has been the most common condition associated with aspergillomas; however, in some areas, sarcoidosis is the most frequent underlying cause. Other predisposing conditions include cavitary neoplasms, cystic (pulmonary) fibrosis, the pneumoconioses, healed abscess cavities, ankylosing spondylitis,

other fungal infections (especially healed coccidioidomycosis), bronchiectasis, congenital cysts, pulmonary infarctions, and bullous emphysema.

The probability of developing an aspergilloma appears to depend on the population. In patients with healed tuberculous cavities, the prevalence of aspergilloma ranges from 15 to 20 percent. In contrast, the incidence in patients with cystic sarcoidosis may be as high as 50 percent.

The mechanism by which the aspergilloma forms within a pulmonary cavity is still a matter of speculation. One explanation is that inhaled *Aspergillus* spores lodge in the wall of a preexisting cavity. Fungal proliferation begins, and a repetitive cycle of growth and death of the organism is established, depending on local intracavitary conditions and the degree of host resistance. Eventually, a tangled mass of living and dead fungal elements, mucus, blood, inflammatory cells, and debris accumulates within the cavity and forms the radiographically visible fungus ball. The wall of the cavity is lined by an extremely vascular granulation tissue. The process also stimulates a response in the surrounding pulmonary parenchyma: marked pleural thickening in the vicinity is common; also characteristic of the inflammatory reaction is a marked increase in collateral circulation to the affected area (Fig. 103-3).

CLINICAL COURSE

Few aspergillomas, i.e., no more than 7 to 10 percent, lyse spontaneously, generally after a bacterial infection. Some fungus balls persist asymptomatically for many years, eventually forming inactive calcified scars. Transition of an aspergilloma to allergic bronchopulmonary aspergillosis or invasive pulmonary disease is unusual.

About 70 percent of patients who have an aspergilloma manifest a chronic cough, malaise, weight loss or, most importantly, hemoptysis. Hemoptysis is usually recurrent and mild. But in some patients (up to 20 percent) the quantity of blood coughed up exceeds 150 ml per 24 h, i.e., the hemoptysis is "severe." Death from massive hemoptysis has been estimated to occur in 5 to 10 percent of patients with aspergillomas. However, in the vast majority of these patients, the underlying pulmonary disease is the most important factor in determining survival outcome. Most deaths in patients with pulmonary aspergillomas are due to chronic respiratory failure or pneumonia.

DIAGNOSIS

The diagnosis of aspergilloma is established by a combination of radiographic and serologic tests; culture of expectorated sputum yields *Aspergillus* in only about half of patients with this disorder.

The characteristic radiographic appearance of an aspergilloma is one or more rounded masses within a round

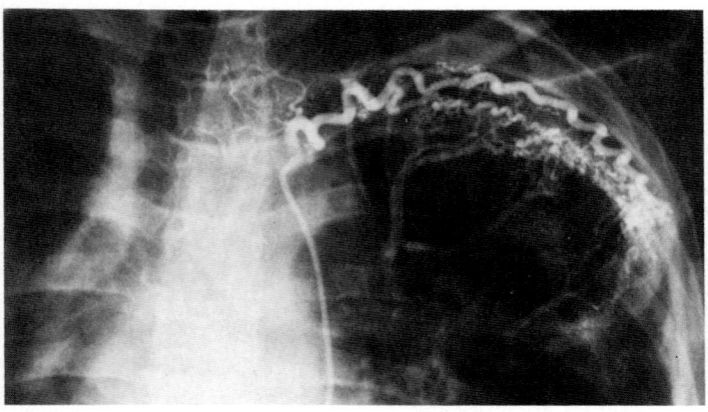
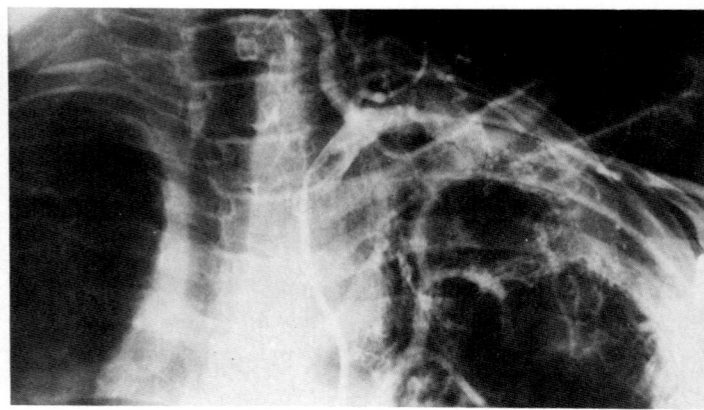

FIGURE 103-3 Arteriography was performed in a 43-year-old female with cystic sarcoidosis and a large left upper lobe aspergilloma because of massive hemoptysis. *A.* Injection of a bronchial artery shows that much of the blood supply of the superior portion of the aspergilloma was supplied by this vessel. *B.* Injection of the left subclavian artery demonstrates additional extensive collateral blood flow through the chest wall via the long thoracic artery.

or ovoid cavity (Fig. 103-4); "classically," the mass is demarcated on one aspect from the wall of the cavity by a crescent-shaped collection of air (Monod's sign). In some patients, the mycelial "ball" moves when the patient shifts position (Fig. 103-4C and D). Most of the cavities are in the upper lobes, reflecting the association with tuberculosis and sarcoidosis; their average diameter is 3 to 6 cm. The wall thickness varies. Adjacent pleural thickening is common and often precedes the characteristic radiologic appearance of a fungus ball. Air-fluid levels are unusual; they denote hemorrhage, concomitant bacterial infection, or liquefaction of the fungal mass. Calcification along the rim or within the fungal mass sometimes occurs in long-standing lesions.

Although a standard chest radiograph usually suffices to identify the presence of a mycetoma, diagnosis can be difficult when the appearance of the lesion is atypical, i.e., when it appears to be a poorly defined upper lobe density or an "empty" cavity. In patients with extensive underlying lung disease, linear or computed tomography generally settles the diagnosis (see Fig. 36-16).

Although the radiographic appearance of a fungus ball is relatively sensitive for detecting an aspergilloma, it is not specific. Differential diagnosis includes bacterial or tuberculous lung abscesses, cavitating tumors, liquefying pulmonary infarcts, or mycetomas due to other fungal organisms. For this reason, serologic confirmation of the diagnosis is important. Almost 100 percent of immunologically normal patients who develop an aspergilloma demonstrate precipitating IgG antibodies against *Aspergillus* antigens; in contrast, the prevalence of a positive test in normal individuals is less than 1 percent. However, the precipitin test may be positive only for the particular *Aspergillus* species infecting the patient. In contrast to the value of the serum precipitating antibody test, skin testing with *Aspergillus* antigens is of relatively little diagnostic value: only about half the patients with aspergillomas manifest skin test reactivity of the immediate type, and only an occasional patient develops a late response to intradermal testing.

TREATMENT

The major clinical concern in patients with pulmonary aspergillomas is massive hemoptysis. Since there is no effective medical therapy for aspergilloma, some clinics recommend surgical removal of all lesions. Indeed, surgical resection of an aspergilloma is the only certain method of cure. Unfortunately, only 20 to 40 percent of patients with mycetomas are candidates for surgical excision of the lesion. The remainder are disqualified on different grounds: bilateral or multiple aspergillomas, severe pulmonary fibrosis, chronic bronchitis and emphysema, or cor pulmonale. Even in those who are judged to be capable of withstanding the surgical procedure, the incidence of surgical complications is high (on the order of 25 percent). The complications include massive bleeding that requires inordinate blood transfusions, bronchopleural fistula, *Aspergillus* empyema, postoperative pneumonia, and difficulty in weaning from mechanical ventilator support. In addition, the surgical mortality rate is 5 to 10 percent. The high morbidity and mortality is generally due to a combination of inadequate pulmonary reserve and the technically difficult surgical procedures arising from obliteration of surgical planes and blurring of anatomic boundaries in the vicinity of the aspergilloma by the intense pleural inflammatory reaction. As a result, the surgeon is constrained to "nonanatomic" resection. The proliferated collateral circulation adds to the complexity of the procedure. Finally, the remaining lung is often diffi-

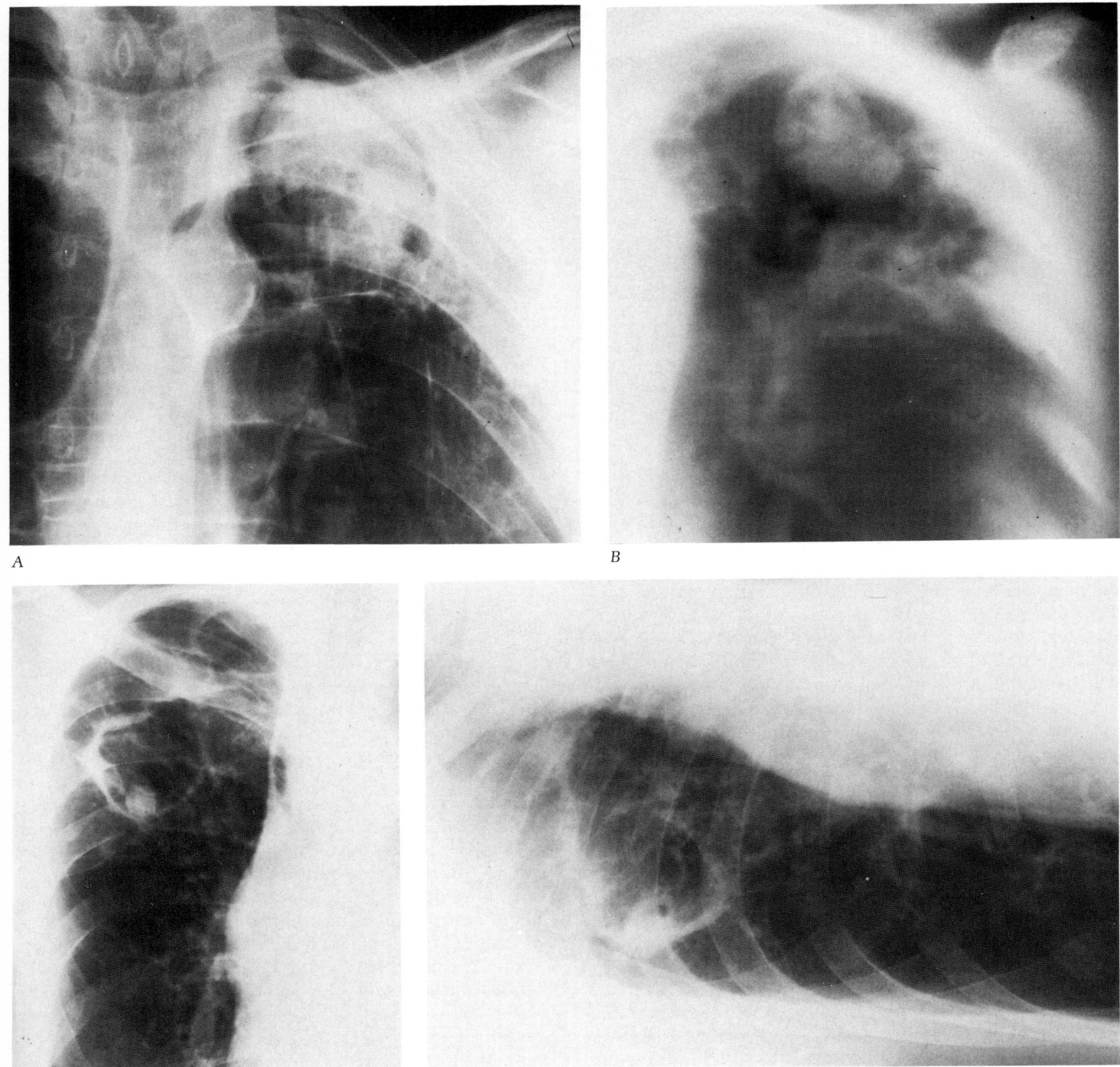

A

B

C

D

FIGURE 103-4 Radiographic appearances of pulmonary aspergillomas. *A.* A 51-year-old male with a history of tuberculosis shows the classic crescent-shaped patch of air (Monod's sign), as well as marked pleural thickening. *B.* Tomogram shows well-defined fungus ball within a thick walled upper lobe cavity. *C.* A 49-year-old male with ankylosing spondylitis who developed an aspergilloma inside a thin-walled cavity. *D.* Decubitus film from same patient shows fungus ball moving when the patient changes position.

cult to reexpand, predisposing the patient to infection and bronchopleural fistula.

Because surgical intervention carries such a high risk, surgical resection is generally reserved for two relatively small groups: symptomatic patients in whom the disease is localized and pulmonary function is good, and desperately ill patients in whom hemoptysis is uncontrollable and life-threatening.

An assortment of "medical" therapies have been tried in symptomatic patients who are poor surgical candidates because of underlying pulmonary disease. These include: (1) amphotericin B administered intravenously; as a rule this treatment is ineffective, probably because of poor penetration of the drug into the fungal mass; (2) direct instillation of antifungal agents (such as sodium iodide, nystatin hydrochloride, natamycin, and amphotericin B) via endobronchial or transthoracic routes; because this approach is only occasionally successful and often evokes systemic symptoms (e.g., fever), it is generally reserved for patients with active hemoptysis; (3) a mixture of amphotericin B and N-acetyl-L-cysteine administered transthoracically directly into the aspergilloma cavity; this technique is also reserved for high-risk surgical patients with massive hemoptysis and is effective in controlling the bleeding even though the aspergilloma persists; and (4) bronchial artery embolization; unfortunately, because of the extensive collateral circulation (Fig. 103-3), this technique is rarely successful in controlling bleeding from an aspergilloma (in contrast to patients with pulmonary bleeding due to tuberculosis or bronchogenic carcinoma).

In summary, the choice of therapy for a particular patient with a pulmonary aspergilloma must be carefully individualized. Often, observation without intervention proves to be the best course of "action."

INVASIVE ASPERGILLOSIS

Invasive Pulmonary Aspergillosis

Invasive pulmonary aspergillosis (IPA) is almost always caused by the inhalation of *Aspergillus* species spores by a susceptible host. However, in a few instances, hematogenous dissemination to the lungs occurs from a cutaneous or gastrointestinal source. Both a susceptible host and exposure to environmental *Aspergillus* spores are essential for the occurrence of IPA.

PATHOPHYSIOLOGY

Where inhaled spores land in the respiratory tract depends on their size and surface characteristics. Since *A. fumigatus* spores are 2 to 4 μm in diameter and *A. flavus*, 3.5 to 4.2 μm, appreciable numbers of either organism would be expected to reach the alveoli. Larger spores, es-

pecially those of *A. flavus*, also deposit in the upper respiratory tract. The size-related difference in sites of deposition may underlie the known propensity of *A. flavus* to cause not only IPA, but also invasive nasal and sinus aspergillosis. Although it has been proposed that a state of nasal colonization precedes the invasive state, careful examination of patients whose nasal cultures grow *A. fumigatus* or *A. flavus* consistently reveals small nasal ulcerations that suggest early invasive disease.

Once *Aspergillus* spores reach the lower respiratory tract, they germinate and develop into invasive hyphae only if local conditions permit. Pulmonary defenses against IPA depend on two independent, but complementary, mechanisms. First, alveolar macrophages ingest inhaled spores and kill them. Studies in nude mice suggest that the function of macrophages that act to eliminate *Aspergillus* spores is enhanced by immunologic mechanisms involving T cells. Impairment of macrophage fungicidal mechanisms, as by corticosteroids, enables spores to develop into invasive hyphae.

Second, germinating spores and hyphae are attacked by polymorphonuclear leukocytes and monocytes. Whereas resting *Aspergillus* spores do not induce neutrophil chemotaxis, stimulated spores attract neutrophils, which kill hyphae, primarily by oxidative microbicidal mechanisms; experimental animals, rendered neutropenic, are markedly susceptible to invasive aspergillosis. Monocytes are also involved; they use both oxidative mechanisms and nonoxidative microbicidal mechanisms to destroy hyphae.

Both quantitative and qualitative defects in macrophage or neutrophil function enhance the prospects for developing IPA (Table 103-5). The defect may stem from the underlying disease [e.g., chronic granulomatous disease (CGD)] or from medical therapy (e.g., corticosteroids, radiation therapy or from cytotoxic chemotherapy). In acute leukemia, the duration of neutropenia constitutes a major risk factor. The role of antibiotic therapy in the pathogenesis of IPA remains uncertain: carbenicillin, which eradicates normal nasal flora, has been postulated to enhance the development of IPA; alternatively, antibiotic therapy may simply permit patients to survive long enough for invasive fungal disease to occur.

Rarely, individuals who are apparently normal develop IPA. On occasion, they have been exposed to overwhelming amounts of environmental *Aspergillus* spores. However, the reason often remains unclear; in these, it can be postulated that one or more subtle defects in anti-*Aspergillus* defenses—defects that defied recognition despite extensive testing—are responsible for the IPA.

The propensity of pathogenic *Aspergillus* species for vascular invasion produces vascular inflammation and infarction distal to the vasculitis. Although most manifestations of IPA are presumed due to invasion of tissues and blood vessels by the organisms, soluble products that are

TABLE 103-5
Risk Factors for the Development of Invasive Pulmonary Aspergillosis

Host Defense Defect	Patient Populations at Risk
Quantitative neutrophil defect (neutropenia)	Acute leukemia during chemotherapy-induced nadir
	Bone marrow transplantation
	Aplastic anemia
	Lymphoma/carcinoma (during neutropenia)
Qualitative neutrophil defect	Corticosteroid therapy
	Renal transplantation
	Cardiac transplantation
	Severe hepatic disease
	Endogenous hypercortisolism (Cushing's syndrome)
	Chronic abnormalities of neutrophil microbicidal function (e.g., chronic granulomatous disease of childhood)
Pulmonary macrophage defect (qualitative or quantitative)	Diffuse lung infection
	Influenza
	? Cytomegalovirus
	Other causes of diffuse lung damage
	Bone marrow transplantation
	? Chemotherapy, e.g., cytosine arabinoside
	Corticosteroid therapy

elaborated by the organism may contribute to the pathogenesis of the IPA. For example, *A. flavus* produces aflatoxin that might contribute to the hemorrhagic tendencies of these patients. In addition, some strains of *A. fumigatus* produce an elastase which increases the pathogenicity of the organism in mice.

The pathologic features of IPA include both suppurative and infarctive components. The relative contribution of each depends on the immune status of the patient and the massiveness of the infection. In those patients in whom local necrosis rather than suppuration predominates, the lesions resemble either hemorrhagic infarcts or pyemic abscesses. Bronchi within the area or in the vicinity sometimes contain mycelia, presumably reflecting the portal of entry of the fungus into the pulmonary parenchyma. Occasionally, hemorrhagic infarction (Fig. 103-5) can be shown to be secondary to mycotic invasion and thrombosis of a pulmonary arterial branch. These individuals, who cannot mount an adequate tissue reaction to the invading fungus, are likely candidates for overwhelming dissemination of the organism by bloodstream, occasionally in conjunction with bacterial septicemia, e.g., with *Pseudomonas aeruginosa*.

Patients capable of a neutrophilic response develop either an acute pneumonia or local abscess (Fig. 103-6C). The cavity of the abscess contains fungal hyphae and polymorphonuclear leukocytes surrounded by chronic inflammatory cells and foreign body giant cells. In the pneumonic type, polymorphonuclear leukocytes generally predominate; but, on occasion, an eosinophilic pneumonia ensues.

Other tissue responses also occur, presumably reflecting the immune status and massiveness of the infection. Thus, tuberculoid lesions of the parenchyma, granulomatous lesions of the bronchi, and invasive tracheobronchitis have also been reported.

CLINICAL COURSE

The presenting clinical manifestations of IPA can be subtle when severe qualitative or quantitative neutrophil abnormalities impair the host's inflammatory response. In hospitalized neutropenic patients, persistent fever is often the sole presenting manifestation. In time, a mild nonproductive cough may develop, reflecting bronchitis without pulmonary parenchymal invasion. Alternatively, patients may develop acute pleuritic chest or upper abdominal pain, which may be so severe as to require narcotic analgesia. As the disease progresses, fever worsens, rales develop, and pulmonary infiltrates appear.

In patients with acute leukemia, the clinical manifestations of IPA often evolve as the patient's neutrophil count recovers from the nadir induced by chemotherapy. Cough often worsens and becomes productive. Hemoptysis, which occurs in up to 40 percent of patients, is usually minor (20 ml or less of blood), but on occasion may be massive. Massive hemoptysis appears to coincide with the resolution of the neutropenia. It is apparently a consequence of the formation of abscesses and necrosis as granulocytes move into infected areas of the lung. In support of this proposed mechanism is the observation that some patients expectorate plugs of necrotic lung laden with *Aspergillus* hyphae.

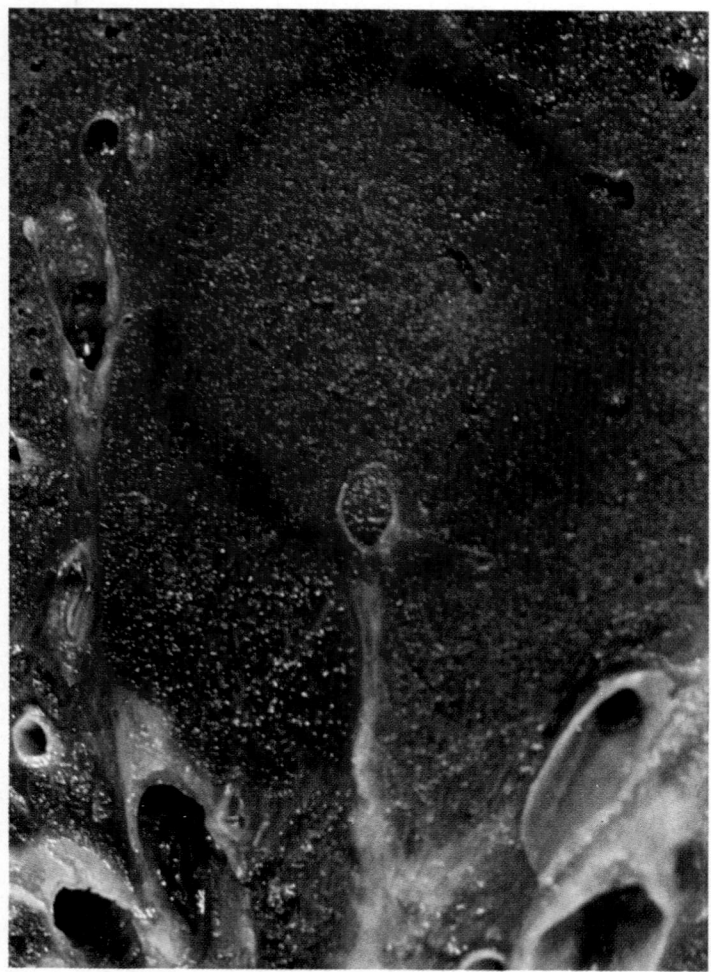
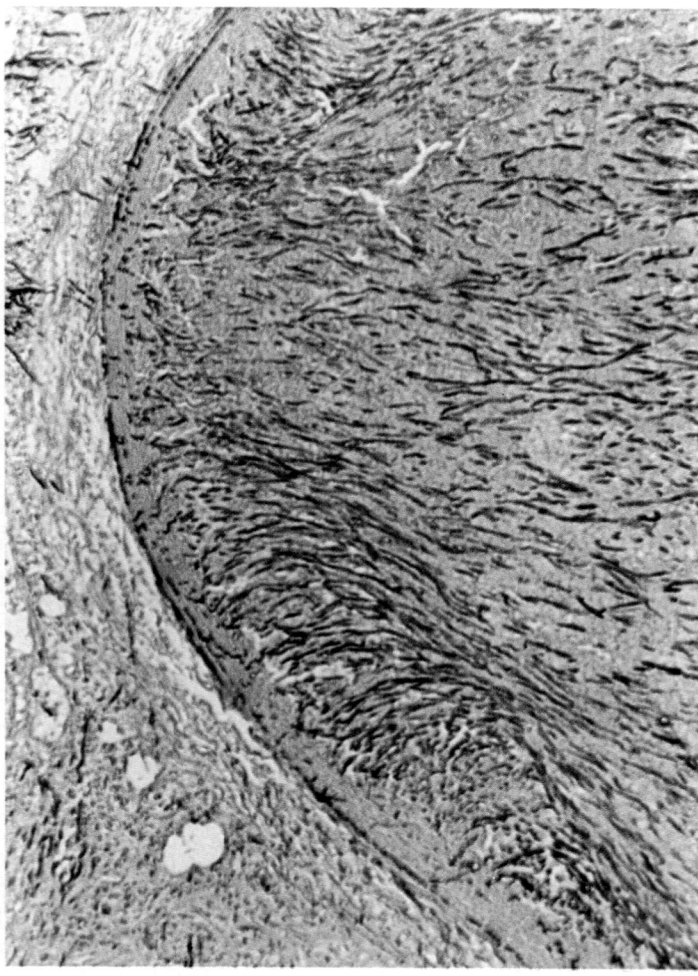

A   B

FIGURE 103-5 A 62-year-old male with acute leukemia who developed invasive pulmonary aspergillosis.   A. Gross appearance of fungal lesion. A central necrotic area is surrounded by a lining of hemorrhagic infarction.   B. Grocott stain shows characteristic appearance of aspergilli in tissue. *(Courtesy of Dr. G. G. Pietra.)*

Although the lower respiratory tract is the only site of involvement in 60 percent of patients with invasive aspergillosis, in 30 percent the disease is both pulmonary and extrapulmonary. Among the extrapulmonary sites are the highly vascular organs, such as the gastrointestinal tract, the brain, the liver, the kidneys, and the thyroid. On occasion, *Aspergillus* is also found in the heart, the diaphragm, the testes, and the skin.

IPA is sometimes preceded by invasive aspergillosis of the *upper* respiratory tract. Although epiglottitis and oropharyngeal involvement occasionally occur, invasive disease of the nose and paranasal sinuses is more common, especially when the causative agent is *A. flavus.* Epistaxis and nasal stuffiness may herald the development of localized nasal ulceration, with or without eschar formation. Although not pathognomonic of invasive aspergillosis, the combination of nasal ulceration and a pulmonary infiltrate in the profoundly neutropenic host is

highly suggestive of the diagnosis. However, mucormycosis, trauma, bacterial infection, and infection with the herpes simplex virus must be included in the differential diagnosis.

Nasal aspergillosis may be accompanied by invasive aspergillosis of the paranasal sinuses, but sinusitis can occur without antecedent nasal aspergillosis; the maxillary, sphenoid, and/or ethmoid sinuses may be involved. Complaints of paranasal pain and congestion with tenderness on palpation are followed by facial swelling and discoloration over the affected sinus.

DIAGNOSIS

The unequivocal diagnosis of IPA requires both the pathologic demonstration of tissue invasion by hyphae that are morphologically consistent with *Aspergillus* species and the recovery of the organism on culture. Morphologic criteria, per se, can be misleading because of the organism's

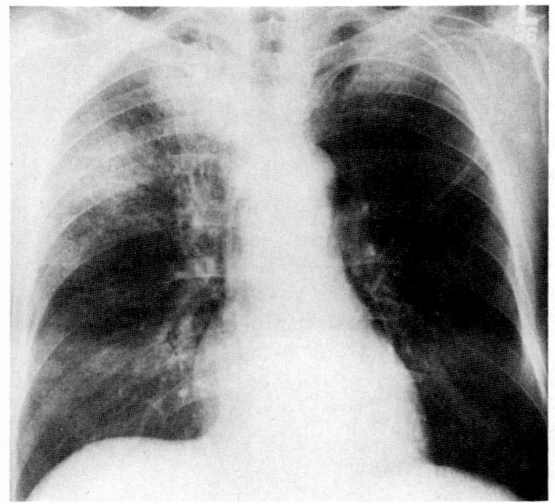

A

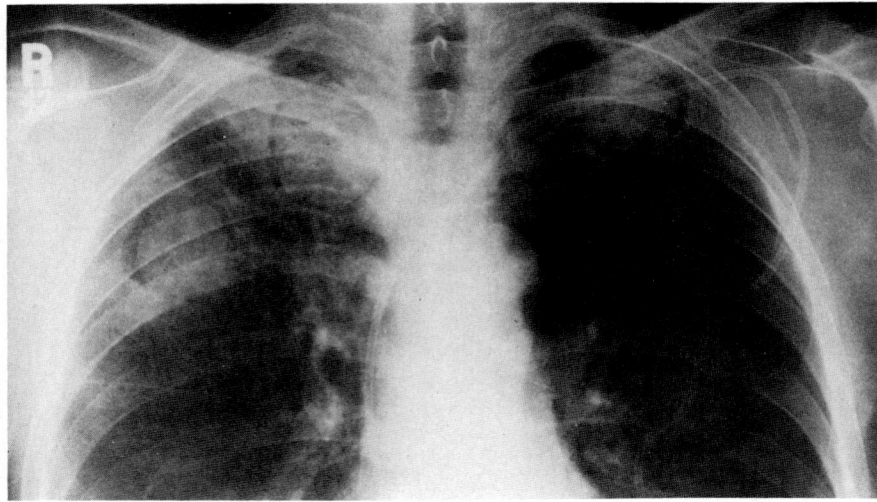

B

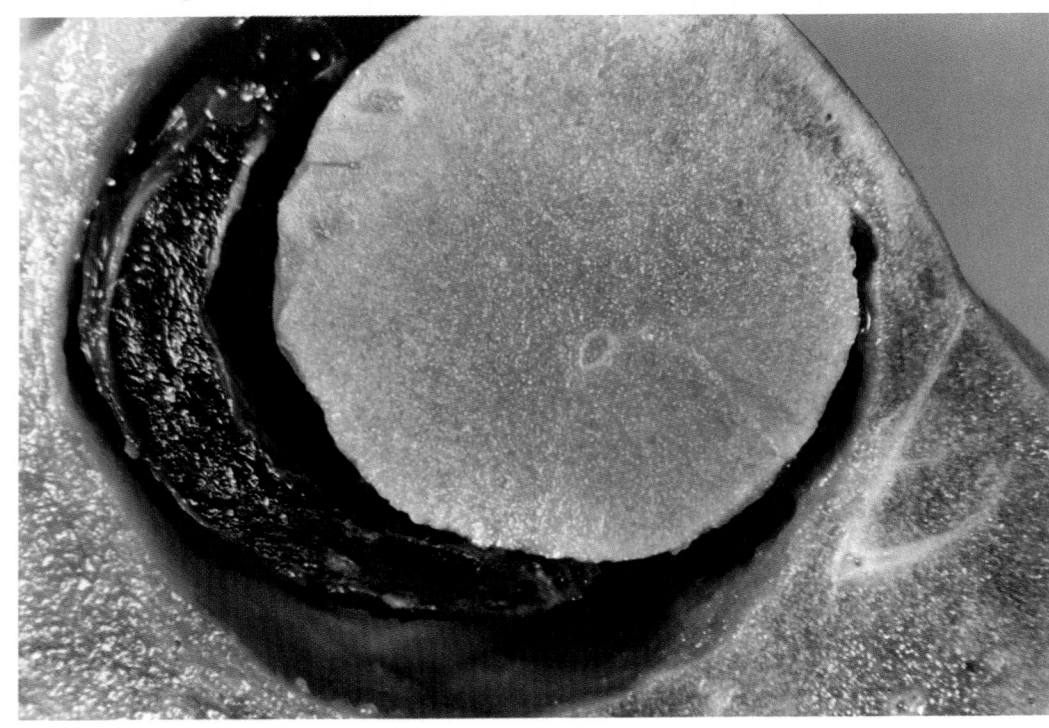

C

FIGURE 103-6 The characteristic pathologic and radiographic features of invasive pulmonary aspergillosis are illustrated in this 56-year-old man with acute leukemia. *A.* Multiple hazy nodular infiltrates appear after 2 weeks of chemotherapy-induced neutropenia. *B.* As the neutrophil count begins to rise, the lesions become more "discrete" and nodular in appearance. Two days after the neutrophil count exceeded 500 cells per cubic millimeter, all the lesions have cavitated, creating "air crescents." *C.* Gross appearance of one of the lesions shows the necrotic "lung ball" surrounded by hemorrhage and a crescent of air. *(By permission of Gefter WB, et al., Radiology 157:607, 1985.)*

resemblance to other fungi, primarily to *Pseudoallescheria boydii* and *Penicillium* and *Fusarium* species.

A variety of invasive diagnostic techniques are used in different clinics to establish the diagnosis of IPA. The diagnostic yield from each procedure varies with the experience of those performing the procedure, the patient population studied, the timing of the procedure, and the definitions used to categorize diseases caused by *Aspergillus* infection. Bronchoscopy is a common procedure. Brushings and washings obtained by bronchoscopy or bronchoalveolar lavage fluid are helpful in diagnosis when *Aspergillus* is identified morphologically or by cul-

ture. However, failure to find the organism does not exclude IPA and false-positive results do occur. Transbronchial biopsy is falsely negative in approximately 50 percent of patients. Brushings and washings performed later in the course of disease are more apt to be positive than in the earlier stages.

Transthoracic needle biopsy is helpful when organisms are demonstrated histologically, but false-negative results occur. Surprisingly, falsely negative results have also been obtained by open lung biopsy, presumably due to sampling error.

Unfortunately, the severely immunocompromised

patient who is at highest risk for IPA is also least likely able to tolerate invasive diagnostic procedures. Therefore, efforts have focused on noninvasive clinical and laboratory techniques to establish the diagnosis of IPA. An understanding of the patient populations at risk for developing IPA, plus awareness of its presenting signs and symptoms, should permit the clinician to suspect the diagnosis of IPA antemortem. The specificity of clinical signs and symptoms is increased substantially if clustering of IPA has occurred in a particular hospital or hospital ward.

The chest radiograph may be entirely normal despite fever and pleuritic chest pain. When an infiltrate does appear, it may be subtle, so that several days are lost before the radiographic diagnosis is made. The initial infiltrate may be lobar or a patchy bronchopneumonia. However, bilateral or multilobed unilateral infiltrates occur in approximately 50 percent of patients (Fig. 103-6A). Infiltrates characteristically become nodular, except during persistent neutropenia or when coexisting candidiasis causes diffuse lung disease. As neutropenia resolves, pulmonary cavitation develops de novo in 75 percent of cases; multiple nodules may cavitate simultaneously (Fig. 103-6B and C). Although the "air crescent" sign also occurs in mucormycosis, nocardiosis, bacterial lung abscess, malignancy, and tuberculosis, IPA is the most likely cause in a patient with a qualitative or quantitative deficiency of neutrophils. Unfortunately, air crescents do not develop soon enough to facilitate early diagnosis and therapy.

Blood cultures rarely yield *Aspergillus,* even when endothelium in heart valves or vessels has been seeded with the organism. In patients at low risk for IPA, cultures of expectorated sputum for *Aspergillus* are unreliable due to a high frequency of both false positives and false negatives. However, in patients at high risk for IPA, sputum cultures are highly sensitive and specific. Exceedingly relevant for interpretation of sputum cultures is the *Aspergillus* species that is isolated: *A. flavus* or *A. fumigatus* is much more likely to be related to IPA than is recovery of other, less pathogenic, *Aspergillus* species. Isolation of *A. flavus* or *A. fumigatus* from even a single expectorated sputum from a patient at high risk for IPA strongly suggests invasive aspergillosis; multiple positive cultures for these organisms reinforce the diagnosis. The major limitation of the forced reliance on cultures is the inevitable delay before results become available and the inability of some patients to produce sputum for culture.

Recovery of *A. flavus* or *A. fumigatus* from nasal swab specimens raises the prospect that the oropharynx, nose, and sinuses may be involved. Nasal surveillance cultures may be especially useful in epidemic situations, but even in these circumstances the inherent delay in obtaining results of cultures diminishes their practical utility.

The value of detecting *Aspergillus* antibodies for the immunodiagnosis of IPA is limited, presumably because of the impaired immune status of these severely compromised patients. A solid-phase radioimmunoassay technique reported in 1979 was promising, but neither this method nor others have become widely available. As a result, attention has turned to detection of circulating *Aspergillus* antigen. Both radioimmunoassay and enzyme-linked immunosorbent assay appear to be of diagnostic value. In addition, the radioimmunoassay has been employed to detect *Aspergillus* antigen in bronchoalveolar lavage fluid. However, neither test is yet available commercially.

TREATMENT

The critical variables affecting the prognosis of patients with IPA are the severity and outcome of the underlying disease. In neutropenic patients, antifungal therapy may delay progression of IPA, but cure is virtually impossible unless the bone marrow recovers. In contrast, antifungal therapy may cure patients with chronic granulomatous disease, in which the immunologic defect is less severe. Early treatment of IPA is essential, since patients with overwhelming infection may succumb even though normal host defenses are restored.

Amphotericin B, administered intravenously, is the mainstay of treatment. However, successful treatment using amphotericin B is limited by the toxicity of the drug and the organism's intrinsic resistance to its antifungal activity. The minimum inhibitory concentration of amphotericin B for various *Aspergillus* species ranges from 0.5 μg/ml or less to 3 μg/ml or more. Since peak serum concentrations of amphotericin B following conventional intravenous doses rarely exceed 1 to 2 μg/ml, the therapeutic index of amphotericin B is small. Treatment failures occur even though the drug is concentrated in the liver, spleen, kidneys, and lungs. Few data exist as a basis for correlating the susceptibility of the organism in vitro with the response to antifungal chemotherapy.

Despite these limitations, amphotericin B is administered intravenously when IPA is proved or strongly suspected. For clinically evident disease, the patient receives on the first day a test dose of 1 mg followed by a total of 0.2 to 0.3 mg/kg; the next dose, 0.5 to 0.6 mg/kg, is given within 12 to 24 h. A daily maintenance dose of 0.6 to 0.7 mg/kg per day often suffices, but higher doses, i.e., up to 1.0 to 1.5 mg/kg per day, are sometimes used. Doses in the higher range can be complicated by nephrotoxicity. Patients receiving amphotericin B must also be monitored closely for other predictable adverse reactions, including phlebitis, hypokalemia, hypomagnesemia, and anemia. Although the optimal total dose of amphotericin B is not settled, a dose of 1 to 2 g is generally recommended.

Neither miconazole, 5-fluorocytosine (5-FC), nor ketoconazole is, per se, an acceptable substitute for amphotericin B. However, experimental data do afford a ra-

tionale for using 5-FC, rifampin, or tetracycline in combination with amphotericin B; presumably, the second agent enters the organism when fungal cell wall synthesis is interrupted by amphotericin B. Although anecdotal accounts have been encouraging, no controlled data are available to prove the efficacy of these combinations. Observations in vitro and animal experiments suggest that administration of ketoconazole before amphotericin B is given causes antagonism between the two agents. A second antifungal agent, such as rifampin, is sometimes used empirically when the condition of a patient with IPA worsens in the face of maximal amphotericin B therapy.

Among the agents being investigated with respect to the treatment of IPA are liposomal amphotericin B and itraconazole; the latter is an oral imidazole that has excellent in vitro activity against a variety of *Aspergillus* species.

White blood cell transfusions have been used successfully in some patients with chronic granulomatous disease who develop IPA. However, no controlled data exist to support this approach. Because of uncertain effectiveness of white blood cell transfusions in the treatment of proved bacterial infection, and because of the possible interaction of the transfused cells with concurrently administered amphotericin B, no recommendation can yet be made concerning the use of white blood cell transfusion in IPA.

Surgical resection of a localized area is indicated in the patient with IPA who develops massive hemoptysis *if* the site of bleeding can be identified and *if* the patient's prognosis warrants intervention. Surgery is also curative in some patients with chronic granulomatous disease and localized IPA. An essential preoperative consideration is whether the disease is truly localized so that surgical resection can be curative. The multicentric nature of IPA makes it ill-advised to assume that resection of a single segment, or lobe, will result in cure.

PREVENTION

Prevention can be achieved either by (1) eliminating, or abbreviating, the duration of high risk engendered by the underlying defect in host defenses or (2) preventing, or reducing, exposure of susceptible patients to *Aspergillus* spores. Unfortunately, intensely myelosuppressive chemotherapy remains an essential part of treatment for many forms of acute leukemia, lymphoma, and carcinoma. More feasible is shortening of the period of risk in patients undergoing organ transplantation; the use of cyclosporin in these patients has reduced the requirement for high-dose, prolonged corticosteroid therapy.

Although elimination of environmental sources of *Aspergillus* and improvement in hospital air filtration systems may decrease airborne spore counts, complete elimination of spores from most hospital rooms and corridors is virtually impossible since they may enter through open windows, on clothes, and on other materials. Installation of laminar airflow systems is an expensive, logistically difficult solution not available to most hospitals. Self-contained, in-room, high efficiency filtration units are a less expensive option that may be helpful.

Accordingly, prophylactic antifungal chemotherapy would be valuable if a suitable agent could be found. Unfortunately, the potential toxicities of amphotericin B administered intravenously preclude its use as a prophylactic agent. A nasal spray containing amphotericin B has recently been advocated as effective in prophylaxis of aspergillosis in neutropenic patients. However, the observations were uncontrolled and the underlying assumption to this approach is that IPA is a consequence of nasal aspergillosis. Other available antifungal agents do not have sufficient in vitro or in vivo activity against *Aspergillus* to be effective. New antifungal agents with both efficacy against *Aspergillus* species organisms and lack of severe toxicities is needed.

At present, the most reasonable approach to early intervention is empirical amphotericin B treatment of neutropenic patients who develop a fever that is unresponsive to antibacterial antibiotics. Seven days of fever is one generally accepted starting time. This approach seems to strike a proper balance between the need on the one hand to minimize the likelihood of drug toxicity (that is apt to ensue if treatment with amphotericin B is started prematurely) and on the other hand to prevent the accumulation of fungi in the body to a level that would preclude effective therapy. Institution of amphotericin B therapy empirically after 7 days of fever affords the added advantage of treating occult systemic candidiasis. Development of newer immunodiagnostic techniques is expected to facilitate the early institution of antifungal therapy.

Chronic Necrotizing Pulmonary Aspergillosis

Patients with chronic necrotizing pulmonary aspergillosis are less severely immunocompromised than are those with "classic" invasive pulmonary aspergillosis. Accordingly, their disease runs a more indolent course. It begins with fever and productive cough of a 1- to 6-month duration. Affected individuals are usually middle-aged and mildly compromised by diabetes mellitus, malnutrition, connective tissue disease, corticosteroid therapy, or chronic lung disease. The chest radiograph reveals an infiltrate that involves one or more lobes and is often cavitary. Cavitation may be accompanied by appearance of a fungus ball similar to that seen in IPA but distinctly different from an aspergilloma. The diagnosis is suggested by recovery of *Aspergillus* from sputum cultures in the appropriate clinical setting; it is established by pathologic

confirmation of tissue invasion. Amphotericin B, administered intravenously, cures some patients, but pulmonary resection may be necessary in individuals with extensive disease.

PLEURAL ASPERGILLOSIS

In addition to the various forms of pulmonary disease caused by *Aspergillus*, pleural involvement also occasionally occurs. The most common form of pleural aspergillosis is an *Aspergillus* empyema that results from secondary infection of a preexisting chronic pleural effusion. Nearly 90 percent of these effusions are related to underlying tuberculosis, and most occur in patients in whom the effusions are associated with bronchopleural, or pleurocutaneous, fistulas. In almost every instance, the use of multiple antibiotics antecedes the development of the pleural aspergillosis. Other conditions associated with *Aspergillus* infection of the pleura include bacterial empyemas, open or closed pleural drainage procedures, and lung resection.

Pleural *Aspergillus* infection that is secondary to pulmonary aspergillosis is quite unusual. However, infection due to spillage of the contents of an aspergilloma during surgery or spontaneous rupture of an aspergilloma into the pleural cavity do occur. In immunocompromised hosts, pleural infection and a pneumothorax occasionally result from extension of invasive pulmonary aspergillosis.

The optimal treatment of pleural aspergillosis is not well established. Pleural drainage, open or closed, appears to be a cornerstone of therapy. Most successfully treated patients have received amphotericin B intravenously, often for prolonged periods. If the disease is circumscribed and the patient can tolerate surgery, resection of the involved area may hasten recovery. Intrapleural administration of amphotericin B has been suggested. However, there are few data to document the efficacy of this approach.

BIBLIOGRAPHY

Aisner J, Murillo J, Schimpff SC, Steere AC: Invasive aspergillosis in acute leukemia: Correlation with nose cultures and antibiotic use. Ann Intern Med 90:4–9, 1979.
   Ten of eleven patients with nose cultures growing A. flavus or A. fumigatus had invasive pulmonary aspergillosis.

Albelda SM, Gefter WB, Epstein DM, Miller WT: Bronchopleural fistula complicating invasive pulmonary aspergillosis. Am Rev Respir Dis 126:163–165, 1982.
   Describes first case of pleural involvement in invasive aspergillosis disease and reviews the literature on pleural aspergillosis.

Albelda SM, Talbot GH, Gerson SL, Miller WT, Cassileth PA: Pulmonary cavitation and massive hemoptysis in invasive pulmonary aspergillosis. Influence of bone marrow recovery in patients with acute leukemia. Am Rev Respir Dis 131:115–120, 1985.
   In patients with acute leukemia and invasive pulmonary aspergillosis, recovery of the neutrophil count to greater than 500 per cubic milliliter was associated with pulmonary cavitation and, on occasion, with massive hemoptysis.

Gerson SL, Talbot GH, Hurwitz S, Strom BL, Lusk EJ, Cassileth PA: Prolonged granulocytopenia: The major risk factor for invasive pulmonary aspergillosis in patients with acute leukemia. Ann Intern Med 100:345–351, 1984.
   Granulocytopenia persisting longer than 3 weeks was the major risk factor for invasive pulmonary aspergillosis; neither antibiotic nor corticosteroid therapy was a significant risk factor.

Gerson SL, Talbot GH, Lusk E, Hurwitz S, Strom BL, Cassileth PA: Invasive pulmonary aspergillosis in adult acute leukemia: Clinical clues to its diagnosis. J Clin Oncol 3:1109–1116, 1985.
   The clinical picture of 15 patients with invasive pulmonary aspergillosis complicating acute leukemia in adults is compared with that of 45 patients without this complication.

Glimp RA, Bayor AS: Pulmonary aspergilloma: Diagnostic and therapeutic considerations. Arch Intern Med 143:303–308, 1983.
   Recent, thorough, well-referenced review article.

Gustafson TL, Shaffnner W, Lavely GP, Stratton CW, Johnson HK, Hutcheson RH: Invasive aspergillosis in renal transplant recipients: Correlation with corticosteroid therapy. J Infect Dis 148:230–238, 1983.
   In renal transplant recipients, an average daily prednisone dose of ≥1.25 mg/kg was the best predictor of subsequent invasive aspergillosis.

Hargis JL, Bone RC, Stewart J, Rector N, Hiller FC: Intracavitary amphotericin B in the treatment of symptomatic pulmonary aspergillomas. Am J Med 68:389–394, 1980.

Report of six patients with symptomatic aspergillomas who were treated with intracavitary amphotericin B. Four of the six showed improvement.

Israel HL, Lenchner GS, Atkinson GW: Sarcoidosis and aspergilloma—the role of surgery. Chest 82:430–432, 1982.

Documents the problems with surgical treatment of aspergilloma in sarcoid patients.

Kahn FW, Jones JM, England DM: The role of bronchoalveolar lavage in the diagnosis of invasive pulmonary aspergillosis. Am J Clin Pathol 86:518–523, 1986.

Cultures and histochemical stains for fungi were performed on concentrated, cytocentrifuged bronchoalveolar lavage (BAL) samples from 82 immunocompromised patients undergoing bronchoscopic evaluation of new pulmonary infiltrates. Aspergillus hyphae was identified in 9 of 17 BAL samples from patients with invasive pulmonary aspergillosis and from 3 of the remaining 65 study patients without this diagnosis. BAL is a valuable first procedure for diagnosing invasive pulmonary aspergillosis in the compromised host.

Katzenstein AL, Liebow AA, Friedman PJ: Bronchocentric granulomatosis, mucoid impaction, and hypersensitivity reactions to fungi. Am Rev Respir Dis 111:497–537, 1975.

Proposes interrelationships between the various hypersensitivity reactions to Aspergillus with emphasis on the clinical and pathologic features of bronchocentric granulomatosis.

Kuhlman JE, Fishman EK, Burch PA, Karp JE, Zerhouni EA, Siegelman SS: Invasive pulmonary aspergillosis in acute leukemia. The contribution of CT to early diagnosis and aggressive management. Chest 92:95–99, 1987.

Computed tomography played an important role in early diagnosis of invasive pulmonary aspergillosis. Over 80 percent of patients with this disorder who underwent intensive antileukemic chemotherapy survived the pulmonary infection as a result of early diagnosis and aggressive therapy with high-dose amphotericin B and 5-flurocytosine.

Lee SH, Barnes WG, Schaetzel WP: Pulmonary aspergillosis and the importance of oxalate crystal recognition in cytology specimens. Arch Pathol Lab Med 110:1176–1179, 1986.

The presence of calcium oxalate crystals in pulmonary biopsy and cytology specimens can be regarded as an important diagnostic aid in the diagnosis of pulmonary aspergillosis due to A. niger.

Patterson R, Greenberger PA, Radin RC, Roberts M: Allergic bronchopulmonary aspergillosis: Staging as an aid to management. Ann Intern Med 96:286–291, 1982.

First paper to describe clinical staging system for allergic bronchopulmonary aspergillosis. Five stages of disease were identified in 40 patients studied for several years.

Rosenberg M, Patterson R, Roberts M, Wang J: The assessment of immunological and clinical changes occurring during corticosteroid therapy for allergic bronchopulmonary aspergillosis. Am J Med 64:599–606, 1978.

Original paper outlining the use of total serum IgE to monitor disease activity during treatment of allergic bronchopulmonary aspergillosis.

Ruutu P, Valtonen V, Tiitanen L, Elonen E, Volin L, Veijalainen P, Ruutu T: An outbreak of invasive aspergillosis in a haematologic unit. Scand J Infect Dis 19:347–351, 1987.

Within a period of 15 months, 8 cases of invasive pulmonary aspergillosis were seen in a hematologic unit. Environmental sanitation, including cleaning of the ventilation ducts and change of filters in the ventilation system, stopped the outbreak.

Sider L, Davis T: Pulmonary aspergillosis: Unusual radiographic appearance. Radiology 162:657–659, 1987.

Three cases of pulmonary aspergillosis are reported in which the pulmonary lesion was a stable, well-defined nodule.

Talbot GH, Weiner MH, Gerson SL, Provencher M, Hurwitz S: Serodiagnosis of invasive aspergillosis in patients with hematologic malignancy: Validation of the A. fumigatus antigen radioimmunoassay. J Infect Dis 155:12–27, 1987.

Over six hundred sera were screened by radioimmunoassay for A. fumigatus antigen. The sensitivity was 74%, the specificity 90%, and the positive predictive value 90%.

Treger TR, Visscher DW, Bartlett MS, Smith JW: Diagnosis of pulmonary infection caused by Aspergillus: Usefulness of respiratory cultures. J Infect Dis 152:572–576, 1985.

Eight of nine patients with two or more positive cultures for A. fumigatus or A. flavus had proved disease, versus 1 of 81 who were uninfected (p < .001).

Young RC, Bennett JE, Vogel CL, Carbone PP, Devita VT: Aspergillosis: The spectrum of the disease in ninety-eight patients. Medicine 49:147–173, 1970.

A classic review of autopsied patients with invasive aspergillosis.

Chapter 104

Protozoan Infections of the Lung

Jay A. Fishman

The protozoa comprise a group of about 45,000 single-celled eukaryotic species, of which approximately 10,000 are parasitic for humans. Protozoa are worldwide in distribution. Although these organisms account for extrapulmonary disease in 10 to 20 percent of the world population, few cause pulmonary disease in the immunologically normal host. Recognition that a pneumonia is caused by a protozoan should automatically prompt a search for a defect in host immunity and for the coexistence of other infections, either pulmonary or extrapulmonary. For example, pulmonary *Pneumocystis* infection may be associated with infection of the lungs by *Aspergillus* or cytomegalovirus, of the intestine by *Cryptosporidium*, or of the central nervous system by *Toxoplasma*. The protozoa that cause pulmonary disease should be considered in the differential diagnosis of certain clinical syndromes even if the patient has not traveled in areas where their occurrence is endemic.

The distribution and relevant clinical aspects of the major species of protozoa involved in pulmonary infection are summarized in Table 104-1. Since early diagnosis enhances the prospects for successful therapy, the handling of tissue and sputum specimens is directed at detecting the organism as quickly as possible. For example, before freezing or fixing a lung biopsy for routine histopathologic or special examination, impression smears ("touch preparations") are made by pressing the cut surface of the fresh lung tissue against labeled, sterile microscope slides; some of the slides are air-dried for prompt examination using stains (see below); a few can be examined for fungi under water or after adding iodine. The remainder are fixed in fresh absolute methanol for additional stains, e.g., Gram-Weigert, fluorescent antibody, or repeat examinations.

PNEUMOCYSTIS CARINII

Pneumocystis carinii is classified as a protozoan for three reasons: (1) the morphology of its cyst and trophozoite forms resembles that of conventional protozoa, e.g., *Toxoplasma*; (2) prevention and treatment of an infection with *P. carinii* can be accomplished by medications that have proved successful against unquestionable protozoa; and (3) attempts to treat *Pneumocystis* infections as though the organism were a fungus—a proposed taxonomic alternative to its classification as a protozoan—have been consistently unsuccessful. Nonetheless, the organism stains like a fungus with the silver and periodic acid-Schiff stains.

Pneumonitis caused by *P. carinii* characteristically occurs in the immunocompromised host (Table 104-2). The prevalence of this disease has increased greatly during the past decade, largely on three accounts: (1) the prolonged survival of patients with neoplastic disease, (2) the increasing use of immunosuppressive therapy, and (3) development of the acquired immunodeficiency syndrome (AIDS) in homosexuals, intravenous drug abusers, blood product recipients, and others who lack known causes of immune deficiency.

Although the organism has been known for about 75 years, remarkable uncertainty still prevails not only about its taxonomy, but also about its mode of transmission, its mechanism of producing tissue damage, and its epidemiology. The cyst form was first recognized by Chagas (1909) and Carini (1910), who misinterpreted it as a stage in the life cycle of the trypanosome; this error was corrected by Delanoe and Delanoe in 1912. Interest in the organism

TABLE 104-1
Principal Protozoan Infections Involving the Lung

Organism	Distribution	Reservoir/Vector	Diagnostic Approach	Pulmonary Pathology	Organism Stains	Comments
Pneumocystis carinii	Worldwide	Unknown (? species specific)	Bronchoalveolar lavage, brushing and biopsy, lung biopsy, impression smear, induced sputum	Adult: alveolitis, interstitial infiltrate; Neonatal: interstitial plasma cells	Cysts: toluidine blue O, methenamine silver; Trophs: Giemsa, Wright, methylene blue	Latent infection? ICH, AIDS
Toxoplasma gondii	Worldwide	Cat feces, undercooked meats	Impression smear, serology, biopsy	Interstitial pneumonitis, organisms in MØ	Cysts: Silver, PAS; Trophs: Giemsa, Wright	Disseminated disease: ICH CNS infection
Entamoeba histolytica	Worldwide	Fecal-oral	Liver ultrasound, serology	Abscess, empyema, "anchovy paste"	PAS iodine, iron hematoxylin	Liver abscess Fluid overload
Plasmodium falciparum	Tropics, subtropics	Anopheles mosquito, needles, transfusion	Blood smear, thick/thin films	Edema, effusion, microvascular congestion	Giemsa	Fluid overload
Leishmania donovani	Worldwide (except North America)	Phlebotomus (sandfly): dog, rodent, fox, and humans	Bone marrow biopsy	Organisms in MØ, alveolar cells	Giemsa, H&E Leishman's	Kala azar
Cryptosporidium	Worldwide (especially tropical, rural)	Fecal-oral (calves, farm animals), inhalation, zoonotic	Sputum, impression smear, biopsy	Organisms on alveolar brush border, interstitial infiltrate	Modified Kinyoun acid-fast, auramine-rhodamine, Sheather's	AIDS, ICH, gastrointestinal disease; ? aspiration

NOTE: H&E = hematoxylin and eosin; PAS = periodic acid-Schiff; ICH = immunocompromised host; MØ = alveolar macrophages; AIDS = acquired immunodeficiency syndrome; Trophs = trophozoites.

was rekindled after World War II when outbreaks of "plasma cell interstitial pneumonitis" occurred in malnourished, premature, and debilitated infants living under crowded conditions in European orphanages. The cyst forms of Pneumocystis in the lungs were felt to be the cause of the diffuse pneumonia. Similar outbreaks of epidemic disease were described among war orphans from Vietnam. In the 1950s, an association was recognized between Pneumocystis carinii pneumonia and congenital immunodeficiency syndromes (B- and T-cell). In the 1960s and 1970s, as the use of chemotherapy for carcinoma became widespread, P. carinii was implicated as the cause of a sporadic, diffuse pneumonia that occurred exclusively in immunocompromised hosts of all ages (Table 104-2). In the 1980s, interest in Pneumocystis peaked when pneumonia caused by P. carinii reached epidemic proportions in adults who had not received immunosuppressive agents and had no apparent basis for immunodeficiency. These observations culminated in the identification of AIDS, a syndrome that affects certain populations without overt cause or prior history of immunodeficiency and that are particularly susceptible to opportunistic infection. Most often the infection is a pneumonia caused by P. carinii, sometimes in association with other infections or tumors including Kaposi's sarcoma and B-cell lymphoma. The causative virus of AIDS, the human immuno-

TABLE 104-2
Conditions Associated with Pneumocystis Carinii Pneumonitis

Chemotherapy (corticosteroids)
Radiation therapy
Organ transplantation
Acquired immunodeficiency syndrome (AIDS)
Prematurity
Malnutrition (protein and calorie)
Malignancies (leukemia, lymphoma, Hodgkin's disease, solid tumors)
Primary immune deficiency diseases (cellular, humoral, and combined)
Collagen vascular disease
Hematologic disorders (autoimmune hemolytic anemia, aplastic anemia, hemophilia, thrombocytopenic purpura, Henoch-Schönlein disease)
Cushing's syndrome
Nephrotic syndrome

deficiency virus or HIV, is a lymphotropic retrovirus. The particular immune lesion(s) of AIDS allows a variety of protozoan infections of usually minor significance to develop into life-threatening infections. More than two-thirds of the over 40,000 AIDS victims in the United

States have developed *P. carinii* pneumonia. Thus, over the last 35 years, *P. carinii* pneumonia has been transformed from a medical curiosity to an important respiratory infection that affects four distinct categories of immunocompromised hosts: (1) *congenital*, caused by inborn defects in antibody synthesizing capacity and/or in the cellular mechanisms responsible for delayed hypersensitivity; (2) *induced*, as by immunosuppressive therapy, especially corticosteroids, in the setting of hematopoietic malignancies; (3) *acquired*, occurring as part of AIDS in individuals who were previously healthy; and (4) *nutritional*, in neonates and infants. It has become evident that defects in cellular immune mechanisms predominate over humoral mechanisms in predisposing to overt infection with *P. carinii*.

The Organism

In humans and animals, three forms of the organism have been identified: trophozoite, cyst, and sporozoite. The trophozoite, 2 to 5 μm in diameter, is either round or sickle-shaped and contains a nucleus, mitochondria, and vacuoles; it also includes pseudopodia and filopodia that suggest motility. The cyst usually measures between 3 and 6 μm in diameter. Its cell wall consists of three layers, and its cytoplasm contains eight small pleomorphic intracystic (oval) bodies (*sporozoites*). Two other cystic forms have been described, but these are probably intermediates.

The cyst wall can be displayed by a variety of staining techniques: of these, the Gomori methenamine silver nitrate method (brown or black) is the more reliable, even though it is susceptible to artifacts and does not stain intracellular bodies (Fig. 104-1C). Sporozoites and trophozoites are stained by polychrome stains, particularly the Giemsa stain. The Giemsa, Wright, toluidine blue O, or Grocott's rapid silver stain techniques are most useful in dealing with lung imprints, bronchial lavage fluid, or pulmonary aspirates. When a silver stain is used, a counterstain such as Gram, Wright, Giemsa, hematoxylin, or trichrome may be required to identify intracystic bodies and to distinguish cysts from red blood cells and yeasts.

The life cycle of *Pneumocystis* is still poorly understood. It is now believed that the sporozoites (daughter forms) emerge from the cyst to develop into trophozoites. Some of the trophozoites mature to form cysts and then repeat the cycle in vitro. However, this sequence is far from settled, and both sexual and asexual intermediate stages have been postulated. Although the organisms have not been well characterized genotypically and phenotypically, the likelihood is great that some differences exist between the murine and human species. In principle, *P. carinii* would be a fitting designation for the rodent organism and *P. jiroveci* for the human organism, the latter in honor of an investigator who first convincingly associated cysts with the human disease. However, by tradi-

tion, the clinical syndrome is still referred to as *P. carinii* pneumonia.

Research on *Pneumocystis* has long been hampered by difficulties in propagating the organism in cell culture. Studies have been performed on organisms derived from immunosuppressed rodents, which "spontaneously" develop *P. carinii* pneumonia. Hughes and coworkers have used this model to demonstrate the aerosol transmission of *P. carinii*. Recently "feeder cells" of different types have been used to enhance the growth of *P. carinii* from rat lungs in vitro. One intriguing insight that this approach has provided is that the type of feeder cell plays a critical role in determining the ratio of cyst to trophozoite forms. Unfortunately, cell culture techniques have not yet become useful diagnostically because of the difficulty in culturing the organism from infected human tissues. *Pneumocystis* is occasionally grown as a "contaminant" in viral cultures of bronchial lavage fluid on a variety of feeder cell lines.

Pathology

To identify the organisms, tissue sections are customarily stained by the Gomori methenamine silver nitrate method or a modification of it. By light microscopy, trophozoites predominate numerically, but cysts are more readily identified. In the adult immunosuppressed rat model, the organism appears to adhere to and injure exclusively the surface of type I alveolar epithelial cells, while the adjacent type II cells undergo hyperplasia.

In the lung, the reaction to *Pneumocystis* involves interstitium and alveoli and is usually distinctive enough to be diagnostic even when organisms cannot be found; in the adult, the disease appears to be predominantly alveolar: the airspaces are filled with a foamy, eosinophilic exudate and appear honeycombed; at the same time, the alveolar interstitium is infiltrated by polymorphonuclear leukocytes and lymphocytes (Fig. 104-1B). Patchiness in the distribution of disease within the lungs is common. In contrast to the adult form, the infantile form has a major interstitial component: the interstitium is filled with fluid, plasma cells, cysts, and lymphocytes; these formed elements seem to overflow into the airspaces which are also filled with a frothy eosinophilic exudate (Fig. 104-1A). In both forms, the organisms usually appear intermingled with alveolar macrophages in the alveolar exudate (Fig. 104-1C). In AIDS, the interstitial inflammation is less marked than in other adult forms, and greater numbers of both cysts and trophozoites are seen in the alveoli. Although hyaline membranes may line alveoli, they are not diagnostic of infection with *Pneumocystis*, since oxygen toxicity or the adult respiratory distress syndrome can evoke similar changes and either, or both, may coexist with *Pneumocystis* infection. In pediatric AIDS, lymphocytic interstitial pneumonitis, without evidence of an infectious etiology, is second only to *P. carinii* as a pulmonary manifestation.

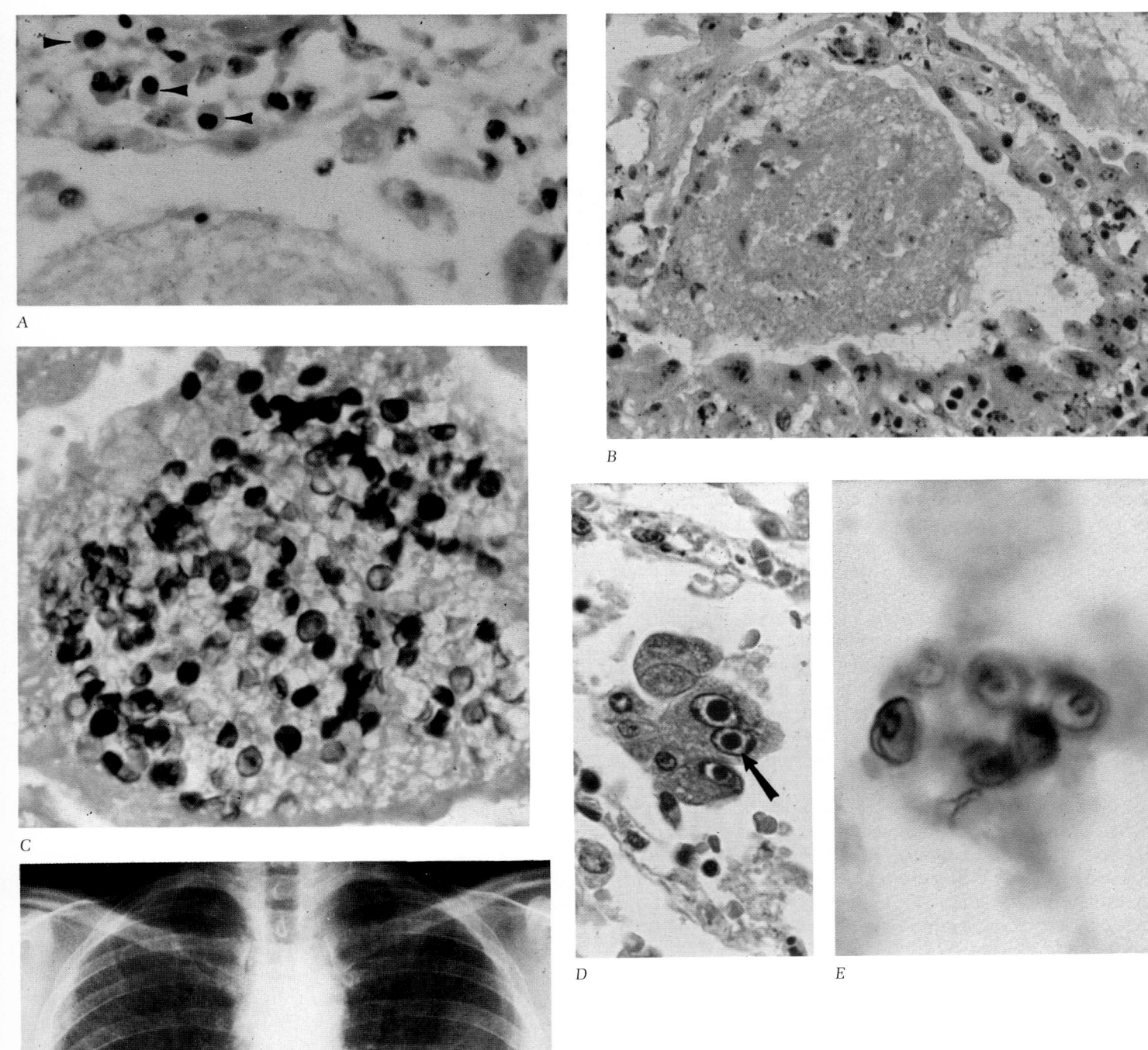

FIGURE 104-1 *Pneumocystis carinii.* *A.* Lung of a malnourished infant showing an intra-alveolar foamy exudate and plasma cell infiltrate (arrowheads) in the interstitium. (H&E, ×620.) *B.* Lung of an adult showing swelling of alveolar epithelial cells and intra-alveolar exudate. Inflammatory response in interstitium is minimal. (H&E, ×500.) *C. Pneumocystis* in the form of thick-walled cysts within the foamy exudate. Displayed by Gomori's methenamine-silver nitrate stain and brilliant green counterstain. (×1250.) *D.* Cytomegalovirus inclusion bodies in alveolar macrophages. (H&E, ×720.) *E. Pneumocystis* cysts in cytologic preparation of induced sputum from AIDS patient. (Silver stain, ×1250.) *F. Pneumocystis* pneumonitis. Typical chest radiograph showing bilateral, diffuse interstitial infiltrates extending from hilar area.

Even when chest radiography indicates that *P. carinii* pneumonia has cleared, interstitial fibrosis is likely to be found at rebiopsy or autopsy. Unfortunately, the contribution of *Pneumocystis* to the residual fibrosis is often obscured by the tendency of superimposed infection, therapeutic agents, or intervening radiation therapy to elicit inflammatory responses in the interstitium. Extrapulmonary organisms have occasionally been identified in pulmonary lymphoid tissue and in blood, liver, spleen, heart, kidney, pancreas, adrenal, mesentary, ear, and eye tissue. In extrapulmonary sites, care must be taken to avoid confusing yeast forms with *Pneumocystis*.

Epidemiology

Asymptomatic pulmonary infection with *P. carinii* is widespread in normal humans and in other mammals. The natural habitat of the organism is unknown, but the frequency of infection varies with geography and locale. Based on finding cyst forms in the lungs, autopsy studies indicate that the incidence is high in immunosuppressed individuals and relatively less common in normals. The prevalence of exposure to *P. carinii* is indicated by the demonstration that, in the Netherlands, virtually all normal children have serologic evidence of infection during the first 2 years of life. In the United States about 75 percent of normal children have evidence of infection by age 4, and 78 percent of adults' lymphocytes proliferate when exposed to *P. carinii* antigen. Despite the high incidence of exposure to *Pneumocystis*, disease caused by this organism is virtually confined to immunocompromised hosts. The prevalence of infection with *P. carinii* in patients with AIDS has prompted a large effort to develop diagnostic serologic tests that might be applied to this population: some tests are concerned with detecting antigenemia; others with antibodies, even though the hosts are immunosuppressed to varying degrees. Among the serologic tests being investigated are immunofluorescence, enzyme-linked immunosorbent assays (ELISA), and counterimmunoelectrophoresis (CIE). Although serologic testing for *Pneumocystis* infection is in its infancy and the results are inconsistent, current data reinforce the view that subclinical infection is common and that a reactivation of latent infection is involved in the pathogenesis of *P. carinii* pneumonia. Newer serologic methods may allow the development of noninvasive methods useful in the screening of asymptomatic populations at risk of infection and in the diagnosis and management of active disease.

P. carinii is an organism of low virulence. Commonly, infection with *Pneumocystis* is associated with other infections. Among these, the cytomegalovirus (CMV) has attracted the most attention as a likely predisposing agent for *Pneumocystis* infection (Fig. 104-1*D*). Whether CMV directly stimulates the proliferation of *Pneumocystis*, or acts indirectly as an immunosuppressive agent, or is simply a fellow traveler in the immunocompromised host, remains to be settled. In the murine model of *P. carinii* pneumonia, CMV infection does not appear to enhance *Pneumocystis* infection. However, this does not necessarily negate the proposed CMV-*Pneumocystis* interplay in humans since, as was pointed out above, there is still some uncertainty about whether the *Pneumocystis* in rodent and human are the same species.

How the disease is acquired is obviously of paramount concern. In the epidemic form of the disease, usually affecting malnourished infants less than 6 months of age and living under crowded conditions, airborne transmission is likely. A similar mechanism has been demonstrated in immunocompromised rats exposed to air from animals infected with *Pneumocystis*. However, even in the infantile form, an alternative explanation is that infection in early life is quite common and that malnutrition (and the resultant immunosuppression) converts latent infection into disease. Horizontal transmission may also explain the occurrence of clusters of disease, in adults and children, in medical centers that house immunosuppressed patients with neoplastic disease or organ transplants; physicians taking care of these patients have also developed serologic evidence of infection with *Pneumocystis*. However, in these instances, it has generally proved difficult to judge whether clustering is attributable to spread between individuals, to activation of latent infection by induced immunosuppression, or both. Nor has the recent epidemic of *P. carinii* infection in AIDS patients distinguished between the respective roles of activation and person-to-person transmission of the infective agent. The current consensus seems to be that, in AIDS, infection with a transmissible, immunosuppressive agent (HIV) may act, as does chemotherapy, to either set the stage for new infection by the *Pneumocystis* or for reactivation of latent infection.

The range of diseases associated with *P. carinii* pneumonia is broad (Table 104-2). Although immunosuppression undoubtedly plays a critical pathogenetic role in these infections, the specific nature of the prerequisite immune lesion(s) is not clear. For example, the immunosuppression induced by treatment (e.g., by corticosteroids) may be more important than the intrinsic immunosuppression induced by the malignancy for which treatment is being administered. Also, the severity of infection with *Pneumocystis* seems related to the degree and duration of immunosuppression. In AIDS, in which the primary defect appears to be in T-lymphocyte-mediated immunity and in the generation of immunity to novel antigens, abnormalities in humoral defenses against *Pneumocystis* infection and in the process of opsonization and phagocytosis of organisms by alveolar macrophages may also be involved.

Clinical Manifestations

In the adult, *P. carinii* pneumonia is usually gradual in onset, manifesting itself insidiously over a few days to weeks by progressive dyspnea, tachypnea, cyanosis, and a nonproductive cough; auscultatory findings at the onset are minimal, generally no more than scattered rales and somewhat diminished breath sounds. In AIDS the manifestations of the initial episode of *P. carinii* pneumonia (usually dyspnea and fever) evolve over 2 to 4 weeks. Subsequent relapses may evolve more rapidly, especially in the setting of simultaneous infection with cytomegalovirus or the *Mycobacteria* (*M. tuberculosis* or *M. avium-intracellulare* complex).

By the time of hospitalization, despite hyperventilation, arterial hypoxemia is generally moderate to severe and the alveolar-arterial O_2 gradient is considerably widened; the degree of arterial hypoxemia is inordinate for the physical and radiologic findings. Indeed, dyspnea and arterial hypoxemia may occur despite a normal chest radiograph. Fever is common, usually low grade, and precedes the development of respiratory symptoms. In the patient undergoing chemotherapy, clinical manifestations of pulmonary disease often intensify after the immunosuppressive agents are discontinued and pulmonary infiltrates appear on the chest radiograph as the host's inflammatory response reemerges.

The chest radiograph plays a central role in the diagnosis of *P. carinii* pneumonia (Fig. 104-1F). The radiographic pattern depends on the patient's underlying or accompanying disease, the state of immunosuppression, and the duration of infection. No radiographic appearance is specific for the diagnosis of *P. carinii* pneumonia. Sometimes the chest radiograph is normal despite overt pulmonary disease. But, more often, the early stage of *P. carinii* pneumonia is manifested by fine, bilateral, perihilar, diffuse infiltrates that progress to an interstitial-alveolar butterfly pattern; from the hilar regions, the infiltrates spread to the apices or bases. Despite therapy, this pattern is often succeeded in 3 to 5 days by progressive consolidation, the appearance of air bronchograms, and complete opacification of the lung fields. As in many of the "atypical pneumonias," unusual courses and patterns are seen: nodules, unilateral infiltrates, or even lobar consolidations. Small pleural effusions also occur. Distortions in pattern are commonly produced by prior radiation, drug-induced pulmonary injury, or concurrent infection with another organism.

The infant with the disease tends to be underweight for age and to have decreased serum albumin levels. Early signs of disease include diarrhea, poor feeding, and coryza; the respiratory manifestations then progress to nasal flaring, intercostal retraction, and cyanosis. Fever is variable. As in the adult, arterial blood is generally hypoxemic and shows evidence of a respiratory alkalosis (pH of 7.45 to 7.60; P_{CO_2} from 20 to 40 mmHg).

Diagnosis

A wide array of other pulmonary disturbances can coexist with or mimic *P. carinii* pneumonia: neoplasms, edema, and pneumonia caused by all sorts of infectious agents (Fig. 104-2) (e.g., viruses, fungi, bacteria, mycoplasma), drug reactions, and radiation. Identification of *Pneumocystis* as the etiologic agent requires the demonstration of the organism in lung washings, secretions, impressions, or histologic sections. Tests measuring antibodies to *P. carinii* do not have the specificity needed for reliable diagnosis. Noninvasive measures in the non-AIDS patient, such as collection of sputum aspirated from endotracheal tubes or induced sputum specimens (Fig. 104-1E), are often tried, but these techniques only inconsistently yield organisms and will not diagnose dual infection. In the AIDS patient, by contrast, the greater number of organisms present in the lungs has allowed the diagnosis of *P. carinii* pneumonia to be made in 30 to 60 percent of cases by the examination of induced sputum specimens. Such specimens may be collected after 20 to 30 min of exposure to aerosolized saline or water. Smears are prepared from the mucoid, nonpurulent portion of the specimen and stained with either Giemsa or silver stains. Smears may be improved through use of a mucolytic agent (Mucomyst) just prior to preparation. A negative smear does not indicate the absence of *P. carinii*. Although gallium scans often become abnormal before the radiographic appearance of disease, they are not diagnostic of *Pneumocystis* infection. Some centers make a presumptive diagnosis of *P. carinii* pneumonia in the patient with AIDS when a decrease in diffusing capacity ($D_{L_{CO}}$) is coupled with an abnormal chest radiograph and gallium scan. The clearance of radiolabeled, inhaled DTPA (diethylenetriamine penta-acetate) is also increased in *P. carinii* pneumonia (as in other pneumonitides). Although these tests are usually abnormal in *P. carinii* pneumonia, they lack specificity.

At present, accurate diagnosis in the non-AIDS patient relies on invasive procedures. One element in the choice of procedure depends on the clinical state of the patient: patients who have an uncontrollable bleeding diathesis are poor candidates for either bronchoscopy or open lung biopsy. Another determinant of the invasive procedure to be used is the experience and practice of the institution: if the bronchoscopist is unfamiliar with the proper technique for sampling or handling specimens for the diagnosis of *Pneumocystis* infection, open lung biopsy is apt to be the more rewarding procedure, particularly if it is done by an experienced thoracic surgeon and the tissue is handled by a surgical pathologist familiar with the disease. Because disease caused by *P. carinii* pneumonia progresses rapidly, the likelihood of success in treatment is greatest at the outset. Therefore, invasive procedures to disclose the organism and any secondary infections should be undertaken early in the course of the disease.

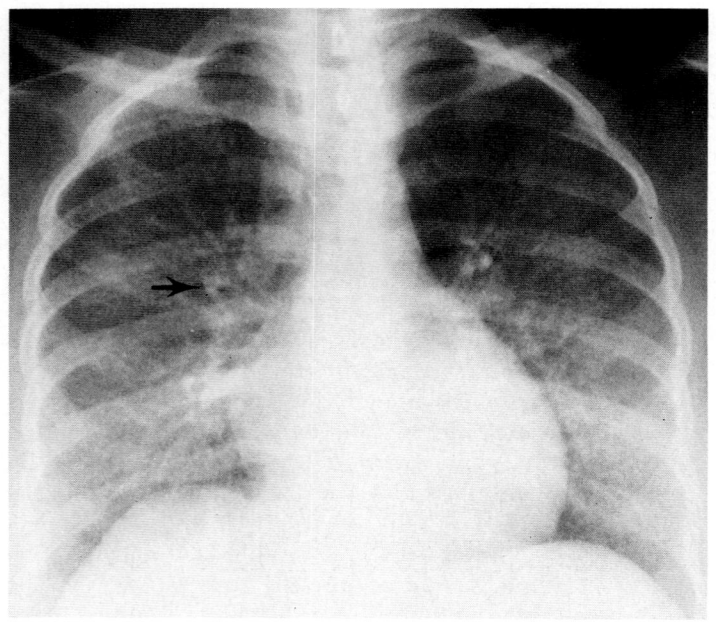

A

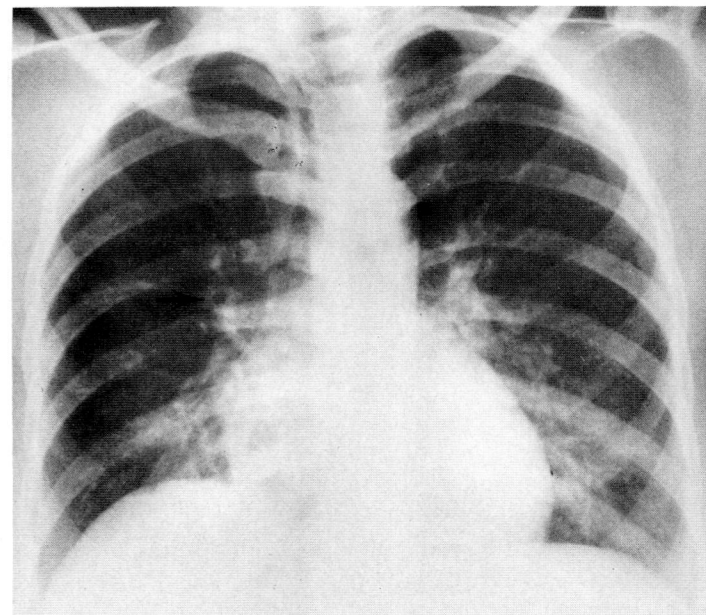

B

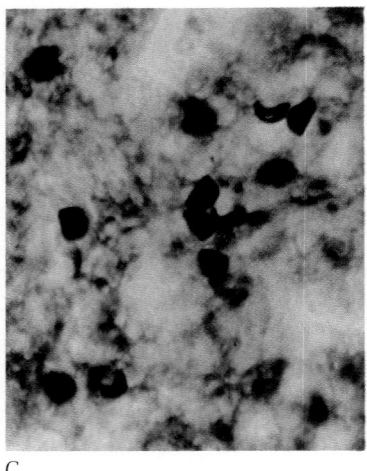

C

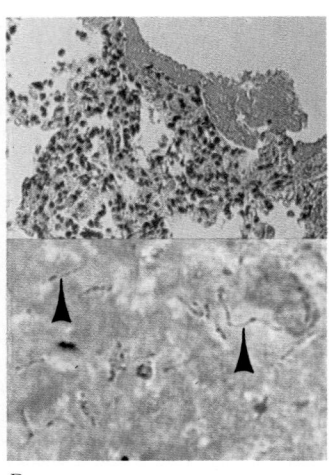

D

FIGURE 104-2 *Pneumocystis* and *Mycobacterium avium-intracellulare.* Haitian woman with AIDS (see also Fig. 104-6). *A.* Diffuse pulmonary infiltrates before treatment of *Pneumocystis* infection. Arrow indicates small abscess. *B.* After treatment for *Pneumocystis,* multiple cavitary nodules remain (arrow). *C.* Lung biopsy after treatment for *Pneumocystis* (B, above) reveals *Pneumocystis* cysts. (Silver, ×760.) *D.* Lung biopsy included areas of pneumonitis atypical for *Pneumocystis* (*upper*) and containing *Mycobacterium avium-intracellulare* (arrowheads, *lower*). (Kinyoun acid-fast stain, ×950.)

Invasive procedures for the diagnosis of *P. carinii* pneumonia fall into several categories: tracheal aspiration; fiberoptic bronchoscopy; transthoracic aspiration; and open lung biopsy. Attempts to avoid invasive procedures by resorting to empiric therapy run a great risk of inappropriate medications and undesirable side effects.

1. *Tracheal aspiration:* The yield from this procedure is generally low, and the hazards, particularly in inexperienced hands, are high. In intubated patients, respiratory secretions should be carefully smeared on slides, stained, and examined. If the physician or the microbiology technician has had little experience with *Pneumocystis* smears, fiberoptic bronchoscopy or open lung biopsy is indicated, followed by methenamine silver staining of the tissue sections.

2. *Fiberoptic bronchoscopy:* The importance of knowing the success rate of the institution as a basis for selecting the proper invasive diagnostic approach is illustrated by published reports of diagnostic yields from fiberoptic bronchoscopy. In proven instances of *P. carinii* pneumonia in non-AIDS immunocompromised hosts, the reported yields range from 5 to 95 percent. As a rule, those institutions that have had a large experience with bronchoscopy and with *P. carinii* pneumonia have been very successful in uncovering the organism. Indeed, when bronchial lavage, brushing, and transbronchial lung biopsies are part of the diagnostic procedure, the success rate has exceeded 90 percent. The yield has been even higher in AIDS. In these patients, lavage specimens must be gathered from a wedged bronchoscope with at least 50 ml of physiolog-

ical saline for alveolar washings. Trophozoites predominate in bronchial washings. In general, lung biopsy is not essential for the diagnosis of *P. carinii* pneumonia in AIDS. Patients suspected of harboring multiple pathogens may still benefit from the more invasive procedure. Although bleeding from the biopsy site is common, i.e., in up to 25 percent of patients, it is rarely threatening if the coagulation indices are normal.

3. *Percutaneous needle aspiration:* High success rates in finding *P. carinii* have also been reported in patients with *P. carinii* pneumonia (up to 60 percent), particularly when aspiration is performed under fluoroscopic guidance. The incidence of pneumothorax during the procedure is high, i.e., in up to one-third of patients; in about 20 percent of these, pneumothorax requires insertion of a chest tube.

4. *Lung biopsy:* Thoracotomy followed by lung biopsy affords the most unequivocal avenue for diagnosis. Although the patients may be quite ill by the time that this step is taken, in the hands of skilled surgeons thoracotomy has proved remarkably safe, even in the intubated patient.

Biopsies and aspirates should be utilized for fungal, bacterial, mycobacterial, or viral cultures and to make slides for rapid staining with toluidine blue O, Gomori, Giemsa, or Wright stains. Early diagnosis is frequently made and therapy initiated on the basis of such smears, especially in AIDS.

Therapy and Outcome

Even though the infection is incompletely understood and diagnosis often depends on invasive procedures, considerable progress has been made in treating and preventing the disease. As indicated above, the keystone for treating *P. carinii* pneumonia successfully is early and accurate diagnosis. Once the diagnosis is established, attention is directed at any immunosuppressive therapy that the patient is receiving with an eye toward reducing the dosage or even discontinuing the medication. The next essential step is eradicating the infection; 50 percent of infants with *P. carinii* pneumonia and more than 90 percent of adults who have the disease will die if not treated.

Two agents are currently available for treating *P. carinii* pneumonia: pentamidine and co-trimoxazole. The older of the two, pentamidine isethionate (Table 104-3), was first administered intramuscularly during an epidemic of the infantile form of the disease. It decreased mortality from 50 to 3.5 percent of those affected. Subsequently, less-dramatic effects were obtained using this agent in older children and adults: survival rates of 25 to 85 percent have since been reported following its use. Pentamidine is now judged to be about 70 percent effec-

TABLE 104-3
Antibiotic Therapy and Prophylaxis: Pneumocystis Carinii Pneumonia*

Agent	Route of Administration	Dosage, mg/kg per day	Duration of Treatment, days	Adverse Reactions	Remarks
Pentamidine methanesulfonate *or*	IM (IV)	2.3	12–14	Common, including hypoglycemia, renal and hepatic disturbances, local reactions at injection site, hypotension, hematologic disturbances, pain, and sterile abscess at injection site	Either form of pentamidine appropriate for therapy; 3–6 weeks in AIDS; relapse common in AIDS; inhalation therapy under study
Pentamidine isethionate	IM (IV)	4	12–14		
Trimethoprim-sulfamethoxazole in 1:5 combination (co-trimoxazole)	Oral or IV in 4 equal doses/day	Trimethoprim: 20; sulfamethoxazole: 100	14	Skin rash, fever, gastrointestinal upsets; bone marrow suppression (leukopenia); hepatic dysfunction (transaminase); common in AIDS	As effective as pentamidine with fewer side effects in non-AIDS patients; Require 3–6 weeks of therapy in AIDS; high relapse rate in AIDS
Prophylaxis					
Co-trimoxazole	Oral	5	Indefinite	Low incidence of adverse reactions in non-AIDS patients	Administered orally in 2 equal doses per day or 150 mg/m^2 per day

*Investigational agents used in AIDS are described in text.

tive. Complications are common, i.e., in up to 50 percent of patients. Until recently, pentamidine isethionate was distributed by the Centers for Disease Control as an investigational drug (Table 104-3). Pentamidine isethionate and methanesulfonate are now available commercially. These agents may be administered either intravenously or intramuscularly, but in differing dosages depending on the formulation used. Pentamidine achieves therapeutic levels in the lungs slowly (5 to 7 days) owing to high levels of extrapulmonary tissue binding. Slow accumulation of pentamidine in pulmonary tissue may account for the delayed onset of activity when compared with co-trimoxazole. However, increased serum levels and a long serum half-life may play a role in its continued effect after the cessation of therapy. Studies of inhalation and endotracheal administration of pentamidine for therapy and for prophylaxis are ongoing.

Pentamidine has largely been supplanted by co-trimoxazole for the therapy of *Pneumocystis* infection in the non-AIDS patient. But pentamidine continues to be used in infection refractory to co-trimoxazole or in patients allergic to trimethoprim or sulfonamides. Partly because of the high incidence of adverse reactions to co-trimoxazole in patients with AIDS, pentamidine has been widely adopted as the drug of choice for starting treatment of *P. carinii* pneumonia in these patients. Patients treated intravenously with pentamidine (the same daily dosage given over 2 h in 250 to 500 cm³ of 5% dextrose solution) have done as well or better than those treated by intramuscular injection.

For the non-AIDS patients with *P. carinii* pneumonia, initial treatment with a combination of trimethoprim and sulfamethoxazole (co-trimoxazole) is preferred because the combination evokes fewer side effects than pentamidine (about 15 percent) (Table 104-3). Both trimethoprim and sulfamethoxazole interfere with folate metabolism. Two weeks of treatment with co-trimoxazole have proved adequate if the dosage of immunosuppressive agents being used to treat the underlying disease can be reduced. Oral therapy has proved to be as successful as intravenous therapy as long as gastrointestinal absorption is adequate, e.g., ileus does not develop. Peak levels of trimethoprim in the serum are reached within 1 to 1.5 h after ingestion and are maintained in the range of 5 to 15 μg/ml. The toxic side effects of co-trimoxazole are generally those of a sulfonamide; however, trimethoprim allergy is not uncommon. Leukopenia, thrombocytopenia, and anemia elicited by co-trimoxazole are generally relieved by folinic acid, whereas drug rash, fever, azotemia, and increased blood levels of transaminase will reverse only when therapy is stopped. Folinic acid should not be used in patients with acute leukemia.

Clinical improvement in response to treatment with either pentamidine or trimethoprim-sulfamethoxazole is often delayed for up to 1 week, usually for 4 to 7 days. If the patient fails to respond in 4 to 7 days to initial therapy with co-trimoxazole, or if toxic manifestations supervene, pentamidine therapy can be used as a replacement. Adding pentamidine to co-trimoxazole offers no advantage over simply switching agents. Indeed, animal experiments suggest the possibility of antagonism between these agents when used in combination. As a rule, those patients who need to be switched from co-trimoxazole to pentamidine, or vice versa, do not fare as well as those who can be treated for 12 to 14 days with either agent alone. The success rate using either pentamidine or trimethoprim-sulfamethoxazole for initial treatment is of the order of 60 to 70 percent. Switching from one drug regimen to another because of a poor response to therapy gains another 10 percent.

AIDS patients do as well in response to *initial* therapy for *Pneumocystis* as do comparable groups of patients with induced immunosuppression. But, in AIDS patients, prolonged therapy (3 to 6 weeks) is required for remission, and the rate of relapse or recurrence is high (greater than 50 percent). Frequently, AIDS patients who appear to respond clinically to treatment with co-trimoxazole are found to have residual cysts and trophozoite forms in their lungs at rebiopsy or at autopsy. The incidence of relapse does not, however, appear to be related to the presence or absence of residual organisms.

The effectiveness of pentamidine and of co-trimoxazole therapy decreases during subsequent episodes of *P. carinii* pneumonia. In AIDS patients, the incidence and severity of drug reactions to co-trimoxazole is much higher, and occurs sooner, than in other immunosuppressed hosts (50 to 75 percent versus 15 percent). Indeed, the frequency of toxic reactions is the same as, or greater than, that seen with pentamidine (40 to 55 percent). Skin rashes occur 10 times more often in AIDS patients than in other patients with *P. carinii* pneumonia, and hepatic toxicity occurs in up to 20 percent of AIDS patients. Thus, therapy may be initiated with either agent in AIDS. Many of the minor reactions (rash, fever) are due to trimethoprim. Reduction of the trimethoprim dosage by half and/or administration of diphenhydramine may allow the trimethoprim-sulfamethoxazole combination to be continued.

In AIDS patients who are either allergic or unresponsive to both co-trimoxazole and pentamidine, the combination of diaminodiphenylsulfone (Dapsone, Jacobus, 100 mg orally per day) and trimethoprim (20 mg/kg per day in four intravenous doses) has proven useful for therapy. Dapsone has been well tolerated even in patients with sulfa-drug allergy to co-trimoxazole. Care must be exercised, however, when sulfa-containing agents are used in any patient with a history of hypersensitivity to this group of agents.

Supportive therapy is largely in the form of measures to improve hydration, nutrition, and arterial oxygenation.

As the pneumonia spreads, patients often need supplemental oxygen by mask or by tracheal intubation and mechanical ventilation. But, when inspired oxygen concentrations exceed 50 percent, especially if continued for more than a day or two, the risk of oxygen toxicity, and its effect in increasing pulmonary microcirculatory permeability, is added to the damage caused by the *Pneumocystis* organism, thereby predisposing to the adult respiratory distress syndrome (ARDS). The administration of gamma globulin is reserved for those with documented humoral immune deficiency.

Because associated pulmonary infections are common, a continuing alert is necessary for bacterial or fungal infections (Fig. 104-2). Regular chest radiographs and sputum examinations are indispensible for this purpose. Nutritional support is critical in patients with *P. carinii* pneumonia. In AIDS patients, treatment of coexisting cytomegalovirus infection with DHPG {investigational agent 9-[2-hydroxy-1-(hydroxymethyl) ethoxymethyl] guanine} may improve the clinical response to therapy for *P. carinii*. In AIDS patients failing to respond to antibiotics alone, a short course of high dose corticosteroids may reduce pulmonary inflammation and improve oxygenation until the pulmonary infection abates. Steroid therapy is not recommended for the non-AIDS patient or for routine use in AIDS.

Prevention

In the hospital, the patient with *P. carinii* pneumonia should be isolated from other immunocompromised patients, but neither laminar airflow rooms nor gown-and-glove precautions are necessary. However, the hospitalized patient in whom *P. carinii* pneumonia is part of AIDS should be managed so as to avoid exposure of physicians, technicians, and service staff to body fluids and excreta, including blood, feces, and saliva. The guarding of personnel is not against the *Pneumocystis* organism but against contact with other pathogens.

Chemoprophylaxis, using trimethoprim-sulfamethoxazole, is useful in protecting patients at risk against developing *P. carinii* pneumonia. The drug has been effective as a prophylactic agent in hospitalized pediatric oncology patients who are at risk of *Pneumocystis* infection, in patients with severe combined immunodeficiency (SCID) syndrome, and in immunocompromised adults with and without AIDS. Prophylaxis lasts only as long as the medication is continued and should be reserved for centers that are known to have a fixed high incidence of disease (i.e., of the order of 3 to 5 percent of susceptible hosts), or for individuals with recurrent *Pneumocystis* disease. Oral administration of 5 mg/kg per day of trimethoprim (as co-trimoxazole) divided into two daily doses, or of 150 mg/m² per day, has proved effective for prophylaxis. On this regimen, the incidence of toxicity is less

than 10 percent. Because of the slow growth rate of *P. carinii*, intermittent prophylaxis (three consecutive days per week) with co-trimoxazole appears to be adequate to prevent *P. carinii* pneumonia while reducing the incidence of drug toxicity.

Prophylaxis of *Pneumocystis* infections in patients with AIDS is on less-firm footing than in non-AIDS patients. Without prophylaxis, relapse is almost universal. However, the incidence of side effects to the agents used has made practitioners wary. Oral co-trimoxazole, as above, has been useful in those who tolerate its use. Sulfa toxicity is reduced if prophylaxis is begun immediately after the completion of the course of therapy. Some success has also been achieved using pyramethamine-sulfadoxine (Fansidar, Roche) given weekly or diamino-diphenyl-sulfone given daily (with or without trimethoprim). However, Fansidar has been implicated in cases of severe hepatitis in a small number of individuals. Pentamidine isethionate (4 mg/kg per month) intravenously or by injection has been effective in small groups of patients with AIDS. Aerosolized pentamidine may prove to be useful in prophylaxis and as an adjunct to intravenous therapy. Investigation of the utility of inhaled aerosolized pentamidine in the prevention and therapy of *P. carinii* pneumonia in AIDS is underway.

Other agents are currently being tested against *Pneumocystis* in vitro, in animals and in clinical trials. α-Difluoromethylornithine (DFMO, Merrell Dow) has been used in patients with AIDS and *P. carinii* pneumonia who were unresponsive to, or intolerant of, other agents. According to protocol, initial therapy with 100 mg/kg intravenously every 6 h for 14 days (up to a maximum of 30 mg per day) is followed by 75 mg/kg orally every 6 h for 4 weeks. Alternatively, 6 to 8 weeks of oral α-difluoromethylornithine [6 g/m² of BSA (body surface area) per day in three doses] have been given. Prospective trials with DFMO have been disappointing. Successful therapy with this agent appears to depend on residual tissue levels from prior pentamidine therapy. Trials with a lipid soluble dihydrofolate reductase inhibitor, trimetrexate, are promising despite the consistent bone marrow toxicity from this chemotherapeutic agent. It is worth noting that in AIDS patients treated with AZT (azidothymidine, zidovudine, or Retrovir, Burroughs Wellcome Co.) the incidence of opportunistic infections is reduced by up to 50 percent. The incidence of specific pathogens among those who become infected is unchanged.

ENTAMOEBA HISTOLYTICA

Endemic infection with *Entamoeba histolytica* is common in tropical and subtropical regions of the world, notably southeast Asia, southern Africa, and Latin America. In the United States, there are more than 3500 cases per

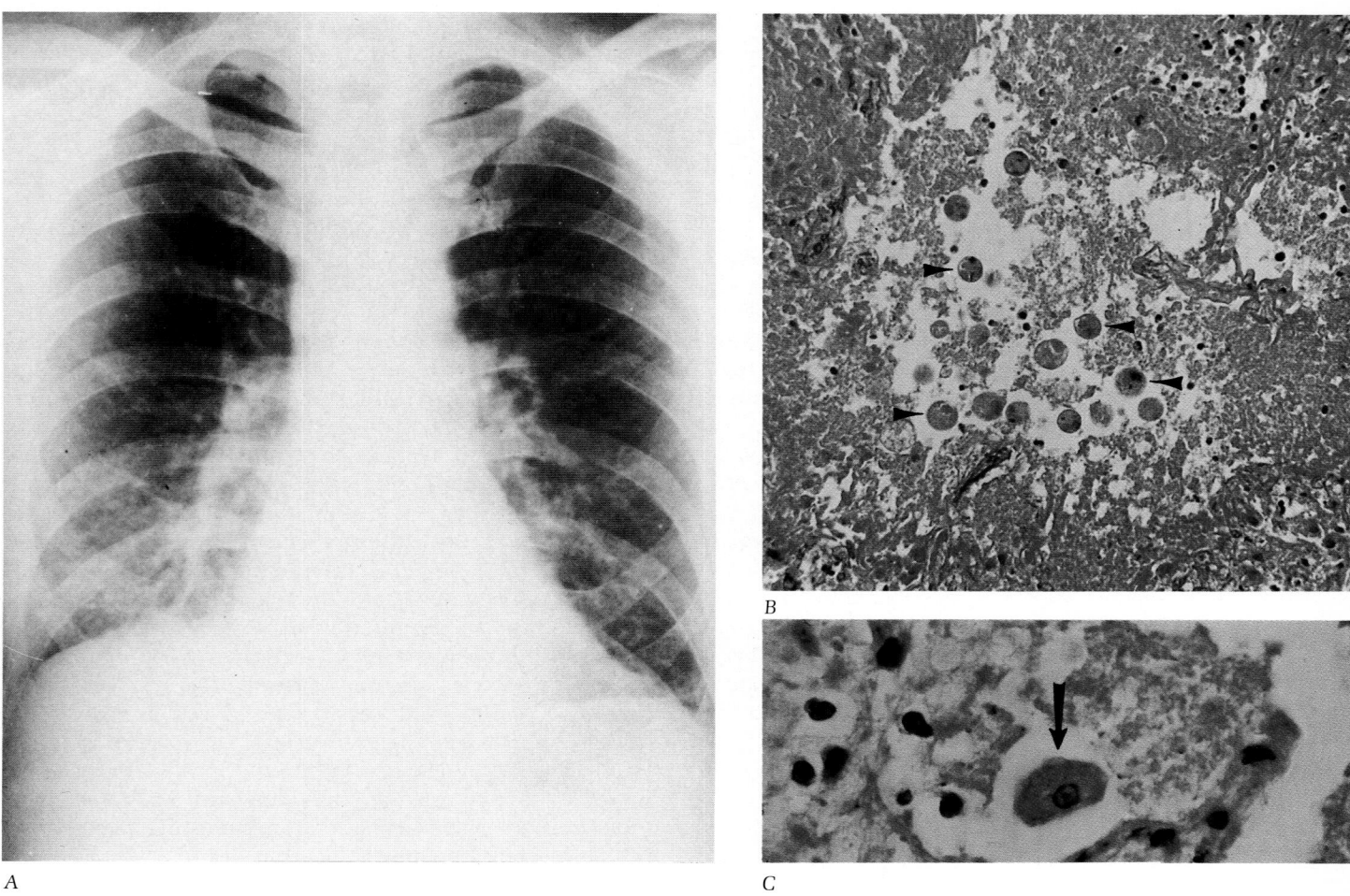

A   *C*

FIGURE 104-3 *Entamoeba histolytica* involving lung after rupture of a hepatic abscess through the right hemidiaphragm. A. Chest radiograph shows elevated right hemidiaphragm, right lower lobe infiltrate, and effusion. *(Courtesy of Armed Forces Institute of Pathology.)* B. Alveolar spaces are filled with amebic cysts (arrowheads). *(Iron hematoxylin, ×300.)* *(Courtesy of Dr. Y. Gutierrez.)* C. Trophozoites (arrow) and necrotic debris.

year. More than 95 percent of amebic infections do not extend beyond the bowel wall of the lower ileum and cecum, and most infected individuals are virtually asymptomatic carriers.

The overall incidence of amebic involvement of the lungs and pleura as a complication of amebic intestinal disease is low, but in any particular area it is a function of the incidence of amebic dysentery in that population. In the United States, occasional instances of amebic pleuropulmonary disease turn up in travelers returning from endemic areas, in immigrants from endemic zones, and in homosexual patients. Small outbreaks are occasionally encountered in chronic care facilities such as orphanages and mental health hospitals.

The Organism

Nonpathogenic and invasive amebas coexist as commensals within the intestinal tract. But *E. histolytica*, the cause of amebic dysentery and amebic liver abscess, is the only one of the amebae inhabiting the alimentary tract that has been shown to be pathogenic for humans.

E. histolytica exists in two forms: trophozoite and cyst. Cysts (7 to 20 μm) are the thick-walled transmissive stage carried in the stools of nondysenteric, but infected, individuals (Fig. 104-3*B*). Cysts can survive for months in a warm, moist environment and are spread via contaminated food and water, by flies and cockroaches, and, rarely, by sexual contact. Ingestion of cysts causes them to evolve into trophozoites that mature, become motile, and multiply by binary fission within the mucosal crypts. Trophozoites (15 to 40 μm) are noninfectious. Typically, they are ameboid in appearance, are motile, and undergo spontaneous changes in shape and feeding habits (Fig. 104-3C). They can ingest red blood cells (which are often seen in the endoplasm) and cellular debris (that is sequestered in vacuoles). Before penetrating the intestinal mu-

cosa, trophozoites increase in size (30 to 40 μm in diameter) and become more motile. They are agglutinated by concanavalin A and have a distinctive pattern of isoenzymes (see below). The stools of nondysenteric individuals episodically contain millions of cysts, whereas only individuals with dysentery shed trophozoites in their stools. In amebic dysentery, the trophozoites are large and often contain erythrocytes.

Whether invasiveness is an intrinsic attribute (e.g., surface "lectins" or secretory hormones) of special populations of *E. histolytica* or is due to the conversion of avirulent to virulent strains is unknown. However, certain conditions seem to favor the likelihood of invasion: malnutrition arising from protein-deficient diets, the male gender, genetic predisposition, immunosuppression, and cytotoxic agents. For example, in nonendemic regions, where amebic dysentery is often misinterpreted as ulcerative colitis, the immunosuppression associated with administration of corticosteroids—locally as well as systemically—has resulted in disseminated infection.

In invasive disease of the bowel, trophozoites penetrate the mucosa presumably through the tight intercellular junctions of mucosal cells to form distinctive flask-shaped ulcers. Trophozoites have been shown to be capable of direct lysis of host tissues and neutrophils. Tissue necrosis may be the result of the release of the contents of acid vesicles by invasive organisms. Trophozoites that erode into portal venules or lymphatics seed the liver, brain, or lung; in the liver, amebic hepatitis and amebic abscess may ensue. Pleural or pulmonary involvement occurs either via rupture of a liver abscess through the diaphragm, embolic seeding via the bloodstream, or via lymphatics traversing the diaphragm. About 15 percent of liver abscesses invade the thorax directly. Pulmonary disease is uncommon without concurrent hepatic or pleural involvement.

The Host

In the majority of patients with a hepatic abscess, the lesion is solitary, massive, and confined to the upper part of the right lobe. Most patients with hepatic abscess either cannot recall an antecedent episode of dysentery or recall a bout of diarrhea for 1 to 2 weeks that underwent spontaneous resolution. Other amebic complications, such as peritonitis, appendicitis, amebomas (colonic obstruction), or cutaneous lesions, may coexist with an amebic hepatic abscess.

An amebic hepatic abscess is generally manifested by hepatomegaly and tenderness over the liver. Jaundice is rare. The patient often complains of pain in either the right upper quadrant, epigastrium, or right shoulder; occasionally, the pain is pleural in nature. Fever, cough, dyspnea, anorexia, malaise, sweating, and hiccoughing often occur. Radiography characteristically shows that the right diaphragm is abnormally high and has decreased motility

(Fig. 104-1A). Sometimes a serous right pleural effusion is present in association with basal atelectasis or infiltrate. Leukocytosis, without eosinophilia, and the "anemia of chronic disease" are the rule in amebic abscess. Serologic tests for the presence of amebas are positive in about 90 percent of patients with amebic hepatic involvement. Except for mild hyperbilirubinemia and high levels of alkaline phosphatase in blood attributable to the mass lesion(s), liver function tests are often normal since the abscess(es) is a local lesion that is generally unaccompanied by widespread hepatitis.

As the hepatic abscess enlarges upward, adhesions are generally formed between the surface of the liver and the diaphragm. As a result, a subdiaphragmatic abscess is uncommon. Instead, the amebic infection generally burrows into the pleural space or the lung, causing (1) amebic empyema, (2) pneumonitis, or (3) pulmonary abscess and, occasionally, (4) a hepatobronchial fistula. Therefore, the signs and symptoms of entry into the thorax depend on the extent to which the subdiaphragmatic and pleural spaces have been obliterated by the advancing disease: an acute rupture into the pleural space may evoke excruciating pain in the back, right shoulder, or abdomen, accompanied by an exacerbation of fever, dyspnea, and even circulatory collapse; the liver may shrink in size as the abscess empties into the pleural space. A hepatobronchial fistula is associated with the production of large quantities of "anchovy paste" sputum consisting of red cells and necrotic liver tissue debris. The perforating abscess may choose alternative routes: into the peritoneum where it causes peritonitis or into the pericardial sac—commonly from the left lobe of the liver—to cause suppurative amebic pericarditis that may progress to cardiac tamponade.

Diagnosis

In the individual with amebic hepatic abscess, other than evidence of hepatic dysfunction, liver scanning, using isotopic gallium or technetium-colloid, discloses a filling defect. Noninvasive techniques have reduced the need for hepatic aspiration to clinch the diagnosis. Ultrasound examination of the liver reveals a thick-walled cyst(s) with internal echoes. When scanning and ultrasound are inconclusive, computed tomography may be useful in outlining the hepatic lesion(s). Aspiration yields bacteria-free, almost odorless material that, depending on the age of the abscess, ranges from chocolate brown to creamy in color.

Identification of the organism is the sine qua non for the diagnosis of amebiasis. In amebic pneumonitis and abscess, wet mounts from sputum can be searched for trophozoites. Staining with eosin or with iodine solution of an emulsion of a bit of sputum makes cysts stand out against the background. In hepatobronchial fistula, the thick red-brown sputum contains few organisms. Organisms in tissue or empyema fluid are more easily demon-

strated using permanent stains after fixation. Fixation is done in Schaudinn's fixing fluid or formalin; the usual stains are PAS trichrome, iron hematoxylin, or Lawless, stain (Fig. 104-3B). The other *Entamoeba* species that commonly need to be distinguished from *E. histolytica*, i.e., *E. coli* and *E. hartmanni* in fecal material, pose no problem since they do not appear in sputum.

In the lung, tissue trophozoites are the hallmark of invasive amebiasis. Organisms are best seen at the viable tissue margin. They are ameboid, amphiphilic and, if well fixed, will have a sharp border, central "ground glass" nucleus and a central karyosome (Fig. 104-1C). Organisms stained by PAS may be confused with alveolar macrophages unless counterstained with hematoxylin and eosin. Similarly, *E. histolytica* may be distinguished from degenerating parenchymal cells by searching for ingested red blood cells. The last portion of fluid aspirated from the abscess, i.e., that closest to the perimeter of the abscess, has the largest number of recognizable organisms. In only 60 percent of patients with hepatic amebiasis can *E. histolytica* be found in the stool; zinc sulfate flotation often increases the diagnostic yield.

Serologic tests have proved positive in over 90 percent of patients with either hepatic or pleuropulmonary amebiasis. Antibodies are present 1 week into an acute infection. However, a positive serology does not distinguish between ongoing tissue invasion and past infection. Serologic tests may be positive for 2 years or more after effective treatment. Most sensitive of the available tests are indirect hemagglutination, ELISA, indirect immunofluorescence, and counterimmunoelectrophoresis. A latex agglutination slide test is available commercially and is useful for quick and easy screening. Negative serologic tests render unlikely the diagnosis of hepatic and/or pleuropulmonary amebiasis; infection with other amebae may cause false-positive serologies. A determination of the pathogenicity of isolated enteric organisms can be made by "zymodeme" (isozyme) analysis. A number of dot-ELISA and DNA probe hybridization tests have also been developed to improve the diagnosis of acute *E. histolytica* infection.

Therapy

Asymptomatic and mild dysenteric forms of the disease should be treated prophylactically, especially in patients who are to become pregnant or immunosuppressed (Table 104-4). Therapy for liver abscess using metronidazole

TABLE 104-4
Antibiotic Therapy: Entamoeba Histolytica

Patient	Drug	Dose, mg PO	Duration, days	Comments
Asymptomatic Cyst Passer	Diloxanide furoate	500 tid	10	Not available in U.S.
	or Iodoquinol	650 tid (max 2 g per day)	21	(di-iodohydroxyquin) Nausea, rash, thyroid size increase, optic atrophy
	or Metronidazole	750 tid	10	Nausea, vomiting, diarrhea, paresthesias, neutropenia, urticaria, possible carcinogen, *avoid alcohol*
Intestinal Nondysenteric	Metronidazole followed by Iodoquinol	750 tid 650 tid	5 21	
Intestinal Dysenteric	Metronidazole and Iodoquinol	750 tid 650 tid	10 21	(Alternative: Tetracycline 250 mg PO qid × 10 d and emetine HCl 1 mg/kg IM × 5 d)
Extraintestinal	Metronidazole with Iodoquinol or Chloroquine base	750 tid 650 qd 600 qd 300 bid	14 21 2 14	Abscess drainage (alternative: emetine HCl 60 mg IM qd × 10 d or dihydroemetine di-HCl 90 mg IM qd × 10 d with chloroquine as noted)

alone is successful in over 85 percent of patients. Those who fail to respond are at increased risk of abscess growth and rupture. Rupture of a liver abscess into the pleural cavity or pericardium requires surgical intervention: the liver abscess calls for aspiration and the amebic empyema or pericarditis requires prompt drainage, particularly in the setting of cardiac tamponade. Because of the gravity of thoracic amebiasis, combined treatment is instituted using metronidazole, 750 mg by mouth, three times daily for 10 to 15 days, in conjunction with either iodoquinol (650 mg PO bid for 10 to 20 days) or chloroquine base (600 mg PO bid for 2 days, then 300 mg PO bid for 14 days) (Table 104-4). Metronidazole acts to destroy amebae in tissues and in the intestinal lumen. It should not be given during pregnancy nor ingested along with alcoholic beverages. The more common side effects of metronidazole are anorexia, nausea, and dizziness; prolonged courses can cause leukopenia, peripheral neuropathy, and possibly oncogenesis. Chloroquine or iodoquinol may cause rash, pruritis, diarrhea, and minor electrocardiographic changes; optic neuritis has been reported as a rare complication.

Emetine and synthetic racemic 2-dehydroemetine remain the most potent tissue amebicides known. Dehydroemetine has a lower toxicity than emetine, but the side effects are qualitatively similar: local pain at the site of intramuscular or deep subcutaneous injection, gastrointestinal upsets, autonomic blockade with resultant hypotension, peripheral neuropathy, cardiac arrhythmia, or cardiomyopathy. Because of these untoward prospects, patients receiving emetine or its derivative require bed rest during treatment. Despite these reservations, dehydroemetine may be required in thoracic amebiasis. It is given intramuscularly, 1.5 mg/kg per day for up to a maximum of 90 mg per day for 5 days, in conjunction with chloroquine (as above).

Other Amebae

Pulmonary infections caused by amebae other than *E. histolytica* are uncommon. Rare instances of aspiration pneumonitis have been attributed to *Trichomonas vaginalis* and *T. tenax*. *Naegleria* and *acanthamoeba* species occasionally evoke disease of the upper respiratory passages by gaining entry via nasal or aural routes from lakes, pools, and dusts. Although these organisms are generally localized as commensals in the upper respiratory tract and sinuses, immunosuppression may permit dissemination via olfactory tracts to cause meningoencephalitis. Extraintestinal spread of *Balantidium coli* in immunocompromised patients has been observed via blood or lymph resulting in metastatic seeding of pleura, lungs, liver, and hilar lymph nodes.

TOXOPLASMA GONDII

Toxoplasmosis is a worldwide protozoan disease caused by *Toxoplasma gondii*, an obligate intracellular coccidian parasite. It affects humans, animals, and birds, and is transmitted exclusively by cats, its definitive host. Except for immunosuppressed hosts, clinically important disease occurs only in neonates and children. Significant pulmonary disease is observed only in the individual who is immunocompromised.

The Organism

The multiple developmental stages of *T. gondii* are important to the clinical expressions of the disease. These stages are the infective *oocyst* from cats, the invasive *sporozoites*, the motile and proliferative *trophozoites* (often called *tachyzoites*), and the long-lived tissue *cyst*.

The life cycle begins when cats (or other *Felidae*), previously unexposed to *Toxoplasma*, ingest infected meats containing tissue cysts or oocysts (Fig. 104-4). After disruption of cysts or oocysts, asexual (schizogony) and sexual (gametogony) reproduction occurs throughout the small intestine. Self-propagating infection (the *enteroepithelial cycle*) within the cat's intestinal epithelial cells generates the millions of oocysts excreted daily in cat feces. Fecal oocysts 10 to 20 μm in diameter may survive more than a year in moist soil and undergo sporulation over 2 to 3 days after excretion, becoming infective. Infective oocysts are killed by boiling or adequately cooking (over 65°C) meats or vegetables.

Ingestion by humans or other animals (the intermediate hosts) of cyst-containing meats, or foods contaminated by oocysts from cat feces, initiates the infection. The cysts are disrupted by gastric enzymes, whereas the oocysts undergo a further cycle of sporulation in the intestine, releasing the motile sporozoites. These penetrate the intestinal epithelial cells and spread throughout the body via the bloodstream and lymphatics. Within the vacuoles of reticuloendothelial cells and other tissues, sporozoites mature into trophozoites. Trophozoites are 4- to 8-μm-long, crescentic, and nucleated forms which move by body flexion without flagella (Fig. 104-5D). They multiply within the cell by internal division (*endodyogeny*) until the cell ruptures, thereby enabling invasion of adjacent tissues. Unless the invasion is arrested by a specific immune response, parasitization of tissues continues. In some instances, infection is circumscribed by a membrane that bounds intracellular and relatively inactive colonies of trophozoites, i.e., the tissue cyst.

Cysts are large (up to 200 μm) and contain up to 3000 slowly dividing trophozoite forms sometimes termed *bradyzoites* to underscore their relatively inactive state

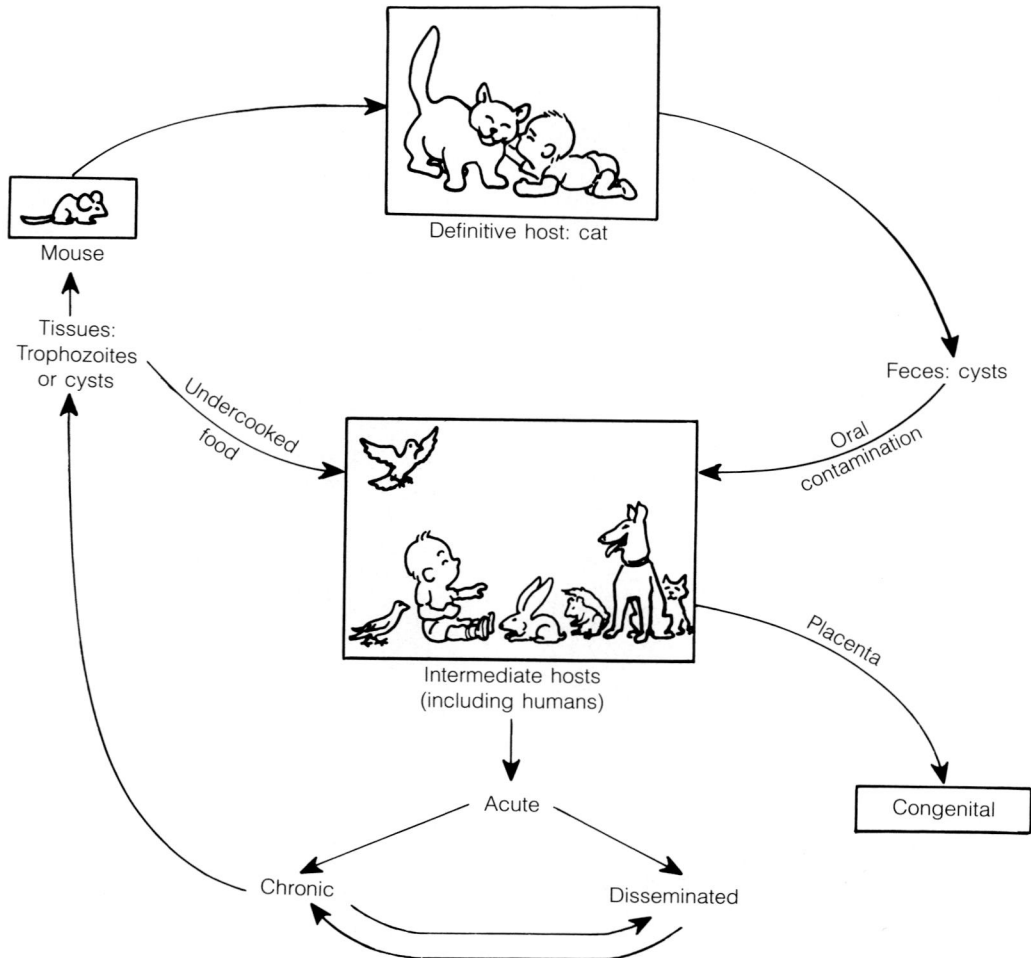

FIGURE 104-4 Life cycle of *Toxoplasma gondii*. The enteroepithelial cycle in the cat releases oocysts in cat feces. These become infectious and are passed to humans via infected meat or water.

(Fig. 104-5C). Cysts persist in host tissues as a potential reservoir of infection throughout the life of the host. Rupture of cysts due to ingestion of undercooked meats or to immunosuppression of the host allows another cycle of local infection to ensue.

Parasitization is generally most marked in the brain, heart, lung, and lymphoid tissues with active infection with trophozoites and cyst formation coexisting. The factors responsible for cyst formation are unclear. The host's immune response may play a role. However, multiple subpopulations of *Toxoplasma* exist which differ in virulence and may also have differing developmental dispositions. It is not known whether pulmonary infection in toxoplasmosis is due to local cyst rupture or to dissemination of extrapulmonary disease to the lungs. The determinants of pulmonary involvement are also not known.

The Host

The disease is manifested in one of four clinical forms: congenital, acquired in nonimmunocompromised individuals, disseminated in immunocompromised individuals, and reactivation of latent infection within the eye (ocular toxoplasmosis). Only in the disseminated form of the disease is pulmonary involvement a prominent feature.

CONGENITAL

This form occurs in infants as a complication of an *acute* maternal infection during pregnancy. Although pneumonitis does occur, the predominant manifestations are of central nervous system disease, particularly chorioretinitis and hydrocephaly.

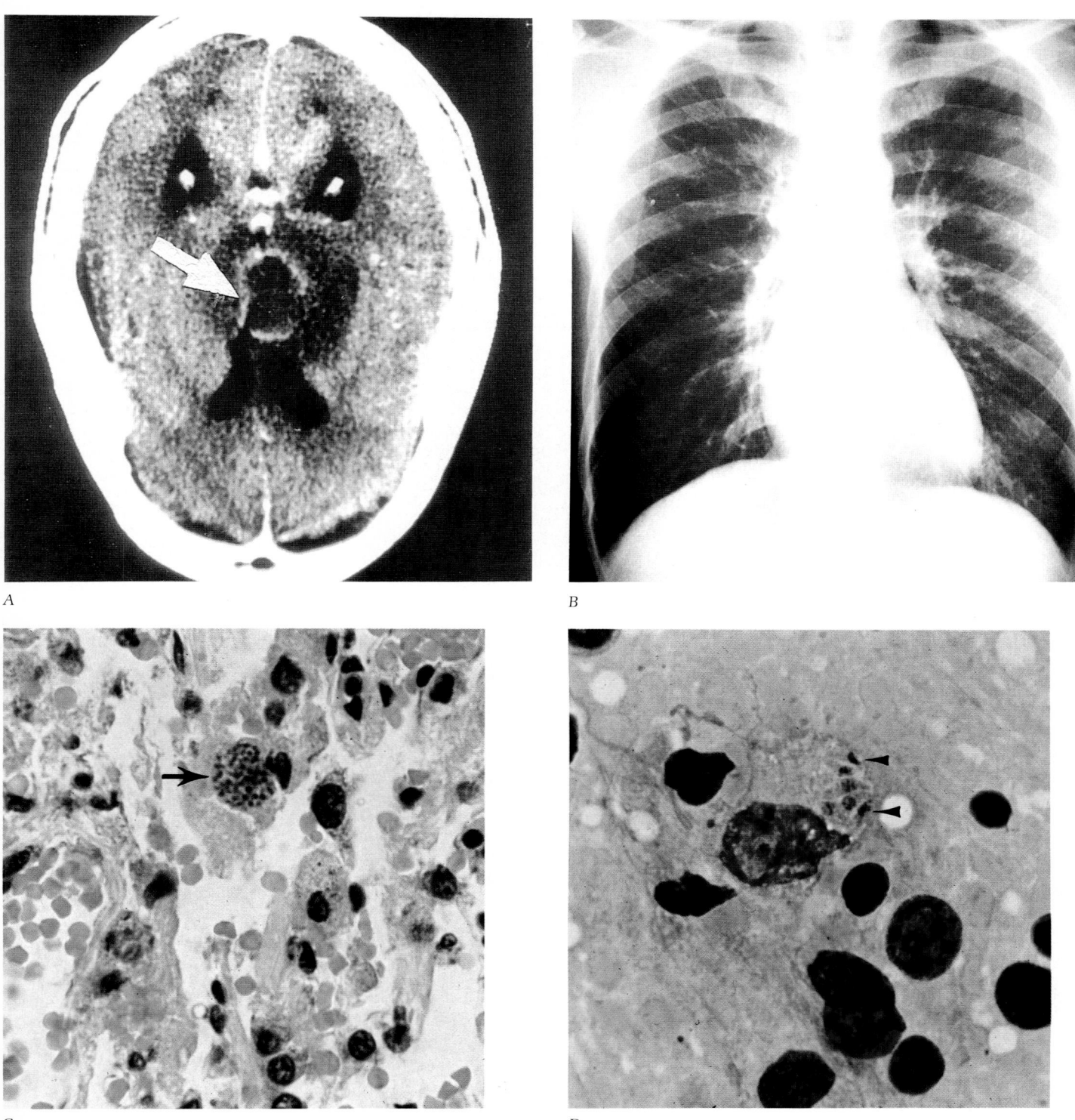

A

B

C

D

FIGURE 104-5 *Toxoplasma gondii* in brain and lung in a patient with AIDS. *A*. Brain, computed tomography shows *Toxoplasma* abscess as a contrast enhancing lesion (arrow). *B*. Chest radiography. Diffuse bilateral infiltrates and hilar adenopathy. *C*. Lung biopsy shows *Toxoplasma* cyst forms. (H&E, ×1000.) *D*. Impression smear of brain biopsy shows five intracellular trophozoites (arrowheads). (Giemsa stain, ×1500.) *(C and D are courtesy of Dr. Y. Gutierrez.)*

ACQUIRED IN NONIMMUNOCOMPROMISED INDIVIDUALS

Most individuals with acquired toxoplasmosis have no clinical signs or symptoms of their infection. A few develop lymphadenopathy, sometimes with a syndrome resembling infectious mononucleosis. Waxing and waning of the disease may suggest lymphoma. Pneumonitis is not a conspicuous part of the syndrome which may last for weeks to months—usually with full recovery. Humoral and cellular immunity limit the infection without eliminating tissue cysts.

REACTIVATION (OCULAR TOXOPLASMOSIS)

This form occurs in immunologically normal young adults, almost invariably as a sequel to congenital infection. Characteristically it affects the retina and underlying choroid and presents as a chorioretinitis of one or both eyes. The process heals by local scarring but may recur years later as encysted colonies of *T. gondii* rupture to produce fresh chorioretinitis. The ocular process is not accompanied by systemic manifestations of toxoplasmosis.

DISSEMINATED IN IMMUNOCOMPROMISED INDIVIDUALS

In this category, clinically important pneumonitis caused by *T. gondii* occurs primarily in patients with a defect in cell-mediated immunity such as those with Hodgkin's disease or other hematopoietic neoplasias who are also being immunosuppressed by corticosteroids, alkylating agents, or radiation therapy. Also vulnerable are patients receiving granulocyte or organ transplants, or chemotherapy or radiation therapy as part of the management of systemic lupus erythematosus or other connective tissue disease. A recent addition to the susceptible populations are patients with AIDS. Almost invariably, pneumonia due to *T. gondii* in these patients is associated with central nervous system disease.

Pneumonitis due to *T. gondii* probably occurs in over half of immunocompromised individuals who die of disseminated toxoplasmosis. The patient may present with signs of encephalitis or with primary pulmonary symptoms. Like other "atypical pneumonias," the patient will often have fever and dyspnea with minimal sputum production and few clinical or radiographic findings. Lymphadenopathy and a maculopapular rash are occasionally noted. The brain disease generally is in the form of either a meningoencephalitis or encephalomyelitis on the one hand, or a localized mass lesion (abscess) on the other. The cerebrospinal fluid shows a marked mononuclear pleocytosis with elevated protein. The pneumonia is discussed below. The heart is often the seat of either myocarditis or conduction defects. Myositis is frequent. Infection of the liver, spleen, bone marrow, adrenals, lymph nodes, and kidneys may produce a typhuslike syndrome.

In contrast to the focal lesions produced in other organs, *T. gondii* usually evokes diffuse disease in the lungs, presumably because of the role played by the lungs as a filter of circulating organisms and its extensive phagocyte population. Interstitial infiltrates may progress to bronchopneumonia, necrotizing pneumonia, and pulmonary infarction. Death may follow hepatic necrosis, cardiomyopathy, and secondary pulmonary edema. Not infrequently, infection with other organisms, such as cytomegalovirus and *P. carinii*, coexists with *T. gondii* pneumonitis. In some instances, *T. gondii* is a superinfecting agent on an underlying bacterial pneumonia.

Diagnosis

Diagnosis of infection due to *Toxoplasma* is usually difficult, most notably in the disseminated form of the disease. It begins with the suspicion that the disease may be present; proof depends on the demonstration of invasive organisms in tissue and/or serologic testing. Culture methods are still in their infancy. Encysted organisms in tissue, particularly in lymph nodes, are not proof of active infection since cysts can survive in tissues for years after the initial infection: cysts have been found in brain, lymph nodes, lung, liver, and spleen of adults more than 1 year after an acute infection (Fig. 104-5C). Therefore, the diagnosis of active infection is based on either the demonstration of trophozoites in body fluids (e.g., cerebrospinal fluid) or tissue or, if organisms cannot be found, on a positive serology (see below) in an individual with an appropriate clinical syndrome.

T. gondii tachyzoites have been found in bronchoalveolar lavage and lung biopsy samples from some patients who have radiographic evidence of pneumonitis. However, while biopsy or bronchoscopy are useful when positive, a number of autopsies have revealed active pulmonary toxoplasmosis missed antemortem by these procedures. These patients may undergo a lung biopsy in the face of nondiagnostic aspiration or pulmonary bronchoscopy. Early in its course, the pneumonitis is predominantly interstitial and characterized by an infiltrate of macrophages, lymphocytes, plasma cells, and occasionally polymorphonuclear leukocytes. The local inflammatory response is usually mild, owing both to defects in the host's immune response and to immune suppression induced by the organism itself. Areas of bronchopneumonia, arteriolar endarteritis and occlusion, or necrosis may develop. Proliferating stages of *T. gondii* are found not only in the macrophages but also free in alveoli.

Because brain disease features so prominently in the disseminated form of the disease that affects the immunosuppressed patient, brain biopsy has become increasingly important in obtaining tissue for detection of trophozoites, particularly in AIDS patients (Fig. 104-5C). Computed tomography has been helpful in identifying a brain

lesion, establishing its size and location (Fig. 104-5A). In AIDS patients, presumptive diagnosis may be made in the presence of multiple and bilateral contrast enhancing lesions on CT scan or cranial magnetic resonance imaging scans. Early diagnosis by brain biopsy is rewarding not only because of the possibility of favorably influencing the course of toxoplasmosis in the brain and lungs but also because of uncovering other fungal or viral infections, or a lymphoma of the brain in AIDS patients. The chest radiograph is nonspecific in pulmonary toxoplasmosis. There is prominent hilar lymphadenopathy (easily confused with lymphoma) with a diffuse interstitial infiltrate (Fig. 104-5B). Unilateral and nodular radiographic patterns are also seen. Pleural effusions or cavitation are uncommon. A therapeutic trial for 10 to 14 days should be accompanied by improvement on radiologic imaging. Such an improvement is not meaningful diagnostically if corticosteroid therapy is employed.

As noted previously organisms are generally not identifiable in sputum, bronchopulmonary brushings, or lavage specimens; occasionally, they can be identified in cytology specimens obtained by pulmonary abscess aspiration—either by needle or bronchoscopically—or by open lung biopsy. Occasionally, organisms may be grown on tissue culture "feeder" cells from blood, tissue, or bronchial lavage fluid and, like *Pneumocystis*, may be grown accidentally in viral cell cultures of these fluids. Touch preparations of infected lung that are treated with Giemsa stain demonstrate both cyst and trophozoite forms (Fig. 104-5). Cyst walls are nicely outlined by periodic acid-Schiff stain, whereas trophozoites are better seen with either Wright or Giemsa stain or with fluorescent or peroxidase-tagged antibody to *Toxoplasma* on histologic sections. The presence of multiple cyst forms of *T. gondii* in areas of active inflammation and in the absence of other pulmonary pathogens may be used for a presumptive diagnosis of toxoplasmosis. Organisms are often difficult to detect. The newer peroxidase-antiperoxidase tissue staining method is able to localize *Toxoplasma* organisms or antigen not visualized by histologic stains. Mouse inoculation with biopsy or aspiration material has the greatest sensitivity for detection of *T. gondii* infection. This method is, however, impractical in most clinical centers.

The diagnosis of active toxoplasmosis usually relies on serologic tests that are often positive during infection even in the face of severe cellular immune dysfunction (Table 104-5). The Sabin-Feldman dye test is based on the ability of the immunoglobulin G antibodies from immune sera to block methylene blue staining of live organisms. This test requires the use of live organisms and does not differentiate present from past infection. Its use is hampered by the fact that it is positive (at serum dilutions of 1:1000 or greater) in over 35 percent of all normal adults in the United States. Tests to detect antibodies to *Toxoplasma* include the indirect fluorescent antibody (IFA, for both IgG and IgM antibodies), complement fixation, hemagglutination and ELISA. These have become generally available, most laboratories using IFA or ELISA.

Many patients have peak antibody titers by the time that the disease is first suspected. Nevertheless, "acute"

TABLE 104-5
Serologic Assays Used in the Diagnosis of Toxoplasma Gondii Infection*

Test	Acute Titer	Chronic Titer	Comments
Sabin-Feldman dye test (IgG)	≥1:1000	1:4–1:2000	Remains elevated; onset 7–10 days
IFA-IgG (Indirect fluorescent antibody)	≥1:1000	1:4–1:2000	Remains elevated; onset 2–3 weeks
IFA-IgM†	≥1:64	0–1:20	Negative in months; first positive acutely (1 week)
Indirect hemagglutination (IHA) (IgG)	≥1:1000	1:16–1:256	Remains elevated; onset 2–3 weeks
Complement fixation (IgG)	≥1:16	0–1:8	Remains elevated; onset 2–3 weeks
ELISA†-double sandwich-IgM	≥1:256	0–1:256	Remains elevated; early onset

*Reviewed in McCabe and Remington, 1985, and Ruskin, 1981; two-tube fourfold rise in titer to "acute" level is diagnostic for any test.

†May give false-positive value in presence of rheumatoid, antinuclear, or other autoantibodies; single high titer is diagnostic of acute infection.

NOTE: Positive/diagnostic values for the various tests will vary between clinical laboratories, and some patients will fall outside these ranges.

and "convalescent" serum antibody titers should be drawn for both IgG and IgM; the IgM titer is a better reflection of acute infection (Table 104-5). Immunocompromised individuals may not manifest elevated serum antibody titers in the face of active infection. In these patients, pulmonary or brain lesions should be biopsied to establish a pathologic diagnosis. In interpreting serologic tests, it is relevant to recall that some antibodies that bind *T. gondii* may be elicited by *Trichomonas* organisms. Also, tests for IgM antibody may be false-positive in the presence of antinuclear antibodies or rheumatoid factor. Finally, the more recent tests to detect *Toxoplasma* antigens (e.g., ELISA) and the IgM immunosorbent assay (IgM-ISA) are sensitive, have fewer false positives, and are helpful diagnostically in the immunosuppressed host with dampened antibody responses. Sera from patients with AIDS or from patients about to receive immunosuppressive chemotherapy or organ transplantation should be stored as "preimmune" controls.

Therapy

Because the disseminated form of the disease is usually fatal without treatment, suspicion of the clinical syndrome coupled with serologic testing usually suffices as the springboard for therapy. As a rule of thumb, treatment for toxoplasmosis is generally begun in a likely clinical candidate in whom both IgG and IgM serum antibody levels are elevated: clinical infection should be assumed when the IgG titer exceeds 1:1000 and the IgM titer is greater than 1:64 or when a fourfold rise in IgG antibody titer is observed (Table 104-5).

Cellular immunity is needed to eradicate intracellular *T. gondii* since antibody in conjunction with complement kills only extracellular organisms. In the normal host, monocyte myeloperoxidase-containing granules play a role in killing phagocytosed *T. gondii*. The initial therapy for *T. gondii* infection should therefore include a reduc-

tion in immunosuppressive therapy where possible. The cysts are resistant to antibiotic therapy. Drug therapy of disseminated toxoplasmosis consists of a synergistic combination of pyrimethamine with a sulfonamide (Table 104-6). Pyrimethamine is given in two 50-mg oral loading doses followed by 25 or 50 mg by mouth daily or every other day, depending on the severity of the disease. In order to combat bone marrow suppression induced by the drugs, as well as by the underlying disease, folinic acid (calcium Leukovorin, 5 mg every other day) is administered. This agent should be omitted during therapy for acute leukemia as folinic acid may accelerate tumor growth. A sulfonamide, either trisulfapyrimidines or sulfadiazine, is given orally as a 4-g load followed by 1 to 1.5 g (75 to 100 mg/kg per day), four times each day. In those allergic to sulfonamides or during pregnancy, spiramycin may be preferable to sulfonamide. Spiramycin is a macrolide antibiotic similar to erythromycin which has been a useful adjunct to therapy in AIDS. It is available as Rovamycine (Rhone-Poulene Pharma, Montreal, Canada) and can be given in dosages of 2 to 4 g per day. Spiramycin can be obtained in the United States on a "compassionate" basis from the Food and Drug Administration. Combination therapy should be maintained for 3 to 6 weeks. Preliminary experiences with clindamycin and co-trimoxazole or pyrimethamine are also encouraging. Vaccines are being developed for use in cats to prevent carriage of the organisms. Prevention of infection in humans is based on properly cooking or curing meats, on the total avoidance of cats, and potentially, by prophylactic treatment of susceptible hosts. Prophylaxis in the AIDS population has been successful using sulfadoxine and pyrimethamine (Fansidar, one tablet orally once or twice per week), co-trimoxazole (160 mg trimethoprim and 800 mg sulfamethoxazole per day) or low-dose pyrimethamine with sulfadiazine given on alternate days. These therapies are lifelong and are used to prevent relapse of *Toxoplasma* in the central nervous system. In general,

TABLE 104-6
*Antibiotic Therapy: Toxoplasma Gondii**

Drug	Dose	Duration	Comments
Pyrimethamine and	100 mg (then) 25 mg to 50 mg PO qd or qod	Load 3–6 weeks	Bone marrow suppression: may give folinic acid 5 mg PO or IM qod except in acute leukemia
Sulfonamide or	4 g PO (then) 1–1.5 g PO qid (75–100 mg/kg per day)	Load 3–6 weeks	Sulfadiazine or trisulfa-pyrimidine: decrease dose for neutropenia; sulfa-allergy common
Spiramycin	1g PO tid or qid	3–6 weeks	In pregnancy or sulfa allergy with pyrimethamine

* Active infection; twice weekly blood counts are necessary to detect bone marrow suppression due to therapy. Lifelong prophylaxis after therapy for acute infection is recommended in AIDS patients.

prophylactic regimens including either or both pyrimeth-amine and sulfadiazine have been more successful than those regimens not including these agents. Fansidar has caused severe hepatic toxicity in some individuals. AIDS patients may develop hypersensitivity to sulfa-containing antibiotics beyond that expected in other patient populations.

CRYPTOSPORIDIUM

Cryptosporidium species are intestinal protozoan parasites that belong to the Coccidia as do *Toxoplasma* and *Isospora*. It is well known both as a commensal and as a cause of diarrhea in a wide range of animal species, including rabbits, chickens, lambs, cattle, turkeys, geese, snakes, dingoes, monkeys, rodents, and birds. Current understanding is that a single species of *Cryptosporidium* affects these diverse hosts as well as humans. *Cryptosporidium* occurs in asymptomatic individuals as well as in up to 5 percent of immunologically normal individuals experiencing gastroenteritis or chronic malabsorption. In neonatal or immunocompromised animals, infection results in a fatal diarrheal illness. In humans, the outcome of infection with *Cryptosporidium* depends on the immunologic status of the host: in otherwise normal individuals, the gastrointestinal disease caused by *Cryptosporidium* is self-limited; in the immunocompromised individual, the disease is more serious and potentialy life-threatening.

The picture of clinical infection with *Cryptosporidium* is that of a flulike syndrome that resolves in 1 to 2 weeks. In the individual with diarrhea who is identified as harboring *Cryptosporidium* in the gastrointestinal tract, the organism is often associated with other pathogens, e.g., amebae, cytomegalovirus, *Giardia lamblia*, *Isospora belli*, or adenovirus. Outbreaks of cryptosporidial infection have occurred in day-care centers and in the families of the affected children. Immunocompromised individuals, notably recipients of bone marrow, patients undergoing chemotherapy after renal transplantation, individuals with immunoglobulin deficiency, and patients with AIDS, are candidates for severe and generally unremitting gastrointestinal and gallbladder infections. In 1984, more than 200 infections with *Cryptosporidium* were identified in patients with AIDS. Often the diarrhea was uncontrollable.

The Organism

Cryptosporidium is transmitted by the fecal-oral route and undergoes both asexual and sexual reproduction in the human host. After ingestion, the small oocysts (2 to 6 mm) excyst in the stomach or small intestine releasing their sporozoites. These attach to the brush border of the small intestine (Fig. 104-6) and mature into merozoites

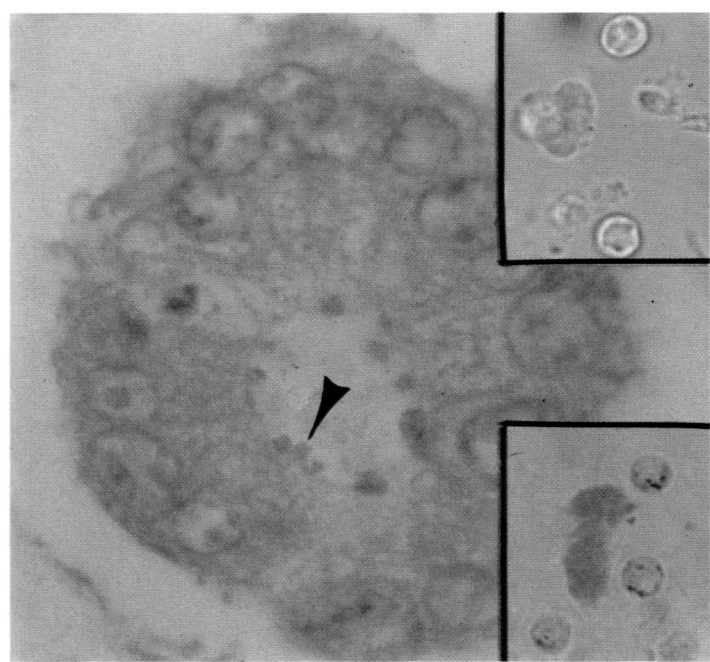

FIGURE 104-6 Cryptosporidiosis (patient from Fig. 104-2). *Cryptosporidium* (arrowhead) is adherent to the intestinal epithelium. (H&E, ×25.) *Insets:* Organisms isolated from feces: *upper* = Sheather's sugar flotation, ×1360; *lower* = Giesma-Jenner stain, ×1360.

that attach to, or lodge just inside of, the enterocyte. The number of organisms and the rapidity of its life cycle depend on the age, immune status, and species of the host. Both calves and lambs serve as a reservoir for zoonotic infection of humans; person-to-person transmission occurs by fecal-oral route. Direct pulmonary transmission has been demonstrated in turkeys. The autoinfectious cycle, which has been described by Current and Reese, explains the basis of a small inoculum of *Cryptosporidium* causing life-threatening disease in the absence of a normal immune response.

The Host

As indicated above, *Cryptosporidium* is an established cause of disease in domestic and wild animals. Before 1982, only eight instances of infection had been reported in humans. However, since then the number of reported cases has increased exponentially because of both the increasing occurrence of AIDS and the advent of efficient screening methods. *Cryptosporidium* has been found both in animal handlers and in individuals drinking surface water contaminated with animal feces. The clinical manifestations of cryptosporidial infection depend in large measure on the immune status of the patient. Although the normal host can either be an asymptomatic carrier or manifest a flulike syndrome, life-threatening diarrhea or cholecystitis may develop in the immunosuppressed host.

Pulmonary infection with *Cryptosporidium* has been observed only in patients with AIDS and is often complicated by concomitant infection with other pathogens: protozoa (*P. carinii, T. gondii, E. histolytica*), viruses (cytomegalovirus, herpes simplex), fungi (*Candida*), *Legionella*, atypical *Mycobacterium*, or intestinal *Cryptosporidium*. In individuals with AIDS, infection occurs year-round. In contrast, infection in the noncompromised host is seasonal: diarrhea due to the organism occurs primarily in the summer or fall seasons; no special relation exists between the occurrence of the disorder and age or sex. How the organism reaches the lungs in humans is unknown, but aspiration of gastrointestinal organisms or airborne transmission are the likely mechanisms.

Diagnosis

Some uncertainty exists about the etiologic role of the organism in producing pneumonitis in the immunocompromised host: the causative agent, a superinfecting fellow traveler, or none at all. However, in the patient with pulmonary cryptosporidiosis, dyspnea and cough are generally prominent and heavy, frothy sputum is produced. Physical examination may reveal only scattered rales. Chest radiography demonstrates a mild diffuse increase in bronchial markings unless other organisms are also involved in producing the pneumonitis. *Cryptosporidium* is identified in the sputum (as in stools) by a modified (cold) acid-fast Kinyoun stain (see below). Care must be taken to identify other infecting agents.

Diagnosis of cryptosporidiosis depends on the identification of oocysts in the stools and sputum of patients. When stool organisms are sparse, oocysts can be concentrated by using Sheather's sugar cover-slip flotation method and phase contrast microscopy; the cryptosporidia appear as refractile bodies without internal structures (Fig. 104-6). Detection of organisms in stool specimens is enhanced by the use of a concentrator that also reduces handling. Endoscopic biopsy of the large and small intestines may also be useful in demonstrating the parasite, but this procedure is usually not necessary to make the diagnosis.

Cryptosporidia are identified on either wet-mount or fixed preparations of sputum or stool (Fig. 104-7). They must be distinguished from the colonizing yeasts that are common both in stool specimens and in the sputum of AIDS patients (with thrush or cryptococcosis). The oocysts do not stain with iodine on wet mounts and are orange with Truant's auramine-rhodamine stain. Yeasts are brown with iodine and do not stain with Truant's. On fixed smears, oocysts stain red with dense internal granules on cold Kinyoun stain, whereas yeasts stain green. The typical morphology of cryptosporidia will also be revealed by Giemsa staining (see Fig. 104-7) with a light green counterstain.

Serologic tests hold promise for establishing the diagnosis, especially when illness is protracted. But current assays, such as indirect immunofluorescence or ELISA systems, are not useful for the diagnosis of *acute* gastrointestinal disease even though they do correlate well with the presence or history of infection. In immunologically normal hosts, positive antibody titers (>1:20) take up to 2 weeks to develop and reach their peak 8 to 10 weeks after the start of infection; positive titers may persist for more than a year after infection. In the immunocompromised patient, serology may never turn positive. The basis of protective immunity to this organism is not understood.

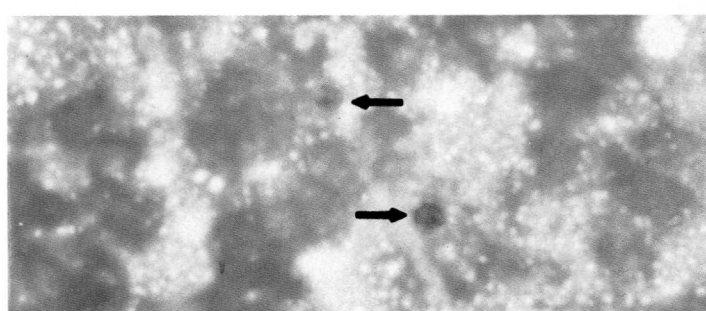

A

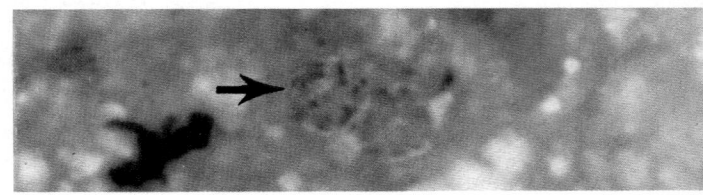

B

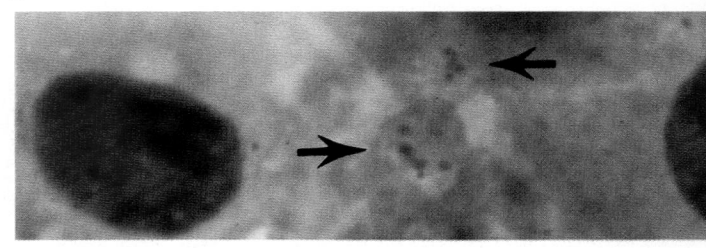

C

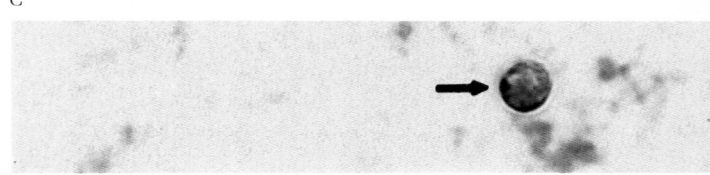

D

FIGURE 104-7 Cryptosporidiosis in "touch preparation" and sputum. *A.* Touch preparation from lung biopsy of AIDS patient. *Cryptosporidium* shown by modified cold Kinyoun (MCK) technique that stains organisms red (arrows). (×880.) *B.* Same preparation and stain as *A* showing internal dense red granules characteristic of the oocyst (arrow). (×375.) *C.* Same preparation as *A* showing similar morphology with rapid Giemsa Hemacolor stain. (Arrows indicate organisms.) (×375.) *D. Sputum* stained with MCK technique reveals organism (arrow). (×990.) *(A to D courtesy of Dr. P. Ma.)*

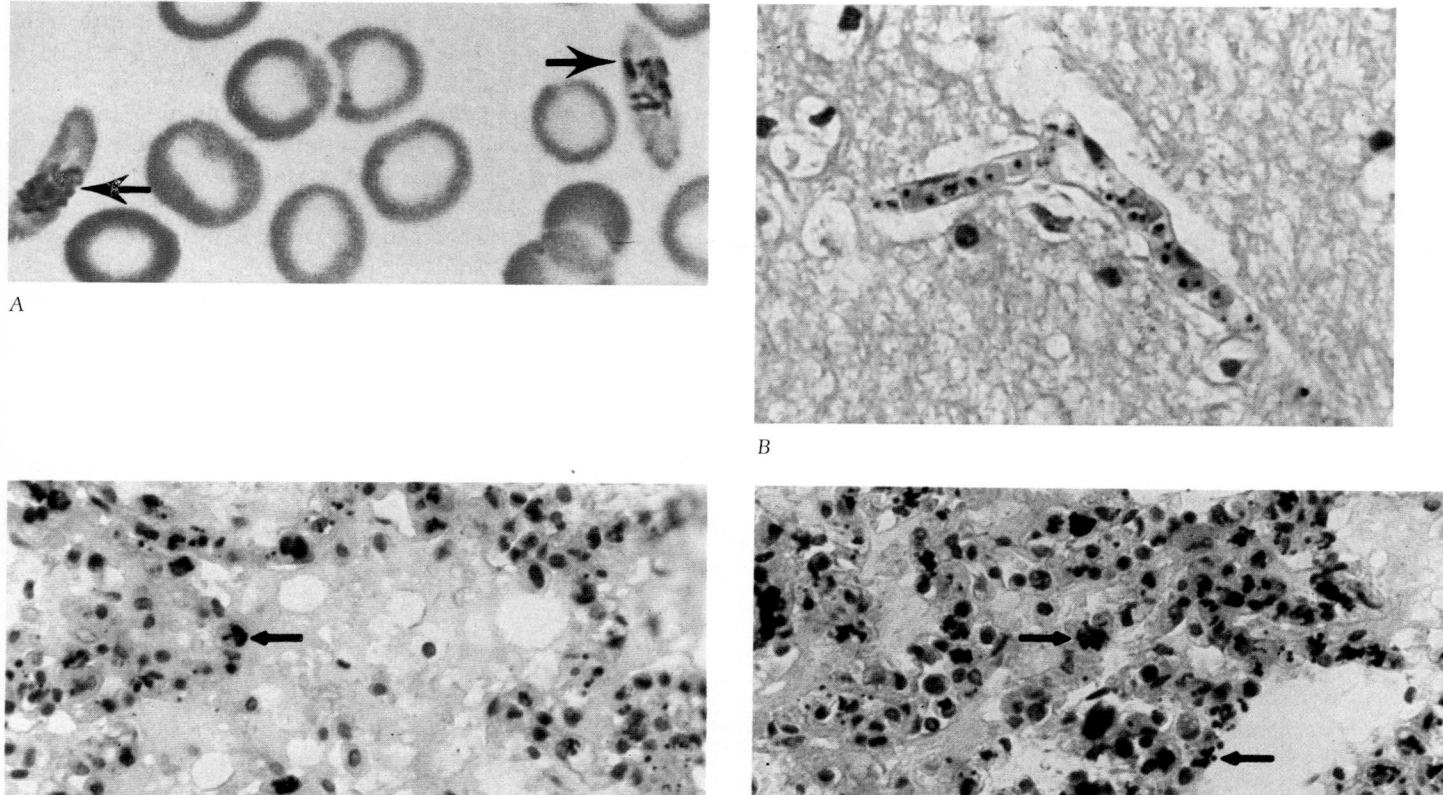

FIGURE 104-8 *Plasmodium falciparum.* A. Banana-shaped microgametocytes on peripheral blood smear (arrows). (Wright stain, ×1375.) B. Cerebral vessels obstructed by parasitized red blood cells and surrounding edema. (H&E, ×1375.) C. Acute pulmonary edema due to pulmonary venular occlusion (organism at arrow). (H&E.) D. Deposition of malarial pigment (arrows) in vicinity of occluded pulmonary vessels.

Therapy

No antibiotic treatment has proved effective for cryptosporidiosis in the immunocompromised host. The list of ineffective agents includes trimethoprim-sulfamethoxazole, pentamidine, metronidazole, quinacrine, chloroquine, and tetracycline. As a result, treatment is largely symptomatic. In immunocompetent individuals, the disease is self-limited. However, in the immunocompromised host, supportive therapy is essential, especially if diarrhea dominates the clinical picture. Parenteral nutrition and fluids are administered and immunosuppressive therapy is reduced or discontinued. Coexisting pulmonary or extrapulmonary infections should be identified and treated. Even if the diarrhea should stop, the immunocompromised patient often continues to pass oocysts in stools for up to 3 months. Some AIDS patients have experienced symptomatic relief from spiramycin (Rovamycine, Rhone-Poulenc Pharma, Montreal, Quebec, Canada, 1 g orally, three or four times a day). This medication is available in the United States through the Food and Drug Administration. Treatment with this agent is continued for 3 to 4 weeks. Although stools and intestinal biop-

sies sometimes do become parasite-free, most patients relapse when the drug is stopped. Other agents that have been used with apparent success on rare occasions are furazolidone (100 to 300 mg, orally, four times a day) or diloxanide furoate (500 mg, orally, three times a day).

Other Coccidians

Other ways by which the lungs may be affected in coccidian infections warrant brief mention. *Plasmodium falciparum* malaria is sometimes complicated by pulmonary edema, especially with excessive intravenous fluid administration. Patients with high-grade parasitemias may develop central nervous system injury (Fig. 104-8). Organisms have also been found attached to pulmonary vascular (venous) endothelium causing increased permeability and obstruction. Chloroquine phosphate is the drug of choice, but the possibility of chloroquine resistance should be considered in patients with exposures obtained in southeast Asia, central and eastern Africa, and in Central or South America. Falciparum malaria is a medical emergency. In kala azar, *Leishmania donovani* are seen in macrophages in lungs, lymph nodes, and myocardium. A

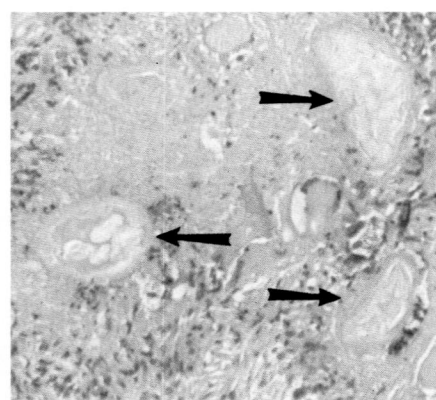

FIGURE 104-9 Lentil pneumonia. An aspiration syndrome occasionally confused with parasitic infection. Arrows indicate aspirated lentil seeds. (H&E, ×500.)

few cases of visceral leishmaniasis have been reported in AIDS patients. Such patients fail to develop a cellular or humoral immune response to the organism. Acute respiratory failure has been described in this setting. In Chagas' disease (American trypanosomiasis), the lungs are often affected by emboli secondary to cardiomyopathy and cardiac mural thrombi. Finally, aspirated vegetable matter may simulate parasitic infection. Notable in this category is the "lentil pneumonia" caused by aspiration of lentil seeds (Fig. 104-9).

BIBLIOGRAPHY

Blumenfeld W, Wagar E, Hadley WK: Use of transbronchial biopsy for diagnosis of opportunistic pulmonary infections in acquired immunodeficiency syndrome (AIDS). Am J Clin Pathol 81:1–5, 1984.
> Emphasizes the role of invasive diagnosis and of Giemsa-stained "touch preparations" in the correct, early, and complete diagnosis of pneumonitis in AIDS.

Broaddus C, Dake MD, Stulbarg MS, Blumenfeld W, Hadley WK, Golden JA, Hopewell PC: Bronchoalveolar lavage and transbronchial biopsy for the diagnosis of pulmonary infections in the acquired immunodeficiency syndrome. Ann Intern Med 102:747–752, 1985.
> The combination of bronchoalveolar lavage and transbronchial biopsy gave a 98 percent yield for all pathogens in 171 patients with AIDS. The incidence of dual pulmonary infections in AIDS is notable.

Current WL, Reese NC: A comparison of endogenous development of three isolates of Cryptosporidium in suckling mice. J Protozool 36:98–108, 1986.
> A demonstration of the autoinfectious life cycle of Cryptosporidium by electron microscopy.

Current WL, Reese NC, Ernst JV, Bailey WS, Heyman MB, Weinstein WM: Human cryptosporidiosis in immunocompetent and immunodeficient persons. N Engl J Med 308:1252–1257, 1983.
> Distinguishes between self-limited infection in normal hosts and the prolonged and severe infection in the immunodeficient patient. Zoonosis occurs through contact with infected calves.

Duarte MIS, Corbett CEP, Boulos M, Amato Neto V: Ultrastructure of the lung in falciparum malaria. Am J Trop Med Hyg 34:31–35, 1985.
> Vascular endothelial injury dominates the pathologic appearance of pulmonary edema due to malaria.

Fischl MA, Richman DD, Grieco MH, Gottlieb MS, Volberding PA, and the AZT Collaborative Working Group: The efficacy of Azidothymidine (AZT) in the treatment of patients with AIDS and AIDS-related complex. N Engl J Med 317:185–191, 1987.
> A summary of the initial results of AZT therapy in AIDS and ARC.

Furuta T, Veda K, Fujiwara K, Yamanouchi K: Cellular and humoral immune responses of mice subclinically infected with Pneumocystis carinii. Infect Immunol 47:544–548, 1985.
> Transfer of immunity to P. carinii in nude mice achieved with T lymphocytes.

Gal AA, Klatt Ec, Koss MN, Strigle SM, Boylen CT: The effectiveness of bronchoscopy in the diagnosis of Pneumocystis carinii and cytomegalovirus pulmonary infections in acquired immunodeficiency syndrome. Arch Pathol Lab Med 111:238–241, 1987.
> In autopsy-proved cases of Pneumocystis carinii pneumonia, the organism was correctly identified antemortem in 22 (88%) of 25 cases, including 95% of adequate transbronchial bronchoscopic biopsy specimens, 95% and 88% of bronchoalveolar lavage cell blocks and smears, respectively, and 79% of brushing. The diagnosis of cytomegalovirus infection was made bronchoscopically in only 55% of autopsy-proved cases.

Garcia LS, Bruckner DA, Brewer TC, Shimizu RY: Techniques for the recovery and identification of Cryptosporidium oocysts from stool specimens. J Clin Microbiol 18:185–190, 1983.
 Discusses concentration and staining of stool specimens for the diagnosis of cryptosporidiosis. Recommends a modified acid-fast stain as most consistently helpful.

Golden JA, Hollander H, Stulbarg MS, Gamsu G: Bronchoalveolar lavage as the exclusive diagnositc modality for Pneumocystis carinii pneumonia. A prospective study amont patients with acquired immunodeficiency syndrome. Chest 90:18–22, 1986.
 Bronchoalveolar lavage detected Pneumocystis carinii pneumonia in 36 of 37 patients and cytomegalovirus in 15 of 38 patients.

Gottlieb MS, Schroff R, Shanker HM: Pneumocystis carinii pneumonia and mucosal candidiasis in previously healthy homosexual men: Evidence of a new acquired cellular immunodeficiency. N Engl J Med 305:1425–1431, 1981.
 The first few reported cases of Pneumocystis in previously healthy homosexual men.

Haverkos HW: Assessment of therapy for Pneumocystis carinii pneumonia. Am J Med 76:501–508, 1984.
 Multicenter retrospective analysis for 282 biopsy-proved cases of P. carinii pneumonia reveals need for prolonged therapy and high relapse rate in AIDS patients. Failure of initial therapy was a poor prognostic sign.

Hofflin JM, Potasman I, Baldwin JC, Oyer PE, Stinson EB, Remington JS: Infectius complications in heart transplant recipients receiving cyclosporine and corticosteroids. Ann Intern Med 106:209–216, 1987.
 In two groups of heart transplant recipients who received different immunosuppressive regimens, patients treated with cyclosporine had a lower rate of infectious complications than did those who underwent conventional immunosuppression and the contribution of infection to mortality was lower.

Hughes WT: Five-year absence of Pneumocystis carinii pneumonitis in a pediatric oncology center. J Infect Dis 150:305–306, 1984.
 Large and successful experience with co-trimoxazole prophylaxis against Pneumocystis in the face of fixed annual attack rate of 3 percent.

Hughes WT, Bartley DL, Smith BM: A natural source of infection due to Pneumocystis carinii. J Infect Dis 147:595, 1983.
 Demonstrates respiratory transmission of infection with P. carinii in rats and suggests need for isolation of immunocompromised patients from others with P. carinii pneumonitis.

Hughes WT, Rivera GK, Schell MJ, Thornton D, Lott L: Successful intermittent chemoprophylaxis for Pneumocystis carinii pneumonitis. N Engl J Med 316:1627–1632, 1987.
 Intermittent prophylaxis with co-trimoxazole in patients with acute lymphocytic leukemia may reduce the incidence both of P. carinii and of superinfection with fungal pathogens when compared with daily administration.

Ibarra-Perez C, Selman-Lama M: Diagnosis and treatment of amebic "empyema." Am J Surg 134:283–287, 1977.
 Experience with 409 cases of pleuropulmonary amebiasis emphasizing the need for surgical drainage of empyema, nutritional support, and amebicidal antibiotics.

Lanken PN, Minda M, Pietra GG, Fishman AP: Alveolar response to experimental Pneumocystis carinii in the rat. Am J Pathol 99:561–578, 1980.
 Pneumocystis binds specifically to type I alveolar epithelial cells causing cell injury and hyperplasia of type II cells.

Leoung GS, Mills, J, Hopewell PC, Hughes W, Wofsy C: Dapsonetrimethoprim for Pneumocystis carinii pneumonia in the acquired immunodeficiency syndrome. Ann Intern Med 105:45–48, 1986.
 Compared with trimethoprim-sulfamethoxazole or pentamidine used to treat P. carinii pneumonia, oral dapsone-trimethoprim is at least as effective, seems to be better tolerated, and may have a lower frequency of serious side effects. However, the incidence of skin rashes is high.

Long EG, Smith JS, Meier JL: Attachment of Pneumocystis carinii to rat pneumocytes. Lab Invest 54:609–615, 1986.
 Electron microscopic observations that may help explain why P. carinii can attach tenaciously to lung epithelium without cell-membrane fusion, production of a glycocalyx, or invasion of host cells.

Luft BJ, Kansas G, Engleman EG, Remington JS: Functional and quantitative alterations in T-lymphocyte subpopulations in acute toxoplasmosis. J Infect Dis 150:761–767, 1984.
Toxoplasma induces an elevation in host "suppressor" T lymphocytes and may modulate host immunity to infection.

Luft BJ, Naot Y, Araujo FG, Stinson EB, Remington JS: Primary and reactivated *Toxoplasma* infection in patients with cardiac transplants. Ann Intern Med 99:27–31, 1983.
Seroconversion of patients transplanted with a heart from seropositive donors was accompanied by life-threatening toxoplasmosis in a few patients. Emphasizes spectrum of serologic responses in immunosuppressed host.

Ma P: Laboratory diagnosis of coccidiosis, in Leive L, Schlessinger D (eds), *Microbiology 1984*. Washington, D.C., American Society for Microbiology, 1984, pp 224–231.
A review of diagnostic methods for Cryptosporidium, Toxoplasma, Isospora, and Pneumocystis species.

Ma P, Villaneuva TG, Kaufman D, Gillooley JF: Respiratory cryptosporidiosis in the acquired immune deficiency syndrome. JAMA 252:1298–1301, 1984.
Patients with pulmonary cryptosporidiosis had concurrent infections with other viruses, protozoa, or mycobacteria. The pathophysiological role of these organisms is unclear. Reviews stains for diagnosis.

McCabe RE, Remington JS: *Toxoplasma gondii*, in Mandell GL, Douglas RG, Bennett JE (eds), *Principles and Practice of Infectious Diseases*, 2d ed. New York, Wiley, 1985, pp 1540–1548.
Excellent overview of clinical syndromes caused by T. gondii.

McGowan K, Guerina V, Wicks J, Danowitz M: Secretory hormones of *Entamoeba histolytica*, in Evered D, Whelan J (eds), *Microbial Toxins and Diarrhoeal Disease*. London, Pitman, 1985, pp 139–150.
E. histolytica contains neurohumoral substances that affect intestinal secretion. Illustrates the complex mechanisms by which the organism exerts its effects.

Meuwissen JHET, Tauber I, Leeuwenberg ADEM, Beckers PJA, Seiben M: Parasitologic and serologic observations of infection with *Pneumocystis* in humans. J Infect Dis 136:43–49, 1977.
Classic study demonstrating that nearly 100 percent of all children in the Netherlands have serologic evidence of infection with Pneumocystis by age 2 years. Significant disease was found by tissue histology only in immunocompromised patients.

Mills J: *Pneumocystis carinii* and *Toxoplasma gondii* infections in patients with AIDS. Rev Infect Dis 8:1001–1011, 1986.
Pneumocystis carinii and Toxoplasma gondii are the commonest protozoans causing infections in patients with acquired immunodeficiency syndrome (AIDS).

Morbidity and Mortality Weekly Report (MMWR): Pentamidine methanesulfonate to be distributed by CDC: 33:225–226, 1984.
Two forms of pentamidine are now available for use in treating Pneumocystis carinii. Pentamidines no longer need to be obtained from the CDC.

Morbidity and Mortality Weekly Report (MMWR): Update: Treatment of cryptosporidiosis in patients with acquired immunodeficiency syndrome (AIDS): 33:117–119, 1984.
Review of the generally disappointing clinical experience with various modalities of therapy.

Pifer LL, Hughes WT, Murphy MJ: Propagation of *Pneumocystis carinii* in vitro. Pediatr Res 11:305–316, 1977.
The first cultivation of P. carinii in vitro allowing description of the life cycle of the organism.

Portnoy D, Whiteside ME, Buckley E, MacLeod CL: Treatment of intestinal cryptosporidiosis with spiramycin. Ann Intern Med 101:202–204, 1984.
Successful small, clinical trial of spiramycin in AIDS patients.

Robbins JB, deVita VT, Dutz W (eds): Symposium on *Pneumocystis carinii* infection. NCI Monograph #43. Washington, National Cancer Institute, 1976.
Summary of a symposium describing the state of the art of the understanding of infections with P. carinii in the 1970s. A valuable reference.

Ruskin J: Toxoplasmosis, in Rubin RH, Young LS (eds), *Clinical Approaches to Infection in the Compromised Host*. New York, Plenum, 1981, pp 311–323.
A useful review of diagnostic approaches to toxoplasmosis in the adult.

Sargeaunt PG, Williams JE: Electrophoretic isozyme patterns of *Entamoeba histolytica* and *Entamoeba coli*. Trans R Soc Trop Med Hyg 72:164–166, 1978.
  A description of laboratory methods capable of differentiating between pathogenic and nonpathogenic amoebas in humans.

Sepulveda B: Amebiasis: Host-pathogen biology. Rev Infect Dis 4:836–842, 1982.
  Characterization of the immunopathology of invasive amebiasis with a discussion of vaccine development.

Sharma SD, Hofflin JM, Remington JS: In vivo recombinant interleukin 2 administration enhances survival against a lethal challenge with *Toxoplasma gondii*. J Immunol 135:4160–4163, 1985.
  Administration of recombinant interleukin 12 (rIL-2) resulted in a statistically significant decrease in mortality in mice infected with T. gondii that killed 100 percent of infected mice. The results are provocative in suggesting that rIL-2 may afford unusual protection against intracellular parasites.

Thompson JE, Forlenza S, Verma R: Amebic liver abscess: A therapeutic approach. Rev Infect Dis 7:171–179, 1985.
  Patients unresponsive to metronidazole therapy within 72 h may need alternative therapy or surgical drainage. All patients who developed amebic empyema were nonresponders in this retrospective review of 48 cases.

Tzipori S: Cryptosporidiosis in animals and humans. Microbiol Rev 47:84–96, 1983.
  Extensive review of microbiology of Cryptosporidium in humans and other animals.

Wanke C, Tuazon CU, Kovacs A, Dina T, Davis DO, Barton N, Katz D, Lunde M, Levy C, Conley FK, Lane HC, Fauci AS, Masur H: *Toxoplasma* encephalitis in patients with acquired immune deficiency syndrome: Diagnosis and response to therapy. Am J Trop Med Hyg 36:509–516, 1987.
  Mouse inoculation was needed to demonstrate toxoplasmosis of the brain even with brain biopsy material. Lifelong therapy with pyrimethamine and/or sulfadiazine recommended in AIDS.

Wharton JM, Coleman DL, Wofsy CB, Luce JM, Blumenfeld W, Hadley WK, Ingram DL, Volberding PA, Hopewell PC: Trimethoprim-sulfamethoxazole or pentamidine for *Pneumocystis carinii* pneumonia in the acquired immunodeficiency syndrome. A prospective randomized trial. Ann Intern Med 105:37–44, 1986.
  In 40 patients with AIDS and the first episode of Pneumocystis carinii pneumonia, trimethoprim-sulfamethoxazole and pentamidine did not have statistically significant differences in efficacy or frequency of adverse reactions.

Wolfson JS, Richter JM, Waldron MA, Weber DJ, McCarthy DM, Hopkins CC: Cryptosporidiosis in immunocompetent patients. N Engl J Med 312:1278–1282, 1985.
  Cryptosporidiosis is a seasonal illness with self-limited symptoms in the immunologically normal host.

Young JA, Stone JW, McGonigle RJ, Adu D, Michael J: Diagnosing *Pneumocystis carinii* pneumonia by cytological examination of bronchoalveolar lavage fluid: Report of 15 cases. J Clin Pathol 39:945–949, 1986.
  Of the 5 stains applied to bronchial lavage fluid for the diagnosis of Pneumocystis carinii pneumonia, the Papanicolaou and the Grocott methenamine silver techinques were most effective.

Chapter 105

The Acquired Immunodeficiency Syndrome

Stuart M. Garay

Almost simultaneously, in late 1980 and early 1981, physicians in New York City, Los Angeles, and San Francisco recognized an unusual pattern of opportunistic diseases occurring in predominantly young homosexual men and notified the Centers for Disease Control (CDC) in Atlanta. The initial two reports of 26 previously healthy young homosexual men diagnosed with Kaposi's sarcoma and 15 diagnosed with Pneumocystis carinii pneumonia were published by the CDC in its Morbidity and Mortality Weekly Report during June and July of 1981. Since that time, there has been an extraordinary escalation in the number of reported cases reaching epidemic proportions with over 62,000 reported cases occurring in 160 countries as of December 1987. By 1991, the number of cases in the United States is expected to reach between 175,000 to 225,000.

The acquired immunodeficiency syndrome (AIDS) represents the severe end of the clinical spectrum of infection with a retrovirus, the human immunodeficiency virus (HIV), originally referred to as the human T-cell lymphocyte virus type III (HTLV-III) or AIDS-related virus (ARV) in the United States and lymphadenopathy-associated virus (LAV) in France. This retrovirus belongs to a group of RNA viruses that infect mammalian cells and is closely related to the simian retrovirus that infects an African nonhuman primate without apparent evidence of disease (Fig. 105-1). This chapter will focus on the pulmonary manifestations associated with AIDS.

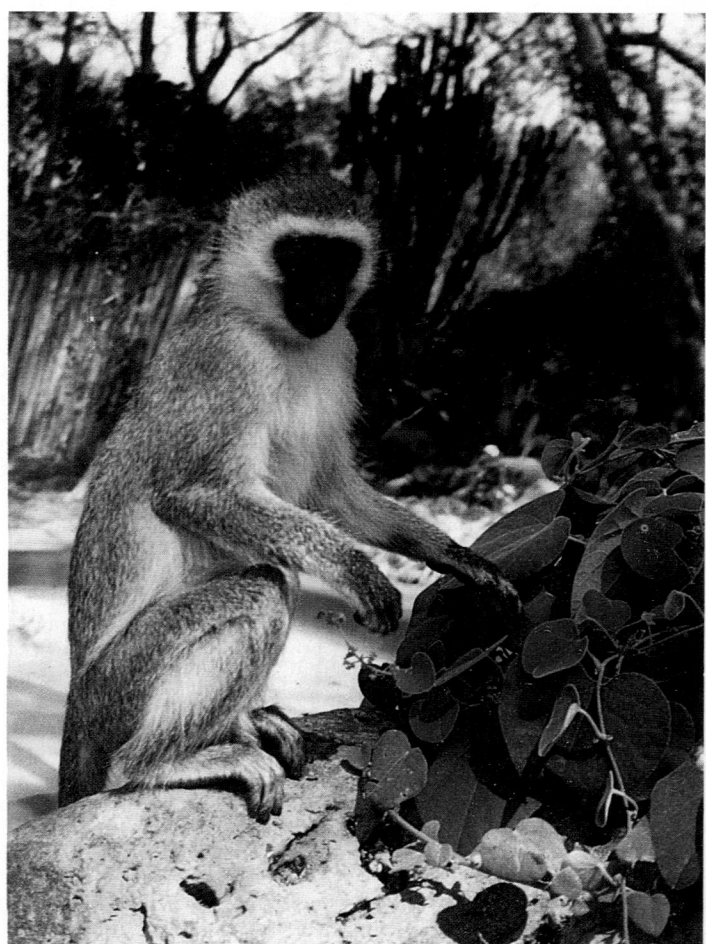

FIGURE 105-1 African Green monkey (Cercopithecus aethiops), a small primate found throughout most of sub-Saharan Africa. This animal is naturally infected with a virus related to the AIDS virus of humans. The human AIDS virus in Africa may have arisen from this group of simian retroviruses. (Courtesy of Dr. P. J. Kanki.)

TABLE 105-1

1987 Revision of Case Definition for AIDS for Surveillance Purposes

For national reporting, a case of AIDS is defined as an illness characterized by one or more of the following "indicator" diseases, depending on the status of laboratory evidence of HIV infection, as shown below.

I. **Without laboratory evidence regarding HIV infection:** If laboratory tests for HIV were not performed or gave inconclusive results and the patient had no other cause of immunodeficiency listed in Section I.A, below, then any disease listed in Section I.B indicates AIDS if it was diagnosed by a definitive method.

    A. Causes of immunodeficiency that disqualify diseases as indicators of AIDS in the absence of laboratory evidence for HIV infection.

        1. High-dose or long-term systemic corticosteroid therapy or other immunosuppressive-cytotoxic therapy ≤3 months before the onset of the indicator disease.

        2. Any of the following diseases diagnosed ≤3 months after diagnosis of the indicator disease: Hodgkin's disease, non-Hodgkin's lymphoma (other than primary brain lymphoma), lymphocytic leukemia, multiple myeloma, any other cancer of lymphoreticular or histiocytic tissue, or angioimmunoblastic lymphadenopathy.

        3. A genetic (congenital) immunodeficiency syndrome or an acquired immunodeficiency syndrome atypical of HIV infection, such as one involving hypogammaglobulinemia.

    B. Indicator diseases diagnosed definitively.

        1. Candidiasis of the esophagus, trachea, bronchi, or lungs.

        2. Cryptococcosis, extrapulmonary.

        3. Cryptosporidiosis with diarrhea persisting >1 month.

        4. Cytomegalovirus disease of an organ other than liver, spleen, or lymph nodes in a patient >1 month of age.

        5. Herpes simplex virus infection causing a mucocutaneous ulcer that persists longer than >1 month; or bronchitis, pneumonitis, or esophagitis for any duration affecting a patient >1 month of age.

        6. Kaposi's sarcoma affecting a patient <60 years of age.

        7. Lymphoma of the brain (primary) affecting a patient >60 years of age.

        8. Lymphoid interstitial pneumonia and/or pulmonary lymphoid hyperplasia (LIP/PLH complex) affecting a child <13 years of age.

        9. *Mycobacterium avium* complex or *M. kansasii* disease, disseminated (at a site other than or in addition to lungs, skin, or cervical or hilar lymph nodes).

        10. *Pneumocystis carinii* pneumonia.

        11. Progressive multifocal leukoencephalopathy.

        12. Toxoplasmosis of the brain affecting a patient >1 month of age.

II. **With laboratory evidence for HIV infection:** Regardless of the presence of other causes of immunodeficiency (I.A), in the presence of laboratory evidence for HIV infection any disease listed above (I.B) or below (II.A or II.B) indicates a diagnosis of AIDS.

    A. Indicator diseases diagnosed definitively.

        1. Bacterial infections, multiple or recurrent (any combination of at least two within a 2-year period), of the following types affecting a child <13 years of age: septicemia, pneumonia, meningitis, bone or joint infection, or abscess of an internal organ or body cavity (excluding otitis media or superficial skin or mucosal abscesses), caused by *Haemophilus, Streptococcus* (including *Pneumococcus*), or other pyogenic bacteria.

        2. Coccidioidomycosis, disseminated (at a site other than or in addition to lungs or cervical or hilar lymph nodes).

        3. HIV encephalopathy (also called HIV dementia, AIDS dementia, or subacute encephalitis due to HIV).

        4. Histoplasmosis, disseminated (at a site other than or in addition to lungs or cervical or hilar lymph nodes).

        5. Isosporiasis with diarrhea persisting >1 month.

        6. Kaposi's sarcoma at any age.

        7. Lymphoma of the brain (primary) at any age.

        8. Other non-Hodgkin's lymphoma of B-cell or unknown immunologic phenotype and the following histologic types:

            a. Small noncleaved lymphoma (either Burkitt or non-Burkitt type).

            b. Immunoblastic sarcoma (equivalent to any of the following, although not necessarily all in combination: immunoblastic lymphoma, large-cell lymphoma, diffuse histiocytic lymphoma, diffuse undifferentiated lymphoma, or high-grade lymphoma).

            NOTE: Lymphomas are not included here if they are of T-cell immunologic phenotype or their histologic type is not described or is described as "lymphocytic," "lymphoblastic," "small cleaved," or "plasmacytoid lymphocytic."

        9. Any mycobacterial disease caused by mycobacteria other than *M. tuberculosis*, disseminated (at a site other than or in addition to lungs, skin, or cervical or hilar lymph nodes).

        10. Disease caused by *M. tuberculosis*, extrapulmonary (involving at least one site outside the lungs, regardless of whether there is concurrent pulmonary involvement).

        11. Salmonella (nontyphoid) septicemia, recurrent.

        12. HIV wasting syndrome (emaciation, "slim disease").

    B. Indicator diseases diagnosed presumptively (without histopathology or culture).

        1. Candidiasis of the esophagus.

        2. Cytomegalovirus retinitis with loss of vision.

        3. Kaposi's sarcoma.

TABLE 105-1 *(continued)*

II. With laboratory evidence for HIV infection *(continued)*

    4. Lymphoid interstitial pneumonia and/or pulmonary lymphoid hyperplasia (LIP/PLH complex) affecting a child <13 years of age.

    5. Mycobacterial disease (acid-fast bacilli with species not identified by culture), disseminated (involving at least one site other than or in addition to lungs, skin, or cervical or hilar lymph nodes).

    6. *Pneumocystis carinii* pneumonia.

    7. Toxoplasmosis of the brain affecting a patient >1 month of age.

III. With laboratory evidence against HIV infection: With laboratory test results negative for HIV infection a diagnosis of AIDS for surveillance purposes is ruled out unless:

    A. All the other causes of immunodeficiency listed above, in Sec. I.A, are excluded **and**

    B. The patient has had either:

        1. *P. carinii* pneumonia diagnosed by a definitive method **or**

        2.   **a.** Any of the other diseases indicative of AIDS listed above in Sec. I.B diagnosed by a definitive method **and**

            b. A T-helper/inducer (CD4) lymphocyte count <400 per cubic millimeter.

SOURCE: Centers for Disease Control. MMWR (suppl. 1S)36:3S–15S, 1987.

DEFINITION

The acquired immunodeficiency syndrome was defined by the Centers for Disease Control for the purpose of national reporting in 1981 before its cause was known. The definition encompassed only certain secondary conditions that reflected the presence of severe cellular immune dysfunction and occurred in a person without known cause for reduced resistance. This definition has been revised in light of the discovery that AIDS is caused by the human immunodeficiency virus. In the absence of the opportunistic diseases required by the original surveillance definition, any of the following diseases are also considered indicative of the syndrome if the patient has positive serology for HIV: (1) disseminated histoplasmosis, diagnosed by culture, histology, or antigen detections; (2) isosporiasis, causing chronic diarrhea (over 1 month), diagnosed by microscopy or by presence of characteristic white plaques grossly on the bronchial mucosa (not by cultures alone); (4) non-Hodgkin's lymphoma of high-grade pathologic type (diffuse, undifferentiated) and of B-cell or unknown immunologic phenotype, diagnosed by biopsy; (5) histologically confirmed Kaposi's sarcoma in patients who are 60 years old or older when diagnosed; and (6) a histologically confirmed diagnosis of chronic lymphoid interstitial pneumonitis in a child (under 13 years of age). The most recent revision (August 1987) by the Centers for Disease Control of the case definition expands the definition to include clinical syndromes attributable to HIV infection (e.g., the chronic wasting syndrome and HIV dementia complex) in the absence of secondary pathogens (Table 105-1). In addition, the new case definition allows for the presumptive diagnosis of indicator diseases (e.g., the diagnosis of Kaposi's sarcoma based on gross appearance of the skin or the diagnosis of *P. carinii* pneumonia based on clinical and radiographic findings) without confirmatory evidence. The goal of these changes is to enable public health departments to track HIV-related morbidity by increasing the number of reported cases and including previously unreported groups. It is hoped that this will improve our understanding of the natural history of this disease. The need on an individual patient basis for specific diagnoses and exact therapy is still warranted and is the justification for much of the remainder of this chapter. In May 1986, the Centers for Disease Control issued a comprehensive classification system for categorizing patients infected with HIV according to certain clinical characteristics. The classification incorporates the previous surveillance definition as well as the above modifications and includes the range of identified associated conditions as well as asymptomatic infection (Table 105-2). Presently recognized pulmonary complications due to HIV infection are listed in Table 105-3.

EPIDEMIOLOGY

As of December 1987, over 48,000 patients have been diagnosed with AIDS in the United States; more than 27,000 patients have died. Race, age, and sex distribution in adult AIDS patients have remained relatively constant over time. Ninety-three percent of all patients have been men. Among adult male AIDS patients, 61 percent have been white, 24 percent black, 14 percent Hispanic, and 1 percent other or unknown. Almost 90 percent have ranged in age from 20 to 49 years old (mean = 36.8 years). *P. carinii* pneumonia (PCP) has been the most frequent opportunistic infection. Among male AIDS patients, 64 percent have been diagnosed with PCP, 21 percent had other opportunistic diseases without PCP, and 15 percent had Kaposi's sarcoma alone. Recently, the incidence of Kaposi's sarcoma has decreased. Eighty-eight percent of women with AIDS have been 20 to 49 years of age, 27 percent white, 52

TABLE 105-2
CDC Classification of HIV Infection

Group I: Acute infection
Mononucleosislike syndrome associated with seroconversion.

Group II: Asymptomatic infection
Positive HIV antibody or viral culture. May be subclassified on basis of laboratory evaluation (CBC, platelet count, T-cell subset studies).

Group III: Persistent generalized lymphadenopathy
Palpable lymphadenopathy (>1 cm) at two or more extrainguinal sites for more than 3 months in the absence of a concurrent illness or infection to explain the findings. May be subclassified on the basis of laboratory evaluation (see above).

Group IV: Other HIV disease
Subgroup A: Constitutional disease
One or more of the following: fever or diarrhea persisting more than 1 month or involuntary weight loss greater than 10% of baseline; and absence of a concurrent illness or infection to explain the findings.

Subgroup B: Neurologic disease
One or more of the following: dementia, myelopathy, or peripheral neuropathy; and absence of a concurrent illness or condition.

Subgroup C: Secondary infectious diseases
Infectious disease associated with HIV infection and/or at least moderately indicative of a defect in cell-mediated immunity.

Category C-1
Symptomatic or invasive disease due to one of 12 specified diseases listed in the surveillance definition of AIDS: *P. carinii* pneumonia, chronic cryptosporidiosis, toxoplasmosis, extraintestinal strongyloidiasis, isosporiasis, candidiasis (esophageal, bronchial, or pulmonary), histoplasmosis, cryptococcosis, mycobacterial infection (*M. avium* complex or *M. kansasii*), cytomegalovirus infection, chronic mucocutaneous or disseminated herpes simplex virus infection, and progressive multifocal leukoencephalopathy.

Category C-2
Symptomatic or invasive disease due to one of six other specified diseases: oral hairy leukoplakia, multidermatomal herpes zoster, recurrent *Salmonella* bacteremia, nocardiosis, tuberculosis, and oral candidiasis (thrush).

Subgroup D: Secondary cancers
Diagnosis of one or more cancers known to be associated with HIV infection as listed in the surveillance definition of AIDS and at least moderately indicative of a defect in cell-mediated immunity: Kaposi's sarcoma, non-Hodgkin's lymphoma (small, noncleaved lymphoma or immunoblastic sarcoma), or primary lymphoma of the brain.

Subgroup E: Other conditions of HIV infection
Clinical findings or diseases, not classified above, that may be attributable to HIV infection and are indicative of a defect in cell-mediated immunity; symptoms attributable to either HIV infection or a coexisting disease not classified elsewhere; or clinical illnesses that may be complicated or altered by HIV infection. These include chronic lymphoid interstitial pneumonitis and constitutional symptoms, secondary infectious diseases, and neoplasms not listed above.

SOURCE: Centers for Disease Control. MMWR 35:334–339, 1986.

TABLE 105-3
Pulmonary Complications of HIV Infection

A. Opportunistic infections diagnostic of AIDS
1. *P. carinii* pneumonia
2. Pulmonary toxoplasmosis
3. Pulmonary strongyloidosis
4. Bronchopulmonary candidiasis
5. Pulmonary cryptococcosis
6. Disseminated histoplasmosis
7. Disseminated *M. avium* complex
8. Cytomegalovirus pneumonia
9. Herpes simplex pneumonia

B. HIV-related pulmonary infections
1. Tuberculosis
2. Nocardiosis

C. Presumed HIV-related pulmonary disorders
1. Pyogenic bacterial pneumonia
2. Lymphoid interstitial pneumonitis

D. AIDS-related pulmonary neoplasia
1. Kaposi's sarcoma
2. Non-Hodgkin's lymphoma

percent black, 20 percent Hispanic, and 1 percent other or unknown. Sixty-seven percent of women had PCP, 31 percent had other opportunistic diseases with PCP, and 2 percent had Kaposi's sarcoma alone. The distribution among risk groups has not changed significantly throughout this epidemic: homosexual or bisexual men (66 percent); homosexual or bisexual men with a history of using intravenous drugs (8 percent); heterosexual intravenous drug abusers (16 percent); hemophiliac patients (1 percent); heterosexual sex partners of persons with AIDS or at risk for AIDS (4 percent); and recipients of transfused blood or blood components (2 percent). Approximately 3 percent of patients have had no indentifiable risk factors for AIDS.

The epidemiology of AIDS is somewhat different in New York City, which has contributed almost 30 percent of the nationally reported cases. The proportion of white subjects is 47 percent, that of black subjects 30 percent, and that of Hispanic subjects 23.0 percent. The percentage of homosexual men is 58 percent, that of intravenous drug users 28.5 percent, and that of subjects classified as both homosexual men and intravenous drug users 5.0 percent. Female cases (84% black or Hispanic) represent 11% of the cumulative New York City cases and 42% of all adult female cases reported nationally. Risk factors for women include intravenous drug use in 61% and sexual intercourse with men of high risk. *Pneumocystis carinii* pneumonia has been the major opportunistic manifestation, though occurring in a lower percentage of patients (44 percent).

In addition, reported tuberculosis cases in New York City have increased substantially, in large part related to coexisting HIV and *Mycobacterium tuberculosis* infection. From 1984 to 1986, reported *M. tuberculosis* cases increased by 30 percent, or 593 cases (from 1630 to 2223

cases), a numerical increase greater than that for any state or city in the nation. By comparison, during that same period, reported cases for the entire nation increased 2 percent, or 513 (from 22,255 to 22,768). Thus the increase in New York City cases exceeded the numerical increase in the entire nation. During these same years 27 percent of the nation's cumulative reported cases were New York City residents. This association of M. tuberculosis with AIDS has also been found in communities with large AIDS populations such as Dade County, Florida, Newark, and San Francisco.

Soon after AIDS was reported in the United States, several countries in Central Africa as well as Haiti also began recognizing cases. HIV serology has demonstrated the presence of this virus in frozen blood and tissue from Africa as early as the 1960s. In Central Africa, the distribution of AIDS cases is equal among males and females, reflecting the predominantly heterosexual mode of transmission in that region.

In the United States, the rate of HIV seropositivity among healthy blood donors ranges between 0.02 and 0.04 percent. A seroprevalence of 1.5/100 in civilian recruits for military service who were systematically subjected to mandatory HIV testing has been reported. In contrast, the prevalence of HIV infection in members of the various risk groups is significantly higher. Cohort studies of homosexual men in San Francisco have identified an HIV seroprevalence of 65 percent. Similarly, the rate of positive HIV antibodies among intravenous drug users approximates 50 percent. Hemophiliacs receiving factor VIII concentrates have an HIV seroprevalence approaching 70 percent. A recent cohort study of homosexual men from San Francisco reported at the Third International Conference on AIDS in June 1987 has enhanced our understanding of the natural history of HIV infection. The risk of developing AIDS following HIV infection was 15 percent at 60 months, 24 percent after 72 months, and 36 percent at 88 months of followup.

HUMAN IMMUNODEFICIENCY VIRUS

The initial epidemiology of AIDS strongly suggested that the etiologic agent was a virus that could be transmitted by sexual contact, blood and blood products, sharing of contaminated needles, and placental transmission of maternal blood. In 1984, investigators in the United States and France proposed a retrovirus, now known as the human immunodeficiency virus, as the inciting agent for this syndrome.

During the 3 years since the discovery of HIV, much has been learned concerning its method of infection and replication (Figs. 105-2 and 105-3). The envelope of HIV consists of the externalized gp120 and the transmembrane gp41 molecules. Initially, the HIV envelope binds specifically to the CD4 molecule that is expressed on the surface of CD4+ T lymphocytes, monocytes, and some cells of the central nervous system but not CD8+ T lymphocytes. The interaction of the CD4 glycoprotein receptor with the HIV envelope contributes to the cytopathic effects during infection, including cell fusion and cell death. After binding, the virus enters the cell, where it loses its envelope coat and releases its single strand of RNA into the cytoplasm. Utilizing its own special DNA polymerase, reverse transcriptase, the virus "reverse transcribes" the RNA into double-stranded DNA. The DNA copy of the virus is circularized soon after its formation and can remain unintegrated or become integrated into the host cell genome. The integrated viral genome, known as a provirus, may remain latent until the host cell is stimulated, possibly by another infection (such as cytomegalovirus). The proviral DNA is then transcribed into mRNA, which directs with synthesis of viral proteins. The newly formed viral proteins are cleaved and glycosylated and are assembled with the genomic RNA at the cell membrane to form new HIV particles, which then bud from the cell (Fig. 105-2). The unusual regulatory genes, tat and trs/art, are found in retroviruses such as HIV; they code for small proteins which enhance the transcription of proviral DNA and the synthesis of viral proteins.

The features of retroviruses—T-helper lymphocyte tropism, ability to induce immunodeficiency syndromes in animals, and cytopathic effect on lymphocytes infected in vitro—are the same characteristics necessary to produce the clinical and laboratory abnormalities of AIDS. The evidence linking human immunodeficiency virus to AIDS is the following: this virus has been isolated from blood and lymph nodes of patients with AIDS but not from members of risk-free groups; antibody to the virus can be found in 90 percent of patients with AIDS but not in members of risk-free groups; antibodies to the virus appeared in many areas coincident with the onset of AIDS in those areas. Simian AIDS is induced by the simian T-lymphotropic virus (STLV-III), a retrovirus related to HIV, lending further support for the disease-inducing potential of this class of virus. The spectrum of disease associated with HIV infection ranges from subclinical disease to the full-blown syndrome involving the central nervous system, gastrointestinal tract, bone marrow skin, and lungs.

With the discovery of the AIDS retrovirus as the etiologic agent, much interest has focused on the development of drugs that might interrupt the viral life cycle and thus inhibit replication. If viral replication can be inhibited, perhaps immune function will subsequently improve. Because of its unique role in retroviral replication and its irrelevance to the host cell, reverse transcriptase has been the leading target for antiviral therapy (Fig. 105-3). Several drugs have been shown to reduce the activity of reverse transcriptase in vitro, including suramin (an antiparasitic agent), antimoniotungstate (also called HPA-23), phosphonoformate, and a new class of nucleo-

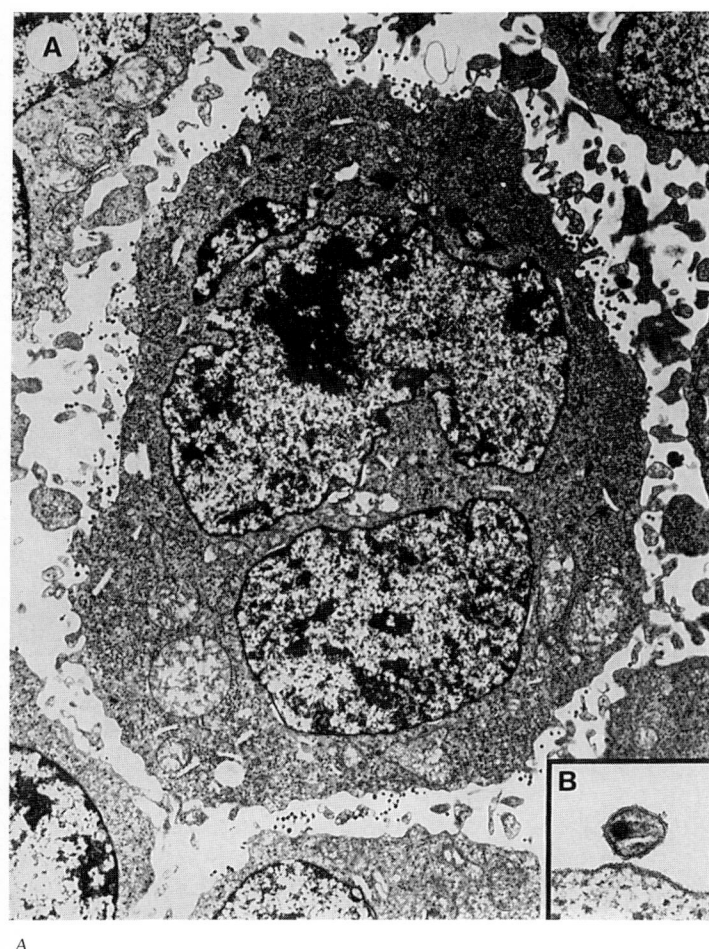

A

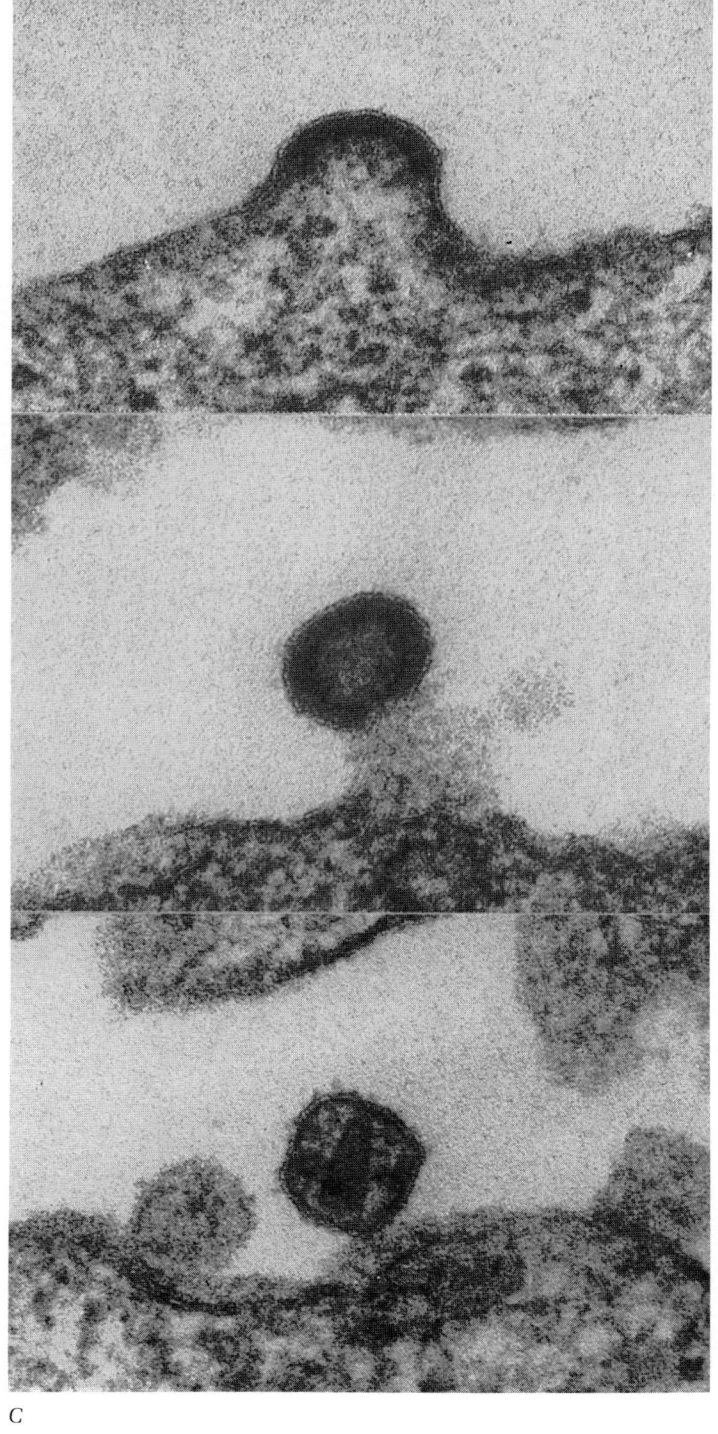

FIGURE 105-2 Electron microscopy of the AIDS virus. *A.* A multinucleated leukocyte producing particles of the AIDS retrovirus. Large numbers of virus particles can be seen along the margin of the cell. *B.* A mature virus particle with the characteristic cylindrical core. *C. Top:* The earliest visible stage of virus replication. Viral proteins accumulate beneath the cell membrane in a process called budding. *Middle:* A later stage of budding. The crescent-shaped early bud has constricted, forming a membrane-encapsulated sphere with a dense center called the *viral nucleoid. Bottom:* Continuation of the constricting process causes the virus to pinch off and become a free, extracellular infectious virus. At this stage, the dark circular nucleoid condenses into a bar, a morphologic feature that is useful in discriminating between the AIDS retrovirus and related viruses. *(Courtesy of Dr. M. A. Gonda.)*

C

side analogues called dideoxynucleotides, which act by being chain terminators of DNA. These drugs are currently undergoing clinical trials. Azidothymidine (AZT), a nucleoside analogue, has already proved it has some clinical efficacy, although it has shown to be considerably toxic to the bone marrow. A recent randomized, multicenter, placebo-controlled trial was instituted in a total of 280 patients with either a successfully treated first episode of *P. carinii* pneumonia or a history of AIDS-related complex (ARC). After a median of 5 months, there were a total of 16 deaths (11 AIDS, 5 ARC) in the placebo group and one (AIDS) in the AZT-treated group. There were measured

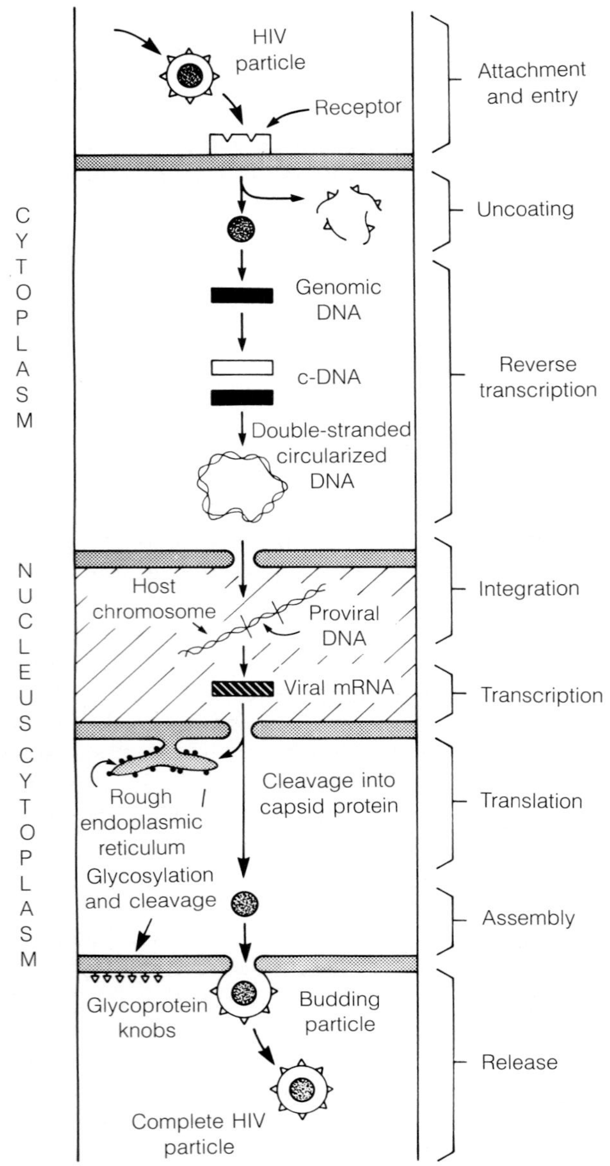

HIV particle
Receptor
Attachment and entry
C Y T O P L A S M
Uncoating
Genomic DNA
c-DNA
Double-stranded circularized DNA
Reverse transcription
N U C L E U S
Host chromosome
Proviral DNA
Integration
Viral mRNA
Transcription
C Y T O P L A S M
Rough endoplasmic reticulum
Cleavage into capsid protein
Translation
Glycosylation and cleavage
Assembly
Glycoprotein knobs
Budding particle
Release
Complete HIV particle

FIGURE 105-3 The proposed steps for HIV infection of T4 lymphocytes as well as mechanisms of action for antiviral therapy.

improvements in CD4+ T-cell counts and circulating p24 antigen levels in the drug recipients. Furthermore, drug recipients exhibited significantly fewer opportunistic infections as compared to the placebo group, and a four- to sixfold reduction in mortality. This agent is given orally at 4-h intervals because of a short serum half-life. It penetrates the blood-brain barrier well, achieving 50 percent of the serum levels in the cerebrospinal fluid. Macrocytic anemia is the most commonly observed side effect, necessitating transfusion in 25 percent of those receiving AZT. Whether this drug will have long-term benefit for patients is unknown.

Other steps in HIV replication may also prove to be successful targets for antiviral agents. Ribavarin, which acts as a guanosine analogue, interferes with the 5′-capping of viral mRNA; its clinical efficacy remains to be proven. Human interferon α, which inhibits the production of viral mRNA, the synthesis of viral proteins, as well as the assembly and release of new particles, slows HIV replication in vitro. Drugs that interfere with the binding and penetration of HIV onto the CD4 lymphocytes are the latest to be promulgated. "Peptide-T" is an octapeptide derived from a small segment of the HIV envelope protein (gp120). It potentially blocks the binding of the intact virus to the CD4 antigen on the T-helper cell membrane. Early studies have yielded conflicting results, but further testing is planned. AL721 may inhibit HIV-CD4 antigen binding. The lipid components (glycerides, phosphatidylcholine, and phosphatidyl ethanokimine are in a 7:2:1 ratio) extract cholestrol from cellular membranes and thus alter the HIV binding sites. Various clinical studies have been initiated, but results are not available. Finally, when CD4 protein, produced by recombinant techniques, is juxtapositioned to HIV, the protein attracts the virus and prevents it from entering nearby cells. This novel therapy is first being tested in animals, and no human data concerning efficacy or toxicity are available.

Antiviral therapy must theoretically be employed indefinitely because it would be inactive against latent HIV that is nonreplicative. The combining of antiviral agents with immune stimulants would be desirable since stimulation of HIV-infected CD4 lymphocytes promotes viral replication. Future antiviral research will explore the combination of two or more antivirals with different sites of action. Development of an effective vaccine is difficult, because of the antigenic heterogeneity of HIV and the capacity for cell-to-cell spread of HIV through syncytial cell formation. Suggested target antigens are HIV envelope glycoprotein (gp120) and the transmembrane glycoprotein (gp41), both of which have neutralizing epitopes. Initial attempts at vaccine development are currently underway.

IMMUNOLOGIC DEFECT

The primary deficit in AIDS appears to be an almost total destruction of the CD4+ T-helper-cell population. The resulting cellular immune defect includes: cutaneous anergy, lymphopenia, decreased helper-to-suppressor ratio (smaller than 1.5:1), and poor in vitro proliferative responses of peripheral blood lymphocytes. Immunologic defects are not restricted to the cellular immune system but profoundly involve the humoral immune system as well. The humoral immune abnormalities include hypergammaglobulinemia with associated autoimmune phenomena (thrombocytopenia, hemolytic anemia, granulocytopenia, a lupuslike syndrome), intact anamnestic antibody responses, and impaired primary antibody responses. Patients with opportunistic infections have an

absolute decrease in CD4+ T cells as well as reduced helper-to-suppressor cell ratios compared to patients with Kaposi's sarcoma.

Analysis of alveolar lavage cells and immunoglobulins in AIDS patients infected with *Pneumocystis* has revealed an increased cellular content with a predominance of lymphocytes as well as significantly more neutrophils. In addition, the lymphocytes in lavage fluid demonstrate a decreased CD4+/CD8+ ratio due to an increase in total CD8+ T cells. There is often a normal total CD4+ cell count, despite a significant decrease in numbers of CD4+ cells in the peripheral blood. These data suggest a sequestration or local proliferation of lymphocytes occurring in alveolar structures with preferential expansion of CD8+ T lymphocytes. Increased IgG-releasing cells and higher IgG levels than controls are also found in lavage fluid of AIDS patients because of immunoglobin transudation from intra-alveolar spaces into the lung and increased local production by airway plasma cells.

Many of the infections seen in patients with AIDS represent endogenous reactivation of previously dormant organisms, which are unmasked by the defect in cellular immunity. For example, there is evidence that *Pneumocystis* is acquired as an asymptomatic infection by large numbers of healthy people, often at a young age; a clinical pneumonia may develop with the onset of immunosuppression. Another example relates to the finding that a high percentage of Haitians as well as intravenous drug abusers who develop AIDS present with *M. tuberculosis* as the initial manifestation of their immune defect: the incidence of tuberculous infection is high among non-AIDS Haitians as well as intravenous drug abusers. The histologic analogue of the reduction in cellular immunity is the absence of granuloma formation in tissues involved with infection by organisms that usually elicit a granulomatous response in persons with normal immunity. Such is the case in AIDS-related mycobacterial infections. Deficient cellular immunity may also be important for the development of Kaposi's sarcoma, as has been suggested by the transplant- and chemotherapy-associated cases in non-AIDS patients. The polyclonal B-cell activation in AIDS patients results in a nonspecific overproduction of immunoglobulins that may account for the high frequency of hypersensitivity reactions to drugs, particularly trimethoprim-sulfamethoxazole. The decreased inability to mount a specific response to newly encountered antigens may explain the higher incidence of pneumococcal and salmonella septicemia in AIDS patients.

DIAGNOSTIC APPROACH TO PULMONARY DISEASE

The non-AIDS immunocompromised patient with an abnormal chest radiograph presents a diagnostic dilemma.

While extension of an underlying malignancy and chemotherapy-related lung disease are diagnostic considerations, pulmonary infection is responsible for the majority of complications in such patients. An aggressive diagnostic approach utilizing fiberoptic bronchoscopy or open lung biopsy usually proves necessary. In the pre-AIDS era, the diagnostic yield from fiberoptic bronchoscopy (utilizing transbronchial biopsy, bronchial washings, and brush biopsy) was approximately 50 percent compared to 70 percent from open lung biopsy. Even at autopsy, an exact etiologic diagnosis could not be made in 15 to 20 percent of cases with the final diagnosis being *nonspecific pneumonitis*.

In light of this background, the National Heart, Lung, and Blood Institute (NHLBI) convened a workshop in October 1983 to assess methods for diagnosis and treatment of pulmonary complications in AIDS patients. The six participating medical centers from New York, Los Angeles, and San Francisco had seen a total of 1067 patients with the diagnosis of AIDS (representing approximately half of the total AIDS patients in the United States at that time) between November 1980 and July 1983. From this group, 441 patients (41 percent) were found to have pulmonary disorders. *P. carinii* pneumonia, either alone or coexisting with one or more infections, was the most common complication. This was seen in over three quarters of patients. Approximately one quarter of all patients had pulmonary opportunistic infections other than *P. carinii* pneumonia. A small percentage (8 percent) of patients had pulmonary involvement with Kaposi's sarcoma. Fiberoptic bronchoscopy proved to be an effective means for diagnosing infections. Ninety-one percent of pulmonary opportunistic infections were diagnosed by fiberoptic bronchoscopy: *P. carinii* (95 percent); *Mycobacterium avium-intracellulare* (78 percent); cytomegalovirus (85 percent); *Legionella* (95 percent); and fungal pneumonias (82 percent). The yield from various aspects of the bronchoscopic procedure was assessed with respect to the diagnosis of *P. carinii* pneumonia: transbronchial biopsy had the highest yield (93 percent), whereas brush biopsy had the lowest (39 percent). Bronchoalveolar lavage had a yield of 79 percent. Subsequent studies have shown alveolar lavage to be an extremely sensitive bronchoscopic technique for the diagnosis of *P. carinii* pneumonia with sensitivity approaching that of transbronchial biopsy. The lavage technique instills significantly greater quantities of fluid than the usual bronchial washings. The bronchoscope is wedged in a middle or lower lobe subsegmental bronchus, and 100 to 150 ml of sterile, nonbacteriostatic, room temperature saline is instilled in 20- to 40-ml aliquots. Suctioning after each aliquot recovers 50 to 75 percent of the total instillate. Most patients tolerate the procedure with only transient worsening of gas exchange and chest radiograph. The yield for *P. carinii* from combined bronchoscopic techniques approaches 95 percent; sepa-

rately, lavage and transbronchial biopsy sensitivities range between 85 and 95 percent.

Because the organism load in AIDS patients appears to be overwhelming, less "invasive" diagnostic approaches have been sought: induction of sputum as well as utilization of a fiberoptic suction catheter have proved effective. Initial reports of induced sputum suggest a diagnostic sensitivity ranging from 50 to 78 percent for *Pneumocystis*. Both Giemsa (which stains trophozoites) and silver methenamine (which stains cysts) stains have been used on sputum specimens. Cresyl violet has been a recently suggested alternative, because it readily stains both cysts and trophozoites. The recent development of a monoclonal antibody for *P. carinii* may further improve the yield from induced sputum as well as alveolar lavage. The issue of specificity and sensitivity as well as the ability of these techniques to identify multiple infectious agents (up to 25 percent of patients may have concurrent pulmonary infections) needs further evaluation. However, utilization of these noninvasive techniques may reduce the need for bronchoscopy, a need that has become increasingly difficult to fulfill in hospitals with large numbers of AIDS patients.

An updated approach to diagnosis suggested by participants of the second NHLBI workshop on the pulmonary complications of AIDS (convened in May 1986) is found in Fig. 105-4. In addition, an approach to the differential diagnosis of the radiographic manifestations is provided in Table 105-4.

The problem of a nondiagnostic bronchoscopy in an AIDS patient and/or one at risk for AIDS occurs in approximately 10 to 20 percent of proven AIDS cases. The role of open lung biopsy is limited and should be considered only in the following settings: patients with progressive pulmonary disease in whom both alveolar lavage and transbronchial biopsy are unrevealing; patients with co-

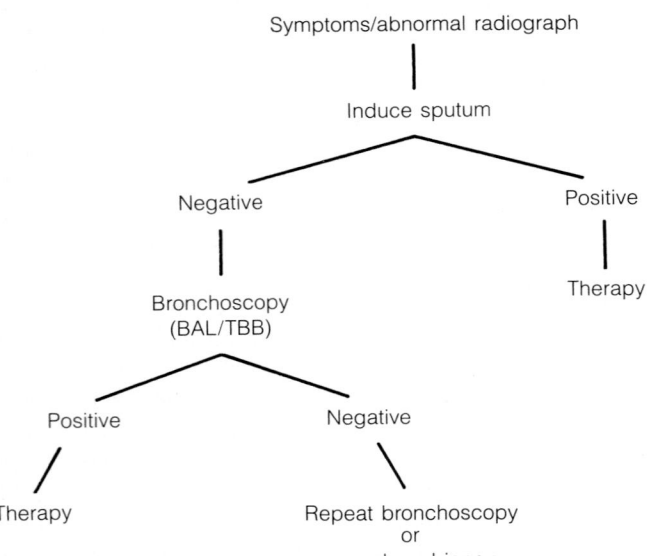

FIGURE 105-4 Suggested approach by the second NHLBI workshop for diagnosis of pulmonary complications in AIDS patients. See text for role of sputum induction and open lung biopsy. BAL = bronchoalveolar lavage; TBB = transbronchial biopsy.

TABLE 105-4
Radiographic Signs: Differential Diagnosis

A. Diffuse infiltrates
    Common: PCP
               PCP + other infections (CMV, MAI, MTB, *Candida, Toxoplasma*, fungi)
               PCP + KS
               Idiopathic interstitial fibrosis
               TB
               KS
    Uncommon: Lymphocytic interstitial pneumonitis
B. Focal infiltrates
    Common: Pyogenic bacterial pneumonia
               PCP
               MTB
    Uncommon: Non-Hodgkin's lymphoma
                    KS
         Rare: *Legionella*
               Nocardia
C. Cavitation
    Common: Septic emboli (addicts)
               PCP
    Uncommon: Fungi
         Rare: MTB/MAI
               Nocardia
D. Nodules
    Common: KS
               Fungi
               Septic emboli
    Uncommon: Lymphoma
        Rare: PCP
E. Adenopathy
    Common: MTB/MAI
               Fungi
               KS
               Lymphoma
        Rare: PCP
F. Miliary disease
    Common: Histoplasmosis
               Cryptococcosis
               MTB
    Uncommon: Foreign body granulomas (addicts)
         Rare: PCP
G. Pleural disease
    Common: KS
               Pyogenic bacterial pneumonia
    Uncommon: Lymphoma
                    Cryptococcus
                    MTB
        Rare: PCP

NOTE: PCP = *Pneumocystis carinii pneumonia*; CMV = cytomegalovirus; MAI = *Mycobacterium avium-intracellulare*; KS = Kaposi's sarcoma; MTB = *Mycobacterium tuberculosis*.

agulopathies or those requiring mechanical ventilation in whom alveolar lavage is nondiagnostic. When open lung biopsies have been performed, *P. carinii* pneumonia (30 percent), "nonspecific interstitial pneumonitis" (30 percent), and pulmonary Kaposi's sarcoma (25 percent) have been the most frequent findings. Less commonly, cytomegalovirus and mycobacterial infections have been found. Rarely, lymphocytic interstitial pneumonitis (LIP) has been found. At present, clinicians are divided in their belief as to whether open lung biopsies should be performed in this patient population in light of the limited treatable yield and the overall poor prognosis.

The first NHLBI workshop also addressed the diagnostic approach to patients at risk for AIDS, who present with nonspecific symptoms of fever, malaise, and dyspnea and a normal chest radiograph: noninvasive procedures should be initially attempted. Measurement of the alveolar-arterial O_2 gradient, single-breath diffusing capacity for carbon monoxide, and gallium lung scanning may distinguish which patients require further diagnostic procedures such as induction of sputum or fiberoptic bronchoscopy. In the NHLBI series, most patients with proven *Pneumocystis* had an increased alveolar-arterial O_2 gradient (mean = 47 mmHg), even those with a normal chest radiograph. Some investigators have found that exercise may increase the $P(A-a)_{O_2}$ gradient in patients with *Pneumocystis* but usually not in other AIDS-associated opportunistic infections. Although an abnormal diffusing capacity is highly sensitive for the diagnosis of *Pneumocystis*, it is not specific. Thus, intravenous drug abusers, a high-risk group for the development of AIDS, have low diffusing capacity values in the absence of AIDS. Data from the first NHLBI workshop also revealed that gallium lung scanning had a sensitivity of 98 percent for *Pneumocystis*; however, the specificity was only 47 percent. Several subsequent studies have demonstrated the utility of gallium lung scanning, especially when the chest radiograph is normal. Diffuse uptake suggests *Pneumocystis*; focal uptake suggests mycobacterial or bacterial infection; lack of gallium uptake in the presence of a diffusely abnormal chest radiograph is most suggestive of pulmonary Kaposi's sarcoma; and uptake limited to hilar or mediastinal nodes usually suggests mycobacterial or fungal disease or lymphoma. A graded scoring system improves the specificity for *Pneumocystis* to 90 percent. Images are graded for intensity of pulmonary uptake: grade 1, normal (intensity less than or equal to adjacent soft tissues); grade 2, minimally abnormal (intensity greater than adjacent soft tissue but less than hepatic uptake); grade 3, abnormal (intensity equivalent to hepatic uptake); and grade 4, significantly abnormal (intensity greater than hepatic uptake). Patients with grade 1 or 2 uptake do not usually have *Pneumocystis* pneumonia, while grades 3 to 4 uptake are highly suggestive for the pneumonia.

OPPORTUNISTIC INFECTIONS

Pneumocystis carinii Pneumonia

CLINICAL PRESENTATION

Pneumonia due to *P. carinii* is the most common life-threatening infection in patients with AIDS. It occurs at least once in 60 percent of patients, and approximately one quarter of these initial episodes are fatal. Statistics compiled by the New York City Department of Health reveal that the median survival for AIDS patients presenting with *Pneumocystis* was 318 days (mean = 317 days) in comparison with a median survival of 750 days (mean = 568 days) for those presenting with only extrapulmonary Kaposi's sarcoma. The diagnosis of *Pneumocystis* pneumonia requires a high index of suspicion, since it often presents in a subacute fashion in previously healthy subjects. Fever, cough, and dyspnea are nonspecific and may occur greater than 2 weeks in duration prior to presentation. In a comparative study of AIDS and non-AIDS immunosuppressed patients, the median duration of symptoms was 28 days versus 5 days. Occasional findings include chills, chest tightness, and scanty sputum. The physical findings on admission are usually unremarkable except for tachypnea and a mean temperature elevation to 39°C. Various nonpulmonary findings typical of AIDS patients may be present including diffuse lymphadenopathy, oral candidiasis, perianal ulcers, and cutaneous Kaposi's sarcoma lesions. Laboratory studies are usually unrevealing except for lymphopenia and abnormalities in gas exchange. Analysis of the first 200 patients with *P. carinii* pneumonia who presented to New York University Medical Center revealed the mean admission arterial P_{O_2} was 73 ± 6 mmHg with a mean $P(A-a)_{O_2}$ gradient of 44 ± 8 mmHg. Although hypoxemia is usually present, it is often milder than in non-AIDS patients. An unexpected laboratory finding in our experience in patients with *Pneumocystis* has been an increase in admission serum lactic dehydrogenase (mean serum LDH = 465 ± 67 IU/L), probably secondary to alveolar damage. The chest radiograph typically shows diffuse bilateral interstitial infiltrates, although infiltrates may be confined to upper and lower lobes and may be unilateral at the time of presentation (Figs. 105-5 to 105-7). Apical infiltrates may simulate tuberculosis. Rarely, cavitation has been reported, although fungal, tuberculous, and *Legionella* infection are more likely etiologies. Between 5 and 10 percent of patients present with normal chest radiographs. While enlarged hilar or mediastinal lymph nodes have been described in many patients, these findings are probably due to associated tuberculous or fungal infections or Kaposi's sarcoma. Spontaneous pneumothoraxes and pleural effusions have also rarely been described; the latter are more likely due to associated infections or Kaposi's

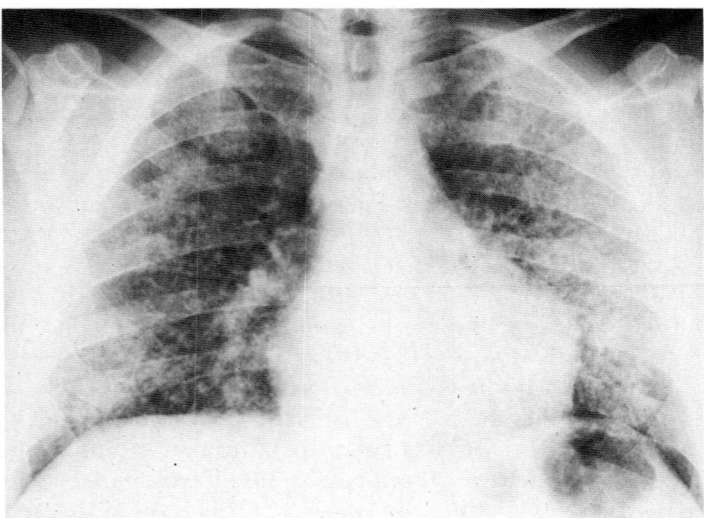

FIGURE 105-5   Chest radiograph of a 33-year-old homosexual male with *P. carinii* pneumonia. Bilateral reticulonodular infiltrates.

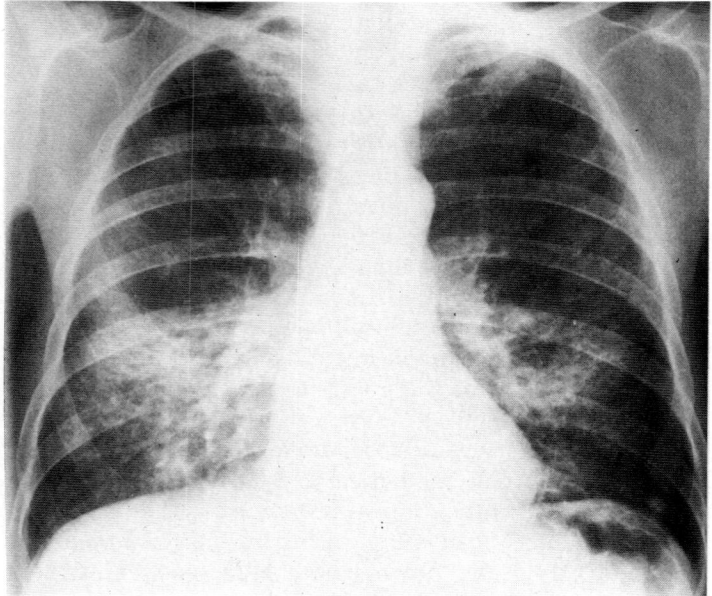

FIGURE 105-6   Chest radiograph of a 28-year-old male intravenous drug abuser with *P. carinii* pneumonia. Predominantly bilateral perihilar reticular interstitial infiltrates.

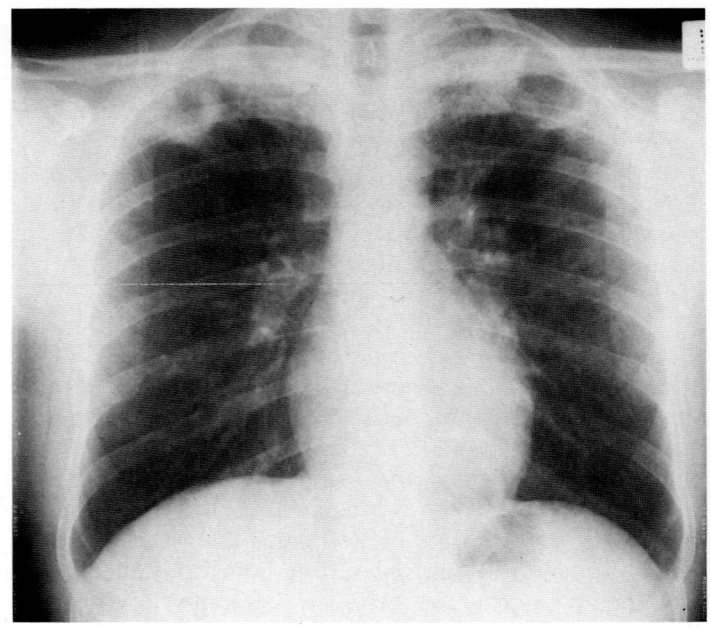

FIGURE 105-7   Chest radiograph of a 48-year-old bisexual male with proven *P. carinii* pneumonia. Bilateral apical infiltrates simulating *M. tuberculosis.*

TREATMENT

In the pre-AIDS era, trimethoprim-sulfamethoxazole was the drug of choice for *P. carinii* pneumonia. As of December 1987, it remains the drug initially chosen by most clinicians. However, as much as 50 percent of patients initially treated with this drug cannot complete their course of treatment owing to toxicity and/or failure to improve. The toxicity due to trimethoprim-sulfamethoxazole usually occurs between 7 and 10 days after initiation of therapy and has included leukopenia, diffuse erythematous skin rashes including Stevens-Johnson syndrome, hepatotoxicity, thrombocytopenia, azotemia, and drug fever. These complications have occurred in 18 to 65 percent of patients. This is in sharp contrast to the toxicity reported in non-AIDS immunosuppressed patients. The dosage of trimethoprim-sulfamethoxazole is 20 mg/kg of trimethoprim and 100 mg/kg of sulfamethoxazole daily, divided into four doses. It is usually administered intravenously initially, but can be administered orally at the same dosage. While there are no studies demonstrating the intravenous route to be superior to oral administration, the intravenous route is often initially preferred, because failure in non-AIDS immunosuppressed patients has been attributed to inadequate blood levels. Furthermore, gastrointestinal intolerance present in many AIDS patients may limit oral therapy. With clinical improvement, patients may complete therapy with oral administration. Folinic acid is not given routinely to patients receiving trimethoprim-

sarcoma. Even endobronchial *Pneumocystis* (not appreciated by chest radiograph) has recently been described. We have seen rare cases of extrapulmonary *Pneumocystis*, involving skin as well as ear. The lung biopsy specimen demonstrates the classic acellular intra-alveolar exudate that is almost pathognomonic of *Pneumocystis*. Upon special staining this exudate proves to be composed chiefly of organisms, primarily trophozoites.

sulfamethoxazole, since there is no evidence that the vitamin prevents or reverses the cytopenia observed in AIDS patients. The cytopenias which occur with trimethoprim-sulfamethoxazole in AIDS patients appear to have an immunologic rather than a metabolic basis. Although both trimethoprim-sulfamethoxazole and pentamidine cause leukopenia, the mechanism is probably different with the two agents; experience has shown that it is safe to switch patients to pentamidine despite a leukopenia that develops with trimethoprim-sulfamethoxazole.

Most patients who do not tolerate trimethoprim-sulfamethoxazole because of toxicity can complete a 2- to 3-week course of pentamidine. However, in our experience almost half of the patients who fail to improve with trimethoprim-sulfamethoxazole also fail to improve with pentamidine. The toxicity due to pentamidine includes azotemia, hepatoxicity, hypoglycemia, orthostatic hypotension, drug fever, and occasional leukopenia. With the change in route of administration from intramuscular to intravenous, sterile abscesses are no longer a complication. Pentamidine isethionate is administered at a once-daily dose of 4 mg/kg per day. A recent prospective, randomized trial comparing trimethoprim-sulfamethoxazole to pentamidine revealed both drugs to be equally effective for *P. carinii* pneumonia. No significant differences were seen in rates of improvement, pulmonary function tests, or gallium uptake by the lungs in survivors at completion of therapy. The rates of complications were similar (approximately 50 percent with each), although the types of complications differed. Patients at risk for AIDS with suspected *P. carinii* pneumonia should be started on therapy even prior to diagnostic bronchoscopy, since organisms persist for at least 72 h after initiation of therapy. Therapy with either trimethoprim-sulfamethoxazole or pentamidine should be administered for at least 4 to 6 days before considering a change of treatment. Since the rate of response is slower in AIDS patients, change should be considered only if there is clinical deterioration in the first 4 to 6 days or failure to show signs of improvement within 6 to 8 days. If treatment with the first drug fails, it should be discontinued. Simultaneous treatment with both drugs does not improve survival, and toxicities are often additive.

Because of the significant drug toxicity as well as drug failure rate, three additional drugs, diaminodiphenylsulfone (Dapsone), an anti-leprosy drug, difluoromethylornithine (DFMO), a polyamine synthesis inhibitor used to treat trypanosomiasis, and trimetrexate, a methotrexate analogue, are currently being investigated for their efficacy against *P. carinii*, their potential in refractory cases, and their possible lower incidence of side effects. Dapsone is a sulfone that competes with *p*-aminobenzoic acid in folate synthesis. Dapsone alone has not proved more effective than standard therapy. Dapsone in combination with trimethoprim has been shown in a limited trial to be as effective as trimethoprim-sulfamethoxazole, but nearly 65 percent of patients had adverse reactions and in 18 percent this therapy was discontinued. DFMO competitively inhibits ornithine decarboxylase and has proven efficacy in protozoan diseases such as trypanosomiasis. Although it has been reported successful in a limited number of patients, its true efficacy cannot be determined because most patients have received previous or concomitant standard therapy. Recently, the lipid-soluble trimetrexate, a dihydrofolate reductase inhibitor, has proved effective against *Pneumocystis*. It appears to be significantly more potent than trimethroprim. The associated myelosuppression and intestinal epithelial toxicity can be prevented by leucovorin administration. A novel approach to therapy has been the administration of pentamidine by aerosol. It appears to be effective and minimally toxic. Crucial to the success of this form of therapy has been the utilization of a nebulizer capable of producing droplet particles 1.5 to 3.0 μm in diameter. High levels of pentamidine are achieved in lung tissue as well as bronchoalveolar lavage fluid with minimal intravenous and renal (a site of potential toxicity) concentrations. Aerosol administration delivers greater concentrations of pentamidine to the airspaces than intravenous delivery. All these new therapies await further clinical testing.

The rate of response to therapy appears to be slower in AIDS patients than in non-AIDS patients. Patients defervesce after 5 to 8 days of treatment; they increase their arterial P_{O_2} by 10 mmHg between 7 and 13 days; and their chest radiographs show significant clearing of infiltrates between 10 and 15 days after therapy. Treatment with either trimethoprim-sulfamethoxazole or pentamidine should be continued for at least 14 to 21 days. The optimal duration for therapy is uncertain, since it is not clear what constitutes a "cure" of *Pneumocystis* infection in these patients. The relapse rate for *Pneumocystis* pneumonia in AIDS patients has ranged from 20 to 30 percent within 6 to 9 months. Repeat bronchoscopic analysis has revealed persistent cyst organisms even after 3 weeks of treatment. It is not known whether persistence of these organisms represents an increased risk for relapse, but has been correlated with decreased long-term survival.

Observations from a recently concluded study at New York University Medical Center in a group of 150 consecutive cases of *P. carinii* pneumonia, suggest that admission arterial P_{O_2}, alveolar-arterial O_2 gradient, and serum lactate dehydrogenase levels have prognostic implications. When survivors are compared to those who died, the former demonstrate a mean admission arterial P_{O_2} of 72 versus 56 mmHg, a mean admission alveolar-arterial O_2 gradient of 42 ± 6 versus 55 ± 6 mmHg, and a mean admission serum LDH of 394 ± 45 versus 717 ± 51 IU/L. Other investigators have found higher serum albumin levels, higher absolute lymphocyte counts, and higher admission arterial P_{O_2} values in survivors. In addition, mild

abnormalities on the initial chest radiograph and minimal interstitial edema on the initial transbronchial biopsy have been promulgated as more favorable prognostic findings.

Because of the significant relapse rate, effective prophylaxis is needed. Chemoprophylaxis utilizing low dosage trimethoprim-sulfamethoxazole has been effective in preventing overt *Pneumocystis* infection in non-AIDS immunosuppressed patients. Unfortunately, a significant percentage of AIDS patients do not tolerate trimethoprim-sulfamethoxazole. Those who do should receive 5 mg/kg daily (usually one double strength tablet twice daily). Pyrimethamine-sulfadoxine (Fansidar) and aerosolized pentamidine have also been proposed as effective prophylactic agents with fewer side effects. The former has been utilized on a weekly basis with good results, although some investigators have reported such toxic side effects as the Stevens-Johnson syndrome. Prophylaxis with aerosolized pentamidine appears to be minimally toxic, but its true efficacy is still being evaluated. Confirmation of chemoprophylaxis regimens in AIDS patients awaits controlled, prospective studies.

MYCOBACTERIAL INFECTIONS

Mycobacterium tuberculosis infection occurs in about 10 percent of AIDS patients. This appears to be more common in intravenous drug abusers, black and Haitian patients (the latter no longer considered a risk group), as well as African patients as opposed to those patients who are homosexual or bisexual males. A significant number of patients are diagnosed with *M. tuberculosis* several months prior to, or concomitant with, the diagnosis of AIDS. Although the clinical presentation is variable, there is a consistent lack of apical and/or cavitary disease on chest radiograph, despite a high yield from cultured sputum. Histologic examination of the lung usually does not reveal acid-fast organisms or granulomata, despite positive cultures from these sites. In half of the patients, *M. tuberculosis* grows from at least one extrapulmonary site. Most patients can be treated with conventional therapy, i.e., isoniazid and rifampin, although an initial three-drug regimen is advocated pending the results of cultures (because of potential resistant organisms). Unlike AIDS patients with other infections, those who acquire *M. tuberculosis* usually respond to therapy, if treated early and for a prolonged period.

M. avium-intracellulare infection in AIDS patients is quite different from that in nonimmunocompromised patients. In normal hosts, the infection is primarily a pulmonary process characterized by slowly progressing local lesions which appear radiologically as cavities or patchy nodular infiltrates. Most patients are between 50 and 60 years of age, have a high prevalence of chronic obstructive

pulmonary disease, and have mild or nonspecific symptoms, shortness of breath or cough. In contrast, this infection is usually disseminated in AIDS patients. In contrast to *Pneumocystis*, this infection occurs late in the patient's clinical course. While the initial portal of entry is the lung, the most important clinical involvement is often nonpulmonary. Biopsy from lymph nodes and bone marrow is often more revealing than from the lung. Blood, bone marrow, stool, and urine cultures are also of value. Alveolar lavage cultures frequently grow *M. avium* in the absence of any histologic evidence of infection in the lung. When there is existing pathology, it is usually in the form of poorly formed granulomata without caseating necrosis. The radiographic findings may be normal or may demonstrate mediastinal adenopathy, miliary patterns, pulmonary nodules, and patchy lower lobe alveolar and interstitial infiltrates. No therapeutic regimen has shown clinical or microbiologic efficacy. Both ansamycin, a rifampicin derivative, and clofazamine, a riminophenzaine derivative which has antileprosy properties, have in vitro activity and are administered with at least two other antituberculous drugs.

Other typical mycobacteria (including *M. kansasii*, *M. fortuitum*, *M. gordonae*, and *M. xenopi*) have rarely caused disseminated disease with pulmonary involvement in patients with AIDS.

CYTOMEGALOVIRUS

Cytomegalovirus is the most frequent infectious organism found in autopsied AIDS patients in some series. Premortem, approximately 25 percent of bronchoscopic lavage specimens contain cytomegalovirus as demonstrated by culture or cytologic methods, often in association with *P. carinii*. Pneumonia as opposed to infection is less frequent. Evidence for disease should be based on histology with demonstration of typical inclusion bodies rather than culture, since viremia is frequent and tissue specimens may be contaminated by blood. Radiographically, the bilateral interstitial infiltrates are indistinguishable from those of *Pneumocystis*. When extensive cytomegalovirus pneumonia is present, it is usually a terminal complication and histologic evidence of dissemination to other organs is present. In contrast to extrapulmonary infection, there is still no effective treatment for the pneumonitis. The results of therapy with the acyclic nucleotide gancyclovir (DHPG), as well as with phosphonoformate (foscarnet), are promising.

MISCELLANEOUS PULMONARY INFECTIONS
Fungi

Fungal pneumonias are unusual, often accompany a disseminated infection, and occur in less than 5 percent of

AIDS patients. *Cryptococcus neoformans* is most common, though this may vary geographically. When presenting as an isolated pneumonia, a lobar infiltrate may be seen radiographically; with dissemination (usually meningitis), an interstitial or miliary pattern is observed. Rarely, it has caused pleural effusions. *C. neoformans* may be recovered from alveolar lavage fluid culture; histopathologic evidence of infection is variable but has been observed on transbronchial biopsy as well as open lung biopsy specimens. When cryptococcal infection is found in the lungs, a search for disseminated disease must be undertaken. Prolonged amphotericin B therapy (0.6 mg/kg/day intravenously for 42–70 days) has been recommended in AIDS patients owing to the high rates of relapse.

The occurrence of progressive disseminated histoplasmosis (with pulmonary findings in one-third of patients) has ranged from 2.7 percent in Houston to 21 percent and 53 percent in Alabama and Indianapolis of all cases of AIDS. However, the finding of pulmonary infection with *H. capsulatum* has not been confined to endemic areas. At New York University Medical Center, 18 patients with pulmonary histoplasmosis (2 percent of our pulmonary AIDS patients) have been recently diagnosed, most of whom originated from an endemic area. The clinical presentation is usually subacute, consisting of fever, weight loss, and splenomegaly, although rare presentations have included cutaneous and gastrointestinal histoplasmosis. Respiratory symptoms are less prominent. Normal chest radiographs are observed in approximately one-third of patients; miliary nodules or diffuse interstitial infiltrates are most frequently found when the chest radiograph is abnormal. Lung biopsy demonstrates mild interstitial inflammation of the alveolar septae with focal nodules of chronic inflammatory cells containing histiocytes. Staining with Gomori's methenamine-silver reveals small (3 to 5 μm), black, round structures that may be misinterpreted as *P. carinii* cysts. Culture of lavage fluid or lung tissue, however, yields colonies of *H. capsulatum*. Serologies do not develop in all patients with progressive disseminated histoplasmosis. Unless a fourfold rise is observed, a single positive titer does not establish the diagnosis. Confirmation of dissemination is made by culture and microscopic review of bone marrow aspirate and biopsy as well as blood culture (10 percent yield). Amphotericin B in 2.0- to 2.5-g total dosages is the treatment of choice, although relapses may occur.

Like histoplasmosis, disseminated coccidioidomycosis occurs in AIDS patients living in endemic areas. Following inhalation of airborne arthrospores, pulmonary infection ensues with hematogenous dissemination to extrapulmonary sites. Single or multiple thin-walled cavities may be seen radiographically. Widespread fungemic dissemination in AIDS patients has recently been reported in endemic areas such as Tucson. Patients present with vague constitutional signs, dyspnea, and a nonproductive cough. The chest radiographic pattern in these patients demonstrates diffuse bilateral reticulonodular infiltrates. Typical lesions of dissemination such as cutaneous lesions, joint effusions, or bone destruction are not found. Biopsy specimens demonstrate poorly formed granulomata with thick-walled, 30- to 60-μm spherules containing numerous endospores, which are identified by periodic acid-Schiff stain. Cultures of alveolar lavage fluid grow *C. immitis*. Initial serology is usually positive. Amphotericin B is the treatment for coccidioidomycosis, though it usually is not curative. Long-term ketoconazole therapy should probably be started after the disease has been stabilized.

Surprisingly, nocardiosis, invasive candidiasis, and aspergillosis are extremely rare in AIDS patients, which accounts for their infrequent pulmonary involvement. *Nocardia* presents as a unilateral lobar or segmental cavitating infiltrate and is often associated with mycobacterial disease. Diagnosis is obtained by culture of lavage fluid as well as histopathologic examination of the biopsy specimen. Spores and pseudohyphae of *Candida* species may invade bronchial walls and pulmonary parenchyma without significant inflammatory reaction. *Aspergillus* results in a hyphal pseudomembrane covering the mucosa of the entire bronchial tree with underlying transmural necrotizing bronchitis. Associated peribronchial and vascular invasion is present.

Bacteria

Community-acquired bacterial pneumonias are unusual in patients with the acquired immunodeficiency syndrome. The data from the first NHLBI workshop revealed that only 11 of 441 patients had a primary bacterial pneumonia. However, since 1983 a number of investigators have reported certain bacterial pneumonias occurring in greater frequency in AIDS patients compared to the normal population. These pneumonias have resulted from *Streptococcus pneumoniae*, *Hemophilus influenzae*, *Branhamella catarrhalis*, and *Staphylococcus aureus*. Recurrent bacterial infection may be an early marker of immune deficiency and has been found in higher incidences in ARC and AIDS patients. Bacterial pneumonias are often associated with bacteremia. During a brief 9-month period in 1983, *Legionella* pneumonia was reported with increased frequency in AIDS patients in New York City. Since that time, *Legionella* pneumonia has rarely been seen. It should be remembered that AIDS patients, like normal hosts, may encounter infectious agents which occur sporadically in a given city or environment; such may have been the case with *Legionella*.

Other Infections

Rarely, pulmonary infections in AIDS patients have included *Toxoplasma gondii*, *Cryptosporidium*, *Strongyloides stercoralis*, adenovirus, herpes simplex, and

varicella. When *Pneumocystis*, mycobacteria, cytomegalovirus, and fungal infections have been excluded as diagnostic possibilities, these unusual infections should be considered. Alternatively, Kaposi's sarcoma, pulmonary lymphoma, lymphocytic interstitial pneumonia, or pulmonary infection due to HIV may be responsible for the respiratory complaints and radiographic findings.

PLEURAL INVOLVEMENT IN AIDS PATIENTS

Clinically apparent pleural involvement is unusual. If an effusion is present, the most likely cause is Kaposi's sarcoma, which is also evident either in the lung or in extrapulmonary sites (see below). Rarely, pleural effusions may be due to *C. neoformans*, *Aspergillus species*, *M. tuberculosis*, or *Legionella*. Several documented cases of *Pneumocystis* presenting with spontaneous pneumothorax or as a pleural-based mass have recently been reported.

LYMPHOCYTIC INTERSTITIAL PNEUMONIA

First described in 1966 by Carrington and Liebow, lymphocytic interstitial pneumonia is a pathologic term used to describe an intense interstitial infiltration of the lung by lymphocytes, plasma cells, and immunoblasts. Often LIP is associated with defined clinical entities such as Sjögren's syndrome or, rarely, systemic lupus erythematosus. It has also been described in association with a number of other disorders considered to be of immune origin: myasthenia gravis, pernicious anemia, chronic active hepatitis, and the auto-erythrocyte sensitization syndrome. Lymphocytic interstitial pneumonia has now been reported in association with the acquired immunodeficiency syndrome, more commonly found in children. In adults, its clinical and radiographic presentation is indistinguishable from that of pulmonary opportunistic infections in patients with AIDS. Transbronchial biopsy is often nondiagnostic; the diagnosis is obtained by open lung biopsy. Pathologic examination reveals diffuse infiltration of the alveolar septa and peribronchiolar areas by lymphocytes, plasma cells with Russell bodies, plasmacytoid lymphocytes, and immunoblasts. Vascular involvement occurs without necrosis or angiodestruction. Nodular aggregates of lymphoid cells with germinal centers are seen. A viral etiology may be responsible for this entity in both the AIDS and non-AIDS patients. Preliminary evidence suggests either the Epstein-Barr virus or HIV as the inciting agent in AIDS patients. Studies utilizing in situ molecular hybridization techniques have demonstrated HIV-RNA in lung tissue, suggesting a role in the development of LIP and perhaps the nonspecific interstitial pneumonitis that has been observed. While some patients have improved without specific therapy, others have responded to immunosuppressive agents including cyclophosphamide and/or prednisone.

RESPIRATORY FAILURE

Many patients with AIDS develop respiratory failure at some time during the course of their illness. The NHLBI workshop evaluated the outcome of endotracheal intubation and mechanical ventilation. Most patients had advanced *Pneumocystis* pneumonia with severe and refractory hypoxemia; the mortality rate was 86 percent. Several recent studies have confirmed this high mortality rate in intubated AIDS patients (ranging from 85 to 100 percent mortality). The poor prognosis of patients with AIDS who require mechanical ventilation has raised difficult ethical and economic questions regarding the appropriateness of intensive-care intervention. The inherent uncertainty regarding the outcome of any individual patient precludes any standard recommendation.

Patients with AIDS and *P. carinii* pneumonia manifest a clinical syndrome of hypoxemic respiratory failure indistinguishable from other forms of the *acute respiratory distress syndrome*. Pathologically, the spectrum of lung injury and response is also similar to ARDS. Physiologically, these patients require high inspired oxygen concentrations. They develop significant anatomic shunting (usually greater than 25 percent) as well as ventilation-perfusion mismatch and demonstrate significantly low static thoracic compliance (usually less than 20 cmH$_2$O). As with other forms of ARDS, the use of positive end-expiratory pressure (PEEP) should be utilized to maintain adequate oxygen saturation and avoid toxic inspired oxygen concentrations. Barotrauma and hemodynamic problems are frequently experienced in AIDS patients. Preterminally, patients often develop progressive hypercapnia with increased dead-space-to-tidal-volume ratios. Preliminary reports have claimed an improved survival rate due to administration of corticosteroids, which supposedly reduces the inflammation and ultimate fibrosis resulting from *Pneumocystis* infection. These claims await prospective, randomized, blinded clinical trial confirmation.

KAPOSI'S SARCOMA

Approximately 15 to 20 percent of AIDS patients have proven epidemic Kaposi's sarcoma. This multifocal, factor VIII producing vascular tumor of the skin was first described in 1872 by the Hungarian dermatologist, Moriz Kaposi. In its classic form, it presents as reddish-brown plaques and nodules on the lower extremities, especially the ankles and soles. Visceral involvement occurs rarely and usually late in the course of the disease. The disorder is a chronic, eventually fatal cutaneous disorder of adult men occurring most often in persons aged 50 years and older with a male-female ratio of 15:1; most patients are of Jewish or Italian ancestry.

In the 1950s, renewed interest in this disease developed with the recognition that Kaposi's sarcoma also occurred in Africans, especially the Bantu tribe of South

Africa and in an endemic belt located in equatorial Africa (which includes Uganda, Zaire, Rwanda, Burundi, Tanzania, Zimbabwe, Zambia, and Kenya). African Kaposi's sarcoma is most commonly seen in young adults between the ages of 25 and 45, with a male-female ratio of 17:1. A third category of Kaposi's sarcoma has been reported in immunosuppressed patients. This form usually presents following renal transplants, but also occurs in patients with lupus erythematosus treated with chemotherapy as well as patients treated with corticosteroids for other disorders.

Epidemic Kaposi's Sarcoma

Epidemic Kaposi's sarcoma differs markedly from the classic disease seen in the United States before the AIDS epidemic. In many respects, it tends to resemble the lymphadenopathic and visceral forms of the disease seen in young African patients. Homosexual men of Mediterranean extraction do not appear to have a particular predisposition to the neoplasm. Onset is usually in the fourth decade, and males outnumber females with the disease by a ratio of 50:1. The incidence of Kaposi's sarcoma is variable among the groups at risk for AIDS. The highest incidence is found among homosexual or bisexual men (95 percent), while intravenous drug abusers account for only 4 percent of cases. Kaposi's sarcoma is infrequently diagnosed among women (3 percent of cases) and children (4 percent of cases). At the onset, skin lesions may be faint, flat, macular and even overlooked. New lesions continue to appear throughout the course of the disease. The flat lesions become elevated and develop into red or blue papules or plaques, occurring on the skin of the face, trunk, or extremities as well as in the occipital region behind the ears and ear lobes. Oropharyngeal lesions are seen on the hard and soft palates, the gingival and buccal mucosa, and the tonsils. Most patients with lymph node involvement are asymptomatic. The nodes are firm, usually 1 to 2 cm in diameter, movable, nontender, and not fixed to one another. Involvement of the upper airway has been observed and occasionally requires emergency irradiation to prevent impending upper airway obstruction. Gastrointestinal involvement occurs in up to 50 percent of patients, but most patients remain asymptomatic; massive upper gastrointestinal bleeding occurs rarely. Although epidemic Kaposi's sarcoma is often an aggressive disease, most patients succumb to opportunistic infections rather than the tumor.

Pulmonary Kaposi's Sarcoma

CLINICAL PRESENTATION

Prior to the onset of AIDS, pulmonary Kaposi's sarcoma was an extremely rare finding. The NHLBI workshop found pulmonary Kaposi's sarcoma an unusual premor-

tem finding despite the frequency of cutaneous and lymph nodal Kaposi's sarcoma. In contrast, several autopsy studies have shown that Kaposi's sarcoma is often present in the lungs. The discrepancy is most likely due to the difficulty in achieving a premortem diagnosis. The NYU Medical Center experience has found clinical pulmonary involvement in approximately 20 percent of patients with epidemic Kaposi's sarcoma. In half of these patients, the diagnosis of AIDS is less than 5 months. Most patients have previous and/or concurrent pulmonary opportunistic infections and are usually bisexual or homosexual males. The mean age at the time of initial diagnosis of AIDS is 38 years.

The presentation of pulmonary Kaposi's sarcoma may be indistinguishable from that of pulmonary opportunistic infection with respect to symptoms, physical findings, chest radiographs, and gas exchange. Most patients present with a fever, nonproductive cough, and dyspnea. Occasionally, patients present with hoarseness and hemoptysis. The physical examination usually reveals cutaneous sarcomatous lesions, while the chest exam is unremarkable. While most patients are hypoxemic, the gas exchange abnormalities may be due to previous or concurrent opportunistic pneumonias.

In the pre-AIDs era, radiographic descriptions of Kaposi's sarcoma noted hilar and mediastinal adenopathy, nodular infiltrates, and pleural effusions. Reports involving AIDS patients have confirmed similar radiographic findings as well as suggested a nonspecific, diffuse interstitial pattern, indistinguishable from *P. carinii* pneumonia (Figs. 105-8 and 105-9). The most common

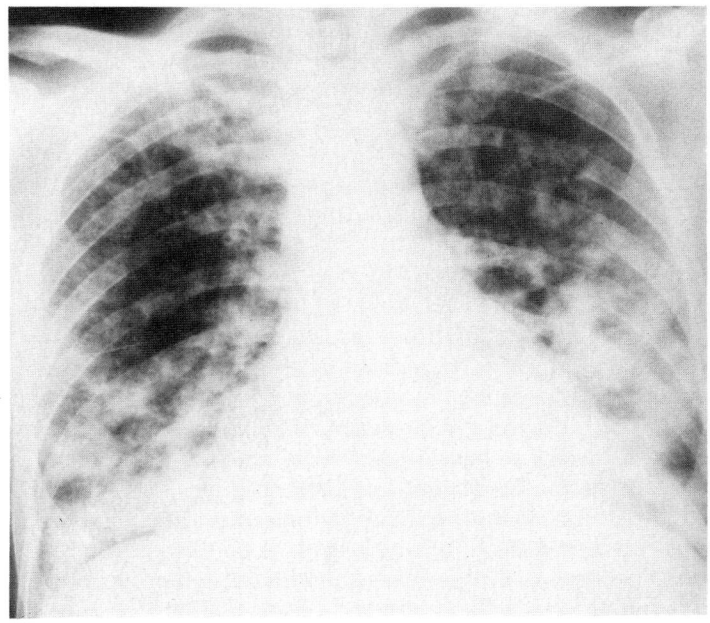

FIGURE 105-8 Chest radiograph of a 36-year-old homosexual male with pulmonary Kaposi's sarcoma. Bilateral nodular infiltrates.

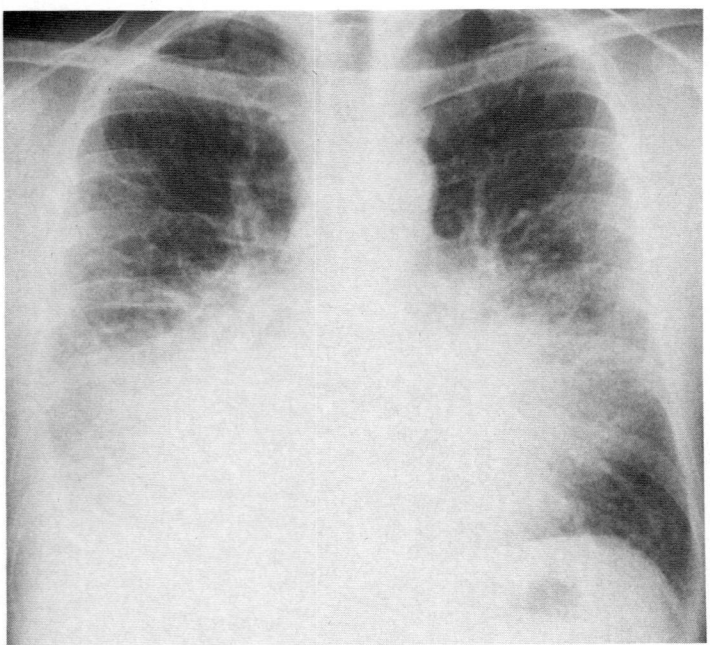

FIGURE 105-9 Chest radiograph of a 31-year-old homosexual male with biopsy-proven parenchymal and pleural Kaposi's sarcoma. Bilateral perihilar interstitial disease and pleural effusions due solely to Kaposi's sarcoma.

findings are either bilateral fluffy nodular infiltrates or mixed interstitial and alveolar infiltrates. Occasionally, a unilateral interstitial infiltrate, an alveolar process, or an entirely normal chest radiograph is present. In contrast to opportunistic infection, gallium scanning of the lung reveals little or no uptake. Pleural effusions are found in approximately 30 percent of patients and may be unilateral or bilateral. They are usually exudative and serosanguinous; cytologic examination is nondiagnostic. Pleural biopsy is also unrevealing, since the lesions occur sporadically on the pleural surface. Mediastinal nodal involvement may be due to Kaposi's sarcoma, but may also be caused by mycobacterial infection or a concurrent non-Hodgkin's lymphoma.

As previously noted, it is difficult to achieve a premortem diagnosis of pulmonary Kaposi's sarcoma. In contrast to the experience with opportunistic infections in AIDS patients, fiberoptic bronchoscopy has a low diagnostic yield (25 percent). When present, endobronchial tumors appear as multiple red or violaceous lesions which are slightly raised and vascular. Visual appearance provides a tentative diagnosis. These lesions are often quite difficult to biopsy and occasionally lead to profuse bleeding. The difficulties encountered with transbronchial biopsy may be due to the fact that the sarcomatous lesions are focal, less cellular than most tumors, and scattered throughout the pulmonary interstitium. Similarly, open lung biopsy may fail to provide the diagnosis. Thus, autopsy will often reveal unsuspected Kaposi's sarcoma.

PATHOLOGIC FINDINGS

The pulmonary lesions seen in biopsy or autopsy specimens are less cellular than classic cutaneous Kaposi's sarcoma. The tumor consists of loosely aggregated spindle cells and often contains atypical nuclei with occasional mitoses (Fig. 105-10). Spindle cells surround small bronchi and vessels and extend into the interstitium. Endobronchial lesions reveal tumor cells in tight bundles beneath the respiratory epithelium. Vascular slits are less prominent, and hemosiderin may also be present. The presence of extravasated erythrocytes and the evidence of hemosiderin pigment between the spindle cells distinguish Kaposi's sarcoma lesions from low grade fibrosarcomas. Pleural-based lesions have similar histologic characteristics. It should be noted that unequivocal Kaposi's sarcoma lesions can be recognized only in large tissue specimens.

CLINICAL COURSE

Once the diagnosis of pulmonary Kaposi's sarcoma has been established, the mean duration of survival varies from 5 to 8 months. Most patients have already received chemotherapy for previously diagnosed cutaneous or visceral involvement. While chemotherapy may be responsible for prolonged survival in some patients during their nonpulmonary phase, it is less successful when pulmonary involvement has been documented. However, despite the progressive nature of pulmonary Kaposi's sarcoma, there may be some short-lived (2 to 4 months) palliation due to chemotherapy. Combination chemotherapy has consisted of adriamycin, vinblastine, bleomycin, vincristine, VP-16, and interferon. Death is not always due to pulmonary involvement with sarcoma; patients often succumb to a concurrent or subsequent pulmonary opportunistic infection.

INFECTION CONTROL PRECAUTIONS

Patients with AIDS pose special problems because of potential individual and environmental contamination from their blood and other body fluids. As a result, they are a cause of severe anxiety to many of the health professionals caring for them. Appropriate educational programs regarding modes of transmission of the disease and institutional preventive measures will allay most of these fears. The major pathogens of concern regarding transmission to medical personnel are HIV, hepatitis B virus, and *M. tuberculosis*. HIV is susceptible to physical or chemical disinfection measures and is readily killed by all mycobactericidal methods. In contrast, hepatitis B virus is much less susceptible than HIV. Patients with hepatitis B are highly infectious by the parenteral route. It has been shown that 1 ml of blood infected with hepatitis B con-

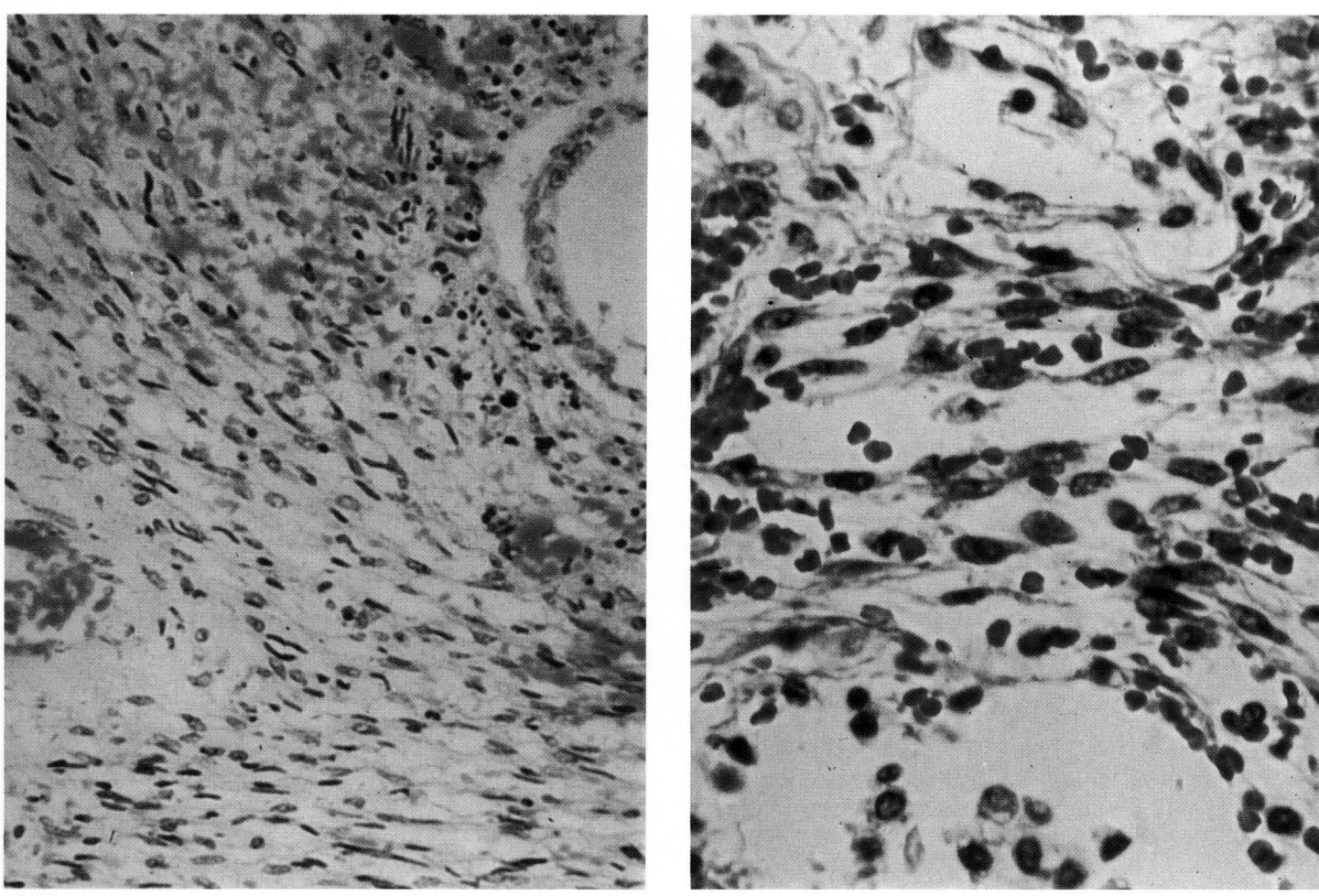

FIGURE 105-10 Histologic appearance of Kaposi's sarcoma. A. Loosely aggregated spindle cells surrounding a small bronchus and pulmonary artery branch and extending into the interstitium. H&E, ×30. B. Higher magnification. Atypical and mitotically active spindle cells with irregular cleftlike spaces and many extravasated erythrocytes. H&E, ×188.

tains more than 10^{13} viral particles compared with only 10^4 for HIV. Radiation, heat (autoclaving, boiling), activated glutaraldehyde (Cidex), sodium hypochlorite (bleach), alcohol, and other commonly used disinfection and sterilization procedures are effective for inactivating HIV. Several hospital epidemiologic surveys have documented that transmission of HIV from patients to hospital personnel is extraordinarily rare, in marked contrast to hepatitis B virus. The exceptional cases of HIV transmission have resulted from gross parenteral contamination (i.e., inadvertent injection of a small amount of blood from an infected patient). Transmission has also occurred with prolonged mucocutaneous exposure to blood, wound fluid, and stool. Personnel caring for AIDS patients should wear gloves and gowns when in contact with blood, stool, and respiratory tract secretions. Physicians performing fiberoptic bronchoscopy should exercise the same precautions, as well as wear masks and protective eyewear. The bronchoscope should be cleaned with high level disinfection or gas sterilization after each use. Some institutions fear the destruction of the fiberoptic fibers by gas sterilization. Alternatively, bronchoscopes should be thoroughly cleaned with soap and water, and then immersed in freshly activated 2% glutaraldehyde (Cidex) for 30 to 60 min, followed by rinsing prior to use. Expired air from mechanical ventilators may disseminate airborne pathogens; a filter should be placed in the expired gas line. Contaminated surfaces can be disinfected with alcohol, sodium hypochlorite, the detergent NP-40, H_2O_2, phenolics, or paraformaldehyde.

Patients with documented or suspected pulmonary AIDS may have tuberculosis and, thus, should be kept in respiratory isolation until a diagnosis has been established. *P. carinii, M. avium* complex, *C. neoformans,* and

most other opportunistic pathogens are not infectious for normal hosts. Routine respiratory isolation for patients with these infections is unnecessary. However, AIDS patients with active pulmonary infection should not be placed adjacent to other immunosuppressed patients, because of isolated reports of apparent transmission of some of these pathogens to immunosuppressed patients.

Pulmonary function laboratories must be concerned with contamination of equipment by saliva, which may contain HIV, hepatitis B virus, and tuberculosis. Whenever possible, sterilization of individual parts with activated glutaraldehyde should be attempted. Disposable mouthpieces and tubing should be used. Care must be taken when drawing arterial blood to avoid accidental needle sticks and surface contamination.

CONCLUSION

During the first 7 years of the AIDS epidemic, certain patterns have emerged with respect to the pulmonary manifestation of AIDS. Many unanswered questions still re-main. The predominance of *P. carinii* pneumonia has become apparent; the reason for this has not. Why some patients respond to trimethoprim-sulfamethoxazole, pentamidine, or neither, as well as the excessive morbidity associated with therapy, remains a perplexing daily clinical problem. Furthermore, the role and form of prophylactic therapy to prevent *Pneumocystis* still need to be addressed. Other infectious organisms, e.g., *M. tuberculosis*, *M. avium-intracellulare*, cytomegalovirus, fungi, and pyogenic bacteria, make empiric antibiotic therapy unsatisfying and potentially dangerous. Improved means to diagnose and treat pulmonary Kaposi's sarcoma await further research. While noninvasive means to diagnosis must be stressed, more invasive approaches must not be forsaken. Because this epidemic is still evolving, caution must be taken not to preclude diagnostic means that may recognize changing patterns of infection as well as discover new pathologic entities; the recent awareness of LIP and HIV-associated interstitial disease are examples of this. Finally, the devastating prognosis for AIDS patients with respiratory failure must be dealt with on an individual and realistic basis by patient, family, and physician.

BIBLIOGRAPHY

Allegra CJ, Chabner BA, Tuazon CV, Ogata-Arakaki D, Baird B, Drake JC, Simmons JT, Lack EE, Shelhamer JH, Balis F, Walker R, Kovacs JA, Lane HC, Masur H.: Trimetrexate for the treatment of *Pneumocystis carinii* pneumonia in patients with the acquired immunodeficiency syndrome. N Engl J Med 317:978–985, 1987.
  This lipid-soluble potent dihydrofolate reductase inhibitor was administered to 49 patients with PCP with simultaneous administration of the reduced folate leucovorin (to protect host tissues without affecting the antipneumocystis action of trimetrexate) and achieved a response rate of over 63 percent in various patient populations with minimal toxicity.

Baker JL, Kelen GD, Silverson KT, Quinn TC: Unsuspected human immunodeficiency in critically ill emergency patients. JAMA 275:2609–2611, 1987.
  Three percent of critically ill patients presenting to an emergency room with no history of HIV infection were HIV-seropositive; infection control precautions are indicated in this setting for all patients.

Barrio JL, Harcup C, Baier HJ, Pitchenik AE: Value of repeat fiberoptic bronchoscopies and significance of nondiagnostic bronchoscopic results in patients with the acquired immunodeficiency syndrome. Am Rev Respir Dis 135:422–425, 1987.
  Repeat bronchoscopy (within 30 days of the initial procedure) in patients with persistent fever and radiographic abnormalities yielded a new treatable diagnosis in 5 percent of patients. The most commonly missed diagnoses were cytomegalovirus pneumonia and Kaposi's sarcoma.

Bigby TD, Margolskee D, Curtis JL, Michael PF, Sheppard D, Hadley WK, Hopewell PC: The usefulness of induced sputum in the diagnosis of *Pneumocystis carinii* pneumonia in patients with the acquired immunodeficiency syndrome. Am Rev Respir Dis 133:515–518, 1986.
  Extremely high yield (78 percent sensitivity) for diagnosing Pneumocystis utilizing induced sputum.

Brenner M, Ognibene FP, Lack EE, et al.: Prognostic factors and life expectancy of patients with acquired immunodeficiency syndrome and *Pneumocystis carinii* pneumonia. Am Rev Respir Dis 136:1199–1206, 1987.
  Severe abnormalities on initial chest radiographs and $P(A - a)_{O_2} > 30$ mmHg are associated with higher mortality during the acute episode. Decreased long-term survival with PCT correlates with severity of interstitial edema on initial biopsy, elevation of initial $P(A - a)_{O_2}$, and persistence of Pneumocystis cysts after three weeks of therapy.

Broaddus C, Dake MD, Stulbarg MS, Blumenfeld W, Hadley WK, Golden JA, Hopewell PC: Bronchoalveolar lavage and transbronchial biopsy for the diagnosis of pulmonary infections in the acquired immunodeficiency syndrome. Ann Intern Med 102:747–752, 1985.
   Lavage and biopsy are extremely sensitive and specific for diagnosing infections in AIDS.

Bronnimann DA, Adam RD, Galgiani JN, Habib MP, Peterson EA, Porter B, Bloom JW: Coccidioidomycosis in the acquired immunodeficiency syndrome. Ann Intern Med 106:372–379, 1987.
   Widespread fungemic dissemination is common in AIDS patients in contrast to other immunocompromised patients.

Centers for Disease Control: *Pneumocystis* pneumonia—Los Angeles. Morbidity and Mortality Weekly Report (MMWR) 30:250–252, 1981.
   The initial CDC report concerning Pneumocystis in AIDS.

Centers for Disease Control: Kaposi's sarcoma and *Pneumocystis* pneumonia among homosexual men—New York City and California. MMWR 30:305–308, 1981.
   The initial CDC report concerning Kaposi's sarcoma in AIDS. One month following the first CDC alert, spread to New York as well as the association of Kaposi's sarcoma was reported.

Centers for Disease Control: Classification system for human T-lymphotropic virus type III/lymphadenopathy-associated virus infections. MMWR 35:334–339, 1986.
   This classification is reproduced in Table 105-2.

Centers for Disease Control: Diagnosis and management of mycobacterial infection and disease in persons with human immunodeficiency virus infection. Ann Intern Med 106:254–256, 1987.
   Extrapulmonary disease and noncavitary, nonapical pulmonary tuberculosis is seen and requires initial treatment with at least three standard antituberculosis drugs with continued therapy for a minimum of 9 months.

Centers for Disease Control: Revision of the CDC surveillance case definition for acquired immunodeficiency syndrome. MMWR(suppl. 1S) 36:3S–15S, 1987.
   This revised definition is reproduced in Table 105-1.

Centers for Disease Control: Recommendations for prevention of HIV transmission in health care settings. MMWR(suppl. 2S) 36:3S–18S, 1987.
   Outline of CDC recommendations on precautionary measures.

Chaisson RE, Schecter GF, Thever CP, Rutherford GW, Echenberg DF, Hopewell PC: Tuberculosis in patients with the acquired immunodeficiency syndrome. Am Rev Respir Dis 136:570–574, 1987.
   Twelve percent (35 of 287) of tuberculosis cases in San Francisco involving non-Asian born males ages 15 to 60 between 1981 through 1985 also had AIDS. These patients were mostly nonwhite, intravenous drug abusers with 51 percent having the diagnosis of tuberculosis prior to AIDS and 37 percent having the diagnosis of AIDS at least one month prior to that of tuberculosis.

Chayt KJ, Harper ME, Marselle LM, Lewin EB, Rose RM, Oleske JM, Epstein LG, Wong-Staal F, Gallo RC: Detection of HTLV-III RNA in lungs of patients with AIDS and pulmonary involvement. JAMA 256:2356–2359, 1986.
   Evidence that HIV may be responsible for LIP.

Coleman DL, Hattner RS, Luce JM, Dodek PM, Golden JA, Murray JF: Correlation between gallium lung scans and fiberoptic bronchoscopy in patients with suspected *Pneumocystis carinii* pneumonia and the acquired immunodeficiency syndrome. Am Rev Respir Dis 130:1166–1169, 1984.
   Graded gallium scans are sensitive and more specific for diagnosing Pneumocystis.

Conte JE, Hollander H, Golden JA: Inhaled or reduced dose intravenous pentamidine for *Pneumocystis carinii* pneumonia. Ann Intern Med 107:495–498, 1987.
   A nonrandomized pilot study demonstrating that nebulized pentamidine (4 mg/kg) as well as a reduced dose of intravenous pentamidine (3 mg/kg) was effective in 10 of 13 patients with inhaled pentamidine and 9 of 10 patients with the reduced dose intravenous pentamidine.

DeLorenzo LJ, Huang CT, Maguire GP, Stone DJ: Roentgenographic patterns of *Pneumocystis carinii* pneumonia in 104 patients with AIDS. Chest 91:323–326, 1987.
   While bilateral interstitial infiltrates are most commonly observed, unusual radiographic patterns may be seen including localized infiltrates, cystic or honeycomb lesions, and spontaneous pneumothorax.

DeLorenzo LJ, Maguire GP, Wormser GP, Davidian MM, Stone DJ: Persistence of *Pneumocystis carinii* pneumonia in the acquired immunodeficiency syndrome: Evaluation of therapy by follow-up transbronchial lung biopsy. Chest 88:79–82, 1985.
   Persistence of Pneumocystis after treatment may account for a high recurrence rate.

Fitzgerald W, Bevelaqua FA, Garay SM, Aranda C: The role of open lung biopsy in patients with the acquired immunodeficiency syndrome. Chest 91:659–661, 1987.
  Open lung biopsy in patients with AIDS is rarely indicated but occasionally may yield a treatable diagnosis.

Friedland GH, Lein RS: Transmission of the human immunodeficiency virus. N Engl J Med 317:1125–1135, 1987.
  A definitive overview of the subject, which should be read by all health care workers to allay unwarranted fears.

Friedman-Kien AE, Laubenstein LJ, Rubinstein P, Buimovici-Klein E, Marmor M, Stahl R, Spigland I, Kim SK, Zolla-Pazner S: Disseminated Kaposi's sarcoma in homosexual men. Ann Intern Med 96:693–700, 1982.
  Clinical and immunologic description of disseminated epidemic Kaposi's sarcoma.

Garay SM: Respiratory failure in AIDS. Am Rev Respir Dis 133:A344, 1986.
  During a 3-year period, 65 patients (mostly with P. carinii pneumonia) required mechanical ventilation because of hypoxemic respiratory failure with a physiological pattern indistinguishable from ARDS: only eight patients survived.

Garay SM, Belenko M, Fazzini E, Schinella R: Pulmonary manifestations of Kaposi's sarcoma. Chest 91:39–43, 1987.
  Pulmonary Kaposi's sarcoma is extremely difficult to diagnose premortem and is associated with a rapidly progressive deterioration.

Garay SM, Greene JB: Diagnostic and prognostic implications of elevated serum lactic dehydrogenase (LDH) and AIDS-related *Pneumocystis carinii* pneumonia. Am Rev Respir Dis 135:A172, 1987.
  Mean admission serum LDH in patients with P. carinii pneumonia is 465 ± 67; mean admission LDH for patients who survived their initial episode of P. carinii pneumonia is 394 ± 45 versus 717 ± 51 in patients who died.

Gordin FM, Simon GL, Wofsy CB, Mills J: Adverse reactions to trimethoprim-sulfamethoxazole in patients with the acquired immunodeficiency syndrome. Ann Intern Med 100:495–499, 1984.
  Rash, drug fever, and leukopenia occur in up to 65 percent of patients.

Gottlieb MS, Schroff R, Schanker HM, Weisman JD, Fan PT, Wolf RA, Saxon A: Pneumocystis carinii pneumonia and mucosal candidiasis in previously healthy homosexual men: Evidence of a new acquired cellular immunodeficiency. N Engl J Med 305:1425–1431, 1981.
  One of the initial reports on AIDS in Los Angeles.

Greene JB, Sidhu GS, Lewin S, Levine JF, Masur H, Simberkoff MS, Nicholas P, Good RC, Zolla-Pazner SB, Pollock AA, Tapper ML, Holzman RS: *Mycobacterium avium-intracellulare:* A cause of disseminated life-threatening infection in homosexuals and drug abusers. Ann Intern Med 97:539–546, 1982.
  Initial description of M. avium-intracellulare infection in AIDS.

Grieco MH, Chinoy-Acharya P: Lymphocytic interstitial pneumonia associated with the acquired immunodeficiency syndrome. Am Rev Respir Dis 131:952–955, 1985.
  Report of adults with lymphocytic interstitial pneumonia.

Johnson PC, Sarosi GA, Septimus EJ, Satterwhite TK: Progressive disseminated histoplasmosis in patients with the acquired immunodeficiency syndrome: A report of 12 cases and a literature review. Semin Respir Infect 1:1–8, 1986.
  Histoplasmosis with pulmonary involvement may be the initial presentation in AIDS patients, especially in endemic regions.

Joshi, VV, Oleske JM, Minnefor AB, Saad S, Klein KM, Singh R, Zabala M, Dadzie C, Simpser M, Rapkin RH: Pathologic pulmonary findings in children with the acquired immunodeficiency syndrome: A study of ten cases. Hum Pathol 16:241–246, 1986.
  Opportunistic infections, lymphocytic interstitial pneumonia, and desquamative interstitial pneumonia are seen in children.

Kanki PJ, Alroy J, Essex M: Isolation of T-lymphotropic retrovirus related to HTLV-III/LAV from wild-caught African Green monkeys. Science 230:951–954, 1985.
  AIDS is pictured as a new disease that originated in Central Africa in recent decades. This report describes the isolation of a simian retrovirus closely related to the human AIDS retrovirus (HIV).

Kovacs JA, Gill V, Swan et al: Prospective evaluation of a monoclonal antibody in diagnosis of Pneumocystis carinii pneumonia. Lancet 2:1–2, 1986.
  An important technique that may prove extremely useful when applied to induced sputum.

Kovacs JA, Hiemenz JW, Macher AM: Pneumocystis carinii pneumonia: A comparison between patients with the acquired immunodeficiency syndrome and patients with other immunodeficiencies. Ann Intern Med 100:663–671, 1984.
Pneumocystis has a subacute presentation and a slower resolution in AIDS patients.

Kramer EL, Sanger JJ, Garay SM, Greene JB, Tiu S, Banner H, McCauley DI: Chest gallium scans in patients with acquired immunodeficiency syndrome. J Nucl Med 28:1107–1114, 1987.
Diffuse uptake is consistent with P. carinii but is occasionally found with other infections; focal nodal uptake suggests M. avium-intracellulare or lymphoma; a negative scan with an abnormal chest radiograph suggests Kaposi's sarcoma.

Louie E, Rice LB, Holzman RS: Tuberculosis in non-Haitian patients with acquired immunodeficiency syndrome. Chest 90:542–545, 1986.
A reminder that M. tuberculosis may herald the clinical onset of AIDS; extrapulmonary sites are common.

Mangura BT, Reichman LB: Treatment of tuberculosis in human immunodeficiency virus infection. Semin Respir Infect 1:239–241, 1986.
A pithy discussion regarding the therapy of M. tuberculosis infections in AIDS patients.

Masur H, Michelis MA, Green JB, Onorato I, Vande Stouwe RA, Holzman RS, Wormser G, Brettman L, Lange M, Murray HW, Cunningham-Rundles S: An outbreak of community-acquired Pneumocystis carinii pneumonia: Initial manifestation of cellular immune dysfunction. N Engl J Med 305:1431–1439, 1981.
One of the early reports on AIDS from New York City.

Maxfield RA, Sorkin IB, Fazzini EP, Rapoport DM, Stenson WM, Goldring RM: Respiratory failure in patients with acquired immunodeficiency and Pneumocystis carinii pneumonia. Crit Care Med 14:443–449, 1986.
Physiological assessment of ARDS in AIDS patients.

McFadden DK, Hyland RH, Inouye T, Edelson JD, Rodriguez CH, Rebuck AS: Corticosteroids as adjunctive therapy in treatment of Pneumocystis carinii pneumonia in patients with acquired immunodeficiency syndrome. Lancet 1:1477–1479, 1987.
A small nonrandomized, unblinded study (which awaits confirmation) which shows a dramatic survival rate (9 of 10) in patients with P. carinii-related respiratory failure treated with corticosteroids as opposed to the low survival rate with conventional antibiotic therapy (2 of 8).

Montgomery AB, Luce JM, Turner J, Lin ET, Deb RJ, Corkery KJ, Brunette EN, Hopewell PC: Aerosolized pentamidine as sole therapy for Pneumocystis carinii pneumonia in patients with acquired immunodeficiency syndrome. Lancet 2:480–483, 1987.
This pilot study involved 15 patients with first episodes of PCP who received a daily 20-min inhalation of aerosolized pentamidine as sole therapy for 21 days; 13 of 15 patients responded, with cough being the only adverse side effect in 12 patients.

Murray JF, Felton CP, Garay SM, Gottlieb MS, Hopewell PC, Stover DE, Teirstein AS: Pulmonary complications of the acquired immunodeficiency syndrome. N Engl J Med 310:1682–1688, 1984.
The first NHLBI workshop.

Murray JF, Garay SM, Hopewell PC, Mills J, Snider GL, Stover DE: Pulmonary complications of the acquired immunodeficiency syndrome: An update. Am Rev Respir Dis 135:504–509, 1987.
Update of the first NHLBI workshop emphasizing new findings such as the increasing frequency of bacterial pneumonias, M. tuberculosis, LIP, and nondiagnostic biopsies. Role of newer diagnostic techniques such as sputum induction is discussed.

Naidich DP, Garay SM, Leitman BS, McCauley DI: Radiographic manifestations of pulmonary disease in the acquired immunodeficiency syndrome. Semin Roentgenol 22:14–30, 1987.
An extensive review of the plain film and CT scan findings in AIDS.

Niedt GW, Schinella RA: Acquired immunodeficiency syndrome: Clinicopathologic study of 56 patients. Arch Pathol Lab Med 109:727–734, 1985.
Cytomegalovirus, Pneumocystis, and Kaposi's sarcoma are most often found on autopsy.

Ognibene FP, Steiss RG, Macher AM, Liotta L, Gellmann E, Pass HI, Lane CH, Fauci AS, Parrillo JE, Masur H, Shelhamer J: Kaposi's sarcoma causing pulmonary infiltrates and respiratory failure in the acquired immunodeficiency syndrome. Ann Intern Med 102:471–475, 1985.
Pulmonary Kaposi's sarcoma is difficult to diagnose premortem.

Rosen MJ, Cucco RA, Teirstein AS: Outcome of intensive care in patients with the acquired immunodeficiency syndrome. J Intens Care Med 1:55–60, 1986.
Respiratory failure requiring mechanical ventilation carries a mortality rate of 87 percent.

Rothenberg R, Woelfel M, Stoneburner R, Milberg J, Parker R, Truman B: Survival with the acquired immunodeficiency syndrome. N Engl J Med 317:1297–1302, 1987.

An important cohort study of 5833 subjects with AIDS diagnosed prior to 1986 revealing: (1) mean cumulative and probability survival of 49 percent at 1 year and 15 percent at 5 years; (2) most favorable survival rate occurred in white homosexual males 30 to 34 years old with Kaposi's sarcoma only; (3) there was a significant improvement in 1-year cumulative probability of survival among subjects with Pneumocystis based on the year of diagnosis (1981 through 1985), probably due to earlier recognition and treatment.

Salzman SH, Smith RL, Aranda CP: Histoplasmosis in patients at risk for the acquired immunodeficiency syndrome in a non-endemic setting. Chest (in press), 1988.

Histoplasmosis occurs in nonendemic areas (see text, p. 1696).

Shelhamer JH, Ognibene FP, Macher AM, Tuazon C, Steiss R, Longo D, Kovacs JA, Parker MM, Natanson C, Lane HC, Fauci AS, Parrillo JE, Masur H: Persistence of *Pneumocystis carinii* in lung tissue of acquired immunodeficiency syndrome patients treated for pneumocystis pneumonia. Am Rev Respir Dis 130:1161–1165, 1984.

P. carinii cysts often persist despite 2 weeks of therapy.

Simberkoff MS, El Sadr W, Schiffman G, Rahal Jr JJ: *Streptococcus pneumoniae* infections and bacteremia in patients with acquired immunodeficiency syndrome, with a report of a pneumococcal vaccine failure. Am Rev Respir Dis 130:1174–1176, 1984.

A higher than expected incidence of pneumococcal pneumonia is seen in AIDS patients.

Smith RL, El-Sadr WM, Lewis ML: Correlation of bronchoalveolar lavage cell populations with clinical severity of Pneumocystis carinii pneumonia. Chest 92:60–64, 1988.

Increased lavage granulocytes are associated with severity of respiratory compromise in PCT.

Stover DE, White DA, Romano PA, Gellene RA, Robeson WA: Spectrum of pulmonary diseases associated with the acquired immune deficiency syndrome. Am J Med 78:429–437, 1985.

Clinical presentation, chest radiograph, and pulmonary function in AIDS: exercise blood-gas analysis may differentiate Pneumocystis from other pulmonary opportunistic processes.

Wachter RM, Luce JM, Turner J, Volberding P, Hopewell PC: Intensive care of patients with the acquired immunodeficiency syndrome: Outcome and changing patterns of utilization. Am Rev Respir Dis 134:891–896, 1986.

A sobering discussion of the poor prognosis associated with intubated AIDS patients.

Wallace JM, Barbers RG, Oishi JS, Prince H: Cellular and T-lymphocyte subpopulation profiles in bronchoalveolar lavage fluid from patients with acquired immunodeficiency syndrome and pneumonitis. Am Rev Respir Dis 130:786–790, 1984.

Decreased CD4+/CD8+ secondary to decreased T-helper cells in lavage fluid.

Wallace JM, Hannah J: Cytomegalovirus pneumonitis in AIDS: Findings in an autopsy study. Chest 92:198–203, 1987.

CMV pneumonitis occurs in 80 percent of patients with CMV infection; rarely is CMV the only causative agent identified in patients with severe pulmonary disease.

Wharton JM, Coleman DL, Wofsy CB, Luce JM, Blumenfeld W, Hadley WK, Ingram-Drake L, Volberding PA, Hopewell PC: Trimethoprim-sulfamethoxazole or pentamidine for *Pneumocystis carinii* pneumonia in the acquired immunodeficiency syndrome. Ann Intern Med 105:37–44, 1986.

Forty patients with the acquired immunodeficiency syndrome (AIDS) and their first episodes of Pneumocystis carinii pneumonia were assigned at random to receive either trimethoprim-sulfamethoxazole or pentamidine isethionate. In patients with AIDS, trimethoprim-sulfamethoxazole and pentamidine do not have statistically significant differences in efficacy or frequency of adverse reactions.

White DA, Gellene RA, Gupta S, Cunningham-Rundles C, Stover DE: Pulmonary cell populations in the immunosuppressed patient. Bronchoalveolar lavage findings during episodes of pneumonitis. Chest 88:352–359, 1985.

There is lavage fluid lymphocytosis but no characteristic cell profile diagnostic of any specific pneumonitis in AIDS.

Young KR Jr, Rankin JA, Naegel GP, Paul ES, Reynolds HY: Bronchoalveolar lavage cells and proteins in patients with the acquired immunodeficiency syndrome. Ann Intern Med 103:522–533, 1985.

Increased lymphocytes, decreased CD4+/CD8+, and increased IgG are found in lavage fluid.

Chapter 106

Hypersensitivity Reactions to Fungi

Anna-Luise A. Katzenstein

Hypersensitivity reactions to fungi that occur in the lung can be broadly classified into two categories: eosinophilic lung disease and hypersensitivity pneumonia. *Eosinophilic lung disease* includes allergic bronchopulmonary aspergillosis (ABPA) and similar reactions caused by fungi other than *Aspergillus*; these disorders occur almost exclusively in asthmatics, and eosinophilia is a prominent feature. Patchy airspace opacities are usually seen radiographically. Although the pathologic manifestations vary somewhat, in general they include tissue eosinophilia often with parenchymal necrosis.

The second category, *hypersensitivity pneumonia*, also known as extrinsic allergic alveolitis, is characterized radiographically by diffuse interstitial infiltrates and pathologically by a chronic inflammatory cell infiltrate often with granuloma formation. Eosinophilia is usually not a feature. The differing manifestations of these two diseases reflect different types of immunologic responses, probably related to both the nature of the antigen and the host responsiveness.

ALLERGIC BRONCHOPULMONARY ASPERGILLOSIS

Clinical Features

Allergic bronchopulmonary aspergillosis was first described in Great Britain in 1952. Although the disorder was initially considered rare in the United States, numerous cases have been reported since the first description in this country in 1968. Cumulative experience since then suggests that the paucity of earlier cases was probably due to lack of recognition rather than to the absence of the disease.

Almost all patients with ABPA have episodic airways obstruction (asthma). Many patients have had previous bouts of pneumonia or pulmonary infiltrates. Fever, chest pain, productive cough, and hemoptysis are common during the acute episode of ABPA. In some patients, the asthmatic symptoms worsen, whereas a few are asymptomatic. Expectoration of mucous plugs is common. These plugs are composed of tenacious mucus and cellular debris that often retain the elongated, cylindrical shape of the parent bronchi (Fig. 106-1).

Radiographic Findings

The most frequent chest radiographic findings in active ABPA are patchy airspace densities or evidence of mucoid impaction. The airspace densities are most common in the upper lung fields and may involve an entire lobe or a portion of a lobe. Migratory infiltrates are common (Fig. 106-2). Mucoid impaction causes several radiographic patterns, most commonly shadows that resemble gloved fingers when the affected bronchi are viewed in longitudinal section or clusters of grapes when viewed in cross section. This appearance is related to bronchial filling and distention by mucus. The lesions may resolve completely fol-

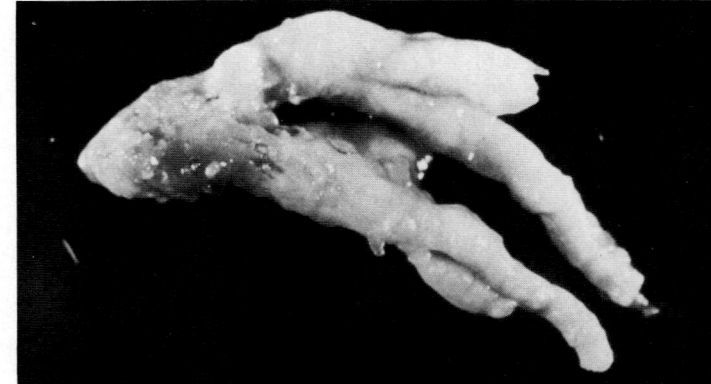

FIGURE 106-1 Mucous plug expectorated by a patient with ABPA. Note the tapering, cylindrical shape with branching characteristic of the parent bronchi. *(Photograph courtesy of Dr. Frederic Askin, Chapel Hill, N.C.)*

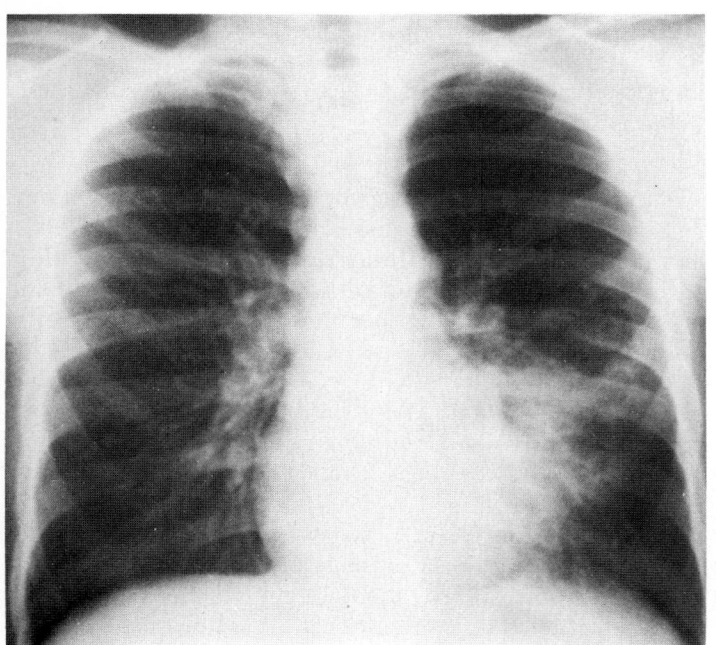 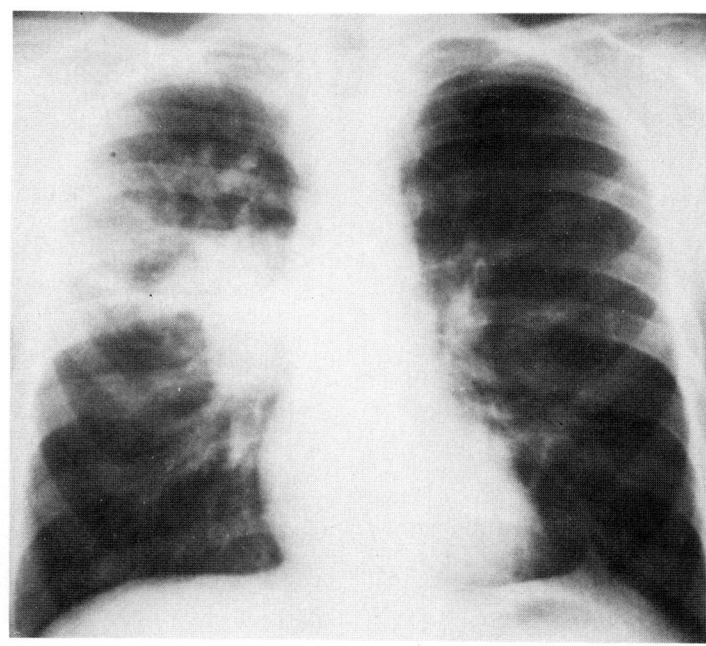

A   B

FIGURE 106-2 Serial chest radiographs from a patient with ABPA. *A.* Initial radiograph showing a lingular infiltrate. *B.* Radiograph taken 7 months later showing resolution of the lingular infiltrate and a new infiltrate in the right upper lobe.

lowing therapy, or they may leave permanent lung damage as residua (see "Staging and Treatment of ABPA," below).

Permanent radiographic changes occur secondary to bronchial damage from repeated episodes of inflammation; they include tram-line, parallel-line, and ring shadows. Tram-line shadows represent thickened walls in bronchi of normal diameter, whereas parallel-line and ring shadows reflect the presence of bronchiectasis. Proximal bronchiectasis is common and is considered pathognomonic of ABPA. This lesion is characterized by proximal dilatation of bronchi that taper into normal diameter distally. Proximal bronchiectasis is best demonstrated by bronchography. However, this procedure is not undertaken lightly in patients with ABPA because of the high risk of adverse reactions. Tomography generally suffices in demonstrating the presence of bronchiectasis.

Diagnosis

There are seven primary diagnostic criteria for ABPA: asthma, blood eosinophilia, immediate cutaneous reactivity to *Aspergillus* antigens, precipitating antibodies against *Aspergillus* antigens, increase in the concentration of total IgE in serum, a history of pulmonary infiltrates, and proximal bronchiectasis. According to Rosenberg et al., the presence of all seven criteria makes the diagnosis certain; the diagnosis is very likely when six of the seven are present. Additional secondary criteria include the finding of *Aspergillus* in sputum, a history of

expectorating mucous plugs, and late skin reactivity to *Aspergillus*. With the exception of the proximal bronchiectasis, none of these criteria is specific for ABPA. Although proximal bronchiectasis is thought to be a specific diagnostic criterion, it may be difficult to demonstrate and often is absent early in the disease. Conversely, other features, such as serum precipitins and immediate skin reactivity to *Aspergillus*, may be found in atopic asthmatic patients who do not have ABPA.

Recently, determination of the serum concentrations of specific IgG and IgE antibodies to *Aspergillus fumigatus* has been reported to be useful in the diagnosis of ABPA. The proposed value of this test is in distinguishing patients with ABPA from atopic asthmatics, in whom the skin test is immediately positive or whose serum contains precipitating antibodies to *Aspergillus*, or in whom the concentration of total IgE in serum is increased. However, caution is required in applying this approach. Although specific IgG and IgE antibodies to *A. fumigatus* may be present in the atopic asthmatics, the level of antibody activity is lower than in most patients with ABPA. Therefore, antibody levels in a known control population of allergic asthmatics without ABPA must be known in order to evaluate the significance of levels found in patients suspected of having ABPA. Conversely, in some patients with ABPA, antibody levels may be no higher than in allergic asthmatics, so that the absence of increased levels of specific antibodies does not exclude the diagnosis of ABPA.

Measurement of specific IgG and IgE antibodies can be useful also for the diagnosis of ABPA in the occasional

patient in whom the concentration of total IgE in serum is normal. This situation may occur in persons receiving corticosteroids for asthma: the corticosteroids suppress asthma symptoms, eosinophilia, and levels of total IgE in serum but may fail to prevent exacerbations of ABPA.

Staging and Treatment of ABPA

A staging system has been proposed for ABPA that aids in clinical management and helps to define the natural history of the disease. Five stages have been identified: *acute, remission, exacerbation, corticosteroid-dependent asthma,* and *fibrotic.* The *acute stage* corresponds to the classic form of the disease as outlined in the previous sections. These patients have asthma, eosinophilia, increased concentrations of total IgE in serum, pulmonary infiltrates, immediate cutaneous reactivity, and serum precipitins to *Aspergillus.* The acute stage is treated with prednisone (0.5 mg/kg body weight) daily for 2 weeks, and then on alternate days until the infiltrates clear and the level of total IgE in serum decreases. The dosage of prednisone is tapered after 3 months and is discontinued after another 3 months. Prolonged and even permanent *remission* may occur after treatment of the acute stage, although recurrences (exacerbation stage) are common.

The *exacerbation stage* may have all the characteristics of the *acute stage,* or it may be unassociated with symptoms. Frequent monitoring of the total IgE in serum and serial chest radiographs are necessary to avoid overlooking an asymptomatic exacerbation. *Exacerbations* are treated like the *acute stage.*

The *corticosteroid-dependent asthma stage* is characterized by a continued need for corticosteroids to control the symptoms of asthma. It may precede or follow the initial diagnosis of ABPA. Difficulty in managing these patients arises because the dose of steroids that suppresses asthma symptoms may not be sufficient to prevent *exacerbation.* Also, it may be difficult to distinguish worsening asthma from *exacerbation.* Monitoring of the concentration of total IgE in serum is helpful since it is usually high in this stage. Also, determinations of the levels of specific IgG and IgE antibodies to *Aspergillus,* as discussed previously, may aid in diagnosis.

The *fibrotic stage* occurs in long-standing, chronic ABPA. It is characterized by permanent fibrotic changes on the chest radiograph and by irreversible obstructive defects on pulmonary function testing. Neither of these features responds to prednisone therapy.

Pathology

The pathologic findings in ordinary instances of ABPA are difficult to assess since most patients do not undergo biopsy. If they are biopsied, transbronchial rather than open lung biopsies are often done. However, based on reports in the literature and personal experience, there appear to be three major pathologic manifestations of ABPA: eosinophilic pneumonia, mucoid impaction of bronchi (MIB), and bronchocentric granulomatosis (BCG). One or a combination of two or all three of these lesions may be present in a given patient. Of the three, eosinophilic pneumonia is probably the most common pathologic finding. When present in a diagnostic lung biopsy or in a surgical specimen, these conditions should raise the suspicion of ABPA even though they are not pathognomonic and do occur in situations other than ABPA (see below).

EOSINOPHILIC PNEUMONIA

Eosinophilic pneumonia is a descriptive pathologic term for a pneumonic process in which eosinophils are predominant inflammatory cells. The lesion has been divided on clinical grounds into three categories: (1) *Loeffler's syndrome,* an asymptomatic and self-limited form that by definition resolves within 1 month; the etiology is usually not known. (2) *Chronic eosinophilic pneumonia,* a variant that lasts longer than 1 month, is generally associated with severe constitutional symptoms and is steroid responsive. Radiographically, there are peripheral, often migratory, infiltrates that may have an unusual distribution resembling the photographic negative of pulmonary edema. Most cases of chronic eosinophilic pneumonia are idiopathic, although reactions to certain drugs or inhalants and hypersensitivity to parasites and fungi are etiologic in some cases. ABPA is one of the most important identifiable causes of chronic eosinophilic pneumonia. (3) *Tropical eosinophilic pneumonia,* a form that, as the name implies, occurs almost exclusively in the tropics. It is thought to be caused by hypersensitivity to microfilaria.

The histologic appearance is identical for all three clinical forms of eosinophilic pneumonia, and there is nothing specific to suggest one etiology over another. Therefore, whenever eosinophilic pneumonia is found on a lung biopsy, efforts should be made to identify a cause, especially drugs, inhalants, parasites, and fungal hypersensitivity, before concluding that the disease is idiopathic. Failure to recognize the etiologic agent may predispose the patient to recurrences and to eventual irreversible lung damage.

The histopathologic findings in chronic eosinophilic pneumonia include a combination of airspace and interstitial abnormalities. The airspace component generally predominates and is characterized by the filling of alveolar spaces by eosinophils usually admixed with variable numbers of alveolar macrophages (Figs. 106-3 and 106-4). Multinucleated giant cells are often found, and Charcot-Leyden crystals (see "Mucoid Impaction of Bronchi," below) may be numerous. Eosinophils may also fill distal bronchioles; when this lesion is widespread, it is termed *eosinophilic bronchiolitis.* So-called eosinophilic abscesses may also be found. These lesions are characterized by central zones of necrotic eosinophils surrounded by

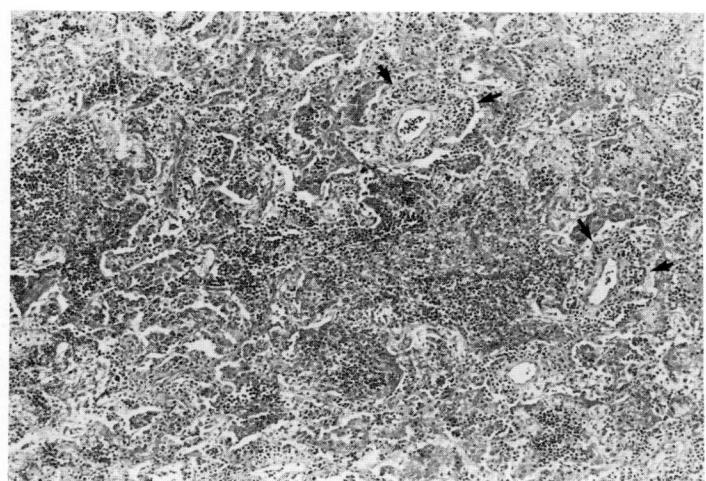

FIGURE 106-3 Low-magnification photomicrograph of eosinophilic pneumonia showing airspace filling by eosinophils and macrophages. Note also the perivascular chronic inflammatory cell infiltrate (arrows). H&E, ×67.

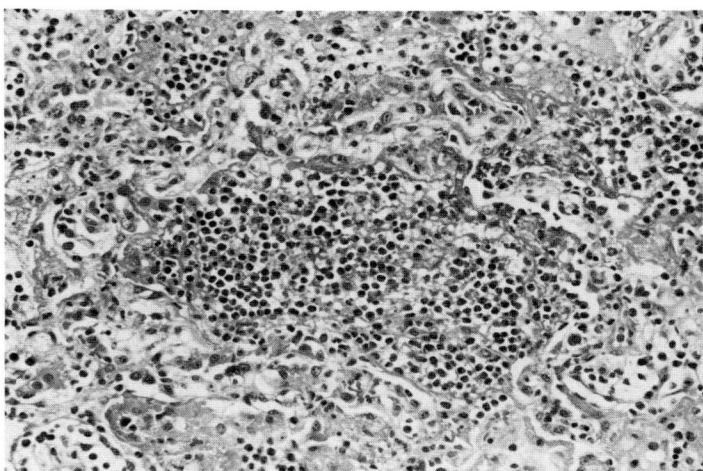

FIGURE 106-4 Higher-magnification view of eosinophilic pneumonia showing numerous eosinophils within alveolar spaces. The alveolar septa are thickened by edema and a chronic inflammatory cell infiltrate. H&E, ×187.

epithelioid histiocytes often arranged in a palisading pattern. These abscesses are always microscopic in size and cannot be appreciated radiographically. The alveolar septa in the region of the airspace inflammation are thickened by edema and an infiltrate of eosinophils, lymphocytes, and plasma cells. Type II pneumocytes are often hyperplastic and appear as enlarged, hobnail-shaped cells lining alveolar septa. Perivascular infiltrates of eosinophils and chronic inflammatory cells may be prominent (Fig. 106-3), and a similar infiltrate may surround small bronchioles. Occasional bronchioles may show evidence of bronchiolitis obliterans. Despite the dense inflammatory cell infiltrate, there is relatively little tissue destruction, and the lung can be expected to return to normal following treatment.

MUCOID IMPACTION OF BRONCHI

Mucoid impaction of bronchi refers to a condition where bronchi are dilated and packed with inspissated mucoid material and cellular debris. It may occur as an isolated phenomenon of unknown etiology, or it may be one manifestation of ABPA. A similar lesion also occurs in patients with cystic fibrosis. The term does not encompass the more common causes of mucous plugging distal to bronchial obstruction, as may be caused, for example, by endobronchial tumors, aspirated foreign material, or lithiasis.

Grossly, MIB is characterized by dilated bronchi with thinned walls, roughened mucosal surfaces, and atrophic cartilage. The impacted mucus is firm, glassy and tan to gray; it has been described as agarlike in consistency. It often has a laminated configuration.

The microscopic features of MIB are distinct and, when fungi are present, are diagnostic of ABPA. The impacted mucus is composed of sheets of degenerating eosinophils and bronchial epithelial cells that are usually arranged in a characteristic layered pattern (Figs. 106-5 and 106-6). Mucus and proteinaceous debris that stain pale blue to pink are present between the cellular zones, and clusters of orange-staining Charcot-Leyden crystals are easily visible within the mucus (Fig. 106-7). These crystals are thought to originate from the aggregation of eosinophil granules under certain abnormal physicochemical conditions. They vary considerably in size and are hexagonal in cross section and bipyramidal in longitudinal section. Fragments of fungal hyphae are also scattered within the mucus (Fig. 106-7). Although most hyphae demonstrate the typical morphology of *Aspergillus* species—including long thin filaments, septa, and dichotomous branching—abnormal degenerating forms may be numerous. These variants are characterized by marked dilatation of organisms with irregularity and folding of cell walls. Tissue invasion by the fungi is absent; i.e., the hyphae are located only within the impacted mucus and are not seen invading the bronchial wall. The bronchial wall is thin and contains islands of atrophic cartilage; the number of bronchial glands is decreased. The mucosa may be ulcerated, show foci of squamous metaplasia, or contain increased numbers of goblet cells. Usually the submucosa is the seat of a dense chronic inflammatory cell infiltrate that contains many eosinophils.

BRONCHOCENTRIC GRANULOMATOSIS

Bronchocentric granulomatosis was first described by Liebow in 1973, based on the morphologic finding of granulomatous destruction of bronchioles. Approximately one-half the original series of 23 patients had

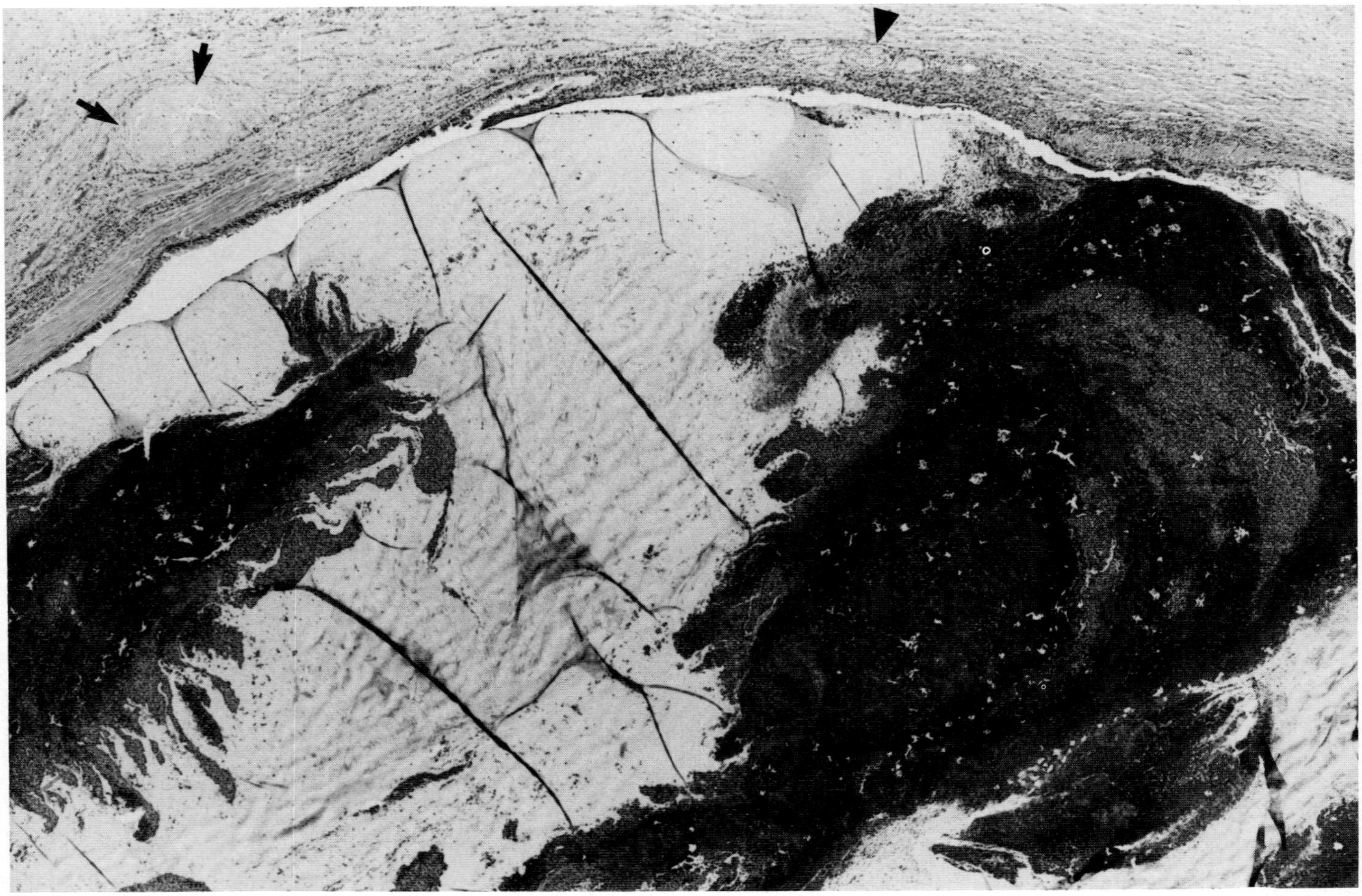

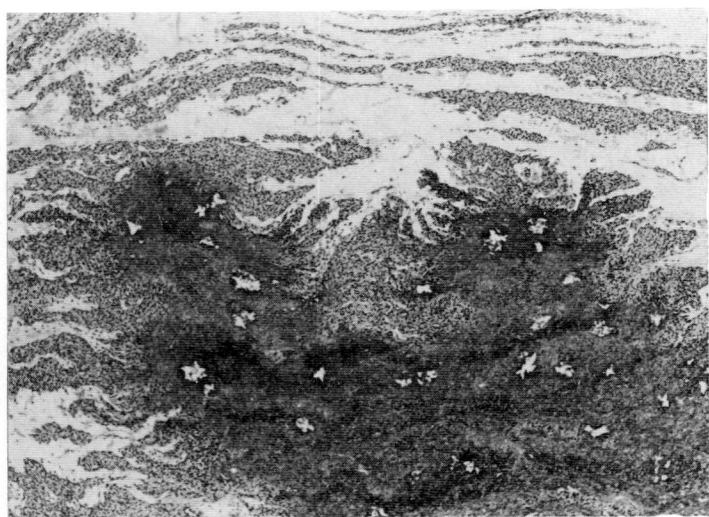

FIGURE 106-5 Low-magnification photomicrograph of a bronchus involved by MIB. The bronchus is markedly dilated and its lumen packed with mucus (light stained material) and cellular debris (dark staining foci). Note remnant of atrophic cartilage at top left (arrows) and bronchial mucous glands at top right (arrowhead). H&E, ×64.

FIGURE 106-6 Photomicrograph of impacted mucoid material in MIB demonstrating the characteristic lamellated configuration of the necrotic cellular debris. H&E, ×86.

asthma, and fungal hyphae were usually found in their tissue specimens. These individuals were believed to have ABPA. Subsequent reports in the literature have reinforced the diagnosis of ABPA using appropriate laboratory methods in similar cases.

Those patients with BCG who did not have asthma composed a more heterogeneous group for whom an etiology could not be identified; they lacked certain histologic features that are prominent in asthmatics, most notably tissue eosinophilia. Recent studies have suggested that examples of BCG occurring in nonasthmatics lacking tissue eosinophilia may in fact represent infectious granulomas, even though organisms are difficult to identify. Therefore, the diagnosis of BCG should be limited to asthmatics, in whom the lesion most likely represents a pathologic manifestation of ABPA or some other fungal hypersensitivity reaction. The diagnosis of BCG in nonasthmatics should be viewed with skepticism.

Grossly, BCG affects in the distal pulmonary paren-

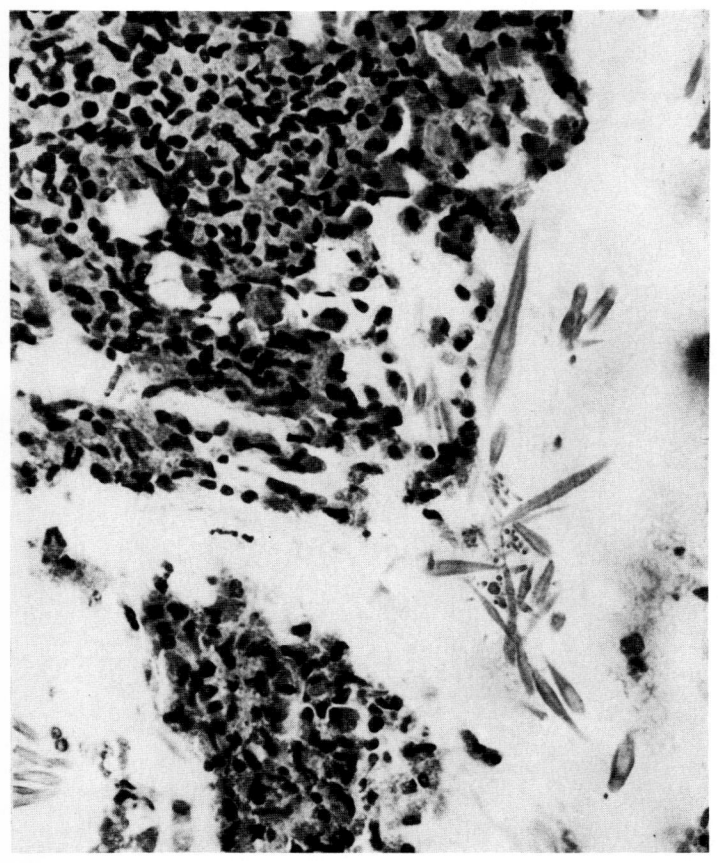
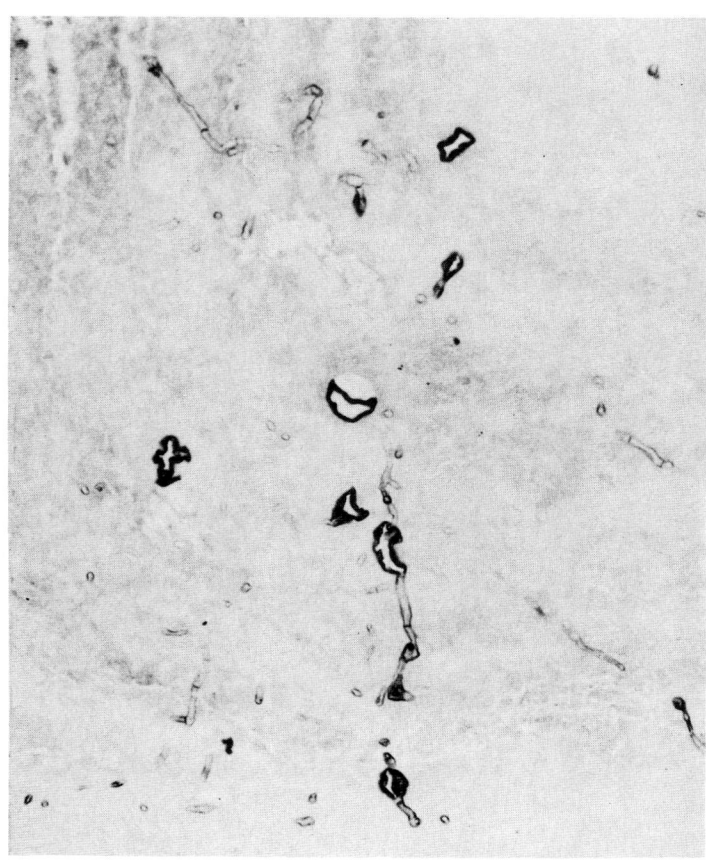

A   B

FIGURE 106-7   High-magnification photomicrograph of inspissated mucus in MIB.   A. Groups of Charcot-Leyden crystals adjacent to clusters of necrotic eosinophils. H&E, ×520.   B. Aspergillus hyphae. Note transition from regular, thin septate hyphae to dilated, often folded degenerating forms. H&E, ×354.

chyma. It is characterized by the presence of linear to nodular areas of lung destruction by yellow, cheesy material resembling ordinary necrotizing granulomas. The unusual feature is the distribution of the changes along bronchioles, thereby imparting an elongated or serpiginous shape to the lesions.

Microscopically, the necrotizing granulomas in BCG center upon and destroy bronchioles. This bronchocentric distribution can be recognized in two ways. In early lesions, there may be only partial destruction of the bronchioles (Fig. 106-8). In such cases, remnants of residual bronchiolar epithelium can be identified within the wall of the granuloma and the epithelium appears to be abruptly replaced by palisading histiocytes. In more advanced lesions, bronchiolar epithelium is no longer identifiable. However, the location of the necrotizing granuloma adjacent to a pulmonary artery, a position normally occupied by a bronchiole, confirms that the granuloma is bronchocentric (Fig. 106-9). Elastic tissue stains can be helpful in evaluating the nature of the lesions since they can identify a vessel as an artery by the presence of two elastic tissue layers. Sometimes the stain demon-

strates remnants of the single, interrupted elastic tissue layer characteristic of bronchioles around the granuloma. The centers of the granulomas usually contain necrotic neutrophils and eosinophils surrounded by palisading histiocytes. Special stains often reveal fungal hyphae within the necrotic centers, but as in MIB, the fungi do not invade the pulmonary parenchyma. Although at first glance the presence of fungi within lung granulomas may suggest tissue invasion, the fungi prove to be within lumens of bronchioles that have been replaced by granulomas. The parenchyma surrounding the granulomas also shows changes, usually consisting of a dense chronic inflammatory cell infiltrate that contains numerous eosinophils and is associated with extensive scarring. Frequently, a foreign body giant cell reaction surrounds cellular debris; it is believed to represent a reaction to necrotic eosinophils.

BCG is the most severe manifestation of ABPA, and it probably results from long-standing untreated disease. Unlike eosinophilic pneumonia, it is associated with extensive parenchymal destruction that is probably not reversible even with corticosteroid therapy.

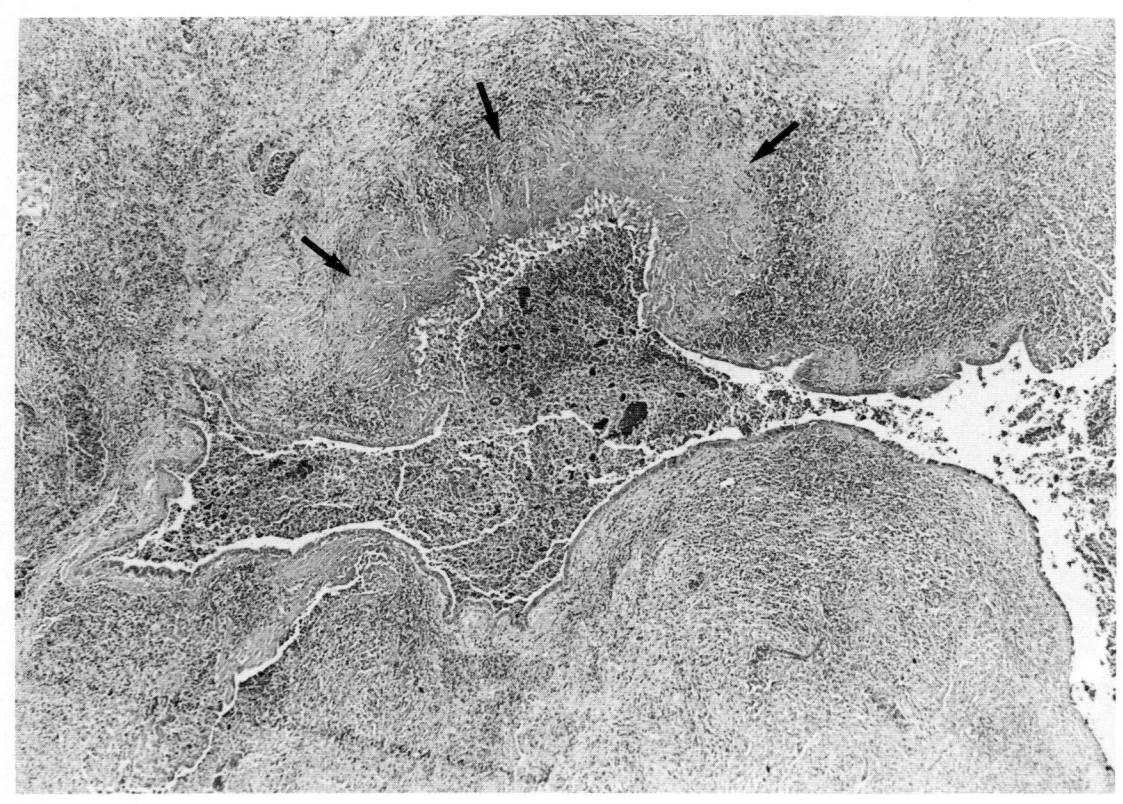

FIGURE 106-8 Low-magnification photomicrograph of BCG showing partial replacement of bronchiolar mucosa by palisading histiocytes (arrows). H&E, ×55.

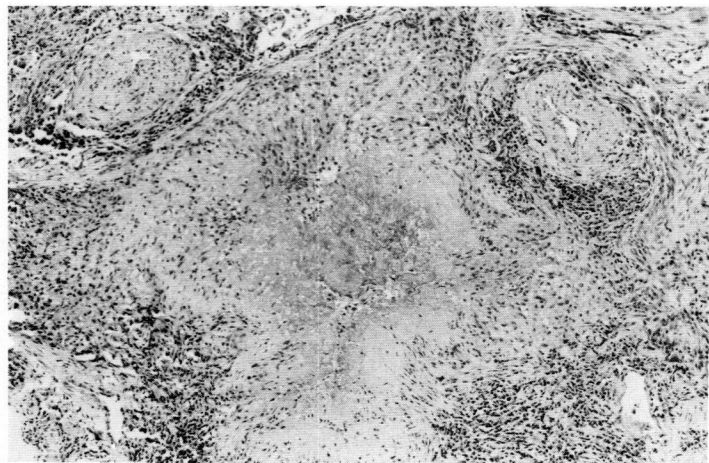

FIGURE 106-9 Necrotizing bronchocentric granuloma (center) in BCG that has totally destroyed the bronchiole wall. The granuloma is inferred to be bronchocentric because of its location adjacent to branches of a pulmonary artery (top right and top left). H&E, ×68.

Pathogenesis

The pathogenesis of ABPA is thought to be related to a combination of type I and type III immunologic reactions against *Aspergillus* antigens within bronchi. Participation of the type I mechanism is reflected in the elevated IgE levels; eosinophilia of blood, sputum, and tissue; and immediate skin reactivity to *Aspergillus*. Evidence for involvement of type III reactivity includes the presence of late (Arthus) skin and bronchial reactivity to *Aspergillus*. Also, experimentally some features of ABPA have been reproduced by serum transfer studies. Lymphocyte transformation in response to *Aspergillus* has been documented in some patients with ABPA. This finding as well as the granulomatous inflammation seen in some patients suggests that type IV immunity may also play a role in the pathogenesis of ABPA.

Allergic Bronchopulmonary Disease Caused by Fungi Other Than *A. Fumigatus*

On rare occasions, reactions that are clinically identical with ABPA are caused by fungi other than *A. fumigatus*. Instances have been reported that were related to *Aspergillus terreus*, *Candida albicans*, *Torulopsis glabrata*, *Drechslera hawaiiensis*, *Stemphylium lanuginosum*, *Curvalaria lunata*, and *Helminthosporium* species. These rare occurrences have prompted some investigators to suggest the broader terms, *allergic bronchopulmonary fungal disease* or *allergic bronchopulmonary mycosis*.

HYPERSENSITIVITY PNEUMONIA

Hypersensitivity pneumonia, also known as extrinsic allergic alveolitis, refers to a group of lung diseases caused

by hypersensitivity to inhaled organic antigens. The disease generally affects nonatopic individuals and is characterized by inflammation involving the interstitium of the distal pulmonary parenchyma. The antigens most commonly implicated in producing the disease include thermophylic actinomycetes, as in farmer's lung, or humidifier–air-conditioner lung and avian proteins as in pigeon breeder's lung. Less often, fungal antigens are etiologic, and malt worker's lung and maple bark disease are examples of this form of the disease. Other fungal organisms have been occasionally implicated as well; they are listed in Table 106-1.

Clinical Features

Two clinically distinct forms of hypersensitivity pneumonia exist, the classic acute form and the chronic variant. In the acute form, fever, chills, cough, dyspnea, and chest infiltrates develop 4 to 6 h following exposure to the antigen. Farmer's lung or pigeon breeder's lung are the classic examples of this form of the disease. Most cases of hypersensitivity pneumonia caused by fungal antigens also present acutely. The chronic form of the disease differs in that the onset is insidious with gradually worsening dyspnea and cough, and the relationship of symptoms to an exposure source may not be obvious. Bilateral interstitial infiltrates are seen radiographically in both forms, although fibrosis, volume loss, and even honeycomb change

may be evident in the chronic form (Fig. 106-10). The treatment of choice is to remove the patient from the source of exposure, since continued exposure may lead to irreversible lung destruction. Corticosteroids may hasten resolution of both symptoms and chest infiltrates.

Diagnosis

In the acute form of hypersensitivity pneumonia, the relation of symptoms to antigen exposure is usually obvious, and the diagnosis is easily established from the clinical history. Precipitating antibodies to the offending antigen are found in most patients. Skin tests can be performed with avian proteins and show late (Arthus) reactivity. Cutaneous reactivity, however, cannot be assessed using fungal or bacterial antigens, since these substances cause local irritation that obscures immunologic reactions. Bronchoprovocation tests also show late bronchial reactivity, but they are usually not necessary and are not routinely performed.

The diagnosis is more difficult in the chronic form of the disease where the relation of symptoms to antigenic source is usually not apparent. The clinical presentation of these patients may mimic chronic interstitial lung disease, and the possibility of hypersensitivity pneumonia may not be suspected until after lung biopsy. The mainstay of diagnosis is to identify a source of exposure, to demonstrate a relationship of symptoms to exposure, and

TABLE 106-1
Hypersensitivity Pneumonia Related to Fungal Antigens

Disease	Source	Organism
Malt worker's lung	Germinating barley	*Aspergillus clavatus*
Maple bark disease	Maple bark, sycamore trees	*Cryptostroma corticale*
Wood pulp worker's disease	Wood dust	*Alternaria* species
Sequoiosis	Moldy sawdust	*Graphium, Aureobasidium*
Cheese washer's lung	Cheese mold	*Penicillium casei*
Cheese worker's lung	Blue cheese	*Penicillium roqueforti*
Suberosis	Cork dust	*Penicillium frequentens*
Hypersensitivity pneumonia	Leaky heating system	*Penicillium chrysogenum Penicillium cyclopium*
Hypersensitivity pneumonia	Contaminated humidifier	*Penicillium* species
Hypersensitivity pneumonia	Moldy wood chips	*Penicillium* species
Hypersensitivity pneumonia	Leaky sewage, contaminated humidifier	*Cephalosporium*
Hypersensitivity pneumonia	House dust, bird droppings	*Trichosporon cutaneum*
Hypersensitivity pneumonia	Moldy straw	*Sporobolomyces*
Hypersensitivity pneumonia	Moldy hay, home humidifier	*Aspergillus fumigatus, Aspergillus umbrosus, Penicillium* species

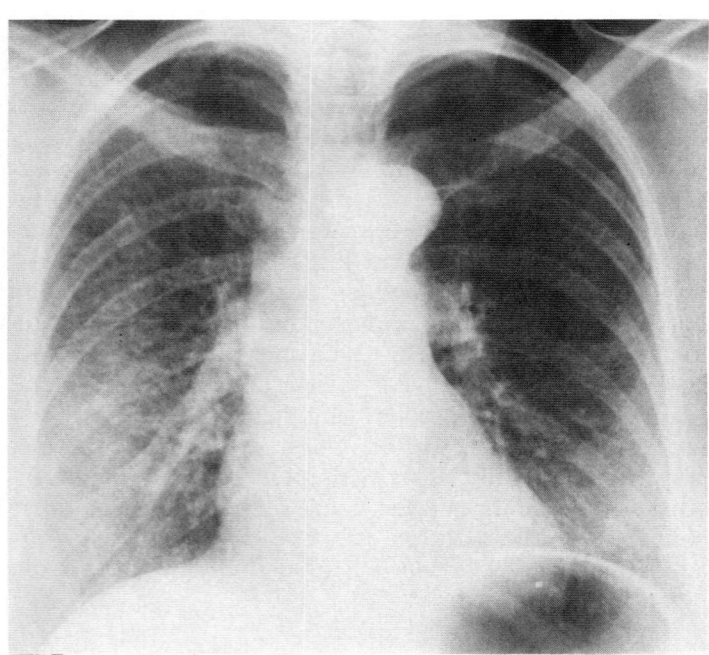

FIGURE 106-10 Chest radiograph from a patient with hypersensitivity pneumonia showing bilateral interstitial infiltrates.

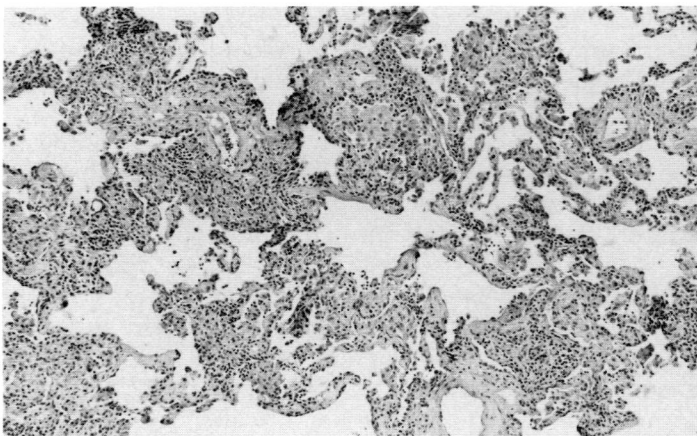

FIGURE 106-11 Low-magnification photomicrograph of hypersensitivity pneumonia showing a cellular infiltrate affecting predominantly the interstitium. H&E, ×67.

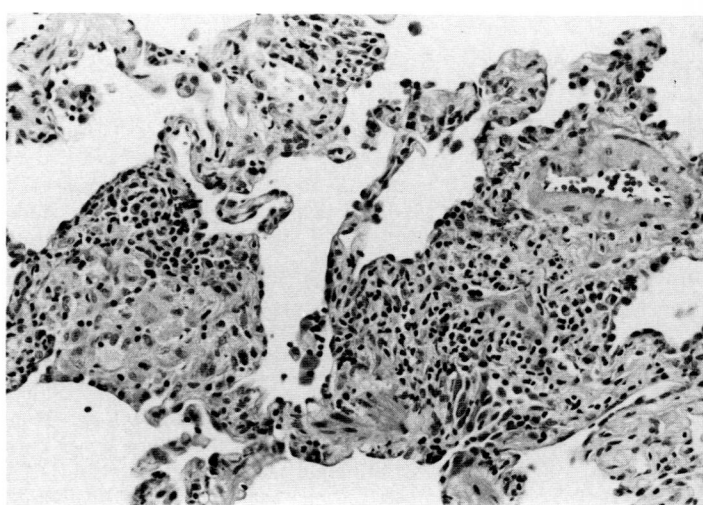

FIGURE 106-12 Higher-magnification view of hypersensitivity pneumonia showing numerous lymphocytes and histiocytes within the alveolar septa. A loose, poorly formed, noncaseating granuloma is seen on the left. H&E, ×187.

to observe the patient improving when exposure stops. The presence of serum precipitins to a suspected antigen supports the diagnosis but is not pathognomonic, since precipitins are commonly found in exposed but asymptomatic individuals. Conversely, precipitins may be absent in some patients with the disease.

As in the acute form, bronchial inhalation challenges with the antigen are helpful in diagnosis. However, they are not done routinely largely because of the possibility of adverse effects. Bronchoalveolar lavage studies can be useful in separating hypersensitivity pneumonia from other chronic interstitial lung diseases: increased numbers of T lymphocytes are found in bronchoalveolar lavage fluids from patients with hypersensitivity pneumonia in contrast to increased numbers of neutrophils in the idiopathic interstitial pneumonias. Although the number of T lymphocytes is also increased in patients with sarcoidosis, most lymphocytes in hypersensitivity pneumonia are suppressor T cells, whereas helper T cells predominate in sarcoidosis. In most patients with hypersensitivity pneumonia specific antigens can be shown to stimulate proliferation of lymphocytes obtained by bronchoalveolar lavage, but this phenomenon is not specific since it also occurs in exposed but asymptomatic individuals.

Pathology

The pathologic findings are identical in both the acute and the chronic form of hypersensitivity pneumonia, and there are usually no specific features to suggest an etio-

logic agent. One exception is maple bark stripper's disease in which spores of *Cryptostroma corticale* can be identified in tissue specimens.

The usual pathologic abnormality in hypersensitivity pneumonia is a distinct type of chronic interstitial pneumonia that differs in appearance from idiopathic interstitial pneumonia. This lesion is characterized by expansion of alveolar septa by numerous plasma cells and lymphocytes, with varying numbers of epithelioid histiocytes (Fig. 106-11). The histiocytes are organized into loose, noncaseating granulomas in two-thirds of cases (Fig. 106-12). These granulomas are poorly circumscribed and usually contain many lymphocytes. Eosinophils are occasionally seen in the interstitium, but these cells are generally not prominent. The interstitial process is patchy and

tends to be accentuated around distal bronchioles with intervening areas of relatively normal lung. Interstitial fibrosis may occur late in the disease but is usually not a prominent feature.

Various airspace abnormalities can also be found in hypersensitivity pneumonia; these are usually most prominent in the vicinity of the interstitial process. A fibrinous exudate containing neutrophils and chronic inflammatory cells is sometimes present within alveolar spaces, and this exudate may undergo organization. In about half of the patients with hypersensitivity pneumonia, bronchiolitis obliterans accompanies the interstitial pneumonia. Foamy macrophages are frequently present within both the interstitium and the airspaces. Although these macrophages were once believed to be specific for pigeon breeder's disease, it turns out that they can be found in all forms of hypersensitivity pneumonia; probably, they are related to bronchiolar obstruction caused by the bronchiolitis obliterans.

Pathogenesis

The immunopathogenesis of hypersensitivity pneumonia has not been completely elucidated. However, most evidence suggests a combination of type III and type IV immunologic reactions. A role for the former mechanism is suggested by the finding of serum precipitating antibodies to specific antigens, late bronchial reactivity in bronchoprovocation tests, late skin test reactivity, and delayed onset of symptoms following exposure. The participation of type IV reactivity is supported by the finding of granulomatous inflammation in tissue specimens as well as reactivity of bronchoalveolar lavage and peripheral blood lymphocytes to specific antigens. The fact that precipitating antibodies and activated lymphocytes can be found in asymptomatic individuals without evidence of hypersensitivity pneumonia suggests that other factors may also contribute to the pathogenesis. For example, nonspecific activation of complement by inhaled organic dust could be an initiating factor.

BIBLIOGRAPHY

Bosken C, Myers J, Greenberger P, Katzenstein A: Pathologic features of allergic bronchopulmonary aspergillosis. Lab Invest 56:8A, 1987.
   Describes the pathologic features in 19 cases of ABPA. Suggests that the finding in asthmatic patients of MIB, BCG, or eosinophilic pneumonia alone or in combination, along with fungal hyphae is diagnostic of allergic bronchopulmonary fungal disease.

Costabel U, Bross KJ, Marxen J, Matthys H: T-lymphocytosis in bronchoalveolar lavage fluid of hypersensitivity pneumonitis. Changes in profile of T-cell subsets during the course of disease. Chest 85:514–522, 1984.
   Describes the predominance of T-suppressor lymphocytes in bronchoalveolar lavage fluid of hypersensitivity pneumonia versus T-helper cells in sarcoidosis.

Haslam PL, Dewar A, Butchers P, Primett ZS, Newman-Taylor A, Turner-Warwick M: Mast cells, atypical lymphocytes, and neutrophils in bronchoalveolar lavage in extrinsic allergic alveolitis. Comparison with other interstitial lung diseases. Am Rev Respir Dis 135:35–47, 1987.
   Documents increased numbers of mast cells in addition to lymphocytes in bronchoalveolar lavage fluids from patients with extrinsic allergic alveolitis compared to sarcoidosis and interstitial pneumonias.

Henderson AH: Allergic aspergillosis: Review of 32 cases. Thorax 23:501–512, 1968.
   Good description of clinical and radiographic features of ABPA. Emphasizes the frequency of recurrence and the fibrotic complications that can occur in late stages of the disease.

Hinson KFW, Moon AJ, Plummer NS: Bronchopulmonary aspergillosis. A review and report of eight new cases. Thorax 7:317–333, 1952.
   Classic article first describing ABPA. Three cases of ABPA are contrasted with five cases of saprophytic or invasive aspergillosis.

Irwin RS, Thomas HM III: Mucoid impaction of the bronchus. Diagnosis and treatment. Am Rev Respir Dis 108:955–959, 1973.
   Brief review of clinical and pathologic features of MIB, including etiology and speculation on pathogenesis.

Jelihovsky T: The structure of bronchial plugs in mucoid impaction, bronchocentric granulomatosis and asthma. Histopathology 7:153–167, 1983.
   Describes in detail the pathologic appearance of mucous plugs in various conditions and emphasizes their distinctive features in ABPA.

Katzenstein A-LA, Askin FB: Surgical Pathology of Non-Neoplastic Lung Disease. Philadelphia, Saunders, 1982, pp 108–138.
   Describes the pathologic findings in allergic bronchopulmonary aspergillosis and hypersensitivity pneumonia.

Katzenstein A-LA, Liebow AA, Friedman PJ: Bronchocentric granulomatosis, mucoid impaction and hypersensitivity reactions to fungi. Am Rev Respir Dis 111:497–537, 1975.
  Early series describing the clinical and pathologic features of 23 cases of bronchocentric granulomatosis and suggesting fungal hypersensitivity in the pathogenesis of some.

Kawanami O, Basset F, Barrios R, Lacronique JG, Ferrans VJ, Crystal RG: Hypersensitivity pneumonitis in man. Light and electron-microscopic studies of 18 lung biopsies. Am J Pathol 110:275–289, 1983.
  Discusses the light- and electron-microscopic features of 18 open lung biopsies from patients with hypersensitivity pneumonia. Emphasizes the presence of airspace as well as interstitial inflammation.

Koss MN, Robinson RG, Hochholzer L: Bronchocentric granulomatosis. Hum Pathol 12:632–638, 1981.
  Presents the clinical and pathologic findings in 15 patients with BCG.

Leatherman JW, Michael AF, Schwartz BA, Hoidal JR: Lung T cells in hypersensitivity pneumonitis. Ann Intern Med 100:390–392, 1984.
  Contrasts the finding of predominantly suppressor T lymphocytes in bronchoalveolar lavage fluid in hypersensitivity pneumonia with predominantly helper T cells in sarcoidosis.

Lee TM, Greenberger PA, Patterson R, Roberts M, Liotta JL: Stage V (fibrotic) allergic bronchopulmonary aspergillosis. A review of 17 cases followed from diagnosis. Arch Intern Med 147:319–323, 1987.
  A review of the course and management of patients in the fibrotic stage of ABPA.

Liebow A: Pulmonary angiitis and granulomatosis. J Burns Amberson Lecture. Am Rev Respir Dis 108:1–18, 1973.
  Classic review of pulmonary angiitis and granulomatosis, containing the first description of BCG.

Malo JL, Hawkins R, Pepys J: Studies in chronic allergic bronchopulmonary aspergillosis. 1. Clinical and physiological findings. Thorax 32:254–261, 1977.
  Describes the clinical and physiological features of 50 patients with ABPA of long duration (mean follow-up 11 years).

Malo JL, Pepys J, Simon G: Studies in chronic allergic bronchopulmonary aspergillosis. 2. Radiological findings. Thorax 32:262–268, 1977.
  Emphasizes the frequency of recurrent infiltrates and the development of permanent lung damage in patients with long-standing ABPA.

McCarthy DS, Pepys J: Allergic bronchopulmonary aspergillosis. Clinical immunology: 1. Clinical features. Clin Allergy 1:261–286, 1971.
  Describes the clinical and laboratory features in a large series of 111 patients with ABPA.

McCarthy DS, Simon G, Hargreave FE: The radiological appearances in allergic broncho-pulmonary aspergillosis. Clin Radiol 21:366–375, 1970.
  Detailed radiographic description of findings in 111 patients with ABPA.

Mendelson EB, Fisher MR, Mintzer RA, Halwig JM, Greenberger PA: Roentgenographic and clinical staging of allergic bronchopulmonary aspergillosis. Chest 87:334–339, 1985.
  Describes the radiologic manifestations seen in the various stages of ABPA in 24 patients with long-term follow-up. Emphasizes the importance of demonstrating proximal bronchiectasis for diagnosis and the use of chest radiographs to confirm recurrent disease.

Mintzer RA, Rogers LF, Kruglik GD, Rosenberg M, Neiman HL, Patterson R: The spectrum of radiologic findings in allergic bronchopulmonary aspergillosis. Radiology 127:301–307, 1978.
  Describes radiographic changes seen in 20 patients with ABPA. Perihilar infiltrates simulating adenopathy and air-fluid levels, although not emphasized in previous studies, were present in 40 percent. Three patients had normal chest radiographs with abnormalities identifiable only by bronchography.

Moore VL, Pedersen GM, Hauser WC, Fink JN: A study of lung lavage materials in patients with hypersensitivity pneumonitis: In vitro response to mitogen and antigen in pigeon breeder's disease. J Allergy Clin Immunol 65:365–370, 1980.
  Reports increased numbers of T lymphocytes in bronchoalveolar lavage fluid from patients with pigeon breeder's disease. Also notes a response of lymphocytes to phytohemagglutinin (PHA) and pigeon antigen in most patients. Similar responses were present in a few asymptomatic pigeon breeders as well.

Morrissey WL, Gaensler EA, Carrington CB, Turner HG: Chronic eosinophilic pneumonia. Respiration 32:453–468, 1975.
   Reviews the classification, etiology, and therapy of eosinophilic pneumonia.

Myers JL, Katzenstein A: Granulomatous infection mimicking bronchocentric granulomatosis. Am J Surg Pathol 10:317–322, 1986.
   Describes four nonasthmatic patients with granulomatous lung infections pathologically resembling BCG. Suggests that the diagnosis of BCG should be made rarely, if at all, in nonasthmatics.

Patterson R, Greenberger PA, Halwig JM, Liotta JL, Roberts M: Allergic bronchopulmonary aspergillosis. Natural history and classification of early disease by serologic and roentgenographic studies. Arch Intern Med 146:916–918, 1986.
   In a series of 84 patients, the authors identify a group with the serologic characteristics of ABPA but no central bronchiectasis. Presumably this is the earliest stage at which ABPA can be diagnosed.

Patterson R, Greenberger PA, Radin RC, Roberts M: Allergic bronchopulmonary aspergillosis: Staging as an aid to management. Ann Intern Med 96:286–291, 1982.
   The five stages of ABPA are described in 40 patients. The usefulness of measuring specific IgE and IgG antibodies to Aspergillus in diagnosing ABPA is emphasized.

Reyes CN, Wenzel FJ, Lawton BR, Emanuel DA: The pulmonary pathology of farmer's lung disease. Chest 81:142–146, 1982.
   Reviews the pathologic findings in open lung biopsies from 60 patients with farmer's lung. Granulomas were present in two-thirds and bronchiolitis obliterans in one-half of cases.

Roberts RC, Moore VL: Immunopathogenesis of hypersensitivity pneumonitis. Am Rev Respir Dis 116:1075–1090, 1977.
   Review article emphasizing immunologic mechanisms responsible for hypersensitivity pneumonia. Experimental hypersensitivity pneumonia in animal models is also discussed.

Rosenberg M, Patterson R, Mintzer R, Cooper BJ, Roberts M, Harris KE: Clinical and immunologic criteria for the diagnosis of allergic bronchopulmonary aspergillosis. Ann Intern Med 86:405–414, 1977.
   Defines primary and secondary diagnostic criteria for ABPA.

Safirstein BH, D'Souza MF, Simon G, Tai EH-C, Pepys J: Five-year follow-up of allergic bronchopulmonary aspergillosis. Am Rev Respir Dis 108:450–459, 1973.
   Includes 50 patients with ABPA followed for 5 years. Emphasizes the chronic nature of the disease with frequent recurrences and often lung destruction.

Schatz M, Patterson R, Fink J: Immunological lung disease. N Engl J Med 300:1310–1320, 1979.
   Review of basic immunologic mechanisms and their relationship to various immune-mediated lung diseases.

Sutinen S, Reijula K, Huhti E, Karkola P: Extrinsic allergic bronchiolo-alveolitis: Serology and biopsy findings. Eur J Respir Dis 64:271–282, 1983.
   Open lung biopsies from 14 patients with hypersensitivity pneumonitis were studied. Granulomas were present in all. The authors emphasize that the histologic appearance of hypersensitivity pneumonia is similar, regardless of the nature of the antigen.

Urschel HC, Paulson DL, Shaw RR: Mucoid impaction of the bronchi. Ann Thorac Surg 2:1–16, 1966.
   Reviews the clinical, radiographic, and pathologic findings in 85 cases of MIB.

Wang JLF, Patterson R, Roberts M, Ghory AC: The management of allergic bronchopulmonary aspergillosis. Am Rev Respir Dis 120:87–92, 1979.
   Outlines a therapy protocol for ABPA and emphasizes the usefulness of serial measurements of total serum IgE to monitor disease activity.

Wang JLF, Patterson R, Rosenberg M, Roberts M, Cooper BJ: Serum IgE and IgG antibody activity against Aspergillus fumigatus as a diagnostic aid in allergic bronchopulmonary aspergillosis. Am Rev Respir Dis 117:917–927, 1978.
   Found that specific IgE and IgG antibodies to A. fumigatus were elevated in patients with ABPA compared with controls. This test may help in diagnosing difficult cases as well as in recognizing early cases.

Chapter 107

Helminthic Diseases of the Lungs

Adel A. F. Mahmoud

Biology and Immunology
    Biology of Helminths
    Host-Parasite Relationship in Pulmonary Helminthiases

Approach to the Patient with Helminthic Infection
of the Lungs

Diseases Due to Nematodes (Roundworms)
    Ascariasis, Hookworms, and Strongyloidiasis
    Pulmonary Filariasis (Tropical Pulmonary Eosinophilia)
    Toxocariasis (Visceral Larva Migrans)

Diseases Due to Cestodes (Segmented Worms)
    Echinococcosis

Diseases Due to Trematodes
    Schistosomiasis
    Paragonimiasis

Parasitic helminths are a distinct group of infectious agents that are responsible for worldwide morbidity and mortality in humans. Individuals with helminthic infec-

tions of the lungs often seek medical advice because of one or more common chest complaints, i.e., cough, pain, or breathlessness. They pose a diagnostic challenge, particularly in areas where helminthic infections are not endemic, in that other more common causes of chest complaints have to be excluded, because a history of residence in certain geographic locations has to be elicited, and because the proper procedures for making the diagnosis of helminthiasis have to be selected.

In humans, worms produce a variety of pulmonary parenchymal and vascular diseases (Table 107-1). Because only certain stages in the life cycle of the parasite are infectious for humans, and because pulmonary lesions occur at a particular phase of the life cycle, familiarity with the biologic behavior of the organisms is essential for proper diagnosis and treatment.

BIOLOGY AND IMMUNOLOGY

Biology of Helminths

Worms are multicellular organisms that vary considerably in size (from a few millimeters to several meters). They are among the most developed and elaborate of human parasites. Their parasitic capabilities are such that they often parasitize more than one host and survive different hostile environments. Despite their relatively large size, the infective stages of worms invade human tissues either by ingestion, penetration of skin, or insect vectors. Furthermore, parasitic helminths have developed a myriad of mechanisms by which they can evade the protective mechanisms of the host.

A basic biologic generalization about helminthic infections is that the worms, as a rule, cannot multiply within the mammalian host. This phenomenon is impor-

TABLE 107-1
Pulmonary Parenchymal and Vascular Diseases Produced by Worms

Major Pulmonary Presentation	Infection	Causative Organism	Infective Stage	Pathogenic Stage
Loeffler-like syndrome	Ascariasis	*Ascaris lumbricoides*	Embryonated eggs in soil	Migrating larvae
	Hookworms	*Ancylostoma duodenale* *Necator americanus*	Larvae in soil Larvae in soil	Migrating larvae
	Strongyloidiasis	*Strongyloides stercoralis*	Larvae in soil	Migrating rhabditiform larvae
	Hyperinfection with *S. stercoralis*	*Strongyloides stercoralis*	Larvae in bowel	Migrating filariform larvae
Pulmonary eosinophilia	Lymphatic filariasis	*Wuchereria bancrofti* *Brugia malayi*	Larvae in mosquito	Microfilariae
Space-occupying lesions	Echinococcosis	*Echinococcus granulosus*	Eggs in soil	Hydatid cysts
	Paragonimiasis	*Paragonimus westermani*	Metacercariae	Adult worms
Vascular obstruction	Schistosomiasis	*Schistosoma mansoni,* *Schistosoma japonicum,* *Schistosoma haematobium*	Cercariae in fresh water	Eggs

tant for the understanding of the dynamics of helminthic infection and of the relationship between the intensity of a particular worm load within the host and its pathologic consequences. However, there are exceptions to this rule. For example, several of the worms that infect human lungs, such as *Strongyloides stercoralis* and *Echinococcus granulosus*, can increase their numbers within an individual even though the individual is not exposed to additional infective forms. This ability of *S. stercoralis* to autoinfect the same individual and cause a hyperinfection syndrome is of considerable clinical significance, especially in immunosuppressed patients, and often proves fatal. A different example is that of echinococcosis in which dissemination is usually a consequence of leakage or rupture of a hydatid cyst, thereby releasing its contents which seed sites elsewhere and initiate similar lesions.

Another biologic characteristic of worm infections, particularly of those affecting internal organs such as the lungs, is their association with eosinophilia in the peripheral blood and tissue. When eosinophilia is marked, this association provides a clinically useful sign of a migratory worm infection. The prominent peripheral blood eosinophilia of tissue migratory worm infections contrasts with the much more modest eosinophilia in individuals in whom the worm infection is confined to the gut lumen or in whom the infection is due to other agents, e.g., viruses or bacteria. The mechanism and specificity of this eosinophilic response depends on the integrity of the *cellular* immune response of the host: sensitized T lymphocytes produce mediators that induce differentiation in the bone marrow or progenitor cells into mature eosinophils; this is done either directly or via other cell products from mononuclear phagocytes. Eosinophilia does not occur in athymic nude mice infected with *Trichinella spiralis* or *Schistosoma mansoni*. Similarly, eosinophilia often does not feature prominently when strongyloidiasis occurs in immunosuppressed individuals. Although some of the specific mediators responsible for inducing proliferation and increasing production of eosinophils have been partially characterized, the specific helminth antigens responsible for initiating this response are unknown.

Recent investigations suggest that the increased eosinophil level that occurs in experimental animals or humans with helminthiasis is related to their biologic role as an integral component of host defenses. In vitro, eosinophils along with antibodies or complement kill the larval forms of several helminths. The killing of parasites is accompanied by a respiratory burst in these cells and evacuation of the contents of their granules onto the surface of the helminth. In vivo, depletion of eosinophils in experimental animals leads to loss of their acquired resistance to several helminth infections, such as *T. spiralis* and *S. mansoni*. Both oxidative and nonoxidative products of eosinophil granules have been implicated in target killing, but the specific effector molecules have not yet been de-

fined. The helminth-killing capability of human eosinophils is regulated by several effector mediators. Eosinophils obtained from individuals with high peripheral blood cell counts are known to be metabolically active. Recently, several products of helminth-T-lymphocyte-monocyte interaction have been shown to cause metabolic activation of eosinophils and to enhance their ability to kill extracellular helminth targets. It remains to be seen if activation or modulation of eosinophil function during the course of helminthic infections has a biologically meaningful role.

Host-Parasite Relationship in Pulmonary Helminthiases

Human disease caused by pulmonary helminthiases results from a heterologous group of factors. Several classes of helminths reside in human lungs during one or more of their parasitic stages. They include nematodes (roundworms), trematodes (flatworms), and cestodes (segmented worms). The stage of the life cycle that causes human pulmonary disease also varies, e.g., larvae of nematodes, eggs of schistosomes, and adult worms in paragonimiasis. The multiplicity and complex structure of these etiologic agents leads to a heterogenous set of responses, both immunologic and nonimmunologic. Moreover, disease may result from either the mechanical presence of worms (space-occupying lesions) and the associated inflammatory responses, or as a by-product of the host immune responses, or both. For example, in echinococcosis, hydatid cysts displace lung tissues, but in pulmonary schistosomiasis, the vascular obstructive lesions are predominantly the outcome of the delayed-hypersensitivity granulomatous response of the host. The understanding of host-parasite relationship in pulmonary helminthiasis is, therefore, based on appreciating the heterogeneity of etiologic agents and the corresponding host responses.

An additional and biologically relevant factor concerning helminthic infections and their role in etiology of human disease is the intensity of infection. Since most worm infections in humans cannot increase their population without additional exposure to the infective stages, the worm load generally determines to a large extent the degree of pathologic sequelae. For example, the number of schistosome eggs reaching the pulmonary circulation is an essential determinant of the severity of the induced disease. Although the number of eggs reaching the lungs may be influenced by several factors, the most important determinant is the number of adult worms in the infected individual.

The immune responses of the host often feature prominently in shaping the pathologic consequences of helminthic infection of the lungs. In experimental animals, the degree of tissue injury and host responsiveness to several helminthiases has been shown to be regulated by modulatory antibody and cellular responses.

Whether humans acquire resistance to helminthic infection and whether resistance can be induced has not been settled. Resistance against several helminths occurs in experimental animals after primary infection, and it can be induced by exposing the host to irradiated larval forms of the parasite. However, in most instances the resistance is only partial. The recent introduction of monoclonal antibodies and the technology for genetic engineering has made it possible to induce equivalent degrees of partial resistance by using special helminth components. Whether any of these candidate vaccines will reach the stage of practical application in humans remains to be seen.

APPROACH TO THE PATIENT WITH HELMINTHIC INFECTION OF THE LUNGS

As indicated above, the major symptoms and signs of pulmonary disease are common to most etiologic agents, noninfectious as well as infectious. Although helminth infections are, in general, particularly common in temperate and hot areas of the world, some are transmitted in the United States and in other colder and developed areas. A history that the patient has lived overseas or in certain parts of the United States is helpful in alerting the examiner to the possibility of a helminth infection. The geographic distribution of the major helminthic infections is roughly known. Also, some infections, such as with *E. granulosus*, are common in sheep-raising countries and in certain sheep-raising areas in the United States. Knowledge of the immunologic status of the patient is valuable in suspecting helminth infection, e.g., the hyperinfection syndrome caused by *S. stercoralis*.

Eosinophilia in peripheral blood, sputum, or pulmonary tissue is a helpful clue in directing the diagnostic workup. Although increased eosinophil counts do occur in several other pulmonary diseases, the close association with helminthic infections necessitates appropriate diagnostic procedures to define if a worm is involved. Definitive diagnosis of helminthic infections of the lungs requires isolation and identification of diagnostic stages in the life cycle of the parasite which routine examination of appropriate specimens may miss. Therefore, the appropriate laboratory personnel should be alerted to the possibility of a worm infection so that proper samples can be obtained and preserved for special examinations.

DISEASES DUE TO NEMATODES (ROUNDWORMS)

Ascariasis, Hookworms, and Strongyloidiasis

Human infections with *Ascaris lumbricoides*, with the hookworms *Ancylostoma duodenale* and *Necator americanus*, and with *S. stercoralis* are among the most preva-

lent helminthiases worldwide. Transmission also occurs in the southeastern United States.

ETIOLOGY

Human ascariasis (Fig. 107-1) results from ingestion of embryonated *A. lumbricoides* eggs that are contained in feces-contaminated soil. The disease follows ingestion of contaminated vegetables and fruits that have not been properly washed. *Ascaris* eggs hatch in the gastrointestinal tract, there producing larvae that penetrate the gut wall and migrate via venous blood and the right side of the heart to the lungs. Hookworms (*A. duodenale* and *N. americanus*) and *S. stercoralis* infect humans when infective larvae, found in soil, penetrate intact skin. Larvae of hookworms or of *S. stercoralis* travel via the bloodstream to the lungs (Fig. 107-1). The parasite larvae migrate via pulmonary capillaries into alveolar spaces. They then ascend toward the trachea to be swallowed en route to their final habitat in the small intestines. Although larvae are sometimes found in the sputum of infected individuals, more often the eggs (*A. lumbricoides*, *A. duodenale*, and *N. americanus*) or the larvae (*S. stercoralis*) are found in stools. Passage to the outside environment completes their life cycle, and they develop into stages infective for humans.

PATHOGENESIS AND PATHOLOGY

In nematode infections, the most prominent pulmonary pathologic changes occur in individuals with ascariasis or with the hyperinfection syndrome of strongyloidiasis. *Ascaris* pneumonia may occur 1 to 2 weeks after infection. Portions of larvae are seen in the pulmonary parenchyma surrounded by patchy infiltrate of neutrophils and eosinophils. The alveoli contain a serous exudate; the production of bronchial mucus is increased. Later, migrating larvae are destroyed within aggregates of eosinophils. The nature of the inflammatory process in *Ascaris* pneumonia suggests hypersensitivity. The intensity of the reaction depends on the number of parasite larvae and on previous sensitization. In areas in which transmission of *Ascaris* eggs occurs seasonally, pulmonary reactions are usually more in evidence during these periods.

In *immunocompetent individuals*, pulmonary disease caused by hookworms or *S. stercoralis* is unremarkable. However, infection with *S. stercoralis* can be life-threatening in *immunocompromised* individuals. Filariform larvae seem to develop prematurely in immunocompromised individuals and invade the gut wall and/or the perianal skin. Tissue migration occurs through most body organs, including the lungs. Initially, the pulmonary lesions resemble those of *Ascaris* pneumonia. In some patients, bronchopneumonia and lung abscesses develop. The lungs of fatal cases show intra-alveolar hemorrhages and inflammatory changes.

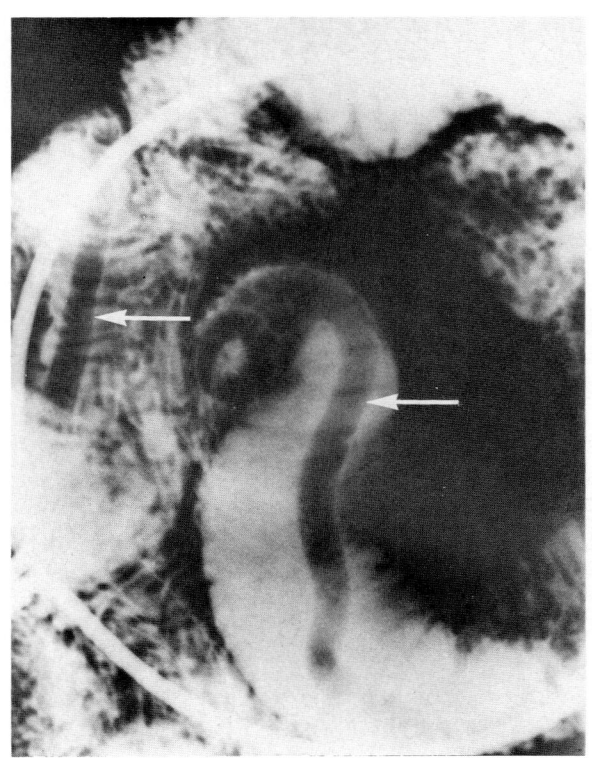
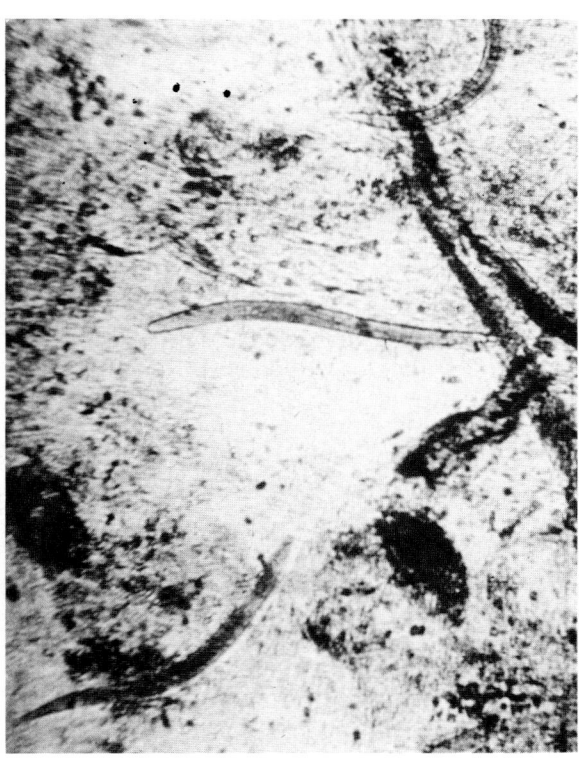

A

B

FIGURE 107-1 Nematodes. *A.* Ascariasis. Barium in the small intestine outlines two *Ascaris* worms (arrows). *(From Shaba, 1980.)* *B. Strongyloides stercoralis.* Rhabditiform larvae. *(Courtesy of Dr. Stanley H. Abadie.)*

CLINICAL FEATURES

The major clinical manifestations caused by infection of the lungs with the larval forms of intestinal nematodes resemble those of Loeffler's syndrome; these manifestations occur typically in patients with seasonal or *Ascaris* pneumonia. The symptoms include persistent, irritating and nonproductive cough, substernal pain, and, in the severely ill, hemoptysis and dyspnea. Eosinophilia is the most consistent laboratory finding. Radiographic signs, e.g., patchy or miliary infiltrate, are sometimes seen.

The onset of the Loeffler-like syndrome caused by intestinal nematodes usually occurs 2 to 3 weeks after infection, coincident with larval migration from the pulmonary circulation to the alveoli. This coincidence was illustrated by the occurrence of the syndrome in a group of students exposed to eggs of the pig roundworm *(Ascaris suum)*. Typical symptoms occurred 10 to 15 days later; some individuals developed marked respiratory failure. In locations where transmission of ascariasis is cyclical because of environmental factors, pneumonitis occurs seasonally. Mild symptoms are occasionally encountered in individuals with hookworm infection or in immunocompetent individuals who have strongyloidiasis.

The most clinically significant pulmonary syndrome induced by intestinal nematodes is caused by hyperinfec-

tion with *S. stercoralis* (Fig. 107-2). As a rule, the syndrome occurs in patients with compromised cell-mediated immunity although it is occasionally encountered in normal individuals. Immunosuppression is usually caused by neoplastic diseases, such as Hodgkin's, other lymphomas and leukemias, or nonmalignant conditions that are being treated by corticosteroids, e.g., organ transplantation. The sequence of events in immunosuppressed patients indicates that a change has occurred in the reproductive cycle of the parasite: in nonimmunosuppressed individuals, the rhabditiform larvae have to go to the outside world to transform into the infective filariform organisms; in immunosuppressed patients, the change to infective larvae occurs within the host. The organisms penetrate the intestinal mucosa resulting in massive invasion of almost every organ including the lungs. The major clinical features include asthma, pulmonary opacities and cavitation, consolidation, and diffuse focal infiltrates. Usually widespread dissemination of the nematode is accompanied by secondary infection caused by gram-negative organisms carried along with *S. stercoralis*. Eosinophilia is often absent in patients with the *S. stercoralis* hyperinfection syndrome, probably because of defective cell-mediated immunity. The *S. stercoralis* hyperinfection syndrome is highly fatal: the mortality is up to 77 percent.

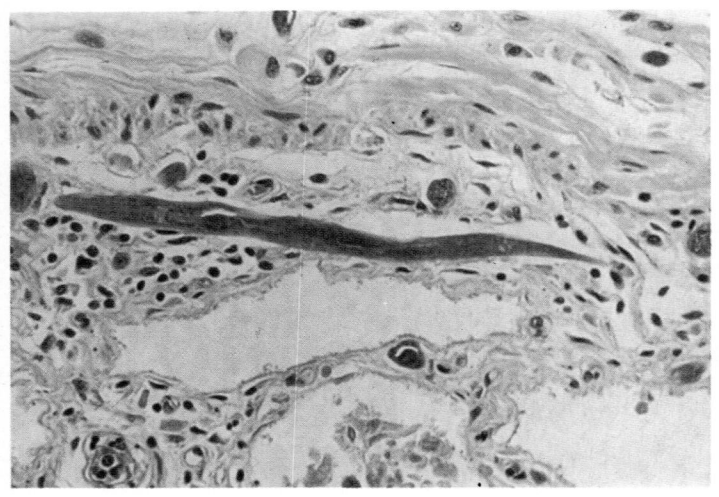
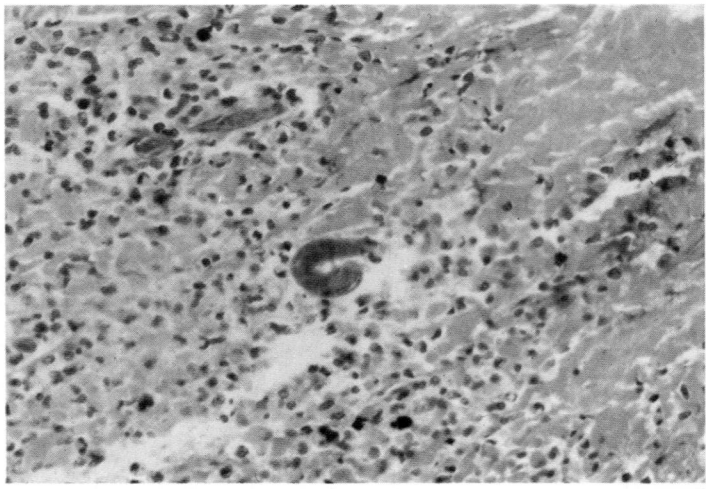

A   B

FIGURE 107-2   Strongyloidiasis.   A. 55-year-old man with chronic lymphocytic leukemia who presented with abdominal discomfort and weight loss. The patient developed progressive pulmonary congestion and edema with dyspnea, fever to 103°, and progressive hypotension before death. Blood cultures revealed *Escherichia coli*. Histologic section of colon at autopsy shows adult *Strongyloides stercoralis* in wall. B. 24-year-old male with AIDS who developed diarrhea, weight loss, and, finally, shock with *E. coli* bacteremia and strongyloidiasis. The larval form is shown in the jejunum. *(Courtesy of Dr. Jay A. Fishman.)*

MANAGEMENT

Diagnosis of infection with intestinal nematodes that causes Loeffler-like syndrome can be difficult. Only occasionally is the search for parasite larvae in sputum rewarding. Indeed, not infrequently definitive diagnosis is delayed for weeks until the adult worms mature in the small intestine. At this stage, fecal examination will disclose the characteristic eggs of hookworms or *Ascaris* or the larvae of *S. stercoralis*. The management of patients with the pulmonary manifestations of these parasitic worms is nonspecific and symptomatic. Reduction of exposure in areas where transmission of ascariasis is seasonal will decrease the prevalence and severity of clinical presentations. Specific antihelminthic therapy is ineffective during the pulmonary stage but can cure the infection once the parasites reach maturity in the small intestines.

Mebendazole is the drug of choice for treating ascariasis and hookworms. It is given orally, 100 mg per day for 2 to 3 days. Thiabendazole, 25 mg/kg body weight, twice daily for 2 days, is the recommended treatment for intestinal strongyloidiasis. In patients suspected of having the hyperinfection syndrome, early diagnosis, modification of the immunosuppressive therapy, and prompt antistrongyloides chemotherapy are the important elements in averting a fatal outcome. A high degree of suspicion that strongyloidosis is also present is needed in dealing with pulmonary disease associated with bacteremia in immunosuppressed patients. Most instances of strongyloidiasis in these patients are diagnosed at autopsy or shortly before death. Aggressive efforts at demonstrating *S. stercoralis* larvae entail repeated examination of stools and duodenal aspirates. Parasite larvae are also searched for in sputum and bronchial washings. In these patients, thiabendazole is started as early as possible and continued for 10 to 15 days.

Pulmonary Filariasis (Tropical Pulmonary Eosinophilia)

Persons living in areas endemic for *Wuchereria bancrofti* and *Brugia malayi* may present with an acute or chronic lung disease usually referred to as *tropical pulmonary eosinophilia*. This is still a poorly defined clinical entity. Its main features are a history of residence in filaria-endemic areas, particularly India, chronic nocturnal paroxysmal cough, marked eosinophilia, and a therapeutic response to the administration of diethylcarbamazine.

ETIOLOGY

Human infection with the tissue nematodes *W. bancrofti* or *B. malayi* can cause several amicrofilaremic syndromes, including tropical pulmonary eosinophilia. Infection is transmitted by the bite of several species of mosquitos, thereby introducing the infective third-stage larvae. These organisms undergo ill-defined maturational stages that culminate in the development of adult male and female worms that are usually situated in lymphatic vessels and lymph nodes. Mature worms deposit microfilariae that appear in peripheral circulation, often at maximum numbers at specific times of the day. However, some filariae show no periodicity with respect to the appearance of their microfilariae in peripheral blood. Microfilariae are taken up by mosquitos during their bites, thereby completing the life cycle of the parasite.

The life span of adult filariae is not known. Nonetheless, serologic or histopathologic evidence of infection can be obtained in the syndrome known collectively as *amicrofilaremic states*, even though larvae cannot be found in the blood. For example, in tropical pulmonary eosinophilia, high concentrations of antifilarial IgG and IgE in serum have been demonstrated despite invariably negative blood examinations for parasites. Also, despite the negative blood examinations, microfilariae have been found in lung and lymph node biopsies confirming the filarial etiology of this syndrome.

PATHOGENESIS AND PATHOLOGY

Patients with pulmonary filariasis *(tropical pulmonary eosinophilia)* show evidence of humoral hyperreactivity manifested as increased serum levels of total IgE and antifiliarial IgG and IgE. The possibility has been raised that these antibodies play a causal role in producing the pulmonary symptoms by inducing clearance of microfilariae and acute IgE-mediated responses which are manifested clinically as asthma and eosinophilic pulmonary infiltrates. Histopathologically, the earliest lesions are histiocytic infiltrates in the interstitium and alveolar spaces. In established cases, the cell infiltrate consists predominantly of eosinophils, lymphocytes, and histiocytes and it assumes a nodular configuration.

CLINICAL FEATURES

Young males are predominantly afflicted with tropical pulmonary eosinophilia. The syndrome is characterized by episodes of dry night cough, low grade fever, and general fatigue. Examination of the chest may reveal coarse rales and rhonchi along with wheezing. In many patients, pulmonary function tests disclose a restrictive pattern in which vital and total lung capacity and residual volumes are all decreased. Some patients with chronic disease have perfusion impairment. Radiographically, the syndrome may be associated with reticulonodular opacities and increased bronchovascular markings. The sera of these patients usually demonstrate high IgE levels and specific antibodies to the parasite. Eosinophil counts in peripheral blood generally exceed 3000 per cubic millimeter.

MANAGEMENT

Diagnosis is based on the typical clinical, radiographic, functional, and immunologic findings in the setting of an appropriate epidemiologic history, i.e., previous residence in a filaria-endemic area. A favorable response to diethylcarbamazine therapy confirms the diagnosis. The drug is usually administered as 5 mg/kg body weight per day in divided doses for 2 to 3 weeks. Recurrences of tropical pulmonary eosinophilia are rare. If they do occur, a second course of antihelminthic chemotherapy is indicated.

DIROFILARIASIS

Another filarial parasite, *Dirofilaria immitis* (dog heartworm), may accidentally be transmitted to humans via the bites of the mosquito intermediate vector (Fig. 107-3). Several cases have been reported in the United States. In most, the condition was discovered as a coin lesion on the chest radiograph. In some, cough, chest pain, hemoptysis, and eosinophilia were manifested. Definitive diagnosis is usually obtained by microscopic examination of excised lesions.

Toxocariasis (Visceral Larva Migrans)

Toxocariasis is due to human infection with animal parasites (dog or cat ascarids). It is most commonly encountered in children. The invading parasite larvae migrate in human tissues, but cannot mature to adult worms. *Toxocara canis* and *Toxocara catis* are the two recognized etiologic agents of human visceral larva migrans. They both are widely distributed, both in developing and developed countries.

ETIOLOGY

The eggs of *T. canis* and *T. catis* are passed in the stools of dogs and cats, respectively. Transmission to humans occurs by ingestion of embryonated eggs in the soil or by contamination of food. Larvae hatch in the small intestine, penetrate the gut wall, migrate to the liver, and are then carried via systemic veins to the systemic arterial circulation for distribution throughout the body. Larval migration through the host tissues and the associated inflammatory responses are considered responsible for the manifestations of disease in toxocariasis. Most of these manifestations relate to liver pathology, eosinophilia, and pulmonary involvement. The concentrations in serum of total and specific immunoglobulins are also increased.

PATHOGENESIS AND PATHOLOGY

Toxocara larvae remain viable in humans for many years. It is not clear whether tissue injury results from the invasion of different organs by the parasite larvae or from death and encapsulation of some organisms by an eosinophilic response by the host. The most commonly affected organ is the liver where granulomas surround parasite larvae. Similar lesions can be induced in experimental animals (Fig. 107-4). In the few fatal cases of toxocariasis, autopsy revealed that the major pathologic lesions were in the central nervous system.

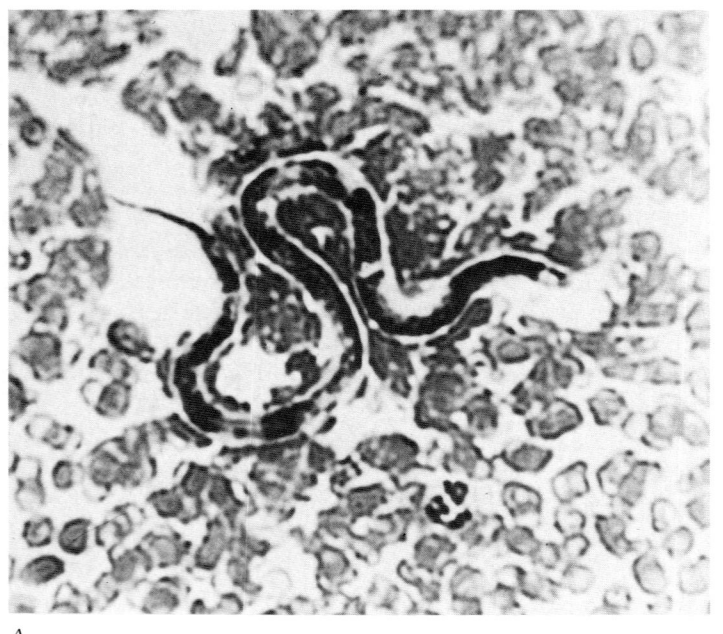

A

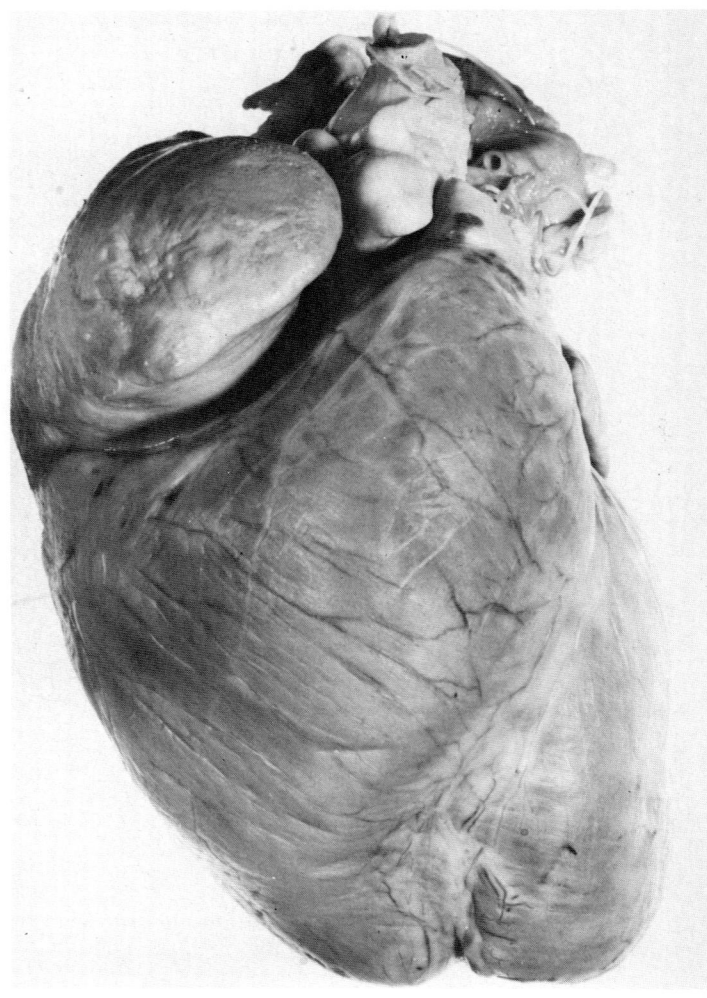

B

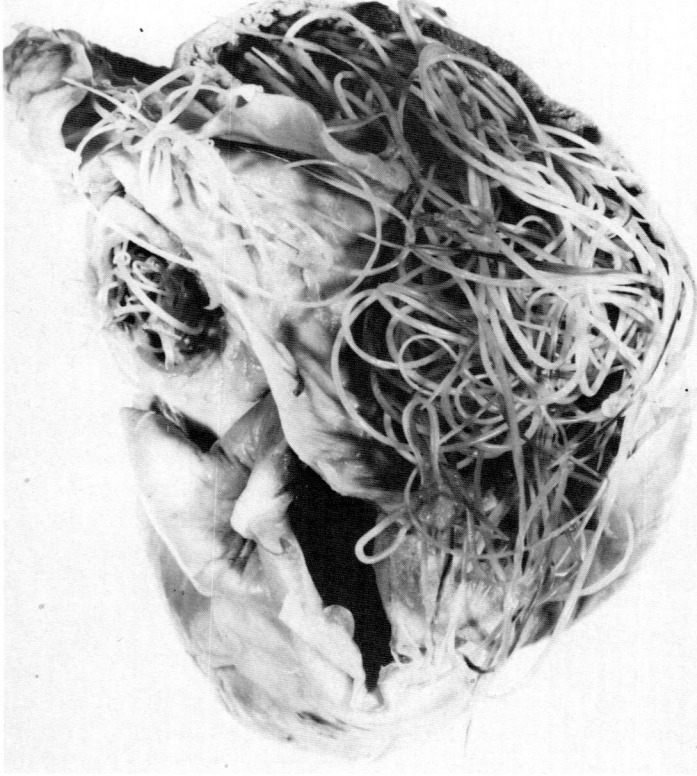

C

FIGURE 107-3 Pulmonary dirofilariasis in the dog. A. Microfilaria (D. immitis) in blood. B. Right ventricular hypertrophy due to dirofilariasis. C. Heartworms filling the right atrium and protruding through the pulmonary valve. (Courtesy of Dr. David H. Knight; from Shaba, 1980.)

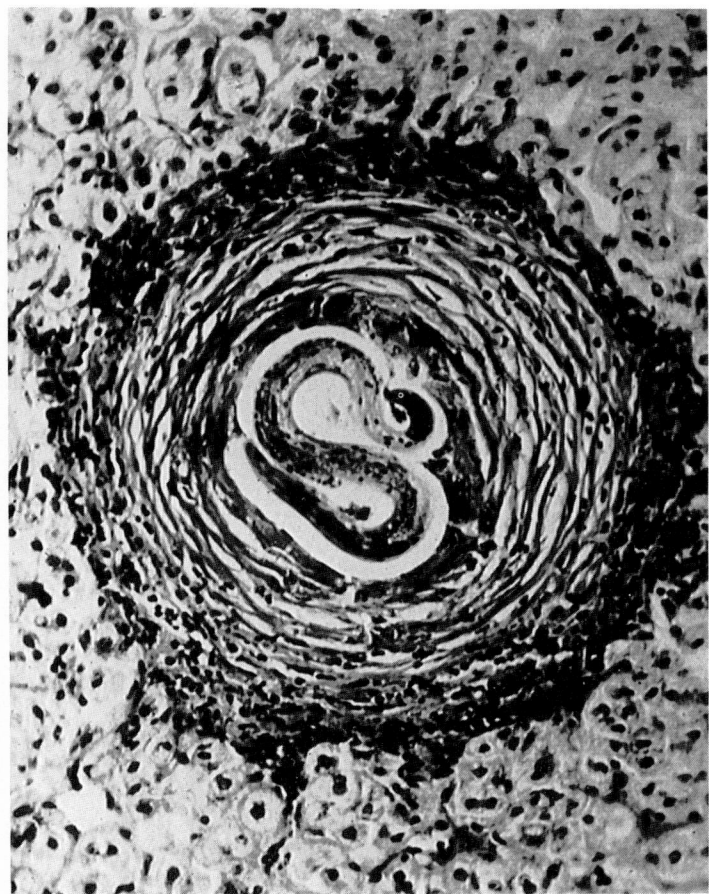

FIGURE 107-4 *Toxocara canis.* Granulomatous response to larvae in the liver. *(Courtesy of the American Society of Pathologists.)*

CLINICAL FEATURES

Toxocariasis is a disease of children 1 to 4 years of age. It is particularly common in those with a history of pica. The two main presenting features relate to the chest and abdomen. Pulmonary complaints, such as cough and wheezing, and pulmonary infiltrates occur in over one-third of symptomatic children. Peripheral eosinophilia is usually marked and may persist for years. In one study of serologically proven toxocariasis, hepatomegaly was present in 25 percent of patients.

MANAGEMENT

Toxocariasis is a cosmopolitan infection of children. Diagnosis is suspected because of the clinical presentation and serologic evidence of antitoxocara antibodies. Since the disease is usually benign and self-limiting and since the efficacy of most antihelminthics against *Toxocara* infection is doubtful, no specific therapy is recommended. Corticosteroids may be necessary to limit the inflammatory response in patients with extensive disease of the lungs or central nervous system.

RARE NEMATODE INFECTIONS

In severe human *T. spiralis* infection, pneumonitis occurs accompanied by eosinophilia. The pulmonary syndrome follows the intestinal phase of infection and is usually associated with other allergic manifestations of trichinosis, including periorbital edema, muscle swelling, and weakness.

Anisakiasis in humans results from infection with the larval forms of a nematode of marine mammals. The disease has been reported in Japan and Western Europe. Although it is usually manifested as an intestinal eosinophilic disorder, it has also been implicated as the probable cause of cough, eosinophilia, and pleural effusion.

DISEASES DUE TO CESTODES (SEGMENTED WORMS)

Echinococcosis

Human infection with the larval stage of the canine tapeworm *Echinococcus granulosus* is one of the most important helminthic pulmonary diseases. *E. granulosus* is worldwide in distribution; it occurs most commonly in sheep- and cattle-raising countries, particularly in Australia, South America, the Mediterranean, and some parts of Africa. The infection has also been reported in the United States.

ETIOLOGY

Adult *E. granulosus* is manifested by small tapeworms found in the intestines of dogs and wolves; they release eggs from their gravid segments which are passed in the feces. Humans acquire the infection by ingesting the eggs; embryos are then released and migrate to the liver, where most cysts in humans are found. Embryos may also migrate to the lungs or other tissues. Once the parasite has lodged in human tissues, it may develop in a space-occupying hydatid cyst. The inner lining of these cysts is a germinal layer capable of producing daughter cysts that may seed other organs upon spontaneous rupture or surgical manipulation of the original cyst (Fig. 107-5).

PATHOGENESIS AND PATHOLOGY

Hydatid cysts are more frequently found in the lungs of children than of adults. In most instances, the slowly enlarging, space-occupying lesion is well tolerated. Cysts in the lungs are usually discovered early in the course of the disease because radiographic examinations of the chest are now so common. Pulmonary cysts are usually solitary, in 72 percent of cases affecting one lobe. The classic unilocular hydatid cyst is usually fertile: its contents can seed other sites and start new cysts. The cyst is surrounded early in the course of infection by a granulomatous reaction on the part of the host; later, the inflammatory reaction is succeeded by fibrosis. Rupture of a fertile

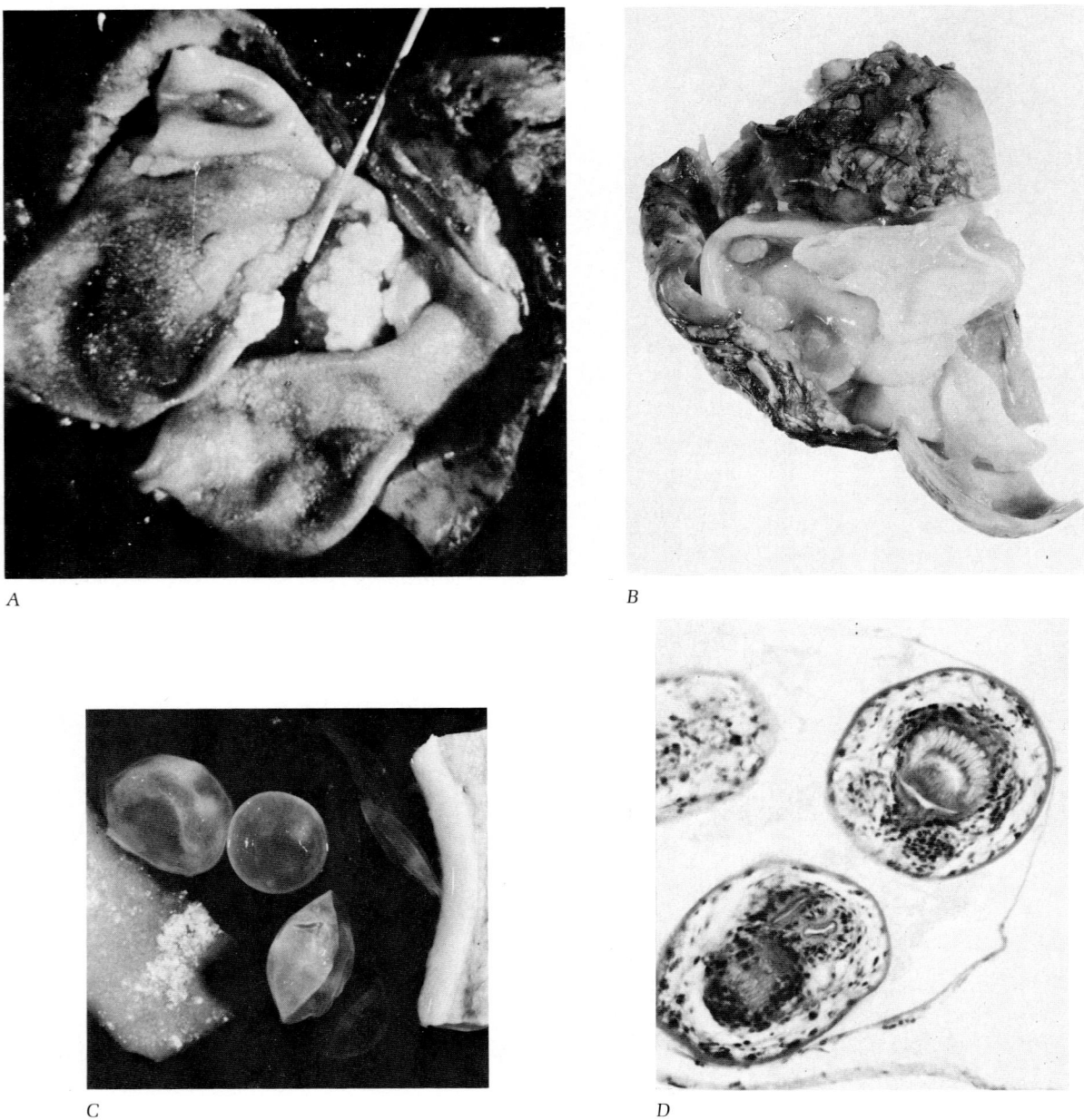

A

B

C

D

FIGURE 107-5   Echinococcosis.   A. Hydatid cyst in the lung. The glistening membrane constitutes the wall of the cyst.   B. Hydatid cysts in mesentary. Note similarity to appearance in the lung.   C. Fragment of liver on the right is lined with *Echinococcus* membrane. Brood capsules are on the left.   D. Three scoleces of *Echinococcus granulosus*. The upper right scolex shows the hooklets of the organism. *(A, courtesy of Dr. Stanley H. Abadie; B to D, courtesy of Dr. Daniel H. Connor, Armed Forces Institute of Pathology, illustration nos. 63-1059 and 70-4279 and accession no. 70-6734, respectively.)*

hydatid cyst may occur through a bronchus, leading to expectoration of scoleces in the sputum. Rupture into the mediastinum or pleural cavity can lead to secondary implantations. The fluid content of a hydatid cyst is believed to be immunogenic, and leakage of the cyst may evoke an anaphylactic response. Although eosinophilia has been reported to accompany hydatid disease of the lung, its frequency is not known.

CLINICAL FEATURES

Hydatid cysts are usually asymptomatic; approximately half of the clinically diagnosed cysts are in the lungs. Most patients with pulmonary hydatid disease are children. In about three quarters of the patients, the cysts are in one lung lobe. Approximately half of the patients present with cough; smaller fractions present with dyspnea or

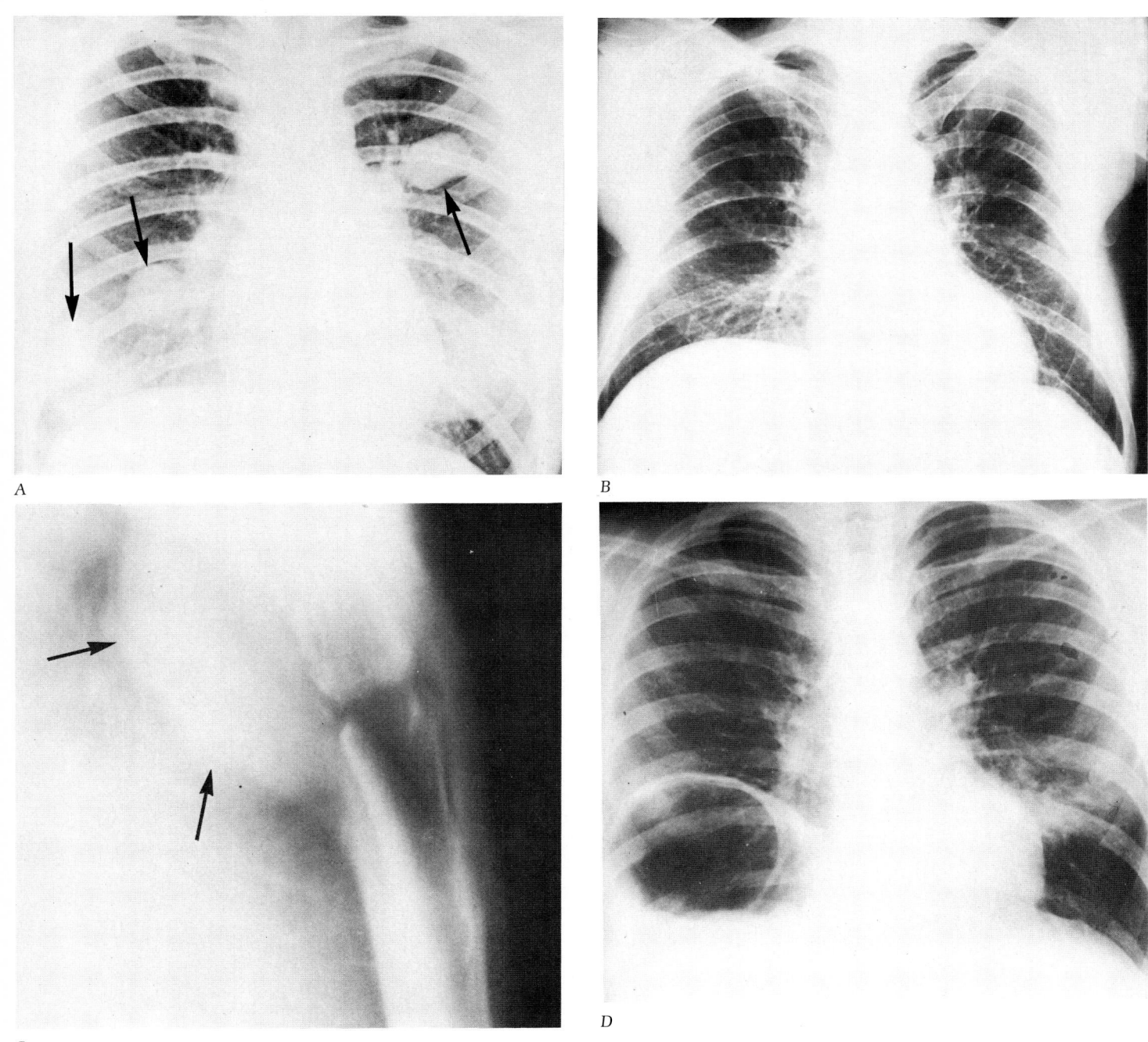

FIGURE 107-6 Echinococcosis. *A.* Multiple pulmonary cysts (arrows). *(Courtesy of Dr. Carl Heitz.)* *B.* Another patient with echinococcus cyst behind the sternum. The retrosternal mass is difficult to discern on the posteroanterior radiograph. *C.* Lateral view. Mass (cyst) is seen (arrows). *D.* Hydatid cyst, right lower lobe. *(Courtesy of Dr. Philip Lerner.)*

chest pain. On chest radiograph, the lesions vary in diameter from 1 to 20 cm; sometimes the cyst is surrounded by an area of pneumonitis or atelectasis. Less often, a fluid level, "water lily sign" (Fig. 107-6), or calcification is seen. Other diagnostic procedures, e.g., computed tomography, may be useful in improving characterization of the lesions.

MANAGEMENT

In most instances, diagnosis of the hydatid nature of a pulmonary cyst depends on immunologic procedures. The double diffusion test which detects arc-5 is the most sensitive and specific. Surgery is the treatment of choice for hydatid disease of the lungs. The Barrett procedure is

currently recommended for small- or moderate-size cysts; the open method, in which the parasite cyst is removed but the cavity is left draining to the pleural space, is preferred for large cysts. More extensive procedures, such as lobectomy and segmental resection, may not be necessary for most pulmonary hydatid cysts.

There is no satisfactory medical treatment for hydatid disease in humans. Mebendazole and albendazole have been tried experimentally. Although albendazole does show promise, further evaluation is needed before it can be recommended, particularly in treating patients with recurrent or multiple cysts.

DISEASES DUE TO TREMATODES

Schistosomiasis

Schistosomal infections of humans represent one of the major endemic helminthiases in Southeast Asia, the Middle East, Africa, the Caribbean, and South America. Three species represent the most common and clinically significant infections: *Schistosoma haematobium*, *S. mansoni*, and *S. japonicum*.

ETIOLOGY

The schistosomes are blood flukes; in humans, they inhabit the venous system around the urinary bladder or the small and large intestine. Human infection is initiated by penetration of intact skin by the free-living cercariae that are shed by specific freshwater snails. The cercariae change within a few hours into schistosomula, which migrate from the subcutaneous tissues to the lungs and then the liver where they mature into adult worms. Fecund adult parasites then migrate to their final habitat: the veins around the ureters and urinary bladder (*S. haematobium*) and the mesenteric veins (*S. mansoni* and *S. japonicum*). Adult worms deposit eggs that are intended to pass via the lumen of ureters or gut to the outside environment in order to complete the life cycle of the parasite. However, some of these ova may be trapped in the host tissues. Other ova may be carried by the venous circulation to the heart and then lungs. In *S. haematobium* infection, schistosome eggs reach the pulmonary circulation via the inferior vena cava. Eggs of the other two species (*S. mansoni* and *S. japonicum*) reach the systemic circulation after the development of portal hypertension and portosystemic anastomosis.

PATHOGENESIS AND PATHOLOGY

Schistosome eggs reach the pulmonary circulation via routes that depend on the species of the parasite, their final habitat, and the stage of infection. Because *S. haematobium* worms parasitize the vesicle plexus which connects directly with the inferior vena cava, egg seeding to the lungs may occur at any phase of infection. In contrast, the anatomic location of *S. mansoni* and *S. japonicum* adult worms in the mesenteric veins does not allow parasite ova to travel through the portal to the hepatic, and subsequently systemic, circulations. Eggs of these two species are believed to reach the lungs only in the late stages of infection after portal hypertension develops and anastomotic channels open between the portal and systemic circulations.

Upon reaching the pulmonary circulation, schistosome eggs usually impact in small arterioles where they induce the formation of granulomas made up of eosinophils, lymphocytes, and macrophages (Fig. 107-7). In addition, deposition of fibrous tissue causes narrowing, thickening, and occlusion of pulmonary arterioles. In a recent autopsy study of 32 cases of *S. mansoni* cor pulmonale, two characteristic histopathologic lesions were identified: (1) focal changes related directly to the presence of schistosome eggs; these were located either within the alveolar tissue or within the pulmonary arteries or arteri-

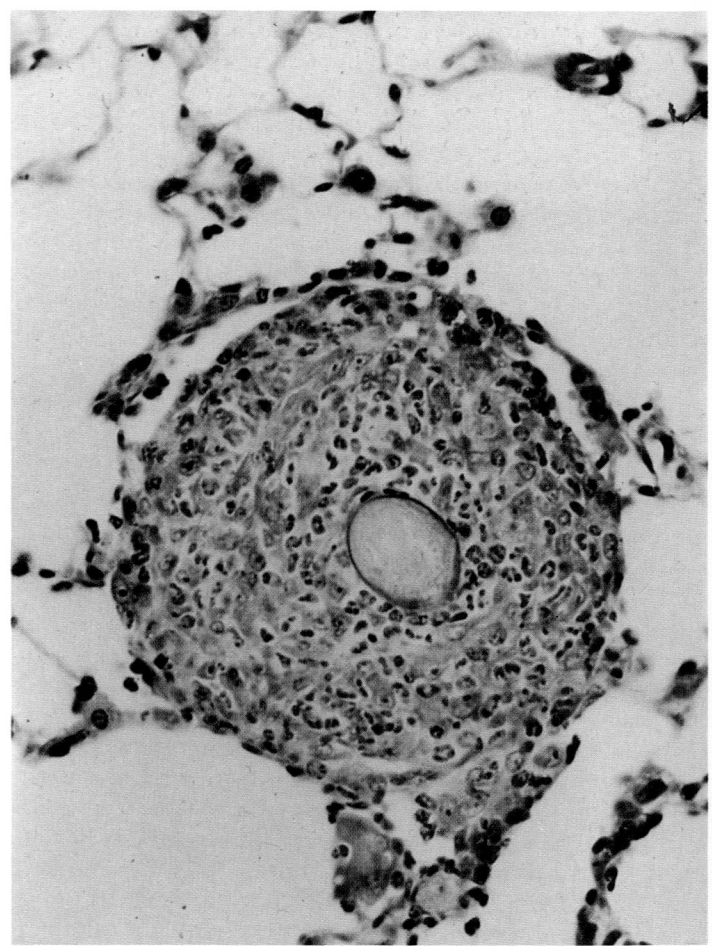

FIGURE 107-7 Schistosomal granuloma. (*Courtesy of Dr. Jay A. Fishman.*)

oles; and (2) plexiform or angiomatoid lesions consisting of several thin-walled and dilated vessels. The most prominent vascular lesions were associated with the focal changes surrounding mature schistosome eggs in the lumen of pulmonary arteries or arterioles. These were accompanied by fibrin deposition and remarkable proliferation of endothelial cells. Fibrosis surrounds most focal lesions. Because of the curtailment of the pulmonary vasculature and the decreased distensibility caused by the perivascular fibrosis, pulmonary hypertension and cor pulmonale ensue. Pulmonary function tests are predominantly restrictive in nature and accompanied by a decrease in the diffusing capacity.

CLINICAL FEATURES

It is not clear whether schistosome infection during its early phases in humans is associated with appreciable pulmonary disease. Migration of schistosomula through human lungs is not known to cause detectable symptoms or signs. In contrast, after the onset of oviposition, some ova may reach the lungs, particularly in S. haematobium infection. Furthermore, chronic infection with either S. mansoni or S. japonicum may be associated with sufficient deposition of eggs in the lungs to cause the development of cor pulmonale. The clinical features and radiographic findings in schistosomal pulmonary hypertension and cor pulmonale are not distinctive (see Chapter 64). The prevalence of the pulmonary hypertensive syndrome in schistosome-infected patients is not known. In Egypt, 7.5 percent of patients hospitalized with schistosomal hepatomegaly had cor pulmonale; in Brazil, 23 percent of similar patients had pulmonary hypertension, i.e., pulmonary arterial blood pressure higher than 20 mmHg.

MANAGEMENT

Diagnosis of pulmonary disease due to schistosomiasis may be achieved by finding the parasite eggs in urine or stools of individuals with suggestive clinical manifestations. However, pulmonary disease may occur several years after infection, and finding parasite ova may be difficult. Under these circumstances, demonstrating the characteristic pathologic changes and ova in tissues may settle the diagnosis.

Active schistosome infections are treated with praziquantel which kills adult worms and stops further tissue destruction of tissue by ova deposition. The drug is administered as a single oral dose of 40 mg/kg body weight for S. mansoni and S. haematobium infection and in a dose of 20 mg/kg body weight tid for S. japonicum infection. However, reversal of pathologic lesions in the lungs after antischistosomal chemotherapy has not been documented.

Paragonimiasis

Human infection with species of the lung fluke *Paragonimus* is prevalent in the Far East, Africa, and South and Central America. Infection is maintained in endemic areas through contamination of water sources with feces or sputum of infected individuals resulting in infection of the intermediate snail and crustacean hosts. Symptomatic paragonimiasis is initially characterized by cough and bloody sputum that may lead to bronchiectasis or lung abscesses.

ETIOLOGY

Human infection with *Paragonimus* is acquired by eating raw or pickled crustacea (freshwater crayfish and crabs) that harbor the infective parasite stage (metacercariae). These forms excyst in the duodenum, penetrate the intestinal wall, and migrate via the diaphragm and pleural cavity to the lungs where they mature into adult worms (12 × 6 × 5 mm). Adult *Paragonimus* worms are hermaphroditic; they produce golden brown eggs which are coughed up and voided either through sputum or feces. The life cycle of the parasite outside the human host goes through a specific snail intermediate host; metacercariae then encyst on freshwater crustacea.

PATHOGENESIS AND PATHOLOGY

The primary site of infection in humans is the lungs. The worm is also found in the brain in 25 percent of patients and less often in many other tissues. During invasion of the lungs by the maturing adult worms, parasite tunnels in the pulmonary parenchyma can usually be demonstrated, particularly in peripheral areas. The tunnels and parasites are surrounded by a granulocytic reaction made of eosinophils and neutrophils. Charcot-Leyden crystals are often seen. In patients with encysted worms, the parasites are enclosed with cystic lesions that may communicate with each other or with a bronchus. Death of the worms usually leads to collapse of the cyst, disintegration of the parasite, and fibrosis or calcification. The surrounding pulmonary tissue may show evidence of atelectasis, bronchiectasis, or compensatory emphysema. In some patients, secondary infection and lung abscess develop in the cystic lesions surrounding adult parasites. The radiographic changes correspond roughly to the three stages of parasite development within the lungs: maturing worms upon arrival in the lungs are associated with the development of radiographic opacities; these are succeeded by nodules that correspond to the parasite cysts; finally, fibrosis or calcification ensues.

CLINICAL FEATURES

The incubation period between infection and the development of maturing adults in the lungs is 2 to 20 days. Few

specific symptoms have been described during this stage. In individuals with established infection, the worm load seems to determine the extent of clinical features. Light infection is invariably asymptomatic. Moderate-to-heavy worm loads, complaint of cough and respiratory discomfort particularly upon rising in the morning, rusty blood-tinged sputum containing parasite eggs, necrotic material, and Charcot-Leyden crystals are common. Frank hemoptysis, sometimes severe, also occurs in patients with pulmonary paragonimiasis.

The chest radiograph is normal in 10 to 20 percent of infected individuals. The radiographic signs in the others include infiltrate, cavitation, fibrosis, and pulmonary thickening. The characteristic ring shadow with a crescent corona occurs in some infected individuals.

MANAGEMENT

The diagnosis of paragonimiasis is made by detection of the characteristic eggs in the sputum or stools of infected individuals. Serologic testing may be helpful in egg-negative cases. The drug of choice for treating paragonimiasis is praziquantel. It is administered orally, 75 mg/kg per day for 2 days. Chemotherapy usually leads to cessation of egg passage in sputum and stools, some clearing of the chest radiograph in almost two-thirds of treated patients, and a decrease in serum IgG antibodies against the parasite.

BIBLIOGRAPHY

Adkins RB, Dao AH: Pulmonary dirofilariasis: A diagnostic challenge. South Med J 77:372–374, 1984.
    A description of a patient presenting with right lower lobe pulmonary nodule due to D. immitis infection. A discussion of the parasitologic and clinical aspects of the syndrome is included.

Al-Omeri M, Wasif SN: Surgical management of hydatid disease of the lung. J R Coll Surg (Edinburgh) 29:218–220, 1984.
    A report on the experience of two surgeons in treating 346 cases of hydatid disease of the lung.

Aytac A, Yurdakul Y, Ikizler C, Olga R, Saylam A: Pulmonary hydatid disease: Report of 100 patients. Ann Thorac Surg 23:145–151, 1977.
    A detailed description of 100 patients with hydatid disease of the lungs and experience in surgical treatment. Immunologic diagnosis included is outdated.

Gelpi AP, Mustafa A: Ascaris pneumonia. Am J Med 44:377–389, 1968.
    A good clinical description of Ascaris pneumonia as it occurs in an area with seasonal transmission of infection. Investigations and chemotherapy may be outdated.

Giannoulis E, Arvanitakis C, Zaphiropoulos A, Nakos V, Karkavelas G, Haralambidis S: Disseminated strongyloidiasis with uncommon manifestations in Greece. J Trop Med Hyg 89:171–178, 1986.
    This report describes an unusual case of severe disseminated strongyloidiasis, with intestinal, pulmonary and neurological manifestations, in a previously healthy male. Response to mebendazole treatment was prompt and complete.

Igra-Siegman Y, Kapila R, Sen P, Kaminski ZC, Louria DB: Syndrome of hyperinfection with Strongyloides stercoralis. Rev Infect Dis 3:397–407, 1981.
    Description of the course of hyperinfection with S. stercoralis in two immunosuppressed patients. The article includes a review of 103 previously reported cases and examines the underlying conditions and role of secondary bacterial infection in morbidity and mortality.

Johnson JR, Falk A, Iber C, Davies S: Paragonimiasis in the United States. A report of nine cases among immigrants. Chest 82:168–171, 1982.
    Clinical and laboratory features of paragonimiasis in infected Laotian immigrants. Cases were treated before the introduction of praziquantel.

Johnson RJ, Jong EC, Dunning SB, Carberry WL, Minshew BH: Paragonimiasis: Diagnosis and the use of praziquantel in treatment. Rev Infect Dis 7:200–206, 1985.
    Praziquantel is a new safe effective broad-spectrum antihelminth. The article evaluates clinical and parasitologic findings in eight patients with paragonimiasis treated with praziquantel. It also includes a review of the epidemiologic and clinical aspects of pulmonary paragonimiasis.

Lal RB, Paranjape RS, Briles DE, Nutman TB, Ottesen EA: Circulating parasite antigen(s) in lymphatic filariasis: Use of monoclonal antibodies to phosphocholine for immunodiagnosis. J Immunol 138:3454–3460, 1987.
    A sensitive monoclonal antibody (CA101)-based ELISA for measuring circulating parasite antigen detected antigen in the sera of 93% of patients with microfilaremia, 46% of those with lymphatic obstruction, and 56% of patients with the tropical pulmonary eosinophilia syndrome.

Mahmoud AAF: The ecology of eosinophils in schistosomiasis. J Infect Dis 145:613–622, 1982.
A detailed review of the mechanisms of eosinophilia and the functional role of these cells in antihelminth immunity.

Mahmoud AAF: Schistosomiasis, in Warren KS, Mahmoud AAF (eds), *Tropical and Geographical Medicine.* New York, McGraw-Hill, 1984, pp 433–457.
A detailed description of human schistosomes, and the corresponding clinical syndromes in individual patients and in populations of endemic communities.

Mahmoud AAF: Praziquantel for the treatment of helminthic infections. Adv Intern Med 32:193–206, 1987.
This new broad-spectrum antihelminthic agent has been a significant addition to the chemotherapy of these infections. The article details the pharmacology and clinical applications of praziquantel.

Mariano EG, Borja SR, Vruno MJ: A human infection with *Paragonimus kellicotti* (lung fluke) in the United States. Am J Clin Pathol 86:685–687, 1986.
A first case of Paragonimus kellicotti infection in the United States, involving a nonimmigrant adult, is reported.

Milder JE, Walzer PD, Kilgore G, Rutherford I, Klein M: Clinical features of *Strongyloides stercoralis* infection in an endemic area in the United States. Gastroenterology 80:1481–1488, 1981.
A recent description of strongyloidiasis in a group of 56 patients with no apparent immunosuppression. The presenting feature is mainly gastrointestinal, and response to therapy is uniformly excellent.

Miller TA: Hookworm infection in man. Adv Parasitol 17:315–383, 1979.
A complete and fairly critical review of the parasitologic and clinical aspects of hookworm infection and disease in humans.

Neva FA, Ottesen EA: Current concepts in parasitology. Tropical (filarial) eosinophilia. N Engl J Med 298:1129–1131, 1978.
A critical evaluation of the clinical and pathophysiological aspects of tropical pulmonary eosinophilia and its filarial etiology.

Novick RJ, Tchervenkov CI, Wilson JA, Munro DD, Mulder DS: Surgery for thoracic hydatid disease: A North American experience. Ann Thorac Surg 43:681–686, 1987.
The clinical course of 20 patients with 22 thoracic hydatid cysts operated on from 1957 to 1984, is reviewed. The prevalence of ruptured cysts and infected hepatic cysts involving the lung was higher than in most other series.

Ottesen EA: Filariasis and tropical eosinophilia, in Warren KS, Mahmoud AAF (eds), *Tropical and Geographical Medicine.* New York, McGraw-Hill, 1984, pp 390–410.
A detailed examination of the syndromes caused by human filarial infections. The classification of disease manifestations during microfilaremic and amicrofilaremic phases is important for understanding the etiology and pathophysiology of tropical filarial eosinophilia.

Pan American Zoonoses Center, PAHO/WHO: The arc-5 double diffusion test or the immunodiagnosis of human hydatid disease. Ramos Mejia. Buenos Aires (Tech. Note 22).
Description and evaluation of the echinococcosis immunodiagnostic method involving detection of arc-5.

Pawlowski ZS: Ascariasis: Host pathogen biology. Rev Infect Dis 4:806–814, 1982.
A summary of host-parasite relationship in ascariasis.

Phills JA, Harrold AJ, Whiteman GV, Perelmutter L: Pulmonary infiltrates, asthma, and eosinophilia due to *Ascaris suum* infestation in man. N Engl J Med 286:965–970, 1972.
Description of the clinical course in a group of male students who had been exposed to a massive dose of A. suum eggs.

Prata A: Infection with *Schistosoma mansoni,* in Jordan P, Webbe G (eds), *Schistosomiasis: Epidemiology, Treatment and Control.* London, Heinemann Medical Books, 1982, pp 105–127.
General description of the clinical syndromes associated with S. mansoni infection in humans.

Rausch RL, Wilson JF, McMahon BJ, O'Gorman MA: Consequences of continuous mebendazole therapy in alveolar hydatid disease—with a summary of a ten-year clinical trial. Ann Trop Med Parasitol 80:403–419, 1986.
A ten-year clinical trial of continuous therapy in eight patients provided evidence of a significant therapeutic effect of mebendazole on alveolar hydatid disease.

Romeo DP, Pollock JJ: Pulmonary paragonimiasis: Diagnostic value of pleural fluid analysis. South Med J 79:241–243, 1986.
Pleural fluid with a glucose content of less than 10 ml/dl and LDH level greater than 1000 IU/L, eosinophilia, a high protein value, and low pH are characteristic of paragonimiasis.

Sadigursky M, Andrade ZA: Pulmonary changes in schistosomal cor pulmonale. Am J Trop Med Hyg 31:779–784, 1982.
Careful histopathologic and plastic vascular castings of the lung lesions in 32 autopsy cases of schistosomal cor pulmonale.

Saksouk FA, Fahl MH, Rizk GK: Computed tomography of pulmonary hydatid disease. J Comput Assist Tomogr 10:226–232, 1986.
Certain pathognomonic features of ruptured or complicated hydatid cysts can be better visualized by CT than by conventional radiography. These include detached or collapsed endocyst membrane(s), collapsed daughter cyst membranes, and intact daughter cysts.

Schad GA, Banwell JG: Hookworms, in Warren KS, Mahmoud AAF (eds), *Tropical and Geographical Medicine*. New York, McGraw-Hill, 1984, pp 359–372.
An up-to-date examination of the problem of hookworm infection in humans from the parasitologic, clinical, and population aspects.

Shaba JK: Protozoan and metazoan infections, in Fishman AP (ed), *Pulmonary Diseases and Disorders*. New York, McGraw-Hill, 1980, pp 1182–1201.
A review of protozoan and metazoan diseases of the lungs as opportunistic infections, as part of extrapulmonary parasitic infections and as a consequence of spread from beneath the diaphragm.

Singh TS, Mutum SS, Razaque MA: Pulmonary paragonimiasis: Clinical features, diagnosis and treatment of 39 cases in Manipur. Trans R Soc Trop Med Hyg 80:967–971, 1986.
Thirty-nine cases of pulmonary paragonimiasis due to Paragonimus westermani were identified in Manipur, India. Bithionol [2,2'-thiobis (4,6-dichlorophenol)] orally, 40 mg/kg body weight/day, 10 to 25 doses, cured all patients and, except in one, side effects were minimal.

Warren KS: Experimental pulmonary schistosomiasis. Trans R Soc Trop Med Hyg 58:228–233, 1964.
Pulmonary schistosomiasis can be induced in mice following partial ligation of the portal vein early in the course of infection. This results in the development of collateral circulation, and approximately 20 percent of the eggs were recovered from the lungs. Granuloma formation resulted with arteritis, and many of the animals developed systemic venous hypertension.

Warren KS, Mahmoud AAF: Tropical and Geographical Medicine. New York, McGraw-Hill, 1984.
A reference textbook on the infections and nutritional diseases of the developing world. Special emphasis is given to the biology of causative agents and clinical disease in individual patients and populations in endemic areas.

Warren KS, Mahmoud AAF: *Geographical Medicine for the Practitioner*, 2d ed. New York, Springer-Verlag, 1985.
A concise description of the most common parasitic, bacterial and viral infections that may be imported to the United States. Emphasis is on developing a step-by-step approach to diagnosis and management.

Webster LT Jr: Drugs used in the chemotherapy of helminthiasis, in Gilman AG, Goodman LS, Raal TW, Murad F (eds), *The Pharmacological Basis of Therapeutics*, 7th ed. New York, Macmillan, 1985, pp 1009–1028.
An up-to-date examination of the pharmacology and efficacy of drugs used in the treatment of helminthiases.

Yarzabal LA, Leiton J, Lopez-Lemes MH: The diagnosis of human pulmonary hydatidosis by the immunoelectrophoresis test. Am J Trop Med Hyg 23:662–666, 1974.
Evaluation of sera from 111 individuals with suspected pulmonary hydatid cysts including 54 subsequently confirmed at surgery. The immunoelectrophoresis was used to demonstrate the specificity of arc-5 and evaluate its sensitivity as a diagnostic method.

Chapter 108

Principles Governing Use of Antibiotics in Pulmonary Infections

Harold C. Neu

Selection of an Antimicrobial Agent
  Testing Susceptibility and Efficacy
  Bacteriostatic versus Bactericidal

Pharmacologic Considerations

Pharmacokinetics of Antimicrobial Agents
in Respiratory Secretions

Special Considerations in Using Antimicrobial Agents
Failure of Chemotherapy

The chemotherapy of pulmonary infections dates from the 1930s with the introduction of the sulfonamides. By the mid-1940s, the value of penicillin G in the therapy of pneumococcal pneumonia was clear. In 1961 the newer semisynthetic penicillins were developed in response to the specter of penicillinase-producing staphylococci. Cephalosporin antibiotics and the aminoglycosides were synthesized in the 1960s. Under study are the 4-quinolones which hold great promise for certain respiratory infections.

Concomitant with the development of this array of antibacterial agents has been the emergence of an increasing resistance of bacteria to the drugs. This has prompted further search for structural modifications of antibiotics to overcome the resistance.

The chemotherapy of tuberculosis has progressed with the availability of drugs of low toxicity, such as ethambutol and rifampin, but progress in the development of agents to treat pulmonary fungal infections in the ever-increasing number of immunocompromised hosts has been slow. Indeed, the few agents available have defects from the standpoints of both inhibitory activity and their pharmacology in human beings. *Pneumocystis carinii* pneumonia in patients with AIDS has been a major target for use of trimethoprim-sulfamethoxazole and of the antiparasitic agent pentamidine. Mebendazole and albendazole have been used to treat echinococcosis of the lung, and praziquantel has been useful in schistosomiasis.

SELECTION OF AN ANTIMICROBIAL AGENT

The selection of the appropriate antibacterial agent for a pulmonary infection is based on knowledge of the infecting organism, which is derived from clinical and epidemiologic clues as well as appropriate stains and culture. Experience with anaerobic pleuropulmonary infections and with fungal and parasitic infections of the lung has taught that, unless adequate material for culture or tissue examination is obtained, it is impossible to select a rational chemotherapeutic program. Initial therapy of pulmonary infection is often based on the triad of purulent sputum, infiltrate noted on a chest radiograph, and fever. Therapy may subsequently be modified by results of culture if the organisms are found not to be those originally anticipated. Unlike infections of the bloodstream or even the urinary tract, in which isolation of a single pathogenic species is the rule, cultures of the respiratory tract often yield numerous organisms, many of which may not be the significant pathogen. Furthermore, except in situations such as the aspiration of pleural fluid, culture of material from the lung usually is contaminated by organisms of the oropharynx. Use of antimicrobial agents changes the oral flora. Hospitalization, per se, results in colonization of the oropharynx with gram-negative enteric species. These factors must always be considered when determining which antimicrobial agent is most appropriate. It is crucial to remember that the pulmonary signs of infection need not resolve in the same way as do urinary or wound infections. Accordingly, neither radiographic evidence of disease nor the repeated isolation of bacteria from sputum constitutes an absolute indication for prolonging, or continuing, a chemotherapeutic program.

Antibiotics are usually selected for the chemotherapy of infection on the basis of three factors: known susceptibility of the infecting species (Table 108-1), the lowest degree of toxicity, and expense, particularly in the outpatient setting. At one time, some organisms, such as *Streptococcus pneumoniae*, were consistently sensitive to penicillin G. Others, such as *Hemophilus influenzae*, were inhibited by ampicillin. This is no longer true.

Testing Susceptibility and Efficacy

A number of different methods are available for testing susceptibility to antibiotics. The most commonly used method is a filter paper disk impregnated with the antibiotic (Kirby-Bauer method). Zones of inhibition of bacteria growth on an agar plate reflect the inhibitory level of the antibiotic, which is related in turn to the serum levels that can be achieved by administering the particular agent to the patient. In general, susceptibilities determined using disks apply to pulmonary infections, since the lung is a highly perfused organ, so that serum levels probably reflect pulmonary tissue levels. Agar disk diffusion studies

TABLE 108-1
Pharmacokinetic Data and Antibacterial Activity of Agents Commonly Used to Treat Pulmonary Infections*

Antibiotic	Dose	Route	Average Peak Serum Level, µg/ml	Average Serum Half-Life, h	Range of Sputum Bronchial Levels µg/ml	Antibiotic Concentrations, µg/ml, to Inhibit Gram-Positive	Gram-Negative
Benzyl penicillin	600,000 U	IM	6	1.0	0.06–0.5		
	600,000 U	IV	35	0.5			
	4 × 10^6 U	IV	270	0.5	0.1–1.0	0.05–0.5	
Procaine penicillin	600,000 U	IM	1	18			
Benzathine penicillin	1.2 × 10^6 U	IM	0.12	92			
Penicillin V	0.5 g	PO	3–4	1			
Ampicillin	0.5 g	PO	4	1	0.02–0.85		
	1 g	IM	9	1		0.05–0.5	1–8
	2 g	IV	70	0.5	4.8		
Amoxicillin	0.5 g	PO	7.5	1	0.06–0.5		
Bacampicillin	0.8 g	PO	8	1	0.2–0.5		
Methicillin	2 g	IV	75	0.5			
Oxacillin-nafcillin	1g	IV	10–40	1		0.1–0.3	
Cloxacillin-dicloxacillin	0.250 g	PO	5–20	1			
Carbenicillin	5 g	IV	300	1	3–20	0.1–1.0	1–128
Ticarcillin	3 g	IV	300	1	3–12	0.1–1	1–128
Azlocillin	3 g	IV	300	1	5–40	0.1–2	1–64
Mezlocillin	3 g	IV	300	1	5–40	0.1–2	1–64
Piperacillin	3 g	IV	300	1	5–40	0.1–2	1–64
Cephalothin	2 g	IV	70	0.6	0.5–2	0.05–1	1–16
Cefazolin	1 g	IM	80	1.9		0.05–1	1–16
	1 g	IV	180	1.9			
Cefuroxime	0.75 g	IM	35	1.1	1–4	0.05–1	1–16
	1 g	IV	180				
Cefamandole	1 g	IM	20	0.6		0.05–1	1–16
	1 g	IV	70	0.6			
Cefoxitin	1 g	IV	70	0.8	1.0–4	1–3	1–16
Cephalexin-cephradine	0.250 g	PO	10	1	0.4	0.5–3	1–16
Cefotetan	1 g	IV	150	3	0.75–12	0.1–4	0.1–16
Cefotaxime	1 g	IV	65	1	1–3	0.1–4	0.1–16
Ceftizoxime	1 g	IV	80	1.6	1–3	0.1–4	0.1–16
Ceftriaxone	1 g	IV	150	7	1–5	0.1–4	0.1–16
Cefoperazone	2 g	IV	200	2	1–6	0.1–4	0.1–16
Ceftazidime	1 g	IV	120	1.9	1–9	0.1–4	0.1–16
Aztreonam	1 g	IV	100	1.6	1–10		0.1–16
Imipenem	0.5 g	IV	35	1	1–3	0.1–4	0.1–4
Erythromycin	0.5 g	PO	1.4–2	1.5	1.3–5	0.05–1	
Clindamycin	0.3 g	PO	4–6	2–3	0.7–2.5	0.02–1.5	
	0.3 g	IM	4–6	2–3			
	0.6 g	IV	10	2–3	1.5–7		
Tetracycline	0.250 g	PO	2–4	8			
	0.250 g	IV	1–3	8	0.01–0.05	0.5–1	
Minocycline	0.1 g	PO	1–3	12–16			
	0.1 g	IV	8	12–16	<3	0.1–1	0.4–2
Doxycycline	0.1 g	PO	2	18			
	1.1 g	IV	1–3	20	<3	0.1–1	0.4–2
Chloramphenicol	50 mg/kg	PO	10–20	1.5–3	5–10	0.5–2	1–8
		IV	5–15	2–3			

TABLE 108-1 (continued)

Antibiotic	Dose	Route	Average Peak Serum Level, μg/ml	Average Serum Half-Life, h	Range of Sputum Bronchial Levels μg/ml	Antibiotic Concentrations, μg/ml, to Inhibit	
						Gram-Positive	Gram-Negative
Kanamycin	7.5 mg/kg	IM	15–25	2			1–6
Gentamicin	1.5 mg/kg	IM,IV	6–10	2	1–4		1–8
Tobramycin	1.5 mg/kg	IM,IV	6–10	2	1–4		1–8
Amikacin	7.5 mg/kg	IM,IV	15–25	2			1–8
Netilmicin	2 mg/kg	IM,IV	6–10	2			1–8
Trimethoprim	0.16 g	PO	1.5	10	2	0.03–1	0.1–4
Sulfamethoxazole	0.8 g	PO	40	9	2		
Rifampin	0.6 g	PO	15	1.5–5			
Vancomycin	0.5 g	IV	10–20	6		0.5–6	
Ofloxacin	0.4 g	PO	4	8	3–5	0.5–4	0.1–2
Enoxacin	0.4 g	PO	4	5	3–5	0.5–16	0.1–2
Pefloxacin	0.4 g	PO	4	8	5–10	0.5–16	0.1–2
Ciprofloxacin	0.75 g	PO	3	4	1.5–3	0.5–2	0.1–2

*Data in this table are given as averages. Intravenous therapy is usually given over 20 to 30 min, and the peak value given is that which would be attained at the end of infusion. Serum levels and half-lives are for individuals with normal renal function. Antibiotic concentrations are given for organisms for which the agent would be appropriate therapy.

require 18 to 24 h for completion. Direct testing for sensitivity using sputum is unreliable because a small number of organisms in the original sample can overgrow the specimen, thereby suggesting resistance falsely. More rapid methods of antibiotic testing, such as those that yield results in 3 to 4 h, have not proved completely reliable. The determination of the actual inhibitory concentration needed for a particular organism can be done using microtiter methods. Based on minimal inhibitory concentrations (MICs), the dose of antibiotic or the route of administration can be adjusted. The results of the disk and microtiter methods are generally comparable since both depend on inhibition of growth over a set time period using a concentration of antibiotic similar to that which is achieved in the serum while on standard therapeutic programs.

The determination of the minimal bactericidal concentration (MBC) may be useful in distinguishing between an inhibitory level and a bactericidal level. This determination is rarely needed for the treatment of aerobic gram-positive infections due to streptococci or anaerobic mouth flora. But, occasionally it is useful in infections caused by *Staphylococcus aureus* or certain gram-negative species. For example, a *S. aureus* isolate may have an MIC for oxacillin of 0.5 μg/ml, but an MBC of 32 μg/ml. In this instance, a major difference exists between the inhibitory and the bactericidal levels. The same situation could occur for *Pseudomonas aeruginosa* and antipseudomonas compounds, e.g., an MIC of 16 μg/ml and an MBC > 128 μg/ml.

Another approach to using an antibiotic regimen effectively is the determination of serum bactericidal levels. These levels are often used as guides in the treatment of bacterial endocarditis; concentrations of antibiotics in serum should be at least eightfold greater than that required to inhibit the infecting microorganism in vitro. In performing this test, serial dilutions of serum are made using a standard inoculum of bacteria, and the dilution is determined at which bacterial growth fails to occur. Although there is little evidence that, in pulmonary infections, bactericidal titers in serum correlate with successful outcome, in general the outcome in neutropenic patients is unfavorable if bactericidal titers in serum are greater than 1:8.

Many factors, including pH, ionic strength, osmolality, and growth phase of the bacteria, alter the antibacterial activity of the available antibiotics and complicate the prognostic value of in vitro tests done on isolated pure cultures. Nonetheless, in vitro resistance usually does correlate with therapeutic failure.

Bacteriostatic versus Bactericidal

Antibacterial agents are divided into those that are *bactericidal*, i.e., kill organisms, and those that are *bacteriostatic*, i.e., inhibit bacterial growth. For the individual in whom immunologic and phagocytic defenses are normal, pulmonary infections can be treated using antibiotics of either class. Thus, a tetracycline or erythromycin, both of which are bacteriostatic, will cure a *Streptococcus pneu-*

moniae infection as readily as penicillin G, which is bactericidal. However, it is wise to use a bactericidal agent whenever possible, particularly in the compromised host, to prevent the development of metastatic foci of infection and to minimize the destruction of pulmonary tissue. Unfortunately, it is not known if bactericidal agents are more effective than bacteriostatic agents in treating chronic pulmonary diseases such as acute bacterial bronchitis or bronchiectasis. Structural abnormalities in the pulmonary defense system in these chronic infections are probably more important than the particular antibiotic that is used.

PHARMACOLOGIC CONSIDERATIONS

An antibiotic may have an extensive antibacterial spectrum in vitro, but its pharmacologic properties may render it inappropriate for therapy of infection in the lungs and pleural space. After an antibiotic is administered by any route—oral, intramuscular, or intravenous—it mixes with plasma where it is bound to proteins. It is distributed to various extravascular tissues where it may also be bound; the distribution results in a peak concentration in plasma followed by a rapid fall. The time that peak level is achieved varies with the route of administration; after intravenous injection, it generally occurs when the infusion is stopped; after intramuscular injection, the peak is at 30 to 60 min; after oral ingestion, the peak is at 1 to 2 h. Subsequent decreases in serum levels depend on renal and biliary excretion, and for some antibiotics, on metabolism.

Although antibiotic concentrations in the lung generally correspond to those of plasma, in areas that are not well perfused, such as abscesses within the lung, bronchial secretions, and pleural effusions, peak levels of antibiotics are achieved several hours after the peak blood levels. Furthermore, the concentration of antimicrobial agent in the poorly perfused areas of the lung are less than that in the blood. However, the level of antibiotic persists in these extraparenchymal locations for 4 to 6 h after the serum level has fallen below the effective level.

Antimicrobial agents differ in their ability to cross the tissue-blood barriers. These pharmacologic differences may be of therapeutic significance. Concentrations in extravascular tissue depend on the concentration gradient from serum to tissue fluid, the degree of binding in serum and tissues, and the diffusivity of the agent, which is determined by its molecular size, its pK, and its lipid solubility, as well as by the extent of inflammation.

The effect of protein binding on the efficacy of antibiotics is poorly understood. By acting to temporarily store the agent, protein binding prevents large fluctuations in the concentration of the free agent in body fluids. The affinity constants of the antibiotics for serum-tissue proteins determine the extent to which the agent is free to exert its antibacterial effect.

Antibiotics differ greatly in protein binding from class to class and within a class. Antimicrobial agents that are less than 90 percent protein-bound produce adequate concentrations in pulmonary tissues. For example, oxacillin is 94 percent protein bound. A serum level of 70 μg/ml yields adequate pulmonary tissue and bronchial levels for *S. pneumoniae* and *S. aureus* (MICs 0.12 and 0.5 μg/ml, respectively) but not for *H. influenzae* (MIC 16 μg/ml) since the levels of free drug are 4 μg/ml. Leakage of serum into an area of inflammation probably increases the level of drug in that area beyond that achieved by diffusion of unbound drugs in the normal state, but the easier access to the area is advantageous only if the binding affinity of the antibiotic to protein is low, and if the drug is released and unbound so that it can enter the bacterial cells. Maintenance of high serum levels for a long period is easier to achieve with agents that bind to protein. Should the level of free drug that is needed to inhibit a pathogen be low, adequate levels in the interstitium can be achieved for hours even if the agent is highly bound to protein. In essence, no substantial bases exist for predicting the extent to which protein binding of an antibiotic determines its effectiveness in treating a pulmonary infection.

Body tissues can bind antibiotics and render them inactive. This is particularly true for the polymyxin class of antibiotics, polymyxin B and colistimethate sodium, which bind to phospholipids in tissue, resulting in inadequate levels at wound sites. Polyene agents, such as amphotericin, that bind to sterols and are taken up by the reticuloendothelial system are at a similar disadvantage. Aminoglycosides can be inactivated by purulent material by binding to nucleic acid debris and to acid nucleoproteins. Gentamicin, tobramycin, and amikacin have decreased activity against *Pseudomonas* and *Serratia* species when high levels of magnesium, calcium, and sodium are present in purulent tissue. These agents are also less active in an acid environment, as exists in infected areas of the lung, and they are inactive under anaerobic conditions.

PHARMACOKINETICS OF ANTIMICROBIAL AGENTS IN RESPIRATORY SECRETIONS

In principle, the concentration of antimicrobial agent in pulmonary tissue is similar to that in interstitial fluid. Interstitial fluid concentrations are calculated on the basis of blister fluid concentrations of antibiotics or upon lymph concentrations. Conversely, the amount of antibiotic in bronchial secretions is much more difficult to calculate. In general, we assume that antibiotics are distributed into bronchial compartments by passive diffusion and active transport, and that there is removal of drug by the flow of sputum. One problem in the use of antibiotics in the treatment of bronchopulmonary infection is that in

inflamed areas of the tracheobronchial tree the concentrations of antibiotics do not equilibrate fully with those in the "central compartment" that is more available for rapid entry and distribution.

In general, the molecular weights of antibiotics are less than 1000. As a result, they can readily cross normal capillary walls as part of bulk flow. But, in normal pulmonary parenchyma, junctions between alveolar epithelial cells are tighter than those of the alveolar capillaries (see Chapter 60) so that most antibiotics cannot pass. Also, passage may be strongly influenced by ionic charge: as a rule, β lactams are weak anions, whereas aminoglycosides are cations. Highly lipid-soluble agents such as chloramphenicol, erythromycin, most tetracyclines, and rifampin readily cross normal pulmonary cellular barriers.

Inflammation undoubtedly influences permeability of normal barriers, generally enhancing passage of molecules of all sizes. In addition, among the factors that influence the penetration of antibiotics into an area of infection and inflammation are ionization, lipid solubility, and protein binding. The local characteristics of pulmonary tissue, such as the state of the inflammatory process, the presence of fibrosis and edema, and the vascularity of the affected tissue, can all enhance or reduce the amount of antibiotic that penetrates the infected area.

As a rule, the concentrations of antibiotics in the airways depend on blood levels since they cross blood-tissue barriers by diffusion; i.e., higher concentrations in the lungs are achieved by higher doses. Also, the concentrations of antibiotics in bronchial secretions increase more slowly than in blood regardless of whether the intravenous, intramuscular, or oral route is used to administer the drug. Finally, peak concentrations in the bronchi are less than in blood, but half-lives are longer; appreciable concentrations of antibiotics probably persist in the lungs after blood levels are no longer detectable.

The extent to which antimicrobial agents penetrate into bronchial secretions and sputum is controversial. One of the problems is the contamination of one secretion by another. For example, sputum is readily contaminated with saliva. Admixture with sputum of saliva that is rich in antibiotic artificially increases the level of the antibiotic in the sputum; conversely, dilution of sputum by saliva artificially decreases the concentration of antibiotic in sputum. Bronchial secretions can be contaminated by aspiration of pharyngeal secretions. Nonhomogeneities in vascular supply and different degrees of inflammation also influence levels greatly. Consequently, reported results of concentrations of antibiotics in bronchial secretions differ widely: some researchers find that bronchial concentrations equal those in serum, whereas others find that concentrations in bronchial secretions are only 10 to 25 percent of those in the serum.

Many other problems are inherent in attempts to assess the levels of antimicrobial agents in sputum or bronchial secretions. For example, sampling techniques, the bronchial level of sampling, the storage of samples, the assay methods, all affect the results. Another problem is that methods used to homogenize secretions may damage the antibiotic or fail to accomplish complete homogenization. Microbiologic assays or high-performance liquid chromatography methods need not measure the same active drug. Finally, the extraction method may liberate drug from bronchial secretions that have rendered it inactive.

Even after all due precautions, including that of dilution, have been taken, the ranges of concentration of the penicillins, tetracyclines, and aminoglycosides in sputum are wide. Penicillin V and ampicillin, 250 to 500 mg taken orally, are undetectable in sputum until 2 to 3 h have elapsed; at 2 to 3 h, levels range from nil to 1 μg/ml with mean values of 0.2 μg/ml. Little difference exists between the concentrations achieved in sputum after a 250- or 500-mg dose, whereas a dose of 1 g increases concentration in sputum considerably. Amoxicillin, an aminopenicillin analogous to ampicillin, produces higher levels in sputum than those produced by an equivalent dose of ampicillin. This observation correlates well with the higher serum levels that amoxicillin produces. Bacampicillin also produces higher serum and bronchial levels of active ampicillin.

The concentration of a penicillin required to inhibit most *S. pneumoniae* and *Hemophilus* species ranges between 0.06 and 0.25 μg/ml. If the site of infection in chronic bronchitis is assumed to be just below the surface of the bronchi, and if sputum levels of antibiotics are a reflection of levels in lung tissue, then large doses of ampicillin, or doses of amoxicillin equal to one-half of the ampicillin dose, should achieve the needed concentrations in the bronchi.

Levels of carbenicillin and ticarcillin in sputum are only 3 to 5 percent of the serum levels. The same is true of ureidopenicillins such as mezlocillin and piperacillin. Nonetheless, all the agents cure bacterial pneumonia due to susceptible streptococci, Enterobacteriaceae, and *Pseudomonas*. Cephalexin and cephradine reach mean peak sputum levels of 0.4 μg/ml 2 to 3 h after a dose of 500 mg. It is noteworthy that the concentration of cephalexin required to inhibit 90 percent of pneumococci is 4 μg/ml; to inhibit *Hemophilus* it is 8 μg/ml. The same is true for cephradine, but lower concentrations of cefaclor are needed for *Hemophilus*. These observations on penicillins and cephalosporins underscore that the concentrations of penicillins and cephalosporins in sputum are determined by diffusion and not by active transport. In order to achieve large concentration gradients for diffusion, large doses of antibiotic should be used early in infection to cause a rapid decline in the bacterial population.

Tetracycline concentrations in sputum are generally low and do not seem to vary with the degree of purulence.

In the first 24 h, all tetracyclines, tetracycline-HCl, minocycline, and doxycycline, are poorly transported into sputum and even into bronchial secretions. Only after 48 h are appreciable levels attained. The levels in sputum usually range from nil to 2.1 μg/ml, with mean levels of 0.2 to 0.5 μg/ml. Nonetheless, despite the low absolute values in sputum, the ratio of bronchial to serum concentrations is of the order of 20 to 40 percent. In contrast to the low levels in sputum or in bronchial secretions, levels in bronchial epithelium and pulmonary parenchyma are of the order of 2 to 5 μg/ml. The mean inhibitory level of tetracycline for *S. pneumoniae* is 0.2 μg/ml and for *Hemophilus* 1 μg/ml.

Aminoglycosides and penicillins appear in bronchial secretions within 5 min after an intravenous injection and reach peak concentration in 1 to 2 h. Levels decrease more slowly in the respiratory tract than in the serum. After intravenous infusions, the concentrations of ampicillin in bronchial secretions are less than 10 percent of serum levels, usually less than 4 μg/ml. Cephalothin concentrations are 25 percent or less of serum levels, usually less than 2.5 μg/ml. New agents, such as cefuroxime and cefotaxime, produce bronchial concentrations that are 20 to 30 percent of serum levels. Bronchial levels of aminoglycosides, gentamicin, tobramycin, sisomicin, and amikacin in bronchial secretions range from 20 to 60 percent of serum levels.

Chloramphenicol, because of its lipid solubility, achieves high concentrations in sputum and bronchial secretions. Trimethoprim also has chemical properties that favor passage across interstitial barriers; concentrations in sputum and bronchial secretions exceed serum levels. Quinolone antibiotics such as ciprofloxacin and ofloxacin produce sputum levels above the MICs of *H. influenzae* and *Branhamella catarrhalis*. They also produce bronchial tissue levels that exceed by several fold the serum levels. Ciprofloxacin also produces sputum levels above the MICs of most *P. aeruginosa*. Aztreonam, a monobactam, produces sputum and lung tissue levels above the MICs of most *Enterobacteriaceae* and *Pseudomonas*.

The concentrations of penicillins or cephalosporins in bronchial secretions are adequate to inhibit most grampositive coccal species such as *S. pneumoniae*, *S. aureus*, anaerobic streptococci, fusobacteria, and *Bacteroides melaninogenicus*. New cephalosporins such as cefotaxime, ceftizoxime, ceftriaxone, and ceftazidime achieve bronchial and pulmonary concentrations adequate to inhibit most Enterobacteriaceae. Although the levels of aminoglycosides in bronchial secretions inhibit many Enterobacteriaceae and *Pseudomonas*, results of therapy are poor because of their limited ability to penetrate secretions that are dense with bacteria; pulmonary secretions protect bacteria from the therapeutic agents. Conversely the penetration of drugs such as clindamycin into mucous material could contribute to effectiveness in pulmonary infections

even though it is a bacteriostatic, rather than a bactericidal agent.

SPECIAL CONSIDERATIONS IN USING ANTIMICROBIAL AGENTS

Combination chemotherapy is used either for a life-threatening infection, to prevent emergence of bacterial resistance, to treat a known mixed infection, to enhance antibacterial activity, or as a strategy by which the dosage of a toxic drug can be decreased. With few exceptions, two drugs are not superior to a single one as long as the one is bactericidal. For example, although the combination of cephalosporin and an aminoglycoside has been advocated for serious *Klebsiella* infection, there is no proof that this combination is superior to the new cephalosporins, such as cefotaxime, ceftizoxime, ceftazidime, aztreonam, or imipenem. The prime exception is *Pseudomonas* pulmonary infection in a compromised host when the combination of an antipseudomonas penicillin and an aminoglycoside is required for treatment. Also, since Enterobacteriaceae and *Serratia* species seem to develop resistance to cephalosporins rapidly, combination therapy using an aminoglycoside and a cephalosporin is advisable for the first few days of treatment. Hospital-acquired aspiration is another indication for combination chemotherapy if both mouth flora and *Pseudomonas* are involved; in this case, clindamycin can be combined with aztreonam or ceftazidime to minimize the risk of nephrotoxicity.

As a rule, in patients who have adequate host defenses, neither morbidity nor mortality is decreased by administering large doses of antibiotic. However, in patients with serious staphylococcal disease, or infection due to virulent gram-negative species, or advanced anaerobic pleuropulmonary disease, as well as in the host in whom white blood cell function is depressed, it may be circumspect to use large doses in the attempt to minimize destruction of pulmonary parenchyma since decreased blood flow to an affected area impairs the delivery of drug to the site of infection.

The optimal duration of therapy for most respiratory infections is unknown. It is probable that 2 days of therapy with penicillin would be curative for pneumococcal pneumonia in a healthy young individual. Many hospitalized individuals are probably overtreated because it is not the infection, per se, that causes a high morbidity and mortality, but the respiratory insufficiency or failure to maintain adequate drainage of secretions that produces much of the morbidity and mortality. Most pulmonary infections can be adequately treated in 7 to 10 days, except for staphylococcal infections which require 3 to 4 weeks and *Nocardia* infections which often require up to 6 months of therapy. Sputum will not be cleared of orga-

nisms, nor will the chest radiograph return to normal in patients with underlying structural disease of the lungs.

The use of aerosolized antibiotics in chemotherapy remains highly controversial. There are several objections to its use: sensitization of the patient, production of resistance bacteria in the environment, and failure to deliver the agent to the infected site, either because of inability to produce a fine enough aerosol or because of airways obstruction: the aerosolized agent remains on the outside plugs of mucus, while the bacteria proliferate inside. At one time polymyxin B seemed ideal for use as an aerosol to prevent colonization and subsequent infection. It acts essentially as a detergent on gram-negative bacteria, has no gram-positive activity, is highly soluble, is minimally absorbed, and does not select R-factor-carrying bacteria. However, subsequent study has shown that use of the drug sometimes results in bronchospasm and in an overgrowth of *S. aureus*, *Proteus*, or fungi such as *Candida albicans*.

Aerosolization of aminoglycosides, in particular gentamicin and sisomicin, has been used in the intensive-care setting. Although this usage was reported to be successful in preventing infection, the possibility exists that this practice has contributed to the increase in plasmid-carrying bacteria that are resistant to aminoglycosides. For this reason this technique is not recommended. In certain circumstances, instillation of an aminoglycoside into the lung of the tracheotomized patient via the flexible bron-

choscope may be useful. This technique offers particular promise in the case of the individual in whom reduced renal function is associated with inadequate blood flow to one region of the lung.

Prevention of pulmonary infections by administering antibiotics has usually been disappointing. Emergence of a drug-resistant flora is the usual outcome. Administration of antibiotics to patients who are unconscious, or to those in congestive heart failure, has not prevented the development of pneumonia. The use of antibiotics to prevent bacterial superinfection in patients with viral pneumonitis also has been unsuccessful.

FAILURE OF CHEMOTHERAPY

A common apology for failure of chemotherapy in infection is inadequate duration of therapy, or failure to use a correct dosage, or failure to use ancillary measures. Defects in host resistance and structural problems are the major cause of failure in the chemotherapy of pulmonary infections. Dosage is a minor consideration in dealing with gram-positive infections, such as *S. pneumoniae*; in contrast, the prospect of suboptimal therapy has to be weighted much more seriously in gram-negative infections. But, in either case, preoccupation with dosage is doomed to fail unless adequate drainage is achieved.

BIBLIOGRAPHY

Bakker-Woudenberg IAJM, VandenBerg JC, Michel MF: Therapeutic activities of cefazolin, cefotaxime and ceftazidime against experimentally induced *Klebsiella pneumoniae* pneumonia in rats. Antimicrob Agents Chemother 22:1042–1050, 1982.
    An animal model of pneumonia illustrating the correlation of antimicrobial activity and pharmacokinetics.

Barza M: Principles of tissue penetration of antibiotics. J Antimicrob Chemother 8(Suppl C):7–28, 1981.
    A detailed analysis of the kinetics of tissue penetration of antibiotics into different body tissues.

Bergogne-Berezin E: Penetration of antibiotics into the respiratory tree. J Antimicrob Chemother 8:171–174, 1981.
    A review of the concentrations of many antibiotics in respiratory secretions.

Bergogne-Berezin E: Pharmacokinetics of antibiotics, in Pennington JE (ed), *Respiratory Infections: Diagnosis and Management*. New York, Raven, 1983, pp 461–479.
    A review of kinetics of transfer of antibiotics into respiratory secretions.

Blummer JL, Stern RC, Klinger JD, Yamashita TS, Meyers CM, Blum A, Reed MD: Ceftazidime therapy in patients with cystic fibrosis and multiple-resistant *Pseudomonas*. Am J Med 79(2A):37–46, 1985.
    A review of the use of ceftazidime in the treatment of Pseudomonas infections in cystic fibrosis patients.

Bodern CR, Lampton LM, Miller DP, Tarka EF, Evertt ED: Endobronchial relevance to aminoglycoside activity in gram-negative bacillary pneumonia. Am Rev Respir Dis 127:39–41, 1983.
    Provides details of pH in areas of lung during infection.

Bodey GP, Elting L, Kassamali H, Lim, BP: *Escherichia coli* bacteremia in cancer patients. Am J Med 81:85–95, 1986.

> During a 10-year period, 621 episodes of Escherichia coli bacteremia occurred in 575 cancer patients. The infection was most common in patients with acute leukemia and genitourinary and gastrointestinal malignancies. The response rate was 71 percent for patients who received appropriate antibiotics, 38 percent for patients who received inappropriate antibiotics, and 8 percent for patients who received no antibiotics. A single appropriate antibiotic was as effective as a combination.

Dummer JS, Montero CG, Griffith BP, Hardesty RL, Paradis IL, Ho M: Infections of heart-lung transplant recipients. Transplantation 41:725–729, 1986.

> In 14 heart-lung transplant recipients who survived more than one week after transplantation, the rates of infection were higher than in the heart transplant recipients; more than 90% of the infections were potentially life-threatening. A total of 67% of the infections involved the lungs or thoracic cavity as a primary site; most of the rest were disseminated viral or fungal infections.

Feeley TW, DuMoulin GC, Hedley-Whyte J, Bushnell LS, Gilbert JP, Feingold DS: Aerosol polymyxin and pneumonia in seriously ill patients. N Engl J Med 293:471–475, 1975.

> Analysis of problems of aerosol antibiotic use in an intensive-care unit.

Gentry LO, Zeluff BJ: Diagnosis and treatment of infection in cardiac transplant patients. Surg Clin North Am 66:459–465, 1986.

> Infectious complications in transplant patients occur in two phases: the first, 30–60 days after transplantation, nosocomial bacterial infections are then most common; and the second, usually more than a month after transplantation when immunosuppression is high, opportunistic infections are then common.

Klastersky J, Thys JP, Monbelli G: Comparative studies of intermittent and continuous administration of aminoglycosides in the treatment of bronchopulmonary infections due to gram-negative bacteria. Rev Infect Dis 3:74–83, 1981.

> A review of studies of endotracheal use of aminoglycosides.

Lambert HP: Clinical significance of tissue penetration of antibiotics in the respiratory tree. Scand J Infect Dis Suppl 14:262–266, 1978.

> An analysis of the role of pulmonary tissue concentrations of antibiotics and the influence on therapeutic results.

Neu HC: Tetracycline: A major appraisal. Bull NY Acad Med 54:141–155, 1978.

> A complete review of the microbiology and pharmacology of tetracycline.

Neu HC: Optimal antibiotic therapy in bronchopulmonary infections. Infection 8(Suppl 1):62–69, 1980.

> A review of the data on the use of antimicrobial agents in respiratory infections with reference to antimicrobial activity and pharmacology.

Neu HC: Current mechanisms of resistance to antimicrobial agents in microorganisms at risk for infection. Am J Med 76(Suppl 5A):11–27, 1984.

> A complete discussion of the biochemical mechanisms of bacterial resistance with particular reference to new agents.

Neu HC: Antimicrobial activity, bacterial resistance and antimicrobial pharmacology. Am J Med 78(6B):17–22, 1985.

> An analysis of how in vitro activity of antimicrobial agents and pharmacokinetics can be correlated.

Neu HC: Structure-activity relations of new beta-lactam compounds and *in vitro* activity against common bacteria. Rev Infect Dis 5(Suppl 2):319–336, 1986.

> A major review of new penicillins and cephalosporins which correlates structure with in vitro activity and pharmacology.

Neu HC: The pharmacology and toxicology of antimicrobial agents, in Braude AI (ed), *Infectious Diseases and Medical Microbiology*, 2d ed. New York, Saunders, 1986, pp 219–235.

> Comprehensive review of all antimicrobial agents with particular stress on potential toxic reactions during therapy.

Pennington JE: Kinetics of penetration and clearance of antibiotics in respiratory secretions, in Kirkpatrick CH, Reynolds HY (eds), *Immunologic and Infectious Reactions of the Lung*. New York, Dekker, 1976, pp 355–374.

> Analysis of the pulmonary distribution and clearance of antibiotics.

Perkins RL: Clinical trials of cefotaxime for the treatment of bacterial infections of the lower respiratory tract. Rev Infect Dis 4(Suppl):421–431, 1982.
A review of clinical studies with an extended spectrum of cephalosporin in the treatment of pneumonia.

Rondanelli R, Dionigi RV, Regazzi MB, Maurelli M, Calvi M, Mapelli A: Ceftazidime in the treatment of *Pseudomonas* infections in intensive-care patients. Int J Clin Pharmacol Ther Toxicol 24:457–459, 1986.
Ceftazidime was effective as a single antiinfective agent in Pseudomonas sp. infections. Plasma concentrations were an important predictor of bacteriological and clinical response.

Roselle GA: Nosocomial and nursing home-acquired pneumonia. Recent therapeutic advances. Postgrad Med 81:131–132, 135–136, 1987.
For the treatment of complex pneumonia, the author urges circumspect use of the new antibiotics as monotherapy rather than the multiple-drug combinations.

Salata RA, Gebhart RL, Palmer DL, Wade BH, Scheld WM, Groschel DHM, Wenzel RP, Mandel GL, Duma RJ: Pneumonia treated with imipenemcilastatin. Am J Med 78(6A):104–109, 1985.
An example of the problem of resistance development in gram-negative pneumonia even with a highly potent antimicrobial agent.

Salata RA, Lederman MM, Shlaes DM, Jacobs MR, Eckstein E, Tweardy D, Toossi Z, Chmielewski R, Marino J, King CH, et al.: Diagnosis of nosocomial pneumonia in intubated, intensive care unit patients. Am Rev Respir Dis 135:426–432, 1987.
Based on experience with 51 intubated patients in the intensive care unit, the authors conclude that patients with infection can be identified if they have new or progessive pulmonary infiltrates plus 1 of the following: positive blood cultures, radiographic evidence of cavitation or histologic evidence of pneumonia or 2 or more of the following: new fever, new leukocytosis or grossly purulent tracheal aspirates.

Schiff JB, Small GJ, Pennington JE: Comparative activities of ciprofloxacin, ticardillin and tobramycin against experimental *Pseudomonas aeruginosa* pneumonia. Antimicrob Agents Chemother 26:1–4, 1984.
An animal model of pneumonia illustrating the effect of three classes of antibiotic on survival and pneumonia.

Scully BE, Neu HC: Use of aztreonam in the treatment of serious infections due to multiresistant gram-negative organisms, including *Pseudomonas aeruginosa*. Am J Med 78:251–261, 1985.
A report of the use of monobactam in various infections including respiratory infections due to Pseudomonas.

Scully BE, Neu HC, Parry MF, Mandell W: Oral ciprofloxacin therapy of infections due to *Pseudomonas aeruginosa*. Lancet 1:819–822, 1986.
A report of the use of ciprofloxacin, an oral quinolone, in treatment of infections including respiratory infections due to Pseudomonas.

Smith BB, LeFrock JL: Bronchial tree penetration of antibiotics. Chest 83:904–908, 1983.
Data on the concentrations of antimicrobial agents in sputum and lung tissue.

Young LS: Treatment of respiratory infections in the patient at risk. Am J Med 76(5A):61–68, 1984.
A review of the use of antimicrobial agents in the treatment of gram-negative bacillary infections of the respiratory tract.

Chapter 109

Pneumonia in the Immunocompromised Host

Robert H. Rubin

Pneumonia is the most common life-threatening infection for the immunocompromised individual. There are several reasons for this special vulnerability: deficient host defenses, a vast array of potential pathogens, unusual epidemiologic exposures, and attenuation of the clinical response to infection because of altered inflammatory response. The abnormal inflammatory response not only blunts the early clinical and radiographic signs of pneumonia, but also promotes the rapid development of sepsis because the infection is poorly contained. Therefore, it is not surprising that pneumonia accounts for 40 percent or more of the deaths in such widely disparate patient populations as those with the acquired immunodeficiency syndrome (AIDS) or leukemia or those who have undergone organ transplantation.

Compounding the diagnostic problem is the fact that about 25 percent of the episodes of fever and pneumonia in the immunocompromised person (the *febrile pneumonitis syndrome*) are noninfectious in nature: atypical pulmonary edema in association with fever from another source, pulmonary hemorrhage, pulmonary embolic disease, radiation lung injury, drug reactions, leukostasis, or a leukoagglutinin transfusion reaction. As shown in Table 109-1, the clinical problem is not only the differential diagnosis of pulmonary infection in the compromised host, but rather the differential diagnosis of fever and pulmonary infiltrates.

Despite these difficulties, certain clues have proved helpful in expediting early diagnosis and prompt institution of therapy in the immunocompromised patient with the febrile pneumonitis syndrome: the epidemiologic and clinical settings in which the pulmonary process is occurring, the nature of the defect(s) in host defense, the rate of progression of the illness, and the pattern of pulmonary abnormality on the chest radiograph. It is worth emphasizing that an expeditious diagnosis and treatment is essential for minimizing morbidity and mortality in immunocompromised patients with the febrile pneumonitis syndrome.

EPIDEMIOLOGIC ASPECTS OF PULMONARY INFECTION IN THE IMMUNOSUPPRESSED PATIENT

Whether an immunocompromised patient will develop pneumonia depends on two competing processes: (1) the delivery of infectious organisms to the lower respiratory tract in a form and in numbers adequate to initiate the infectious process and (2) the ability of the host's defenses to mount an effective attack against these potential invaders. The first of these processes is assessed by considering the epidemiologic factors that appear to relate to the pneumonia in the immunocompromised host. These epidemiologic factors can be divided into three categories: (1) remote factors, (2) contact in the community and hospital, and (3) hospital exposure.

Remote Factors

Four major considerations are included in this category. First is whether the patient has been exposed to a systemic mycotic infection that asymptomatically infects most denizens of a circumscribed geographic area (blastomycosis, coccidioidomycosis, and histoplasmosis are the prime concerns in North America). Primary pulmonary infections have occurred in immunocompromised hosts within weeks to months of travel in an endemic area. But much more common is the reactivation of a dormant in-

TABLE 109-1

Etiology of the Febrile Pneumonitis Syndrome in 100 Cancer Patients and 51 Renal Transplant Patients at the Massachusetts General Hospital*

Etiology	No. of Cancer Patients	No. of Transplant Patients	Total Patients	
			Number	Percent
Infectious causes				
Conventional bacterial infection	26	10	36	23.8
Viral infection	11	9	20	13.2
Fungal infection	10	6	16	10.6
Nocardia asteroides	5	8	13	8.6
Pneumocystis carinii	6	2	8	5.3
Mycobacterium tuberculosis	1	0	1	0.7
Mixed infections	14	1	15	9.9
Total	73	36	109	72.1
Noninfectious causes				
Pulmonary emboli	3	9	12	7.9
Recurrent tumor	8	0	8	5.3
Radiation pneumonitis	7	0	7	4.6
Pulmonary edema	1	6	7	4.6
Drug-induced pneumonitis	5	0	5	3.3
Leukoagglutinin reaction	2	0	2	1.3
Pulmonary hemorrhage	1	0	1	0.7
Total	27	15	42	27.7

*Modified after Rubin, 1981.

fection due to the breakdown in the normal cell-mediated immune defenses.

The second consideration is whether the patient has been exposed to active tuberculosis or is known to have had a positive tuberculin test. Again, although progressive primary infection in the immunocompromised host is a familiar entity, reactivation disease is far more common. A controversial issue, both in the case of mycotic infection and tuberculosis, is whether exogenous reinfection occurs in immunocompromised individuals who have long dormant tuberculosis or fungal infection.

The third consideration is whether the patient has been exposed to *Strongyloides stercoralis* infection recently or in the remote past. *S. stercoralis* is the one intestinal nematode with an autoinfection cycle that can take place completely within the gastrointestinal tract of the host. Because of this capability, chronic gastrointestinal infestation can persist for decades after the individual leaves an endemic area. In recent years, problems with *S. stercoralis* have been particularly common in immigrants from Southeast Asia and Central America who become immunosuppressed. Should the individual develop a systemic immunosuppressed state that involves the cell-mediated immune system, systemic infection with this organism may ensue and be devastating. Hemorrhagic pulmonary infiltrates or diffuse, bilateral alveolar infiltrates can occur, with or without accompanying gastrointestinal complaints. Systemic strongyloidiasis can even give rise to the adult respiratory distress syndrome.

Finally, it is important to determine if the patient has received blood transfusions. Posttransfusion episodes of pneumonitis due to leukoagglutinin reactions or to cytomegalovirus infection (see below) have long been recognized. What is new is the appreciation of the entity of posttransfusion AIDS in an individual who had received blood transfusion(s) some time back. For example, if a transfusion has transmitted the virus to a patient with a blood dyscrasia, the patient will turn to the physician not because of the original hematologic disorder but because of manifestations of infection with *Pneumocystis carinii* or some other opportunistic pneumonia that heralds the onset of transfusion-acquired AIDS.

Contact in the Community and Hospital

The epidemiologic setting within which the immunocompromised patient acquires pneumonia is an important clue to its likely etiology. Infections acquired in the hospital are heavily weighted toward antibiotic-resistant, gram-negative bacilli, fungi, *Nocardia*, *Legionella* species, *Pneumocystis*, and herpes group viruses. Community-acquired pneumonias are of two general kinds: (1) those due to *P. carinii* and/or cytomegalovirus, or some other opportunistic pathogen; this type of infection is usually

seen in the immunosuppressed patient with AIDS, far-advanced Hodgkin's disease, or recent intensive antirejection therapy post-organ transplant; and (2) those due to *Streptococcus pneumoniae, Hemophilus influenzae* type B, and *Mycoplasma pneumoniae*; these infections are apt to affect the stable cancer or transplant patient. The incidence of pneumonia with common pathogens, such as *S. pneumoniae* and *H. influenzae* type B, is also high in AIDS patients because of their defect in B-lymphocyte function.

Patients with pneumococcal and influenzal infection (Fig. 109-1) differ in several important historical respects from those with opportunistic infections: (1) the pneumonia was acquired in the community while the primary disease was in remission or relatively quiescent; (2) when the pneumonia began, immunosuppressive therapy was at a minimum; (3) at the same time, the incidence of viral respiratory infections, particularly influenza, in the community and in their families was high; and (4) while in the hospital, they were in contact primarily with patients who had stable renal transplants, solid tumors, or collagen disease, and with few patients who were being treated either for acute allograft rejection or acute leukemia.

Hospital Exposure

Nosocomial pulmonary infection, a problem for any hospitalized patient, is of particular concern for the hospitalized, immunosuppressed patient. The most common infections are due to aerobic or facultative, gram-negative bacilli: Enterobacteriaceae, *Pseudomonas aeruginosa,* and

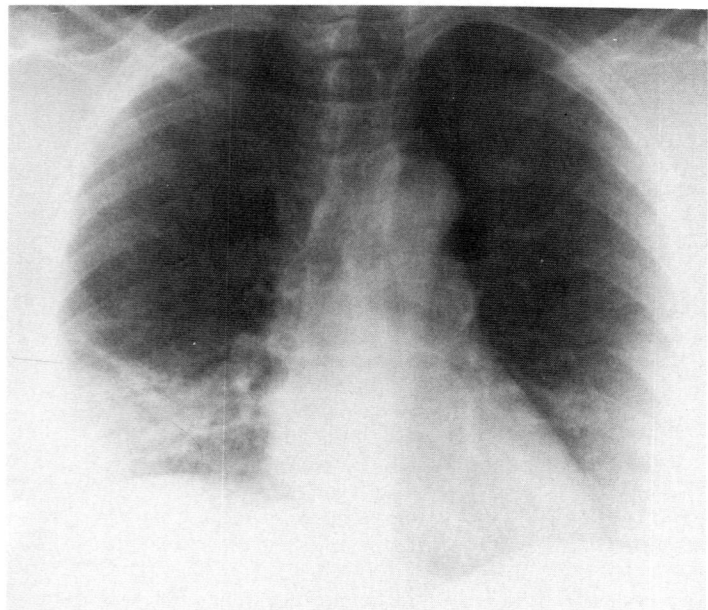

FIGURE 109-1 Community-acquired pneumonia in a patient with lymphoma.

Acinetobacter. These infections are thought to follow the aspiration of the bacterial flora colonizing the upper respiratory tract.

In normal individuals, the flora of the upper respiratory tract is primarily gram-positive, relatively nonvirulent, and antibiotic-sensitive; the flora persists in large part because of a selective advantage provided by specific interaction between ligands on the surface of these bacteria and specialized receptors on the surfaces of upper respiratory epithelial cells. This specific interaction normally prevents the colonization of the respiratory tract with gram-negative bacilli.

In seriously ill individuals, such as hospitalized immunocompromised patients undergoing acute immunosuppressive therapy, this ecologic system is disturbed, resulting in a high rate of colonization of the upper respiratory tract with gram-negative organisms. The increased rate of gram-negative colonization is due to an alteration in the epithelial cell surface that favors the adherence of gram-negative bacteria at the expense of the normal flora. Aspiration then results in the delivery of virulent, relatively antibiotic-resistant bacteria to the lungs. Thus, the gravity of the patient's illness influences the type of bacteria that adhere, the nature of the colonizing flora, and the subsequent rate of gram-negative pneumonia. In addition, the contaminated hospital environment can accelerate gram-negative colonization.

Aspergillus species and *Legionella* species are other organisms that are of major importance in immunosuppressed patients as a cause of hospital-acquired pulmonary infection. Both of these types of infection have been associated with hospital construction or renovation: in the case of *Aspergillus* species, spores have contaminated materials used for weatherproofing and fireproofing; in the case of *Legionella*, organisms have contaminated cooling towers, shower baths, ultrasonic nebulizers, and other sources of standing and potable water, with both *L. pneumophila* and *L. micdadei* (the Pittsburgh pneumonia agent) posing major problems.

Most instances of epidemic nosocomial infection are due to contamination of the air in the patients' rooms, so-called domiciliary epidemics. Such epidemics can be prevented or greatly limited by keeping immunocompromised patients in rooms supplied with HEPA-filtered air. Recently, a second type of epidemic has occurred: an outbreak of invasive *A. fumigatus* infection among immunocompromised patients housed in widely disparate parts of the hospital; the epidemic was due to construction in the radiology suite that these patients visited for radiographic studies, i.e., a *nondomiciliary, common source* epidemic. Such epidemics are probably not uncommon. Their sources are often difficult to detect, and they illustrate the need for unflagging surveillance of the immunocompromised patient population.

RELATION OF INFECTION TO DEFECTS IN HOST DEFENSE

Children with congenital abnormalities in host defense, i.e., in the number and function of granulocytes, antibody formation, or cell-mediated immunity, have relatively "pure" syndromes in which specific defects in host defense can be related to a high risk of infection with a relatively few microorganisms (Table 109-2). In contrast, most immunocompromised adult patients have multiple defects. For example, although the predominant defect in untreated patients with Hodgkin's disease is in cell-mediated immunity, the addition of splenectomy, chemotherapy, and aggressive radiation therapy superimposes a profound defect in antibody synthesis; the latter is manifested by low levels of serum IgM and of specific antibody against *H. influenzae* type B, poor response to pneumococcal vaccine, and an increased risk of life-threatening infection with these two organisms. Similarly, although untreated Hodgkin's disease is associated with a defect in cell-mediated immunity, it is only after chemotherapy is added, particularly in the form of corticosteroids, that opportunistic infections such as *P. carinii* become major problems. In addition to the roles played by the underlying disease and its treatment in the pathogenesis of the *net state of immunosuppression*, certain metabolic factors, particularly malnutrition, uremia, and hyperglycemia, potentiate infection in the compromised host.

Critically important in promoting infection by causing defects in the host defenses are immune-modulating effects of certain infectious agents, particularly viruses. The most notable example of this phenomenon is the profound immunodeficiency state initiated by infection with the human T-cell lymphotropic virus HIV which preferentially infects lymphocytes of the helper-inducer phenotype, thereby initiating the chain of events culminating in the acquired immunodeficiency syndrome (see Chapter 105). Other viruses, which are more widespread among immunocompromised patients, can also exert important immunosuppressing effects. The most important of these

TABLE 109-2

Relationship between Types of Pulmonary Infection and Defects in Host Defenses in the Immunocompromised Patient

Host Defense Defect	Conditions Commonly Associated	Pulmonary Infection to Which Patient Is Predisposed
Impaired antibody formation	Congenital and acquired hypoglobulinemias, chronic lymphocytic leukemia, multiple myeloma, B-cell lymphoma, acquired immunodeficiency syndrome	*Streptococcus pneumoniae*, *Hemophilus influenzae* type B
Depressed cell-mediated immunity	Lymphoma, acquired immunodeficiency syndrome, transplantation, prolonged corticosteroid therapy	Typical and atypical mycobacteria, *Nocardia asteroides*, fungi, herpes group viruses, measles virus, *Pneumocystis carinii*, *Toxoplasma gondii*, *Strongyloides stercoralis*
Decrease in the number of fully functional granulocytes	Myeloproliferative disorders, cytotoxic chemotherapy, congenital defects	Oral bacterial flora, *Staphylococcus aureus*, Enterobacteriaceae, *Pseudomonas aeruginosa*, *Acinetobacter*, *Aspergillus* species
Defects in complement	Congenital and acquired hypocomplementemic states, hypocomplementemic vasculitis	*Streptococcus pneumoniae*, *Hemophilus influenzae* type B
Oral and tracheobronchial ulcerations and/or obstructions	Tumors of respiratory tract, cytotoxic chemotherapy	Oral bacterial flora, Enterbacteriaceae

is the cytomegalovirus (CMV). CMV is ubiquitous among transplant populations and patients with AIDS and is not uncommon among other immunosuppressed patients. In addition to causing a variety of different syndromes of infectious disease, including interstitial pneumonia, CMV markedly predisposes to potentially lethal superinfection with a wide variety of infectious agents, including *P. carinii,* fungi, and bacteria. Other viral infections that appear to contribute significantly to the net state of immunosuppression are Epstein-Barr virus and non-A, non-B hepatitis.

The final element in considering the net immunosuppressed state present is time. Even though the dosage of immunosuppressive therapy is at its peak in the first month after transplantation, or after the start of either corticosteroids in asthmatics or chemotherapy in cancer patients, opportunistic infection is unusual at this time. Figure 109-2 illustrates for the renal transplant patient a timetable that indicates when certain forms of infection can be expected. The same can be done for each broad category of immunosuppressed patients. This information is useful in two ways: (1) for the diagnostic evaluation of the individual patient, and (2) as a clue to unusual epidemiologic hazards. Failure of the patient's course to adhere to this timetable suggests the occurrence of an unusual, often correctable, exposure. For example, invasive aspergillosis or Legionnaires' disease that occurs during the first month after transplantation should trigger a search for an unusual nosocomial hazard.

RADIOLOGIC ASPECTS OF THE FEBRILE PNEUMONITIS SYNDROME IN THE IMMUNOCOMPROMISED PATIENT

The impaired inflammatory response of the immunocompromised host may greatly modify or delay the appearance of a pulmonary infiltrate on the chest radiograph. This is most evident in patients with severe neutropenia (absolute granulocyte count < 500 per cubic millimeter): when severe neutropenia is present, atelectasis may be the only radiographic clue to the presence of important pulmonary infection; radiographic evidence of infection with organisms such as fungi, which normally excite a less exuberant inflammatory response than do ordinary bacterial pathogens, is typically very slow to appear on chest radiographs. For example, the first evidence of invasive aspergillosis emanating from a pulmonary focus may be metastatic infection of the brain or skin. In patients recovering from neutropenia, the radiographic findings sometimes increase paradoxically, because of an increase in the granulocyte count, despite a good clinical response to treatment.

Despite these limitations, the chest radiograph remains the major signpost of pneumonitis. Although no radiographic pattern of pneumonitis is specific either for a particular process in the lungs or for a particular microbial invader, etiologic-radiographic correlations are more characteristic of some processes than of others. By relating this etiologic-radiographic categorization to rate of pro-

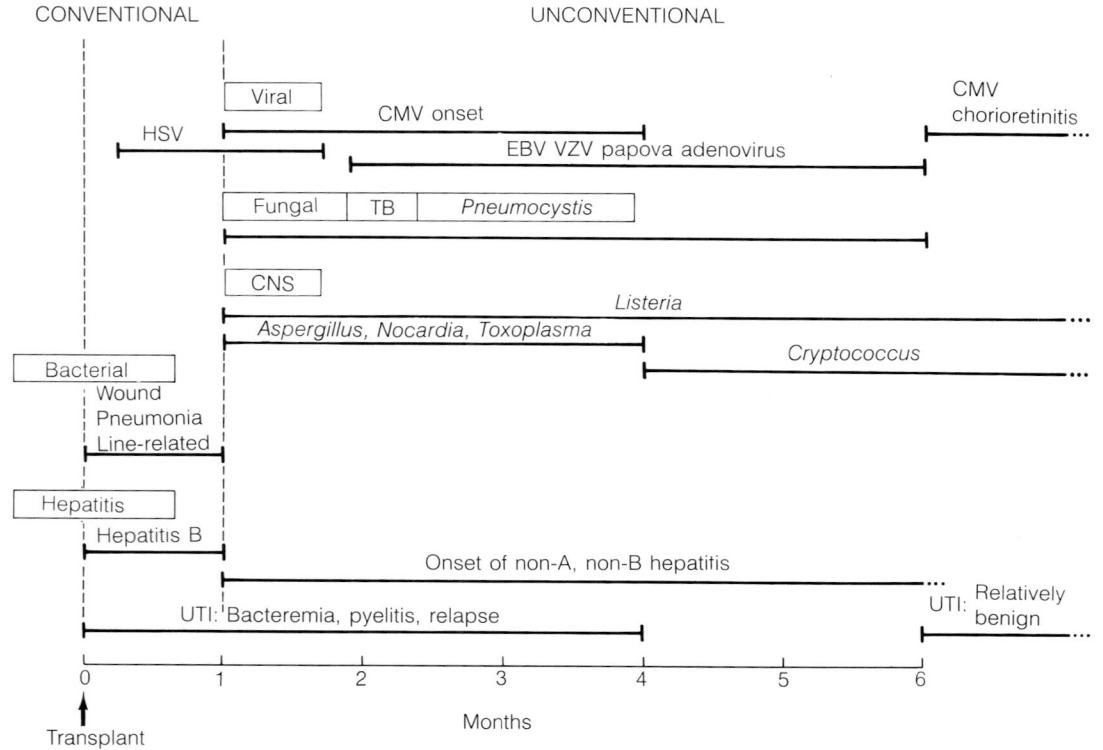

FIGURE 109-2 Timetable of the occurrence of infection in the renal transplant patient. Opportunistic infection is absent during the first month posttransplant, and the peak incidence of infection is 1 to 6 months posttransplant. HSV = herpes simplex virus; CMV = cytomegalovirus; EBV = Epstein-Barr virus; PAPVA = papovavirus; CNS = central nervous system; UTI = urinary tract infection; VZV = varicella-zoster virus. (*From Rubin et al., 1981.*)

TABLE 109-3

Etiologies of the Febrile Pneumonitis Syndromes in the Compromised Host Based on the Chest Radiograph and the Rate of Progression of the Illness*

Abnormality on the Chest Radiograph	Rate of Progression of the Illness	
	Acute†	Subacute-to-Chronic‡
Consolidation	Bacterial (including *Legionella*), thromboembolism, hemorrhage (pulmonary edema)	Fungal, nocardial, mycobacterial, tumor, (viral *Pneumocystis*, radiation, drug-induced)
Interstitial (peribronchovascular) infiltrate	Pulmonary edema, leukoagglutinin reaction (bacterial)	Viral *Pneumocystis*, radiation, drug-induced, (fungal, nocardial, mycobacterial, tumor)
Nodules	(Bacterial, pulmonary edema)	Tumor, fungal, nocardial, mycobacterial, (*Pneumocystis*, cytomegalovirus)

*Modified from Rubin et al., 1981.

†An *acute* illness is one developing and requiring medical attention in less than 24 h.

‡A *subacute-to-chronic* illness develops over several days to weeks. Unusual causes of a process are indicated in parentheses.

gression of the illness (*acute* versus *subacute-chronic*), the process of differential diagnosis can be greatly simplified (Table 109-3).

DIAGNOSTIC APPROACH TO THE FEBRILE PNEUMONITIS SYNDROME IN THE IMMUNOSUPPRESSED HOST

The approach outlined above usually circumscribes the diagnostic possibilities. However, identification of the etiologic agent, i.e., specific diagnosis, is still necessary to avoid drug toxicity and to minimize the risk of superinfection. The rapidity with which specific diagnosis is made and effective therapy instituted is the most important, controllable variable in determining the patient's outcome. Specific diagnosis may be accomplished by one of several approaches: conventional examination of expectorated sputum, immunologic assays, invasive procedures designed to sample secretions from the lower respiratory tract and/or lung tissue, and biopsy either of the lung or of more accessible metastatic sites.

Conventional Sputum Examination

Examination of expectorated sputum specimens by Gram stain and culture is the cornerstone of diagnosing pulmonary infection. The Gram stain is helpful in the immunocompromised host even if it only distinguishes between sputum that contains a few epithelial cells and that which contains many polymorphonuclear leukocytes (more than 25 per low power field). Unfortunately, in the immunocompromised patient, particularly one who is granulocytopenic, this approach often provides inadequate or confusing information for several reasons: (1) even when the infection is caused by conventional pathogens, but particularly when such opportunists as *P. carinii* or *A. fumigatus* are present, inadequate amounts of sputum for diagnosis are produced; (2) the upper respiratory tracts of many of these patients are frequently colonized by a large number of possible pathogens, ranging from such viruses as cytomegalovirus and herpes simplex virus to gram-negative bacilli and *Staphylococcus aureus* and potentially invasive fungi; delineation of the causative organism in this morass of colonizing flora, particularly in the neutropenic patient, is usually very difficult; and (3) the noninfectious causes of the febrile pneumonitis syndrome cannot be identified by these techniques (although some may be suggested by cytologic examination of the sputum). Because of these limitations, other diagnostic techniques must usually be employed to determine the etiology of the febrile pneumonitis syndrome in the immunocompromised host.

Immunologic Techniques

The traditional immunologic techniques for diagnosing invasive infection are skin testing and the identification of an antibody response to a specific microbial antigen. Unfortunately, such tests are of limited usefulness for the evaluation of the immunosuppressed patient for at least two reasons: (1) the immunologic response to microbial invasion may be delayed or even totally abrogated in the immunocompromised individual; since a high priority is given to rapidity of diagnosis, the delays inherent in these tests, particularly in this population, are unacceptable; and (2) many of the opportunistic organisms that cause life-threatening infection in the compromised host are saprophytic colonizers that elicit immunologic response but no symptoms in the general population; accordingly, the incidence of false-positive tests in applying the traditional immunologic techniques is unacceptably high.

Far more promising are attempts to detect microbial antigens, DNA, or unique metabolites in body fluids or tissues. For example, immunofluorescent staining for the antigens of *Legionella* in sputum, pleural fluid, or lung tissue usually yields the appropriate diagnosis before culture results become available. In situ DNA hybridization

using specific viral probes on lung tissue can also enable prompt diagnosis. Also helpful can be the detection of circulating *Cryptococcus neoformans* capsular antigen in the serum of patients with interstitial pulmonary disease. Although it is anticipated that the newer specific direct tests for microorganisms will obviate the present need for invasive techniques used in diagnosing the febrile pneumonitis syndrome, at present, proper application of such techniques as transtracheal aspiration, percutaneous lung aspiration, fiberoptic bronchoscopy, and open lung biopsy constitutes the major reliable approach to diagnosis in the immunocompromised host with pneumonia.

Transtracheal Aspiration

A relatively simple technique that is generally well tolerated for sampling lower respiratory tract flora with minimal contamination from the oropharynx is transtracheal aspiration (TTA). It is particularly useful in diagnosing acute bacterial infection in the patient who is not producing adequate amounts of evaluable sputum, although viral infection and, occasionally (10 to 20 percent of cases), *Pneumocystis* and *Aspergillus* infection can be diagnosed with this technique. There have been several reports of prolonged hemorrhage or cervical cellulitis in immunocompromised patients subjected to TTA. However, in more than 500 such procedures on immunocompromised patients (primarily organ transplant patients and leukemia patients), this procedure has been carried out with a complication rate of less than 1 percent and no deaths. The following precautions were observed: (1) TTA was not done in uncooperative individuals, those with anatomic abnormalities that obscure local anatomic landmarks in the neck, and those with uncorrectable bleeding diatheses; (2) anesthetizing the area over the cricothyroid membrane where the lavage needle and catheter were inserted, a small 25-gauge needle was used both to deliver the local anesthesia and to delineate the track that the larger needle would follow; (3) in neutropenic patients, broad-spectrum antibacterial therapy was initiated immediately after the procedure and was continued for a minimum of 48 h postprocedure; and (4) in patients subject to bleeding difficulties, such as those with leukemia, appropriate clotting studies and platelet counts were done and abnormalities corrected, for 48 h post-TTA. Even in patients with acute leukemia or other causes of severe thrombocytopenia, this procedure can be safely carried out *if platelet transfusions are available, if they can sustain a platelet count of greater than 50,000 per cubic millimeter for more than 24 h after the procedure, and if other causes of bleeding are not present.* In our clinic, TTA is done routinely on immunocompromised patients with *acute* pneumonias that fail to be diagnosed by examination of expectorated sputum.

Invasive Diagnosis of the Febrile Pneumonitis Syndrome

If the diagnosis remains obscure after the initial evaluation, then more invasive techniques are resorted to promptly. Extrapulmonary metastatic lesions that are readily accessible are given first priority.

With respect to direct sampling of the lesions in the lungs, the technique applied depends on several factors: the severity of the illness, the rate of progression of the disease, the type of infiltrate present on the chest radiograph, and the specialized skills and techniques that are available at the institution caring for the patient. The definitive diagnostic procedure is open lung biopsy, which should be carried out as expeditiously as possible if arterial hypoxemia is intensifying and the pulmonary infiltrates are spreading rapidly. Despite the need for general anesthesia, thoracotomy, and a postoperative chest tube, the procedure is remarkably well tolerated, especially in those patients in whom a treatable disorder is identified. A specific diagnosis is made in approximately 70 to 80 percent of immunosuppressed patients who come to open lung biopsy. The undiagnosed cases probably represent instances of unrecognized pulmonary drug toxicity, the effects of antecedent antimicrobial therapy in modifying the disease process, or even some new pathologic process. Recent experiences with *Legionella pneumophila* and *Legionella micdadei* suggest that there are previously undiagnosed pathogens causing human disease and that immunocompromised individuals are the ones most likely to be infected with such agents.

If the problem is more of a diagnostic dilemma than a therapeutic emergency, one of the less invasive, "middle-level" techniques is tried first, reserving open lung biopsy for those instances in which the initial procedure fails to establish the diagnosis. Of the "middle level" techniques (all of which should be carried out under fluoroscopic control), percutaneous lung aspiration using a thin-walled, 18- to 20-gauge needle is particularly useful for the diagnosis of focal, peripherally based nodular lesions, especially those that have undergone cavitation. The material obtained with this procedure is suitable for microbiologic and cytologic analysis and provides the diagnosis in about 90 percent of the bacterial or fungal lesions of this type. Approximately 10 percent of individuals develop hemoptysis after this procedure, and an additional 10 to 20 percent develop pneumothoraxes. However, these are usually mild and require no special intervention.

Unfortunately, the aspirating needle is generally inadequate for the evaluation of diffuse pulmonary infiltrates, such as that caused by *P. carinii*. In these patients, the middle level procedure of choice entails fiberoptic bronchoscopy. *In expert hands,* the combination of fiberoptic bronchoscopy and transbronchial biopsy, plus bron-

chial brushing, has been successful in establishing the diagnosis of *P. carinii* infection in approximately 90 percent of proven cases and in yielding sufficient biopsy material for the diagnosis of radiation and drug-induced disease in about the same percentage. Bacterial pneumonias can be diagnosed with the bronchoscope by introducing a special telescoping cannula that is protected against contamination by upper respiratory bacteria.

The complication rates of fiberoptic bronchoscopy with biopsy and brushing are 5 percent for pneumothorax, and 1 to 2 percent for significant hemorrhage; the mortality rate is of the order of 0.2 percent. Particularly at risk for complications is the severely granulocytopenic patient who is apt to develop life-threatening bacteremia and/or pneumonia following the procedure. To guard against this complication, a 48- to 72-h course of broad spectrum antibacterial therapy is begun as soon as specimens for bacterial culture are obtained.

Recently, particularly in the AIDS patient, there has been increasing interest in the use of bronchoalveolar lavage in the diagnosis of pneumonia in the immunocompromised host. This requires the wedging of the bronchoscope into a diseased segment of lung, lavaging the segment with 200 ml of sterile saline, and then submitting the lavage fluid for appropriate studies. This technique has been successful in diagnosing up to 95 percent of *Pneumocystis* infections, about 80 percent of opportunistic infections in other immunocompromised hosts (who usually carry less of a microbial burden than do AIDS patients) and less than half of the cases of drug toxicity or malignancy. The chief advantage of bronchoalveolar lavage is its lower rate of complications, particularly in less experienced hands.

One final technique that merits comment is thoracoscopy-guided biopsy. In this procedure, a flexible endoscope is inserted between the periosteal and visceral pleura under fluoroscopic guidance, and biopsies of the pulmonary parenchyma are carried out under direct vision. A chest tube is required for 24 to 48 h postprocedure. Although the complication rate is similar to that for transbronchial biopsy, better specimens for pathologic analysis are generally obtained. This procedure is aimed at the diagnosis of peripheral, focal infiltrates or diffuse lung processes.

Whatever invasive diagnostic procedure is employed, a detailed analysis of the material is carried out: the sample is cultured aerobically and anaerobically for bacterial pathogens, in appropriate media for mycobacteria, fungi, viruses, mycoplasmas, and *Legionella* species. In addition, materials are processed to enable methenamine silver staining for *Pneumocystis*, immunofluorescent staining for *Legionella*, routine staining by the Ziehl-Neelsen and Gram techniques, and cytologic and fungal examination using wet mounts. A sample of any biopsy material should be prepared for staining with hematoxylin and eosin, methenamine silver, Gram, auramine-rhodamine, and other stains as indicated. Recently, some laboratories have been utilizing specific immunofluorescent reagents and DNA probes on frozen sections of tissue, looking for *Legionella*, cytomegalovirus, and other organisms that are difficult to culture. When limited material is available for study, highest priority should be given to the technique indicated by previous noninvasive assessment.

Empiric Therapy

Under certain circumstances, empiric therapy rather than specific treatment based on the results of invasive diagnostic procedures is mandatory. These circumstances include (1) far-advanced AIDS or relapsing acute myelogenous leukemia, in which life expectancy is limited because of the gravity of the primary illness; (2) leukemia that has not been managed by chemotherapy so that there is only a low probability of opportunistic infection; (3) an uncorrectable bleeding diasthesis or such impaired pulmonary function that invasive diagnostic techniques would not be tolerated; and (4) unwillingness of the patient to undergo invasive diagnostic studies. Under such circumstances, the choice of empiric therapy is based on the indirect clues outlined previously: the epidemiologic and clinical setting, the nature of the immune defect(s) present, the pace of the pulmonary process, and the radiographic pattern.

ETIOLOGIES OF THE FEBRILE PNEUMONITIS SYNDROME IN THE IMMUNOSUPPRESSED PATIENT

Several different etiologies can elicit the febrile pneumonitis syndrome in the immunosuppressed patient.

Infectious Causes

BACTERIAL AND VIRAL INFECTION

Gram-negative bacilli, particularly *Klebsiella, Pseudomonas,* and *Serratia,* aspirated from a colonized upper respiratory tract, are the most common causes of bacterial pneumonia in the compromised host, particularly of pneumonia developing in-hospital. This form of infection is most common in patients with hematologic malignancy undergoing chemotherapy, especially those with profound granulocytopenia. In more stable patients, such as long-term, organ transplant patients, those with solid tumors, and even some AIDS patients, pulmonary infection is usually acquired in the community and the bacterial etiologies reflect this source, i.e., *S. pneumoniae, H. influenzae* type B, and *S. aureus* (Fig. 109-1).

Three other types of pulmonary bacterial infection that are more "opportunistic" in character can occur in

significantly immunocompromised patients: (1) The most important is infection with two of the *Legionella* species— *L. pneumophila* and *L. micdadei*. The incidence of sporadic community-acquired pneumonia due to these organisms in the immunosuppressed patient does not appear to differ appreciably from that of the general population. However, epidemic infection, particularly that associated with the hospital environment, has a much greater impact on immunosuppressed patients. (2) *Corynebacterium equi*, rarely a pathogen in normal hosts, can produce a subacute focal or cavitary pneumonia in patients with lymphoma or in organ transplant recipients. An important clue regarding *C. equi* infection is that these organisms are acid-fast and can be mistaken for mycobacteria on smear. (3) Bacteremic and/or cavitary pneumonia due to *Bacillus cereus* can occur in leukemic patients. It is important not to dismiss the finding of *Bacillus* species on blood culture of such individuals as a contaminant.

NOCARDIAL AND MYCOBACTERIAL INFECTION

Nocardia asteroides, *Mycobacterium tuberculosis* (and the atypical mycobacteria), and such fungi as *Aspergillus*, *Cryptococcus*, and *Mucor* produce pneumonias in the immunocompromised patient that share the following characteristics: (1) The production of a focal or multifocal, often cavitary pneumonitis with a subacute-chronic rate of progression, that is particularly common in patients with defects in cell-mediated immunity. (2) Diversion of pulmonary blood flow away from the involved alveolar portions of the lung, thereby minimizing ventilation-perfusion ($\dot{V}A/\dot{Q}$) mismatches; this automatic adjustment is responsible for the clinical observation that arterial oxygenation usually remains high despite extensive pulmonary involvement on the chest radiograph. This observation affords a useful clue in the differential diagnosis of the immunosuppressed patient with a focal pulmonary lesion, since bacterial infection is usually associated with disordered ventilation-blood flow relationships and appreciable arterial hypoxemia early in the clinical course. (3) The incidence of hematogenous spread is high. Indeed, the likelihood of metastatic spread is so great that part of the routine workup of each patient with an infection due to one of these organisms is a "metastatic workup" akin to that commonly carried out in cancer patients. Particular attention in such a workup is paid to the central nervous system, skeletal system, skin, and subcutaneous tissue. Such metastatic sites of infection can be the tipoff to previously unsuspected pulmonary infection and should be pursued vigorously.

Nocardial infection has been observed in a broad range of immunocompromised patients, including those with AIDS and hematologic malignancy. However, it has been particularly prominent in organ transplant recipients, especially heart transplant patients. An important

clue to the presence of nocardial infection is its predilection for spreading to the pleural space. Although mortality rates due to nocardial infection in immunosuppressed patients as high as 80 percent have been reported, early diagnosis and prolonged courses of therapy (6 to 12 months in many instances), *before extensive dissemination has occurred*, can result in survival rates of better than 80 percent.

Mycobacterial infection is particularly prominent in two groups of immunosuppressed patients—those with hairy cell leukemia and patients with AIDS. In patients with hairy cell leukemia, either typical or atypical pulmonary infection may occur. Although disseminated *Mycobacterium avium-intracellulare* infection with minimal impact on the lungs has been observed among all types of patients with AIDS, typical pulmonary or disseminated *M. tuberculosis* infection can also occur, particularly in AIDS patients of Haitian background.

FUNGAL INFECTION

The fungal infections that occur in the immunosuppressed patient may be divided into three categories: (1) opportunistic infections caused by organisms that primarily invade the lung, e.g., *Aspergillus* species and *Cryptococcus neoformans*; (2) opportunistic infections that reach the lung either by way of hematogenous spread from another site or as organisms superinfecting a lung that was previously injured by a viral or bacterial process, e.g., *Candida* species and *Aspergillus* species; and (3) systemic mycoses that resemble tuberculosis by lying dormant for many years after the initial infection but subsequently undergo reactivation during the development of the immunosuppressed state, e.g., blastomycosis, coccidioidomycosis, and histoplasmosis.

Of all the fungal pulmonary infections that occur in immunosuppressed patients, invasive aspergillosis is by far the most important in terms of both incidence and clinical impact. The *Aspergillus* species most commonly associated with invasive infections are *A. fumigatus* and *A. flavum*; in contrast, *A. niger* (a very common laboratory contaminant) rarely causes invasive infection. A typical clinical setting for the development of invasive aspergillosis is the patient with severe granulocytopenia or the patient under treatment with high doses of corticosteroids who has received broad-spectrum antibiotics in the last month. Invasive pulmonary aspergillosis causes a necrotizing bronchopneumonia, with or without hemorrhagic infarction. The most characteristic radiographic picture is one that reveals a rapidly progressing nodular infiltrate, often cavitating, that frequently crosses lung fissures (Fig. 109-3).

The most challenging aspect of *Aspergillus* infection is the fact that metastatic spread, particularly to the central nervous system, occurs early in the disease process,

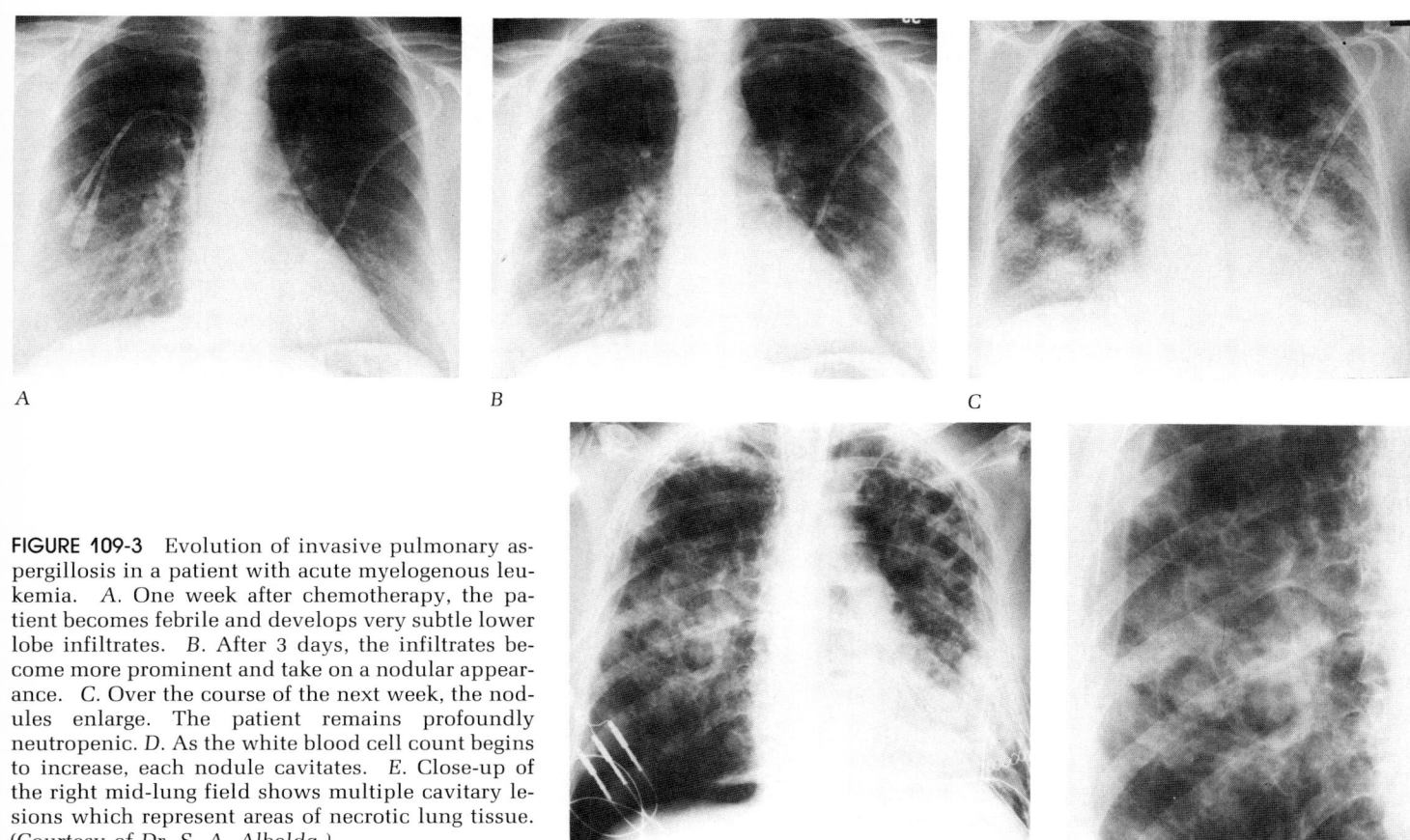

FIGURE 109-3 Evolution of invasive pulmonary aspergillosis in a patient with acute myelogenous leukemia. *A.* One week after chemotherapy, the patient becomes febrile and develops very subtle lower lobe infiltrates. *B.* After 3 days, the infiltrates become more prominent and take on a nodular appearance. *C.* Over the course of the next week, the nodules enlarge. The patient remains profoundly neutropenic. *D.* As the white blood cell count begins to increase, each nodule cavitates. *E.* Close-up of the right mid-lung field shows multiple cavitary lesions which represent areas of necrotic lung tissue. (*Courtesy of Dr. S. A. Albelda.*)

even while the primary pulmonary site of infection is relatively asymptomatic. Therefore, the major emphasis is on early diagnosis, a formidable task since skin tests and serologic tests are of little use in this circumstance. Typically, the diagnosis requires either needle aspiration or open lung biopsy. However, presumptive therapy can be initiated in the immunosuppressed patient who has a clinically compatible syndrome and radiographic picture, and has either *A. fumigatus* or *A. flavus* (but not *A. niger*) isolated from respiratory secretions.

C. neoformans tends to occur predominantly in patients with defects in cell-mediated immunity rather than granulocytopenia, and tends to be relatively asymptomatic. The unique feature of cryptococcal infection is the high incidence of spread to the meninges. It is not uncommon in patients who are hospitalized because of symptomatic cryptococcal meningitis to discover a seemingly innocuous cryptococcal pulmonary lesion on the chest radiograph.

Whereas *Aspergillus* and cryptococcal infections invade the normal lung of the immunosuppressed patient, *Candida* rarely does so. Although commonly isolated from expectorated sputum specimens, *Candida* cannot be

accepted as an adequate explanation for the febrile pneumonitis syndrome unless it is isolated directly from lung biopsy. If it is isolated from the lung biopsy, then hematogenous spread from some other primary site (such as a contaminated central venous catheter) should be the first thought and an appropriate search for the primary portal of entry should be undertaken. In contrast to its rarity as a primary agent in pneumonia, *Candida* species are very common superinfecting agents.

VIRAL INFECTION

Viral infections in the immunosuppressed host can be divided into two categories: those, such as influenza, respiratory syncytial virus, and adenovirus infections, which occur in the general population and which may be acquired in the community as part of a community-wide outbreak; and those, primarily caused by the *herpesvirus* group, which selectively affect immunosuppressed patients. It is the latter with which we are primarily concerned.

Pulmonary infection occasionally develops as part of a disseminated varicella-zoster or herpes simplex viral

infection in the patient in whom cell-mediated immunity is depressed. Herpes simplex pneumonia after prolonged endotracheal intubation is also not uncommon in this type of patient. Nonetheless, the viral agent most often associated with pneumonia in the immunosuppressed host is cytomegalovirus. It is the most important single cause of pneumonia in transplant patients, is commonly present in AIDS patients with pneumonia, and occurs not uncommonly in patients with hematologic malignancy and in those treated with intensive immunosuppression for a variety of disease states.

The diagnosis of a pulmonary infection due to CMV begins with a patient at risk for CMV, e.g., a patient who underwent organ transplantation 1 to 4 months prior. The chest radiograph reveals an interstitial process that is characteristically symmetric and involves both lower lobes (Fig. 109-4). In addition, there is evidence of involvement of multiple organs, i.e., hepatic dysfunction, atypical lymphocytes, leukopenia, and/or thrombocytopenia. In such an individual, the critical question is not whether CMV is present; instead, the critical question is whether a more treatable process is also present. In the AIDS patient and the transplant recipient, the additional process is most commonly *P. carinii* (Fig. 109-4).

PARASITIC INFECTION

Three parasites can produce the febrile pneumonitis syndrome in the immunosuppressed host: *P. carinii, Toxo-plasma gondii,* and *Strongyloides stercoralis.* By far the most important is *P. carinii* (see Chapter 104). Important factors that predispose to *Pneumocystis* infection are infection with the causative agent of AIDS and/or cytomegalovirus, therapy with corticosteroids or cyclophosphamide, and protein malnutrition.

The typical radiographic appearance of *Pneumocystis* infection in the lungs is that of a diffuse interstitial alveolar pneumonia that often becomes confluent as it progresses. Usually, the disease affects the lower lobes and is bilateral and symmetric (Fig. 109-4). Occasionally, the radiographic findings are atypical, i.e., unilateral predominance, lobar or segmental consolidation, cavitation, or a pseudonodular appearance. Particularly in AIDS patients, a nonproductive cough, tachypnea, arterial hypoxemia, and findings of a restrictive defect on pulmonary function testing can be due to active *Pneumocystis* infection even though the chest radiograph is normal. In such patients, a positive gallium scan can be useful in suggesting the presence of a treatable *Pneumocystis* infection.

Toxoplasmosis is an uncommon cause of pneumonia in the immunosuppressed host. As a rule, its most important effect in this population is on the central nervous system. Although *Toxoplasma gondii* does occasionally infect the lungs, almost invariably other pathogens, particularly one or more of the herpes groups of viruses or *Pneumocystis,* are also present.

As noted above, hyperinfection with *Strongyloides*

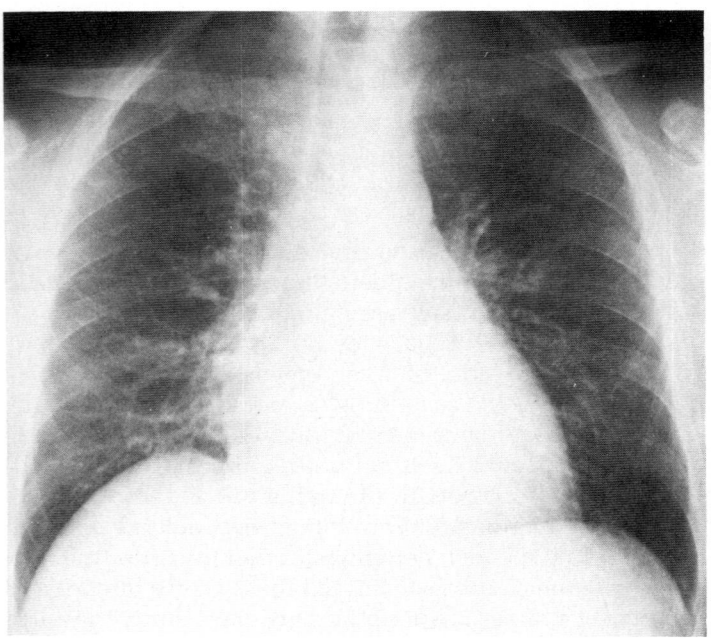
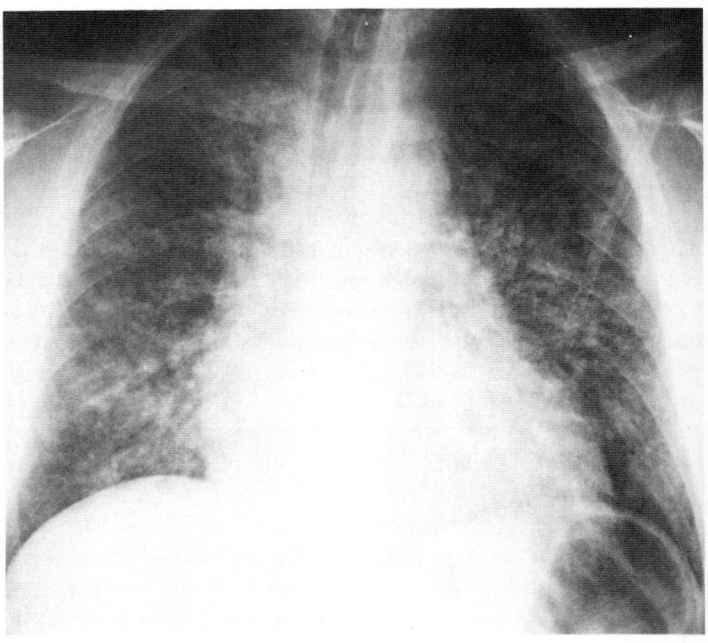

A   *B*

FIGURE 109-4 Dual infection due to cytomegalovirus and *P. carinii* in a renal transplant patient. *A.* Early peribronchovascular changes 6 weeks after renal transplantation. The patient had a 5-day history of fever, nonproductive cough, and leukopenia. *B.* Four days later, the pulmonary process has progressed rapidly. Bronchoalveolar lavage yielded both cytomegalovirus and *P. carinii.* Therapy with trimethoprim-sulfamethoxazole was successful.

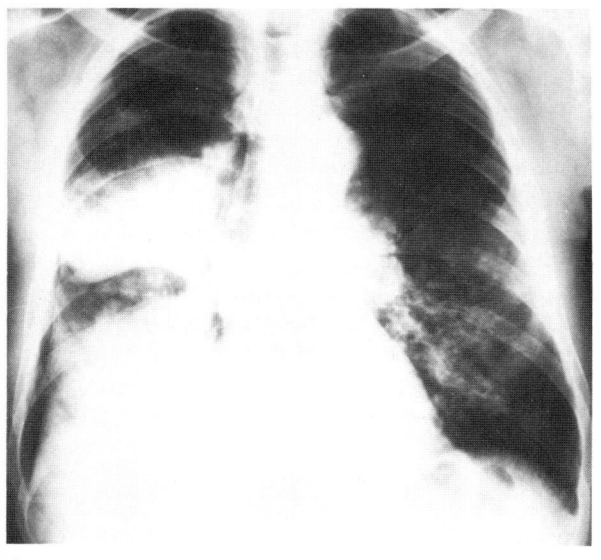

A

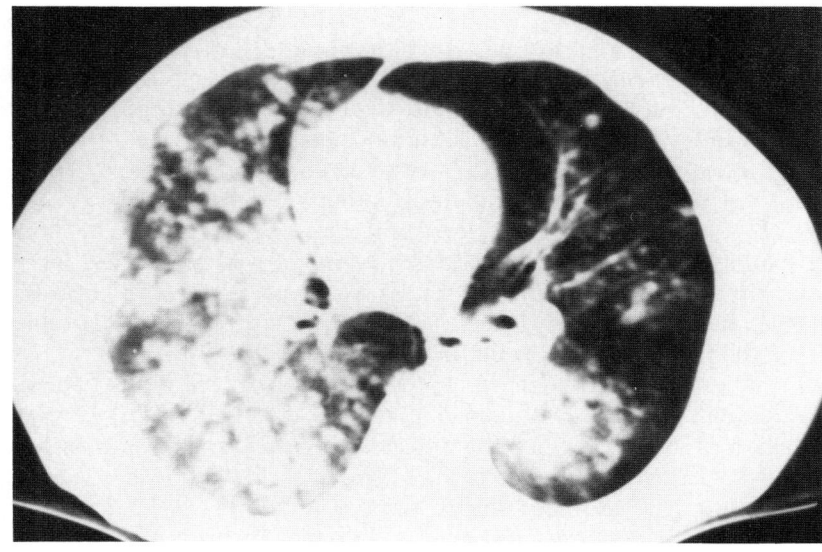

B

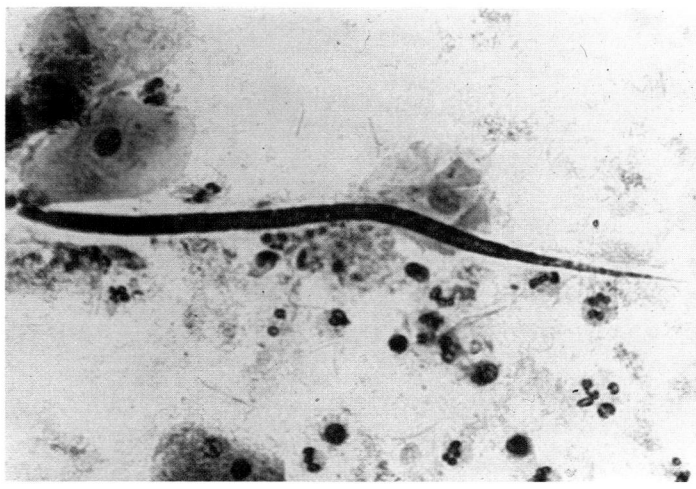

C

FIGURE 109-5 *S. stercoralis* larva in sputum. A 65-year-old male veteran of World War II who complained for 1 month of anorexia, cough, and weight loss. *A.* Chest radiograph reveals a pneumothorax on the right after needle biopsy that disclosed adenocarcinoma of right upper lobe. Etiology of nodules in lower lobe unknown. *B.* Computed tomography demarcated nodules more clearly. *C.* Sputum cytology revealed larvae of S. *stercoralis*, suggesting the possibility of parasitic, rather than neoplastic, etiology for the nodules. *(Courtesy of Dr. R. A. Panettieri, Jr.)*

stercoralis may occur in the immunosuppressed host (Fig. 109-5). Pulmonary involvement due to this helminth may be suggested by the combination of hemorrhagic pulmonary infiltrates with enterocolitis in an immunosuppressed patient with the appropriate epidemiologic background.

Noninfectious Causes

RADIATION PNEUMONITIS

Among the noninfectious causes of the febrile pneumonitis syndrome are radiation pneumonitis, drug-induced pneumonitis, and a variety of other etiologies. The acute phase of radiation lung injury, *radiation pneumonitis*, usually begins 1 to 6 months following the completion of a course of radiation therapy (see Chapter 51). It is characterized histologically by edema and engorgement and thrombosis of capillaries and arterioles on the one hand,

and by atypia, hyperplasia, and desquamation of alveolar epithelial cells on the other. Protein-rich alveolar fluid and hyaline membranes are common.

Clinically, radiation pneumonitis begins insidiously with fever, nonproductive cough, and progressive dyspnea—closely resembling a viral or *Pneumocystis* pneumonia. Radiographically, the characteristic feature is a centrally located infiltrate with sharp margins that almost always conforms to the radiation portals.

Symptomatic radiation injury of the lung is most common in patients receiving radiotherapy for breast cancer, lymphoma, and cancer of the lung. The incidence and severity of radiation lung injury are determined, in large part, by the characteristics of the radiation therapy, i.e., the volume of lung exposed to the radiation, the total dosage of radiation that is administered, and the rate of administration. The greater the volume of lung exposed to the radiation, the higher the dose and the shorter the pe-

riod of time over which the therapy is administered, the greater the chance of severe lung injury. In addition, individual susceptibility to radiation injury is quite variable, in part because of certain modifying factors that increase the risk of radiation lung injury: previous exposure of the lungs to radiation therapy, abrupt withdrawal of corticosteroid therapy, concomitant administration of such cytotoxic drugs as adriamycin, actinomycin D, cyclophosphamide, and vincristine, and, possibly, preexisting asbestosis.

DRUG-INDUCED PNEUMONITIS

A variety of cytotoxic agents, used either for the treatment of cancer or as immunosuppressive agents, can cause pulmonary injury that closely resembles that produced by radiation. Although bleomycin and busulfan have been the major causes of this syndrome, other agents such as cyclophosphamide and chlorambucil have been occasionally implicated. Probably all alkylating agents can produce such injury, because of their radiomimetic and mutagenic properties. As in radiation lung injury, the pathologic effects are most evident in the epithelium of the alveolar lining and in the capillary endothelium. It has been proposed that the mechanism of lung injury is drug-induced production of oxygen radicals such as hydrogen peroxide and superoxide anions, an event that also occurs during irradiation. Such injuries are minimally influenced by corticosteroid administration.

The chemotherapeutic agents which have been associated with drug-induced pneumonitis are identified in Table 109-4. In addition to the cytotoxic drugs previously mentioned, noncytotoxic drugs, such as methotrexate, can also cause pulmonary injury. The noncytotoxic reactions are characterized by a pathologic picture suggesting a

TABLE 109-4
*Cytotoxic and Noncytotoxic Chemotherapeutic Agents Known to Induce Pulmonary Disease**

Cytotoxic	Noncytotoxic
Azathioprine	Bleomycin sulfate
Bleomycin sulfate	Cytosine arabinoside
Busulfan	Methotrexate sodium
Chlorambucil	Procarbazine hydrochloride
Cyclophosphamide	
Hydroxyurea	
Melphalan	
Mitomycin	
Nitrosourea (BCNU, CCNU, methyl-CCNU)	
Procarbazine hydrochloride	

* Modified from Rosenow, Wilson, and Cockerill, 1985. Although both bleomycin and procarbazine are associated primarily with cytotoxic reactions, noncytotoxic reactions have also been observed, albeit uncommonly.

hypersensitivity reaction: noncaseating granulomas, giant cells, interstitial lymphocytes, and plasma cell infiltrates, not infrequently associated with a peripheral eosinophilia. This form of reaction does not appear to be influenced by prior radiation therapy and does appear to respond to corticosteroids.

Two clinical syndromes of drug-induced pneumonitis are recognized. The first is a subacute, progressive interstitial pneumonitis that is characterized by fever, nonproductive cough, and dyspnea. This form begins weeks to months after drug therapy is begun and resembles viral or *Pneumocystis* pneumonia both clinically and radiographically. The second is a chronic interstitial fibrosis that either follows symptomatic inflammatory disease or occurs insidiously without a previous warning syndrome. Not surprisingly, preceding radiation therapy increases the incidence and severity of the lung disease caused by these agents. Gallium scans are usually positive in the inflammatory form of the disease. Pulmonary function tests reveal progressive pulmonary restriction and a decrease in diffusing capacity. Transbronchial or open lung biopsy is usually required for diagnosis.

The agents listed in Table 109-4 are probably not the only ones capable of producing fever and pneumonitis. As indicated previously, 20 percent or more of immunosuppressed patients with this clinical problem remain undiagnosed even at autopsy. It is likely that many of these represent drug reactions, either to single agents not currently recognized as causes of this syndrome or to the combination of drugs that would be innocuous individually.

OTHER NONINFECTIOUS CAUSES OF THE FEBRILE PNEUMONITIS SYNDROME

Among the less common causes of the febrile pneumonitis syndrome in immunosuppressed patients are pulmonary edema, emboli, neoplastic invasion, leukoagglutinin reactions, and hemorrhage. It is important to note that any of these can be complicated by superinfection in this group of patients, particularly if the patient has undergone endotracheal intubation.

Occasionally, the combination of neoplastic invasion of the lung and fever mimics opportunistic pulmonary infection, especially in patients with lymphoma. Occasionally, patients with leukemia (particularly chronic lymphocytic leukemia and acute monocytic leukemia) also have pulmonary leukemic infiltrates in association with fever. However, since infection and hemorrhage are far more likely in this clinical situation, biopsy proof of leukemic infiltrates is required before accepting this diagnosis. In addition, a "leukemic cell lysis pneumopathy" beginning 12 h to 4 days after aggressive chemotherapy can occur in patients with acute nonleukocytic leukemia who have inordinately increased leukocyte counts

(>200,000 per cubic millimeter). Finally, the febrile pneumonitis syndrome is occasionally mimicked by atelectasis and infection distal to an endobronchial carcinoma, primary or metastatic. The important clue to this possibility is segmental atelectasis on the chest radiograph and/or localized wheeze on auscultation of the chest.

An unusual cause of the febrile pneumonitis syndrome is a leukoagglutinin reaction. The syndrome is characterized by the abrupt onset of fever, rigors, tachypnea, nonproductive cough, and respiratory distress in the first 24 h following transfusion of a blood product. The clinical picture stems from the interaction in the blood between preformed agglutinating antibodies and antigens, probably HLA and non-HLA in type, on the leukocyte surfaces. These antibodies can be preformed in the patient's serum as a result of previous sensitization, e.g., from previous transfusions or pregnancies, and can be directed against the leukocytes being transfused. Alternatively, they can be present in plasma being transfused and directed against the patient's leukocytes. Leukoagglutinin reactions are best avoided by using for transfusions washed, packed red blood cells or frozen red blood cell preparations that are relatively free of both exogenous white cells and preformed leukoagglutinins. Not unexpectedly, these reactions are most common after granulocyte transfusions.

MULTIPLE INFECTIONS

The final consideration in dealing with the immunocompromised patient with fever and pneumonitis is that multiple processes may be present. For example, sequential infection with fungal or nocardial infection following initial lung injury from viruses or conventional bacteria is not uncommon, particularly if the first process resulted in endotracheal intubation. Even more challenging is the fact that multiple processes may be present simultaneously, particularly in the AIDS patient but in as many as 10 percent of transplant or lymphoma patients with pneumonia. The major clues to the possible presence of more than one pathogen are the following: the presence of different types of infiltrates or the development of new infiltrates on the chest radiograph during therapy, failure to respond to appropriate therapy, and recurrence of symptoms after an initial response to treatment.

BIBLIOGRAPHY

Cheson BD, Samlowski WE, Tang TT, Spruance SL: Value of open-lung biopsy in 87 immunocompromised patients with pulmonary infiltrates. Cancer 55:453–459, 1985.
  The authors performed a retrospective analysis of 87 consecutive immunocompromised patients who underwent open lung biopsy. Eleven significant operative complications were encountered, but no deaths were attributable to the biopsy. An open lung biopsy in immunocompromised patients is a relatively safe and accurate diagnostic procedure.

Dijkman JH, van der Meer JWM, Bakker W, Wever AMJ, van der Broek PJ: Transpleural lung biopsy by the thoracoscopic route in patients with diffuse interstitial pulmonary disease. Chest 82:76–83, 1982.
  Thoracoscopy was carried out in 81 patients with diffuse pulmonary disease—26 of whom were immunocompromised—to obtain lung tissue for biopsy. Results were extremely helpful.

Emanuel D, Peppard J, Stover D, Gold J, Armstrong D, Hammerling U: Rapid immunodiagnosis of cytomegalovirus pneumonia by bronchoalveolar lavage using human and murine monoclonal antibodies. Ann Intern Med 104:476–481, 1986.
  Bronchoalveolar lavage material from 54 immunocompromised patients with interstitial pneumonia was examined by immunofluorescence with cytomegalovirus-specific monoclonal antibodies. The method is a sensitive, rapid, and quantifiable approach to the detection of cytomegalovirus.

Erice A, Jordan MC, Chace BA, Fletcher C, Chinnock BJ, Balfour HH Jr: Ganciclovir treatment of cytomegalovirus disease in transplant recipients and other immunocompromised hosts. JAMA 257:3082–3087, 1987.
  Thirty-one immunocompromised patients with severe cytomegalovirus (CMV) disease were treated with intravenous ganciclovir. The agent exerted an antiviral effect against CMV.

Fanta CH, Pennington JE: Fever and new lung infiltrates in the immunocompromised host. Clin Chest Med 2:19–39, 1981.
  Comprehensive review of the diagnostic considerations and techniques with particular reference to the patient with leukemia or lymphoma.

Hall CB, Powell KR, MacDonald NE, Gala CL, Menegus ME, Suffin SC, Cohen HJ: Respiratory syncytial viral infection in children with compromised immune function. N Engl J Med 315:77–81, 1986.

For ten winters, 608 children (5 years old or younger) who were hospitalized with respiratory syncytial virus (RSV) infection were prospectively studied to evaluate the relation between their immune status and the severity of their infection. Children receiving chemotherapy for cancer and those with immunodeficiency disease are at risk for complicated or fatal infections from RSV.

Johanson WG, Pierce AK, Sanford JP: Changing pharyngeal bacterial flora of hospitalized patients: Emergence of gram-negative bacilli. N Engl J Med 281:1137–1140, 1969.

A landmark paper calling attention to an important problem.

Kaplan MH, Armstrong D, Rosen P: Tuberculosis complicating neoplastic disease: A review of 201 cases. Cancer 33:850–858, 1974.

An important review of the problem in patients with different types of cancer.

Levine AS, Schimpff SC, Graw RG Jr, Young RC: Hematologic malignancies and other marrow failure states: Progress in the management of complicating infections. Semin Hematol 11:141–202, 1974.

Still the classic paper on this subject.

Masur H, Rosen PP, Armstrong D: Pulmonary disease caused by *Candida* species. Am J Med 63:914–920, 1977.

An important paper that established the true role of Candida in the causation of pulmonary infection in the compromised host.

Masur H, Shelhamer J, Parrillo JE: The management of pneumonias in immunosuppressed patients. JAMA 253:1769–1773, 1985.

Candida species rarely cause significant pulmonary disease. When such improvement is extensive, the patient is usually terminally ill from multiple other factors.

McCabe RE, Brooks RG, Mark JBD, Remington JS: Open lung biopsy in patients with acute leukemia. Am J Med 78:609–616, 1985.

Based on the results of open lung biopsy in 15 patients with acute leukemia, pulmonary infiltrates, neutropenia, and fever, the authors conclude that open lung biopsy is often of little help in directing medical therapy or influencing clinical outcome in this type of patient.

Murray JF, Felton CP, Garay SM, Gottlief MS, Hopewell PC, Stover DE, Teirstein AS: Pulmonary complications of the acquired immunodeficiency syndrome. N Engl J Med 310:1682–1688, 1984.

An important review of the diagnostic considerations in patients with AIDS.

Myerowitz RL, Pasculle AW, Dowling JN, Pazin GJ, Peurzer M, Yee RB, Rinaldo CR, Hakala TR: Opportunistic lung infection due to "Pittsburgh pneumonia agent." N Engl J Med 301:953–958, 1979.

The report of the discovery of L. micdadei as a cause of a hospital outbreak of pneumonia in compromised hosts. Eight immunosuppressed patients had pneumonia due to Pittsburgh pneumonia agent (PPA), a gram-negative, weakly acid-fast bacterium cultivatable only in embryonated eggs and guinea pigs and distinct from L. pneumophila. The diagnosis was established by isolation of the agent from lung or visualization of the organism in lung tissue.

Myers TJ, Cole SR, Klatsky AU, Hild DH: Respiratory failure due to pulmonary leukostasis following chemotherapy of acute non-lymphocytic leukemia. Cancer 51:1808–1813, 1983.

Four patients with acute nonlymphocytic leukemia and leukocyte counts of more than 200,000 per cubic millimeter developed respiratory distress due to pulmonary leukostasis within 10 to 48 h after initiation of chemotherapy.

Ramsey PG, Rubin RH, Tolkoff-Rubin NE, Cosimi AB, Russell PS, Greene R: The renal transplant patient with fever and pulmonary infiltrates: Etiology, clinical manifestations, and management. Medicine 59:206–222, 1980.

A comprehensive review of the pulmonary problems of the renal transplant patient.

Rhame FS, Striefel AJ, Kersey JH Jr, McGlave PB: Extrinsic risk factors for pneumonia in the patient at high risk of infection. Am J Med 76:42–52, 1984.

A consideration of epidemiologic factors in the occurrence of pneumonia in the compromised host. Particular attention is paid to three exceptional pathogens: Aspergillus, P. carinii, and Legionella.

Rosenow EC III: Chemotherapeutic drug-induced pulmonary disease. Semin Respir Med 2:89–96, 1980.
> An excellent review of this subject.

Rosenow EC III, Wilson WR, Cockerill FR III: Pulmonary disease in the immunocompromised host. Mayo Clinic Proc 60:473–487, 1985.
> First part of a review of differential diagnosis and treatment, with particular reference to early intervention. (Second part appears in same journal, 60:610–631, 1985.)

Rubin RH: The cancer patient with fever and pulmonary infiltrates: Etiology and diagnostic approach. Cur Clin Topics Infect Dis 1:288–303, 1980.
> Comprehensive review of infection-, drug-, and radiation-induced pulmonary injury in the cancer patient.

Rubin RH: Infection in the immunosuppressed host, in Rubenstein E, Federman DD (eds), Scientific American Textbook of Medicine. New York, Scientific American, 1985, sec 7, pp 1–24.
> A textbook overview, with particular concentration on epidemiology and clinical aspects.

Rubin RH, Wolfson JS, Cosimi AB, Tolkoff-Rubin NE: Infection in the renal transplant recipient. Am J Med 70:405–411, 1981.
> A consideration of the major types of infection according to the time period posttransplant in which they occur: postsurgical bacterial infection in the first month after transplantation; opportunistic infection, with cytomegalovirus playing a major role, and transplant pyelonephritis in the period 1 to 4 months posttransplant; and a mixture of conventional and opportunistic infections in the last posttransplant period.

Ruskin J: Parasitic disease in the compromised host, in Rubin RH, Young LS (eds), A Clinical Approach to Infection in the Compromised Host, 2d ed. New York, Plenum, 1987, pp 253–304.
> A monograph devoted to parasitic infection in the compromised host, with a particular emphasis on pulmonary infection.

Schooley RT, Hirsch MS, Colvin RB, Cosimi AB, Tolkoff-Rubin NE, McCluskey RT, Burton RC, Russell PS, Herrin JT, Delmonico FL, Giorgi JV, Henle W, Rubin RH: Association of herpes virus infections with T-lymphocyte-subset alterations, glomerulopathy, and opportunistic infections after renal transplantation. N Engl J Med 308:307–313, 1983.
> Clinical documentation of the contributions of viruses to the net state of immunosuppression and the value of T-cell subset monitoring in providing early evidence of herpesvirus infections, based on experience with 28 recipients of renal allografts.

Springmeyer SC, Hackman RC, Holle R, Greenberg GM, Weems CE, Myerson D, Meyers JD, Thomas ED: Use of bronchoalveolar lavage to diagnose acute diffuse pneumonia in the immunocompromised host. J Infect Dis 154:604–610, 1986.
> The authors compared the diagnostic information obtained by bronchoscopy and needle aspiration of the lung with information obtained concurrently by open lung biopsy in 15 marrow transplant recipients. The diagnostic sensitivity of the bronchoscopy was 89 percent and 17 percent for needle aspiration; there were no complications.

Stover DE, Zamov MB, Hajdu SI, Lange M, Gold J, Armstrong D: Bronchoalveolar lavage in the diagnosis of diffuse pulmonary infiltrates in the immunosuppressed host. Ann Intern Med 101:1–7, 1984.
> Based on experience with 97 patients, the authors conclude that bronchoalveolar lavage is a valuable procedure for evaluation of pulmonary disease in the immunosuppressed host.

Tenholder MF, Hooper RG: Pulmonary infiltrates in leukemia. Chest 78:468–473, 1980.
> A careful analysis of the causes of pulmonary infiltrates in 139 adult patients with leukemia at different points in their clinical course.

Van Etta LL, Felice GA, Ferguson RM, Gerding DN: Corynebacterium equi: A review of 12 cases of human infection. Rev Infect Dis 5:1012–1018, 1983.
> A review of diagnosis and treatment of infection with C. equi, an aerobic, variably acid-fast, gram-positive "diphtheroid" that is an unusual cause of pulmonary infection in immunosuppressed patients. Initially, infection with C. equi may be mistaken for a mycobacterial infection.

Williams DM, Krick JA, Remington JS: Pulmonary infection in the compromised host. Am Rev Respir Dis 114:359–392, 593–627, 1976.
> A two-part review of the wide variety of opportunistic pathogens that cause pulmonary infection in the immunocompromised host; particularly useful summary of opportunistic infections in the pre-AIDS era.

Fungal Infections in the Immunocompromised Host

Robert H. Rubin

In the immunocompromised host there are few forms of infection that represent as much of a challenge to the clinician as do invasive fungal infections. The clinical presentation can be insidious, diagnosis is difficult, and therapy is prolonged and associated with a high rate of toxicity. Despite these problems, increasing numbers of immunocompromised patients with invasive fungal infection of the lungs are being recognized and successfully treated. No longer does such a diagnosis have to be tantamount to a death sentence.

The fungal agents that invade the lungs of immunocompromised patients may be divided into three general categories:

1. Fungal agents, such as *Histoplasma capsulatum*, *Coccidioides immitis*, and *Blastomyces dermatitidis*, that are found only in certain circumscribed geographic areas where they usually produce asymptomatic infection in large numbers of normal individuals and uncommonly cause symptomatic pulmonary disease in these people but can be important causes of morbidity and mortality in immunocompromised patients.

2. Fungal agents, such as *Aspergillus* species, the Mucoraceae, and *Cryptococcus neoformans*, that are ubiquitous in the environment and rarely produce invasive infection in the normal host but are the major causes of *primary* fungal pulmonary infection in the immunocompromised individual.

3. Fungal agents, such as *Candida* species, *Trichosporon beigelii*, *Sporothrix schenckii*, and *Petriellidium boydii*, that are ubiquitous in the environment and rarely produce primary pulmonary infection even in the immunocompromised patient. These may, however, produce *secondary* pulmonary infection following either hematogenous seeding of the lungs or superinfection of a lung previously injured by some other microbial agent or process.

Figure 110-1 presents an example of the first of these categories: disseminated histoplasmosis in a renal transplant patient resident in an area endemic for *H. capsulatum*, who presented with fever, nonproductive cough, and abnormal chest radiograph. Increasing numbers of immunocompromised individuals, particularly patients with acquired immunodeficiency syndrome (AIDS), are being recognized with this form of fungal pulmonary infection. This entity is discussed in Chapter 105. The primary concerns of this chapter are those fungal processes in the second and third categories, which are largely restricted to the immunocompromised patient population.

INVASIVE PULMONARY ASPERGILLOSIS (IPA)

Aspergillus species are ubiquitous dimorphic fungi that grow throughout the world as saprophytes in decaying organic material. The term *aspergillosis* encompasses a diverse group of clinical syndromes caused by this fungus, all of which have a major clinical impact on the lungs (see Chapter 103). These include a variety of allergic disorders, mycetoma (in which the aspergilli colonize a preexisting pulmonary cavity or area of bronchiectasis), and invasive pulmonary aspergillosis. This last is the single most important cause of invasive pulmonary infection in the immunocompromised individual.

Epidemiology

Invasive pulmonary aspergillosis is the result of the inhalation of spores of *Aspergillus* species into the lower res-

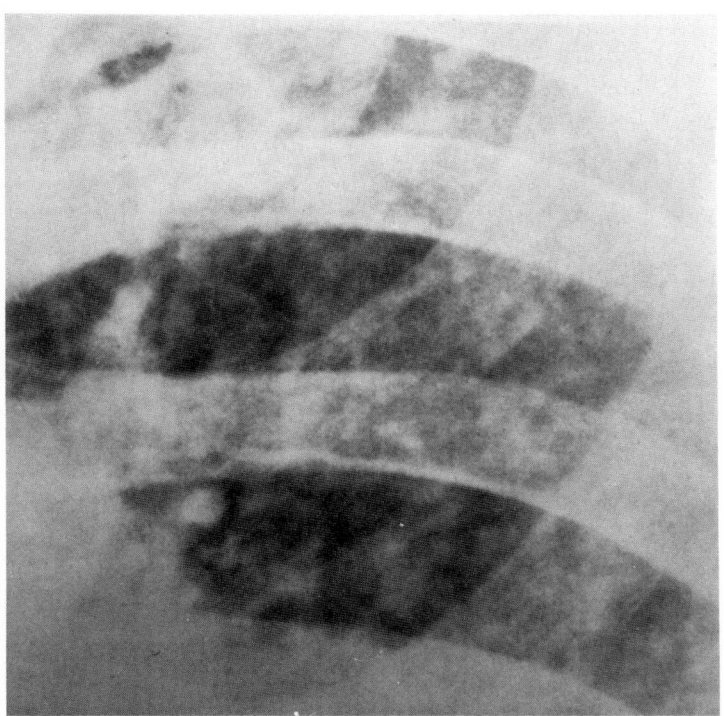
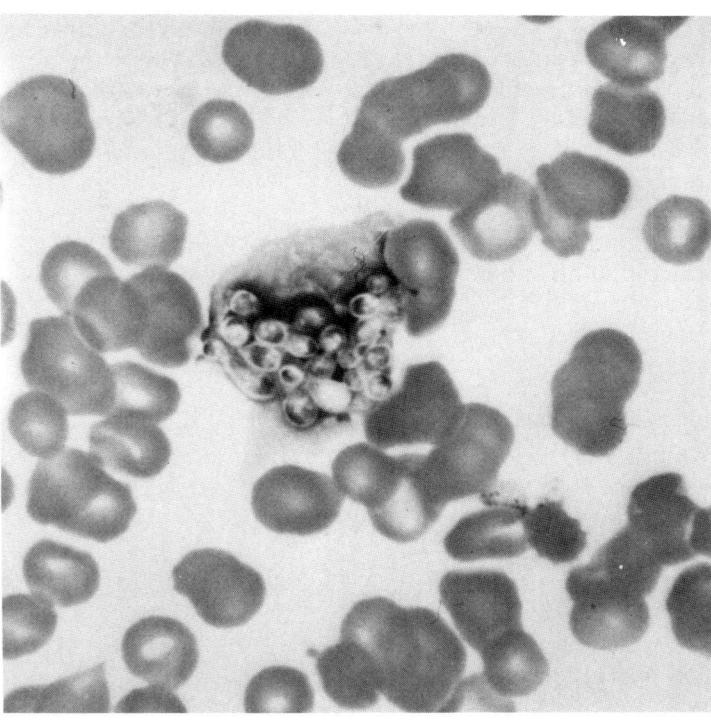

A   B

FIGURE 110-1 *Histoplasma capsulatum.* A 56-year old man, lifelong resident of Kansas, presented 2½ years post-renal transplant with fever, nonproductive cough, and 3-month weight loss. The chest radiograph was diffusely abnormal. *A.* Close-up reveals extensive micronodular disease. *B.* Peripheral blood smear on which the diagnosis of disseminated histoplasmosis was made showing macrophage laden with *Histoplasma capsulatum.* Treatment with a total of 2.5 g of amphotericin B resulted in total clearing of the radiograph and blood, and cure of the infection.

piratory tract of susceptible individuals. Although rare cases of invasive aspergillosis have been reported in apparently normal individuals and patients with such minimally immunosuppressing conditions as influenza, hepatic failure, psittacosis, and diabetic ketoacidosis, the great majority of cases have occurred among three groups of patients: those rendered severely leukopenic by cytotoxic therapy for leukemia or lymphoma, those with functional neutrophil disorders such as those with chronic granulomatous disease, and those, such as transplant patients, receiving high dose corticosteroids. Clinical infection is the result of the interaction of two factors: *epidemiologic* factors, which determine the risk of encountering this organism, and the *net state of immunosuppression,* which defines the susceptibility of the individual once the organisms have been delivered to the lower respiratory tract.

The ubiquity of aspergilli in nature is related to three factors: their simple metabolic requirements, their ability to withstand a broad range of metabolic and temperature conditions, and their capability of being widely dispersed in the air. Each mycelial growth of *Aspergillus* liberates into the air thousands of 1.5- to 6-μm spores (a size favorable for delivery to the lower airways). Although intermittent low level *Aspergillus* contamination probably occurs

not infrequently, even more important is the fact that large numbers of *Aspergillus* spores are routinely liberated into the air during any construction project. When such heavily contaminated air is inhaled by susceptible patients, epidemic disease will occur. This is particularly important within the hospital. Two forms of epidemic nosocomial invasive aspergillosis have been observed among immunocompromised patients: so-called *domiciliary* epidemics, in which *Aspergillus* spore-laden air is delivered to the rooms of susceptible individuals, there to be inhaled and to initiate disease; and *nondomiciliary,* "common source" epidemics, in which the contamination occurs at a central site such as a radiology suite or operating rooms, to which patients travel from widely disparate portions of the hospital for essential procedures. Although the clustering of cases in one geographic area of a hospital has led to the frequent identification of domiciliary epidemics, it is likely that nondomiciliary exposures are at least as important in the occurrence of nosocomial aspergillosis.

The most effective means of preventing invasive pulmonary aspergillosis, either of the sporadic or epidemic variety, is by ensuring that all air delivered to susceptible individuals is passed through properly functioning, high-efficiency particulate air (HEPA) filters. Such filters can

eradicate domiciliary acquisition of infection on units caring for immunocompromised individuals. Unfortunately, the provision of HEPA-filtered air throughout the hospital environment is impractical at most institutions, and nondomiciliary acquisition of infection remains a problem whenever other portions of the hospital that these patients visit undergo construction. It has been suggested that the careful construction of physical barriers of floor-to-ceiling plastic or dry walls across all openings between construction areas and patient care areas can decrease the risk, particularly when combined with the careful application of the fungicide copper-8-quinolinolate to the areas in question. Needless to say, careful surveillance of immunocompromised patients for the occurrence of invasive aspergillosis during periods of construction activity is essential.

One other potential source of *Aspergillus* infection is the smoking of marijuana. Aspergilli can be cultured from the majority of marijuana samples, *Aspergillus* precipitins have been found in approximately half of immunologically normal marijuana smokers, and invasive aspergillosis has developed in immunosuppressed marijuana smokers without other exposures.

Pathogenesis and Pathology

In more than 90 percent of cases of invasive pulmonary aspergillosis, the portal of entry is the lung, following the inhalation of spore-laden air (most of the remaining cases begin similarly from the inhalation of contaminated air, but with the initial lesion developing on the palate, epiglottis, or nasal sinuses). The first event in the lungs is the endobronchial invasion of hyphal forms of the germinating spores, thus producing a necrotizing bronchopneumonia. Very rapidly invasion of blood vessels, including both medium- and large-sized pulmonary vessels, occurs, which has three significant effects: occlusion of vessels with tissue *infarction*; destruction of vessels with resulting *hemorrhage*; and access to the circulation, resulting in a high rate of *metastatic spread*, particularly to organs with a rich blood supply such as the brain, heart, kidneys, liver, and spleen (Fig. 110-2).

When *Aspergillus species* invade tissues such as the lung, a characteristic hyphal form which branches dichotomously at a 45° angle is observed (Fig. 110-2). A single species, *A. fumigatus*, accounts for one-half to two-thirds of all cases of invasive aspergillosis, with *A. flavus* producing most of the rest. Uncommonly, invasive infection may be caused by *A. terreus*, *A. niger*, and *A. glaucus*, and only rarely by other *Aspergillus* species.

Two important host defenses against the invasion of the lung have been identified: the bronchoalveolar macrophage and the neutrophil. The bronchoalveolar macrophages are the first phagocytic cells to encounter the inhaled *Aspergillus* spores. These cells act to kill the spores

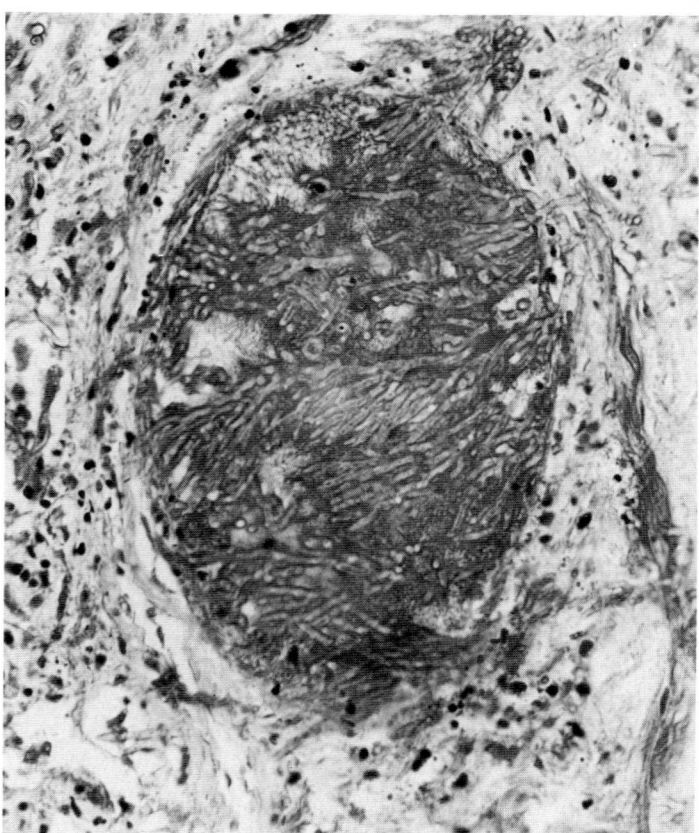

FIGURE 110-2 *Aspergillus fumigatus.* The fungus is invading the wall and filling the lumen of a pulmonary blood vessel of a leukemic patient with invasive pulmonary aspergillosis. Note the characteristic hyphal form which branches dichotomously at a 45° angle. H&E, ×520.

and to inhibit spore germination. Studies in mice have shown that this defense mechanism is greatly depressed by the administration of corticosteroids. Neutrophils, in contrast, have little sporicidal effect, are moderately effective against germinating spores, and are quite fungicidal against the invading hyphal forms. This fungicidal activity of neutrophils is dependent on the neutrophils' production of superoxide anion, hydrogen peroxide, hypochlorous acid and myeloperoxidase-dependent iodination following phagocytosis of the organisms. It is predictable, then, that patients receiving corticosteroids, those with inadequate numbers of circulating neutrophils (usually less than 500 per cubic millimeter), and those with functional neutrophil defects (such as chronic granulomatous disease in which there is an inadequate generation of oxidants) would be susceptible to invasive infection with this organism.

In contrast, hypoglobulinemia plays no role in the pathogenesis of invasive aspergillosis. Similarly, prior or concomitant antibacterial therapy, despite widespread belief to the contrary, does not appear to play a significant role in the evolution of this infection.

Clinical Manifestations

The usual presenting symptoms of invasive pulmonary aspergillosis are well explained by the prime features of the pulmonary pathology, necrotizing bronchopneumonia and hemorrhagic pulmonary infarction: nonproductive cough, pleuritic chest pain, hemoptysis, fever and chills, and, occasionally, dyspnea and tachypnea. Other than fever, most patients with infection restricted to the lungs have little in the way of physical findings. Fever is observed in more than 90 percent of patients, pleural pain in some 50 percent, and hemoptysis in approximately 30 percent. Hemoptysis is usually minor, although occasionally life-threatening pulmonary hemorrhage may occur due to fungal invasion of a major pulmonary vessel. In addition, IPA may be associated with a systemic bleeding disorder characterized by a prolonged thrombin time, but without the classic features of disseminated intravascular coagulation. It is hypothesized that this coagulopathy is due to the release of proteolytic enzymes by the fungus into the circulation. Two not uncommon thoracic complications of invasive pulmonary aspergillosis are the development of a bronchopleural fistula and pericardial disease with or without tamponade. The bronchopleural fistula is due to the necrotizing, tissue infarcting nature of the pulmonary infection, whereas the pericardial involvement is due to direct extension from an adjoining pulmonary site of infection or a metastatic myocardial focus.

Less commonly, the primary focus of infection in the lungs may be relatively asymptomatic, and the symptom complex that brings the patients to medical attention is due to metastatic infection. Thus, necrotizing skin papules or focal neurologic deficits due to hematogenous dissemination of the *Aspergillus* infection (Fig. 110-3) from the pulmonary portal of entry may be the major presenting complaint.

Although the patient is frequently quite ill and toxic when first seen, the clinical presentation is a subacute one, taking days to a few weeks to evolve. Indeed, a more acute course suggests the presence of simultaneous infection with other organisms or that vascular invasion and infarction have occurred—events highly associated with bloodstream dissemination.

The preceding descriptions have been that of *primary* invasive pulmonary aspergillosis. Particularly in intubated patients who are immunosuppressed or during the course of a nosocomial epidemic, secondary invasive aspergillosis can also occur; that is, invasive aspergillosis developing sequentially in a lung previously injured by viral (particularly cytomegalovirus) or bacterial pneumonia. In these patients, many of the same symptoms as in primary infection may be present, but not uncommonly a more insidious clinical syndrome is present, characterized by persistent fevers, new chest radiograph abnormalities, and increasing respiratory distress.

Recently, a less virulent form of IPA has been defined and termed *chronic necrotizing pulmonary aspergillosis* or *semi-invasive pulmonary aspergillosis*. The affected patients include those with a chronic pulmonary disease, such as inactive tuberculosis, a pneumoconiosis, or

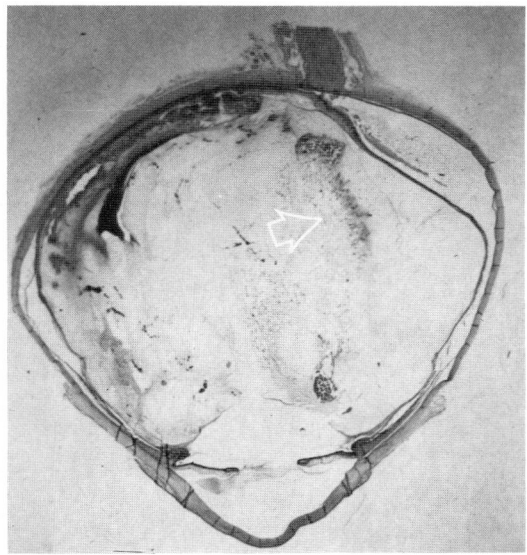
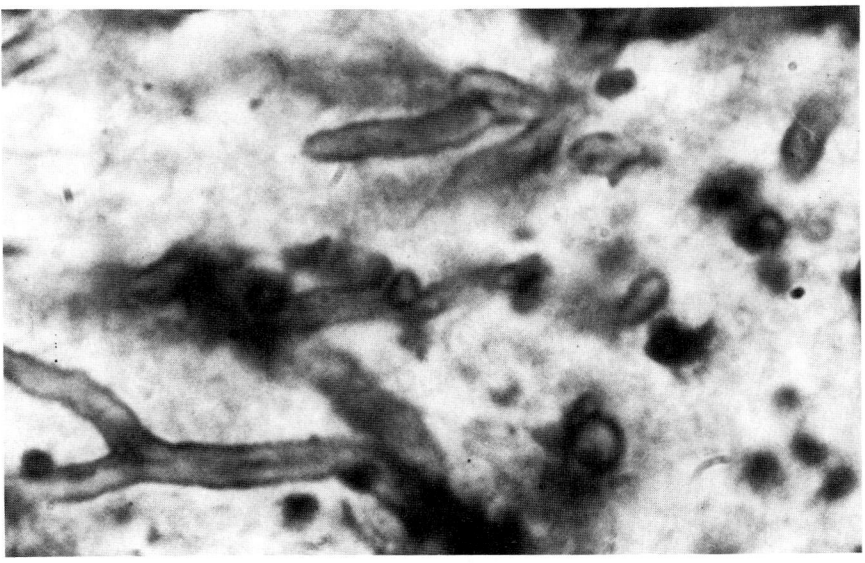

A   *B*

FIGURE 110-3 Metastatic infection with *Aspergillus fumigatus* involving the eye. The removed eye of a 32-year-old woman, 3 months post-renal transplant, who presented with fever, nonproductive cough, and normal chest radiograph accompanied by increasing pain and loss of vision in one eye. All vision was lost in that eye during the next 3 days. The eye was removed for relief of pain and for diagnosis. *A.* Low-power photomicrograph (×7) of the eye reveals areas of increased inflammation (arrow). *B.* High power (×425) of the area of inflammation reveals the metastatic invasive *Aspergillus* infection.

chronic obstructive airways disease; the net state of immunocompromise is mild to moderate, such as that caused by malnutrition and low dose corticosteroid therapy. The clinical illness is chronic, starting after weeks or months of fever, weight loss, and cough—a presentation quite similar to that of reactivation tuberculosis, an anaerobic lung abscess, or progressive pulmonary histoplasmosis. Typically, the chest radiograph reveals a slowly progressive infiltrate of an upper lobe that may go on to cavitation.

Radiographic Findings

The radiographic findings in *primary* invasive pulmonary aspergillosis can be quite variable. In as many as 25 percent of patients, the conventional chest radiograph is normal in the face of symptoms or even metastatic disease. In such patients, the ventilation-perfusion nuclear scan is sometimes helpful in suggesting the diagnosis. As a rule, the earliest findings are single or multiple nodules or patchy areas of bronchopneumonia. The lesions may cross lung fissures and are usually located peripherally. The subsequent course can vary: an increase in size and diffuseness, with the frequent development of cavitation; increasing bronchopneumonia; or, less often, a diffuse interstitial process.

The radiographic appearance that has received most attention in recent years, particularly in leukemic patients, is the "air crescent sign," i.e., a nodular infiltrate with central necrosis and peripheral crescentic or circumferential cavitation (Fig. 110-4). Until recently, this sign was identified primarily with a mycetoma or fungal ball in an old pulmonary cavity in patients with previous tuberculosis or bronchiectasis. It was also known to occur in such conditions as echinococcal cysts, nocardial or anaerobic bacterial lung abscesses, and malignancies. In the leukemic patient with IPA, the typical progression is from normal lung through poorly defined infiltrate to cavitation and the appearance of an air crescent sign (Fig. 110-4). Unlike the mycetoma that develops in immunocompetent individuals with preexisting cavities—in whom the material in the cavity is a mat of fungal forms bearing conidiophores—the "mycetomas" seen in immunocompromised patients represent autoamputated, infarcted spheres of lung tissue containing invading *Aspergillus* hyphae—pulmonary sequestra.

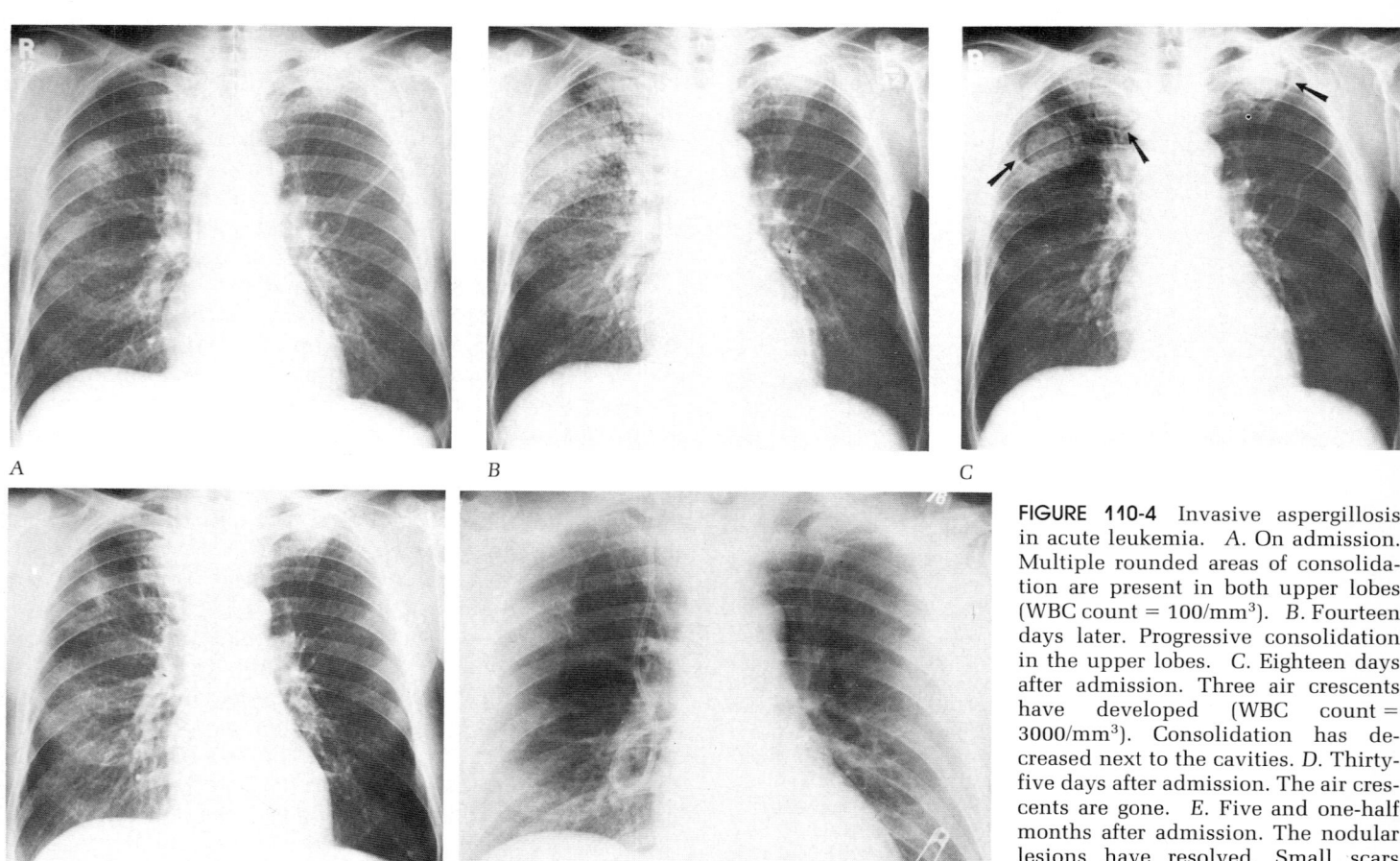

A

B

C

D

E

FIGURE 110-4 Invasive aspergillosis in acute leukemia. *A.* On admission. Multiple rounded areas of consolidation are present in both upper lobes (WBC count = 100/mm³). *B.* Fourteen days later. Progressive consolidation in the upper lobes. *C.* Eighteen days after admission. Three air crescents have developed (WBC count = 3000/mm³). Consolidation has decreased next to the cavities. *D.* Thirty-five days after admission. The air crescents are gone. *E.* Five and one-half months after admission. The nodular lesions have resolved. Small scars persist. (*Courtesy of Dr. Warren Gefter.*)

Approximately 50 percent of leukemic patients with invasive pulmonary aspergillosis develop pulmonary cavitation; some 80 percent of these have air crescents (Fig. 110-4). The air crescents are accompanied by a return of circulating neutrophils and are a positive prognostic sign, even though massive hemorrhage is a serious risk in a few of these: despite this risk, the likelihood of survival is eight times greater in those who develop air crescent than in those whose lesions fail to cavitate. In the latter, the pulmonary process usually proceeds to diffuse disease, and less than 10 percent survive (Fig. 110-5). The number and effectiveness of functioning neutrophils are implicated in the pathogenesis of the cavities, the development of air crescent, and clinical recovery.

Cavitation usually is not observed on conventional chest radiographs for at least 10 to 14 days after the appearance of the infiltrate—a period too delayed for this to be a useful *early* diagnostic sign. However, computed tomography (CT) may be diagnostically helpful earlier in the disease by identifying small lesions and the onset of cavitation.

The radiographic findings in patients with *secondary* invasive pulmonary aspergillosis, i.e., a form that develops as a superinfection in an individual with a primary pneumonia of other causes, are quite subtle. Increasing infiltrate or the development of a nodular character to the infiltrate in an immunocompromised patient can suggest

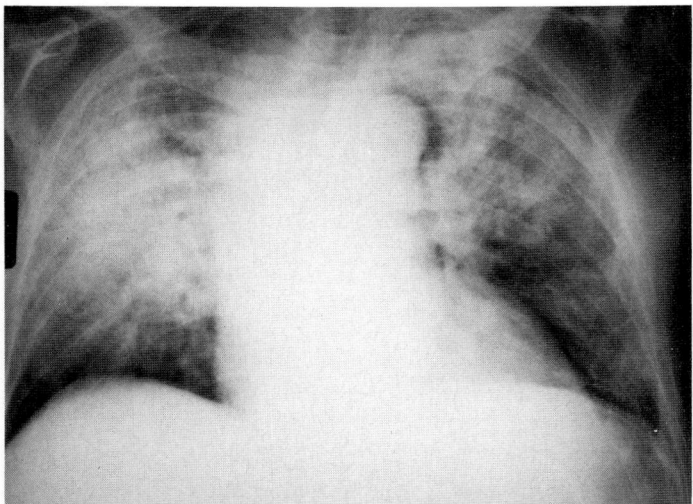

FIGURE 110-5 Invasive pulmonary aspergillosis after liver transplantation. A diffuse *Klebsiella* pneumonia had been treated with cephalothin and gentamicin, and the initial clinical response was favorable. However, after 2 days of being afebrile, fever returned and was accompanied by increasing shortness of breath while the chest radiograph remained unchanged. One day after this radiograph was taken, the patient died. Autopsy revealed two processes in the lungs: a diffuse gram-negative pneumonia and focal areas of invasive aspergillosis restricted to the right lower and middle lobes. This figure illustrates the difficulty in differentiating the focal areas of *Aspergillus* superinfection from the primary bacterial process.

this diagnosis. Again, early CT scanning can be quite helpful.

Diagnosis

Survival of patients with invasive pulmonary aspergillosis is directly related to the rapidity with which the diagnosis is made and effective therapy instituted. The definitive diagnostic method is the histopathologic and/or cultural identification of the fungus in pulmonary tissue. Open lung biopsy remains the most reliable method for making the diagnosis. However, because the prognosis of immunosuppressed patients, such as the leukemics, is quite poor, there is increasing reluctance to resort to open lung biopsy. Therefore, less invasive diagnostic procedures are usually attempted first. Fiberoptic bronchoscopy, with transbronchial biopsy, bronchial washings, and brushings, yields the diagnosis in approximately 50 to 60 percent of patients with invasive pulmonary aspergillosis. Pleural-based disease is better approached by percutaneous needle lung aspiration, which has yielded the diagnosis in more than 85 percent of such patients.

However, even the less-invasive procedures are undesirable in many patients, and attention has turned to noninvasive, indirect methods of diagnosis. Determination of antibodies to *Aspergillus* is not helpful—measurement gives a high rate of both false-positive and false-negative results. More promising have been attempts to identify *Aspergillus* antigens in either serum or bronchoalveolar lavage fluid by immunoassay. These studies have revealed a high specificity and a sensitivity of approximately 50 to 70 percent. At present, however, this remains only a promising investigative procedure.

Many attempts have been made to correlate the results of sputum and/or nasal cultures with the presence of IPA. The problem is that while transient colonization with *Aspergillus* species occurs in as many as 15 percent of individuals without invasive infection, it will be grown from the sputum in only 8 to 34 percent of patients with proven disease. This is not to say, however, that sputum culture results should be ignored. When *A. fumigatus* or *A. flavus* are isolated alone, not as part of a mixture of *Aspergillus* species, when two or more cultures are positive, and/or when nasal cultures are also positive in an immunocompromised patient with a clinically compatible syndrome, this is sufficient information to initiate antifungal chemotherapy. The problem here is less specificity than sensitivity; that is, the absence of these findings does not rule out invasive pulmonary aspergillosis.

The final approach to the diagnosis of IPA relies on the clinical presentation and setting and starts therapy on the basis of statistical argument rather than on a definitive diagnosis. For example, in patients with granulocytopenia secondary to treatment of leukemia, the risk of developing invasive *Aspergillus* infection is approximately 1 percent

per day in the first few weeks and increases to 4.3 percent per day by the 24th day; those in whom the granulocytopenia has lasted for 28 or more days have 50 to 60 percent risk of developing IPA. By combining this information with other clinical characteristics that are frequently associated with this infection makes it possible to develop a discriminant scorecard (Table 110-1): a high score is correlated with a high probability of infection with this fungus and is an indication for therapy.

A reasonable approach to these therapeutic options is that if the underlying disease is one for which the overall prognosis is poor, e.g., acute nonlymphocytic leukemia, empiric therapy is undertaken based on indirect diagnostic clues such as the discriminant scorecard. However, in those who have a much greater potential for survival, if recovery from invasive infection can be accomplished, e.g., transplant patients, it is preferable to resort to invasive techniques to establish a definitive diagnosis, first by percutaneous needle aspiration or fiberoptic bronchoscopy and then, if necessary, open lung biopsy.

Therapy

The cornerstone of therapy for invasive pulmonary aspergillosis remains amphotericin B. The imidazole drugs miconazole and ketoconazole and the oral agent 5-fluorocytosine are not alternatives. In particular, ketoconazole not only is ineffective, but it may also select for *Aspergillus* infection, and, when given together with amphotericin, ketoconazole appears to antagonize amphotericin's therapeutic effects.

The first step in treatment is to initiate amphotericin therapy, quickly reaching a daily dose of 0.4 to 0.75 mg/kg per day to reach a total dose of 2 to 2.5 g per day. If the patient's clinical course stabilizes, much of this therapy can be given as an outpatient on alternate days, giving a dose of 0.8 mg/kg thrice weekly. It is also wise to "stage the patient," i.e., to search for metastatic infection using a cranial CT scan and nuclear bone and liver scans. The definition of sites of metastatic infection affords important guidelines in determining the dose and duration of antifungal therapy and the possible use of adjunctive surgical treatment.

Although amphotericin treatment of IPA has become increasingly successful in recent years, the therapy of metastatic infection—particularly to the brain—has remained very disappointing. Because of this, there has been considerable interest in the *addition* of such drugs as 5-fluorocytosine or rifampin to the amphotericin regimen in the hopes of effecting cure with synergistic therapy. In vitro data and some animal studies have suggested that this might be a promising approach. However, there are only anecdotal experiences in humans with this approach at present. Because of the increased incidence of toxicity with the combined regimens, amphotericin B is used alone for infection restricted to the lungs and the use of the combined regimens is reserved for patients with metastatic infection (prescribing rifampin at a dose of 300 mg thrice daily or 5-fluorocytosine 37.5 mg/kg four times a day in addition to full dose amphotericin).

Surgery can occasionally be useful in patients with a single residual site of infection, in those with relapsing disease in a single pulmonary segment, in patients with residual cavities or mycetomas following completion of treatment and control of their underlying illnesses, or in patients with a single site of metastatic infection. Surgical intervention is particularly attractive in individuals whose course of amphotericin therapy must be abbreviated because of unacceptable levels of toxicity. It must be emphasized, however, that surgery is not primary treatment, but rather only adjunctive to effective chemotherapy.

TABLE 110-1
Discriminant Scorecard* for Invasive Pulmonary Aspergillosis for Patients with Leukemia

Parameter	Criteria Control (Score = 0)	Case (Score = 1)
Temperature, F°	< 100	> 101
Granulocytopenic days (granulocyte count = 500 mm⁻³)	< 22	≥ 30
Febrile episodes without a source	None	≥ 2
Febrile days without a source	< 6	≥ 14
Febrile days during antibiotic therapy	< 13	≥ 19
Rales on physical examination without volume overload	Absent	Present
Nasal-sinus abnormality on examination	None	Nasal eschar or discharge plus epistaxis plus sinus tenderness
Pleuritic chest pain	Absent	Present
Days of onset of pulmonary infiltrate	Before 7th day	After 14th day
Pulmonary infiltrate on chest radiography	None or unilobed	Multilobed
Cavitary or nodules on chest radiography	Absent	Present

*Each parameter in the control range is given a value of 0; each parameter in the case range is given a value of 1. A parameter within an intermediate range or for which there is no information receives no score. The cumulative discriminant scorecard value is defined as the average of all score values that were neither missing nor intermediate. A score greater than 0.4 is highly associated with the presence of invasive pulmonary aspergillosis in patients undergoing treatment of leukemia.

SOURCE: Modified from Gerson et al., 1985.

PULMONARY MUCORMYCOSIS

Pulmonary mucormycosis is an invasive, opportunistic pulmonary infection caused by fungi of the family Mucoraceae. *Rhizopus*, *Mucor*, and *Absidia* species are the ones most commonly associated with human infection, although *Cunninghamella* and *Saksenaea* have also been occasionally noted to produce significant disease in severely immunocompromised hosts. Although Mucoraceae are taxonomically distinct from *Aspergillus* species, the invasive pulmonary infection produced by the two groups or organisms is very similar.

Epidemiology

Mucoraceae, like *Aspergillus* species, are dimorphic fungi that grow saprophytically on decaying vegetation and other organic matter. Pulmonary mucormycosis begins with the inhalation of spores of the fungus into the lower respiratory tract of susceptible individuals. As with *Aspergillus* infection, person-to-person spread does not occur; unlike *Aspergillus* infection, epidemic disease does not appear to be a significant problem. Because of this, pulmonary mucormycosis is quantitatively much less important than aspergillosis among immunocompromised individuals. Although rarely seen in normal hosts, pulmonary mucormycosis is observed primarily among three groups of patients: diabetics, especially those with ketoacidosis; patients with leukemia or lymphoma; and those receiving high dose corticosteroid therapy over a prolonged period of time. Surprisingly, unlike the situation with *Aspergillus* infection, pulmonary mucormycosis appears to be an uncommon problem in transplant patients, unless neutropenia and unstable diabetes are also present.

Pathogenesis and Pathology

The spores of Mucoraceae that are inhaled appear to be resistant to host defenses, but germination of the spores—the critical step in the initiation of invasive infection—is strongly inhibited by normal bronchoalveolar macrophages. This host defense has been shown in experimental models to be markedly impaired by the induction of diabetes or by the administration of corticosteroids. (In contrast, *Aspergillus* infection in these same models is unaffected by the induction of the diabetic state.) In addition, normal human serum, but not serum from diabetic patients with ketoacidosis, will inhibit hyphal growth of Mucoraceae. This serum effect is not due to the presence of antispore or antihyphal antibodies. Normally functioning granulocytes in adequate numbers are capable of destroying germinating spores that escape the bronchoalveolar macrophages and develop into the tissue-invasive hyphal forms. Thus, within the lung an exuberant polymorphonuclear leukocyte response occurs in patients capable of generating such a response.

The outstanding pathologic characteristic of mucormycosis is the invasion of blood vessels by broad, nonseptate hyphae that branch at right angles, thereby producing tissue infarction and a characteristic blackish inflammatory exudate. Although tissue infarction is the most important result of this vascular invasion, significant hemorrhage is not uncommon, and hematogenous dissemination can occur. When compared with invasive aspergillosis, pulmonary mucormycosis has certain subtle differences: blood vessel invasion with infarction and progressive gangrene is more marked with Mucoraceae infection, while metastatic infection is less common.

Clinical Manifestations

The clinical manifestations of pulmonary mucormycosis are indistinguishable from those of invasive aspergillosis: fever and chills, nonproductive cough, pleuritic chest pain, hemoptysis, and, as the disease progresses, dyspnea and tachypnea. Again, physical examination, with the occasional exception of a pleural rub, is usually not very helpful.

Radiographic Findings

Typically, the chest radiograph of a patient with pulmonary mucormycosis is that of an enlarging nodular infiltrate that cavitates, with the not-infrequent development of the air crescent sign. Alternatively, typical peripherally located infiltrates consistent with pulmonary infarction may develop. Disease may be unifocal or multifocal, and there is no particular predilection for any particular lobe of the lung (Fig. 110-6). In short, the findings are identical with those seen in invasive pulmonary aspergillosis.

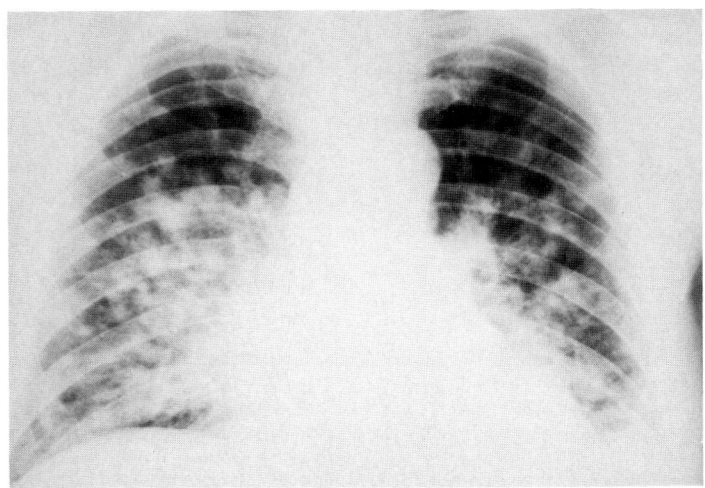

FIGURE 110-6   Invasive mucormycosis in lymphoma. Multifocal, nodular pulmonary lesions are due to invasive mucormycosis.

Diagnosis

The only method currently available for diagnosing pulmonary mucormycosis is histologic demonstration of the fungus on lung biopsy material. Cultures of sputum and even biopsy material have a high false-negative rate. There are no serologic methods for measuring either antibody to the organism or antigen.

Therapy

Amphotericin B is the only drug currently available with any efficacy against infection with Mucoraceae. However, even this drug is relatively ineffective for two reasons: because of the vascular obstruction provided by this organism, delivery of the drug to the site of infection may be greatly compromised; many of the isolates are significantly more resistant to amphotericin than are other fungal species. Therefore, although an occasional patient has been reported to be cured with medical therapy alone, if at all possible, surgical resection with adjuvant chemotherapy should be regarded as the ideal method of therapy with the greatest chance of cure. An appropriate analogy is to lung cancer—the best chance of cure is with complete surgical resection, with chemotherapy reserved to deal with any microscopic foci of disease. Because of the relative resistance of the organism, dosages of amphotericin required are higher than with other fungal infections: 0.5 to 1.0 mg/kg per day, with a total dose of at least 2.5 to 3.0 g.

PULMONARY CRYPTOCOCCOSIS

Cryptococcosis is a systemic fungal infection caused by *Cryptococcus neoformans*, an encapsulated yeastlike organism, which is commonly found throughout the world, particularly at sites contaminated with pigeon and other bird excreta. The portal of entry for cryptococcal infection is the lung, where the organism may cause subclinical or symptomatic infection, and from which dissemination can occur. Although infection with *C. neoformans* can occur in apparently normal individuals, the majority of cases today are observed among immunocompromised individuals.

Epidemiology

Cryptococcal infection is thought to be initiated by the inhalation of aerosolized organisms growing in nature. Neither person-to-person nor animal-to-person transmission of the infection occurs. Outbreaks of cryptococcosis are rarely observed, occupational associations with clinical disease are not apparent, and histories of heavy exposure to pigeons and dust do not correlate well with clinical illness. Instead, it is believed that inhalation of this organism is a relatively common event, as documented by the not-infrequent finding of asymptomatic subpleural nodules containing *C. neoformans* in the lungs of individuals dying of other causes. The development of clinical disease appears to be primarily related to inadequacies in host responses to the inhalation of the organism, with individuals having defects in cell-mediated immunity being at highest risk. These include patients with Hodgkin's and non-Hodgkin's lymphomas; those, such as transplant recipients, receiving prolonged corticosteroid therapy; and patients with AIDS. These last are in greatest jeopardy, with 5 to 10 percent of AIDS patients developing cryptococcal infection, not uncommonly as the first manifestation of this illness.

Pathogenesis and Pathology

Many cryptococci growing in nature are unencapsulated, but shortly after inhalation many organisms begin to form a polysaccharide capsule. This occurrence is an important event, since unencapsulated organisms are rather easily phagocytosed and destroyed by both macrophages and neutrophils. The capsular polysaccharide has been shown to interfere with attachment of phagocytic cells to intact cryptococci, impair phagocytosis, and induce T-cell suppression of both the cell-mediated and antibody response to the organism. As a result, bronchoalveolar macrophages can wall off the infection but do not kill the encapsulated organisms. Although granulocytes can phagocytize and kill the unencapsulated cryptococci, there is little evidence that granulocytopenia or impaired granulocyte function plays a significant role in the pathogenesis of this infection. Similarly, humoral immunity appears to play a minor role. The major host defense against invasive cryptococcal infection, then, is an intact cell-mediated immune system, which itself can be suppressed by infection with encapsulated organisms. Hence not only do the immunocompromised patients with cryptococcosis have defects in cell-mediated immunity, but even apparently normal individuals with the infection can be shown to have subtle defects in this limb of host defense.

Cryptococcus neoformans is an unusual pathogen in that it produces no toxins and is relatively inert as a stimulus to tissue reaction, often provoking little or no inflammatory response. Four basic histopathologic patterns of pulmonary cryptococcal infection are observed: one or more peripheral pulmonary granulomas, sometimes associated with hilar lymph node involvement—a "cryptococcal primary complex" considered by some to be similar in pathogenesis to the primary Ghon complex of tuberculosis; granulomatous pneumonitis, with intra-alveolar proliferating organisms and an inflammatory response that can vary from an acute granulocytic infiltrate to diffuse intra-alveolar granulomas with giant cells; and

diffuse pneumonia with organisms present within alveolar capillaries and interstitial tissues, and overwhelming infection, with both intra-alveolar and intravascular organisms present in massive numbers. These last are associated with the greatest amount of systemic dissemination and are observed in patients with the most profound defects in cell-mediated immune function.

Clinical Manifestations

Of all the primary opportunistic infections of the lungs occurring in immunocompromised patients, cryptococcal infection is the one associated with the least amount of systemic toxicity or reaction. It is subacute-chronic in presentation and often relatively asymptomatic even in instances in which extensive pulmonary disease is demonstrable on chest radiograph. Among immunocompromised patients with pulmonary cryptococcosis, fully 20 percent are totally asymptomatic, fever and malaise are present in only 60 percent of patients, chest discomfort in 40 percent, weight loss in 35 percent, dyspnea and night sweats in 25 percent, and cough in 20 to 40 percent. Hemoptysis is quite rare. A similar lack of symptoms is noted in normal individuals with active pulmonary cryptococcosis. Even those patients who are symptomatic have such minor symptoms that there is frequently a long delay, during which systemic dissemination can occur, before they come to medical attention. In our experience, the most frequent sequence of events is the recognition of a new lesion on a routine chest radiograph with patients then admitting that perhaps they have minor symptoms.

The major significance of pulmonary cryptococcosis is not that this is a disabling illness, but that it can lead to disseminated infection with a particularly striking effect on the central nervous system. Progressive pulmonary cryptococcosis is a rare cause of death, even in the AIDS patient whose major problem is the disseminated infection. On the other hand, once pulmonary cryptococcosis is identified, the search for metastatic infection is obligatory. Even subtle symptoms referrable to the central nervous system, such as headache, lethargy, and personality change, in this setting should be carefully evaluated, as such symptoms with infection localized to the lungs are most uncommon.

Radiographic Findings

The range of radiographic findings observed in patients with pulmonary cryptococcosis is quite broad, with some patients, particularly those with AIDS, having negative chest films in the face of extensive disease. The most common pattern observed is one of uni- or multifocal nodular lesions, with or without cavitation (Fig. 110-7). In addition, alveolar or interstitial infiltrates, or a miliary pattern may be observed. Hilar lymph node enlargement may be seen in approximately 10 percent of patients, with a simi-

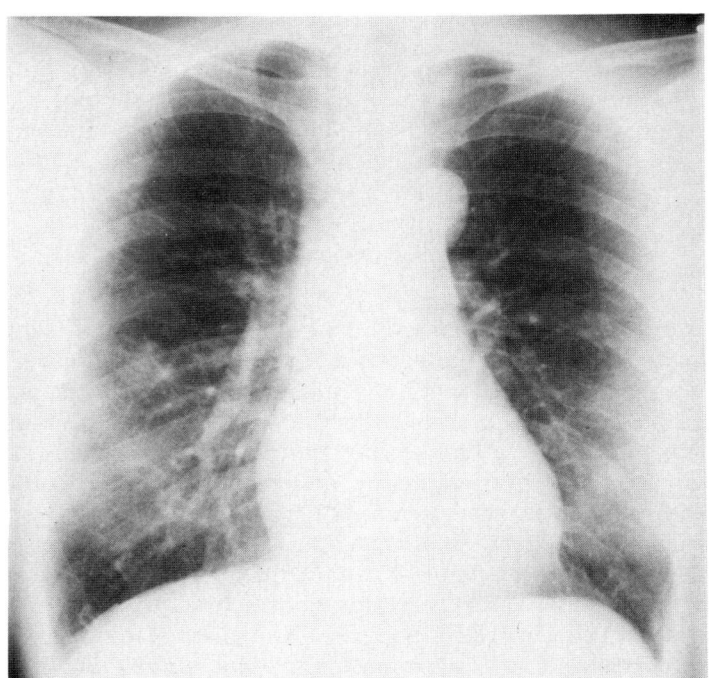

FIGURE 110-7 *Cryptococcus neoformans.* Asymptomatic renal transplant patient. The nodular lesion in the right mid-lung field was discovered on routine screening. Percutaneous needle aspiration of this lesion yielded *Cryptococcus neoformans* on fungal culture.

lar percentage of patients having evidence of pleural effusion. This last is highly associated with the presence of disseminated disease.

Diagnosis

The diagnosis of pulmonary cryptococcosis depends on the isolation of the organism or the demonstration of cryptococcal antigen in a bodily fluid. Cultures of expectorated sputum, transtracheal aspirates, or bronchial brushings are variably positive in patients with pulmonary cryptococcosis. However, *C. neoformans* may be isolated from the sputa of as many as 20 percent of normal individuals and immunocompromised individuals without invasive pulmonary infection. Therefore, unless the organisms or cryptococcal antigens are identified at extrapulmonary sites, a biopsy procedure is necessary. Although fiberoptic bronchoscopy with transbronchial biopsy can be useful in this setting, we have found that percutaneous needle aspiration will yield the diagnosis in more than 90 percent of patients with focal cryptococcal disease. If this fails, then open lung biopsy may be necessary.

Serum of patients with pulmonary cryptococcosis may occasionally be positive for the presence of cryptococcal antigen, particularly in patients with disseminated disease. A negative result, however, in no way rules out this diagnosis. Extrapulmonary sites that can yield the

diagnosis on culture include skin lesions, bone marrow, urine, blood, and cerebrospinal fluid. Conversely, any patient with proven pulmonary cryptococcosis should have all these sites sampled to determine the extent of dissemination. Lumbar puncture (with the cerebrospinal fluid being tested for cryptococcal antigen as well as culture for the organisms) and cranial CT scanning should be carried out in all such patients, as the intensity of therapy and the long-term prognosis is to a great extent determined by the presence or absence of dissemination to the central nervous system.

Therapy

Every immunocompromised patient with proven pulmonary cryptococcosis merits therapy, even if the individual is asymptomatic, because of the risk of extrapulmonary dissemination. Such therapy should consist of amphotericin B alone or combined with 5-fluorocytosine. Choosing between these two regimens cannot be done at present based on controlled studies, but many investigators in this field argue that since the big concern is silent dissemination to the central nervous system, the best treatment regimen should include a regimen designed to treat the brain as well. Hence, if tolerated, amphotericin B at a dose of 0.3 mg/kg per day intravenously plus 5-fluorocytosine at a dose of 37.5 mg/kg every 6 h by mouth for a period of 6 weeks is prescribed. Ketoconazole is reserved for the treatment of individuals who cannot tolerate amphotericin therapy; it is only a second-line drug here. Surgical resection is reserved for the patient with localized disease who either will not tolerate amphotericin therapy or has relapsed after an adequate course of treatment.

The AIDS patient with cryptococcal infection represents a particular challenge. As with other forms of opportunistic infection in this patient population, cure of cryptococcal infection appears to be impossible. The aim here should be control of symptoms with acceptable levels of toxicity, using repeated courses of antifungal therapy.

CANDIDAL INFECTION IN THE LUNG

Candida species are isolated from the respiratory secretions of immunocompromised patients more often than all other fungal organisms combined. For example, sputum cultures performed on patients receiving corticosteroids and antibiotics revealed the presence of *Candida* species in more than 40 percent of cultures. Despite this, primary candidal pneumonia is exceedingly rare, even in the most immunocompromised of patients. When *Candida* are found in lung biopsy specimens, one of the following clinical situations is usually present: (1) the most important consideration is hematogenous delivery of the organism to the lung as part of a disseminated candidiasis syndrome. Between 20 and 40 percent of patients with disseminated candidiasis will seed their lungs, although it is unusual for these pulmonary candidal lesions to be an important determinant of the patient's course. (2) Immunocompromised patients with acute or chronic pulmonary disease who are debilitated and whose posterior pharynx is colonized with *Candida* species will occasionally aspirate these organisms and develop secondary or superinfecting areas of candidal pneumonitis. Again, the impact of such pulmonary infection is usually minimal, as these are usually late events in the terminal stages of the patient's illness. (3) Similarly, intubated, immunocompromised patients whose sputum is colonized with *Candida* species may develop areas of candidal superinfection. Perhaps the best study of the overall significance of candidal pneumonia in the immunocompromised host is the report from Memorial-Sloan-Kettering Cancer Center of 30 immunocompromised patients with histopathologic evidence of candidal pulmonary infection. All but one case was found at autopsy, and in only three cases was the candidal infection felt to have played a significant role in the patients' course.

When *Candida* species do invade the lung, microabscesses, nodular lesions, focal consolidations, or, rarely, a miliary pattern may be observed. Because of the rarity of candidal pneumonia as an important clinical entity and the high rate of isolation from sputum cultures, the only diagnostic procedure of value is the histopathologic and/or cultural identification of the organism within lung tissue obtained at biopsy. True candidal pulmonary infection is treated like disseminated candidiasis and cryptococcosis—amphotericin B, with or without 5-fluorocytosine.

RARE CAUSES OF FUNGAL PNEUMONIA IN THE IMMUNOCOMPROMISED HOST

Invasive pulmonary infection caused by a variety of saprophytic fungi is occasionally seen in immunocompromised patients. These fungal species include *Sporothrix schenckii, Petriellidium boydii, Trichosporon beigelii, Penicillium* and *Fusarium* species, and *Geotrichum candidum*. These all share certain general characteristics: a clinical picture that resembles other invasive fungal pneumonias in this population—fever, nonproductive cough, pleurisy, and the not-infrequent occurrence of metastatic infection; a pathologic picture that reveals a high rate of vascular invasion and hemorrhagic infarction, particularly with *T. beigelii, Penicillium,* and *Fusarium* infections; a similar range of radiographic findings; and a need for biopsy to establish the diagnosis. It is important to note that such organisms as *T. beigelii* and *P. boydii* are resistant to amphotericin B in vitro, while being sensitive to miconazole. Therefore, distinguishing at least these two organisms from the other fungal invaders carries important therapeutic implications.

BIBLIOGRAPHY

Adam RD, Paquin ML, Petersen EA, Saubolle MA, Rinaldi MG, Corcoran JG, Galgiani JN, Sobonya RE: Phaeohyphomycosis caused by the fungal genera *Bipolaris* and *Exserohilum*. A report of 9 cases and review of the literature. Medicine 65:203–217, 1986.
> *The authors report seven new cases of Bipolaris infection and two of Exserohilum infection. Amphotericin B appears to be the treatment of choice for invasive infections caused by Bipolaris/Exserohilum species. The role of ketoconazole and other imidazole derivatives has yet to be defined.*

Bigby TD, Serota ML, Tierney LM Jr, Matthay MA: Clinical spectrum of pulmonary mucormycosis. Chest 89:435–439, 1986.
> *This review emphasizes clinical and pathologic characteristics of pulmonary mucormycosis. The most common clinical presentation of pulmonary mucormycosis is a rapidly progressive pneumonia in a patient with underlying hematologic malignancy treated with immunosuppressive drugs. Patients with diabetes mellitus may develop a distinctive endobronchial form of this disease.*

Cairns MR, Durack DT: Fungal pneumonia in the immunocompromised host. Semin Respir Infect 1:166–185, 1986.
> *An excellent review of the subject with a complete bibliography.*

Cohen MS, Isturiz RE, Malech HL, Root RK, Wilfert CM, Gutman L, Buckley RH: Fungal infection in chronic granulomatous disease. The importance of the phagocyte in defense against fungi. Am J Med 71:59–66, 1981.
> *The landmark paper documenting the importance of normal microbicidal function of phagocytic cells in defending against such invasive fungal infections as invasive aspergillosis.*

Drouhet E, Dupont B: Evolution of antifungal agents: Past, present, and future. Rev Infect Dis 9(Suppl 1):S4–14, 1987.
> *A review of the development of the various antifungal agents and of the indications for their use.*

Gefter WB, Albelda SM, Talbot GH, Gerson SL, Cassileth PA, Miller WT: Invasive pulmonary aspergillosis and acute leukemia. Limitations in the diagnostic utility of the air crescent sign. Radiology 157:605–610, 1985.
> *A careful analysis of the sequential radiologic findings in patients with invasive pulmonary aspergillosis.*

Gerding DN: Treatment of pulmonary sporotrichosis. Semin Respir Infect 1:61–65, 1986.
> *A review of the management of pulmonary infection with Sporothrix schenckii. Three modalities are considered: saturated solution of potassium iodide, amphotericin B, and resective surgery.*

Gerson SL, Talbot GH, Hurwitz S, Lusk EJ, Strom BL, Cassileth PA: Discriminant scorecard for diagnosis of invasive pulmonary aspergillosis in patients with acute leukemia. Am J Med 79:57–64, 1985.
> *A useful clinical approach to the diagnosis of invasive pulmonary aspergillosis in patients poorly suited for definitive biopsy studies.*

Gerson SL, Talbot GH, Hurwitz S, Strom BL, Lusk EJ, Cassileth PA: Prolonged granulocytopenia: The major risk factor for invasive pulmonary aspergillosis in patients with acute leukemia. Ann Intern Med 100:345–351, 1984.
> *A careful documentation of the importance of granulocytes in the pathogenesis of and recovery from invasive aspergillosis.*

Hadfield TL, Smith MB, Winn RE, Rinaldi MG, Guerra C: Mycoses caused by *Candida lusitaniae*. Rev Infect Dis 9:1006–1012, 1987.
> *Candida lusitaniae, a fungus that has a low incidence of infection in immunocompetent people, is emerging as an opportunistic pathogen in immunocompromised hosts.*

Hawkins C, Armstrong D: Fungal infections in the immunocompromised host. Clin Haematol 13:599–630, 1984.
> *An excellent overview of this subject with a very useful bibliography.*

Jensen WA, Rose RM, Hammer SM, Karchmer AW: Serologic diagnosis of focal pneumonia caused by *Cryptococcus neoformans*. Am Rev Respir Dis 132:189–191, 1985.
> *A careful review of the possible utility of serologic testing for cryptococcal antigen in the diagnosis of pulmonary cryptococcus.*

Kahn FW, Jones JM, England DM: The role of bronchoalveolar lavage in the diagnosis of invasive pulmonary aspergillosis. Am J Clin Pathol 86:518–523, 1986.

Cultures and histochemical stains for fungi were performed on concentrated, cytocentrifuged bronchoalveolar lavage (BAL) samples from 82 immunocompromised patients undergoing bronchoscopic evaluation of new pulmonary infiltrates. Aspergillus hyphae were identified in 9 of 17 BAL samples from patients with invasive pulmonary aspergillosis. The presence of A. hyphae in BAL samples had a 53% sensitivity, 97% specificity, and 75% positive predictive value for the diagnosis of invasive pulmonary aspergillosis. BAL fungal cultures were positive in only 4 of 17 cases (23% sensitivity). However, a combination of fungal stains and cultures yielded a diagnostic sensitivity of 58% and a specificity of 92%.

Klotz SA, Penn RL, George RB: Antigen detection in the diagnosis of fungal respiratory infections. Semin Respir Infect 1:16–21, 1986.

A review of current techniques used for the detection of fungal antigens, including their sensitivity and specificity, and their use in diagnosing human infections.

Kuhlman JE, Fishman EK, Siegelman SS: Invasive pulmonary aspergillosis in acute leukemia: Characteristic findings on CT, the CT halo sign, and the role of CT in early diagnosis. Radiology 157:611–614, 1985.

A useful delineation of the role of CT scans in the diagnosis of invasive pulmonary aspergillosis.

Lehrer RI, Howard DH, Sypherd PS, Edwards J, Segal G, Winston D: Mucormycosis. Ann Intern Med 93:93–108, 1980.

An excellent review with a complete bibliography on pathogenesis and clinical, diagnostic, and therapeutic aspects of mucormycosis.

Levitz SM, Diamond RD: Changing patterns of aspergillosis infections. Adv Intern Med 30:153–174, 1984.

An excellent review of all aspects of aspergillosis with a complete bibliography.

Levitz SM, Diamond RD: Mechanisms of resistance of *Aspergillus fumigatus* conidia to killing by neutrophils in vitro. J Infect Dis 152:33–42, 1985.

A useful presentation of the host defenses against invasive aspergillosis.

Linder J, Vaughan WP, Armitage JO, Ghafouri MA, Hurkman D, Mroczek EC, Miller NG, Rennard SI: Cytopathology of opportunistic infection in bronchoalveolar lavage. Am J Clin Pathol 88:421–428, 1987.

Silver- or Papanicolaou-stained slides from 604 lavage specimens from 344 patients were evaluated for the presence of fungal, parasitic, and viral organisms. Yeast, pseudohyphae, or hyphae occurred in 155 specimens (25.7%). Candida was the most frequent opportunistic fungus in immunosuppressed hosts.

Martin WJ II, Smith TF, Sanderson DR, Brutinel WM, Cockerill FR III, Douglas WW: Role of bronchoalveolar lavage in the assessment of opportunistic pulmonary infections: Utility and complications. Mayo Clin Proc 62:549–557, 1987.

A review of the value of bronchoalveolar lavage in diagnosing opportunistic infections, including fungal infections.

Masur H, Rosen PP, Armstrong D: Pulmonary disease caused by *Candida* species. Am J Med 63:914–925, 1977.

The best article currently available for assessing the true role of candidal infection of the lung in causing morbidity and mortality on the compromised host, taken from the experience at Memorial-Sloan Kettering Cancer Center.

McDonnell JM, Hutchins GM: Pulmonary cryptococcosis. Hum Pathol 16:121–128, 1985.

An excellent review of the pathology of pulmonary cryptococcosis and its correlation with compromised host defenses.

Meyer RD, Rosen P, Armstrong D: Phycomycosis complicating leukemia and lymphoma. Ann Intern Med 77:871–879, 1972.

A careful delineation of invasive mucormycosis in patients with leukemia and lymphoma.

Nishioka G, Schwartz JG, Rinaldi MG, Aufdemorte TB, Mackie E: Fungal maxillary sinusitis caused by Curvularia lunata. Arch Otolaryngol Head Neck Surg 113:665–666, 1987.

The second known published case of maxillary sinusitis caused by Curvularia lunata in an immunocompetent patient.

Opal SM, APS AA, Cannady PB, Morse PL, Burton LJ, Hammer PG II: Efficacy of infection control measures during a nosocomial outbreak of disseminated aspergillosis associated with hospital construction. J Infect Dis 153:634–637, 1986.
> *Control measures for preventing epidemic, nosocomial invasive aspergillosis.*

Rhame FS, Streifel AJ, Kersey JH Jr, McGlave PB: Extrinsic risk factors for pneumonia in the patient at high risk of infection. Am J Med 76:42–52, 1984.
> *Excellent overview on the epidemiology of nosocomial pneumonia in the compromised host.*

Sherertz RJ, Belani A, Kramer BS, Elfenbein GJ, Weiner RS, Sullivan ML, Thomas RG, Samsa GP: Impact of air filtration on nosocomial *Aspergillus* infections. Unique risk of bone marrow transplant recipients. Am J Med 83:709–718, 1987.
> *Bone marrow transplant recipients were found to have a tenfold greater incidence of nosocomial Aspergillus infection than other immunocompromised patient populations when housed outside a high-efficiency particulate air (HEPA) filtered environment. This risk could be eliminated by using HEPA filters with horizontal laminar airflow.*

Sutton S, Lum BL, Torti FM: Possible risk of invasive pulmonary aspergillosis with marijuana use during chemotherapy for small cell lung cancer. Drug Intell Clin Pharm 20:289–291, 1986.
> *Bacterial and fungal contaminants have been identified in marijuana samples and thus are a potential risk factor in the immunocompromised patient using it as an antiemetic.*

Ventura GJ, Kantarjian HM, Anaissie E, Hopfer RL, Fainstein V: Pneumonia with *Cunninghamella* species in patients with hematologic malignancies. A case report and review of the literature. Cancer 58:1534–1536, 1986.
> *A patient with chronic myelogenous leukemia in blastic crisis who developed pulmonary and systemic infection with Cunninghamella species is described.*

Waldorf AR, Levitz SM, Diamond RD: In vivo bronchoalveolar macrophage defense against *Rhizopus oryzae* and *Aspergillus fumigatus*. J Infect Dis 150:752–760, 1984.
> *An important article delineating the critical role of the bronchoalveolar macrophage in protecting against invasive aspergillosis and mucormycosis.*

Weiner MH, Talbot GH, Gerson SL, Filice G, Cassileth PA: Antigen detection in the diagnosis of invasive aspergillosis. Utility in controlled, blinded trials. Ann Intern Med 99:777–782, 1983.
> *A careful study of the possible utility of antigen detection in the noninvasive diagnosis of invasive aspergillosis.*

Williams DM, Krick JA, Remington JS: Pulmonary infection in the compromised host (Parts I and II). Am Rev Respir Dis 114:359–394; 593–627, 1976.
> *After 10 years, still the most complete review of pulmonary infection, especially fungal infection, in the compromised host.*

Zuger A, Louie E, Holzman RS, Simberkoff MS, Rahal JJ: Cryptococcal disease in patients with the acquired immunodeficiency syndrome. Diagnostic features and outcome of treatment. Ann Intern Med 104:234–240, 1986.
> *A careful delineation of the importance of cryptococcal infection in the AIDS patient.*

Chapter 111

Histoplasmosis

George A. Sarosi / Scott F. Davies

History and Epidemiology

Pathogenesis

Clinical Manifestations

Progressive Disseminated Histoplasmosis

Diagnosis

Treatment

Histoplasmosis is the illness caused by the thermal dimorphic fungus, *Histoplasma capsulatum*. The spectrum of disease caused by the fungus ranges from the asymptomatic acquisition of a positive histoplasmin skin test to a rapidly fatal pulmonary or disseminated illness.

HISTORY AND EPIDEMIOLOGY

The first cast of histoplasmosis was recognized by Samuel Darling in Panama in 1905. Darling, a U.S. Army pathologist, performed an autopsy on a man who had died of a progressive systemic infection. He identified an organism which he assumed was protozoan and named it *H. capsulatum*. During the next 2 years, Darling found two similar cases at autopsy examination in Panama, after which the disease was nearly forgotten.

C. J. Watson, then a first-year resident in pathology, found the next case in 1926 in Minneapolis in an autopsy of a lifelong resident of Minnesota. Only his diligent search of the literature rescued Darling's seminal observation from obscurity. The disease was first diagnosed antemortem by Tompkins in 1933. She identified intracellular organisms in polymorphonuclear leukocytes (PMN) in the blood smear of a child dying of a febrile illness with hepatosplenomegaly and anemia. DeMonbreum then successfully isolated the organism from blood cultures of this child and confirmed deRocha-Lima's hypothesis that the organism was indeed a fungus. Moreover, he demonstrated the temperature-dependent dimorphism of *H. capsulatum*.

During the general mobilization for World War II, many young men inducted into the U.S. Army had pulmonary calcification on the chest radiograph and negative tuberculin skin tests. These cases were initially thought to discredit tuberculin skin testing. However, Christie and Peterson reasoned that these pulmonary calcifications in tuberculin-negative individuals might be caused by another infection, perhaps due to *H. capsulatum*. Using the original DeMonbreum isolate, they prepared histoplasmin, a complex skin test antigen, and showed that almost all tuberculin-negative persons in Nashville, Tennessee, who had calcifications on the chest radiograph reacted to this antigen.

Large skin test surveys subsequently showed that skin test reactions to histoplasmin were very common throughout the central United States. The highest percentage of positive skin tests was found in residents in the Ohio and Mississippi River Valleys. In some areas, more than 90 percent of residents had positive skin tests.

The results of the skin test surveys challenged the prevailing concept that histoplasmosis was a rare and uniformly fatal illness. By the end of World War II, it was known that the central United States is a highly endemic area for histoplasmosis, that the infection is very common, and that it is usually mild and self-limited. It is now estimated that 50 million people in the United States have been infected by *H. capsulatum*. As many as 500,000 new infections may occur yearly.

Shortly after the extent of the endemic area was defined by the surveys using skin tests, the fungus was grown from soil, especially from soil enriched by bird droppings. It is now established that *H. capsulatum* is a soil-dwelling fungus that requires organic nitrogen for growth; this requirement accounts for its frequent isolation from soil heavily contaminated by bird or bat feces. It grows as an aerial mycelium in nature, and in the laboratory at 23°C, producing large numbers of infective spores, 2 to 5 μm in size. When these infectious particles are disturbed, an aerosol is formed. If inhaled, the aerosolized spores are almost the perfect size to reach the alveoli, so that exposure often causes infection.

For many years, chicken houses were important in the epidemiology of histoplasmosis. Numerous small outbreaks were linked to exposure to chicken houses, usually to those that had been abandoned. The shift of the United States population from predominantly rural to urban and suburban, and the abandonment of household raising of chickens, led to a striking change in the epidemiology of histoplasmosis. Most recent outbreaks of histoplasmosis have occurred in urban settings and frequently in areas of relatively low endemicity, such as Montreal, Canada, and Mason City, Iowa. These outbreaks have been associated with construction projects that disturbed large amounts of contaminated soil. The most recent (and perhaps the largest) epidemic occurred in Indianapolis, Indiana, during

construction of a swimming pool and tennis court complex. Indianapolis is within the endemic area for histoplasmosis, where lifelong residents would be expected to have had histoplasmosis. Yet, judging by the large numbers of new cases during the epidemic, one would have to assume that urban dwellers are no longer exposed to the infection as a matter of routine, even in endemic areas, and thus remain susceptible when exposed to large numbers of spores during construction.

PATHOGENESIS

The lung is the portal of entry for the fungus. Even though spores may be swallowed, there is no evidence that direct invasion of the gastrointestinal tract occurs. Direct percutaneous inoculation of the spores may occur, but only a few such cases have been reported. Clinical manifestations of inoculation histoplasmosis include an ulcer or nodule at the site and regional lymphadenopathy, similar to sporotrichosis.

When spores of *H. capsulatum* are inhaled, some reach the alveoli and begin to germinate. Conversion to the yeast phase takes place, and multiplication occurs by binary fission. The initial tissue response to the organism is an exudation of PMNs followed by the rapid accumulation of alveolar macrophages. The yeasts are phagocytosed by the macrophages. They multiply within the cells and spread to regional lymph nodes and then are spread via the bloodstream, throughout the body. During this stage of preimmune fungemia, foci of infection develop in many organs, such as the liver and spleen.

When lymphocyte-mediated cellular immunity develops, usually 2 to 3 weeks after the original infection, intense cellular inflammation occurs and is followed by necrosis; the necrosis is often caseous in nature, frequently indistinguishable from tuberculosis. These areas of caseation necrosis occur not only in the lung, but also in draining lymph nodes and at the extrapulmonary sites of infection.

Healing is accompanied by peripheral fibrosis. Foci of encapsulated, necrotic material frequently calcify, especially in young children. Calcified foci of histoplasmosis frequently mimic the classic Ghon complex of tuberculosis, manifesting peripheral and hilar calcifications on the chest radiograph. Similar calcified lesions are often seen in the liver and spleen.

CLINICAL MANIFESTATIONS

In individuals who are otherwise normal, most remain asymptomatic; when symptoms do occur, they are so nonspecific that sporadic, mild infections are seldom diagnosed. Most of what is known about symptomatic human histoplasmosis comes from the study of epidemics of histoplasmosis. The infectious particle is the microconidium or spore from the mycelial phase of growth. The yeast form which grows in the body (and in the laboratory at 37°C) is not aerosolized and is not infectious except by inoculation. There is no person-to-person transmission.

Most of the early reports of outbreaks dealt with small numbers of patients. Exposure to the fungus usually occurred in confined places, such as storm cellars, chicken houses, or bat caves. Many patients were symptomatic. The severity of illness ranged from mild respiratory illness to overwhelming, occasionally fatal pneumonia.

In the more recent, community-wide outbreaks exposure to the fungus has occurred in open air via wind-borne spread of spores. Presumably the number of particles inhaled was fewer and more random. In these groups the frequency of symptomatic illness was lower and the severity of symptoms less. In general, in wind-borne epidemics less than 50 percent of infected individuals (as determined by skin test or serologic conversion) have any symptoms.

The incubation time of acute histoplasmosis in previously nonimmune individuals, determined from published series, is between 9 and 17 days. In a recent open-air outbreak in Minneapolis, an area of low background endemicity, the mean incubation time was 14 days, identical to the peak calculated by Goodwin who summarized data from a number of previous reports. In the Minneapolis outbreak the day (and the hour) of exposure was known since all patients visited the site for a defined period of time; therefore, the incubation time was determined precisely. Symptoms vary from brief periods of malaise to severe, life-threatening illness. In a typical patient the illness resembles influenza: the illness begins abruptly, with fever, chills, and substernal chest discomfort; a harsh, nonproductive cough develops along with headache, arthralgias, and myalgias.

More than 90 percent of normal hosts who develop primary pulmonary histoplasmosis recover uneventfully. Occasionally, especially when the infective dose is unusually high, severe pulmonary illness may develop which may progress rapidly to the adult respiratory distress syndrome (ARDS). Death may then follow quickly from respiratory insufficiency unless the diagnosis is established early and treatment with amphotericin B is begun (Fig. 111-1).

Even though the lungs are the portal of entry, in many patients (even some with respiratory symptoms), the chest radiograph is normal. When the chest radiograph is abnormal, the characteristic finding is a single (occasionally multiple) area of pneumonitis, usually in the better-ventilated lower zones of a lung. The draining hilar and mediastinal lymph nodes are often enlarged on the ipsilateral side (Fig. 111-2). Unfortunately, this parenchymal-hilar node complex may be incomplete, either component

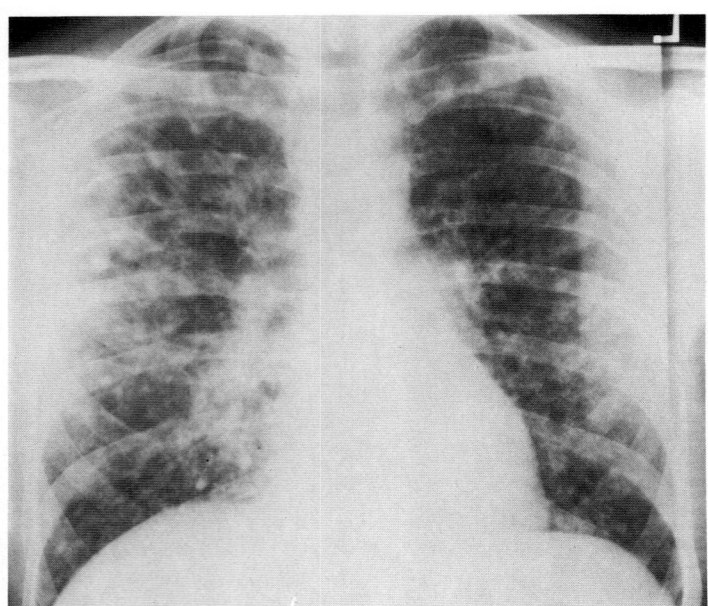

FIGURE 111-1 Severe pulmonary histoplasmosis in a 23-year-old man. Infection occurred in a closed space (attic remodeling). In spite of severe disease, he did not require intubation and recovered.

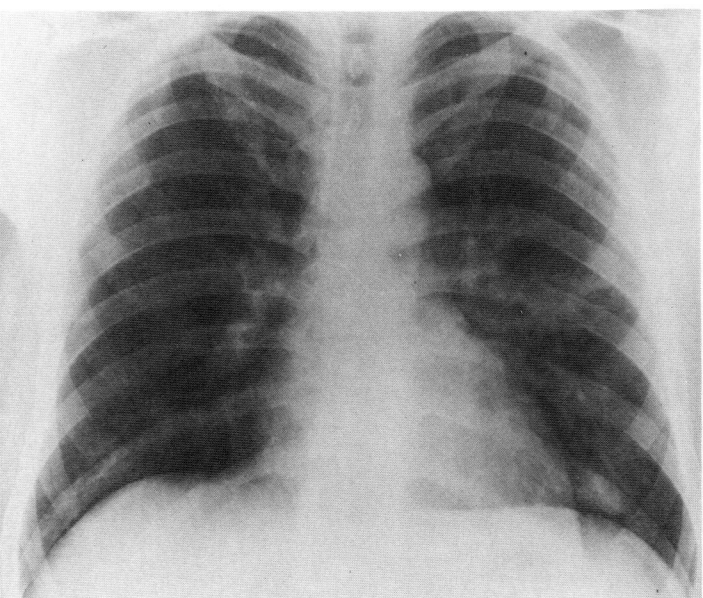

FIGURE 111-2 Arthralgia-erythema nodosum complex in a 40-year-old man. Infiltrates are seen on the left in the lower and mid-zones. Hilar adenopathy is also present.

being absent, rendering the radiographic diagnosis more difficult. Furthermore, these abnormalities on the chest radiograph occur frequently in asymptomatic individuals in whom they are discovered accidentally.

Healing of histoplasma pulmonary lesions usually results in complete resolution of the areas of pneumonitis. However, in some patients, the area of pneumonitis "hardens" and contracts, leaving a residual nodular lesion. Fibrous encapsulation occurs, but a caseous necrosis is present in the center of the lesion; the necrotic center sometimes becomes densely calcified, leaving a "coin" lesion. In endemic areas, these residual coin lesions are common and are often difficult to distinguish from carcinoma of the lung, especially when they slowly enlarge (Fig. 111-3). In children and young adults, the lesions calcify more readily than in older individuals. This difference is unfortunate since the differential diagnosis between bronchogenic carcinoma and histoplasmosis is more apt to be required in older individuals in whom a histoplasmoma is least likely to calcify and, thereby, to indicate its benignity. Many thoracotomies are done to remove such uncalcified lesions as the only way to exclude carcinoma when previous chest radiographs are not available.

Calcification may also occur in hilar and mediastinal lymph nodes as a result of the healing of caseation necrosis. Nodal calcifications tend to be scattered, uneven foci within enlarged nodes. The calcifications are usually larger than nodal calcification in tuberculosis and are frequently referred to as "mulberry" calcifications.

Diffuse nodular infiltrates often develop after heavy exposure. The chest radiograph then resembles miliary tuberculosis, but the individual lesions are usually larger. The mechanism of infection is inhalation rather than hematogenous spread. Caseation necrosis and subsequent calcification in each nodular area produce the "buck shot" calcifications characteristic of healed primary histoplasmosis.

The literature regarding reinfection in histoplasmosis is somewhat confusing. Two circumstantial arguments suggest that reinfection may occur in humans. First, skin test reactivity to histoplasmin wanes with age, reaching a peak during early adulthood and decreasing thereafter. However, in endemic areas many older patients maintain a positive skin test to histoplasmin. Goodwin has implicated repeated asymptomatic reexposure to the fungus followed by reestablishment of adequate lymphocyte-mediated cellular immunity in the maintenance of a positive skin test in older individuals.

Second, the incubation time for patients in reported epidemics follows a biphasic distribution. Most patients become symptomatic between the 12th and 19th days after infection. A smaller group, found only in outbreaks involving endemic areas, becomes symptomatic between the fifth and seventh days. Goodwin and others have suggested that this second group is undergoing symptomatic reinfection, which is responsible for the earlier onset of illness. Attractive as the hypothesis may be, the occurrence of reinfection histoplasmosis is not firmly established.

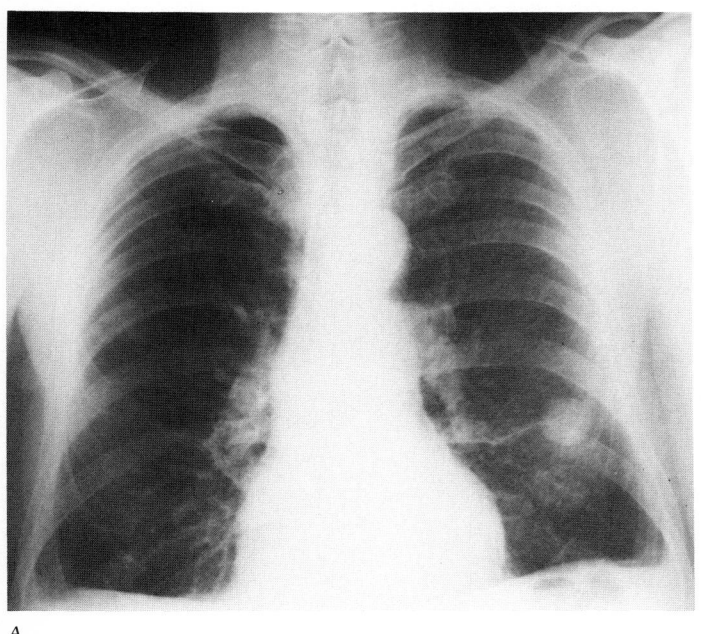

A

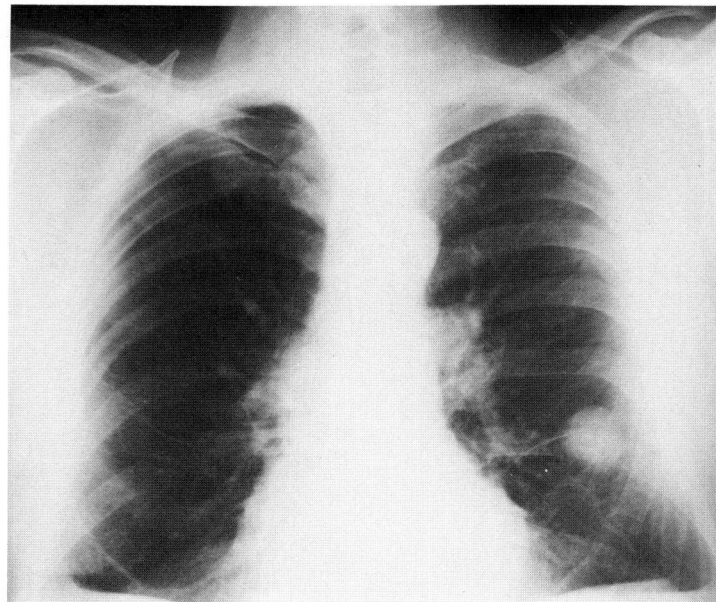

B

C   D

FIGURE 111-3 *A* to *C*. Asymptomatic "coin" lesion in a 55-year-old man. *A*. The lesion is clearly seen on the left in the lower lung field. *B*. Six years later, the nodule has increased in size. The central calcification is readily seen. *C*. Tomogram of lesion seen in *A* shows dense nodule with central calcifications. *D*. Tomogram of "coin" lesion in a 32-year-old woman. The characteristic laminated calcifications common in histoplasmosis can be seen.

In addition to respiratory symptoms, several systemic syndromes are associated with acute histoplasmosis. Arthralgias are common and may be sufficiently severe to interfere with walking and other activities; although the arthralgia usually resolves within several days, it may last for weeks or more. Erythema nodosum and erythema multiforme may accompany arthralgias; the skin lesions are more common in women than in men. It has been estimated that erythema nodosum and/or erythema multiforme occur in 1 of 200 primary infections. These manifestations are presumably allergic and may occur in patients in whom the chest radiographs are normal.

Pericarditis in histoplasmosis was once believed to be quite rare. But during the recent large outbreak of histoplasmosis in Indianapolis, Indiana, pericarditis was quite common: 45 of 712 (6.3 percent) individuals with primary histoplasmosis developed pericarditis. The pericarditis is probably due to involvement of adjacent mediastinal structures by *Histoplasma* rather than to hematogenous spread of the fungus to the pericardium. The pericardial fluid is usually a nonspecific sterile exudate.

Acute histoplasmosis in normal hosts is benign and self-limited. However, it may also lead to serious compli-

cations, usually due to involvement of strategically situated structures in the thorax. For example, paratracheal lymph node enlargement may compress the trachea or one of the main-stem bronchi, causing an irritative cough or dyspnea. Dysphagia may result from impingement of enlarged nodes on the esophagus; the nodes may adhere to the esophagus, contracting as they heal, creating traction diverticula. Healed, calcified nodes may also erode into various adjacent tissues; erosion of such nodes into the tracheobronchial tree causes broncholithiasis, which may lead to obstructive pneumonitis, expectoration of stones, or hemoptysis. On rare occasions, exuberant fibrosis accompanies the healing of involved mediastinal lymph nodes, entrapping many mediastinal structures. Vascular compression may cause the superior vena cava syndrome. In fact, histoplasmosis is probably the most common benign cause of this syndrome.

Structural abnormalities in the lungs affect the distribution of the histoplasmosis lesions. For example, in patients with centrilobular emphysema, the infection often involves the upper lobes, and the chest radiograph frequently resembles that of reinfection-type tuberculosis (Fig. 111-4). Infiltration surrounding airspaces mimics

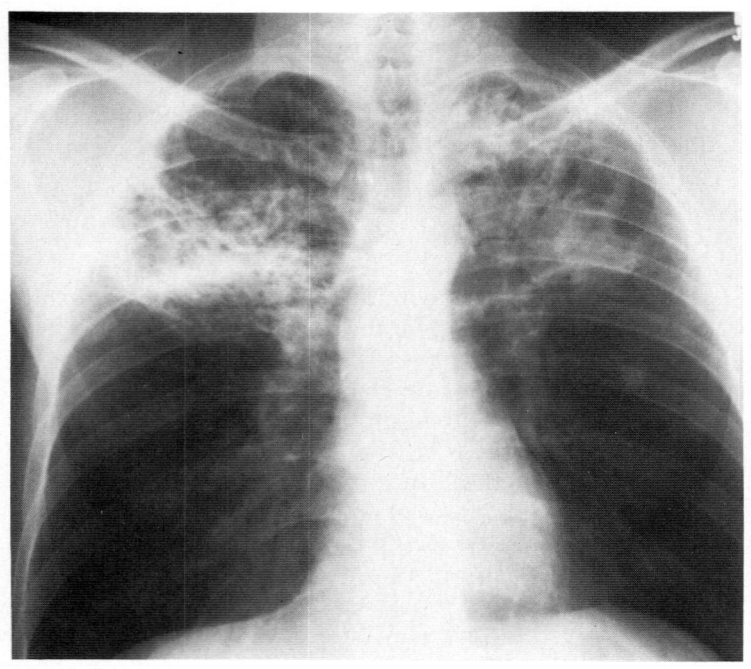
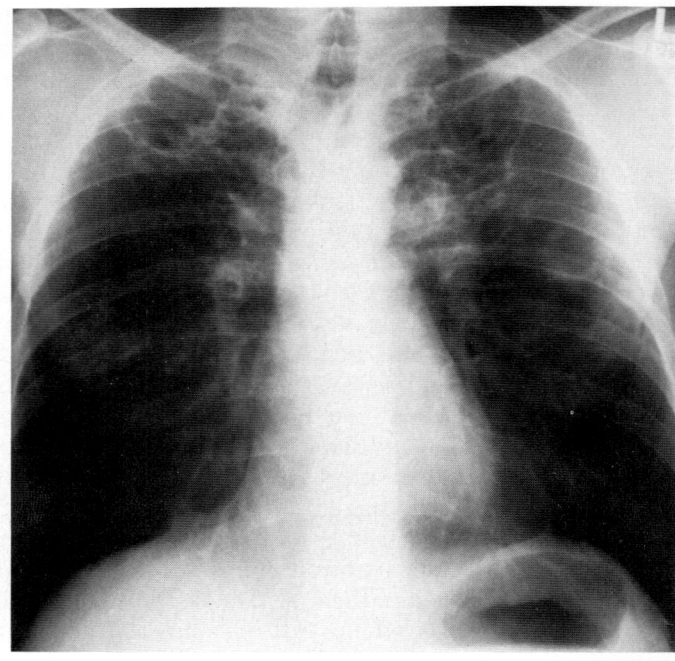

FIGURE 111-4 Chronic pulmonary histoplasmosis in a 44-year-old heavy smoker. A. Before ketoconazole therapy. B. After 6 months of ketoconazole therapy, the patient improved and the chest radiograph was clearing, but the sputum was still positive for *H. capsulatum*.

cavitary disease. This form of histoplasmosis resembles tuberculosis both clinically and radiographically. Many patients manifest chronic cough, weight loss, low grade fevers and night sweats. In the early reports, survival rates were low, suggesting that this form of histoplasmosis was a severe, usually fatal illness. However, not all such patients undergo a relentlessly progressive pulmonary disease. Although acute histoplasmosis in patients with obstructive airways disease tends to persist longer than in normal individuals, with symptoms and infiltrates that last for weeks or even a few months, as a rule the disease resolves spontaneously.

In a few patients, infection persists in the abnormal airspaces and spreads to involve adjacent areas of the lung; if the disease is untreated, it may spread, eventually involving much of the lung and culminating in the death of the patient even though spread to distant sites is uncommon.

PROGRESSIVE DISSEMINATED HISTOPLASMOSIS

Following inhalation of the fungus into the terminal airspaces, germination begins; multiplication occurs by binary fission, and the organism gains access to the hilar lymph nodes and then to the systemic circulation. Fungemia occurs in most patients. Postmortem studies performed in endemic areas show that more than 70 percent of persons dying of other causes have healed *Histoplasma*

granulomas in their spleens. The designation *progressive disseminated histoplasmosis* refers only to progressive infection in extrapulmonary sites and not to the self-limited fungemia which accompanies acute pulmonary histoplasmosis.

During the fungemia that accompanies acute histoplasmosis, circulating yeasts are phagocytosed by cells of the reticuloendothelial system. Before the development of lymphocyte-mediated cellular immunity, the reticuloendothelial cells cannot kill the fungi, and intracellular multiplication continues. When specific T-lymphocyte-mediated cellular immunity does develop, the macrophages are "armed"; granulomas form, and fungal multiplication is checked. This sequence occurs in normal persons. Calcifications of such foci serve as markers of remote histoplasmosis but have no other significance. In contrast, when the lymphocyte-mediated cellular immune response is poor or absent, the intracellular yeasts continue to grow and multiply and additional macrophages are recruited and parasitized. Unchecked growth of the fungus results in a severe systemic illness which, if untreated, invariably leads to death.

Physical examination usually shows high fever, and the patient is often acutely ill. Hepatosplenomegaly is common. In at least half of the patients, laboratory evaluation shows anemia, leukopenia, and thrombocytopenia. The level of alkaline phosphatase in serum is frequently increased. Extremely ill patients sometimes develop the syndrome of disseminated intravascular coagulation. The

chest radiograph is variable, ranging from normal to diffuse interstitial infiltrates. Bone marrow biopsy shows collections of macrophages full of intracellular yeasts or, in the more severely ill, widespread necrosis with large numbers of organisms in the extracellular debris. In patients with severe and rapidly progressive illness, histopathologic examination of involved tissues usually does not show well-formed granulomas.

Before immunosuppressive and glucocorticoid therapy became widespread, the progressive disseminated form of histoplasmosis was most common in young children; for this reason, it is frequently still referred to as the *infantile form* of the disease. Today, virtually all patients with progressive disseminated histoplasmosis have some degree of T-cell defect, either due to an underlying disease such as Hodgkin's disease or to treatment with glucocorticoids and/or cytotoxic agents. Perhaps the most severe form of progressive disseminated histoplasmosis occurs in patients with the acquired immunodeficiency syndrome (AIDS), the paradigm of T-cell dysfunction; indeed, in many areas where histoplasmosis is endemic, progressive disseminated histoplasmosis is most often seen in patients with AIDS. In some individuals the onset of the illness is temporarily related to the starting of immunosuppressive therapy, most often with glucocorticoids, suggesting reactivation of dormant foci of histoplasmosis, especially when the illness occurs in a nonendemic area in a patient who had previously lived in a highly endemic area. In other instances, exposure of an immunosuppressed patient to an infected aerosol is the mechanism of infection. In the recent large outbreak of histoplasmosis in Indianapolis, most immunosuppressed patients who were infected with *H. capsulatum* developed progressive disseminated histoplasmosis.

Progressive disseminated histoplasmosis also occurs in a more chronic form. Frequently these individuals have no obvious reason for T-cell dysfunction: when tested after recovery from histoplasmosis, T-cell function appears normal. Goodwin postulated that transient T-cell dysfunction, perhaps related to an intercurrent viral infection, rendered these patients susceptible to progressive disseminated histoplasmosis; however, this proposal remains speculative. The chronic form of progressive disseminated histoplasmosis is an indolent wasting disease with anorexia, weight loss, and low grade fever. Mucosal and mucocutaneous junction ulcers occur in the mouth, oropharynx, rectum, and glans penis. Adrenal involvement is common and may cause Addison's disease. Histopathology of involved tissues shows well-formed epithelioid granulomas; organisms are difficult to find. Special stains are needed to demonstrate the fungus.

Symptomatic involvement of the central nervous system in progressive disseminated histoplasmosis is rare and may present as chronic meningitis or as an intracranial histoplasmoma. Endocarditis is also rare. It may involve either the aortic or mitral valves; the valves may have been previously normal. The vegetations are usually large and emboli are frequent. *Histoplasma* involvement of abnormal aortic aneurysms also occurs occasionally in the chronic form of progressive disseminated histoplasmosis.

DIAGNOSIS

Direct examination of sputum digested in 10% potassium hydroxide is not useful for the diagnosis of histoplasmosis because of the intracellular location and the small size of *H. capsulatum*. The gold standard of diagnosis is the recovery in culture of the fungus from biologic material obtained from a patient with clinical manifestations of the disease. Although sputum cultures are positive in less than 10 percent of cases of acute pulmonary histoplasmosis, they are usually positive in patients with progressive cavitary histoplasmosis of the upper lobes. The fungus is hardy and survives prolonged trips via the mail. Since shedding of the organism is intermittent, daily sputum specimens should be obtained for six consecutive days. When the patient cannot cough up secretions, sputum should be induced by nebulizing 10 percent saline before proceeding to more invasive methods, such as bronchoscopy for brushings, washings, and transbronchial biopsies.

When progressive disseminated histoplasmosis is suspected, sampling of the reticuloendothelial system is necessary. Bone marrow biopsy is the best and safest diagnostic method. Liver biopsy is also an excellent way to sample this system, but is more hazardous, especially in patients who are thrombocytopenic. Some patients with the chronic form of progressive disseminated histoplasmosis have mucosal lesions which can be easily biopsied.

Recovery of the fungus by culture is not difficult, but it is slow. Final mycologic diagnosis may take up to 30 days, depending on the size of the inoculum. The laboratory should be informed that histoplasmosis is suspected, since often a tentative diagnosis can be ventured if large tuberculate conidiospores are seen in a mycelial isolate. Final, definite diagnosis requires conversion to the yeast phase at 37°C and then back to the mycelial form.

Histopathologic examination of bone marrow (or other tissues) is an excellent and rapid method to establish the diagnosis. In heavily parasitized samples, a direct smear of the marrow, stained with a supravital stain, e.g., the Giemsa stain, is often diagnostic. Occasionally the organism can be visualized directly in a peripheral blood smear, or better still, in a buffy coat preparation; they are found within PMNs or macrophages.

Special stains are necessary to visualize the organism in tissue sections, since the standard hematoxylin and eosin stain is inadequate. Most laboratories use a modification of the silver stain; unfortunately, the silver stain

tends to obscure important morphologic details and also stains nuclear material and other debris, often causing diagnostic confusion. The periodic acid-Schiff (PAS) stain provides good morphologic definition and does not stain nuclear debris. Special stains are especially important when well-formed granulomas are present because there are only a few organisms in these lesions: in general, the more the granulomas resemble those of sarcoidosis, the harder the organisms are to find.

Skin testing with 0.1 ml of histoplasmin identifies individuals who have, or have had, histoplasmosis. As mentioned above, skin testing was the main tool used in the epidemiologic investigations which defined the high incidence of infection over the extensive endemic area in the central United States. Unfortunately, the skin test cannot be used to diagnose current infection in individual patients. Unless the previous skin test status of a given patient is known, a positive skin test is not helpful. A positive skin test only means that the individual, sometime during the past, has been infected with the fungus. In endemic areas, skin test positivity is nearly universal by the time the individual reaches adulthood. To complicate matters further, in many patients with progressive disseminated histoplasmosis, the skin test is negative because of either the underlying T-cell defect or the infection itself. Thus, a positive skin test does not establish the diagnosis, nor does a negative skin test exclude it. Therefore, although the histoplasmin skin test is an invaluable epidemiologic tool, it should not be relied on to establish the diagnosis in individual patients.

Because recovery of the fungus from sputum culture is rarely possible in acute histoplasmosis, and because a positive skin test is not helpful, serologic tests are extremely important for diagnosis. Currently, three methods are available for the serodiagnosis of histoplasmosis. The standard method is the complement fixation test: this test becomes positive 3 to 6 weeks after exposure and remains positive for months or occasionally years in diminishing titer. A fourfold rise in titer, or a titer of 1:32 or higher on a single determination, suggests recent infection. Unfortunately, the complement fixation test is negative in about 30 percent of patients with acute histoplasmosis and in up to 50 percent of patients with progressive disseminated histoplasmosis. Patients with established chronic upper lobe pulmonary histoplasmosis frequently have titers of 1:8 or 1:16 which do not increase during a period of observation.

Immunodiffusion (ID) testing for precipitating antibodies to the H & M antigens is easy to perform and is specific for histoplasmosis. Regrettably, it is negative in up to 50 percent of patients with acute histoplasmosis and does not become positive for 4 to 6 weeks after exposure.

A recently developed radioimmunoassay (RIA) appears to be more sensitive than either the complement fixation or the immunodiffusion tests. In a recent outbreak of histoplasmosis it was the best test: it became positive before the others, and almost 80 percent of the patients had diagnostic levels. It is not yet available commercially.

The serologic tests are helpful in establishing that an acute illness was histoplasmosis. However, the tests generally do not become positive until the patient has been symptomatic for at least 2 or 3 weeks; often another week or two of additional delay supervenes while waiting for the serum specimen to be sent and processed by a reference laboratory. By the time results are available, the vast majority of patients have recovered. The others have required invasive diagnostic tests because the illness was severe and rapidly progressing.

TREATMENT

The great bulk of patients with acute histoplasmosis are either asymptomatic or have rapidly resolving, self-limited disease; they require no treatment. In the rare patients with severe acute histoplasmosis who have diffuse infiltrates and progress toward respiratory failure, amphotericin B is used in full doses as soon as the diagnosis is established; this prompt intervention may be lifesaving. Some seasoned clinicians recommend a dose of 500 mg of amphotericin B for patients with acute histoplasmosis even though it is not immediately life-threatening but is more severe or more presistent than usual, e.g., fever lasts longer than 2 weeks. This practice has never been evaluated critically. Ketoconazole is generally not appropriate for treatment of acute pulmonary histoplasmosis. If the patient is critically ill, amphotericin B should be used. The response time for ketoconazole is sufficiently slow (usually 3 weeks or more) that almost all patients with acute histoplasmosis recover before any drug effect could reasonably be expected.

Progressive cavitary upper lobe pulmonary disease can be treated successfully using 400 mg daily of ketoconazole; if necessary, the dose may be increased to 800 mg daily. Treatment is continued for 6 to 12 months, and relapses may occur when it is stopped. Alternatively, amphotericin B in a total dose of 35 mg/kg may be administered for 12 to 16 weeks; this course of therapy has been very successful.

The patient who is critically ill with progressive disseminated histoplasmosis is treated aggressively with amphotericin B. The total dose should be 40 mg/kg. Hospitalized, seriously ill patients are usually given rapidly escalating daily doses of 10, 20, 30, and then 40 or 50 mg. If, after the first several weeks, the patient has improved clinically, the 40- or 50-mg dose is continued while he or she is an outpatient, three times weekly, until the desired cumulative dose is reached. In patients with more chronic forms of progressive disseminated histoplasmosis who are not critically ill, ketoconazole has also been used successfully.

BIBLIOGRAPHY

Baughman RP, Kim CK, Vinegar A, Hendricks DE, Schmidt DJ, Bullock WE: The pathogenesis of experimental pulmonary histoplasmosis. Correlative studies of histopathology, bronchoalveolar lavage, and respiratory function. Am Rev Respir Dis 134:771–776, 1986.
   A murine model of acute pulmonary histoplasmosis was employed to study the pathogenesis of the disease process by means of histopathology, bronchoalveolar lavage, and respiratory function tests.

Bunnell IL, Furcolow ML: A report on ten proved cases of histoplasmosis. U.S. Public Health Rep 63:299–316, 1948.
   The first description of chronic pulmonary histoplasmosis as seen in tuberculosis sanitoria.

D'Alessio DJ, Heeren RH, Hendricks SL, Ogilvie P, Furcolow ML: A starling roost as the source of urban epidemic histoplasmosis in an area of low incidence. Am Rev Respir Dis 92:731–925, 1965.
   One of the classics of epidemic investigation pertaining to a large, community-wide outbreak of urban histoplasmosis.

Davies SF, Khan M, Sarosi GA: Disseminated histoplasmosis in immunologically suppressed patients. Am J Med 64:94–100, 1978.
   This is the first large study showing that disseminated histoplasmosis usually occurs in immunocompromised hosts.

Davies SF, McKenna RW, Sarosi GA: Trephine biopsy of the bone marrow in disseminated histoplasmosis. Am J Med 67:617–622, 1979.
   A large study on the value of bone marrow biopsies in the diagnosis of disseminated histoplasmosis. Bone marrow biopsy is shown to be the best way to sample the reticuloendothelial system, which is the characteristic feature of histoplasmosis.

Davies SF, Sarosi GA: Acute cavitary histoplasmosis. Chest 73:103–105, 1978.
   Description of acute pulmonary histoplasmosis in a smoker—giving a reasonable proof of a previous hypothesis as to the different nature of acute histoplasmosis in smokers versus nonsmokers.

Dismukes W, Cloud G, Bowles C, Sarosi GA, Gregg CR, Chapman SW, Scheld WM, Farr B, Gallis HA, Marier RL, Karam GH, Bennett JE, Kauffman CA, Medoff G, Stevens DA, Kaplowitz LG, Black JR, Roselle GA, Pankey GA, Kerkering TM, Fisher JF, Graybill JR, Shadomy S: Treatment of blastomycosis and histoplasmosis with ketoconazole: Results of a prospective randomized clinical trial. Ann Intern Med 103:861–872, 1985.
   A carefully done multicenter study on the use and value of ketoconazole in histoplasmosis (and blastomycosis).

Garrett HE Jr, Roper CL: Surgical intervention in histoplasmosis. Ann Thorac Surg 42:711–722, 1986.
   The cases of 94 recently treated patients are presented, and a review of the American surgical literature is given.

Goodwin RA Jr, DesPrez RM: Histoplasmosis: State of the art. Am Rev Respir Dis 117:929–956, 1978.
   The most comprehensive review of histoplasmosis. The authors go into great detail of epidemiology and pathogenesis, as well as the various manifestations of the disease.

Goodwin RA Jr, Loyd JE, DesPrez RM: Histoplasmosis in normal hosts. Medicine 60:231–266, 1981.
   The most comprehensive description of the disease as seen in normal individuals. Contains an excellent description of the natural history of this common infection.

Goodwin RA Jr, Owens FT, Snell JD, Hubbard WW, Buchanan RD, Terry RT, DesPrez RM: Chronic pulmonary histoplasmosis. Medicine 55:413–452, 1976.
   A careful and painstaking description of this illness, distilled from a large personal experience.

Goodwin RA Jr, Shapiro JL, Thurman GH, Thurman SS, DesPrez RM: Disseminated histoplasmosis: Clinical and pathologic correlations. Medicine 59:1–33, 1980.
   A comprehensive review of clinical, epidemiologic, and pathologic features of disseminated histoplasmosis. The authors' contention is that disseminated histoplasmosis is usually a sign of an immunocompromised host.

Graybill JR, Palou E, Ahrens J: Treatment of murine histoplasmosis with UK 49,858 (fluconazole). Am Rev Respir Dis 134:768–770, 1986.
> *Fluconazole, ketoconazole, and amphotericin B were equally effective in the treatment of induced pulmonary histoplasmosis in immunologically intact mice and in congenitally athymic nude mice.*

Lambert RS, George RB: Evaluation of enzyme immunoassay as a rapid screening test for histoplasmosis and blastomycosis. Am Rev Respir Dis 136:316–319, 1987.
> *Enzyme immunoassay is a useful screening test for serum antibodies to H. capsulatum and B. dermatitidis.*

Medeiros AA, Marty SD, Tosh FE, Chin TD: Erythema nodosum and erythema multiforme as clinical manifestations of histoplasmosis in community outbreak. N Engl J Med 274:415–420, 1966.
> *A carefully performed epidemiologic survey, describing the clinical manifestations of these common skin lesions and their relationship to histoplasmosis.*

Naylor BA: Low dose amphotericin B. Therapy for acute pulmonary histoplasmosis. Chest 71:404–406, 1977.
> *An uncontrolled study on the value of low-dose amphotericin B treatment in acute histoplasmosis.*

Negroni R, Palmieri O, Koren F, Tiraboschi IN, Galimberti RL: Oral treatment of paracoccidioidomycosis and histoplasmosis with itraconazole in humans. Rev Infect Dis 9(Suppl 1): S47–50, 1987.
> *Twenty-five patients with paracoccidioidomycosis and 17 patients with histoplasmosis were treated with itraconazole. All infections were clinically cured or showed striking improvement.*

Parker JD, Sarosi GA, Doto IL, Bailey RE, Tosh FE: Treatment of chronic pulmonary histoplasmosis. N Engl J Med 283:225–229, 1970.
> *This is the largest series where amphotericin B was used as a sole form of treatment for chronic pulmonary histoplasmosis. It establishes the value of 35 mg/kg as the minimum standard.*

Paya CV, Roberts GD, Cockerill FR III: Transient fungemia in acute pulmonary histoplasmosis: Detection by new blood-culturing techniques. J Infect Dis 156:313–315, 1987.
> *A report of two cases of acute pulmonary histoplasmosis in which transient fungemia was detected by the lysiscentrifugation blood-culture technique.*

Sacks JJ, Ajello L, Crockett LK: An outbreak and review of cave-associated histoplasmosis capsulati. J Med Vet Mycol 24:313–325, 1986.
> *Three male college students who had been "spelunking" (cave exploring) developed acute onsets of fever, chills, shortness of breath and cough within one day of each other, and all were eventually hospitalized for 4 to 29 days. A review of 42 reported outbreaks of cave-associated histoplasmosis and the approach to environmental control of infected caves are included.*

Sarosi GA: Histoplasmosis outbreaks: Their patterns, in Balows A (ed), *Histoplasmosis.* Springfield, IL, Charles C Thomas, 1971, pp 123–128.
> *A comparison of histoplasmosis outbreaks in the classic years of histoplasmosis versus more recent, large, community-wide outbreaks.*

Sarosi GA, Voth DW, Dahl BA, Doto IL, Tosh FE: Disseminated histoplasmosis: Results of long term follow up. Ann Intern Med 75:511–516, 1971.
> *The results of long-term treatment follow-up of a large group of patients with disseminated histoplasmosis, collected mostly prior to the use of large doses of glucocorticoids and cytoxic agents. The article further points out the frequent occurrence of adrenal gland destruction in chronic disseminated histoplasmosis.*

Wheat LJ, French MLU, Kohler RB: The diagnostic laboratory tests for histoplasmosis. Analysis of experience in a large urban outbreak. Ann Intern Med 97:680–685, 1982.
> *A carefully done comparison study of the values of the various diagnostic tests routinely available to clinicians for the diagnosis of histoplasmosis.*

Wheat LJ, Slama TG, Eitzen HE, Kohler RB, French ML, Biesecker JL: A large outbreak of histoplasmosis: Clinical features. Ann Intern Med 94:331–337, 1981.
> *The results of the investigation of the latest large urban outbreak of histoplasmosis.*

Wheat LJ, Slama TG, Norton JA, Kohler RB, Eitzen HE, French ML, Sathapatayavongs B: Risk factors for disseminated or fatal histoplasmosis: Analysis of a large urban outbreak. Ann Intern Med 96:159–163, 1982.

Describes and discusses the risks for disseminated histoplasmosis during the large urban outbreak in Indianapolis. It confirms the fact that immunocompromised patients will frequently develop disseminated disease when exposed to histoplasmosis.

Wheat LJ, Slama TG, Zeckel ML: Histoplasmosis in the acquired immune deficiency syndrome. Am J Med 78:203–210, 1985.

This is the first large series documenting that patients with AIDS are uniquely susceptible to disseminated histoplasmosis.

Wheat LJ, Stein L, Corya BC, Wass JL, Norton JA, Grider K, Slama TG, French ML, Kohler RB: Pericarditis as a manifestation of histoplasmosis during two large urban outbreaks. Medicine 62:110–118, 1983.

Description of the pericarditis and other rheumatologic manifestations during an outbreak of histoplasmosis.

Chapter *112*

Coccidioidomycosis

John N. Galgiani / Elizabeth E. Wack

Coccidioidomycosis is a systemic fungal infection endemic to the southwestern United States. It is caused by the soil saprophyte *Coccidioides immitis*. Valley fever, desert rheumatism, and San Joaquin fever are common names for symptom complexes associated with infection. The first cases of coccidioidomycosis, recognized near the beginning of this century, were characterized by progressive skin destruction. It was not until the 1930s that the more common, self-limited forms of infection were attributed to *C. immitis*. Since the occasional visitor may develop symptoms on returning to nonendemic regions, it is important that physicians everywhere have some familiarity with this disease.

EPIDEMIOLOGY

C. immitis has been found in the soil in localized areas throughout North and South America. In the United States, it is endemic to parts of California, Arizona, New Mexico, Texas, Nevada, and Utah. Coccidioidal infections diagnosed elsewhere can usually be traced to contact with contaminated agricultural products from the endemic areas, travel through the endemic areas, or laboratory accidents. The fungus is found in the ecosystem of the Lower Sonoran Life Zone, which is characterized by low altitude, dry climate, hot summers, mild winters, and alkaline soil.

Approximately 50,000 persons become infected yearly. In susceptible populations, approximately 0.4 percent/year seek medical attention for their infections. Twenty percent of the population in some regions have skin test evidence of prior infection. Approximately 50 infections per year result in death. Cases are diagnosed throughout the year, although the dry months have the highest incidence of infection.

PATHOGENESIS AND IMMUNOLOGY

Life Cycle

C. immitis exists in the soil as mycelia. Hyphal fragments (arthroconidia), approximately 5 μm long, become airborne, especially during dry, windy seasons. If inhaled, arthroconidia penetrate into lung alveoli, where they transform into spherules of 30 μm or larger in diameter. The inner wall of each spherule invaginates, forms septa, and creates multiple endospores within the spherule. When the spherule ruptures, hundreds of clustered endospores are released, each of which is capable of propagating the spherule cycle. Although spherules are the predominant phase of fungal growth in tissue, hyphae can occasionally be seen, especially in pulmonary cavities.

Cellular Response

NEUTROPHILS AND ACUTE INFLAMMATION

The initial inflammatory response to fungal proliferation is an influx of neutrophils, probably as a result of chemotactic stimuli. Evidence of acute inflammation, including eosinophilia, is associated with each wave of spherule rupture. These host responses may slow fungal proliferation and thereby modify the course of infection.

T-LYMPHOCYTE-MEDIATED IMMUNITY

Cellular immunity is an important defense against *C. immitis*. Delayed hypersensitivity is frequently present in patients who resolve their illness and absent in those who do not. In addition, T cells appear to be crucial in transfer of resistance against infection in mice. Spherule propagation ceases, and well-organized granulomata develop only after sensitization and subsequent macrophage activation has occurred. Nonetheless, in quiescent lesions, including

pulmonary nodules, *C. immitis* often remains viable, suggesting that competent host responses may not need to be fungicidal.

Humoral Immunity

Although humoral antibodies do not in themselves appear to mediate protection, antibodies are formed to many coccidioidal antigens. Detection of these antibodies is the basis of several diagnostic tests. There is also evidence that circulating antigens or antigen-antibody complexes may be responsible for some of the systemic symptoms.

Host Susceptibility Factors

The spectrum of disease seen in infection with *C. immitis* is primarily attributable to differences in host immunity. The clearest predisposition to dissemination is immunosuppression as occurs with malignancy, cytotoxic therapy, or acquired immunodeficiency syndrome (AIDS). Certain blood types, specifically B and AB, are also associated with increased risk of dissemination. Dissemination of infection is more likely in men than in pregnant women. Published reports indicate that coccidioidal infections during the third trimester of pregnancy are extremely severe. However, surveys of obstetricians within the endemic regions have not corroborated this view. Racial predilections have been suggested for blacks, Hispanics, American Indians, and Filipinos. Most of these associations are controversial, but taken together, they implicate host factors as important determinants of coccidioidal infections.

CLINICAL MANIFESTATIONS

Approximately two-thirds of infections due to *C. immitis* are asymptomatic and are recognized only by reactive skin tests. The other third of infections cause a spectrum of disease from a flulike illness to frank pneumonia.

Primary Pneumonia

Symptoms associated with primary infection are cough, fever, and chest pain. These are seen in 70 to 90 percent of cases. The cough typically produces scant, occasionally blood-streaked sputum. Fever is sometimes associated with night sweats, and chest pain is usually pleuritic. Marked fatigue and lethargy are common complaints. Other symptoms of the primary infection are headache, sore throat, myalgias, and anorexia.

Infection is associated frequently with skin manifestations. Erythema nodosum is especially common in adult women. Erythema multiforme and a diffuse maculopapular rash known as toxic erythema also commonly accompany infection. The complex of symptoms known as *valley fever,* or *desert rheumatism,* consists of E. nodosum or E. *multiforme* plus arthralgias, arthritis, and occasionally mild conjunctivitis.

A high percentage of patients with primary coccidioidomycosis have abnormal chest radiographs. Alveolar infiltrates are most frequent, usually involve single segments or lobes, and appear soft, hazy, and homogeneous. Areas of associated atelectasis are common. Hilar adenopathy is seen in 20 percent of these patients and is usually ipsilateral to the infiltrate. Small pleural effusions are detected in approximately 20 percent of patients; larger effusions are found in 2 to 6 percent. An effusion is usually unilateral and represents a parapneumonic process rather than evidence of extrathoracic dissemination. Forty to sixty percent of patients with primary coccidioidomycosis have positive sputum culture.

Peripheral eosinophilia (greater than 5 percent) is common in primary coccidioidomycosis with peak counts noted in the second and third weeks. A persistent peripheral count greater than 20 percent may be associated with a poor prognosis.

The majority of patients with primary coccidioidomycosis resolve their infection without sequelae or complications in 6 to 8 weeks. Adenopathy and effusions usually resolve spontaneously.

Pulmonary Sequelae

Approximately 4 percent of patients with primary coccidioidomycosis develop radiographically detectable sequelae. These most frequently consist of nodules and cavities which form in areas of previous infiltrates. Fortunately, the course of these sequelae is usually benign, although their presence is often the focus of considerable attention.

NODULES

Granulomatous nodules usually cause no symptoms and are often discovered by chest radiographs obtained for other purposes. Only about one half of patients with nodules have recognized histories of coccidioidomycosis. Although these lesions rarely cause the patient difficulty, they may be impossible to distinguish from malignancy without aggressive diagnostic evaluation, often including thoracotomy.

Nodules are usually single, 1 to 4 cm in size, and in the mid-lung, within 5 cm of the hilus. Coccidioidal granulomas generally do not calcify densely. This makes reliable differentiation from malignancy by computerized tomography difficult. Most patients with nodules are skin test positive and 60 to 70 percent have low or undetectable antibody levels. *C. immitis* is rarely cultured from the sputum. However, spherules can be found in approximately two-thirds of resected nodules, and cultures of surgical tissue are frequently positive. Most nodules are radiographically stable. If enlargement does occur, doubling times are greater than 1 year.

CAVITIES

As with nodules, coccidioidal cavities usually cause no symptoms. However, in some patients, fever and hemoptysis develop. Generally, cavities measure 2 to 4 cm on chest radiographs; only 7 percent are larger than 6 cm. Seventy percent are in the upper lung fields, 5 percent cross fissures. Typically, the cavity wall appears thin with very little surrounding infiltrate. If the infection is unusually destructive, the cavity is likely to have a shaggy border and be filled with fluid (Fig. 112-1). Sixty to seventy percent of patients have reactive coccidioidal skin tests, concentrations of antibodies in serum are often low, and sputum cultures are usually positive. The majority of cavities resolve spontaneously within 2 years, and most of the others remain radiologically static.

There are three major complications of coccidioidal cavities, all of which occur infrequently. First, the cavities may become secondarily colonized with other fungi which form mycetomas. This may produce persistent coughing, fever, and hemoptysis. Second, cavities may rupture and cause a pyopneumothorax. Most frequently, this complication occurs in otherwise healthy young men and produces acute pleuritic chest pain and dyspnea. The initial chest radiograph will almost always disclose an air-fluid level in the pleural space (Fig. 112-2), which distinguishes a ruptured coccidioidal cavity from spontaneous pneumothorax or a ruptured bulla. Third, life-threatening hemorrhage has occurred.

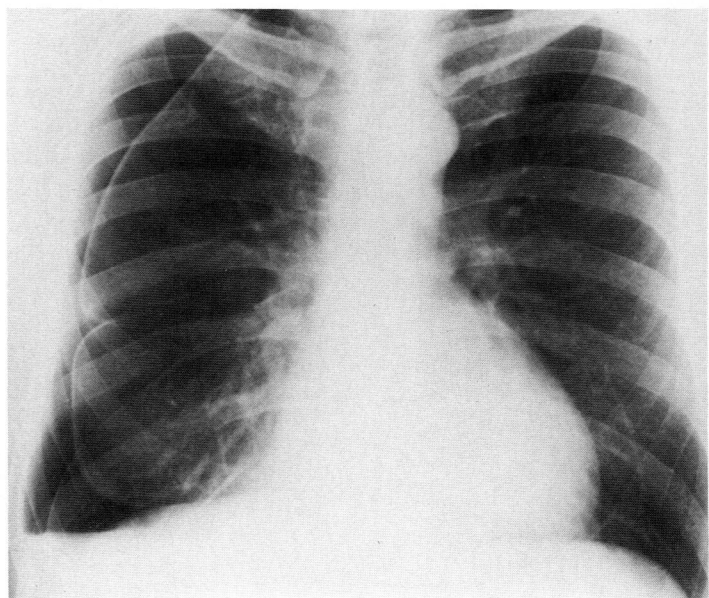

FIGURE 112-2 Pyopneumothorax from a ruptured coccidioidal cavity that developed as the first manifestation of infection in an otherwise healthy young male physician. The cavity can be seen in the right upper lung field.

Persistent and Chronic Progressive Pneumonia

If the symptoms of primary coccidioidomycosis do not resolve within 8 weeks, the disease is considered "persistent." In immunocompetent patients, the course may still be one of gradual improvement over a period of several months. However, as will be discussed, therapy may be considered for this group. In a very few patients, the infection may never resolve, progressively involving more pulmonary parenchyma. This form of the disease is referred to as *chronic progressive coccidioidal pneumonia*, and its manifestations are similar to those of chronic pulmonary tuberculosis. Symptoms include low-grade fevers, productive cough, and weight loss. Radiographs of the chest usually show biapical fibronodular lesions and multiple cavities with retraction. Cultures of sputum from such patients persistently yield *C. immitis*.

Miliary Coccidioidomycosis

Approximately 4 percent of patients hospitalized with coccidioidomycosis have miliary infections (Fig. 112-3). It may be the first presentation of infection or may occur later in a complicated course. It is thought to reflect widespread blood-borne infection, is often associated with dissemination, and carries a mortality of 50 percent. Miliary coccidioidomycosis occurs most often in immunosuppressed patients and is a very common presentation in patients with AIDS. Coccidioidal serology is usually reactive, but cultures of sputum are positive in fewer than 40 percent of the patients.

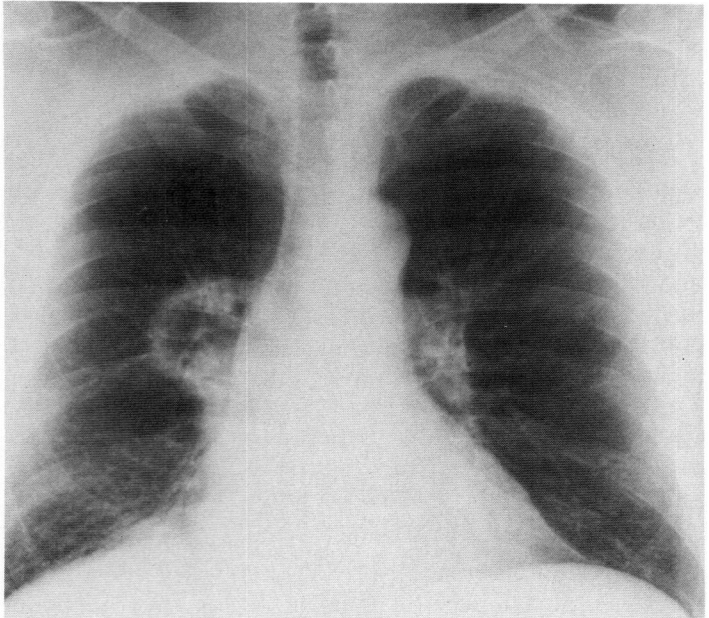

FIGURE 112-1 Thick-walled coccidioidal cavity which recurred many months after the initial infection resolved. This lesion was treated with amphotericin B before and after surgical resection.

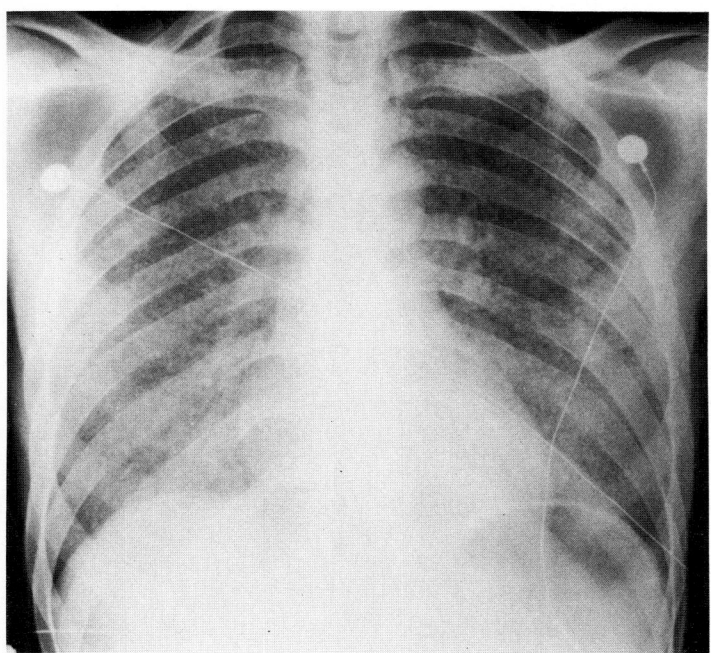

FIGURE 112-3 Fatal miliary coccidioidomycosis in a 32-year-old IV drug abuser.

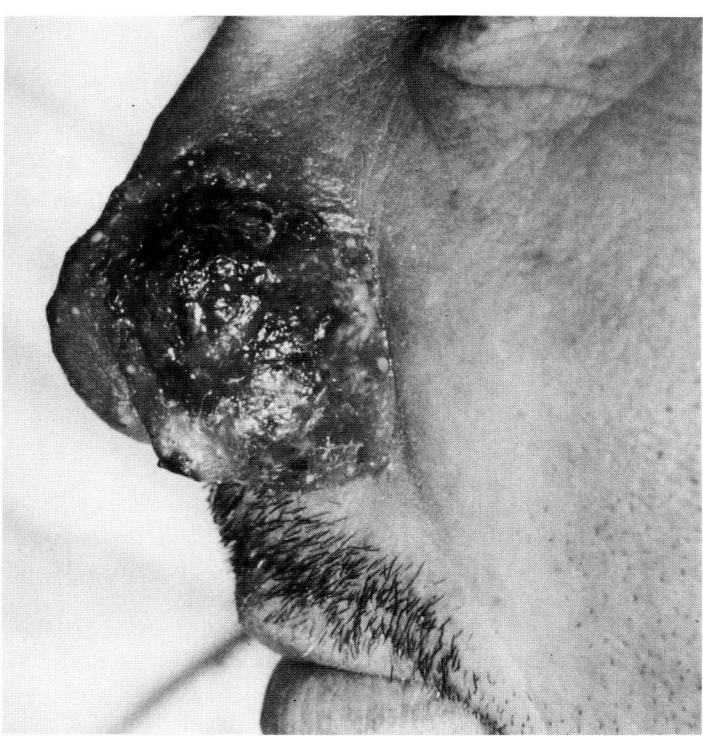

FIGURE 112-4 Coccidioidal dissemination to the skin. This lesion healed completely during treatment with ketoconazole. *(Courtesy of Dr. B. Friedman, Tucson, Arizona.)*

Dissemination

Subclinical fungemia may be common during the initial phases of coccidioidal infections as is the case with histoplasmosis. Asymptomatic coccidioidal chorioretinal scars and *C. immitis* in urine cultures have been demonstrated in approximately 10 percent of patients who resolved their infections without antifungal therapy. However, destructive lesions outside the chest occur in less than 1 percent of infections. In these patients, common sites of involvement are skin, joints, bones, and meninges (Fig. 112-4). Other sites of infection include the eye, peritoneum, middle ear, upper airways, myocardium, endocardium, pericardium, liver, spleen, adrenals, and thyroid. Infection of the urinary bladder is extremely rare, and intestinal involvement has not been reported. Although disseminated infection is most likely the result of hematogenous spread from an original pulmonary focus, dissemination often occurs in the absence of abnormalities referable to the chest.

DIAGNOSIS

Coccidioidomycosis should be considered in patients with pulmonary lesions or granulomatous disease in other organs. A careful travel history is important to avoid missing the occasional patient in nonendemic regions of the country.

Sputum Examination and Culture

The diagnosis of coccidioidomycosis is established by identifying spherules in, or recovering *C. immitis* from, clinical specimens.

EXAMINATION OF CLINICAL SPECIMENS

Spherules can be identified in sputum or other body fluids by examination of wet mount preparations with addition of 10 percent KOH. Spherules are relatively large, and their walls are doubly refractile. They can also be detected by Papanicolaou staining of bronchoscopy specimens and, in fixed tissue, with hematoxylin and eosin staining. However, they are not seen on Gram stain.

FUNGAL CULTURES

C. immitis will grow on most media available in a clinical microbiology laboratory. The typical colony is flat and nonpigmented and grows within 1 week of incubation at ambient temperatures. However, *C. immitis* sometimes displays unusual growth characteristics. To avoid laboratory accidents, any mold recovered in culture should be handled with considerable care until identification is complete.

Invasive Pulmonary Procedures

FLEXIBLE FIBEROPTIC BRONCHOSCOPY

If sputum specimens are nondiagnostic, cultures of bronchoscopy specimens may produce *C. immitis*. This approach is most useful in the evaluation of pulmonary infiltrates and is least helpful in patients with nodules. Bronchoscopy may also be useful in the evaluation of cavitary lesions, although sputum specimens, serology, and radiographic findings may provide sufficient information for practical purposes.

PERCUTANEOUS NEEDLE BIOPSY

Spherules can frequently be identified in smears of needle aspirates in patients with nodules. Cultures of biopsy specimens slightly increase the diagnostic yield of the procedure, and it is recommended that thoracotomy be delayed until the results of cultures are known.

PLEURAL BIOPSY AND THORACENTESIS

Cultures of pleural biopsy specimens are generally more likely to diagnose this infection than is culture of the pleural fluid. Coccidioidal effusions are usually exudative with a modest mononuclear pleocytosis (a white blood cell count of 5000).

Serology

Serologic tests for antibodies against coccidioidal antibodies were first developed in the mid 1940s and have been proven to show very few false-positive reactions from other systemic mycoses such as blastomycosis or histoplasmosis. By current techniques, any detectable antibody in serum is considered presumptive evidence of a coccidioidal infection.

TUBE PRECIPITIN TEST

Originally a precipitation reaction performed in test tubes, the tube precipitin test measures IgM and usually demonstrates a rapid early rise and fall (Fig. 112-5). Results are not quantified and are generally reported as positive or negative. In primary infections, the test is positive in over 90 percent of patients by the second week of illness. Reactivity may reappear if dissemination occurs. This test should not be applied to cerebrospinal fluid specimens because false-positive results are frequent.

LATEX AGGLUTINATION TEST

The latex agglutination test presumably also measures IgM and is more sensitive, convenient, and available than the tube precipitin test. It is useful as a screening test which, if positive, may be confirmed by the more specific tube precipitin test.

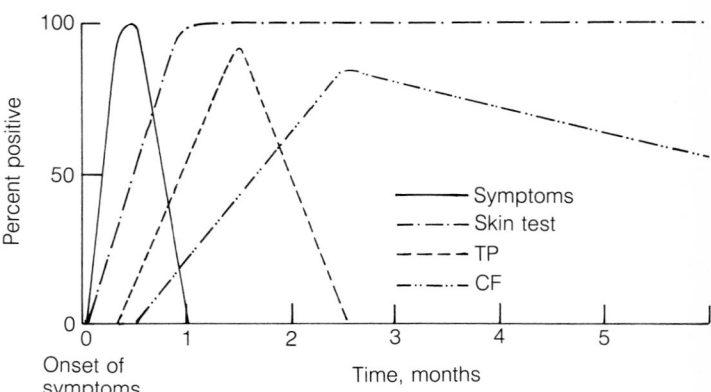

FIGURE 112-5 Temporal relationship of symptoms with prevalence of immunologic markers of infection in primary coccidioidomycosis. Skin test = delayed hypersensitivity to coccidioidin; TP = tube precipitating antibodies; CF = complement fixing antibodies.

COMPLEMENT FIXATION TEST

The complement fixation test measures IgG. Reactivity develops more slowly after infection than does that of the tube precipitin test. However, by the eighth week of illness, sera from greater than 90 percent of patients are positive. Antibody titers correlate with the extent of disease, although quantitative results of this test vary among laboratories. In the absence of a parameningeal focus, complement-fixing antibodies in the cerebrospinal fluid indicate meningitis.

IMMUNODIFFUSION TEST

Another test available commercially for detection of IgG uses an agar-gel immunodiffusion technique. This test is easier for laboratories to perform than the complement fixation test. However, results may require three or more days to be completed, whereas the complement fixation test is performed in 1 to 2 days. Immunodiffusion tests are especially useful for serum that is anticomplementary.

Skin Testing

In general, skin test results are most useful as epidemiologic tools or as a way of assessing a patient's immune response after a coccidioidal infection has been diagnosed by other means. The skin test usually becomes positive within 4 weeks of the primary infection and, in most persons, remains positive for life. Thus, a positive test is helpful diagnostically only if it was recently negative. Even in this circumstance, other explanations such as booster phenomena may confuse interpretation.

Coccidioidin, derived from filtrates of mycelial growth, was the antigen first used for skin testing. One-tenth of a milliliter of antigen is injected intradermally. A test is positive if there is a 5- by 5-mm area of induration

after 1 or 2 days. Spherulin, which is made from a lysate of spherules, is administered and interpreted in the same way as coccidioidin. It is slightly more sensitive than coccidioidin. In patients with erythema nodosum, it is suggested to first test with diluted antigen to avoid exaggerated reactions and local necrosis.

MANAGEMENT

Available Chemotherapies

The currently available drugs for coccidioidal treatment are amphotericin B, miconazole, and ketoconazole. All inhibit *C. immitis* in vitro, are effective in treating experimental murine coccidioidomycosis, and have published support for efficacy in patients. Comparative studies between these drugs have not been performed. Thus, it is not possible to confidently rank their relatively efficacy.

AMPHOTERICIN B

Amphotericin B is an intravenously administered antifungal agent which has been in use for more than 20 years. Drug clearance is slow so that therapy can be administered on alternate days without loss of effectiveness. The major problems with amphotericin B relate to drug toxicity. These include phlebitis at the injection site, nausea, high fevers, hypotension, marrow suppression, and a variety of electrolyte disturbances, most of which are secondary to renal damage. In some patients who receive a cumulative dose of more than 3 g, nephrotoxicity becomes irreversible.

MICONAZOLE

Like amphotericin B, miconazole must be administered intravenously and has a number of significant side effects, although they all remit when the drug is discontinued. Administration is often accompanied by fever, nausea, vomiting, and phlebitis. Rapid infusion has been associated with cardiac arrhythmias. Miconazole is occasionally used when amphotericin B fails, but currently is used infrequently to treat coccidioidal infections.

KETOCONAZOLE

Ketoconazole is an antifungal agent which was released in 1981. It is administered orally although intestinal absorption is variable. The most common side effects are nausea and vomiting which has led to discontinuation of therapy in 5 percent of patients receiving 400 mg per day. Gynecomastia and other results of hypogonadism also occur, especially when doses above 400 mg per day are used. Although mild elevations of liver enzymes are not infrequent, clinical hepatitis is rare.

Therapeutic Strategies

PRIMARY PNEUMONIA

Symptoms from the initial infection are nearly always self-limited. Parapneumonic pleural effusions do not change this prognosis. Despite the fact that the pleural space is usually infected, effusions need not be drained except for relief of symptoms. Because most primary infections follow a self-limited course, there is no indication to treat most of these patients with intravenous and highly toxic agents such as amphotericin B.

Important exceptions to this pattern are immunocompromised patients in whom dissemination is very frequent and the occasional immune competent patient who does not seem to be controlling the infection satisfactorily. For the latter, criteria sometimes considered when determining the need for treatment are as follows: extensive, enlarging, or persisting involvement of pulmonary parenchyma; persistent fever; persistently high or rising concentrations of complement-fixing coccidioidal antibodies; persistently reactive tube precipitin test; persistently nonreactive coccidioidal skin tests; or concurrent diseases likely to be adversely affected by coccidioidal infection. A short course of amphotericin B (total dose of 500 mg) is sometimes used for such patients.

Recently, with the advent of orally administered and less toxic agents such as ketoconazole, there has been a new interest in the possible benefit from treating patients with less severe forms of the primary pneumonia. Unfortunately, data are not yet available to generally recommend such therapy.

CHRONIC PNEUMONIA

Treatment is usually employed to limit the symptoms of exacerbations. Five hundred to one thousand milligrams of amphotericin B will generally result in improvement of symptoms and transient sterilization of sputum. Ketoconazole has also been reported to improve symptoms, although prompt relapses have been frequent when this drug has been discontinued. Whether prolonged use of ketoconazole will alter the overall course of chronic pneumonia is not yet known.

PULMONARY NODULES

No interventions are normally required other than to allay concerns about other possible causes of the lesion, such as malignancy. If the nodule is resected for purposes of diagnosis, antifungal therapy is not necessary either before or following the procedure.

PULMONARY CAVITIES

In patients with small cavities and no symptoms, no intervention is usually required. It is advisable to obtain repeat

chest radiographs several times during subsequent years to reassess the cavity's appearance. Patients whose cavities are associated with symptoms such as cough, sputum production, or mild hemoptysis may be considered for treatment with 500 to 1000 mg of amphotericin B or ketoconazole, although these treatments will not speed cavity closure. Recurrence of cavities years after the original infections, significant enlargement of activities, and massive hemoptysis are findings that suggest the need for surgical resection. Resection of active cavities is usually performed with approximately 500 mg of amphotericin B administered perioperatively. Even if the lesion appears fairly circumscribed on radiographs, it is likely that satellite lesions will be found at the time of surgery and wide resections seem to minimize the risk of postoperative complications. It should be emphasized that such procedures carry no assurance of cure. Unfortunately, recurrence of new lesions in other lobes is common.

Ruptured cavities require prompt surgical correction with wide excision of involved areas. The need for concurrent antifungal therapy in such patients is not established, but is recommended for those with other debilitating conditions such as diabetes, for those with suspected residual disease, or for those whose surgery is delayed. One gram of amphotericin B, started before and continued after the surgical procedure, is recommended.

MILIARY INFECTIONS

Miliary or diffuse reticulondular infiltrates are caused by life-threatening infections and should be treated aggressively. In such circumstances, parenteral therapy is most appropriate. Amphotericin B should be rapidly advanced to a dose of approximately 0.4 mg/per day.

DISSEMINATED INFECTIONS

Disseminated infections are often chronic, and patients can appropriately be treated on an outpatient basis. For patients with nonmeningeal dissemination, it is rational to attempt therapy with ketoconazole at a dose of at least 400 mg per day. After a year, if the disease is quiescent, the drug should be stopped and the patient watched. If relapse occurs, ketoconazole can be resumed for an indefinite length of time. For patients with more progressive lesions, amphotericin B is indicated. Optimally, any treatment should result in clinical improvement, a fall in complement fixation titers, and a return of skin test reactivity.

Patients with coccidioidal meningitis should be treated with intrathecal amphotericin B. Although there is current interest in substituting or adding ketoconazole at doses of 1200 to 2000 mg per day, these approaches have insufficient experience to be considered standard therapy.

BIBLIOGRAPHY

Bayer AS: Fungal pneumonias: Pulmonary coccidioidal syndromes (Part I). Chest 79:575–583, 1981.
  A comprehensive review of primary and progressive coccidioidal pneumonia including diagnostic, therapeutic, and prognostic considerations. Also addresses the role of surgery.

Bronnimann DA, Adam RD, Galgiani JN, Habib MP, Petersen EA, Porter B, Bloom JW: Coccidioidomycosis in the acquired immunodeficiency syndrome. Ann Intern Med 106:372–329, 1987.
  Of 27 patients with the acquired immunodeficiency syndrome (AIDS) in Tucson, Arizona, 7 had concurrent coccidioidomycosis. Early manifestations of infection in six patients included diffuse nodular pulmonary infiltrates and Coccidioides immitis in many extrathoracic sites.

Catanzaro A, Einstein H, Levine B, Ross B, Schillaci R, Fierer J, Friedman PJ: Ketoconazole for treatment of disseminated coccidioidomycosis. Ann Intern Med 96:436–440, 1982.
  Twenty seven of twenty nine selected patients with disseminated coccidioidomycosis were treated with ketoconazole for at least 6 months, in dosages of 200 to 600 mg per day, administered orally. These doses seem to suppress but not eradicate C. immitis.

Cunningham RT, Einstein H: Coccidioidal pulmonary cavities with rupture. J Thorac Cardiovasc Surg 84:172–177, 1982.
  The clinical and laboratory findings, medical and surgical treatment, and complications are presented for 23 patients with coccidioidal pulmonary cavities in whom the cavities underwent spontaneous rupture followed by a pyopneumothorax. Prompt surgical intervention is recommended when the diagnosis is suspected. The criteria for using amphotericin B are detailed.

DeFelice R, Galgiani JN, Campbell SC, Palpant SD, Friedman BA, Dodge RR, Weinberg MG, Lincoln LJ, Tennican PO, Barbee RA: Ketoconazole treatment of nonprimary coccidioidomycosis. Am J Med 72:681–687, 1982.
  Sixty patients with coccidioidomycosis were treated with ketoconazole in dosages of 200 mg per day (soft tissue lesions) or 400 mg per day (skeletal and pulmonary lesions). Improvement oc-

curred in 12 of 19 patients with chronic pulmonary infections, in 20 of 23 with soft tissue lesions and in 6 of 11 with skeletal complications. Recurrences and complications are described.

Drutz DJ, Catanzaro A: Coccidioidomycosis. Am Rev Respir Dis 117:559–585,727–771, 1978.
  A two-part review of the various aspects of the disease, including historical perspective, ecology, epidemiology, immunology, serology, and pathology.

Echols RM, Palmer DL, Long GW: Tissue eosinophilia in human coccidioidomycosis. Rev Infect Dis 4:656–664, 1982.
  Although it has been suggested that peripheral blood eosinophilia is a good prognostic sign in coccidioidomycosis, a blood eosinophilia >20 percent and the presence of eosinophilic micro-abscesses carries a poor prognosis, i.e., of progressive or disseminated infection.

Greendyke WH, Resnick DL, Harvey WC: The varied roentgen manifestations of primary coccidioidomycosis. Am J Roentgenol Rad Ther Nucl Med 109:491–499, 1970.
  The radiographic manifestations of coccidioidomycosis are presented based on 59 patients seen at a U.S. Air Force Base during 1 year. Pneumonia was the most common presentation.

Harvey WC, Greendyke WH: Skin lesions in acute coccidioidomycosis. Am Fam Physician 2:81–85, 1970.
  In 44 patients with acute coccidioidomycosis, skin lesions were noted in 27. The predominant specific lesions were erythema multiforme and erythema nodosum.

Kerrick SS, Lundergan LL, Galgiani JN: Coccidioidomycosis at a university health service. Am Rev Respir Dis 131:100–201, 1985.
  At a single university health service within an endemic area, 172 cases of coccidioidomycosis were respectively identified by fungal cultures, serologic studies, or intercurrent conversions of the skin test. Coccidioidomycosis was diagnosed about half as frequently as mononucleosis but required more protracted medical care.

Lonky SA, Catanzaro A, Moser KM, Einstein H: Acute coccidioidal pleural effusion. Am Rev Respir Dis 114:681–688, 1976.
  In more than 90 percent of 28 patients with acute coccidioidal effusions, direct extension of contiguous parenchymal infection, rather than hematogenous dissemination, seemed to explain the pathogenesis of the effusion. In most patients, the prognosis of this type of pleural effusion proved to be excellent. Pleural biopsies were the most rewarding source of material for culture.

Ross JB, Levine B, Catanzaro A, Einstein H, Schillag, R, Friedman PJ: Ketoconazole for treatment of chronic pulmonary coccidioidomycosis. Ann Intern Med 96:440–443, 1982.
  In most of 21 patients with chronic pulmonary coccidioidomycosis, clinical and radiographic improvements occurred and were associated with culture conversion and serologic improvement. Further experience is needed to evaluate the proper place of this agent in treating chronic pulmonary coccidioidomycosis.

Sarosi GA, Parker JD, Doto IL, Tosh FE: Chronic pulmonary coccidioidomycosis. A National Communicable Disease Center Cooperative Mycoses Study. N Engl J Med 283:325–329, 1970.
  Of 109 patients with proven coccidioidomycosis, in 20 the chest radiographs and clinical findings were indistinguishable from either chronic pulmonary histoplasmosis or chronic pulmonary tuberculosis.

Stevens DA: Coccidioidomycosis. A Text. New York, Plenum, 1980.
  A multiauthored monograph on coccidioidomycosis that deals with its microbiology, epidemiology, serology, immunology, pathology, and clinical manifestations.

Wallace JM, Catanzaro A, Moser KM, Harrell JH: Flexible fiberoptic bronchoscopy for diagnosing pulmonary coccidioidomycosis. Am Rev Respir Dis 123:286–290, 1981.
  In about half of 30 patients who had proven coccidioidomycosis and abnormal chest radiographs, flexible fiberoptic bronchscopy provided diagnostic specimens. In none of eight patients with a solitary pulmonary nodule due to coccidioidomycosis was the biopsy established by bronchoscopy.

Yoshino MT, Hillman BJ, Galgiani JN: Coccidioidomycosis in renal dialysis and transplant patients: Radiologic findings in 30 patients. AJR 149:989–992, 1987.
  The radiographic manifestations of pulmonary coccidioidomycosis in renal transplant and dialysis patients are highly variable. Interstitial and alveolar patterns of disease are equally likely to occur.

NOTES

NOTES

Appendixes

Appendix *A*

Respiratory Questionnaire

Name _____   Social security no. _____   Date _____

Plant _____   Sex ____ Date of birth _____   Age _____

Questionnaire administered by _____

_____

I. Occupational history: Please list entire work history starting with present job and going back to first job. (Use extra sheet if necessary.)

Industry (or company) and location	From	To	Specific job

	Yes	No	Number of years
A. Have you ever worked in a dusty job?			
1. In a mine?			
2. In a quarry?			
3. In a foundry?			
4. In a pottery?			
5. In a cotton, flax, or hemp mill?			
6. With asbestos?			
7. In a brick plant?			
8. As a sandblaster?			
9. In the manufacture of glass, ceramics, or abrasives?			
10. In other dusty jobs?			
Specify _____			
B. Have you ever worked with chemicals?			
1. Solvents?			
Specify _____			
2. Acids?			
Specify _____			
3. Lead?			
4. Plastics?			
Specify _____			
5. TDI?			

	Yes	No

II. Previous illnesses
    A. Have you ever had any of the following problems?
        1. Asthma?
        2. Emphysema?
        3. Chronic bronchitis?
        4. Pneumonia?
        5. Tuberculosis?
        6. Pleurisy?
        7. Heart trouble of any type?

III. Symptoms
    A. Cough
        1. Do you usually cough first thing in the morning?
        2. Do you usually cough at other times during the day or night?

Skip 3 to 6 if answer to 1 and 2 is "no." Answer if "yes."

        3. Do you cough on most days for as much as 3 months of the year?
        4. For how many years have you had this cough?
           Less than 2 years _____
           2 to 5 years _____
           5 years or more _____
        5. Do you cough more on any particular day of the week?
           If yes, which day? _____
        6. Do you cough during any particular season of the year?
           If yes, which season? _____

    B. Sputum
        1. Do you usually bring up phlegm, sputum, or mucus from your chest first thing in the morning?
        2. Do you usually bring up phlegm, sputum, or mucus from your chest at other times of the day or night?

Skip 3 and 4 if answer to 1 and 2 is "no." Answer if "yes."

        3. Do you bring up phlegm, sputum, or mucus from your chest on most days for as much as 3 months of the year?
        4. For how many years have you raised phlegm, sputum, or mucus from your chest
           Less than 2 years _____
           2 to 5 years _____
           5 years or more _____

    C. Wheezing
        1. Does your breathing ever sound wheezy?
        2. Have you ever had attacks of shortness of breath with wheezing?
        3. Have you ever had a feeling of tightness in your chest?

Skip 4 to 6 if answer to 1, 2, or 3 is "no." Answer if "yes."

        4. At what age did wheezing first occur? ____
        5. How frequently does wheezing occur?
           Daily _____
           Nightly _____
           A few times per week _____
           A few times per month _____
           A few times per year _____
        6. Is it worse on any particular day of the week?
           What day? _____

D. Breathlessness
   1. Do you get short of breath when walking on level ground?
   2. Do you get short of breath while walking up stairs?
   3. How many flights of stairs can you climb up without stopping?
      1 to 2? _____
      2 to 3? _____
      More than 3? _____
E. Hemoptysis
   1. Have you ever coughed up blood from your chest? If yes, when was the last time this happened? _____
IV. Smoking
   A. Smoking (currently)
      1. Do you now smoke regularly (cigarettes, pipe, cigars)?

Skip 2 to 6 if answer to 1 is "no." Answer if "yes."

   2. How old were you when you started smoking?
      _____

   3. For how many years have you smoked regularly?
      _____

   4. How many cigarettes do you now smoke each day?
      _____

   5. How much pipe tobacco do you now smoke each week?
      _____

   6. How many cigars do you now smoke each day?
      _____

   B. Smoking (formerly)
      1. Have you ever smoked regularly?

Skip 2 to 7 if answer to 1 is "no." Answer if "yes."

   2. How old were you when you started smoking regularly?
      _____

   3. For how many years did you smoke regularly?
      _____

   4. How long ago did you last quit smoking?
      Months _____
      Years _____
   5. How many cigarettes did you usually smoke per day?
      _____

   6. How much pipe tobacco did you usually smoke per week?
      _____

   7. How many cigars did you usually smoke per day?
      _____

V. Additional comments

Appendix *B*

Normal Values

TYPICAL VALUES FOR A 20-YEAR-OLD, SEATED MAN*

Ventilation (BTPS)

Tidal volume, L	0.50
Frequency, breaths/min	12
Minute volume, L/min	6.00
Respiratory dead space, ml	150
Alveolar ventilation, L/min	4.20

Lung Volumes (BTPS)

Inspiratory capacity (IC), L	3.00
Expiratory reserve volume (ERV), L	1.50
Vital capacity (VC), L	4.50
Residual volume (RV), L	1.50
Functional residual capacity (FRC), L	3.00
Total lung capacity (TLC), L	6.00
Residual volume/total lung capacity $\times$ 100 (RV/TLC%)	25

Mechanics of Breathing

Maximum voluntary ventilation (MVV), L/min	170
Forced expiratory volume in 1 s (FEV_1/FVC%)	83
Forced expiratory volume in 3 s (FEV_3/FVC%)	97
Forced expiratory flow during middle half of FVC ($FEF_{25-75\%}$), L/s	4.7
Forced inspiratory flow during middle half of FIVC ($FIF_{25-75\%}$), L/s	5.0
Static compliance of the lungs (Cst,L), L/cmH_2O	0.2
Compliance of lungs and thoracic cage, L/cmH_2O	0.1
Airway resistance at FRC (Raw), cmH_2O/L/s	1.5
Pulmonary resistance at FRC, cmH_2O/L/s	2.0
Airway conductance at FRC (Gaw), L/s/cmH_2O	0.66
Specific conductance (Gaw/V_L)	0.22
Work of quiet breathing, (kg $\cdot$ m)/min	0.5
Maximum work of breathing, (kg $\cdot$ m)/breath	10
Maximum inspiratory pressure, mmHg	75
Maximum expiratory pressure, mmHg	120

Distribution of Inspired Gas

Single-breath N_2 test (ΔN_2 from 750 to 1250 ml in expired gas), % N_2	<1.5
Alveolar N_2 after 7 min of breathing O_2, % N_2	<2.5
Closing volume (CV), ml	400
CV/VC $\times$ 100%	9
Closing capacity (CC), ml	1900
CC/TLC $\times$ 100%	32
Slope of phase III in single-breath N_2 test, % N_2/L	<2

*Height = 165 cm; weight = 64 kg; body surface area = 1.7 m².

Pulmonary Blood Flow

Cardiac output, L/min	5.40
Virtual venous admixture/cardiac output $\times$ 100%	<7
Anatomic venous admixture/cardiac output $\times$ 100%	<3

Gas Exchange

O_2 consumption at rest (STPD), ml/min	240
CO_2 output at rest (STPD), ml/min	192
Respiratory exchange ratio (R), CO_2 output/O_2 uptake	0.8

Alveolar Gas

$P_{A_{O_2}}$, mmHg	105
$P_{A_{CO_2}}$, mmHg	40

Arterial Blood

Pa_{O_2}, mmHg	95
Sa_{O_2}, %	98
pH	7.41
Pa_{CO_2}, mmHg	40
Pa_{O_2} while breathing 100% O_2, mmHg	640
$P(A\text{-}a)_{O_2}$, mmHg	10

Alveolar Ventilation-Perfusion

Alveolar ventilation, L/min	4.20
Pulmonary capillary blood flow, L/min	5.40
Alveolar ventilation/blood flow ($\dot{V}_A/\dot{Q}$)	0.8
Physiological dead space/tidal volume $\times$ 100 (V_D/V_T, %)	<30
Alveolar-arterial P_{O_2}, mmHg	10

Diffusion

Diffusing capacity at rest for CO, single-breath ($DL_{CO_{sb}}$), ml CO/min/mmHg	32

Control of Ventilation

Ventilatory response to hypercapnia, L/min/mmHg	>0.5
Ventilatory response to hypoxia, L/min per ΔS_{O_2} (%)	>0.2
Arterial blood P_{O_2} during moderate exercise, mmHg	95

Pulmonary Hemodynamics

Pulmonary blood flow (cardiac output), L/min	5.40
Pulmonary artery pressure, mmHg	25/8
Pulmonary capillary blood volume, ml	100
Pulmonary "capillary" blood pressure (wedge), mmHg	<10

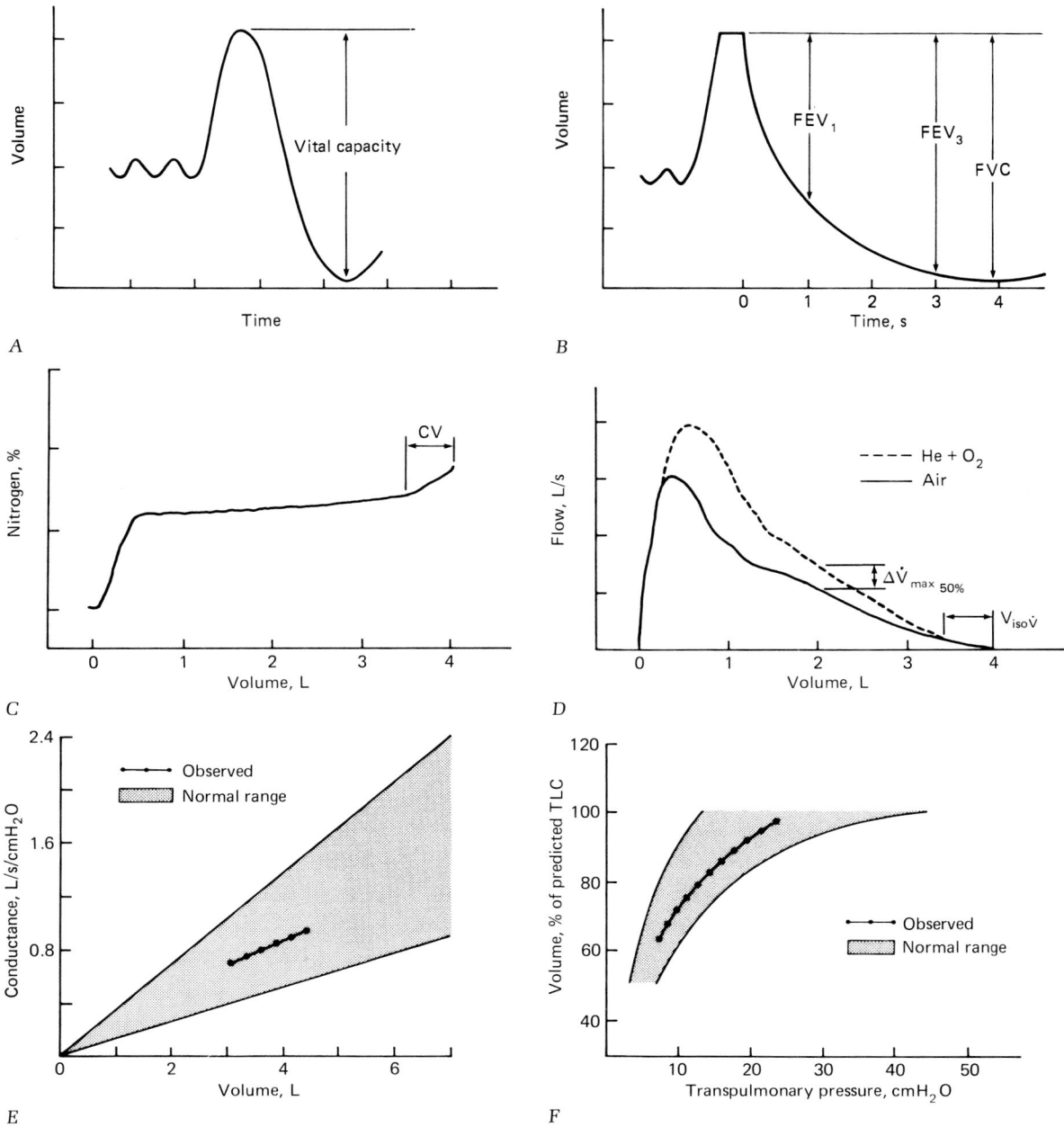

FIGURE B-1 Representative tracings and graphs commonly used in assessing pulmonary function. A. Lung volumes (vital capacity). B. Mechanics of breathing (forced expiratory volumes). C. Distribution (closing volumes). D. Flow-volume curves for breathing air and a helium-oxygen mixture. E. Mechanics of breathing (airway conductance). F. Mechanics of breathing (compliance of lungs).

Appendix *C*

Prophylaxis for Influenza and Pneumococcal Pneumonia

Influenza Vaccine
  The Viruses
  Individuals at Risk
  Options for Preventing Influenza

Pneumococcal Vaccine

Vaccines are now available to prevent influenza and pneumococcal pneumonia in individuals who might have difficulty in coping with them under conventional medical management or are particularly vulnerable to respiratory infection.

INFLUENZA VACCINE

In May 1986, the Immunization Practices Advisory Committee (ACIP) of the Centers for Disease Control (CDC) issued its annual advisory concerning Recommendations for the Use of the Influenza Vaccine During the Year 1986–1987. The following draws heavily on the CDC report. Even though the nature of the vaccine is destined to change somewhat almost from year to year, the general guiding principles for the use of this vaccine will probably remain unchanged. The CDC report for each year should be consulted for changes and details.

Influenza is a major threat to life among certain high-risk patients. It is responsible for about 10,000 patients in a nonepidemic year and for more than 30,000 after a severe epidemic. Killed influenza vaccine can prevent the illness if the viruses represented in the vaccine correspond closely in antigenic structure to the anticipated wild-type strain: the vaccine has proved to be completely effective in about two-thirds of recipients and has attenuated the disease in others whom it failed to protect completely.

The Viruses

Influenza A viruses are classified into subtypes based on two antigens: hemagglutinin (H) and neuraminidase (N). Three subtypes of hemagglutinin (H1, H2, H3) and two

subtypes of neuraminidase (N1, N2) are recognized among influenza A viruses that have caused widespread human disease. Immunity to these antigens, especially hemagglutinin, reduces the likelihood of infection and the severity of disease if infection does occur. However, there may be sufficient antigenic variation (antigenic drift) within the same subtype over time, so that infection or vaccination with one strain may not induce immunity to distantly related strains of the same subtype. Although influenza B viruses have shown much more antigenic stability than influenza A viruses, antigenic variation does occur. For these reasons, major epidemics of respiratory disease caused by new variants of influenza continue to occur, and the antigenic characteristics of current strains provide the basis for selecting virus strains included in each year's vaccine.

Individuals at Risk

"High-risk" persons may become deathly ill during a bout of influenza because of either associated health problems or age. Not only are they apt to require hospitalization for their illness but mortality rates are apt to be inordinate. The high mortality is due not only to the pneumonia but also to the final strain that the disease imposes on the underlying chronic pulmonary or cardiopulmonary disease. Influenza is a serious epidemiologic problem for the increasing number of elderly and for certain groups of younger individuals who are particularly susceptible to the disease, e.g., neonates who have survived respiratory intensive care, patients with cystic fibrosis, and individuals who have undergone organ transplantation.

Options for Preventing Influenza

Two measures are available to prevent influenza: (1) immunoprophylaxis using vaccines; and (2) chemoprophylaxis (as well as chemotherapy) using the antiviral drug amantadine hydrochloride (Symmetrel).

VACCINATION

The best protection for the high-risk individuals is vaccination, *each year*, before the start of the influenza season. High-risk individuals include those for whom influenza would have dire consequences and those who have an inordinate potential for infection. Vaccination is also used for individuals with a strong interest in avoiding influenza, in reducing the severity of disease if it should befall them, or minimizing chances of transmitting infection to high-risk individuals in their environments.

Inactivated Vaccine

Influenza vaccines are made from highly purified egg-grown viruses that have been rendered noninfectious ("inactivated"). Influenza vaccine contains three virus strains (two type A and one type B) that represent influ-

enza viruses currently circulating in the world and believed likely to occur in the United States in the winter ahead. The potency of the vaccine is adjusted with two goals in mind: (1) to evoke minimal systemic and febrile reactions; and (2) to elicit hemagglutinin-inhibition antibody titers that probably would protect them against infection by strains like those in the vaccine or by related variants. Although the elderly, the very young, and patients with certain chronic diseases may develop lower postvaccination antibody titers than young adults—and thus be more susceptible to upper respiratory tract infection—influenza vaccine can still be effective in preventing lower respiratory tract involvement or other complications of influenza.

Recommendations for Use of Inactivated Vaccine
Influenza vaccine is recommended for individuals at high risk who are 6 months of age or older, for the medical personnel who care for them, for primary providers of care in the home setting, for children receiving long-term aspirin therapy, and for other persons who wish to decrease their chances of acquiring influenza illness. Vaccine composition for 1987–1988 and doses are given in Table C-1. Guidelines for the use of vaccine are given below for different segments of the population. Any vaccine left over from the previous year should not be used: although the current influenza vaccine often contains one or more antigens used in previous years, immunity declines during the year following vaccination. Therefore, a history of vaccination in any previous year with a vaccine containing one or more antigens included in the current vaccine does not preclude the need for revaccination for the 1987–1988 influenza season to provide optimal protection.

TABLE C-1

Influenza Vaccine Dosage by Age of Patient— United States, 1987–1988 Influenza Season*

Age Group	Product†	Dosage‡, ml	No. Doses	Route§
6–35 months	Split virus only	0.25	2¶	IM
3–12 years	Split virus only	0.5	2¶	IM
Older than 12 years	Whole or split virus	0.5	1	IM

* Vaccine contains 15 μg each of influenza A/Taiwan/1/86 (hemagluttinin 1, neuraminidase 1); influenza A/Leningrad/360/86 (hemagluttinin 3, neuraminidase 2); and influenza B/Ann Arbor/1/86 hemagluttin antigens in each 0.5 ml. Manufacturers include Connaught Laboratories (Swiftwater, Pennsylvania) (Fluzone, whole or split; distributed by E. R. Squibb, Princeton, New Jersey), Parke-Davis (Fluogen; Morris Plains, New Jersey), and Wyeth Laboratories (Influenza Virus Vaccine, Trivalent, split; Philadelphia, Pennsylvania). Manufacturer's phone numbers for further information are Connaught, (800) 822-2463; Parke-Davis, (800) 223-0432; and Wyeth, (800) 321-2304.

†Because of the lower potential for causing febrile reactions, only split (subvirion) vaccine should be used in children. When used according to the recommended dosage, split and whole virus vaccines produce similar immunogenicity and side effects in adults.

‡Because children are accessible when pediatric vaccines are administered, it may be desirable to administer influenza vaccine to high-risk children simultaneously with routine pediatric vaccine or pneumococcal polysaccharide vaccine, but in a different site. Although studies have not been done, no diminution of immunogenicity or enhancement of adverse reactions should be expected.

§The recommended site of vaccination is the deltoid muscle for adults and older children. The preferred site for infants and young children is the anterolateral aspect of the thigh.

¶Two doses are recommended for maximum protection with at least 4 weeks between doses. However, if the individual received at least one dose of influenza vaccine between the 1978 to 1979 and 1986 to 1987 influenza seasons, one dose is sufficient.

NOTE: IM = intramuscular.

SOURCE: Prevention and Control of Influenza. Recommendations of the Immunization Practices Advisory Committee. Centers for Disease Control. Ann Intern Med 107:521–525, 1987.

TABLE C-2

Influenza Vaccination: High-Priority Target Groups for Special Vaccination Programs

Greatest medical risk of influenza-related complications

Adults and children with chronic disorders of the cardiovascular or pulmonary systems that are severe enough to have required medical follow-up or hospitalization during the preceding year.

Residents of nursing homes and other chronic-care facilities (i.e., institutions housing patients of any age with chronic medical conditions).

Moderate medical risk of influenza-related complications

Otherwise healthy individuals 6 years of age or older.

Adults and children with chronic metabolic diseases (including diabetes mellitus), renal dysfunction, anemia, immunosuppression, or asthma severe enough to require regular medical follow-up or hospitalization during the preceding year.

Children receiving long-term aspirin therapy, who may be at risk of developing Reye's syndrome following influenza infection.

Potentially capable of nosocomial transmission of influenza to high-risk persons

Physicians, nurses, and other personnel who have extensive contact with high-risk patients (e.g., primary-care and certain specialty clinicians, staff of intensive-care units, particularly neonatal intensive-care units).

Providers of care to high-risk persons in the home setting, e.g., family members, visiting nurses, volunteer workers.

Other groups

Any person who wishes to reduce the likelihood of acquiring influenza infection.

A pregnant woman with a medical condition that increases her risk of complications from influenza should be vaccinated as long as she has no egg allergy. Waiting until after the first trimester is a reasonable precaution to minimize the theoretical possibility of teratogenicity. However, it may be undesirable to delay vaccination of a pregnant woman with a high-risk condition who will be in the first trimester of pregnancy when the "influenza season" usually begins.

The preferred route of vaccination is intramuscular. The recommended site of vaccination is the deltoid muscle for adults and older children and the anterolateral aspect of the thigh for infants and young children.

High-Priority Target Groups

The highest priority for vaccination is directed toward the two high-risk groups in Table C-2.

Persons Who Should Not Be Vaccinated

Inactivated influenza vaccine should not be given to persons who have an anaphylactic sensitivity to eggs. Persons with acute febrile illnesses usually should not be vaccinated until their temporary symptoms have abated.

Timing of Influenza Vaccination Activities

For high-risk persons who are readily accessible, such as those in chronic-care facilities or work sites, vaccination is optimally undertaken in November. Earlier vaccination, i.e., in September and October, is warranted if (1) regional experience indicates earlier-than-normal epidemic activity, (2) hospitalized high-risk patients are discharged between September and the time that influenza activity begins to decline in their community, or (3) persons have been recommended for vaccination but will not be seen again until after November.

Children who have not been previously vaccinated require two doses of vaccine with at least 1 month between doses. Programs for childhood influenza vaccination should be scheduled so the second dose can be given before December. Vaccine can be given to both children and adults up to and even after influenza virus activity is documented in a region, although temporary chemoprophylaxis using amantadine may be indicated when influenza outbreaks are occurring.

Side Effects and Adverse Reactions

Because vaccines contain only noninfectious viruses, they cannot cause influenza. The most frequent side effect of vaccination, which occurs in fewer than one-third of vaccines, is soreness around the vaccination site for up to 1 to 2 days. Systemic reactions have been of two types:

1. Fever, malaise, myalgia, and other systemic symptoms of toxicity that, although infrequent, most often affect persons such as young children who have had no exposure to the influenza virus antigens contained in the vaccine. These reactions begin 6 to 12 h after vaccination and can persist for 1 to 2 days.

2. Immediate, presumably allergic, responses, such as flare and wheal or various respiratory tract symptoms of hypersensitivity, which may occur extremely rarely after influenza vaccination. These symptoms probably result from sensitivity to some vaccine component—most likely residual egg protein. Although current influenza vaccines contain only a small quantity of egg protein, the vaccine is presumed capable of inducing hypersensitivity reactions in individuals with anaphylactic hypersensitivity to eggs, and such persons should *not* be given influenza vaccine. This includes individuals who, after eating eggs, develop swelling of the lips or tongue or experience acute respiratory distress or collapse, or persons who have a documented IgE-mediated hypersensitivity reaction to eggs, including those who, from occupational exposure to egg protein, have developed evidence of occupational asthma or other allergic response. Unlike the 1976 swine influenza vaccine, subsequent vaccines, which have been prepared from other virus strains, have not been associated with an increased frequency of Guillain-Barré syndrome.

Simultaneous Administration of Other or Childhood Vaccines

There is considerable overlap in the target groups for influenza and pneumococcal vaccination. Pneumococcal and influenza vaccines can be given at the same time at different sites without increased side effects, but it should be emphasized that, whereas influenza vaccine is given annually, pneumococcal vaccine should be given only once.

AMANTADINE HYDROCHLORIDE (SYMMETREL)

Specific therapy for influenza A by treatment with amantadine is indicated for individuals who seek medical attention promptly after the abrupt onset of troublesome symptoms of an acute respiratory infection during an influenza A epidemic. For high-risk individuals for whom influenza vaccine has not been used or has not prevented infection, early treatment with amantadine should help to reduce the severity and duration of illness.

Amantadine is the only drug currently approved in the United States for the specific prophylaxis and therapy of influenza virus infections. This drug appears to interfere with the uncoating step in the virus replication cycle and also reduces virus shedding. Amantadine is 76 to 90 percent effective in preventing illnesses caused by circulating strains of type A influenza viruses, but it is not effective against type B influenza. When administered within 24 to 48 h after onset of illness, amantadine reduces the duration of fever and other systemic symptoms, allowing for a more rapid return to routine daily activities and improvement in peripheral airway function. Although it may not prevent infection, persons who take the drug may still develop immune responses that will protect them when exposed to antigenically related viruses.

Although amantadine chemoprophylaxis is effective against influenza A, under most circumstances, it should not be used in lieu of vaccination for two reasons: (1) it confers no protection against influenza B; and (2) patient compliance could be a problem for continuous adminis-

tration throughout epidemic periods, which generally last 6 to 12 weeks.

Recommendations for Amantadine Prophylaxis
Amantadine prophylaxis is particularly recommended to control outbreaks presumably due to influenza A. The drug should be given as early as possible after recognition of an outbreak in an effort to reduce the spread of the infection. When the decision is made to give amantadine for outbreak control, it is desirable to administer the drug to all residents of the affected institution. Amantadine prophylaxis should also be offered to unvaccinated staff who provide care to high-risk residents of chronic-care institutions or hospitals experiencing a presumed influenza A outbreak.

Amantadine prophylaxis is also recommended in the following situations:

1. As an adjunct to late immunization of high-risk individuals. It is not too late to immunize even when influenza A is known to be in the community. However, since the development of an antibody response following vaccination takes about 2 weeks, amantadine should be used in the interim. The drug does not interfere with antibody response to the vaccine.

2. To reduce spread of virus and maintain care for high-risk persons in the home setting. Persons who play a major role in providing care for high-risk persons in the home setting (e.g., family members, visiting nurses, volunteer workers) should also receive amantadine for prophylaxis when influenza A virus outbreaks occur in their communities, if such persons have not been appropriately immunized.

3. For immunodeficient persons. To supplement protection afforded by vaccination, chemoprophylaxis is also indicated for high-risk patients who may be expected to have a poor antibody response to influenza vaccine, e.g., those with severe immunodeficiency.

4. For persons for whom influenza vaccine is contraindicated. Chemoprophylaxis throughout the influenza season is appropriate for those few high-risk individuals for whom influenza vaccine is contraindicated because of anaphylactic hypersensitivity to egg protein or prior severe reactions associated with influenza vaccination.

5. For prophylactic use in other situations (e.g., unimmunized members of the general population who wish to avoid influenza A illness). This decision should be made on an individual basis.

Recommendations for Amantadine Therapy
Amantadine should be considered for therapeutic use, particularly for persons in the high-risk groups who develop an illness compatible with influenza during known or suspected influenza A activity in the community. The drug should be given within 24 to 48 h of onset of illness and should be continued until 48 h after resolution of signs and symptoms.

Precautions in Using Amantadine
Special precautions should be taken when amantadine is administered to persons with impaired renal function or those with an active seizure disorder (see "Dosage" below). The safety and efficacy of amantadine for children under 1 year of age have not been fully established.

Dosage
The usual adult dosage of amantadine is 200 mg per day; splitting the dose into 100 mg twice daily may reduce the incidence of side effects (Table C-3). Amantadine is not

TABLE C-3
Amantadine Hydrochloride Dosage, by Age of Patient and Level of Renal Function*

Age Group	Dosage†
No recognized renal disease	
1–9 years‡	4.4–8.8 mg/kg/day once daily or divided twice daily. Total dosage should not exceed 150 mg/day.
10–64 years§	200 mg once daily or divided twice daily.
≥65 years	100 mg once daily.¶

Creatinine clearance, ml/min 1.73 m²	Dosage
Recognized renal disease	
≥80	100 mg twice daily
60–79	200 mg/100 mg on alternate days
40–59	100 mg once daily
30–39	200 mg twice weekly
20–29	100 mg thrice weekly
10–19	200 mg/100 mg alternating every 7 days

* Amantadine hydrochloride (Symmetrel®) is manufactured and distributed by E.I. DuPont de Nemours and Company [Medical Department phone number (800) 441-9861, or in Delaware (302) 992-3273].

† For prophylaxis, amantadine must be taken each day for the duration of influenza A activity in the community (generally 6 to 12 weeks). For therapy, amantadine should be started as soon as possible after onset of symptoms and should be continued for 24 to 48 h after the disappearance of symptoms (generally 5 to 7 days).

‡ Use in children under 1 year has not been evaluated adequately.

§ Reduction of dosage to 100 mg per day is also recommended for persons with an active seizure disorder, because such persons may be at risk of experiencing an increase in the frequency of their seizures when given amantadine at 200 mg per day.

¶ The reduced dosage of 100 mg per day for persons 65 years of age or older without recognized renal disease is recommended to minimize the risk of toxicity, because renal function normally declines with age, and because side effects have been reported more frequently in the elderly when a daily dose of 200 mg has been used.

metabolized and is excreted unchanged in the urine. Because renal function normally decreases with age, and because side effects have been reported more frequently among older persons, a reduced dosage of 100 mg per day is generally advisable for persons aged 65 years or older to minimize the risk of toxicity. Persons 10 to 64 years old with an active seizure disorder may also be at risk of increased frequency of seizures when given amantadine at 200 mg per day rather than 100 mg per day.

Side Effects and Adverse Reactions
Five to ten percent of otherwise healthy adults taking amantadine report side effects such as insomnia, lightheadedness, irritability, and difficulty concentrating. These and other side effects may be more pronounced among patients with underlying diseases, particularly those common among the elderly; provisions for careful monitoring are needed for these individuals so that adverse effects may be recognized promptly and the drug reduced in dosage or discontinued, if needed. Since amantadine is not metabolized, toxic levels can occur in individuals in whom renal function is sufficiently impaired.

PNEUMOCOCCAL VACCINE

The original vaccine against disease caused by *Streptococcus pneumoniae* (pneumococcus) was licensed in 1977 and contained 14 serotypes. It was succeeded in 1983 by a 23-valent polysaccharide vaccine. The increase in efficacy afforded by the 23-valent vaccine is modest. Although virtually all epidemiologic studies to date are based on the 14-valent vaccine, the results are considered to be applicable to the 23-valent vaccine. There is still no consensus about the efficacy of the pneumococcal vaccine. Nonetheless, evidence is mounting in favor of vaccinating high-risk patients. The following material and recommendations draw heavily on the Report of the Immunization Practices Advisory Committee of the Centers for Disease Control.

The estimated number of cases of pneumococcal pneumonia per year ranges from 150 to 750 per 1000, and the case-fatality rate is about 5 percent. *S. pneumoniae* is the most common cause of pneumonia, meningitis, and otitis media in the western world. Bacteremia, which occurs in about 20 to 25 percent of all patients, is associated with a high mortality. Before antibiotics became available, mortality from bacteremia was about 75 percent, approaching 100 percent in the elderly. Since the advent of antibiotics, mortality has decreased, and leveled off, at about 25 to 30 percent (reports vary from 13 to 52 percent). The two principal factors that predispose to pneumococcal pneumonia are underlying disease and old age. However, pneumococcal pneumonia occurs in all age groups: in adults, its incidence increases gradually among those over 40 years old, with a twofold increase in incidence among those over 60 years old.

Patients with certain chronic conditions are clearly at increased risk of developing pneumococcal infection, as well as experiencing more severe pneumococcal illness. These conditions include: sickle cell anemia, Hodgkin's disease, multiple myeloma, cirrhosis, alcoholism, nephrotic syndrome, renal failure, chronic pulmonary disease, splenic dysfunction, and history of splenectomy or organ transplant. Other patients may be at greater risk of developing pneumococcal infection or having more severe illness because of diabetes mellitus, congestive heart failure, or conditions associated with immunosuppression. Patients with cerebrospinal fluid (CSF) leakage complicating skull fractures or neurosurgical procedures can have recurrent pneumococcal meningitis.

The importance of preventing pneumococcal bacteremia is underscored by the increasing frequency of penicillin resistance and by failure of sophisticated management in the intensive-care setting to improve survival. However, the extent to which the vaccine will be effective in this regard remains to be settled.

Pneumococcal Polysaccharide Vaccines
The new pneumococcal vaccine is composed of purified, capsular polysaccharide antigens of 23 types of *S. pneumoniae* (Danish types 1, 2, 3, 4, 5, 6B, 7F, 8, 9N, 9V, 10A, 11A, 12F, 14, 15B, 17F, 18C, 19A, 19F, 20, 22F, 23F, and 33F). Each polysaccharide is extracted separately and combined into the final product. Each dose of the new vaccine contains 25 μg of each polysaccharide antigen.

The 23 bacterial types represented in the current vaccine are responsible for 87 percent of bacteremic pneumococcal disease in the United States reported to the CDC in 1983, compared with 71 percent for the previous 14-valent formulation. Studies of the cross reactivity of human antibodies against related types suggest that cross protection may occur among some of these types (e.g., 6A and 6B).

Although the new polysaccharide vaccine contains only 25 μg of each antigen, compared with 50 μg of antigen in the old 14-valent vaccine, a study of 53 adults reveals comparable levels of immunogenicity of the two vaccines. Most healthy adults show a twofold or greater rise in type-specific antibody, as measured by radioimmunoassay, within 2 to 3 weeks after vaccination. In contrast, the vaccine is generally less antigenic for children under 2 years old than are other vaccinees. However, because the precise protective titers of antibody for any of these serotypes have not been established, measuring antibody levels in vaccinated persons is not indicated.

Effectiveness of Pneumococcal Polysaccharide Vaccines
In the 1970s, two randomized controlled trials were conducted in populations with a high incidence of disease in

South Africa and New Guinea using newly formulated pneumococcal vaccine. Both studies demonstrated significant reductions in the occurrence of pneumonia in these young, healthy populations.

However, other subsequent randomized controlled trials of pneumococcal vaccine in older-aged U.S. adults showed less satisfactory results. One was of outpatients over 45 years old; the second, of inpatients of a chronic-care psychiatric facility. In neither study was there any difference in the occurrence of respiratory morbidity and mortality between those vaccinated and those given a placebo. Nor did a Veterans' Administration Cooperative Study using high-risk ambulatory patients support the use of vaccine.

A major difficulty in comparing the results of epidemiologic studies is the different populations used, the different criteria for identification of pneumococcal infections, and the varied statistical treatment of the data. Methodologies are also far from uniform. For example, one recent approach assessed the efficacy of pneumococcal vaccine by comparing the distribution of serotypes of pneumococci isolated from the blood of vaccinated and unvaccinated persons, i.e., S. pneumoniae isolates from the blood of persons who receive the 14-valent vaccine were compared with blood isolates from unvaccinated persons. Among individuals more than 60 years old without either underlying illness or chronic pulmonary disease, chronic heart disease, or diabetes mellitus, the estimated efficacy of the vaccine ranged between 60 and 80 percent; the efficacy was lower among individuals with cirrhosis or renal failure.

Few studies of the efficacy of pneumococcal vaccine have been conducted in children. However, in one small, nonrandomized study of children and young adults 2 to 25 years old who had sickle cell anemia or who had undergone splenectomy, the occurrence of bacteremic pneumococcal disease was significantly reduced by immunization with an 8-valent vaccine.

The duration of protection induced by vaccination is unknown. Although antibody titers remain high 5 years after immunization, how long the high titers will persist after vaccination is not known.

Recommendations for Use of Inactivated Vaccine

Mounting evidence favors the more extensive use of pneumococcal vaccine.

Adults

Vaccination is particularly recommended for the following:

1. Adults with chronic illnesses, especially cardiovascular disease and chronic pulmonary disease, who are seriously compromised by respiratory infections.

2. Adults with chronic illnesses specifically associated with an increased risk for pneumococcal disease or its complications. These include splenic dysfunction or anatomic asplenia, Hodgkin's disease, multiple myeloma, cirrhosis, alcoholism, renal failure, CSF leaks, and conditions associated with immunosuppression.

3. Older adults, especially those aged 65 and over, who are otherwise healthy.

Children

Vaccination is particularly recommended for the following:

1. Children aged 2 years and older with chronic illnesses specifically associated with increased risk for pneumococcal disease or its complications. These include anatomic or functional asplenia, such as sickle cell disease or splenectomy, nephrotic syndrome, CSF leaks, and conditions associated with immunosuppression.

2. Recurrent upper respiratory diseases, including otitis media and sinusitis, are not considered indications for the use of vaccine in children.

General Considerations

When elective splenectomy is being considered, pneumococcal vaccine should be given, if possible, at least 2 weeks before the operation. Similarly, when immunosuppressive therapy is being planned, as in patients who are candidates for organ transplants, the interval between vaccination and initiation of immunosuppressive therapy should be as long as possible.

Although vaccine failures have been reported in some of these groups, especially those who are immunocompromised, vaccination is still recommended for such persons because they are at high risk of developing severe disease.

Adverse Reactions

About half of those given pneumococcal vaccine develop mild side effects, such as erythema and pain at the injection site. In less than 1 percent of those given pneumococcal vaccine, fever, myalgias, and severe local reactions have been reported. Severe adverse effects, such as anaphylactoid reactions, have rarely been reported—about 5 per million doses administered.

Revaccination

It should be emphasized that pneumococcal vaccine should be given only once to adults. Arthus' reactions and systemic reactions have been common among adults given second doses and are thought to result from localized antigen-antibody reactions involving antibody induced by previous vaccination. Therefore, second or "booster" doses are not recommended, at least at this time. Data on revaccination of children are not yet sufficient to provide a basis for comment.

Persons who have received the 14-valent pneumococcal vaccine should not be revaccinated with the 23-valent

vaccine, as the modest increase in coverage does not warrant the possible increased risk of adverse reactions. However, when there is doubt or no information on whether a person has ever received pneumococcal vaccine, the vaccine should not be given.

Precautions
The safety of pneumococcal vaccine for pregnant women has not been evaluated. It should not be given to otherwise healthy pregnant women. Women at high risk of pneumococcal disease ideally should be vaccinated before pregnancy.

BIBLIOGRAPHY

American Lung Association: Update: Pneumococcal polysaccharide vaccine usage—United States. ATS News, Spring, 1985.
A strong endorsement, by the Subcommittee on Prevention of Pneumonia and Influenza of the American Thoracic Society, of the Immunization Practices Advisory Committee, United States Public Health Service. The new 23-valent vaccine should be given to individuals either at high risk of developing pneumococcal pneumonia or who would be in serious jeopardy if pneumococcal pneumonia supervened on an underlying chronic disorder, including chronic pulmonary disease.

Bolan G, Broome CV, Fracklam RR, Plikaytis BD, Fraser DW, Schlech WF III: Pneumococcal vaccine efficacy in selected populations in the United States. Ann Intern Med 104:1–6, 1986.
In an analysis of 1634 bacteremic infections, the pneumococcal vaccine proved to be efficacious, to some degree, in all the immunocompetent groups. This study supports the use of pneumococcal vaccine.

Health and Public Policy Committee, American College of Physicians: Pneumococcal vaccine. Ann Intern Med 104:118–120, 1986.
Endorses the use of pneumococcal vaccine.

LaForce FM, Eickhoff TC: Pneumococcal vaccine: The evidence mounts. Ann Intern Med 104:110–112, 1986.
In favor of vaccinating high-risk patients.

Prevention and control of influenza. Recommendations of the Immunization Practices Advisory Committee. Centers for Disease Control. Ann Intern Med 107:521–525, 1987.
An update of information on the vaccine and antiviral agent available for prevention and control of influenza. It extends the 1985 report in several different ways: (1) updating of the influenza strains in the vaccine for 1986–1987; (2) immunization and amantadine prophylaxis for household members who provide home care for high-risk persons; (3) optimal time for conducting routine vaccination programs; (4) concurrent administration of influenza vaccine and childhood vaccines; (5) immunization of children receiving long-term aspirin therapy; and (6) other sources of information about influenza and control measures. It also includes a selected but comprehensive bibliography.

Simberkoff MS, Cross AP, Al-Ibrahim M, Baltch AL, Geiseler PJ, Nadler J, Richmond AS, Smith RP, Schiffman G, Shepard DS et al: Efficacy of pneumococcal vaccine in high-risk patients: Results of a Veterans' Administration Cooperative Study. N Engl J Med 315:1318–1327, 1986.
A report of a cooperative study to test the effectiveness of pneumococcal vaccine in preventing vaccine-serotype Streptococcus pneumoniae infections in high-risk ambulatory patients (not hospitalized bacteremic patients). The study was unable to prove efficacy of pneumococcal vaccine in this high-risk population. The authors suggest that chronically ill patients, who are most susceptible to infection, may have an impaired immune response to the pneumococcal vaccine. (See also Letters to the Editor, N Engl J Med 316:1272–1273, 1987.)

Update: Pneumococcal polysaccharide vaccine usage—United States. MMWR 33:273–281, 1984.
Recommends pneumococcal vaccine for adults with chronic illnesses "who sustain increased morbidity with respiratory infections" and for those "with chronic illnesses specifically associated with an increased risk for pneumococcal disease or its complications."

Appendix **D**

Terms and Symbols in Respiratory Physiology

GENERAL SYMBOLS

P	Partial pressure in blood or gas.
	P_{O_2} = partial pressure of O_2
$\overline{X}$	A bar over the symbol indicates a mean value.
	$\overline{P}$ = mean pressure, as distinct from instantaneous pressure
$\dot{X}$	A time derivative (rate) is indicated by a dot above the symbol.
	$\dot{V}_{O_2}$ = O_2 consumption per unit time
	$\dot{V}_{CO_2}$ = CO_2 production per unit time
% X	Percent sign preceding a symbol indicates percentage of the predicted normal value.
X/Y %	Percent sign following a symbol indicates a ratio function with the ratio expressed as a percentage. Both components of the ratio must be designated.
	FEV_2/FVC % = $100 \times FEV_1/FVC$
X_A, X_a	A small capital letter or a lowercase letter on the same line following a primary symbol is a qualifier to further define the primary symbol. When small capital letters are not available on typewriters or to printers, subscript capital letters may be used.
	$X_A = X_A$
$P_{E_{CO_2}}$, $\dot{V}_{D_{an}}$	Additional qualifiers of the primary symbol may be identified as shown.

GAS PHASE SYMBOLS

Primary Symbols

V	Volume of gas.
$\dot{V}$	Flow of gas.
F	Fractional concentration of a gas.

Common Qualifying Symbols

I	Inspired.
	V_I = inspired volume
E	Expired.
	V_E = expired volume
A	Alveolar.
	V_A = alveolar volume
	$\dot{V}_A$ = alveolar ventilation per unit time
T	Tidal.
	V_T = tidal volume

D-1

D   Dead space.

> V_D = volume of dead space
>
> $\dot{V}_D$ = dead space ventilation per unit time

B   Barometric.

> P_B = barometric pressure

L   Lung.

STPD   Standard conditions: temperature 0°C, pressure 760 mmHg, and dry (0 mmHg water vapor).

BTPS   Body conditions: body temperature and ambient pressure, saturated with water vapor at these conditions.

ATPD   Ambient temperature and pressure, dry.

ATPS   Ambient temperature and pressure, saturated with water vapor at these conditions.

an   Anatomic.

p   Physiological.

f   Respiratory frequency, per minute.

max   Maximum.

t   Time.

BLOOD PHASE SYMBOLS

Primary Symbols

Q   Volume of blood.

$\dot{Q}$ Blood flow.

> $\dot{Q}$ = cardiac output, L/min

C   Concentration in the blood phase.

> C_{N_2} = concentration of N_2 in blood, ml of N_2 per 100 ml of blood

S   Saturation in the blood phase.

> S_{O_2} = saturation of hemoglobin with O_2, percent

Qualifying Symbols

b   Blood, in general.

> Cb_{O_2} = concentration of O_2 in blood, ml of O_2 per 100 ml of blood

a   Arterial.

> Ca_{O_2} = concentration of O_2 in arterial blood, ml of O_2 per 100 ml of blood

c   Capillary.

> Cc_{O_2} = concentration of O_2 in capillary blood, ml of O_2 per 100 ml of blood

c′   Pulmonary end-capillary.

> Pc'_{CO_2} = partial pressure of CO_2 in end-capillary blood, mmHg

v   Venous.

> Cv_{O_2} = concentration of O_2 in venous blood, ml of O_2 per 100 ml of blood

$\overline{v}$ Mixed venous.

$$C\overline{v}_{O_2} = \text{concentration of } O_2 \text{ in mixed venous blood, ml of } O_2 \text{ per 100 ml of blood}$$

VENTILATION AND LUNG MECHANICS TESTS AND SYMBOLS

Static Lung volumes[1]

PRIMARY COMPARTMENTS (SEE FIG. 163-1)

RV	Residual volume. Volume of air remaining in the lungs after maximum expiration.
CV	Closing volume. Volume of air remaining in the lungs at onset of airways closure (see Fig. 163-30). Often expressed as a fraction of VC, that is, CV/VC %.
ERV	Expiratory reserve volume. Maximum volume of air expired from the resting end-expiratory level.
V_T	Tidal volume. Volume of air inspired or expired with each breath during quiet breathing. When tidal volume is used in gas-exchange formulations, this symbol is used. When indicating a subdivision of lung volumes, the symbol TV may be used.
IRV	Inspiratory reserve volume. Maximum volume of air inspired from the resting end-inspiratory level.
V_L	Volume of the lung, including the conducting airways.

Lung Capacities[2]

IC	Inspiratory capacity. The sum of IRV and TV.
IVC	Inspiratory vital capacity. Maximum volume of air inspired from the point of maximum expiration.
VC	Vital capacity. Maximum volume of air expired from the point of maximum inspiration.
FRC	Functional residual capacity. Sum of RV and ERV. FRC is the volume of air remaining in the lungs at the resting end-expiratory position.
TLC	Total lung capacity. Volume of air in the lungs after maximum inspiration. Also, the sum of all volume compartments of the lungs.
RV/TLC %	Residual volume to total lung capacity ratio, expressed as a percentage.
CC	Closing capacity. Closing volume plus residual volume, often expressed as a ratio of TLC, that is, CC/TLC %.

Forced Respiratory Maneuvers during Spirometry[3]

FVC	Forced vital capacity. The maximum volume of air forcibly expired from the maximum inspiratory position.
FIVC	Forced inspiratory vital capacity. Maximum volume of air forcibly inspired starting from a maximum expiration.
FEV_t	Timed forced expiratory volume. Volume of air expired in a specified time in the course of the forced vital capacity maneuver.

$$FEV_1 = \text{volume of air expired during the first second of the FVC}$$

FEV_t/FVC %	Ratio of time forced expiratory volume to forced vital capacity, expressed as a percentage.
FEF_x	Forced expiratory flow, related to some portion of the FVC curve. Modifiers refer to the amount of the FVC that has been expired at the time of measurement.
$FEF_{200-1200}$	Forced expiratory flow between 200 and 1200 ml of the FVC (formerly called the maximum expiratory flow rate).
$FEF_{25-75\%}$	Forced expiratory flow during middle half of the FVC (formerly called the maximum midexpiratory flow rate).
PEF	Peak expiratory flow. Highest value for expiratory flow.
$\dot{V}max_{x\%}$	Maximum flow when x percent of the FVC has been expired.

$$\dot{V}max_{75\%} = \text{flow (instantaneous) when 75 percent of the FVC has been expired}$$

[1] Expressed at BTPS unless otherwise specified. Asterisks indicate values obtainable by spirometry.

[2] Combinations of volumes for practical purposes.

[3] All values at BTPS unless otherwise specified.

$\dot{V}max_{x\%TLC}$	Maximum flow when x percent of the TLC remains.

$\dot{V}max_{75\%TLC}$ = flow (instantaneous) when the lungs contain 75 percent of the TLC

FET_x	Forced expiratory time required to expire a specified FVC.

$FET_{95\%}$ = time required to expire the first 95 percent of the FVC

$FET_{25-75\%}$ = time required to expire the $FET_{25-75\%}$

FIF_x	Forced inspiratory flow. As in the case of the FEF, appropriate modifiers designate the volume at which flow is being measured. Unless otherwise specified, the volume qualifiers indicate the volume inspired from RV at the point of measurement.

$FIF_{25-75\%}$ = forced inspiratory flow during the middle half of the FIVC

$I\dot{V}max_{x\%}$	Maximum inspiratory flow (instantaneous) when x percent of the FIVC has been inspired.
$I\dot{V}max_{x\%TLC}$	Maximum inspiratory flow (instantaneous) when the lungs contain x percent of the TLC.
MVV	Maximum voluntary ventilation. Volume of air breathed during maximum breathing efforts during a specified time period. Formerly called maximum breathing capacity. If breathing frequency is set by the examiner, it is indicated by the qualifier.

MVV_{60} = MVV at a breathing frequency of 60 per minute

Measurements Related to Ventilation

$\dot{V}E$	Expired volume per minute (BTPS).
$\dot{V}I$	Inspired volume per minute (BTPS).
$\dot{V}_{CO_2}$	Carbon dioxide production per minute (STPD).
$\dot{V}_{O_2}$	Oxygen consumption per minute (STPD).
R	Respiratory exchange ratio, the ratio of CO_2 output to O_2 intake in the lungs.
$\dot{V}A$	Alveolar ventilation per minute (BTPS).
$\dot{V}D$	Ventilation per minute of the physiological dead space (BTPS) defined by the equation

$$\dot{V}D = \dot{V}E \frac{Pa_{CO_2} - PE_{CO_2}}{Pa_{CO_2} - PI_{CO_2}}$$

VD	Volume of the physiological dead space, calculated as $\dot{V}D/f$.
$\dot{V}D_{an}$	Ventilation per minute of the anatomic dead space, that portion of the conducting airway in which no significant gas exchange occurs (BTPS).
VD_{an}	Volume of the anatomic dead space (BTPS).
$\dot{V}D_A$	Ventilation of the alveolar dead space (BTPS), defined by the equation

$$\dot{V}D_A = \dot{V}D - \dot{V}D_{an}$$

VD_A	The alveolar dead space volume, defined as

$$VD_A = \dot{V}D_A/f$$

Mechanics of Breathing[1]

Paw	Pressure at any point along the airways.
Pao	Pressure at the airway opening.
Ppl	Pleural pressure.
PA	Alveolar pressure.
Pbs	Pressure at the body surface.
Pes	Esophageal pressure; used to estimate Ppl.
$PA - Ppl$	Transpulmonary pressure.

[1] All pressures expressed relative to ambient pressure unless otherwise specified.

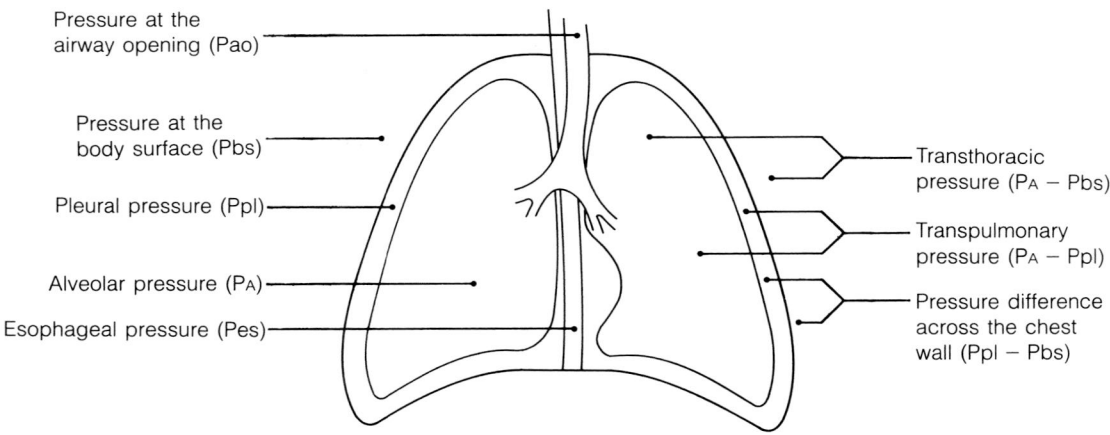

Pressure at the airway opening (Pao)

Pressure at the body surface (Pbs)

Pleural pressure (Ppl)

Alveolar pressure (PA)

Esophageal pressure (Pes)

Transthoracic pressure (PA − Pbs)

Transpulmonary pressure (PA − Ppl)

Pressure difference across the chest wall (Ppl − Pbs)

Ppl − Pbs	Transthoracic pressure, pressure difference across the chest wall.
Paw − Ppl	Transbronchial pressure, estimated as difference between airway and pleural pressures.

FLOW-PRESSURE RELATIONSHIPS[1]

R	General symbol for frictional resistance, defined as the ratio of pressure difference to flow.
Raw	Airway resistance, calculated from pressure difference between airway opening (Pao) and alveoli (PA) divided by the airflow, $cmH_2O/L/s$.
RL	Total pulmonary resistance, measured by relating flow-dependent transpulmonary pressure to airflow at the mouth.
Rti	Tissue resistance (viscous resistance of lung tissue), calculated as difference between RL and Raw.
Rus	Resistance of the airways on the upstream (alveolar) side of the point in the airways where intraluminal pressure equals Ppl, i.e., equal pressure point. Measured during a forced expiration.
Rds	Resistance of the airways on the downstream (mouth) side of the point in the airways where intraluminal pressure equals Ppl, i.e., equal pressure point. Measured during a forced expiration.
Gaw	Airway conductance, reciprocal of Raw.
Gaw/VL	Specific conductance, airway conductance, expressed per liter of lung volume at which Gaw is measured.
$\dot{W}$	Rate of work or power. Expressed either in kpm/min or J/s (watt).

VOLUME-PRESSURE RELATIONSHIPS

C	General symbol for compliance of the lungs, chest wall, or total respiratory system. Volume change per unit change in applied pressure. For the lungs, the applied pressure is the pressure difference across the lungs, or transpulmonary pressure, Pao − Ppl; for the chest wall, the applied pressure is the transthoracic pressure, Ppl − Pbs; for the entire respiratory system the applied pressure is Pao − Pbs.
Cdyn	Dynamic compliance. Value for compliance determined at time of zero gas flow at the mouth during uninterrupted breathing. The respiratory frequency appears as a qualifier.

$$Cdyn_{40} = \text{dynamic compliance at a respiratory frequency of 40 per minute}$$

Cst	Static compliance, value for compliance determined on the basis of measurements made during a period of zero airflow.
C/VL	Specific compliance. Compliance divided by the lung volume at which it is determined, usually FRC.
E	Reciprocal of compliance (elastance).
Pst	Static pulmonary pressure at a specified lung volume.

$$Pst_{TLC} = \text{static recoil pressure of the lung measured at TLC (maximum recoil pressure)}$$

W	Mechanical work of breathing.

[1]Unless otherwise specified, all resistance measurements assumed to be made at lung FRC.

DIFFUSING CAPACITY TESTS AND SYMBOLS

DL_X, D_X	Diffusing capacity of the lung expressed as volume (STPD) of gas (x) uptake per minute per unit alveolar-capillary pressure difference for the gas used. A modifier can be used to designate the technique:

$$DL_{CO_{sb}} = \text{single-breath CO diffusing capacity}$$
$$DL_{CO_{ss}} = \text{steady-state CO diffusing capacity}$$

DM	Diffusing capacity of the alveolar-capillary membrane (STPD).
θ	Reaction rate coefficient for red blood cells. Determined as the volume of gas (STPD) which will combine per minute with 1 unit volume of blood per unit of gas tension. If the specific gas is not stated, θ is assumed to refer to CO and is a function of existing O_2 tension.
Vc	Capillary blood volume. This should be Qc for consistency with other symbols, but Vc is entrenched in the literature. In the equation which follows for $1/DL$, Vc represents the effective pulmonary capillary blood volume, i.e., capillary blood volume in intimate association with alveolar gas.
$1/DL$	Total resistance to diffusion, including resistance to diffusion of test gas across the alveolar-capillary membrane, through plasma in the capillary, and across the red blood cell membrane ($1/DM$), the resistance to diffusion with the red cell arising from the chemical reaction of the test gas and hemoglobin ($1/\theta Vc$), according to the formulation

$$\frac{1}{DL} = \frac{1}{DM} + \frac{1}{\theta Vc}$$

DL/VA	Diffusion per unit of alveolar volume. DL is expressed STPD, and VA is expressed in liters, BTPS.

BLOOD GAS SYMBOLS

Symbols for these values are readily composed by combining general symbols. Some examples include the following.

Pa_{CO_2}	Arterial CO_2 tension, torr (mmHg)
Sa_{O_2}	Arterial O_2 saturation, percent
Cc'_{O_2}	Oxygen content of pulmonary end-capillary blood, ml of O_2 per 100 ml of blood
$PA_{O_2} - Pa_{O_2}$, $P(A-a)_{O_2}$	Alveolar-arterial difference in the partial pressure of O_2 mmHg
$Ca_{O_2} - Cv_{O_2}$	Arteriovenous O_2 content difference, ml of O_2 per 100 ml of blood

PULMONARY SHUNT SYMBOLS

$\dot{Q}s$	Flow of blood via shunts. Usually determined as percent of cardiac output ($\dot{Q}$) while breathing 100% O_2, according to the equation

$$\frac{\dot{Q}s}{\dot{Q}} = \frac{Cc' - Ca}{Cc' - C\overline{v}}$$

where

$$\frac{\dot{Q}s}{\dot{Q}} = \text{``anatomic'' venous admixture}$$

and

$$Cc'_{O_2} = O_2 \text{ content of end-capillary blood}$$
$$Ca_{O_2} = O_2 \text{ content of arterial blood}$$
$$C\overline{v}_{O_2} = O_2 \text{ content of mixed venous blood, usually assumed to be 4.5 to 5.0 ml/100 ml of blood}$$

NOTES

Index

Abdomen: motion of, 2273
Abdominal muscles and expiration, 2269–2270, 2272
Abdominal surgery
  and pleural effusions, 2147–2148
  pulmonary function effects of, 2415
ABPA (see Aspergillosis, allergic bronchopulmonary)
Abscess
  hepatic: from *E. hystolitica*, 1668–1670
  lung (see Lung abscess)
  mediastinal, 2075
  peritonsillar, 1453
  subphrenic
    and pleural effusions, 2148
    and spontaneous pneumothorax, 2175
  tuboovarian, 1618
Absidia: infection with (see Mucormycosis)
Acanthamoeba: aspiration pneumonitis from, 1670
Acanthosis nigricans, 367, 384
  and neoplasms, 384
Acceleration in lungs, 177
  convective, 177
  local, 177
Acclimatization to altitude, 140–141, 251–252, 255
Acebutolol: small vessel vasculitis induced by, 1146
Acetaminophen sodium salicylate: asthma and, 1303
Acetazolamide
  for alveolar hypoventilation, 1343
  and bicarbonate excretion, 1191
  in chronic hypercapnia, 287, 1197
  in cor pulmonale therapy, 1015
  effects of, 166–167
  and sleep apnea, 1356
Acetone, 207
Acetylcholine
  in airway smooth muscle regulation, 123
  as neurotransmitter, 134
  and sleep, 147
  as vasodilator, 985
Acetylcysteine
  in acute respiratory failure treatment, 2294
  for cystic fibrosis, 1284, 1285
Acetylene, 207
Acetylsalicylic acid (see Aspirin)
Acid anhydrides: asthma induced by, 857
Acid-base balance, 1189–1194
  kidneys in, 1190–1192
  monitoring in mechanical ventilation, 2363
Acid-base disturbances (see Metabolic acid-base disturbances; Respiratory: acid-base disturbances)
Acid-base map, 1192

Acid-fast stains for Mycobacteria, 1812–1813
Acidosis (see Metabolic acidosis; Respiratory acidosis)
Acidphosphatase in alveolar macrophages, 705
Acinar adenocarcinoma, 1915, 1921, 1924, 1935
  (See also Adenocarcinoma)
Acinar capillary sheet: blood flow through, 44
Acinar pathway: length of, 54–55
Acinetobacter spp.
  antibiotics for, 1403
  nosocomial infection with, 1436, 1747
  stains of, 1399
  A. antritatus: nosocomial pneumonia from, 1491
  A. lwoffi: nosocomial pneumonia from, 1491
Acini
  anatomy of, 17, 1250
  development of, 62, 64
  function in parenchyma, 33
  number of, 29
  plasma cells in, 27
Acinic cell tumors, 2017
Acne: drug-induced, 374
Acquired immunodeficiency syndrome (AIDS)
  antiviral research, 1687–1689
  and ARDS, 1697
  AZT for, 1666, 1688–1689
  bacterial infections in, 1696
  bronchoalveolar lavage in, 433, 1405, 1690, 1752
  bronchoscopy in, 453, 1405, 1467, 1690, 1700
  candidal infection in, 1684, 1686, 1692, 1696
  case definition for surveillance purposes, 1684–1685
  CDC classification of HIV infection, 1686
  coccidioidomycosis in, 1696, 1786, 1787
  cryptococcosis in, 1421, 1453, 1460, 1696, 1769–1771
  Cryptosporidium infection in, 1676–1679, 1684, 1686, 1696
  cytomegalovirus infection in, 1395, 1397, 1421, 1460, 1661, 1666, 1672, 1684, 1685, 1687, 1690, 1691, 1695, 1701, 1749, 1755
    coexistent with *P. carinii*, 1460, 1661, 1666, 1672, 1755
  dementia in, 1684, 1685, 1686
  diagnostic approach to pulmonary disease, 1690–1692
  differential diagnosis: radiography, 1691, 1692
  among drug abusers, 1456, 1467, 1686–1687, 1690, 1695, 1698

Acquired immunodeficiency syndrome (AIDS) *(Cont.)*
  endoscopist risk, 462
  and eosinophilic pneumonia, 686
  epidemiology of, 1685–1687
    in Africa, 1687, 1695, 1697–1698
    in New York City, 1686–1687
  etiology of, 1687–1689
    (See also Human immunodeficiency virus)
  fungal infections in, 1421, 1453, 1460, 1684–1686, 1691, 1695–1696, 1761, 1769–1771, 1780
  gallium lung scanning in, 1691, 2553, 2554
  among hemophiliacs, 1686, 1687
  among heterosexuals, 1686–1687
  histoplasmosis in, 1684, 1685, 1686, 1691, 1696, 1780
  among homosexuals, 1683, 1686–1687, 1698
  immunologic defect in, 1689–1690
  incidence of, 1683, 1685
  infection control precautions, 1699–1701
  Kaposi's sarcoma in, 1467, 1658, 1683, 1684, 1685, 1686, 1690, 1691, 1692, 1697–1700, 2025, 2026, 2028
    epidemic, 1698
    pulmonary, 1698–1699
    (See also Kaposi's sarcoma)
  Legionella infection in, 1395, 1421, 1696, 1697
  leishmaniasis, 1679
  lymphomas, primary malignant lung, 2050, 2052
  mycobacterial infection and disease in, 1395, 1421, 1467, 1684, 1686, 1691, 1695, 1701, 1753, 1800, 1812, 1817, 1838–1839, 1858, 1859, 1863, 1864, 1867
  nocardial infections in, 1696, 1753
  nonHodgkin's lymphoma and, 1684, 1685, 1686, 1691
  open lung biopsy in, 1691–1692
  pleural involvement in, 1697
  pneumonia in, 1393, 1394–1395, 1397, 1460, 1538, 1745–1747, 1749, 1752–1753, 1755, 1758
    bacterial, 1696
    diagnostic approach, 1690–1692
    diagnostic studies, 1400, 1401, 1402, 1690–1692
    fungal, 1695–1696
    lymphocytic interstitial, 1684, 1685, 1686, 1691, 1692, 1697
    P. carinii, 1394–1395, 1397, 1421, 1460, 1657–1666, 1683, 1684, 1685, 1686, 1690, 1691, 1692–1695, 1697, 1700, 1701, 1752, 1755
    treatment for, 1664–1666, 1693–1695

Bronchial circulation *(Cont.)*
  and cardiac disease, 1121–1123
    bronchopulmonary anastomoses,
      1121–1123
    clinical importance of, 1123
  in disease, 995–996
  hemoptysis, 1123
  shunts, 1123
Bronchial cysts, 73, 2087, 2089, 2090–
    2091, 2105, 2107
  congenital, 1556, 1557, 1558, 1560,
    1572, 1951
  radiography of, 514
  solitary nodules, 511
Bronchial cytology, 433
  bronchoalveolar lavage, 433
  brushing and washing, 433
Bronchial epithelial cells (BEC) in spu-
    tum, 416
Bronchial metastases, 1900, 2013, 2018
Bronchial mucosa: tissue of, 17
Bronchial mucous: discharge of, 17
Bronchial obstruction
  and ARDS, 2203
  and bronchiectasis, 1561–1562
  mediastinitis and, 2076, 2077, 2079,
    2081
  and premalignant pleural effusions,
    2159
Bronchial stenosis, 73
Bronchial veins, 20, 1121
Bronchial venules: and water exchange,
    922
Bronchiectasis, 1258, 1553–1577
  acquired, 1559–1560
  and allergic bronchopulmonary as-
    pergillosis, 1642, 1708
  and anaerobic infection, 1506, 1512
  and aspergillomas, 1646
  atelectatic, 1561–1562
  bilateral, 1555
  bronchial obstruction and, 1561–
    1562
    allergic bronchopulmonary asper-
      gillosis, 1559, 1562
    chronic obstructive airways dis-
      ease, 1562
    foreign body, 1559, 1561–1562
    mucoid impaction, 1559, 1562
    neoplasms, 1562
  bronchography of, 1571–1572, 1574
    chronic bronchitis, bronchographic
      changes in, 1572
    pseudobronchiectasis (reversible
      bronchiectasis), 1572
  bronchoscopy in, 444, 1249–1250,
    1554
  chronic: clubbing and, 395
  and ciliary dyskinesia syndrome,
    1559, 1563–1565, 1568, 1576
  classification of, 1555–1556
    cylindrical, 1554, 1555, 1557, 1571
    saccular (cystic), 1556, 1557, 1572
    varicose, 1555–1556, 1557, 1571
  clinical features of, 1569–1570
  clubbing in, 1570

Bronchiectasis *(Cont.)*
  collateral circulation and, 1006,
    1554–1555
  complications and prognosis of,
    1575–1576
  congenital anatomic defects and,
    1558–1560, 1562–1563
    lymphatic, 1559, 1563
    Mounier-Kuhn syndrome, 1559,
      1562–1563
    tracheobronchial, 1559, 1562–1563
    vascular, 1559, 1563
    Williams-Campbell syndrome,
      1559, 1562
    yellow-nail syndrome, 1559, 1563
  congenital bronchial cysts, 1558,
    1560
  and cor pulmonale, 1573–1574, 1575
  CT scan of, 1572, 1574
  cystic, 1556, 1557, 1572
    multiple nodules from, 1951
  in cystic fibrosis, 1275, 1285, 1286,
    1559, 1567–1568, 1569, 1570,
    1573, 1575, 1576
  diagnosis of, 1574–1575
    bacteriologic findings, 1574–1575
    bronchography, 1571–1572, 1574
    bronchoscopy, 444, 1249–1250,
      1574
    computed tomography, 1572, 1574
    sputum stains, 422, 1569–1570,
      1575
  differential diagnosis, 1575
  among drug abusers, 1468
  elastase and proteases in airway
    damage, role of, 1569
  follicular, 1558, 1560
  hemoptysis and, 347, 350, 1570,
    1575, 1590
  hereditary abnormalities and, 1559,
    1563–1568
    α_1-antitrypsin deficiency, 1559,
      1567
    ciliary defects of respiratory mu-
      cosa, 1559, 1563–1565, 1576
    cystic fibrosis (mucoviscidosis),
      1275, 1285, 1286, 1559, 1567–
      1568, 1569, 1570, 1575, 1576
    dyskinetic cilia syndrome, 1559,
      1563–1565, 1576
    Kartagener's syndrome, 1559,
      1565–1566
  immunodeficiency states and, 1559,
    1563
    bare lymphocyte syndrome, 1563
    IgA deficiency, 1563
    IgG deficiency, 1559, 1563
  infections and, 1559, 1560–1561
    measles, 1559, 1560, 1574
    mycotic, 1559, 1561
    necrotizing pneumonia from anaer-
      obic bacteria, 1559, 1561, 1574
    pertussis, 1559, 1560
    tuberculosis, 1559, 1561
  intralobar bronchopulmonary seques-
    tration, 1558, 1559, 1560, 1563

Bronchiectasis *(Cont.)*
  and nontuberculous mycobacteriosis,
    1838
  pathogenesis and predisposing fac-
    tors for, 1385, 1558–1569
  pathology of, 1385, 1554–1558
  pathophysiological changes, 1572–
    1574
    hemodynamic changes, 1573–1574
    pulmonary function, 1572–1573
  and pneumococcal pneumonia, 1559,
    1560–1561, 1574
  prevalence of, 1553–1554
  pulmonary circulation in, 1554–1555
  radiography of, 488, 1045, 1570–
    1572, 1574
    bronchography, 1571–1572, 1574
    chest, 1570–1571, 1574
    computed tomography, 1572, 1574
  reversible, 1572
  sputum in, 422, 428, 1569–1570,
    1575
  and staphylococcal pneumonia, 1559,
    1560–1561, 1574, 1576
  treatment of, 1576–1577
    surgical, 1577
  Young's syndrome and, 1568–1569
  (See also Bronchiolectasis)
Bronchiolectasis, 1258
  and ARDS, 2205
  cough in, 345–346
  (See also Bronchiectasis)
Bronchioles
  in aged, 81
  anatomy of, 12, 17–18, 28, 33
  development of, 69–70, 72
  and respiratory immunity, 595–596,
    1411
Bronchiolitis, 1251–1252, 1588–1591
  acute, 1251
  chronic, 1251
  clinical presentation of, 1589
  control and prevention of, 1591
  definition of, 1247, 1248
  diagnosis of, 1590
  drug-induced: in rheumatoid arthritis
    therapy, 651
  early infancy presentation, 1590
  epidemiology of, 1588–1589
  etiology of, 1588
  in heart-lung transplantation, 2463
  in interstitial lung disease, 2244
  laboratory studies of, 1590
  management of, 1590–1591
  pathophysiology of, 1589
  in spectrum of obstructive airways
    disease, 1162, 1167, 1247,
    1248
  and ulceration, 1257
Bronchiolitis obliterans
  and ARDS, 2211, 2212, 2224
  causes of, 853
  and collagen-vascular diseases, 741
  differential diagnosis
    from bronchiectasis, 1575
    from pulmonary infections, 1379

Lymph nodes (*Cont.*)
  regional, of lung, 904–905
    development of, 904–905
    distribution of, 905–906
  resection in NSCLC surgery, 1994
  and respiratory immunity, 595, 1414
  in sarcoidosis, 632, 635
  tuberculosis in, 1832–1833
Lymphadenitis, tuberculous, 1855–1856
Lymphadenopathy
  mediastinal: CT scanning of, 535
  in sarcoidosis, 632
  (*See also* Sarcoidosis)
Lymphadenopathy-associated virus
      (LAV) (*see* Human immunode-
      ficiency virus)
Lymphangiogram dye, oil-based
  and pulmonary hemorrhage, 796
  and pulmonary vasculitis, 795
Lymphangiography contrast medium:
      ARDS induced by, 2207
Lymphangioleiomyomatosis (*see* Lym-
      phangiomyomatosis)
Lymphangiomyomatosis, 966–970,
      2025, 2027
  chylothorax in, 967, 969, 2152
  clinical features of, 967
  as heart-lung transplantation indica-
      tion, 2459
  and interstitial distortion, 714
  pathology of, 967
  pulmonary performance in, 967–969
  and spontaneous pneumothorax,
      2174
  treatment of, 969
Lymphangitic carcinoma, 2025, 2026
Lymphatic drainage: pleural, 2117–
      2119
Lymphatic obstruction and premalig-
      nant pleural effusions, 2159
Lymphatic system, pulmonary, 901–
      907, 926–927, 2045–2047
  intrapulmonary, 902–904, 906, 909–
      910
    of animals, 904
    bronchi and lymphatics, 903
    efferent lymphatics, 909–910
    interlobular lymphatics, 902–903
    lymph flow of, 904, 906
    pulmonary arteries and lymphat-
      ics, 903–904
    pulmonary veins and lymphatics,
      903
    subpleural lymphatics, 902
    terminal lymphatics, 909–910
  intrathoracic lymphatics, 906–907
    diaphragm, 906–907
    heart, 907
    parietal pleura, 907
  regional lymph nodes, 904–906
    development of, 904–905
    distribution of, 905–906
    hilar, 905–906
    intrapulmonary, 906
    mediastinal, 905
  tissue fluid pathway, 901

Lymphatics
  mediastinal, 2069–2073
  in metastases
    from lung, 1937–1938, 1940
    to lung, 2024
  and respiratory immunity, 595, 596
Lymphocyte activation factor (*see* Inter-
      leukin 1)
Lymphocyte localization in respiratory
      immunity, 581
Lymphocytes
  in bronchoalveolar lavage fluid, 591–
      593
  in defense system of lungs, 27,
      1414–1418
  deficiency in: and pneumonia, 1421
  in delayed hypersensitivity granulo-
      mas, 614–615
  imbalances of: in AIDS, 1421, 1689–
      1690, 1839
  in immune response, 589–591
  radiation injury to, 774
  and respiratory immunity, 581, 582,
      584, 585, 593, 596, 614–615,
      719, 720–724, 2045–2047
  in sarcoidosis, 623, 624–625
  sieving by lungs, 206
  and tuberculous lesions, 1821–1822
  (*See also* B cells; T cells)
Lymphocytic angiitis and granulomato-
      sis, benign, 1137–1138
  differential diagnosis, 1138
Lymphocytic interstitial pneumonia
      (LIP), 756, 1380
  and AIDS, 1684, 1685, 1686, 1691,
      1692, 1697
  and Sjögren's syndrome, 661–662
  in systemic lupus erythematosus,
      660–661
Lymphoid tissue (*see* Bronchial-associ-
      ated lymphoid tissue)
Lymphokines
  in immune response, 590–591, 615,
      1821–1822
  and tuberculous lesions, 1821–1822
Lymphomas
  in AIDS, 2050, 2052
  biopsy of, 465, 467
  chylothorax and, 2152
  CT scanning of, 548
  hilar adenopathy due to: NMR imag-
      ing, 558
  histiocytic, 2095
  Hodgkin's (*see* Hodgkin's disease)
  immunologic markers in identifica-
      tion of, 2046–2047
  and invasive aspergillosis suscepti-
      bility, 1762
  lymphoblastic, 2097
  lymphocytic, 2095
  malignant
    differential diagnosis from lympho-
      matoid granulomatosis, 2057
    of lung, 2049–2053
      primary, 2050–2052
      secondary, 2052–2053

Lymphomas: malignant (*Cont.*)
    radiation therapy, pulmonary fibro-
      sis and, 773
    and Sjögren's syndrome, 661–662
    in thoracic wall, 2040
    and malignant pleural effusions,
      2131, 2159–2161, 2166
    mediastinal, 2087, 2089, 2090–2091,
      2092, 2095–2097
    metastatic to lung, 2052–2053
    mucormycosis and, 1768
    multiple nodules from, 1951
    nonHodgkin's (*see* NonHodgkin's
      lymphoma)
    and pneumonitis in immunocompro-
      mised, 1757
    pseudo (*see* Pseudolymphomas)
    and pulmonary cavities, 1386
    skin lesions in, 384–385
    tracheal, 1178–1179
Lymphomatoid granulomatosis, 1134,
      1136–1137, 2056–2057
  clinical presentation of, 1136–1137,
      2057
  course of, 1137
  differential diagnosis: from We-
      gener's granulomatosis and
      nonHodgkin's lymphoma, 2057
  and interstitial distortion, 714
  laboratory tests for, 1137
  pathology of, 1137, 2057
  radiologic findings in, 2057
  skin lesions in, 370, 383, 1136–1137
  therapy and prognosis for, 2057
Lymphoproliferative disorders of lungs,
      2045–2057
  Hodgkin's disease of lungs, 2053–
      2055
  (*See also* Hodgkin's disease)
  lymphoid system, 2045–2047
  lymphomas (*see* Lymphomas)
  lymphomatoid granulomatosis, 1134,
      1136–1137, 2056–2057
  malignant lymphomas, 2049–2053
  plasmacytoma of lungs, 1951, 2055–
      2056
  pseudolymphoma, 2045, 2046, 2047–
      2049
  (*See also* Pseudolymphoma)
  Waldenström's macroglobulinemia,
      2055
Lymphotoxin, 1451
Lysosomes in alveolar macrophages,
      705–706
Lysozyme and respiratory immunity,
      582

M cells, 580
M proteins: and bacterial binding, 1444
Macleod's syndrome, 495, 1252, 1267–
      1268, 1575, 2550–2551
α_2-Macroglobulin, 726
Macroglobulinemia, Waldenström's,
      2055

Muscles *(Cont.)*
  endurance of, 235–236
  malnutrition effects on, 2388, 2389
  metabolism of, 236–238
  mitochondria in, 48–49, 51
  power: in exercise performance,
    235–236
  respiratory *(see* Respiratory muscles)
  in sarcoidosis, 634
  strength of, 235–236
Muscular dystrophies
  and inspiratory muscle fatigue, 2281,
    2306
  respiratory failure in, 2306
Musculoskeletal disorders from *M.*
    pneumoniae, 1616–1617
Musculoskeletal pain in chest, 355
Mushroom worker's lung, 667–673
Mustard gas and lung cancer, 1910
Myasthenia gravis
  airway management in, 2340
  alveolar hypoventilation and, 1335,
    1339, 2303, 2304, 2340
  and aspiration susceptibility, 878,
    2340
  carcinomatous, 1965
  and hypercapnic respiratory failure,
    2186, 2303, 2304, 2366
  and inspiratory muscle fatigue, 2281,
    2303, 2304
  mechanical ventilation for, 2377
  and mediastinal thymomas, 543,
    2089, 2092, 2095
Mycetomas
  multiple, 1951
  pulmonary *(see* Aspergilloma; Fun-
    gus ball)
Mycobacteria
  acid-fast stains for, 1812–1813
  atypical, 1836–1839, 1857–1859
    identification of, 1816–1818
    surgery for infections, 2420
    (See also Tuberculosis, atypical)
  bacteremia caused by, 1443
  bronchoscopic diagnosis, 454
  culturing, 1813–1815
    Bactec system, 1814–1816, 1819
    Lowenstein-Jensen media, 1813–
      1814
  drug susceptibility testing, 1818–
    1819
  identification of, 1815–1818
  in immunocompromised host, 1753,
    1837–1839, 1858, 1859
  Kinyoun stain, 1812
  mediastinal granulomas from,
    2078
  microscopy of, 1812–1813
  nontuberculous *(see* atypical, *above)*
  obtaining samples, 182–1813
  in sputum, identification of, 421
  Ziehl-Neelsen stain, 1812
  (See also specific mycobacteria)
Mycobacteriosis
  atypical tuberculosis *(see* Tuberculo-
    sis, atypical)
  tuberculosis *(see* Tuberculosis)

Mycobacterium abscessus, 1857
  treatment against, 1864
M. africanum: identification of, 1816
M. aquae (see M. gordonae)
M. asiaticum: identification of, 1817,
    1857
M. avium-intracellulare
  diagnostic smears for, 1400, 1401
  drug-resistance, 1819
  identification of, 1817, 1857
  infection and disease, 1857, 1859,
    1865–1868
    in AIDS, 1395, 1421, 1467, 1684,
      1686, 1691, 1695, 1701, 1753,
      1800, 1812, 1817, 1838–1839,
      1859, 1863, 1864, 1867
    bronchoscopic diagnosis in, 453
    disseminated, 1838–1839, 1859
    histopathologic evidence of, 1838
    treatment against, 1865–1868, 2414
  PPD-B test, 1802
  relative virulence of, 1863
M. bovis
  identification of, 1816
  infection with, 1802, 1857–1858
M. chelonae
  identification of, 1815, 1817, 1818,
    1857
  mediastinitis from, 2075
  opportunistic infection with, 1837
  treatment against, 1864
M. faeni and macrophage proliferation,
    758, 761
M. flavescens: identification of, 1818
M. fortuitum
  histopathologic evidence of infection
    with, 1838
  identification of, 1817, 1818, 1837
  mediastinitis from, 2075
  opportunistic infection with, 1695,
    1837
  PPD-F test, 1802
  relative virulence of, 1863
  treatment against, 1864
M. gastri: identification of, 1817
M. gordonae, 1813, 1837
  histopathologic evidence of infection
    with, 1838
  identification of, 1817
  opportunistic infection with, 1695,
    1837
  relative virulence of, 1863
M. haemophilum: identification of,
    1818
M. kansasii
  disease due to, 1695, 1836, 1837,
    1857–1859, 1864
  identification of, 1815, 1816–1817
  PPD-Y test, 1802
  relative virulence of, 1863
  treatment against, 1819, 1864
M. kansassi: histopathologic evidence
    of infection with, 1838
M. leprae, 1857, 1863, 1865
M. malmoense
  identification of, 1817, 1857
  opportunistic infection with, 1837

M. marianum (see M. scrofulaceum)
M. marinum
  disease due to, 1858, 1864
  identification of, 1815, 1817–1818
  relative virulence of, 1863
  treatment against, 1864
M. scrofulaceum
  disease caused by, 1857, 1858–1859,
    1865–1868
  histopathologic evidence of infection
    with, 1838
  identification of, 1817
  opportunistic infection with, 1837
  PPD-G test, 1802
M. shimoidei: identification of, 1817
M. simiae
  disease due to, 1858, 1868
  identification of, 1817, 1857
  opportunistic infection with, 1837
  relative virulence of, 1863
  treatment against, 1868
M. smegmatis, 1854
M. szulgai
  identification of, 1817, 1818, 1857
  opportunistic infection with, 1837
  relative virulence of, 1863
  treatment against, 1868
M. terrae, 1813
  identification of, 1817
  relative virulence of, 1863
M. tuberculosis
  culturing, 1401, 1813–1815
  diagnostic smears for, 1400
  identification of, 1815–1816
    Bactec system, 1815–1816
    hydroxylamine (HA), 1815–1816
    NAP, 1815–1816
  obtaining specimens, 1811–1812
  relative virulence of, 1863
  smears, 1812–1813
  in sputum, 421, 1401
  (See also Tuberculosis)
M. tyzeraelons in AIDS, 1421
M. ulcerans: identification of, 1818,
    1857
M. xenopi
  identification of, 1815, 1817, 1857
  opportunistic infection with, 1695,
    1837
  relative virulence of, 1863
  treatment against, 1819, 1868
Mycolog cream: skin reactions and, 388
Mycoplasma pneumoniae
  and acute respiratory failure, 2291
  asthma and, 1300–1301
  bacteremia from: in sickle cell
    anemia, 1460
  binding by, 1427, 1614
  and chronic bronchitis exacerbation,
    1547
  and ciliary defects, 102
  extrapulmonary complications from,
    1616–1618
    cardiac, 1616, 1617
    dermatologic, 376–377, 1616, 1617
    gastrointestinal, 1617
    hematologic, 1616–1617

Nonsmall cell carcinoma
  biology of, 1885–1896
    DNA and chromosome analysis, 1886
    in vitro growth of specimens, 1886–
      1896
      antigen expression, 1893
      class 1 histocompatibility antigens,
        1893
      common stem cell evidence, 1894–
        1896
      differential expression of
        biomarkers, 1890–1892
      intermediate cell filaments, 1893
  medical management of, 1983–1987
    adjuvant chemotherapy, 1987
    efficacy of chemotherapy, 1983–
      1986
    immunotherapy, 1987
    quality of life, 1983, 1986
    recommendations for, 1986–1987
    survival rates, 1984–1986
    toxicity, 1986
    tumor size, 1983–1984
  metastases, 1937–1938
  pathology of, 1885–1886
  radiation therapy for inoperable,
    2002–2004
    for cure, 2002–2003
    effect on normal tissue, 2003–2004
  surgical treatment of, 1991–1997
    adjuvant, 1997
    bronchoscopy, 1995
    clinical staging, 1991–1993
    complications, 1993
    computed tomography, 1995
    expectations, 1997
    mediastinoscopy, 1995
    operability, 1993
    pneumonectomy vs. lobectomy,
      1994
    pulmonary function evaluation,
      1993–1994
    for stage III disease, 1995–1997
    technical resectability, 1994–1997
  TNM staging of, 1976, 1991–1993
    new international definitions,
      1992–1993
  (See also Adenocarcinoma; Large cell
    carcinoma; Squamous cell car-
    cinoma)
Nonspecific bronchial hyperresponsive-
    ness (NSBH), 855, 2488–2490
  (See also Asthma)
Nonsteroidal anti-inflammatory drugs
  and airways disease, 797
  asthma and, 1303
  and hypersensitivity syndrome, 802
  for small vessel vasculitis, 1147
  in thromboembolism prophylaxis,
    1053
Norepinephrine
  and alpha receptor stimulation, 1097
  as local hormone, 213
  and pulmonary edema, 795
  as vasoconstrictor, 984
  (See also Catecholamines)

North American blastomycosis, 315
Nose
  and airway resistance, 176
  and airway stabilization, 105
  cleansing function of, 95–96, 1412–
    1413
  conditioning function of, 96
  diseases of, 98–99
  foreign bodies in, 99
  function of, 95–98
  morphology of, 91–94
  mucociliary function of, 96
  reflexes between lung and, 98
  viral infections of, 1413
  (See also entries commencing with
    term Nasal)
Nosocomial infections, 1431
  and bacterial adhesion/colonization,
    1444
  (See also Nosocomial pneumonia)
Nosocomial pneumonia, 1431–1438
  anaerobic, 1436
  antibiotics for: initial, 1403
  and ARDS, 1437, 2230
  bronchoscopy and, 461–462
  as complication of mechanical venti-
    lation, 1432, 1436, 1438, 2381
  cost of, 1431
  diagnosis of, 1375, 1391–1392, 1437
  differential diagnosis, 1437
  domiciliary epidemics, 1747, 1762–
    1763
  environmental factors, 1432, 1436
  etiology of, 1391–1392, 1436
  gram-negative bacteria, 1496–1497
    clinical features, 1497
    epidemiology, 1496–1497
    (See also Gram-negative bacteria,
      pneumonia from)
  host factors, 1431–1432, 1433–1435
  in immunocompromised host, 1746–
    1747, 1762
  incidence of, 1391, 1431
  nondomiciliary epidemics, 1747, 1762
  pathophysiology of, 1431
  pleural fluid analysis in, 1437, 1438
  and postsurgical respiratory failure,
    2433, 2434, 2436
  predisposing factors, 1431–1436
  prevention of, 1432, 1438
  treatment of, 1438
NREM-REM cycle, 145–147
NREM sleep, 145–147
  alterations
    in apnea threshold, 148–149
    in respiratory mechanics, 149–150
    in set point and chemosensitivity,
      147–148
  and central sleep apnea, 1355
  changes in stability of ventilation,
    149
  and obstructive sleep apnea, 1349–
    1350
  response to mechanical loads, 149–
    150
  ventilatory control in, 147–150

NSBH (see Nonspecific bronchial hy-
    perresponsiveness)
NSCLC (see Non-small cell carcinoma)
Nuclear magnetic resonance (NMR),
    485, 549–563
  in atelectasis, 559–560
  clinical applications, 552–563
    chest wall, 560–562
    future prospects, 562–563
    heart, 555–559
    mediastinal neoplasms and cysts,
      2092
    mediastinum, 513, 517, 519, 520,
      552–557
    pleura, 560–562
    in pulmonary embolism, 1075
    pulmonary hili, 558, 559
    pulmonary parenchyma, 559–560
    pulmonary vessels, 559
    radiation fibrosis, 784–785, 787,
      788
    in valvular heart disease, 1091
  concepts and techniques, 549–551
    hazards, 551
    MR imager, 550
    respiratory and cardiac motion, 551
Nursing homes: tuberculosis in, 1799,
    1804–1805, 1880
Nutrition
  and acute respiratory failure, 2387–
    2394, 2440
    assessment and indications for
      support, 2389–2390
    caloric requirements, 2390–2391,
      2392
    delivery techniques, 2392–2393
    metabolic changes, 2388–2389
    minerals, trace elements, and vita-
      mins, 2391, 2392
    nutrient prescription, 2390–2392,
      2392
    protein requirements, 2391, 2392
    refeeding effects, 2392
    respiratory efects of starvation,
      2387–2388
  deficiencies in: and tuberculosis sus-
    ceptibility, 1836
  and oxygen tolerance, 2336
  and respiratory immunity, 581
  support
    in ARDS, 2229
    for cystic fibrosis patients, 1284
  total parenteral (TPN), 2388, 2391,
    2392–2393
  (See also Malnutrition)
Nutritive vessels of lung, 20

Oat cell carcinoma, 1915, 1935, 1971,
    1972
  of airways, 1178
  biopsy of, 466, 1918, 1920
  combined, 1915, 1971, 1972
  sputum in, 431, 432, 1918
  (See also Small cell carcinoma)

Pollution *(Cont.)*
  indoor
    and asthma, 1303
    and chronic bronchitis and emphysema, 1240
Polonium 218 and lung cancer, 1910
Polyangiitis overlap syndrome: differential diagnosis from pulmonary infections, 1379
Polyarteritis nodosa, 1127–1128, 1134, 1145
  alveolar hemorrhage and, 959
  differential diagnosis
    Churg-Strauss syndrome, 696
    lymphomatoid granulomatosis, 2057
  and eosinophilic pneumonia, 696
  and Goodpasture's syndrome, 675, 681
  microscopic, 1128
  upper airway involvement, 102
Polychondritis, relapsing, 1174, 1180, 1181
  lung scanning, 2554
Polycyclic aromatic hydrocarbons: carcinogenic properties of, 859
Polycythemia and diffusing capacity of lungs, 2497
Polycythemia vera, 1045, 2062
  thrombotic tendency in, 1050, 1062
Polymorphous reticulosis, 1138
Polymyositis
  cancer association of, 1965–1966
  and dermatomyositis (PM-DM), 646, 656–657
    clinical features of, 646
    Hamman-Rich type, 646, 657
    interstitial lung disease in, 646, 657
    pulmonary manifestations of, 646
    skin lesions in, 646, 656
    vasculitis in, 1146, 1148–1150
    ventilatory insufficiency in, 646, 657
  and inspiratory muscle fatigue, 2281, 2299
Polymyxins, 1738, 1741
  neuromuscular dysfunction from, 800
Polypoid neoplasms (see Endobronchial neoplasms)
Polyps
  "allergic": in Churg-Strauss syndrome, 1142
  nasal, 95, 100
Polysomnography, 1352–1353, 1355, 1356–1357
  variables measured during, 1352
Polyurethane: asthma from, 1301
Pompe's disease: lungs in, 871
Pontiac fever from *Legionella*, 1629, 1632, 1633
Portable chest examination, 525–526
Portal vein: metastases via, 2024
Positive end-expiratory pressure (PEEP)
  for acute respiratory failure, 2194
  for ARDS, 2201, 2204, 2205, 2225–2226, 2227, 2234

Positive end-expiratory pressure (PEEP) *(Cont.)*
  for arterial hypoxemia, 2379–2380
  auto, 2368, 2378, 2381
  best, 2368, 2379
  cardiac output and, 2378, 2379
  in combined cardiac-pulmonary disease, 1116–1117
  for drug overdosage, 1467
  for flail chest, 2449
  increasing intrathoracic pressure, 2356–2357
  and inspiratory muscle fatigue, 2280
  monitoring, 2362
  optimum, 2368
  and pulmonary artery wedge pressure measurement, 2355
  for pulmonary edema, 947
  and pulmonary hemodynamics, 982–983
  in RDS, 2259
  (See also Mechanical ventilation)
Postcommissurotomy syndrome, 355
Postinspiration phase of breathing, 137–138, 139
Postnatal lung development, 66–70
  alveolar stage, 66–70
  stage of, of microvascular maturation, 66–70
Postoperative management (see Respiratory failure, acute, postoperative; Surgery)
Postpartum state: thromboembolism and, 1050, 1051
Postpericardiotomy syndrome, 355
Postsynaptic inhibition (hyperpolarization) and atonia in REM sleep, 151
Posttussive syncope, 346
Posture: effect on perfusion, 190
Potassium bisulfite: astma and, 1303–1304
Potassium iodide: skin reactions to, 388
Potassium iodine: small vessel vasculitis induced by, 1146
Potassium metabisulfite: asthma and, 1303–1304
Potassium-sparing diuretics, 1198
Pott's disease, 2300
Praziquantel
  for paragonimiasis, 1731
  for schistosomiasis, 1730, 1735
Predisposing influences in respiratory disorders, 313–318
Prednisolone (see Corticosteroids)
Prednisone (see Corticosteroids)
Pregnancy
  antituberculous therapy during, 1880–1881
  asthma in: therapy for, 1320–1321
  coccidioidomycosis in, 1786
  complications in cystic fibrosis, 1290
  and influenza vaccine, 1587
  maternal oversedation, and postpartum neonate apnea, 1369, 1370

Premature atrial contractions during sleep, 156
Premature infants
  apneas in, 305, 306
    (See also Apneas, neonate)
  RDS in (see Respiratory distress syndrome of newborn)
  SIDS and near-SIDS in, 1363, 1369–1370
  and surfactant synthesis, 25
Premature ventricular contractions: asthma and, 1307
Pressure
  distending, 979
  luminal, 979
  pleural (see Pleural pressure)
  pulmonary vascular, 977–979
  transmural, 979
  transpulmonary, 171–172, 175, 180–181
Pressure support (PS) ventilation for postoperative respiratory failure, 2438
Pressure-volume curves of lung, 173–174, 176–178, 2477–2482
  in aged, 82–83
  dynamic normal, 2374, 2375
  effects of lung disease on, 2374–2376, 2480, 2481
  elastin and, 1202
  in interstitial lung disease, 740–741, 747
  isovolume, 179
  monitoring
    in mechanical ventilation, 2363
    postoperatively, 2436–2437
  normal, 2374, 2477–2480
  in optimizing mechanical ventilation, 2367
  relaxation, 175–176
  static normal, 2374, 2375, 2480–2481
Pressure-volume symbols, D5
Pretest probability in diagnostic reasoning, 400, 404–406
Priestley, Joseph, 5
Primary pulmonary hypertension (see Hypertension, pulmonary, primary)
Primary septa, 66
Prisons: tuberculosis in, 1800, 1805
Procainamide
  pulmonary disorders induced by, 1378
  SLE induced by, 800
  small vessel vasculitis induced by, 1146
Procaine penicillin: pharmacokinetic data and antibacterial activity of, 1736
Procarbazine
  and hypersensitivity syndrome, 802
  and pleural disease, 798, 2150, 2159
  pulmonary disorders induced by, 1379, 1757
  for small cell carcinoma, 1977
Procoagulant factors, 1049–1050

Respiratory Disease Librar